LIVER AND BILIARY DISEASE

Pathophysiology · Diagnosis · Management

LIVER AND BILIARY DISEASE

Pathophysiology · Diagnosis · Management

EDITED BY

RALPH WRIGHT

K.G.M.M. ALBERTI STEPHEN KARRAN

G.H. MILLWARD-SADLER

1979

W. B. Saunders Company Ltd London · Philadelphia · Toronto

W. B. Saunders Company Ltd: 1 St Anne's Road
Eastbourne, East Sussex BN21 3UN

West Washington Square
Philadelphia, PA 19105

1 Goldthorne Avenue
Toronto, Ontario M8Z 5T9

Library of Congress Cataloging in Publication Data

Main entry under title:

Liver and biliary disease.

Includes index.
1. Liver—Diseases. 2. Liver. 3. Biliary tract—Diseases. I. Wright, Ralph, MD
[DNLM: 1. Biliary tract diseases. 2. Liver diseases WI700.3 L784]
RC845.L57 616.3′6 79-1531

ISBN 0-7216-9609-0

Printed by The Whitefriars Press Ltd, Tonbridge, Kent.

Print No.: 9 8 7 6 5 4 3

Contributors

D.M. ACKERY, MA, MB, MSc, Consultant in Nuclear Medicine, Southampton University Hospitals, Southampton.

K.G.M.M. ALBERTI, MA, DPhil, BM, BCh, MRCPath, FRCP, Professor of Clinical Biochemistry, The University of Newcastle upon Tyne; Honorary Consultant Chemical Pathologist, Newcastle Area Health Authority (Teaching), Newcastle upon Tyne.

M. BALASEGARAM, MB, FRCS, FRCS(Ed), FACS, FRACS, FPCS, Kehormat Professor of Surgery, Faculty of Medicine, National University of Malaysia; Senior Consultant Surgeon, Ministry of Health, Malaysia; Head, Department of Surgery, General Hospital, Kuala Lumpur, Malaysia; Hunterian Professor of Surgery 1969, Royal College of Surgeons, England.

JOSEPH BENICHOU, MD, Fellow in Transplantation, Department of Surgery, University of Colorado Medical Center, Denver, Colorado; Chef de Clinique Assistant, South Paris University, Centre Hôpitalier–Kremlin Bicetre, Paris.

I.S. BENJAMIN, BSc, MB, ChB, FRCS, Lecturer in Surgery, University of Glasgow; Honorary Registrar, Royal Infirmary, Glasgow.

GEORGE BERCI, MD, FCSH, Associate Clinical Professor of Surgery, University of California, Los Angeles; Associate Director, Department of Surgery, Cedars-Sinai Medical Center, Los Angeles, California.

D.M. BISSELL, MD, Assistant Professor of Medicine, University of California, San Francisco; Attending Physician, University of California Medical Center and San Francisco General Hospital, San Francisco, California.

L.H. BLUMGART, MD, FRCS(Engl, Ed, Glas), Director and Professor of Surgery, Royal Postgraduate Medical School, Hammersmith Hospital, London.

NANCY L.R. BUCHER, MD, Associate Professor of Medicine (Oncology), Harvard Medical School, Boston; Associate Biologist, Massachusetts General Hospital, Boston, Massachusetts.

R.Y. CALNE, MA, MS, FRCS, FRS, Professor of Surgery, University of Cambridge; Honorary Consultant Surgeon, Addenbrooke's Hospital, Cambridge.

MORAG CHISHOLM, MD, MRCPath, Senior Lecturer in Haematology, The University of Southampton; Consultant Haematologist, Southampton University Hospitals, Southampton.

M. CLASSEN, MD, Professor of Medicine, University of Hamburg; Chief of the Department of Internal Medicine, Barmbek General Hospital, Hamburg, West Germany.

RUSSELL E. COWAN, MB, MRCP, Clinical Research Fellow, University of Southern California, Los Angeles, California.

J.L. DAWSON, MS, FRCS, Consultant Surgeon, King's College Hospital, London, King Edward VII Hospital for Officers, London, and Bromley Hospital, Bromley, Kent.

RICHARD C. DAY, BA, MB(Cantab), MRCP, Prophit Scholar and Honorary Lecturer in Medicine, Academic Department of Medicine, The Royal Free Hospital, London.

K.C. DEWBURY, BSc, MBBS, FRCR, Consultant Radiologist, Southampton University Hospitals, Southampton.

R. DICK, MB, BS, MRACR, FRCR, Teacher in Radiology, The Royal Free Hospital School of Medicine, London; Consultant Radiologist, The Royal Free Hospital and The London Clinic, London.

CAROL EAGLES, BSc, Research Associate, Department of Surgery, Southampton University Hospitals, Southampton.

JOSEF E. FISCHER, MD, Associate Professor of Surgery, Harvard Medical School, Boston; Associate Visiting Surgeon, Massachusetts General Hospital, Boston; Chief of the Hyperalimentation Unit and the Surgical Physiology Laboratory, Massachusetts General Hospital, Boston, Massachusetts.

CHARLES F. GEORGE, MD, BSc, FRCP, Professor of Clinical Pharmacology, The University of Southampton; Consultant Physician, Southampton University Hospitals, Southampton.

JOHN GOLLAN, MD, PhD, FRACP, MRCP, Assistant Professor of Medicine, University of California, San Francisco; Attending Physician, University of California Medical Center, San Francisco, California.

DAVID S. HARRY, BTech, PhD, Honorary Lecturer in Biochemistry, The Royal Free Hospital School of Medicine, London; Senior Biochemist, Academic Department of Medicine, The Royal Free Hospital, London.

K.W. HEATON, MA, MD, FRCP, Reader in Medicine, University of Bristol; Honorary Consultant Physician, Bristol Health District (Teaching), Bristol.

K.E.F. HOBBS, ChM, FRCS, Professor of Surgery, The Royal Free Hospital School of Medicine, London; Honorary Consultant Surgeon, The Royal Free Hospital, London.

GREG HOLDSTOCK, MB, MRCP, Research Fellow and Honorary Senior Registrar, Southampton University Hospitals, Southampton.

J.E. HUSBAND, MRCP, FRCP, Research Fellow in Radiology and Honorary Senior Lecturer, The Royal Marsden Hospital and Institute of Cancer Research, Sutton, Surrey.

C.W. IMRIE, BSc, MB, FRCS, Consultant Surgeon, Royal Infirmary, Glasgow.

KURT J. ISSELBACHER, MD, Mallinckrodt Professor of Medicine, Harvard Medical School, Boston; Chief of the Gastrointestinal Unit, Massachusetts General Hospital, Boston, Massachusetts.

A.M. JEZEQUEL, MD, Professor of Cell Pharmacology, University of Ancona School of Medicine, Ancona, Italy.

D.G. JOHNSTON, MRCP, Lecturer in Medicine, The University of Newcastle upon Tyne; First Assistant in Endocrinology, The Royal Victoria Infirmary, Newcastle upon Tyne.

A.E.A. JOSEPH, MBBS, MSc, FRCR, Honorary Senior Lecturer, St George's Hospital Medical School, London; Consultant Radiologist and Head of the Department of Nuclear Medicine and Ultrasound, St George's Hospital, London.

STEPHEN KARRAN, MA, FRCS, FRCS(Ed), Senior Lecturer in Surgery, The University of Southampton; Honorary Consultant Surgeon, Southampton University Hospitals, Southampton.

R.E. KIRSCH, MD, FCP(SA), Senior Lecturer, University of Cape Town; Principal Physician, Groote Schuur Hospital, Cape Town, South Africa.

J. THOMAS LAMONT, MD, Assistant Professor of Medicine, Harvard Medical School, Boston; Associate in Medicine, Peter Bent Brigham Hospital, Boston, Massachusetts.

R.H.S. LANE, FRCS, Lecturer in Surgery, The University of Southampton.

CHARLES S. LIEBER, MD, Professor of Medicine and Pathology, Mount Sinai School of Medicine (CUNY); Director, Alcohol Research Center, and Chief, Section of Liver Disease and Nutrition, Veterans Administration Hospital, New York.

J.A. LYNN, MS, FRCS, Lecturer in Surgery, Westminster Medical School, University of London; Honorary Senior Surgical Registrar, Westminster Hospital, London.

WILLIAM V. MCDERMOTT, MD, FACS, David W. and David Cheever Professor of Surgery, Harvard Medical School, Boston; Director, Harvard Surgical Service, New England Deaconess Hospital, Boston; Director, Cancer Research Institute, New England Deaconess Hospital, Boston, Massachusetts.

JOAN A. MCGOWAN, PhD, Research Fellow in Medicine, Massachusetts General Hospital, Boston, Massachusetts.

NEIL M. McINTYRE, BSc, MD, FRCP, Professor of Medicine, The Royal Free Hospital School of Medicine, University of London; Honorary Consultant Physician, The Royal Free Hospital, London.

H.B. MEIRE, MBBS, FRCR, Consultant in Ultrasound, Clinical Research Centre, Northwick Park Hospital, London.

G.H. MILLWARD-SADLER, BSc, MB, ChB, MRCPath, Senior Lecturer, Southampton University Medical School; Consultant Pathologist, Southampton University Hospitals, Southampton.

MARSHA Y. MORGAN, MB, MRCP, Lecturer in Medicine, The Royal Free Hospital Medical School, University of London; Honorary Senior Registrar, The Royal Free Hospital, London.

ALEX P. MOWAT, MB, ChB, DCH(Lond), FRCP(Lond), Honorary Clinical Lecturer, King's College Hospital Medical School, London; Consultant Paediatrician, King's College Hospital, Bethlem Royal Hospital and Maudsley Hospital, London.

H. HOMEWOOD NIXON, MA, MB, BChir, FRCS, FAAP(Hon), Consultant Paediatric Surgeon, The Hospital for Sick Children and Paddington Green Children's Hospital, London.

G.B. ONG, FRCS(Ed), FRCS, FRACS, FRSE, FPCS(Hon), FACS(Hon), FCS(SA)(Hon), FRCPS(Glas), FRCS(C)(Hon), Professor of Surgery, University of Hong Kong; Head of University Surgical Unit, Queen Mary Hospital, Hong Kong.

F.W. OSSENBERG, MD, Senior Lecturer, University of Hamburg; Senior Registrar, Barmbek General Hospital, Hamburg, West Germany.

HANS POPPER, MD, PhD, Gustave L. Levy Distinguished Service Professor, Mount Sinai School of Medicine, City University of New York, New York.

L.W. POWELL, MD, PhD, FRACP, Professor of Medicine, University of Queensland; Consultant Physician, Royal Brisbane Hospital, Brisbane, Australia.

C.P. PRICE, BSc, PhD, MCB, MRIC, Honorary Senior Lecturer in Chemical Pathology and Human Metabolism, Southampton University Medical School; Top Grade Biochemist, Southampton General Hospital, Southampton.

ALAN E. READ, MD, FRCP, Professor of Medicine, University of Bristol; Consultant Physician, Bristol Health District (Teaching), Bristol.

TELFER B. REYNOLDS, MD, Clayton G. Loosli Professor of Medicine, University of Southern California, Los Angeles, California.

MIKKO P. SALASPURO, MD, Lecturer in Medicine, University of Helsinki; Chief, Gastroenterological Unit, Second Department of Medicine, University of Helsinki, Helsinki, Finland.

S.J. SAUNDERS, MD, FRCP, FCP(SA), Professor and Head, Department of Medicine, and Co-Director, MRC/UCT Liver Research Group, University of Cape Town, Groote Schuur Hospital, Cape Town, South Africa.

FENTON SCHAFFNER, MD, George Baehr Professor of Medicine and Chief, Division of Liver Disease, Mount Sinai School of Medicine, City University of New York, New York.

I. HERBERT SCHEINBERG, MD, Professor of Medicine and Head, Division of Genetic Medicine, Albert Einstein College of Medicine, New York; Visiting Physician, Bronx Municipal Hospital Center, New York.

RUDI SCHMID, MD, PhD, Professor of Medicine, University of California, San Francisco; Director, Liver Center, and Chief, Gastroenterology Unit, University of California, San Francisco, California.

M.M. SCHONLAND, MD, Former Senior Lecturer in Pathology, University of Natal, Natal, South Africa.

JANET SEGGIE, BSc(Hons), MB, MRCP(UK), Medical Registrar, Department of Medicine, University of Cape Town, Groote Schuur Hospital, Cape Town, South Africa.

SHEILA SHERLOCK, DBE, MD, Professor of Medicine and Chairman, Department of Medicine, University of London; Consultant Physician, The Royal Free Hospital, London.

J. MANNY SHORE, MD, FACS, Attending Surgeon, Cedars-Sinai Medical Center, Los Angeles, California.

D.B.A. SILK, MD, MRCP, Senior Lecturer and Consultant, Liver Unit, King's College Hospital, London.

THOMAS E. STARZL, MD, PhD, Professor and Chairman, Department of Surgery, University of Colorado Medical Center, Denver, Colorado.

IRMIN STERNLIEB, MD, Professor of Medicine and Associate Director, Liver Research Center, Albert Einstein College of Medicine, New York; Visiting Physician, Bronx Municipal Hospital Center, New York.

LEO STRUNIN, MD, FFARCS, Professor of Anaesthetics, King's College Hospital Medical School, London; Honorary Consultant Anaesthetist, King's College Hospital, London.

A.S. TAVILL, MD, FRCP, Professor of Medicine, Case Western Reserve University, Cleveland; Director of Gastroenterology, Cleveland Metropolitan General Hospital, Cleveland, Ohio.

J. TERBLANCHE, ChM, FRCS, FCS(SA), Professor of Surgery and Co-Director, MRC/UCT Liver Research Group, Department of Surgery, University of Cape Town, Groote Schuur Hospital, Cape Town, South Africa.

D.R. TRIGER, MA, BM, BCh, DPhil, MRCP, Senior Lecturer in Medicine, University of Sheffield; Honorary Consultant Physician, United Sheffield Hospitals, Sheffield.

ALEXANDER J. WALT, MB, ChB, MS(Minn), FRCS, FRCS(C), FACS, Professor and Chairman, Department of Surgery, Wayne State University School of Medicine, Detroit; Chief of Surgery, Harper-Grace Hospitals and Detroit General Hospital, Detroit, Michigan.

PETER J. WATT, MD, MRCP, Professor of Microbiology, The University of Southampton; Honorary Consultant Microbiologist, Hampshire Area Health Authority, Southampton.

P.J. WHORWELL, BSc, MB, BS, MRCP, Lecturer in Medicine, The University of Southampton and Southampton University Hospitals, Southampton.

S.P. WILKINSON, BSc, MB, MRCP, Senior Medical Registrar, Liver Unit, King's College Hospital, London.

ROGER WILLIAMS, MD, FRCP, Director and Consultant Physician, Liver Unit, King's College Hospital, London.

D.H. WRIGHT, MD, FRCPath, Professor of Pathology, University of Southampton Medical School; Consultant Pathologist, Southampton General Hospital, Southampton.

RALPH WRIGHT, MA, MD, DPhil, FRCP, Professor of Medicine, University of Southampton Medical School and Medical Unit; Honorary Consultant Physician, Southampton General Hospital, Southampton.

Contents

Preface

Hepatology, like other branches of clinical medicine, has increasingly become the province of many special interests involving the clinician, biochemist, immunologist and fundamental cell biologist.

In the new Medical School at Southampton, emphasis is placed on an interdisciplinary approach to teaching and research. It is therefore natural for a physician, a biochemist, a surgeon and a pathologist to adopt a combined pathophysiological approach to diagnosis and management when editing a book on liver disease.

In the first part of the book, we have covered the normal structure and functions of the liver and the way in which they might be deranged in broad basic terms. These include areas such as nutritional and endocrine aspects of liver disease and drug metabolism by the liver which have received little attention in other textbooks. In the second part we have covered the diagnosis and management of specific disorders affecting the liver.

Over the past decade, advances in our knowledge of the basic pathophysiology, diagnosis and management of liver disease have been rapid. During this time, the viruses causing the common forms of viral hepatitis have been identified, their causal relationship to chronic liver disease established and the association of alpha-1-antitrypsin deficiency with liver disease has been recognized. Ultrasonography, computerized tomography and endoscopic retrograde cholangiopancreatography have greatly accelerated diagnosis in the jaundiced patient. New staining techniques and interpretation have improved morphological diagnosis. New approaches to the management of gallstones include endoscopic extraction as well as dissolution by medical means.

A comprehensive textbook is inevitably not fully up to date at the time of publication and this applies particularly in these areas where advances have been so rapid. It is a tribute to our distinguished contributors and the publishers, W.B. Saunders, that this first edition has appeared within three years of its initiation.

Our thanks are due to many others who helped in the preparation of this book. Opinions are inevitably influenced by discussion with colleagues and students for whose stimulus we are greatly indebted. The excellent facilities and the help of the Wessex Medical Library and the Department of Teaching Media have made our task much easier. Much of the histological material in our own chapters has been produced with the assistance of Mr Brian Mepham and Mr

Ray Griffin and staff. We wish to thank our secretaries, particularly Mrs Jill Clark and Mrs Isabella Strachan, as well as Mrs Clare Bright, Miss Phillipa Boston and Mrs Marjorie Slack, who have provided administrative and secretarial help most efficiently and cheerfully coped with our excessive demands. Miss Patricia Terry, manuscript editor, and Mr David Inglis of W.B. Saunders have provided us with friendly and patient but highly professional guidance.

Finally, we wish to dedicate this book to our wives and families for their forbearance and support.

1979

RALPH WRIGHT
K.G.M.M. ALBERTI
STEPHEN KARRAN
G.H. MILLWARD-SADLER

Liver and Biliary Disease

PART ONE

Pathophysiology

Chapter 1

Normal Anatomy

J.L. DAWSON

Functionally the liver is a bilobed organ: each lobe has separate afferent and efferent blood vessels.[6,9] The contiguous surfaces of the two lobes are closely applied and lie within a common capsule, so that there is no external evidence of this important lobar division. The true division between right and left lobes is also called the principal plane of the liver; it corresponds with a line which runs from the fundus of the gallbladder to the vena cava (Figure 1.1). The afferent vessels to the two lobes of the liver enter the organ at the hilum and branch in a recognizable pattern within the liver substance. They are accompanied by the branches of the bile ducts. The regular branching pattern of the portal vein within the hepatic parenchyma allows each lobe of the liver to be subdivided into four functional segments.[6] Knowledge of the intrahepatic segmental anatomy is especially important in the interpretation of selective angiograms and for the planning of hepatic resections. The efferent vessels are the hepatic veins which run quite separately from the afferent vessels within the liver substance and drain directly into the inferior vena cava. None of the hepatic veins has any significant extrahepatic course.

EXTERNAL APPEARANCE

The liver is the largest solid organ in the body and normally weighs between 1.2 and 1.8 kg. It is roughly wedge shaped and the base of the wedge occupies the right side of the upper part of the peritoneal cavity. The right side of the liver is closely applied to the costal fibres and the central tendon of the right leaf of the diaphragm. The left lobe (the apex of the wedge) reaches for a variable distance into the left upper part of the abdominal cavity, abutting the left leaf of the diaphragm. The posterior, upper and anterior surfaces of the liver are convex and the underside to the right of the midline is slightly concave.

Most of the liver substance is covered by peritoneum which, apart from a small area on the underside of the left lobe, is related to the greater sac. The peritoneal attachments are asymmetrical and best understood by considering the development of the liver (see below).

SURFACE ANATOMY

The upper border of the right lobe reaches to the right fifth rib about 2 cm medial to the mid-clavicular line. This is usually 1 cm below the right nipple. The left lobe reaches to the left sixth rib in the mid-clavicular line. This point is about 2 cm below the left nipple. The oblique inferior margin passes from the highest point on the left downwards to the right, passing through the fundus of the gallbladder. This latter point is where the transpyloric plane crosses the costal margin.

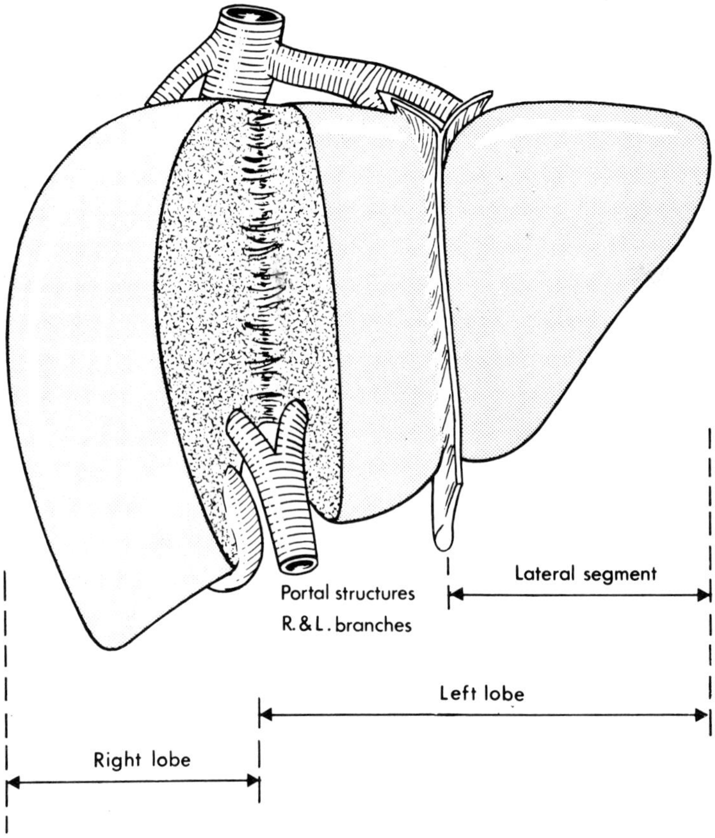

Figure 1.1. Diagram to show the two functional halves of the liver. The three hilar structures are represented by a single tube with right and left elements. The hepatic veins are shown with a long extrahepatic course for the sake of clarity. The functional division into right and left lobes is not related to the attachment of the falciform ligament.

DEVELOPMENT

In the developing embryo the gut is suspended dorsally by a double fold of peritoneum. Between the two layers of this fold run three arteries, the coeliac, the superior mesenteric and the inferior mesenteric. The area of gut supplied by each of these vessels is known as the foregut, midgut and hindgut respectively. In addition to a dorsal mesentery the foregut is also attached ventrally by a ventral mesogastrium which develops from the caudal part of the septum transversum. Initially, the ventral mesogastrium contains a mass of anastomosing veins into which drain the vitelline veins from the yolk sac. The vitelline veins later form the portal system and the yolk sac becomes the gut.

The liver first appears as a hollow endodermal bud from the foregut. This bud grows into the ventral mesogastrium and the end bifurcates and produces epithelial trabeculae which are called the hepatic cylinders. Extensive branching takes place and the cells proliferate to produce a meshwork. These cells become the liver cells and the spaces between them become the sinusoids of the liver. Thus the hepatic cell in the adult comes to lie in close contact with blood draining from the portal venous system. The gallbladder develops as a separate bud from the main diverticulum. It is solid at first but later in development becomes hollow. Initially, the blood from the yolk sac is drained through right and left vitelline veins which also have numerous cross channels. During development, complicated changes take place, with the disappearance of some segments and persistence of some communicating veins, until the normal adult arrangement of a single portal vein dividing into right and left branches of the hilum of the liver is achieved. On the cephalic side of the liver, part of the vitelline venous system persists as the terminal segment of the inferior vena cava.

Early in development there are two umbilical veins but the right soon disappears. The left runs in the free edge of the ventral mesogastrium and drains into the left branch of the portal vein. In the fetus there is a further venous channel, the ductus venosum, which connects the left branch of the portal vein to the inferior vena cava. This channel allows oxygenated

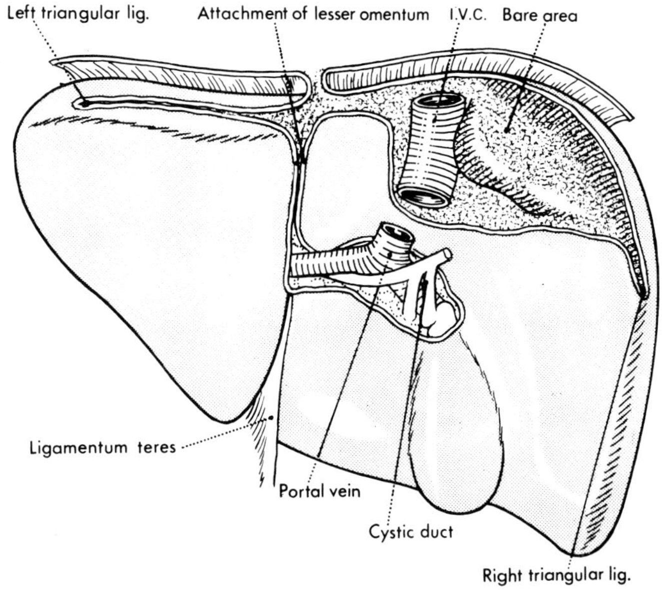

Figure 1.2. Sketch of the posterior aspect of the liver to show the arrangement of the peritoneal attachments. Note the horizontal course of the left branch of the portal vein and the comparatively short course of the right branch.

blood from the placenta to bypass the liver and gain direct access to the inferior vena cava. The umbilical vein closes soon after birth and the adult remnant is known as the ligamentum teres. The ductus venosus closes and becomes the ligamentum venosum which, in the adult, is found in the region of the attachment of the lesser omentum to the under surface of the liver (Figure 1.2). Even in the adult it is possible to dilate up the obliterated umbilical vein to gain access to the portal venous system through the left branch of the portal vein, e.g. for radiological investigations. As the development of the fetus proceeds, the viscera in the upper abdomen rotate and an enormous growth of the liver occurs. The two leaves of peritoneum, which make up the ventral mesogastrium, are taken up over the liver, almost completely covering it. In the adult, only the lesser omentum and falciform ligament remain as a double leaf of peritoneum, and the ligamentum teres notches the inferior border of the liver.

PERITONEAL ATTACHMENTS

In the adult the falciform ligament stretches from the body wall to the liver. The line of its ventral attachment runs from the umbilicus along the posterior aspect of the anterior abdominal wall and the diaphragm in the midline as far back as the inferior vena cava opening just above the liver. Its attachment to the liver is to the right of the midline; thus the falciform ligament lies in an oblique plane with its right surface facing anteriorly and its left surface facing posteriorly. The left leaf of the falciform ligament is continued laterally and to the left over the surface of the liver where superiorly it becomes the left triangular ligament of the liver. This ligament consists of the two layers of peritoneum, from the anterior and posterior aspect of the left lobe of the liver, which have been fused together and which suspend the lateral part of the left lobe of the liver to the under surface of the diaphragm. The left phrenic vessels run close to the diaphragmatic attachment of this ligament. Division of the left triangular ligament of the liver renders the lateral part of the left lobe of the liver freely mobile. The medial end of the posterior aspect of the triangular ligament is continued into the two layers of the lesser omentum.

The lesser omentum is a double layer of peritoneum and represents that part of the ventral mesogastrium between the stomach and the liver; in its free lower margin run the three structures of the portal triad, the bile ducts anteriorly to the right, the hepatic artery anteriorly slightly to the left and the portal vein immediately posterior to both structures. On the liver the right posterior leaf of the lesser omentum is reflected inferiorly over the front of the inferior cava and passes to the right. The two layers of the peritoneum here are widely separated to encompass the bare area of the liver, except at the extreme right where they fuse to become the right triangular ligament of the

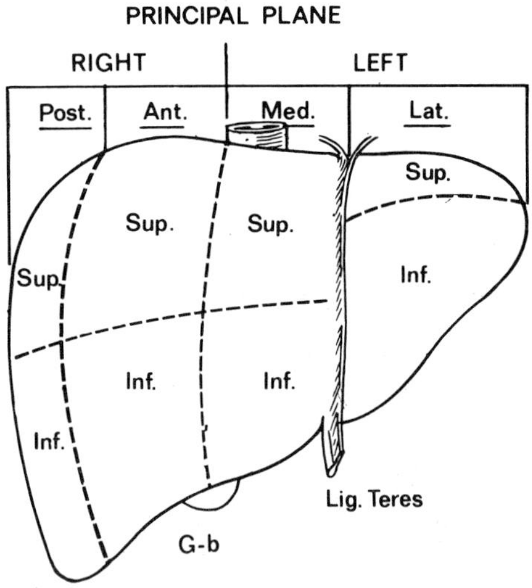

Figure 1.3. The surface markings of the eight segments of the liver.

liver (Figure 1.2). The upper reflection of the peritoneum is continued until it reaches the right lateral leaf of the falciform ligament. Division of the right triangular ligament and the two diverging peritoneal reflections on the right lobe of the liver, as far medially as the inferior vena cava, is required to mobilize the right lobe of the liver and gain access to its posterior aspect.

THE LOBES OF THE LIVER

For the clinician the division of the liver into two functional parts called right and left lobes is of considerable practical importance (Figure 1.1). The left lobe is further subdivided by the attachment of the falciform ligament into medial and lateral segments.

Before the bilateral nature of the liver was appreciated[9] the liver was arbitrarily divided into various parts according to the peritoneal attachments, e.g. quadrate and caudate lobes. These names are purely descriptive and do not have much practical significance.

The regular branching pattern of the 'afferent structures' (i.e., portal vein, hepatic artery and bile ducts) allows the right and left lobes of the liver to be further subdivided into four parts or segments. The right lobe is divided into anterior and posterior parts, each of which is subdivided into superior and inferior parts.

The left lobe is divided by the line of the umbilical fissure into medial and lateral parts, each of which is subdivided into superior and inferior segments. The surface marking of these eight segments of the liver is shown in Figure 1.3. Surface fissures, corresponding to the division of the right lobe into anterior and posterior parts, are sometimes seen in the liver at operation, but usually the external capsule gives no clue to the segmental arrangement of the parenchyma.

ARTERIAL BLOOD SUPPLY

The hepatic artery supplies arterial blood to the liver; it is responsible for approximately 25 to 30 per cent of the total afferent blood flow but carries about 50 per cent of the available

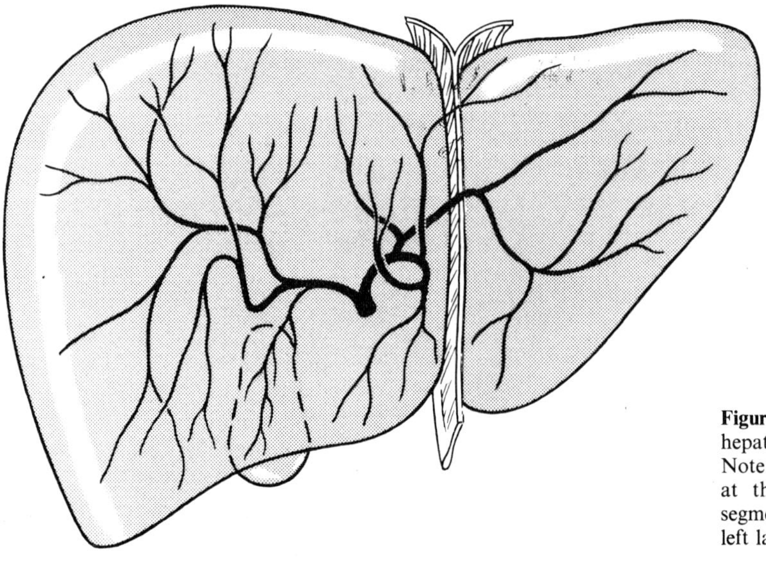

Figure 1.4. Diagram to show the intrahepatic distribution of the hepatic artery. Note the 'returning loop' of the left branch at the junction of medial and lateral segments. It is liable to injury here during left lateral segmentectomy.

oxygen. The hepatic artery most commonly arises as a branch of the coeliac axis and passes forwards and to the right to gain access to the lesser omentum. As it does so it raises a small fold of peritoneum, the right or inferior gastropancreatic fold, which lies at the lower margin of the inner aspect of the aditus to the lesser sac. Before it passes upwards to the hilum of the liver the hepatic artery gives off the right gastric and gastroduodenal arteries. It divides at the hilum of the liver into right and left branches. The intrahepatic course of these arteries and their branches is shown in Figure 1.4. The division takes place at a variable level, sometimes being high in the hilum, sometimes being comparatively low down in the free edge of the lesser omentum. The right and left hepatic arteries usually lie on a plane posterior to the bile ducts at the hilum of the liver. The cystic artery which supplies the gallbladder is usually given off in the lesser omentum from the right branch of the hepatic artery and passes behind the bile ducts to reach the anterior surface of the gallbladder. Variations in the arrangement of the arterial supply to the liver are common and a completely normal arrangement is found in only 50 per cent of subjects.[10] Part or all of the left lobe of the liver may be supplied by an abnormal left hepatic artery which arises from the left gastric artery. All or part of the territory normally supplied by the right branch of the hepatic artery may come from a vessel which arises from the superior mesenteric artery. Such an abnormal right hepatic artery passes up to the hilum of the liver, lying at first posterior to the portal vein, and often winds around its right margin in the lesser omentum. This arrangement may sometimes cause difficulty when the portal vein is being dissected free in the course of a portacaval shunt operation. Sometimes the superior mesenteric artery may share a common origin with the coeliac axis. All of these abnormal vessels are end arteries, not accessory vessels, and their division results in lack of arterial supply to that part of the liver to which they are distributed. The branching of the hepatic artery within the liver is very similar to the pattern of the portal vein (Figures 1.4 and 1.5).

THE PORTAL VEIN

The portal vein drains blood from the splanchnic area and carries approximately 75 per cent of the total liver blood flow. It is formed behind the neck of the pancreas as an upward continuation of the superior mesenteric vein after this vessel has been joined by the splenic vein. It then lies posterior to the bile ducts and hepatic artery in the free edge of the lesser omentum. At the hilum of the liver the vein divides into right and left branches which run with the right and left hepatic arteries and the

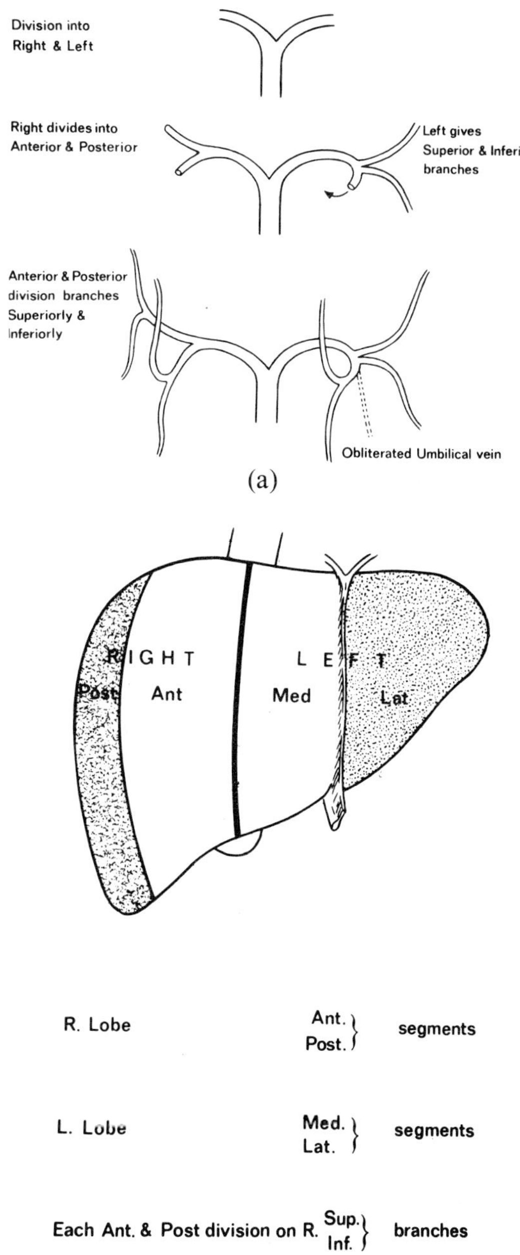

(b)

Figure 1.5. Diagrams showing the progressive branching of the intrahepatic portal vein and its distribution to the lobes of the liver.

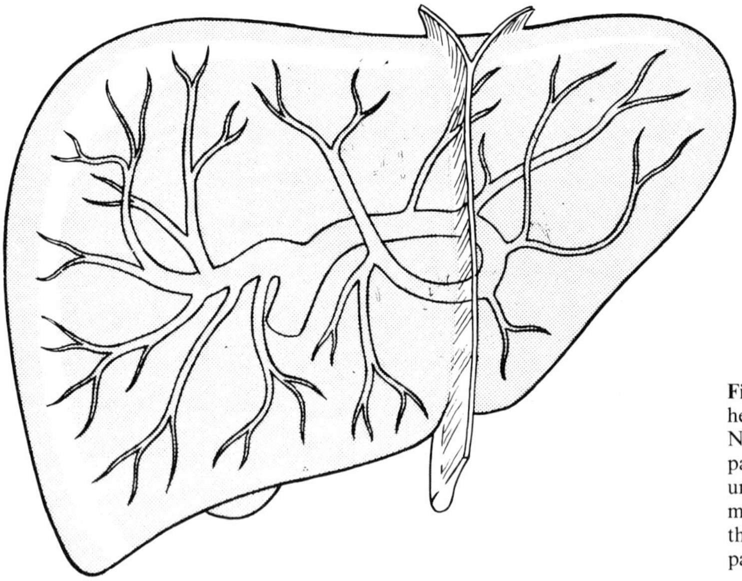

Figure 1.6. Diagram to show the intrahepatic distribution of the portal vein. Note that the left branch has a horizontal part which turns forwards towards the umbilical fissure. The branches to the medial segment of the left lobe come from the right side of this part of the vessel (the pars umbilicalis).

right and left hepatic ducts. The right branch of the portal vein is shorter than the left and runs more vertically. It is therefore much more difficult to dissect than the left.

The portal vein has a recognizable pattern of branching within the liver and, unlike the hepatic arterial supply, anomalies are rare. Each branch of the portal vein within the liver is accompanied by divisions of the hepatic artery and bile ducts. The regular intrahepatic branching pattern allows the liver to be divided into eight segments (see Figure 1.5a). However, the vascular pedicle of each of these segments lies within hepatic parenchyma so that resection of a single segment is difficult.

The main right and left branches of the portal vein supply the right and left lobes of the liver. The right branch of the portal vein is usually less than 3 cm long. It divides into anterior and posterior branches which supply the anterior and posterior parts of the right lobe. Each of these vessels divides again into superior and inferior branches. The right lobe is thus divided into four segments (see Figures 1.5b and 1.3).

The left branch of the portal vein passes horizontally to the left (Figure 1.6) to give branches to supply the superior and inferior parts of the lateral part of the left lobe. The vein is then joined by the obliterated umbilical vein as it turns medially. The terminal part of the vessel divides into superior and inferior branches which supply the superior and inferior segments of the medial part of the left lobe.

This arrangement of blood supply to the medial segment of the left lobe may lead to inadvertent devascularization of either the medial or lateral segment of the left lobe during trisegmentectomy or lateral segmentectomy.[2,11]

THE HEPATIC VEINS

All the hepatic veins drain into the inferior vena cava (Figure 1.7). None of them has any significant extra-hepatic course. Three large hepatic veins lie posterosuperiorly just below the diaphragm and a number of smaller ones drain from the posterior aspect of the right lobe directly into the vena cava which is lying in a groove in the liver substance. The branches of the hepatic vein ramify in the hepatic parenchyma in a distribution that is quite separate from the rest of the vascular and biliary structures. The right hepatic vein drains most of the true right lobe of the liver, namely all the posterior segment and part of the anterior segment. The vein itself lies in the plane between the anterior and posterior segment. The surface marking of this plane is approximately the line of the eighth intercostal space. The middle hepatic vein lies in the principal plane between the true right and left lobes and drains approximately one-third of the liver substance, namely part of the anterior segment of the right lobe and the whole of the medial segment of the left lobe, the latter being that part which lies between the falciform ligament and the principal plane. The middle hepatic vein drains into

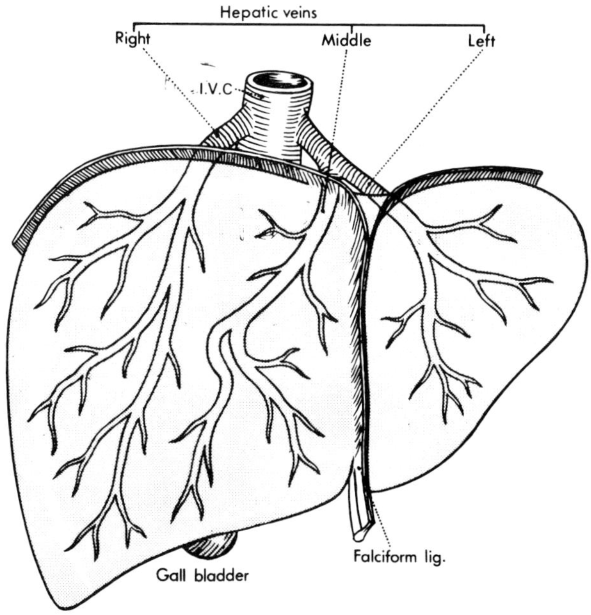

Figure 1.7. Diagram to show the usual arrangement of the main hepatic veins (the small veins draining the posterior aspect of the right lobe into the inferior vena cava are not shown). For the sake of clarity the right and left hepatic veins are shown as having an extrahepatic course (which they do not).

the left hepatic vein or, sometimes, it opens separately into the inferior vena cava (Figure 1.7). The left hepatic vein drains the left lateral segment of the liver (i.e., that part which lies lateral to the falciform ligament) and it drains directly into the inferior vena cava. The number of small veins varies but may reach 15, and these pass from the posterior aspect of the right lobe of the liver into the inferior vena cava (not shown in Figure 1.7). Usually the most caudal ones are the largest. These veins are particularly thin walled and great care has to be taken during their dissection in a right hemihepatectomy.[8]

THE GALLBLADDER

The gallbladder is pear shaped and lies on the under surface of the liver. It holds 50 to 75 ml of bile and is connected to the common hepatic duct by the cystic duct. The blind end, or fundus, usually projects beyond the lower end of the liver and is the lowest point. The body of the gallbladder is applied to the sloping under surface of the liver by the peritoneum; thus it passes upwards and medially before tapering to join the cystic duct. About two-thirds of the circumference of the gallbladder are usually visible. They are covered by peritoneum. The body of the gallbladder sometimes lies in a deep bed of liver tissue and is hardly visible. Alternatively, the peritoneal covering may be fused between the liver and the gallbladder, thus creating a mesentery which allows the gall-bladder to undergo torsion. In adult life a dilatation of the gallbladder at the point where the neck joins the cystic duct (Hartmann's pouch) is often seen at operation. This dilatation is probably the result of pathology and is not a normal anatomical structure.

The cystic duct runs downwards with a sinuous course before joining the common hepatic duct to form the common bile duct. Its lumen contains a spiral valve of Heister and this 'concertinaed' part of the cystic duct is surrounded by connective tissue and autonomic nerves. The cystic duct usually enters from the right side to form a T-junction but the manner of this junction varies greatly. For example, the cystic duct may run anterior or posterior to the bile duct, spiralling round it before joining it on its medial side (Figure 1.8). Sometimes the bile duct joins the common bile duct and runs parallel with it for some distance before entering its lumen. From the outside there may be no obvious sulcus and the duct system is double barrelled for a short distance. This arrangement may occasionally give rise to confusion during attempted exploration of the common bile duct. The cystic artery pursues a straight course to the gallbladder and until it is divided at operation the cystic duct cannot be dissected free and 'straightened out'. The tortuous course of the

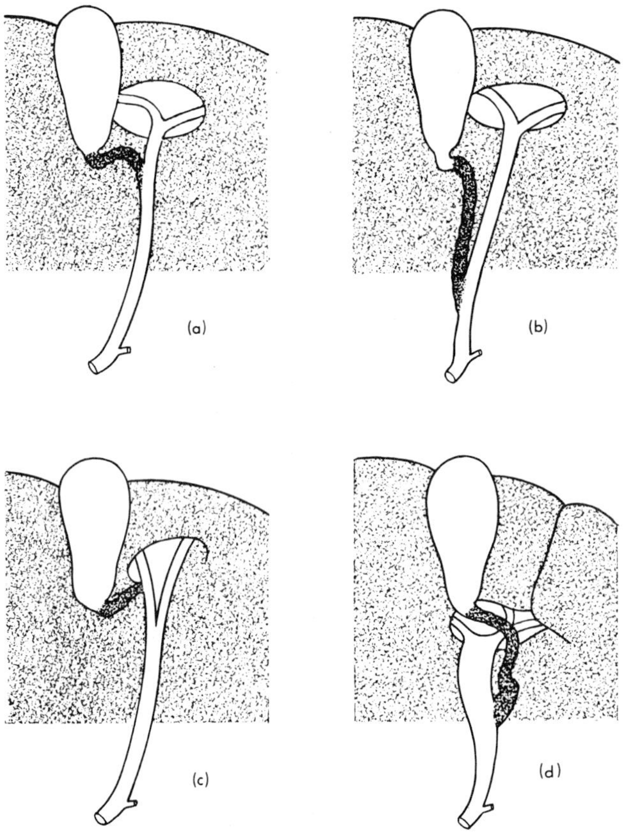

Figure 1.8. Sketches to show some of the common variations in the mode of the junction between the cystic duct and the common hepatic duct (CHD): (a) a high union with the CHD; (b) low union with the CHD. The ducts may be 'double-barrelled', i.e. share a common covering with no sulcus visible externally; (c) union with the right hepatic duct. This is often associated with a low union of the right and left hepatic ducts; (d) entry of the cystic duct low on the left side of the CHD. The cystic duct may cross either in front of or behind the CHD. After Grant (1947) *An Atlas of Anatomy* (Williams and Wilkins, Baltimore).

cystic duct is not often seen when the gallbladder is damaged by severe inflammatory disease.

BILE DUCTS

Bile ducts drain bile from the bile ductular and canalicular network of the lobule (see below). These ducts run with the branches of the portal vein and hepatic artery between the liver lobules. The smallest interlobular ducts eventually join to form septal bile ducts and these finally form the right and left hepatic ducts draining the true right and left lobes of the liver. These ducts usually fuse at the hilum of the liver as they emerge from the capsule to form the common hepatic duct which runs caudally in the free edge of the lesser omentum. The common hepatic duct is joined at a variable level by the cystic duct to form the common bile duct, normally about 2.5 cm above the duodenum. Variations in the anatomy of the biliary tree are common. The junction of right and left hepatic ducts may be low, e.g. 2 to 5 cm below the hilum of the liver. The cystic duct may join the right hepatic duct rather than the common bile duct. The common bile duct passes downwards behind the first part of the duodenum and the head of the pancreas. This part of the duct is often completely buried in the pancreas. The duct then inclines to the right to pass through the duodenal wall to open into the lumen about 10 cm from the pylorus. The lumen of the common duct is considerably reduced as it passes through the duodenal wall. A characteristic notch is seen on the operative cholangiogram and this represents the upper border of the choledochal sphincter which surrounds the distal duct and extends upwards around the duct, reaching more proximally than the duodenal wall itself.[4] The pancreatic duct lies in close apposition to the narrow segment of bile duct and is also surrounded by the fibres of the choledochal sphincter. The common bile duct and pancreatic ducts have a common channel, from 2 to 7 mm long, which is usually called the ampulla of Vater although there is in fact no dilatation or ampulla. The distal part of the duct is surrounded by the choledochal muscle and lies in the medial wall of the second part of the duodenum. The opening is recognized by a small elevation, the papilla, which can be seen and felt.

BLOOD SUPPLY OF GALLBLADDER AND BILE DUCTS

The gallbladder is supplied by the cystic artery which is normally a branch of the right hepatic artery. The latter usually passes laterally behind the common hepatic duct before giving off the cystic artery which reaches the gallbladder on the superior aspect of its neck. At this point the right hepatic artery turns cephalad to enter the liver. The cystic lymph node is closely related to the cystic artery on the wall of the gallbladder. The artery usually divides into two vessels on the surface of the gallbladder. These divide again so that four vessels run towards the fundus, giving off tiny lateral branches to produce a reticular pattern.[3] However, the origin and course of the cystic artery are variable. It may reach the gallbladder by passing caudal to the union of the cystic and common hepatic ducts. It may pass in front of the common hepatic duct and there may be two cystic arteries (see Chapter 53). The common bile duct is supplied by small twigs derived from the hepatic artery as well as from the gastroduodenal artery.

The veins draining the gallbladder show no constant pattern and drain directly into the liver; they also communicate with the meshwork of veins, the choledochal plexus, which surrounds and drains the bile ducts. This plexus communicates with the duodenal, pancreatic and gastric venous drainage.

The lymphatics of the gallbladder drain through the cystic and superior pancreatic and duodenal lymph nodes. The latter is constant and is sometimes known as the common duct node because it lies immediately to the right of the common bile duct at the junction of the first and second parts of the duodenum. It is sometimes a useful landmark during re-exploration of the common bile duct. As the cystic gland lies in close proximity to the cystic artery on the wall of the gallbladder it is a useful landmark for the surgeon seeking the cystic artery.

NERVE SUPPLY

The nerve supply of the liver and biliary tree is derived from the hepatic plexus which is formed by sympathetic fibres from thoracic segments 7 to 10, parasympathetic fibres from both right and left vagi and a few fibres from the right phrenic nerve.[1] The branches from the left vagus run in the upper part of the lesser omentum towards the hilum of the liver. Branches of the sympathetic and the right vagus travel with the hepatic arteries to reach the viscera. Afferent impulses from the liver and common duct travel in the sympathetic nerves.

LYMPH DRAINAGE OF THE LIVER

Lymph from the liver drains through superficial and deep channels. The convex surface drains into nodes along the falciform ligament, coeliac axis and oesophageal nodes. Some passes through the diaphragm into the xiphisternal nodes.

The under surface of the liver drains to nodes on the inferior vena cava and the common bile duct. The deep channels surround each branch of the portal vein and pass to the biliary and hepatic artery nodes. The nodes in the porta are arranged in an asymmetrical fashion and lie posterior to the portal vein and its left branch. On the right, nodes occur infrequently and are small. Nodal enlargement is an unlikely cause of obstruction to bile flow.[5]

REFERENCES

1. Burnett, W., Cairns, F.W. & Bacsich, P. (1964) Innervation of the extrahepatic biliary system. *Annals of Surgery*, **123**, 8–26.
2. Goldsmith, N.A. & Woodburne, R.T. (1957) The surgical anatomy pertaining to liver resection. *Surgery, Gynecology and Obstetrics*, **105**, 310–318.
3. Gordon, K.C.D. (1967) Cystic arterial patterns in diseased human gall bladders. *Gut*, **8**, 565–568.
4. Hand, B.H. (1973) Anatomy and function of the extra hepatic biliary system. *Clinics in Gastroenterology*, **2**, 3–29.
5. Hardy, K.J., Wheatley, I.C., Anderson, A.I.E. & Bond, R.J. (1976) The lymph nodes of the porta hepatis. *Surgery, Gynecology and Obstetrics*, **143**, 225–228.

6. Healey, J.E. (1954) Clinical anatomic aspects of radical hepatic surgery. *Journal of the International College of Surgeons,* **22,** 542.
7. Healey, J.E., Schroy, P. & Sorensen, R. (1953) The intrahepatic distribution of the hepatic artery in man. *Journal of the International College of Surgeons,* **20,** 133.
8. Longmire, W.P. & Cleveland, R.J. (1972) Surgical anatomy and blunt trauma of the liver. *Surgical Clinics of North America,* **52,** 687–689.
9. McIndoe, A.H. & Counseller, V.S. (1927) The bilaterality of the liver. *Archives of Surgery,* **15,** 589–611.
10. Michels, N.A. (1960) Newer anatomy of liver: variant blood supply and collateral circulation. *Journal of the American Medical Association,* **172,** 125.
11. Starzl, T.E., Bell, R.H., Beart, R.W. & Putnam, C.W. (1975) Hepatic trisegmentectomy and other liver resections. *Surgery, Gynecology and Obstetrics,* **141,** 429–437.

Chapter 2

Normal Histology and Ultrastructure

G.H. MILLWARD-SADLER
A.M. JEZEQUEL

LIVER MICROANATOMY AND HISTOLOGY

G.H. MILLWARD-SADLER

The commonly accepted basic unit of the liver is the lobule. This is identified from the microscopic anatomical features of the liver and is composed of a central efferent vein surrounded by parenchyma with portal tracts at the periphery. It does not correspond to the acinus which is the functional unit of the liver.[85] An acinus is composed of a portal tract and that mass of parenchyma dependent on the blood flow arriving through the vessels within the tract. It is not well defined anatomically without injection studies.

Because of long-established usage as well as the pragmatic identification of an anatomical substructure in liver biopsies we shall continue to use the term 'lobule' throughout this book. Nonetheless, the concept of the acinus often allows better understanding of disease mechanisms and their relationship to the morphological features produced so that both entities will be described before individual features are considered.[87]

HEPATIC ARCHITECTURE

The Lobule

The lobule is the classical microscopic unit of the liver and is an efferent vein centrally positioned and surrounded by radially orientated sinusoids alternating with anastomosing columns of hepatocytes. Spaced around the periphery are up to five or six portal tracts, although rarely more than three or four tracts are seen in human liver (Figure 2.1). The lobule is occasionally emphasized, as in the pig, by fibrous tissue which links the portal tracts and so highlights the central position of the efferent vein.[34]

In this lobular concept, the unit vessel to which the parenchyma is related is not the portal vein or hepatic artery but the central hepatic vein which receives blood from several portal tracts. In addition, despite the enlarge-

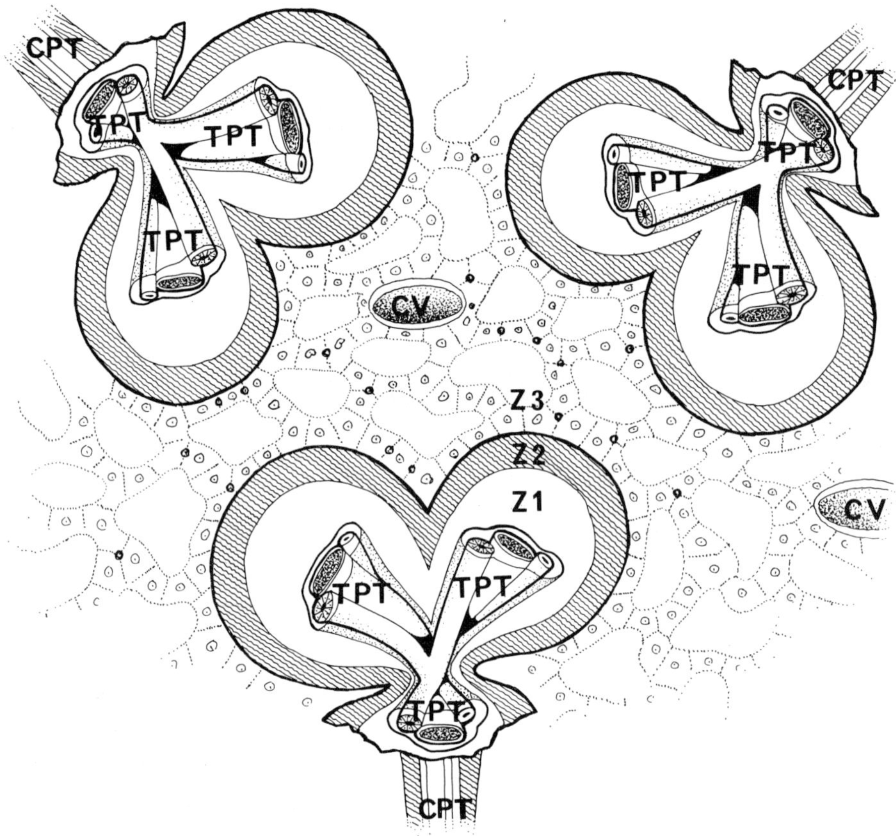

Figure 2.1. This is a diagrammatic representation of a lobule with the centrally positioned vein (CV) surrounded by parenchyma and with the portal tracts (TPT) at the periphery. Note that the portal tracts normally arise at differing heights and angles from the conducting tract and not, as represented here, by simultaneous division. Thus there may be as few as three or as many as six portal tracts visualized around any one lobule.

Three conducting portal tracts (CPT) here each split into three terminal portal tracts (TPT). The parenchyma has been diagrammatically represented as three zones which do not have a morphologically visible counterpart in routine histology. Zone 1 (Z1) is immediately around the terminal portal tract. Zone 2 (Z2) surrounds zone 1 and zone 3 (Z3), drawn in as hepatocytes and sinusoids, fills in the spaces between the zone 2s down to the central efferent vein (CV).

Each terminal portal tract is surrounded by zoned parenchyma and constitutes an acinus. Each group of three acini with their conducting portal tract form a complex acinus. Nine potential acini are illustrated, of which six are more fully detailed to include zone 3 hepatocytes. No acinus is complete because each will drain to more than one central vein.

Note also that one lobule is formed from between three and six acini with approximately half of any one acinus contributing to the lobule.

ment of the central veins as they unite to drain into the hepatic veins, the lobule is the basic microanatomical structure and there is no compounding of units to form a lobular complex.

The Acinus

The acinus is the functional unit of the liver and conceptually is a mass of parenchyma dependent upon a unit blood supply which is provided through the portal tracts. Therefore, the acinus has a central portal tract of the smallest calibre which when transversely sectioned may be identified in a liver biopsy as a small round portal tract. The blood flows from the artery and portal vein of this terminal portal tract into the sinusoids, supplies the intervening parenchyma and then drains into two or three peripheral efferent veins (the central veins of the lobule). Each efferent vein receives blood from several acini. The hepatocytes of the acinus are zoned or graded relative to the terminal portal tract. Those nearest the tract are zone 1 and those farthest away zone 3 (Figure 2.1). This grading cannot be histologically identified by standard methods but it reflects, for instance, the distribution of oxygenated blood to hepatocytes and the distribution of intracellular metabolic functions.

Hepatocytes adjacent to the portal tract receive blood with the highest content of oxygen, insulin and glucagon. This increased oxygen and nutrient content of the blood may explain the higher metabolic ability of zone 1 hepatocytes and also the fact that the earliest signs of regeneration are found here. Autoradiographic studies using ^{3}H-leucine have demonstrated that protein synthesis occurs predominantly in the periportal hepatocytes corresponding to zone 1.[50] The microanatomical distribution of intracellular enzymes supports the concept of the Rappaport acinus. Thus, transaminases,[98] glutamyl transpeptidase[68] and alcohol dehydrogenase[32] are most readily demonstrated in periportal, zone 1 hepatocytes while the NADH and NADPH reductases and esterases are likewise seen in zone 3 hepatocytes.[68]

Complex acinus

This is the term used for groups of three or more simple acini served by the common vascular bundle of a larger conducting portal tract.[86] The latter has a triangular outline on liver biopsy. Both the portal vein and hepatic artery within this conducting portal tract subdivide into branches, each of which is terminal and supplies one acinus. In addition to the simple acini, a complex acinus has a sheath of hepatocytes around the conducting portal tract which does not belong to any acinus but which is supplied by vascular twigs arising directly from the vessels of the conducting tract. This sheath is a composite of small groups of hepatocytes and each group is called an acinulus. A tiny vascular twig supplies each acinulus. The grade III hepatocytes from the simple acini abut on to this acinular sleeve of hepatocytes. Consequently, necrosis of zone 3 hepatocytes will appear not only as centrilobular necrosis but also may be found approximating to some of the larger portal tracts, exaggerating the severity of the lesion. Such necrosis often has a stellate configuration and this is more easily explained using the concept of the acinus.

Acinar agglomerate

A further enlargement of the multi-acinar concept has also been described in which three or more of these complex acini are grouped together to form an acinar agglomerate. This likewise has a directly supplied sleeve of hepatocytes around the basic vascular core. These complicated acinar agglomerates are not visualized fully in routine histological sections because their divisions branch to produce a three-dimensional network that is being examined in only two dimensions. Their complete demonstration requires the use of vascular injection studies and cleared thick sections of liver.[86]

Biliary Tree

So far, no mention has been made of the biliary tree but in essence the features are the same although the flow pattern is reversed. Consequently, bile produced by hepatocytes of one acinus drains through the canalicular network to the appropriate portal tract and is then excreted through the supra-acinar organization in the variously graded interlobular and, finally, septal bile ducts. As there are components of several drainage pathways in a *lobule*, functional disturbance in hepatocytes of one *acinus* may result in an eccentric distribution of bile around the central vein. The intrahepatic canaliculi do not simply run between hepatocytes in a straight line from efferent vein to portal tract but form a complicated three-dimensional network.[36,103] The anastomoses are so extensive that focal mechanical obstruction at this level does not usually result in blockage of bile flow.

HISTOLOGY

Portal Tracts (see Figure 2.2)

The stromal trabeculae of the liver are continuous with its capsule and extend from the porta hepatis into the organ by repeated branching. The various branches of the portal vein, hepatic artery and bile ducts, as well as lymphatics and nerve fibres, are carried within these trabeculae. The stroma is a tightly woven meshwork of type I collagen bundles and elastic fibres with the elongated spindle nuclei of the fibroblast interspersed. The stroma is condensed into a concentrically orientated cuff around the bile ducts, especially those of septal calibre. Basement membrane is found around the various arterial, portal venous and bile duct branches in the portal tract.

In biopsy specimens the majority of portal

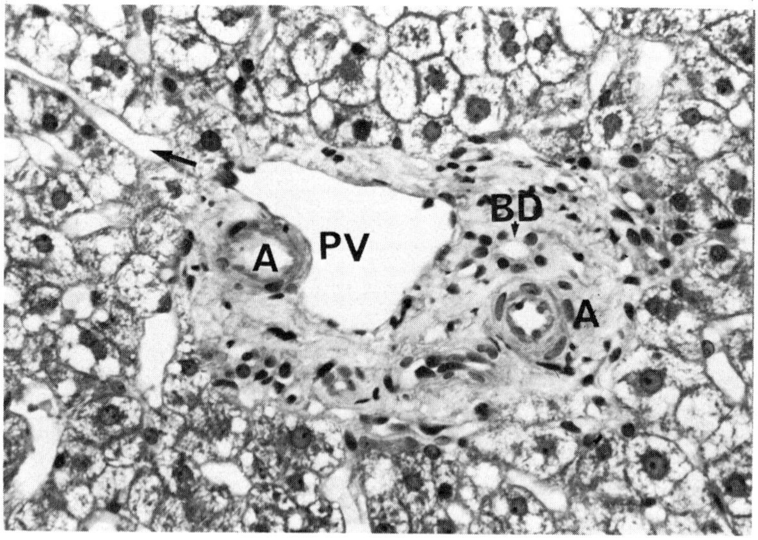

Figure 2.2. An oval cross-section of a terminal portal tract. The portal vein is the largest vascular space (PV) and a tributary has directly entered the sinusoid (arrow). Two arterioles are present (A). The endothelium and double layer of smooth muscle cells are clearly demonstrated in the arteriole on the right. A small interlobular bile duct (BD) is present just above this arteriole and small bile ductules are present along the lower margin of the tract.

tracts will be terminal structures or their preterminal trunks. The former are the smallest divisions and are visualized as round or oval tracts when cut in cross-section (Figure 2.2). Their preterminal trunks are larger and in cross-section are the smallest angular, frequently triangular, tracts. This appearance is created by the branching of the trunks into their terminal divisions. Consequently, a longitudinal section of these trunks may show a bifurcating portal tract. All three branches are rarely identified in the plane of a single section in routine histological preparations.

Hepatic artery

Branches of the hepatic artery are intimately related to the corresponding branch of the portal vein. As well as branching, the artery spirals around the portal vein (Figure 2.3) and thus may appear as several unconnected arteries adjacent to a portal vein.

Arteries and arterioles that are commonly visualized in biopsy material have at most an intima, an internal elastic lamina and two or three layers of smooth muscle cells in the media (Figures 2.2 and 2.3). A cuff of adventitia surrounds the media and contains numerous unmyelinated nerve fibres. The terminal arterioles are much smaller, lack an internal elastic lamina and have intima surrounded by a single layer of smooth muscle. They produce a leash of capillaries that encircles the accompanying bile duct and is termed the 'peribiliary plexus'.[59] This is thought to help to regulate the concentration of bile excreted. Drainage of the plexus is directly into the sinusoids.[63] Another leash of capillaries from the arteriole supplies other portal tract structures and drains either directly into the sinusoidal network or may join the terminal portal venule immediately before it enters this network. A smooth muscle sphincter has been described around these latter capillaries so that the volume and pressure of arterial blood can be controlled.[89]

Portal vein

In microscopic sections, branches of the portal vein are usually the largest blood-containing, endothelial-lined space within the portal tract (Figures 2.2 and 2.3). Smooth muscle surrounds the endothelium in the largest veins but such branches are rarely identified within biopsy material. Mostly, veins are composed of a layer of endothelium surrounded by a thin basement membrane. Both the 'conducting' and 'axial distributing' veins, as described by Elias,[21] produce a large number of venules which empty into periportal sinusoids. Many, if not all, of these venules, as well as those arising from terminals of the portal vein, regulate the rate of flow of portal blood into the sinusoids.[86] However, as there are no muscle cells it has been suggested that this is possible only through swelling and shrinking of reticuloendothelial cells at the junction of venules with sinusoids.[57] The mechanisms by which this postulated sphincter is controlled are not understood but a response to vasodilators such as adenine nucleotides was noted.[57] As these vasodilators are postulated to arise locally from hypoxic

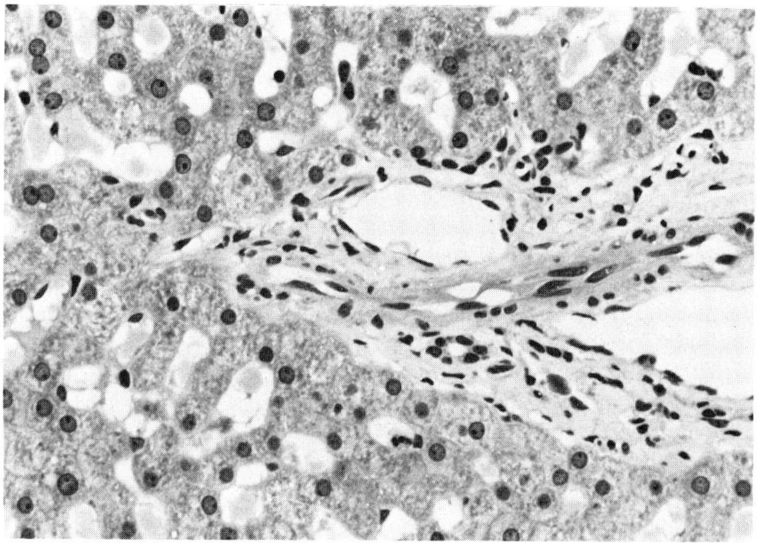

Figure 2.3. A terminal portal tract cut obliquely. The hepatic arteriole runs longitudinally from right to centre and, in spiralling around the portal vein, appears to separate it into the two branches. The limiting plate of hepatocytes is clearly defined along the lower margin of the portal tract as the layer of hepatocytes parallel to the edge of the tract and at right angles to the other plates of hepatocytes.

hepatocytes and as oxygenated blood is provided predominantly by the arterioles a complex interrelationship may exist in the regulation of sinusoidal blood flow.

A second mechanism may be present. Arteriolar vasodilatation will increase the arteriolar blood contribution in the sinusoids. Thus a higher pressure will be transmitted into the sinusoid effectively reducing portal venous flow. McCuskey[57] has described types of arterioportal anastomoses, one of which may be very effective in this respect. The arteriolar blood empties directly into the sinusoid just beyond the portal vein inlet but is directed against the flow of blood entering the sinusoid from the portal venule. Arteriolar vasodilatation will therefore be a very effective means of reducing portal blood flow.

Bile ducts

The largest intrahepatic branches are the septal bile ducts (Figure 2.4) which, after repeated branching, diminish in calibre to interlobular bile ducts. The smallest interlobular bile duct is present in the terminal portal tracts (Figure 2.2) and communicates by bile ductules and the canal of Hering with the canalicular network (Figure 2.23) between hepatocytes. All branches of the biliary tree, down to the junction of ductule with hepatocytes, have a basement

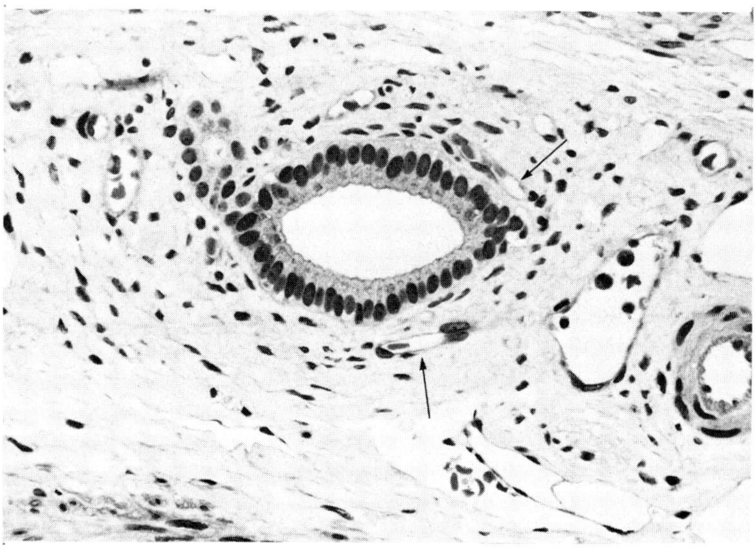

Figure 2.4. Septal bile duct lined by tall columnar epithelium with oval nuclei at the basal pole of the cell. The stroma immediately around the bile duct is more condensed and contains capillaries (arrows) which are part of the peribiliary plexus.

membrane. This is a homogeneous layer of a gel containing mucopolysaccharides and mucoprotein in contact with the duct epithelium on one surface and closely associated with fine reticular fibres on the other surface. It is classified as type IV collagen. Because of its mucopolysaccharide component it can be well demonstrated by oxidation–aldehyde techniques such as periodic acid-Schiff or methenamine-silver.[75] Bile duct basement membrane may be antigenically distinct from capillary basement membrane.[80]

Septal bile ducts are readily recognized by their large calibre although the greatest has a diameter two to three times that of the smallest. Characteristically, the epithelium is formed by tall columnar mucus-secreting cells resting on a basement membrane. These have abundant clear cytoplasm and a small round or oval nucleus situated at the basal pole of the cell (Figure 2.4). The cytoplasm and apical border stain positively with the periodic acid-Schiff (PAS) technique and the cytoplasmic contents can be stained by alcian blue. Around these ducts is the basement membrane and then a concentric layering of collagen. In this cuff of connective tissue is the peribiliary plexus derived from the hepatic arterioles.

Interlobular bile ducts are those found in the smaller portal tracts. They occupy a central position in the tract and are lined by a cuboidal epithelium resting on a basement membrane. The cells have a slightly smaller round nucleus but the cytoplasm is, by comparison, scanty and eosinophilic. Usually no PAS-positive staining or glycocalyx can be identified although on occasions a transition zone, where a positively stained brush border occurs in a cuboidal epithelium, can be found. The cytoplasm is usually negative with alcian blue pH 2.5.

The smallest interlobular duct is formed by the amalgamation, rarely visualized, of bile ductules. These ductules are seen in the periphery of the tracts usually as an elongated double column of flattened cells (Figure 2.5). The nucleus is similar to those in other bile duct epithelium. The cytoplasm is even more scanty and has no special staining properties. The ductules link up directly with the hepatocytes and at this point the basement membrane ceases. This is the region sometimes referred to as the canal of Hering.

Other portal tract structures

These include lymphatics and nerves. Lymphatics are present in all portal tracts and surround the artery and vein. They are also present in the wall of the larger branches of

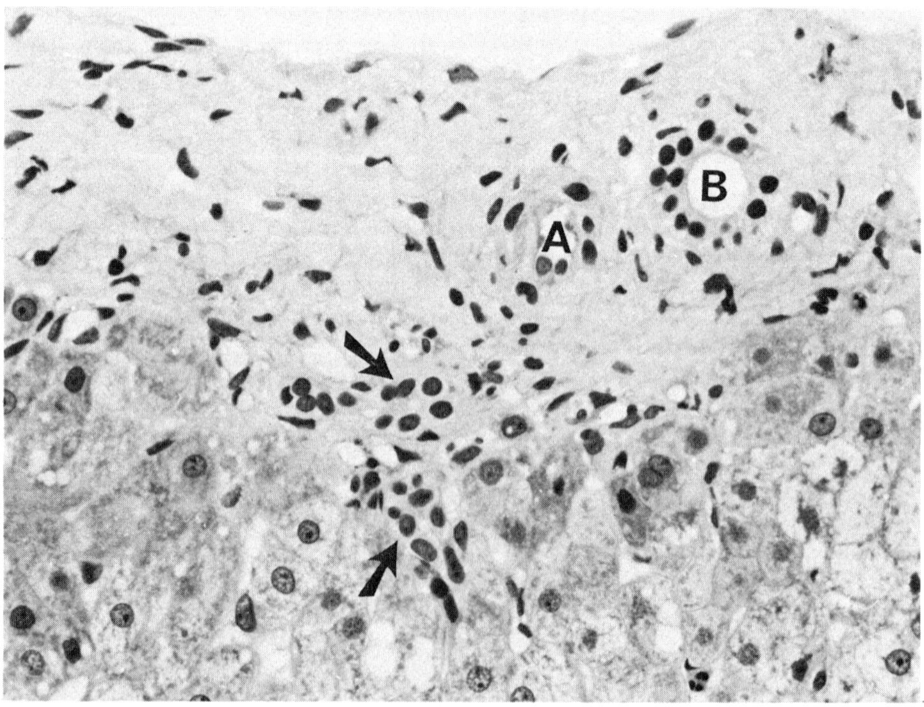

Figure 2.5. Bile ductules at the edge of a portal tract (arrows). It is an elongated double column of epithelial cells which have scanty cytoplasm. A tiny lumen can be seen. In the centre is an interlobular bile duct (B) with an hepatic arteriole (A).

portal and hepatic veins. Nerve bundles are usually only identified in the largest portal tracts of a wedge biopsy but unmyelinated fibres can be identified around the hepatic arterioles by the electron microscope.

Parenchyma

The cell plates on standard microscopy appear as anastomosing Indian file cords of polygonal hepatocytes which pass in radial manner from portal tract to central vein. Around the portal tract is a concentric but discontinuous layer of hepatocytes from which these cords arise (Figure 2.3). This layer forms the limiting plate of the lobule and is a feature frequently altered in the many diseases affecting the liver. There is no morphological change in either the portal tract collagen at its interface with the limiting plate or in the hepatocytes of the limiting plate when compared with their immediate neighbours. Communications between portal vessels and the sinusoids of necessity breach the plate and so produce the discontinuity.

The Indian file arrangement of hepatocytes between portal tracts and central veins is only a two-dimensional representation of the architecture. The constancy of this arrangement in histological sections, despite the plane of the liver in which they are examined, indicates a symmetrical meshwork of hepatocytes. This is formed by a fenestrated series of cell plates that are both anastomosing and continually curving (Figure 2.6). An analogy with a sponge can be made in which the air spaces represent intercommunicating sinusoids and the matrix the anastomosing cell plates (Figure 2.7).

In babies and small children, the cell plates are double and the adult single cell plate pattern is slowly acquired, usually by the age of five years. Over this age twinning of cell plates is generally regarded as evidence of regeneration.

Hepatocytes

These are large polygonal cells 20 to 30 μm across which have clearly defined cell margins and a prominent nucleus. This is round, has

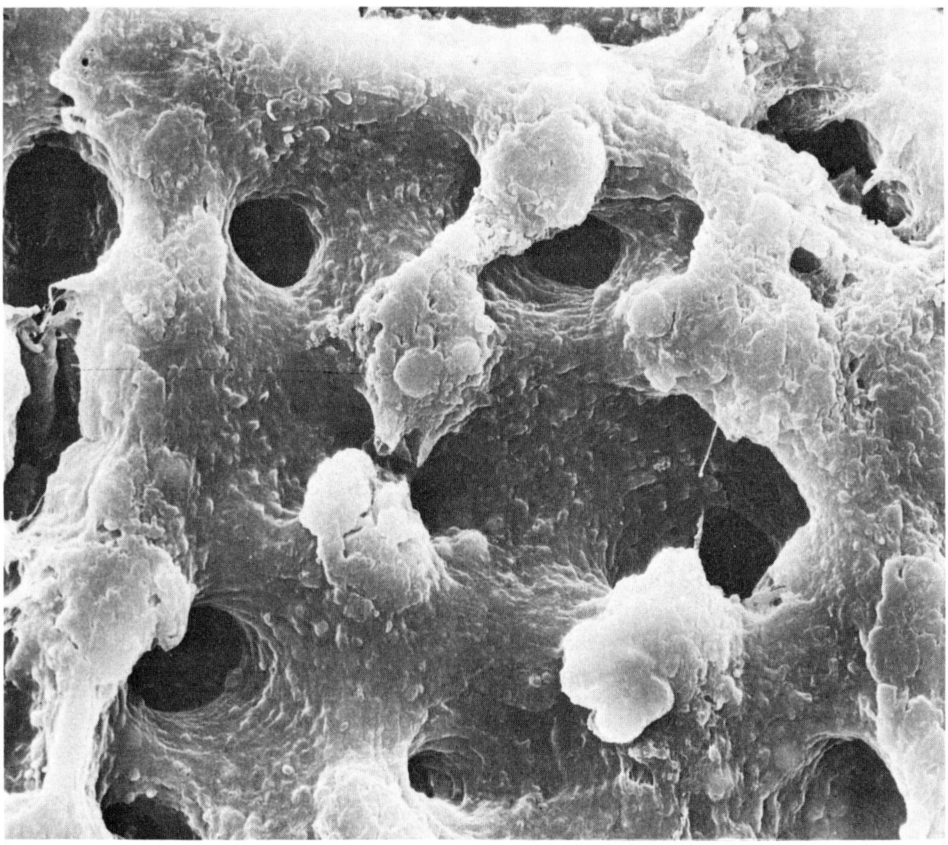

Figure 2.6. Scanning electron microscopy of human liver biopsy with a normal architecture. Note the continually curving nature of the cell plates.

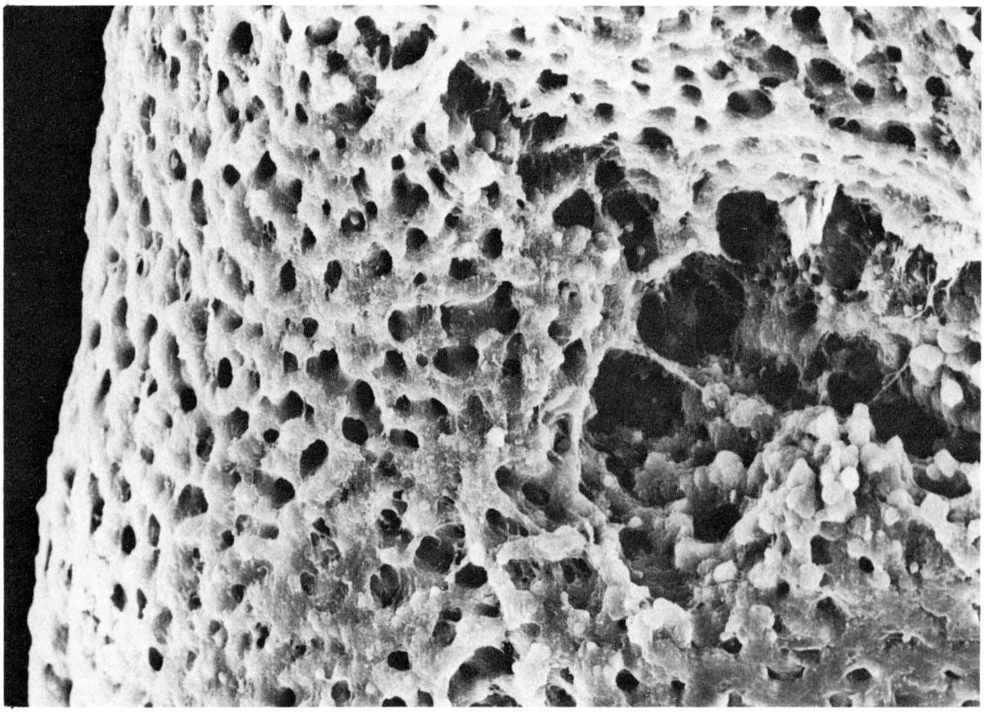

Figure 2.7. Scanning electron microscopy of normal human liver. The portal tract (right) is dividing into branches but the stroma has been torn out. The parenchyma shows a sponge-like arrangement of intercommunicating sinusoids and anastomosing cell plates.

finely dispersed chromatin condensed slightly around the nuclear envelope and contains a large nucleolus. Occasional hepatocytes are binucleate and the proportion increases with age or any stimulus to regeneration. Most cells also have diploid nuclei but again there are occasional tetraploid and polyploid nuclei to be found. Polyploidy is represented morphologically by a large, denser, more haematoxyphilic nucleus. This anisonucleosis also increases with age or with stimuli to regeneration. Vacuoles can sometimes be identified within nuclei of hepatocytes from apparently normal biopsies and are formed by cytoplasmic invaginations (Figure 2.8). They are most frequent in periportal hepatocytes and usually enlarge the nucleus considerably.

The abundant eosinophilic cytoplasm frequently shows a basophilic stippling due to the haematoxyphilia of the RNA in the rough endoplasmic reticulum. It may also contain a centrilobular brown granular pigment which is likely to be lipofuscin. Lipofuscin, a normal 'wear and tear' pigment, must be differentiated from intrahepatic and canalicular bile pigment which indicates cholestasis and is a pathological change. Lipofuscin granules are more uniform in size, refractile and golden to dark brown.

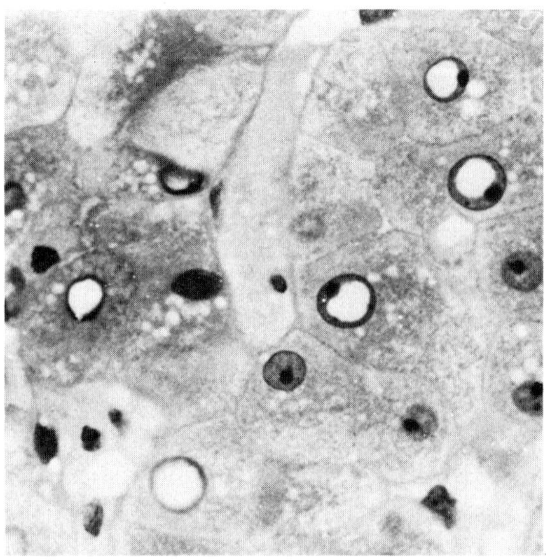

Figure 2.8. Periportal hepatocytes with vacuolated 'empty' nuclei. A membrane usually demarcates the vacuole which in the electron microscope can be identified as invagination of the nucleus by cytoplasm.

They cluster around but are never seen within the canaliculus. Although it is a 'normal' pigment there are pathological conditions in which it is in excess (see Chapter 18).

By using histochemical, autoradiographic and immunological techniques a variety of other normal cell constituents can be demonstrated. These include glycogen, the bile canalicular network,[114,115] albumin[24,28] and a wide variety of enzymes.[32,68,98,114]

Sinusoids

The sinusoids are wide vascular channels lined by endothelial cells (Figures 2.9 and 2.12). Gaps between, but more particularly in, these cells (the sieve plates or fenestrations) allow ready access of plasma to the space of Disse (see Figure 2.13). This contains the reticulin fibrils (type III collagen) which constitute the framework of the lobule and are present along the sinusoidal surfaces of all hepatocytes (Figures 2.10 and 2.26). There is no basement membrane (type IV collagen) in a normal sinusoid.

The sinusoids also contain sporadically distributed Kupffer cells, usually positioned at the junction of two sinusoids (Figures 2.9 and 2.11). These are macrophages and are larger with more cytoplasm that extends out into, and sometimes across, the sinusoid. The nucleus of the Kupffer cell is elongated but has a plumper, slightly more irregular outline than the slimmer, smoother, elongated nucleus of the endothelial cell. There has been controversy about the

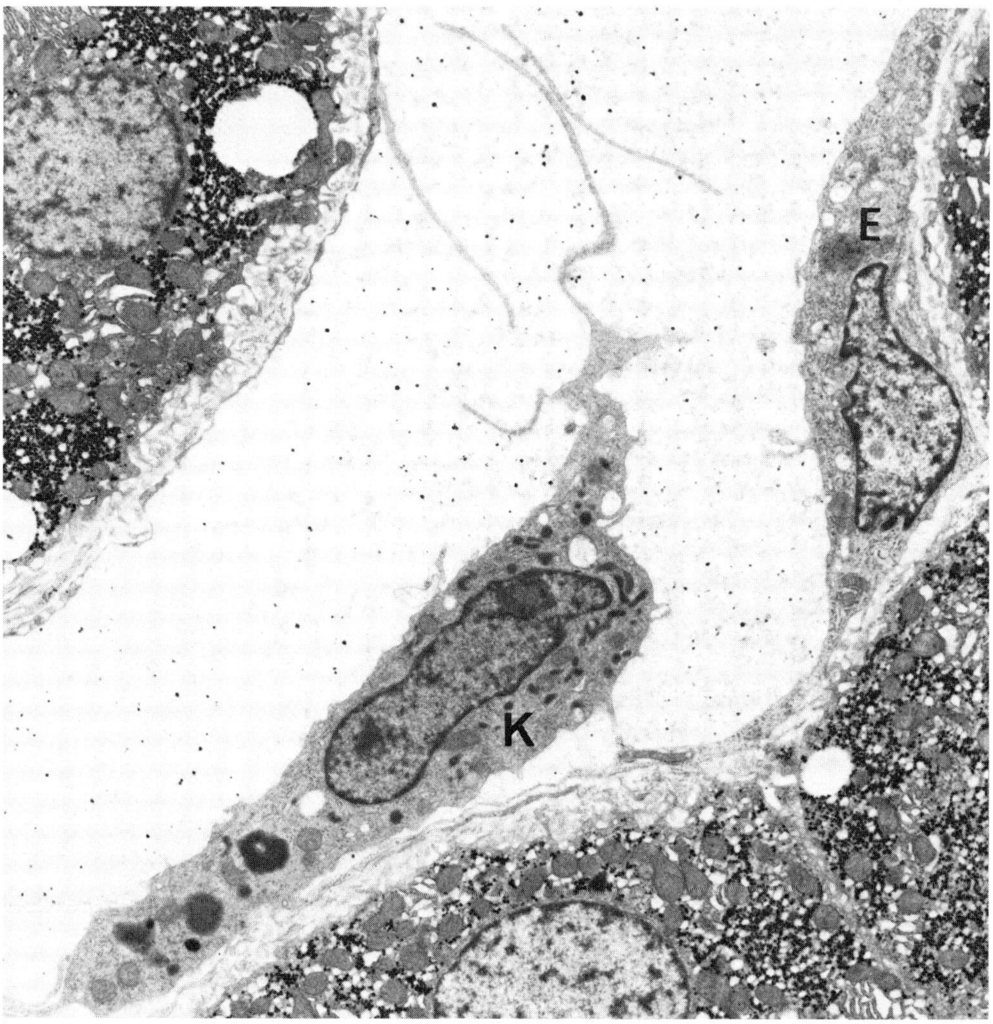

Figure 2.9. Transmission electron microscopy of human liver. A Kupffer cell (K) is demonstrated with elongated cytoplasmic processes extending into the sinusoid. Phagosomes are present as large dark intracytoplasmic bodies bottom left. Note the adjacent endothelial cell (E) with its attenuated cytoplasm extending between the Kupffer cell and subjacent hepatocyte.

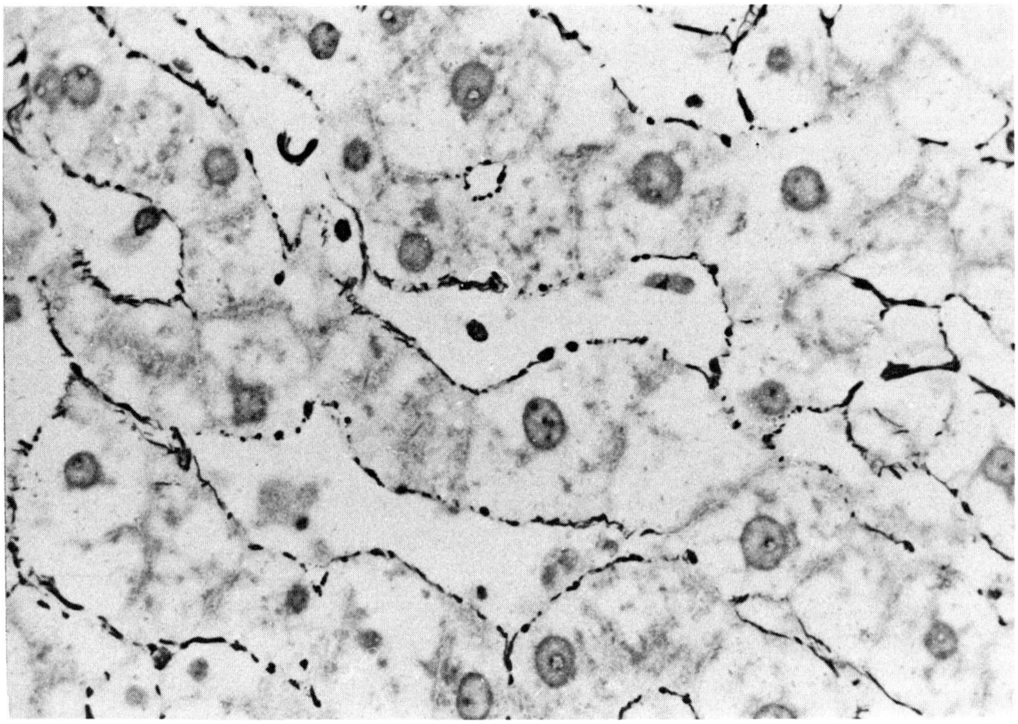

Figure 2.10. Reticulin architecture of liver. Wilder's reticulin on 2 μm methacrylate section of human liver to demonstrate the continuously intermittent deposit of silver along the sinusoidal surfaces of hepatocytes.

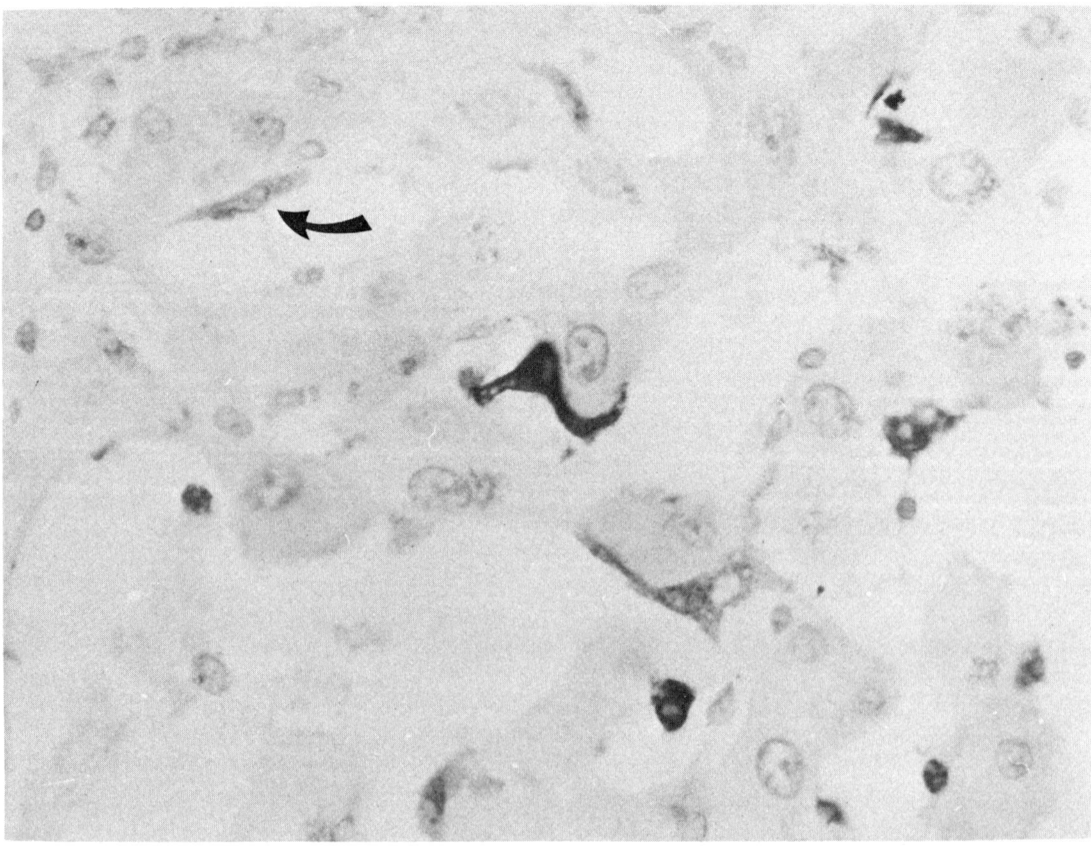

Figure 2.11. Demonstration of muramidase in a Kupffer cell using the peroxidase-antiperoxidase technique with primary antibody diluted at 1/1000. Note the negative endothelial cell (arrow).

interchangeability of endothelial and Kupffer cells. It is now mostly accepted that the two are separate entities[122] and that transitions from one to the other do not occur. Distinction between the two cell types can be made if phagocytosis occurs but otherwise involves the histochemical demonstration in Kupffer cells of non-specific esterase or peroxidase, the immunological demonstration of alpha-1-antitrypsin or muramidase in Kupffer cells (Figure 2.11)[58] or electron microscopy. The distinction on electron microscopy is discussed later.

Central (Efferent) Veins

The smallest are little more than a slightly dilated sinusoid but the larger ones are surrounded by a fenestrated wall of collagen. Smooth muscle cells and lymphatics have been demonstrated in this wall.[82]

ULTRASTRUCTURE

A.M. JEZEQUEL

The first comprehensive ultrastructural study of liver cells was published by Fawcett in 1955.[23] Since then progress in the preparation of material for electron microscopy, the use of autoradiography, cytochemistry and immunocytochemistry, and the study of cell fractions have improved our knowledge of the functional organization of the hepatic parenchyma. In the last few years, a new dimension has been added with the application of stereological techniques to the study of the liver in animals or in man. Application of this technique has established baseline 'reference' data useful in the interpretation of pathological situations and in the correlation of morphological and biochemical data. The meaning of a 'normal' liver cell and the variety of selection criteria adopted in different studies have already been extensively discussed[74] and the difficulties – practical and ethical – of selecting a reference population in human studies have been emphasized.

With the electron microscope, the one cell thick plates formed by the parenchymal cells appear separated from the sinusoids by a thin endothelial lining. Bile canaliculi are seen as spaces between the hepatocytes and do not show communications with the subendothelial space or space of Disse. This arrangement is evident in transmission (Figure 2.12) as well as in scanning electron microscopy (Figure 2.13).

THE HEPATOCYTE

Stereological studies show that hepatocytes account for about 78 per cent of the volume in normal adult rats with about 6 per cent for non-hepatocytes and 16 per cent for intracellular spaces.[8] In man, the hepatocytes represent 80 to 88 per cent of the parenchymal volume.[74,91]

The Nucleus

The nucleus is separated from the cytoplasm by a double membrane and accounts for 7 to 8 per cent of the parenchymal volume in animals and in man.[8,74,91] The space between the two leaflets of the nuclear membrane is considered to be part of the granular endoplasmic reticulum, although continuity is rarely found in thin sections. The outer membrane of the nucleus is studded with ribosomes and may extend into the cytoplasm as brief segments of rough endoplasmic reticulum. The inner membrane is smooth and in close contact with small clumps of heterochromatin which are also seen around the nucleolus. At intervals, the outer and inner membranes of the nucleus show close apposition to form the nuclear pores (Figure 2.14). These have been demonstrated in thin sections, negative staining, freeze etching, scanning electron microscopy, in whole tissue, in isolated nuclei or in nuclear 'ghosts'.[37,49,94] The outer diameter of the nuclear 'pore complex' varies from 85 to 100 nm (850 to 1000 Å) and the inner diameter measures from 25 to 40 nm (250 to 400 Å), depending on the different techniques. A granule is sometimes evident in the centre of the pore complex, especially in nuclear ghosts sectioned parallel to the membrane surface. Besides the central granule, other structures or 'diaphragm material' such as fibres or tubules are seen inside the annulus but their significance has not been elucidated. No significant differences have been noted between the pore complexes from nuclei of normal rat liver or from hepatomas.[37]

The general and enzymatic composition of the nuclear envelope has been studied mainly on rat and bovine liver but this is difficult because of its close association with DNA, RNA and various proteins on the inner side and with cytoplasmic ribosomes and proteins on the outer side. Most, if not all, enzymes of the nuclear envelope are microsomal enzymes.[76] Some of them, such as nucleoside diphosphatase[70] or glucose-6-phosphatase,[30] have

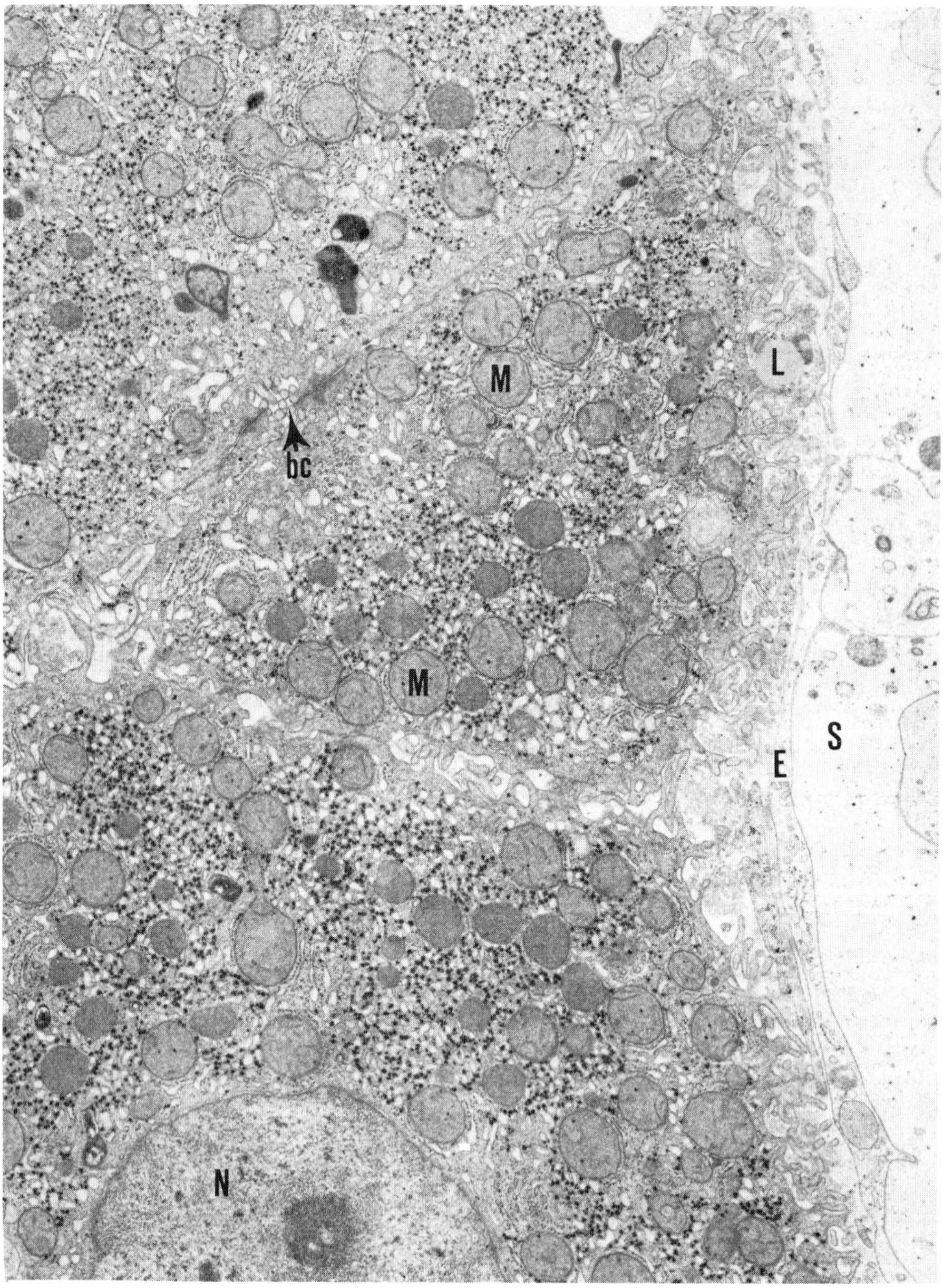

Figure 2.12. Low-power electron micrograph of normal human liver. Three hepatocytes are present in the field. They are separated from the sinusoidal lumen (S) by a thin layer of endothelium (E). A small lipid droplet (L), visible in the space of Disse, probably belongs to a lipocyte. The nucleus (N) and nucleolus of an hepatocyte are evident at the bottom of the illustration. In the cytoplasm, numerous mitochondria (M) and peroxisomes are present. The rough endoplasmic reticulum is preferentially located around the nucleus, the sinusoidal border and around mitochondria. The smooth endoplasmic reticulum is diffusely distributed throughout the cytoplasm. It shows a finely vesicular pattern and is associated with rosettes of glycogen. Some elements of the Golgi apparatus are present, together with lysosomes, next to a small bile canaliculus (bc). The junctional complexes on either side of the bile canaliculus are evident. × 9900.

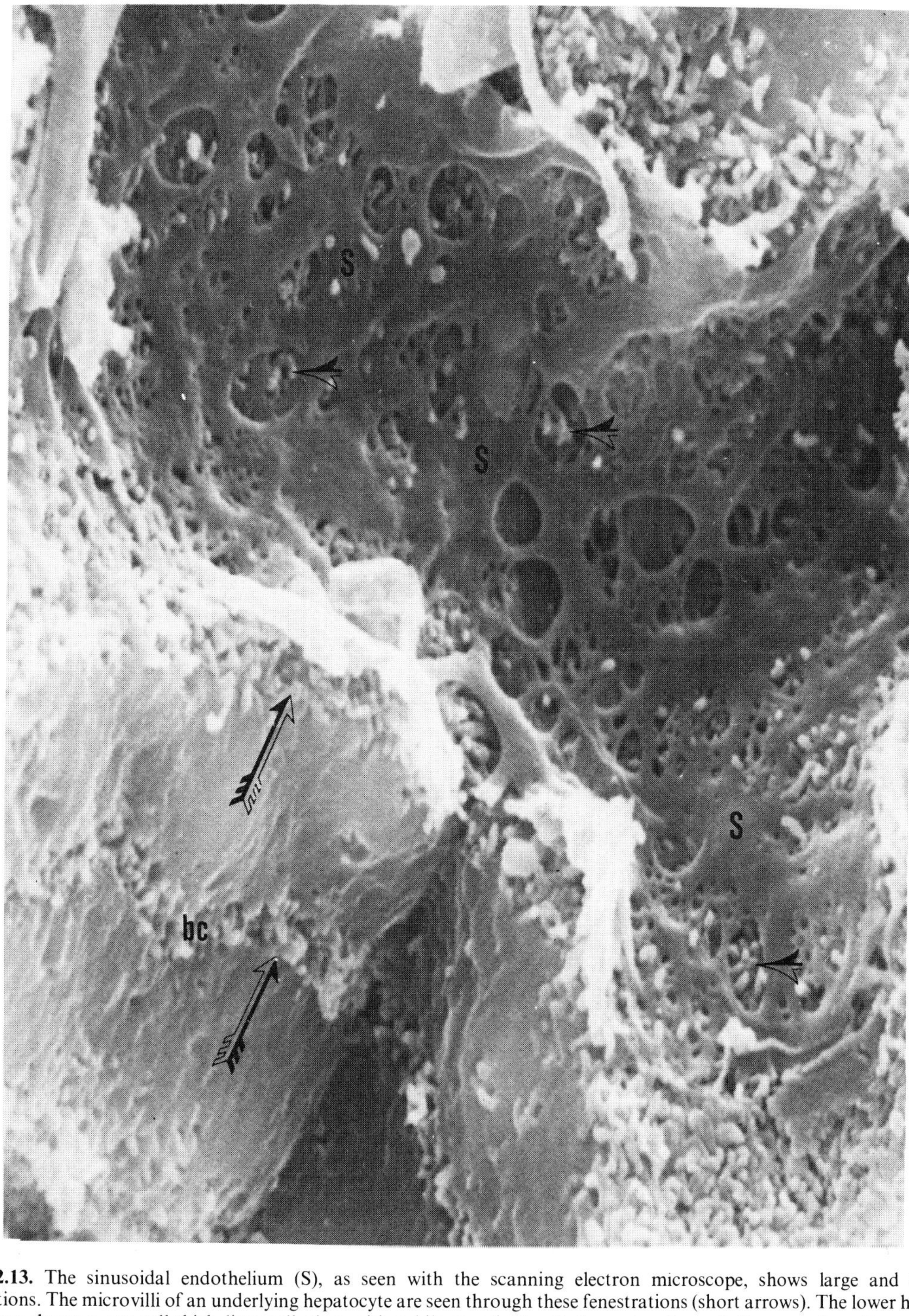

Figure 2.13. The sinusoidal endothelium (S), as seen with the scanning electron microscope, shows large and small fenestrations. The microvilli of an underlying hepatocyte are seen through these fenestrations (short arrows). The lower half of the picture shows a one-cell-thick liver cell plate with a bile canaliculus (bc) running through the central portion of the hepatocytes. Microvilli are seen along the bile canaliculus and along the sinusoidal surface of hepatocytes (long arrows). × 8500.

Courtesy of Dr K. Miyai, Department of Pathology, University of California, San Diego.

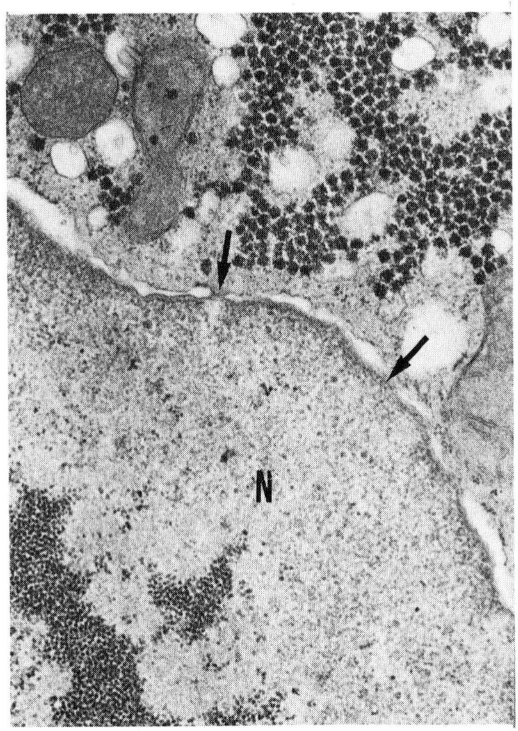

Figure 2.14. Part of an hepatocyte showing the perinuclear space interrupted by the nuclear pores (arrows). Some monoparticulate glycogen is present in the nucleus (N) whereas the intracytoplasmic glycogen has a rosette-like appearance. × 25000.

been demonstrated in situ by histochemical techniques.

In the nucleoplasm, most of the chromatin is present as euchromatin but the appearance varies with the mode of fixation. Clumps of heterochromatin are more evident when the fixation with aldehydes (formaldehyde, acrolein or glutaraldehyde) precedes osmium tetroxide than when osmium is used alone. Next to the clumps of chromatin and separated from them by a clear halo are the perichromatin granules, about 40 nm (400 Å) in diameter (Figure 2.14). Enzymic digestion shows that they contain proteins and RNA fibrils, possibly a type of messenger RNA.[4] Clusters of small interchromatin granules 20 to 25 nm (200 to 250 Å) in diameter, are dispersed in the nucleoplasm and are thought to be ribonucleoproteins.[4]

The nucleolus appears as a spongy network, roughly circular in shape, not limited by a membrane (Figures 2.12 and 2.15). It is composed of 15 nm (150 Å) granules and 5 to 8 nm (50 to 80 Å) fibrils – both containing RNA – embedded in a protein matrix.[55] Transport of messenger RNA and other macromolecules to the cytoplasm is believed to be through the nuclear pores. There is also evidence that macromolecular complexes are transported from the cytoplasm to the nucleus. No visible transport of material across the nuclear membrane has yet been detected.

Nuclear inclusions are unusual in normal conditions, except for glycogen. The intranuclear glycogen is always in the form of isolated particles, about 30 nm (300 Å) in diameter, as opposed to the large rosette-like aggregates present in the cytoplasm (Figure 2.14). It occupies large areas, well circumscribed but without a limiting membrane, save for small dense deposits which are often encircled by a thick, finely fibrillar envelope. Although intranuclear glycogen is common in diabetes[20] and in various other conditions, including glycogen storage diseases,[5,92,99] it can also be an occasional finding in normal human liver.[54]

Small cytoplasmic areas occasionally containing lipid droplets may be entrapped in invaginations of the nuclear membrane and, depending on the plane of section, may appear as intranuclear inclusions. These are more frequently observed in old animals and in some pathological situations.[2,68]

The Cytoplasm

The cytoplasm of the hepatocytes contains a variety of organelles and membrane systems, which occupy roughly half of the cell volume.[8,39,74,91] The membranous system divides the cytoplasm into two compartments, cytoplasmic and intracisternal, and it also surrounds the various organelles, isolating areas where specialized functions can be carried out.

Endoplasmic reticulum

The endoplasmic reticulum is made up of the rough endoplasmic reticulum, with membranes studded with ribosomes, 15 nm (150 Å) in diameter, and the agranular or smooth endoplasmic reticulum which lacks ribosomes (Figure 2.16). The total density of endoplasmic reticulum is about 3.8 m^2/cm^3 of parenchyma with 62 per cent and 38 per cent respectively for the rough and smooth endoplasmic reticulum in adult rats.[8] In this species the two-cell layer adjacent to the central vein has approximately equal proportions of rough and smooth.[53] The relative proportion of the two aspects of the endoplasmic reticulum varies according to the species: in dogs, the rough and smooth endoplasmic reticulum represent

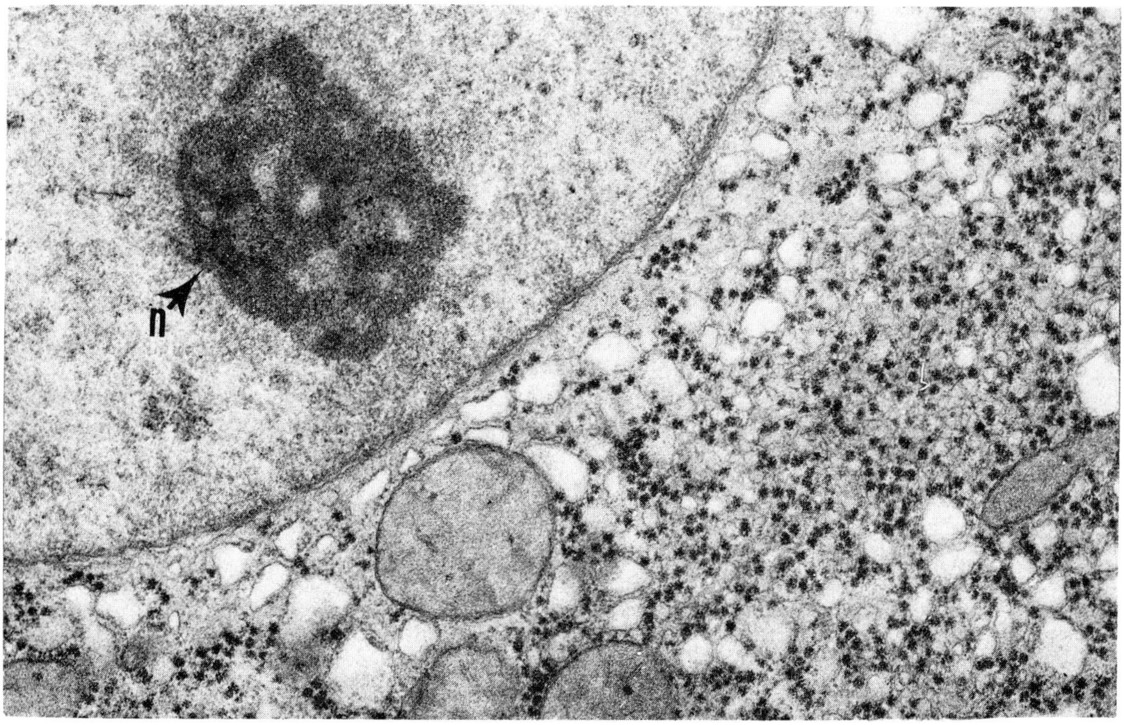

Figure 2.15. The sponge-like appearance of the nucleolus (n) is evident on this electron micrograph. The chromatin is slightly denser around the nucleolus and along the nuclear membrane than in the remaining nucleoplasm. × 25000.

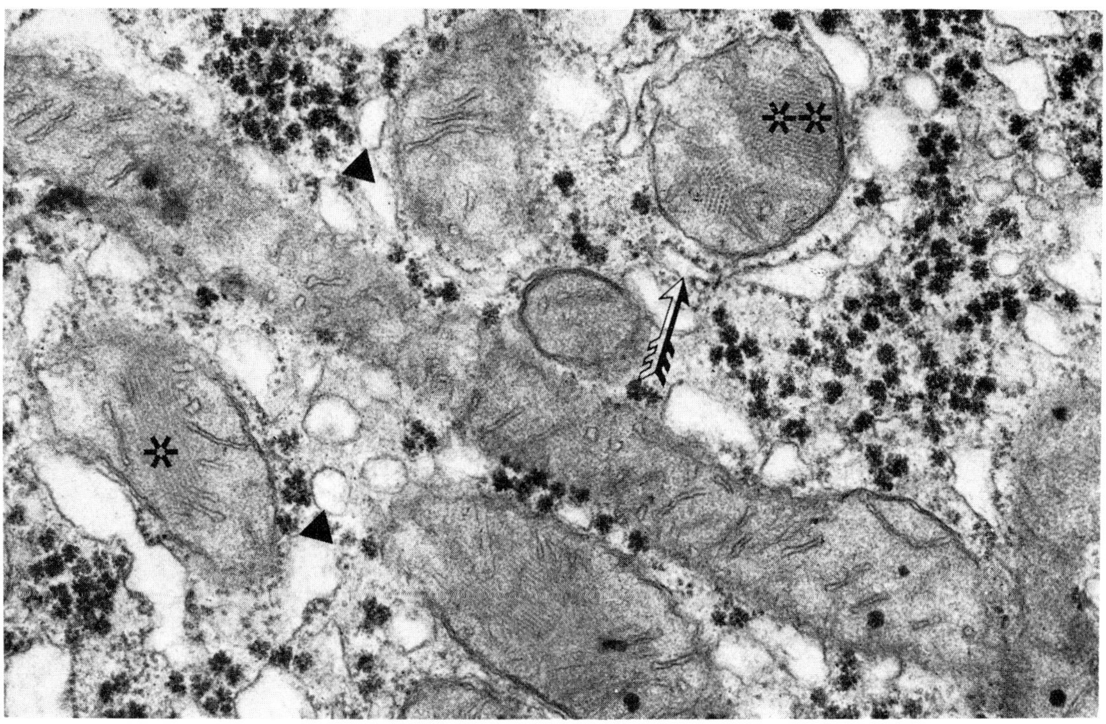

Figure 2.16. Part of the cytoplasm of an hepatocyte of a normal subject showing cisternae of rough (long arrow) and smooth (short arrow) endoplasmic reticulum. Electron-dense rosettes of glycogen are dispersed throughout the cytoplasm. The mitochondria contain crystalline formations seen in longitudinal (single asterisk) or in cross-sections (double asterisk). × 37 500.

respectively 40 and 60 per cent of the total[39] whereas in adult man the values are around 25 and 75 per cent.[48,91] These species differences have not always been taken into account, especially in studies on humans, and numerous reports of 'hypertrophy' of the smooth endoplasmic reticulum in human hepatocytes should be interpreted with caution.

Rough endoplasmic reticulum. This is arranged in flattened cisternae often grouped around the nucleus and mitochondria and along the sinusoidal border at the margin of areas of smooth endoplasmic reticulum with glycogen. This disposition is more evident in human liver, especially in the hepatocytes surrounding the central vein. Also, in human hepatocytes the cisternae of the rough endoplasmic reticulum appear more fragmented than in those of animals. Ribosomes are attached on the cytoplasmic side of the rough endoplasmic reticulum but can also be seen free in the cytoplasm, either isolated or arranged along a fine thread of messenger RNA in spirals or rosettes to constitute the polysomes, the functional unit of protein synthesis. Polysomes are also associated with the membrane of the endoplasmic reticulum but can be seen as such only in tangential sections of the membranous sheet. Synthesis of protein takes place at the level of the rough endoplasmic reticulum. Morphological demonstration of albumin synthesis in the liver has been achieved by autoradiography[28] and by immune electron microscopy.[24] The heterogeneous distribution of the reaction product in human liver had suggested that only a small number of hepatocytes are engaged in albumin synthesis. This may be due to the low turnover of human serum albumin rather than a specialization of some liver cells. In fact, the use of different fixation techniques on rat liver tissue tends to demonstrate that all hepatocytes are engaged in albumin production.[41] Enzyme proteins and phospholipids are not randomly distributed in the endoplasmic reticulum but are concentrated at the inner or the outer surface of the membrane.[13,65]

Smooth endoplasmic reticulum and glycogen. The smooth endoplasmic reticulum is distributed throughout the hepatocyte, mainly as small vesicles associated with glycogen. The glycogen has a stellate shape or a rosette-like appearance and is arranged in clusters of granules each 10 to 20 nm (100 to 200 Å) in diameter (Figures 2.14 and 2.16). In man, the smooth endoplasmic reticulum is more diffusely distributed than in rat, dog or rabbit hepatocytes. Moreover, two types occur; the more common form, type I, has a finely vesicular honeycomb pattern and accounts for 77 per cent of the smooth membranes while the other, type II, is made up of densely packed membranes without a cavitary system and accounts for 23 per cent (Figure 2.17).[47] Until now this dual configuration has been observed only in human liver. Its significance is suggested by the modifications occurring when there are changes of microsomal enzyme activity (see Chapter 19).

It is known that the smooth endoplasmic reticulum is mainly concerned with the synthesis of lipids, the accumulation of glycogen and the metabolism of drugs and endogenous hormones.[29] It also contains enzymes for the synthesis of cholesterol and the formation of bile acids. Uridine diphosphate (UDP) glucuronyl transferase is also associated with the smooth endoplasmic reticulum.[101] Some enzymes of the endoplasmic reticulum have been demonstrated by ultrastructural histochemistry and include glucose-6-phosphatase,[30] nucleoside diphosphatase[70] and acetyl CoA carboxylase.[126] Glucose-6-phosphatase is evenly distributed throughout the endoplasmic reticulum, including the nuclear envelope, but seems to develop asynchronously in the hepatocyte population.[52]

Studies in rats and mice on the endoplasmic reticulum during the perinatal period show that rough and smooth endoplasmic reticula are present at birth. Little variation in the rough endoplasmic reticulum is observed thereafter, but the smooth endoplasmic reticulum increases in association with the maturation of some microsomal enzymes.[13,14,15] However, the enzymes of the endoplasmic reticulum do not rise in parallel with the membranous compartment.[14,52] In rats the maximum increase in the smooth endoplasmic reticulum occurs 24 to 72 hours after birth but this continues to rise thereafter.[18,38,90,97] In human liver, a small amount of smooth endoplasmic reticulum has been found in young children up to nine months of age with an increase up to 18 years.[18,111] These data make it clear that the limits of 'normal' vary and that age should be carefully considered.

The Golgi apparatus

The Golgi apparatus is a specialized area of the smooth endoplasmic reticulum, located in the

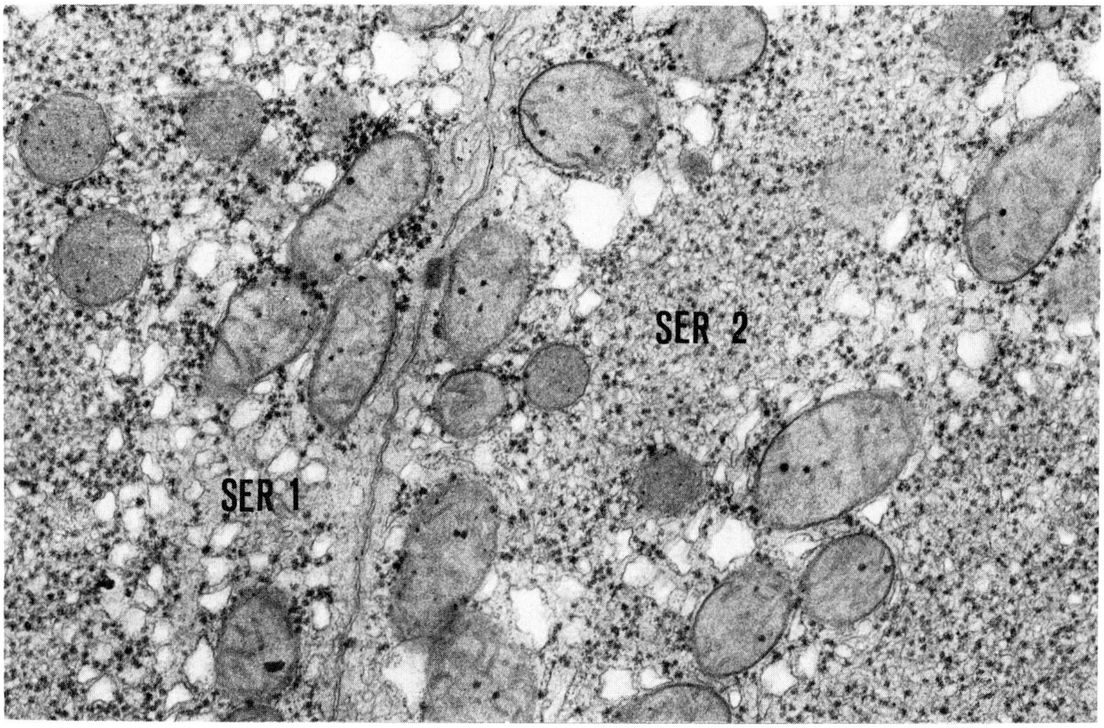

Figure 2.17. Part of two hepatocytes in human liver showing the variable pattern of distribution of the smooth endoplasmic reticulum. The SER type 1 (SER 1) has a grossly vesicular appearance, with vesicles varying in size and shape. The SER type 2 (SER 2) is formed of densely packed membranes concentrated in various areas of the cytoplasm and shows little or no evidence of a cavitary system. × 21000.

vicinity of the bile canaliculi (Figure 2.18). It is arranged as a group of flattened saccules, vacuoles and small vesicles. These are sometimes seen budding off the extremities of the saccules. Multivesicular bodies and lysosomes are frequently associated with the Golgi areas. The cisternae usually appear empty but in liver perfused with free fatty acids may be filled with dense particles 30 to 100 nm (300 to 1000 Å) in diameter. These have been identified as very low density lipoproteins, later secreted in the space of Disse and the sinusoids.[35] The name of GERL has been proposed to designate a specialized area of the endoplasmic reticulum which, together with the innermost elements of the Golgi apparatus, contributes to the formation of lysosomes. It is identified by acid phosphatase cytochemistry.[67] In normal animals, GERL is not conspicuous but it becomes enlarged and swollen in some experimental situations. The Golgi apparatus is a site for assembly and packaging of lipoproteins and glycoproteins which are then exported or incorporated into intracellular components. It has been shown to participate in the intracellular migration of albumin.[28] A specific role of the Golgi complex in the transport of biliary lipids seems to be excluded.[82] In adult rats the density of the Golgi membranes is 0.17 m^2/cm^3 of liver parenchyma, and these contribute 4 per cent to the membranes of the endoplasmic reticulum in hepatocytes.[8] In adult man, the Golgi contributes about 6 per cent to the membranes of the endoplasmic reticulum with a density of 0.23 $\mu m^2/\mu m^3$ of cytoplasm.[48,74] This appears to be higher in younger individuals.[18] In rats the maximum values are observed around five weeks of age[111] and a significant decrease of Golgi membranes occurs with ageing.[97]

Mitochondria

The mitochondria account for about 23 per cent of the cytoplasmic volume in adult rat hepatocytes,[118] 24 per cent in dogs[39] and 14 to 19 per cent in adult man.[74,102] They measure 0.4 to 0.5 μm by 0.5 to 1 μm. Small intralobular differences have been observed, the mitochondria being longer, thinner and more numerous in centrilobular areas than in periportal areas of rat liver;[53] the variation in mitochondrial number means that the mitochondrial volume density remains constant throughout the lo-

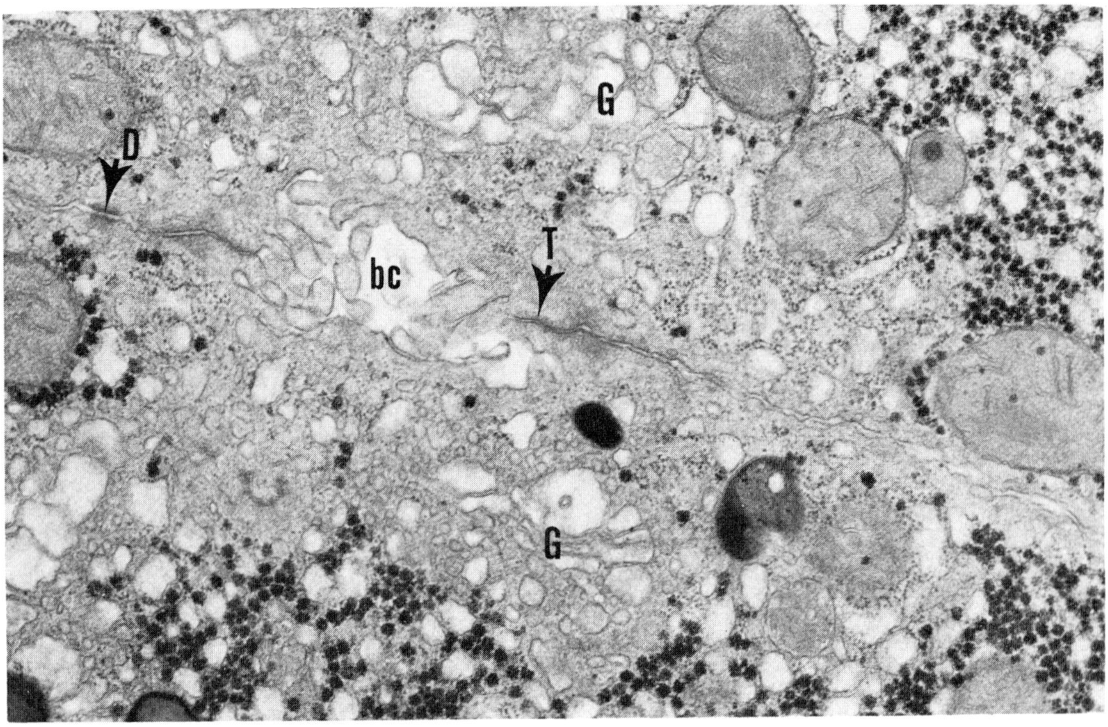

Figure 2.18. Part of two hepatocytes showing the specializations of the cell surface at the level of bile canaliculi. Microvilli of various sizes project into the lumen of the canaliculus (bc) and the Golgi apparatus (G) is evident in both hepatocytes at a short distance from the cell border. T = tight junctions, D = desmosomes. × 25000.

bule.[3] The mitochondria are limited by a double membrane. The outer membrane is closely apposed to the rough endoplasmic reticulum and the inner membrane is folded in numerous invaginations to form the cristae (Figure 2.16). Negative staining reveals club-shaped particles associated with the inner membrane: the head, about 9 nm (90 Å) in diameter, is thought to represent molecules of ATPase while the stalk contains the components of the electron transfer system.[84] The matrix contains naked DNA, a small amount of RNA and ribosomes.[62] The dense granules, about 10 to 25 nm (100 to 250 Å) in diameter, often present in the matrix have been shown to bind various cations, especially calcium and phosphorus.[9,62] The mitochondria are involved in a variety of metabolic pathways, mainly citric acid cycle, fatty acid activation and oxidation, steroid metabolism, respiration, nucleic acid and protein synthesis and haem biosynthesis. Ultrastructural cytochemistry has localized NADH2-TNBT reductase activity to the mitochondria in all hepatocytes, with a higher activity in portal areas.[54] The activity of cytochrome-*c* and -*b* has also been demonstrated in situ by various techniques.[54,69,113] No major qualitative differ-

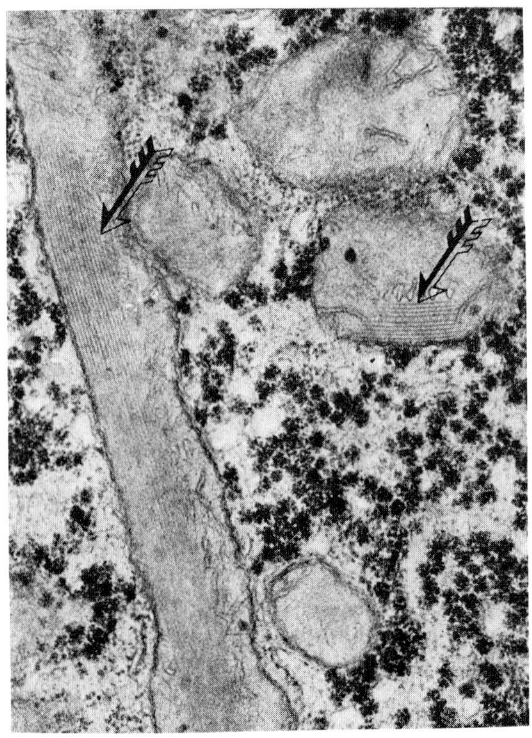

Figure 2.19. Group of mitochondria containing crystals shown in longitudinal sections (arrows) in the hepatocytes of a normal subject. × 27500.

ences are evident in the structure of mitochondria in different species. The variety of profile shapes seen in thin sections is due to the morphological heterogeneity of mitochondria. Serial section analysis reveals V-shaped or club-shaped mitochondria, disks, cylinders or spheres.[3,105] Giant mitochondria, up to 5 μm, are occasionally observed in human hepatocytes and often contain bundles of filaments arranged in an orderly fashion (Figure 2.19). These were originally described as a pathological finding but are now well established as an occasional feature of human liver.[44,54,61,92,102,120] By optical diffraction these inclusions are crystalline and made either of phospholipid micelles or of relatively large protein molecules.[108] A protein component in these crystals is also suggested by ultrastructural histochemistry.[95,96] Giant mitochondria seem to be frequently associated with steatosis. A light microscopic study has shown that in normal or pathological liver tissue giant mitochondria have a heterogeneous distribution and are found in clusters of a few hepatocytes,[77] which explains why they can be missed or overestimated in the electron microscope. Stacks of mitochondrial cristae are occasionally observed in human hepatocytes and have also been noted in livers of pathogen-free dogs.[27] In monkey liver, mitochondria show an intricate fibrillar pattern which in cross-section appears as groups of dots sometimes arranged as annulets 65 nm (650 Å) in diameter.[93] The significance of these formations is still unknown.

The greatest pleomorphism and the greatest individual mitochondrial volume are found in the first 24 hours after birth.[91,105] In ageing rats and mice, the volume and shape of the average mitochondrion remain constant[97,112] but the number of mitochondria and the surface density of mitochondrial cristae appear to decrease.[112]

Lysosomes

The heterogeneous class of organelles known as lysosomes actually represents residual bodies or secondary lysosomes, made up of particles limited by a single membrane, containing a variety of inclusions and showing acid phosphatase and β-glucuronidase activity.[54,66] These secondary lysosomes are a storage form – temporary or definitive – of degradation products of normal cell metabolism, auto- or heterophagocytosis. In the hepatocytes, most residual bodies are preferentially located around the bile canaliculi (Figures 2.12 and 2.18). They include autophagic vacuoles, multivesicular bodies, ferritin-containing granules and lipofuscin granules (the most common residual body in human hepatocytes) (Figure 2.20). Lipofuscin granules are irregularly lobulated and show a complex structure with electron lucid regions, dense lipid-containing globules and ferritin-

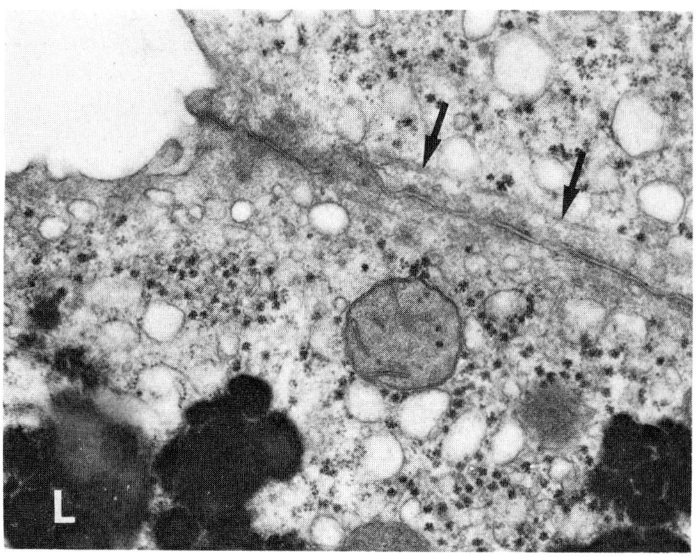

Figure 2.20. Part of two hepatocytes showing lipofuscin granules (L) in the lower left corner and a bundle of microfilaments (arrows) running parallel to the cell membrane. × 25000.

containing areas.[22,54] They have been considered as a member of the lipolysosome (lipid-containing lysosomes) family, to which also belong the electron-lucent lipid inclusions seen in golden hamsters.[64] The volume occupied by the residual bodies in hepatocytes of adult rats varies from 0.3 to 0.9 per cent of cytoplasmic volume, without significant differences in volume density in various parts of the lobule.[54,118] However, the number of particles seems to be higher in the centrilobular areas.[53] In dog liver, the volume occupied by lysosomes is around 0.7 per cent of the cytoplasmic volume[39] whereas in man the values vary from 1.33 per cent[73] to 2 per cent of cytoplasmic volume.[91]

The maximal volume density of dense bodies is found at 24 hours after birth[90] in association with the formation of numerous autophagic vacuoles in the cytoplasm of hepatocytes.[47] The volume returns rapidly to adult values which are reached by the third day post-partum.[90] Little difference in relative volume of lysosomes seems to occur thereafter, although a moderate but significant increase has been found in old virgin rats compared with old breeder rats.[97] Thus, except for the perinatal period, it appears that no gross changes in the volume density of residual bodies occur in normal individuals. This probably reflects the steady state in cell metabolism and turnover of the various cell components.

Peroxisomes

The peroxisomes (microbodies) are made up of granules about 0.25 to 1 μm in diameter, limited by a single membrane. The largest ones – up to 1.50 μm – are found in human liver.[72,109] They are occasionally arranged in clusters and are usually distributed in close proximity to the smooth endoplasmic reticulum and glycogen areas (Figures 12 and 14). Slender communications between smooth endoplasmic reticulum and peroxisomes have been observed in rat and human liver. These have suggested that hepatic peroxisomes may arise as dilatations of smooth endoplasmic reticulum cisternae.[72] The matrix of peroxisomes is homogeneous, of moderate electron density, and in some species contains a crystalline inclusion or core made up of the enzyme urate oxidase. This core is lacking in peroxisomes of human hepatocytes[42,72,100] but marginal plates and a variety of matrical inclusions are irregularly observed.[109] Histochemical reactions based on the demonstration of catalase activity using 3′,3′-diaminobenzidine[69,71] helped to characterize this group of organelles and the term 'microperoxisomes' has been proposed for 'anucleoid' peroxisome-like structures in a variety of tissues.[72] In adult rats, the mean volume density of peroxisomes represents about 1.5 per cent of cytoplasmic volume[53,118] with higher values in centrilobular areas.[53] The highest volume, 3.7 per cent, is found in dog liver[39] compared with 0.97 to 1.33 per cent in man.[74,91] Adult values seem to be reached very rapidly following the sharp increase in volume density of peroxisomes noted in neonatal rats.[91] Little is known about the function of peroxisomes. They have been involved in the metabolism of hydrogen peroxide, in lipid metabolism and gluconeogenesis.[17,42,88] A number of situations are known to be accompanied by alterations in their shape or number (see Chapter 19).

Crystalline structures

The presence of crystalline formations in the cytoplasm of hepatocytes is irregularly observed. These formations occupy large areas of the hyaloplasm, often interspersed with rosettes of glycogen, and are not limited by a membrane (Figure 2.21). They measure 1 to 7 μm in length by 1 to 2.5 μm.[12,46,61,110] There is a variable internal arrangement: a regular honeycomb pattern is sometimes evident, with occasional cross-sections of filamentous components 6 nm (60 Å) thick with a spacing of 19 nm (190 Å). The periodicity may also give a 'herring-bone' appearance in some sections.[12] The intracytoplasmic crystals are occasionally seen together with intramitochondrial crystals in the same cell but the former are more rarely observed. Proteins are the most likely constituent of intracytoplasmic crystals as shown by optical diffraction analysis.[110]

Lipids

In normal conditions, the hepatocytes may also contain some lipid droplets. These account for 0.37 per cent of the hepatocyte volume in normal rats,[8] 0.14 per cent in dogs[39] and 0.3 to 2.1 per cent in man.[74,91]

The Plasma Membrane

The hepatocyte is in contact with three

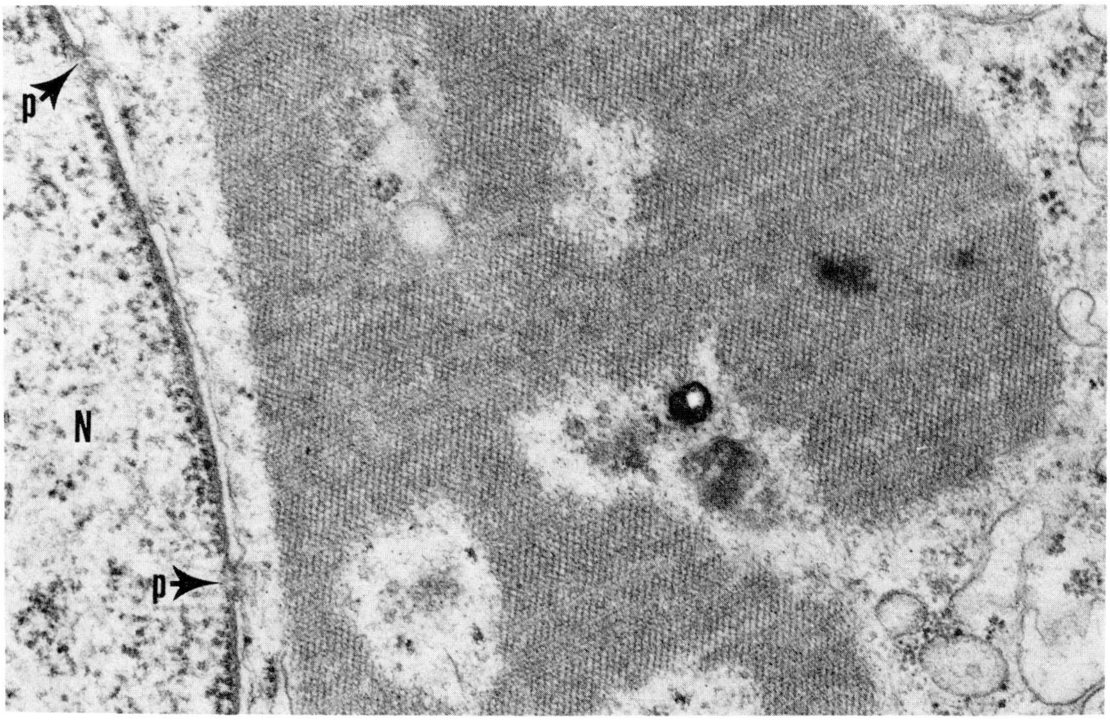

Figure 2.21. Large crystalline inclusion in the cytoplasm of a liver cell. The inclusion has no limiting membrane and is complex in shape with numerous cytoplasmic invaginations. The organization of the crystal shows a regular, honeycomb pattern in this plane of section. p = nuclear pore, N = nucleus. × 36000.

compartments: the perisinusoidal space or space of Disse, the intercellular space and the bile canaliculi. The membrane facing the perisinusoidal space forms numerous microvilli (Figure 2.22) and represents 72 per cent of the whole plasma membrane in rats.[8] In man, the membranes facing the sinusoidal and the intercellular spaces represent together 83.3 per cent of the total plasma membrane.[74] The sinusoidal surface exhibits an intense alkaline phosphatase and nucleoside monophosphatase activity while the nucleoside di- and tri-phosphatase activity is weak. No zonal differences are evident.[54] The functional differentiation of the liver plasma membrane is best demonstrated by the studies on isolated membrane subfractions which show that glucagon-stimulated adenylate-cyclase activity is highest at the sinusoidal membrane and lacking at the bile canalicular surface.[121] The microvilli which project into the space of Disse are occasionally in contact with the sinusoidal lumen through fenestrae in the endothelial cells. These are evident in transmission as well as in scanning electron microscopy (Figure 2.13). At the base of microvilli small regular invaginations of the cell membrane are often seen. These 'bristle-coated' vesicles of micropinocytosis have a constant diameter, around 0.1 μm, and are easily identified by their dense outline (Figure 2.22), apparent even on unstained sections.[54, 92] In normal conditions, the pinocytic activity of the hepatocyte is low: the pinocytic vesicles represent only 0.08 per cent of the cell volume in rats.[8]

Along the lateral cell membranes, desmosomes are inconstantly observed. These are focal specializations of the cell membrane situated at a variable distance from the bile canaliculi. They are characterized by the apposition of short, straight segments of the membranes of adjacent cells, separated by a gap of about 25 nm (250 Å), filled with homogeneous electron dense material and reinforced by a plaque on the cytoplasmic side of the membrane.[6] Microfilaments often originate from the desmosomes: they may be seen expanding fan-wise into the cytoplasm or running along the cell membranes and around the bile canaliculi as part of the microfilamentous network of the hepatocyte (see below).

The membrane lining the canalicular spaces

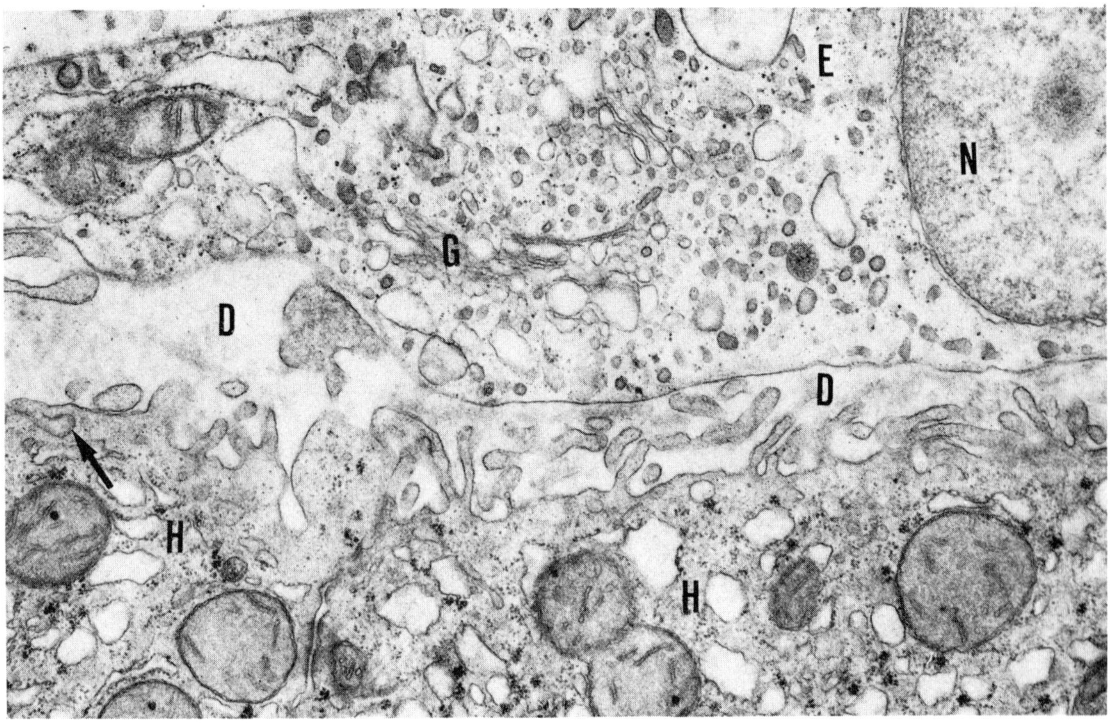

Figure 2.22. The space of Disse (D) is defined on one side by the hepatocytes (H) and on the other side by the sinusoidal lining cells. Part of an endothelial cell (E) is shown here with a large pale nucleus (N). The cytoplasm lacks phagocytic inclusions and shows some elements of the Golgi apparatus (G). Some pinocytic vesicles can be seen along the cell surface (arrow). × 21 000.

forms the initial segment of the biliary tree.

THE BILIARY TREE

The biliary tree includes the bile canaliculi (or bile capillaries), the ducts of Hering (preductules or intermediary portion), the bile ductules and larger bile ducts located in the portal tracts.[103,104]

Canaliculi

The bile canaliculi are spaces formed by separation of adjacent cells (Figure 2.18). Numerous microvilli project into their lumen but extended areas may be deprived of microvilli even in normal conditions. The anastomosing network of bile canaliculi running between hepatocytes is well shown by scanning electron microscopy (Figure 2.13).[33] The four different types of canaliculi which have been distinguished in fetal and neonatal rat liver might represent various stages of maturation of the biliary pole of the liver cell, characterized by an increase in the surface/volume ratio of canaliculi.[19] In adult liver, the width and shape of the canaliculi are variable; altogether they represent 0.4 per cent of the parenchymal volume.[8] The canaliculi of the centrilobular zone seem to have fewer microvilli and a narrower lumen than those in the periportal areas.[54] Both transmission electron microscopy[103] and scanning electron microscopy have failed to reveal any direct connection between the canaliculi and the perisinusoidal spaces.[33] A strong cohesion between hepatocytes is provided by the tight junctions (zonula occludens) which separate the intercellular spaces or perisinusoidal recesses from the canalicular lumen. These junctions are formed by the fusion of the outer leaflet of adjacent cellular membranes and are of variable size, from 0.1 to 0.4 μm. They extend over the whole length of bile canaliculi.[6] The cell attachment appears to be provided by single fibrils shared by the membranes of adjacent cells.[116] The bond provided by the tight junctions resists mechanical disruption and permits isolation of intact segments of the bile canalicular network from the rest of the parenchyma.[79] Next to the tight junctions, the lateral cell membranes form the intermediate junction with an intercellular gap of about 20 nm (200 Å). The staining of the bile canalicular membrane by phosphotungstic acid[103] or by ruthenium red[73] may be due to the presence of a fuzzy coat on the cell surface. A high 5′-nucleotidase and ATPase activity is present at the canalicular level but in normal conditions the alkaline phosphatase activity is low.[54] On the cytoplasmic side, a zone of condensed cytoplasm or 'pericanalicular ectoplasm' reinforces the bile canalicular wall. It may be considered a differentiated area of the cytoplasm similar to the terminal web of intestinal columnar cells. Filamentous structures have been demonstrated in this area[6,31,125] and thin (5 nm [50 Å]) and thick (10 nm [100 Å]) filaments have been identified in association with isolated bile canaliculi. These filaments are distributed around the canaliculi and extend into the microvilli.[73] There is evidence that an actin-like protein is present at this site,[25,41,78] suggesting that the microfilaments are contractile and have a role in intracellular transport, bile flow and tone of the canalicular wall. The microfilaments are also the site of binding of smooth muscle autoantibody – identified as anti-actin antibody – present in patients with chronic liver disease.[26] Besides the pericanalicular area, microfilaments can be seen in the cytoplasm, along the lateral cell membrane (Figure 2.20) and along the sinusoids, in association, or not, with microtubules.[11,25,106]

Ductules

The ducts of Hering or preductules are spaces limited by both hepatocytes and biliary epithelial cells without an intermediate cell type[1,104] (Figure 2.23). They can be found in both adult and newborn liver.[47,103] They represent a very short segment of the biliary tree which communicates at one end with the bile canaliculi and at the other end with the bile ductules. The latter are surrounded only by biliary epithelial cells or 'ductular cells'. The ductular cells are cuboidal, with a cytoplasm lighter and more homogeneous than the cytoplasm of hepatocytes (Figure 2.24). Occasional 'dark' cells can be observed between the light ductular cells.[103] Whether at the level of the duct of Hering or at the ductular level, the biliary epithelium rests on a basement membrane (Figures 2.23, 2.24 and 2.25) which takes up phosphotungstic acid and appears more complex, with branching structures, in humans than in animals. The basement membrane can also be stained with periodic acid silver methenamine in methacrylate-embedded material. This reaction has been attributed to a high glycoprotein content.[103] On the apical surface of the ductular cells, numerous microvilli project into the ductular lumen and occasional cilia have been observed.[107] The basal surface is straight and the lateral membranes may show complex interdigitations (Figure 2.24) or be separated from each other by wide gaps, especially towards the basal pole of the cells. Near the apical pole, strong cohesion is provided by junctional complexes which are also seen at the point of contact between hepatocytes and ductular cells (Figures 2.23 and 2.24). The nucleus is located towards the basal pole of the cell while the Golgi apparatus is located towards the luminal or the lateral surface (Figure 2.23). Small round or elongated mitochondria are dispersed in the cytoplasm. The endoplasmic reticulum is scarce and mainly of the smooth type. The cytoplasm also contains some lysosomes, a few lipid droplets and a rich network of filaments originating from the junctional complexes. These filaments probably represent a contractile system involved in intracellular transport.

Blood vessels and lymphatics are closely apposed to the ductules in the portal tracts and unmyelinated nerve fibres are sometimes seen next to the basement membrane of venules (Figure 2.25).[107]

THE SINUSOID

The sinusoidal wall consists of three types of cells: endothelial cells, Kupffer cells and fat-storing cells or lipocytes. Kupffer cells and endothelial cells are littoral cells in contact with the lumen of the sinusoids while the lipocytes are located in the space of Disse between the hepatocyte and the littoral cells.

Thin cytoplasmic extensions covering the microvilli of hepatocytes characterize the endothelial cells (Figures 2.22 and 2.26) while the Kupffer cells are voluminous with a prominent nucleus and numerous phagocytic inclusions.[122] Cytochemically, the cells may be distinguished by the lack of both peroxidase and phagocytic activity in endothelial cells.[119,123] No transitional stages have been observed between the two types of cells.[122]

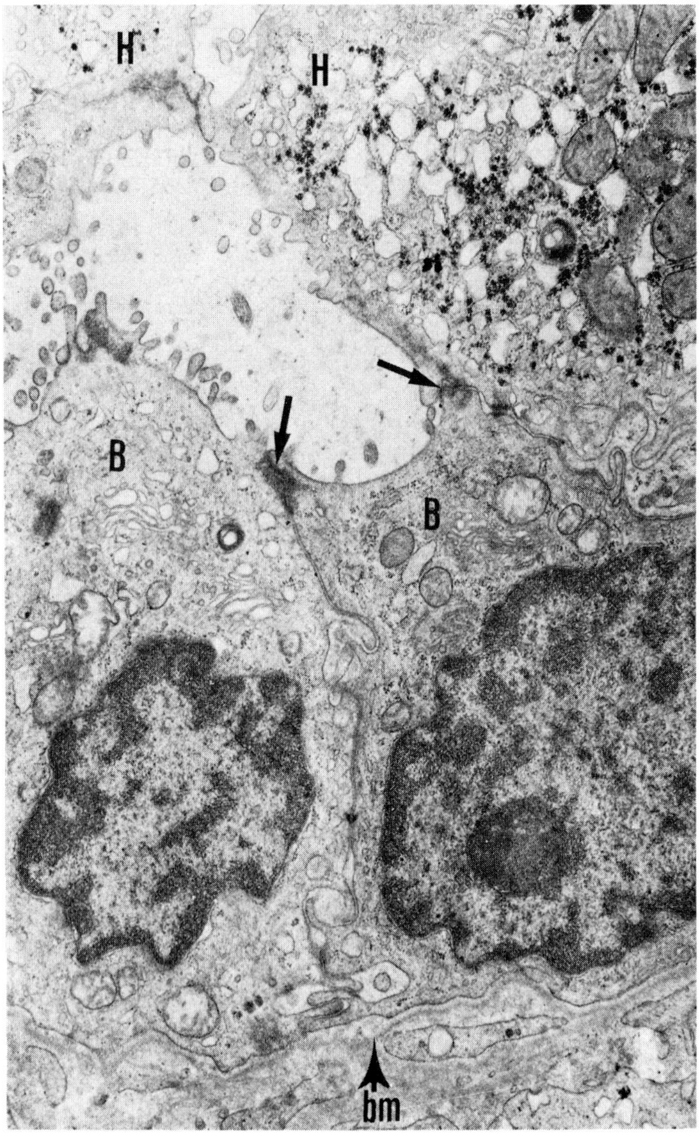

Figure 2.23. The lumen of a duct of Hering is surrounded by both hepatocytes (H) and biliary epithelial cells (B). Tight junctions are evident around the lumen, and also between cells of different types (arrows). A basement membrane (bm) runs along the basal pole of the ductular cells. × 14000.

Endothelial Cells

These form a 'fenestrated' endothelium well demonstrated by scanning electron microscopy (Figure 2.13).[33] In rat liver, endothelial cells account for 2.8 per cent of the parenchymal volume, roughly equivalent to that of the Kupffer cells.[8] Their cytoplasm (Figure 2.22) contains small mitochondria which represent only 0.53 per cent of the total mitochondrial volume of the hepatic parenchyma. The cisternae of the rough endoplasmic reticulum are connected with an anastomosing network of smooth membranes. The relative proportion is 60 per cent of rough and 40 per cent of smooth membranes. Together they represent only 3.3 per cent of the total area of the endoplasmic reticulum of the parenchyma.[8] The Golgi apparatus represents 11.9 per cent of the total Golgi membranes. Lysosomes are not prominent and constitute 7 per cent of the cell volume.[8] Contrary to rat liver, human liver often shows large amounts of monoparticulate glycogen inside endothelial cells. A measure of the high process of pinocytosis in endothelial cells is given by the volume density of pinocytic vesicles – 2.51 per cent of the cell volume.[8] The luminal surface of the endothelial cells, including the pinocytic vesicles, intracytoplasmic tubules and the mature face of the Golgi complex, stains with phosphotungstic acid, suggesting common physicochemical properties,

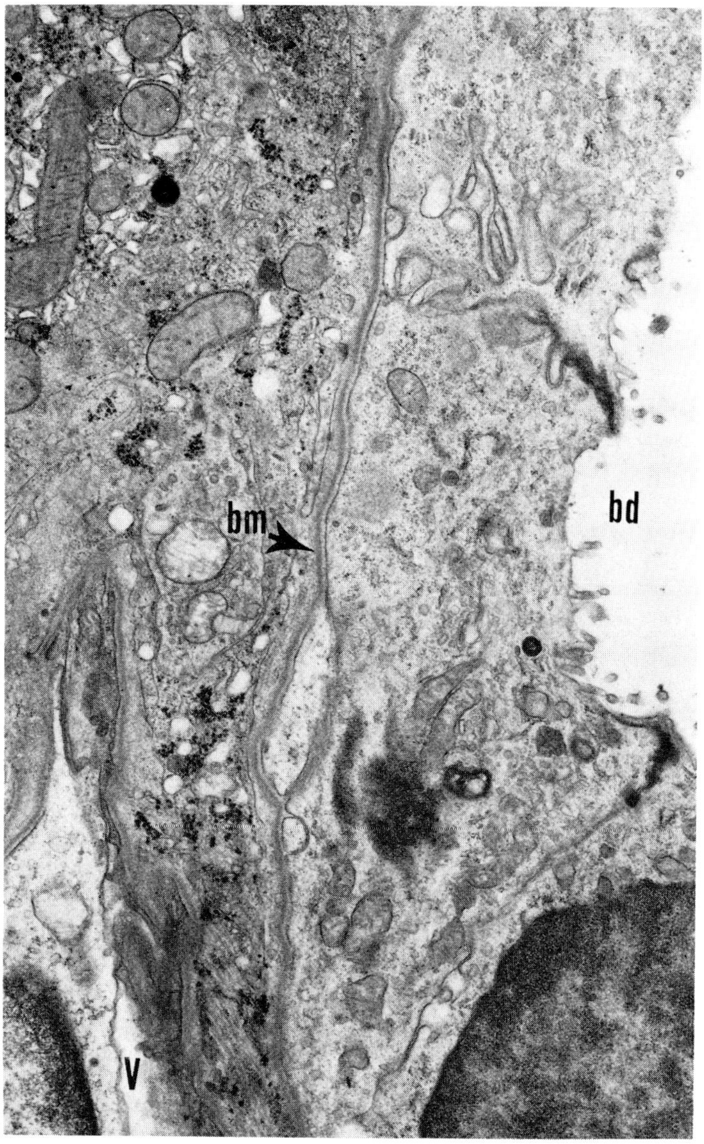

Figure 2.24. Part of a small portal tract showing the close apposition between the parenchymal cells and the bile ductule (bd). The ductular cells rest upon a thick basement membrane (bm) showing evidence of branching structure. Part of a venule (V) with an endothelial cell is also visible. × 10 500.

perhaps related to a transfer process operating through membrane fusion between the cell surface and the inner cellular compartments.[16]

Kupffer Cells

The Kupffer cells constitute 2.1 per cent of the parenchymal volume in adult rat liver.[8] Their cytoplasm is more abundant than that of the endothelial cells. It contains numerous phagocytic inclusions which represent 14 per cent of the cell volume. The endoplasmic reticulum is scarce and is mainly found as rough endoplasmic reticulum.[8] Microtubules and microfilaments are commonly observed.[123] In rats, peroxidase activity is present in the perinuclear space, endoplasmic reticulum and also in occasional annulate lamellae. This has been linked with the clearing of living microorganisms from the blood.[119,123] The surface of the Kupffer cells is sometimes indented to form peculiar worm-like structures about 140 nm (1400 Å) in diameter with an irregular dense line in the centre. They form a complex system communicating with the vascular space and they appear to be engaged in a so-called process of 'micropinocytosis vermiformis'.[56,119,123] Erythrocyte catabolism is one of the main functions of the Kupffer cell but it appears to be limited to a specialized subpopulation (about 30 per cent) of sinusoidal cells. This erythrophago-

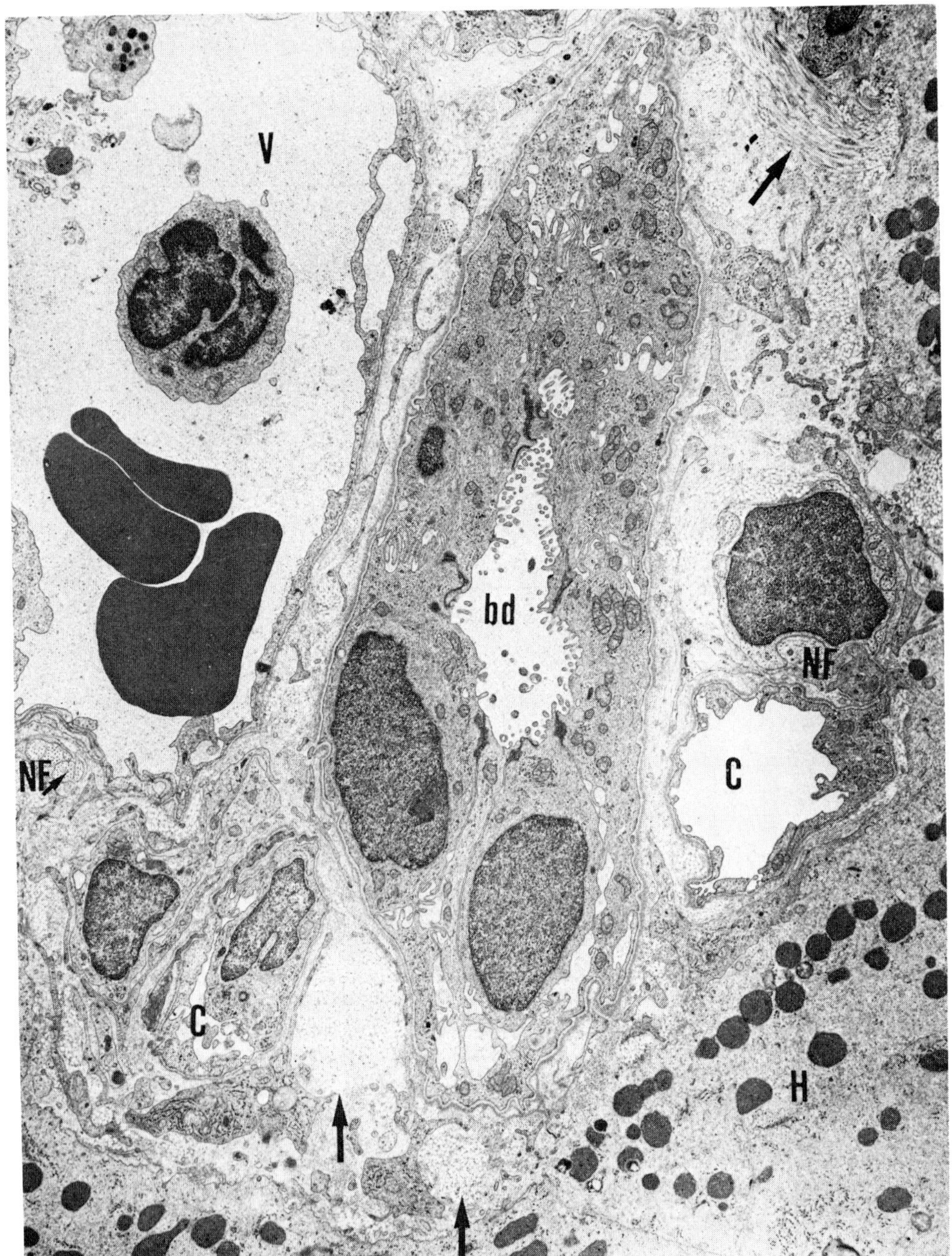

Figure 2.25. Low power view of a small portal tract, showing the bile ductule (bd) surrounded by a basement membrane, venules (V) and capillaries (C). Bundles of collagen fibres are present (arrows) around the bile ductule and in close contact with hepatocytes (H). Small unmyelinated nerve fibres (NF) are seen close to the venule and a capillary. × 4000.
From Sternlieb,[107] with kind permission of the author and Williams and Wilkins Co.

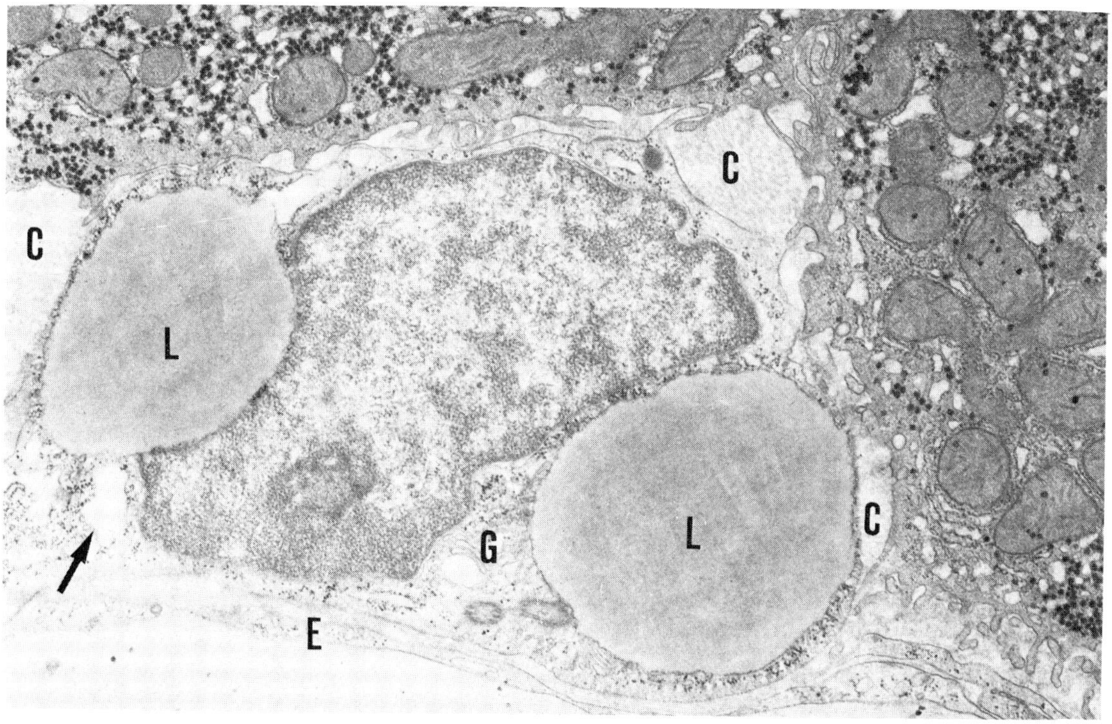

Figure 2.26. A lipocyte is located in the space between the endothelium (E) and the hepatocytes. Two large lipid droplets (L) occupy most of the cytoplasm of the lipocyte, and one of them is pressing against the nucleus. The cytoplasm contains little rough endoplasmic reticulum (arrow), and a small Golgi apparatus (G) next to two centrioles. Bundles of collagen fibres (C) are closely apposed to the lipocyte. × 14000.

cytic property would be directly related to the cellular content of microsomal haem oxygenase.[7]

Fat-storing Cells

The fat-storing cells or lipocytes located in the perisinusoidal space have received a variety of names: Ito cells, interstitial cells, and fat-laden perisinusoidal cells.[10,43,117] They are located beneath the endothelium, in close contact with hepatocytes, and sometimes project into perisinusoidal recesses between hepatocytes. Small bundles of collagen fibrils are often evident between the lipocytes and the hepatocytes (Figure 2.26). The lipocytes appear to be present in the liver of all species and they account for 1.40 per cent of the parenchymal volume in normal adult rat liver [8] and 1.88 per cent in man.[45] Their cytoplasm contains a few profiles of rough endoplasmic reticulum, monoparticulate glycogen isolated or in small clumps, and small mitochondria with a light matrix and short cristae. Centrioles are frequently observed. The lipocytes do not show evidence of phagocytosis, and pinocytic vesicles are rarely seen. The cytoplasm also contains a variable number of large round or star-shaped lipid droplets, which sometimes displace the nucleus. These droplets react intensely with gold chloride and exhibit intense vitamin A fluorescence.[117] The role of lipocytes is still a matter of speculation: they have been implicated in fat transport, vitamin A storage and fibrogenesis. They probably represent undifferentiated mesenchymal cells or resting fibroblasts.[81] No relationship between lipocytes and parenchymal steatosis has been found in adult human liver.[45] Although uncommon in normal liver, cells resembling mature fibroblasts are occasionally seen in the space of Disse. They are morphologically similar to the lipocytes except for the absence of lipid droplets in their cytoplasm.

Pit Cells

Recently, a new type of cell, the 'pit' cell, has been described in the sinusoidal wall of rat liver. These cells are infrequent and have a dense nucleus and an electron-lucent cytoplasm. They are in contact with both the hepatocytes and the sinusoidal lumen and may replace the endothelium over a large area. They are also found in other locations in the body. The pit cells are characterized by the presence of intracytoplasmic granules, about 0.3 μm in diameter, and this has suggested that pit cells might have an endocrine function.[124]

REFERENCES

1. Albot, G. & Jezequel, A.M. (1962) Le passage entre les canalicules biliaires trabéculaires et les canaux biliaires interlobulaires chez l'homme. *Presse Médicale*, **70,** 1485–1498.
2. Andrew, W. (1962) An electron microscope study of age changes in the liver of the mouse. *American Journal of Anatomy*, **110,** 1–18.
3. Berger, E.R. (1973) Two morphologically different mitochondrial populations in the rat hepatocyte as determined by quantitative three dimensional electron microscopy. *Journal of Ultrastructure Research*, **45,** 303–327.
4. Bernhard, W. (1971) Drug effects on the nucleus. In *Advances in Cell Pharmacology* (Ed.) Clementi, F. & Ceccarelli, B. Vol. 1, pp. 49–67. New York: Raven Press.
5. Biava, C. (1963) Identification and structural forms of human particulate glycogen. *Laboratory Investigation*, **12,** 1179–1197.
6. Biava, C. (1964) Studies on cholestasis. A reevaluation of the fine structure of normal human bile canaliculi. *Laboratory Investigation*, **13,** 840–864.
7. Bissell, D.M., Hammaker, L. & Schmid, R. (1972) Liver sinusoidal cells. Identification of a subpopulation for erythrocyte catabolism. *Journal of Cell Biology*, **54,** 107–119.
8. Blouin, A., Bolender, R.P. & Weibel, E.R. (1977) Distribution of organelles and membranes between hepatocytes and non hepatocytes in the rat liver parenchyma. *Journal of Cell Biology*, **72,** 441–455.
9. Bonucci, E., Derenzini, M. & Marinozzi, V. (1973) The organic-inorganic relationship in calcified mitochondria. *Journal of Cell Biology*, **59,** 185–212.
10. Bronfenmajer, S., Schaffner, F. & Popper, H. (1966) Fat-storing cells (lipocytes) in human liver. *Archives of Pathology*, **82,** 447–453.
11. Bruni, C. & Porter, K. (1965) The fine structure of the parenchymal cell of the normal rat liver. I. General observations. *American Journal of Pathology*, **46,** 691–755.
12. Burns, W.A., Vanderweide, G., Goldstein, L.I. & Chan, C.H. (1974) Cytoplasmic crystalline regions in hepatocytes of liver biopsy specimens. *Archives of Pathology*, **97,** 43–45.
13. Dallner, G. & Ericsson, J.L.E. (1976) Molecular structure and biological implication of the liver endoplasmic reticulum. In *Progress in Liver Diseases* (Ed.) Popper, H. & Schaffner, F. Vol. 5, pp. 35–50. New York: Grune & Stratton.
14. Dallner, G., Siekevitz, P. & Palade, G.E. (1966) Biogenesis of endoplasmic reticulum membranes. I. Structural and chemical differentiation in developing rat hepatocyte. *Journal of Cell Biology*, **30,** 73–96.
15. Dallner, G., Siekevitz, P. & Palade, G.E. (1966) Biogenesis of endoplasmic reticulum membranes. II. Synthesis of constitutive microsomal enzymes in developing rat hepatocyte. *Journal of Cell Biology*, **30,** 97–118.
16. De Bruyn, P.P.H., Michelson, S. & Becker, R.P. (1977) Phosphotungstic acid as a marker for the endocyticlysosomal system (vacuolar apparatus) including transfer tubules of the lining cells of the sinusoids in the bone marrow and liver. *Journal of Ultrastructure Research*, **58,** 87–95.
17. De Duve, C. (1966) Peroxisomes (microbodies) and related particles. *Physiological Reviews*, **46,** 323–357.
18. De La Iglesia, F.A., Sturgess, J.M., McGuire, E.J. & Feuer, G. (1976) Quantitative microscopic evaluation of the endoplasmic reticulum in developing human liver. *American Journal of Pathology*, **82,** 61–70.
19. De Wolf-Peeters, C., De Vos, R., Desmet, V., Bianchi, L. & Rohr, H.P. (1974) Electron microscopy and morphometry of canalicular differentiation in fetal and neonatal rat liver. *Experimental and Molecular Pathology*, **21,** 339–350.
20. Dominici, G. & Orlandi, F. (1961) Ultrastructural and microanalytical observations on human hepatic tissue removed by puncture biopsy in diabetic subjects. *Proceedings of the International Congress of Gastroenterology*, pp. 125–128. Amsterdam: Excerpta Medica.
21. Elias, H. (1949) A re-examination of the structure of the mammalian liver. II. The hepatic lobule and its relations to the vascular and biliary system. *American Journal of Anatomy*, **85,** 379.
22. Essner, E. & Novikoff, A.B. (1960) Human hepatocellular pigments and lysosomes. *Journal of Ultrastructure Research*, **3,** 374–391.
23. Fawcett, D.W. (1955) Observations on cytology and electron microscopy of hepatic cells. *Journal of the National Cancer Institute*, **15,** 1475–1503.
24. Feldmann, G., Penaud-Laurencin, J., Crassous, J. & Benhamou, J.P. (1972) Albumin synthesis by human liver cells. Its morphological demonstration. *Gastroenterology*, **63,** 1036–1048.
25. French, S.W. & Davies, P.L. (1975) Ultrastructure localization of actin-like filaments in rat hepatocytes. *Gastroenterology*, **68,** 765–774.
26. Gabbiani, G., Ryan, G.B., Lamelin, J.P., Vassali, P., Majno, G., Bouvier, C.A., Cruchaud, A. & Luschner, E.F. (1973) Human smooth muscle auto antibody. Its identification as antiactin antibody and a study of its binding to 'non-muscular' cells. *American Journal of Pathology*, **72,** 473–488.
27. Givan, K. & Jezequel, A.M. (1969) Infectious canine hepatitis. A virological and ultrastructural study. *Laboratory Investigation*, **20,** 36–45.
28. Glaumann, H. & Ericsson, J.L.E. (1970) Evidence for the participation of the Golgi apparatus in the intracellular transport of nascent albumin in the liver cell. *Journal of Cell Biology*, **47,** 555–567.
29. Goldblatt, P.J. (1969) The endoplasmic reticulum. In *Handbook of Molecular Cytology* (Ed.) Lima de Faria, A. pp. 1101–1129. New York: North Holland.
30. Goldfischer, S., Essner, E. & Novikoff, A.B. (1964) The localization of phosphatase activity at the level of ultrastructure. *Journal of Histochemistry and Cytochemistry*, **12,** 72–95.
31. Goodenough, D.A. & Revel, J.P. (1971) The permeability of isolated and in situ mouse hepatic gap junctions studied with enzymatic tracers. *Journal of Cell Biology*, **50,** 81–91.

32. Greenberger, N.J., Cohen, R.B. & Isselbacher, K.J. (1965) The effect of chronic ethanol administration on liver alcohol dehydrogenase activity in the rat. *Laboratory Investigation,* **14,** 264–271.
33. Grisham, J.W., Nopanitaya, W. & Compagno, J. (1976) Scanning electron microscopy of the liver: a review of methods and results. In *Progress in Liver Diseases* (Ed.) Popper, H. & Schaffner, F. Vol. 5, pp. 1–23. New York: Grune & Stratton.
34. Ham, A.W. (1974) In *Histology,* 7th ed. Philadelphia: J.B. Lippincott.
35. Hamilton, R.L., Regan, D.M., Gray, M.E. & Le Quire, V.S. (1967) Lipid transport in liver. I. Electron microscopic identification of very low density lipoproteins in perfused rat liver. *Laboratory Investigation,* **16,** 305–319.
36. Hanzon, V. (1952) Liver cell secretion under normal and pathologic conditions studied by fluorescence microscopy on living rats. *Acta Physiologica Scandinavica* (Suppl. 101), **28,** 1–268.
37. Harris, J.R., Price, M.R. & Willison, M. (1974) A comparative study on rat liver and hepatoma nuclear membranes. *Journal of Ultrastructure Research,* **48,** 17–32.
38. Herzfeld, A.M., Federman, M. & Greengard, O. (1973) Subcellular morphometric and biochemical analyses of developing rat hepatocytes. *Journal of Cell Biology,* **57,** 475–483.
39. Hess, F.A., Weibel, E.R. & Preisig, R. (1973) Morphometry of dog liver. Normal baseline data. *Virchows Archiv Abteilung B.,* **12,** 303–317.
40. Holborow, E.J., Trenchev, P.S., Dorling, J. & Webb, J. (1975) Demonstration of smooth muscle contractile protein antigens in liver and epithelial cells. *Annals of the New York Academy of Sciences,* **254,** 489–504.
41. Horikawa, M., Chisaka, N., Yokoyama, S. & Onoe, T. (1976) Effect of stirring during fixation upon immunofluorescence results with distribution of albumin-producing cells in liver. *Journal of Histochemistry and Cytochemistry,* **24,** 926–932.
42. Hruban, Z. & Rechcigl, M.J. (1969) *Microbodies and Related Particles.* New York: Academic Press.
43. Ito, T. & Nemoto, M. (1952) Ueber die Kupfferschen Sternzellen und die 'Fettspeicherungszellen' ('fat-storing cells') in der Blutkapillarenwand der menschlichen Leber. *Okajimas Folia Anatomica Japonica,* **24,** 243–258.
44. Jezequel, A.M. (1959) Dégénérescence myélinique des mitochondries de foie humain dans un épithélioma du cholédoque et un ictère viral. *Journal of Ultrastructure Research,* **3,** 210–215.
45. Jezequel, A.M. (1978) (In press).
46. Jezequel, A.M. & Orlandi, F. (1972) Fine morphology of the liver as a tool in clinical pharmacology. In *Liver and Drugs* (Ed.) Jezequel, A.M. & Orlandi, F. pp. 145–192. London: Academic Press.
47. Jezequel, A.M., Arakawa, K. & Steiner, J.W. (1965) The fine structure of the normal neonatal mouse liver. *Laboratory Investigation,* **14,** 1894–1930.
48. Jezequel, A.M., Koch, M. & Orlandi, F. (1974) A morphometric study of the endoplasmic reticulum in human hepatocytes. *Gut,* **15,** 737–747.
49. Kirschner, R.H., Rusli, M. & Martin, T.E. (1977) Characterization of the nuclear envelope, pore complexes and dense lamina of mouse liver nuclei by high resolution scanning electron microscopy. *Journal of Cell Biology,* **72,** 118–132.
50. LeBouton, A.V. (1968) Heterogeneity of protein metabolism between liver cells as studied by autoradiography. *Currents in Modern Biology,* **2,** 111–114.
51. LeBouton, A.V. (1969) Relations and extent of the zone of intensified protein metabolism in the liver acinus. *Currents in Modern Biology,* **3,** 4–8.
52. Leskes, A., Siekevitz, P. & Palade, G.E. (1971) Differentiation of endoplasmic reticulum in hepatocytes. I. Glucose-6-phosphatase distribution in situ. *Journal of Cell Biology,* **49,** 264–287.
53. Loud, A.V. (1968) A quantitative stereological description of the ultrastructure of normal rat liver parenchymal cells. *Journal of Cell Biology,* **37,** 27–46.
54. Ma, M.H. & Biempica, L. (1971) The normal human liver cell. Cytochemical and ultrastructural studies. *American Journal of Pathology,* **62,** 353–390.
55. Marinozzi, V. (1964) Cytochimie ultrastructurale du nucléole. RNA et proteines intranucléolaires. *Journal of Ultrastructure Research,* **10,** 433–456.
56. Matter, A., Orci, L., Forssmann, W.G. & Rouiller, C. (1968) The stereological analysis of the fine structure of the 'micropinocytosis vermiformis' in Kupffer cells of the rat. *Journal of Ultrastructure Research,* **23,** 272–279.
57. McCuskey, R.A. (1966) A dynamic and static study of hepatic arterioles and hepatic sphincters. *American Journal of Anatomy,* **119,** 455–477.
58. Millward-Sadler, G.H. (1978) Personal observations.
59. Mitra, S.K. (1966) The terminal distribution of the hepatic artery with special references to arterio-portal anastomosis. *Journal of Anatomy,* **100,** 651–663.
60. Miyai, K., Abraham, J.L., Linthicum, D.S. & Wagner, R.M. (1976) Scanning electron microscopy of hepatic ultrastructure: secondary, back-scattered and transmitted electron imaging. *Laboratory Investigation,* **35,** 369–376.
61. Mugnaini, E. (1964) Filamentous inclusions in the matrix of mitochondria from human livers. *Journal of Ultrastructure Research,* **11,** 525–544.
62. Munn, E.A. (1974) *The Fine structure of Mitochondria.* London: Academic Press.
63. Nakata, K. & Kanbe, A. (1966) The terminal distribution of the hepatic artery and its relationship to the development of focal liver necrosis following interruption of the portal blood supply. *Acta Pathologica Japonica,* **16,** 313–321.
64. Nehemiah, J.L. & Novikoff, A.B. (1974) Unusual lysosomes in hamster hepatocytes. *Experimental and Molecular Pathology,* **21,** 398–423.
65. Nilsson, O. & Dallner, G. (1977) Enzyme and phospholipid asymmetry in liver microsomal membranes. *Journal of Cell Biology,* **72,** 568–583.
66. Novikoff, A.B. (1973) Lysosomes: a personal account. In *Lysosomes and Storage Diseases* (Ed.) Hers, H.G. & Van Hoof, F. pp. 1–42. New York: Academic Press.
67. Novikoff, A.B. (1976) The endoplasmic reticulum. A cytochemist's view. A review. *Proceedings of the National Academy of Sciences of the United States of America,* **73,** 2781–2787.
68. Novikoff, A.B. & Essner, E. (1960) The liver cell: Some new approaches to its study. *American Journal of Medicine,* **29,** 102–131.
69. Novikoff, A.B. & Goldfischer, S. (1969) Visualization of peroxisomes (microbodies) and mitochondria with diaminobenzidine. *Journal of Histochemistry and Cytochemistry,* **17,** 675–680.
70. Novikoff, A.B., Essner, E., Goldfischer, S. & Heus, M. (1962) Nucleoside phosphatase activities of cytomembranes. In *The Interpretation of Ultrastructure* (Ed.) Harris, R.J.C. pp. 149–192. New York: Academic Press.

71. Novikoff, A.B., Novikoff, P.M., Davis, C. & Quintana, N. (1972) Studies on microperoxisomes. II. A cytochemical method for light and electron microscopy. *Journal of Histochemistry and Cytochemistry,* **20,** 1006–1023.
72. Novikoff, P.M., Novikoff, A.B., Quintana, N. & Davis, C. (1973) Studies on microperoxisomes. III. Observations on human and rat hepatocytes. *Journal of Histochemistry and Cytochemistry,* **21,** 540–558.
73. Oda, M., Price, V.M., Fisher, M.M. & Phillips, M.J. (1974) Ultrastructure of bile canaliculi with special reference to the surface coat and the pericanalicular web. *Laboratory Investigation,* **31,** 314–323.
74. Orlandi, F. & Koch, M. (1976) The fine structure of liver cells. In *The Hepatobiliary System* (Ed.) Taylor, W. pp. 145–177. New York: Plenum Press.
75. Pearse, A.G.E. (1968) *Histochemistry: Theoretical and Applied,* 3rd ed., Vol. 1, pp. 294–380. London: J. & A. Churchill.
76. Pederson, T. (1975) Nuclei. In *Cell Biology* (Ed.) Altman, P.L. & Katz, D.D. Vol. 1, pp. 363–400. Bethesda, Maryland: Federation of American Societies for Experimental Biology.
77. Perrin, C., Oudea, M.C., Lenne, Y. & Oudea, P. (1970) Les mitochondries géantes. Appréciation au microscope photonique de leur fréquence en pathologie humaine. *Pathologie Biologie (Paris),* **18,** 613–618.
78. Phillips, M.J., Oda, M., Mak, E. & Fisher, M.M. (1975) Bile canalicular structure and function. In *Jaundice* (Ed.) Goresky, C. & Fisher, M.M. pp. 367–382. New York: Plenum.
79. Phillips, M.J., Oda, M., Mak, E., Edwards, V., Yousef, I. & Fisher, M.M. (1976) The bile canalicular network in vitro. *Journal of Ultrastructure Research,* **57,** 163–167.
80. Pierce, G.B. Jr, Midgeley, A.R. Jr & SriRam, J. (1963) The histogenesis of basement membranes. *Journal of Experimental Medicine,* **117,** 339–348.
81. Popper, H. & Udenfriend, S. (1970) Hepatic fibrosis. *American Journal of Medicine,* **49,** 707–721.
82. Popper, H., Elias, H. & Petty, D.E. (1952) Vascular pattern of cirrhotic liver. *American Journal of Clinical Pathology,* **22,** 717–729.
83. Prugh, M.F., Gregory, D.H., Vhlacevic, Z.R. & Swell, L. (1976) Role of the 'microtubular-Golgi' network in the hepatocellular transport of biliary lipids. *Gastroenterology,* **70,** A-132/990.
84. Racker, E. & Horstman, L.L. (1967) Partial resolution of the enzymes catalyzing oxidative phosphorylation. XIII. Structure and function of submitochondrial particles completely resolved with respect to coupling factor. *Journal of Biological Chemistry,* **242,** 2547–2551.
85. Rappaport, A.M. (1958) The structural and functional unit in the human liver (liver acinus). *Anatomical Record,* **130,** 673–689.
86. Rappaport, A.M. (1973) The microcirculatory hepatic unit. *Microvascular Research,* **6,** 212–228.
87. Rappaport, A.M. & Hiracki, G.Y. (1958) Histopathological changes in the structural and functional unit of the human liver. *Acta Anatomica,* **32,** 240–255.
88. Reddy, J.K. (1973) Possible properties of microbodies (peroxisomes): microbody proliferation and hypolipidemic drugs. *Journal of Histochemistry and Cytochemistry,* **21,** 967–972.
89. Rhodin, J.A.G. (1967) The ultrastructure of mammalian arterioles and precapillary sphincters. *Journal of Ultrastructure Research,* **18,** 181–223.
90. Rohr, H.P., Wirz, A., Henning, L.G., Reide, U.N. & Bianchi, L. (1971) Morphometric analysis of the rat liver cell in the perinatal period. *Laboratory Investigation,* **24,** 128–139.
91. Rohr, H.P., Luthy, J., Gudat, F., Oberholzer, M., Gysin, C. & Bianchi, L. (1976) Stereology of liver biopsies from healthy volunteers. *Virchows Archiv Abteilung A,* **371,** 251–263.
92. Rouiller, C. & Jezequel, A.M. (1963) Electron microscopy of the liver. In *The Liver* (Ed.) Rouiller, C. Vol. 1, pp. 195–264. New York: Academic Press.
93. Ruebner, B.H., Aguirre, J., Brayton, M.A. & Watanabe, K. (1971) Inclusions with helical substructure in hepatocytic mitochondria of Rhesus monkey. *Journal of Ultrastructure Research,* **35,** 499–507.
94. Sadowski, P. & Steiner, J.W. (1968) Electron microscopic and biochemical characteristics of nuclei and nucleoli isolated from rat liver. *Journal of Cell Biology,* **37,** 147–161.
95. Schaff, S., Lapis, K. & Andre, J. (1974) Study of the tridimensional structure of intramitochondrial crystalline inclusions. *Journal of Microscopy,* **20,** 259–264.
96. Schaff, S., Lapis, K. & Andre, J. (1974) Effect of proteolytic digestion on mitochondrial crystalline inclusions in Gilbert's syndrome. *Journal of Microscopy,* **20,** 265–270.
97. Schmucker, D.L. (1976) Age related change in hepatic fine structure: a quantitative analysis. *Journal of Gerontology,* **31,** 135–143.
98. Shank, R.E., Morrison, G., Cheng, C.H., Karl, I. & Schwartz, R. (1959) Cell heterogeneity within the hepatic lobule: quantitative histochemistry. *Journal of Histochemistry and Cytochemistry,* **7,** 237–239.
99. Sheldon, H., Silverberg, M. & Kerner, I. (1962) On the differing appearance of intranuclear and cytoplasmic glycogen in liver cells in glycogen storage disease. *Journal of Cell Biology,* **13,** 468–473.
100. Shnitka, T.K. (1966) Comparative ultrastructure of hepatic microbodies in some mammals and birds in relation to species differences. *Journal of Ultrastructure Research,* **16,** 598–625.
101. Siekevitz, P. (1976) Endoplasmic reticulum, microsomes, ribosomes and Golgi. In *Cell Biology* (Ed.) Altman, P.L. & Katz, D.D. pp. 231–313. Bethesda, Maryland: Federation of American Societies for Experimental Biology.
102. Slabodsky-Brousse, N., Feldmann, G., Brousse, J. & Dreyfus, P. (1974) Étude stéréologique de la fréquence des mitochondries géantes hépatiques dans la maladie de Gilbert. Comparaison avec le sujet normal. *Biologie et Gastroenterologie (Paris),* **7,** 179–186.
103. Steiner, J.W. & Carruthers, J.S. (1961) Studies on the fine structure of the terminal branches of the biliary tree. *American Journal of Pathology,* **38,** 639–661.
104. Steiner, J.W., Jezequel, A.M., Phillips, M.J., Miyai, K. & Arakawa, K. (1965) Some aspects of the ultrastructural pathology of the liver. In *Progress in Liver Diseases* (Ed.) Popper, H. & Schaffner, F. Vol. 2, pp. 303–372. New York: Grune & Stratton.
105. Stempak, J. & Laurencin, M. (1976) Mitochondrial forms in hepatic parenchymal cells in rats of several ages. *American Journal of Anatomy,* **145,** 261–281.
106. Sternlieb, I. (1965) Perinuclear filaments and microtubules in human hepatocytes and biliary epithelial cells. *Journal of Microscopy,* **4,** 551–558.
107. Sternlieb, I. (1972) Functional implication of human portal and bile ductular ultrastructure. *Gastroenterology,* **63,** 321–327.
108. Sternlieb, I. & Berger, J.E. (1969) Optical diffraction

studies of crystalline structures in electron micrographs. *Journal of Cell Biology*, **43**, 448–455.

109. Sternlieb, I. & Quintana, N. (1977) The peroxisomes of human hepatocytes. *Laboratory Investigation*, **36**, 140–149.
110. Sternlieb, I., Berger, J.E., Biempica, L., Quintana, N. & Hodge, T. (1971) Cytoplasmic crystals in human hepatocytes. *Laboratory Investigation*, **25**, 503–508.
111. Sturgess, J.M. & De La Iglesia, F.A. (1972) Morphometry of the Golgi apparatus in developing liver. *Journal of Cell Biology*, **55**, 524–530.
112. Tate, E.L. & Herbener, G.H. (1976) A morphometric study of the density of mitochondrial cristae in heart and liver of ageing mice. *Journal of Gerontology*, **31**, 129–134.
113. Tsou, K.C., Mela, L., Gupta, P.D. & Lynm, D. (1976) Mitochondrial ultrastructure study with the new cytochrome *c* binding agent 4,4′diamino-2,2′-bipyridyl ferrous chelate. *Journal of Ultrastructure Research*, **54**, 235–242.
114. Wachstein, M. (1959) Enzymic histochemistry of the liver. *Gastroenterology*, **37**, 525–537.
115. Wachstein, M. & Meisel, E. (1957) Histochemistry of hepatic phosphatases at a physiological pH with special reference to the demonstration of bile canaliculi. *American Journal of Clinical Pathology*, **27**, 13–23.
116. Wade, J.B. & Karnovsky, M. (1974) The structure of the zonula occludens. A single fibril model based on freeze-fracture. *Journal of Cell Biology*, **60**, 168–180.
117. Wake, K. (1971) 'Sternzellen' in the liver: perisinusoidal cells with special reference to storage of vitamin A. *American Journal of Anatomy*, **132**, 429–462.
118. Weibel, E.R., Staubli, W., Gnagi, H.R. & Hess, F.A. (1969) Correlated morphometric and biochemical studies on the liver cell. *Journal of Cell Biology*, **42**, 68–91.
119. Widman, J.J., Cotran, R.S. & Fahimi, H.D. (1972) Mononuclear phagocytes (Kupffer cells) and endothelial cells. Identification of two functional cell types in rat liver sinusoids by endogenous peroxidase activity. *Journal of Cell Biology*, **52**, 159–170.
120. Wills, E.J. (1965) Crystalline structures in the mitochondria of normal human liver parenchymal cells. *Journal of Cell Biology*, **24**, 511–514.
121. Wisher, M.H. & Evans, W.H. (1975) Functional polarity of the rat hepatocyte surface membrane. Isolation and characterization of plasma-membrane subfractions from the blood–sinusoidal, bile canalicular and contiguous surfaces of the hepatocyte. *Biochemical Journal*, **146**, 375–388.
122. Wisse, E. (1972) An ultrastructural characterization of the endothelial cell in the rat liver sinusoid under normal and various experimental conditions, as a contribution to the distinction between endothelial and Kupffer cells. *Journal of Ultrastructure Research*, **38**, 528–562.
123. Wisse, E. (1974) Observation on the fine structure and peroxidase cytochemistry of normal rat liver Kupffer cells. *Journal of Ultrastructure Research*, **46**, 393–426.
124. Wisse, E., Van't Noordende, J.M., Van Dermeulen, J. & Daems, W. (1976) The Pit cell: description of a new type of cell occurring in rat liver sinusoids and peripheral blood. *Cell and Tissue Research*, **173**, 423–435.
125. Wood, R.L. (1961) Some structural features of the bile canaliculus in calf liver. *Anatomical Record*, **140**, 207–216.
126. Yates, R.D., Higgins, J.A. & Barrnett, R.J. (1969) Fine structural localization of acetylcoenzyme A carboxylase in rat liver hepatocytes. *Journal of Histochemistry and Cytochemistry*, **17**, 379–385.

Chapter 3

Carbohydrate Metabolism in Liver Disease

K.G.M.M. ALBERTI
D.G. JOHNSTON

The liver is of prime importance in the regulation of carbohydrate metabolism.[15] It receives the majority of ingested carbohydrates via the portal circulation and plays a critical role in homeostasis by damping down sudden surges in the concentrations of fuels, thus preventing excessive fluctuations in systemic osmolality. Man is an intermittent feeder but uses glucose continuously and the liver is the major organ which prevents blood glucose levels falling in these periods of fasting. Indeed the blood glucose level in normal man shows surprisingly small fluctuations, less than 10 per cent of the mean level.[6] Perhaps the most important role of the liver in metabolism is in preserving this constancy, thus ensuring a fixed, even and predictable supply of carbohydrate to extra-hepatic tissues.

The metabolic functions of the liver are outlined in Table 3.1. It can be seen that not only do many important reactions take place in the liver, but many of these are virtually unique to the liver. In addition, many hormones exert regulatory roles on these metabolic reactions in the liver, and the liver degrades several of these hormones, in certain cases being the only important site of their catabolism (see Chapter 7). It can also be seen from Table 3.1 that the main actions of the liver with regard to carbohydrate metabolism can be divided into

Table 3.1. *Metabolic Actions of the Liver.*[a]

Substrate metabolism:	
Carbohydrates	Glucose storage as glycogen Glycogenolysis Gluconeogenesis[b] Glucose clearance Lactate clearance Non-glucose hexose metabolism[c]
Lipids	Triglyceride production (in part from glucose) VLDL production[c] Cholesterol synthesis NEFA synthesis and degradation Ketogenesis[c]
Proteins	Amino acid degradation Ureagenesis[c] Plasma protein synthesis[c]
Hormones:	
Major action on the liver	Insulin, glucagon, growth hormone, glucocorticoids, catecholamines, thyroxine
Catabolized by the liver	Insulin,[c] glucagon, growth hormone,[c] glucocorticoids,[c] thyroxine

[a] Adapted from Alberti[3] and Alberti, Johnston and Sutton.[7]
[b] Takes place in liver and kidney.
[c] Primarily occurs in liver only.

glucose producing functions, glucose storage functions, and metabolism of hexoses and sugars other than glucose, which are ingested but not utilized to any major extent elsewhere in the body.

In view of these critical roles of the liver in carbohydrate homeostasis it would be surprising if carbohydrate metabolism were not disturbed in liver disease. What *is* perhaps surprising is that the disturbance is not greater than that commonly found. This reflects the large reserve capacity of the liver parenchyma.

In this chapter we shall first review briefly the role of the normal liver in carbohydrate metabolism with emphasis on the contrasts between the fed and starved states. The effects of different disorders of the liver on these processes will then be described. Most studies in man have concentrated on measurements of metabolites in blood, but where possible reference will be made to changes in intracellular enzymes and metabolites in diseased liver and relevant animal data will be discussed. Hormonal changes will be referred to only in so far as they impinge directly on regulatory processes in carbohydrate metabolism, as hormones in general are referred to in more detail in Chapter 7. Similarly the metabolism and acute effects of ethanol are described in detail elsewhere in this volume (Chapter 32) and will not be described here.

The reader is referred to several reviews which have appeared in the last decade for further information on the general metabolic aspects of liver disease[2, 3, 7, 32, 47, 72, 136] and on the role of the liver in carbohydrate homeostasis.[46, 107, 108, 161]

THE REGULATION OF HEPATIC CARBOHYDRATE METABOLISM IN NORMAL MAN

The Fasted State

In short-term starvation certain tissues have an obligatory requirement for glucose. These include the central nervous system, peripheral nerves, red blood corpuscles, white blood cells and fibroblasts with a total requirement of some 160 g/day in normal man.[17] Other tissues can use substrates such as fatty acids and ketone bodies with brain able to use the latter on adaptation to starvation. Only liver and to a lesser extent kidney contain the key enzyme glucose-6-phosphatase which allows glucose to be formed in the tissue and released into the circulation for use by other tissues. As ingested glucose disappears so the liver releases glucose with the result that blood glucose concentration falls only slightly.

After an overnight fast approximately 75 per cent of the released glucose is derived from glycogenolysis, with approximately 25 per cent coming from gluconeogenesis.[45, 68] The liver contains, however, only 70 to 80 g of glycogen after an overnight fast, so that the contribution of glycogenolysis to glucose production falls rapidly after the first 18 to 24 hours of fasting.[88] As starvation continues the total body glucose requirement falls due to the adaptation of the brain to ketone body utilization.[112] Thus after five to six weeks' fasting only 40 g glucose/day are required[113] and about half of this requirement is produced by the kidney.

The precursors for gluconeogenesis are lactate, pyruvate, glucogenic amino acids (mainly alanine) and glycerol. Lactate is quantitatively the most important, providing about half of non-glycogen glucose and approximately 20 per cent of total glucose after an overnight fast. Total lactate turnover is some 140 g/day.[82] However, more than half of this lactate is derived in turn from glucose metabolism (the Cori cycle) in extrahepatic tissues and from muscle glycogen, much of which is also derived originally from glucose released from the liver. This role of muscle glycogen as a glucose precursor has been elegantly demonstrated in the rat by Sugden, Sharples and Randle.[166] It can thus be considered that although lactate is a useful (albeit energetically wasteful) means whereby extrahepatic tissues can conserve glucose and divert fuels to other tissues via the liver, it is hardly, in the long term, a means for de novo glucose synthesis. This role must be reserved for amino acids which are irreversibly converted to glucose and contribute 6 to 12 per cent of total glucose production after an overnight fast but a much greater proportion with prolongation of the fast.

The importance of alanine as a gluconeogenic precursor was first formalized in 1970 by Felig and his colleagues[52] who had studied arteriovenous differences of amino acids across muscle during fasting. Alanine and glutamine accounted for more than 50 per cent of the amino acids released. Felig and Wahren[48] then showed that alanine is taken up in significant quantities by the splanchnic bed. Subsequently it has been shown that glutamine released by muscle is taken up mainly by gut and kidney while the alanine is taken up by the liver and converted to glucose.

Alanine is formed in peripheral tissues by transamination of pyruvate, the amino groups deriving from the other amino acids, particularly the branched chain amino acids. It is immediately obvious that if, as was first postulated by Felig,[45] the carbon skeleton derived primarily from glucose then, again, no de novo glucose synthesis would be taking place. Garber, Karl and Kipnis[55] have now shown that much of the carbon skeleton of alanine derives from the carbon skeleton of the other amino acids. Thus (after Levenson[88]):

$$\text{amino acid} + \text{2-oxoglutarate} \rightleftarrows \alpha\text{-oxoanalogue} + \text{glutamate} \qquad [1]$$

$$\text{or amino acid} \rightarrow$$

$$\rightarrow \alpha\text{-oxoanalogue} + NH_3;\ NH_3 + \text{2-oxoglutarate} \rightarrow \text{glutamate} \qquad [2]$$

$$\text{From [1] and [2]: } \alpha\text{-oxoanalogue} \rightarrow \text{malate; malate} \rightarrow \text{pyruvate} \qquad [3]$$

$$\text{From [1], [2] and [3]: pyruvate} + \text{glutamate} \rightarrow \text{alanine} + \text{2-oxoglutarate} \qquad [4]$$

$$\text{Net: amino acid} \rightarrow \text{alanine} \qquad [5]$$

The whole process can be considered as a molecular reorganization whereby many different amino acids reach the liver in the form of a single amino acid which undoubtedly simplifies the regulatory processes required in the liver. Further amino groups in peripheral tissues will combine with glutamate to give glutamine which will be disposed of in the gut and kidney. Much of this glutamine will then be converted to alanine and delivered to the liver.[50] In the liver alanine is again transaminated, this time with oxaloacetate, forming pyruvate and aspartate. The latter participates in the urea cycle yielding urea while the pyruvate passes up the usual gluconeogenic pathway.

It is worth pointing out the key regulatory steps in gluconeogenesis as these are most likely to be affected by disorders of the liver. They are:

$$\text{pyruvate} + CO_2 + \text{ATP} \underset{}{\overset{\text{Pyruvate carboxylase}}{\rightleftarrows}} \text{oxaloacetate} + \text{ADP} + \text{Pi} \qquad [6]$$

$$\text{oxaloacetate} + \text{GTP} \underset{\text{PEP-carboxykinase}}{\rightleftarrows} \text{phosphoenolpyruvate} + \text{GDP} + CO_2 \qquad [7]$$

$$\text{fructose-1,6-diphosphate} \xrightarrow{\text{fructose-1,6-diphosphatase}} \text{fructose-6-phosphate} + \text{Pi} \qquad [8]$$

$$\text{glucose-6-phosphate} + H_2O \rightarrow \text{glucose} + \text{orthophosphate} \qquad [9]$$

The fine regulation of gluconeogenesis and its integration with the regulation of glycogenolysis are obviously important in the maintenance of a constant blood glucose. Glucose, glucose precursors and hormones are all important in this regulation. The autoregulation of hepatic glucose production by glucose availability has been discussed since the classic early studies of Soskin and Levine.[159] In experimental studies several authors have shown that the liver no longer takes up glucose when portal vein levels fall below approximately 7 mmol/l (120 mg/dl).[27] As pointed out by Newsholme[107] glucose enters the liver cell extremely rapidly and is converted by glucokinase to glucose-6-phosphate. This, together with glucose-6-phosphatase, forms a sensitive substrate cycle. Glucose-6-phosphate will influence glycogenesis while glucose itself has a direct inhibitory effect on liver phosphorylase.[161] These effects of glucose are more important, however, in regulating glucose uptake (see below) than output by the liver.

Substrate availability appears to be important in determining the contribution of gluconeogenesis to glucose output. Both Dietze and his co-workers[41] and Lundholm and Schersten[91] have shown that gluconeogenesis in man increases with increasing precursor supply. Release of these precursors from the periphery will thus be all important. A more detailed account of the regulation of gluconeogenesis can be found in Söling and Kleineke.[158]

In fasting man most of the changes in carbohydrate metabolism can be explained by changes in circulating hormone levels superimposed on these endogenous regulatory mechanisms. Thus as blood glucose concentration falls so insulin secretion will decrease and glucagon secretion will rise. There will also be a relative increase in the concentrations of glucocorticoids, growth hormone and catecholamines when compared with insulin. The effect of insulin on amino acid transport and amino acid synthesis within peripheral tissues will be decreased and glucocorticoid effects will predominate. More amino acids, particularly alanine, will be released into the circulation. At the same time there will be increased extraction of alanine, due to increased glucagon, as well as enhanced extraction of other glucose precursors, by the liver. The normal constraints of insulin on gluconeogenesis will be lost and gluconeogenesis will increase. The importance of this hepatic extraction is shown by the observation that alanine levels in the circulation fall rather than rise on fasting.[120] Glycogenolysis will increase, due partly to the lack of inhibition by both glucose and insulin. Recent studies have shown that the liver is exquisitely sensitive to small increments in portal insulin concentration with glycogenolysis being more sensitive than gluconeogenesis.[21,46] Glycogenolysis will also be enhanced through activation of adenyl cyclase by glucagon and catecholamines. Recently it has been suggested that other hormones, such as vasopressin and parathormone, also exert acute effects on hepatic glucose metabolism.[62]

In the longer term lipolysis will increase, again due to the relative lack of insulin. Increased non-esterified fatty acid (NEFA) supply to the liver in the presence of a relative increase in glucagon will result in enhanced ketogenesis. Ketone bodies thus become available as an alternative fuel. The brain then adapts to ketone body utilization with a resultant fall in total body glucose requirement. This is synchronized with an inhibitory effect of ketone bodies on muscle amino acid release, thereby conserving protein.[150]

The Fed State

The main roles of the liver in the fed state are to prevent violent oscillations in peripheral substrate concentrations and to conserve, store and convert into suitable storage forms fuels which are ingested in excess of requirements at the time.

The main carbohydrates ingested by man are sucrose, which yields equimolar amounts of glucose and fructose, lactose, which yields glucose and galactose, and starch which is broken down in the gut to glucose. Quantitatively glucose and fructose are the most important.

Glucose

Even after ingestion of large amounts of glucose there is relatively little fluctuation in blood glucose concentration. It can be calculated that if 100 g of glucose were infused and all remained in the circulation blood glucose concentration would rise by 37 mmol/l (670 mg/dl) where the measured rise is rarely more than 4 mmol/l (72 mg/dl). Glucose must therefore be disposed of rapidly and in large quantities. The liver is obviously important in this disposal, a fact recognized by Bernard more than a hundred years ago, but arguments still rage as to the exact distribution of this ingested glucose between the liver and the periphery.

All ingested glucose passes through the liver before reaching the peripheral circulation. It has always been assumed that much of this glucose will be sequestered and metabolized by the liver and will not reach the peripheral circulation. There have, however, been wide discrepancies in the estimates of the amount which actually passes through the liver between those using radioactive glucose turnover methods and those using catheterization techniques. Both methods are fraught with difficulties, the former because of recycling or exchange of the radioactive label, and the latter because of the inexact methods available for measuring blood flow and the stressful nature of the experiments.

The primary exponents of the catheterization technique have been Felig and his co-workers.[46, 49] They showed that after oral ingestion of 100 g of glucose only 40 g appeared in the hepatic vein over the next 180 minutes. At the same time hepatic glucose production was decreased from the expected 25 g to near zero. They concluded that there was a net uptake of 85 per cent or a real uptake of 60 per cent of the glucose load. This agrees with the estimates of others.[117] In contrast, if glucose is slowly infused directly into the portal vein no uptake can be demonstrated.[89] These observations are not inconsistent in that oral ingestion of glucose is associated with stimulation of the entero-insular axis[97] with a resulting surge of insulin secretion due to stimulation by both glucose and probably glucose-1-phosphate.[43] The liver is extremely sensitive to small amounts of insulin in both man[48] and dog,[19] the effects being both direct, and indirect through lowering the threshold for glucose autoregulation.[161] Bergman[14] has suggested that although autoregulation may be important for minute-to-minute adjustment of hepatic glucose metabolism this effect is of short duration and insulin is required for the sustained uptake of glucose seen after oral glucose loading. Thus the effect of portal infusion of glucose will depend purely on the relatively insensitive autoregulatory process while oral glucose loading will be assisted by simultaneous insulin secretion into the portal vein.

The discrepancies between hepatic catheterization studies and turnover data have been more serious. Steele et al,[163] working with anaesthetized dogs, estimated that 72 per cent of an oral U-^{14}C-glucose load entered the peripheral circulation in the three hours following glucose ingestion. Hepatic glucose output decreased 42 per cent while peripheral glucose utilization increased by 58 per cent. It was estimated that about 16 per cent of the glucose load was taken up on first passage through the liver. Since that time several thoughtful accounts of radioactive turnover methodology and its problems have appeared.[42, 123] An excellent study by Radziuk et al[125] has now been published in which they examine the problem of hepatic glucose uptake in normal man. They show convincingly that on first passage of glucose through the liver a maximum of 8 per cent is taken up directly, with 92 per cent appearing in the peripheral circulation. By use of different labels they are able to show that little if any glucose is sequestered in the liver either as such or as glycogen. They also demonstrate a 66 per cent suppression of endogenous glucose production.

As Radziuk points out these data are not inconsistent with catheterization studies. The latter provide estimates of total hepatic glucose uptake while the radioactive studies indicate only that amount of glucose extracted on the first pass through the liver. In fact, extrapolation of these studies gives an estimate of total hepatic uptake of 40 to 50 g glucose of a 100 g load, and this is not dissimilar to the conclusions of Felig.[46] These data are also consistent with the findings of Mosora et al,[103] who used a stable isotope method, that some 10 per cent of an administered glucose load is oxidized within the first three hours of ingestion. It is important to realize, however, that the importance of the liver in taking up an oral glucose load is not because of its anatomical location astride the portal vein, but rather because of the sensitivity of the liver to insulin. The importance of oral rather than intravenous glucose feeding is due to the potentiation of insulin secretion by gut hormones.

It is thus apparent that the liver is important in glucose disposal and that both autoregulation by glucose and insulin are important determinants of this disposal. The role of other hormones is less clear. Glucagon has been emphasized by Unger[170] and he has suggested that the ratio of glucagon to insulin is an important determinant of glucose metabolism. Glucagon has only short-term effects on glycogen breakdown but has a more sustained stimulatory effect on gluconeogenesis.[5] After glucose ingestion glucagon levels fall and its effects are almost certainly overcome entirely by insulin plus glucose. Indeed, the importance of glucagon in glucoregulation when insulin is present has been severely questioned.[152]

Other hormones such as glucocorticoids are probably more important than glucagon in counteracting the effects of insulin on glucose disposal in the liver. In the presence of excess amounts of glucocorticoids glucose disposal is impaired, partly as a peripheral effect but also by a direct effect on the liver which is thought to be due to enhanced activity of the substrate cycle between glucose and glucose-6-phosphate[70] as well as to a direct stimulation of gluconeogenesis.[4]

As stated above, glucose diffuses rapidly into the liver and is then phosphorylated to glucose-6-phosphate with glucokinase. The majority of the glucose is stored as glycogen. Glycolysis, either from glucose or from glycogen, is relatively inactive in the liver and less than 10 per cent of glucose is disposed of via this route.[142] Glucose will also be disposed of via the hexose monophosphate shunt. Both this and the glycolytic pathways will direct glucose towards glycerol and fatty acid synthesis for subsequent release as very low-density lipoprotein (VLDL)-triglyceride.

After glucose ingestion changes in circulating concentrations of carbohydrate intermediates are found. These include a 50 per cent rise in blood lactate and pyruvate concentrations, which follows the rise in blood glucose concentration by 10 to 20 minutes.[146] The rise in lactate is not due to enhanced peripheral lactate production[71] and is unlikely to be due to enhanced hepatic glycolysis because of the relative inactivity of this pathway. It is most likely secondary to an insulin-induced inhibition of gluconeogenesis with a consequent decrease in hepatic uptake of gluconeogenic precursors. Blood citrate and 2-oxoglutarate concentrations also rise after oral glucose loading but the source and significance of these changes are unclear.

Most emphasis has been placed on the changes which occur after glucose feeding. Precise studies of hepatic carbohydrate metabolism after mixed feeding are more difficult to interpret. Obviously the hormonal milieu after a mixed meal is different from that following glucose alone, in that insulin secretion is likely to be enhanced while glucagon levels will tend to rise rather than fall. Surprisingly, however, using continuous in vivo glucose monitoring we have shown that blood glucose profiles were superimposable when 50 g glucose were taken alone or an equivalent amount of carbohydrate was taken in a mixed meal.[146] It is probably fair to assume that disposal of glucose will in principle be similar to that shown for pure glucose feeding.

Other hexoses

Quantitatively fructose forms an important caloric source in western society. There is little doubt that the majority of ingested fructose is taken up by and metabolized in the liver. It is phosphorylated rapidly to fructose-1-phosphate and subsequently enters the glycolytic/gluconeogenic pathway.[54] In normal liver approximately 70 per cent of a fructose load appears as lactate with the rest converted to glycogen. Fructose administration can also lead to a fall in hepatic ATP concentration and hyperuricaemia[173] but these changes are minor with oral ingestion of the normal dietary amounts of fructose.

Galactose and other rarer hexoses are also metabolized almost exclusively by the liver, being in the main converted to glucose or glycogen.

THE REGULATION OF HEPATIC CARBOHYDRATE METABOLISM IN PATIENTS WITH LIVER DISEASE

The Fasted State

Blood glucose

Despite the importance of the liver in glucose production fasting hypoglycaemia is surprisingly rare in liver disease.[136, 177] There are two possible reasons for this. Firstly, the liver has a large reserve capacity and it has been suggested that normal glucose homeostasis can be maintained with as little as 20 per cent of parenchymal cells functional. Secondly, the kidney is capable of gluconeogenesis and it is possible that this organ could take over a significant proportion of glucose production in chronic liver damage as it does in starvation. There is argument about this as Owen et al[114] showed little net renal glucose exchange after overnight or three-day fasts in cirrhotic subjects. These patients, however, had only mild cirrhosis.

Hypoglycaemia when it occurs is generally found in acute fulminant hepatic disease (Table 3.2). Hypoglycaemia has been reported in acute viral hepatitis[51, 90] although this has not been corroborated in our own studies (Table 3.3) where subjects were in a better nutritional state.[129] Hypoglycaemia has also been reported in association with toxic liver damage secondary to overdosage of agents such as chloroform and paracetamol. Ethanol-induced hypoglycaemia should be regarded as a separate case in that there is a specific biochemical reason for the hypoglycaemia and it occurs in normal as well as in diseased liver (see Chapter 32). Other causes of hepatogenous hypoglycaemia are shown in Table 3.2. It can be seen that most of these are acute disorders apart from rare instances of hypoglycaemia in cirrhosis and in association with primary hepatic carcinoma. In this latter case the mechanism may be similar to that found in other large tumours such as mesenchymal tumours.[84] In other cases of chronic liver disease there is often mild hyperglycaemia after an overnight fast[8] (Table 3.2) and even after a three-day fast Owen et al[114] were unable to provoke hypoglycaemia in their cirrhotic subjects.

The possible causes of hepatogenic hypoglycaemia include (a) impaired glycogen synthesis and breakdown and (b) impaired gluconeogenesis. It should be pointed out that these processes may be impaired in hepatic disease even without overt hypoglycaemia occurring provided that the disturbance is mild or that compensatory mechanisms have come into play. These latter could include increased renal gluconeogenesis (see above) and provision of alternative substrates such as fatty acids, the levels of which are often increased in liver disease.[102]

Glycogen metabolism

A primary defect in many forms of liver disease may be a defect in the capacity to store glycogen. Owen et al[114] with elegant catheterization studies showed that after an overnight fast only about one-third of glucose production was derived from glycogen in

Table 3.2. *Fasting Hypoglycaemia in Liver Disease.*[a]

Cause	Authors
Acute viral hepatitis	Felig et al[51]; Lindner[90]
Fulminant hepatitis	Samson et al[137]; Moore, O'Farrell & Heandon[101]
Primary hepatic carcinoma	Krönig & Bass[83]; McFadzean & Young[95]
Metastatic carcinoma	Keating & Wilder[78]
Cirrhosis	Samols & Holdsworth[136]
Cholangitis	Conn et al[30]; Marks & Rose[94]
Hepatic 'congestion'	Mellinkoff & Tumulty[100]; Block et al[16]
Hepatotoxins, general	
Chloroform	Stander[162]
Neoarsphenamine	Cross & Blackford[34]
Paracetamol	Record et al[130]
Phosphorus	McIntosh[96]
Hepatotoxins, specific	
Ethanol	See Chapter 32
Hypoglycin (ackee fruit)	Hassall & Reyle[59]

[a] Based on Samols and Holdsworth.[136]

Table 3.3. *Fasting Values for Metabolites in Liver Disease.*

Metabolite*	Cirrhosis		Hepatic coma	
	Patient	Control	Patient	Control
Glucose (mmol/l [mg/dl])	5.17±0.33 (93±6) 4.59±0.48 (83±9) 5.17±0.17 (93±3) 5.44±0.17 (98±3)	3.94±0.33 (71±6)[a] 4.58±0.48 (82±9)[b] 5.12±0.11 (92±2)[c] 5.44±0.39 (98±7)[d]	5.83±0.50 (105±9)	5.44±0.39 (98±7)[d]
Lactate (mmol/l)	0.97±0.12 1.02±0.08	0.68±0.05[c] 0.69±0.06	3.01 (1.03–15.4)‡	1.18±0.05[i]
Pyruvate (mmol/l)	0.092±0.008 0.124±0.040 0.112 (0.06–0.16)	0.071±0.005[c] 0.118±0.020[b] 0.089 (0.045–0.160)[f]	0.225 (0.120–0.350) 0.305±0.110 0.203 (0.053–0.643)‡	0.089 (0.045–0.160)[f] 0.120±0.010[j] 0.106±0.004[i]
2-Oxoglutarate (mmol/l)	0.011 (0.010–0.013) 0.009±0.002§ 0.021 (0.018–0.030)	0.010 (0.006–0.021)[g] 0.004±0.003[h] 0.012 (0.008–0.018)[f]	0.040 (0.020–0.086) 0.020±0.006	0.012 (0.008–0.018)[f] 0.010 (0.006–0.021)[g]
Glycerol (mmol/l)	0.116±0.011	0.058±0.012[c]		
Alanine (mmol/l)	0.307±0.026 0.33±0.02	0.309±0.024[c] 0.38±0.02[s]	1.036±0.444† 0.48±0.10	0.412 (0.273–0.565)[k] 0.38±0.02[s]

Table adapted from Johnston and Alberti.[72]
Values are the median and range: mean ± s.e. mean.
* Values for metabolites are given for whole blood except where otherwise stated.
† Values expressed as mmol/l plasma.
‡ Patients and controls had both received I.V. glucose; values are for arterial blood.
§ 38 patients with liver disease studied, 33 of whom had cirrhosis.

Metabolite*	Acute viral hepatitis		Untreated chronic active hepatitis		Paracetamol poisoning	
	Patient	Control	Patient	Control	Patient	Control
Glucose (mmol/l[mg/dl])	3.31±0.16 (60±3)†	4.26±0.06 (77±1)[l] 3.84±0.10 (69±2)[m] 4.61±0.39 (83±7)[n]	4.22±0.17 (76±3)	3.67±0.17 (66±3)[p]	2.60±0.20 (47±4)	3.80±0.10 (68±2)[r]
Lactate (mmol/l)	0.96±0.13	0.72±0.04[m]	0.76±0.11	0.74±0.05[p]	1.47±0.24	0.72±0.04[r]
Pyruvate (mmol/l)	0.116±0.016 0.078±0.009 0.091±0.026	0.120±0.010[j] 0.072±0.005[m] 0.073±0.016[o]	0.064±0.009	0.070±0.006[p]	0.137±0.026	0.072±0.005[r]
2-Oxoglutarate (mmol/l)	0.013±0.002 0.024±0.012	0.009±0.001[m] 0.013±0.002[o]	0.013±0.001	0.011±0.001[p]	0.015±0.002	0.009±0.001[r]
Glycerol (mmol/l)	0.087±0.014	0.074±0.005[m]	0.112±0.013	0.077±0.006[p]		
Alanine (mmol/l)	0.322±0.034†	0.343±0.021[l]	0.261±0.016	0.309±0.024[q]		

[a] Greco et al[57]
[b] Amatuzio et al[11]
[c] Johnston, Alberti and Wright[74]
[d] Sestoft and Rehfield[148]
[e] Klassen, Aronoff and Karpati[81]
[f] Summerskill, Wolfe and Davidson[167]
[g] Walshe[172]
[h] Dawson et al[36]
[i] Record et al[131]
[j] Amatuzio and Nesbitt[10]
[k] Wu, Bollman and Butt[175]
[l] Felig et al[51]
[m] Record et al[129]
[n] Nieschlag, Kremer and Mussgnug[109]
[o] Seligson, McCormick and Sborov[147]
[p] Alberti et al[8]
[q] Johnston, Alberti and Wright[73]
[r] Record et al[130]
[s] Rosen et al[133]

cirrhotic subjects while 70 to 80 per cent came from glycogen in normal subjects. The same conclusions can be drawn from studies where glucagon was administered. Thus Felig et al[51] showed a diminished glycaemic response to glucagon in viral hepatitis patients and Yeung and Wang[176] obtained the same results in patients with postnecrotic cirrhosis, as did de Moura and Cruz[38] in a group of cirrhotic patients of varied aetiology. In Yeung and Wang's series those subjects with the lowest glucose response had the most severe liver disease.[176] There is also suggestive evidence of impaired glycogen metabolism in patients with acute hepatic failure secondary to paracetamol poisoning.[130] Against these positive reports are the negative findings of Strange et al[165] and Van Itallie and Bentley[171] who could show no abnormality in the glucose response to glucagon in most patients with cirrhosis. These discrepancies may have been due to differing patient populations or to different nutritional states of the patients.

An impaired glucose response to glucagon could be explained in several ways. Thus there may indeed be decreased hepatic glycogen. This could be due either to parenchymal damage per se, or to chronically increased glycogenolysis. The latter is a real possibility as patients with liver disease have chronically elevated portal and peripheral glucagon levels with hyperresponsiveness to different physiological stimuli.[58, 153] Alternatively, there may be damage to glucagon receptors in liver disease. The report by Davies, Prudhoe and Douglas[35] of an increased plasma cyclic AMP response to glucagon infusion in patients with cirrhosis, and extrahepatic and intrahepatic cholestasis, is of interest. It suggests that glucagon receptors are fully functional in these states although the glucose response to glucagon was also normal in these patients. Davies and his colleagues also found that the cyclic AMP response was diminished in six of eight patients with portacaval shunts and that these patients had a somewhat lowered glucose response. This was also found by Sherwin et al[153] and their patients had the highest glucagon values. It is worth pointing out that Sherwin's cirrhotic patients with normal hepatic blood flow had an exaggerated glucose response to glucagon infusion. Shunting is, therefore, important as a possible mechanism for diminished delivery of appropriate stimuli to glycogen breakdown, and may result in an inaccurate picture of glycogen reserves.

Obviously, more direct studies of glycogenolysis and glycogenesis in man are required, particularly in view of the discrepant results obtained by different groups and the strikingly suggestive results of Owen et al referred to above.[114]

Gluconeogenesis

Gluconeogenesis in patients with liver disease has been examined in four ways: indirectly by measurement of circulating gluconeogenic precursor concentrations and by measuring clearance of exogenous loads of these precursors; and directly by measuring transhepatic substrate balances or by using radioactive turnover techniques.

Precursor concentrations. The main gluconeogenic precursors are lactate, pyruvate, alanine and glycerol. Table 3.3 shows blood concentrations of these substrates after an overnight fast in a broad spectrum of hepatic disorders. Lactate concentrations are moderately elevated in acute viral hepatitis,[129] cirrhosis,[2, 76, 167] and paracetamol poisoning[130] although values rarely exceed 2 mmol/l (18 mg/dl). In acute hepatic failure values may be higher.[131] Impaired hepatic clearance may be contributory but it should also be recognized that increased production may occur. This could be secondary to impaired pyruvate oxidation[126] due to the raised circulating fatty acid concentrations.[102] Pyruvate concentrations tend to parallel those of lactate.

Alanine concentrations are more variable. We could show no change in fasting whole blood concentrations in patients with cirrhosis, viral hepatitis or chronic active hepatitis, although Rosen et al[133] showed a small decrease in cirrhotic subjects. In acute hepatic necrosis[133] or fulminant hepatic failure[132, 175] alanine values were elevated, as were concentrations of the other glucogenic amino acids, glycine, glutamate and glutamine. The reason for the lack of abnormality of fasting alanine concentrations in all but the most severe forms of liver disease may be sought both in the peripheral tissues and in the liver. Systemic plasma insulin concentrations are raised in most forms of liver disease (See Chapter 7) and this will tend to drive alanine back into peripheral tissues, particularly muscle. Alternatively, glucagon levels are raised in liver disease and in normal man glucagon enhances hepatic alanine uptake,[20] although Felig et al[51] suggested that this mechanism was impaired in viral hepatitis.

Fasting concentrations of glycerol are also raised in approximately 50 per cent of patients with liver disease.[3] Enhanced adipose tissue lipolysis may of course contribute to this and the relative roles of liver and periphery have yet to be established.

Clearance studies. Interpretation of blood metabolite concentrations in terms of mechanisms and the role of individual tissues is difficult if not impossible. By infusing known amounts of precursors which are metabolized mainly in the liver more information can be gained, although it will reveal more about maximal metabolic capacity than subtle alterations in regulatory processes.

Impaired hepatic lactate clearance in cirrhotic subjects was first demonstrated more than 40 years ago.[24, 156] This has been elegantly reaffirmed recently by Connor et al.[31] The authors showed that, albeit in the fed state, lactate clearance was decreased from the normal of 0.018 ± 0.002 l/min/kg bodyweight to 0.014 ± 0.001 l/min/kg bodyweight in 35 patients with assorted liver diseases. Endogenous production rate of lactate was unaltered (1.59 ± 0.29 v. 1.58 ± 0.13 mol/70 kg/24 hr or 143 ± 26 v. 142 ± 12 mg/70 kg/24 hr).

Lactate has the disadvantage that it can be used by many different tissues, particularly if blood levels are increased. Many patients with liver disease have disturbances of other organs so that impaired clearance of lactate, although suggestive of hepatic impairment, cannot be taken as total proof. We have instead used glycerol which is particularly attractive as an experimental substrate in that more than 90 per cent is metabolized by the liver. It is non-ionic, therefore does not generate acid-base disturbances, and can be given safely in relatively high doses. Using a steady state infusion technique we have estimated metabolic clearance and disappearance rates in normal and stable cirrhotic subjects. Half-disappearance time was increased from 5.9 ± 0.4 minutes to 16.0 ± 2.3 minutes in the cirrhotics, while metabolic clearance rate was decreased from 0.039 to 0.024 l/min/kg. Disappearance could be divided into slow and fast components, and the major change occurred in the latter. We would suggest that the fast component, which represented 80 to 90 per cent of total clearance, was the hepatic component, and the data give clear evidence of impaired hepatic handling of a relatively large load of a gluconeogenic substrate.

In contrast to these clear-cut findings we were unable to show any alteration in alanine handling in cirrhotic subjects when using a continuous infusion protocol similar to that used for glycerol. This may have been due to the excessive glucagon response to alanine which is found in cirrhotic subjects[151] and which would tend to compensate any defect by stimulating hepatic alanine uptake.

Catheterization studies. All the results outlined so far give an indirect measure of hepatic gluconeogenetic capacity in liver disease. Direct measurement of hepatic gluconeogenic precursor uptake and glucose output is obviously preferable, but few data are available due to the technical problems involved and ethical considerations.

In early studies Myers[104] showed a 25 per cent decrease in hepatic glucose production in cirrhotic subjects after an overnight fast. He did not establish the relative impairment of glycogenolysis and gluconeogenesis. More recently Feruglio et al[53] have studied hepatosplanchnic glucose and lactate balances in normal and cirrhotic subjects. In the post-absorptive state there was no difference in glucose production between the two groups and similarly splanchnic lactate balances were not different (uptake of 26.9 ± 18 mg/min [0.30 ± 0.20 mol/min] in normals and 33.9 ± 47.2 mg/min [0.38 ± 0.52 mol/min] in cirrhotics). However, on infusion of 1.5 mg glucagon over 30 minutes (a pharmacological dose) there was a twofold greater output of glucose from the liver in the normal subjects. In addition, lactate uptake doubled in normals but was unaltered in the cirrhotic patients. Too much weight should not be placed on these results as there was considerable between- and within-patient variation.

The best executed study to date has been that of Owen et al.[114] They studied six cirrhotic subjects and it should be noted that these patients had only a mild degree of metabolic disturbance. Arterial lactate, pyruvate, glycerol, alanine and glucose concentrations were normal after an overnight fast. However, splanchnic glucose release was decreased by more than half. The contributions of the gluconeogenic precursors were normal, apart from a slightly elevated fractional extraction of glycerol, and the major defect was an 80 per cent decrease in the contribution of glycogenolysis. With further provocation in a three-day fast, there was a marked decrease in the contribution of alanine with a fractional extraction of only 14 per cent compared with 39 per cent in normal subjects. There is a striking similarity, as pointed out by Owen, between the results found in cirrhotics and those reported by Nilsson, Furst and Hultman[110] for subjects receiving a carbohydrate restricted diet, where liver glycogen content was decreased.

Providing that the nutritional status of the cirrhotic subjects was normal it can be concluded that in mild degrees of liver disease there is indeed decreased hepatic glucose production but this is due to impaired glycogenolysis, not decreased gluconeogenesis. It will be of major interest to study patients with more severe hepatic disease to establish how much damage is required before gluconeogenesis is also impaired.

Glucose turnover studies. In one of the few studies which have examined glucose turnover in cirrhotic subjects Perez et al[116] were unable to demonstrate any abnormality in glucose output, uptake or metabolic clearance rate. It should be noted that at the time of study both peripheral plasma glucagon and insulin concentrations were twice normal. After injection of insulin plasma glucose concentration showed a similar fall in both normal and cirrhotic subjects. There was, however, a marked decrease in both glucose production and glucose uptake in response to hypoglycaemia in the cirrhotics. Insulin levels were similar in both groups but the glucagon response was markedly enhanced in the cirrhotics. The latter has also been found in cirrhotic dogs when similar tracer techniques have been used.[124] The authors[124] suggest that the studies demonstrate both peripheral insulin resistance and hepatic glucagon insensitivity. Adlung et al,[1] using ^{14}C-glucose, have shown that glucose production starts when blood glucose concentration falls below 7 mmol/l (125 mg/dl) in normal subjects but only at 4.4 mmol/l (80 mg/dl) in patients with cirrhosis. This again could be due to hepatic insensitivity to glucagon, secondary perhaps to depleted glycogen stores.

Techniques such as these should be useful in the future. More studies are required, particularly in different forms of liver disease.

Animal studies. Animal models of liver disease have been used to determine more precisely the nature of the impairment in hepatic glucose production. Unfortunately there are major problems in relating animal models of alcoholic cirrhosis to the human condition. Studies have, however, been performed in rats with diet-produced cirrhosis.[63] When livers from such rats were isolated and perfused there was a decrease in gluconeogenesis from both lactate and alanine. This was associated with a lower oxygen consumption and lower Krebs cycle activity. Fatty acids also failed to stimulate gluconeogenesis in the usual way, perhaps because of limited pyruvate carboxylase activity.

Galactosamine hepatitis has proved useful as a model for acute hepatitis.[80] Using this model we have shown increased blood lactate concentrations as in human hepatitis.[127] Perfused liver experiments revealed impaired gluconeogenic capacity from lactate, and direct measurement showed a marked decrease in activity of the key gluconeogenic enzyme, phosphoenolpyruvate carboxykinase, as well as of alanine aminotransferase.[128] Impaired gluconeogenesis has also been reported after bile duct ligation in the rat.[86, 127] More work is required to validate these animal models as useful guides to human disease.

The Fed State

Normal feeding

Most studies of patients with liver diesease have concentrated on the fasted state or on provocative tests such as glucose tolerance tests. Relatively little is known of circulating glucose and metabolic intermediates under normal conditions.

In an attempt to rectify this we have measured circulating hormones and metabolites over a 12-hour period in patients with differing degrees of alcoholic liver disease.[72, 164] Reasonable nutritional state was ensured before testing. In normal subjects blood glucose concentration varied little through the 12 hours with increments of 1 to 2 mmol/l (18 to 36 mg/dl) after meals. These meal time responses were exaggerated (a rise of 4 to 5 mmol/l [72 to 90 mg/dl]) in patients with mild alcoholic liver disease while in subjects with severe cirrhosis glucose values rose from normal fasting levels to a mean of 11 mmol/l (198 mg/dl) with breakfast and remained there throughout the day. This hyperglycaemia was associated with marked fasting and postprandial peripheral hyperinsulinism (see Chapter 7), suggesting both insulin resistance and impaired degradation and/or increased secretion.

Diurnal patterns of gluconeogenic precursors were also distorted. Blood lactate concentrations showed exaggerated postprandial rises in mildly affected subjects. In patients with the more severe cirrhosis fasting levels were already raised (Table 3.3) and after breakfast rose to more than 2 mmol/l (36 mg/dl) and remained elevated for the rest of the day. Surprisingly, the extent of hyperlactataemia in these cirrhotic patients showed a close correlation with two unrelated aspects of liver function, the rise in serum bilirubin and the fall in serum albumin. Pyruvate changed in a similar way to lactate although the lactate/pyruvate ratio was mildly increased, suggesting perhaps an increased intrahepatic (free NADH/free NAD) ratio, although these ratios should be interpreted with caution.[22] The increase in lactate is mainly due to inhibition of hepatic lactate uptake in normal subjects (see above) with perhaps some contribution from hepatic fructose metabolism, derived from dietary sucrose. In the cirrhotic subjects, presumably, there is defective lactate clearance which will be exaggerated in the fed state. This point is of practical clinical importance in that lactic acidosis can be provoked relatively easily in patients with severe liver disease.

In contrast, diurnal levels of alanine were lowered in both mild and severe cirrhotic groups. This could be related to both the peripheral hyperinsulinism and to a selective increase in hepatic extraction secondary to the hyperglucagonaemia although the results of Felig et al (1970) make this hypothesis doubtful.[51]

Glucose loading

Glucose intolerance in liver disease has been recognized since the first description of so-called 'hepatogenous diabetes' by Naunyn.[106] It occurs commonly in cirrhosis,[9, 18, 25, 61, 65, 69, 77, 93, 99, 160] active chronic hepatitis,[8] acute viral hepatitis,[56, 79, 109, 129] obstructive liver disease,[157] and toxic hepatitis.[130] Many of these studies could be criticized in that patients were inadequately prepared in a nutritional sense. Adequate precautions were taken, however, in many other studies and the incidence of oral glucose intolerance of 50 to 100 per cent is impressive. One common finding is that more patients show intolerance to oral than to intravenous glucose.[32] This could be due partly to portasystemic shunting of glucose[37] although, as shown by Radziuk et al,[125] only 8 per cent of portal vein glucose is extracted at first pass. Thereafter all glucose, whether derived from the oral or the intravenous route, will reach the liver by the same routes. Alternatively, there could be defective gut hormone release.

Peripheral insulin levels have been measured in many of the above studies. Hyperinsulinaemia after glucose loading appears to be associated particularly with hepatic cirrhosis and acute severe liver damage, while hypoinsulinaemia appears to be more characteristic of chronic active hepatitis and prolonged-course hepatitis. This is discussed in detail in Chapter 7, as is the problem of distinguishing hepatogenous diabetes from maturity-onset diabetes.

Intermediary metabolite changes after glucose loading. Measurements of lactate and pyruvate have been made during glucose tolerance tests in several different diseases of the liver. In alcoholic liver disease the lactate response to intravenous glucose is increased,[76] although we found a diminished rise in patients with cryptogenic cirrhosis.[3] No consistent change was found in cases of viral hepatitis or paracetamol poisoning while a consistently lowered response was found in patients with chronic active hepatitis.[8] In this latter group there was a close correlation with the initial insulin response to glucose. Amatuzio et al[11] showed an increased pyruvate response to intravenous glucose in hepatic failure. The mechanism of these changes remains unclear, and it should be noted that overall there was no correlation between glucose tolerance and change in blood lactate concentration. Similarly there were no consistent changes in 2-oxoglutarate, glycerol or the lipid metabolites, non-esterified fatty acids (NEFA) and ketone bodies.

Mechanism of glucose intolerance in liver disease. This remains a largely unsolved problem. Some suggestions which have been put forward are shown in Table 3.4 (see also Samols and Holdsworth;[136] Felig and Sherwin[47]). There is always the problem of impaired nutritional status in any group of diseased subjects but this is unlikely to be important in many of the more careful studies. The possibility of potassium depletion as a cause of impaired insulin secretion and glucose intolerance in cirrhotic patients has also been raised.[28, 119] However, improved glucose tolerance on potassium repletion was not found in all patients, and in any case it is unlikely that all patients with liver disease are potassium depleted.

Impaired insulin secretion may contribute to glucose intolerance in some liver diseases such as chronic active hepatitis[8] although in most liver disorders hyperinsulinaemia rather than

Table 3.4. *Possible Causes of Glucose Intolerance in Hepatic Disease.*

General factors
Poor nutritional state
Potassium deficiency
Hepatic factors
Decreased parenchymal mass
Portasystemic shunting
Decreased glycogen synthetic capacity
Impaired insulin action, e.g. decreased insulin receptors
Increased glucagon secretion
Increased cortisol secretion
Increased growth hormone secretion
Haemosiderosis
Hypoinsulinaemia
Extrahepatic factors
Peripheral insulin resistance
Increased NEFA levels
Circulating antagonists
Increased cortisol secretion

hypoinsulinaemia is the rule. It should be noted that this is systemic hyperinsulinism and actual secretion may be normal or even depressed (see Chapter 7), although in general the liver will be receiving normal amounts of insulin. It is therefore difficult to implicate defective insulin secretion as the primary cause of the glucose intolerance seen in so many cases of liver disease.

The other suggested mechanisms of the intolerance can be divided into those involving primarily the liver, and those affecting peripheral tissues (Table 3.4). Of the hepatic factors a decrease in parenchymal mass was the first major suggestion although this was disabused nearly 40 years ago.[115] The second major suggestion was that portasystemic shunting dumped portal vein glucose directly into the peripheral circulation.[37] If one accepts the view of Radziuk et al[125] that the liver would have extracted only 8 per cent of this glucose on first pass then this hypothesis carries little credibility. Portasystemic shunting alone probably alters glucose tolerance little,[155] but portasystemic shunting associated with or due to liver parenchymal damage may be more important. Obviously, if hepatic architecture is distorted in such a way that glucose and hormones cannot reach the appropriate cells, then glucose uptake will be impaired. It is difficult to interpret many of the earlier studies of the effects of portasystemic shunting in that severe parenchymal damage was generally present before the shunt operation took place and the careful studies of Holdsworth and his colleagues[66, 67] showed impaired glucose tolerance preoperatively which did not change after the operation, despite a further increase in peripheral insulin levels (see also Megyesi, Samols and Marks[99]). In contrast to this are the findings of Lickley et al[89] in conscious normal dogs. They have shown that although portal delivery of glucose is not particularly important there is none the less some gut factor which must be delivered via the portal system to achieve normal glucose tolerance.

Impaired ability to store and synthesize glycogen has been described above and this must remain a major candidate for the 'intolerance' factor. This could be related to either increased glucagon or decreased insulin sensitivity due perhaps to destruction of or damage to insulin receptors. Certainly insensitivity of plasma glucose concentration to exogenous insulin infusions is well established in cirrhosis.[26, 33] What is not known is whether this insensitivity is primarily hepatic or peripheral.

Anti-insulin hormones could also contribute to glucose intolerance by driving gluconeogenesis and/or glycogenolysis. Glucagon has already been referred to. Glucocorticoids are potential but doubtful candidates. Thus, although glucocorticoid catabolism may be impaired circulating concentrations are rarely raised[3] (see also Chapter 7). Growth hormone could be more important. High levels have been reported by several authors,[12, 64] and there is often an inappropriate rise following glucose in cirrhotic subjects.[3, 29] However, there is little relation between growth hormone levels and the degree of disturbance of carbohydrate metabolism.[93]

Extrahepatic mechanisms have also been suggested as a cause for glucose intolerance. The insulin resistance referred to above has been suggested as being primarily extrahepatic in origin. Few systematic studies have been made of this. Hed et al[60] showed diminished forearm glucose uptake after a glucose load in alcoholic subjects which improved on withdrawal of alcohol. Insulin concentrations remained the same on both occasions. In a similar study in patients with cryptogenic cirrhosis we found glucose intolerance in the patients but the same forearm glucose uptake as in control subjects.[85] In the cirrhotics, however, peripheral insulin and glucose concentrations were higher. The results can be construed as indicating either impaired insulin action or the possibility that peripheral glucose uptake mechanisms were already saturated at the lower insulin and glucose levels found in the control subjects. This interesting problem awaits further elucidation.

The final putative causes of the glucose intolerance are the presence of circulating antagonists or the lack of a 'glucose tolerance factor' supposedly synthesized by the liver.[145] Dzúriková et al[44] have reported the partial purification of a substance from cirrhotic blood which inhibits glucose utilization. The finding remains to be confirmed. The commonest suggestion, however, has been that NEFA inhibit peripheral glucose oxidation in liver disease. Again, the validity of this hypothesis is doubtful. Certainly plasma fatty acid levels may be raised in patients with liver disease,[102] but as Descos and his colleagues, amongst many others, have pointed out there is little relation between the NEFA levels and the degree of carbohydrate intolerance.[39]

It can be seen that there is no single simple answer to the question: 'what causes glucose intolerance in liver disease?' The cause probably varies between different liver diseases and may indeed be multifactorial. The most likely of the many possibilities seems to be a diminished ability of the damaged liver to retain glycogen, but the mechanism remains to be established.

Other carbohydrates

Less work has been done with other carbohydrates than with glucose, although it has been known for many years that galactose, for example, is cleared less readily in liver disease.[149] It is rational to consider that measurement of specific hexoses such as galactose could be used as tests of liver function in that these are metabolized primarily in the liver. However, there has been only sporadic interest, due no doubt to a combination of problems in measurement of these hexoses and the need for exogenous administration (see Chapter 17). Recently Nakamura et al[105] have reported the use of D-galactose-1-^{14}C in the assessment of degree of intrahepatic shunting while Tygstrup and Lundquist[169] have used galactose measurements in their investigations of the effect of ethanol on hepatic metabolism. Tengström[168] has published a thoughtful account of the use of the IV galactose tolerance test compared with other liver function tests, and it has no clear advantage over the more common tests. Royle et al[134] have now suggested the use of an intravenous galactose test as a measure of hepatic glucose output, but the clinical application of this has not yet been established.

More attention has been paid to fructose than galactose because of its potentially injurious effects. Approximately 70 per cent of fructose is converted rapidly to lactate in the liver. Normally this lactate would be metabolized rapidly but this does not occur with severe parenchymal damage. The amounts of fructose ingested normally as sucrose may contribute to the hyperlactataemia that we have noted in cirrhosis[164] but are probably not harmful. Problems arise when fructose is given intravenously as part of an intravenous feeding regimen. In this situation we have reported fatal lactic acidosis in patients with acute hepatic failure given fructose,[173] a problem which has been well reviewed by Cohen and Woods.[23] Sorbitol is also potentially hazardous as it follows the same metabolic route as fructose. One interesting point is that fructose causes hepatic adenine nucleotide depletion.[92] This could well compromise hepatic regeneration after and during damage in that ATP and total adenine nucleotide levels are already low in the regenerating liver, at least in the experimental situation.[75]

There has also been some interest in the metabolism of xylose and xylulose in patients with liver disease, less from a pathophysiological viewpoint than in their use as liver function tests. The conversion of D-xylose to threitol, which normally occurs in liver and kidney, is diminished in patients with cirrhosis[118] but not to an extent sufficient to cause abnormal results in the oral D-xylose tolerance test. Similarly there is diminished metabolism of xylulose after IV loading and fasting levels are raised in cirrhotic subjects.[111]

It is not surprising that metabolism of many non-glucose hexoses and pentoses is disturbed in hepatic disease. Specific information is still required, however, on the exact nature of the lesions and the effect of different hepatic diseases on these processes. The metabolism of ethanol itself in liver disease is dealt with elsewhere in this volume (see Chapter 32).

Biopsy Studies

Most of the work described above has been performed indirectly through studies in blood and urine. There is a paucity of direct information on the metabolism of liver in human liver disease due to obvious technical and ethical problems. As stated above more information is available using animal models but the absolute relevance of this remains to be proven. Some biopsy studies have been published. It should be remembered, however, that if the disease process is not uniformly distributed through the liver there could be gross errors due to sampling problems. Thus a biopsy may contain a disproportionate amount of fat or fibrous tissue as pointed out by Schmidt and Schmidt.[143] Kupffer cells may also show markedly different changes from biliary tract or parenchymal cells, as elegantly shown by Wootton, Neale and Moss.[174] Thus after experimental bile duct ligation 5′-nucleotidase activity increased in parenchymal cells but fell in Kupffer cells.

Schersten[139] has summarized many of the differences in metabolic activity between liver from patients with hepatitis and those with cholestasis. Amongst the earliest studies was that of Schmidt, Schmidt and Wildhirt[144] who showed decreased activity of alpha-glycerophosphate dehydrogenase, aldolase and glutamate dehydrogenase together with an increase in glucose-6-phosphate dehydrogenase in patients with viral hepatitis. This suggests increased pentose phosphate shunt activity. At the same time there may be decreased transport of NADH equivalents into the mitochondria because of the decreased alpha-glycerophosphate dehydrogenase activity. This would tend to increase intrahepatic lactate levels and may explain the accumulation of lactate in blood in such patients. Liver mitochondria from hepatitis patients may also be abnormal. Both a low oxygen uptake and uncoupled oxidative phosphorylation have been found.[141] Gross disturbances of endoplasmic reticular function have also been described in hepatitis[139] but these have less relevance to carbohydrate metabolism.

In biopsies from patients with cholestatic jaundice there is similar evidence of decreased oxygen uptake by isolated mitochondria.[140, 141] This may be due to a direct effect of bile acids and/or bilirubin.[87, 121]

The problems of uneven biopsy in patients with hepatic cirrhosis are more severe. Diaz Gil et al[40] found that cirrhotic livers appear to contain fewer mitochondria, however, and these authors also found decreased mitochondrial respiratory control together with a marked fall in the levels of cytochrome-b_5 and cytochrome P-450. Others have reported more variable changes in cytochrome-b_5 but a distinct fall in the level of cytochrome-aa_3 with a decreased $aa_3/c+c_1$ ratio.[138] These data are consistent with a change in respiratory control and may explain the earlier finding of Benga and Muresan[13] that cirrhotic livers had reduced ATP synthesizing ability. Sato et al[138] also studied biopsies from patients with hepatoma, where similar but more pronounced changes were found, and from patients with chronic hepatitis where the changes were extremely variable.

A considerable amount of work has been done on the effects of acute and chronic ethanol intake on hepatic cell function. Thus Rubin and Lieber[135] demonstrated directly the induction of a microsomal enzyme system by ethanol. These studies are not immediately relevant to carbohydrate metabolism and are described in Chapter 32.

The work reported to date has been somewhat disappointing, mainly due to technical problems. Studies of substrate levels, as well as of enzyme activities, will be of interest and may be aided by the application of newer techniques such as isotachophoresis.

CONCLUSIONS

It can be seen from the above that a great deal of factual information has now been obtained on carbohydrate metabolism in patients with liver disease. Abnormalities have been described in fasting glucose and gluconeogenic precursor concentrations. Glucose intolerance is abnormal in the majority of cases although there are still occasional difficulties in distinguishing liver disease associated with glucose intolerance from liver disease in patients who also have maturity onset diabetes. Aberrations in circulating concentrations of lactate and other carbohydrate moieties are also found during glucose tolerance tests and in the fed state. Information on mechanisms as well as direct studies of metabolism in the diseased liver remain sparse.

Emphasis in the future should be placed on turnover and catheterization techniques together with biopsy studies, particularly in conditions other than hepatic cirrhosis.

Finally, it might be reasonable to suggest a world-wide embargo on glucose tolerance tests in patients with alcoholic cirrhosis. This would undoubtedly save much time and work, would not cause any significant loss of knowledge, and might indeed stimulate workers to have new thoughts and approaches.

REFERENCES

1. Adlung, J., Kelch, L., Peters, J. & Grazikowske, H. (1977) Leberglukosebildung und Insulinresistenz bei der Leberzirrhose. Untersuchungen mit ^{14}C-glukose. *Zeitschrift für Gastroenterologie*, **15**, 553–564.
2. Alberti, K.G.M.M. (1972) Gluconeogenesis in liver disease. *Connecticut Medicine*, **36**, 568–571.
3. Alberti, K.G.M.M. (1974) In *Some Metabolic Aspects of Liver Disease* (Ed.) Truelove, S.C. & Trowell, J. pp. 341–359. Oxford: Blackwell.
4. Alberti, K.G.M.M. & Johnston, D.G. (1977) Cortisol: a new perspective. *Clinical Science and Molecular Medicine*, **52**, 333–336.
5. Alberti, K.G.M.M. & Nattrass, M. (1977) The physiological functions of glucagon. *European Journal of Clinical Investigation*, **7**, 151–154.
6. Alberti, K.G.M.M., Dornhorst, A. & Rowe, A.S. (1975) Metabolic rhythms in normal and diabetic man. *Israeli Journal of Medical Science*, **11**, 571–580.
7. Alberti, K.G.M.M., Johnston, D.G. & Sutton, G. (1979) Some aspects of carbohydrate metabolism in liver disease. In *Diabetes, Hyperlipidaemia and Obesity* (Ed.) Crepaldi, G., Lefebvre, P.J. & Alberti, K.G.M.M. In press.
8. Alberti, K.G.M.M., Record, C.O., Williamson, D.H. & Wright, R. (1972) Metabolic changes in active chronic hepatitis. *Clinical Science*, **42**, 591–605.
9. Althausen, T.L., Gunther, L., Lagen, J.B. & Kerr, W.J. (1930) Modification of dextrose tolerance test as index of metabolic activity of liver. *Archives of Internal Medicine*, **46**, 482–493.
10. Amatuzio, D.S. & Nesbitt, S. (1950) A study of pyruvic acid in the blood and spinal fluid of patients with liver disease with and without hepatic coma. *Journal of Clinical Investigation*, **29**, 1486–1490.
11. Amatuzio, D.S., Schrifter, N., Stutzman, F.L. & Nesbitt, S. (1952) Blood pyruvic acid response to intravenous glucose or insulin in the normal and in patients with liver disease and with diabetes mellitus. *Journal of Clinical Investigation*, **31**, 751–755.
12. Becker, M.D., Cook, G.C. & Wright, A.D. (1969) Paradoxical elevation of growth hormone in active chronic hepatitis. *Lancet*, **ii**, 1035–1039.
13. Benga, G. & Muresan, L. (1974) Human liver mitochondria. III. ATPase activity as an index of mitochondrial damage. *Medicine*, **10**, 131–139.
14. Bergman, R.N. (1977) Integrated control of hepatic glucose metabolism. *Federation Proceedings*, **36**, 265–270.
15. Bernard, C. (1876) Critique expérimentale sur la glycémie. Des conditions physiologiques à remplir pour constater la présence du sucre dans le sang. *Comptes Rendus Hebdomadaires des Séances de l'Académie des Sciences* (*Paris*), **82**, 1405–1410.
16. Block, M.B., Gambetta, M., Resnekov, L. & Rubinstein, A.H. (1972) Spontaneous hypoglycaemia in congestive heart failure. *Lancet*, **ii**, 736–738.
17. Cahill, G.F. & Owen, O.E. (1968) Some observations on carbohydrate metabolism in man. In *Carbohydrate Metabolism and its Disorders* (Ed.) Dickens, F., Randle, P.J. & Whelan, W.J. pp. 497–522. London and New York: Academic Press.
18. Campbell, J.A. & Tagnon, H.J. (1946) Intravenous glucose tolerance test in liver disease. *New England Journal of Medicine*, **234**, 216–221.
19. Camu, F. (1975) Hepatic balances of glucose and insulin in response to physiological increments of endogenous insulin during glucose infusions in dogs. *European Journal of Clinical Investigation*, **5**, 101–108.
20. Chiasson, J.L., Liljenquist, J.E., Sinclair-Smith, B.C. & Lacy, W.W. (1975) Gluconeogenesis from alanine in normal postabsorptive man. Intrahepatic stimulatory effect of glucagon. *Diabetes*, **24**, 574–584.
21. Chiasson, J.L., Liljenquist, J.E., Finger, F.E. & Lacy, W.W. (1976) Differential sensitivity of glycogenolysis and gluconeogenesis to insulin infusions in dogs. *Diabetes*, **25**, 283–291.
22. Cohen, R.D. (1976) Disorder of lactic acid metabolism. *Clinics in Endocrinology and Metabolism*, **5**, 613–625.
23. Cohen, R.D. & Woods, H.F. (1976) *Clinical and Metabolic Aspects of Lactic Acidosis*. Oxford: Blackwell Scientific Publications.
24. Cohn, C. (1942) Sodium D-lactate tolerance as test of hepatic function. *Archives of Internal Medicine*, **70**, 829–835.
25. Coller, F.A. & Troost, F.L. (1929) Glucose tolerance and hepatic damage. *Annals of Surgery*, **90**, 781–793.
26. Collins, J.R., Lacy, W.W., Stiel, J.N. & Crofford, O.B. (1970) Glucose intolerance and insulin resistance in patients with liver disease. II. A study of etiological factors and evaluation of insulin actions. *Archives of Internal Medicine*, **126**, 608–614.
27. Combes, B., Adams, R.H., Strickland, W. & Madison, L.L. (1961) The physiological significance of the secretion of endogenous insulin into the portal circulation. IV. Hepatic uptake of glucose during glucose infusion in non-diabetic dogs. *Journal of Clinical Investigation*, **40**, 1706–1718.
28. Conn, H.O. (1970) Cirrhosis and diabetes. IV. Effect of potassium chloride administration on glucose and insulin metabolism. *American Journal of Medical Science*, **259**, 394–404.
29. Conn, H.O. & Daughaday, W.H. (1970) Cirrhosis and diabetes. V. Serum growth hormone levels in Laennec's cirrhosis. *Journal of Laboratory and Clinical Medicine*, **76**, 678–688.
30. Conn, J.W., Newburgh, L.H., Johnston, M.W. & Sheldon, J.M. (1938) Study of deranged carbohydrate metabolism in chronic infectious hepatitis. *Archives of Internal Medicine*, **62**, 765–782.
31. Connor, H., Woods, H.F., Murray, J.D. & Ledingham, J.G.G. (1978) The kinetics of elimination of a sodium L-lactate load in man: the effect of liver disease. *Clinical Science and Molecular Medicine*, **54**, 33–34.
32. Creutzfeldt, W., Frerichs, H. & Sickinger, K. (1970) Liver diseases and diabetes mellitus. In *Progress in Liver Diseases* (Ed.) Popper, H. & Schaffner, F. Vol. 3, pp. 371–407. London: Heinemann.
33. Creutzfeldt, W., Wille, K. & Kaup, H. (1962) Intravenöse belastung mit glucose, insulin und tolbutamid bei gesunden, diabetikern, leberzirrhotikern und insulom trägern. *Deutsche Medizinische Wochenschrift*, **87**, 2189–2195.
34. Cross, J.B. & Blackford, L.M. (1930) Fatal hepatogenic hypoglycemia following neoarsphenamine. *Journal of the American Medical Association*, **94**, 1739–1742.
35. Davies, T.F., Prudhoe, K. & Douglas, A.P. (1976) Plasma cyclic adenosine-3′, 5′-monophosphate response to glucagon in patients with liver disease.

British Medical Journal, **i**, 931–933.

36. Dawson, A.M., Rosenthal, W.S., deGroote, J. & Sherlock, S. (1957) Blood pyruvic acid and alpha-ketoglutaric-acid levels in liver disease and hepatic coma. *Lancet*, **i**, 392–396.
37. Débry, G. & Charles, J. (1965) Étude des perturbations due métabolisme des glucides chez les sujets atteints de cirrhose hépatique. *Diabète*, **13**, 151–168.
38. de Moura, M.C. & Cruz, A.G. (1968) Carbohydrate metabolism studies in cirrhosis of the liver. *American Journal of Digestive Diseases*, **13**, 891–906.
39. Descos, L., M'Bendi, S., Sassolas, G., Audigier, J.-C., Sidiqian, N., Faure, A. & Bizollon, C.-A. (1974) Dosage de l'insuline et de l'hormone de croissance plasmatiques au cours de l'épreuve d'hyperglycémie provoquée par voie orale dans la cirrhose alcoolique. *Archives Française des Maladies de L'Appareil Digestif*, **63**, 17–24.
40. Diaz Gil, J., Rossi, I., Escartin, P., Segovia, J.M. & Gosalvez, M. (1977) Mitochondrial functions and content of microsomal and mitochondrial cytochromes in human cirrhosis. *Clinical Science and Molecular Medicine*, **52**, 599–606.
41. Dietze, G., Wicklmayr, M., Hepp, K.D., Bogner, W., Mehnert, H., Czempiel, H. & Henftling, H.G. (1976) On gluconeogenesis of human liver. Accelerated hepatic glucose formation induced by increased precursor supply. *Diabetologia*, **12**, 555–561.
42. Dunn, A., Chenoweth, M. & Bever, K. (1977) Use of ^{3}H and ^{14}C doubly labeled glucose and amino acids in the study of hormonal regulation of gluconeogenesis in rats. *Federation Proceedings*, **36**, 245–252.
43. Dupre, J., Ross, S.A., Watson, D. & Brown, J.C. (1973) Stimulation of insulin secretion by gastric inhibitory polypeptide in man. *Journal of Clinical Endocrinology and Metabolism*, **37**, 826–828.
44. Dzúriková, V., Černáček, P., Niederland, T.R. & Dzúrik, R. (1974) Isolation of an inhibitor responsible for abnormal glucose utilisation in liver disease. *Acta Diabetologica Latina*, **11**, 277–282.
45. Felig, P. (1973) The glucose–alanine cycle. *Metabolism*, **22**, 179–207.
46. Felig, P. (1976) The liver in glucose homeostasis in normal man and in diabetes. In *Diabetes, its Physiological and Biochemical Basis* (Ed.) Vallance-Owen, J. pp. 93–123. Lancaster: MIP Press.
47. Felig, P. & Sherwin, R. (1976) Carbohydrate homeostasis, liver and diabetes. In *Progress in Liver Diseases* (Ed.) Popper, H. & Schaffner, F. Vol. 5, pp. 149–171. New York: Grune & Stratton.
48. Felig, P. & Wahren, J. (1971) Influence of endogenous insulin secretion on splanchnic glucose and amino acid balance in man. *Journal of Clinical Investigation*, **50**, 1702–1711.
49. Felig, P., Wahren, J. & Hendler, R. (1975) Influence of oral glucose ingestion on splanchnic glucose and gluconeogenic substrate metabolism in man. *Diabetes*, **24**, 468–475.
50. Felig, P., Wahren, J. & Räf, L. (1973) Evidence of inter-organ amino-acid transport by blood cells in humans. *Proceedings of the National Academy of Sciences of the United States of America*, **70**, 1775–1779.
51. Felig, P., Brown, W.V., Levine, R.A. & Klatskin, G. (1970) Glucose homeostasis in viral hepatitis. *New England Journal of Medicine*, **283**, 1436–1440.
52. Felig, P., Pozefsky, T., Marliss, E. & Cahill, G.F. (1970) Alanine: key role in gluconeogenesis. *Science*, **167**, 1003–1004.
53. Feruglio, F.S., Greco, F., Cesano, L., Colongo, P.G., Sardi, G. & Chiandussi, L. (1966) The effects of glucagon on systemic and hepatosplanchnic haemodynamics and on net peripheral and hepatosplanchnic balance of glucose, lactic and pyruvic acids in normal subjects and cirrhotics. *Clinical Science*, **30**, 43–50.
54. Froesch, R. (1976) Disorders of fructose metabolism. *Clinics in Endocrinology and Metabolism*, **5**, 599–611.
55. Garber, A.J., Karl, I.E. & Kipnis, D.M. (1976) Alanine and glutamine synthesis and release from skeletal muscle. *Journal of Biological Chemistry*, **251**, 836–843.
56. Gioannini, I.P. & Scalise, G. (1971) Glucose tolerance in viral hepatitis. *Acta Diabetica Latina*, **8**, 932–948.
57. Greco, A.V., Fedeli, G., Ghirlanda, G., Manna, R. & Patrono, C. (1974) Behaviour of pancreatic glucagon, insulin and HGH in liver cirrhosis, after arginine and I.V. glucose. *Acta Diabetologica Latina*, **11**, 330–339.
58. Greco, A.V., Crucitti, F., Ghirlanda, G., Manna, R., Altomonte, L., Rebuzzi, A. & Bertoli, A. (1978) Insulin and glucagon concentrations in portal and peripheral veins in patients with hepatic cirrhosis. *Diabetologia*. In press.
59. Hassall, C.H. & Reyle, K. (1955) Hypoglycin A and B, two biologically active peptides from Blighia sapida. *Biochemical Journal*, **60**, 334.
60. Hed, G., Lindblad, L.E., Nygren, A. & Sundblad, L. (1977) Forearm glucose uptake during glucose tolerance tests in chronic alcoholics. *Scandinavian Journal of Clinical and Laboratory Investigation*, **37**, 229–233.
61. Hed, R. (1958) Clinical studies in chronic alcoholism. II. Carbohydrate metabolism in chronic alcoholism with particular reference to glucose and insulin tolerances. *Acta Medica Scandinavica*, **162**, 195–202.
62. Hems, D.A. (1977) Short-term hormonal control of hepatic carbohydrate and lipid metabolism. *FEBS Letters*, **80**, 237–245.
63. Henley, K.S., Laughrey, E.G. & Clancy, P.E. (1974) Gluconeogenesis in the fatty and cirrhotic liver of the rat. The effect of oleate and ethanol. In *Regulation of Hepatic Metabolism* (Ed.) Lundquist, F. & Tygstrup, N. pp. 401–413. Copenhagen: Munksgaard.
64. Hernandez, A., Zorilla, E. & Gershberg, H. (1969) Decreased insulin production, elevated growth hormone levels, and glucose intolerance in liver disease. *Journal of Laboratory and Clinical Medicine*, **73**, 25–33.
65. Hillemand, B., Joly, J.-P., Brunelle, P., Legueult, L. & Huet, P. (1974) Étude comparative des taux de glucose et d'insuline dans le sang veineux péripherique et le liquide d'ascite du cirrhotique éthylique, au cours de l'hyperglycémie provoquée orale. *Annales de Médecine Interne*, **125**, 395–402.
66. Holdsworth, C.D. (1969) The gut and oral glucose tolerance. *Gut*, **10**, 422–427.
67. Holdsworth, C.D., Nyc, L. & King, E. (1972) The effect of portacaval anastomosis on oral glucose tolerance and on plasma insulin levels. *Gut*, **13**, 58–63.
68. Hultman, E. & Nilsson, L.H. (1971) Liver glycogen in man. Effect of different diets and muscular exercise. *Advances in Experimental Medicine and Biology*, **11**, 143.
69. Ishii, H., Mamori, H., Takahashi, H., Muraoka, M., Arai, M., Shigeta, Y., Saito, H. & Tsuchiya, M.

(1975) Klinsche untersuchungen zur pathogenese des hepatogenenen diabetes. *Leber Magen Darm*, **5**, 52–57.

70. Issekutz, B. (1977) Studies on hepatic glucose cycles in normal and methyl prednisolone-treated dogs. *Metabolism*, **26**, 157–170.
71. Jackson, R.A., Advani, U., Perry, G., Rogers, J., Peters, N., Day, S. & Pilkington, T.R.E. (1973) Forearm glucose uptake during the oral glucose tolerance test in normal subjects. *Diabetes*, **22**, 442–458.
72. Johnston, D.G. & Alberti, K.G.M.M. (1976) Carbohydrate metabolism in liver disease. *Clinics in Endocrinology and Metabolism*, **5**, 675–702.
73. Johnston, D.G., Alberti, K.G.M.M. & Wright, R. (1976) Unpublished observations.
74. Johnston, D.G., Alberti, K.G.M.M. & Wright, R. (1979) Metabolic response to oral glucose in hepatic cirrhosis. In preparation.
75. Johnston, D.G., Johnson, G.A. & Alberti, K.G.M.M. (1978) Hepatotrophic factors: implications for diabetes mellitus. In *Hepatotrophic Factors*. Ciba Symposium 55, pp. 357–373. Amsterdam: Elsevier.
76. Johnston, D.G., Hinks, L., Smythe, P., Wright, R. & Alberti, K.G.M.M. (1976) Metabolic effects of oral glucose loading in hepatic cirrhosis. *Clinical Science and Molecular Medicine*, **51**, p. 18.
77. Kato, K., Kikuchi, S., Ito, M., Hidano, S., Oya, T., Banno, H., Tomura, A., Koyama, T., Komatsu, T., Takei, T., Tomimura, K. & Yamauchi, M. (1973) Clinical investigation on glucose tolerance in liver cirrhosis. *Nagoya Journal of Medical Science*, **35**, 91–101.
78. Keating, F.R. & Wilder, J.M. (1941) Spontaneous hypoglycemia: report of cases. *Southern Medical Surgery*, **103**, 125–131.
79. Kelly, M., Walsh, H., Doyle, C., O'Sullivan, D.S., O'Regan, S. & Whelton, H. (1972) Glucose homeostasis in viral hepatitis. *Digestion*, **6**, 286.
80. Keppler, D., Lesch, R., Reutter, W. & Decker, K. (1968) Experimental hepatitis induced by D-galactosamine. *Experimental and Molecular Pathology*, **9**, 279–290.
81. Klassen, G.A., Aronoff, A. & Karpati, G. (1969) Forearm metabolism in patients with chronic liver disease. *Clinical Science*, **37**, 455–470.
82. Kreisberg, R.A. (1972) Glucose–lactate interrelations in man. *New England Journal of Medicine*, **287**, 132–137.
83. Krönig, B. & Bass, E.U. (1973) Paraneoplastische hypoglykämie bei leberzellkarzinom. *Deutsche Medizinische Wochenschrift*, **98**, 322–325.
84. Laurent, J., Debry, G. & Floquet, J. (1971) *Hypoglycaemic tumours*. Amsterdam: Excerpta Medica.
85. Leatherdale, B.A., Record, C.O., Chase, R.A., Rogers, J., Alberti, K.G.M.M. & Davies, P. (1979). In preparation.
86. Lee, E., Ross, B.D. & Haines, J.R. (1972) The effect of experimental bile duct obstruction on critical biosynthetic functions of the liver. *British Journal of Surgery*, **59**, 564–568.
87. Lee, M.J. & Whitehouse, M.W. (1965) Inhibition of electron transport and coupled phosphorylation in liver mitochondria by cholanic (bile) acids and their conjugates. *Biochimica et Biophysica Acta*, **100**, 317–328.
88. Levenson, S.M. (1977) Starvation. In *Nutritional Aspects of Care of the Critically Ill* (Ed.) Richards, J.R. & Kinney, J.M. pp. 3–94. Edinburgh: Churchill Livingstone.
89. Lickley, H.L.A., Chisholm, D.J., Rabinowitch, A., Wexler, M. & Dupre, J. (1975) Effects of portacaval anastomosis on glucose tolerance in the dog: evidence of an interaction between the gut and the liver in oral glucose disposal. *Metabolism*, **24**, 1157–1168.
90. Lindner, W. (1975) Hypoglykämie-Aglykämie bei virushepatitis. *Münchener Medizinische Wochenschrift*, **117**, 855–860.
91. Lundholm, K. & Schersten, T. (1976) Gluconeogenesis in human liver tissue. An in vitro method for evaluation of gluconeogenesis in man. *Scandinavian Journal of Clinical and Laboratory Investigation*, **36**, 339–346.
92. Maenpaa, P.H., Raivio, K.O. & Kekomaki, M.P. (1968) Liver adenine nucleotides: fructose-induced depletion and its effect on protein synthesis. *Science*, **161**, 1253–1254.
93. Maranon, A., Duran, S., Sanjose, G. & Romero, E. (1974) Tolerancia a la glucosa, insulin secrecion, nivelles de acidos grasos libres y de hormona de crecimiento en la cirrosis hepatico. *Revista Clinica Espanola*, **132**, 299–306.
94. Marks, V. & Rose, C.F. (1965) *Hypoglycaemia*. pp. 166–172. Oxford: Blackwell.
95. McFadzean, A.J.S. & Young, T.T. (1956) Hypoglycaemia in primary carcinoma of the liver. *Archives of Internal Medicine*, **98**, 720–731.
96. McIntosh, R. (1927) Acute phosphorus poisoning. Report of a case with recovery. *American Journal of Diseases of Children*, **34**, 595–602.
97. McIntyre, N., Holdsworth, C.D. & Turner, D.S. (1964) New interpretation of oral glucose tolerance. *Lancet*, **ii**, 20–21.
98. McIntyre, N., Turner, D.S. & Holdsworth, C.D. (1970) The role of the portal circulation in glucose and fructose tolerance. *Diabetologia*, **6**, 593–596.
99. Megyesi, C., Samols, E. & Marks, V. (1967) Glucose tolerance and diabetes in chronic liver disease. *Lancet*, **ii**, 1051–1056.
100. Mellinkoff, S.M. & Tumulty, P.A. (1952) Hepatic hypoglycemia. Its occurrence in congestive heart failure. *New England Journal of Medicine*, **247**, 745–750.
101. Moore, H., O'Farrell, W.R. & Heandon, M.F. (1934) Spontaneous hypoglycaemia associated with hepatitis. *British Medical Journal*, **i**, 225–226.
102. Mortiaux, A. & Dawson, A.M. (1961) Plasma free fatty acid in liver disease. *Gut*, **2**, 204–209.
103. Mosora, F., Lefebvre, P., Pirnay, F., Lacroix, M., Luyckx, A. & Duchesne, J. (1976) Quantitative evaluation of the oxidation of exogenous glucose load using naturally labeled C-glucose. *Metabolism*, **25**, 1575–1582.
104. Myers, J.D. (1950) Net splanchnic glucose production in normal man and in various disease states. *Journal of Clinical Investigation*, **29**, 1421–1429.
105. Nakamura, S., Sasaki, K., Takezawa, Y., Yoshida, G. & Sato, T. (1974) Physiological measurement of intrahepatic shunted blood flow by method of continuous infusion of D-galactose-1-C^{14}. *Angiology*, **25**, 484–489.
106. Naunyn, B. (1906) Der diabetes Mellitus. In *Nothnagels Handbuch* (Ed.) Holder, A. Vol. 7.2. Vienna.
107. Newsholme, E.A. (1976) Role of the liver in integration of fat and carbohydrate metabolism and clinical implications in patients with liver disease. In *Progress in Liver Diseases* (Ed.) Popper, H. &

Schaffner, F. Vol. 5, pp. 125–135. New York: Grune & Stratton.

108. Newsholme, E.A. (1976) Carbohydrate metabolism in vivo: regulation of the blood glucose level. *Clinics in Endocrinology and Metabolism*, **5**, 543–578.
109. Nieschlag, E., Kremer, G.J. & Mussgnug, U. (1970) Insulin, Glucosetoleranz und freie Fettsauren wahrend und nach akuter Hepatitis. *Klinische Wochenschrift*, **48**, 381–383.
110 Nilsson, L.H., Furst, P. & Hultman, E. (1973) Carbohydrate metabolism of the liver in normal man under varying dietary conditions. *Scandinavian Journal of Clinical and Laboratory Investigation*, **32**, 331–337.
111. Oka, H., Suzuki, S., Suzuki, H. & Oda, T. (1976) Increased urinary excretion of L-xylulose in patients with liver cirrhosis. *Clinica Chimica Acta*, **67**, 131–136.
112. Owen, O.E., Morgan, A.P., Kemp, H.G., Sullivan, J.N., Herrera, M.G. & Cahill, G.F. (1967) Brain metabolism during fasting. *Journal of Clinical Investigation*, **46**, 1589–1595.
113. Owen, O.E., Felig, P., Morgan, A.P., Wahren, J. & Cahill, G.F. (1969) Liver and kidney metabolism during prolonged fasting. *Journal of Clinical Investigation*, **48**, 574–583.
114. Owen, O.E., Patel, M.S., Block, B.S.B., Kreulen, T.H., Reichle, F.A. & Mozzoli, M.A. (1976) Gluconeogenesis in normal, cirrhotic and diabetic humans. In *Gluconeogenesis: its Regulation in Mammalian Species* (Ed.) Hanson, R.W. & Mehlman, M.A. pp. 533–558. New York: Wiley.
115. Pachmann, D.J. (1940) Oral and intravenous dextrose tolerance tests in cases of acute (catarrhal) hepatitis. *American Journal of Diseases of Children*, **60**, 1277–1288.
116. Perez, G., Trimarco, B., Ungaro, B., Rengo, F. & Sacca, L. (1978) Glucoregulatory response to insulin-induced hypoglycemia in Laennec's cirrhosis. *Journal of Clinical Endocrinology and Metabolism*, **46**, 778–783.
117. Perley, M.J. & Kipnis, D.M. (1967) Plasma insulin responses to oral and intravenous glucose: studies in normal and diabetic subjects. *Journal of Clinical Investigation*, **46**, 1954–1962.
118. Pitkänen, H. (1977) The conversion of D-xylose into D-theitol in patients without liver disease and in patients with portal liver cirrhosis. *Clinica Chimica Acta*, **80**, 49–54.
119. Podolsky, S., Zimmerman, H.J., Burrows, B.A., Cardarelli, J.A. & Pattavina, C.G. (1973) Potassium depletion in hepatic cirrhosis. *New England Journal of Medicine*, **288**, 644–648.
120. Pozefsky, T., Tancredi, R.G., Moxley, R.T., Dupre, J. & Tobin, J.D. (1976) Effects of brief starvation on muscle amino acid metabolism in non obese man. *Journal of Clinical Investigation*, **57**, 444–449.
121. Pressman, B.C. & Lardy, H.A. (1956) Effect of surface active agents on the latent ATPase of mitochondria. *Biochimica et Biophysica Acta*, **100**, 317–328.
122. Rabinowitch, I.M. (1929) Biochemical finding in a rare case of acute yellow atrophy of the liver with particular reference to the origin of urea in the body. *Journal of Biological Chemistry*, **83**, 333–335.
123. Radziuk, J. & Vranic, M. (1977) Estimating rapid changes in the rates of glucose production from glycogenolysis and recycling through lactate. *Federation Proceedings*, **36**, 236–238.
124. Radziuk, J., Dupre, J., McDonald, T.J., Levy, M. & Wexler, M. (1977) Decreased sensitivity of glucose turnover in hepatic cirrhosis in dogs. *Clinical Research*, **25**, 397.
125. Radziuk, J., McDonald, T.J., Rubenstein, D. & Dupre, J. (1978) Initial splanchnic extraction of ingested glucose in normal man. *Metabolism*, **27**, 657–669.
126. Randle, P.J., Garland, P.B., Hales, C.N. & Newsholme, E.A. (1963) The glucose and fatty acid cycle. Its role in insulin sensitivity and the metabolic disturbance of diabetes mellitus. *Lancet*, **ii**, 785–789.
127. Record, C.O. & Alberti, K.G.M.M. (1973) Glucose tolerance and blood metabolite changes in galactosamine hepatitis and obstructive jaundice in the rat. *European Journal of Clinical Investigation*, **3**, 130–135.
128. Record, C.O., Alberti, K.G.M.M. & Williamson, D.H. (1972) Metabolic studies in experimental liver disease resulting from D(+)-galactosamine administration. *Biochemical Journal*, **130**, 37–44.
129. Record, C.O., Alberti, K.G.M.M., Williamson, D.H. & Wright, R. (1973) Glucose tolerance and metabolic changes in human viral hepatitis. *Clinical Science and Molecular Medicine*, **45**, 677–690.
130. Record, C.O., Chase, R.A., Alberti, K.G.M.M. & Williams, R. (1975) Disturbances in glucose metabolism in patients with liver damage due to paracetamol overdose. *Clinical Science and Molecular Medicine*, **49**, 473–479.
131. Record, C.O., Iles, R.A., Cohen, R.D. & Williams, R. (1975) Acid-base and metabolic disturbances in fulminant hepatic failure. *Gut*, **16**, 144–149.
132. Record, C.O., Buxton, B., Chase, R.A., Curzon, G., Murray-Lyon, I.M. & Williams, R. (1976) Plasma and brain amino acids in fulminant hepatic failure and their relationship to hepatic encephalopathy. *European Journal of Clinical Investigation*, **6**, 387–394.
133. Rosen, H.M., Yoshimura, N., Hodgman, J.M., Fischer, J.E. (1977) Plasma amino acid patterns in hepatic encephalopathy of differing etiology. *Gastroenterology*, **72**, 483–487.
134. Royle, G., Kettlewell, M.G.W., Ilic, V. & Williamson, D.H. (1978) The metabolic response to galactose as a measure of hepatic glucose release in man. *Clinical Science and Molecular Medicine*, **54**, 107–109.
135. Rubin, E. & Lieber, C.S. (1968) Hepatic microsomal enzymes in man and rat. Induction and inhibition by ethanol. *Science*, **162**, 690–691.
136. Samols, E. & Holdsworth, D. (1968) Disturbances in carbohydrate metabolism: liver disease. In *Carbohydrate Metabolism and its Disorders* (Ed.) Dickens, F., Randle, P.J. & Whelan, W.J. Vol. 2, pp. 289–336. London: Academic Press.
137. Samson, R.I., Trey, C., Timme, A.H. & Saunders, S.J. (1967) Fulminating hepatitis with recurrent hypoglycemia and hemorrhage. *Gastroenterology*, **53**, 291–300.
138. Sato, N., Kamada, T., Abe, H., Suematsu, T., Kawano, S., Hayashi, N., Matsumura, T. & Hagihara, B. (1977) Simultaneous measurement of mitochondrial and microsomal cytochrome levels in human liver biopsy. *Clinica Chimica Acta*, **80**, 243–251.
139. Schersten, T. (1972) Metabolic differences between hepatitis and cholestasis in human liver. In *Progress in Liver Diseases* (Ed.) Popper, H. & Schaffner, F. Vol. 4, pp. 133–150. New York: Grune & Stratton.
140. Schersten, T., Bjorkerud, S., Jakoi, L. & Bjorntorp, P. (1966) Oxidation and phosphorylation reactions in isolated liver mitochondria in normal and icteric

conditions. *Scandinavian Journal of Gastroenterology*, **1**, 284–291.

141. Schersten, T., Bjorntorp, P., Bjorkerud, S., Smeds, S. & Ekholm, R. (1970) Liver cell function in infectious hepatitis in man. *Acta Hepato-Splenologica*, **17**, 375–392.
142. Schimassek, H., Walli, A.K., Langhans, W. & Mayer, P. (1974) Glycolysis and gluconeogenesis in the rat liver. In *Regulation of Hepatic Metabolism* (Ed.) Lundquist, F. & Tygstrup, N. pp. 92–104. Copenhagen: Munksgaard.
143. Schmidt, E. & Schmidt, F.W. (1962–1963) Die Auswirkungen verschiedener Extraktions-Arten auf Enzym-Aktivitats-Bestimmungen in Lebergewebe. *Enzymologia Biologica et Clinica*, **2**, 223–232.
144. Schmidt, E., Schmidt, F.W. & Wildhirt, E. (1958) Aktivitats-bestimmungen von enzymen des engergieliefeinden stoffwechsels in der menschlichen leber bei der akuten hepatitis und ihren ausheilungs zustanden. *Klinische Wochenschrift*, **36**, 227–233.
145. Schwarz, K. & Mertz, W. (1957) A glucose tolerance factor and its differentiation from factor 3. *Archives of Biochemistry and Biophysics*, **72**, 515–518.
146. Selam, J.-L., Noy, G. & Alberti, K.G.M.M. (1978) Unpublished observations.
147. Seligson, D., McCormick, G.J. & Sborov, V. (1952) Blood ketoglutarate and pyruvate in liver disease. *Journal of Clinical Investigation*, **31**, 661 (abstract).
148. Sestoft, L. & Rehfield, J.F. (1970) Insulin and glucose metabolism in liver cirrhosis and in liver failure. *Scandinavian Journal of Gastroenterology* (Suppl.), **7**, 133–136.
149. Shay, H., Schloss, E.M. & Bell, M.A. (1931) Metabolism of galactose; considerations underlying use of galactose in tests of function of liver. *Archives of Internal Medicine*, **47**, 391–402.
150. Sherwin, R.S., Hendler, R.G. & Felig, P. (1975) Effect of ketone infusions on amino acid and nitrogen metabolism in man. *Journal of Clinical Investigation*, **55**, 1382–1390.
151. Sherwin, R.S., Joshi, P., Hendler, R., Felig, P. & Conn, H.O. (1974) Hyperglucagonaemia in Laennec's cirrhosis, the role of portal–systemic shunting. *New England Journal of Medicine*, **290**, 239–242.
152. Sherwin, R.S., Fisher, M., Hendler, R. & Felig, P. (1976) Hyperglucagonaemia and blood glucose regulation in normal, obese and diabetic subjects. *New England Journal of Medicine*, **294**, 455–461.
153. Sherwin, R.S., Fisher, M., Bessoff, J., Snyder, N., Hendler, R., Conn, H.O. & Felig, P. (1978) Hyperglucagonaemia in cirrhosis: altered secretion and sensitivity to glucagon. *Gastroenterology*, **74**, 1224–1228.
154. Shoemaker, W.C., Yanof, H.M., Turk, L.N. & Wilson, T.H. (1963) Glucose and fructose absorption in the unanesthetized dog. *Gastroenterology*, **44**, 654–663.
155. Smith-Laing, G. (1978) Personal communication.
156. Soffer, L.J., Dantes, D.A., Newburger, R. & Sobotka, J. (1937) Metabolism of sodium D-lactate by patients with acute diffuse parenchymal injury of liver. *Archives of Internal Medicine*, **60**, 822–886.
157. Soler, N.G., Exon, P.D. & Paton, A. (1974) Carbohydrate tolerance and insulin responses in obstructive jaundice. *British Medical Journal*, **iv**, 447–451.
158. Söling, H.-D. & Kleineke, J. (1976) Species dependent regulation of hepatic gluconeogenesis in higher animals. In *Gluconeogenesis: its Regulation in Mammalian Species* (Ed.) Hanson, R.W. & Mehlman, M.A. pp. 369–462. New York: Wiley.
159. Soskin, S. & Levine, R. (1946) *Carbohydrate Metabolism*. Chicago: University of Chicago Press.
160. Soskin, S. & Mirsky, I.A. (1935) Influence of progressive toxemic liver damage upon dextrose tolerance curve. *American Journal of Physiology*, **112**, 649–656.
161. Stalmans, W. (1976) The role of the liver in the homeostasis of blood glucose. *Current Topics in Cellular Regulation*, **11**, 51–97.
162. Stander, H.J. (1924) A chemical study of a case of chloroform poisoning. *Johns Hopkins Medical Bulletin*, **35**, 46–49.
163. Steele, R., Bjerknes, C., Rathgeb, I. & Altzuler, N. (1968) Glucose uptake and production during the oral glucose tolerance test. *Diabetes*, **17**, 415–421.
164. Stewart, A., Alberti, K.G.M.M., Lloyd, B., Johnston, D.G., Nattrass, M. & Wright, R. (1979) Metabolic rhythms in alcoholic liver disease. In preparation.
165. Strange, R.C., Mjøs, O.D., Hendon, T. & Jynge, P. (1977) The effect of glucagon on plasma cyclic AMP and glucose concentrations in patients with alcoholic cirrhosis. *Acta Medica Scandinavica*, **202**, 87–88.
166. Sugden, M.C., Sharples, C. & Randle, P.J. (1976) Carcass glycogen as a potential source of glucose during short-term starvation. *Biochemical Journal*, **160**, 817–819.
167. Summerskill, W.H.J., Wolfe, S.J. & Davidson, C.S. (1957) The metabolism of ammonia and aketo-acids in liver disease and hepatic coma. *Journal of Clinical Investigation*, **36**, 361–372.
168. Tengström, B. (1966) An intravenous galactose tolerance test with an enzymatic determination of galactose. A comparison with other diagnostic aids in hepatobiliary disease. *Scandinavian Journal of Clinical and Laboratory Investigation*, **18** (Suppl. 92), 132–142.
169. Tygstrup, N. & Lundquist, F. (1962) The effect of ethanol on galactose elimination in man. *Journal of Laboratory and Clinical Medicine*, **59**, 637–644.
170. Unger, R.H. (1971) Glucagon and the insulin:glucagon ratio in diabetes and other catabolic illnesses. *Diabetes*, **20**, 834–838.
171. Van Itallie, T.B. & Bentley, W.B.A. (1955) Glucagon-induced hyperglycemia as an index of liver function. *Journal of Clinical Investigation*, **34**, 1730–1737.
172. Walshe, J.M. (1955) Glutamic acid in hepatic coma. *Lancet*, **i**, 1235–1239.
173. Woods, H.F. & Alberti, K.G.M.M. (1972) Dangers of intravenous fructose. *Lancet*, **ii**, 1354–1357.
174. Wootton, A.M., Neale, G. & Moss, D.W. (1977) Enzyme activities of cells of different types isolated from livers of normal and cholestatic rats. *Clinical Science and Molecular Medicine*, **52**, 585–590.
175. Wu, C., Bollman, J.L. & Butt, H.R. (1955) Changes in free amino acids in the plasma during hepatic coma. *Journal of Clinical Investigation*, **34**, 845–849.
176. Yeung, R.T.T. & Wang, C.C.L. (1974) A study of carbohydrate metabolism in postnecrotic cirrhosis of liver. *Gut*, **15**, 907–912.
177. Zimmerman, H.J., Thomas, L.J. & Scherr, E.H. (1953) Fasting blood sugar in hepatic disease with reference to infrequency of hypoglycemia. *Archives of Internal Medicine*, **91**, 577–584.

Chapter 4

Plasma Lipoproteins and the Liver

RICHARD C. DAY
DAVID S. HARRY
NEIL McINTYRE

The major lipids carried in plasma are cholesterol and cholesteryl esters, phospholipids and triglycerides. Cholesterol is present in all mammalian plasma membranes and is a precursor of bile acids and steroid hormones. Apart from the hydroxyl group at C_3 and the double bond between C_5 and C_6 it is a fully saturated non-polar hydrocarbon, chemically unreactive and insoluble in water. It is thus admirably suited to its role as a structural component of membranes. The cholesterol of membranes and of bile is free sterol but in plasma and in tissues such as liver, adrenal and skin, cholesteryl esters are also present; in these the 3β-OH group of cholesterol is esterified with the carboxyl group of a long chain fatty acid. Cholesteryl esters are even less soluble in water than free cholesterol.

There are many types of phospholipid. They all contain one or more phosphoric acid groups and all except phosphatidic acid have another polar group; this may be a nitrogenous base such as choline, ethanolamine or sphingosine, an amino acid, serine, or the polyalcohol inositol. In the glycerophosphatides one or more long chain fatty acids are attached to a glycerol backbone. The phospholipids are major constituents of membranes and take part in many important biochemical reactions. The most abundant phospholipid in plasma and in most membranes is lecithin or phosphatidylcholine.

In the triglycerides fatty acids are esterified with the three hydroxyl groups of glycerol. A variety of different fatty acids are found in naturally occurring triglycerides which store energy and transport it from the gut and liver to other tissues.

LIPOPROTEINS

The water-insoluble lipids are present in plasma in lipid–protein complexes called lipoproteins.[88] In 1945 Blix and his colleagues identified two major groups of lipoproteins. One migrated in an electrical field with alpha-1 globulins and the other with beta globulins. Subsequently, with paper electrophoresis a lipoprotein with pre-beta mobility was discovered.

Lipoproteins have average hydrated densities of between 0.93 and 1.16 g/ml while those of other serum proteins range between 1.27 and 1.37 g/ml.[130] Lipoprotein sub-groups can be separated in the ultracentrifuge and on this basis the normal beta-lipoproteins are also known as low-density lipoproteins (LDL), alpha-lipoproteins as high-density lipoproteins (HDL) and the pre-beta fraction as very low-density lipoproteins (VLDL). A fourth class of lipoproteins, the chylomicrons, float readily in plasma without centrifugation and remain at the origin on paper or agarose electrophoresis. They are not normally found in fasting plasma but are large enough to be recognized by dark ground microscopy in postprandial plasma; they were first identified by Gage in 1920.[58]

The physicochemical characteristics of lipoproteins depend on their lipid and protein composition (Tables 4.1 and 4.2). LDL have been subdivided into LDL_1 (intermediate-density lipoprotein, IDL; S_f 12 to 20, density 1.006 to 1.019) and the major component LDL_2 (S_f 0 to 12, density 1.019 to 1.063): LDL_1 contains more triglyceride, and less cholesterol and protein than LDL_2. There are also two HDL: HDL_2 ($S_{f1.21}$ 3.6 to 9, density 1.063 to 1.125) and HDL_3 ($S_{f1.21}$ 0 to 3.5, density 1.125 to 1.21); HDL_2 is the larger of the two and is richer in lipid.

The lipoproteins normally found in plasma seem to be spherical on electron microscopy, with a surface appearance suggesting subunits, but this interpretation is still hypothetical. They appear to have an inner electron-deficient core consisting of triglyceride and cholesteryl ester and an electron-dense coat of protein, phospholipid and free cholesterol.

Apoproteins

The protein components of lipoproteins are called apoproteins and several groups have been identified. They are now classified alphabetically[5] but were originally classified according to their C-terminal amino acids.[136] All lipoprotein fractions, with the possible exception of LDL_2, contain more than one type of apoprotein (Table 4.3).

Apo B, the apoprotein of LDL_2, is difficult to study because it is insoluble in water; estimates of its molecular weight have ranged from 8000 to 275 000. In about 90 per cent of normal subjects the LDL_2 fraction contains small amounts of another lipoprotein Lp(a). This has a distinct apoprotein, apo Lp(a),[6,15] which differs from apo B only in its content of carbohydrate.[41] Its presence seems to be determined genetically. Its physiological significance is unknown but a strong association with ischaemic heart disease is claimed, particularly in young people.[36]

There are at least three different types of apo C (C-I, C-II and C-III) and they are the major apoproteins of VLDL and chylomicrons. Apo

Table 4.1. *Physical Characteristics of Major Lipoprotein Classes.*

Lipoprotein	S_f[a]	Solvent density of isolation (g/ml)	Mobility[b]	Molecular wt	Diameter[c] (nm)
Chylomicrons	>400	<0.95	origin	4×10^8	75–100
VLDL	20–400	<1.006	pre-β	$5–10 \times 10^6$	25–80
LDL	0–20	1.006–1.063	β	$2–4 \times 10^6$	20–25
HDL	–	1.063–1.21	α	$2–4 \times 10^5$	5–10

[a] S_f = lipoprotein flotation rate in Svedberg units in a sodium chloride solution of density 1.063 g/ml (26°C).
[b] Electrophoretic mobility on paper, agarose or starch gel.
[c] As determined by electron microscopy.

Table 4.2. *Composition (% by Weight) of the Major Classes of Human Serum Lipoprotein and Concentration in Normal Fasting Plasma.*

	Chylomicrons	VLDL	LDL	HDL
Protein	1–2	8–10	21–23	48–54
Triglyceride	80–90	50–55	8–10	3–4
Cholesterol (unesterified)	1–2	7–10	8–9	2–5
Cholesteryl ester	2–5	10–14	36–38	14–18
Phospholipid	5–7	15–20	21–23	25–30
Concentration of whole lipoprotein mg/dl fasting plasma	None	20–400	200–400	150–420 males 250–600 females

Table 4.3. *Apo Lipoproteins of Human Plasma Lipoproteins.*

Apoprotein	Lipoprotein	C-terminal	N-terminal	Molecular wt	Carbohydrate (% wt)
A-I	HDL	Glutamine	Aspartic acid	28 000	0
A-II	HDL	Glutamine	Proline	17 000[a]	0
B	LDL, VLDL	?	Glutamic acid	unknown	3–4
C-I	VLDL, HDL	Serine	Threonine	7000	0
C-II	VLDL, HDL	Glutamic acid	Threonine	10 000	0
C-III	VLDL, HDL	Alanine	Serine	8764	2–3
D(A-III)	HDL	Serine	–	20 000	0
Apo E (arginine rich)	VLDL, HDL	? Alanine	? Lysine	? 33 000	0

[a] Dimeric form.

C-I is an activator of lecithin cholesterol acyltransferase (LCAT). Apo C-II is necessary for the activation of extrahepatic lipoprotein lipase.[76,84] Apo C-III has strong phospholipid binding properties and seems to be an inhibitor of lipoprotein lipase. Apo C-III contains 3 per cent of carbohydrate by weight and has three polymorphic forms, apo C-III-0, apo C-III-1 and apo C-III-2, which contain 0, 1 and 2 mol of sialic acid per mol of protein respectively.[22]

The major HDL proteins are apo A-I and apo A-II; both have a C-terminal glutamine residue. Apo A-I is the chief activator of LCAT. The function of apo A-II is not clear. It consists of two identical polypeptide chains and seems to be a more avid binder of lipid than apo A-I.

There are several other apoproteins in plasma. Apo E (arginine-rich apoprotein) is present in VLDL and HDL and has several polymorphic forms. Its biological significance is unknown. Apo D (apo A-III or thin line peptide) is a minor constituent of HDL. Its function is not known but it has been implicated in the activation of LCAT.[44]

Synthesis and Secretion of Lipoproteins

Most studies of lipoprotein synthesis and secretion have been done in the rat and other experimental animals, but the mechanisms are probably similar in the human.[154]

Only the intestine and liver appear to synthesize and secrete plasma lipoproteins. Chylomicrons are made in the mucosal cells of the small intestine but only during dietary fat absorption. VLDL are produced in the liver and intestine. HDL are made in the liver; there is evidence that they may also come from the intestine.[161] LDL is produced mainly, perhaps entirely in man, within the plasma as a result of the catabolism of VLDL (see below).

Studies on the subcellular aspects of synthesis and secretion have been confined largely to VLDL and chylomicrons. Apoproteins are synthesized on the ribosomes and linked to lipid in the smooth endoplasmic reticulum where the enzymes for lipogenesis are found. Particles which look like VLDL and chylomicrons can be seen in vesicles of the smooth endoplasmic reticulum. They are transferred to the Golgi organelles, where carbohydrate is attached to them by the enzyme glycoprotein glycosyl transferase,[86] and then accumulate in secretory vesicles derived from the Golgi; these migrate to the lateral cell membrane and fuse with the lateral plasmalemma. In the small intestine particles are discharged into the intercellular space and in the liver into the space of Disse.[127]

The secretory vesicles have a protuberance of thickened membrane, the 'coated pit', which first makes contact with the cell membrane. The secretory vesicle membrane fuses with the membrane but the coated pit retains its identity. Movement of the secretory vesicle appears to be guided by the microtubular system. Colchicine disrupts the microtubular system without interfering with lipoprotein synthesis[143] and lipoproteins remain in the secretory vesicles until the microtubules have re-formed. It is of interest that fibroblasts have coated pits on their cell membranes which apparently contain receptors for LDL.[8] In this situation, however, the coated pits are involved in the endocytosis of LDL rather than exocytosis of newly formed lipoprotein (see below).

The VLDL found in the Golgi organelles of rat liver and intestine have a similar composition to circulating VLDL but contain less apo C and more phospholipid.[91,71] When they are incubated with plasma or HDL their composition becomes closer to that of circulating VLDL which suggests transfer of protein and lipid between VLDL and HDL (see below).

A lipoprotein with alpha mobility has been isolated from the Golgi apparatus of rat liver and it reacts with immunological identity to the major apoprotein of HDL.[91] The composition of HDL before secretion is unknown but 'nascent' HDL, isolated from the perfusate of an isolated rat liver system, are markedly different from circulating HDL.[71] Nascent HDL are small discs, 20 nm in diameter and 4 nm thick, which are made up of a single lipid bilayer. They are composed almost exclusively of polar lipids and protein and are particularly rich in apo E.[48] These discs assume the composition and spherical shape of 'normal' HDL when incubated with plasma containing LCAT.[65]

We have some understanding of the factors controlling the production of chylomicrons and VLDL. Chylomicron production depends on the amount of dietary fat presented for absorption. Individual particles also tend to be larger with large fat loads, presumably to reduce the amount of surface material (especially apoproteins) which mucosal cells have to synthesize. The size of intestinal VLDL particles may vary with the types of fatty acid absorbed. VLDL production by the liver is increased when the liver is presented with a large energy load, either as preformed fatty acids or as carbohydrates which are converted to fatty acids and then incorporated into triglycerides.

There is no evidence that chylomicron and VLDL production is regulated through the production of apoproteins. If, however, apoprotein synthesis is inhibited the synthesis and secretion of lipoproteins may be impaired. This can be demonstrated experimentally[43] and in the rare inherited disorder abetalipoproteinaemia. In the latter condition there is failure of synthesis of apo B; neither chylomicrons nor VLDL are synthesized, and the enterocytes of the small intestine become engorged with fat droplets.

Little is known about the factors regulating the production of HDL. HDL levels are higher in premenopausal women than in men and are increased by oestrogens and reduced by androgens. They are decreased with high carbohydrate diets but increased by alcohol.[77] Tangier disease is a familial disorder characterized by deficiency of HDL, and plasma levels in homozygotes are less than 5 per cent of normal.[53] Apo-II is the only apoprotein found in this HDL. Apo A-I is present in plasma in small amounts but it is confined to the fraction of density > 1.2 g/l. Morphologically, Tangier HDL consists of large spherical particles, stacked discs and small (5 to 7 nm) spherical particles. Only the small spherical particles migrate with alpha mobility on electrophoresis and their gross chemical composition is similar to normal HDL.[9]

We stated earlier that LDL are produced in plasma as a consequence of the intravascular catabolism of VLDL but some believe that LDL can be made by the liver. Data suggesting that this occurs in homozygous familial hypercholesterolaemia have been put forward by Soutar et al.[140] However, LDL-like particles have not been seen in the Golgi apparatus and they are not released by the isolated perfused rat liver. Recently, Nakaya and colleagues[99] reported that the pig liver can remove LDL from the plasma and return it to the circulation together with newly synthesized LDL. Whether this is true of other species is unknown.

The Metabolism of Plasma Lipoproteins

Two types of enzyme play key roles in the metabolism of plasma lipoproteins: the lipoprotein lipases (EC 3.1.1.3) and lecithin cholesterol acyltransferase or LCAT (EC 2.3.1.43).

LCAT is synthesized by the liver and probably by the gut.[32] It is secreted into plasma where it catalyses the transfer of a long chain fatty acid from the β-position of lecithin to the 3β-hydroxyl position of free cholesterol; cholesteryl ester and lysolecithin are produced. The reaction appears to take place on the surface of HDL particles and it is activated by apo A-I, apo C-I and possibly by apo E.

Lipoprotein lipases are bound to the capillary wall of various tissues by a heparin-like substance which also acts as an activator.[80] These enzymes are barely detectable in normal human plasma but they are released into the circulation following the intravenous injection of heparin and can be measured as post-heparin lipolytic activity (PHLA). At least two lipases are responsible for PHLA, one of hepatic origin (hepatic triglyceride lipase, HTGL) and peripheral lipoprotein lipase (LPL) found in adipose tissue, muscle and other tissues. Both have a molecular weight of approximately 65 000.[42] LPL requires apo C-II as cofactor for maximal activity and is inhibited by protamine sulphate and a high salt concentration.[42, 85] HTGL does not require a cofactor, is insensitive to protamine sulphate and shows maximal activity at sodium chloride concentrations between 0.5 and 1.0 mol/l.

The activity of LPL is influenced by a number

of hormones. It is increased by insulin and decreased by hormones such as glucagon, ACTH and TSH which are increased during fasting.[124]

Chylomicrons have a half-life of about 15 minutes. Their triglyceride is hydrolysed by LPL and remnant particles rich in cholesteryl ester, phospholipid and protein remain in plasma.[121] These are rapidly cleared by the liver and it seems likely that HTGL is involved in remnant removal.

VLDL triglyceride is also hydrolysed by LPL but it has a half-life of several hours. As VLDL is catabolized the core of triglyceride becomes depleted. Apo C subunits from the surface are transferred to HDL together with free cholesterol and phospholipid.[44] Partially degraded VLDL are found in the circulation as the short-lived intermediate-density lipoprotein (IDL). Compared with VLDL, IDL is rich in cholesteryl ester, but it still contains 20 to 30 per cent of the triglyceride present in the original VLDL; its main apoprotein is apo B. IDL particles interact again with LPL and possibly HTGL, becoming smaller in size as they lose triglyceride and excess surface coat; apo B remains. Eventually LDL is formed which has only one apoprotein in its surface coat, apo B, and a core rich in cholesteryl esters.

The source of this cholesteryl ester is not certain; available evidence suggests that some comes from HDL following the action of LCAT on free cholesterol and lecithin picked up either from plasma membranes or from the surface coat of VLDL. Apolar cholesteryl esters enter the disc like 'nascent' HDL, so producing spherical HDL particles with a core rich in cholesteryl esters. Once HDL has its complement of cholesteryl ester it is likely that further action of LCAT results in a transfer of cholesteryl ester to IDL (perhaps in exchange for polar lipids and apo C) and this process eventually leads to the formation of LDL.

The fate of LDL and HDL is ill understood. Certain peripheral tissues such as skin fibroblasts have receptors for LDL. These receptors, found in coated pits on the cells, bind LDL and take it into the cell where it is catabolized by lysosomal enzymes.[67,68] The evidence for LDL uptake by peripheral tissues is strong but it is not certain that it can account fully for LDL turnover in vivo. LDL might also be removed by the liver; its cholesteryl ester could be used for the synthesis of bile acids and this would reduce the demand for hepatic cholesterol biosynthesis. However, the rate of disappearance of plasma LDL is increased in the pig following hepatectomy[139] and this casts doubt on the role of hepatic removal.

Data on the metabolic fate of HDL are scarce. Experiments with ^{125}I-HDL in the human suggests that apo A-I and apo A-II are metabolized together.[19] Furman et al[57] reported a direct relationship between plasma triglyceride levels and the rate of decay of ^{125}I-HDL but the reason for this relationship is not known. However, it does suggest that increased VLDL concentrations may be linked to an increased catabolism of HDL.

THE EFFECT OF LIVER DISEASE ON PLASMA LIPIDS AND LIPOPROTEINS

Clearly, the liver plays a key role in the production and metabolism of plasma lipids and lipoproteins and it is not surprising that with liver damage there are changes in the plasma content of lipids and lipoproteins.

It is over a hundred years since Austin Flint[50] found a high blood cholesterol in three jaundiced patients; he attributed this to failure of the diseased liver to remove cholesterol from the blood. Flint is often given the credit for describing the hypercholesterolaemia of obstructive jaundice but there is little doubt that his patients suffered from parenchymal liver disease. Widal, Weill and Laudat[160] studied two deeply jaundiced patients with extrahepatic obstruction (one with gallstones and one with pancreatic carcinoma). Not only did they find hypercholesterolaemia but noted that it was due predominantly to an elevation of free cholesterol; they contrasted it with the hypercholesterolaemia of renal disease which was characterized by an increase in ester.

In 1932 Epstein[46] confirmed that an elevation of free cholesterol, often to very high levels, was characteristic of obstructive jaundice; ester cholesterol was also raised in many of his obstructed patients but in some the ester fell even when the total cholesterol was greatly increased. A low ester content was also seen in severe parenchymal liver disease and falling ester levels in both types of liver disease were attributed to liver cell damage.

There have been fewer studies on other plasma lipids in liver disease. Phospholipids were, and still are, estimated by measuring the phosphorus content of plasma lipids but triglycerides were originally measured more crudely, by subtracting the fatty acids of phospholipids (assuming a phospholipid mixture of a given composition) from the total non-cholesteryl ester fatty acids of plasma.[112] Later it was possible to separate plasma lipids by chromatography but Phillips in 1960 still measured triglyceride by subtracting the serum cholesteryl ester fatty acids from the total non-phospholipid fatty acids.

Man and his colleagues[92] found 'neutral fat' to be normal in most patients with liver disease but occasionally it was greatly elevated, as in obstructive jaundice or early in the course of infectious hepatitis; it fell when the obstruction was relieved or when the hepatitis subsided. Phillips confirmed that serum triglyceride levels were elevated in patients with biliary obstruction and hepatitis and commented that the plasma remained clear despite the triglyceride increase. He also found a high triglyceride in three patients with biliary fistula.

Man and his colleagues[92] demonstrated that lipid phosphorus rose in obstructed patients and noted that the levels tended to follow those of cholesterol; above a certain level the relationship between the two compounds was virtually linear. They subsequently demonstrated that this relationship depended on the association between phospholipid and *free* cholesterol, and postulated that lecithin was the phospholipid involved.[7] These studies confirmed the experimental findings of Chanutin and Ludewig[30] who showed in the rat that plasma lipid phosphorus rose in direct proportion to free cholesterol following bile duct ligation.

Man et al[92] also found that serum phospholipids were often reduced with parenchymal liver disease although they rose in some patients with infectious hepatitis. Phillips[113] found little change in total plasma phospholipid in parenchymal liver disease but more was present as lecithin in some patients. There was less lysolecithin in jaundiced patients and Phillips suggested that it fell, like cholesteryl ester, because liver function was impaired. Gjone and Orning[61] confirmed and extended these findings. They showed that lysolecithin was lowest in patients with the greatest degree of liver damage and commented on the low lysolecithin found with markedly elevated lecithin in patients with obstructive jaundice.

Studies on the lipid composition of whole plasma provide an incomplete picture of the plasma lipid changes which occur with liver disease. More information can be obtained by measuring the lipid content of the individual lipoprotein fractions but methods for separating lipoproteins are costly and time consuming and progress has been slow.

Gofman and his colleagues[66] pioneered the ultracentrifugal separation of plasma lipoproteins. They were interested in the changes found in liver disease, and particularly in the striking hyperlipidaemia sometimes seen with obstructive jaundice. This emphasis on the study of obstructive jaundice has persisted to the present day; by comparison, the lipoprotein changes of parenchymal liver disease have been neglected.

Lecithin:Cholesterol Acyltransferase (LCAT) and Triglyceride Lipase Activity

The reduced plasma cholesteryl ester level in liver disease was originally attributed to decreased production by the damaged liver. The fall in plasma ester levels after hepatectomy in animals[55] and the demonstration of a cholesterol-esterifying system in liver homogenates[96] seemed to support this explanation.

There is another explanation. It has been known for many years that plasma can esterify free cholesterol in vitro[141] and that this activity is reduced in patients with liver disease.[29,153] The full significance of these observations was not recognized until Glomset's[63,64] demonstration of the quantitative importance of plasma LCAT in the formation of plasma cholesteryl ester, and the discovery by Norum and Gjone[102] of the rare disorder, familial LCAT deficiency, in which plasma cholesteryl esters are extremely low.

Evidence for the hepatic origin of LCAT has been obtained from animal experiments. In rats, plasma cholesteryl ester fell following hepatectomy[55] and evisceration was associated with a decrease of in vitro plasma cholesterol esterifying activity.[21] Rats with a liver damaged by carbon tetrachloride,[145] ethionine[87] or partial hepatectomy[49] showed reduced plasma LCAT activity. The best evidence, however, for the hepatic origin of this enzyme is the demonstration of a linear increase in LCAT activity in the perfusate from an isolated rat liver system[106,137] and the appearance of LCAT in the medium surrounding isolated rat hepatocytes.[101]

Following the early papers of Glomset and of Norum and Gjone several groups reported decreased plasma LCAT activity in human liver disease[27,60,62,138,147] which correlated with the percentage of plasma cholesterol present as ester. The low activity was due to a reduced plasma concentration of enzyme and not to the presence of inhibitors, the absence of activators, or a lack of suitable substrate lipoproteins.[27,138] It was suggested that the low LCAT activity was due to defective synthesis, or impaired release of the enzyme from the damaged liver.

Hypertriglyceridaemia may be present in acute and chronic hepatitis and in cholestasis[94,111] and it is associated with abnormal triglyceride-rich LDL particles.[1,94] Triglycerides are normally cleared from the plasma by peripheral and hepatic triglyceride lipases. Müller et al[94] and Bolzano et al[20] have demonstrated that although peripheral lipase activity is normal in patients with liver disease the hepatic lipase is often strikingly reduced. It has been argued that the large amounts of triglyceride in the LDL fraction may therefore be a consequence of decreased hepatic lipase activity (but see below).

The Lipoproteins of Obstructive Jaundice

Many lipoprotein studies have been carried out on plasma from patients with primary biliary cirrhosis who may have cholesterol and phospholipid levels far higher than those seen with extrahepatic biliary obstruction. Kunkel and Ahrens,[82] using electrophoretic separation, showed that the increases were mainly in the beta-globulin fraction and that they were disproportionately large compared to the increase in protein. Gofman and his colleagues[66] confirmed the massive elevation of LDL in six patients with chronic biliary obstruction and hinted that these LDL might differ chemically from those found in other conditions. In five patients there was a marked decrease in HDL.

Eder and his colleagues[40] first presented convincing evidence that the LDL of obstructive jaundice were indeed abnormal in composition. In a Cohn fraction which normally contained HDL running with alpha-mobility they found large amounts of LDL with beta-mobility; almost all of its cholesterol was unesterified. These studies were extended on plasma from one patient with primary biliary cirrhosis.[126] The unusual LDL was shown to have a low cholesterol:phospholipid ratio and a low protein content; it did not react to antisera against normal LDL. Russ and her colleagues thought that several abnormal LDL were present in their patient's plasma, and heterogeneity of LDL with obstructive jaundice was also postulated by Furman and Conrad.[56]

Lipoprotein-X (LP-X)

A major breakthrough in our understanding of the hyperlipidaemia of obstructive jaundice came with the isolation and characterization of 'LP-X'. In 1967 Switzer used antibodies to 'normal' LDL to remove it from the LDL fraction of patients with primary biliary cirrhosis. A lipoprotein remained which was rich in phospholipid and free cholesterol; triglyceride and cholesteryl ester were virtually absent. There was little protein present but what there was had an amino acid pattern like that of VLDL; an antiserum against this material reacted with VLDL but did not react with normal LDL or HDL.

Switzer's findings were confirmed and extended by Seidel and his colleagues[132,134] who called the abnormal lipoprotein LP-X, believing that it contained a specific apolipoprotein, Apo X, with an extraordinary lipid-binding capacity. After delipidation, however, Apo X appeared by several methods to be identical with Apo C, the group of peptides associated with VLDL.

On electron microscopy whole sera containing LP-X show abnormal particles which look like coins or discs and which tend to form rouleaux.[72] Their major axis is about 40 to 60 nm and they are about 10 nm thick. They appear to be partially flattened vesicles with walls which are a continuous lipid bilayer (Figure 4.1). These sera may also contain larger structures in the form of stacked layers or lamellar whorls and these often appear to be continuous with the rouleaux.[119] Free cholesterol and lecithin are present in this material in a 1 : 1 molar ratio and similar structures can be produced artificially by mixing free cholesterol and phospholipid in similar proportions.

Patsch and his colleagues[109] suggested that more than one type of LP-X may be present in the plasma of patients with obstructive jaundice. Their LP-X_1 had a higher phospholipid to protein ratio than LP-X_2 and a lower hydrated density. It was cleared more slowly from the plasma than LP-X_2 following the relief of biliary obstruction. The functional significance of their findings is not yet clear.

Several techniques are now available for the detection of LP-X in plasma or serum and several groups of workers have claimed that they are of practical clinical use. Seidel and his colleagues[133] claimed that LP-X could be detected in 99 per cent of patients with

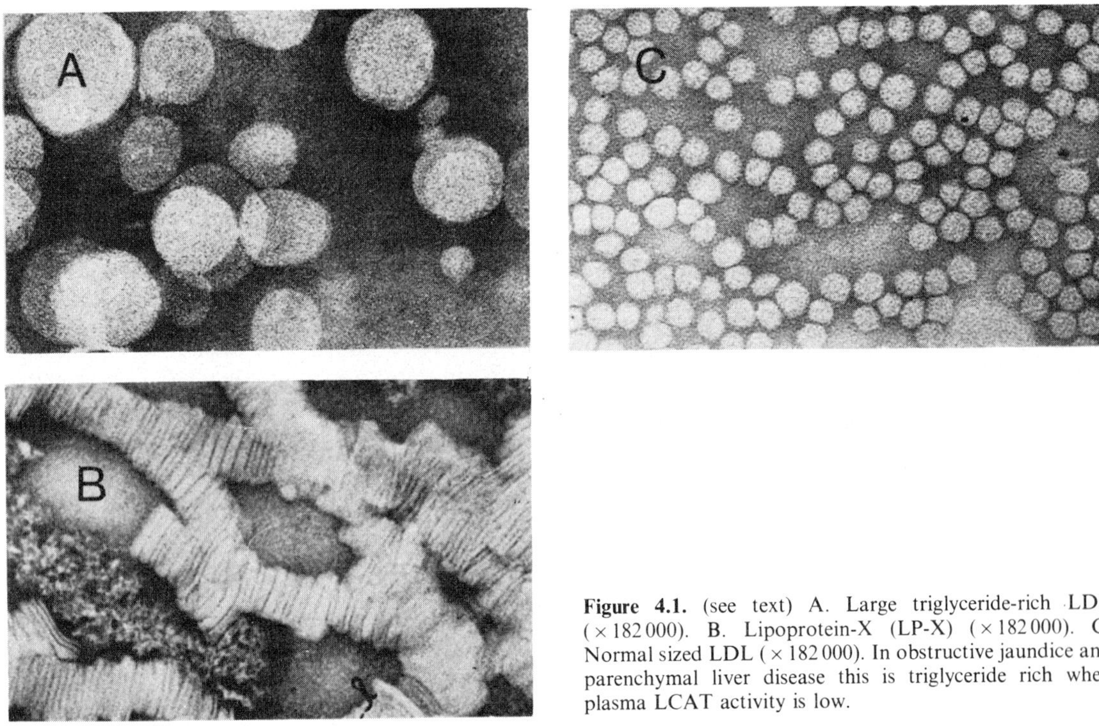

Figure 4.1. (see text) A. Large triglyceride-rich LDL (× 182 000). B. Lipoprotein-X (LP-X) (× 182 000). C. Normal sized LDL (× 182 000). In obstructive jaundice and parenchymal liver disease this is triglyceride rich when plasma LCAT activity is low.

histological evidence of cholestasis and that it was undetectable in about 97 per cent of those without cholestasis; others have reported similar findings.[95] In itself this observation is of little *diagnostic* value as 'cholestasis' may be found in parenchymal liver diseases such as hepatitis and cirrhosis. From our own experience (see below) it is clear that LP-X may be undetectable in patients with surgical obstruction to the biliary tree and review of the literature reveals other patients with 'obstruction' and a negative test for LP-X.[39, 89, 123, 125, 133, 159] This limits the value of LP-X as a *screening* procedure.

Magnani and Alaupovic[89] and Ritland[122] measured the amount of LP-X in plasma and claimed that this helps in differential diagnosis if the direction of change is also plotted. Inspection of their data makes it clear that the valuable distinction between 'extrahepatic' and 'intrahepatic' obstruction could not be made on the basis of plasma LP-X levels. The measurement of trends was also unreliable and it cannot be considered as a simple method of diagnosis. It does not justify delay in applying more precise techniques for assessing the patency of the biliary tree. We believe that the LP-X test is of little clinical value in the management of jaundice in adults.

In children the test may be more useful. Poley et al[116] compared 14 children having surgically proved extrahepatic biliary obstruction with 14 who had intrahepatic cholestasis (11 with neonatal hepatitis, three with other causes). All of the children with extrahepatic block had LP-X in the serum and in all of them the level rose after the administration of cholestyramine (4 g/day) for two weeks. Six of the patients with neonatal hepatitis had no LP-X in the plasma before or after cholestyramine, while the remainder of those with intrahepatic cholestasis showed either a fall in LP-X (seven patients) or no change (one patient). The true value of this test in infants remains to be established.

A commonly used test for LP-X ('Rapidophor all in for LP-X' test, Immuno AG Vienna) is based on the assumption that LP-X is the only lipoprotein in serum which migrates towards the cathode on agar electrophoresis. Following the application of a polyanion solution a precipitate on the cathode side is considered to indicate the presence of LP-X.

Using this test almost all of 270 neonates were found to have LP-X in plasma at some stage during the first 16 weeks of life;[83] it is of interest that a naturally occurring heparin-like anticoagulant has been found in the blood of neonates[97] because fibrinogen also migrates cathodally and false positive results are obtained in adults if plasma is used instead of serum. In another series there was a very high incidence of positive results in adults with a variety of haematological disorders;[39] no information was presented about their liver function. Unfortunately, neither in this series nor in the neonates was any other evidence (e.g. chemical analysis or electron microscopy) presented that the cathodally migrating material was indeed lipoprotein-X.

Other lipoprotein changes in obstructive jaundice

LDL. In patients with obstructive jaundice there is more lipid than usual in the LDL fraction but its composition depends on the level of plasma LCAT activity. When LCAT activity is normal or high the LDL is virtually normal and on electron microscopy it looks like the LDL found in normal subjects, i.e. small spheres with a diameter of approximately 20 nm.

With a fall in LCAT activity the picture becomes more complex. LP-X appears and this accounts for most of the striking increase in free cholesterol and phospholipid which is often seen in patients with obstructive jaundice. A large (30 to 70 nm) triglyceride-rich particle is also present in patients who have an elevated plasma triglyceride[1,81,98] (Figure 4.1). This particle contains both B and C apoproteins. Müller and his colleagues suggested that it results from reduced hepatic lipase activity but a similar particle is present in patients with familial LCAT deficiency who have normal hepatic and peripheral lipase activity.[70]

The excess plasma triglyceride found in many patients with obstructive jaundice is not present in VLDL, the fraction which we might expect to carry it. Some is present in the large LDL particles described in the last paragraph; the remainder is found in normal sized (20 nm) LDL particles. These are found on electron microscopy of the LDL fraction regardless of plasma LCAT activity. When LCAT is normal or high the composition of these particles is also normal but as LCAT activity falls their triglyceride content increases and their cholesteryl ester falls. The cause of this abnormality is not certain. Both triglyceride and cholesteryl ester are non-polar lipids and must form the core of the spherical LDL particle. If the particle size is to remain constant an increase in one of these lipids must be accompanied by a decrease in the other. Lipoprotein lipase removes triglyceride from VLDL during its conversion to LDL. Cholesteryl ester, produced by LCAT, seems to be incorporated into LDL. LDL with a high triglyceride:cholesteryl ester ratio might therefore result if the apoprotein carried more triglyceride than usual from its parent VLDL particle (perhaps because lipase activity was reduced). Alternatively, reduction of plasma LCAT activity could have the same effect on the ratio if, as a result, less cholesteryl ester was transferred to the beta-apoprotein. The normal sized LDL in familial LCAT deficiency is also triglyceride rich and in these patients hepatic and peripheral lipase activity is normal. This suggests that reduced LCAT activity is probably the cause in obstructive jaundice, a hypothesis supported by the significant correlation which exists between the cholesteryl ester:triglyceride ratio of these particles and the plasma LCAT activity.

VLDL. When the plasma LCAT activity is normal or high with obstructive jaundice the lipoprotein pattern on paper or agarose electrophoresis is also normal. A pre-beta band is seen and this VLDL has a normal composition. When the LCAT level falls the marked increase in plasma lipids which usually occurs is reflected only in a broad densely staining beta band. Although no distinct pre-beta band is seen VLDL is present and can be isolated by preparative ultracentrifugation. The electrophoretic mobility is abnormal and it runs in the broad beta band.[135] The reason for this change in mobility is not clear but it may be due to an altered apoprotein composition.[119] When LCAT activity is low the composition of VLDL is abnormal and it has a high protein, phospholipid and free cholesterol while cholesteryl ester and triglyceride are reduced. The total amount of VLDL present is correlated with plasma LCAT activity.

HDL. Gofman and his colleagues[66] called attention to the 'wipe out' of HDL which may occur with chronic biliary obstruction and which they observed in studies using preparative and analytical ultracentrifugation. Absence of alpha-lipoprotein (HDL) is also found on electrophoresis of the plasma of most patients with obstructive jaundice. The electrophoretic pattern depends on the plasma LCAT activity and when it is normal or high a prominent alpha band is visible. Although the band is absent when LCAT activity is low this does not mean that there is no HDL in the plasma; it can be isolated by preparative ultracentrifugation.

There have been relatively few studies on the composition and the physicochemical characteristics of HDL in obstructive jaundice and the results have been conflicting.[17,51,119] In our studies we found HDL virtually normal in patients with high LCAT levels;[1] only one peak was seen on column chromatography and it had a normal appearance on electron microscopy (Figure 4.2). There were two major peaks when LCAT levels were low. One peak looked like normal HDL on electron microscopy but its triglyceride and free cholesterol content was higher than normal and cholesteryl ester and phospholipid lower. The other peak was richer in free cholesterol and phospholipid and contained less cholesteryl ester and protein. On electron microscopy this fraction contained 'stacked discs' (Figure 4.2). These discs (4 nm thick and 15 to 20 nm in diameter) resemble those found in familial LCAT deficiency[104] and in cholestasis[51,155] and are like the 'nascent' HDL described by Hamilton et al.[73]

In some patients with low LCAT we found small amounts of HDL in a third peak. This peak was rich in triglyceride and phospholipid. Similar particles have been described in familial LCAT deficiency and in cholestasis; they may be a minor component of normal HDL or may be artefacts of preparation.

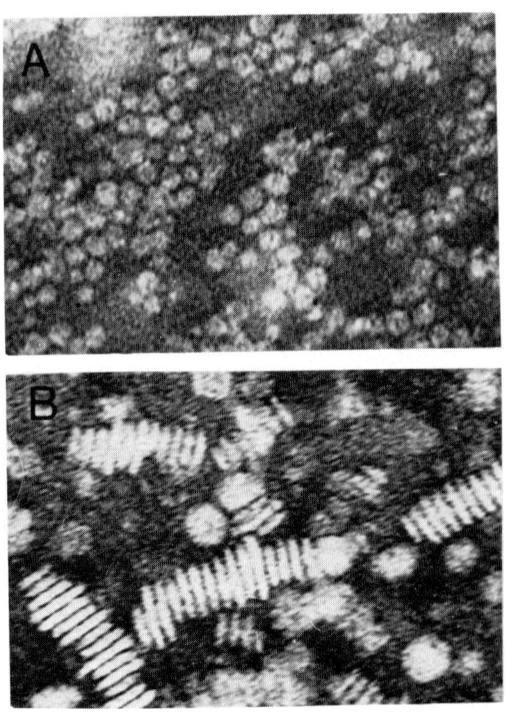

Figure 4.2. A. Normal HDL (×220 000). B. Abnormal 'nascent' HDL, found in obstructive jaundice and parenchymal liver disease when plasma LCAT activity is low (×220 000).

The Hyperlipidaemia of Obstructive Jaundice[94]

In preceding sections we have pointed out that high plasma lipids are characteristic of obstructive jaundice even when, in the presence of high LCAT levels, the individual lipoprotein fractions appear to be virtually normal in composition. What is the reason for this hyperlipidaemia?

Flint[50] suggested that hypercholesterolaemia resulted because the liver failed to remove cholesterol from the blood. But subsequently it became clear that with severe parenchymal liver disease there is a fall in total cholesterol due to a fall in ester. Although free cholesterol tends to rise under these circumstances the levels found with straightforward parenchymal damage are never very high and it seems unlikely that Flint's hypothesis could account for the striking increase in free cholesterol often seen with obstructive jaundice.

When bile ducts are occluded canaliculi become distended and may rupture.[13,45] Epstein[46] therefore argued that hypercholesterolaemia results from the regurgitation of bile, rich in free cholesterol, into the blood stream. This is an attractive hypothesis but in rats cholesterol of biliary origin could not account for more than a third of the excess sterol found in the plasma 24 hours after experimental biliary obstruction.

The most widely accepted explanation for the hypercholesterolaemia of obstructive jaundice is based on the study of Fredrickson and his colleagues[54] who showed that cholesterol synthesis in rat liver was strikingly increased following ligation of the bile duct. This hypothesis does not explain all the facts, however. The increase in cholesterol synthesis in 'obstructed' rat liver can be prevented by the administration of cycloheximide but this does not prevent the marked rise in plasma-free cholesterol.[75] Furthermore, increased cholesterol synthesis does not account for the equally impressive rise in plasma phospholipid and there is no agreement that phospholipid synthesis increases following biliary obstruction.[69,142] Nor does this hypothesis explain how cholesterol enters plasma in such large amounts. The cholesterol, being insoluble, would presumably need to be transferred in a lipoprotein or complexed with phospholipid as in biliary micelles or in LP-X. There are no data to suggest that more cholesterol is secreted in normal lipoproteins and electron microscopic studies of the liver early in obstructive jaundice did not show LP-X awaiting secretion.[34,144]

Recently, Felker and Hamilton[47] claimed that LP-X can be seen in the bile canaliculi, cytosol and in the spaces of Disse of the isolated perfused rat liver with bile duct obstruction, and that LP-X is found in the perfusate. It is not clear whether the perfusate LP-X was 'secreted' from the hepatocyte or resulted from regurgitation from the biliary tree.

The discovery of familial LCAT deficiency suggested another explanation for the hypercholesterolaemia of liver disease, one which accounted for other lipid and lipoprotein changes. Patients with this rare condition show a hyperlipidaemic pattern similar to that found with obstructive jaundice and lipoprotein changes which are almost identical.[103] They even have 'target' erythrocytes in the blood, a common finding in obstructive jaundice and one which appears to be secondary to the lipoprotein abnormalities.[35]

Low values for LCAT activity were found in early studies on obstructive jaundice[27,59] and this suggested that reduced LCAT activity might be implicated in the production of the plasma lipid and lipoprotein abnormalities. But it was recognized from the beginning that reduced LCAT activity alone could not account for the changes.[93] With obstructive jaundice and *low* LCAT activity free cholesterol is often far higher than with familial *absence* of the enzyme. Secondly, plasma cholesteryl ester levels may be low, normal or even elevated with obstructive jaundice; they are invariably low in familial LCAT deficiency. This variation in plasma cholesteryl ester levels seems to be related to variable LCAT activity which may be low, normal or markedly elevated in obstructive jaundice and there is a good correlation between the two variables.[78]

Our recent studies suggest that reduced LCAT activity may contribute to increased plasma lipid levels of obstructive jaundice as the total plasma lipids were higher in patients with low LCAT (mean 24.3 mmol/l) than in obstructed patients with normal or high LCAT activity (19.5 mmol/l).[1] It can be seen that the effect is not a striking one and both groups of patients had far higher plasma lipid levels than normal subjects (8.8 mmol/l). Clearly, a factor other than LCAT activity was operating in these patients.

We believe that the best explanation for the hyperlipidaemia of obstructive jaundice is the regurgitation of lecithin from the obstructed biliary tree into the blood. Byers and Friedman[23] suggested that some factor in bile was important because plasma cholesterol rose when the bile duct of the rat was anastomosed to the inferior vena cava. Initially, bile salts were incriminated but subsequently these workers concluded that retention of biliary phospholipid caused the hypercholesterolaemia of obstructive jaundice. Following the infusion of phospholipid (brain lecithin) plasma cholesterol:phospholipid ratios were almost identical to those found in rats following bile duct ligation.[24]

More recently, Quarfordt and his colleagues[120] obstructed the bile duct in cholecystectomized dogs and sampled bile through a catheter. As plasma-free cholesterol and lecithin rose in plasma their concentration fell in the stagnant bile and the regurgitation of phospholipid normally excreted in the bile accounted for the phospholipid accumulating in plasma. When purified egg lecithin was infused into the biliary tree almost all of it appeared in plasma, and as the plasma lecithin increased so did the plasma cholesterol. These studies give strong support to the conclusions of Byers and Friedman.[24]

But where does the extra cholesterol come from? Byers and his colleagues[25,26] believed that the liver was not the only source as hypercholesterolaemia occurred if phospholipid was infused into hepatectomized animals. Their experiments in this field were not conclusive but eventually they suggested that the cholesterol accumulating in blood was derived partly from the partitioning of pre-existing tissue cholesterol into the excess phospholipid in the plasma, and that the rest was derived from an increase in cholesterol synthesis.

It seems likely that some of the cholesterol does normally come from the liver as Quarfordt and Jakoi[118] found a significant increase in hepatic cholesterol synthesis following phospholipid infusion; this did not occur when an equimolar amount of cholesterol was given with the lecithin. Presumably, lecithin removed cholesterol from the liver and cholesterol synthesis increased as a compensatory mechanism. This observation is of particular interest as it offers a partial explanation for the increased cholesterol synthesis found with biliary ligation (but see Cooper and Ockner[33]).

There have been few studies on cholesterol synthesis in humans with obstructive jaundice. Ahrens[3] calculated total body synthesis from the results of cholesterol balance studies; with chronic biliary obstruction synthesis appeared to be reduced. His data fit those of Nicolau et al[100] who found reduced activity of hepatic HMG CoA reductase (the rate-limiting enzyme of cholesterol biosynthesis) in biopsies from patients with extrahepatic biliary obstruction. In contrast, Orlandi[105] found an increased rate of cholesterol synthesis (measured as incorporation into digitonin precipitable sterols) in several patients with obstructive jaundice. Further work must be done to clarify this point.

The regurgitation of phospholipid and secondary accumulation of free cholesterol can obviously account for the appearance in plasma of LP-X in which these two compounds are present in a 1:1 molar ratio. It is unclear why phospholipid regurgitation should increase the concentration of apparently normal lipoproteins. There is some experimental evidence bearing on this point. Thompson et al[151] infused phospholipid intravenously into human volunteers with normal plasma lipids (and presumably with normal LCAT). They observed an increase of cholesteryl ester and of LDL. This suggests that normal lipoproteins might accumulate if the patient has enough plasma LCAT to cope with the extra substrate. They also found a transient accumulation of phospholipid suggesting that LCAT might have been temporarily overloaded. High rates of regurgitation from the biliary tree might similarly exceed the esterification capacity in obstructed patients with normal or high LCAT levels and this could explain why LP-X is found in some of these patients.[18] Such results fit with our earlier study in rats:[28] following bile duct ligation we found not only a marked rise of plasma-free cholesterol and phospholipid (which was presumably in LP-X) but also an increase in LCAT activity, and in plasma cholesteryl ester which we subsequently found to be present in the LDL fraction.

Liver function becomes impaired with severe and prolonged obstruction; LCAT levels fall and are inversely related to the level of plasma bilirubin. Free cholesterol, lecithin and LP-X should then accumulate in plasma as they do in LCAT deficiency, although the amount present would not depend only on LCAT activity. If there was a large amount of regurgitation from bile, plasma lecithin and free cholesterol would be able to reach the very high levels found in some patients with chronic obstruction. But if the liver cells fail, bile flow and, presumably, regurgitation would fall and this might account for the drop in plasma lecithin and cholesterol seen with end stage biliary obstruction.

The Lipoproteins of Parenchymal Liver Disease

The plasma lipid changes in parenchymal liver disease were described earlier in this chapter. Relatively few studies have been carried out on the corresponding lipoprotein abnormalities. Pierce and Gofman[114] found minor changes in plasma LDL concentration in cirrhosis and in a later study Pierce et al[115] found significant elevations of LDL in patients with viral hepatitis; in the latter condition there was a fall in VLDL (of S_f 100 to 400).

In early acute hepatitis Eder and his colleagues[40] found that the lipoprotein fractions were abnormal; they ran with abnormal electrophoretic mobility and the cholesteryl ester:free cholesterol ratio was low. The lipoproteins returned to normal with recovery. The changes were similar to those found with biliary obstruction. Different results were found with cirrhosis. Unfortunately, the results of Eder et al,[40] like those of Pierce and Gofman,[114] are difficult to interpret in retrospect.

More recent studies with agarose gel electrophoresis have shown that the alpha and pre-beta bands disappear early in acute viral hepatitis and reappear with recovery.[62,108,111,135] Early in the attack the beta band is broader, stains more densely and migrates slightly faster than normal. Thalassinos et al[148] studied 57 patients with viral hepatitis using paper electrophoresis. In mild or moderate cases alpha-lipoprotein was usually absent in the early stages and gradually reappeared with recovery. In severe cases it was absent for a longer period and did not reappear in those who eventually died.

In our own studies on parenchymal liver disease such changes appear to relate to LCAT activity.[38] When LCAT is normal or high the lipoprotein electrophoretic pattern is normal; with moderate reduction of LCAT activity there is loss of the pre-beta band, and with severe reduction both the pre-beta and alpha bands disappear.

Seidel et al[135] studied patients with parenchymal and obstructive liver disease and observed similar changes. Despite the absence of pre-beta and alpha bands both VLDL and HDL were obtained with ultracentrifugation. The concentration of VLDL was normal[98] and it had a normal composition, lipid:protein ratio and particle size; its abnormal electrophoretic mobility was attributed to the absence of apo A. HDL in these patients was found to have an increased protein:lipid ratio and this, and its abnormal mobility, was attributed to an impaired ability of apo A to bind lipid though apo A was thought to be present in normal amounts (but see below).

Pearson et al[108] studied plasma lipids and lipoproteins serially in 11 cases of acute viral hepatitis. High plasma triglyceride levels were common initially, but the triglyceride was found not in VLDL but in LDL which contained less cholesteryl ester than usual. With recovery, the cholesteryl ester content of LDL rose and the triglyceride fell reciprocally. HDL were present in reduced amounts and on analytical ultracentrifugation there were at least two HDL components.

Müller et al[98] found, as in obstructive liver disease, that hypertriglyceridaemia in patients with parenchymal liver disease was associated with the appearance of a large (30 to 70 nm) triglyceride-rich particle in the LDL fraction, which they called beta-2-lipoprotein. On this basis they explained the increased LDL triglyceride found by other workers;[79,110,111] the triglyceride content of the normal sized (20 nm) LDL was not recorded.

Sabesin et al,[129] in a serial study of patients with acute alcoholic liver disease (characterized by massive fatty liver, alcoholic hepatitis and intrahepatic cholestasis), found striking abnormalities of plasma lipoproteins associated with a marked decrease in plasma LCAT activity. The predominant lipoprotein was the triglyceride-rich LDL described by Müller et al.[98] LP-X was also present as a minor component of LDL. Most of the HDL consisted of long chains of bilamellar discs. Sabesin et al[128] found a similar picture with galactosamine-induced hepatic injury in the rat.

The patients studied by Müller et al[98] and by Sabesin et al[129] had evidence of cholestasis and it is difficult to distinguish the effects of parenchymal disease from those of biliary obstruction. We have recently studied plasma lipoproteins in patients with parenchymal liver disease of varying severity and with a wide range of plasma LCAT activity.[38] None had obvious evidence of intra- or extrahepatic cholestasis. Patients with normal or high LCAT activity had lipoproteins of normal structure, electrophoretic mobility and composition. Patients with low LCAT activity showed a number of abnormalities. Their HDL were decreased in amount, were of abnormal composition, and consisted largely of stacked discs on electron microscopy, similar to those in low LCAT obstructive jaundice and in familial deficiency. The similarity of these HDL changes in obstructive and parenchymal liver disease suggests that they are due to LCAT deficiency per se, presumably because the enzyme is not available to act on the nascent HDL released from the liver. The percentage protein content of the HDL was reduced and our findings, and those of Blomhoff[17] and Pearson et al,[111] do not support the suggestion of Seidel et al[135] that lipid binding by the apo A of HDL is decreased in liver disease.

Our most interesting findings were in the LDL fraction. In contrast to patients with obstructive jaundice only one peak was found on gel filtration regardless of plasma LCAT activity; but when LCAT activity was low the particles in this peak, which were the same size and shape as normal LDL, had an abnormal composition. Like the 'normal sized' LDL particles found in low LCAT obstructive jaundice and in familial LCAT deficiency they were deficient in cholesteryl ester and rich in triglyceride. The appearance in plasma of triglyceride-rich LDL in all these low LCAT states also seems to be a direct consequence of LCAT deficiency, perhaps because less cholesteryl ester is produced to take the place of triglyceride in the core of the particle during the catabolism of VLDL to LDL. Our findings also show that an increased triglyceride content of LDL in liver disease is not necessarily due to the presence of beta-2-lipoprotein as suggested by Müller et al.[98]

Our patients with parenchymal liver disease and low LCAT levels had low total plasma lipids but, surprisingly, the plasma concentration of LDL was normal. The markedly reduced levels of its precursor, VLDL, suggest that LDL catabolism may be markedly reduced, but this hypothesis needs to be tested by LDL turnover studies.

The mechanism and site of LDL removal from the plasma have not been established but are of obvious importance in view of the relationship between plasma LDL levels and the risk of ischaemic heart disease. The liver has been considered as the major site of LDL breakdown but it is now recognized that fibroblasts and arterial smooth muscle cells can take up and catabolize LDL in vitro.[68] Removal by extrahepatic tissues may therefore be of quantitative importance in vivo. Sniderman et al[139] showed that the catabolism of injected iodinated LDL is actually increased in the hepatectomized pig. However, van Tol et al[158] found that partial hepatectomy in the rat slowed the rate of LDL catabolism. Further studies of lipoproteins and their metabolism in patients with impaired liver function may help to clarify this fascinating problem.

THE CLINICAL IMPLICATIONS OF THE PLASMA LIPOPROTEIN ABNORMALITIES OF LIVER DISEASE

The overt clinical consequences of the plasma lipoprotein abnormalities found with liver disease are few. When plasma lipid levels are very high, as in chronic obstructive jaundice, cutaneous xanthomas may appear.[4] These may be scanty or there may be a widespread eruption with a characteristic distribution in the palmar creases, in the skin of the palms and soles, around the eyes, and over the elbows, buttocks and knees. Areas subject to pressure or to trauma are also frequently involved.

When palmar and plantar xanthomatosis is severe there may be tenderness of the affected skin due to a mild sensory neuropathy associated with xanthomatous deposits in the peripheral nerves.[150] Involvement of other tissues appears to be rare.

There are few good descriptions of the histology of the xanthomas of biliary obstruction and we are not aware of any electron-microscopic observations. The chemical composition of these deposits has received little attention. Thannhauser and Magendantz[149] analysed one and, surprisingly, all of the cholesterol was present in the form of ester. We have analysed several and found a large proportion of ester, although free cholesterol was also present.

Ahrens[2] studied the incidence of aortic atheroma in patients with the hyperlipidaemia of primary biliary cirrhosis. Paradoxically, the extent of atheroma seemed to be inversely related to plasma lipid levels. In four patients with marked cutaneous xanthomatosis there was minimal evidence of atheroma but in three patients in the prexanthomatous stage of the disease arterial lesions were present which were disproportionately severe in relation to the age and sex of the patients.

Despite these observations of Ahrens it has been generally accepted that ischaemic heart disease is uncommon in patients with primary biliary cirrhosis. Schaffner[131] has cast doubt on this assumption. In a review of the literature he quotes three series in which ischaemic heart disease had been found in a small number of patients; in his own series of over 50 patients four had suffered a myocardial infarct and two had severe angina. This problem deserves further study.

The disfigurement caused by cutaneous xanthomas and the disabling effects of the peripheral neuropathy have led many workers to try to treat the elevated plasma cholesterol levels in patients with chronic obstruction. There is little to suggest that dietary measures would be of value. Steroids have been given without obvious benefit.[131] Cholestyramine and clofibrate have both been tried. Cholestyramine reduces plasma cholesterol in patients with familial hypercholesterolaemia.[52] When given to patients with obstructive jaundice (in order to reduce itching) it has been observed that serum cholesterol levels fall and that there may be some clearing of xanthomas.[37, 157] The changes are not striking and cholestyramine would be an unsatisfactory treatment if it were used only for its effect on serum cholesterol and on xanthomas.

Schaffner[131] gave clofibrate to several patients with primary biliary cirrhosis hoping that it would decrease plasma cholesterol concentrations. Paradoxically, the cholesterol rose or there was an increase in the size of the cutaneous lesions. We have also seen patients in whom cholesterol rose after clofibrate had been given. To study the mechanism of this effect we administered clofibrate to rats following bile duct ligation.[117] They showed a much greater rise in free cholesterol and phospholipid than animals subjected only to biliary ligation; ester cholesterol and triglyceride concentrations were lower and there were other differences in the plasma lipoproteins. The results are difficult to explain. They might fit with the hypothesis (mentioned earlier) that hypercholesterolaemia is a consequence of regurgitation of biliary phospholipid from damaged ductules; it has been claimed that in the rat clofibrate enhances biliary lecithin output but in man this effect was not found consistently.[74] Further studies of this phenomenon are clearly indicated as they might shed light not only on the mechanism of obstructive hypercholesterolaemia but also on the way in which clofibrate produces its *hypolipidaemic* effect.

Because conventional methods of reducing plasma cholesterol levels are so unsatisfactory, Turnberg and his colleagues used mechanical methods to reduce cholesterol levels in two patients with severe xanthomatous neuropathy.[152] In one, plasmaphoresis was used; the other patient was treated with plasma exchange using a blood cell separator. In both patients there was a striking fall in plasma cholesterol, symptoms improved and xanthomas regressed. These mechanical methods of treatment are both time-consuming and inconvenient for the patient but they are effective. At present the only indications for their use appear to be severe neuropathic symptoms and possibly disfiguring xanthomas.

Obstructive hypercholesterolaemia creates problems in the interpretation of some laboratory tests. Commonly, lipoprotein electrophoresis is used to type the observed hyperlipidaemia. Because a broad, densely-staining beta band is found in association with high cholesterol and increased triglyceride, a diagnosis of type IIa or type III hyperlipoproteinaemia is made[14] and dietary and other advice may be given on this basis. Such advice is inappropriate. The lipoprotein abnormalities of liver disease are quite different from conventional hyperlipoproteinaemias and there is no evidence that the same approaches to management are useful (see above).

It has long been recognized that sera from patients with liver disease inhibit the haemolytic effect of streptolysin 0 and that falsely high titres of antistreptolysin 0 may be recorded as a result. The protective effect of these sera seems to be related to their increased content of free cholesterol.[10] A true measurement of the antistreptolysin 0 content can be made following pre-treatment of serum with isoamyl alcohol.[11]

Other haemolytic agents are also inhibited by an excess of free cholesterol, perhaps because they act by binding with the free cholesterol of the erythrocyte membrane. Charache and Margolis[31] found that saponin used to prepare samples for white cell counting by electronic particle counter failed to haemolyse all the red cells in four patients with extreme hypercholesterolaemia secondary to liver disease. This caused falsely high 'leucocytosis'. They postulated that a stable complex formed between saponin and the free cholesterol in the plasma and that the action of the saponin on red cells was thus prevented.

Patients with liver disease have abnormal red cells which contain more cholesterol, or more cholesterol and phospholipid, than those of normal subjects.[35] This increase of membrane lipids leads to an expansion of the surface area without a corresponding change in volume and as a result there is a change in shape. In wet preparations the erythrocytes are 'bowl' shaped but the drying procedure used for making conventional blood films distorts them and as a result they appear as 'target' cells.[12] Target cells may result from the failure of plasma lipoproteins to handle lecithin and free cholesterol added to the plasma; this explanation would also account for their appearance in familial LCAT deficiency.[103] It is possible that an excess of lipid may be deposited in the membrane of other cells and this may play a part in the production of the generalized metabolic disturbance found in the jaundiced patient.

Recently, we have shown that the erythrocyte membrane abnormalities found with liver disease are associated with an impaired transport of sodium across the membrane.[107] The erythrocyte membrane is considered to be a satisfactory model for the lipid bilayer of all plasma membranes.[156] It is thus possible that excess lipid is deposited in membranes of cells other than the erythrocyte. If a similar functional disturbance is produced it might contribute to the general cellular disturbance which characterizes serious liver disease of many kinds. This is an exciting concept as it might be possible to reverse these membrane changes in vivo.

REFERENCES

1. Agorastos, J., Fox, C., Harry, D.S. & McIntyre, N. (1978) Lecithin:cholesterol acyltransferase and the lipoprotein abnormalities of obstructive jaundice. *Clinical Science and Molecular Medicine*, **54**, 369–379.
2. Ahrens, E.H. Jr (1950) The lipid disturbance in biliary obstruction and its relationship to the genesis of arteriosclerosis. *Bulletin of the New York Academy of Medicine*, **26**, 151–162.
3. Ahrens, E.H. Jr (1975) personal communication.
4. Ahrens, E.H. Jr & Kunkel, H.G. (1949) The relationship between serum lipids and skin xanthomata in eighteen patients with primary biliary cirrhosis. *Journal of Clinical Investigation*, **28**, 1565 1574.
5. Alaupovic, P. (1971) Apolipoproteins and lipoproteins. *Atherosclerosis*, **13**, 141–146.
6. Albers, J.J. & Hazzard, W.R. (1974) Immunochemical quantification of human plasma Lp(a) lipoprotein. *Lipids*, **9**, 15–26.
7. Albrink, M.J., Man, E.B. & Peters, J.P. (1950) Serum lipids in infectious hepatitis and obstructive jaundice. *Journal of Clinical Investigation*, **29**, 781–788.

8. Anderson, R.G.H., Goldstein, J.C. & Brown, M.S. (1977) A mutation that impairs the ability of lipoprotein receptors to localise in coated pits on the cell surface of human fibroblasts. *Nature*, **270**, 695–699.
9. Assmann, G., Herbert, P.N., Fredrickson, D.S. & Forte, T. (1977) Isolation and characterisation of an abnormal high density lipoprotein in Tangier disease. *Journal of Clinical Investigation*, **60**, 242–252.
10. Badin, J. & Barillee, A. (1968) Effet des lipides de la β-lipoprotéine humaine normale sur le pouvoir hémolytique de la streptolysine O et de la digitonine. *Annales de Biologie Clinique*, **26**, 213–229.
11. Badin, J. & Barillee, A. (1969) Dosage spécifique de l'antistreptolysine O sérique après élimination des lipoprotéines par l'alcohol isoamylique. *Annales de Biologie Clinique*, **27**, 395–402.
12. Barrett, A.M. (1938) A special form of erythrocyte possessing increased resistance to hypotonic saline. *Journal of Pathology and Bacteriology*, **46**, 603–618.
13. Barron, E.S.G. & Bumstead, J.H. (1928) The pathogenesis of early obstructive jaundice. *Journal of Experimental Medicine*, **47**, 999–1012.
14. Beaumont, J.L., Carlson, L.A., Cooper, G.R., Fejfar, Z., Fredrickson, D.S. & Strasser, T. (1970) Classification of hyperlipidaemias and hyperlipoproteinaemias. *Bulletin of the World Health Organisation*, **43**, 891–915.
15. Berg, K. (1963) A new serum type system in man – the Lp system. *Acta Pathologica et Microbiologica Scandinavica*, **59**, 369–382.
16. Blix, G., Tiselius, A. & Svensson, H. (1945) Lipids and polysaccharides in electrophoretically separated blood serum proteins. *Journal of Biological Chemistry*, **137**, 485–494.
17. Blomhoff, J.P. (1974) High density lipoproteins in cholestasis. *Scandinavian Journal of Gastroenterology*, **9**, 591–596.
18. Blomhoff, J.P., Skrede, S. & Ritland, S. (1974) Lecithin:cholesterol acyltransferase and plasma proteins in liver disease. *Clinica Chimica Acta*, **53**, 197–207.
19. Blum, C.B., Levy, R.I., Eisenberg, S., Hall, M., Goebel, R.H. & Berman, M. (1977) High density lipoprotein metabolism in man. *Journal of Clinical Investigation*, **60**, 795–807.
20. Bolzano, K., Krempler, F. & Sandhofer, F. (1975) Hepatic and extrahepatic triglyceride lipase activity in post-heparin plasma of normals and patients with cirrhosis of the liver. *Hormone and Metabolic Research*, **7**, 238–241.
21. Brot, N., Lossow, W.J. & Chaikoff, I.L. (1962) In vitro esterification of cholesterol by plasma: the effect of evisceration. *Journal of Lipid Research*, **3**, 413–415.
22. Brown, W.V., Levy, R.I. & Fredrickson, D.S. (1969) Studies of the proteins in human plasma very low density lipoproteins. *Journal of Biological Chemistry*, **244**, 5687–5694.
23. Byers, S.O. & Friedman, M. (1952) The relation of biliary retention of cholesterol, distension of the biliary tract, the shunting of bile to the vena cava, and the removal of the gastro-intestinal tract to the hypercholesterolemia consequent on biliary obstruction. *Journal of Experimental Medicine*, **95**, 19–24.
24. Byers, S.O. & Friedman, M. (1957) Cholesterol and phospholipid concentration in hepatic lymph and bile during phosphatide-induced hypercholesterolemia. *Proceedings of the Society for Experimental Biology and Medicine*, **96**, 702–705.
25. Byers, S.O. & Friedman, M. (1969) Probable sources of plasma cholesterol during phosphatide-induced hypercholesterolemia. *Lipids*, **4**, 123–128.
26. Byers, S.O., Friedman, M. & Sugiyama, T. (1962) Mechanism underlying phosphatide-induced hypercholesterolemia. *Journal of Biological Chemistry*, **237**, 3375–3380.
27. Calandra, S., Martin, M.J. & McIntyre, N. (1971) Plasma lecithin:cholesterol acyltransferase activity in liver disease. *European Journal of Clinical Investigation*, **1**, 352–360.
28. Calandra, S., Martin, M.J., O'Shea, M.J. & McIntyre, N. (1972) The effect of experimental biliary obstruction on the structure and lipid content of rat erythrocytes. *Biochimica et Biophysica Acta*, **260**, 424–432.
29. Castro Mendoza, H. & Diaz, C.J. (1949) The cholesterase of the serum (Sperry's enzyme) under normal and pathological conditions. *Bulletin of the Institute of Medical Research (Madrid)*, **2**, 81–93.
30. Chanutin, A. & Ludewig, S. (1936) The blood plasma cholesterol and phospholipid phosphorus in rats following partial hepatectomy and following ligation of the bile duct. *Journal of Biological Chemistry*, **115**, 1–7.
31. Charache, S. & Margolis, S. (1969) Effect of plasma from patients with liver disease on resistance of red blood cells to lysis by saponin. *Journal of Laboratory and Clinical Medicine*, **73**, 951–955.
32. Clark, S.B. & Norum, K.R. (1977) The lecithin–cholesterol acyl transferase activity of rat intestinal lymph. *Journal of Lipid Research*, **18**, 293–300.
33. Cooper, A.D. & Ockner, R.K. (1974) Studies of hepatic cholesterol synthesis in experimental acute biliary obstruction. *Gastroenterology*, **66**, 586–595.
34. Cooper, A.D., Jones, A.L., Koldinger, R.E. & Ockner, R.K. (1974) Selective biliary obstruction: a model for the study of lipid metabolism in cholestasis. *Gastroenterology*, **66**, 584–585.
35. Cooper, R.A. (1970) Lipids of human red cell membrane: normal composition and variability in disease. *Seminars in Hematology*, **7**, 296–322.
36. Dahlen, G., Berg, K. & Frick, M.H. (1976) Lp(a) lipoprotein/pre β lipoprotein, serum lipids and atherosclerotic disease. *Clinical Genetics*, **9**, 558–566.
37. Datta, D.V. & Sherlock, S. (1963) Treatment of pruritus of obstructive jaundice with cholestyramine. *British Medical Journal*, **i**, 216–219.
38. Day, R.C., Harry, D.S., Owen, J.S. & McIntyre, N. (1978) Plasma lecithin:cholesterol acyl transferase activity and the lipoprotein abnormalities of parenchymal liver disease. *Clinical Science and Molecular Medicine*, **54**, 36.
39. Eder, G., Weiss, W., Neumayr, A., Schüller, J. & Baumgartner, G. (1977) Conclusions of LP-X determinations in more than 2500 patients. In *Protides of Biological Fluids* (Ed.) Peeters, H. Vol. 25, pp. 341–347. Oxford: Pergamon Press.
40. Eder, H.A., Russ, E.M., Rees Pritchett, R.A., Wilber, M.M. & Barr, D.P. (1955) Protein-lipid relationships in human plasma: in biliary cirrhosis, obstructive jaundice and acute hepatitis. *Journal of Clinical Investigation*, **34**, 1147–1162.
41. Ehnholm, C., Garoff, H., Renkonen, O. & Simons, K. (1972) Protein and carbohydrate composition of Lp(a) lipoprotein from human plasma. *Biochemistry*, **11**, 3229–3232.

42. Ehnholm, C., Shaw, W., Greten, H., Brown, W.V. (1975) Purification from human plasma of a heparin released lipase with activity against triglyceride and phospholipid. *Journal of Biological Chemistry*, **250**, 6756–6761.
43. Eisenberg, S. (1973) In *Dietary Lipids and Postnatal Development* (Ed.) Galli, C., Jacini, G. & Pecile, A. p. 57. New York: Raven Press.
44. Eisenberg, S. & Levy, R.I. (1975) Lipoprotein metabolism. *Advances in Lipid Research*, **13**, 1–89.
45. Eppinger, H. (1902) Beiträge zur normalen und pathol Histologie der menschlichen Gallencapillaren mit bes. Berücksichtigung der Pathogenese des Ikterus. *Beiträge zur Pathologischen Anatomie*, **31**, 230–295.
46. Epstein, E.Z. (1932) Cholesterol of the blood plasma in hepatic and biliary disease. *Archives of Internal Medicine*, **50**, 203–222.
46. Felker, T.E. & Hamilton, R.L. (1977) Secretion of plasma lipoproteins by perfused livers of cholestatic rats. *Journal of Cell Biology*, **75**, 375a (abstract).
48. Felker, T.E., Fainarua, M., Hamilton, R.L. & Havel, R.J. (1977) Secretion of the arginine-rich and A-I apolipoproteins by the isolated perfused rat liver. *Journal of Lipid Research*, **18**, 465–473.
49. Fex, G. & Wallinder, L. (1973) Liver and plasma cholesteryl ester metabolism after partial hepatectomy in the rat. *Biochimica et Biophysica Acta*, **316**, 91–97.
50. Flint, A. Jr (1862) Experimental researches into a new excretory function of the liver: consisting in the removal of cholesterine from the blood, and its discharge from the body in the form of stercorine. *American Journal of Medical Science*, **44**, 305–365.
51. Forte, T., Nichols, A., Glomset, J. & Norum, K. (1974) The ultrastructure of plasma lipoproteins in lecithin : cholesterol acyl transferase deficiency. *Scandinavian Journal of Clinical and Laboratory Investigation*, **33** (Suppl. 137), 121–132.
52. Fredrickson, D.S. & Levy, R.I. (1972) Familial hyperlipoproteinemia. In *The Metabolic Basis of Inherited Disease* (Ed.) Stanbury, J.B., Wyngaarden, J.B. & Fredrickson, D.S. 3rd ed., Ch. 28, pp. 545–614. New York: McGraw-Hill.
53. Fredrickson, D.S., Gotto, A.M. & Levy, R.I. (1972) Familial lipoprotein deficiency (abetalipoproteinemia, hypobetalipoproteinemia, and Tangier disease). In *The Metabolic Basis of Inherited Disease* (Ed.) Stanbury, J.B., Wyngaarden, J.B. & Fredrickson, D.S. 3rd ed. pp. 493–530. New York: McGraw-Hill.
54. Fredrickson, D.S., Loud, A.V., Hinkelman, B.T., Schneider, H.S. & Frantz, I.D. Jr (1954) The effect of ligation of the common bile duct on cholesterol synthesis in the rat. *Journal of Experimental Medicine*, **99**, 43–53.
55. Friedman, M. & Byers, S.O. (1955) Observations concerning the production and excretion of cholesterol in mammals. XVI. The relationship of the liver to the content and control of plasma cholesterol ester. *Journal of Clinical Investigation*, **34**, 1369–1374.
56. Furman, R.H. & Conrad, L.L. (1957) Ultracentrifugal characterization of the lipoprotein spectrum in obstructive jaundice: studies of serum lipid relationships in intra- and extrahepatic biliary obstruction. *Journal of Clinical Investigation*, **36**, 713–722.
57. Furman, R.H., Sanbar, S.S., Alaupovic, P., Bradford, R.H. & Howard, R.P. (1964) Studies on the metabolism of radio-iodinated human serum alpha lipoprotein in normal and hyperlipidemic subjects. *Journal of Laboratory and Clinical Medicine*, **63**, 193–204.
58. Gage, S.H. (1920) The free granules (chylomicrons) of the blood as shown by the dark-field microscope. *Cornell Veterinarian*, **10**, 154–158.
59. Gjone, E. & Blomhoff, J.P. (1970) Plasma lecithin–cholesterol acyltransferase in obstructive jaundice. *Scandinavian Journal of Gastroenterology*, **5**, 305–308.
60. Gjone, E. & Norum, K.R. (1970) Plasma lecithin–cholesterol acyltransferase and erythrocyte lipids in liver disease. *Acta Medica Scandinavica*, **187**, 153–161.
61. Gjone, E. & Orning, O.M. (1966) Plasma phospholipids in patients with liver disease. *Scandinavian Journal of Clinical and Laboratory Investigation*, **18**, 209–216.
62. Gjone, E., Blomhoff, J.P. & Wiencke, I. (1971) Plasma lecithin : cholesterol acyltransferase activity in acute hepatitis. *Scandinavian Journal of Gastroenterology*, **6**, 161–168.
63. Glomset, J.A. (1962) The mechanism of the plasma cholesterol esterification reaction: plasma fatty acid transferase. *Biochimica et Biophysica Acta*, **65**, 128–135.
64. Glomset, J.A. (1968) The plasma lecithin : cholesterol acyltransferase reaction. *Journal of Lipid Research*, **9**, 155–167.
65. Glomset, J.A., Norum, J.R., Nichols, A.V., King, W.C., Mitchell, C.D., Applegate, K.R., Gong, E.L. & Gjone, E. (1975) Plasma lipoproteins in familial lecithin :cholesterol acyltransferase deficiency: effects of dietary manipulation. *Scandinavian Journal of Clinical and Laboratory Investigation*, **35** (Suppl. 142), 1–55.
66. Gofman, J.W., De Lalla, O., Glazier, F., Freeman, N.K., Lindgren, F.T., Nichols, A.V., Strisower, B. & Tamplin, A.R. (1954) The serum lipoprotein transport system in health, metabolic disorders, atherosclerosis and coronary heart disease. *Plasma*, **2**, 413–484.
67. Goldstein, J.L. & Brown, M.S. (1973) Familial hypercholesterolemia: identification of a defect in the regulation of 3-hydroxy-3-methylglutaryl coenzyme A reductase activity associated with overproduction of cholesterol. *Proceedings of the National Academy of Science of the United States of America*, **70**, 2804–2808.
68. Goldstein, J.L. & Brown, M.S. (1977) Atherosclerosis: the low density lipoprotein receptor hypothesis. *Metabolism*, **26**, 1257–1275.
69. Gregory, P.B. & Beck, R. (1973) Lecithin metabolism during experimental cholestasis in the rat. *Gastroenterology*, **65**, 543 (abstract).
70. Greten, H., Degrella, R., Klose, G., Rascher, W., de Gennes, J.L. & Gjone, E. (1976) Measurement of two plasma triglyceride lipases by an immunochemical method: studies in patients with hypertriglyceridemia. *Journal of Lipid Research*, **17**, 203–210.
71. Hamilton, R.L. (1972) Synthesis and secretion of plasma lipoproteins. *Advances in Experimental Biology and Medicine*, **26**, 7–24.
72. Hamilton, R.L., Havel, R.J., Kane, J.P., Blaurock, A.E. & Sata, T. (1971) Cholestasis: lamellar structure of the abnormal human serum lipoprotein. *Science*, **172**, 475–478.
73. Hamilton, R.L., Williams, M.C., Fielding, C.J. & Havel, R.J. (1976) Discoidal bilayer structure of

nascent high density lipoproteins from perfused rat liver. *Journal of Clinical Investigation,* **58,** 667–680.

74. Hanson, K.C., Deal, J., Schmidt, G. & Brunworth, D. (1974) Effect of clofibrate on hepatic, biliary and serum lipids in the rat. *Gastroenterology,* **64,** 740 (abstract).
75. Harry, D.S., Dini, M. & McIntyre, N. (1973) Effect of cholesterol feeding and biliary obstruction on hepatic cholesterol biosynthesis in the rat. *Biochimica et Biophysica Acta,* **296,** 209–220.
76. Havel, R.J., Shore, V.G., Shore, B. & Bier, D.M. (1970) Role of specific glycopeptides of human serum lipoproteins in the activation of lipoprotein lipase. *Circulation Research,* **27,** 595–600.
77. Johansson, B.G. & Medhus, A. (1974) Increase in plasma α-lipoproteins in chronic alcoholics after acute abuse. *Acta Medica Scandinavica,* **195,** 273–277.
78. Kepkay, D.L., Poon, R. & Simon, J.B. (1973) Lecithin : cholesterol acyl transferase and serum cholesterol esterification in obstructive jaundice. *Journal of Laboratory and Clinical Medicine,* **81,** 172–181.
79. Klor, U., Ditschuneit, H.H., Rakow, D. & Ditschuneit, H. (1972) Further characterisation of dyslipoproteinaemia in hepatic disease. *European Journal of Clinical Investigation,* **2,** 291 (abstract).
80. Korn, E.D. (1955) Clearing factor, a heparin-activated lipoprotein lipase. *The Journal of Biological Chemistry,* **215,** 1–14.
81. Kostner, G.M., Laggner, P., Prexl, H.J. & Holasek, A. (1976) Investigation of the abnormal low-density lipoproteins occurring in patients with obstructive jaundice. *Biochemical Journal,* **157,** 401–407.
82. Kunkel, H.G. & Ahrens, E.H. Jr (1949) The relationship between serum lipids and the electrophoretic pattern, with particular reference to patients with primary biliary cirrhosis. *Journal of Clinical Investigation,* **28,** 1575–1579.
83. Lachmann, D. & Eder, G. (1977) LP-X in mature and premature newborn infants. In *Protides of Biological Fluids* (Ed.) Peeters, H. Vol. 25, pp. 337–340. Oxford: Pergamon Press.
84. La Rosa, J.C., Levy, R.I., Hervert, P.N., Lux, S.E. & Fredrickson, D.S. (1970) A specific apoprotein activator for lipoprotein lipase. *Biochemical and Biophysical Research Communications,* **41,** 57–62.
85. La Rosa, J.C., Levy, R.I., Windmueller, H.G. & Fredrickson, D.S. (1972) Comparison of the triglyceride lipase of liver, adipose tissue, and postheparin plasma. *Journal of Lipid Research,* **13,** 356–363.
86. Lo, C.-H. & Marsh, J.B. (1970) Biosynthesis of plasma lipoproteins. Incorporation of 14C-glucosamine by cells and subcellular fractions of rat liver. *Journal of Biological Chemistry,* **245,** 5001–5006.
87. Lossow, W.J., Shah, S.N., Brot, N. & Chaikoff, I.L. (1963) Effect of ethionine treatment on esterification in vitro of free (4–^{14}C) cholesterol by rat plasma. *Biochimica et Biophysica Acta,* **70,** 593–595.
88. Machebouef, M.M.A. (1929) Recherches sur les phosphoaminolipides et les stérides du sérum et du plasma sanguins: entraînement des phospholipides, des stérols et des stérides par les diverses fractions au cours du fractionnement des protéides du sérum. *Bulletin Société de Chimie et de Biologie,* **11,** 268–293.
89. Magnani, H.N. & Alaupovic, P. (1976) Utilisation of the quantitative assay of lipoprotein-X in the differential diagnosis of extrahepatic and intrahepatic diseases. *Gastroenterology,* **71,** 87–93.
90. Mahley, R.H., Bersot, T.P. & Lequire, V.S. (1970) Identity of very low density lipoprotein apoproteins of plasma and liver Golgi apparatus. *Science,* **168,** 380–382.
91. Mahley, R.W., Bennett, B.D., Morre, D.J., Gray, M.E., Thistlethwaite, W. & Lequire, V.S. (1971) Lipoproteins associated with the Golgi apparatus isolated from epithelial cells of rat small intestine. *Laboratory Investigation,* **25,** 435–444.
92. Man, E.B., Kartin, B.L., Durlacher, S.H. & Peters, J.B. (1945) The lipids of serum and liver in patients with hepatic diseases. *Journal of Clinical Investigation,* **24,** 623–643.
93. McIntyre, N., Calandra, S. & Pearson, A.J.G. (1974) Lipid and lipoprotein abnormalities in liver disease: the possible role of lecithin : cholesterol acyltransferase deficiency. *Scandinavian Journal of Clinical and Laboratory Investigation,* **33** (Suppl. 137), 115–120.
94. McIntyre, N., Harry, D.S. & Pearson, A.J.G. (1975) The hypercholesterolaemia of obstructive jaundice. *Gut,* **16,** 379–391.
95. Milewski, B. & Palynyczko, Z. (1975) Evaluation of the usefulness of serum lipoprotein-X (LP-X) detection test for the diagnosis of cholestasis in chronic liver diseases. *Polish Archives of Medicine,* **53,** 445–452.
96. Mukherjee, S., Kunitake, G. & Alfin-Slater, R.B. (1958) The esterification of cholesterol with palmitic acid by rat liver homogenates. *Journal of Biological Chemistry,* **230,** 91–96.
97. Muller, A.D., van Doorm, J.M. & Hemker, H.C. (1977) Heparin-like inhibitor of blood coagulation in normal newborn. *Nature,* **267,** 616–617.
98. Müller, P., Fellin, R., Lambrecht, J., Agostini, B., Wieland, H., Rost, W. & Seidel, D. (1974) Hypertriglyceridaemia secondary to liver disease. *European Journal of Clinical Investigation,* **4,** 419–428.
99. Nakaya, N., Chung, B.H., Patsch, J.R., Taunton, D.D. (1977) Synthesis and release of low density lipoprotein by the isolated perfused pig liver. *Journal of Biological Chemistry,* **252,** 7530–7532.
100. Nicolau, G., Shefer, S., Salen, G. & Mosbach, E.H. (1974) Regulation of cholesterol and bile acid synthesis in patients with gallstones and biliary obstruction. *Hepatologie,* **5,** 231 (abstract).
101. Nordby, G., Berg, T., Nilsson, M. & Norum, K.R. (1976) Secretion of lecithin : cholesterol acyltransferase from isolated rat hepatocytes. *Biochimica et Biophysica Acta,* **450,** 69–77.
102. Norum, K.R. & Gjone, E. (1967) Familial plasma lecithin : cholesterol acyltransferase deficiency. Biochemical study of a new inborn error of metabolism. *Scandinavian Journal of Clinical and Laboratory Investigation,* **20,** 231–243.
103. Norum, K.R., Glomset, J.A. & Gjone, E. (1972) Familial lecithin:cholesterol acyltransferase deficiency. In *The Metabolic Basis of Inherited Disease* (Ed.) Stanbury, J.B., Wyngaarden, J.B. & Fredrickson, D.S. 3rd ed. Ch. 27, pp. 531–544. New York: McGraw-Hill.
104. Norum, K.R., Glomset, J.A., Nichols, A.V. & Forte, T. (1971) Plasma lipoproteins in familial lecithin : cholesterol acyltransferase deficiency: physical and chemical studies of low and high density lipoproteins. *Journal of Clinical Investigation,* **50,** 1131–1140.
105. Orlandi, F. (1975) personal communication.

106. Osuga, T. & Portman, O.W. (1971) Origin and disappearance of plasma lecithin : cholesterol acyltransferase. *American Journal of Physiology*, **220**, 735–741.

107. Owen, J.S. & McIntyre, N. (1978) Erythrocyte lipid composition and sodium transport in human liver disease. *Biochimica et Biophysica Acta*, **510**, 168–176.

108. Papadopoulos, N.M. & Charles, M.A. (1970) Serum lipoprotein patterns in liver disease. *Proceedings of the Society for Experimental Biology and Medicine*, **134**, 797–799

109. Patsch, J.R., Patsch, W., Sailor, S. & Braunsteiner, H. (1976) Isolation and partial characterization of two abnormal human plasma lipoproteins: LP-X_1 and LP-X_2. *Biochimica et Biophysica Acta*, **434**, 419–427.

110. Pearson, A.J.G. (1972) Triglycerides in obstructive liver disease. *Abstracts of the 5th meeting of the International Association for the Study of the Liver, Versailles*, p. VI.

111. Pearson, A.J.G., Pyrovolakis, J. & McIntyre, N. (1974) Plasma lipids and lipoprotein changes in acute viral hepatitis. *Digestion*, **10**, 322 (abstract).

112. Peters, J.P. & Man, E.B. (1943) The inter-relations of serum lipids in normal persons. *Journal of Clinical Investigation*, **22**, 707–714.

113. Phillips, G.B. (1960) The lipid composition of serum in patients with liver disease. *Journal of Clinical Investigation*, **39**, 1639–1650.

114. Pierce, F.T. & Gofman, J.W. (1951) Lipoproteins, liver disease and atherosclerosis. *Circulation*, **4**, 25–28.

115. Pierce, F.T., Kimmel, J.R. & Burns, T.W. (1954) Lipoproteins in infectious and serum hepatitis. *Metabolism*, **3**, 228–239.

116. Poley, J.R., Alaupovic, P., Magnani, H.N., Bhatia, M., Smith, E.I. & Campbell, D.P. (1974) Quantitative serum lipoprotein-X (LP-X) before and after cholestyramine (CSM) in the diagnosis of extra-hepatic biliary atresia (EBA). *Gastroenterology*, **66**, 761 (abstract).

117. Pyrovolakis, J., Pearson, A.J.G., Harry, D.S., Martin, M.J. & McIntyre, N. (1975) Elevation of plasma cholesterol by clofibrate in rats with biliary obstruction. In *Drugs and the Liver* (Ed.) Gerok, W. & Sickinger, K. pp. 381–386. Stuttgart: Schattauer Verlag.

118. Quarfordt, S.H. & Jakoi, L. (1973) Alterations of hepatic cholesterol synthesis in rats by lecithin and lecithin cholesterol mesophase infusions. *Gastroenterology*, **65**, 566 (abstract).

119. Quarfordt, S.H., Oelschlaeger, H. & Krigbaum, W.R. (1972) Liquid crystalline lipid in the plasma of humans with biliary obstruction. *Journal of Clinical Investigation*, **51**, 1979–1988.

120. Quarfordt, S.H., Oelschlaeger, H., Krigbaum, W.R., Jakoi, L. & Davis, R. (1973) Effect of biliary obstruction on canine plasma and biliary lipids. *Lipids*, **8**, 522–530.

121. Redgrave, T.G. (1970) Formation of cholesteryl ester-rich particulate lipid during metabolism of chylomicrons. *Journal of Clinical Investigation*, **49**, 465–471.

122. Ritland, S. (1975) Quantitative determination of the abnormal lipoprotein of cholestasis, LP-X, in liver disease. *Scandinavian Journal of Gastroenterology*, **10**, 5–15.

123. Ritland, S., Blomhoff, J.P. & Gjone, E. (1973) Lecithin : cholesterol acyltransferase and lipoprotein-X in liver disease. *Clinica Chimica Acta*, **49**, 251–259.

124. Robinson, D.S. & Wing, D.R. (1971) Studies on tissue clearing factor lipase related to its role in the removal of lipoprotein triglyceride from the plasma. In *Plasma Lipoproteins* (Ed.) Smellie, R.M.S. pp. 123–135. London: Academic Press.

125. Ross, A., Murphy, G.M., Wilkinson, P.A., Mills, G.L. & Sherlock, S. (1970) Occurrence of an abnormal lipoprotein in patients with liver disease. *Gut*, **11**, 1035–1037.

126. Russ, E.M., Raymunt, J. & Barr, D.P. (1956) Lipoproteins in primary biliary cirrhosis. *Journal of Clinical Investigation*, **35**, 133–144.

127. Sabesin, S.M. & Frase, S. (1977) Electron microscopic studies of the assembly, intracellular transport, and secretion of chylomicrons by rat intestine. *Journal of Lipid Research*, **18**, 496–511.

128. Sabesin, S.M., Kuiken, L.B. & Ragland, J.B. (1975) Lipoprotein and lecithin : cholesterol acyltransferase in galactosamine-induced rat liver injury. *Science*, **190**, 1302–1304.

129. Sabesin, S.M., Hawkins, H.L., Kuiken, L. & Ragland, J.B. (1977) Abnormal plasma lipoproteins and lecithin–cholesterol acyltransferase deficiency in alcoholic liver disease. *Gastroenterology*, **72**, 510–518.

130. Scanu, A.M., Edelstein, C. & Klim, P. (1975) Serum lipoproteins. In *The Plasma Proteins* (Ed.) Putman, F.W. Vol. 1, pp. 317–391. New York: Academic Press.

131. Schaffner, F. (1969) Paradoxical elevation of serum cholesterol by clofibrate in patients with primary biliary cirrhosis. *Gastroenterology*, **57**, 253–255.

132. Seidel, D., Alaupovic, P. & Furman, R.H. (1969) A lipoprotein characterizing obstructive jaundice. I. Method for quantitative separation and identification of lipoproteins in jaundiced subjects. *Journal of Clinical Investigation*, **48**, 1211–1223.

133. Seidel, D., Gretz, H. & Ruppert, C. (1973) Significance of the LP-X test in differential diagnosis of jaundice. *Clinical Chemistry*, **19**, 86–91.

134. Seidel, D., Alaupovic, P., Furman, R.H. & McConathy, W.J. (1970) A lipoprotein characterizing obstructive jaundice. II. Isolation and partial characterization of the protein moieties of low-density lipoproteins. *Journal of Clinical Investigation*, **49**, 2396–2407.

135. Seidel, D., Greten, H., Geisen, H.P., Wengeler, H. & Wieland, H. (1972) Further aspects on the characterisation of high and very low density lipoproteins in patients with liver disease. *European Journal of Clinical Investigation*, **2**, 359–364.

136. Shore, B. & Shore, V. (1969) Isolation and characterization of polypeptides of human serum lipoproteins. *Biochemistry*, **8**, 4510–4516.

137. Simon, J.B. & Boyer, J.L. (1971) Production of lecithin : cholesterol acyltransferase by the isolated perfused rat liver. *Biochimica et Biophysica Acta*, **218**, 549–551.

138. Simon, J.B. & Schieg, R. (1970) Serum cholesterol esterification in liver disease: importance of lecithin : cholesterol acyltransferase. *New England Journal of Medicine*, **283**, 841–846.

139. Sniderman, A.D., Carew, T.E., Chandler, J.G. & Steinberg, D. (1974) Paradoxical increase in rate of catabolism of low-density lipoproteins after hepatectomy. *Science*, **183**, 526–528.

140. Soutar, A.K., Myant, N.B. & Thompson, G.R. (1977) Simultaneous measurements of apolipoprotein B

turnover in very low and low density lipoproteins in familial hypercholesterolaemia. *Atherosclerosis*, **28**, 247–256.

141. Sperry, U.M. (1935) Cholesterol esterase in blood. *Journal of Biological Chemistry*, **111**, 467–478.

142. Stakeberg, H., Lundborg, H. & Schersten, T. (1974) Rate of in vitro incorporation of precursors into hepatic lipids and proteins in patients with extrahepatic cholestasis. *European Journal of Clinical Investigation*, **4**, 399–403.

143. Stein, O. & Stein, Y. (1973) Colchicine-induced inhibition of very low density lipoprotein release by rat liver in vivo. *Biochimica et Biophysica Acta*, **306**, 142–147.

144. Stein, O., Alkan, M. & Stein, Y. (1973) Obstructive jaundice lipoprotein particles studied in ultrathin sections of livers of bile duct-ligated mice. *Laboratory Investigation*, **29**, 166–172.

145. Sugano, M., Hori, K. & Wada, M. (1969) Hepatotoxicity and plasma cholesterol esterification by rats. *Archives of Biochemistry*, **129**, 588–596.

146. Switzer, S. (1967) Plasma lipoproteins in liver disease: 1. Immunologically distinct low-density lipoproteins in patients with biliary obstruction. *Journal of Clinical Investigation*, **46**, 1855–1866.

147. Takahashi, Z. & Muto, Y. (1968) The importance of lecithin: cholesterol acyltransferase in diseases of the liver and biliary tree (in Japanese). *Japanese Journal of Gastroenterology*, **65**, 1139–1142.

148. Thalassinos, N., Hatzioannou, J., Scliros, Ph., Kanaghinis, T., Anastasiou, C., Crocos, P., Thomopoulos, D. & Gardikas, C. (1975) Plasma α-lipoprotein pattern in acute viral hepatitis. *American Journal of Digestive Diseases*, **20**, 148–155.

149. Thannhauser, S.J. & Magendantz, H. (1938) The different clinical groups of xanthomatous diseases: a clinical physiological study of 22 cases. *Annals of Internal Medicine*, **11**, 1662–1746.

150. Thomas, P.K. & Walker, J.G. (1965) Xanthomatous neuropathy in primary biliary cirrhosis. *Brain*, **88**, 1079–1088.

151. Thompson, G.R., Jadhav, A., Nava, M. & Gotto, A.M. Jr (1976) Effects of intravenous phospholipid on low-density lipoprotein turnover in man. *European Journal of Clinical Investigation*, **6**, 241–248.

152. Turnberg, L.A., Mahoney, M.P., Gleeson, M.H., Freeman, C.B. & Gowenlock, A.H. (1972) Plasmaphoresis and plasma exchange in the treatment of hyperlipaemia and xanthomatous neuropathy in patients with primary biliary cirrhosis. *Gut*, **13**, 976–981.

153. Turner, K.B., McCormack, G.H. & Richards, A. (1953) The cholesterol-esterifying enzymes of human serum. I. In liver disease. *Journal of Clinical Investigation*, **32**, 801–806.

154. Tytgat, G.N., Rubin, C. & Saunders, D.R. (1971) Synthesis and transport of lipoprotein particles by intestinal absorptive cells in man. *Journal of Clinical Investigation*, **50**, 2065–2078.

155. Utermann, G., Schoenborn, W., Langer, K.H. & Dicker, P. (1972) Lipoproteins in LCAT-deficiency. *Humangenetik*, **16**, 295–306.

156. Van Deenen, L.L.M. & de Gier, J. (1974) Lipids of the red cell membrane. In *The Red Blood Cell* (Ed.) Surgenor, D.M. Ch. 4, pp. 147–211. New York: Academic Press.

157. Van Itallie, T.B., Hashim, S.A., Crampton, R.S. & Tennent, D.M. (1961) The treatment of pruritus and hypercholesterolemia of primary biliary cirrhosis with cholestyramine. *New England Journal of Medicine*, **265**, 469–474.

158. Van Tol, A., van Gent, T. & van't Hooft, F.M. (1977) Low density lipoprotein catabolism in the liver: decrease of fractional catabolic rate after partial hepatectomy. In *Protides of Biological Fluids* (Ed.) Peeters, H. Vol. 25, pp. 197–200. Oxford: Pergamon Press.

159. Vergani, C., Pietrogrande, M. & Grondona, M.C. (1973) Study of the abnormal lipoprotein-X in obstructive and non-obstructive jaundice. *Clinica Chimica Acta*, **48**, 243–248.

160. Widal, F., Weill, A. & Laudat, M. (1912) La lipémie des brightiques: rapports de la rétinite des brightiques avec l'azotémie et la cholestérolémie. *Semaine Médicale*, **32**, 529–531.

161. Windmueller, H.G., Herbert, P.N. & Levy, R.I. (1973) Biosynthesis of lymph and plasma lipoprotein apoproteins by isolated perfused rat liver and intestine. *Journal of Lipid Research*, **14**, 215–233.

Chapter 5

Protein Metabolism and the Liver

A.S. TAVILL

The liver is of importance in protein and amino acid metabolism by virtue of a number of fundamental structural and functional properties. Located astride the portal vein it is uniquely subjected to large fluxes in dietary amino acid supply. These amino acids are processed to meet the needs of protein synthesis by the liver itself and by the peripheral tissues, predominantly muscle. In addition, it is a recipient of amino acids returning from the periphery which participate in transamination reactions, in gluconeogenesis and in metabolic degradation. Ureagenesis which is the concomitant reaction of gluconeogenesis from amino acids is a unique hepatic function whereby a non-toxic, rapidly filterable product of obligatory tissue and dietary nitrogen catabolism can be eliminated from the body. The quantitative analysis of the foregoing reactions indicates a remarkable capacity of the liver to modulate protein turnover and amino acid metabolism in response to changes in dietary nitrogen supply. In this way it imposes a high degree of control on plasma and tissue amino acid fluxes, and thereby on protein synthesis and gluconeogenesis. In both acute and chronic liver disease this control may be disturbed by hepatocyte dysfunction and portasystemic shunting. The resultant changes in amino acid metabolism may play a role in portasystemic encephalopathy and have prompted a rational approach to parenteral amino acid therapy in such patients.[2]

This chapter will attempt to deal with the quantitative and qualitative aspects of the hepatic role in protein metabolism in the context of dietary nitrogen supply, overall body protein metabolism and carbohydrate–protein interactions. It will also cover some of the special functions of the liver in plasma protein metabolism and will address itself to both specific and non-specific mechanisms of regulation of their synthesis and degradation. Since the liver makes a major contribution to protein synthesis by way of secretion into the plasma compartment, the concepts of control of protein synthesis as it may be exerted at transcriptional, translational, post-translational and secretory sites will be summarized for certain selected proteins. This section will include a discussion of major factors responsible for regulation in the normal state and of certain injurious agents which may disturb normal homeostasis in disease states. Thus recent research on the effects of alcohol on protein metabolism has revealed defects in the secretory pathway in addition to ribosomal changes. In particular, specific proteins have been selected because of their relevance to the pathogenesis or diagnosis of certain human disease states and because changes in their plasma concentrations and pool masses have recently been explained in molecular terms. This is also the case for some which are not usually regarded as plasma proteins but which are present in the plasma as a result of active synthetic and secretory processes rather than of release from damaged cells. These proteins have also been shown to be of diagnostic value in hepatic disease and recent advances have been made in our understanding of their molecular pathophysiology.

QUANTITATIVE ASPECTS OF BODY PROTEIN METABOLISM

Hepatic Amino Acid Fluxes: Role of Dietary, Gastrointestinal and Tissue Nitrogen

Total body protein in an average 70 kg adult is approximately 12 kg turning over at a rate of about 200 to 300 g/day.[52,192,204] In the steady state this represents the synthesis and degradation of an equal amount of protein with the attendant fluxes of amino acids utilized and released by these processes. As will be discussed later, part of these fluxes occurs locally at a tissue level. Thus in conditions of normal dietary supply both liver and muscle utilize amino acids released by local protein degradation for up to 50 per cent of their synthetic requirements. When dietary nitrogen is restricted this may be increased to 90 per cent.[43,44]

As discussed by Fauconneau and Michel,[36] the body amino acid pool receives contributions from the degradation of about 250 g of body protein plus dietary protein which is completely hydrolysed to amino acids in the process of digestion and intestinal absorption. In addition, total body protein turnover includes endogenous secretion of enzyme proteins, exfoliated cellular protein and a relatively small exudative loss of plasma protein into the lumen of the gastrointestinal tract. These largely undergo enterohepatic recycling by way of the common digestive–absorptive pathway, the resultant amino acids mixing and losing their identity with those derived from dietary protein. Amino acids entering the portal vein originate from approximately 90 g of dietary protein, 50 g of exfoliated cellular protein, 16 g of secreted enzyme protein and 1 to 2 g of exuded plasma protein.

The liver plays a special role in the utilization and processing of dietary amino acids by virtue of its unique position in the portal venous circulation. Following a protein meal there are large changes in amino acid concentration in portal venous blood which are not mirrored by those occurring in the peripheral blood. Dogs fed a casein meal increased portal venous leucine concentration by 450 per cent in the absorptive period with only a 40 per cent increase in peripheral blood.[25] As indicated above there are selective differences in hepatic amino acid uptake and metabolism with a relative barrier to branched chain amino acids (BCAA) which are metabolized predominantly by muscle. These amino acids are valine, isoleucine and leucine which account for more than 60 per cent of the total amino acids appearing in the systemic blood although they represent only 20 per cent of amino acids in dietary protein.[187]

The fate of the amino acids arriving via the portal vein has been evaluated experimentally by Elwyn[32] in dogs by means of selective cannulation of the portal and hepatic veins and the hepatic artery. Total amino acid fluxes were measured in both the non-absorptive (12 midnight to 12 noon) period and in the absorptive period following a large protein meal (12 noon to 12 midnight). Calculation of net balance of nitrogen in this system indicated that 57 per cent of incoming nitrogen in the absorptive period is converted to urea, 6 per cent is utilized for plasma protein synthesis, 14 per cent is utilized for endogenous hepatic protein synthesis and 23 per cent is passed on to the peripheral blood as amino acids. In the non-absorptive period the picture changes. Since there is still enterohepatic recycling of amino acids from secreted and exfoliated protein, inflow via the portal vein continues at about one-sixth of the absorptive level. Urea synthesis falls to about one-third and net amino acid release virtually ceases. In fact, there is net uptake from the periphery, largely as alanine. Hepatic tissue protein now goes into a catabolic phase and together with amino acids released from muscle makes a contribution to gluconeogenesis and ureagenesis. Plasma protein synthesis, on the other hand, seems to be relatively well buffered from these major short-term changes in amino acid supply and continues at a normal rate with little circadian variation (Table 5.1).[32,124]

The events related to a protein meal outlined above are mediated through a variety of enzymes concerned with intermediary amino acid metabolism.[72] These are concerned largely with gluconeogenesis, ureagenesis, transamination and synthesis of non-essential amino acids. For example, it has been shown that parallel

Table 5.1. *Hepatic Amino Acid Economy.*

Process	Dietary phase Absorptive mmol (g)	Non-absorptive mmol (g)
Hepatic uptake:		
Portal vein	1700 (23.8)	300 (4.20)
Hepatic artery	0	50 (0.70)
Hepatic release:		
Free amino acids	400 (5.60)	0
Urea	970 (13.6)	300 (4.20)
Plasma proteins	100 (1.40)	100 (1.40)
Hepatic protein anabolism (+) or catabolism (−)	230 (3.22)	−50 (−0.70)

Disposition of absorbed amino acids (mmol [g] N/kg of liver) by the dog liver. The absorptive phase after a high protein intake at midday (12 midday to 12 midnight) is compared to the non-absorptive phase (12 midnight to 12 midday). During the absorptive period there is no amino acid uptake from the hepatic arterial blood. Rather there is release into the hepatic vein for utilization by peripheral tissues. There is net utilization of absorbed amino acids for hepatic protein synthesis. In the non-absorptive period there is hepatic arterial uptake and release to the hepatic vein ceases. Urea synthesis falls to one-third and hepatic protein goes into a catabolic phase releasing amino acid to the periphery (hence the negative sign). Utilization of amino acids for plasma protein synthesis remains relatively unaffected by circadian variations in amino acid fluxes. Adapted from Elwyn.[32]

changes occur for the hepatic activity of amino acid degradative enzymes such as serine dehydratase (which catalyses the non-oxidative deamination of serine to pyruvate and ammonia) and a number of gluconeogenic enzymes concerned with the utilization of pyruvate. These changes may be induced by a high protein, low carbohydrate intake and glucagon, both of which are powerful promoters of gluconeogenesis. Enhanced gluconeogenesis is also associated with increased activity of hepatic glutamic-alanine transaminase and glutamic-aspartic transaminase. These effects are largely suppressed by feeding of glucose. Another example is tyrosine transaminase which undergoes fluctuations of 600 per cent in activity in relation to the ingestion of a high protein meal.[191]

Similarly, the influences of diet on ureagenesis can be related to changes in the activity of the various enzymes of the urea cycle. Four of these, carbamyl phosphate synthetase, ornithine transcarbamylase, arginino-succinate synthetase and arginino-succinase, are concerned with synthesis of arginine and their synthesis is induced by dietary protein, while the fifth, arginase, which is concerned with arginine breakdown to urea, is increased in activity under the influence of dietary protein by virtue of inhibition of its degradation.[155] These changes are contrasted with the decreased activity of branched chain amino acid (BCAA) transaminase in muscle with increases in dietary protein.[103] This transaminase is a single enzyme for all three BCAA, is present in high specific activity in muscle and is responsible for the initial step in BCAA degradation.

As indicated by Munro,[113] the absence of large changes in systemic plasma amino acid concentrations in response to the major influx of amino acids from the gut, and a total plasma pool of amino acids which is about 1/200 the size of this influx indicate a rapid turnover of plasma amino acids. In contrast, the tissue amino acid pool is about half the size of the absorbed amino acid load and consists mainly of glutamic acid, glutamine, alanine and glycine, indicating that the turnover of plasma amino acids is associated with rapid transamination as well as utilization for protein synthesis.

Protein–Carbohydrate Interactions in Liver and Muscle

The integration of carbohydrate and protein metabolism by the mutual interaction of liver and muscle has been described by Felig and his group[40,41] (Figure 5.1; see also Chapter 3). Although the pathological state investigated most fully by these workers was that of the diabetic, their observations have provided insight into the normal handling of dietary protein and the specific fluxes of amino acids between liver and muscle and vice versa.

In the post-absorptive state, for example during an overnight fast, there is net release of amino acids from the protein reservoir in the muscles. Alanine and glutamine are the predominant amino acids released, but since they constitute a relatively small proportion of the amino acid residues in muscle protein their predominance in muscle venous outflow indicates in situ synthesis by transamination of pyruvate. The major nitrogen sources for transamination are the BCAA, leucine, isoleucine and valine. These amino acids are oxidized almost exclusively in muscle, the liver being unable to do this efficiently, and their rate of degradation is quantitatively sufficient to account for all the nitrogen required for alanine synthesis.[116] This explains why the BCAA are released in disproportionately low concentrations from muscle during an overnight fast. In addition, although 60 per cent of the

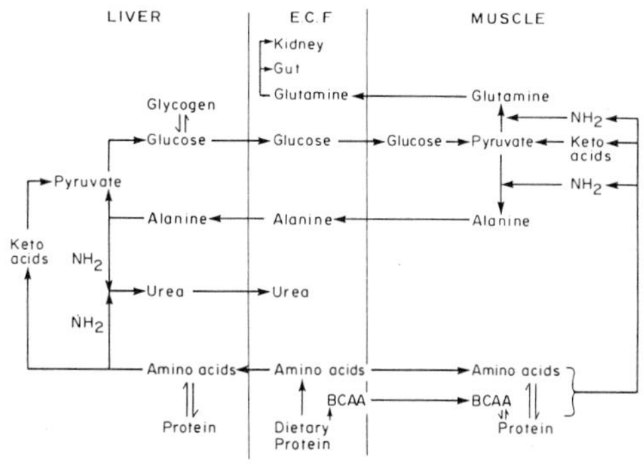

Figure 5.1. Carbohydrate–protein exchange between muscle and liver in normal humans (based upon data presented by Felig[39] and Felig et al[41]). After an overnight fast there is net release of amino acids by muscle predominantly as alanine and glutamine. These are derived by transamination of pyruvate, the carbon skeletons being provided by both degraded amino acids and glucose. Branched chain amino acids (BCAA) are particularly important in the provision of nitrogen for alanine synthesis, and also possibly the carbon skeletons. Alanine is utilized for gluconeogenesis by the liver and urea is formed as a by-product. The kidney and the gut are the main sites of uptake of glutamine where it is used for ammonia production and as a possible source of energy respectively. Following dietary protein ingestion muscle goes into an anabolic phase, there is selective hepatic escape and muscle uptake of dietary BCAA, reduced muscle output of alanine and glutamine, and a reduced rate of hepatic gluconeogenesis. Hepatic tissue protein also goes into an anabolic phase following protein ingestion. However, although about 14 per cent of dietary amino acids are used for hepatic protein synthesis up to 50 to 60 per cent may be deaminated to urea and keto acid analogues.

pyruvate required for alanine synthesis is provided by glycolysis, there is a contribution from BCAA. It is apparent that BCAA undergo degradation as a source of energy for muscle, for the provision of both the carbon skeletons for pyruvate and the nitrogen required for its transamination to alanine. The net flux of alanine is largely mopped up by the liver where its carbon skeleton becomes a source of glucose[17] and its nitrogen undergoes transamination or ureagenesis. In calorie deprivation alanine is rate-limiting in gluconeogenesis. The glutamine released by muscle during an overnight fast is largely taken up by the kidney as a source of ammonia, and the gut for energy.

Repletion of muscle protein occurs after protein feeding. Again, the BCAA play a unique role in reversing the negative nitrogen balance induced by fasting. As mentioned above, although they constitute only 20 per cent of dietary amino acids they account for more than 60 per cent of the amino acids entering the systemic circulation after a protein meal and subsequently are the predominant source of amino acid uptake by muscle.[187] As with dietary protein they comprise only 20 per cent of the amino acid residues in muscle. These findings indicate that there is selective exclusion by the liver of BCAA derived from dietary protein, together with selective uptake by muscle where they provide a source not only for repletion of protein but also for energy. The observations outlined above have led Felig[39] to propose the concept of the glucose–alanine cycle in which glucose released by the liver is first converted to pyruvate and thence transaminated to alanine. In turn, alanine released by muscle is taken up by the liver where it is the major amino acid source for gluconeogenesis and ureagenesis. During fasting, however, this cycle alone cannot account for net synthesis of glucose. In these circumstances, there is breakdown of muscle protein which becomes a major source of gluconeogenic amino acids, and transamination of incoming amino acids to alanine and glutamine.[23,45] It has been calculated by Daniel, Pratt and Spargo[24] that in order to account for the release of gluconeogenic amino acids during the post-absorptive period there must be net loss of 39 ± 4 g/day of muscle protein in a 70 kg man.

From observations in the diabetic it has been possible to formulate a role for insulin in the overall schema outlined above. The negative nitrogen balance and excessive protein catabolism of the insulin-dependent diabetic is associated with exaggerated gluconeogenesis. Evidence has been provided that the liver of the fasted diabetic takes up alanine at an excessive rate which contributes up to 40 per cent to gluconeogenesis compared with 20 per cent normally. This is associated with an accelerated rate of BCAA catabolism in muscle. During protein feeding there is impaired uptake of BCAA by muscle, excessive alanine release, and a concomitant aggravation of hyperglycaemia because of inappropriate hepatic glucose production. In this way, insulin deficiency has inevitable consequences for muscle anabolism and catabolism, for disposition of dietary amino acids and for hepatic gluconeogenesis. In these respects, glucagon has virtually opposite effects to insulin, possibly contributing to excessive and inappropriate gluconeogenesis and ureagenesis and to tissue protein catabolism.

Dietary Protein Requirements

Guidelines for human dietary protein requirements, reviewed by Munro[114] and Waterlow and Payne,[193] have been set down by expert committees of the FAO/WHO on the basis of two methods of calculation. The 'factorial' method is based upon addition of all the factors of obligatory nitrogen loss from the body at zero nitrogen intake. The second method quantifies the minimum requirements for achievement of nitrogen balance (plus optimal growth rates in children). Reasonably close agreement has been observed between the two techniques; the average minimum requirement for adults is 0.45 g protein/kg body weight. Greatly increased needs occur in infancy and childhood and at all ages during stress. Furthermore, the required ratio of essential : non-essential amino acids changes from about 20 per cent in the adult to 40 per cent in the growing infant and up to as much as 50 per cent in the postoperative state in order to provide for replacement of wasted, diseased or damaged tissue proteins (Table 5.2). The low requirements of essential amino acids for maintenance reflect their efficient recycling.

Table 5.2. *Human Dietary Protein and Essential Amino Acid Requirements as a Function of Age and Disease.*

Category	Protein requirements (mg/kg/day) As total amino acid	As essential amino acid	Essential as % of total
Infant	1700	680	40
Child (10–12 y)	700	260	36
Adult	450	85	19
Disease:			
Adult (postoperative)	2000–3000	500–1500	25–50
Adult (uraemia)	400	100–200	25–50

Adapted from Munro.[114]

Another consideration in the calculation of protein requirements is the utilization value of dietary protein. Egg protein with an ideal balance of amino acids has the maximum utilization value of close to 100 per cent. On a typical western diet containing proteins of mixed animal and vegetable origin averaging 75 to 80 per cent utilization, the minimum intake needed to maintain nitrogen balance is about 42 g for a 70 kg adult. This may be decreased deliberately under special circumstances by providing a diet of high utilization value. This is the basis of the Giordano–Giovanetti diet, for patients with chronic renal failure which aims to reduce intake to about 32 g/day for a 70 kg patient (Table 5.2).

The factorial method for calculation of protein requirements gives an indication of the adaptation to protein restriction (Table 5.3). The main response occurs within about 7 to 10 days of total protein withdrawal; namely, there is a reduction in urinary nitrogen excretion to an

Table 5.3. *Dietary Protein Requirements Based upon Factorial Method of Calculation.*[a]

Source	Losses (N/kg b.w.) mmol (mg)
Urine	2.64 (37)
Faeces	0.86 (12)
Skin	0.21 (3)
Miscellaneous	0.14–0.21 (2–3)
Total loss at zero intake =	3.86 (54)

[a] From total losses of nitrogen from the body at zero nitrogen intake.
Adapted from Munro.[114]

average of 2.64 mmol/kg (37 mg/kg) body weight which is the amount released by total catabolism of 16 g of protein in a 70 kg adult. This is about one-fifth of that lost via the kidneys when dietary protein intake is 90 g/day. In contrast, there is little change in faecal nitrogen excretion which represents residual endogenous losses arising from bacterial proteins, exfoliated intestinal cells and unabsorbed secretions. Using the data given by Young and Scrimshaw[203] and Calloway and Margen[19] these add up to about 0.85 mmol (12 mg) of nitrogen/kg body weight. Losses through the skin show some adaptation, plateauing at about 0.21 mmol/kg (3 mg/kg), while miscellaneous losses through other minor routes make up the total of 3.86 mmol (54 mg) N/kg. Translated into dietary protein this comes to 24 g/day for a 70 kg adult. Since this is an average figure with a coefficient of variation of ±15 per cent, it has been increased by 30 per cent to provide guidance for the needs of the majority of the population. In this way, figures of 5.0 mmol (70 mg) N/kg, 0.45 g protein/kg and 32 g protein for a 70 kg adult have been reached for minimum requirements, and such levels of intake guarantee a high margin of safety.

The second technique for evaluation of protein requirements also provides estimates of the requirements for individual amino acids, in particular the essential amino acids. By feeding diets adequate in all other nutrients it is possible to titrate the intake of the essential amino acid under investigation against nitrogen balance and determine the point at which positive balance is just achieved. As pointed out by Munro[111] this technique must make allowance for the influence of other dietary constituents on nitrogen balance, in particular caloric intake. With the changing needs for essential amino acids during development and for recovery from hypercatabolic processes it is comforting to know that most sources of dietary protein, with the exception of wheat flour, will provide an excess of essential amino acids when fed in amounts sufficient to meet total dietary protein needs.

Waterlow and Payne[193] have emphasized that although kwashiorkor is undeniably partly a protein deficiency state there is strong evidence that energy deprivation coexists as part of overall food deprivation. The difference between kwashiorkor and marasmus lies in the relatively increased requirements of malnourished children for protein or energy respectively depending on the presence of various coexisting debilitating diseases. These workers have indicated that most cereal diets available in developing countries where kwashiorkor is common, if consumed in quantities sufficient to satisfy energy requirements, would automatically provide enough protein. Unfortunately, these diets are frequently not consumed in sufficient quantities and the childhood victim of malnutrition is deprived of calories as well as receiving insufficient protein to provide for growth and replacement of obligatory nitrogen losses.

Anabolic Role of Urea

Another potential source of nitrogen available for anabolic purposes by the liver is that which is enterohepatically recycled in the form of urea. Following the demonstration by Walser and Bodenlos[189] that about 20 per cent of the urea synthesized by normal man is degraded in the gastrointestinal tract, several studies have indicated that ammonia nitrogen released by intestinal urease hydrolysis can be utilized for protein synthesis and may play a role in the maintenance of nitrogen balance in patients receiving a minimum amount of dietary essential amino acids.[49,167] Since uraemic patients on a low protein diet adequate in essential amino acids may have a relative deficiency in non-essential amino acids and an increased endogenous supply of ammonia nitrogen derived from hydrolysed urea,[49,135] it is possible that this source of nitrogen may be potentially useful if the efficiency of hepatic recapture is high. This hypothesis has been evaluated in uraemic patients and normal subjects on a restricted protein intake by means of double-labelling of the body urea pool with (^{15}N) urea and (^{14}C) urea.[185] Simultaneous identification of the dynamics of albumin metabolism enabled the calculation to be made of the efficiency of utilization of released urea nitrogen for albumin synthesis. Although the body urea pool was expanded by about fivefold in uraemic patients, the absolute rate of urea degradation in the gut was increased by just over 50 per cent. The rate of utilization of urea nitrogen for albumin synthesis was low and provided on average about 2.4 per cent of the requirements for nitrogen for this purpose, compared with 0.13 per cent in normal subjects. In those patients with renal failure restricted to 30 g of protein per day this rose to 3.1 per cent re-utilization for albumin synthesis. On the assumption that the liver has priority for fixation of ammonia nitrogen and on the basis that albumin constitutes about 25 per cent of all hepatic protein synthesis it appears that utilization of nitrogen from this source is quantitatively an inefficient process and is nutritionally relatively unimportant.

REGULATION OF PROTEIN TURNOVER WITH PARTICULAR EMPHASIS ON ALBUMIN

Concepts and Normal Rates of Turnover

The concept of turnover as it relates to proteins of hepatic origin has been reviewed in detail elsewhere.[177,178] The latter reference also deals with the methods available for measurement of protein synthesis and degradation both in vivo and in vitro. These will not be reviewed in this chapter except where consideration of techniques influences the interpretation of data. However, it is necessary to re-examine the process in this chapter in order to place the liver in its appropriate perspective, namely as an organ undergoing dynamic changes in its protein constituents, and subjected to continuous interaction with other organs which are also carrying out synthesis and degradation of protein, as well as with routes of supply of amino acids and sites of elimination of products of protein breakdown.

Although it was Magendie in 1829 who pointed out the evanescent nature of all living matter, with every organ of the body breaking down and replacing its constituent molecules,[91,110] it was Schoenheimer and his colleagues who, with the aid of the newly available stable isotopes of nitrogen and hydrogen, provided the most precise quantitative data of protein turnover. This group was the first to identify the random turnover of serum proteins and to distinguish it from life-span turnover which occurs in certain body proteins such as haemoglobin and possibly in myofibrillar protein, in which the rate of degradation is governed by the survival of the specialized cell or organelle in which the protein is contained.[157] In contrast, random degradation of both circulating and fixed tissue proteins takes place from a mixed heterogeneous pool of young and old molecules into which synthesis is continually replenishing new protein at a rate adequate to maintain constancy of the pool size.

For didactic purposes turnover will be regarded as consisting of both synthesis and degradation. However, it should be understood that modulation of turnover may stem primarily either from changes in rates of synthesis or of degradation. This varies depending on the modulating factor and on the tissue and even differs from protein to protein within a tissue. Random kinetics of degradation, as demonstrated for serum proteins, imply a first order process[89] which may remain as such even when the system is perturbed by exogenous expansion or contraction of the pool or by change in the rate of synthesis. Under certain circumstances for some proteins fractional rates of degradation may change, suggesting a second order response to perturbation of the system. This occurs for albumin and IgG when depletion is severe enough to produce a fall in plasma concentration. Synthesis, on the other hand, is a zero order process which may respond by relatively abrupt steps when called upon to replace losses or when increased by specific inducing agents. Homeostasis is primarily geared to restoration of steady state metabolic conditions, namely a re-attainment of the balance between synthesis and degradation. As reviewed by Tavill,[177] if synthesis in absolute terms is adjusted to breakdown and the latter occurs at a constant fractional rate, perturbation of either side of the metabolic equation will evoke a response in the opposite side in absolute terms such that a new equilibrium will be established at a lower or higher pool size. In this way the effects of environmental changes, whether these are physiological, such as circadian variations in amino acid supply, or pathological, such as sustained dietary protein deprivation, will be contained and limited by the adjustments evoked in either synthesis or degradation or in both processes. Therefore, in teleological terms the apparent energy wasting mechanisms of degradation provide one means of adaptation to the vagaries of environmental changes which exert effects primarily on synthesis.[156] By the same reasoning the synthetic process is endowed with the potential for dynamic responses to pathological alterations in degradation.

Protein turnover in individual organs can also be thought of as a means of providing amino acids when dietary supply is limited. Either rapidly-turning-over proteins or proteins whose degradation rates can be promptly increased may be regarded as a labile source of amino acids during protein-calorie malnutrition, either for gluconeogenesis or for maintenance of synthesis of priority proteins in the same or different tissues. Likewise, growth is not simply the accretion of protein but involves also qualitative changes in the tissues and alterations in the balance of metabolic activity between organs. Relatively rapid protein turnover in the growing organism is a means for making such developmental changes. Regulatory mechanisms in protein turnover which are responsive to dietary energy or protein supply and to hormonal influences can be predicted for the most part on the basis of the tissue or organ location. Some of these mechanisms will be discussed below in contrast to more specific mechanisms of synthesis and degradation for individual proteins which show unique responses to substrates, drugs, prosthetic groups and ligands. These responses may occasionally have a function-related effect and some of these will be discussed for specialized proteins of hepatic origin.

On a fractional basis the liver is one of the most active protein synthetic organs of the body, surpassed only by intestinal mucosa and pancreas. However, muscle protein with a much lower fractional rate of turnover accounts for the major mass of protein undergoing synthesis and degradation. Total export proteins comprise about 50 per cent of the liver's protein synthesis.[195] The average synthesis of albumin of 12 g/day (in a 70 kg man)[158] constitutes about 25 per cent of total hepatic protein synthesis, i.e., half of the total export protein synthesis.[198] These figures should be compared with those for muscle proteins. Muscle contains approximately 45 per cent of the total body protein, that is about 5.5 kg.[102] Recent data in humans obtained by direct needle biopsies of muscle following a continuous infusion of ^{15}N-labelled lysine have yielded fractional synthetic rates for sarcoplasmic proteins of 3.8 per cent/day and for myofibrillar structural proteins of 1.5 per cent/day.[52] From these data figures were derived for total muscle protein synthesis of 53.2 per cent of total body protein synthesis, which gave an absolute synthesis rate of 130 g/day for a 70 kg body weight, or about three times that of the liver.

Mechanisms of Albumin Synthesis and Secretion

Human plasma albumin is the most abundant circulating protein and exists as a single chain of 575 amino acid residues devoid of a significant carbohydrate component.[123] It functions as the principal transport protein for organic anions of both metabolic and exogenous origin, cations, hormones, tryptophan and fatty acids, in addition to being quantitatively the most important mediator of the plasma colloid osmotic pressure. In spite of these identifiable functional roles it is possible for rare individuals with a congenital inability to synthesize albumin to live relatively normal lives, troubled only by the excessive but variable accumulation of extravascular fluid.[12,42,188] Evidence based upon isolated perfused liver studies and experiments in the hepatectomized dog confirm that the liver is the exclusive site of albumin synthesis.[81,101] The parameters of normal albumin metabolism in humans have been summarized by Rothschild, Oratz and Schreiber.[137] A normal adult synthesizes 120 to 200 mg/kg/day into a total exchangeable pool of 3.5 to 5.0 g/kg body weight, of which 38 to 45 per cent is located intravascularly. The plasma albumin concentration varies between 35 and 45 g/l and is subject to the additional factors modulating distribution as well as those affecting synthesis and degradation.

Mechanisms of synthesis. The polyribosomes attached to the membranes of the rough endoplasmic reticulum are the principal sites of synthesis of albumin destined for export from the hepatocyte.[59,131,176] Although nascent immunoreactive albumin has been identified on free (non-membrane-bound) polyribosomes,[61] it is evident that this represents a minority commitment to overall hepatic albumin production as identification of specific mRNA for albumin has demonstrated that 98 per cent of such sequences is located in membrane-bound polyribosomes.[200] However, under circumstances of short-term fasting this predominant association of albumin mRNA with polyribosomes is drastically reduced and is then found in the cytosol disassociated from polyribosomes and from membrane structures.[201] These workers speculate that this cytosolic albumin mRNA may represent a storage form of ribonucleoprotein available for uptake into reassembled membrane-bound polyribosomes. This suggestion would be in keeping with observations on the relative stability and long half-life of albumin mRNA observed by other workers.[197,198]

The synthesis of albumin is regulated by many of the control mechanisms identified for eukaryotic cells in general. These have been summarized by Munro[113] and Swain and Tavill,[174] and limitations of space prevent comprehensive discussion in this chapter. However, they include the rate of transcription of specific mRNA and availability of rRNA and tRNA. In turn, these may be regulated by activity of polymerases and ribonucleases. At the translational level the integrity and activity of polyribosomes may be regulated by factors affecting initiation, elongation and release as well as by the supply of high energy phosphates, ATP and GTP, and Mg^{++} ions. In the case of secreted proteins like albumin, post-translational factors such as those which govern the ultimate three-dimensional form of the protein may also influence the synthetic process; while the addition of carbohydrate residues to the majority of plasma proteins (other than albumin) may subsequently influence the secretory process. The secretory process itself may come under a variety of regulatory influences and there is progressively accumulating evidence that the events of polypeptide elongation and assembly and those of secretion may be independently controlled. In certain circumstances, however, the formation of a precursor protein within the hepatocyte (which cannot be detected in the plasma) may provide a means for integrating synthesis and secretion. Such an intracellular precursor form of albumin, termed 'proalbumin' has been identified by chromatographic techniques, and has been shown to be formed by an amino-terminal peptide consisting of five or six amino acid residues.[71,129,153,184]

Pathway of secretion. While the 40S ribosomal subunit translates the messenger RNA, the propagating polypeptide chain of the protein is protruded through the larger 60S subunit which is attached to the membrane of the rough endoplasmic reticulum (RER). In this way the amino-terminal completed portion of the nascent protein lies within the cisternae of the endoplasmic vesicle. It takes about 1 to 2 minutes for the ribosome to complete the translation of the 575 nucleotide triplets before the complete protein appears at the membrane of the RER. It subsequently traverses the smooth endoplasmic reticulum and reaches the Golgi apparatus in 15 to 20 minutes.[50,125] Although the liver lacks the capacity to store large quantities of plasma proteins in readiness for secretion, there is evidence that the volume of the Golgi bodies may vary in response to factors which regulate protein synthesis.[50,125] This may account for the bulk of hepatic intracellular albumin (equivalent to about 750 mg in an average 1500 g human liver, as indicated by Rothschild, Oratz and Schreiber).[137] However, calculation of turnover time of this amount of albumin indicates that about two-thirds of functional hepatocytes are probably not engaged in albumin synthesis. These biochemical data are consistent with histochemical and immunocytochemical studies showing that only 10 to 35 per cent of parenchymal cells contain albumin at any point in time.[37,55] It is possible that hepatocytes rotate their synthetic and secretory activity and lie fallow for some time after a burst of synthetic output.

The final phase of secretion involves transport of completed protein from the Golgi body to the plasma membrane. In the case of plasma glycoproteins, the carbohydrate units will have been added sequentially, beginning while the polypeptide is still attached to the ribosome and not reaching completion until it is ready to leave the Golgi body. Vesicles derived from the Golgi apparatus encapsulate the protein and are guided to the periphery by the contraction of the filaments of the microtubular apparatus.[117] Colchicine specifically interferes with this stage of secretion and leads to accumulation of plasma proteins as far back as the cisternae of the RER.[38,132] Although the drug interacts with the microtubules and may bind to the contractile protein, tubulin, it has not been possible to correlate secretory inhibition with depolymerization of tubulin.

Factors which influence total delivery of protein into the circulation may affect the processes of synthesis and secretion quite independently. As will be discussed later in this chapter, alcohol administered acutely to the perfused rabbit liver profoundly affects net synthesis without prolonging intracellular transit time.[138] However, alcohol administered chronically to the rat leads to an accumulation of secretory protein within the hepatocyte, diminished net secretion, but an increase in synthesis as evidenced by enhancement of amino acid incorporation into secretory protein.[10]

Although hepatic lymph of the space of Disse provides a potential milieu for the newly released albumin, it has been shown by differential labelling of newly synthesized albumin and the albumin already equilibrated throughout intravascular and extravascular compartments that the plasma of the sinusoid is the immediate recipient of newly secreted protein.[165] In cirrhosis, although rates of hepatic lymph flow are greatly increased, newly synthesized albumin bypasses both the thoracic duct lymph and the plasma and is lost directly into ascites.[206]

Finally, albumin distributes itself throughout plasma and interstitial fluid, and may appear in a number of secretions. The intravascular : extravascular distribution ratio is approximately 2 : 3. The interstitial spaces of the muscles and skin contain the bulk of extravascular albumin with only about 1 per cent located in the liver.[145] Available interstitial water is also limited by the presence of protein–polysaccharide complexes which prevent homogeneous distribution of soluble macromolecules of the size of albumin.[84] Nevertheless, it has been shown that the small hepatic interstitial albumin compartment is probably the mediator of colloid osmotic control of albumin synthesis.

Osmotic regulation of albumin synthesis. The liver responds to reductions in extravascular colloid osmotic pressure by increasing its rate of synthesis of albumin. The reverse effect can be produced by infusions of gamma globulin and dextran in vivo. Both these manoeuvres lead to a relative increase in extravascular albumin with resultant increase in interstitial oncotic pressure.[143,144] Since only about one-tenth of the hepatic interstitial volume is available for distribution of albumin, this restricted space enhances the effects of translocation of osmotically active macromolecules in terms of modulating the osmotic environment of the hepatocyte. This has been shown to be the mechanism of the rapidly mediated effects of changing the osmotic pressure of the perfusate circulating through the isolated rabbit or rat liver.[27,145] It is possible that the failure to suppress albumin synthesis in patients with cirrhosis and hypoalbuminaemia by intravenous infusions of salt-poor albumin which were sufficient to raise the plasma albumin concentration was based upon the lack of a significant effect upon hepatic interstitial fluid oncotic pressure due to rapid degradation and distribution in non-functional compartments of the extravascular space, for example, ascites.[180]

Role of Amino Acid Supply

It has been shown in both the experimental rat and in man that the total flux of amino acids calculated from the rate of disappearance from the plasma of a constantly infused radioactive amino acid is about four times greater than the daily input to the system from dietary protein intake.[192,194] Reduction of the exogenous supply by low protein feeding over a period of six weeks produced a 30 per cent reduction in body protein turnover when measured by this method.[195] This relative stability in overall protein turnover rate in the face of protein deprivation may be indicative of mutually compensating changes which occur in the major metabolic areas, namely the liver and the muscles.

In the liver a distinction has to be made between effects upon fixed tissue protein and secreted proteins, between the effects of short-term or long-term deprivation and between fasting (calorie restriction) and protein restriction. Evidence based upon comparison of specific activities of intracellular and extracellular amino acids indicates that 50 per cent of available precursor amino acid arises by degradation of hepatic cellular protein.[43] Protein deprivation increases this contribution to 90 per cent, suggesting that reduction of exogenous supply is associated with an increased rate of degradation of endogenous protein. The early classical data of Addis, Poo and Lew,[1] in which there was evidence for loss of up to 40 per cent of hepatic protein after two days of fasting, may be explained on this basis rather than by a reduction in the fractional rate of synthesis. More sophisticated techniques utilizing constant infusion of radioactively labelled amino acids[46,195] confirm that there is no reduction in synthesis expressed on a fractional basis. However, as excessive degradation results in 'wasting' of the mass of hepatic tissue protein, so does the absolute rate of synthesis fall. Eventually, a new equilibrium is established, set at lower rates for synthesis, degradation and pool mass. Studies in the isolated perfused rat liver have shown that the increased degradation can be prevented by restoring amino acid supply or adding insulin in vitro[108,199] while glucagon increases degradation as judged by rates of glucose production, ureagenesis and amino acid metabolism.[99] A disturbance in the normal insulin : glucagon concentration ratio in the blood perfusing the liver in vivo may therefore be relevant to the pathogenesis of disturbed hepatic protein metabolism during amino acid deprivation.

In the case of proteins secreted by the liver into the plasma, there is considerable evidence that amino acid supply is a fundamental factor regulating their synthesis. By the same token, there is good correlation between dietary protein requirements and protein turnover rates during the human life span.[204] Garrow[47] has indicated the positive correlation between dietary protein supply and the plasma concentration of albumin, transferrin and caeruloplasmin. Interestingly, immunoglobulins which are largely of extrahepatic origin are not reduced in concentration under similar circumstances, again demonstrating the differential effects of regulatory factors in various tissues.

Studies in man based upon measurement of catabolic rates of albumin labelled with radioactive iodine under steady state circumstances have shown that limitation of dietary protein intake is associated with low fractional rates of degradation.[21,60,64] In the presence of depleted albumin pools this was indicative of a primary reduction in hepatic synthesis followed by reduction in degradation. Studies in the experimental rat have confirmed this sequence of events. Early in the course of dietary protein restriction there was a fall in the rate of synthesis of albumin, as measured directly by the (^{14}C)-carbonate method. Normal catabolic rates were maintained for a latent period. Only when the imbalance between synthesis and degradation had exerted an effect on plasma albumin concentration was there a reduction in catabolic rate. Refeeding of a diet adequate in protein reversed these effects. An early response in synthesis to reach supranormal rates was followed by a gradual increase in catabolic rate *pari passu* with the rise in plasma albumin concentration.[78] These findings in the intact animal have been confirmed by studies in the isolated perfused rabbit or rat liver. Isolated perfused livers from fasted rats and rabbits show a profound reduction in the rate of synthesis of albumin as measured by the (^{14}C)-carbonate method, by quantitative immunoassay, or by the rate of incorporation of a labelled amino acid.[74,107,146] In these circumstances it was possible to show rapid reversal of the synthetic defect by refeeding in vivo or by supplying the perfused liver with high concentrations of amino acids, and also to confirm the supranormal rates of synthesis previously seen in vivo in response to dietary protein restoration. These workers could show no such induction by supplying supranormal amounts of amino acids to the perfused livers isolated from fed animals. In the case of the rabbit, it was shown that supplying tryptophan alone was equally effective in promoting synthesis of albumin in livers from fasted animals.[147] Evidence in humans for a response in albumin synthesis to amino acid supply is available from relatively short-term studies in postoperative patients fed parenterally with a mixture of essential and non-essential amino acids. Synthetic rates on the fourth postoperative day were significantly higher than in a control group fed with only a source of calories.[164]

A similar rate-limiting role for tryptophan in the synthesis of albumin and other protein has been demonstrated in the mouse, rat and rabbit.[112,148,163] This observation has led Munro[113] to speculate on the special rate-limiting role for tryptophan in regulation of protein synthesis at a translational level. Tryptophan is the least well represented and least abundant amino acid in fixed hepatic tissue protein and is therefore least available for re-utilization for protein synthesis by endogenous turnover. At times when the liver is most dependent upon recycling for supply of amino acids for protein synthesis, namely during starvation or protein deprivation, the amount of available activated tryptophan tRNA is limiting for translation of messenger RNA. Depending upon the position of tryptophan in the particular growing polypeptide chain it will be possible or not to complete the protein already nascent on the polyribosome. Those that do not require tryptophan for completion will be able to complete translation and be released from the polyribosome. Those that do will show inhibition of translation and retention of incomplete polypeptide chains on the mRNA. Of course, other essential amino acids will also be rate-limiting in extreme circumstances but require relatively greater exogenous deprivation to become manifested because they are proportionately better represented in endogenous protein. There is also evidence that tryptophan has a unique effect on the rate of synthesis of both mRNA and rRNA[58,186] and is not solely involved with the translational phase of synthesis. Rare examples of the role of tryptophan resulting in hypoproteinaemia in man have been provided by excessive diversion of free tryptophan to metabolic pathways other than protein synthesis. This may occur in the carcinoid syndrome in which diversion of tryptophan to serotonin biosynthesis may result in insufficient availability for either protein or nicotinic acid synthesis.[175]

The effects of repletion with amino acids differ depending upon whether deprivation has been short-term or long-term. The low albumin and transferrin synthesis resulting from long-term deprivation of dietary protein in the rat could not be reversed by supplying amino acids to the isolated perfused liver at high concentrations.[181] In these circumstances short-term translational effects of amino acid deprivation operating at the level of the polyribosome were probably reinforced by long-term and less rapidly reversible effects occurring at a transcriptional level. Indeed, the synthesis of ribosomal, messenger and transfer RNA may become limited in these circumstances.[33,115] and longer periods of repletion are required for reversal of the effects of their deficiency. Deficiency of specific template activity for albumin synthesis has been observed in the livers of rats subjected to prolonged protein deficiency,[77] while in acutely starved rats there is a shift of albumin mRNA from membrane-bound polyribosomes into the cytoplasm where it can be stored as non-translated mRNA–protein complexes.[202]

Munro (1970) has pointed out that long-term responses in the synthesis of specific protein may be mediated by varying the number of cells devoted to the synthesis of that particular protein.[113] Stimulation of synthesis would involve derepression of dormant genomes and recruitment of cells to synthesis. Suppression of synthesis would reverse the process. Evidence based upon specific immunofluorescence has shown that the number of hepatic cells staining for albumin could be varied from 0 to 10 to 60 per cent when rats were changed from a zero protein intake to normal stock diet to a high protein diet.[20] Unfortunately, this is a technique which provides a static view of a dynamic process, the amount of albumin in the hepatocyte being a function of the sum of synthesis and secretion. Only secretory proteins which have completed translation and assembly and are in the process of secretion within the channels of the endoplasmic reticulum or Golgi apparatus are likely to give positive immunofluorescence. This quantity cannot necessarily be equated with rates of synthesis since regulatory mechanisms may be operative at the level of secretion. In these circumstances, inhibition of secretion without change in rate of translation would be interpreted as recruitment of cells to the synthesis of a specific protein and would clearly be erroneous. For this reason it is probably better to rely upon dynamic measurement of synthesis and secretion for the identification of control mechanisms.

Role of Hormones

Hormonal influences on hepatic protein metabolism are closely integrated with nutritional ones and the outcome as far as the prototype export protein albumin is concerned represents the combined effects on synthesis, degradation and distribution. Furthermore, different effects on the metabolism of fixed (tissue) proteins and secreted proteins make it difficult to assign specific anabolic or catabolic roles for individual hormones. Therefore, it has been necessary to identify individual hormone actions in the isolated perfused liver and other tissue preparations, including cell-free systems, in order to suggest mechanisms for observed phenomena in the intact organism. Finally, it should be added that such an analytical approach may ultimately fail to take into account complex hormonal interactions which occur as an integrated response to individual endocrine disturbances in vivo.

Insulin is an anabolic hormone for both tissue and export protein synthesis. It is necessary for maximum synthesis of albumin in the isolated perfused rat liver[69] and isolated rat hepatocytes.[26,68] In addition, it has anticatabolic effects on the degradation of tissue proteins.[104] While there is evidence that it plays a role in preserving the capacity for hepatic regeneration and DNA synthesis following portacaval shunt-induced atrophy,[170] it also clearly has a translational effect upon polyribosome structure and function.[48,120] Nevertheless, it has not been possible to identify defective synthesis of albumin in insulin-dependent or maturity onset diabetes in man although excessive extravascular distribution has been noted.[98]

Glucagon has profound effects upon intermediary metabolism manifested as promotion of gluconeogenesis and ureagenesis, derived partially by enhanced degradation of both tissue and secretory proteins.[51,100] A direct anti-anabolic role has also been identified in the synthesis of both types of protein which can be explained in part at least by disaggregation of polyribosomes. It is likely that these responses are mediated by cyclic AMP in the light of observed inhibition of amino acid incorporation into protein by liver slices exposed to cyclic AMP.[15] Since a fall in the plasma insulin : glucagon ratio is observed in a number of hypercatabolic/hypoanabolic states in man,[182,183] it is possible to offer a plausible explanation for the disturbances in protein metabolism on the basis of the combined effects of insulin deficiency and glucagon excess upon protein synthesis and degradation.

Corticosteroids have a stimulatory effect upon hepatic protein synthesis at both transcriptional and translational levels.[22,28,34,65,69] Administration or excess secretion of corticosteroids in man is associated with increased synthesis and degradation of albumin.[18,141,142,172]

Briefly, growth hormone appears to play an anabolic role in albumin synthesis in vivo.[75] Although it has not been possible to demonstrate such a role in albumin synthesis by the isolated perfused rat liver,[69] fibrinogen synthesis did show a synthetic response in vitro.[65] Thyroid hormone in the context of hyperthyroidism and hypothyroidism is stimulatory to both albumin synthesis and degradation with little change in the total exchangeable pool, although it does result in marked distribution changes in favour of extravascular albumin.[11,85,140] Thyroid hormone has stimulatory effects upon transcription in the form of promotion of mRNA and rRNA synthesis as well as translational effects in enhancing polyribosome integrity and function, as reviewed by Rothschild, Oratz and Schreiber.[137]

In summary, it is apparent that hormonal control of protein metabolism is complex and, in vivo, other factors may complicate the outcome of endocrine disturbances, such as changes in nutrition and amino acid supply and disturbances in fluid distribution, as well as the responses in secretion by other endocrine glands.

Effects of Liver Disease

Patients with chronic liver disease and hypoalbuminaemia show a prolonged half-life of survival of radio-iodine-labelled albumin even though the intravascular pool and total exchangeable pool masses of albumin are not invariably reduced.[13,31,171,180,196] Calculations derived from this type of data indicate that a reduced rate of degradation in both fractional and absolute terms has compensated partly for a primary reduction in the rate of albumin synthesis by the liver. Additionally, in patients with ascites there is an abnormal intravascular : extravascular distribution of albumin with a greater proportion of the total exchangeable pool located in the extravascular space. In these circumstances, the low fractional rate of degradation is related more closely to the plasma albumin concentration than to the intravascular pool mass; the absolute rate of degradation, and also by implication the absolute rate of synthesis, may be normal. The mechanism of reduction in rates of albumin degradation in liver disease is unknown and is not a feature that is shared by all liver-produced plasma proteins. Thus decreased fibrinogen and prothrombin synthesis may be associated with excessive degradation in consumptive coagulopathy, while the C3 component of complement may be reduced by defective hepatic synthesis and degradation by virtue of immune complex deposition, particularly in primary biliary cirrhosis.

Alcoholic cirrhotic subjects with hypoalbuminaemia and ascites may have normal or elevated rates of hepatic albumin synthesis when measured directly by the (^{14}C) carbonate method.[136,149] In these circumstances the low plasma albumin concentration is presumed to reflect dilution by salt and water retention, and the high plasma and extravascular fluid volumes seen in such patients are compatible with this mechanism. In other studies in patients without detectable clinical ascites, low rates of albumin synthesis also measured directly with (^{14}C) carbonate were observed in association with low intravascular and total exchangeable albumin pool masses.[180] Similar measurements made in chronic active hepatitis have yielded reduced or normal rates of synthesis. Repeated measurements after a period of treatment with corticosteroids demonstrated greatly enhanced rates of synthesis, without a proportional increase in plasma albumin concentration or intravascular pool mass, suggesting concomitant and counterbalancing effects on degradation.[18] Simultaneous determination of fibrinogen synthesis in these patients did not show any parallel enhancement of fibrinogen synthesis, attesting to the differences in control mechanisms and pharmacological responses by the various plasma proteins.

Patients with cirrhosis have elevated plasma concentrations of glucagon in response to infusions of arginine and alanine, as well as in the basal state[93,161] (see also Chapter 7). Several explanations have been offered, including inadequate hepatic degradation, excessive and inappropriate alpha cell secretion, and portasystemic shunting of hormone. However, since Sherwin et al[161] observed that patients with extensive portacaval shunting have higher increments in plasma glucagon than those without, in the absence of demonstrable differences in liver function it seems unlikely that inadequate degradation is the sole explanation. Also, since insulin levels were also elevated, although not to the same degree, it seems probable that a combination of hypersecretion plus shunting can explain the prevailing hyperglucagonaemia. The relative increase in plasma concentrations of aromatic amino acids compared to branched chain amino acids in cirrhosis is evidence of the continued efficient metabolic ability of the muscles in contrast to that of the diseased liver. However, it has been suggested that the absolute decrease in concentration of the BCAA is the consequence of the hyperinsulinaemia which is evident, particularly in cirrhosis with portasystemic shunting. While it is likely that the reduction in the insulin : glucagon ratio contributes to glucose intolerance in cirrhosis, its relevance to the abnormalities in protein metabolism remains speculative. However, in the light of the observed effects of insulin and glucagon on protein synthesis and degradation in vitro, a potential role for this particular hormonal imbalance in the aggravation of the protein disturbances of liver disease must be considered.

Direct sampling of thoracic duct lymph and hepatic venous blood in dogs labelled with intravenous (^{14}C)-carbonate has indicated that newly synthesized albumin is secreted directly into the sinusoidal circulation.[165] However, in patients with cirrhosis, portal hypertension and ascites, the increased post-sinusoidal resistance to portal venous flow appears to be associated with diversion of newly synthesized albumin directly into thoracic duct lymph and ascites. This occurs prior to mixing with the pool of intravascular albumin and attests to the role of hepatic lymph dynamics in the pathogenesis of ascites.[206] It does not explain, however, why a priority exists in cirrhotics for secretion of albumin directly into lymph. It is possible that shunting of blood around regenerating nodules and inadequate sinusoidal perfusion is associated with relative hypertrophy of the lymphatic circulation.

In addition to quantitative deficiencies in protein synthesis and aberrant pathways of secretion, patients with hepatobiliary disease may produce qualitatively abnormal plasma proteins. This has been suggested for fibrinogen (see 'Pathophysiology of specialized proteins', below), thyroid binding globulin[94] and for other glycoproteins. The presence of high concentrations of many types of desialylated glycoproteins in the circulation of patients with acute and chronic parenchymal liver disease may be explained on the basis of either abnormal biosynthesis and sialylation or on defective uptake by the diseased liver.[95,96] Since the liver usually binds desialylated glycoproteins with avidity,[106] it is possible that the liver plasma membrane-binding sites of patients with cirrhosis are partially blocked, reduced in number or relatively inaccessible to circulating desialylated glycoproteins.

The maximal rates of urea synthesis (MRUS) of patients with cirrhosis ingesting 37.8 mmol (0.53 g) protein N/kg body weight are reduced from 4.64 mmol (65 mg) urea N/hr/kg in controls to an average of 1.93 mmol (27 mg) urea N/hr/kg.[152] The MRUS at all levels of protein intake correlated inversely with blood levels of ammonia and amino acids and the occurrence of encephalopathy, while the extent of depletion of three of the urea cycle enzymes, as measured in operative liver biopsies, correlated directly with the MRUS.[76] Although all the urea cycle enzymes were depressed in cirrhosis, other workers have observed only selective reductions in alcoholic hepatitis[92] and in experimental cirrhosis in the rat,[73] the magnitude of which was not rate limiting for urea synthesis.

Although there is evidence that the urea cycle is operating at only 60 per cent capacity under normal circumstances,[57] and the enzymes of the cycle can be considerably induced by feeding a high protein diet,[154] it is evident that the reduction in MRUS seen in parenchymal liver disease represents a significant limitation in adaptive ability which manifests itself by elevation in plasma amino acids and ammonia and encephalopathy.[159] Although adaptation to protein intake is curtailed in chronic liver disease, it does appear that treatment with corticosteroids in appropriate patients is associated with promotion of urea synthesis.[70]

In Reye's syndrome the severe reduction in ornithine transcarbamylase and carbamyl phosphate synthetase in mitochondria has suggested that the preceding viral illness results in selective mitochondrial injury which is responsible for defective urea synthesis and hyperammonaemia.[166]

Effects of Alcohol (see also Chapter 32)

Many explanations have been offered for the hepatic metabolic disturbances produced by alcohol. The effects of ethyl alcohol per se, its principal degradation products acetaldehyde and hydrogen ions, and associated nutritional deprivation have variously been proposed as factors either individually or in combination.

Under various defined conditions ethanol can inhibit, accelerate or produce no major changes in gluconeogenesis from alanine. However, when ornithine is added with alanine to the isolated perfused liver preparation ethanol greatly accelerates gluconeogenesis. In contrast, in the presence of ammonia and lactate ethanol causes a major accumulation of amino acids, especially aspartate and alanine.[80] The latter situation reflects the observed failure of gluconeogenesis from pyruvate and amino acids, particularly from alanine, thereby potentially contributing to the hypoglycaemic syndrome of the alcoholic. It also suggests, in addition to the inability to metabolize amino acids, a relative reduction in their utilization for protein synthesis.

When administered acutely to isolated rat hepatocytes, to rat liver slices, to the isolated perfused rat or rabbit liver or to rats in vivo, ethanol produces a measurable, significant reduction in albumin, transferrin, glycoprotein and tissue protein synthesis but not in fibrinogen synthesis.[66,79,105,122,148,169] The inhibition of albumin synthesis is preventable in the liver of a fed donor rabbit by the addition of tryptophan to the perfusate, while in the rat it is largely prevented by the previous or acute administration of large amounts of all amino acids. Although the suppression of albumin synthesis produced by alcohol was similar to that observed in response to fasting and was also associated with disaggregation of membrane-bound polyribosomes it did not share the nutritional mechanism of reduction of hepatic total RNA concentration. It has subsequently been shown that livers from fed rabbit donors exposed to alcohol were able to reverse the reduction in albumin synthesis and membrane-bound polyribosome disaggregation in response to a number of amino acids, namely arginine, ornithine and lysine in addition to tryptophan. The combination of both a 24-hour fast and exposure to 220 mg/dl of alcohol in the perfusate resulted in disaggregation of both free and membrane-bound polyribosomes, loss of hepatic RNA and a failure to respond to the high concentrations of amino acids which were effective with either stress alone.[138] However, the combination of spermine, a polyamine, and arginine was effective in restoring aggregation of free and bound polyribosomes and in maintaining rates of albumin synthesis in perfused liver from fasted rabbits exposed to alcohol.[118] In contrast to these animal studies, acute alcohol administration to well-fed alcoholic patients failed to produce any consistent effects on albumin synthesis.[67]

The effects of alcohol administration may also differ after acute or chronic administration. Although ultrastructural examination has revealed a reduction in the membranes of the rough endoplasmic reticulum following chronic alcohol consumption in man,[62,83,87,151] it has been reported that synthesis of ribosomal and mitochondrial proteins may actually be enhanced in experimental animals.[82,134] While earlier reports suggest that alcohol inhibits lipoprotein synthesis and the incorporation of labelled glucosamine into the carbohydrate moiety of lipoproteins,[105] more recent studies have shown enhanced incorporation of both radioactive lipid and amino acids into lipoproteins and increased lipoprotein secretion after both acute and chronic alcohol administration in the rat, suggesting a mechanism for the hyperlipaemia of the chronic alcoholic[7,8] (see also Chapter 4).

The primate model of alcohol dependence and liver injury and a satisfactory alcohol diet for the rat has made it possible to follow the evolution of hepatic pathophysiology during the time of exposure to alcohol. It has been suggested that the accentuation of hepatic fat deposition is associated with failure of lipoprotein secretion as the disease progresses, and the early compensatory role of enhanced lipoprotein synthesis and secretion is lost.[16,86] Support for this hypothesis has been provided in man by the observation that blood lipids decrease with progression of disease to alcoholic hepatitis and cirrhosis.[97]

Recent studies have been carried out in order to differentiate the effects of alcohol from the potential deleterious actions of its principal metabolite acetaldehyde. Since the metabolism of acetaldehyde to acetate is reduced in the alcoholic, the former substance is a putative candidate for some of the observed inhibition of protein synthesis. The separate effects of ethanol and acetaldehyde on hepatic albumin synthesis have been studied in the isolated perfused liver from fed and fasted rabbits.[119] The previous nutritional state profoundly affects the outcome in terms both of net albumin synthesis and of the degree of polyribosome disaggregation induced by alcohol in the perfusate. It is apparent that ethanol perfused at a concentration of 200 mg/dl depresses albumin synthesis in livers from both fed and fasted donors and also produces polyribosome disaggregation. On the other hand, acetaldehyde at a concentration of 2 mg/dl inhibits albumin synthesis only in fed livers but in neither circumstance does it affect the degree of polyribosome integrity. When oxidation of ethanol is prevented by 4-methylpyrazole, albumin synthesis in fed livers remains suppressed to the same degree but polyribosome disaggregation is no longer evident. However, in the fasted liver inhibition of oxidation of ethanol did prevent the reduction of albumin synthesis. Oratz and his colleagues[119] speculate that it is the *process* of ethanol oxidation which is responsible for polyribosome disaggregation, and that neither ethanol nor acetaldehyde are directly the mediators of this effect on the protein synthesizing machinery. Furthermore, both ethanol and acetaldehyde are capable of inhibiting protein synthesis in the fed state, but only ethanol seems to have this potential in the fasted state. Since most of the effects of ethanol in the fasted state are inhibited by 4-methylpyrazole, and since acetaldehyde is not toxic under these circumstances, these data support the concept of the metabolic degradation of ethanol contributing to inhibition of protein synthesis as well as polyribosome degradation, at least under the circumstances of fasting.

In contrast to these observations on the mechanism of inhibition of albumin synthesis, a defect in the synthesis of hepatic glycoproteins produced by ethanol is due to inhibition of glycosylation which has been attributed to acetaldehyde rather than to ethanol itself or to an alteration in the redox state.[169] These effects of acetaldehyde persisted for at least three hours in rat liver slices exposed previously but then subsequently incubated in an acetaldehyde-free medium.[168]

Studies in the rat fed 36 per cent of its energy intake in the form of alcohol have demonstrated progressive development of hepatomegaly, fatty liver and hepatocyte hypertrophy over a four- to eight-week period. Livers from alcohol-fed rats increased by 30 per cent in volume and net weight. Fat accounted for only 50 per cent of the increase in dry weight, the remainder being made up of protein. Since hepatic protein concentration did not change it was apparent that water content increased in proportion to the increase in protein. Similarly, the absence of any change in DNA content indicated that cellular hypertrophy and not hyperplasia was the basis for hepatomegaly. The protein accumulation was found predominantly in the cytosolic compartment although smaller increases in mitochondrial and microsomal protein were also observed. Analysis of the intracellular protein content after alcohol feeding identified a predominant accumulation of export proteins, albumin and transferrin, with a relative and absolute decrease in intracellular protein exemplified by ferritin.[9] Dynamic studies of hepatic synthesis of export and tissue proteins in chronically alcohol-fed rats showed that synthesis of liver protein, proalbumin and transferrin were increased but that there was delayed transport of newly labelled albumin and transferrin into the plasma. It was also apparent that alcohol feeding reduced the absolute amount of total and polymerized tubulin in the liver, contributing to a postulated defect in microtubular structure and secretory function.[10] It was clear from these studies that accumulation of two major export proteins, albumin and transferrin, could not in themselves account for the total accumulation of soluble proteins in the hepatocyte. The identification of other retained or induced proteins is awaited.

PATHOPHYSIOLOGY OF SPECIALIZED PROTEINS

This section will attempt to identify a number of situations in which regulatory mechanisms controlling the synthesis, secretion and degradation of hepatic secretory proteins may be related to a specific function of some of those proteins. In addition, it has been possible in the case of certain glycoproteins to identify potential catabolic pathways related to alterations in the structure of the carbohydrate moiety of the protein. Finally, the appearance in the circulation of certain proteins which are usually present in only minute quantities or the alternative finding of a deficiency of a protein provides an opportunity to discuss a number of disease processes in terms of molecular mechanisms. Limitations of space prevent comprehensive coverage and only references to more detailed reviews will be provided.

Transferrin

The role of the iron-binding function of transferrin in iron metabolism and the functions of the liver in transferrin metabolism have been reviewed recently.[3,179] The liver is the principal but not the only site of transferrin synthesis. Evidence has been provided that the elevated concentrations of plasma transferrin observed in iron deficiency states can be explained on the basis of enhanced hepatic synthesis.[109] Experimental manipulations in iron deficient rats demonstrated a significant negative correlation between hepatic iron stores in the form of ferritin and the rate of transferrin synthesis. One could not, however, demonstrate a role for anaemia, for the plasma iron concentration or for plasma ferritin as the mediator of the synthetic response in iron deficiency anaemia, nor could a reduction in the rate of degradation be incriminated from studies of radio-iodinated transferrin turnover in iron deficient patients. The latter observation is in keeping with those of other workers who have shown dissociation between the half-lives of plasma iron and plasma transferrin. In summary, it appears that synthesis plays the predominant role in governing the plasma transferrin concentration. However, in certain toxic and infectious states, enhanced degradation does seem to be responsible for the observed reduction in plasma iron-binding capacity. Although ferritin has not been conclusively shown to modulate transferrin synthesis at a molecular level, its close contiguity together with other forms of storage iron to the site of transferrin synthesis within the hepatocyte provides an ideally situated regulatory mechanism which enables transferrin, the unique iron transport protein, to respond rapidly to changes in body iron status.

Caeruloplasmin[174]

While several physiological actions of caeruloplasmin have been described, no single major biological function has been assigned to it. Roles have been proposed for copper transport and homeostasis, polyamine oxidase and ferroxidase activity.

In Wilson's disease, low plasma caeruloplasmin concentrations are associated with high tissue copper concentrations. Studies of copper turnover and biliary kinetics suggest that the high tissue copper (at least in the liver) is due to diminished biliary excretion. Turnover time of intrahepatic copper is greatly prolonged. However, it is difficult to incriminate the deficient caeruloplasmin in the pathogenesis of these phenomena. The kinetics of turnover of the copper moiety of caeruloplasmin are too sluggish for the protein to regulate either copper absorption or tissue copper uptake. Furthermore, about 5 per cent of patients with Wilson's disease have normal plasma caeruloplasmin concentrations, and the protein in these patients and also in those with profound deficiency is apparently structurally normal. Although desialylation of caeruloplasmin results in rapid hepatic uptake and degradation, there is no evidence for an acceleration of this potential pathway in patients with Wilson's disease. Finally, it has not been possible to accelerate copper excretion by administration of caeruloplasmin to deficient patients. It may be that Wilson's disease is the result of a defect in intracellular transfer of copper and that the caeruloplasmin changes are secondary. In fact, the usual response to copper loading of the liver is an increase in plasma caeruloplasmin concentration. This is true of the experimental rat and of human disease states characterized by prolonged cholestasis. Since there are eight copper atoms covalently incorporated into the protein, it is not difficult to suggest a regulatory role for copper in the synthesis of the apoprotein.

Alpha-l-antitrypsin[160] (see also Chapter 35)

Alpha-l-antitrypsin (AlAT) is a serine protease inhibitor with an attributed function of inactivation of proteases released from intracellular sites. It is synthesized by the liver and its synthesis is stimulated by acute stress situations in company with the acute phase reactants. It is responsible for 90 per cent of the protease inhibitory capacity of normal human plasma.

A deficiency state associated with the development of cirrhosis has been described in childhood. In these circumstances there is usually less than 15 per cent of normal protease inhibitory activity in plasma. In the case of the homozygous deficiency state (PiZZ), the phenotypic variant protein has been shown to differ in carbohydrate content and structure from the most prevalent phenotype, PiM. However, this does not affect the protease inhibitory capacity of the protein, so that the consequences of the deficiency can be related to a critical quantitative deficiency in the ability to bind proteases rather than a qualitatively defective protein. Likewise, it is also evident that degradation of the variant protein in deficiency states is also normal, suggesting that the deficiency state is based upon a reduction in hepatic synthesis of a functionally normal protein.

Ultrastructural studies of the liver in patients with AlAT deficiency have identified granules of PAS-positive amorphous proteinaceous material within dilated vesicles of the rough endoplasmic reticulum (RER), rather than in the Golgi bodies or lysosomes. Although these deposits have been shown to be antigenically identical with A1AT, they lack sialic acid and differ in amino acid content. It has been suggested that an anomalous primary protein structure leads to defective glycosylation, a failure to negotiate the normal secretory pathway and ultimate aggregation of the protein within the RER. In this way, a post-translational malfunction (secretion) is superimposed upon a primary defect in the synthesis of a genetic variant protein. Recently, there has been a report of successful transplantation of a liver from a PiMM phenotype to a PiZZ recipient with reversal of the quantitative plasma deficiency of A1AT, conversion to the donor phenotype and absence of PAS-positive granules in the liver over two years following transplantation.[128]

Prothrombin[173]

Prothrombin is discussed as an example of a protein whose biosynthesis is regulated at a post-translational level within the liver; modifications of the end product of synthesis lead to the generation of an active coagulation protein from an inactive precursor. The conversion of the precursor pool of inactive prothrombin requires vitamin K. The precursor protein differs from active prothrombin by the absence of γ-carboxyglutamic acid which is found as a modification of the first 10 of the 33 glutamic acid residues. The carboxylase enzyme responsible for this modification is dependent upon the presence of the reduced form of vitamin K and can be inhibited by the anticoagulant warfarin. Failure of carboxylation by reason of vitamin K deficiency also leads to failure of Ca^{++} binding, and inability to bind to phospholipid membranes.

Fibrinogen[130,133]

The liver is involved in the process of haemostasis by virtue of both its anabolic and catabolic functions. It is responsible for the synthesis of many of the coagulation factors, namely fibrinogen (factor I), prothrombin (factor II), and factors V, VII, IX and X. All of these, except fibrinogen, have vitamin K-dependent biosynthetic mechanisms. The liver is also responsible for the synthesis and degradation of fibrinolytic factors and, finally, it clears activated clotting factors from the circulation. While severe liver disease depresses the plasma concentrations of factors II, V, VII, IX and X, with the one-stage prothrombin time measuring all except IX, it is unusual for fibrinogen to be significantly reduced unless there is associated disseminated intravascular coagulation.

Under normal circumstances, intravascular fibrinogenolysis or fibrin formation is not quantitatively the most important mechanism of fibrinogen degradation. Fibrinogen degradation is normally a first-order process, the absolute amount catabolized being proportional to the plasma concentration. Under pathological circumstances cleavage of fibrinogen to fibrin monomers may account for a major route of degradation.

In severe liver disease, low molecular weight forms of fibrinogen may be found in the plasma in association with diminished concentrations of plasminogen inactivators. It has been suggested that these low molecular weight fibrinogens represent partial degradation products of native fibrinogen, with prolonged thrombin times which may contribute to a bleeding diathesis.[88] Others have described the presence of functionally abnormal fibrinogens with reduced clotting ability based upon a defect in fibrin monomer polymerization.[121] This appears to be an intrinsic property of the molecule synthesized by the diseased liver, although it is possible that the molecular alterations leading to the phenomenon may take place in the circulation or as a result of post-translational modifications within the hepatocyte.

Alpha-1-fetoprotein[4]

The presence of alpha-1-fetoprotein (AFP) in the circulation is an example of carcinofetal reversion in which proliferating malignant cells recapitulate some of the metabolic features of developing fetal tissues. The molecular basis is speculated to be a derepression of fetal genomes which are normally repressed as differentiation occurs.

AFP is a normal secretory product of human fetal liver, as well as originating in intestinal and yolk sac cells. About 80 to 90 per cent of human hepatocellular carcinomas are capable of synthesizing AFP, but the range of plasma AFP concentrations that results varies widely. The quantitative variation has necessitated the use of highly sensitive techniques for detection. Histopathological evidence of carcinogenesis is by no means always present. The concentration of AFP is a function of other factors as well as size of tumour; for example, the nature of the carcinogen, the degree of differentiation of the tumour and the age of the patient. It may also appear in response to acute hepatic injury of either viral or toxic origin. High concentrations have been observed in massive hepatic necrosis, and it has been suggested that these reflect normal hepatic regeneration. However, regeneration itself is not the prerequisite for AFP synthesis. Rather, it is the type of injurious agent, together with a distinctive form of regeneration. Thus it has been reported recently that sera from patients recovering from partial hepatectomy were consistently negative for AFP.[5] Derepression of the AFP genome is therefore probably a very specific response to a limited number of stimuli.

Ferritin[56]

Ferritin is located intracellularly in many tissues and constitutes the principal form of available storage iron. However, by sensitive radioimmunoassay techniques it is detectable in the plasma of all normal individuals where it provides good correlation with total body iron stores. There is evidence that serum ferritin represents a secreted plasma protein, originating partly at least in the liver. Tissue ferritins demonstrate microheterogeneity which, it has been suggested, is due to the different proportions of heavy and light subunits of apoferritin which constitute the protein shell of ferritin.[30]

Apoferritin synthesis is stimulated by the administration of iron. The stimulation is not prevented by blocking DNA-directed mRNA synthesis, nor is it inhibited in cell-free systems by the administration of cycloheximide.[29] In part, at least, the role of iron may be in assembly or release of subunits. More recently it has been shown that apoferritin subunits inactivate specific mRNA for apoferritin. Iron prevents this inactivation and makes mRNA functionally available for translational activity.[205] Iron also has a stabilizing effect on degradation of tissue ferritin in vivo, although iron-containing ferritin in the circulation is rapidly removed by the tissues.

Serum ferritin correlates well with iron stores at all levels and provides a good screening test for iron deficiency and iron overload states. In primary haemochromatosis and transfusional haemochromatosis serum ferritin resembles natural apoferritin of liver origin, in terms of iron content, isoelectric focusing and immunological properties.[6] The observation that serum ferritin contains far less iron than coexisting tissue ferritin is evidence against the concept that it originates solely by leakage from damaged cells. However, in the special circumstances of acute liver disease, or ongoing chronic active liver damage, it may indeed originate in this way. It is possible to make allowance for necrosis and to show that there is good correlation between the serum ferritin : aspartate transaminase ratio and body iron stores.[127] In most other circumstances, however, it is possible that serum ferritin is synthesized afresh on membrane-bound polyribosomes and, as with tissue ferritins which originate on free-polyribosomes, is subjected to regulation by iron supply even though iron is not incorporated into the secreted protein. The value of serum ferritin in detecting iron overload in asymptomatic relatives of patients with haemochromatosis has been questioned by the finding of normal values in subjects with elevated iron stores.[190] More recently, however, an Australian study has shown excellent correlation between serum ferritin and iron stores in the vast majority of relatives of such patients.[53]

Tissue isoferritin patterns on isoelectric focusing change with iron status in patients with haemochromatosis treated by venesection. High degrees of iron overload produce an isoferritin pattern characteristic of liver ferritin in all tissues which revert to those of the tissue of origin as iron is removed.[126] Serum ferritin also shows a shift from relatively basic to more acidic isoferritins during therapy.[54] It is therefore possible that the relative proportion of heavy and light subunits assembled into the different isoferritins is partially governed by iron supply.

Ferritin provides an intriguing example of a protein originally thought of exclusively as a tissue protein. Recent evidence indicates that it may also be a secreted plasma protein sharing some but not all of the regulatory mechanisms of tissue ferritin. Its function as a circulating protein remains elusive.

SUMMARY

This chapter has attempted to provide some insight into the many roles of the liver in protein metabolism. As a major processor of dietary protein and reprocessor of nitrogen recycled from amino acids released by muscle protein degradation, it has both an important quantitative and unique qualitative role in nutrition. As the site of origin of virtually all the plasma proteins except immunoglobulins, it is responsible for the maintenance of the many functions of these proteins, and in certain disease states and congenital disorders there may be resultant quantitative and qualitative deficiencies. The molecular basis of some of these disorders has been elucidated but many await additional data on pathogenesis. While control mechanisms for the synthesis and degradation of liver-produced proteins are subjected to non-specific nutritional and hormonal influences, many are specific and function-related. The identification of some of these specific mechanisms has yielded new concepts of control, not merely of transcription and translation, but also of post-translational modifications and secretory pathways. As is frequently the case, the study of pathogenesis of disease phenomena has clarified physiological concepts.

ACKNOWLEDGMENTS

This work was supported in part by Grant HD11089 from the National Institutes of Health. I would like to express my gratitude to my secretary Ms Kathy Kane for expert secretarial assistance.

REFERENCES

1. Addis, T., Poo, L.J. & Lew, W. (1936) Protein loss from liver during a 2-day fast. *Journal of Biological Chemistry,* **115,** 117–118.
2. Aguirre, A., Funovics, J., Wesdorp, R.I.C. & Fischer, J.E. (1976) Parenteral nutrition in hepatic failure. In

Total Parenteral Nutrition (Ed.) Fischer, J.E. pp. 219–230. Boston: Little, Brown.

3. Aisen, P. & Brown, E.B. (1977) The iron-binding function of transferrin in iron metabolism. *Seminars in Hematology*, **14**, 31–53.
4. Alpert, E. (1976) Human alpha 1-fetoprotein. In *Progress in Liver Diseases*, Vol. 5 (Ed.) Popper, H. & Schaffner, F. pp. 337–349. New York: Grune & Stratton.
5. Alpert, E. & Feller, E.R. (1978) α-fetoprotein (AFP) in benign liver disease. Evidence that normal liver regeneration does not induce AFP synthesis. *Gastroenterology*, **74**, 856–858.
6. Arosio, P., Yokota, M. & Drysdale, J.W. (1977) Characterization of serum ferritin in iron overload: possible identity to natural apoferritin. *British Journal of Haematology*, **36**, 199–207.
7. Baroana, E. & Lieber, C.S. (1970) Effects of chronic ethanol feeding on serum lipoprotein metabolism in the rat. *Journal of Clinical Investigation*, **49**, 769–778.
8. Baroana, E., Pirola, R.C. & Lieber, C.S. (1973) Pathogenesis of postprandial hyperlipemia in rats fed ethanol-containing diets. *Journal of Clinical Investigation*, **52**, 296–303.
9. Baroana, E., Leo, M.A., Borowsky, S.A. & Lieber, C.S. (1975) Alcoholic hepatomegaly: accumulation of protein in the liver. *Science (Washington)*, **190**, 794–795.
10. Baroana, E., Leo, M.A., Borowsky, S.A. & Lieber, C.S. (1977) Pathogenesis of alcohol-induced accumulation of protein in the liver. *Journal of Clinical Investigation*, **60**, 546–554.
11. Bauman, A., Rothschild, M.A., Yalow, R.S. & Berson, A. (1955) Distribution and metabolism of I^{131} labeled human serum albumin in congestive heart failure with and without proteinuria. *Journal of Clinical Investigation*, **34**, 1359–1368.
12. Bennhold, H. & Kallee, E. (1959) Comparative studies on the half-life of I^{131}-labeled albumin and non-radioactive human serum albumin in a case of analbuminemia. *Journal of Clinical Investigation*, **38**, 863–872.
13. Berson, S.A. & Yalow, R.S. (1954) The distribution of I^{131}-labeled human serum albumin introduced into ascitic fluid: analysis of the kinetics of a three compartment quaternary transfer system in man and speculation on possible sites of degradation. *Journal of Clinical Investigation*, **33**, 377–387.
14. Berson, S.A., Yalow, R.S., Schreiber, S.S. & Post, J. (1953) Tracer experiments with I^{131}-labeled human serum albumin. Distribution and degradation studies. *Journal of Clinical Investigation*, **32**, 746–768.
15. Bloxham, D.P. & Akhtar, M. (1972) An anti-anabolic role of adenosine 3′,5′-cyclic monophosphate in the control of liver metabolism. A hypothetical mechanism for gluconeogenesis. *International Journal of Biochemistry*, **3**, 294–308.
16. Borowsky, S.A., Perlow, W., Baroana, E. & Lieber, C.S. (1976) Disappearance of alcoholic hyperlipemia as a sign of advancing liver damage. *Gastroenterology*, **70**, 978 (abstract).
17. Cahill, G.F., Herrera, M.G., Morgan, A.P., Soeldner, J.S., Steinke, J., Levy, P.L., Reichard, G.A. & Kipnis, D.M. (1966) Hormone fuel interrelationships during fasting. *Journal of Clinical Investigation*, **45**, 1751–1769.
18. Cain, G.D., Mayer, G. & Jones, E.A. (1970) Augmentation of albumin but not fibrinogen synthesis by corticosteroids in patients with hepatocellular disease. *Journal of Clinical Investigation*, **49**, 2198–2204.
19. Calloway, D.H. & Margen, S. (1971) Variation in endogenous nitrogen excretion and dietary nitrogen utilization as determinants of human protein requirement. *Journal of Nutrition*, **101**, 205–216.
20. Chandrasakharam, N., Fleck, A. & Munro, H.N. (1967) Albumin content of rat hepatic cells at different levels of protein intake. *Journal of Nutrition*, **92**, 497–502.
21. Cohen, S. & Hansen, J.D.L. (1962) Metabolism of albumin and γ-globulin in kwashiorkor. *Clinical Science*, **23**, 351–359.
22. Cox, R.F. & Matthias, A.P. (1969) Cytoplasmic effects of cortisol in liver. *Biochemical Journal*, **115**, 777–787.
23. Daniel, P.M., Pratt, O.E. & Spargo, E. (1977) The mechanism by which glucagon induces the release of amino acids from muscle and its relevance to fasting. *Proceedings of the Royal Society (London) (Biol.)*, **196**, 347–365.
24. Daniel, P.M., Pratt, O.E. & Spargo, E. (1977) The metabolic homeostatic role of muscle and its function as a store of protein. *Lancet*, **ii**, 446–448.
25. Denton, A.E. & Elvehjem, C.A. (1954) Amino acid concentration in the portal vein after ingestion of amino acids. *Journal of Biological Chemistry*, **206**, 455–460.
26. Dich, J. & Gluud, C.N. (1975) Effect of insulin on albumin production and incorporation of ^{14}C-leucine into proteins in isolated parenchymal liver cells from normal rats. *Acta Physiologica Scandinavica*, **94**, 236–243.
27. Dich, J., Hansen, S.E. & Thieden, H.D. (1973) Effect of albumin concentration and colloid osmotic pressure on albumin synthesis in the perfused rat liver. *Acta Physiologica Scandinavica*, **89**, 352–358.
28. Drews, J. & Braverman, G. (1967) Alterations in the nature of ribonucleic acid synthesized in rat liver during regeneration and after cortisol administration. *Journal of Biological Chemistry*, **242**, 801–808.
29. Drysdale, J.W. & Shafritz, D.A. (1975) In vitro stimulation of apoferritin synthesis by iron. *Biochimica et Biophysica Acta*, **383**, 97–105.
30. Drysdale, J.W., Arosio, P., Adelman, T., Hazard, J.T. & Brooks, D. (1975) Isoferritins in normal and diseased states. In *Proteins of Iron Storage and Transport in Biochemistry and Medicine* (Ed.) Crichton, R.R. pp. 359–366. Amsterdam: North Holland.
31. Dykes, P.W. (1968) The rates of distribution and catabolism of albumin in normal subjects and in patients with cirrhosis of the liver. *Clinical Science*, **34**, 161–183.
32. Elwyn, D.H. (1970) The role of the liver in regulation of amino acid and protein metabolism. In *Mammalian Protein Metabolism*, Vol. IV (Ed.) Munro, H.N. pp. 523–558. New York: Academic Press.
33. Enwonwu, C.O. & Munro, H.N. (1970) Rate of RNA turnover in rat liver in relation to intake of protein. *Archives of Biochemistry and Biophysics*, **138**, 532–539.
34. Enwonwu, C.O. & Munro, H.N. (1971) Changes in liver polyribosome patterns following administration of hydrocortisone and actinomycin. *Biochimica et Biophysica Acta*, **238**, 264–276.
35. FAO/WHO. World Health Organization Technical Reports Series, No. 522 (1973) Geneva: WHO.

36. Fauconneau, G. & Michel, M.C. (1970) The role of gastrointestinal tract in the regulation of protein metabolism. In *Mammalian Protein Metabolism*, Vol. IV (Ed.) Munro, H.N. pp. 481–522. New York: Academic Press.
37. Feldmann, G., Penaud-Laurencin, J., Grassous, J. & Benhamou, J.P. (1972) Albumin synthesis by human liver cells: its morphological demonstration. *Gastroenterology*, **63**, 1036–1048.
38. Feldmann, G., Maurice, M., Sapin, C. & Benhamou, J.P. (1975) Inhibition by colchicine of fibrinogen translocation in hepatocytes. *Journal of Cell Biology*, **67**, 237–243.
39. Felig, P. (1973) The glucose–alanine cycle. *Metabolism*, **22**, 179–207.
40. Felig, P. (1975) Amino acid metabolism in man. *Annual Review of Biochemistry*, **44**, 933–955.
41. Felig, P., Wahren, J., Sherwin, R. & Palaiologos, G. (1977) Amino acid and protein metabolism in diabetes mellitus. *Archives of Internal Medicine*, **137**, 507–513.
42. Freeman, T. (1969) Analbuminemia – a study of albumin and transferrin metabolism. In *Physiology and Pathophysiology of Plasma Protein Metabolism* (Ed.) Birke, G., Norberg, R. & Plantin, L.O. pp. 75–85. New York: Pergamon Press.
43. Gan, J.C. & Jeffay, H. (1967) Origins and metabolism of the intracellular amino acid pools in rat liver and muscle. *Biochimica et Biophysica Acta*, **148**, 448–459.
44. Gan, J.C. & Jeffay, H. (1971) The kinetics of transfer of plasma amino acids to tissues and the turnover rates of liver and muscle proteins. *Biochimica et Biophysica Acta*, **252**, 125–135.
45. Garber, A.J., Karl, I.E. & Kipnis, D.M. (1976) Alanine and glutamine synthesis and release from skeletal muscle. I. Glycolysis and amino acid release. II. The precursor role of amino acids in alanine and glutamine synthesis. *Journal of Biological Chemistry*, **251**, 826–835; 836–843.
46. Garlick, P.J., Millward, D.J. & James, W.P.T. (1973) The diurnal response of muscle and liver protein synthesis *in vivo* in meal-fed rats. *Biochemical Journal*, **136**, 935–946.
47. Garrow, J.S. (1974) Nutrition and plasma proteins. In *Structure and Function of Plasma Proteins*, Vol. 1 (Ed.) Allison, A.C. pp. 283–304. London: Plenum.
48. Gerschenson, L.E., Davidson, M.B. & Andersson, M. (1974) Hormonal regulation of rat liver cells cultured in chemically defined medium. Dexamethasone and insulin effects on different forms of tyrosine 2-oxoglutarate transaminase. *European Journal of Biochemistry*, **41**, 139–148.
49. Giordano, C. (1963) Use of exogenous and endogenous urea for protein synthesis in normal and uremic subjects. *Journal of Laboratory and Clinical Medicine*, **62**, 231–246.
50. Glaumann, H. & Ericsson, J.L.E. (1970) Evidence for the participation of the Golgi apparatus in the intracellular transport of nascent albumin in the liver cell. *Journal of Cell Biology*, **47**, 555–567.
51. Green, M. & Miller, L.L. (1960) Protein catabolism and protein synthesis in perfused livers of normal and alloxan-diabetic rats. *Journal of Biological Chemistry*, **235**, 3202–3208.
52. Halliday, D. & McKeran, R.O. (1975) Measurement of muscle protein synthetic rate from serial muscle biopsies and total body protein turnover in man by continuous intravenous infusion of L-(α-^{15}N)lysine. *Clinical Science and Molecular Medicine*, **49**, 581–590.
53. Halliday, J.W., Cowlishaw, J.L., Russo, A.M. & Powell, L.W. (1977) Serum-ferritin in diagnosis of haemochromatosis. *Lancet*, **ii**, 621–624.
54. Halliday, J.W., McKeering, L.V., Tweedale, R. & Powell, L.W. (1977) Serum ferritin in haemochromatosis: changes in the isoferritin composition during venesection therapy. *British Journal of Haematology*, **36**, 395–404.
55. Hamashima, Y., Harter, J.G. & Coons, A.H. (1964) The localization of albumin and fibrinogen in human liver cells. *Journal of Cell Biology*, **20**, 271–279.
56. Harrison, P.M. (1977) Ferritin: an iron storage molecule. *Seminars in Haematology*, **14**, 55–70.
57. Hems, R., Ross, B.D., Berry, M.N. & Krebs, H.A. (1966) Gluconeogenesis in the perfused rat liver. *Biochemical Journal*, **101**, 284–292.
58. Henderson, A.R. (1970) The effect of feeding with a tryptophan-free amino acid mixture on rat liver magnesium ion-activated deoxyribonucleic acid polymerase. *Biochemical Journal*, **120**, 205–214.
59. Hicks, S.J., Drysdale, J.W. & Munro, H.N. (1969) Preferential synthesis of ferritin and albumin by different populations of liver polysomes. *Science (Washington)*, **164**, 584–585.
60. Hoffenberg, R., Black, E. & Brock, J.F. (1966) Albumin and γ-globulin tracer studies in protein depletion states. *Journal of Clinical Investigation*, **45**, 143–152.
61. Ikehara, Y. & Pitot, H.C. (1973) Localization of polysome-bound albumin and serine dehydratase in rat liver cell fractions. *Journal of Cell Biology*, **59**, 28–44.
62. Iseri, O.A., Lieber, C.S. & Gottlieb, L.S. (1966) The ultrastructure of fatty liver induced by prolonged ethanol ingestion. *American Journal of Pathology*, **48**, 535–555.
63. Isselbacher, K.J. & Greenberger, N.J. (1964) Metabolic effects of alcohol on the liver. *New England Journal of Medicine*, **270**, 351–356; 402–410.
64. James, W.P.T. & Hay, A.M. (1968) Albumin metabolism: effect of the nutritional state and dietary protein intake. *Journal of Clinical Investigation*, **47**, 1958–1972.
65. Jeejeebhoy, K.N., Bruce-Robertson, A., Sodtke, U. & Foley, M. (1970) The effect of growth hormone on fibrinogen synthesis. *Biochemical Journal*, **119**, 243–249.
66. Jeejeebhoy, K.N., Phillips, M.J., Bruce-Robertson, A., Ho, J. & Sodtke, U. (1972) The acute effect of ethanol on albumin, fibrinogen and transferrin synthesis in the rat. *Biochemical Journal*, **126**, 1111–1126.
67. Jeejeebhoy, K.N., Bruce-Robertson, A., Ho, J. & Sodtke, U. (1975) The effect of ethanol on albumin and fibrinogen synthesis in vivo and in hepatocyte suspension. In *Alcohol and Abnormal Protein Biosynthesis: Biochemical and Clinical* (Ed.) Rothschild, M.A., Oratz, M. & Schreiber, S.S. p. 373. New York: Pergamon.
68. Jeejeebhoy, K.N., Phillips, M.J., Bruce-Robertson, A., Ho, J. & Sodtke, U. (1975) Albumin, fibrinogen and transferrin synthesis in isolated rat hepatocyte suspensions. *Biochemical Journal*, **146**, 141–155.
69. John, D.W. & Miller, L.L. (1969) Regulation of net biosynthesis of serum albumin and acute phase

plasma proteins. *Journal of Biological Chemistry*, **244,** 6134–6142.

70. Jones, E.A., Cain, G.D. & Dickinson, G. (1972) Corticosteroid-induced change in urea metabolism in patients with hepatocellular disease. *Gastroenterology*, **62,** 612–617.
71. Judah, J.D., Gamble, M. & Steadman, J.H. (1973) Biosynthesis of serum albumin in rat liver. Evidence for the existence of 'proalbumin'. *Biochemical Journal*, **134,** 1083–1091.
72. Kaplan, J.H. & Pitot, H.C. (1970) The regulation of intermediary amino acid metabolism in animal tissues. In *Mammalian Protein Metabolism*, Vol. IV (Ed.) Munro, H.N. pp. 388–443. New York: Academic Press.
73. Kekomäki, M., Schwartz, A.L. & Pentikäinen, P. (1970) Rate of urea synthesis in normal and cirrhotic rat liver with reference to the arginase synthetase system. *Scandinavian Journal of Gastroenterology*, **5,** 375–380.
74. Kelman, L., Saunders, S.J., Wicht, S., Frith, L., Corrigall, A., Kirsch, R.E. & Terblanche, J. (1972) The effect of amino acids on albumin synthesis by the isolated perfused rat liver. *Biochemical Journal*, **129,** 805–809.
75. Kernoff, L.M., Pimstone, B.L., Solomon, J. & Brock, J.F. (1971) The effect of hypophysectomy and growth hormone replacement on albumin synthesis and catabolism in the rat. *Biochemical Journal*, **124,** 529–535.
76. Khatra, B.S., Smith, R.B., Millikan, W.J., Sewell, C.W., Warren, W.D. & Rudman, D. (1974) Activities of Krebs–Henseleit enzymes in normal and cirrhotic human liver. *Journal of Laboratory and Clinical Medicine*, **84,** 708–715.
77. Kido, H., Shimazu, Y., Ueki, M. & Ogata, K. (1973) Effects of protein deficiency on serum albumin synthesizing activity with special reference to the presence of transcriptional controls. *Journal of Biochemistry (Tokyo)*, **74,** 747–756.
78. Kirsch, R., Frith, L., Black, E. & Hoffenberg, R. (1968) Regulation of albumin synthesis and catabolism by alteration of dietary protein. *Nature (London)*, **217,** 578–579.
79. Kirsch, R.E., Frith, L.O., Stead, R.H. & Saunders, S.J. (1973) Effect of alcohol on albumin synthesis by the isolated perfused rat liver. *American Journal of Clinical Nutrition*, **26,** 1191–1194.
80. Krebs, H.A., Hems, R. & Lund, P. (1973) Accumulation of amino acids by the perfused rat liver in the presence of ethanol. *Biochemical Journal*, **134,** 697–705.
81. Kukral, J.C., Kerth, J.D., Pancner, R.J., Cromer, D.W. & Henegar, G.C. (1961) Plasma protein synthesis in the normal dog and after total hepatectomy. *Surgery, Gynecology and Obstetrics*, **113,** 360–372.
82. Kuriyama, K., Sze, P.Y. & Rauscher, G.E. (1971) Effects of acute and chronic ethanol administration on ribosomal protein synthesis in mouse brain and liver. *Life Sciences*, **10** (Part II), 181–189.
83. Lane, B.P. & Lieber, C.S. (1966) Ultrastructural alterations in human hepatocytes following ingestion of ethanol with adequate diets. *American Journal of Pathology*, **49,** 593–603.
84. Laurent, T.C. & Ogston, A.G. (1963) The interaction between polysaccharides and other macromolecules. IV. The osmotic pressure of mixtures of serum albumin and hyaluronic acid. *Biochemical Journal*, **89,** 249–253.
85. Lewallen, C.G., Rall, J.E. & Berman, M. (1959) Studies of iodoalbumin metabolism. II. The effects of thyroid hormone. *Journal of Clinical Investigation*, **38,** 88–101.
86. Lieber, C.S. & DeCarli, L.M. (1974) An experimental model of alcohol feeding and liver injury in the baboon. *Journal of Medical Primatology*, **3,** 153–163.
87. Lieber, C.S. & Rubin, E. (1968) Alcoholic fatty liver in man on a high protein and low fat diet. *American Journal of Medicine*, **44,** 200–206.
88. Lipinski, B., Lipinska, I., Nowak, A. & Gurewich, V. (1977) Abnormal fibrinogen heterogeneity and fibrinolytic activity in advanced liver disease. *Journal of Laboratory and Clinical Medicine*, **90,** 187–194.
89. London, I.M. (1950) Studies on the rates of formation of serum proteins in men. In *Symposia on Nutrition, Vol. 2. Plasma Proteins*. pp. 72–82. Springfield, Illinois: Thomas.
90. Madsen, N.P. (1969) Reduced serum very low-density lipoprotein levels after acute ethanol administration. *Biochemical Pharmacology*, **18,** 216–262.
91. Magendie, F. (1829) *An Elementary Compendium of Physiology for the Use of Students* (trans. Milligan, E.) 3rd ed. Edinburgh: Carfrae. London: Longmans Green.
92. Maier, K.P., Volk, B., Hoppe-Seyler, G. & Gerok, W. (1974) Urea cycle enzymes in normal liver and in patients with alcoholic hepatitis. *European Journal of Clinical Investigation*, **4,** 193–195.
93. Marco, J., Diego, J., Villaneuva, M.L., Diaz-Fierros, M., Valverde, I. & Segovia, J.M. (1973) Elevated plasma glucagon levels in cirrhosis of the liver. *New England Journal of Medicine*, **289,** 1107–1111.
94. Marshall, J.S., Pensky, J. & Green, A.M. (1972) Studies on human thyroxine-binding globulin. VI. The nature of slow thyroxine-binding globulin. *Journal of Clinical Investigation*, **51,** 3173–3181.
95. Marshall, J.S., Green, A.M., Pensky, J., Williams, S., Zinn, A. & Carlson, D.M. (1974) Measurement of circulating desialylated glycoproteins and correlation with hepatocellular damage. *Journal of Clinical Investigation*, **54,** 555–562.
96. Marshall, J.S., Williams, S., Jones, P. & Hepner, G.W. (1978) Serum desialylated glycoproteins in patients with hepatobiliary dysfunction. *Journal of Laboratory and Clinical Medicine*. **92,** 30–37.
97. Marzo, A., Ghirardi, P. & Sardini, D. (1970) Serum lipids and total fatty acids in chronic alcoholic liver disease at different stages of cell damage. *Klinische Wochenschrift (Berlin)*, **48,** 949–950.
98. McPherson, I.G. (1973) Albumin metabolism in diabetes mellitus. *Clinica Chimica Acta*, **49,** 261–275.
99. Miller, L.L. (1960) Glucagon: a protein catabolic hormone in the isolated perfused rat liver. *Nature (London)*, **185,** 248.
100. Miller, L.L. (1961) Some direct actions of insulin, glucagon and hydrocortisone on the isolated perfused rat liver. *Recent Progress in Hormone Research*, **17,** 539–568.
101. Miller, L.L. & Bale, W.F. (1954) Synthesis of all plasma protein fractions except gamma globulins by the liver: the use of zone electrophoresis and lysine E-C^{14} to define the plasma proteins synthesized by the isolated perfused liver. *Journal of Experimental Medicine*, **99,** 125–132.
102. Miller, S.A. (1969) Protein metabolism during growth and development. In *Mammalian Protein*

Metabolism Vol. 3 (Ed.) Munro, H.N. pp. 183–233. New York: Academic Press.

103. Mimura, T., Yamada, C. & Swenseid, M.E. (1968) Influence of dietary protein levels and hydrocortisone administration on the branched chain transaminase activity in rat tissues. *Journal of Nutrition,* **95,** 493–498.
104. Mondon, C.E. & Mortimore, G.E. (1967) Effects of insulin on amino acid release and urea formation in perfused rat liver. *American Journal of Physiology,* **212,** 173–178.
105. Mookerjea, Y. & Chow, A. (1969) Impairment of glycoprotein synthesis in acute ethanol intoxication in rats. *Biochimica et Biophysica Acta,* **184,** 83–92.
106. Morell, A.G., Gregoriadis, G., Scheinberg, I.H., Hickman, J. & Ashwell, G. (1971) The role of sialic acid in determining the survival of glycoproteins in the circulation. *Journal of Biological Chemistry,* **246,** 1461–1467.
107. Morgan, E.H. & Peters, T. (1971) The biosynthesis of rat serum albumin. V. Effect of protein depletion and refeeding on albumin and transferrin synthesis. *Journal of Biological Chemistry,* **246,** 3500–3507.
108. Mortimore, G.E. & Mondon, C.E. (1970) Inhibition by insulin of valine turnover in liver. *Journal of Biological Chemistry,* **245,** 2375–2383.
109. Morton, A.G. & Tavill, A.S. (1977) The role of iron in the regulation of hepatic transferrin synthesis. *British Journal of Haematology,* **36,** 383–394.
110. Munro, H.N. (1964) Historical introduction: the origin and growth of present concepts of protein metabolism. In *Mammalian Protein Metabolism, Vol. 1* (Ed.) Munro, H.N. & Allison, J.B. pp. 1–29. New York: Academic Press.
111. Munro, H.N. (1964) General aspects of the regulation of protein metabolism by diet and by hormones. In *Mammalian Protein Metabolism, Vol. 1* (Ed.) Munro, H.N. & Allison, J.B. pp. 384–481. New York: Academic Press.
112. Munro, H.N. (1968) Role of amino acid supply in regulating ribosome function. *Federation Proceedings,* **27,** 1231–1237.
113. Munro, H.N. (1970) A general survey of mechanisms regulating protein metabolism in mammals. In *Mammalian Protein Metabolism,* Vol. IV (Ed.) Munro, H.N. pp. 3–130. New York: Academic Press.
114. Munro, H.N. (1972) Basic concepts in the use of amino acids and protein hydrolysates for parenteral nutrition. In *Parenteral Nutrition* (Ed.) Wilkinson, A.W. pp. 34–67. Edinburgh: Churchill Livingstone.
115. Munro, H.N., Hubert, C. & Baliga, B.S. (1975) Regulation of protein synthesis in relation to amino acid supply – a review. In *Alcohol and Abnormal Protein Synthesis, Biochemical and Clinical* (Ed.) Rothschild, M.A., Oratz, M. & Schreiber, S.S. pp. 33–66. New York: Pergamon.
116. Odessey, R., Khairallah, E.A. & Goldberg, A.L. (1974) Origin and possible significance of alanine production by skeletal muscle. *Journal of Biological Chemistry,* **249,** 7623–7629.
117. Olmsted, J.B. & Borisy, G.G. (1973) Microtubules. *Annual Review of Biochemistry,* **42,** 507–540.
118. Oratz, M., Rothschild, M.A. & Schreiber, S.S. (1976) Alcohol, amino acids and albumin synthesis. II. Alcohol inhibition of albumin synthesis reversed by arginine and spermine. *Gastroenterology,* **71,** 123–127.
119. Oratz, M., Rothschild, M.A. & Schreiber, S.S. (1978) Alcohol, amino acids and albumin synthesis. III. Effects of ethanol, acetaldehyde and 4-methylpyrazole. *Gastroenterology,* **74,** 672–676.
120. Pain, V.M., Lanoix, J., Bergeron, J.J.M. & Clemens, M.J. (1974) Effects of diabetes on the ultrastructure of the hepatocyte and on the distribution and activity of ribosomes in the free and membrane-bound populations. *Biochimica et Biophysica Acta,* **353,** 487–498.
121. Palascak, J.E. & Martinez, J. (1977) Dysfibrinogenemia associated with liver disease. *Journal of Clinical Investigation,* **60,** 89–95.
122. Perin, A., Scalabrino, G., Sessa, A. & Arnaboldi, A. (1974) *In vitro* inhibition of protein synthesis in rat liver as a consequence of ethanol metabolism. *Biochimica et Biophysica Acta,* **366,** 101–108.
123. Peters, T. Jr (1970) Serum albumin. *Advances in Clinical Chemistry,* **13,** 37–41.
124. Peters, T. & Peters, J.C. (1972) The biosynthesis of rat serum albumin. VI. Intracellular transport of albumin and rates of albumin and liver protein synthesis *in vivo* under various physiological conditions. *Journal of Biological Chemistry,* **247,** 3858–3863.
125. Peters, T. Jr, Fleischer, B. & Fleischer, S. (1971) The biosynthesis of rat serum albumin. IV. Apparent passage of albumin through the Golgi apparatus during secretion. *Journal of Biological Chemistry,* **246,** 240–244.
126. Powell, L.W., Alpert, E., Isselbacher, K.J. & Drysdale, J.W. (1974) Abnormality in tissue isoferritin distribution in idiopathic haemochromatosis. *Nature,* **250,** 333–335.
127. Prieto, J., Barry, M. & Sherlock, S. (1975) Serum ferritin in patients with iron overload and with acute and chronic liver diseases. *Gastroenterology,* **68,** 525–533.
128. Putnam, C.W., Porter, K., Peters, R.L., Ashcavai, M., Redeker, A.G. & Starzl, T.E. (1977) Liver replacement for alpha$_1$-antitrypsin deficiency. *Surgery,* **81,** 258–261.
129. Quinn, P.S., Gamble, M. & Judah, J.D. (1975) Biosynthesis of serum albumin in rat liver. Isolation and probable structure of 'proalbumin' from rat liver. *Biochemical Journal,* **146,** 389–393.
130. Ratnoff, O.D. (1975) Disordered hemostasis in hepatic disease. In *Diseases of the Liver* (Ed.) Schiff, L. pp. 184–203. Philadelphia: Lippincott.
131. Redman, C.M. (1969) Biosynthesis of serum proteins and ferritin by free and attached ribosomes of rat liver. *Journal of Biological Chemistry,* **244,** 4308–4315.
132. Redman, C.M., Bannerjee, D., Howell, K. & Palade, G.E. (1975) Colchicine inhibition of plasma protein release from rat hepatocytes. *Journal of Cell Biology,* **66,** 42–59.
133. Regoeczi, E. (1974) Fibrinogen. In *Structure and Function of Plasma Proteins,* Vol. 1 (Ed.) Allison, A.C. pp. 133–167. London: Plenum.
134. Renis, M., Giovine, A. & Bertolino, A. (1975) Protein synthesis in mitochondrial and microsomal fractions from rat brain and liver after acute and chronic ethanol administration. *Life Sciences,* **16,** 1447–1458.
135. Richards, P., Metcalfe-Gibson, A., Ward, E.E., Wrong, O. & Houghton, B.J. (1967) Utilization of ammonia nitrogen for protein synthesis in man, and the effect of protein restriction and uraemia. *Lancet,* **ii,** 845–849.
136. Rothschild, M.A., Oratz, M. & Schreiber, S.S. (1970) Changing concepts of albumin metabolism and

distribution in cirrhosis of the liver. *Scandinavian Journal of Gastroenterology* (Suppl. 7), **5,** 17–23.

137. Rothschild, M.A., Oratz, M. & Schreiber, S.S. (1972) Albumin synthesis. *New England Journal of Medicine,* **286,** 748–757; 816–821.
138. Rothschild, M.A., Oratz, M. & Schreiber, S.S. (1974) Alcohol, amino acids and albumin synthesis. *Gastroenterology,* **67,** 1200–1213.
139. Rothschild, M.A., Bauman, A., Yalow, R.S. & Berson, S.A. (1955) Tissue distribution of I^{131} labeled human serum albumin following intravenous administration. *Journal of Clinical Investigation,* **34,** 1354–1358.
140. Rothschild, M.A., Bauman, A., Yalow, R.S. & Berson, S.A. (1957) The effect of large doses of desiccated thyroid on the distribution and metabolism of albumin I^{131} in euthyroid subjects. *Journal of Clinical Investigation,* **36,** 422–428.
141. Rothschild, M.A., Schreiber, S.S., Oratz, M. & McGee, H.L. (1958) The effects of adrenocortical hormones on albumin metabolism studied with albumin-I^{131}. *Journal of Clinical Investigation,* **37,** 1229–1235.
142. Rothschild, M.A., Oratz, M., Wimer, E. & Schreiber, S.S. (1961) Studies on albumin synthesis. Effects of dextran and cortisone on albumin metabolism in rabbits studied with ^{131}I-albumin. *Journal of Clinical Investigation,* **40,** 545–554.
143. Rothschild, M.A., Oratz, M., Franklin, E.C. & Schreiber, S.S. (1962) The effect of hyperglobulinemia on albumin metabolism in hyperimmunized rabbits studied with albumin-I^{131} *Journal of Clinical Investigation,* **41,** 1564–1571.
144. Rothschild, M.A., Oratz, M., Evans, C. & Schreiber, S.S. (1964) Alterations in albumin metabolism after serum and albumin infusions. *Journal of Clinical Investigation,* **43,** 1874–1880.
145. Rothschild, M.A., Oratz, M., Evans, C.E. & Schreiber, S.S. (1966) Role of hepatic interstitial albumin in regulating albumin synthesis. *American Journal of Physiology,* **210,** 57–62.
146. Rothschild, M.A., Oratz, M., Mongelli, J. & Schreiber, S.S. (1968) Effects of a short term fast on albumin synthesis studied *in vivo* in the perfused liver and on amino acid incorporation by hepatic microsomes. *Journal of Clinical Investigation,* **47,** 2591–2599.
147. Rothschild, M.A., Oratz, M., Mongelli, J. & Schreiber, S.S. (1969) Amino acid regulation of albumin synthesis. *Journal of Nutrition,* **98,** 395–403.
148. Rothschild, M.A., Oratz, M., Mongelli, J., Fishman, L. & Schreiber, S.S. (1969) Amino acid regulation of albumin synthesis. *Journal of Nutrition,* **98,** 395–403.
149. Rothschild, M.A., Oratz, M., Zimmon, D.S., Schreiber, S.S., Weiner, I. & Van Caneghem, A. (1969) Albumin synthesis in cirrhotic subjects studied with carbonate-^{14}C. *Journal of Clinical Investigation,* **48,** 344–350.
150. Rothschild, M.A., Oratz, M., Mongelli, J. & Schreiber, S.S. (1971) Alcohol-induced depression of albumin synthesis: reversal by tryptophan. *Journal of Clinical Investigation,* **50,** 1812–1818.
151. Rubin, E. & Lieber, C.S. (1967) Early fine structural changes in the human liver induced by alcohol. *Gastroenterology,* **52,** 1–13.
152. Rudman, D., Difulco, T.J., Galambos, J.T., Smith, R.B., Salam, A.A. & Warren, W.D. (1973) Maximal rates of excretion and synthesis of urea in normal and cirrhotic subjects. *Journal of Clinical Investigation,* **52,** 2241–2249.
153. Russell, J.H. & Geller, D.M. (1973) Rat serum albumin biosynthesis: evidence for a precursor. *Biochemical and Biophysical Research Communications,* **55,** 239–245.
154. Schimke, R.T. (1963) Studies on factors affecting the levels of urea cycle enzymes in rat liver. *Journal of Biological Chemistry,* **238,** 1012–1018.
155. Schimke, R.T. (1964) The importance of both synthesis and degradation in the control of arginase levels in rat liver. *Journal of Biological Chemistry,* **239,** 3808–3817.
156. Schimke, R.T. (1970) Regulation of protein degradation in mammalian tissues. In *Mammalian Protein Metabolism,* Vol. IV (Ed.) Munro, H.N. pp. 178–228. New York: Academic Press.
157. Schoenheimer, R. (1942) *The Dynamic State of Body Constituents.* Cambridge, Massachusetts: Harvard University Press.
158. Schultze, H.E. & Heremans, J.F. (1966) *Molecular Biology of Human Proteins,* Vol. I, p. 475. Amsterdam: Elsevier.
159. Shambaugh, G.E. (1978) Urea biosynthesis. II. Normal and abnormal regulation. *American Journal of Clinical Nutrition,* **31,** 126–133.
160. Sharp, H.L. (1976) The current status of alpha-1-antitrypsin, a protease inhibitor, in gastrointestinal disease. *Gastroenterology,* **70,** 611–621.
161. Sherwin, R., Joshi, P., Hendler, R., Felig, P. & Conn, H.O. (1974) Hyperglucagonemia in Laennec's cirrhosis: the role of portal-systemic shunting. *New England Journal of Medicine,* **290,** 239–242.
162. Sidransky, H., Verney, E. & Sarma, D.S.R. (1971) Effect of tryptophan on polyribosomes and protein synthesis in liver. *American Journal of Clinical Nutrition,* **24,** 779–785.
163. Sidransky, H., Sarma, D.S.R., Bongiorno, M. & Verney, E. (1968) Effect of dietary tryptophan on hepatic polyribosomes and protein synthesis in fasted mice. *Journal of Biological Chemistry,* **243,** 1123–1132.
164. Skillman, J.J., Rosenoer, V.M., Smith, P.C. & Fang, M.S. (1976) Improved albumin synthesis in postoperative patients by amino acid infusion. *New England Journal of Medicine,* **295,** 1037–1040.
165. Smallwood, R.A., Jones, E.A., Craigie, S., Raia, S. & Rosenoer, V.M. (1968) The delivery of newly synthesized albumin and fibrinogen to the plasma in dogs. *Clinical Science,* **35,** 35–43.
166. Snodgrass, P.J. & Delong, G.R. (1976) Urea cycle enzyme deficiencies and an increased nitrogen load producing hyperammonemia in Reye's syndrome. *New England Journal of Medicine,* **294,** 855–860.
167. Snyderman, S.E., Holt, L.E., Dancis, J., Roitman, E., Boyer, A. & Balis, M.E. (1962) 'Unessential' nitrogen: a limiting factor for human growth. *Journal of Nutrition,* **78,** 57–72.
168. Sorrell, M.F., Tuma, D.J. & Barak, A.J. (1977) Evidence that acetaldehyde irreversibly impairs glycoprotein metabolism in liver slices. *Gastroenterology,* **73,** 1138–1141.
169. Sorrell, M.F., Tuma, D.J., Schafer, E.C. & Barak, A.J. (1977) Role of acetaldehyde in the ethanol induced impairment of glycoprotein metabolism in rat liver slices. *Gastroenterology,* **73,** 137–144.
170. Starzl, T.E., Porter, K.A., Watanabe, K. & Putnam, C.W. (1976) Effects of insulin, glucagon, and insulin/glucagon infusions on liver morphology and cell division after complete portacaval shunt in dogs. *Lancet,* **i,** 821–825.
171. Sterling, K. (1951) Serum albumin turnover in Laennec's cirrhosis as measured by I^{131}-tagged albumin. *Journal of Clinical Investigation,* **30,** 1238–1242.

172. Sterling, K. (1960) The effect of Cushing's syndrome upon serum albumin metabolism. *Journal of Clinical Investigation,* **39,** 1900–1908.
173. Suttie, J.W. & Jackson, C.M. (1977) Prothrombin structure, activation and biosynthesis. *Physiological Reviews,* **57,** 1–70.
174. Swain, C.P. & Tavill, A.S. (1978) The protein secretory activities of the liver. In *Scientific Basis of Gastroenterology* (Ed.) Wormsley, K.G. & Duthie, H.L. Edinburgh: Churchill-Livingstone. In press.
175. Swain, C.P., Tavill, A.S. & Neale, G. (1976) Studies of tryptophan and albumin metabolism in a patient with carcinoid syndrome, pellagra and hypoproteinemia. *Gastroenterology,* **71,** 484–489.
176. Takagi, M. & Ogata, K. (1968) Direct evidence for albumin biosynthesis by membrane-bound polysomes in rat liver. *Biochemical and Biophysical Research Communications,* **33,** 55–60.
177. Tavill, A.S. (1972) The synthesis and degradation of liver produced proteins. *Gut,* **13,** 225–241.
178. Tavill, A.S. & Hoffenberg, R. (1976) Turnover of plasma proteins. In *Structure and Function of Plasma Proteins,* Vol. 2 (Ed.) Allison, A.C. pp. 107–144. New York: Plenum.
179. Tavill, A.S. & Morton, A.G. (1978) Transferrin metabolism and the liver. In *Metals in the Liver* (Ed.) Powell, L.W. pp. 93–130. New York: Marcel Dekker.
180. Tavill, A.S., Craigie, A. & Rosenoer, V.M. (1968) The measurement of the synthetic rate of albumin in man. *Clinical Science,* **34,** 1–28.
181. Tavill, A.S., East, A.G., Black, E.G., Nadkarni, D. & Hoffenberg, R. (1973) Regulatory factors in the synthesis of plasma proteins by the isolated perfused rat liver. *Ciba Foundation Symposium,* **9** (New Series), 155–180.
182. Unger, R.H. (1971) Glucagon physiology and pathophysiology. *New England Journal of Medicine,* **285,** 443–449.
183. Unger, R.H. (1972) Insulin/glucagon rates. *Israel Journal of Medical Sciences,* **8,** 252–257.
184. Urban, J., Inglis, A.S., Edwards, K. & Schreiber, G. (1974) Chemical evidence for the difference between albumins from microsomes and serum and a possible precursor-product relationship. *Biochemical and Biophysical Research Communications,* **61,** 494–501.
185. Varcoe, R., Halliday, D., Carson, E.R., Richards, P. & Tavill, A.S. (1975) Efficiency of utilization of urea nitrogen for albumin synthesis by chronically uraemic and normal man. *Clinical Science and Molecular Medicine,* **48,** 379–390.
186. Veselý, J. & Cihák, A. (1970) Enhanced DNA-dependent RNA polymerase and RNA synthesis in rat liver nuclei after administration of L-tryptophan. *Biochimica et Biophysica Acta,* **204,** 614–616.
187. Wahren, J., Felig, P. & Hagenfeldt, J. (1976) Effect of protein ingestion on splanchnic and leg metabolism in normal man and in patients with diabetes mellitus. *Journal of Clinical Investigation,* **57,** 987–999.
188. Waldmann, T.A., Gordon, R.S. Jr & Rosse, W. (1964) Studies on the metabolism of the serum proteins and lipids in a patient with analbuminemia. *American Journal of Medicine,* **37,** 960–968.
189. Walser, M. & Bodenlos, L.J. (1959) Urea metabolism in man. *Journal of Clinical Investigation,* **38,** 1617–1626.
190. Wands, J.R., Rowe, J.A., Mezey, S.E., Waterbury, L.A., Wright, J.R., Halliday, J.W., Isselbacher, K.J. & Powell, L.W. (1976) Normal serum ferritin concentrations in precirrhotic hemochromatosis. *New England Journal of Medicine,* **294,** 302–305.
191. Watanabe, M., Potter, V.R. & Pitot, H.C. (1968) Systematic oscillations in tyrosine transaminase and other metabolic functions in liver of normal and adrenalectomised rats on controlled feeding. *Journal of Nutrition,* **95,** 207–227.
192. Waterlow, J.C. (1967) Lysine turnover in man measured by intravenous infusion of L(U-^{14}C)lysine. *Clinical Science,* **33,** 507–515.
193. Waterlow, J.C. & Payne, P.R. (1975) The protein gap. *Nature,* **258,** 113–117.
194. Waterlow, J.C. & Stephen, J.M.L. (1967) The measurement of total lysine turnover in the rat by intravenous infusion of L(U-^{14}C)lysine. *Clinical Science,* **33,** 489–506.
195. Waterlow, J.C. & Stephen, J.M.L. (1968) The effect of low protein diets on the turnover rates of serum, liver and muscle proteins in the rat measured by continuous infusion of L-(U-^{14}C)lysine. *Clinical Science,* **35,** 287–305.
196. Wilkinson, P. & Mendenhall, C.L. (1963) Serum albumin turnover in normal subjects and patients with cirrhosis measured by I^{131}-labelled human albumin. *Clinical Science,* **25,** 281–292.
197. Wilson, S.H. & Hoagland, M.B. (1967) Physiology of rat-liver polysomes. The stability of messenger ribonucleic acid and ribosomes. *Biochemical Journal,* **103,** 556–566.
198. Wilson, S.H., Hill, N.Z. & Hoagland, M.B. (1967) Physiology of rat-liver polysomes. Protein synthesis by stable polysomes. *Biochemical Journal,* **103,** 567–572.
199. Woodside, K.H. & Mortimore, G.E. (1972) Suppression of protein turnover by amino acids in the perfused rat liver. *Journal of Biological Chemistry,* **247,** 6474–6481.
200. Yap, S.H., Strair, S.K. & Shafritz, D.A. (1977) Distribution of rat liver albumin mRNA membrane-bound and free in polyribosomes as determined by molecular hybridization. *Proceedings of the National Academy of Sciences of the United States of America,* **74,** 5397–5401.
201. Yap, S.H., Strair, R.K. & Shafritz, D.A. (1978) Alterations in hepatic mRNA content and subcellular distribution in the fasting state. *Gastroenterology,* **74,** 1168 (abstract).
202. Yap, S.H., Strair, R.K. & Shafritz, D.A. (1978) Effect of a short term fast on the distribution of cytoplasmic albumin messenger ribonucleic acid in rat liver. Evidence for formation of free albumin messenger ribonucleoprotein particles. *Journal of Biological Chemistry,* **253,** 4944–4950.
203. Young, V.R. & Scrimshaw, N.S. (1968) Endogenous nitrogen metabolism and plasma free amino acids in young adults given a 'protein-free' diet. *British Journal of Nutrition,* **22,** 9–20.
204. Young, V.R., Steffee, W.P., Pencharz, P.B., Winterer, J.C. & Scrimshaw, N.S. (1975) Total human body protein synthesis in relation to protein requirements at various ages. *Nature (London),* **253,** 192–194.
205. Zähringer, J., Baliga, B.S. & Munro, H.N. (1976) Novel mechanism for translational control in regulation of ferritin synthesis by iron. *Proceedings of the National Academy of Science,* **73,** 857–861.
206. Zimmon, D.S., Oratz, M., Kessler, R., Schreiber, S.S. & Rothschild, M.A. (1969) Albumin to ascites: demonstration of a direct pathway bypassing the systemic circulation. *Journal of Clinical Investigation,* **48,** 2074–2078.

Chapter 6

Nutritional Aspects of Liver Disease

NEIL McINTYRE
MARSHA Y. MORGAN

The liver plays a key role in the handling of many foodstuffs and in supplying other tissues with the nutrients which they require for normal functioning. Disease of the liver may affect the metabolism of various foodstuffs and normal dietary constituents may then have deleterious effects. Dietary deficiency or excess may damage the liver and it is sometimes injured by toxins present in food. In this chapter we will consider the role of the liver in handling foodstuffs and the nutritional consequences of liver damage. We will discuss nutritional liver injury and the way in which dietary manipulations can be used for the benefit of patients with liver disease.

There is little evidence that liver disease affects the overall energy requirement of the patient, that is the amount which results in no long-term change in body weight. A person's energy requirements depend on body size and composition, on age and physical activity. In normal adults they range from approximately 8 to 15 MJ/24 hr (i.e., from about 2000 to 3600 C) and the major sources of the energy are dietary carbohydrate, protein and fat.

In the United Kingdom most of the dietary carbohydrate (about 60 per cent) is in the form of starch (with small amounts of glycogen) and the remainder is made up of sucrose (about 33 per cent) and lactose. There appears to be no absolute requirement for dietary carbohydrate but a certain amount is necessary to make the diet palatable. 'Roughage' or fibre also seems to be beneficial and this is often associated with carbohydrate-containing foods.

Fat is present in the diet as 'visible' fats, such as butter, margarine, cooking fat and oils and the fat on meat, and as 'invisible' fats which are found in milk, nuts, lean meat and in other animal and vegetable foods. These fats are composed mainly of triglycerides. As with carbohydrate there is no absolute dietary requirement for triglyceride, except that a small amount (about 1 to 2 per cent of energy requirements) of essential fatty acids is required. Fats are important for palatability and in addition are the major source of fat-soluble vitamins.

Protein, the third major source of energy, is essential for normal bodily function and protein malnutrition has serious metabolic consequences at all ages. The amount necessary for normal bodily function has not been established with certainty but probably it should comprise at least 10 per cent of the total energy requirements. In the United Kingdom about a third of dietary protein comes from plant sources and the remainder from animal products.

NUTRITIONAL ROLE OF THE LIVER AND THE CONSEQUENCES OF HEPATOBILIARY DAMAGE

Carbohydrate

Ingested carbohydrate leaves the gut as monosaccharides which travel in the portal vein and reach the liver in relatively high concentration.

They enter the liver freely where all dietary monosaccharides can be assimilated.

The concentration of glucose in hepatic cell water is always relatively high (around 6 mmol/l [110 mg/dl]). In the fasting state glucose, derived from glycogenolysis or gluconeogenesis, diffuses *from* the liver into the blood and is transported to tissues such as the brain which are dependent on glucose for normal functioning. During glucose absorption, when portal venous levels are high, glucose diffuses *into* the liver cells and is phosphorylated by glucokinase: glycogen is synthesized; less glucose is made in the liver and some absorbed glucose may be catabolized by the liver.

The levels of fructose and galactose in hepatic cell water are very low in the fasting state. When these sugars are present in the portal venous blood they diffuse rapidly into hepatic cells to be phosphorylated by fructokinase and galactokinase. Consequently, fructose and galactose in the portal blood are largely removed during their first passage through the liver and peripheral blood levels are very low after an oral load. Some claim that ingested glucose is also largely removed on first passage, but there is evidence to suggest that most of it passes through the liver to be assimilated perhaps by peripheral tissues[49, 54] (see Chapter 3 for full discussion).

Damage to the liver can have striking effects on carbohydrate metabolism. In patients with acute hepatic failure hypoglycaemia is relatively common, presumably because there is a failure of glycogenolysis and gluconeogenesis; this may lead to confusion, coma or other neurological abnormalities. With chronic liver disease, however, hypoglycaemia is uncommon unless provoked by oral hypoglycaemic agents. Instead there is usually a diminished tolerance to oral glucose, with hyperglycaemia, glycosuria and sometimes a frank diabetic syndrome with fasting hyperglycaemia. The reduced tolerance to oral glucose does not result simply from intrahepatic shunting of blood past hepatocytes. There is little or no effect on oral glucose tolerance when the entire portal blood supply is diverted in cirrhotic patients by means of an end-to-side portacaval anastomosis[38] but the same procedure has a striking effect on plasma levels of fructose following oral loading. In patients with chronic liver disease and probably in acute hepatic failure there is insulin resistance but the mechanism for this is not yet clear. The effects of liver disease on carbohydrate metabolism are discussed more fully in Chapter 3.

Protein

Protein presented to the small intestine for absorption arises partly from the diet and partly from desquamated intestinal cells and secretions. The dietary protein intake is highly variable, but in adults should range from 0·5 to 1·5 g/kg body weight/24 hr (see Chapter 5). Dietary protein contains a large number of different amino acids and the amino acid composition of vegetable proteins and of meat is similar except for a significant excess of methionine in the latter.[81] Certain amino acids are considered to be essential because they cannot be manufactured in the human body in adequate amounts. In children and adults isoleucine, leucine, valine, lysine, methionine, phenylalanine, threonine and tryptophan appear to be essential, as is histidine in infants.

In the intestine complex protein molecules are cleaved by intraluminal peptidases with the production of short chain oligopeptides, dipeptides and small amounts of free amino acids. Amino acids are absorbed by a series of active transport systems. Oligo- and dipeptides are either cleaved by brush-border peptidases, and their amino acids then absorbed, or dipeptides may enter the mucosal cells intact for intracellular hydrolysis.[87]

Only free amino acids are transported from the gut into portal blood and thence to the liver. In dogs,[22] rats[98] and sheep[97] the composition of the amino acid mixture leaving the gut is different from that of dietary protein; aspartate and glutamate account for about 20 to 30 per cent of the amino acids of ingested protein, but their concentration is very low in portal blood because the gut converts these amino acids into alanine which is the predominant amino acid presented to the liver.

It is well known that the liver can remove amino acids from the blood, but not all to the same extent. The alanine uptake exceeds that of other amino acids. Serine, threonine and glycine are also taken up, as to a lesser extent are all other glucogenic amino acids. The branched chain amino acids leucine, isoleucine and particularly valine are poorly extracted by the liver, although they are released in large amounts by muscle; it seems that their major site of catabolism is in extrahepatic tissues.[55] Hepatic uptake of branched chain amino acids following protein ingestion is substantially below the amount absorbed from the intestine whereas the uptake of the other amino acids tends to rise in parallel with their concentration in the portal vein. The entry of amino acids into the liver is governed by transport mechanisms which are stereospecific, saturable for certain amino acids, and which may exhibit cross-inhibition.[66]

There are few data in man on the quantitative aspects of amino acid transport from the gut following protein ingestion and the uptake of these amino acids by the liver. When daily protein intake is increased by 50 per cent (from 1 to 1·5 g/kg body weight) there are significant elevations in the peripheral plasma concentrations of proline, cystine, methionine, valine, isoleucine and leucine.[56] There seems to be a relationship between peaks of concentrations and meal times but it is not clear whether the elevations occur because these amino acids are not taken up as well by the liver as are other amino acids.

The concentration of free amino acids in the plasma is, of course, dependent on the net effect of entry of amino acids from the gut, and from other tissues, and their removal by a variety of tissues for many different purposes. Muscle contains about 50 per cent of the total body pool of free amino acids[64] and with the liver it plays a major role in total amino acid metabolism. Alanine appears to play a key role as a precursor of glucose in the liver. Alanine taken up for this purpose not only comes from the diet; it is also synthesized in peripheral tissues, especially muscle, via the transamination of pyruvate.[25]

The role of the liver in other aspects of the intermediary metabolism of amino acids and in hepatic protein synthesis is considered further in Chapter 5.

Damage to the liver may have complex and variable effects on its handling of amino acids. These effects seem to depend on the severity of the damage and possibly on its aetiology.[60] In fulminant hepatic failure plasma amino acid values are increased except for those of branched chain amino acids which are normal or low.[73] This increase occurs even if there is no intake of amino acids or protein and is presumably a reflection both of the release of amino acids from tissues, including the necrotic liver, and the failure of the liver to remove them from the plasma.

In chronic liver disease there is commonly an elevation of one or both of the aromatic amino acids, tyrosine and phenylalanine, together with methionine, and a reduction in the concentration of the three branched chain amino acids, valine, leucine and isoleucine. The reasons for these changes are not clear. The fall in branched chain amino acids may result from the hyperinsulinaemia, found often with chronic liver disease, which suppresses the muscle output of branched chain amino acids;[15] it may also be due to a compensatory increase in their extrahepatic oxidation.

Some of the changes in plasma amino acid concentrations may be a reflection of the liver's inability, due to portasystemic shunting, to handle amino acids absorbed from the intestine and presented to it in the portal vein. In animals the creation of a portacaval shunt results in a rapid elevation of several amino acids, including tyrosine and methionine, and a fall in the branched chain amino acids.[1] In contrast, patients with an extrahepatic portal vein block, who have extensive shunting but little or no liver damage, show no significant change in plasma amino acid values even after a protein load.

Fat

Most dietary lipid is present in the form of triglycerides which contain a variety of different fatty acids. The most important are the long chain fatty acids with chain lengths from 16 carbon atoms upwards. These include the common saturated fatty acids (palmitic [C16] and stearic [C18]), the mono-unsaturated oleic acid (C18Δ9, where Δ signifies the position of the double bond or bonds) and the polyunsaturated fatty acids (linoleic [C18Δ9, 12], linolenic [C18Δ9, 12, 15] and arachidonic [C20Δ5, 8, 11, 14]).

Palmitic, stearic and oleic acids can be synthesized within the body. The three polyunsaturated fatty acids mentioned above cannot be synthesized de novo; they, and other members of their family, are biologically necessary for several reasons, including their role as precursors of prostaglandins. They are therefore called 'essential' fatty acids but only linoleic and linolenic are truly essential because the others can be synthesized from them by mammalian cells.

Some naturally occurring triglycerides contain fatty acids with chain lengths shorter than C16. They are known as medium chain triglycerides and are absorbed by mechanisms different from those for long chain triglycerides; they do not require pancreatic lipase or bile salts for their uptake from the lumen and are transported from the gut in the portal vein, not in the lymphatics. Medium chain triglycerides are synthesized for administration to patients with fat malabsorption.

Following ingestion, lumps of fat containing

long chain triglycerides are emulsified by bile salts. As a result the surface area available for attack by pancreatic lipase is greatly increased. This hydrolytic enzyme attacks the ester linkages at positions 1 and 3 of the glycerol backbone with the production of two fatty acids and a molecule of 2-monoglyceride. The fatty acids and 2-monoglyceride associate with bile acids and phosphatidylcholine to form micelles which incorporate cholesterol and fat-soluble vitamins into their core. Micelles are minute compared with the particles present in an emulsion. When they contact the microvilli of the absorptive cells of the small intestine their fatty acids and monoglyceride and their cholesterol and fat-soluble vitamins are taken up into the enterocyte. The monoglyceride and fatty acids are synthesized into triglyceride. This is packaged into large particles called chylomicrons which also contain cholesterol, cholesteryl esters, phospholipids, apoproteins and fat-soluble vitamins. The chylomicrons leave the gut in intestinal lymph. Details of their subsequent metabolism are presented in Chapter 4. Suffice to say that, although their triglyceride is hydrolysed mainly in peripheral tissues, a large proportion of their fatty acids, including essential fatty acids, is subsequently made available to the liver and to other tissues.

With acute or chronic parenchymal liver damage and with biliary obstruction there is usually a reduction in the flow of bile salts into the intestine. This interferes with emulsification of triglyceride and with the action of pancreatic lipase but even so there may be extensive hydrolysis of triglyceride. Free fatty acids and monoglyceride can still be absorbed from the intestine in relatively large amounts (even in the absence of bile salts) and steatorrhoea is therefore usually modest; its severity is roughly proportional to the degree of hepatocellular damage or biliary obstruction. But when bile salt levels in the intestinal lumen are low, micelle formation tends to be seriously disrupted and, with it, the absorption of fat-soluble vitamins and cholesterol which are dependent on micellar solubility for their uptake.

Vitamins (Table 6.1)

Fat soluble vitamins

Vitamin A.[52] Vitamin A exists in a number of forms. Vitamin A_1 is the primary alcohol retinol, present in animal tissues and in the diet largely as the ester retinyl palmitate. The plant pigment carotene is also an important source of vitamin A; it is cleaved by the small intestinal mucosa into two molecules of the aldehyde retinal which is reduced to retinol; approximately a half of our daily intake of vitamin A is provided as carotene. Fish liver oils are the most concentrated source of vitamin A but substantial amounts are also present in mammalian

Table 6.1. *Daily Adult Vitamin Requirements[a] and the Tests for Vitamin Deficiencies.*

Vitamin	Recommended adult daily requirement	Best test for deficiency
A	2.6 μmol (750 μg) retinol equiv[b]	Serum vitamin A concentration
B_1 (thiamine)	1.0→1.5 mg	Red cell transketolase and thiamine pyrophosphate effect
B_2 (riboflavin)	1.5→2.0 mg	—
Nicotinic acid	13–20 niacin mg equiv[c]	Serum nicotinic acid concentration
B_6 (pyridoxine)	2.0 mg	Serum pyridoxine concentration
Folic acid	200 μg	Serum and red cell folate concentrations
B_{12} (cyanocobalamin)	3 μg	Serum B_{12} concentration
C (ascorbic acid)	50 mg	Leucocyte ascorbic acid concentration
D	2.5 μg	Serum vitamin D concentration
E	15 mg	Serum vitamin E concentration
K	>2.0 μg	Prolonged prothrombin time corrected by intramuscular vitamin K

[a] Department of Health and Social Security Report No. 120 (1969) *Recommended Intakes of Nutrients for the United Kingdom.* London: HMSO.

[b] 1 μg retinol equivalent ≡ 1 μg retinol or 6 μg β-carotene.

[c] Niacin equivalents include dietary sources of the vitamin itself plus 1 mg equivalent for each 60 mg of dietary tryptophan.

liver and kidney, dairy products and eggs. Carotene is found in dark green leafy vegetables such as parsley and spinach, and in carrots.

Vitamin A is readily absorbed from the gastrointestinal tract. It is fat soluble and its absorption is linked to that of lipid and enhanced by bile; when fat absorption is disturbed the uptake of vitamin A is reduced but the vitamin can still be absorbed from water-miscible preparations. Retinyl esters are hydrolysed prior to uptake by the enterocyte; the retinol is largely re-esterified before it leaves the gut. Carotene is less well absorbed than vitamin A and its uptake is more affected by disorders of triglyceride absorption and micelle formation. The retinol resulting from its cleavage is also esterified in the mucosa. Retinyl esters leave the gut in the chylomicron fraction of lymph and are stored largely in the liver in which the concentration of vitamin A is approximately 0·35 μmol/g (100 μg/g) compared with about 0·003 μmol/g (1 μg/g) in tissues such as the kidney, lung or intraperitoneal fat.

Before release into the circulation the hepatic retinyl ester is hydrolysed and the retinol bound to an alpha-l-globulin, retinol binding protein, which circulates in the blood complexed with a pre-albumin protein.

Retinol is an important precursor for the synthesis of the visual pigments rhodopsin, found in rods, and iodopsin, found in cones. It is also important in controlling the differentiation of epithelial cells and the production of epithelial mucus.

Retinol is conjugated to form a β-glucuronide which is excreted in bile and can be reabsorbed. It is also oxidized to retinal and retinoic acid and these, with other water-soluble metabolites, are excreted in the urine and faeces.

Vitamin A absorption may be reduced with biliary obstruction or parenchymal liver disease. Hepatic stores are normally very large and deficiency must be long standing before there are any ill effects. Parenchymal liver damage may also affect vitamin A metabolism by interfering with the release of retinol from the liver into the circulation. The clinical manifestations of vitamin A deficiency are often overlooked. Evidence of impaired adaptation to darkness may be found with special tests but only occasional patients, with severe depletion, complain of night blindness. Vitamin A deficiency is associated with keratinization of epithelia, especially of the conjunctiva and cornea, and there may be an impairment of taste and smell which probably also results from epithelial keratinization. Chronic ingestion of excessive amounts of vitamin A can cause liver damage.[24,83]

Vitamin D.[90] Cholecalciferol, or vitamin D_3, is the principal form of vitamin D found in animal tissues and is produced in skin by the ultraviolet irradiation of 7-dehydrocholesterol. It is also ingested in foods of animal origin such as butter, egg yolks, liver and oily fish. Calciferol, or vitamin D_2, is produced by irradiation of the plant sterol, ergosterol, and is the active principle of commercial preparations such as those added to margarines.

Vitamins D_3 and D_2 are absorbed from the small intestine and depend on micellar solubilization for their uptake.

Most studies on the subsequent metabolism of vitamin D have been undertaken on cholecalciferol. It is now clear that vitamin D_3 requires chemical modification before it has full biological activity on its target organs. Initially it is converted in the liver to 25-hydroxycholecalciferol; this enters the blood stream, circulating with vitamin D-binding globulin, and is then converted by the kidney to 1,25-dihydroxycholecalciferol. The dihydroxy metabolite is many times more active biologically than the monohydroxy compound. The kidney may also hydroxylate the molecule at the 24-position, with the production of 24,25-dihydroxycholecalciferol which also has biological activity. The active forms of vitamin D_2 and D_3 stimulate the absorption of calcium and phosphate from the upper small intestine and so help to promote the normal mineralization of bone. They also promote mobilization of calcium from old bone and probably have a direct action on the kidney to increase calcium and phosphate reabsorption. Vitamins D_2 and D_3 thus play an important role in plasma calcium homeostasis. When vitamin D deficiency exists there is inadequate calcium absorption; plasma levels tend to fall, parathormone secretion increases and bone calcium is removed to maintain plasma values. The resulting changes in bone with widespread decalcification and excessive amounts of uncalcified matrix are called osteomalacia.

Vitamin D absorption is impaired with biliary obstruction and in some patients with parenchymal liver disease. However, stores of vitamin D are normally large (they should last about a year) and vitamin D_3 can also be synthesized in relatively large amounts in the skin. Consequently, osteomalacia is rarely seen except in patients with long-standing biliary cirrhosis or with severe chronic parenchymal disease. The role of skin synthesis of vitamin D_3 may be less important in deeply jaundiced patients as the bilirubin in the skin may interfere with the irradiation of 7-dehydrocholesterol by absorbing ultraviolet rays.

One might expect plasma levels of 25-hydroxycholecalciferol to be reduced in patients with parenchymal liver disease because of reduced 25-hydroxylation within the liver. Levels tend to be low but they correlate poorly with the degree of osteomalacia; presumably this depends more on the availability of 1,25-dihydroxycholecalciferol which has been found to be effective treatment for osteomalacia in patients with normal levels of 25-hydroxycholecalciferol.[51]

The liver is important in the disposal of vitamin D. Some vitamin D is excreted in bile and some is inactivated by microsomal drug-metabolizing enzymes. When these enzymes are induced by phenobarbitone the inactivation of vitamin D is more rapid and in patients on long-term anticonvulsants there is a high incidence of rickets and osteomalacia which can be corrected by vitamin D.

Vitamin K.[13] There are at least two naturally occurring forms of vitamin K: vitamin K_1, or phylloquinone, and vitamin K_2 which represents a series of compounds (the menaquinones) in which the phytyl side chain of phylloquinone has been replaced by a side chain built up of 2 to 13 prenyl units. Vitamin K_1 is found in plants such as spinach, cabbage, cauliflower, peas and cereals, while the menaquinones are synthesized by Gram-positive bacteria. Menadione, or vitamin K_3, is a synthetic quinone derivative which is at least as active as K_1.

Vitamins K_1 and K_2 are dependent for their absorption on their solution in micelles and can be adequately absorbed only if bile salts are present in the intestinal lumen and if there is no other disturbance of fat absorption. Following absorption they enter the circulation in intestinal lymph. Menadione and its water-soluble derivatives can be absorbed in the absence of bile and enter the blood stream directly. After absorption, vitamin K is initially concentrated in the liver but the concentration drops rapidly and very little vitamin K is stored in tissues.

Vitamin K plays a key role in the synthesis of the clotting factors II, VII, IX and X. All of these bind calcium and all bind to the membranes of platelets or disintegrated cells. The binding to membranes is dependent on the presence of calcium. It is now known that the first 10 residues at the amino-terminal end of prothrombin are a new amino acid, γ-carboxyglutamate, while in patients with vitamin K deficiency glutamic acid occupies these positions.[67] The new amino acid is made, after the polypeptide chain of prothrombin has been assembled in the liver, by an enzyme system which adds a second carboxyl group to each of the first 10 glutamates. This enzyme system requires vitamin K as a cofactor. It seems likely that a similar process is involved in the synthesis of factors VII, IX and X.

γ-Carboxyglutamic acid has also been found in a protein in cortical bone, in renal tissue and in a new vitamin K-dependent protein, with unknown function, which has been purified from plasma. These observations suggest that vitamin K may be involved in the synthesis of other proteins besides clotting factors.

Because stores of vitamin K are small, patients with either biliary obstruction or severe parenchymal liver disease rapidly develop hypoprothrombinaemia and when it is severe spontaneous bleeding occurs (see Chapter 8). In uncomplicated biliary obstruction this bleeding disturbance is rapidly corrected by the parenteral administration of vitamin K. Improvement may occur in patients with parenchymal liver disease but in some the response to vitamin K is poor because the liver cells are unable to synthesize prothrombin and the other clotting factors. The response to vitamin K has been used to distinguish between obstructive jaundice and hepatitis but in practice this test has little diagnostic value.

Vitamin E.[13] Vitamin E activity is found in a number of naturally occurring tocopherols of which α-tocopherol is considered to be the most important as it comprises 90 per cent of the tocopherols in animal tissues and shows the greatest biological activity. The main sources of vitamin E are vegetable oils, cereal products and eggs.

The absorption of vitamin E depends on micellar solubilization. It leaves the intestine in the chylomicrons of lymph and is subsequently found associated with the beta-lipoprotein of plasma. Tissue stores of vitamin E are large and animals must be kept on a deficient diet for a long time before signs of deficiency appear.

The functions of vitamin E are not clear. It acts as an anti-oxidant and prevents oxidation of materials such as unsaturated fatty acids.

In patients with biliary obstruction α-tocopherol is not absorbed. The low plasma concentrations of this substance may be associated with a decreased erythrocyte lifetime and an increased red cell sensitivity to hydrogen peroxide. Patients may also develop other abnormalities similar to those seen in animals with vitamin E deficiency, such as muscle weakness, necrosis and creatinuria, but in practice these abnormalities are rarely detected. The creatinuria and red cell changes respond to the administration of vitamin E.

Water-soluble vitamins[32]

Thiamine. Thiamine is easily absorbed from the small intestine both passively and by active transport. Stores are relatively small and when large amounts of thiamine are given the excess is rapidly excreted in the urine. Its active form in tissues is thiamine pyrophosphate, a coenzyme in the decarboxylation of pyruvic and 2-oxoglutaric acids and in the metabolism of pentoses in the hexose monophosphate shunt. The requirement for thiamine is related to metabolic rate and is greatest when carbohydrate is the major source of energy. The main dietary sources in the United Kingdom are bread and flour, wheat, potatoes and meat, but eggs, vegetables and fruit, whole grain cereals and fortified breakfast cereals are also rich sources.

There is no obvious reason why hepatocellular disease should interfere with the handling of thiamine but it has been claimed that patients with cirrhosis have a reduced ability to absorb actively transported thiamine derivatives while allithiamines can be absorbed normally.[92] Patients with alcoholic liver disease are often found to have low values of red cell transketolase, a thiamine pyrophosphate-dependent enzyme, and these are usually attributed to deficient dietary intake and/or increased requirements for the vitamin. In some of these patients the low red cell transketolase activity does not rise with the addition of thiamine pyrophosphate; this suggests a reduction in the amount of apoenzyme rather than a deficiency of thiamine per se. A small number of alcoholics with thiamine deficiency develop a characteristic neuropsychiatric disorder, the Wernicke–Korsakoff syndrome, and in a recent paper Blass and Gibson[7] claimed that subjects developing this syndrome have an abnormal transketolase which binds thiamine poorly.

Clinical evidence of thiamine deficiency is rare in non-alcoholic liver disease and Morgan et al[58] found only one patient out of 31 with cryptogenic cirrhosis or chronic aggressive hepatitis in whom the red cell transketolase activity was low. In contrast, Rossouw et al[101] found evidence of thiamine deficiency in six out of 14 patients with non-alcoholic liver disease. Their patients, however, all showed features of hepatic decompensation and were generally more severely ill than those studied by Morgan and co-workers.

Riboflavin. Riboflavin functions in the body in riboflavin phosphate and in flavin adenine dinucleotide. These are coenzymes for the flavoprotein enzymes which are responsible for a large number of biological oxidations. The requirements for riboflavin seem to be related to energy requirements and are normally met with a reasonable intake of milk, liver, kidney, heart, cheese and green vegetables.

Morgan and his colleagues[58] measured whole blood riboflavin in 25 patients with cirrhosis and chronic hepatitis and in only one was the level slightly abnormal. Overt riboflavin deficiency, with cheilosis and corneal vascularization, is rare in patients with liver disease. One might expect to see riboflavin deficiency in alcoholics with multiple nutritional deficiencies. In the alcoholics studied by Neville and her colleagues,[65] however, the riboflavin intake was usually adequate: the excretion of riboflavin in the urine was either normal or elevated but this finding should be interpreted with caution as urinary riboflavin excretion is increased with negative nitrogen balance.

Nicotinic acid. Nicotinic acid and nicotinamide are readily absorbed from the gastrointestinal tract and are distributed in all tissues. The main dietary sources are meat and meat products, bread and flour, fortified breakfast cereals, vegetables and milk. They are converted in the body into two important substances, nicotinamide adenine dinucleotide (NAD; diphosphopyridine nucleotide or DPN) and nicotinamide adenine dinucleotide phosphate (NADP; triphosphopyridine nucleotide or TPN). NAD and NADP are coenzymes for a wide variety of enzymes involved in tissue respiration; they accept hydrogen from many substrates and are then reoxidized by flavoproteins. Tryptophan can also be converted to NAD via a rather complicated biosynthetic pathway and for this purpose about 60 mg of trytophan are equivalent to 1 mg of nicotinic acid.

Deficiency of nicotinic acid leads to pellagra. This is now an uncommon disease but is sometimes seen in patients with chronic gastrointestinal disease or in alcoholics, when other nutritional deficiencies may coexist.

The principal route of metabolism of nicotinic acid (and nicotinamide) is via *N*-methyl nicotinamide and the urinary excretion of this compound can be used to assess nutritional status.

Pyridoxine. Pyridoxine, pyridoxal and pyridoxamine, the three naturally occurring forms of vitamin B_6, are readily absorbed from the gastrointestinal tract. The main sources are meat and meat products, bread and flour, fortified breakfast cereals, vegetables and milk. All three compounds can be converted to the active compounds pyridoxal 5-phosphate and pyridoxamine phosphate. Pyridoxal 5-phosphate is a coenzyme for many metabolic transformations involving amino acids, including decarboxylation, transamination and racemization; the alanine transaminase activity of erythrocytes has been used to evaluate the availability of pyridoxine.

Plasma levels of pyridoxal 5-phosphate are low in patients with either cirrhosis or obstructive liver diseases and their rise following the intravenous administration of pyridoxine is not as great as in control subjects. The reason is not clear but may be due, at least partly, to an excessively rapid clearance of pyridoxal phosphate from plasma.[57] In addition ethanol may inhibit the conversion of pyridoxine to pyridoxal phosphate.[35]

Deficiency of pyridoxine causes seborrhoeic lesions of the face with glossitis, stomatitis and seizures; it has also been incriminated in the production of an uncommon pyridoxine responsive anaemia. These findings are rare in patients with liver disease.

Ascorbic acid.[10] Ascorbic acid is readily absorbed from the intestine and can be found in all body tissues. Its physiological functions are not clear but it is thought to play a role in biological oxidation and reduction mechanisms. It also seems to be important in the metabolism of large amounts of tyrosine and in the conversion of folic acid to folinic acid. In the blood the ascorbic acid content of leucocytes and platelets is greater than that of plasma and red cells and leucocyte/platelet levels can be used as an index of deficiency.

Morgan and his colleagues[58] found leucocyte ascorbic acid levels to be low in about 35 per cent of their patients with cryptogenic cirrhosis and chronic hepatitis and low plasma levels have also been found with alcoholic liver disease.[48] Beattie and Sherlock[6] studied patients with a variety of liver diseases. Only in patients with alcoholic liver disease and primary biliary cirrhosis was the mean leucocyte ascorbate level significantly lower than in their control group. Like others, they attributed the low levels in alcoholics to poor dietary intake. In the patients with primary biliary cirrhosis, however, they found low levels in patients taking cholestyramine, despite a normal dietary intake, and postulated that this drug interfered with the absorption of ascorbic acid.

Beattie and Sherlock were unable to demonstrate any clear effect of low ascorbate levels on erythrocyte morphology or on plasma cholesterol levels, but did find evidence that ascorbic acid deficiency interfered with antipyrine metabolism and speculated that it might affect the microsomal oxidation of other drugs.

Folic acid (pteroylglutamic acid).[34] Folic acid occurs in many foods, but offal and raw green leafy vegetables are particularly rich sources. Folic acid is also found in pulses, bread, oranges, nuts and bananas; it is readily destroyed by cooking.

Folic acid is normally present in food and tissues in the form of polyglutamates in which reduced pteroylglutamates are conjugated with a small chain of glutamic acid residues. Human cells usually have five glutamate residues in the molecule. Pteroylglutamic acid itself is rapidly absorbed from the small intestine, especially in its upper part, but polyglutamates have to be deconjugated prior to absorption. Food folate is not only deconjugated by mucosal cells but is also fully reduced and methylated and it reaches the blood stream as 5-methyltetrahydrofolate (5-methyl THFA).

Following absorption folic acid can be picked up by all body tissues. Total stores are normally around 11 to 23 nmol/l (5 to 10 mg) and about half of this is present in the liver, mainly as a polyglutamate form of 5-methyl THFA. The various tetrahydrofolates (e.g., 5-formimino THFA; 5,10-methylene THFA) are coenzymes which act as acceptors of one-carbon units; they are involved in the transfer of these units in the synthesis of purine and pyrimidine nucleotides, in a number of amino acid interconversions and in the generation of formate for the 'formate' pool.

The availability of folate in the body is usually assessed by measuring serum or preferably red cell folate. Low levels are often found in patients with liver disease. Morgan et al[58] found low red cell folate in 24 per cent and low plasma folate in 17 per cent of their patients with non-alcoholic liver disease. In alcoholics, folate deficiency is common, presumably because of their inadequate diet. Furthermore, it is claimed that absorption of folate is impaired, that requirements may be increased and that hepatic storage may be reduced. In acute experiments, ethanol causes a sharp fall in serum folate levels.[21] In addition, alcohol directly suppresses haematopoiesis, an effect which may involve blockage of folate metabolism.

Severe hepatic damage from any cause may affect the enzymes involved in folate metabolism and treatment with folic acid may have no effect. If dihydrofolate reductase activity is reduced then the conversion of dihydrofolate to the active tetrahydrofolate will be impaired. This defect can be overcome by the administration of folinic acid which is 5-formyl tetrahydrofolic acid. Some patients with liver disease have megaloblastic anaemia even though plasma levels of B_{12} and folate are normal, and an inability to use these substances, possibly because of abnormal plasma binding, has been suggested.[35] Normally, folate is not strongly bound in plasma and excess folate is excreted in the urine. Some patients with liver disease pass large amounts of folate in the urine, possibly due to release from the liver as a consequence of hepatocellular necrosis and this loss may contribute to subsequent folate deficiency.[75]

Vitamin B_{12} (cyanocobalamin).[34] Vitamin B_{12} is found only in foods of animal origin. Liver is the richest source; eggs, cheese, milk, heart and fish are also good sources. In food, cobalamins are bound to protein and, before absorption, the bond must be broken by proteolysis. They are absorbed from the intestine by two different mechanisms. The more important is mediated by gastric intrinsic factor which binds with vitamin B_{12}; the complex travels to the ileum where it is picked up by receptors on the mucosal surface and after a significant delay vitamin B_{12} is transported from the mucosa to the liver and other organs. Vitamin B_{12} can also be absorbed without intrinsic factor but only if very large amounts are given.

Absorbed vitamin B_{12} binds to a specific B_{12}-binding beta globulin, transcobalamin II, which rapidly transfers the vitamin to the liver, bone marrow and other tissues. Larger amounts are bound to transcobalamin I, which seems to act as a plasma store. The liver contains 50 to 90 per cent of normal body stores which range from 0·7 to 7 μmol (1 to 10 mg) of the vitamin. There is no catabolism of vitamin B_{12} and loss occurs by excretion, largely in the bile.

The vitamin B_{12} in bile (about 2 to 6 nmol/24 hr [3 to 8 μg/24 hr]) is largely reabsorbed in the normal subject. Theoretically, biliary loss might assume greater importance if, due to gastric or small intestinal disease, patients were unable to reabsorb the material secreted with the bile. Surprisingly, loss of radioactive B_{12} from the body is no greater in patients with absorptive defects than it is in vegans who have normal absorption.[37] Normally less than 0·18 nmol (0·25 μg) of vitamin B_{12} is lost in the urine each day.

Cyanocobalamin and hydroxycobalamin are converted in the liver to coenzyme forms, mainly deoxyadenosyl B_{12}, and enter the common storage pool. Cobalamins are involved in many metabolic processes and are necessary for normal growth, haematopoiesis and epithelial cell proliferation because they are essential for nucleic acid synthesis. They are also important for the maintenance of myelin in the nervous system. Vitamin B_{12} helps to keep sulphydryl groups in the reduced form necessary for many enzymatic reactions and with B_{12} deficiency there is a decrease in the glutathione content of liver and erythrocytes. Vitamin B_{12} plays an important role in protein synthesis, partly through the conversion of homocysteine to methionine, and is important in carbohydrate and fat metabolism because deoxyadenosyl B_{12} is involved in the conversion of methylmalonate to succinate.

Abnormalities of vitamin B_{12} metabolism occur in patients with liver disease although absorption and transport of the vitamin appear to be normal.[79] Morgan and his colleagues[58] found low serum levels of vitamin B_{12} in only three of their 73 patients with non-alcoholic liver disease and all three had a megaloblastic marrow. In a number of hepatobiliary disorders, including viral hepatitis, cholangitis, liver abscess, metastatic carcinoma and fatty liver, serum B_{12} levels are elevated. In viral hepatitis this is almost certainly due to release from injured hepatocytes[70] although other mechanisms may play a part. In chronic liver disease hepatic stores of vitamin B_{12} may be reduced even though serum levels are normal or elevated, but serum vitamin B_{12} may not be available for haematopoiesis because of binding to an abnormal protein released from the damaged liver. Patients with pernicious anaemia may have a 'spontaneous' remission if they develop hepatitis, and this suggests that not all of the hepatic stores of vitamin B_{12} in these patients are available for blood formation.[34]

Minerals

Iron[5,34]

The main sources of dietary iron are meat, which supplies about 25 per cent of daily requirements, bread, flour and other cereal products, potatoes and vegetables.

When iron is present in the diet in normal amounts it is absorbed mainly by an active transport system in the upper part of the small intestine, which limits and so controls the amount of iron absorbed. When very large amounts of iron are ingested it is also absorbed by a passive process which can overwhelm the usual control mechanisms. Haem-protein iron can be absorbed in intact haem from which it is split, presumably within the mucosal cell. Elemental iron is absorbed best in the ferrous form and its uptake is increased by reducing agents such as ascorbic acid. Absorption of inorganic iron is reduced by the phytates and phosphates in food, and by antacids.

After absorption iron is transported from the mucosa by transferrin, a beta-1-globulin synthesized in the liver, and becomes available to the bone marrow. In normal man there are about 63 mmol (3·5 g) of total body iron. About two-thirds of it circulate in haemoglobulin; 3 to 4 per cent is found in myoglobin and in the haem enzymes concerned with electron transfer, and the remainder is stored as ferritin and haemosiderin in the reticuloendothelial cells of the liver, spleen and bone marrow. Only a tiny amount is present in transferrin.

Little iron is excreted from the body. In women iron is lost during menstruation (9 to 18 µmol/24 hr [0.5 to 1.0 mg/24 hr] averaged over the menstrual cycle) and pregnancy (9 to 18 mmol [500 to 1000 mg]). Otherwise the main loss is via shedding of epithelial cells from the skin and gastrointestinal tract (9 to 18 µmol/24 hr [0.5 to 1.0 mg/24 hr]).

In patients with hepatocellular disorders serum iron and transferrin levels may be reduced, presumably because of a decrease in transferrin synthesis. This finding is probably of little significance for iron metabolism as the relative amount of iron carried with the transferrin is usually normal.

Serum iron levels are high in 50 to 80 per cent of patients with viral hepatitis.[82] Maximum values are not attained until both transaminase and bilirubin have passed their peak; this suggests that simple release of ferritin from damaged liver cells is not an adequate explanation. Furthermore, although serum ferritin rises with hepatic necrosis, even strikingly elevated levels would not account for the rise in serum iron which occurs in viral hepatitis. Transferrin must also be raised but the reason for this elevation is not clear. Diminished utilization of iron for haemoglobin synthesis, haemolysis, impaired reticuloendothelial uptake and impaired hepatic storage of iron may all play a part.

Patients with cirrhosis and those who abuse alcohol tend to have diminished iron stores. Evidence of iron deficiency was found in about 25 per cent of patients with cryptogenic cirrhosis or chronic hepatitis.[58] In some, blood loss was probably important but many of these patients gave a history of an inadequate diet.

Calcium

Milk and cheese are rich sources of calcium and in the United Kingdom moderately large amounts are present in bread. Some domestic water sources also contain a lot of calcium.

Calcium, from food and gastrointestinal secretions, is absorbed mainly from the upper part of the small intestine. Absorption appears to be carrier mediated and to involve a calcium-binding protein and other components which are stimulated by vitamin D. Parathyroid hormone also seems to stimulate calcium absorption. Food contains substances such as phytates, oxalates and phosphates which form complexes with calcium and interfere with its absorption. Calcium absorption is also decreased by glucocorticoids and by calcitonin and, in rats, alcohol appears to depress duodenal calcium transport.[46]

Following absorption, calcium enters the blood. About a third of plasma calcium is complexed with plasma proteins, especially albumin; about a tenth is diffusible but complexed with anions such as citrate and phosphate; the remainder is free calcium ion and changes in this fraction account for the serious physiological effects of hypo and hypercalcaemia. Although calcium is found in virtually all tissues more than 90 per cent is present in the skeleton.

Patients with liver disease may have diminished calcium absorption due to malabsorption of vitamin D (see earlier) but other factors may also play a part. There may be a deficient dietary intake. When triglyceride absorption is impaired excessive amounts of long chain fatty acids may be present in the intestinal lumen; these may form insoluble soaps with intraluminal ions, thus preventing calcium uptake. For this and other reasons the intake of dietary fat should be reduced in patients with the steatorrhoea of obstructive jaundice. Theoretically, medium chain triglyceride (MCT) would be a useful substitute as it promotes calcium uptake in man and experimental animals. In practice it is rarely necessary to give MCT to patients with obstructive jaundice as the effect of vitamin D on calcium absorption is so pronounced that calcium absorption returns to normal when vitamin D metabolism is corrected.

Some patients with liver disease develop osteoporosis. The cause is not clear. It may be due to a generalized nutritional disturbance, to chronic protein deficiency or to interference with protein metabolism. Osteoporosis is particularly common in patients treated with corticosteroids.

A few patients with primary biliary cirrhosis develop severe bone pain despite long-term treatment with vitamin D. The cause of this bone pain is not certain but it may respond to intravenous infusions of calcium with remission of the pain for several months.[2] The pain does not appear to respond to oral calcium and there is no evidence that it is nutritional in origin.

THE DIET AND OTHER 'NUTRITIONAL' FACTORS IN THE PRODUCTION OF HEPATIC DAMAGE

Alcohol (see also Chapter 32)

Alcohol is the most common cause of liver disease in the USA and ranks high as a cause of liver damage in Great Britain and other western countries. There is now overwhelming evidence that alcohol is hepatotoxic in its own right and that it can damage the liver even when the diet is adequate.[50] Liver disease is not, however, an invariable accompaniment of excessive drinking and occurs in only about 20 per cent of heavy drinkers.

This individual susceptibility to the effects of alcohol has been explained on a genetic basis. Cruz-Coke and Varela[17] found an association between cirrhosis and colour blindness, which is an X-linked trait. This association was challenged by Fialkow and his colleagues[26] and by Reid et al.[74] The latter group, however, claimed that cirrhosis was associated with brown hair and light skin in caucasian alcoholics, and with the Duffy blood group in negroes. Recently, it has been claimed that alcoholic hepatitis in male alcoholics is associated with the presence of the HLA-B8 phenotype.[61] Because of the multiple comparisons made in these studies it is likely that many of the associations are due to chance.

In susceptible individuals liver disease tends to result from the regular and prolonged ingestion of about 80 g or more of alcohol per day (Table 6.2). Overt liver disease may not appear for 20 years but in some it occurs after as little as five years. Alcoholic liver disease appears to progress from fatty infiltration, through alcoholic hepatitis, to cirrhosis. However there is little evidence that fat alone causes serious liver damage and Popper[68] has recently suggested that alcoholic hepatitis is not an essential step in the development of cirrhosis. As many as 14 per cent of alcoholic cirrhotics develop primary liver cell carcinoma as a terminal event.[59]

Abstinence from alcohol is the key to the successful treatment of the patient with alcoholic liver disease (and of patients with other manifestations of alcohol abuse). However, cirrhosis does not disappear after cessation of alcohol intake; the patient may die of its complications and alcoholic hepatitis may still progress to cirrhosis. Even so, the prognosis is greatly improved by abstinence.[9] The short-term effects of abstinence are not impressive; acute exacerbations of alcoholic hepatitis persist

Table 6.2. *Average Alcohol Content of Common Beverages and the Amount of Each Beverage Containing 80 g Ethanol.*

Beverage	Average alcohol content in g/100 ml	Amount of beverage containing 80 g ethanol
Beers		
Draught ale: bitter	3.1	5 pints (Imperial)
Strong ale	6.6	2½ pints
Cider	3.7	3 bottles
Sherry	16.0	⅔ bottle
Table wine: white and red	9.0	1 bottle
Spirit: 70% proof	31.5	⅓ bottle (9 singles)

1 bottle ≃ 780 ml
1 Imperial pint ≃ 570 ml = 1.25 US pints

for weeks or months after stopping and may appear to get worse at this time. Furthermore, large amounts of alcohol can be given to patients with acute alcoholic hepatitis without apparent influence on the rate of recovery.[77]

Women seem to be more susceptible than men to alcohol-induced liver injury and they develop serious liver disease more rapidly. Female alcoholics are more difficult to detect, develop more of the other *medical* complications of alcohol abuse, and are less likely to stop drinking than their male counterparts.[59]

Although it is no longer believed that alcohol-induced liver damage is a consequence of associated nutritional deficiency there can be no doubt, for several reasons, of the importance of nutritional deficiencies in alcoholic subjects. Each gram of ethanol provides 29.8 kJ (7.1 C) so that a bottle (760 ml) of good Scotch whisky (86° proof) provides approximately 6300 kJ (1500 C); this major source of energy contains little in the way of essential nutrients. If the diet is not otherwise adequate deficiencies may result, particularly as the requirement for certain vitamins is thought to be increased in alcoholic subjects. Furthermore, many alcoholics neglect their diet and serious and overt nutritional deficiencies may occur (see above). It is not known whether these deficiencies further interfere with already disturbed liver function but it is clearly sensible to correct deficiencies, and to anticipate their development by giving vitamin supplements to all those at risk.

Phosphate deficiency may occur in malnourished alcoholics with liver disease.[71] The low serum phosphate may be associated with a decrease in erythrocyte 2,3-diphosphoglycerate which plays an important part in oxygen transport. As a result the oxygen dissociation curve is shifted to the right. There may be accompanying mental abnormalities which disappear with phosphate repletion and a shift of the oxygen dissociation curve back to normal.

Malnutrition[14]

Malnutrition has long been incriminated as a causal factor in human cirrhosis. In experimental animals hepatic lesions resembling cirrhosis can be produced by diets deficient in choline, proteins and/or vitamins[33] but these lesions, unlike those of human cirrhosis, are apparently reversible.

The human liver is certainly affected by undernutrition. Kwashiorkor, a disease of children, occurs with protein deficiency in the presence of an adequate energy intake (from carbohydrate). A large fatty liver develops and in some children there is also diffuse fibrosis.[72] Cirrhosis, if it occurs, is a rare complication.

Snapper[88] described an epidemic of cirrhosis, which was thought to result from malnutrition, during the Japanese occupation of Peking. However, the incidence of hepatitis B infection is now known to be high in areas where undernutrition is common, and aflatoxin ingestion, schistosomiasis and a number of other factors might have been contributory. Malnutrition may certainly be associated with the development of chronic liver disease but there is no good evidence that malnutrition per se causes cirrhosis in man.

Obesity

Some authors have claimed that obesity is associated with significant impairment of liver function and histological evidence of liver damage.[95,100] There is undoubtedly an increase in the amount of fat visible on histological examination of the livers of obese subjects but fatty infiltration is rarely gross. Other minor abnormalities are also seen but these are found with fatty infiltration of any cause. The functional impairment of the liver was overemphasized by early workers who stressed minor abnormalities of bromsulphthalein (BSP) retention. It is now known that an 'abnormal' retention of BSP occurs in fat people with an otherwise normal liver and that other criteria must be used for assessing liver function in the obese.[29]

Recent workers have pointed out that biochemical abnormalities in obesity are minimal.[19,80] For practical purposes the liver can be considered to be normal in obese patients.

Jejuno-ileal Bypass

Surgical bypass of much of the small intestine has been used for the treatment of gross obesity since the early sixties. Most obese patients have some fatty infiltration of the liver preoperatively with an increased content of triglycerides. Fatty infiltration becomes more marked postoperatively, during the period of rapid weight loss, and triglycerides may increase severalfold[39] only to regress over the next year or two. Clear evidence of liver damage has been documented in a number of patients. In one

American series two out of 24 patients died of hepatic failure;[96] in another, six out of 36 became jaundiced, one dying in hepatic coma, and two other patients developed portal hypertension and ascites.[8] In a large British series there were 12 deaths in 182 patients;[4] five deaths were associated with liver failure (after reversal of the bypass), severe fatty liver (and Gram-negative septicaemia) and alcoholic cirrhosis, and three other patients developed cirrhosis (one probably due to alcohol).

Maxwell and his colleagues[53] used a modified bypass procedure and observed hepatic dysfunction infrequently. Adverse changes in liver function did occur during the period of weight loss soon after surgery, presumably when the accumulation of fat by the liver was most severe, but this impairment was temporary. There were five deaths in 120 patients but in only two of these were there persistent abnormalities of liver function and frank jaundice. In both patients there was gross fatty liver at autopsy, with cholestasis and some acute inflammatory changes.

The mechanism of hepatic damage with jejuno-ileal bypass is not yet understood but nutritional factors, secondary to interference with small intestine function, may be important. Moxley and his colleagues[63] found reduced plasma amino acid concentrations (except for glycine and serine, which were elevated) in patients following operation. Similar changes have been reported in protein-calorie malnutrition.[84] Moxley et al explained their findings on the basis of impaired absorption of amino acids which, with plasma values, improved one to three years after the operation. Others have explained the hepatic damage on the basis of lithocholate toxicity, claiming increased lithocholate absorption from the colon because more chenodeoxycholate is available for dehydroxylation by colonic bacteria.[19]

It appears that the hepatic disturbances revert to normal if normal intestinal continuity is restored.[8] Regardless of the likely mechanism of the hepatic damage and its potential reversibility it is clear that great caution should be observed in recommending jejuno-ileal bypass for the relief of obesity.

Parenteral Nutrition[47]

In recent years total parenteral nutrition has assumed increasing importance in the management of patients who cannot, or should not, take food through the gastrointestinal tract. Energy is provided as carbohydrate (usually as glucose), as fat (usually as a soybean emulsion – 'Intralipid') and in amino acid mixtures such as 'Vamin' or 'Aminoplex'. Vitamin supplements are usually given at the same time and, when parenteral nutrition is prolonged, trace elements can also be added.

A number of workers have stated that total parenteral nutrition may be accompanied by deleterious effects on liver structure and function. In most American studies only carbohydrate and amino acid mixtures have been given because intravenous fat preparations have not been available. It has been claimed that fatty liver can be induced or aggravated by a carbohydrate/amino acid regimen if the calorie/nitrogen ratio is excessively high, and that postoperative hepatic decompensation is more likely in those with fatty infiltration. Mobilization of the excess fat can be accomplished by giving intravenous regimens which are rich in amino acids. Similar results have been found in animal experiments.[20]

Hepatic damage has also been reported with lipid infusion. The early cottonseed oil preparations seemed to give more trouble than the soybean emulsions now in common use (e.g., Intralipid) but no uniform pattern of damage has been described and histological studies, including electron microscopy, have shown no serious disturbances in hepatic morphology. Transient elevation in alanine and aspartate transaminases have been noted. Many authors have reported the deposition of a pigment in reticuloendothelial cells and hepatocytes in patients receiving prolonged infusions of lipid emulsions (of various types) and this abnormality has also been seen in experimental animals. Its origin and significance is unknown but there is no evidence that this pigment impairs reticuloendothelial or hepatocellular function.[45] Reticuloendothelial blockade and reduced tolerance to certain endotoxins have been described with infusion of cottonseed preparations but similar effects were not obtained with soybean oil emulsion.

Recently, intravenous feeding with glucose and amino acids has been associated with cholestasis in infants. Certainly there were striking changes in bilirubin, aspartate transaminase and alkaline phosphatase which reverted to normal with cessation of the intravenous feeding. Histologically, the liver showed canalicular and/or hepatocellular cholestasis, and varying degrees of local acute inflammation and portal fibrosis.[78,99] Amino acids have been incriminated as the agents responsible, and in animal experiments methionine has been shown to have an anticholeretic effect.[69]

Inborn Errors of Metabolism

In some unfortunate children with inborn errors of metabolism even normal dietary constituents may cause liver damage. Certain of these conditions (hereditary tyrosinaemia, galactose-1-phosphate uridyl transferase deficiency and hereditary fructose intolerance) present soon after birth and successful management is critically dependent on early diagnosis and on the exclusion of offending substances from the diet. The mechanism of liver damage in these conditions is not understood but is assumed to be due to toxic metabolites of tyrosine, galactose or fructose which accumulate because key enzymes for their metabolism are missing. They are rare diseases and readers who wish to learn more about them or about their dietary management should consult the appropriate chapters in the latest edition of *Metabolic Basis of Inherited Disease* edited by Stanbury, Wyngaarden and Fredrickson.

Wilson's disease (hepatolenticular degeneration)

Wilson's disease (see also Chapter 33) is also an inborn error of metabolism but patients with this condition present much later than those with the conditions mentioned above. They have problems in managing copper and large amounts of this element accumulate in the liver, brain, kidney, etc. The mechanism of production of the liver disease is not known. It seems to be secondary to the presence of copper in the liver and when homozygous siblings are treated prophylactically to prevent copper accumulation liver damage may be prevented. Patients with Wilson's disease accumulate copper on a normal diet and dietary copper restriction is of little value for reversing the deleterious effects of copper already deposited in tissues. To remove copper from the body we currently use D-penicillamine which chelates copper; the complex is excreted in the urine. In trying to achieve negative copper balance it is clearly sensible to keep the intake of copper as low as possible; patients should be advised to avoid shellfish, dried fruit, nuts, chocolate, mushrooms and liver and to restrict the amount of salt and pepper they use to flavour their food. If local water supplies contain more than 1.6 μmol/l (0.1 mg/l) of copper, demineralized water should be used. Even with such restrictions it is difficult to keep the intake below 16 μmol (1 mg) a day without severe caloric restriction and it has been suggested that patients should take potassium sulphide with meals in order to reduce copper absorption further.

Idiopathic haemochromatosis

Haemochromatosis, like Wilson's disease, is a condition in which accumulation of a metal, iron, occurs in a number of body tissues (see also Chapter 34). Patients present at a later age than those with Wilson's disease and, except for the presence of cirrhosis and its complications, the clinical features are quite different. The underlying biochemical defect in haemochromatosis is not fully understood, but it seems to be linked with inappropriately high absorption of iron from the gastrointestinal tract.[5]

Patients with haemochromatosis usually ingest a normal diet but it is still possible that dietary factors may accelerate the rate of iron accumulation. Crosby[16] suggests that mandatory fortification of food with iron may lead to an increased incidence of iron storage disease, so it is possible that an intake within the 'normal' range may be significant in those at risk. The role of alcohol may also be relevant. About 30 to 50 per cent of patients with idiopathic haemochromatosis drink large amounts of alcohol. Alcohol may increase iron overload in two ways. Firstly, it can stimulate iron absorption,[12] causing an increase in serum iron concentration and in the percentage saturation of iron binding protein, although this iron does not appear to be used for haematopoiesis. Secondly, alcoholics are often deficient in folic acid, pyridoxine and, less frequently, in vitamin B_{12}. As a result haemopoiesis is defective, less iron is utilized, and absorbed iron is more likely to be deposited in body stores. On this basis Sullivan and Herbert[91] suggested that 'the diagnosis of idiopathic haemochromatosis should not be made in alcoholic patients until it has been shown that the excessive iron stores in the liver are not due to deficiencies of these factors (folate, vitamin B_{12}, pyridoxine) and cannot be reduced by cessation of alcohol and long term therapy with folic acid, vitamin B_{12} and pyridoxine.'

In the management of idiopathic haemochromatosis it has not been considered necessary to use dietary iron restriction because the amount absorbed daily from a normal diet is small in relation to the quantities removed by venesection which is the keystone of treatment. Even so, it would seem sensible that patients should avoid foods rich in iron and which are otherwise of limited nutritional value (such as flour and bread, cereal products and potatoes) and that they should be warned about the dangers of alcohol abuse, not only because it might enhance iron absorption but because it might further affect a liver already damaged by iron.

Nutritional Iron Overload

Tissue damage due to iron accumulation occurs with certain forms of anaemia and can also occur with excessive administration of iron, given ostensibly for 'therapeutic' purposes (see also Chapter 34). Damage from the amount of iron contained in the 'normal' diet is very rare.

In African negroes marked siderosis can occur in association with the chronic ingestion of a diet rich in iron derived from iron cooking pots and from the iron drums in which alcoholic beverages are fermented. Other factors may contribute to the excessive iron absorption and tissue deposition. Venesection is used to get rid of iron but it is clearly sensible in this situation to change cooking utensils and to avoid the ingestion of iron-rich beverages.

Negroes with iron overload present biochemical evidence of ascorbic acid deficiency and frank scurvy is not uncommon.[86] It has been suggested that the presence of excessive amounts of ferric iron leads to the rapid oxidation of ascorbic acid and so deficiency results even when intake is normal.

Lesser degrees of overload with iron of dietary origin occur in alcoholics and in patients with portacaval shunts. The mechanism of hepatic siderosis with shunting is not understood. Nor is it clear why iron deposition should be so marked in some alcoholics, except that some alcoholic beverages, particularly wine, contain large amounts of iron; however, there appears to be no correlation between the iron content of the beverages and the degree of siderosis.[40]

Iron overload is also common in patients with porphyria cutanea tarda. Many of them consume excessive amounts of alcohol and liver damage is commonly found; this is usually mild and cirrhosis is not often seen. Removal of iron by venesection is an effective form of treatment for this condition but the mechanism of action is not clear.

Dangerous Foods and Dietary Contaminants[44]

The consumption of certain foods may result in liver damage. The food itself may be toxic: for example, the mushroom *Amanita phalloides* can cause fatal hepatitis; plants of the genera *Crotalaria* and *Senecio*, which are used to make bush tea, can cause an obstruction of centrilobular hepatic veins due to their content of pyrrolizidine alkaloids. Other foods are contaminated by noxious agents and the associations may be relatively specific. Fascioliasis of the liver results from eating water-cress contaminated with the metacercaria of *Fasciola hepatica*. Epidemics of viral hepatitis have been traced to the ingestion of infected clams and oysters. Peanuts may be contaminated with *Aspergillus flavus*, a fungus which produces aflatoxins; these are hepatotoxic in animals and there is growing evidence to suggest that in certain countries they are a cause of cirrhosis and primary liver cell carcinoma (see Chapter 38).

NUTRITIONAL ASPECTS OF THE MANAGEMENT OF PATIENTS WITH LIVER DISEASE

In this section we shall consider nutritional aspects of the management of several major complications of liver disease including hepatic encephalopathy, oedema and ascites. We will also consider the dietary advice which should be given to patients with hepatitis or cirrhosis and the dietary manipulation which may be necessary in patients with obstructive jaundice.

First we will discuss some general aspects of the subject. Patients with liver disease are often given dietary advice of doubtful value. Even asymptomatic patients are told to take a low fat diet or advised to abstain from alcohol (even if they are not suffering from alcoholic liver disease); more rigorous restrictions may be suggested in some cases. There is no good evidence to support dietary restrictions for patients with few symptoms. Alcoholics, of course, should abstain from alcohol and patients who occasionally suffer nausea, vomiting, abdominal pain or other symptoms after eating should avoid foods which they know will produce symptoms. Anorectic patients should not be given unattractive dishes; they should be encouraged to eat and should be allowed to select foods which appeal to them. Such simple recommendations cover the requirements of most patients in terms of the intake of energy and only weight loss (or weight gain) would suggest a need for intervention. Several workers, however, have found biochemical evidence of malnutrition in patients with liver disease (see earlier) which may not be obvious clinically. This is particularly true of certain vitamins. These biochemical abnormalities may be found despite a normal dietary intake and it is possible that the underlying liver disease may lead to an increased requirement, to increased loss or that it may interfere with the metabolism of a particular substance.

It is useful to know that such biochemical abnormalities are associated with liver disease as it helps in the interpretation of laboratory data. From a more practical point of view it suggests that the common practice of giving 'blunderbuss' vitamin therapy to patients with symptomatic liver disease has a sensible theoretical basis. Although the biochemical defects mentioned may have no serious clinical consequences it is also possible that they have deleterious effects on hepatic function (and on other tissues) which, although unrecognized, may adversely affect prognosis. Furthermore, while it is generally expensive to investigate for vitamin deficiencies, multivitamin therapy is cheap and is assumed to be harmless. From the discussion earlier in this chapter it would seem sensible that, for patients with liver disease, vitamin supplements should include thiamine, riboflavin, pyridoxine, ascorbic acid and folic acid.

Weight loss is the most readily available index of general nutritional status. Nevertheless, body weight alone may be misleading, particularly if there is significant fluid retention. Obvious wasting of skeletal muscle and loss of subcutaneous adipose tissue may occur without weight loss. Only when fluid is lost with treatment can the extent of the nutritional disturbance be assessed. Patients with chronic liver disease who have no loss of fat or lean body mass will gain weight when they develop oedema and/or ascites. Alcoholics, and those patients given steroid therapy, can also develop excess adipose tissue and this may mask loss of lean body mass.

Loss of weight is an important clinical feature in many patients with liver disease. It is due in part to anorexia but other metabolic factors may also be involved. Unfortunately, we have little detailed information on the nature of the weight loss which occurs in either acute or chronic liver disease, and on whether it is due primarily to loss of fat, protein, glycogen or water. It would be of interest to see if the composition of weight loss in response to a weight-reducing regimen is the same in patients with liver disease as in normal individuals, whether obese or non-obese.

In patients with acute or sub-acute hepatitis and in alcoholic patients there may be marked weight loss and profound wasting, particularly of muscle. These patients are often severely anorexic with nausea and vomiting, and malnutrition per se may become a serious problem. It is claimed that prolonged negative nitrogen balance may lead to apathy, increased susceptibility to infection and delayed wound healing, and if more than 30 per cent of body weight is lost during acute metabolic illness the patient's chances of survival are greatly reduced.[47] Unfortunately, it is difficult to increase oral intake of food in patients with severe anorexia and nausea, and vomiting may limit feeding of patients through a nasogastric tube. Intravenous feeding is the logical solution but severe liver disease is considered to be a contraindication to the intravenous administration of lipids, even by the manufacturers.[41] Amino acid mixtures are also considered dangerous because they might exacerbate hepatic encephalopathy. However, Fischer and his colleagues[28] have used a special mixture of amino acids, designed to correct the imbalance between individual plasma amino acids in patients with liver disease, and have found it of benefit in the treatment of encephalopathy (see Chapter 42).

There has been a tendency to give only intravenous glucose or fructose to patients suffering from liver disease because of these strictures on the use of intravenous fat and amino acids. It should be noted, however, that an adequate energy supply is provided only by a daily intake of 400 to 500 g of these substances. Unless highly concentrated solutions are used the hexose has to be given with several litres of water, but since water is poorly tolerated by most patients in need of intravenous feeding profound hyponatraemia may result. Highly concentrated glucose solutions are also difficult to infuse. Fructose has other hazards: it does not protect against hypoglycaemia and should not be used in patients with acute hepatic failure as they are particularly susceptible to this complication, and to lactic acidosis.

Although liver disease is generally considered as a contraindication to the use of intravenous lipid feeding several early reports suggested that I.V. lipids could be given safely to patients with liver disease.[43,85]

Recently, we have fed several patients who have severe liver disease with intravenous soybean oil emulsion (Intralipid), mixed amino acids (Vamin) and glucose. Although they were deeply jaundiced they cleared lipid from the plasma satisfactorily and there appeared to be no ill effects; the infusion of amino acids did not precipitate encephalopathy nor was there any obvious exacerbation of existing precoma. From these preliminary observations we feel that total parenteral nutrition may have an important place in the management of malnourished patients with liver disease, but further studies are needed to establish the indications for its use and the likely benefits. Parenteral nutrition should not be used haphazardly. Proper monitoring requires time and effort. Furthermore, therapy is costly and it is potentially dangerous because of the risks of infection; there are also mechanical dangers if the subclavian route is used for infusion.

Fluid Retention

Many patients with cirrhosis have disturbed renal function and retain salt and water. This excess fluid results in peripheral oedema and/or ascites; both may be uncomfortable and inconvenient for the patient.

The reasons for the fluid retention are poorly understood (see Chapter 46) and this limits our ability to treat it effectively. Empirically it has been established that the manipulation of dietary salt and water may be of therapeutic benefit.

The degree of renal functional disturbance may be assessed arbitrarily from the ability of the kidneys to excrete salt and to clear free water.[3] Some patients with fluid retention pass relatively large amounts of urinary sodium and are able to generate free water (i.e. are 'water tolerant'). It is not always appreciated that such patients may respond to salt restriction alone. It is assumed, erroneously, that all patients with fluid retention are avid salt retainers and diuretics may be given unnecessarily with a low sodium diet.

Although it is possible to reduce dietary sodium to less than 10 mmol/24 hr (10 mEq/24 hr) this cannot be done without an unacceptably low protein intake or the use of artificial protein preparations which are unpalatable. By using unsalted bread and no salt in cooking, and with protein restricted to only 60 to 70 g daily, it is possible to reduce sodium intake to around 20 mmol/24 hr (20 mEq/24 hr). Fortunately, most patients respond adequately to a daily intake of around 40 mmol (40 mEq); this is still severe sodium restriction in dietary terms but it is a more practicable goal for therapy. The low sodium diet used at the Royal Free Hospital is presented in the appendix to this chapter.

The patient and his doctors must be on the look out for foodstuffs which have an unexpectedly high salt content. The patient must avoid alkali preparations, such as Mist. Mag. Trisil., which contain a lot of sodium; sodium-free preparations should be prescribed when alkalis are needed.

Some patients have a very low urinary sodium output but are 'water tolerant'. Diuretics and a low salt diet are usually effective for such patients. The most difficult patients to treat are those with a low urinary sodium who are 'water intolerant'. Their inability to excrete free water is reflected in hyponatraemia. They are usually treated with a low-salt diet and diuretics and by restriction of dietary water intake to around one litre a day. The results of treatment are generally poor and the life expectancy of these patients is short.

Salt restriction is unpleasant for patients and treatment with diuretics may be associated with a number of untoward consequences. It is probably wise not to treat patients with fluid retention unless oedema and/or ascites are causing symptoms which distress the patient; it is certainly unwise to treat too vigorously. It is common practice to restrict salt whenever diuretics are used. Reynolds and his colleagues[76] have shown that patients can be kept comfortable (with a small amount of residual ascites) by the use of intermittent diuretic therapy without salt restriction; with this treatment patients are unlikely to develop azotaemia and/or hyponatraemia. Patients given daily diuretics to clear ascites completely develop azotaemia regardless of dietary salt intake. Hyponatraemia is likely to occur if sodium restriction is added to diuretic therapy, and salt restriction may also increase the risk of diuretic-induced encephalopathy.

Hepatic Encephalopathy

Patients with severe parenchymal liver disease or with shunting of blood from the portal to the systemic circulation may show evidence of cerebral dysfunction. This 'hepatic encephalopathy' may be of several types and these are described in Chapter 42. Although we recognize several precipitants of coma in patients with chronic liver disease we are not yet certain why they suffer intermittent attacks of encephalopathy, often with no obvious cause. A large body of evidence incriminates dietary protein in the production of these attacks, however. If a large amount of protein is given to patients with cirrhosis and/or portasystemic shunting (or to experimental animals with a portasystemic anastomosis) it may cause reversible stupor or coma, often with other neurological manifestations.

It has been suggested that substances toxic to the brain are produced by the action of colonic bacteria on dietary protein; these substances would normally be removed by the liver but would not be cleared from portal blood if the liver was damaged or if there was portasystemic shunting. As dietary protein is almost completely absorbed in the upper small intestine and as intravenous amino acids also cause encephalopathy it is possible that the 'toxin' is produced by the action of intestinal bacteria on a metabolite of dietary protein, produced within the body after absorption of the constituent amino acids, and which is then re-excreted into the intestine.

Many substances, including ammonia, amino acids, mercaptans, short chain fatty acids and false neurochemical transmitters, have been incriminated as the humoral agents of hepatic encephalopathy, and the mechanism is still far from clear. But whatever substance or substances are involved the keystone of nutritional management is the restriction of protein. Sample low protein diets are presented in the appendix.

In acute hepatic failure management of the encephalopathy is only one facet of a complicated regimen which also has to cope with bleeding problems, infections and a variety of other serious metabolic disturbances. Usually little or no food is given orally and conventional amino acid mixtures are avoided as an intravenous source of energy.

In dealing with the acute episodes of encephalopathy which may punctuate the course of chronic liver disease, or with those patients who have chronic encephalopathy, dietary control is extremely important. At the start of the acute episode protein should be removed from the diet altogether. It can be reintroduced gradually in increments of 10 to 20 g; the aim in both types of patient is to give enough protein to prevent negative nitrogen balance but not enough to exacerbate the encephalopathy. Patients with encephalopathy can normally be stabilized on 50 g or more of protein daily. If only first-class protein, rich in essential amino acids, were used it might be possible to make do with a daily protein intake of not more than 30 g. In practice, however, it is difficult to prepare a palatable diet using only protein of high biological value. Recently, it has been suggested that patients with chronic encephalopathy fare better on vegetable protein than on animal protein.[31] The main difference between these proteins is in the methionine content which is significantly higher in animal protein.[81] This amino acid is a precursor of mercaptans which have been incriminated as important factors in the genesis of hepatic encephalopathy.

Dietary protein should be distributed fairly evenly throughout the day as a sudden load may exacerbate encephalopathy; following an oral load of protein the electroencephalographic pattern deteriorates within two hours.[42]

Oral protein cannot be replaced by intravenous infusion of equivalent amounts of conventional amino acid mixtures as these also tend to exacerbate encephalopathy.[27,94] However, encephalopathy may improve with the infusion of an amino acid mixture designed to correct the abnormal amino acid pattern seen in these patients.[28] This mixture contains high concentrations of the branched chain amino acids valine, leucine and isoleucine and very low concentrations of the aromatic amino acids tyrosine and phenylalanine. The results of carefully controlled trials of this amino acid mixture are awaited.

When protein is restricted carbohydrate must be given to reduce endogenous protein catabolism and to promote the anabolic use of the administered protein. A daily carbohydrate load of about 400 g is needed for this purpose and it is often given intravenously as strong glucose solution. Walker et al[93] gave *oral* glucose supplements to cirrhotics taking 40 to 60 g of protein per day in order to increase their circulating insulin and to reduce circulating glucagon values. Oral glucose produces greater changes in circulating insulin than either oral fructose or intravenous glucose. In all of their patients there was a fall in the level of blood ammonia, another factor incriminated as an 'encephalopathic agent'. The implications of their work remain to be explored but it suggests that patients with encephalopathy should, when possible, be given oral glucose or glucose via a nasogastric tube, rather than fructose or intravenous glucose.

Constipation should be prevented as it seems

to precipitate encephalopathy, perhaps by increasing production in the colon of ammonia and other nitrogenous compounds. It would seem sensible for patients at risk to take a high fibre diet although they may still need enemas and purgatives in an acute episode.

The ability to tolerate dietary protein can be enhanced by giving a non-absorbable antibiotic, such as neomycin, which presumably reduces the production of 'cerebral toxins', or the synthetic disaccharide lactulose which may reduce their absorption. Using such compounds patients may be able to tolerate 100 g of protein a day, but it is rarely necessary for them to eat this amount. Tolerance to dietary protein gradually decreases with progression of the disease despite treatment with neomycin or lactulose.

Bleeding from oesophageal varices is sometimes treated by the construction of a portacaval shunt. There is a high incidence of chronic hepatic encephalopathy within three years of the operation. Transient acute encephalopathy may occur in the immediate postoperative period when liver cell function is depressed due to surgery. For this reason we restrict protein immediately after surgery and work up to an eventual intake over a week or so, increasing protein by increments of about 20 g.

Carbohydrate Intolerance

Impaired glucose tolerance commonly occurs in patients with cirrhosis of the liver. It is usually associated with insulin deficiency. Plasma insulin levels tend to be high in cirrhosis and there is a resistance to the action of exogenous insulin. Symptomatic diabetes is less common and when it occurs it can usually be treated by simple dietary restriction of carbohydrates. A few patients with cirrhosis develop insulin-dependent diabetes, which is different from the glucose intolerance usually seen with cirrhosis. The carbohydrate intolerance of liver disease and its dietary control are discussed further in Chapter 3.

The Diet and Hyperbilirubinaemia

Gilbert's syndrome is a chronic, benign, non-haemolytic unconjugated hyperbilirubinaemia secondary to a deficiency of the liver enzyme glucuronyl transferase. In subjects with this condition fasting increases the plasma bilirubin values. The exact mechanism of this effect is not known but it seems to be related more to the amount of fat in the diet than to the caloric intake.[30] Small increases in plasma bilirubin concentrations are also seen with fasting in normal subjects.

The diet-related increase in hyperbilirubinaemia is relatively unimportant in terms of the patient's well-being but it is worthy of recognition as it may be of use diagnostically. Gilbert's syndrome is common, occurring in up to 6 per cent of the population. It usually goes unrecognized but unconjugated hyperbilirubinaemia may be detected when patients in hospital are starved or fed only with intravenous glucose or amino acids. Gilbert's syndrome should be considered as a diagnosis before a vigorous search for other, more sinister, causes of jaundice is undertaken.

Gollan and his colleagues[30] speculated that the low lipid content of certain feeding regimens used for premature infants might exacerbate neonatal hyperbilirubinaemia; they suggested on this basis that a moderate amount of lipid should be included in the diets given to jaundiced neonates. Large amounts of lipid are probably best avoided as they may interfere with protein binding of bilirubin and so exacerbate the effects of neonatal hyperbilirubinaemia.

The Dietary Management of Hepatitis, Cirrhosis and Biliary Obstruction

Three of the commonest disorders of the liver are acute hepatitis, cirrhosis (and chronic hepatitis) and biliary obstruction. Varying degrees of anorexia, nausea, vomiting and food intolerance often accompany them and it is hardly surprising that many dietary measures have been advocated for their management. Little or no evidence has been presented to support most of these dietary regimens.

Viral or drug-induced hepatitis

Patients with hepatitis with few symptoms need no dietary restrictions; they should be encouraged to eat normally. Even when patients have severe anorexia, nausea and vomiting they can usually take small amounts of food by mouth and drink enough to prevent significant dehydration. They should be encouraged to do both and should be tempted with attractive food and drink. It is rarely necessary to give calories

intravenously unless fulminant hepatitis occurs and the patient develops precoma or coma.

Fat should not be restricted. Low fat diets are more bulky for the same caloric load; they are generally unappetizing and may exacerbate anorexia. Hoagland and his colleagues[36] showed in 1946 that patients with hepatitis on a high fat, high protein diet consumed more calories than those given a low fat diet. They gained more weight and appeared to recover more quickly. Other studies also suggest that a high calorie (and high fat) intake may be beneficial in hepatitis. Chalmers and his colleagues[11] force-fed servicemen who had viral hepatitis (using a stomach tube in a small number) to ensure that their diet contained at least 12 600 kJ (3000C) with more than 150 g of both protein and fat. In these patients the clinical illness was shorter, by an average of six days, than in patients who were allowed to eat ad lib, and whose caloric intake was consequently lower. This benefit is relatively small and Chalmers and his colleagues did not believe that it justified the force-feeding of civilians. Even so it seems sensible, on this basis, to advise patients with hepatitis to take a high calorie diet.

A high caloric intake results in increased insulin secretion. Recent animal experiments suggest that insulin and glucagon given intraperitoneally increased the survival of mice with fulminant viral hepatitis; if given prior to viral inoculation they protected against initial cell damage and enhanced regeneration.[23] If a similar effect could be demonstrated in man it would provide a rational treatment for severe hepatitis and would also explain, at least in part, some of the claims for the beneficial effects of glucose in acute hepatitis. As plasma insulin values are higher with oral (i.e. intestinally absorbed) than with intravenous glucose it would seem sensible, even now, to give glucose orally, or by nasogastric tube, whenever possible.

Patients with severe viral hepatitis may not be able to excrete a normal water load[62] and one must be cautious about the amount of water contained in solutions given intravenously.

Patients are often advised to abstain from alcohol during an attack of hepatitis and for six months to a year afterwards. It is harmless advice and focuses attention on the potential hepatotoxicity of alcohol at a time when the patient is introspective about his liver. But there is no good evidence that alcohol in moderation has a deleterious effect on the liver either during an acute attack or during convalescence. Excessive amounts of alcohol are hepatotoxic in their own right and relapse of hepatitis following alcohol abuse has been reported.[18]

Cirrhosis of the liver

The preceding remarks about the dietary management of patients with viral hepatitis are generally applicable to patients with uncomplicated cirrhosis of the liver. Dietary restriction is unnecessary and patients should avoid only foods which upset them.

For patients with certain complications of cirrhosis, such as fluid retention or hepatic encephalopathy, dietary control is very important (see above).

A small number of cirrhotic patients have symptomatic steatorrhoea and require dietary fat restriction. Pancreatic insufficiency may be responsible for the steatorrhoea in some patients, particularly in alcoholics, and they may need pancreatic enzyme supplements.

Patients with cirrhosis often have oesophageal varices and as these are relatively thin walled, it seems sensible to warn patients about the possible risk of ingesting fragments of bone or other hard, sharp-edged foods. Patients who are confused, or who cannot chew their food properly, should be given soft, pulpy foods which are unlikely to cause mucosal damage.

Obstructive jaundice

When the biliary tree is obstructed there is a decrease in the intestinal concentration of bile salts and other substances such as lecithin, and there may be an interference with the flow of pancreatic juice. The severity of the resulting nutritional disturbances depends on the completeness of the obstruction and on the extent to which induced metabolic changes can be reversed by treatment.

Steatorrhoea is common. It is rarely gross because a large amount of fat can be absorbed from the intestine even when a luminal deficiency of bile salts reduces the size of the micellar phase; but severe reduction in micelle formation has serious consequences for the absorption of fat-soluble vitamins (see earlier). Steatorrhoea, and possibly pain of biliary origin, may improve with fat restriction.

When the obstruction is surgically remediable there is little indication for specific dietary measures as the reversible metabolic disturbances will correct themselves rapidly when the obstruction is relieved. Vitamin K deficiency should be corrected preoperatively by the intramuscular injection of phytomenadione in a dose of 10 mg daily. It is, of course, mandatory that dehydration and other obvious metabolic disturbances should be corrected as far as possible before surgery.

In patients with chronic biliary obstruction due to, for example, primary biliary cirrhosis, biliary stricture or biliary atresia, nutritional intervention may be necessary. If steatorrhoea disturbs the patient then the intake of long chain fatty acids should be reduced. Usually the caloric intake will still be adequate but if a large caloric intake must be provided for the purposes of growth, as in young children with biliary atresia, then medium chain triglycerides can be given as they do not require bile salts for their absorption.

Patients with chronic biliary obstruction require supplementation with vitamins A, D and K on a long-term basis. This may be conveniently provided by the monthly intramuscular injection of 10 mg of phytomenadione and 100 000 u each of vitamins A and D (which can be given in one injection if a special preparation is made). Currently, commercial supplies of vitamin A are difficult to obtain.

For reasons which were given earlier it is sensible to give calcium supplements to patients with chronic biliary obstruction, particularly when they are first treated with vitamin D, as their requirements for calcium at this time will be high. Calcium can be given conveniently in several forms in a dose of about 1 g (25 mmol) of elemental calcium daily. Effervescent tablets, such as Calcium Sandoz (which contain calcium lactate gluconate), are more palatable than other preparations; however, effervescent calcium preparations contain relatively large amounts of sodium.

A sample high protein, high energy, low fat diet suitable for patients with steatorrhoea and a low protein diet with added medium chain triglyceride suitable for patients with obstructive jaundice are presented in the appendix.

APPENDIX

Low Sodium Diet (No Salt to be Used in Cooking or Added at Table)

Breakfast	Fruit or fruit juice, if desired
	Shredded Wheat, Puffed Wheat or porridge made without salt
	1 egg, tomatoes, mushrooms
	Salt-free bread, matzos or salt-free crispbread
	Salt-free butter
	Jam, marmalade or honey
	Milk from allowance on cereal and in tea
Mid-morning	Tea or coffee, milk from allowance
Dinner	50 g (2 oz) meat or fish
	Potatoes, rice or pasta, or salt-free bread
	Vegetables or salad
	Fruit, jelly, unsalted pastry
Tea	Tea with milk from allowance
	Salt-free cake or biscuit
Supper	As dinner
Bed-time	Remainder of milk in tea or coffee
	Salt-free bread, salt-free butter and jam or salt-free cake or biscuit
Daily	250 ml ($\frac{1}{2}$ pint) milk for tea, cereal, etc.

This regimen provides approximately 20 mmol (20 mEq) sodium daily. The diet can be increased to 40 mmol (40 mEq) daily by the addition of four slices of ordinary bread instead of salt-free bread. One slice (25 g approx.) ordinary bread contains about 5 mmol (5 mEq) sodium. Salt should not be used in cooking or added at table, and foods forbidden and allowed (given below) are the same for both regimens, apart from bread.

Foods allowed freely

Fruit—fresh, canned, frozen
Fresh or frozen vegetables, except spinach, celery, beetroot, frozen peas
Salt-free bread, matzos, salt-free crispbread
Puffed Wheat, Shredded Wheat, Sugar Puffs, unsalted porridge
Sugar, glucose, honey, marmalade, jam
Boiled sweets, peppermints, chewing-gum
Pepper, herbs, spices, vinegar, powdered mustard
Meat, fish, eggs, milk in limited quantities only.

Salt substances (based on potassium chloride) may be used if serum potassium is normal or low

Foods not allowed

Ordinary bread, biscuits, cakes
Self-raising flour, baking powder
Rice Krispies, Cornflakes, All-Bran
Cheese, yoghourt, ice-cream
Ham, bacon, tinned meats, meat paste
Tinned fish, smoked fish, fish paste
Meat extract, yeast extract
Tinned vegetables
Tinned or packet soups
Sauces, pickles, ready-made mustard
Chocolate, toffees, fudge, golden syrup, fruit gums, fruit pastilles
Fruit squash, Lucozade, soda water
Tomato juice
Sultanas, raisins

Diets Restricted in Protein

It is essential with all restricted protein diets to provide an adequate energy intake to ensure optimal protein utilization. The energy content of the diet can be increased by ensuring the inclusion of non-protein fat and carbohydrate foods (see below). Glucose polymers taken, for example, in fruit juice provide a good source of energy for patients with small appetites.

Foods allowed freely on all diets restricted in protein:

Butter, margarine, lard, oil, double cream
Sugar, glucose, marmalade, jam, honey
Low protein bread, biscuits and pasta
Boiled sweets, fruit juice, squash, carbonated beverages

Minimal protein diet

This diet provides approximately 10 g of protein. Double cream or milk substitutes, such as coffee-mate (Carnation) can be used to replace milk in the diet.

Breakfast	Fruit or fruit juice Fried or grilled tomatoes Low protein bread + butter + marmalade Tea or coffee + sugar + milk substitute or double cream
Mid-morning	Tea or coffee + sugar + milk substitute or double cream Low protein biscuit
Lunch	Fruit juice or clear vegetable soup Low protein vegetable casserole Rice Tinned fruit + sugar + double cream
Tea	As mid-morning Low protein biscuit or cake or low protein bread + tomato sandwich
Supper	Fruit juice or clear vegetable soup Stuffed tomatoes Baked potatoes + butter Blancmange made with double cream
Bed-time	As tea

20 g protein diet

As for minimal protein diet but include:

200 ml milk
1 slice ordinary bread or a small serving breakfast cereal
15 g cooked meat/fish/cheese/$\frac{1}{2}$ egg at lunch and supper

40 g protein diet

Milk allowance 200 ml daily

Breakfast	Fruit or fruit juice Egg – cooked any way 1 slice ordinary bread + butter + marmalade Small serving cereal + milk from allowance (f.a.) Tea or coffee + sugar + milk f.a.
Mid-morning	Tea or coffee + sugar + milk f.a. Plain biscuit
Lunch	Fruit juice or clear vegetable soup 25 g cooked meat/fish/cheese/1 egg Vegetables or salad Potatoes/rice/pasta Tinned fruit + sugar + double cream
Tea	Tea or coffee + sugar + milk f.a. Piece of cake or 1 slice bread + butter + jam
Supper	As lunch
Bed-time	As mid-morning

60 g protein diet

As for 40 g protein diet but include 75 g meat, etc., lunch and supper.

High Protein, High Energy, Low Fat Diet

This provides approx. 80 g protein, 35 g fat, 2400 C (10.8 MJ)

Daily	1 pint skimmed milk (extra skimmed milk powder may be added to increase protein content)
Breakfast	Fruit or fruit juice Cereal or porridge with skimmed milk and sugar 1 egg or lean grilled bacon or lean ham or fish Bread + scrape butter or Outline spread Marmalade, honey or jam Tea or coffee with skimmed milk
Mid-morning	Skimmed milk shake (skimmed milk + skimmed milk powder and flavouring – Nesquick, Crusha, etc.)
Lunch	Average portion lean meat, no visible fat *or* large portion white fish or chicken Potatoes, rice or spaghetti Vegetables or salad, no oil Skimmed milk pudding, fruit or jelly Stewed or tinned fruit

Tea	Tea with skimmed milk
	Plain biscuits
Supper	As lunch
Bed-time	Skimmed milk shake

Energy intake may be increased by fruit drinks plus glucose, or a glucose polymer. The use of high carbohydrate foods such as potatoes, rice and spaghetti should be encouraged. Low fat products such as Carnation Build-up or Cadbury's Two Shakes may make pleasant and useful additions to skimmed milk.

Low Fat Diet with Added Medium Chain Triglyceride

Long chain fat should be restricted, to reduce steatorrhoea, and medium chain triglycerides added to the diet to increase the energy content. Medium chain triglyceride (MCT) should be introduced slowly into the diet over several days, as it may cause gastrointestinal disturbance in the early stages if administered rapidly. The oil should never be given undiluted, as a medicine, but always mixed with at least an equal quantity of fluid or food.

Daily	1 pint skimmed milk, with 1 tablespoon MCT oil added *or* 1 pint reconstituted Cow and Gate MCT milk powder *or* Mead Johnson Portagen
Breakfast	Fruit or fruit juice
	Cereal + MCT milk and sugar
	Bread + scrape butter or Outline spread
	Marmalade, honey, etc.
	Tea or coffee with MCT milk + sugar as desired
Mid-morning	Coffee or tea + MCT milk
	Plain biscuits
Lunch	Lean meat, no visible fat, or white fish
	Potatoes mashed with MCT or fried with MCT *or* bread with scrape butter
	Custard or milk pudding made with MCT milk (see above)
	Tinned or stewed fruit, jelly or jam
Tea	Tea or coffee with MCT milk
Supper	As lunch
Bed-time	MCT milk drink

ACKNOWLEDGEMENTS

We would like to thank Miss Carol Bateman, District Dietitian, Professor Victor Hoffbrand, Professor of Haematology, and Dr Robert Batey, Honorary Lecturer in Medicine, for useful discussions, and Miss Julia Denoon for typing the manuscript.

REFERENCES

1. Aguirre, A., Yoshimura, N., Westman, T. & Fischer, J.E. (1974) Plasma amino acids in dogs with two experimental forms of liver damage. *Journal of Surgical Research,* **16,** 339–345.
2. Ajdukiewicz, A.B., Agnew, J.E., Byers, P.D., Wills, M.R. & Sherlock, S. (1974) The relief of bone pain in primary biliary cirrhosis with calcium infusions. *Gut,* **15,** 788–793.
3. Arroyo, V. & Rodes, J. (1975) A rational approach to the treatment of ascites. *Postgraduate Medical Journal,* **51,** 558–562.
4. Baddeley, R.M. (1976) Results of jejuno-ileostomy for gross refractory obesity. *British Journal of Surgery,* **63,** 801–806.
5. Barry, M. (1974) Iron and the liver. *Gut,* **15,** 324–334.
6. Beattie, A.D. & Sherlock, S. (1976) Ascorbic acid deficiency in liver disease. *Gut,* **17,** 571–575.
7. Blass, J.P. & Gibson, G.E. (1977) Abnormality of a thiamine-requiring enzyme in Korsakoff syndrome. *New England Journal of Medicine,* **297,** 1367–1370.
8. Brown, R.G., O'Leary, J.P. & Woodward, E.R. (1974) Hepatic effect of jejunoileal bypass for morbid obesity. *American Journal of Surgery,* **127,** 53–58.
9. Brunt, P.W., Kew, M.C., Scheuer, P.S. & Sherlock, S. (1974) Studies in alcoholic liver disease in Britain: clinical and pathological patterns related to natural history. *Gut,* **15,** 52–58.
10. Burns, J.J. (1975) Ascorbic acid (vitamin C). In *The Pharmacological Basis of Therapeutics* (Ed.) Goodman, L.S. & Gillman, A. pp. 1564–1569. New York: MacMillan.
11. Chalmers, T.C., Eckhardt, R.D., Reynolds, W.E., Cigarroa, J.G., Deane, N., Reifenstein, R.W. & Smith, C.W. (1955) The treatment of acute infectious hepatitis: studies of the effects of diet, rest, and physical reconditioning on the acute course of the disease and on the incidence of relapse and residual abnormalities. *Journal of Clinical Investigation,* **34,** 1163–1235.
12. Charlton, R.W., Jacobs, P., Seftel, H. & Bothwell, T.H. (1964) Effect of alcohol on iron absorption. *British Medical Journal,* **ii,** 1427–1429.
13. Cohn, V.H. (1975) Vitamin K and vitamin E. In *The Pharmacological Basis of Therapeutics* (Ed.) Goodman, L.S. & Gillman, A. pp. 1591–1600. New York: MacMillan.
14. Conn, H.O. (1975) Cirrhosis. In *Diseases of the Liver* (Ed.) Schiff, L. pp. 833–939. Philadelphia: Lippincott.
15. Creutzfeldt, W., Frerichs, H. & Sickinger, K. (1970) Liver disease and diabetes mellitus. In *Progress in Liver Diseases,* Vol. 3 (Ed.) Popper, H. & Schaffner, F. pp. 371–407. London: Heinemann.
16. Crosby, W.H. (1977) Who needs iron? *New England Journal of Medicine,* **297,** 543–545.
17. Cruz-Coke, R. & Varela, A. (1966) Inheritance of alcoholism. *Lancet,* **ii,** 1282–1284.
18. Damodaran, K. & Hartfall, S.J. (1944) Infective hepatitis in garrison of Malta. *British Medical Journal,* **ii,** 587–590.
19. Drenick, E.J., Simmons, F., Murphy, J.F. (1970) Effect on hepatic morphology of treatment of obesity by fasting, reducing diets and small bowel bypass. *New England Journal of Medicine,* **282,** 829–834.
20. Dudrick, S.J., Macfadyen, B.V., Copeland, E.M. &

Duke, J.H. (1976) Experimental aspects of total parenteral alimentation. In *Total Parenteral Alimentation* (Ed.) Manni, C., Magalini, S.I. & Scrascia, E. pp. 3–7. Amsterdam: Excerpta Medica.

21. Eichner, E.R. & Hillman, R.S. (1971) The evolution of anemia in alcoholic patients. *American Journal of Medicine,* **50,** 218–232.
22. Elwyn, D.H., Parikh, H.C. & Schoemaker, W.C. (1968) Amino acid movements between gut, liver and periphery in unanaesthetized dogs. *American Journal of Physiology,* **215,** 1260–1275.
23. Farivar, M., Bucher, N.L.R., Wands, J. & Isselbacher, K.J. (1976) Beneficial effects of insulin and glucagon on fulminant murine hepatitis. *Gastroenterology,* **70,** 981.
24. Farrell, G.C., Bhathal, P.S. & Powell, L.W. (1977) Abnormal liver function in chronic hypervitaminosis A. *Digestive Diseases,* **22,** 724–728.
25. Felig, P. (1973) The glucose-alanine cycle. *Metabolism,* **22,** 179–207.
26. Fialkow, P.J., Thuline, M.C. & Fenster, R.F. (1966) Lack of association between cirrhosis of the liver and the common types of colour blindness. *New England Journal of Medicine,* **275,** 584–587.
27. Fischer, J.E., Yoshimura, N., Aguirre, A., James, J.H., Cummings, M.G., Abel, R.M. & Deindoerfer, F. (1974) Plasma amino acids in hepatic encephalopathy. *American Journal of Surgery,* **127,** 40–47.
28. Fischer, J.E., Funovics, J.M., Aguirre, A., James, J.H., Keane, J.M., Wesdorp, R.I.C., Yoshimura, N. & Westman, T. (1975) The role of plasma amino acids in hepatic encephalopathy. *Surgery,* **78,** 276–288.
29. Freston, J.W. & Englert, E. (1967) The influence of age and excessive body weight on the distribution and metabolism of bromsulphalein. *Clinical Science,* **33,** 301–312.
30. Gollan, J.L., Bateman, C. & Billing, B.H. (1976) Effect of dietary composition on the unconjugated hyperbilirubinaemia of Gilbert's syndrome. *Gut,* **17,** 335–340.
31. Greenberger, N.J., Carley, J., Schenker, S., Bettinger, I., Stamnes, C. & Beyer, P. (1977) Effect of vegetable and animal protein diets in chronic hepatic encephalopathy. *Digestive Diseases,* **22,** 845–855.
32. Greengard, P. (1975) The vitamin B complex. In *The Pharmacological Basis of Therapeutics* (Ed.) Goodman, L.S. & Gillman, A. pp. 1549–1563. New York: MacMillan.
33. Hartroft, W.S. (1961) Experimental reproduction of human liver disease. In *Progress in Liver Diseases,* Vol. 1 (Ed.) Popper, H. & Schaffner, F. pp. 68–85. New York: Grune & Stratton.
34. Herbert, V. (1975) Drugs effective in megaloblastic anaemias. In *The Pharmacological Basis of Therapeutics* (Ed.) Goodman, L.S. & Gillman, A. pp. 1324–1349. New York: MacMillan.
35. Hines, J.D. (1975) Hematologic abnormalities involving vitamin B_6 and folate metabolism in alcoholic subjects. *Annals of the New York Academy of Science,* **252,** 316–327.
36. Hoagland, C.L., Labby, D.H., Kunkel, H.G. & Shank, R.E. (1946) An analysis of the effect of fat in the diet on recovery from viral hepatitis. *American Journal of Public Health,* **36,** 1287–1292.
37. Hoffbrand, A.V. (1978) Personal communication.
38. Holdsworth, C.D., Nye, L. & King, E. (1972) The effect of portacaval anastomosis on oral carbohydrate tolerance and on plasma insulin levels. *Gut,* **13,** 58–63.
39. Holzbach, R.T., Wieland, R.G., Lieber, C.S., Decarli, L.M., Koepke, K.R. & Green, S.G. (1974) Hepatic lipid in morbid obesity: assessment at and subsequent to jejunoileal bypass. *New England Journal of Medicine,* **290,** 296–299.
40. Jakobovits, A.W., Morgan, M.Y. & Sherlock, S. (1978) Hepatic siderosis in alcoholics. *American Journal of Digestive Diseases.* In press.
41. Kabi Vitrum Limited (1977) In *Data Sheet Compendium.* pp. 381–382. London: Association of the British Pharmaceutical Industry.
42. Kennedy, J. (1978) Personal communication.
43. Kern, F., Jackson, R.G., Martin, T.E., & Mueller, J.F. (1957) Some effects of multiple intravenous infusions of a cottonseed oil emulsion in patients with Laennec's cirrhosis of the liver. *Metabolism,* **6,** 743–757.
44. Klatskin, G. (1975) Toxic and drug induced hepatitis. In *Diseases of the Liver* (Ed.) Schiff, L. pp. 604–710. Philadelphia: Lippincott.
45. Koga, Y., Swanson, V.L. & Hays, D.M. (1975) Hepatic intravenous fat pigment in infants and children receiving lipid emulsion. *Journal of Pediatric Surgery,* **10,** 641–646.
46. Krawitt, E.L. (1975) Effect of ethanol ingestion on duodenal calcium transport. *Journal of Laboratory and Clinical Medicine,* **85,** 665–671.
47. Lee, H.A. (1974) Parenteral nutrition. In *Acute Metabolic Illness* (Ed.) Lee, H.A. London: Academic Press.
48. Leevy, C.M., Baker, H., Tenhove, W., Frank, O. & Cherrick, G.R. (1965) B-complex vitamins in liver disease of the alcoholic. *American Journal of Clinical Nutrition,* **16,** 339–346.
49. Lickley, H.L.A., Chisholm, D.J., Rabinowitch, A., Wexler, M. & Dupre, J. (1975) Effects of portacaval anastomosis on glucose tolerance in dogs: evidence of an interrelationship between gut and liver in oral glucose disposal. *Metabolism,* **24,** 1157–1168.
50. Lieber, C.S. (1975) Liver disease and alcohol: fatty liver, alcholic hepatitis, cirrhosis and their interrelationship. *Annals of the New York Academy of Science,* **252,** 63–84.
51. Long, R.G., Varghese, Z., Meinhard, E.A., Skinner, R.K., Wills, M.R. & Sherlock, S. (1978) Parenteral 1,25-dihydroxycholecalciferol in hepatic osteomalacia. *British Medical Journal,* **i,** 75–77.
52. Mandel, H.G. (1975) Vitamin A. In *The Pharmacological Basis of Therapeutics* (Ed.) Goodman, L.S. & Gillman, A. pp. 1570–1578. New York: MacMillan.
53. Maxwell, J.D., Sanderson, I., Butler, W.H., Gazet, J.C. & Pilkington, T.R.E. (1977) Hepatic structure and function after modified jejunoileal bypass surgery for obesity. *British Medical Journal,* **ii,** 726–729.
54. McIntyre, N., Turner, D.S. & Holdsworth, C.D. (1970) The role of the portal circulation in glucose and fructose tolerance. *Diabetologia,* **6,** 593–596.
55. Miller, L.L. (1961) The role of the liver and non-hepatic tissues in regulation of free amino acid levels in blood. In *Amino Acid Pools* (Ed.) Holden, J.T. pp. 708–721. Amsterdam: Elsevier.
56. Milsom, J.P., Morgan, M.Y. & Sherlock, S. (1979) Factors affecting plasma amino acid concentrations in control subjects. *Metabolism,* **28,** 313–319.
57. Mitchell, D., Wagner, C., Stone, W.J., Wilkinson, G.R. & Schenker, S. (1976) Abnormal regulation of plasma pyridoxal 5-phosphate in patients with liver disease. *Gastroenterology,* **70,** 988.

58. Morgan, A.G., Kelleher, J., Walker, B.E. & Losowsky, M.S. (1976) Nutrition in cryptogenic cirrhosis and chronic aggressive hepatitis. *Gut,* **17,** 113–118.
59. Morgan, M.Y. & Sherlock, S. (1977) Sex-related differences among 100 patients with alcoholic liver disease. *British Medical Journal,* **i,** 939–941.
60. Morgan, M.Y., Milsom, J.P. & Sherlock, S. (1980) Plasma amino acid patterns in liver disease. In preparation.
61. Morgan, M.Y., Ross, M.G.R., Ng, C.M., Adams, D.M., Thomas, H.C. & Sherlock, S. (1980) HLA-B8, immunoglobulins and antibody responses in alcohol related liver disease. *Journal of Clincal Pathology,* in press.
62. Mosley, J.W. & Galambos, J.T. (1975) Viral hepatitis. In *Diseases of the Liver* (Ed.) Schiff, L. pp. 500–593. Philadelphia: Lippincott.
63. Moxley, R.T. III, Pozefsky, T. & Lockwood, D.Y. (1974) Protein nutrition and liver disease after jejunoileal bypass for morbid obesity. *New England Journal of Medicine,* **290,** 921–926.
64. Munro, H.N. (1970) Free amino acid pools and their role in regulation. In *Mammalian Protein Metabolism* Vol. 4 (Ed.) Munro, H.N. & Allison, J.B. pp. 299–388. London: Academic Press.
65. Neville, J.N., Eagles, J.A., Samson, G. & Olson, R.E. (1968) Nutritional status of alcoholics. *American Journal of Clinical Nutrition,* **21,** 1329–1340.
66. Partridge, W.M. & Jefferson, L.S. (1975) Liver uptake of amino acids and carbohydrates on a single circulatory passage. *American Journal of Physiology,* **228,** 1155–1161.
67. Perutz, M. (1976) Fundamental research in molecular biology: relevance to medicine. *Nature,* **262,** 449–453.
68. Popper, H. (1977) The pathogenesis of alcoholic cirrhosis. In *Alcohol and the Liver* (Ed.) Fisher, M.M. & Rankin, J.G. pp. 289–306. New York: Plenum Press.
69. Preisig, R. & Rennert, O. (1977) Anticholeretic effects of amino acids. Abstracts of the 12th meeting of the European Association for the Study of the Liver, Kavouri, 1977. *Archives of the Hellenic Medical Societies,* 3 (Suppl.), p. 62.
70. Rachmilewitz, M., Moshkowitz, B., Rachmilewitz, B., Grosswicz, N. & Gross, J. (1972) Serum vitamin B_{12} binding proteins in viral hepatitis. *European Journal of Clinical Investigation,* **2,** 239–242.
71. Rajan, K.S., Levinson, R. & Leevy, C.M. (1973) Abnormalities in RBC 2,3-DPG in hepatic encephalopathy. *Gastroenterology,* **64,** 191.
72. Ramalingaswami, V. (1964) Perspectives in protein malnutrition. *Nature,* **201,** 546–551.
73. Record, C.O., Buxton, B., Chase, R.A., Curzon, G., Murray-Lyon, I.M. & Williams, R. (1976) Plasma and brain amino acids in fulminant hepatic failure and their relationship to hepatic encephalopathy. *European Journal of Clinical Investigation,* **6,** 387–394.
74. Reid, N.C.R.W., Brunt, P.W., Bias, W.B., Maddrey, W.C., Alonso, B.A. & Iber, F.L. (1968) Genetic characteristics and cirrhosis: a controlled study of 200 patients. *British Medical Journal,* **ii,** 463–465.
75. Retief, F.P. & Huskisson, Y.J. (1969) Serum and urinary folate in liver disease. *British Medical Journal,* **ii,** 150–153.
76. Reynolds, T.B., Lieberman, F.L. & Goodman, A.R. (1978) Advantages of treatment of ascites without sodium restriction and without complete removal of excess fluid. *Gut,* **19,** 549–553.
77. Reynolds, T.B., Redeker, A.G. & Kuzma, O.T. (1965) Role of alcohol in pathogenesis of alcoholic cirrhosis. In *Therapeutic Agents and the Liver* (Ed.) McIntyre, N. & Sherlock, S. pp. 131–142. Oxford: Blackwell.
78. Rodgers, B.M., Hollenbeck, J.I., Donnelly, W.H. & Talbert, J.L. (1976) Intrahepatic cholestasis and parenteral hyperalimentation. *American Journal of Surgery,* **131,** 149–154.
79. Rosenthal, W.S. & Glass, J. (1970) Vitamin B_{12} and the liver. In *Progress in Liver Diseases,* Vol. 3 (Ed.) Popper, H. & Schaffner, F. pp. 118–146. London: Heinemann.
80. Rozental, P., Biava, C., Spencer, H. & Zimmerman, H. (1967) Liver morphology and function tests in obesity and during total starvation. *American Journal of Digestive Diseases,* **12,** 198–208.
81. Rudman, D., Smith, R.B., Salam, A., Warren, W.D., Galambos, J.T. & Wegner, J. (1970) Ammonia content of food. *American Journal of Clinical Nutrition,* **26,** 487–490.
82. Rumball, J.M., Stone, C.M. & Hasset, C. (1959) The behaviour of serum iron in acute hepatitis. *Gastroenterology,* **36,** 219–223.
83. Russell, R.M., Boyer, J.L., Bagheri, S.A. & Hruban, Z. (1974) Hepatic injury from chronic hypervitaminosis A resulting in portal hypertension and ascites. *New England Journal of Medicine,* **291,** 435–440.
84. Saunders, S.J., Truswell, A.S., Barbezat, G.O., Wittman, W. & Hansen, J.D.L. (1967) Plasma free amino acid pattern in protein-calorie malnutrition. *Lancet,* **ii,** 795–797.
85. Schuberth, O. (1963) Clinical results of intravenous fat emulsions. *Nutritio et Dieta (Basel),* **5,** 387–402.
86. Seftel, H.C., Malkin, C., Schmaman, A., Abrahams, C., Lynch, S.R., Charlton, R.W. & Bothwell, T.H. (1966) Osteoporosis, scurvy and siderosis in Johannesburg Bantu. *British Medical Journal,* **i,** 642–646.
87. Silk, D.B.A. (1974) Progress report. Peptide absorption in man. *Gut,* **15,** 494–501.
88. Snapper, I. (1965) Nutritional problems and avitaminosis. In *Chinese Lessons to Western Medicine,* 2nd ed. pp. 9–31. New York: Grune & Stratton.
89. Stanbury, J.B., Wyngaarden, J.B. & Fredrickson, D.S. (1972) *The Metabolic Basis of Inherited Disease.* New York: McGraw Hill.
90. Straw, J.S. (1975) Vitamin D. In *The Pharmacological Basis of Therapeutics* (Ed.) Goodman, L.S. & Gillman, A. pp. 1579–1590. New York: MacMillan.
91. Sullivan, L.W. & Herbert, W. (1964) Suppression of hematopoiesis by ethanol. *Journal of Clinical Investigation,* **43,** 2048–2062.
92. Thomson, A.D., Frank, O., Baker, H. & Leevy, C.M. (1971) Thiamine propyldisulphide: absorption and utilization. *Annals of Internal Medicine,* **74,** 529–534.
93. Walker, C., Peterson, W. & Ungar, R. (1974) Blood ammonia levels in advanced cirrhosis during therapeutic elevation of insulin–glucagon ratio. *New England Journal of Medicine,* **291,** 168–171.
94. Webster, L.T. & Davidson, C.S. (1957) Cirrhosis of the liver: impending hepatic coma and increased blood ammonia concentrations during protein hydrolysate infusion. *Journal of Laboratory and Clinical Medicine,* **50,** 1–10.
95. Westwater, J.O. & Faimer, D. (1958) Liver impairment in the obese. *Gastroenterology,* **34,** 686–693.
96. Winkelman, E.L., Schumacher, O.P. & Hermann, R.E. (1974) Results of the jejunoileal shunt in the treatment of morbid obesity. Abstract 14, *Meeting of American College of Physicians, April 1974.*

97. Wolff, J.E., Bergman, E.N. & Williams, H.H. (1972) Net metabolism of plasma amino acids by liver and portal-drained viscera of fed sheep. *American Journal of Physiology,* **223,** 438–446.
98. Yamamoto, H., Aikawa, T., Matsutaka, H., Okuda, T. & Ishitawa, E. (1974) Interorgan relationship of amino acid metabolism in fed rats. *American Journal of Physiology,* **223,** 438–446.
99. Zarif, M.A., Pildes, R.S., Szanto, P.B. & Vidyasagar, D. (1976) Cholestasis associated with administration of L-amino acids and dextrose solutions. *Biology of the Neonate,* **29,** 66–76.
100. Zelman, S. (1952) The liver in obesity. *Archives of Internal Medicine,* **90,** 141–156.
101. Rossouw, J.E., Labadarios, D., Krasner, N., Davis, M. & Williams, R. (1978) Red blood cell transketolase activity and the effect of thiamine supplementation in patients with chronic liver disease. *Scandinavian Journal of Gastroenterology,* **13,** 133–138.

Chapter 7

The Liver and the Endocrine System

D.G. JOHNSTON
K.G.M.M. ALBERTI

The liver is of key importance in the proper functioning of much of the endocrine system. It is a major organ for metabolic degradation of many hormones (see Table 7.1) and it is therefore to be expected that abnormalities of circulating hormone concentrations will be found in subjects with liver disease. This is of clinical importance in interpretation of laboratory values for blood concentrations of individual hormones, for example thyroid hormones and insulin. The liver is also a prime target organ for action of many hormones, and hepatic disease may be associated with diminished or altered hormone effects despite an apparently normal circulating concentration. In addition, the liver may be necessary for production of a 'secondary messenger' essential for the full effects of a particular hormone to be manifested, for example the somatomedins and growth hormone.

In this chapter we discuss the endocrine abnormalities associated with liver disease; such abnormalities are often similar in hepatic disease of varied aetiology but in certain conditions endocrine changes are either specific or occur with such frequency that they are considered separately, for example in haemochromatosis. In view of the importance of alcohol in the pathogenesis or progression of much of the liver disease seen in western societies, a separate discussion of the endocrine effects of alcohol is included. Finally, we discuss the hepatic disorders observed in patients with primary disease of an endocrine system.

Table 7.1. *Hormones Catabolized by Liver.*

Catabolism primarily by liver:
Insulin
Glucagon (3500-dalton)
Growth hormone
Glucocorticoids
Oestrogens
Progesterone
Parathormone
Some gut hormones
Catabolism by liver and other tissues:
Thyroid hormones
Luteinizing hormone
Antidiuretic hormone
Testosterone
Aldosterone
Oxytocin
Adrenocorticotrophic hormone
Thyroid-stimulating hormone
Thyrotrophin-releasing hormone

ENDOCRINE CHANGES IN LIVER DISEASE

Insulin

Normal physiology

The liver is a major organ in the regulation of carbohydrate, protein and lipid metabolism and as such is an important target tissue for insulin action. It is also important in insulin degradation.

Insulin is secreted directly into the portal venous system, the rate of secretion being influenced by many factors other than blood glucose concentration, for example amino acids, gut hormones and stress. The liver is exquisitely sensitive to small changes in insulin secretion; thus a twofold rise in portal venous insulin concentration in overnight fasted man is sufficient to inhibit hepatic glucose production completely.[67] This fine control of hepatic metabolism is aided by the fact that the liver is exposed to much higher insulin concentrations than are peripheral tissues as a result of direct secretion into the portal venous system.[18] A further factor increasing portal-peripheral venous difference is hepatic degradation of insulin. Most available evidence suggests that approximately 50 per cent of insulin secreted by the pancreas is degraded in the first passage through the liver.[29,114,115,142,163,174,209]

Insulin in liver disease

It is thus to be expected that liver disease will be associated with abnormalities of insulin metabolism. Hepatic cirrhosis is consistently associated with elevated peripheral venous immunoreactive insulin concentrations (Table 7.1) both fasting and in response to normal meals, oral or intravenous glucose, amino acids and tolbutamide.[44,49,89,110,124,154,194] Similar findings have been demonstrated although less consistently in liver failure[143,215,232,265] and in acute viral hepatitis.[68,153,169,200] Liver damage with paracetamol overdose is associated with normal fasting insulin concentrations but an exaggerated insulin response to intravenous glucose.[201] Chronic active hepatitis, on the other hand, is associated with hypoinsulinaemia and a delayed insulin response to intravenous glucose.[6] It is possible that this condition is associated with autoimmune pancreatic damage.

Mechanism of hyperinsulinaemia

Peripheral hyperinsulinaemia is the rule for other forms of liver disease. This may result from either hypersecretion or diminished degradation but recent evidence suggests that the latter is more important.[111,112] In the pancreatic B cell, proinsulin is cleaved to insulin and the connecting peptide, C-peptide, plus some basic amino acids. C-peptide and insulin are released in equimolar quantities[101] but evidence so far suggests that C-peptide is degraded by kidney and not significantly by liver.[116,238] If renal function is normal, peripheral C-peptide levels are unlikely to be influenced by liver disease and will provide a better indication of insulin secretion than measurement of peripheral insulin levels alone. Studies have shown that fasting C-peptide concentrations are normal in hyperinsulinaemic cirrhotics suggesting that despite high peripheral insulin concentrations, insulin secretion is not increased. In addition, after oral glucose, cirrhotics with a high peripheral insulin response have similar C-peptide values to those with normal peripheral insulin values. It therefore appears that hyperinsulinaemia both in fasting and after oral glucose results from diminished degradation rather than hypersecretion of insulin, at least in cirrhotic subjects. Support for this hypothesis comes from recent studies with direct measurement of portal and peripheral venous insulin levels.[90]

Role of portasystemic anastomoses

Diminished insulin degradation in liver cirrhosis may result from parenchymal damage, portasystemic shunting or both. Considerable intrahepatic portasystemic shunting may occur in patients who have no demonstrable large vessel anastomoses. Animal experiments with diversion of portal or pancreatic venous blood into the systemic circulation have produced conflicting results, some workers demonstrating a hyperinsulinaemic effect[133,214,233] while others have not.[41,264] Human studies have shown a rise in basal and stimulated peripheral insulin concentrations in cirrhotic subjects after surgical portacaval anastomosis.[99,154,210,226] This would suggest that portal bypass is an important factor in diminished insulin metabolism but the possibility remains that the bypass procedure itself may produce further liver damage. Evidence against a major role for portal bypass is provided by studies in subjects with long-standing portal venous block who had extensive natural or surgically created portasystemic anastomosis. These subjects had ostensibly normal liver function and normal biopsy to light microscopy.[112] Fasting hyperinsulinaemia did not occur and fasting C-peptide concentrations were normal. Only at high rates of insulin secretion was a defect in insulin degradation observed. Thus significant liver damage is necessary for hyperinsulinaemia to occur and parenchymal damage is likely to be more important than portasystemic anastomosis in the hyperinsulinaemia of cirrhosis.

Glucagon

Normal physiology

In normal man, the importance of the liver in metabolism of glucagon is uncertain, many of the difficulties being attributable to the heterogeneity of total plasma immunoreactive glucagon (IRG). Total plasma IRG is composed of at least four fractions; the 3500-dalton component is the biologically active form of the hormone; the 9000-dalton moiety may be a precursor of the 3500-dalton form but is itself biologically inactive; the significance of the 2000-dalton and 160 000-dalton fractions is uncertain. Thus although the 3500-dalton moiety is the biologically active one, total plasma IRG measures all components and significant changes in 3500-dalton glucagon may occur without a measurable change in total IRG.

Some early studies with total plasma IRG measurement suggested that the kidneys were of major importance in glucagon metabolism, with liver assuming a minor role,[69, 71, 75] whereas other investigators have suggested that the liver was the major site of glucagon metabolism.[23] The importance of gel filtration and measurement of each particular fraction of IRG is illustrated by the recent study of Jaspan and colleagues.[105] Thus in the rat, the liver selectively metabolizes 3500-dalton glucagon with a percentage extraction in fasted animals of 81 ± 5, while extracting only minimal quantities of 9000-dalton and >40 000-dalton glucagon. If these results can be extrapolated to man, hepatic glucagon metabolism may therefore be of major physiological importance.

Glucagon in liver disease

All of the earlier studies in human liver disease give information only about total IRG concentrations. Marco and colleagues[144] found mean fasting plasma glucagon levels of 455 ± 63 pg/ml in cirrhotic patients with a portacaval shunt, 217 ± 23 pg/ml in patients with liver disease but no evidence of portasystemic anastomosis, and 146 ± 10 pg/ml in control subjects. Sherwin and co-workers[222] found elevated plasma IRG concentrations only if portasystemic shunting was present. The importance of portal bypass is further suggested by experiments in normal dogs in which progressive hyperglucagonaemia occurs after surgical portacaval anastomosis.[233] Elevated plasma glucagon concentrations are also found in human subjects with chronic portal venous block and extensive natural or surgically created portasystemic anastomoses, despite normal liver function on routine biochemistry and normal liver biopsy to light microscopy.

The primacy of portal venous bypass in production of hyperglucagonaemia suggests that diminished hepatic breakdown, rather than hypersecretion of glucagon, may be the major factor, a situation analogous to that for insulin. That this is not solely the case is suggested by a recent study of Sherwin and colleagues.[223] Measuring specifically 3500-dalton glucagon, they found a two- to sixfold increase in basal plasma levels in cirrhotics with demonstrable portasystemic anastomoses, but values were normal in cirrhotics without portal venous bypass. Metabolic clearance rate of 3500-dalton glucagon was normal in all subjects, suggesting that the elevated plasma concentrations observed in cirrhotics with portasystemic anastomoses were the result of hypersecretion of glucagon. The stimulus for hypersecretion remains to be established.

Metabolic consequences of hyperglucagonaemia

The pathophysiological importance of hyperglucagonaemia in liver disease is uncertain. The elevated plasma concentrations observed do not fall normally in response to glucose and show abnormal increases after alanine or arginine stimulation.[89, 90] The liver in man is the major organ on which glucagon exerts its glycogenolytic and gluconeogenic actions but portal bypass or hepatic parenchymal damage may serve to decrease the metabolic effect. Exogenous glucagon produces a subnormal glucose response in different forms of liver disease but this may reflect decreased hepatic glycogen stores rather than inadequate metabolic effectiveness of glucagon per se. The glycaemic response to intravenous alanine, a potent stimulus of glucagon release, in normal subjects occurs within 10 to 20 minutes and probably reflects glycogenolysis.[222] In cirrhotic subjects the maximal increase in glucose is similar but delayed to 30 to 60 minutes. This corresponds to the time required for glucagon to stimulate glucose synthesis from ^{14}C-alanine. The hyperglycaemic effect of glucagon in liver disease may therefore be due to a stimulating effect on gluconeogenesis rather than on glycogenolysis.

Plasma cyclic adenosine-3′,5′-monophosphate response to intravenous glucagon has been recently studied.[51, 78] Response may be exaggerated in obstructive jaundice and is claimed to differentiate between extrahepatic and intrahepatic obstruction. Further work is required to establish the usefulness of this as a diagnostic procedure.

Growth Hormone

Normal physiology

Turnover of growth hormone in plasma is rapid with a half-disappearance time of 19 minutes.[175] Secretion is pulsatile and its control is complex; the effects of stress, non-esterified fatty acids, amino acids, glucose deprivation, adrenergic stimulation and deep sleep have been reviewed.[166, 204] There is also suggestive evidence of negative automatic feedback by somatomedins or the growth hormone molecule itself.[1] The liver and kidneys are the major sites of growth hormone degradation.

Growth hormone in liver disease

Basal growth hormone levels may be elevated in various forms of liver disease, particularly cirrhosis (see Table 7.2) and this has been attributed to a decrease in metabolic clearance. Thus Owens and co-workers,[175] using a constant infusion technique to achieve a variety of serum growth hormone levels, showed a decrease in metabolic clearance of unlabelled human growth hormone in 10 of 17 patients with hepatic cirrhosis. Cameron et al,[28] using radiolabelled human growth hormone, obtained similar results. Taylor and colleagues,[243] however, showed that the liver was responsible for 90 per cent of the metabolic clearance of human growth hormone but found normal values in patients with liver disease. In addition, Pimstone et al[187] showed normal clearance of endogenous growth hormone during infusion of somatostatin in four patients with severe liver disease who had elevated basal growth hormone values.

Thus evidence for delayed growth hormone clearance is inconclusive and although in some subjects may contribute to the elevation in basal values, it does not explain the paradoxical rise in growth hormone after oral glucose in some patients with liver disease. Altered hypothalamic–pituitary control of secretion is suggested by the growth hormone response to intravenous thyrotrophin-releasing-hormone which is not observed in normal subjects.[177, 278] Altered dopaminergic control of growth hormone secretion also requires investigation, particularly in patients with hepatic failure in whom a defect in dopaminergic neurotransmission has been postulated.[74]

Somatomedins

Many of the actions of growth hormone are secondary to production of a group of small peptides, the somatomedins. Present evidence suggests that somatomedins are produced by the liver. Somatomedin activity falls after partial hepatectomy in rats and rises as the liver regenerates.[256] Isolated rat liver perfusion experiments have demonstrated an increase in somatomedin activity in the perfusate when growth hormone was added to the perfusion medium.[150, 151] In similar experiments, livers from hypophysectomized rats released less somatomedin activity than livers from intact animals and activity could be increased by addition of growth hormone to the perfusate.[186]

Wu and colleagues[275] studied serum somatomedin activity in a group of patients with chronic liver disease, with the activity assessed by ^{35}S uptake into chick embryo pelvic rudiments. Nine of ten cirrhotics showed low activity which correlated with the degree of liver damage. Elevated basal growth hormone levels were found in seven patients, all of whom had decreased somatomedin activity. Similar findings have been obtained using a somatomedin radioceptor assay.[242] The decreased somatomedin levels probably result directly from liver damage. Abnormal oestrogen metabolism in cirrhotic subjects may contribute as oestrogen administration decreases the somatomedin response to growth hormone both in animals[185] and man.[271, 272]

Metabolic effects

The metabolic effects of a chronic elevation in growth hormone concentration in subjects with liver disease are probably diminished by the decreased somatomedin response. Patients may have raised growth hormone levels for years but do not develop acromegaly. Growth hormone may play some role in the abnormal carbohydrate metabolism observed (see Chapter 3) but levels do not correlate with any index of glucose tolerance.

Cortisol

Normal physiology

Cortisol is the major glucocorticoid hormone and its secretion is influenced by the diurnal rhythm, negative feedback by the cortisol molecule, and stress, of which stress is the most potent stimulus. In the circulation, cortisol is 95 per cent bound to protein, largely cortisol binding globulin and to a lesser extent albumin. It is degraded, primarily in the liver by A-ring reduction to tetrahydrocortisone and subsequent conjugation with glucuronic acid.

Table 7.2. *Basal Values for Hormones in Liver Disease.**

	Cirrhosis		Acute viral hepatitis		Chronic active hepatitis	
	Patient	Control	Patient	Control	Patient	Control
Insulin	17 ± 2.4[a]	8.9 ± 2.1	23.0 ± 9.3[f]	9 ± 4	8.1 ± 0.9[i]	6.4 ± 0.7
(mU/l)	28 ± 7[b]	11 ± 3	10.3 ± 2.1[g]	6.4 ± 0.5		
	16.3[c]	3.8	8.7 ± 1[h]	12.2 ± 1.3ψ		
	12 ± 5[d]	12 ± 2				
	22 ± 2[e]	8 ± 1				
Glucagon	342 ± 28[b]	105 ± 12				
(ng/l)	239 ± 32[e]	146 ± 10				
	243 ± 41[j]	89 ± 16				
	320 ± 15[bb]	90 ± 12				
Growth	6.9 ± 0.9[b]	2.8 ± 0.7	8.6 ± 2.1[g]	6.4 ± 0.5	3.8 ± 1[i]	6.7 ± 2.1
hormone	9.4 ± 7.1[k]	2.5 ± 0.9	3.9 ± 1.7[l]	0.3 – 5		
(μg/l)	10.7 ± 4.6[l]	0.3 – 5				
	8.4 ± 1.4[m]	2.5 ± 0.9				
Thyroxine	97 ± 5[n]	108 ± 3	147 ± 19[p]	111 ± 4	102 ± 6[bb]	46 – 150
(T_4)	94 ± 6[o]	84 ± 3				
(nmol/l)	104 ± 8[p]	111 ± 4				
Tri-iodothyronine	0.51 ± 0.05[n]	1.94 ± 0.05	2.29 ± 0.32[p]	1.94 ± 0.06	1.85 ± 0.10[bb]	1.5 – 3
(T_3)	1.31 ± 0.12[p]	1.94 ± 0.06				
(nmol/l)						
Thyroid-	8 ± 1[n]	4.6 ± 0.3	5.5 ± 0.4[p]	3.1 ± 0.1	10.4 ± 0.8[bb]	8 – 18.7
stimulating	5 ± 0.4[o]	3.6 ± 0.2				
hormone	7.1 ± 0.6[p]	3.1 ± 0.1				
(TSH) (mU/l)						
Testosterone†	7.6	22.6			17.3 ± 3.4[u]	26.4 ± 1.1
(nmol/l)	(3.8–19.1)[q]	(16.7–27.4)				
	17.0 ± 3.1[r]	26.4 ± 2.4			6.9 ± 1.9[v]	8.0 ± 1.1ω
	8.1 ± 1.7[s]	19.7 ± 1.8				
	10.5 ± 0.8[t]	20.8 ± 3.2				
	11.6 ± 1.7[u]	26.4 ± 1.1				
	10.8 ± 2.3[v]	8 ± 1.1ω				
Oestradiol†	109 ± 8[w]	86 ± 7			93 ± 11[u]	70 ± 4
(pmol/l)	115 ± 7[u]	70 ± 4			89 ± 30[v]	85 ± 15
	159 ± 24[x]	84 ± 11				
	174 ± 19[s]	100 ± 7				
	117 ± 16[r]	112 ± 5				
Luteinizing	24.1 ± 2.5[s]	12.1 ± 1.1			18 ± 2[u]	12 ± 1
hormone†	19.5 ± 5.5[y]	11.8 ± 2.5			3.2 ± 0.4[v]	2.4 ± 0.2
(LH)	4 ± 0.4[z]	0.8 – 13.3				
(U/l)	18 ± 1[u]	12 ± 1				
	19.1 ± 3.4[aa]	8.8 ± 1.4				
Follicle-	12.8 ± 2.3[s]	8.4 ± 2				
stimulating	10.1 ± 1.7[y]	5.6 ± 1.7				
hormone†	3.1 ± 0.4[z]	0.2 – 8.3				
(FSH)	20.7 ± 5.1[aa]	11.5 ± 2.9				
(U/l)						

* Values for plasma or serum samples, mean ± standard error of the mean, or range.
† Values are for male subjects.
ψ Values are for a group of hypoglycaemic subjects.
ω Testosterone measured as 17-β-hydroxy androgen, μg/l.

Values are adapted from the following papers:

[a] Johnston et al[111]
[b] Greco et al[89]
[c] West et al[269]
[d] Sestoft and Rehfeld[215]
[e] Marco et al[144]
[f] Nieschlag, Kremer and Mussgnug[169]
[g] Record et al[200]
[h] Felig et al[68]
[i] Alberti et al[6]
[j] Sherwin et al[222]
[k] Conn and Daughaday[44]
[l] Hernandez, Zorilla and Gershberg[97]
[m] Zanoboni and Zanoboni-Muciaccia[278]
[n] Chopra et al[38]
[o] Cuttelod et al[50]
[p] Nomura et al[170]
[q] Coppage and Cooner[46]
[r] Distiller et al[55]
[s] Chopra, Tulchinsky and Greenway[37]
[t] Gordon et al[87]
[u] Kley et al[121]
[v] Galvao-Teles et al[83]
[w] Pentikäinen et al[182]
[x] Korenman, Perrin and McCallum[125]
[y] Schalch et al[212]
[z] Mowat et al[164]
[aa] Van Thiel, Lester and Sherins[260]
[bb] Sheridan, Chapman and Losowsky[219]

Plasma cortisol levels in liver disease

Clinical evidence of cortisol excess, e.g. striae, obesity, facial mooning and acne, may be seen in some patients with liver disease, in particular chronic active hepatitis. Studies of plasma cortisol levels have shown differing results. Peterson[184] and other workers have shown normal values and this is confirmed by our own findings on samples taken from an indwelling cannula throughout a 12-hour period of normal meals and activity. Sholiton, Werk and Marwell,[225] however, showed lower values throughout the day and a loss of the normal diurnal variation has also been described.[253] Absent cortisol response to insulin hypoglycaemia and pseudo-Cushing's syndrome, both recently described in alcoholics (see below), are more likely to result from alcohol ingestion than associated liver disease.

The significance of total plasma cortisol measurements must be questioned in view of the decrease in serum albumin and cortisol binding globulin in subjects with liver disease. Studies which take protein binding into account have clarified this somewhat. McCann and Fulton[149] showed a small (but insignificant) decrease in total 11-hydroxycorticosteroid concentrations throughout the day in a group of patients with a variety of liver diseases. Free hormone levels, however, were normal in the morning and slightly higher than for controls at 2300 hr. Kley et al[121] found normal total levels in liver disease and free hormone concentrations in these subjects were normal. It is likely that, despite known changes in serum proteins, total plasma cortisol estimates continue to be useful and practical in liver disease.

Cortisol metabolism in liver disease

The liver is the major organ of catabolism of adrenal corticosteroids and it is to be expected that abnormalities of clearance be found in liver disease. Radioactive cortisol is cleared more slowly in cirrhotic subjects, and after cortisol or ACTH infusion plasma 17-hydroxycorticosteroids remain elevated longer than normal.[22, 63, 184] Impairment of A-ring reduction has been demonstrated as has impairment of the conjugation mechanism.[279] The decreased metabolic turnover has been postulated as due, at least in part, to decreased transport and binding of cortisol to intracellular metabolic sites.

Normal or near normal plasma cortisol levels in the presence of diminished clearance implies a decrease in cortisol production rate. The two groups to examine this problem, however, have failed to demonstrate a decrease in cortisol secretion rate in cirrhotic subjects[149, 279] and this requires further clarification. Twenty-four-hour urinary free cortisol excretion is diminished[149] as is 17-hydroxysteroid and 17-ketosteroid excretion.[217] This does not necessarily imply diminished adrenal steroid production as urinary excretion may be modified by alterations in glomerular filtration known to occur in cirrhotic patients. The possibility of an increase in extrahepatic hormone metabolism has not been investigated.

Metabolic effects

There is as yet no evidence to suggest that alterations in the amount or action of glucocorticoids are important in production of the metabolic changes observed in subjects with liver disease. The role of cortisol deficiency in pathogenesis of alcoholic hypoglycaemia and cortisol excess in pathogenesis of alcoholic ketosis is discussed in the section 'Endocrine effects of alcohol', below.

Thyroid Hormones

Normal physiology

In normal subjects, the thyroid produces 100 nmol/24 hr (78 μg/24 hr) thyroxine (T_4) of which 20 nmol/24 hr (16 μg/24 hr) is conjugated and excreted in bile or undergoes oxidative deamination.[32, 82] The remaining 80 nmol/24 hr (62 μg/24 hr) is de-iodinated to either tri-iodothyronine (T_3, 35 nmol/24 hr [23 μg/24 hr])[20, 192, 241] or reverse tri-iodothyronine (rT_3, 45 nmol/24 hr [29 μg/24 hr]).[35, 84] rT_3 may be considered biologically inactive at pathophysiological concentrations[191] but T_3 is several times more potent than T_4 on a molar basis[22] so that peripheral conversion of T_4 to T_3 may be considered a form of hormone activation. Only 5 nmol/24 hr (3 μg/24 hr) T_3 is secreted directly by the thyroid.[32, 36]

Hepatectomy in dogs severely impairs production of T_3 but not of rT_3 from exogenously administered T_4.[76] This suggests that the liver is a major organ of T_4 to T_3 conversion but that production of rT_3 occurs in extrahepatic tissues. Thus the liver has a major role in thyroid hormone metabolism, being involved in conjugation, biliary excretion and oxidative deamination of thyroxine and peripheral de-iodination of thyroxine to tri-iodothyronine.

Abnormalities of thyroid hormone metabolism are therefore to be expected in subjects with liver disease.

Liver disease

The majority of patients with liver disease are clinically euthyroid and this view is supported by indirect measures of thyroid hormone action such as Achilles tendon reflex time and indices of myocardial contractility.[38] However, many standard laboratory techniques may give misleading results suggesting hyper- or hypothyroidism.

131-iodine uptake. Patients with acute alcohol-related liver disease may have elevated thyroidal radioactive iodine (^{131}I) uptake and clearance.[224] This has been attributed to iodine deficiency secondary to malnutrition although evidence for this is unconvincing. The elevated ^{131}I uptake, however, does return to normal if these patients are hospitalized and is suppressible with T_3. Accelerated ^{131}I uptakes may also be found in hepatobiliary giardiasis.[131] ^{131}I uptake has been found decreased in acute infective hepatitis, particularly in patients with severe disease.[53, 257] Chronic liver disease, particularly alcoholic cirrhosis, may be associated with increased ^{131}I uptake by a mechanism similar to that of acute alcoholic damage.[165, 224] Uptake may be low in chronic active hepatitis.[219]

Thyroid hormone levels. Serum total and free T_4 levels are normal, slightly increased or slightly decreased in most studies of subjects with a variety of liver diseases [31, 38, 102, 170, 219] (Table 7.2). In occasional patients, however, the total T_4 may be considerably increased or decreased in association with an altered level of thyroxine binding proteins.[102, 219] Estimation of free thyroxine index, calculated from serum thyroxine and thyroid hormone binding level, usually reveals a normal result.[219] Total and free T_3 levels, however, are diminished, sometimes profoundly, and correlate with the degree of liver damage as indicated by serum albumin and bilirubin estimations.[31, 38] Nomura and colleagues[170] have shown T_4 to T_3 conversion in four cirrhotic patients decreased to less than half that seen in normal subjects (15.6 per cent compared with 35.7 per cent). In addition, two convalescing patients with alcoholic hepatitis showed a progressive normalization of serum T_3 levels as liver function improved. Diminished T_4 to T_3 conversion appears the likely mechanism for the low serum T_3 levels observed in liver disease. This reduction in serum T_3 concentration is most marked in, but not specific to, patients with liver disease as similar changes are found in subjects with a variety of other acute and chronic illnesses.[26, 31]

Hepatic cirrhosis is associated with an increase in both total and dialysable rT_3.[38] Again, this is not specific for liver disease, similar changes being observed in acute febrile illness and in patients with disseminated carcinoma.[26] Reciprocal changes in T_3 and rT_3 suggest that the elevated rT_3 levels found in liver disease may result from increased conversion from T_4 although a change in rT_3 clearance has not been excluded.

Thus biochemical assessment of thyroid function will usually yield results appropriate to the clinical status if free thyroid index is measured, but T_3 concentrations may be low and rT_3 levels high. In view of the metabolic potency of T_3, this may suggest hypothyroidism in these subjects although clinical criteria are against this.

Thyroid-stimulating hormone concentration. Estimation of serum thyroid stimulating hormone (TSH) concentration is the most sensitive index of thyroid hypofunction available at present if hypothalamic and pituitary function is normal. In three reports, TSH levels have been elevated to twice normal in chronic liver disease,[38, 50, 170] suggesting mild hypothyroidism. However, there is no correlation between T_3 levels and TSH.[170] In addition, peak TSH response to thyrotrophin releasing hormone (TRH), which is exaggerated in primary hypothyroidism, is normal in liver disease,[38, 193] although TSH clearance may be impaired.

Evidence for hypothyroidism in liver disease is therefore inconclusive and there is no indication for thyroid replacement therapy in those subjects with low circulating T_3 levels if clinical criteria suggest they are euthyroid.

Chronic active hepatitis

Chronic active hepatitis should be considered separately from other forms of liver disturbance in that the incidence of autoimmune thyroid disease is much increased.[57, 219] Thyroid function may be normal, increased or decreased.[199, 247] Primary biliary cirrhosis is also associated with an increased incidence of autoimmune thyroiditis.[58, 220]

Calcium Metabolism

Bone changes in liver disease

Bone thinning and spontaneous fractures occur in patients with chronic cholestatic[11] and alcoholic liver disease,[137] and may result from osteomalacia, osteoporosis or both. Symptomatic bone disease is rare in non-alcoholic, chronic hepatocellular disease.[180] Osteoporosis has long been considered the most common abnormality but recent evidence suggests that osteomalacia may also frequently occur. Thus 75 per cent of a group of patients with primary biliary cirrhosis had histological evidence of osteomalacia and 45 per cent showed evidence of osteoporosis.[137] Alcoholic liver disease may be associated with osteomalacia as well as with osteoporosis.

The high incidence of bone changes, particularly osteomalacia, in recent studies reflects improvement in diagnostic methods. Radiological techniques such as proton absorption bone densitometry are not sufficiently sensitive to distinguish between osteoporosis and osteomalacia; nor is measurement of blood calcium, phosphate and alkaline phosphatase concentration.[137] Bone histology on non-decalcified sections is necessary, preferably with kinetic studies using time-spaced tetracycline markers.[81]

Pathogenesis

Parathyroid hormone. The aetiology of bone changes is multifactorial. The liver appears to be an important organ for metabolism of parathormone[65] in the isolated perfused rat liver but parathormone may be metabolized to products that are biologically active.[30] The importance of this in vivo in man is uncertain, as are the consequences of liver disease on parathormone metabolism. Hypophosphataemia is a frequent finding in hepatic disease but, despite this, immunoassayable parathormone levels are normal and radiological osteitis fibrosa has not been reported. It is therefore unlikely that a major disturbance of parathyroid gland function or parathormone effect is operative in production of bone changes.

Calcium and vitamin D. Many alcoholics have diets low in protein, calcium and most vitamins,[129] and patients with cryptogenic cirrhosis and chronic active hepatitis may be deficient in vitamins A and E and carotene.[161] In addition, calcium malabsorption has been demonstrated in primary biliary cirrhosis and in hepatocellular disease.[2, 117, 270] An increase in non-absorbed gut fat, secondary to diminished bile salt secretion, may allow formation of insoluble calcium soaps in the gut lumen.[270]

Calcium absorption may be further decreased by malabsorption of fat-soluble vitamin D (D_3). Vitamin D given parenterally will correct the defect in calcium absorption but large doses may be necessary, suggesting some resistance to its action. In order to exert its physiological effects, D_3 is hydroxylated in the liver to 25(OH) D_3 and subsequently in the kidney to 1,25(OH) D_3.[79, 196] Blood concentrations of 25(OH) D_3 are decreased in 40 to 50 per cent of patients with a variety of liver diseases.[136, 195] It is therefore possible that resistance to vitamin D action even when given parenterally may result from impaired hydroxylation by the diseased liver.[113] Recent studies in a group of patients with alcoholic cirrhosis, however, suggest that any defect in 25-hydroxylation is mild and insufficient in itself to explain the low plasma 25(OH) D_3 levels found.[138, 195]

A further factor may be interference with the enterohepatic circulation of 25(OH) D_3; one-third of an intravenous dose of 25(OH) D_3 appears in the duodenum over a 24-hour period and, of this, one-quarter is subsequently reabsorbed in the terminal ileum.[9] Malabsorption of enterically secreted 25(OH) D_3[42] may contribute to the lowering of plasma levels in liver disease.

Treatment of bone pathology

Recent studies in a group of subjects with primary biliary cirrhosis suggest that vitamin D given parenterally in large doses (100 000 units monthly for six to 72 months) may produce circulating 25(OH) D_3 concentrations in the normal range.[229] Preliminary evidence suggests that histological osteomalacia may also be reversed by such treatment.[43] In view of such results, expensive synthetic vitamin D analogues such as 1(OH) D_3 and 25(OH) D_3 may not be necessary in those patients requiring treatment. These potent analogues may, however, be of value in patients taking cholestyramine, which interferes with the enterohepatic circulation of 25(OH) D_3, or hepatic microsomal enzyme inducers, e.g. phenobarbitone or spironolactone, which increase vitamin D degradation to inactive products.[42, 203] It seems reasonable, in addition, to provide extra dietary calcium with oral supplements.

Sex Hormones

Male patients with cirrhosis of varied aetiology become feminized and females become masculinized, but only changes in male cirrhotics have been extensively studied.

Normal physiology

Testosterone is the principal androgen secreted by testicular Leydig cells in normal man and requires conversion to a more potent metabolite, dihydrotestosterone, for full effect. Dihydrotestosterone formation can occur both in the circulation and peripheral target tissues. Testosterone has a high affinity for a carrier protein in blood, sex-hormone binding globulin (SHBG), and androgenic activity is believed to be related only to the unbound (free) testosterone concentration. It is degraded particularly in the liver and conjugated with sulphates or glucuronic acid to be excreted in the urine as 17-oxosteroids. Testosterone production is stimulated by interstitial cell-stimulating hormone (ICSH) which is probably the same as luteinizing hormone (LH) in the female, and testosterone exerts negative feedback on ICSH secretion.

The other principal function of the testis is spermatogenesis and spermatogenic activity is closely related to plasma follicle-stimulating hormone (FSH) concentration. It is likely that seminiferous tubules secrete a hormone, inhibin, which is responsible for negative feedback control of FSH secretion. Testosterone is also necessary for normal spermatogenesis and it is likely that the close apposition of the Leydig cells to the tubules may allow high concentrations of androgens to reach the developing spermatogonia.

Primary testicular disease producing androgen deficiency is associated with elevated plasma LH concentrations and, if spermatogenesis is decreased, plasma FSH levels are raised. In hypothalamic–pituitary disease plasma gonadotrophin levels are low. Response to intravenous luteinizing-hormone-releasing hormone (LRH) administration is exaggerated in primary testicular disease and response is diminished, or peak LH and FSH levels delayed, in disease of the pituitary or hypothalamus.

The principal biologically-active naturally occurring oestrogen is oestradiol, with oestrone and oestriol relatively much less potent. Small amounts of oestrogens are produced by the testes and, to a lesser extent, adrenals, in normal man and a further small proportion is derived from peripheral conversion of testosterone. Control of oestrogen secretion and testosterone–oestradiol interconversion in normal man is poorly understood. Oestradiol in blood is bound to SHBG but affinity for SHBG is much lower than that of testosterone. Oestrogens are metabolized largely by the liver, conjugated with glucuronic or sulphuric acid and excreted in bile and urine.

Liver disease

Clinical features. The association of cirrhosis and gynaecomastia was first described in 1835 (Koechling)[123] and documented by Corda[45] and Silvestrini[227] who added testicular atrophy to the pathological complex. Most (80 per cent) cirrhotic males are impotent[13] and seminal fluid may be grossly abnormal in the remainder.[164, 260] More than 50 per cent of cirrhotic men have clinical[13, 135, 197] and histological[17] evidence of testicular atrophy, in particular atrophy of the germinal epithelium with interstitial fibrosis and thickening of the tubular lamina propria. Testicular atrophy is said to be more common in alcoholic than in other forms of cirrhosis,[13, 197] although this is disputed.[258] Secondary sexual characteristics are also diminished with decreased body[13, 64] and facial hair.[260] Benign prostatic hypertrophy occurs less frequently and is delayed in cirrhotic subjects.[17, 239]

Gynaecomastia occurs in 40 per cent of cirrhotic men,[13, 83, 135, 197, 240] and also in young men with active chronic hepatitis. It may be unilateral or bilateral and results from true glandular hyperplasia. It is said to occur more commonly in alcoholic cirrhosis than in other forms of liver disease,[13, 83, 240] although not all studies have found this.[164, 197]

Vascular spider naevi are often considered a consequence of feminization as they occur in normal women with increased frequency in the second to fifth month of pregnancy. However, they frequently occur in normal subjects, especially children, and occasionally in rheumatoid disease. In addition, they are not commonly observed in male patients with prostatic carcinoma given high therapeutic doses of oestrogen. In subjects with liver disease, vascular spider naevi appear and regress with no clinical or biochemical evidence of other endocrine change.[13] It is therefore unlikely that the pathogenesis of vascular naevi in liver disease is related solely to abnormal sex hormone metabolism.

Hormonal changes

Testosterone. Total plasma testosterone concentration is decreased in cirrhotic subjects[13, 37, 46, 119, 121] and the production rate of testosterone is only one-quarter that found in normal subjects.[87, 100] In addition, 15 per cent of circulating testosterone in cirrhotic men is derived not from the testes but from peripheral conversion of androstenedione of adrenal origin.[87] Testosterone output by testes of cirrhotic patients is therefore markedly decreased. Most circulating testosterone is bound to a globulin, sex-hormone-binding globulin (SHBG), and only the small proportion in the free form is biologically active. SHBG concentration is increased in cirrhosis[205, 206, 263] and, as testosterone has a high affinity for SHBG, free testosterone levels are decreased more than would be suggested by total plasma testosterone measurement.

Oestrogens. *Oestradiol* is the most active of the biologically occurring oestrogens. There is little agreement between different studies on total plasma oestradiol concentrations in cirrhotic patients. They have been reported as normal,[83, 85, 92, 258, 260] mildly raised,[13, 125, 182] or markedly increased.[33, 37, 173] Oestradiol, like testosterone, is bound in plasma to SHBG but similarly disparate results have been found when measuring unbound plasma oestradiol as with the total hormone measurements.[13, 37, 83, 92] There are, however, major technical problems in measuring the free hormone concentration and steady-state gel-filtration may be the only accurate method of measurement of non-protein bound oestradiol. Both studies using this technique found normal plasma-free oestradiol concentrations.[83, 92] In addition, metabolic clearance rate of oestradiol is normal in cirrhotic subjects and production rate has been found normal[13] or increased.[173] Variations in total oestradiol concentrations may thus reflect changes in binding protein and not be clinically significant.

Oestrone is a biological precursor of oestradiol but has only one-twelfth the feminizing potency.[98] Plasma oestrone concentrations are raised in cirrhotic patients,[33, 92, 173, 182] as is oestrone production rate.[60, 245]

Oestriol, which is also biologically relatively inactive, is present in raised concentrations in plasma in cirrhotic patients.[92, 182]

The low feminizing potency of oestrone and oestriol makes the pathophysiological significance of these findings doubtful. Oestradiol, which is biologically active, is certainly metabolized by the liver[3, 4] but the Edmondson hypothesis[61] that feminization in liver disease results from diminished oestrogen metabolism is now untenable. Increased peripheral conversion of testosterone to oestradiol occurs in liver disease[13, 246, 262] but as plasma testosterone and testosterone production rate is decreased the quantitative importance of this is unclear.

The pathogenesis of feminization must therefore remain uncertain, although the possibility that masculinization/feminization is related more to the androgen: oestrogen ratio than absolute concentration of either hormone group has not been fully explored.

It is worth adding that, in some cirrhotics, therapy with spironolactone may be a cause of gynaecomastia,[39] as indeed it is in patients with normal liver function.

Gonadotrophins. Studies of urinary gonadotrophin secretion determined by bioassay in male cirrhotic subjects have shown low,[56, 188] normal,[135] or elevated values.[207] Unfortunately, radio-immunoassay of plasma gonadotrophins has shown equally variable results.[13, 37, 83, 85, 119, 164, 260] The largest recent multicentre study[13] showed normal plasma-luteinizing hormone (LH) levels in 64 to 73 per cent of 117 male subjects, elevated levels in 16 to 32 per cent and decreased in 4 to 11 per cent. Follicle-stimulating hormone (FSH) levels were normal in 82 per cent, elevated in 9 to 10 per cent and decreased in 8 to 9 per cent. Almost all subjects with low LH and FSH levels were severely ill with liver failure or alcoholic hepatitis. Thus, in compensated liver cirrhosis, the majority of patients have normal basal gonadotrophin levels.

Decreased plasma testosterone levels, despite normal plasma LH concentrations, suggest primary testicular failure and the Baker study[13] showed an inverse correlation between plasma LH and testosterone levels. LH response to luteinizing-hormone-releasing hormone (LRH) is exaggerated in primary testicular failure and in cirrhotic subjects with compensated disease LH response to LRH has been reported as normal or exaggerated.[13, 55, 164] Interpretation is hampered, however, by delayed clearance of LH in liver disease. Testosterone response to exogenous human chorionic gonadotrophin (which has predominant LH activity) is diminished,[13] which also favours the presence of a primary testicular defect.

However, in the presence of a normal hypothalamus and pituitary, primary testicular failure in other conditions is associated with elevated LH concentrations. Normal LH levels in liver disease suggest a hypothalamic–pituitary defect. Against this are the LH response obtained to LRH, which should be diminished or peak LH value delayed, in hypothalamic–pituitary disease, and the finding of a normal LH response to clomiphene in patients with compensated cirrhosis. Only in patients with uncompensated disease are LH and FSH levels low, and response to LRH and clomiphene diminished.[13, 260]

Thus, evidence for a primary testicular defect in testosterone secretion is strong but there is probably, in addition, a defect in hypothalamic–pituitary control of gonadotrophin secretion, particularly in severely ill patients.

Prolactin. The role of prolactin secretion in production of gynaecomastia and hypogonadism is uncertain. Hyperplasia and hypertrophy of lactotrophs have been described post-mortem in the anterior pituitary of patients with hepatic cirrhosis.[62] Serum prolactin levels have been reported as normal[91, 177, 254] or increased;[261, 277] serum prolactin response to intravenous thyrotrophin-releasing hormone has also been reported as normal[91] or increased.[177, 277] An extensive recent study of 150 patients with a variety of liver diseases showed 12 per cent to have serum prolactin levels above the reference range.[162] Prolactin levels did not correlate with severity of liver disease, or presence of gynaecomastia. Aetiology of liver disease also had no relation to prolactin levels, although Wernze and Schmitz[268] found hyperprolactinaemia in more than 50 per cent of patients with cirrhosis of alcoholic origin.

The mechanism of hyperprolactinaemia in subjects with liver disease is uncertain. Prolactin levels do rise in response to an increase in circulating oestrogen concentrations,[272, 276] but alterations in oestrogen metabolism in liver disease are complex. Alcohol may have a direct effect on prolactin secretion[258] although this is disputed.[251] Irrespective of the mechanism, the lack of correlation with gynaecomastia in male subjects and the absence of galactorrhoea in cirrhotics strongly suggest that prolactin is not of major importance in feminization of male patients.

In summary, there are multiple abnormalities of sex hormones in liver disease, particularly cirrhosis. There is, however, still much disagreement on the extent, nature and aetiology of these changes. Similarly, there is no clear explanation for the clinically common feminization syndrome.

HAEMOCHROMATOSIS

Haemochromatosis is considered separately because endocrine abnormalities occur so frequently.

Diabetes Mellitus

Incidence

Diabetes mellitus occurs in 40 to 50 per cent of subjects with idiopathic haemochromatosis, depending on criteria for diagnosis of both diabetes and haemochromatosis.[16, 59, 171, 218, 237] Of these, 70 per cent ultimately require insulin.[171]

Aetiology

Pancreatic iron content is increased 50- to 100-fold in idiopathic haemochromatosis.[72] Generalized pancreatic fibrosis occurs and the characteristic islet abnormalities are pigmentation, decreased number or absence, and fibrosis.[218] Pigmentation affects only B cells, A cells being normal.[152]

It is uncertain if diabetes is the direct result of excessive iron deposition but the occasional improvement of diabetes with venesection favours this idea. Genetic factors are certainly important; diabetes was found in first-degree relatives of 25 per cent of patients with idiopathic haemochromatosis and diabetes but in first-degree relatives of only 4 per cent of subjects with haemochromatosis without diabetes.[59]

Thus, in addition to the presence of raised serum iron levels or frank haemochromatosis in close relatives, the predisposition to diabetes appears genetically determined. Diabetes is also infrequent in haemochromatotic subjects without frank cirrhosis[237] although this may reflect only the severity of the disease at the time of study. Cirrhosis itself may contribute to the glucose intolerance observed but is unlikely to be a major factor in production of fasting hyperglycaemia and the full syndrome of diabetes mellitus (see Chapter 3).

Insulin secretion and action

The direct cause of diabetes in idiopathic haemochromatosis is deficient insulin secretion. After intravenous glucose, insulin is promptly released but release is not sustained.[237] The average insulin requirement of insulin-dependent subjects is 50 units per day[171] but some patients exhibit remarkable resistance to the effects of exogenous insulin, with daily insulin requirements of up to 4640 units of bovine insulin per day.[59] The mechanism of this resistance is uncertain. Basal glucagon levels are increased in diabetics with haemochromatosis, as is the glucagon response to intravenous arginine,[178] but glucagon levels are similar to those found in idiopathic diabetes.

The effect of venesection on glucose tolerance is variable and is probably dependent on the severity and reversibility of pancreatic damage at the time of treatment. In one major study[59] 20 of 49 patients showed a decrease in insulin requirements and four subjects were able to remain off insulin completely. Other studies have shown results which are much less impressive.

Complications of diabetes

Complications of diabetes occur with the same frequency as in subjects with essential diabetes mellitus. These complications are not seen in haemochromatotic subjects if diabetes is absent. Of 72 patients with haemochromatosis and diabetes, 22 per cent had evidence of nephropathy, neuropathy or peripheral vascular disease.[59] The incidence of retinopathy is also similar to that in essential diabetes.[178]

Fat atrophy with bovine insulin injections occurs more commonly in haemochromatotic subjects than in those with essential diabetes, particularly in male subjects.[59] Again, the mechanism is obscure.

Hypothalamic–Pituitary Function

Hypogonadism

Since the early descriptions of the disease, hypogonadism has been recognized as a feature and subsequent reports suggest that it occurs in 50 to 80 per cent of subjects.[228, 235, 236] Sexual function is decreased in association with testicular atrophy and a decrease in body hair.

Despite earlier reports,[72] there appears to be little correlation with the severity of liver disease. Excessive iron deposition occurs in the pituitary[218] and hypogonadism has been postulated to result from decreased gonadotrophin secretion. Studies so far, however, have produced conflicting results. Stocks and Powell[236] found that 14 of 32 patients showed decreased plasma LH levels and Walsh and colleagues[266] found a decreased LH and FSH response to LRH in two of 12 patients who also had low plasma testosterone levels. Similarly decreased basal gonadotrophin values have been found by other workers,[118, 252] but Simon and colleagues[228] found that basal gonadotrophin levels were normal or elevated in 31 patients and concluded that there was a primary testicular defect. Excess testicular iron deposition has been demonstrated histologically although the effect on testicular function is uncertain.

It is likely that hypogonadism in haemochromatosis is multifactorial in origin. Some patients have deficient secretion of other pituitary hormones in addition to gonadotrophins, and pituitary disease is likely to be of importance. In subjects with raised gonadotrophin levels, primary testicular disease seems likely. Other influences may be severity of cirrhosis, alcohol intake and autonomic neuropathy secondary to diabetes mellitus.

Other aspects of hypothalamic–pituitary function

Other aspects of hypothalamic pituitary function may also be abnormal. Decreased growth hormone response to insulin hypoglycaemia and arginine infusion has been shown in occasional patients.[235, 236] A diminished cortisol response to insulin hypoglycaemia and TSH response to TRH has also been described.

Other Endocrine Glands

Haemosiderin deposits are found in other endocrine glands, e.g. adrenals, thyroid and parathyroids.[190] No specific abnormalities of thyroid or parathyroid function have been demonstrated. In addition, there is no evidence to link the melanin pigmentation and physical weakness often found in haemochromatosis with adrenal insufficiency.

ENDOCRINE EFFECTS OF ALCOHOL

Alcohol ingestion is of such importance in many subjects with liver disease that it is worthy of separate comment. The endocrine effects of alcohol are multiple and the subject has been recently reviewed.[86, 273] Only those effects which are of clinical importance will be discussed.

In assessment of clinical studies of endocrine effects of alcohol, it is important to note the exact experimental conditions and type of subject studied. Thus effects of acute alcohol administration differ considerably from those seen with chronic ingestion; endocrine changes in the habituated may be very different from those seen in alcohol-naive subjects; the effects of alcohol in chronic alcohol abusers must be separated from less specific effects of liver damage.

Adrenocortical Function

Alcohol consumed in moderate doses by normal subjects has little effect on cortisol secretion;[106] only in the presence of intoxication and usually with blood ethanol levels in excess of 217 mmol/l (100 mg/dl) is a rise in plasma cortisol observed.[156, 160] This is probably a non-specific stress effect mediated via the hypothalamic–pituitary–adrenal axis.[106] Alcoholic subjects with tolerance to the intoxicating effects of alcohol may not show a rise in adrenocortical secretion despite blood alcohol levels in excess of 217 mmol/l (100 mg/dl).[160]

Many of the clinical features of chronic alcohol abuse resemble those of Cushing's syndrome, e.g. body habitus, florid complexion and thin skin.[54, 160] Chronic alcoholics have higher morning cortisol levels than normal[159] but this is abolished by alcohol or barbiturate administration, or long-term abstinence[157] and may be related to alcohol withdrawal symptoms. Occasional alcoholic patients, however, present with the clinical and biochemical features of advanced Cushing's syndrome.[77, 181, 202, 230, 231] Plasma cortisol levels are raised and may not suppress adequately with dexamethasone.[231] If alcohol is withdrawn, the biochemical features return to normal during the next two to three weeks. The mechanism for alcohol-induced pseudo-Cushing's syndrome is unknown and further studies with measurement of plasma ACTH levels are necessary. It does not appear to be related to severity of liver damage as most of the subjects described had only mild liver disturbance.

Adrenocortical insufficiency is more common than alcohol-induced pseudo-Cushing's syndrome. The cortisol response to insulin hypoglycaemia is either absent or severely attenuated in more than 25 per cent of chronic alcoholic subjects whether still drinking or recently abstinent.[34, 94, 104, 146] In none of the subjects studied did plasma cortisol rise by more than 137 nmol/l (5 μg/dl) despite adequate hypoglycaemia. The adrenal glands themselves are functionally normal with adequate fasting plasma cortisol levels,[148] cortisol secretion rate[145] and response to ACTH or tetracosactrin,[158] suggesting that the abnormality lies in the hypothalamic–pituitary–adrenal axis. The impairment was reversible in one patient who was studied after six months' abstinence from alcohol. The importance of the deficiency may lie in its role in pathogenesis of alcoholic hypoglycaemia. Similar impairments in growth hormone and prolactin secretion in response to insulin hypoglycaemia have recently been reported.[34]

Sex Hormones

Alcohol has effects on hypothalamic–pituitary and testicular function independent of liver disease, and the effects may be different in habitual drinkers from those in non-drinkers. Short-term feeding of large doses of alcohol to healthy volunteers is associated with dampening of the normal pattern of episodic bursts in testosterone secretion,[88] and the mean plasma testosterone concentration falls after five days. The effect of alcohol in decreasing testosterone production by the testes has been postulated as secondary to an increase in testicular NADH : NAD+ ratio resulting in decreased activity of NAD-dependent enzyme systems involved in steroidogenesis.[258] There may also be competitive inhibition of the alcohol dehydrogenase-dependent conversion of retinol to retinal, the latter being essential for normal spermatogenesis.[259] A decrease in testosterone production rate is already evident after 24 hours.[86] Alcohol may also increase the metabolic clearance of testosterone but in short-term experiments in normal subjects has no effect on peripheral conversion to androstenedione, oestrone or oestradiol. Despite alterations in testosterone secretion, no consistent changes in plasma LH or FSH are observed in normal subjects.

In chronic alcoholics, alcohol ingestion is also associated with a decrease in plasma testosterone levels [134, 155] with a possible rebound in the post-drinking period. Wright and colleagues[274] found basal plasma LH values to be raised in six of 13 actively drinking male alcoholics and these cases showed an exaggerated LH response to LH-releasing hormone. Plasma total 17-hydroxyandrogens were normal in these subjects and showed no correlation with LH values.

Thus the effects of alcohol on sex hormone metabolism are complex and very much dependent on previous ethanol ingestion. It is not surprising therefore that sex hormone studies in subjects with alcoholic liver disease have shown such disparate results (see above).

Alcohol-related Fasting Hypoglycaemia

Hypoglycaemia may occur in severe liver disease, particularly fulminant hepatic failure (see Chapter 3). However, it may also occur in association with alcohol use and abuse in the presence of a normal liver or relatively mild liver dysfunction.

Such patients present with a blood glucose concentration usually 1.5 mmol/l (27 mg/dl) or less.[147] Patients may be children, but are typically chronic alcoholics with a history of ingestion of moderate to large amounts of alcohol six to 36 hours before admission, and are usually malnourished.[141] They may be stuporose or comatose, usually smell of alcohol, and are often hypothermic. Diagnosis is established on the clinical findings, hypoglycaemia and the blood alcohol level (usually less than 21.7 mmol/l [100 mg/l]). Lactic acidosis is not uncommon. Treatment consists of administration of intravenous glucose and hydrocortisone but mortality of 10 to 20 per cent, in spite of glucose therapy, has been reported.[141] It is possible that hypoglycaemia may be a cause of the sudden deaths known to occur in alcoholics.[127]

The mechanism is probably multifactorial. A major factor is likely to be inhibition of gluconeogenesis by alcohol.[70, 80, 125] Plasma insulin levels are low and glucagon levels high,[108, 176, 248] although a recent report with measurement of plasma insulin and C-peptide concentrations[109] suggests that insulin secretion may still be inappropriately high for the blood glucose levels. Growth hormone and cortisol levels are raised but less than might be anticipated in view of the severity of the hypoglycaemia.[8, 108] The importance of the abnormality in the hypothalamic–pituitary–adrenal axis in more than 25 per cent of chronic alcoholics (see above) is suggested by evidence that adrenocortical insufficiency predisposes to development of alcohol-induced hypoglycaemia in experimental situations.[8] A defect in growth hormone secretion to insulin hypoglycaemia[7, 34] may also be of importance.

Alcohol may also be important in the potentiation of drug-induced hypoglycaemia, particularly secondary to insulin,[147] and may induce reactive hypoglycaemia when given with glucose.[172] There is slender evidence that chronic alcoholics may demonstrate reactive hypoglycaemia more than controls.[40, 66, 147, 249, 250]

Alcoholic Ketoacidosis

This uncommon condition occurs in non-diabetic alcoholic patients who almost always have abnormal liver function tests.[45, 107, 132, 198] Females are affected more than males and there is a history of heavy chronic alcohol intake preceded by a drinking 'binge' two to three days before presentation. There is a history of abdominal pain, vomiting and lack of solid food and on examination patients are conscious but tachypnoeic, not grossly salt and water depleted, and usually have diffuse epigastric tenderness. Blood glucose estimation is normal and in one series of six subjects[45] mean arterial pH was 7.25 with an anion gap of 18. Plasma phosphate level may be low and accompanied by red cell haemolysis.[244] Blood ketone body and non-esterified fatty acid concentrations are high. However, testing plasma or urine with a standard nitroprusside reagent (Acetest or Ketostix [Ames]) may reveal mild ketosis only, as 3-hydroxybutyrate is elevated considerably more than acetoacetate and acetone, and 3-hydroxybutyrate is not measured by this method. The principal differential diagnosis is from lactic acidosis, which also occurs in alcoholic liver disease (see Chapter 3) and direct measurement of blood ketone body and lactate concentrations are necessary. Treatment with intravenous glucose, saline and small amounts of sodium bicarbonate lead to prompt recovery.

The mechanism of production of alcoholic ketosis is uncertain. Serum insulin concentrations are low, cortisol markedly increased and growth hormone levels mildly raised.[45]

A ketogenic effect of cortisol in insulin-deficient man has recently been demonstrated[5, 211] and this, combined with increased catecholamine release, may be of importance. It is also possible that there may be direct conversion of alcohol to ketone bodies through acetate. Recent studies in our own laboratory have shown a rise in ketone body concentration within 10 minutes of ingestion of a meal with alcohol, i.e. at a time when fatty acid delivery to the liver was decreased and insulin levels were raised. (J.L. Selam, G.A. Noy and K.G.M.M. Alberti, unpublished observations.) Acetate infusion also causes a rise in ketone body levels. The absolute contribution of this route remains to be established. Finally, fatty acid oxidation may be decreased secondary to the increase in NADH:NAD+ ratio as a result of alcohol oxidation.[73]

HEPATIC DISTURBANCE IN ENDOCRINE DISEASE

Diabetes Mellitus

Hepatotrophic effect of insulin

There is considerable experimental evidence that insulin and possibly other hormones are necessary for maintenance of normal hepatic architecture and for regeneration after injury.

The so-called hepatotrophic effects of substances in the portal blood have been noted under several experimental conditions to include hypertrophy, hyperplasia, glycogen storage and increase of several other synthetic functions. In vitro work has suggested that insulin may have an important role in maintenance of hepatocyte integrity.[130] Extensive in vivo work in dogs by Starzl and colleagues[234] has elaborated on these findings. Experiments in which portal blood was directed at one part of the liver and systemic blood at another have shown the importance of the portal blood in maintenance of normal liver architecture and in the normal regenerative response to injury. The more recent studies by these workers suggest that insulin is the major factor involved although glucagon secretion and the insulin:glucagon ratio may also be of importance.[24, 25] The role of other pancreatic and the numerous gut hormones is at present uncertain.

The liver in diabetes mellitus

The liver in normal man is exposed to much higher insulin concentrations in the portal blood than are found in the systemic circulation.[18] If this is important in maintaining liver structure, it is to be expected that insulin-treated diabetic subjects show a high incidence of hepatic abnormality in that insulin is given systemically rather than portally. Structural abnormalities may even be expected in maturity onset diabetes in which insulin and glucagon are still secreted, as there is a change in their relative proportions, with glucagon preponderant.[255]

Fatty liver

Many pathological changes have been reported in diabetic livers but most are acutely reversible phenomena such as the hepatic enlargement seen in ketoacidosis. Excessive glycogen deposition has been reported[19] but the most consistent change is that of fatty infiltration.

Creutzfeldt, Frerichs and Sickinger[49] in their classic review of 1759 biopsies from different centres reported fatty changes in from 21 to 78 per cent of diabetics. The incidence is lower in juvenile-onset diabetics (25 per cent) than in maturity-onset cases (63 per cent).[96] This difference probably results from the increased number of obese patients in the maturity-onset series. Patients selected for biopsy may also not be representative of diabetics as a whole, as biopsy was performed for a clinical reason such as hepatomegaly or abnormality of liver function. Autopsy studies are also unrepresentative as patients have died from diverse causes and the metabolic status is uncertain, but such studies have shown the incidence of fatty liver to be lower, at 20 to 30 per cent, compared with 15 to 25 per cent in the non-diabetic population.

Fatty change is therefore not specific to diabetes and there is no evidence to suggest a progression to more severe liver damage.[128] In addition, its frequency is lowest in juvenile-onset diabetes, suggesting that insulin lack may not be a major factor in its pathogenesis.

Hepatic cirrhosis

Intolerance to oral or intravenous glucose is a common finding in subjects with liver disease.[110] However, this differs from essential diabetes in that it is usually mild and not associated with fasting hyperglycaemia, and peripheral insulin concentrations are raised. It is therefore vital to distinguish between the glucose intolerance of cirrhosis and the occurrence of cirrhosis in subjects with essential diabetes. Many previous studies have failed to make this distinction.

Standard liver function tests in well-controlled diabetes reveal little difference from the normal population. However, in a review of published autopsy reports, the frequency of cirrhosis in diabetics ranged from 5.7 to 21.4 per cent compared with 2.3 to 13.4 per cent in non-diabetics. In two of the series reported, figures were the same in diabetics and non-diabetics while in four there was a clear preponderance of cirrhosis in diabetic subjects. In the two best clinical studies[48, 167] in the literature, a higher incidence of cirrhosis was found in diabetics (3.7 and 9.2 per cent in diabetics, 1.2 and 1.8 per cent in normals). Even in these studies, however, criteria for distinction between the glucose intolerance of cirrhosis and essential diabetes are questionable and in only 40 per cent of the subjects with both diabetes and cirrhosis was the diabetes diagnosed first.

Evidence for an increased overall incidence of cirrhosis in diabetes is therefore tenuous. There is, nevertheless, a higher incidence of post-necrotic cirrhosis in diabetic subjects,[140] presumably due to the higher incidence of viral hepatitis (type B). Seige and Theirbach[213] have shown that cirrhosis follows viral hepatitis more frequently in diabetics than in non-diabetics. Normal pancreatic secretion may therefore be of importance in the response to viral infection or other liver injury but there is little evidence in man that pancreatic hyposecretion in diabetes leads to a serious loss of hepatic structural integrity in the absence of a further liver insult.

Hyperthyroidism

Histological changes

Many changes in liver histology have been reported in hyperthyroidism, e.g. decreased glycogen content, fatty change, focal necrosis, diffuse or centrilobular necrosis, simple atrophy, nodule formation and cirrhosis with lymphoid infiltration,[15, 27, 189, 216, 267] but most of these findings probably result from cardiac failure or severe weight loss and are not specific to hyperthyroidism. In recent studies of patients with milder disease diagnosed at an earlier stage, histological changes have been unimpressive; in particular severe centrilobular necrosis and cirrhosis are not seen.[10, 183]

Changes in hepatic ultrastructure have been reported in experimental hyperthyroidism, in particular increased size and number of mitochondria with increased cristae formation per mitochondrion.[122] These changes, however, are not specific and are seen after administration of ethanol and other substances.

Chronic active hepatitis[247] and sclerosis of the biliary tree[14, 120] occur more frequently in thyroid disease than would be expected by chance.

Liver function

Despite an increase in cardiac output, hepatic blood flow is not increased in hyperthyroidism.[168] Hepatic oxygen consumption is, however, increased so that hepatocytes extract more oxygen from the blood supplied. Centrizonal areas, which receive their blood supply last, may therefore suffer from diminished oxygen supply and this may contribute to the centrizonal necrosis found occasionally in severely hyperthyroid subjects. There is no correlation between hepatic histology and standard tests of liver function. In a recent series of 570 patients decreased bromsulphthalein excretion was found in only 8 per cent and elevations in aspartate aminotransferase, bilirubin and alkaline phosphatase occurred less frequently.[10] Clinical jaundice is found in hyperthyroidism usually only in the presence of a complication, e.g. infection or cardiac failure, and is seen in 20 to 25 per cent of patients with thyroid crisis.[103] Jaundice in a subject with uncomplicated mild hyperthyroidism, however, should arouse suspicion of coexistent liver disease although thyrotoxicosis may aggravate an underlying defect in bilirubin metabolism such as Gilbert's disease.[93]

Hypothyroidism

Jaundice may be found in neonatal thyroid deficiency but symptoms or signs of disturbed liver function are not usually encountered in adult hypothyroidism. Serum levels of aspartate aminotransferase, lactate dehydrogenase and creatine phosphokinase may, however, be elevated and return to normal after two to four weeks' replacement therapy. These abnormalities are thought to represent altered metabolism of the enzymes rather than liver damage.[52] Exudative ascites and effusions in other body cavities may occur in hypothyroidism, unrelated to liver or cardiac pathology,[208] although centrizonal congestion and fibrosis have been reported on liver biopsy.[12]

Acromegaly

The liver is enlarged in acromegaly as part of the generalized organomegaly. Standard liver function tests are normal but bromsulphthalein excretion time may be increased.[221]

REFERENCES

1. Abrams, R.L., Grumbach, M.M. & Kaplan, S.L. (1971) The effect of intravenous administration of human growth hormone on the plasma growth hormone, cortisol, glucose and free fatty acid response to insulin: evidence for growth hormone auto-regulation in man. *Journal of Clinical Investigation,* **50,** 940–950.
2. Adjukiewicz, A.B., Agnew, J.E., Byers, P.D., Wills, M.R. & Sherlock, S. (1974) The relief of bone pain in primary biliary cirrhosis with calcium infusions. *Gut,* **15,** 788–793.
3. Adlercreutz, H. (1970) Oestrogen metabolism in liver disease. *Journal of Endocrinology,* **46,** 129–163.
4. Adlercreutz, H. (1974) Hepatic metabolism of oestrogens in health and disease. *New England Journal of Medicine,* **290,** 1081–1083.
5. Alberti, K.G.M.M. & Johnston, D.G. (1977) Cortisol and catabolism: a new perspective. *Clinical Science and Molecular Medicine,* **52,** 333–336.
6. Alberti, K.G.M.M., Record, C.O., Williamson, D.H. & Wright, R. (1972) Metabolic changes in active chronic hepatitis. *Clinical Science,* **42,** 591–605.
7. Andreani, D., Tamburrano, G. & Javicoli, M. (1976) Alcohol hypoglycaemia: hormonal changes. In *Hypoglycaemia, Proceedings of the European Symposium, Rome* (Ed.) Andreani, D., Lefebvre, P.J. & Marks, V. pp. 95–105. Stuttgart: Thieme.
8. Arky, R.A. & Freinkel, N. (1966) Alcohol hypoglycaemia. V. Alcohol infusion to test gluconeogenesis in starvation, with specific reference to obesity. *New England Journal of Medicine,* **274,** 426–433.
9. Arnauld, S.B., Goldsmith, R.S. & Lambert, P.W. (1975) 25-Hydroxyvitamin D_3: evidence of an enterohepatic circulation in man. *Proceedings of the Society for Experimental Biology and Medicine,* **149,** 570–572.
10. Ashkar, F.S., Miller, R., Smoak, W.M. & Gilson, A.J. (1971) Liver disease in hyperthyroidism. *Southern Medical Journal,* **64,** 462–465.
11. Atkinson, M., Nordin, B.E.C. & Sherlock, S. (1956) Malabsorption and bone disease in prolonged obstructive jaundice. *Quarterly Journal of Medicine,* **25,** 299–313.
12. Baker, A., Kaplan, M. & Wolfe, H. (1972) Central congestive fibrosis of the liver in myxoedema ascites. *Annals of Internal Medicine,* **77,** 927–929.
13. Baker, H.W.G., Burger, H.G., de Kretser, D.M., Dulmanis, A., Hudson, B., O'Connor, S., Paulsen, C.A., Purcell, N., Rennie, G.C., Seah, C.S., Taft, H.P. & Wang, C. (1976) A study of the endocrine manifestations of hepatic cirrhosis. *Quarterly Journal of Medicine,* **45,** 145–178.
14. Bartholomew, L.G., Cain, J.C., Woolner, L.B., Utz, D.C. & Ferris, D.O. (1963) Sclerosing cholangitis: its possible association with Riedel's struma and fibrous retroperitonitis. Report of two cases. *New England Journal of Medicine,* **269,** 8–12.
15. Beaver, D.C. & Pemberton, J. de J. (1933) The pathologic anatomy of the liver in exophthalamic goitre. *Annals of Internal Medicine,* **7,** 687–708.
16. Becker, D. & Miller, M. (1960) Presence of diabetic glomerulosclerosis in patients with haemochromatosis. *New England Journal of Medicine,* **263,** 367–373.
17. Bennett, H.S., Baggenstoss, A.H. & Butt, H.R. (1950) The testis, breast and prostate of men who die of cirrhosis of the liver. *American Journal of Clinical Pathology,* **20,** 814–828.
18. Blackard, W.G. & Nelson, N.C. (1970) Portal and peripheral vein immunoreactive insulin concentrations before and after glucose infusion. *Diabetes,* **19,** 302–306.
19. Bogoch, A., Casselman, W.G.B., Kaplan, A. & Bockus, H.L. (1955) Studies of hepatic function in diabetes mellitus, portal cirrhosis and other liver diseases; correlation of clinical, biochemical and liver needle biopsy findings. *American Journal of Medicine,* **18,** 354–384.
20. Braverman, L.E., Vagenakis, A., Downs, P., Foster, A.E., Sterling, K. & Ingbar, S.H. (1973) Effects of replacement doses of sodium L-thyroxine on the peripheral metabolism of thyroxine and triiodothyronine in man. *Journal of Clinical Investigation,* **52,** 1010–1017.
21. Brown, H., Willardson, D.G., Samuels, L.T. & Tyler, F.H. (1954) 17-Hydroxycorticosteroid metabolism in liver disease. *Journal of Clinical Investigation,* **33,** 1524–1532.
22. Brown, J., Chopra, J.J., Cornell, J.S., Hershman, J.M., Solomon, D.H., Uller, R.P. & Van Herle, A.J. (1974) Thyroid physiology in health and disease. *Annals of Internal Medicine,* **81,** 68–81.
23. Buchannan, K., Solomon, S., Vance, J., Porter, H. & Williams, R.H. (1968) Glucagon clearance by the isolated perfused rat liver. *Proceedings of the Society for Experimental Biology and Medicine,* **128,** 620–623.
24. Bucher, N.L.R. & Swaffield, M.N. (1975) Regulation of hepatic regeneration in rats by synergistic action of insulin and glucagon. *Proceedings of the National Academy of Sciences of the United States of America,* **72,** 1157–1160.
25. Bucher, N.L.R. & Weir, G.C. (1976) Insulin, glucagon, liver regeneration, and DNA synthesis. *Metabolism,* **25** (Suppl. 1), 1423–1425.
26. Burger, A., Nicod, P., Suter, P., Vallotton, M.D., Vagenakis, A. & Braverman, L. (1976) Reduced active thyroid hormone levels in acute illness. *Lancet,* **i,** 653–655.
27. Cameron, G.R. & Karunaratne, W. (1935) Liver changes in exophthalamic goitre. *Journal of Pathology,* **41,** 267–282.
28. Cameron, D.P., Burger, H.G., Catt, K.J., Gordon, E. & McWatts, J. (1972) Metabolic clearance of human growth hormone in patients with hepatic and renal failure and in the isolated perfused pig liver. *Metabolism,* **21,** 895–904.
29. Camu, F. (1975) Hepatic balances of glucose and insulin in response to physiological increments of endogenous insulin during glucose infusions in dogs. *European Journal of Clinical Investigation,* **5,** 101–108.
30. Canterbury, J.M., Bricker, L.A., Levey, G.S., Kozlovskis, P.L., Rviz, E., Zull, J.E. & Reiss, E. (1975) Metabolism of bovine parathyroid hormone.

Immunological and biological characteristics of fragments generated by liver perfusion. *Journal of Clinical Investigation,* **55,** 1245–1253.

31. Carter, J.N., Eastman, C.J., Corcoran, J.M. & Lazarus, L. (1974) Effect of severe chronic illness on thyroid function. *Lancet,* **ii,** 971–974.
32. Cavalieri, R.R. & Rapoport, B. (1977) Impaired peripheral conversion of thyroxine to triiodothyronine. *Annual Review of Medicine,* **28,** 57–65.
33. Cedard, L., Mosse, A. & Klotz, H.P. (1970) Les oestrogènes plasmatiques dans les gynécomasties et les hépatopathies. *Annales d'Endocrinologie,* **31,** 453–458.
34. Chalmers, R.J., Bennie, E.H., Johnson, R.H. & Masterton, G. (1978) Growth hormone, prolactin and corticosteroid responses to insulin hypoglycaemia in alcoholics. *British Medical Journal,* **i,** 745–748.
35. Chopra, I.J. (1976) An assessment of daily turnover and significance of thyroidal secretion of 3,3′,5′-triiodothyronine (reverse T_3) in man. *Journal of Clinical Investigation,* **58,** 32–40.
36. Chopra, I.J. (1978) Nature, source and biological significance of thyroid hormones in blood. In *The Thyroid* (Ed.) Werner, S.C. & Ingbar, S.H. New York, San Francisco and London: Harper & Row.
37. Chopra, I.J., Tulchinsky, D. & Greenway, F.L. (1973) Estrogen–androgen imbalance in hepatic cirrhosis. *Annals of Internal Medicine,* **79,** 198–203.
38. Chopra, I.J., Solomon, D.H., Chopra, U., Young, R.T. & Chua Teco, G.N. (1974) Alterations in circulating thyroid hormones and thyrotropin in hepatic cirrhosis: evidence of euthyroidism despite subnormal serum triiodothyronine. *Journal of Clinical Endocrinology and Metabolism,* **39,** 501–511.
39. Clark, E. (1965) Spironolactone therapy and gynecomastia. *Journal of the American Medical Association,* **193,** 163–164.
40. Cohen, S. (1976) A review of hypoglycemia and alcoholism with or without liver disease. *Annals of the New York Academy of Sciences,* **273,** 338–342.
41. Collin, J., Taylor, R.M.R. & Johnston, I.D.A. (1977) Carbohydrate tolerance with portal and systemic venous drainage of the pancreas. *British Journal of Surgery,* **64,** 180–182.
42. Compston, J.E. & Thompson, R.P.H. (1977) Intestinal absorption of 25-hydroxyvitamin D and osteomalacia in primary biliary cirrhosis. *Lancet,* **i,** 721–724.
43. Compston, J.E., Horton, L.W.L. & Thompson, R.P.H. (1979) *Gut.* In press.
44. Conn, H.O. & Daughaday, W.H. (1970) Cirrhosis and diabetes v. serum growth hormone levels in Laennec's cirrhosis. *Journal of Laboratory and Clinical Medicine,* **76,** 678–688.
45. Cooperman, M.T., Davidoff, F., Spark, R. & Pallota, J. (1974) Clinical studies of alcoholic ketoacidosis. *Diabetes,* **23,** 433–439.
46. Coppage, W.S. & Cooner, A.E. (1965) Testosterone in human plasma. *New England Journal of Medicine,* **273,** 902–907.
47. Corda, L. (1925) Sulla c.d. reviviscenza della mammella maschile viella cirrosi epatica. *Minerva Medica,* **5,** 1067–1069.
48. Creutzfeldt, W. (1959) Morphologische Befunde an der Leber von Diabetikern nach langfristiger Sulphonylharnstoff behandlung und an verschiedenen Organen nach Synthalin und DBI-Vergiftung beim Tier. In *Diabetes Mellitus,* Proceedings of 3rd Congresse Internationale Diabetes Federation, p. 267. Stuttgart: Thieme.
49. Creutzfeldt, W., Frerichs, H. & Sickinger, K. (1970) Liver diseases and diabetes mellitus. In *Progress in Liver Diseases* (Ed.) Popper, H. & Schaffner, F. Vol. 3, pp. 380–407. New York: Grune & Stratton.
50. Cuttelod, S., Le Marchand-Beraud, T., Magnenat, P., Perret, C., Poli, S. & Vanotti, A. (1974) Effect of age and role of kidneys and liver on thyrotropin turnover in man. *Metabolism,* **23,** 101–113.
51. Davies, T.F., Prudhoe, K. & Douglas, A.P. (1976) Plasma cyclic adenosine-3′,5′-monophosphate response to glucagon in patients with liver disease. *British Medical Journal,* **i,** 931–933.
52. De Groot, L.J. & Stanbury, J.B. (1975) Adult hypothyroid states and myxoedema. In *The Thyroid and its Diseases.* pp. 405–471. New York: Wiley.
53. Desai, K.B., Ganatra, R.D. & Sharma, S.M. (1971) Thyroid uptake studies in infectious hepatitis. *Journal of Nuclear Medicine* (Suppl. 5), **12,** 828–833.
54. Dillon, R.S. (1973) *Handbook of Endocrinology.* Philadelphia: Lea & Febiger.
55. Distiller, L.A., Sagel, J., Dubowitz, B., Kay, G., Carr, P.J., Katz, M. & Kew, M.C. (1976) Pituitary–gonadal function in men with alcoholic cirrhosis of the liver. *Hormone and Metabolic Research,* **8,** 461–465.
56. Dohan, F.C., Richardson, E.M., Bluemle, L.W. & Gyorgy, P. (1952) Hormone excretion in liver disease. *Journal of Clinical Investigation,* **31,** 481–498.
57. Doniach, D., Roitt, I.M., Walker, J.G. & Sherlock, S. (1966) Tissue antibodies in primary biliary cirrhosis, active chronic (lupoid) hepatitis, cryptogenic cirrhosis and other liver diseases and their clinical implications. *Clinical and Experimental Immunology,* **1,** 237–262.
58. Doniach, D., Walker, J.G., Roitt, I.M. & Berg, P.A. (1970) Current concepts: 'autoallergic' hepatitis. *New England Journal of Medicine,* **282,** 86–89.
59. Dymock, I.W., Cassar, J., Pyke, D.A., Oakley, W.G. & Williams, R. (1972) Observations on the pathogenesis, complications and treatment of diabetes in 115 cases of haemochromatosis. *American Journal of Medicine,* **52,** 203–210.
60. Edman, C.D., MacDonald, P.C. & Combes, B. (1975) Extraglandular production of oestrogen in subjects with liver disease. *Gastroenterology,* **69,** A-19/819.
61. Edmondson, H.A., Glass, S.J. & Soll, S.N. (1939) Gynaecomastia associated with cirrhosis of the liver. *Proceedings of the Society for Experimental Biology and Medicine,* **42,** 97–99.
62. El Etreby, M.F. & Günzel, P. (1974) Sex hormones – effects on prolactin cells in the rat, dog, monkey and man. *Acta Endocrinologica* (Suppl.), **189,** 3–15.
63. Englert, E. Jr, Brown, H., Wallach, S. & Simons, L. (1957) Metabolism of free and conjugated 17-hydroxycorticosteroids in subjects with liver disease. *Journal of Clinical Endocrinology,* **17,** 1395–1406.
64. Eppingen (1925) cited in *The Vienna Convention: Diseases of metabolism and of the digestive tract* (Letter). *Journal of the American Medical Association,* **85,** 1572–1574.
65. Fang, V.S. & Tashjian, A.H. Jr (1972) Studies on the role of the liver in the metabolism of parathyroid hormone: effects of partial hepatectomy and incubation of the hormone with tissue homogenates. *Endocrinology,* **90,** 1177–1184.
66. Farmer, R.W., Farrell, G., Pellizzari, E.D. & Fabre, L.F. (1971) Serum insulin levels during oral glucose

tolerance tests in chronic alcoholics. *Federation Proceedings* (abstract), **30,** 250.

67. Felig, P. & Wahren, J. (1971) Influence of endogenous insulin secretion on splanchnic glucose and amino acid balance in man. *Journal of Clinical Investigation,* **50,** 1702–1711.
68. Felig, P., Brown, W.V., Levine, R.A. & Klatskin, G. (1970) Glucose homeostasis in viral hepatitis. *New England Journal of Medicine,* **283,** 1436–1440.
69. Felig, P., Gusberg, R., Hendler, R., Gump, F.E. & Kinney, J.M. (1974) Concentrations of glucagon and the insulin:glucagon ratio in the portal and peripheral circulation. *Proceedings of the Society for Experimental Biology and Medicine,* **147,** 88–90.
70. Field, J.B., Williams, H.E. & Mortimer, G.E. (1963) Studies on the mechanism of ethanol-induced hypoglycaemia. *Journal of Clinical Investigation,* **42,** 497–506.
71. Field, J.B., Bloom, G., Petruska, M., Broskin, K. & Chou, C. (1976) Effects of stimulation of insulin and glucagon secretion on hepatic glucose production, insulin/glucagon ratio and hepatic extraction of insulin and glucagon. *Clinical Research,* **24,** 485A.
72. Finch, S.C. & Finch, C.A. (1955) Idiopathic haemochromatosis and iron storage disease. *Medicine,* **34,** 381–430.
73. Fink, R. & Rosalki, S.B. (1978) Clinical biochemistry of alcoholism. *Clinics in Endocrinology and Metabolism,* **7,** 297–319.
74. Fischer, J.E. & Baldessarini, R.J. (1971) False neurotransmitters and hepatic failure. *Lancet,* **ii,** 75–79.
75. Fischer, M., Sherwin, R.S., Hendler, R. & Felig, P. (1976) Kinetics of glucagon in man: effects of starvation. *Proceedings of the National Academy of Sciences of the United States of America,* **73,** 1735–1739.
76. Flock, E.V., Bollman, J.L., Grindlay, J.H. & Stobie, G.H. (1961) Partial deiodination of L-thyroxine. *Endocrinology,* **69,** 626–637.
77. Frajria, R. & Angeli, A. (1977) Alcohol-induced pseudo-Cushing's syndrome. *Lancet,* **i,** 1050–1051.
78. Francavilla, A., Pansini, F., Sansone, F., Albano, O. & Martellotta, G. (1977) Effect of glucagon infusion on plasma cyclic AMP in patients with cholestatic hepatitis and obstructive jaundice. New test of hepatic cholestasis. *Clinica Chimica Acta,* **75,** 351–357.
79. Fraser, D.R. & Kodicek, E. (1970) Unique biosynthesis by kidney of a biological active vitamin D metabolite. *Nature,* **228,** 764–766.
80. Freinkel, N., Singer, D.L., Arky, R.A., Bleicher, S.J., Anderson, J.B. & Silbert, C.K. (1963) Alcohol hypoglycaemia. 1. Carbohydrate metabolism of patients with clinical alcohol hypoglycaemia and the experimental reproduction of the syndrome with pure ethanol. *Journal of Clinical Investigation,* **42,** 1112–1133.
81. Frost, H.M. (1969) Tetracycline-based histological analysis of bone remodelling. *Calcified Tissue Research,* **3,** 211–237.
82. Galton, V.A. & Nisula, B.C. (1972) The enterohepatic circulation of thyroxine. *Journal of Endocrinology,* **54,** 187–193.
83. Galvao-Teles, A., Anderson, D.C., Burke, C.W., Marshall, J.C., Corker, C.S., Brown, R.L. & Clark, M.L. (1973) Biologically active androgens and oestradiol in men with chronic liver disease. *Lancet,* **i,** 173–177.
84. Gavin, L., Castle, J., McMahon, F., Martin, P., Hammond, M. & Cavalieri, R.R. (1976) Metabolic clearance and production rates of 3,5,3′-triiodothyronine (T_3) and 3,3′,5′-T_3 (reverse T_3) in man. *Clinical Research,* **24,** 427A.
85. Geisthövel, W. & Von zur Mühlen (1975) Studies on the pituitary–testicular axis in patients with chronic hepatic failure (abstract). *Acta Endocrinologica (Copenhagen)* (Suppl.), **199,** 256.
86. Gordon, G.G. & Southren, A.L. (1977) Metabolic effects of alcohol on the endocrine system. In *Metabolic Aspects of Alcohol* (Ed.) Lieber, C.S. Lancaster: Medical and Technical Press.
87. Gordon, G.G., Olivo, J., Rafii, F. & Southren, A.L. (1975) Conversion of androgens to estrogens in cirrhosis of the liver. *Journal of Clinical Endocrinology and Metabolism,* **40,** 1018–1026.
88. Gordon, G.G., Altman, K., Southren, A.L., Rubin, E. & Lieber, C.S. (1976) Effect of alcohol administration on sex-hormone metabolism in normal men. *New England Journal of Medicine,* **295,** 793–797.
89. Greco, A.V., Fedeli, G., Ghirlanda, G., Manna, R. & Patrono, C. (1974) Behaviour of pancreatic glucagon, insulin and HGH in liver cirrhosis after arginine and I.V. glucose. *Acta Diabetologica Latina,* **11,** 330–339.
90. Greco, A.V., Crucitti, F., Ghirlanda, G., Manna, R., Altomonte, L., Rebuzzi, A. & Bertoli, A. (1978) Insulin and glucagon concentrations in portal and peripheral veins in hepatic cirrhosis. *Diabetologia.* In press.
91. Green, J.R.B. (1977) Mechanism of hypogonadism in cirrhotic males. *Gut,* **18,** 843–853.
92. Green, J.R.B., Mowat, N.A.G., Fisher, R.A. & Anderson, D.C. (1976) Plasma oestrogens in men with chronic liver disease. *Gut,* **17,** 426–430.
93. Greenberger, N.J., Milligan, F.D., De Groot, L.J. & Isselbacher, K.J. (1964) Jaundice and thyrotoxicosis in the absence of congestive heart failure. *American Journal of Medicine,* **36,** 840.
94. Greenwood, F.C., Landon, J. & Stamp, T.C. (1966) The plasma sugar, free fatty acid, cortisol, and growth hormone response to insulin. *Journal of Clinical Investigation,* **45,** 429–436.
95. Hagen, T.C., Lawrence, A.M. & Kirsteins, L. (1972) Autoregulation of growth hormone secretion in normal subjects. *Metabolism,* **21,** 603–610.
96. Hanefield, M., Naumann, H.J. & Haller, H. (1967) Statistische Untersuchungen über den Einfluss des Diabetes typs und der Therapieform auf die Ausprägung und Frequenz der Leberverfettung bei Diabetes Mellitus. *Deutsche Zeitschrift für Verdauungs- und Stoffwechselkrankheiten,* **27,** 13–19.
97. Hernandez, A., Zorilla, E. & Gershberg, H. (1969) Decreased insulin production, elevated growth hormone levels, and glucose intolerance in liver disease. *Journal of Laboratory and Clinical Medicine,* **73,** 25–33.
98. Hisaw, F.L. (1959) Comparative effectiveness of estrogens on fluid inbibition and growth of the rat's uterus. *Endocrinology,* **64,** 276–289.
99. Holdsworth, C.D., Nye, L. & King, E. (1972) The effect of portacaval anastomosis on oral carbohydrate tolerance and on plasma insulin levels. *Gut,* **13,** 58–63.
100. Horton, R. & Tait, J.F. (1966) Androstenedione production and interconversion rates measured in peripheral blood and studies on the possible site of its conversion to testosterone. *Journal of Clinical Investigation,* **45,** 301–313.

101. Horwitz, D.L., Starr, J.I., Mako, M.E., Blackard, W.G. & Rubenstein, A.H. (1975) Proinsulin, insulin and C-peptide concentrations in human portal and peripheral blood. *Journal of Clinical Investigation,* **55,** 1278–1283.
102. Inada, M. & Sterling, K. (1967) Thyroxine turnover and transport in Laennec's cirrhosis of the liver. *Journal of Clinical Investigation,* **46,** 1275–1282.
103. Ingbar, S.H. (1978) Thyroid storm or crisis. In *The Thyroid: A Fundamental and Clinical Text* (Ed.) Werner, S.C. & Ingbar, S.H. pp. 800–804. New York: Harper & Row.
104. Jacobs, H.S. & Nabarro, J.D. (1969) Tests of hypothalamic–pituitary–adrenal function in man. *Quarterly Journal of Medicine,* **38,** 475–493.
105. Jaspan, J.B., Huen, A. H.-J., Morley, C.G., Moossa, A.R. & Rubenstein, A.H. (1977) The role of the liver in glucagon metabolism. *Journal of Clinical Investigation,* **60,** 421–428.
106. Jenkins, J.S. & Connolly, J. (1968) Adrenocortical response to ethanol in man. *British Medical Journal,* **ii,** 804–805.
107. Jenkins, D.W., Eckel, R.E. & Craig, J.W. (1971) Alcoholic ketoacidosis. *Journal of the American Medical Association,* **217,** 177–183.
108. Joffe, B.I., Seftel, H.C. & Van As, M. (1975) Hormonal responses in ethanol-induced hypoglycaemia. *Journal of Studies on Alcohol,* **36,** 550–554.
109. Joffe, B.I., Shires, R., Seftel, H.C. & Heding, L.G. (1977) Plasma insulin, C-peptide and glucagon levels in acute phase of ethanol-induced hypoglycaemia. *British Medical Journal,* **ii,** 678–679.
110. Johnston, D.G. & Alberti, K.G.M.M. (1976) Carbohydrate metabolism in liver disease. *Clinics in Endocrinology and Metabolism,* **5,** 675–702.
111. Johnston, D.G., Alberti, K.G.M.M., Faber, O.K., Binder, C. & Wright, R. (1977) Hyperinsulinism of hepatic cirrhosis: diminished degradation or hypersecretion? *Lancet,* **i,** 10–13.
112. Johnston, D.G., Alberti, K.G.M.M., Wright, R., Smith-Laing, G., Stewart, A.M., Sherlock, S., Faber, O. & Binder, C. (1978) C-peptide and insulin in liver disease. *Diabetes,* **27** (Suppl), 201–206.
113. Jung, R.T., Davie, M., Hunter, J.O., Chalmers, T.M. & Lawson, D.E.M. (1978) Abnormal vitamin D metabolism in cirrhosis. *Gut,* **19,** 290–293.
114. Kaden, M., Harding, P. & Field, J.B. (1973) Effect of intraduodenal glucose administration on hepatic extraction of insulin in the anaesthetised dog. *Journal of Clinical Investigation,* **52,** 2016–2028.
115. Kanazawa, Y., Kuzuya, T., Ide, T. & Kosaka, K. (1966) Plasma insulin responses to glucose in femoral, hepatic and pancreatic veins in dogs. *American Journal of Physiology,* **211,** 442–448.
116. Katz, A.I. & Rubenstein, A.H. (1973) Metabolism of proinsulin, insulin and C-peptide in the rat. *Journal of Clinical Investigation,* **52,** 1113–1121.
117. Kehayoglou, A.K., Agnew, J.E., Holdsworth, C.D., Whelton, M.J. & Sherlock, S. (1968) Bone disease and calcium absorption in primary biliary cirrhosis. *Lancet,* **i,** 715–719.
118. Kent, J.R., Aronow, W. & Meister, L. (1969) Hypogonadotrophic hypogonadism in hemochromatosis. *California Medicine,* **111,** 450–452.
119. Kent, J.R., Scaramuzzi, R.J., Lauwers, W., Parlow, A.F., Hill, M., Penardi, R. & Hilliard, J. (1973) Plasma testosterone, estradiol and gonadotrophins in hepatic insufficiency. *Gastroenterology,* **64,** 111–115.
120. Kittredge, R.D. & Nash, A.D. (1974) The many facets of sclerosing fibrosis. *American Journal of Roentgenology,* **122,** 288–298.
121. Kley, H.K., Nieschlag, E., Wiegelmann, W., Solbach, H.G. & Krüskemper, H.L. (1975) Steroid hormones and their binding in plasma of male patients with fatty liver, chronic hepatitis and liver cirrhosis. *Acta Endocrinologica,* **79,** 275–285.
122. Klion, F., Segal, R. & Schaffner, R. (1971) The effect of altered thyroid function on the ultrastructure of the human liver. *American Journal of Medicine,* **50,** 317–324.
123. Koechling, cited by Berzoni, M. (1934) Gynäkomastie und Lebercirrhose. *Virchows Archiv für Pathologie,* **293,** 679–723.
124. Kopetz, K. & Wehrmann, P. (1970) Stoffwechselveränderungen nach glucose und tolbutamidbelastung bei lebercirrhosen und ihr rolle in der pathogenese des hepatogenen diabetes mellitus. *Klinische Wochenschrift,* **48,** 1265–1276.
125. Korenman, S.G., Perrin, L.E. & McCallum, T. (1969) Estradiol in human plasma: demonstration of elevated levels in gynaecomastia and in cirrhosis (abstract). *Journal of Clinical Investigation,* **48,** 45a.
126. Krebs, H.A., Freedland, R.A., Hems, R. & Stubbs, M. (1969) Inhibition of hepatic gluconeogenesis by alcohol. *Biochemical Journal,* **112,** 117–124.
127. Lavrie, W. (1971) Alcohol as a cause of sudden unexpected death. *Medical Journal of Australia,* **1,** 1224–1227.
128. Leevy, C.M. (1952) Fatty liver: a study of 270 patients with biopsy proven fatty liver and a review of the literature. *Medicine (Baltimore),* **41,** 249–278.
129. Leevy, C.M., Thomson, P. & Baker, H. (1970) Vitamins and liver injury. *American Journal of Clinical Nutrition,* **23,** 493–498.
130. Leffert, H.L. (1974) Growth control of differentiated foetal rat hepatocytes in primary monolayer culture. VII. Hormonal control of DNA synthesis and its possible significance to the problem of liver regeneration. *Journal of Cell Biology,* **62,** 792–801.
131. Lepyavko, A.G. (1970) Functional state of the thyroid gland in patients with lambliasis with predominant involvement of the hepatobiliary system. *Klinicheskaia Meditsina (Moscow),* **48,** 83–86.
132. Levy, L.J., Duga, J., Girgis, M. & Gordon, E.E. (1973) Ketoacidosis associated with alcoholism in nondiabetic subjects. *Annals of Internal Medicine,* **78,** 213–219.
133. Lickley, H.L.A., Chisholm, D.J., Rabinowitch, A., Wexler, M. & Dupré, J. (1975) Effects of portacaval anastomosis on glucose tolerance in the dog: evidence of an interaction between the gut and the liver in oral glucose disposal. *Metabolism,* **24,** 1157–1168.
134. Liegel, J., Fabre, L.F., Howard, P.Y. & Farmer, R.W. (1972) Plasma testosterone and sex hormone binding globulin (SBG) in alcoholic subjects (abstract). *Physiologist,* **15,** 918.
135. Lloyd, C.W. & Williams, R.H. (1948) Endocrine changes associated with Laennec's cirrhosis of the liver. *American Journal of Medicine,* **4,** 315–330.
136. Long, R.G., Wills, M.R., Skinner, R.K. & Sherlock, S. (1976) Serum-25-hydroxy-vitamin-D in untreated parenchymal and cholestatic liver disease. *Lancet,* **ii,** 650–652.
137. Long, R.G., Meinhard, E., Skinner, R.K., Varghese, Z., Wills, M.R. & Sherlock, S. (1978) Clinical,

biochemical and histological studies of osteomalacia, osteoporosis and parathyroid function in chronic liver disease. *Gut,* **19,** 85–90.

138. Long, R.G., Skinner, R.K., Wills, M.R. & Sherlock, S. (1978) Formation of vitamin D metabolites from ^{3}H- and ^{14}C-radiolabelled vitamin D-3 in chronic liver diseases. *Clinica Chimica Acta,* **85,** 311–317.

139. Long, R.G., Varghese, Z., Wills, M.R. & Sherlock, S. (1978) Plasma calcium and magnesium fractions in liver disease. *Clinica Chimica Acta,* **84,** 239–245.

140. MacDonald, R.A. & Mallory, G.K. (1958) The natural history of post-necrotic cirrhosis. *American Journal of Medicine,* **24,** 334–357.

141. Madison, L.L. (1968) Ethanol induced hypoglycaemia. In *Advances in Metabolic Disorders* (Ed.) Levine, R. & Luft, R. Vol. 3, pp. 85–109. New York: Academic Press.

142. Madison, L.L., Combes, B., Unger, R.H. & Kaplan, N. (1959) The relationship between the mechanism of action of the sulphonylureas and the secretion of insulin into the portal circulation. *Annals of the New York Academy of Sciences,* **74,** 548–556.

143. Mako, M., Block, M., Starr, J., Nielson, E., Friedman, E. & Rubenstein, A. (1973) Proinsulin in chronic renal and hepatic failure: a reflection of the relative contribution of the liver and kidney to its metabolism. *Clinical Research,* **21,** 631.

144. Marco, J., Diego, J., Villaneuva, M.L., Diaz-Fierros, M., Valverde, I. & Segovia, J.M. (1973) Elevated plasma glucagon levels in cirrhosis of the liver. *New England Journal of Medicine,* **289,** 1107–1111.

145. Margraf, H.W., Moyer, C.A., Ashford, L.E. & Lavelle, L.W. (1967) Adrenocortical function in alcoholics. *Journal of Surgical Research,* **7,** 55–62.

146. Marks, V. (1975) Alcohol and changes in body constituents: glucose and hormones. *Proceedings of the Royal Society of Medicine,* **68,** 377–380.

147. Marks, V. (1978) Alcohol and carbohydrate metabolism. *Clinics in Endocrinology and Metabolism,* **7,** 333–349.

148. Marks, V. & Wright, J. (1977) Endocrinological and metabolic effects of alcohol. *Proceedings of the Royal Society of Medicine,* **70,** 337–344.

149. McCann, V.J. & Fulton, T.T. (1975) Cortisol metabolism in chronic liver disease. *Journal of Clinical Endocrinology and Metabolism,* **40,** 1038–1044.

150. McConaghey, P. (1972) The production of 'sulphation factor' by rat liver. *Journal of Endocrinology,* **52,** 1–9.

151. McConaghey, P. & Sledge, C.B. (1970) Production of 'sulphation factor' by perfused liver. *Nature,* **225,** 1249–1250.

152. McGavran, M.H. & Hartroft, W.S. (1956) The predilection of pancreatic beta cells for pigment deposition in haemochromatosis and haemosiderosis. *American Journal of Clinical Pathology,* **32,** 631.

153. McIlroy, M., Walsh, C.H., Doyle, C., O'Sullivan, D.J. & Whelton, M.J. (1976) Glucose tolerance in viral hepatitis. *Irish Journal of Medical Science,* **145,** 3–6.

154. Megyesi, C., Samols, E. & Marks, V. (1967) Glucose tolerance and diabetes in chronic liver disease. *Lancet,* **ii,** 1051–1056.

155. Mendelson, J.H. & Mello, N.K. (1976) Behavioural and biochemical interrelations in alcoholism. *Annual Review of Medicine,* **27,** 321–323.

156. Mendelson, J.H. & Stein, S. (1966) Serum cortisol levels in alcoholic and non-alcoholic subjects during experimentally induced ethanol intoxication. *Psychosomatic Medicine,* **28,** 616–626.

157. Mendelson, J.H., Ogata, M. & Mello, N.K. (1971) Adrenal function and alcoholism. 1. Serum cortisol. *Psychosomatic Medicine,* **33,** 145–157.

158. Merry, J. & Marks, V. (1969) Plasma hydrocortisone response to ethanol in chronic alcoholics. *Lancet,* **i,** 921–923.

159. Merry, J. & Marks, V. (1972) The effect of alcohol, barbiturate and diazepam on hypothalamic–pituitary–adrenal function in chronic alcoholics. *Lancet,* **ii,** 990–992.

160. Merry, J. & Marks, V. (1973) Hypothalamic–pituitary–adrenal function in chronic alcoholics. In *Alcoholic Intoxication and Withdrawal: Experimental Studies, Advances in Experimental Biology and Medicine* (Ed.) Cross, M.M. p. 167. New York: Plenum Press.

161. Morgan, A.G., Kelleher, J., Walker, B.E. & Losowsky, M.S. (1976) Nutrition in cryptogenic cirrhosis and chronic active hepatitis. *Gut,* **17,** 113–118.

162. Morgan, M.Y., Jakobovits, A.W., Gore, M.B.R., Wills, M.R. & Sherlock, S. (1978) Serum prolactin in liver disease and its relationship to gynaecomastia. *Gut,* **19,** 170–174.

163. Mortimer, G.E. & Tietze, F. (1959) Studies on the mechanism of capture and degradation of insulin I131 by the cyclically perfused rat liver. *Annals of the New York Academy of Sciences,* **82,** 329–337.

164. Mowat, N.A.G., Edwards, C.R.W., Fisher, R., McNeilly, A.S., Green, J.R.B. & Dawson, A.M. (1976) Hypothalamic–pituitary–gonadal function in men with cirrhosis of the liver. *Gut,* **17,** 345–350.

165. Mueller, R., Brausch, C.C., Hirsch, E.Z., Benua, R.S. & Dobyns, B.M. (1954) Thyroid I131 uptake in liver disease. *Journal of Clinical Endocrinology and Metabolism,* **14,** 1287–1299.

166. Müller, E.E. (1974) Growth hormone and the regulation of metabolism. In *MTP International Review of Science. Physiology.* Series One, Vol. 5, *Endocrine Physiology* (Ed.) McCann, S.M. London: Butterworth.

167. Müting, D., Lackas, N., Reikowski, H. & Richmond, S. (1966) Leberzirrhose und Diabetes mellitus. *Deutsche Medizinische Wochenschrift,* **91,** 1433–1438.

168. Myers, J.D., Brannon, E.S. & Holland, B.C. (1950) A correlative study of the cardiac output and the hepatic circulation in hyperthyroidism. *Journal of Clinical Investigation,* **29,** 1069–1077.

169. Nieschlag, E., Kremer, G.J. & Mussgnug, J. (1970) Insulin, Glucose-toleranz und freie Fettsauren Während und nach akuter Hepatitis. *Klinische Wochenschrift,* **48,** 381–385.

170. Nomura, S., Pittman, C.S., Chambers, J.B., Buck, M.W. & Shimizu, T. (1975) Reduced peripheral conversion of thyroxine to triiodothyronine in patients with hepatic cirrhosis. *Journal of Clinical Investigation,* **56,** 643–652.

171. Oakley, W.G. (1968) Pancreatic diabetes and haemochromatosis. In *Clinical Diabetes and its Biochemical Basis* (Ed.) Oakley, W.G., Pyke, D.A. & Taylor, K.W. pp. 663–680. Oxford and Edinburgh: Blackwell.

172. O'Keefe, S.J.D. & Marks, V. (1977) Lunchtime gin and tonic a cause of reactive hypoglycaemia. *Lancet,* **i,** 1286–1288.

173. Olivo, J., Gordon, G.G., Rafii, F. & Southren, A.L. (1975) Estrogen metabolism in hyperthyroidism and cirrhosis of the liver. *Steroids,* **26,** 47–56.

174. Ooms, H.A. (1973) *Emploi des Insulines Radioiodées comme Traceurs en Biologie*. Bruxelles: Arscia Editions.

175. Owens, D., Srivastava, M.C., Tompkins, C.V., Nabarro, J.D.N. & Sonksen, P.H. (1973) Studies on the metabolic clearance rate, apparent distribution space and plasma half-disappearance time of unlabelled human growth hormone in normal subjects and in patients with liver disease, renal disease, thyroid disease and diabetes mellitus. *European Journal of Clinical Investigation*, **3**, 284–294.

176. Palmer, J.P. & Ensinck, J.W. (1975) Stimulation of glucagon secretion by ethanol induced hypoglycaemia in man. *Diabetes*, **24**, 295–300.

177. Panerai, A.E., Salerno, F., Manneschi, M., Cocchi, D. & Müller, E.E. (1977) Growth hormone and prolactin responses to thyrotrophin-releasing hormone in patients with severe liver disease. *Journal of Clinical Endocrinology and Metabolism*, **45**, 134–140.

178. Passa, P., Luyckx, A.S., Carpentier, J.L., Lefebvre, P.J. & Canivet, J. (1977) Glucagon secretion in diabetic patients with haemochromatosis. *Diabetologia*, **13**, 509–513.

179. Passa, P., Rousselie, F., Ganville, C. & Canivet, J. (1977) Retinopathy and plasma growth hormone levels in idiopathic haemochromatosis with diabetes. *Diabetes*, **26**, 113–120.

180. Paterson, C.R. & Losowsky, M.S. (1967) The bones in chronic liver disease. *Scandinavian Journal of Gastroenterology*, **2**, 293–300.

181. Paton, A. (1976) Alcohol-induced Cushingoid syndrome (letter). *British Medical Journal*, **ii**, 1504.

182. Pentikäinen, P.J., Pentikäinen, L.A., Azarnoff, D.L. & Dujoune, C.A. (1975) Plasma levels and excretion of oestrogens in urine in chronic liver disease. *Gastroenterology*, **69**, 20–27.

183. Perin, E. & Sode, J. (1970) The liver in Graves' disease. *Medical Annual DC*, **39**, 563–570.

184. Peterson, R.E. (1960) Adrenocortical steroid metabolism and adrenal cortical function in liver disease. *Journal of Clinical Investigation*, **39**, 320–331.

185. Phillips, L.S., Herington, A.C. & Daughaday, W.H. (1975) Steroid hormone effects on somatomedin. 1. Somatomedin action in vivo. *Endocrinology*, **97**, 780–786.

186. Phillips, L.S., Herington, A.C., Karl, I.E. & Daughaday, W.H. (1976) Comparison of somatomedin activity in perfusates of normal and hypophysectomised rat livers with and without added growth hormone. *Endocrinology*, **98**, 606–614.

187. Pimstone, B.L., Le Roith, D., Epstein, S. & Kronheim, S. (1975) Disappearance rates of plasma growth hormone after intravenous somatostatin in renal and liver disease. *Journal of Clinical Endocrinology and Metabolism*, **41**, 392–395.

188. Pincus, I.J., Rakoff, A.E., Cohn, E.M. & Tumen, H.J. (1951) Hormonal studies in patients with chronic liver disease. *Gastroenterology*, **19**, 735–754.

189. Pipher, J. & Poulsen, E. (1947) Liver biopsy in thyrotoxicosis. *Acta Medica Scandinavica*, **127**, 439.

190. Pirart, J. & Gatez, P. (1958) L'étiologie de l'hémochromatose non transfusionelle: revue de la question; étude de l'hérédité dans 21 familles. *Semaine des hôpitaux de Paris*, **34**, 1044–1051.

191. Pittman, C.S. & Pittman, J.A. (1974) Relation of chemical structure to the action and metabolism of thyroactive substances. *Handbook of Physiology*, **3**, 233–253.

192. Pittman, C.S., Chambers, J.B. & Read, V.H. (1971) The extrathyroidal conversion rate of thyroxine to triiodothyronine in normal man. *Journal of Clinical Investigation*, **50**, 1187–1196.

193. Pokroy, N., Epstein, S., Hendricks, S. & Pimstone, B. (1974) Thyrotrophin response to intravenous thyrotrophin-releasing hormone in patients with hepatic and renal disease. *Hormone and Metabolic Research*, **6**, 132–136.

194. Portugal-Alvarez, J. de, Clamagirand, C.P., Souto, J.M., Catalán, E., Vila, T. & Velasco-Martín, A. (1974) Relationship between growth hormone, insulin and urinary oestrogens in hepatic cirrhosis. *Acta Diabetologica Latina*, **11**, 1–8.

195. Posner, D.B., Russell, R.M., Absood, S., Connor, T.B., Davis, C., Martin, L., Williams, J.B., Norris, A.H. & Merchant, C. (1978) Effective 25-hydroxylation of vitamin D_2 in alcoholic cirrhosis. *Gastroenterology*, **74**, 866–870.

196. Pouchon, G., Kennan, A.L. & De Luca, H.F. (1969) Activation of vitamin D by the liver. *Journal of Clinical Investigation*, **48**, 2032–2037.

197. Powell, L.W., Mortimer, R. & Harris, O.D. (1971) Cirrhosis of the liver – a comparative study of the four major aetiological groups. *Medical Journal of Australia*, **1**, 941–950.

198. Prior, A., Phillips, B.J. & Pain, R.W. (1977) The anion gap (letter). *Lancet*, **ii**, 513.

199. Read, A.E., Harrison, C.V. & Sherlock, S. (1963) 'Juvenile cirrhosis', part of a system disease. The effect of corticosteroid therapy. *Gut*, **4**, 378–384.

200. Record, C.O., Alberti, K.G.M.M., Williamson, D.H. & Wright, R. (1973) Glucose tolerance and metabolic changes in human viral hepatitis. *Clinical Science and Molecular Medicine*, **45**, 677–690.

201. Record, C.O., Chase, R.A., Alberti, K.G.M.M. & Williams, R. (1975) Disturbances in glucose metabolism in patients with liver damage due to paracetamol overdose. *Clinical Science and Molecular Medicine*, **49**, 473–479.

202. Rees, L.H., Besser, G.M., Jeffcoate, W.J., Goldie, D.J. & Marks, V. (1977) Alcohol-induced pseudo-Cushing's syndrome. *Lancet*, **i**, 726–728.

203. Richens, A. (1976) In *Anticonvulsant Drugs and Enzyme Induction* (Ed.), Richens, A. & Woodford, F.P. p. 3. Amsterdam: Elsevier: Excerpta Medica.

204. Root, A.W. (1976) Clinical studies of human growth hormone. *Pharmacology and Therapeutics*, **1**, 19–43.

205. Rosenbaum, W., Christy, N.P. & Kelly, W.G. (1966) Electrophoretic evidence for the presence of an estrogen-binding B-globulin in human plasma. *Journal of Clinical Endocrinology and Metabolism*, **26**, 1399–1403.

206. Rosner, W. (1972) A simplified method for the quantitative determination of testosterone-estradiol-binding globulin activity in human plasma. *Journal of Clinical Endocrinology and Metabolism*, **34**, 983–988.

207. Rupp, J., Cantarow, A., Rakoff, A.E. & Paschkis, K.E. (1951) Hormone excretion in liver disease and in gynaecomastia. *Journal of Clinical Endocrinology*, **11**, 688–699.

208. Sachdev, Y. & Hall, R. (1975) Effusions into body cavities in hypothyroidism. *Lancet*, **i**, 564–566.

209. Samols, E. & Ryder, J.A. (1961) Studies on tissue uptake of insulin in man using a differential immunoassay for endogenous and exogenous

insulin. *Journal of Clinical Investigation,* **40,** 2092–2102.

210. Samols, E. & Turner, M.D. (1968) Disturbances in carbohydrate metabolism liver disease. In *Carbohydrate Metabolism and its Disorders* (Ed.) Dickens, F., Randle, P.J. & Whelan, W.J. p. 298. London: Academic Press.

211. Schade, D.S., Eaton, R.P. & Standefer, J. (1978) The modulation of basal ketone body concentration by cortisol in diabetic man. *Journal of Clinical Endocrinology and Metabolism.* In press.

212. Schalch, D.S., Gonzalez-Barcena, D., Kastin, A.J., Landa, L., Lee, L.A., Zamora, M.T. & Schally, A.V. (1975) Plasma gonadotrophins after administration of LH-releasing hormone in patients with renal or hepatic failure. *Journal of Clinical Endocrinology and Metabolism,* **41,** 921–925.

213. Seige, K. & Thierbach, V. (1959) Posthepatitische Schäden bei Diabetes mellitus. *Verhandlungen der Deutschen Gesellschaft für Innere Medizin,* **65,** 705–709.

214. Sells, R.A., Calne, R.Y., Hadjiyanakis, V. & Marshall, V.C. (1972) Glucose and insulin metabolism after pancreatic transplantation. *British Medical Journal,* **iii,** 678–681.

215. Sestoft, L. & Rehfeld, J.F. (1970) Insulin and glucose metabolism in liver cirrhosis and in liver failure. *Scandinavian Journal of Gastroenterology* (Suppl.), **7,** 133–136.

216. Shaffer, J.M. (1940) Disease of the liver in hyperthyroidism. *Archives of Pathology,* **29,** 20–30.

217. Shedl, H.P. (1965) Steroid hormone metabolism in liver disease. In *Progress in Liver Diseases* (Ed.) Popper, H. & Schaffner, F. New York: Grune & Stratton.

218. Sheldon, J.H. (1935) *Haemochromatosis.* Oxford University Press.

219. Sheridan, P., Chapman, C. & Losowsky, M.S. (1978) Interpretation of laboratory tests of thyroid function in chronic active hepatitis. *Clinica Chimica Acta,* **86,** 73–80.

220. Sherlock, S. (1975) Cholestasis. In *Diseases of the Liver and Biliary System.* pp. 260–304. Oxford: Blackwell.

221. Sherlock, S. (1975) The liver in metabolic disorders. In *Diseases of the Liver and Biliary System.* pp. 506–532. Oxford: Blackwell.

222. Sherwin, R.S., Joshi, P., Hendler, R., Felig, P. & Conn, H.O. (1974) Hyperglucagonaemia in Laennec's cirrhosis, the role of portal-systemic shunting. *New England Journal of Medicine,* **290,** 239–242.

223. Sherwin, R.S., Fisher, M., Bessoff, J., Snyder, N., Hendler, R., Conn, H.O. & Felig, P. (1978) Hyperglucagonaemia in cirrhosis: altered secretion and sensitivity to glucagon. *Gastroenterology,* **74,** 1224–1228.

224. Shipley, R.A. & Chudzik, E.B. (1957) Thyroidal uptake and plasma clearance of I131 and I127 in cirrhosis of the liver. *Journal of Clinical Endocrinology and Metabolism,* **17,** 1229–1236.

225. Sholiton, L.J., Werk, E.E. Jr & Marnell, R.T. (1961) Diurnal variation of adrenocortical function in non-endocrine disease states. *Metabolism,* **10,** 632–646.

226. Shurberg, J.L., Resnick, R.H., Koff, R.S., Ros, E., Baum, R.A. & Pallotta, J.A. (1977) Serum lipids, insulin and glucagon after portacaval shunt in cirrhosis. *Gastroenterology,* **72,** 301–304.

227. Silvestrini, R. (1926) La reviviscenza mammaria nell uomo affeto da cirrosi del Laennec. *Reforma Medica,* **42,** 701–704.

228. Simon, M., Franchimont, P., Murie, N., Ferrant, B., Van Cauwenberge, H. & Bourel, M. (1972) Study of somatotropic and gonadotropic pituitary function in idiopathic haemochromatosis (31 cases). *European Journal of Clinical Investigation,* **2,** 384–389.

229. Skinner, R.K., Long, R.G., Sherlock, S. & Wills, M.R. (1977) 25-hydroxylation of vitamin D in primary biliary cirrhosis. *Lancet,* **i,** 720–721.

230. Smals, A., Kloppenborg, P., Njo, K.T., Knoben, J.M. & Ruland, C.M. (1976) Alcohol-induced Cushingoid syndrome. *British Medical Journal,* **ii,** 1298.

231. Smals, A.G.H., Njo, K.T., Knoben, J.M., Ruland, C.M. & Kloppenborg, P.W.E. (1977) Alcohol-induced Cushingoid syndrome. *Journal of the Royal College of Physicians,* **12,** 36–41.

232. Soeters, P.B. & Fischer, J.E. (1976) Insulin, glucagon, aminoacid imbalance, and hepatic encephalopathy. *Lancet,* **ii,** 880–881.

233. Soeters, P., Weir, G., Ebeid, A.M., James, J.H. & Fischer, J.E. (1975) Insulin and glucagon following porta-caval shunt (meeting abstract). *Gastroenterology,* **69,** 867.

234. Starzl, T.E., Porter, K.A., Francavilla, J.A., Benichou, J. & Putnam, C.W. (1978) A hundred years of the hepatotrophic controversy. In *Hepatotrophic Factors.* Ciba Foundation Symposium 55 (new series). North-Holland, Amsterdam, Oxford and New York: Elsevier, Excerpta Medica.

235. Stocks, A.E. & Martin, F.I.R. (1968) Pituitary function in haemochromatosis. *American Journal of Medicine,* **45,** 839–845.

236. Stocks, A.E. & Powell, L.W. (1972) Pituitary function in idiopathic haemochromatosis and cirrhosis of the liver. *Lancet,* **ii,** 298–300.

237. Stocks, A.E. & Powell, L.W. (1973) Carbohydrate intolerance in idiopathic haemochromatosis and cirrhosis of the liver. *Quarterly Journal of Medicine,* **42,** 733–749.

238. Stoll, R.W., Touber, J.L., Menahan, L.H. & Williams, R.H. (1970) Clearance of porcine insulin, proinsulin and connecting peptide by the isolated rat liver. *Proceedings of the Society for Experimental Biology and Medicine,* **133,** 894–896.

239. Stumpf, H.H. & Wilens, S.L. (1953) Inhibitory effects of portal cirrhosis of liver on prostatic enlargement. *Archives of Internal Medicine,* **91,** 304–309.

240. Summerskill, W.H.J., Davidson, C.S., Dible, J.H., Mallory, G.K., Sherlock, S., Turner, M.D. & Wolfe, S.J. (1960) Cirrhosis of the liver: a study of alcoholic and non-alcoholic patients in Boston and London. *New England Journal of Medicine,* **262,** 1–9.

241. Surks, M.I., Schadlow, A.R., Stock, J.M. & Oppenheimer, J.H. (1973) Determination of iodothyronine absorption and conversion of L-thyroxine (T_4) to L-triiodothyronine (T_3) using turnover rate techniques. *Journal of Clinical Investigation,* **52,** 805–811.

242. Takano, K., Hizuka, N., Shizume, K., Hayashi, N., Motoike, Y. & Obata, H. (1977) Serum somatomedin peptides measured by somatomedin A radio receptor assay in chronic liver disease. *Journal of Clinical Endocrinology and Metabolism,* **45,** 828–832.

243. Taylor, A.L., Upman, R.L., Salam, A. & Mintz, D.H. (1972) Hepatic clearance of human growth hormone. *Journal of Clinical Endocrinology,* **34,** 395–399.

244. Territo, M.C. & Tanaka, K.R. (1974) Hypophosphataemia in chronic alcoholism. *Archives of Internal Medicine,* **134,** 445–447.

245. Thijssen, J.H.H., Lourens, J. & Donker, G.H. (1971) Androstenedione and testosterone production and interconversion rates measured in peripheral blood in male patients with cirrhosis of the liver (abstract). *Acta Endocrinologica (Copenhagen)* (Suppl.), **155,** 116.

246. Thijssen, J.H.H., Lourens, J., Donker, G.H. & Schwartz, F. (1975) The role of the liver in the biogenesis of oestrogens in cirrhosis of the liver (abstract). *Acta Endocrinologica (Copenhagen)* (Suppl.), **199,** 234.

247. Thompson, W.G. & Hart, I.R. (1973) Chronic active hepatitis and Graves' disease. *American Journal of Digestive Diseases,* **18,** 111–119.

248. Tiengo, A., Fedele, D., Dolzani, L., Ancona, E., Muggeo, M. & Crepaldi, G. (1976) Hormonal counterregulation in ethanol-induced hypoglycaemia – glucagon and cortisol secretion in pigs. In *Hypoglycaemia: Proceedings of the European Symposium, Rome* (Ed.) Andreani, D., Lefebvre, P.J. & Marks, V. pp. 105–111. Stuttgart: Thieme.

249. Tintera, J.W. (1966) Stabilising homeostasis in the recovered alcoholic through endocrine therapy: evaluation of the hypoglycaemia factor. *Journal of the American Geriatrics Society,* **14,** 126–150.

250. Tintera, J.W. & Lovell, H.W. (1949) Endocrine treatment of alcoholism. *Geriatrics,* **4,** 274–280.

251. Toro, G., Kolodny, R.C., Jacobs, L.S., Masters, W.H. & Daughaday, W.H. (1973) Failure of alcohol to alter pituitary and target organ hormone levels. *Clinical Research,* **21,** 205.

252. Tourniare, J., Fevre, M., Mazenod, B. & Ponsin, G. (1974) Effects of clomiphene citrate and synthetic LHRH on serum luteinizing hormone (LH) in men with idiopathic haemochromatosis. *Journal of Clinical Endocrinology and Metabolism,* **38,** 1122–1124.

253. Tucci, J.R., Albacete, R.A. & Martin, M.M. (1966) Effect of liver disease upon steroid circadian rhythms in man. *Gastroenterology,* **50,** 637–644.

254. Turkington, R.W. (1972) Serum prolactin levels in patients with gynaecomastia. *Journal of Clinical Endocrinology and Metabolism,* **34,** 62–66.

255. Unger, R.H. (1976) Diabetes and the alpha cell. *Diabetes,* **25,** 136–151.

256. Uthne, K. & Uthne, T. (1972) Influence of liver resection and regeneration on somatomedin (sulfation factor) activity in sera from normal and hypophysectomised rats. *Acta Endocrinologica,* **71,** 255–264.

257. Vanotti, A. & Beraud, T. (1959) Functional relationships between liver, thyroxine-binding protein of serum and the thyroid. *Journal of Clinical Endocrinology and Metabolism,* **19,** 466–477.

258. Van Thiel, D.H. & Lester, R. (1976) Alcoholism: its effect on hypothalamic–pituitary–gonadal function. *Gastroenterology,* **71,** 318–327.

259. Van Thiel, D.H., Gavaler, J. & Lester, R. (1974) Ethanol inhibition of vitamin A metabolism in the testes: possible mechanism for sterility in alcoholics. *Science,* **186,** 941–942.

260. Van Thiel, D.H., Lester, R. & Sherins, R.J. (1974) Hypogonadism in alcoholic liver disease; evidence for a double defect. *Gastroenterology,* **67,** 1188–1199.

261. Van Thiel, D.H., Gavaler, J.S., Lester, R., Loriaux, D.L. & Braunstein, G.D. (1975) Plasma estrone, prolactin, neurophysin, and sex steroid-binding globulin in chronic alcoholic men. *Metabolism,* **24,** 1015–1019.

262. Vermeulen, A., Mussche, M. & Verdonck, L. (1972) Testosterone and estradiol production rates and interconversion in normal males and male cirrhotics. *Proceedings of the 4th International Congress on Endocrinology,* Abstract 305, pp. 123. Amsterdam: Excerpta Medica.

263. Vermeulen, A., Verdonck, L., Van der Straeton, M. & Orie, N. (1969) Capacity of the testosterone binding globulin in human plasma and influence of specific binding of testosterone on its metabolic clearance rate. *Journal of Clinical Endocrinology and Metabolism,* **29,** 1470–1480.

264. Waddell, W.R. & Sussman, K.E. (1967) Plasma insulin after diversion of portal and pancreatic venous blood to vena cava. *Journal of Applied Physiology,* **22,** 808–812.

265. Walker, C., Peterson, W. & Unger, R. (1974) Blood ammonia levels in advanced cirrhosis during therapeutic elevation of the insulin : glucagon ratio. *New England Journal of Medicine,* **211,** 168–171.

266. Walsh, C.H., Wright, A.D., Williams, J.W. & Holder, G. (1976) A study of pituitary function in patients with idiopathic haemochromatosis. *Journal of Clinical Endocrinology and Metabolism,* **43,** 866–872.

267. Weller, C.V. (1930) Hepatic lesions associated with exophthalmic goitre. *Transactions of the Association of American Physicians,* **45,** 71–85.

268. Wernze, H. & Schmitz, E. (1977) Plasma prolactin and prolactin release in liver cirrhosis. *Acta Hepato-Gastroenterologica,* **24,** 97–101.

269. West, T.E.T., Owens, D., Sönksen, P.H., Srivastava, M.C., Tompkins, C.V. & Nabarro, J.D.N. (1975) Metabolic responses to monocomponent human insulin infusions in normal subjects and patients with liver and endocrine disease. *Clinical Endocrinology,* **4,** 573–584.

270. Whelton, M.J., Kehayoglou, A.K., Agnew, J.E., Turnberg, L.A. & Sherlock, S. (1971) Calcium absorption in parenchymatous and biliary disease. *Gut,* **12,** 978–983.

271. Wiedemann, E. & Schwartz, E. (1972) Suppression of growth hormone-dependent human serum sulfation factor by estrogen. *Journal of Clinical Endocrinology and Metabolism,* **34,** 51–58.

272. Wiedemann, E., Schwartz, E. & Frantz, A.G. (1976) Acute and chronic estrogen effects upon serum somatomedin activity, growth hormone and prolactin in man. *Journal of Clinical Endocrinology,* **42,** 942–952.

273. Wright, J. (1978) Endocrine effects of alcohol. *Clinics in Endocrinology and Metabolism,* **7,** 351–367.

274. Wright, J.W., Merry, J., Fry, D. & Marks, V. (1976) Pituitary function in chronic alcoholism. In *Alcohol Intoxication and Withdrawal, Advances in Experimental Medicine and Biology* (Ed.) Cross, p. 253. New York: Plenum Press.

275. Wu, A., Grant, D.B., Hambley, J. & Levi, A.J. (1974) Reduced serum somatomedin activity in patients with chronic liver disease. *Clinical Science and Molecular Medicine,* **47,** 359–366.

276. Yen, S.S.C., Ehara, Y. & Siler, T.M. (1974) Augmentation of prolactin secretion by estrogen in hypogonad women. *Journal of Clinical Investigation,* **53,** 652–655.

277. Zanoboni, A. & Zanoboni-Muciaccia, W. (1975) Gynaecomastia in alcoholic cirrhosis (letter). *Lancet,* **ii,** 876.

278. Zanoboni, A. & Zanoboni-Muciaccia, W. (1977) Elevated basal growth hormone levels and growth hormone response to TRH in alcoholic patients with cirrhosis. *Journal of Clinical Endocrinology and Metabolism,* **45,** 576–578.

279. Zumoff, B., Bradlow, H.L., Gallagher, T.F. & Hellman, L. (1967) Cortisol metabolism in cirrhosis. *Journal of Clinical Investigation,* **46,** 1735–1743.

Chapter 8

Haematological Disorders in Liver Disease

MORAG CHISHOLM

THE PHYSIOLOGICAL ROLE OF THE LIVER IN HAEMOPOIESIS AND HAEMOSTASIS

The liver is the primary site of erythropoiesis in the fetus from the ninth to the twenty-fourth week of gestation, but thereafter the bone marrow becomes the major source of red blood cells. Granulocytes and platelets are produced in the liver from the early weeks of fetal life, but the production of these cells is taken over by the bone marrow as the fetus develops. The potential for haemopoiesis is retained into adult life and in conditions where bone marrow function fails, as for example in myelofibrosis, the liver may again become an active site of haemopoiesis.

The major functions of the liver in relation to the blood are shown in Table 8.1. The major haematinics essential for haemopoiesis are iron, vitamin B_{12} and folate. The liver's role in relation to these will be summarized briefly.

Table 8.1. *Physiological Role of the Liver in Haemopoiesis and Haemostasis.*

1. Production of blood cells in utero
2. Reticuloendothelial function:
   (a) Red cell destruction and breakdown
   (b) Transferrin production
   (c) Clearance of activated coagulation factors and breakdown
3. Bilirubin metabolism and excretion
4. Storage organ for vitamin B_{12}, folate and iron
5. Production of coagulation factors

Red Cell Destruction and Breakdown

Destruction and breakdown of the red cells take place in the liver and other parts of the reticuloendothelial (RE) system. A detailed description is given in Chapter 13. In summary, when the red cell is destroyed, iron and globin are split off and the residual haem is broken down in Kupffer and other RE cells to bilirubin which is then carried in the plasma to the liver, bound to albumin. The bilirubin/albumin complex enters the hepatic cells and undergoes conjugation to glucuronic acid to form a water-soluble compound which passes via the bile duct to the intestine. Urobilinogen is formed and is partly excreted, partly reabsorbed, finally being excreted both in the urine and the faeces.

Iron Metabolism

Transferrin, the major carrier protein for iron, is synthesized in the liver and other reticuloendothelial tissues. To a limited extent the liver acts as a storage organ for iron. The average iron content of a healthy male is about 70 mmol (4 g) and most of this is in the circulating haemoglobin. A small amount (approximately 5.5 mmol [0.3 g]) is stored in the liver either as ferritin, a water-soluble protein iron complex, or in the Kupffer cells as haemosiderin, an insoluble compound easily visible on light microscopy using special stains such as Prussian blue.

Vitamin B_{12} and Folate Metabolism

A large part of the body stores of vitamin B_{12} are present in the liver, the normal content ranging from 0.6 to 1.5 μg vitamin B_{12}/g wet weight. Folic acid is also stored in the liver, with a mean normal level of 7.1 μg/g.[19] The hepatic content of vitamin B_{12} and folate correlate well with blood levels. There would appear to be few haemopoietic consequences of altered metabolism of these essential vitamins by liver disease per se. The changes described result mainly from associated abnormalities such as alcoholism and poor nutrition.

Coagulation Factors

The current hypothesis of blood coagulation proposes that a series of reactions which begins either with activation of factor XII by contact with exposed subendothelial collagen (intrinsic pathway) or with activation of factor VII by tissue substances, known as thromboplastins (extrinsic pathway), leads to the formation of a clot consisting of closely interwoven fibrin and platelets. The coagulation factors are present in the plasma mostly in trace amounts as proenzymes or precursor proteins (zymogens) but during the process of clotting become activated and interact with each other sequentially as shown in Figure 8.1.

The following factors are produced in the liver: fibrinogen, the vitamin K dependent factors II, VII, IX and X, the labile factors V and VIII, the contact factors XI and XII and factor XIII, the fibrin stabilizing factor. Most are produced exclusively in the liver, have a short half-life ranging from a few hours to a few days and are reduced in hepatocellular failure.

Vitamin K dependent factors

The synthesis of factors II, VII, IX and X is dependent both on normal liver function and on an adequate supply of vitamin K. Natural vitamin K is fat soluble and its absorption from the gut is facilitated by bile salts. It is obtained from the diet and from the synthetic activity of intestinal bacteria. Conditions such as malabsorption, obstructive jaundice, antibiotic therapy, and antagonists such as warfarin will lead to vitamin K deficiency. The role of vitamin K in the production of factors II, VII, IX and X has recently been defined.[162] In the first stage the basic precursor proteins are produced in the liver but are non-functional and unable to participate in the clotting cascade. Vitamin K is essential for the second step and directs the insertion of a second carboxyl group into the γ-carbon of glutamic acid residues. This results in a unique amino acid, γ-carboxyglutamic acid, which confers coagulant activity on the precursor proteins[157] enabling them to bind

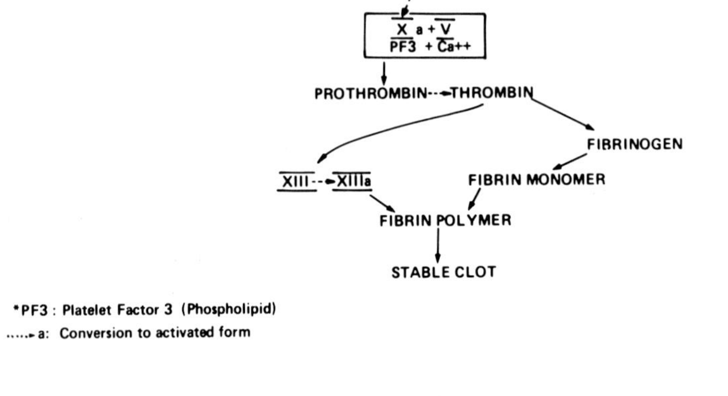

Figure 8.1. The coagulation cascade.

calcium and actively promote coagulation. In vitamin K deficiency the protein precursors known as PIVKA, i.e. protein induced by vitamin K absence or antagonists, accumulate in the plasma and can be detected by coagulation tests in vitro[76] and by immunological techniques.[61]

Other coagulation factors

Fibrinogen is synthesized almost exclusively in the liver where it is produced by the parenchymal cells.[52] Unlike most of the other clotting factors fibrinogen is present in measurable amounts in the plasma (2 to 4 g/l) and has a relatively long half-life of five days.

The site of production of factor VIII has been the subject of much research. It is produced by the liver and spleen and other reticuloendothelial cells, and possibly also by the vascular endothelial cells.[12] It is likely that extrahepatic sites are most important in factor VIII production.

Factor XIII, the fibrin stabilizing factor, is probably synthesized in the liver[176] as well as in the megakaryocytes.[144]

Fibrinolytic and inhibiting factors

A summary of the factors involved in fibrinolysis, the means whereby fibrin clots are broken down, is shown in Figure 8.2. The liver is probably the site of production of plasminogen[145] although bone marrow eosinophils and the kidney have also been suggested. Plasmin is a potent proteolytic enzyme, able to break down fibrin clots, and is produced by the activity of plasminogen activators in the vessel walls and many other tissues.

The role of the liver in the production of inhibitors of coagulation and fibrinolysis is not clear. The inhibitors of plasmin and thrombin, alpha-2-macroglobulin and alpha-1-antitrypsin may alter in liver disease but their physiological role is not defined.[137] A third inhibitor of thrombin and plasmin, antithrombin III, also known as the heparin cofactor, inactivates other coagulation factors including activated forms of factors X, IX, XI and XII and would also appear to be synthesized in the liver.[40]

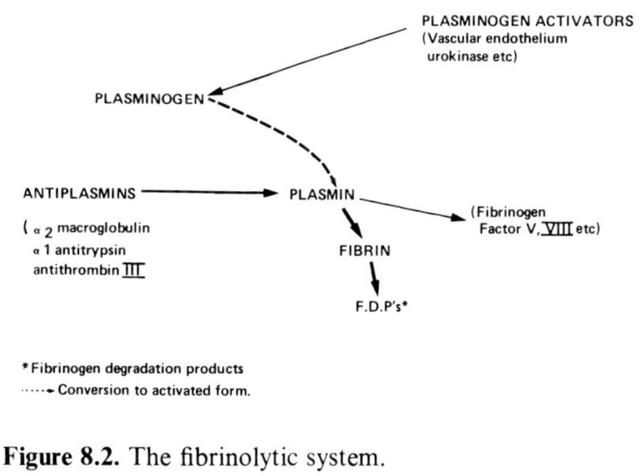

Figure 8.2. The fibrinolytic system.

ABNORMALITIES OF HAEMOPOIESIS

Liver disease may result in abnormalities of haemopoiesis ranging from morphological changes in the red cell to severe anaemia. White cell abnormalities occur but are less striking. Disturbed haemostasis is common and results from thrombocytopenia and impaired synthesis of the coagulation factors or their excessive consumption because of intravascular coagulation or blood loss. Although there is some overlap, it will be convenient to discuss the effects of liver disease on haemopoiesis and haemostasis separately.

Red Cell Abnormalities

General considerations

The normal mature red cell is a bi-concave disc, the shape being maintained by a number of factors including the ratio of the red cell membrane surface area to its volume. A recently proposed international terminology[7] refers to the normal red cell as a discocyte. The red cell membrane is basically structured as a lipid bilayer and cholesterol and phospholipids comprise approximately 90 per cent of the total membrane lipid.[13] The ratio of the membrane cholesterol to the phospholipids (CP ratio) is an important factor determining normal red cell shape. The membrane lipids may undergo a change in composition because of an alteration in plasma lipids as has been shown in vitro by incubating red cells in sera with different lipid constituents.[34] In liver disease the cholesterol and phospholipid content of the plasma may rise, leading to an increased erythrocyte content of both with possibly an altered ratio.[30] As a result of this and other factors as yet poorly understood the morphological changes in the red cell shown in Table 8.2 may occur in liver disease.

Table 8.2. *Morphological Abnormalities of the Red Cell in Liver Disease.*

Macrocytosis
Target cell formation
Stomatocytosis
Acanthocytosis

Morphological abnormalities

Macrocytosis. The macrocytosis associated with liver disease, particularly cirrhosis and obstructive jaundice, has excited much attention. The frequency varies, but approximately 60 to 65 per cent of patients with liver disease will have macrocytic blood films.[8, 9, 177] The erythrocytes are then described as 'thin' macrocytes or leptocytes because they have a diminished thickness but an increased diameter. In an earlier study thin macrocytosis was associated with a macronormoblastic marrow and was noted in just over one-third of patients with various liver diseases, including acute hepatitis and established obstructive jaundice, provided hepatocellular damage was present.[8, 9] The survival of these cells is shortened but there is no clear association with anaemia.[71] This type of macrocytosis resolves after improvement in liver function rather than after treatment with vitamin B_{12} or folate.

Target cells are also thin macrocytes and were noted in one-third of patients in one study.[8, 9] True or 'thick' macrocytosis was seen in less than 10 per cent and was noted only in patients with cirrhosis, mainly alcoholic. Megaloblastic erythropoiesis was common in this group and was almost certainly due to nutritional deficiency of folate.

Thus the underlying pathogenesis of macrocytosis in liver disease varies. Increased membrane cholesterol has been demonstrated in the leptocytes of liver disease[129, 177] and an increased CP ratio in the red cell membrane could cause the broadening and flattening of the red cell. Reticulocytosis in response to haemolysis or blood loss may be a contributory factor[97] and the erythroid hyperplasia and macronormoblastic maturation associated with the bone marrow response to haemolysis also plays a part. It is likely that alcohol has a direct effect on erythropoiesis resulting in macrocytosis. Finally, in a small number of patients macrocytosis will be due to folate deficiency.

Target cell formation. Target cells ('codocytes' according to the international classification) are bell shaped on scanning electron microscopy, but on dried films assume a characteristic target shape. Altered red cell membrane to volume ratio, either due to an absolute increase in membrane content as in liver disease or because of a decrease in intracellular haemoglobin content as in iron deficiency, will result in target cell formation. Target cells in liver disease have an increased content of cholesterol and phospholipid but because of a proportionately greater rise in the membrane lecithin, the CP ratio is not as markedly raised as in acanthocytosis. Target cells are commonly noted in the blood of patients with obstructive jaundice or hepatitis with associated obstruction[34] but the reasons for the development of the defect are not clear. No consistent correlation between the plasma lipids and those of the red cell membrane has been observed.[34, 129] It has been suggested that excess bile salts found in obstructive liver disease may inhibit the enzyme, lecithin cholesterol acyltransferase (necessary for the esterification of cholesterol to lysolecithin), leading to raised plasma cholesterol and associated increase in red cell membrane cholesterol. It is obvious that other factors must also be important since hypercholesterolaemia due to other diseases does not cause increased membrane cholesterol.[130]

Stomatocytosis. Stomatocytes are red cells in which the central circular area is replaced by a 'mouth-like' unstained area due to a dimple on one side. Stomatocytosis, or 'key hole' abnormality, has been defined as more than 4 per cent stomatocytes in the peripheral blood and has been described in chronic liver disease, particularly alcoholic. A variety of agents has been shown to induce stomatocytosis[7] and in hereditary stomatocytosis an elevated membrane lecithin as well as abnormalities in red cell enzyme content have been reported.[179] Douglass and Twomey[42] described stomatocytosis in patients with alcoholic liver disease, but there was no clear correlation between the degree of stomatocytosis, red cell survival and anaemia. The mechanism underlying the phenomenon is not understood.

Acanthocytosis. Acanthocytes (spur cells) are irregularly shaped red cells with multiple spicules (2 to 10) of variable length, projecting from the surface. A markedly increased CP ratio has been noted in the acanthocytes in liver disease[33] and is due to increased membrane cholesterol, the total phospholipid content remaining normal. The defect does not lie in the red cells; normal red cells become abnormal on being transfused into patients with acanthocytosis.[29] Shortened red cell survival with or without haemolytic anaemia is found in association with acanthocytosis and is a feature of established liver disease, usually alcoholic in origin. It is likely that acanthocytosis is irreversible since affected red cells taken from a patient with liver disease continue to have a shortened survival when transfused into normal donors.[31, 153] The spleen has an important role in contributing to the acanthocytosis, shortened survival and haemolytic anaemia.[32] Passage of the cells with their rigid membranes through the filtering system of the spleen leads in time to the development of spiculation and finally destruction by the spleen.

It would seem reasonable to conclude that macrocytes, target cells, acanthocytes and possibly stomatocytes are abnormal red cells found in patients with liver disease which have in common raised membrane lipids and an altered CP ratio. Acanthocytosis is the most severe defect, frequently being associated with haemolytic anaemia.

White Cell Abnormalities

Several leucocyte abnormalities have been described in patients with cirrhosis of the liver,[5] ranging from neutrophilia to neutropenia and lymphopenia. The white count is usually normal but there may be a neutropenia. Hypersplenism is one obvious contributing factor but the degree of splenomegaly and neutropenia does not necessarily correlate. Impaired production has been suggested as a reason but a review of the bone marrow appearance in cirrhosis[5] does not support this.

Leucocytosis as a response to infection, blood loss, haemolysis and malignant infiltration may occur when these complications arise in patients with liver disease. The specific changes associated with acute viral hepatitis and alcohol liver disease will be described under the relevant headings.

Platelet Abnormalities

Moderate thrombocytopenia is a common accompaniment of established liver disease.[41, 47] Severe thrombocytopenia is unusual in uncomplicated cirrhosis, the platelet count usually being above the level associated with spontaneous bleeding (more than 30×10^9/l). There are many reasons for thrombocytopenia in patients with liver disease, but commonly it is secondary to splenomegaly and portal hypertension.[1] Under normal conditions approximately one-third of the circulating platelets are within the spleen, and splenomegaly, whatever its aetiology, can result in thrombocytopenia although the total platelet mass may not be reduced.[1] The platelet half-life in patients with congestive splenomegaly is reported as normal,[1] megakaryocytes are present in normal numbers in the bone marrow[5] and it is not clear why increased platelet production is unable to compensate. It is possible that because the total circulating platelet mass is not reduced there is no increased stimulus to thrombocytopoiesis. Portacaval shunt[69] and splenectomy[118, 159] will improve the thrombocytopenia in a proportion of patients.

Another important cause of thrombocytopenia in liver disease is alcohol which is associated with impaired megakaryocyte response and shortened platelet survival.[35] Other causes include acute severe blood loss, particularly if treated by massive blood transfusion with stored bank blood, and increased consumption secondary to disseminated intravascular coagulation. Rarer causes of thrombocytopenia are acute viral hepatitis[96] and folate deficiency, usually with an associated megaloblastic anaemia and leucopenia.

Abnormal platelet function has been described in association with liver disease. The evidence suggests that the presence of fibrinogen degradation products or fibrin monomer complexes, possibly the result of associated intravascular coagulation and increased fibrinolysis, interferes with platelet aggregation[164] but further study is required.

Anaemia in Liver Disease

While inevitably there must be case selection, surveys of the frequency of anaemia in chronic liver disease indicate that just over one-third of patients with biopsy-documented disease will be anaemic.[39, 91, 100, 102] The anaemia is commonly normochromic, normocytic or macrocytic; a microcytic picture would suggest associated blood loss and resultant iron deficiency or, rarely, a sideroblastic anaemia. Under certain circumstances such as blood loss, acute haemolysis and folic acid deficiency, the anaemia may be marked but it is usually of moderate severity and does not correlate with the degree of hepatocellular failure.

Table 8.3 lists the various types of anaemia found in liver disease whatever the underlying pathology. Rarely, aplastic anaemia occurs in acute viral hepatitis but is not found in chronic liver disease.

Table 8.3. *Anaemia in Liver Disease.*

1. Macrocytic:
   (a) Normoblastic or macronormoblastic
   (b) Megaloblastic
2. Haemolytic
3. Anaemia due to altered iron metabolism:
   (a) iron deficiency
   (b) sideroblastic
   (c) impaired iron utilization
4. Dilutional anaemia and hypersplenism

Macrocytic anaemia

Macrocytosis is reported in up to 65 per cent of patients with various types of liver disease but, in the majority, erythropoiesis is macronormoblastic and the haemoglobin is maintained. The macrocytosis of cirrhosis and obstructive jaundice is not corrected by folic acid or vitamin B_{12}, but may resolve with improved liver function. Disturbances of folic acid and vitamin B_{12} metabolism causing a true megaloblastic anaemia are much less common and are usually due to alcohol abuse and associated nutritional deficiency.

Abnormalities of folic acid and vitamin B_{12} metabolism. Folic acid absorption may be increased,[102] probably because of increased requirements secondary to alcohol excess and haemolysis. Low serum folate levels have been reported in approximately 50 per cent of patients with liver disease, but again mostly in the alcoholic.[39, 78, 100] The serum folate level is a very sensitive index of folate deficiency and falls after three to four weeks on a folate-poor diet;[77] low red cell folate levels indicating folate deficiency of some duration have also been reported.[83] Formimino-glutamic acid excretion is increased in liver disease[78] but this test is not a good one for folate deficiency.[19] Hepatic folate has been measured in a variety of disorders, including alcoholism, where it is commonly reduced and correlates well with the serum folate level.[106]

Disturbances of vitamin B_{12} metabolism are usually of a minor nature. Reduced liver stores are found in patients with a variety of liver disorders[94] but serum levels are usually normal or even raised, particularly in patients with hepatocellular damage.[39, 100, 143] Presumably this is associated with depletion of hepatic stores. In an acute self-limiting disease, such as viral hepatitis, a rapid return to normal serum vitamin B_{12} levels occurs with recovery.[133]

Clinical features. Anaemia is a late development in cirrhosis and is not uncommon; true megaloblastic anaemia is rare (Table 8.4). In one prospective study of 350 patients with cirrhosis bone marrow biopsy was performed in 96 patients with moderately severe anaemia and was only megaloblastic in seven (2 per cent of the total).[102] The erythroid hyperplasia and macronormoblastic picture commonly seen[131] is found in the absence of bleeding and is related to the shortened red cell life. Chronic alcoholism and dietary deficiency are the major causes of folate deficiency and folic acid is the haematinic of choice for megaloblastic anaemia in these patients. Treatment with vitamin B_{12} is not indicated. The diet of alcoholics who develop megaloblastic anaemia may not be obviously different from the diet of those who do not,[90] and other factors, such as an increased requirement for folic acid because of haemolysis, must be important.

Table 8.4. *Incidence of Megaloblastic Anaemia in Liver Disease.*

	Patients studied	Megaloblastic anaemia	
Jarrold and Vilter[91]	30	20	11.8%
Krasnow et al[102]	350	22	
Klipstein and Lindenbaum[100]	40	4	
Deller, Kimber and Ibbotson[39]	46	9	

Haemolytic anaemias

Many of the features of haemolysis, e.g. abnormal red cell morphology, raised serum bilirubin, reduced or absent haptoglobins and shortened red cell survival, are found in liver disease per se without associated anaemia, and their significance should anaemia develop may be difficult to evaluate.

Laboratory findings. A moderate reticulocytosis is a common finding in patients with chronic liver disease.[91] Macrocytes, target cells and acanthocytes due to the altered membrane lipids may be noted but in most patients these findings will not be associated with severe haemolytic anaemia. Spherocytosis and a leucoerythroblastic picture have been described when florid haemolytic anaemia develops.[186]

The bone marrow will show increased cellularity and normoblastic or macronormoblastic maturation, indicating that compensatory haemopoiesis is required to maintain the haemoglobin concentration at near normal levels.[186]

Increased osmotic resistance to saline is a feature of red cells with an increased surface area such as target cells. A mild to moderate shortening of red cell survival is often present in patients with liver disease because of increased membrane lipid and rigidity of the red cell.[136, 158] Increased red cell destruction has been demonstrated using radioactive chromium, and increased splenic radioactivity suggests that the spleen is the site of destruction.[158] The degree to which this occurs is in part related to the spleen size[89, 98] and the role of the spleen in potentiating red cell destruction has been emphasized.[32] However, variable splenic uptake of radio-isotopes and the failure of splenectomy to improve the condition indicates that other factors are involved; reticuloendothelial hyperplasia elsewhere has been suggested but there is no definite evidence for this.

Clinical features. Low grade haemolysis is frequently present in acute and chronic liver disease but anaemia is not common because the bone marrow is able to compensate by increased erythropoiesis. It is difficult to estimate the frequency of anaemia in patients with liver disease from available reports because of the inevitable selection of case material. Factors such as the severity and chronicity of the liver disease, its underlying aetiology, alcohol intake, hyperlipaemia and the degree of splenic enlargement may all play some part in determining the severity of anaemia.

There would appear to be several distinct haemolytic syndromes associated with chronic liver disease (Table 8.5). Self-limiting haemolysis accompanied by hyperlipidaemia and low-grade fever, usually precipitated by alcoholic excess, is known as Zieve's syndrome.[185]

Table 8.5. *Haemolytic Syndromes in Liver Disease.*

Acute viral hepatitis:
Autoimmune
Chronic liver disease:
Hyperlipidaemia
Hypersplenism
'Spur cell' anaemia
Autoimmune

As a group the patients are not acutely ill, hepatomegaly is due to fatty infiltration and spontaneous recovery usually occurs. Zieve[186] distinguished this syndrome from a group of patients who had a significantly enlarged spleen and a much longer history of illness, advanced liver disease and severe cirrhosis on biopsy. Haematologically there was little difference between the two groups except that haemolysis was characteristically brief in the hyperlipidaemic patients; a low platelet and white count were seen in the patients with hypersplenism. No evidence of an autoimmune process was found in either group.

A recent study has shed some light on the mechanisms underlying Zieve's syndrome.[60] The evidence from this study suggests that alcohol-induced vitamin E deficiency together with altered membrane lipid composition leads to pyruvate kinase instability resulting in acute haemolysis. Such a mechanism would be similar to that described in favism where exposure to fava beans precipitates haemolysis in patients with glucose-6-phosphate dehydrogenase deficiency, an inherited metabolic error, and fits with the reports of acute viral hepatitis precipitating haemolysis in patients with this defect.[22, 24]

'Spur' cell anaemia, an acute haemolytic anaemia associated with acanthocytosis, is usually found in patients with advanced alcoholic cirrhosis and a poor prognosis although there have been a few reports in non-alcoholic liver disease.[109] Although there are conflicting reports the defect would appear to be due to the large amount of cholesterol in the red cell membrane and is acquired by normal red cells on contact with the plasma of patients with acanthocytosis. The shortened survival of the acanthocytes seen in the condition persists after transfusion into normal recipients.[29, 153] An interesting report showed that absence of the spleen allows normal red cell survival[32] and it was suggested that the production of 'spur cell' anaemia took place in two stages. Within 12 to 24 hours of contact and acquisition of cholesterol the red cell developed irregular spicules. Subsequently over a period of days in the presence of an intact spleen there was a progressive loss of red cell membrane and the deformity increased, the red cell being finally destroyed in the spleen.

A Coombs positive autoimmune haemolytic anaemia is occasionally described in chronic liver disease, particularly in chronic active hepatitis.[135] The antibody, when it has been characterized, has usually been of the IgG type with Rh specificity but other specificities have been reported.[108]

As is apparent from the foregoing there is considerable overlap between the haemolytic syndromes described in liver disease. Indeed the concept that these are distinct from each other with specific pathogenic mechanisms has been challenged.[109] The practical point of making such a distinction would appear to lie in assessing the prognostic implication of the haemolytic episodes. Treatment has little to offer in this situation: alcohol withdrawal and general measures directed at improving the underlying liver disease will obviously be attempted. The rare autoimmune haemolytic anaemia may respond to corticosteroids and a short course at a high dose (60 mg prednisolone for an initial period of two weeks) is worth trying.

Anaemia due to altered iron metabolism

Many of the abnormalities of iron metabolism associated with liver disease are secondary to other factors such as associated blood loss or alcoholism. In established liver disease uncomplicated by blood loss the serum iron is usually normal or raised,[20] the iron binding capacity (transferrin) normal or low and transferrin saturation increased. In acute liver damage the serum iron and ferritin levels are raised,[138] possibly because of release from liver cells.

Increased iron absorption is documented in patients with cirrhosis.[27, 181] The mechanism is poorly understood. Several possibilities have been suggested, including chronic pancreatitis, a direct effect of alcohol on iron absorption and iron overloading as a consequence of defective erythropoiesis or haemolysis.

Iron deficiency anaemia. The frequency with which signs of iron deficiency (hypochromic anaemia, low serum iron, high transferrin and reduced saturation) are seen in patients with chronic liver disease varies. In chronic liver disease uncomplicated by gastrointestinal haemorrhage or bleeding diathesis iron deficiency is not common. The presence of an iron deficiency anaemia should alert the physician to the likelihood of chronic blood loss which is frequent in advanced liver disease.[98, 152]

Sideroblastic anaemia. Sideroblastic anaemia is an uncommon complication of liver disease and is usually due to alcohol. Severe dietary deficiency may alter the picture, but impaired iron utilization is evident with a rise in serum iron, transferrin saturation and increased iron in the bone marrow erythroblasts and reticuloendothelial cells.[44, 80]

The basic defect which leads to the development of sideroblasts would appear to be in haem synthesis. Interference in the production of pyridoxal phosphate, a cofactor of δ-aminolaevulinic acid synthetase, a mitochondrial enzyme essential for haem production, has been implicated in some cases. As a result of the failure to produce haem, iron accumulates in the red cell where it may lie randomly in the cytoplasm, forming a pathological sideroblast, or in the mitochondria encircling the nucleus, forming a 'ring' sideroblast. On electron microscopy the mitochondria in alcohol-induced sideroblasts are swollen and deformed.[82] Large numbers of ring sideroblasts are found in the bone marrow of chronic alcoholics but the defect may be reversed by abstinence from alcohol or intravenous administration of pyridoxal phosphate.[81]

The association of iron overload and alcoholism has led to controversy regarding the role of alcohol in the aetiology of haemochromatosis.[117] This complex problem is discussed in Chapter 34.

Anaemia due to chronic disease. Chronic disorders such as chronic infection and collagen disease can result in a moderate anaemia and this may rarely be a cause of anaemia in chronic liver disease. The blood picture is usually normochromic normocytic but may be hypochromic microcytic and difficult to distinguish from iron deficiency. The serum iron is low but, unlike the situation in iron deficiency, transferrin levels are also reduced. Bone marrow examination shows some degree of failure and reduced iron in the developing red cells. The defining feature is increased reticuloendothelial iron, indicating the 'RE block' of chronic disease.[113]

The anaemia is usually moderate and the clinical picture is dominated by the underlying disease process. The treatment is control of the underlying disease. Iron therapy should not be given and blood transfusion is not indicated in most cases since there is no evidence that patients benefit from a higher haemoglobin concentration.

Dilutional anaemia and hypersplenism

The anaemia of chronic liver failure is often complicated by portal hypertension and hypersplenism and the increased plasma volume associated with splenomegaly may give a false impression of the degree of anaemia present. In a study of patients with chronic liver disease true anaemia, as defined by a fall in the circulating red cell mass, was present in 40 per cent but an apparent anaemia as defined by a fall in the venous haematocrit was noted in an additional 30 per cent.[152] Lieberman and Reynolds[107] showed in a large number of patients with cirrhosis that an increase in the plasma volume was an important factor contributing to the low haemoglobin. Thus, as in the anaemia of pregnancy, haemodilution contributes to the anaemia of cirrhosis. The pathogenesis of the increased plasma volume is not clear but it must be partly due to portal hypertension.

The shortened red cell survival in this condition correlates with the splenomegaly. When the red cell shape is abnormal prolonged trapping in the spleen may cause significant anaemia.

The leucopenia associated with hypersplenism is mainly due to neutropenia, which may be quite severe.[170] While there is some correlation between splenic size and resultant pancytopenia this is not necessarily predictable and the degree of neutropenia and thrombocytopenia is not always related to the spleen size.

Correction of the portal hypertension by portacaval shunt may reduce the increased plasma volume but it does not usually return to normal.[107] The haematological abnormalities show some improvement in approximately one-third of cases.[118] Splenectomy may succeed in correcting severe pancytopenia and could be combined with a portacaval shunt under certain circumstances.

THE HAEMATOLOGY OF SPECIFIC LIVER DISORDERS

The features associated with particular liver disorders listed in Table 8.6 will now be described.

Acute Viral Hepatitis

Significant anaemia is a rare complication of acute viral hepatitis and leucocyte and platelet abnormalities are noted much more frequently. Mild transient anaemia is not uncommon[28, 48] but occasionally the anaemia is severe and usually either haemolytic or hypoplastic.[99]

Table 8.6. *Liver Disorders with Specific Haematological Features.*

Acute viral hepatitis
Alcoholic liver disease
Non-alcoholic cirrhosis
Hepatocellular carcinoma

Abnormalities in the peripheral blood are common. Macrocytosis is often present by the time jaundice is clinically evident and persists until recovery. Leucopenia develops before the onset of jaundice[75] but by the seventh to fourteenth day the white count returns to normal. Initially there is both a lymphopenia and neutropenia, but by the second week there is often a lymphocytosis.[28] Atypical mononuclear cells seen during the first week are of the type commonly seen in viral infections. Features of these cells, referred to as 'virocytes', include cytoplasmic vacuolation, basophilic cytoplasm and large irregular nucleus occasionally containing nucleoli.[114] The platelet count is usually normal or even raised but transient thrombocytopenia has been reported. The erythrocyte sedimentation rate (ESR) is variable in the early stages of infective hepatitis[128, 172] but by the time the disease is well established the ESR will be moderately elevated in the majority of patients, particularly in HB_sAg negative infections.[172] Raised serum levels of vitamin B_{12} are reported.[139]

Haemolytic anaemia is an uncommon complication of acute viral hepatitis but the frequency is difficult to estimate.[37] Most reports are of small numbers but in one large series of 1200 patients 2 per cent developed this complication.[51] The Coombs' direct antiglobulin test is positive in some cases, and red cell antibodies may be demonstrated. A moderate shortening of the red cell survival is reported but the fragility is normal and a mild reticulocytosis occurs.[28] It usually presents a few weeks after the onset of viral hepatitis, is self-limiting and rarely of clinical significance. Patients with glucose-6-phosphate dehydrogenase deficiency run an increased risk of developing this complication.[22] No treatment is necessary although the use of steroids may be considered if the anaemia is severe. The pathogenesis is unknown but extrinsic factors such as lytic enzymes released from damaged liver cells, direct haemolytic effect of the causative virus, incomplete cold agglutinins and other autoimmune reactions have all been considered.

Prolonged hyperbilirubinaemia following acute viral hepatitis is described and was thought to be in part caused by haemolysis. There is no real evidence to support this and it is possible that impaired hepatocellular function or slow resolution of the hepatitis is the cause.[26]

Aplastic anaemia is a rare and serious complication of viral hepatitis and is associated with a high mortality. The underlying mechanisms are poorly understood; in many reported cases the hepatitis was improving or had resolved when striking pancytopenia developed.[70] Failure of the liver to detoxicate intermediary metabolites or drugs, direct viral-induced bone marrow damage, virally initiated autoimmune mechanisms and individual susceptibility have all been considered. The leucopenia which is an early feature in the course of hepatitis suggests that temporary bone marrow depression can occur and transient pancytopenia must be more common than the full-blown aplasia. Transient red cell aplasia has also been reported.[149] In a review of 195 patients[70] a slightly higher incidence in males was noted and females had a worse prognosis; only 8.5 per cent survived compared with an overall survival for the group of approximately 15 per cent. No other factor of prognostic significance was determined. Eighteen per cent of the patients had been exposed to chloramphenicol. The mean interval between the onset of hepatitis and pancytopenia was 9.3 weeks and the survival time after pancytopenia was 11.3 weeks. The longest interval between the onset of hepatitis and death was 78 weeks. It has been suggested that subclinical hepatitis may be responsible for a significant number of cases of 'idiopathic' aplastic anaemia.

There is no evidence that therapeutic measures alter the course of the aplastic anaemia. Corticosteroids alone or in combination with androgenic agents have been used in the majority of patients but are rarely successful. Bone marrow transplantation for aplastic anaemia associated with viral hepatitis has been attempted in a small number of patients some of whom have benefited.[166] With improving techniques this measure would appear to offer the best chance of cure in this frequently fatal complication.

Alcoholic Liver Disease

Excessive intake of alcohol will have a direct toxic effect on blood and bone marrow and will result in metabolic disturbances and consequent haemopoietic abnormalities (Table 8.7). Red cell, white cell and platelet production may all be affected. Provided caloric and vitamin intake is maintained the haematological sequelae of alcoholism are usually not marked,[111] the major effect being mediated through associated factors such as impaired nutrition, vitamin deficiency and altered liver function.

Table 8.7. *Blood Findings in Alcoholism.*

Peripheral blood

1. Red cells:
   Macrocytosis
   Stomatocytosis
   Target cells
   Acanthocytosis
2. White cells:
   Neutropenia
   Altered granulocyte function
3. Platelets:
   Thrombocytopenia
   Altered platelet function

Bone marrow

1. Vacuolation of precursors
   Variable cellularity
2. Secondary changes due to:
   (a) Folate deficiency
   (b) Haemolysis
   (c) Iron overload with sideroblastosis
   (d) Iron deficiency
3. Impaired megakaryocytopoiesis

Metabolic disturbances

The extent to which the haemopoietic abnormalities reported in alcoholic liver disease are due to direct toxicity of alcohol or to the associated nutritional deficiency has long been debated. It is now clear that both mechanisms operate. A carefully executed study by Sullivan and Herbert[160] showed that alcohol interferes with folate metabolism. In three subjects with megaloblastic anaemia, maintained on a folate-deficient diet, alcohol abstinence was associated with reticulocytosis, a fall in serum iron and a return to normoblastic erythropoiesis, while resumption of alcohol had the opposite effect. An increased dose of folic acid was necessary to prevent the megaloblastic anaemia associated with alcohol, and continued alcohol intake depressed erythropoiesis as well as the white cells and platelets. The metabolic block induced by alcohol has not been defined. Inhibition of the liver enzyme tetrahydrofolate formylase by large doses of alcohol, thus preventing incorporation of ^{14}C-labelled formate into DNA has been reported.[6] In addition, alcohol may block the release of *N*-5-methyltetrahydrofolic acid from storage pools, causing deficiency in the bone marrow.[104] Another mechanism suggested is the direct effect of ethanol on the gut mucosa; ten days of heavy intake is sufficient to cause decreased absorption of labelled folic acid.[73] Further studies by the same workers showed that continued alcohol consumption leads to steatorrhoea in 60 per cent, impaired D-xylose excretion in 76 per cent and abnormal vitamin B_{12} absorption in 53 per cent of patients.[73] Folic acid deficiency per se may have a similar effect so the role of alcohol in producing these abnormalities is not proven.[112]

Alcohol is known to result in significant abnormalities of iron metabolism (see Chapter 34). Severe blood loss or, rarely, dietary deficiency may alter the picture but usually there is an increase in reticuloendothelial iron stores and ring sideroblasts in the bone marrow, a raised serum iron and an increased transferrin saturation. Withdrawal of alcohol rapidly reverses these abnormalities and this suggests that alcohol has a direct toxic effect. A metabolic block in the conversion of pyridoxine to pyridoxal phosphate[81] is suggested by low pyridoxine phosphate serum levels and reversal of the sideroblastic changes by pyridoxal phosphate, whereas intravenous pyridoxine did not have the same effect. The picture is obviously complex; pyridoxine supplements as well as an adequate diet can prevent the sideroblastic change[111] and altered folate metabolism may be a necessary prerequisite.[44]

Laboratory findings

Macrocytosis is the commonest morphological change seen in the peripheral blood of patients with alcoholic liver disease, being reported in nearly 90 per cent of chronic alcoholics.[183] It is suggested that macrocytosis should alert the clinician to the possibility of alcohol abuse;[182] there is usually no associated anaemia. The mean corpuscular volume is moderately raised with Coulter 'S' values of 97 to 105 fl. Most patients have normal folate levels[183] and the macrocytosis disappears on alcohol withdrawal; folate supplementation will not correct the macrocytosis if alcohol abuse continues. The pathogenesis is not clearly established but a direct toxic effect and the membrane changes resulting from increased plasma cholesterol levels are both implicated.

Stomatocytosis is a transient phenomenon associated with acute alcoholism in approximately one-quarter of patients in one study.[42] This is occasionally associated with haemolysis but there is no direct correlation between the degree of stomatocytosis and the occurrence of haemolysis.[109] Target cells are not usually described in alcoholism, their presence suggesting obstructive jaundice and established cirrhosis. Acanthocytosis is the abnormality described when acute haemolytic anaemia complicates alcoholic liver disease. While there is good evidence that increased cholesterol and altered membrane lipids are important in the development of these abnormalities the exact pathogenesis of these changes is not understood.

The bone marrow changes noted in acute alcoholism are quite striking and occur frequently.[123] The overall cellularity of the marrow may be reduced although with the development of cirrhosis the bone marrow usually shows normal or increased cellularity.[98] There is vacuolation of the erythroid precursors and, to a lesser extent, the myeloid precursors which rapidly disappears after alcohol withdrawal. The chemical nature of the vacuoles has not been elucidated by cytochemical techniques[111] and under the electron microscope vacuoles are seen to be formed by a process of red cell membrane invagination,[184] suggesting a direct toxic effect of alcohol on the cells.

Eichner and Hillman[44] studied 65 patients with chronic alcoholism and concluded that the bone marrow changes and development of anaemia takes place in a predictable fashion. Initially, reduced dietary intake and excessive alcohol leads to a negative vitamin balance characterized by a marked drop in the serum folate levels, a finding noted in 80 per cent of alcoholics with cirrhosis. After one to three weeks of continued folate deficiency[78] the red cell folate falls and erythropoiesis becomes megaloblastic, and soon after this sideroblastic changes occur.[111] This effect may be prevented by small doses of pyridoxine. Adequate iron stores are essential for the development of this picture. Recovery rapidly takes place with a normal diet or abstinence from alcohol and erythropoiesis will become normoblastic, vacuolation will disappear and marrow iron stores will decrease. Five to ten days after stopping alcohol the bone marrow will show erythroid hyperplasia and the reticulocyte count will be high. The picture at this stage is indistinguishable from a haemolytic anaemia and if lipaemia is noted an erroneous diagnosis of Zieve's syndrome may be made. Folic acid is the haematinic of choice and will correct the megaloblastic picture.

Haemolytic anaemia and the distinct haemolytic syndromes, i.e. Zieve's syndrome, 'spur' cell anaemia and chronic haemolytic anaemia, have been discussed previously.

Other causes of anaemia such as iron deficiency due to gastrointestinal blood loss, hypersplenism and dilutional anaemia are all described in patients with chronic alcoholic liver disease.[109]

The effect of alcohol on the white cell series is less well described. Vacuolation of the white cell precursors and of the mature cells in the peripheral blood [92] and neutropenia,[115] together with an impaired leucocyte response to infections,[124] have been reported. Patients with alcoholic liver disease may have increased susceptibility to infection and although simple depression of the cough reflex by alcoholic intoxication may explain the frequency of pneumonia[4] an impaired granulocyte response to acute bacterial infection has been demonstrated.[21,124] The reason for this is not clear; neutropenia, if present, is usually mild[45,115] and other factors such as defective reticuloendothelial clearance of organisms,[168] a direct toxic effect of alcohol on granulocyte mobilization[14] and defective cellular immunity[3] have all been suggested.

A direct toxic effect on the marrow has also been suggested as a cause of the thrombocytopenia noted in acute alcoholism. Heavy alcohol intake for only six days will impair megakaryocytopoiesis and accelerated platelet production usually seen after induced thrombocytopenia.[161] Long-standing alcohol intake will cause thrombocytopenia in most patients, counts between 50 and $100 \times 10^9/l$ being common,[36] and indeed Cowan and Hines[36] have suggested that alcoholism is the commonest cause of thrombocytopenia in the United States. Reduced platelet survival may be a contributory factor. On resuming a normal diet with alcohol abstinence the platelet count rises within two to three days, daily increases being of the order of 20 to $30 \times 10^9/l$. Failure of the thrombocytopenia to respond within a week of alcohol withdrawal should suggest some other underlying mechanism. Rebound thrombocytosis is well described.[110]

Clinical features

It is apparent that haematological abnormalities associated with acute intoxication are due both to a direct toxic effect on the bone marrow and to the associated nutritional deficiencies. Anaemia may develop but is usually mild because of the ability of the bone marrow to compensate and will be corrected by alcohol withdrawal. The acute haemolytic anaemia associated with alcoholic excess is similarly self-limiting, requiring no active treatment other than alcohol withdrawal.

The anaemia associated with long-standing alcoholism and cirrhosis is multifactorial; alcohol withdrawal, treatment with folic acid, control of the associated coagulation abnormalities and bleeding problems are obvious therapeutic measures which may result in haematological improvement and amelioration of the patient's general condition. The final factor determining the outcome will be the degree of hepatocellular failure.

Non-alcoholic Cirrhosis

Most clinical and experimental studies of anaemia in patients with chronic liver disease have included a large number of alcoholic patients. While the pathogenesis of the haematological abnormalities in alcoholic and non-alcoholic cirrhosis must be similar to some extent, since haemolysis, hypersplenism, blood loss and the disturbances associated with chronic disease are present in both conditions, there are differences. The metabolic and nutritional consequences of alcoholism are lacking and folic acid deficiency and megaloblastic anaemia are rarely seen in non-alcoholic liver disease.[98,100] The striking sideroblastic change noted in chronic alcoholics is similarly much less evident in non-alcoholic cirrhosis, although it has been described.[82]

Although target cells are described in alcoholic patients, they are usually associated with cholestasis and characteristically are most striking in obstructive jaundice. As mentioned previously, target cells have an increased osmotic resistance but a normal survival, and provided liver function is normal are not associated with anaemia.[33] Their significance lies in drawing attention to the possibility of liver disease. Another interesting feature noted in about one-third of a small group of patients with chronic active hepatitis was a moderate eosinophilia.[180] Increased plasma cells have been reported in the bone marrow of patients with cirrhosis and were proportional to the hypergammaglobulinaemia, a common finding in chronic liver disease.[91]

Autoimmune haemolytic anaemia is a rare complication in patients with chronic active hepatitis or primary biliary cirrhosis (PBC)[85,135] and excites interest because of the association of disease of an autoimmune nature. Typically, the antibody is IgG in type and shows Rh specificity. Treatment with steroids may be successful in reducing haemolysis of this type. In non-immune haemolytic anaemia associated with PBC, the degree of liver dysfunction is an important factor in the production of the anaemia.[85]

Hepatocellular Carcinoma and Erythrocytosis

Erythrocytosis is a rare complication of hepatocellular carcinoma, although well recognized,[66,125,169] the frequency being between 5 and 10 per cent. Most hepatomas are superimposed on pre-existing cirrhosis and because there is often an increased plasma volume in this condition the frequency of an absolute increase in red cell mass may be higher. It has been suggested that at haematocrit levels as low as 48 per cent an increased red cell mass would invariably be present.[95] The clinical features of hepatocellular carcinoma are described in Chapter 38.

The usual features suggestive of polycythaemia vera are of little value in this situation. For example, splenomegaly may be present because of the pre-existing cirrhosis. Leucocytosis is reported in one-third of cases and is usually mild[46] although a leukaemoid reaction is described. An increased platelet count is unusual in the erythrocytosis complicating hepatocellular carcinoma. The oxygen saturation and blood pressure were normal in a small group of patients and raised plasma erythropoietin levels were noted in about half. Attempts to show that increased amounts of erythropoietin are generated by the liver tumour are not convincing[167] and although experimental studies in nephrectomized rats have suggested that the liver is an extrarenal source of erythropoietin, this is not proven.[53] Increased production by rapidly growing liver tissue of a substrate which is converted by the enzymatic renal factor to active erythropoietin has been proposed as one mechanism whereby erythrocytosis develops.[63] No substance with direct erythropoietin activity has been isolated from the normal or neoplastic liver tissue.

COAGULATION DISTURBANCES ASSOCIATED WITH LIVER DISEASE

Effect on Coagulation Factors

Vitamin K dependent factors

Deficiency of the vitamin K dependent factors II, VII, IX and X causes abnormalities in both the extrinsic and intrinsic pathways, resulting in prolongation of the prothrombin time (PT) and the cephalin or partial thromboplastin time (PTT) respectively. Failure to synthesize these factors is an early consequence of liver disease and prolongation of the PT and PTT may be noted while other biochemical tests of liver function are still normal. Two additional tests which are sensitive to deficiency of these factors are (a) the thrombotest, sensitive to the anticoagulant effect of precursor proteins induced by vitamin K absence (PIVKA) and (b) the normotest, which is not affected by PIVKA. These two tests may be used to try to distinguish between hepatocellular failure with impaired production of the precursor protein, and therefore no PIVKA, and vitamin K deficiency with normal protein synthesis and PIVKA in the plasma. In practice these tests are probably no more helpful than the PT alone.[173] The PT is considered the best screening test for coagulation defects in liver disease.[68,101] The PTT is usually also prolonged and occasionally may be abnormal when the PT is within the normal range.[41,105]

Assay of the individual factors has been carried out to see if this is helpful in assessing the degree of liver damage, particularly in acute situations such as paracetamol poisoning and fulminant hepatitis. Factor VII has the shortest half-life (approximately six hours) and severe reduction (below 9 per cent) was shown to carry a poor prognosis in a small group of patients with acute hepatic failure.[43] Of other factors examined only fibrinogen estimation using a clot opacity technique[87] provided a reasonable, but less significant, guide to prognosis.

Factors II, VII, IX and X may be reduced in patients with liver disease because of failed synthesis but will also fall in obstructive jaundice because of impaired absorption of the fat-soluble vitamin K. Treatment with vitamin K can be used to distinguish the underlying mechanism of a coagulation defect in patients with liver disease since this will not correct the coagulation abnormality of hepatocellular failure.[148,155] Not uncommonly, however, there may be a degree of obstruction superimposed on underlying hepatocellular failure and some improvement of the coagulation defect may result from vitamin K injections.

Fibrinogen

Significant fibrinogen deficiency will prolong the thrombin time, a useful screening test which is also sensitive to the presence of fibrin degradation products (FDPs) and an abnormal fibrinogen molecule. The reptilase time[54] is prolonged in hypofibrinogenaemia and shows greater sensitivity to a qualitative abnormality of fibrinogen than the thrombin time. Quantitative methods such as that of Ratnoff and Menzie[142] are most accurate but are time consuming. Semi-quantitative methods such as fibrin clot weight and fibrinogen titre are clinically useful but are also sensitive to FDPs and fibrinolysis.[151]

Fibrinogen is an 'acute phase' reactive protein and is raised in response to a variety of stimuli, including infection, obstruction and neoplasms. Raised levels have been reported in obstructive jaundice[176] and following extensive liver resection. In mild to moderate liver disease fibrinogen levels are normal.[41,171] Reduced fibrinogen levels are described in fulminant hepatic failure[23] and following liver transplantation[50] but intravascular coagulation may be present.

An abnormal fibrinogen molecule suggested by a long thrombin time and a disproportionate increase in the reptilase time has been described in liver disease. A simple colorimetric method with reptilase[68] demonstrated abnormalities of fibrin polymerization in 50 per cent of patients with advanced liver disease. The part played by the dysfibrinogenaemia in the bleeding diathesis associated with severe liver disease is uncertain. In the patients studied by Green and colleagues[68] it appeared to be of prognostic significance; in 13 patients bleeding from oesophageal varices most of those who died had an abnormal fibrinogen whereas it was not detected in those who survived. Fibrin polymerization was normal in their patients with obstructive jaundice, suggesting that this test might help to differentiate obstructive jaundice from severe parenchymal liver disease. The nature of the abnormality is unknown; indeed, it is not certain whether the defective fibrin monomer polymerization is due to a biochemically abnormal fibrinogen molecule. Decreased D-galactose content of fibrinogen and an increase in sialic acid content[154] have been reported and release from damaged liver cells of a precursor of fibrinogen has been suggested.[15] Comparison of the hepatoma-associated dysfibrinogen with the fibrinogen found in fetal plasma shows striking similarities[64] and both have been shown to have increased sialic acid content of the fibrinogen molecule. Reduction of the sialic acid content restored normal function to the hepatoma-associated fibrinogen, suggesting a molecular abnormality although this is not yet proven.

Factor VIII

Factor VIII assays are of little help in clinically evaluating the coagulation defect in liver disease. Raised levels of both factor VIII coagulant activity and factor VIII related antigen have been described in a variety of liver disorders, including acute viral hepatitis[126] (even in a haemophiliac[59]), alcoholic cirrhosis[65] and non-alcoholic cirrhosis.[134] The reason for the raised factor VIII levels is not clear but distinctly argues against the liver being the major site of factor VIII synthesis. In acute hepatitis the rise in factor VIII may be due to release from the hepatocytes, a mechanism thought to account for the raised serum vitamin B_{12} levels in this condition. Increased production of factor VIII, a reactive protein, by the RE system in response to the disease process or impaired denaturation and clearance of the factor VIII molecule by the damaged liver are other possibilities. Factor VIII levels rise significantly during normal pregnancy and the underlying mechanism here may be compensated low-grade intravascular coagulation;[2] low-grade intravascular coagulation in liver disease might similarly result in raised factor VIII levels.

Factor V

Factor V is synthesized by the liver and as it is not vitamin K dependent, theoretically, low levels should help distinguish hepatocellular failure from obstructive jaundice. In practice, factor V assay does not appear to be a useful test for this purpose.[173] This is partly due to the fact that factor V may be raised in patients with acute infections or could be reduced because of disseminated intravascular coagulation.

Other factors

Assay of the contact factors has shown that reduced levels are present in patients with hepatic disease.[141] Technically such assays are difficult and clinically it is unlikely that this observation is significant; even severe congenital deficiency of these factors gives rise to surprisingly few bleeding problems.

Factor XIII is easily assessed by a simple screening test (clot solubility in 5 mol urea or 2 per cent monochloracetic acid). Reduced levels of factor XIII have been reported in hepatocellular disease[119] but not in obstructive jaundice.[176] Low-grade intravascular coagulation might also explain this finding.

Abnormal platelet function has been described in patients with liver disease. Clinically this may be suggested by a prolonged bleeding time. In fulminant hepatic failure impaired aggregation to adenosine diphosphate (ADP) and collagen and structural abnormalities on electron microscopy were demonstrated.[146] Defective aggregation to ristocetin[18] and to ADP and thrombin[164] in cirrhosis may be due to the inhibitory effect of FDPs and fibrin monomers.[163] Control platelet aggregation in patient plasma has given variable results and the pathogenesis and significance of these observations requires further evaluation.

Fibrinolytic activity in liver disease

The basic reactions activating and controlling fibrinolysis are shown in Figure 8.2. Laboratory assessment of fibrinolytic activity is technically difficult, often confusing and would not be within the scope of many laboratories. Tests used to assess fibrinolysis include the measurement of:

1. plasmin and plasminogen activity using fibrin plate methods[38] or lysis of labelled fibrin concentrates;
2. plasminogen activators using the euglobulin clot lysis time;[38]
3. circulating antiplasmin levels, for example antithrombin III;[174]
4. FDPs using techniques such as latex agglutination[56] with the Thrombo-Wellcot kit or haemagglutination inhibition immunoassay.[127]

Various 'paracoagulation' tests such as ethanol gelation or protamine sulphate tests are used to detect the presence of soluble fibrin/FDP complexes.

While much of the evidence is conflicting increased fibrinolytic activity has been frequently noted in cirrhosis of the liver[49,62,103,140] and following surgical resection of the liver[175] and liver transplantation.[156] Decreased fibrinolytic activity has been reported in acute hepatic failure[23] and in obstructive jaundice[93] where it was associated with raised triglyceride levels.

The underlying mechanism leading to changes in the fibrinolytic system in liver disease is controversial. Bleeding as a result of increased fibrinolysis could result from primary activation of fibrinolysis because of impaired clearance of circulating plasminogen activator released following surgery,[49] trauma or other precipitating causes. Alternatively, fibrinolysis could be secondary to underlying disseminated intravascular coagulation (DIC) initiated because of impaired clearance by the liver of activated coagulation products or perhaps decreased synthesis of plasminogen.[23] Plasminogen levels have been reported as normal or low in liver disease.[165] Whether low levels lead to DIC or are a consequence of it is not clear. In the same way, reduced antiplasmins could either predispose to fibrinolysis or could result from activation of the fibrinolytic mechanism. The antiplasmins alpha-1-antitrypsin and alpha-2-macroglobulin have been variously reported as reduced and increased in liver disease and interpretation of these findings is difficult at the present time.[137]

The concept of intravascular coagulation as the primary event is supported by evidence that heparin can reverse such abnormalities as increased breakdown of fibrinogen[171] and hypofibrinogenaemia and thrombocytopenia[84] in patients with cirrhosis.

In summary it would seem possible that primary fibrinolysis is operative in situations of acute liver trauma and surgical stress whereas intravascular coagulation with secondary fibrinolysis is a complication of chronic hepatocellular failure.

Considerable interest has recently been focused on antithrombin III in patients with liver disease, low levels being reported in a variety of liver disorders including chronic liver disease.[121,174] Hereditary deficiency of antithrombin III may lead to the development of a hypercoagulable state[122] and low levels in liver disease could predispose to the development of thrombosis. Reduced levels of antithrombin III have been reported following thrombosis in conditions such as DIC and following surgery and myocardial infarction.[132] Thus interpretation of this observation is difficult.

Clinical Significance of the Coagulation Abnormalities

Patients with established liver disease may bleed for many reasons. Commonly haemorrhage is due to local causes such as oesophageal varices, or gastritis and peptic ulceration. Impaired production of the coagulation factors, especially factors II, VII IX and X, is common and thrombocytopenia and abnormal platelet function may be present. Intravascular coagulation and consumption coagulopathy may contribute to the bleeding problem. Massive transfusion by stored bank blood, low in coagulation factors and platelets, can aggravate and indeed induce a coagulation defect.

Use of coagulation tests to assess function and prognosis

The prothrombin time (PT) and partial thromboplastin time (PTT) are used routinely to screen patients with liver disease and may be considered as liver function tests, occasionally being abnormal while other biochemical tests are within normal limits. With any degree of cellular damage the PT and PTT will be abnormal but bleeding complications will not necessarily be present.[155] In general there is good correlation between coagulation abnormalities and the degree of liver failure; for example, bleeding was noted in three-quarters of patients with acute liver failure[23] and in some was the direct cause of death. Failed synthesis of the clotting factors and disseminated intravascular coagulation are the main reasons for bleeding in such patients, and serial coagulation tests have been used to assess progress and prognosis. In one study of acute liver failure clotting tests rapidly became abnormal and hepatic coma occurred in patients whose PT ratio rose above 2.2.[23] Another group showed that the PT ratio was excessively prolonged (greater than 4.8) in all who died.[43] Similarly, the thrombotest levels are related to prognosis in acute hepatic failure.[79] Of specific factor assays, factor VII appears most significant, levels below 9 per cent being associated with a fatal outcome.[43] In chronic liver disease the factor VII level and the PT correlate well and are equally useful in assessing hepatocellular function. The differential diagnosis of obstructive jaundice and hepatocellular failure is not really helped by detailed coagulation factor analysis. A therapeutic test of vitamin K_1 by parenteral injection (10 mg daily for three days) is helpful, persistent abnormalities indicating functional impairment of the hepatic cells.

Tests such as the PT and PTT are screening tests and may be normal even when specific coagulation factors are as low as 25 to 30 per cent of normal; reductions of this order would be unlikely to lead to bleeding complications. Isolated factor deficiencies have been reported and the association of amyloidosis and factor X deficiency is well recognized.[55]

The clinical significance of laboratory evidence of a coagulation defect is difficult to assess. Many patients with gross abnormalities have little or no spontaneous bleeding. When complications such as oesophageal varices or gastric erosions arise, however, the coagulation defect may prevent normal haemostasis. The greater the coagulation defect the more likely it is that bleeding will occur, but the picture is complex. Bleeding as a result of thrombocytopenia is also a variable phenomenon. As a general rule patients with a platelet count greater than $30 \times 10^9/l$ will not bleed spontaneously but abnormal platelet function may be present. Platelet counts as low as $10 \times 10^9/l$ are rare in patients with liver disease unless there are other complications such as DIC or blood loss; at this level thrombocytopenic bleeding is common, but not necessarily present.

Intravascular Coagulation

Criteria for the diagnosis of significant DIC[17] are marked prolongation of the PT, PTT and thrombin time, evidence of increased lysis and fibrin–fibrinogen breakdown with fibrinogen levels below 1.0 g/l, FDPs greater than 100 g/l and thrombocytopenia (less than $100 \times 10^9/l$). 'Paracoagulation tests' are used in the diagnosis of DIC but a high incidence of false positives has been reported and they do not appear to be helpful in an acute clinical situation.[17] Assay of platelet release factors such as platelet factor IV and beta-thromboglobulin by quantitative radio-immunoassay is a new development which is under investigation.[116] Many of these tests may be abnormal in patients with liver disease for reasons other than DIC and critical evaluation of the significance of laboratory abnormalities is essential.

Evidence of disseminated intravascular coagulation is well documented in patients with liver disease. The pathogenesis is not clear. The combination of release of thromboplastic substances from the diseased liver and impaired hepatic clearance of activated coagulation factors may lead to systemic coagulation. With the generation of thrombin, fibrin and platelet thrombi form and coagulation factors and platelets are consumed. Fibrinolytic mechanisms are activated leading to the formation of plasmin which digests fibrin, fibrinogen and other clotting factors and may lead to further depletion. Fibrin and fibrinogen breakdown leads to FDP formation and impaired fibrin polymerization and the patient may bleed. Clinically significant DIC is rare in uncomplicated cirrhosis of the liver[79] and other trigger factors may be implicated. The commonest cause of DIC is infection[17] and this may be present in some patients with liver disease. Release of endotoxins from the gut may lead to the development of DIC in liver disease.[141] Another situation where DIC may arise is liver transplantation but it has seldom been shown to be a significant cause of bleeding.[50]

The treatment of DIC is unsatisfactory and is difficult. Fortunately most patients with liver disease and DIC do not bleed.[58, 79] The main problem is to assess to what extent the intravascular coagulation is contributing to the bleeding problem. Management of DIC may be summarized as follows:

1. Treat or remove the underlying cause.
2. Replace the missing factors.
3. Take measures to stop continuing thrombosis if necessary.

Trigger factors such as infection, shock, dehydration and vascular stasis must obviously be treated by appropriate methods, and measures which achieve this may be sufficient to control the condition. Serial laboratory assessment will be important to gauge the progress and control of the disease.

No obvious trigger factors may be present and the decision to treat the coagulation defect will depend on the condition of the patient and laboratory evidence of a deteriorating situation.

The bleeding patient with evidence of severe consumption coagulopathy will need to be given replacement therapy. This approach has been questioned on the basis that the bleeding diathesis is due in part to the presence of breakdown products of fibrin and other activated products and their replacement may add 'fuel to the fire'. Such a theory is difficult to prove and if a patient has a severe coagulation defect and is bleeding, specific therapy will be given. If fresh blood, which contains platelets, red cells and coagulation factors, is not available, packed red cells and fresh frozen plasma (FFP) will be given instead. Prothrombin and other concentrates should not be used in DIC. Severe hypofibrinogenaemia may be treated by cryoprecipitate, a rich source of fibrinogen and factor VIII.

If the situation is deteriorating clinically in spite of these measures and there is laboratory evidence of continuing DIC, treatment with heparin will be considered. Since liver disease is often complicated by varices or other gastrointestinal lesions which may bleed, the use of anticoagulants must be viewed with extreme caution. Results of heparin therapy are variable but its value has not yet been proved by any controlled prospective trial. An uncontrolled study of 20 patients with acute hepatic necrosis treated with heparin and fresh frozen plasma suggested this might be beneficial,[23] but a later study in paracetamol-induced hepatic necrosis showed no significant difference when FFP was compared with FFP and heparin.[58]

Increased survival of ^{125}I-labelled fibrinogen was noted in a small group of patients with cirrhosis treated with low dose heparin[25] and this might be a safer alternative to full dosage heparin since its prophylactic use in surgical patients is not followed by significant bleeding.[88] In the absence of convincing evidence that heparin administration leads to significant improvement in DIC[11] the present recommendation would be to reserve this for cases where therapy as outlined previously has failed to reverse life-threatening haemorrhage or thrombosis.

The use of fibrinolytic inhibitors such as epsilon aminocaproic acid and tranexamic acid (Cyclokapron) has been considered for patients where excess fibrinolysis is a major component of the coagulopathy.[137] Such drugs are unphysiological in their action and have theoretical dangers in their use but could be considered, possibly with heparin, when all other measures have failed.

Management of the Coagulation Defect

Non-bleeding patients

In patients about to undergo surgery or liver biopsy, correction of the coagulation defect is necessary. If this cannot be achieved, the decision to proceed with operation or biopsy will depend on its clinical indication.

Vitamin K_1 by intramuscular injection 10 mg daily is given for three days, although maximal correction of the PT is usually achieved within 24 hours. Persistent abnormality beyond this period indicates hepatocellular dysfunction. The use of FFP and prothrombin complex concentrates (PCC) may temporarily correct the defect, the haemostatic effect lasting for a few hours and being sufficient to enable liver biopsy to be carried out safely. Haemostatic control in patients undergoing surgery requires repeated administration of these products over a period of seven to ten days, as is routine for such conditions as Christmas disease.

The decision to use PCC or FFP will depend on the circumstances. FFP must be given in large amounts with the attendant problems of fluid overload and would not be the therapeutic material of choice in patients undergoing surgery. PCC is made up in a small volume of diluent and patients with Christmas disease requiring surgery are treated successfully with these preparations. The multiple deficiencies associated with liver disease are more difficult to correct and complications more likely to occur. Early users of PCC in patients with liver disease reported intravascular coagulation which occasionally proved fatal[10, 58] and it was subsequently shown that concentrates contained activated products. Improved fractionation techniques and exclusion of factor VII has reduced this risk and several of the currently available products contain only factors II, IX and X. With improved in vitro testing for spontaneous thrombin generation[147] concentrates are now considered safe in patients with liver disease even when factor VII is not excluded.[66, 120] Patients with an increased risk of thrombosis should not be treated with such concentrates as they are liable to develop thrombotic complications.[178] Such a hypercoagulable state would be suggested by a history of a previous thrombotic episode or certain coagulation abnormalities such as low levels of antithrombin III.

Even with increased sensitivity of techniques to detect the hepatitis B virus and careful screening of all plasma pooled to make the concentrates, the risk of developing hepatitis still remains (see Chapter 28). Commercial preparations made from plasma taken from paid donors may carry a greater hepatitis risk than concentrates such as the National Health Service concentrate or the Oxford Fractionation Laboratory product which rely on voluntary contributions.

The correction using PCC with either three or four factors has been compared with that achieved using FFP[66, 120] but as yet no definite regimen can be recommended. The latter group showed that a combination of FFP (8 ml/kg body weight) and a four-factor concentrate (12 units/kg body weight) best corrected the defect in patients being prepared for liver biopsy. A single dose of FFP (12 ml/kg) was not effective nor was concentrate lacking factor VII. A current Medical Research Council trial is comparing a three-factor PCC (10 units factor IX/kg body weight) with FFP (5 units factor IX/kg body weight) but limited success has been achieved with this dosage. Maximal correction is usually achieved within 15 minutes of administration of this dose and a second dose can be given with some further improvement. The results of further clinical studies are awaited.

Associated thrombocytopenia is an obvious hazard in patients undergoing liver biopsy but, provided the bleeding time is normal, moderate thrombocytopenia is not a contraindication. The bleeding time is a simple practical manoeuvre which should be performed in any doubtful case; significant prolongation would be considered an absolute contraindication to elective liver biopsy or surgery.

Bleeding patients

Extensive haemorrhage from gastrointestinal lesions such as oesophageal varices and gastric erosions may give rise to a life-threatening situation. Local measures to stem the blood loss such as the use of Sengstaken–Blakemore tubes are discussed in Chapter 43. Any associated coagulation defect will be treated vigorously with the measures described in the foregoing section. The benefit is usually temporary and repeated administration of FFP and or PCC is often necessary to maintain haemostasis. Blood transfusion with fresh whole blood is to be recommended in massive haemorrhage since rapid replacement with stored bank blood may aggravate the coagulation defect. It is often not possible for such requirements to be met but it is recommended that approximately 10 per cent of any massive transfusion should be fresh blood (i.e., less than 24 hours old). If this service is not available. FFP and platelet concentrates should be given. Marked thrombocytopenia may be temporarily corrected by platelet transfusion but it is often difficult to achieve a significant rise in the platelet count. Defects of platelet function are difficult to correct but transfusion with platelet concentrates may be worth trying.

Other measures rarely considered in this situation include the use of plasmapheresis to replace defective plasma which may contain circulating fibrin complexes and FDPs by fresh plasma, without the attendant problems of circulatory overload. Such measures would have a temporary effect but might tide the patient over a life-threatening episode of haemostatic failure associated with acute hepatic necrosis, allowing time for recovery of liver function. On the whole these measures are disappointing, but in desperate situations would be worth trying.

REFERENCES

1. Aster, R.H. (1966) Pooling of platelets in the spleen: role in the pathogenesis of hypersplenic thrombocytopaenia. *Journal of Clinical Investigation,* **45,** 645–657.
2. Bennett, B. & Ratnoff, O.D. (1972) Changes in antihaemophilic factor (AHF factor VIII) procoagulant activity and AHF-like antigen in normal pregnancy and following exercise and pneumoencephalography. *Journal of Laboratory and Clinical Medicine,* **80,** 256–263.
3. Berenyi, M.R., Straus, B. & Cruz, D. (1974) In vitro and in vivo studies of cellular immunity in alcoholic cirrhosis. *American Journal of Digestive Diseases,* **19,** 199–205.
4. Berkowitz, H., Reichel, J. & Shim, C. (1973) The effect of ethanol on the cough reflex. *Clinical Science and Molecular Medicine,* **45,** 527–531.
5. Berman, L., Axelrod, A.R., Horan, T.N., Jacobson, S.D., Sharp, E.A. & Von der Heide, E.C. (1949) The blood and bone marrow in patients with cirrhosis of the liver. *Blood,* **4,** 511–533.
6. Bertino, J.R., Ward, J., Sartorelli, A.C. & Silber, R. (1965) An effect of ethanol on folate metabolism. *Journal of Clinical Investigation,* **44,** 1028.
7. Bessis, M., Weed, R. & Le Blond, P. (1973) *Red Cell Shape: Physiology, Pathology, Ultrastructure.* New York: Springer-Verlag.
8. Bingham, J. (1959) The macrocytosis of hepatic disease. I. Thin macrocytosis. *Blood,* **14,** 244–254.
9. Bingham, J. (1960) The macrocytosis of hepatic disease. II. Thick macrocytosis. *Blood,* **15,** 694–707.
10. Blatt, P.M., Lundblad, R.L., Kingdon, M.S., McLean, G. & Roberts, M.R. (1974) Thrombogenic materials in prothrombin complex concentrates. *Annals of Internal Medicine,* **81,** 766–770.
11. Bloom, A.L. (1975) Annotation: intravascular coagulation and the liver. *British Journal of Haematology,* **30,** 1–7.
12. Bloom, A.L., Giddings, J.C. & Wilks, C.J. (1973) Factor VIII on the vascular intima: possible importance in haemostasis and thrombosis. *Nature New Biology,* **241,** 217–219.
13. Brain, M.C. (1977) Red cell membrane structure and function. In *Recent Advances in Haematology* (Ed.) Hoffbrand, A.V., Brain, M.C. & Hirsh, J. pp. 27–41. Edinburgh, London and New York: Churchill Livingstone.
14. Brayton, R.G., Stokes, P.E., Schwartz, M.S. & Louria, D.B. (1970) Effect of alcohol and various diseases on leukocyte mobilization, phagocytosis and intracellular bacterial killing. *New England Journal of Medicine,* **282,** 123–128.
15. Brodsky, I., Siegel, M.H., Kahn, S.B., Ross, E.M. & Petkov, G. (1970) Simultaneous fibrinogen and platelet survival with (^{75}Se) selenomethionine in man. *British Journal of Haematology,* **18,** 341–355.
16. Brownstein, M.H. & Balliard, H.S. (1966) Hepatoma associated with erythrocytosis. Report of eleven new cases. *American Journal of Medicine,* **40,** 204–210.
17. Cash, J.D. (1977) Disseminated intravascular coagulation. In *Recent Advances in Blood Coagulation* (Ed.) Poller, L. pp. 293–311. Edinburgh, London and New York: Churchill Livingstone.
18. Castillo, R., Maragall, S., Rodés, J., Clemente, C., Profitos, J. & Ordinas, A. (1977) Increased factor VIII complex and defective ristocetin induced platelet aggregation in liver disease. *Thrombosis Research,* **11,** 899–906.
19. Chanarin, I. (1969) *The Megaloblastic Anaemias.* pp. 328–330. Oxford and Edinburgh: Blackwell Scientific Publications.
20. Chiandussi, L., Bianco, A., Massaro, A., Mazza, V. & Cesano, L. (1964) The quantitative determination of iron kinetics and haemoglobin synthesis in anaemia of cirrhosis studies with ^{59}Fe. *Blut,* **10,** 120.
21. Chomet, B. & Gach, B.M. (1967) Lobar pneumonia and alcoholism: an analysis of thirty seven cases. *American Journal of Medical Science,* **253,** 300–304.
22. Choremis, C., Kattamis, Ch. A., Kyriazakou, M. & Gavrillidou, E. (1966) Viral hepatitis in G6PD deficiency. *Lancet,* **i,** 269–270.
23. Clark, R., Rake, M.O., Flute, P.T. & Williams, R. (1973) Coagulation abnormalities in acute liver failure. *Scandinavian Journal of Gastroenterology,* (Suppl. 8) **19,** 63–70.
24. Clearfield, H.R., Brody, J.I. & Tumen, H.J. (1969) Acute viral hepatitis, glucose-6-phosphate dehydrogenase deficiency and hemolytic anemia. *Archives of Internal Medicine,* **123,** 689–691.
25. Coleman, M., Finlayson, N., Bettigole, R.E., Sadula, D., Cohn, M. & Pasmantier, M. (1975) Fibrinogen survival in cirrhosis: improvement by low dose heparin. *Annals of Internal Medicine,* **83,** 79–81.
26. Conrad, M.E. (1969) Persistent haemolysis after infectious hepatitis. *Gut,* **10,** 516–521.
27. Conrad, M.E., Berman, A. & Crosby, W.H. (1962) Iron kinetics in Laennec's cirrhosis. *Gastroenterology,* **43,** 385–390.
28. Conrad, M.E., Schwartz, F.D. & Young, A.A. (1964) Infectious hepatitis – a generalised disease. *American Journal of Medicine,* **37,** 789–801.
29. Cooper, R.A. (1969) Anaemia with spur cells: a red cell defect acquired in serum and modified in the circulation. *Journal of Clinical Investigation,* **48,** 1820–1831.
30. Cooper, R.A. (1970) Lipids of human red cell membrane: normal composition and variability in disease. *Seminars in Hematology,* **7,** 296–322.
31. Cooper, R.A. & Jandl, J.H. (1968) Bile salts and cholesterol in the pathogenesis of target cells in obstructive jaundice. *Journal of Clinical Investigation,* **47,** 809–822.
32. Cooper, R.A., Kimball, D.B. & Durocher, J.R. (1974) Role of the spleen in membrane conditioning and hemolysis of spur cells of liver disease. *New England Journal of Medicine,* **290,** 1279–1284.
33. Cooper, R.A., Diloy-Puray, M., Lando, P. & Greenberg, M.S. (1972) An analysis of lipoproteins, bile acids and red cell membranes associated with target cells and spur cells in patients with liver disease. *Journal of Clinical Investigation,* **51,** 3182–3192.
34. Cooper, R.A., Arner, E.C., Wiley, J.S. & Shattil, S.J. (1975) Modification of red cell membrane structure by cholesterol-rich lipid dispersions. A model for the primary spur cell defect. *Journal of Clinical Investigation,* **55,** 115–126.
35. Cowan, D.H. (1973) Thrombokinetic studies in alcohol related thrombocytopaenia. *Journal of Laboratory and Clinical Medicine,* **81,** 64–76.

36. Cowan, D.H. & Hines, J.D. (1971) Thrombocytopaenia of severe alcoholism. *Annals of Internal Medicine*, **74**, 37–43.

37. Dacie, J.V. (1967) *The Haemolytic Anaemias, Part III – Secondary or Symptomatic Anaemias*. pp. 826–837. London: J. & A. Churchill.

38. Dacie, J.V. & Lewis, S.M. (1975) *Practical Haematology*. Edinburgh, London and New York: Churchill Livingstone.

39. Deller, D.J., Kimber, C.L. & Ibbotson, R.N. (1965) Folic acid deficiency in cirrhosis of the liver. *American Journal of Digestive Diseases*, **10**, 35–42.

40. Denny, G.P. & Minot, G.R. (1915) The origin of antithrombin. *American Journal of Physiology*, **38**, 233.

41. Donaldson, G.W.K., Davies, S.H., Darg, A. & Richmond, J. (1969) Coagulation factors in chronic liver disease. *Journal of Clinical Pathology*, **22**, 199–204.

42. Douglass, C.C. & Twomey, J.J. (1970) Transient stomatocytosis with haemolysis: a previously unrecognised complication of alcoholism. *Annals of Internal Medicine*, **72**, 159–164.

43. Dymock, I.W., Tucker, J.S., Woolf, I.L., Poller, L. & Thomson, J.M. (1975) Coagulation studies as a prognostic index in acute liver failure. *British Journal of Haematology*, **29**, 385–395.

44. Eichner, E.R. & Hillman, R.S. (1971) The evolution of anemia in alcoholic patients. *American Journal of Medicine*, **50**, 218–232.

45. Eichner, E.R., Buchanan, B., Smith, J.W. & Hillman, R.S. (1972) Variations in the hematologic and medical status of alcoholics. *American Journal of Medicine*, **263**, 35–42.

46. Eppstein, S. (1964) Primary carcinoma of the liver. *American Journal of the Medical Sciences*, **247**, 137.

47. Finkbiner, R.B., McGovern, J.J., Goldstein, R. & Bunker, J.P. (1959) Coagulation defects in liver disease and response to transfusion during surgery. *American Journal of Medicine*, **26**, 199–213.

48. Finks, R.M. & Blumberg, R.W. (1945) Epidemic hepatitis with and without jaundice: some clinical studies on two hundred and twenty five patients among troops in a combat zone. *Archives of Internal Medicine*, **76**, 102.

49. Fletcher, A.P., Biederman, D., Moore, D., Alkjaersig, N. & Sherry, S. (1964) Abnormal plasminogen – plasmin system activity (fibrinolysis) in patients with hepatic cirrhosis. *Journal of Clinical Investigation*, **43**, 681–695.

50. Flute, P.T., Rake, M.O., Williams, R., Seaman, M.J. & Calne, R.Y. (1969) Liver transplantation in man. IV. Haemorrhage and thrombosis. *British Medical Journal*, **iii**, 20–23.

51. Fodor, O. & Tanasescu, R. (1962) Anemiile hemolitice immunologice posthepatice. *Medicina Interna (Bucuresti)*, **14**, 1469–1476.

52. Forman, W.B. & Barnhart, M.I. (1964) Cellular site for fibrinogen synthesis. *Journal of the American Medical Association*, **187**, 128–132.

53. Fried, W. (1972) The liver as a source of extrarenal erythropoietin production. *Blood*, **40**, 671–677.

54. Funk, C., Gmur, J., Herold, R. & Straub, P.W. (1971) Reptilase-R. A new reagent in blood coagulation. *British Journal of Haematology*, **21**, 43–52.

55. Galbraith, P.A., Sharma, N., Parker, W.L. & Kilgour, J.M. (1974) Acquired factor X deficiency: altered plasma antithrombin activity and association with amyloidosis. *Journal of the American Medical Association*, **230**, 1658–1660.

56. Garvey, M.B. & Black, J.M. (1972) The detection of fibrinogen/fibrin degradation products by means of a new antibody coated latex particle. *Journal of Clinical Pathology*, **25**, 680–682.

57. Gazzard, B.G., Clark, R., Borirakchanyavat, V. & Williams, R. (1974) A controlled trial of heparin therapy in the coagulation defect of paracetamol-induced hepatic necrosis. *Gut*, **15**, 89–93.

58. Gazzard, B.G., Lewis, M.L., Ash, G., Rizza, C.R., Bidwell, E. & Williams, R. (1974) Coagulation factor concentrates in the treatment of the haemorrhagic diathesis of fulminant hepatic failure. *Gut*, **15**, 993–998.

59. Gazzard, B.G., Clark, R., Flute, P.J. & Williams, R. (1975) Factor VIII levels during the course of acute hepatitis in a haemophiliac. *Journal of Clinical Pathology*, **28**, 972–974.

60. Goebel, K.M., Goebel, F.D., Schubotz, R. & Schneider, J. (1977) Red cell metabolic and membrane features in haemolytic anaemia of alcoholic liver disease (Zieve's syndrome). *British Journal of Haematology*, **35**, 573–585.

61. Goodnight, S.H. Jr, Feinstein, D.I., Østerad, B. & Rapaport, S.I. (1971) Factor VII antibody neutralizing material in hereditary and acquired factor VII deficiency. *Blood*, **38**, 1–8.

62. Goodpasture, E.W. (1914) Fibrinolysis in chronic hepatic insufficiency. *Bulletin of the Johns Hopkins Hospital*, **25**, 330.

63. Gordon, A.S., Zanjani, E.D. & Zalusky, R. (1970) A possible mechanism for the erythrocytosis associated with hepatocellular carcinoma in man. *Blood*, **35**, 151–157.

64. Gralnick, H.R., Givelber, H. & Abrams, E. (1978) Dysfibrinogenaemia associated with hepatoma: increased carbohydrate content of the fibrinogen molecule. *New England Journal of Medicine*, **299**, 221–226.

65. Green, A.J. & Ratnoff, O.D. (1974) Elevated antihaemophiliac factor (AHF factor VIII) procoagulant activity and AHF – like antigen in alcoholic cirrhosis of the liver. *Journal of Laboratory and Clinical Medicine*, **83**, 189–197.

66. Green, G., Dymock, I.W., Poller, L. & Thomson, J.M. (1975) The use of a factor VII rich prothrombin complex concentrate in liver disease. *Lancet*, **i**, 1311–1314.

67. Green, G., Poller, L., Thomson, J.M. & Dymock, I.W. (1976) Factor VII as a marker of hepatocellular synthetic function in liver disease. *Journal of Clinical Pathology*, **29**, 971–975.

68. Green, G., Thomson, J.M., Dymock, I.W. & Poller, L. (1976) Abnormal fibrin polymerization in liver disease. *British Journal of Haematology*, **34**, 427–439.

69. Grossi, C.E., Rousselot, L.M. & Parke, W.F. (1964) Control of fibrinolysis during portocaval shunts. *Journal of the American Medical Association*, **187**, 1005–1008.

70. Hagler, L., Pastore, R.A., Bergin, J.J. & Wrensch, M.R. (1975) Aplastic anaemia following viral hepatitis. *Medicine*, **54**, 139–164.

71. Hall, C.A. (1960) Erythrocyte dynamics in liver disease. *American Journal of Medicine*, **28**, 541–549.

72. Halsted, C.H., Robles, E.A. & Mezey, E. (1971) Decreased jejunal uptake of labelled folic acid (3H PGA) in alcoholic patients: roles of alcohol and nutrition. *New England Journal of Medicine*, **285**, 701–706.

73. Halsted, C.H., Robles, E.A. & Mezey, E. (1973) Intestinal malabsorption in folate deficient alcoholics. *Gastroenterology*, **64,** 526–532.
74. Hardisty, R.M. & Weatherall, D.J. (1974) *Blood and its Disorders*. Oxford, London, Edinburgh and Melbourne: Blackwell Scientific Publications.
75. Havens, W.P. & Marck, R.E. (1946) The leukocytic response of patients with experimentally induced infectious hepatitis. *American Journal of the Medical Sciences*, **212,** 129.
76. Hemker, H.C., Veltkamp, J.J., Hensen, A. & Leoliger, E.A. (1963) Nature of prothrombin biosynthesis: preprothrombinaemia in vitamin K deficiency. *Nature*, **200,** 589–590.
77. Herbert, V. (1962) Experimental nutritional folate deficiency in man. *Transactions of the Association of American Physicians*, **75,** 307.
78. Herbert, V., Zalusky, R. & Davidson, C.S. (1963) Correlation of folate deficiency with alcoholism and associated macrocytosis, anaemia and liver disease. *Annals of Internal Medicine*, **58,** 977–988.
79. Hillenbrand, P., Parbhoo, S.B., Jedrychowski, A. & Sherlock, S. (1974) Significance of intravascular coagulation and fibrinolysis in acute hepatic failure. *Gut*, **15,** 83–88.
80. Hines, J.D. (1969) Reversible megaloblastic and sideroblastic marrow abnormalities in alcoholic patients. *British Journal of Haematology*, **16,** 87–101.
81. Hines, J.D. & Cowan, D.H. (1970) Studies on the pathogenesis of alcohol-induced sideroblastic bone marrow abnormalities. *New England Journal of Medicine*, **283,** 441–446.
82. Hines, J.D. & Grasso, J.A. (1970) The sideroblastic anaemias. *Seminars in Haematology*, **7,** 86–106.
83. Hoffbrand, A.V. (1972) *The Red Cell Folate Assay*. M.D. Thesis, University of Oxford.
84. Horder, M.H. (1969) Consumption coagulopathy in liver cirrhosis. *Thrombosis et Diathesis Haemorrhagica* (Suppl.), **36,** 313–318.
85. Hume, R., Williamson, J.M. & Whitelaw, J.W. (1970) Red cell survival in biliary cirrhosis. *Journal of Clinical Pathology*, **23,** 397–401.
86. Hyman, G.A. & Southworth, H. (1951) Hemolytic anemia associated with liver disease. *American Journal of the Medical Sciences*, **221,** 448–456.
87. Ingram, G.I.C. & Matchett, M.O. (1960) A rapid 'side-room' method for the determination of plasma fibrinogen concentration as fibrin. *Journal of Clinical Pathology*, **13,** 469–474.
88. International Multicentre Trial (1975) Prevention of fatal postoperative pulmonary embolism by low doses of heparin. *Lancet*, **ii,** 45–51.
89. Jandl, J.H. (1955) The anaemia of liver disease: observations on its mechanism. *Journal of Clinical Investigation*, **34,** 390–404.
90. Jandl, J.H. & Lear, A.A. (1956) The metabolism of folic acid in cirrhosis. *Annals of Internal Medicine*, **45,** 1027–1044.
91. Jarrold, T. & Vilter, R.W. (1949) Haematologic observations in patients with chronic hepatic insufficiency. *Journal of Clinical Investigation*, **28,** 286–292.
92. Jarrold, T., Will, J.J. & Davies, A.R. (1967) Bone marrow erythroid morphology in alcoholic patients. *American Journal of Clinical Nutrition*, **20,** 716–722.
93. Jedrychowski, A., Hillenbrand, P., Ajdukiewicz, A.B., Parbhoo, S.P. & Sherlock, S. (1973) Fibrinolysis in cholestatic jaundice. *British Medical Journal*, **i,** 640–642.
94. Joske, R.A. (1963) The vitamin B_{12} content of human liver tissue obtained by aspiration biopsy. *Gut*, **4,** 231–235.
95. Kan, Y.W., McFadzean, A.J.S., Todd, D. & Tso, S.C. (1961) Further observations on polycythaemia in hepatocellular carcinoma. *Blood*, **18,** 592–598.
96. Karpatkin, S., Strick, N., Karpatkin, M.B. & Siskind, G.W. (1972) Cumulative experience in the detection of antiplatelet antibody in 234 patients with idiopathic thrombocytopenic purpura, systemic lupus erythematosus and other clinical disorders. *American Journal of Medicine*, **52,** 776–785.
97. Kilbridge, T.M. & Heller, P. (1969) Determinants of erythrocyte size in chronic liver disease. *Blood*, **34,** 739–746.
98. Kimber, C., Deller, D.J., Ibbotson, R.H. & Lander, H. (1965) The mechanism of anaemia in chronic liver disease. *Quarterly Journal of Medicine*, **34,** 33–64.
99. Kivel, R.M. (1961) Haematologic aspects of acute viral hepatitis. *American Journal of Digestive Diseases* (new series), **6,** 1017–1031.
100. Klipstein, F.A. & Lindenbaum, J. (1965) Folate deficiency in chronic liver disease. *Blood*, **25,** 443–456.
101. Koller, F. (1973) Theory and experience behind the use of coagulation tests in diagnosis and prognosis of liver disease. *Scandinavian Journal of Gastroenterology* (Suppl. 8), **19,** 59–61.
102. Krasnow, S.E., Walsh, J.R., Zimmerman, H.J. & Heller, P. (1957) Megaloblastic anaemia in 'alcoholic' cirrhosis. *Archives of Internal Medicine*, **100,** 870–880.
103. Kwaan, H.C., McFadzean, A.J.S. & Cook, J. (1956) Plasma fibrinolytic activity in cirrhosis of the liver. *Lancet*, **i,** 132–136.
104. Lane, F., Goff, P., McGuffin, R. & Hillman, R. (1973) The influence of ethanol on folate metabolism. *Blood*, **42,** 998.
105. Lee, S., Yip, M. & Sachs, H.J. (1972) Factor IX deficiency in liver disease. *Journal of the American Medical Association*, **221,** 1410–1412.
106. Leevy, C.M., Baker, H., Tenhove, W.W., Frank, O. & Chornick, G.R. (1965) B-complex vitamins in liver disease of the alcoholic. *American Journal of Clinical Nutrition*, **16,** 339–346.
107. Lieberman, F.L. & Reynolds, T.B. (1967) Plasma volume in cirrhosis of the liver. *Journal of Clinical Investigation*, **46,** 1297–1308.
108. Lightwood, A.M. & Scott, G.L. (1973) Auto-immune haemolytic anaemia due to red cell antibodies of different specificities in a patient with chronic hepatitis. *Vox Sanguinis*, **24,** 331–336.
109. Lindenbaum, J. (1977) Metabolic effects of alcohol on the blood and bone marrow. In *Metabolic Aspects of Alcoholism* (Ed.) Leiber, C.S. pp. 215–247. Baltimore: University Park Press.
110. Lindenbaum, J. & Hargrove, R.L. (1968) Thrombocytopaenia in alcoholics. *Annals of Internal Medicine*, **68,** 526–532.
111. Lindenbaum, J. & Lieber, C.S. (1969) Hematologic effects of alcohol in man in the absence of nutritional deficiency. *New England Journal of Medicine*, **281,** 333–338.
112. Lindenbaum, J. & Pezzimenti, J.E. (1972) Effects of B_{12} and folate deficiency on small intestinal function. *Clinical Research*, **20,** 871.
113. Lipschitz, D.A., Cook, J.D. & Finch, C.A. (1974) A clinical evaluation of serum ferritin as an index of

iron stores. *New England Journal of Medicine*, **290,** 1213–1216.

114. Litwins, J. & Liebowitz, S. (1951) Abnormal lymphocytes ('virocytes') in virus diseases other than infectious mononucleosis. *Acta Haematologica*, **5,** 223.

115. Liu, Y.K. (1973) Leukopenia in alcoholics. *American Journal of Medicine*, **54,** 605–610.

116. Ludlam, C.A., Moore, S., Bolton, A.E., Pepper, D.S. & Cash, J.D. (1975) The release of a human platelet specific protein measured by a radioimmunoassay. *Thrombosis Research*, **6,** 543–548.

117. MacDonald, R.A. (1963) Idiopathic haemochromatosis: genetic or acquired? *Archives of Internal Medicine*, **112,** 184–190.

118. MacPherson, A.I.S. & Innes, J. (1953) Peripheral blood picture after operation for portal hypertension. *Lancet*, **i,** 1120–1123.

119. Mandel, E.E. & Gerhold, W.M. (1969) Plasma fibrin stabilizing factor: acquired deficiency in various disorders. *American Journal of Clinical Pathology*, **52,** 547–556.

120. Mannucci, P.M., Franchi, F. & Dioguardi, N. (1976) Correction of abnormal coagulation in chronic liver disease by combined use of fresh frozen plasma and prothrombin. *Lancet*, **ii,** 542–545.

121. Mannucci, L., Dioguardi, N., Del Ninno, E. & Mannucci, P.M. (1973) Value of thrombotest and antithrombin III in the assessment of liver function. *Scandinavian Journal of Gastroenterology*, (Suppl. 8), **19,** 103–107.

122. Marciniak, E., Farley, C.H. & de Simone, P.A. (1974) Familial thrombosis due to antithrombin III deficiency. *Blood*, **43,** 219–231.

123. McCurdy, P.R., Pierce, L.E. & Rath, C.E. (1962) Abnormal bone marrow morphology in acute alcoholism. *New England Journal of Medicine*, **266,** 505–507.

124. McFarland, W. & Leibre, E.P. (1963) Abnormal leukocyte response in alcoholism. *Annals of Internal Medicine*, **59,** 865–877.

125. McFadzean, A.J.S., Todd, D. & Tsang, K.C. (1958) Polycythaemia in primary carcinoma of the liver. *Blood*, **13,** 427–435.

126. Meili, E.O. & Straub, P.W. (1970) Elevation of factor VIII in acute fatal liver necrosis. *Thrombosis et Diathesis Haemorrhagica (Stuttgart)*, **24,** 161–174.

127. Merskey, G., Lalezari, P. & Johnson, A.J. (1969) A rapid, simple, sensitive, method for measuring fibrinolytic split products in human serum. *Proceedings of the Society for Experimental Biology and Medicine*, **131,** 871–875.

128. Miles, J.A.R. (1945) The erythrocyte sedimentation rate in infective hepatitis. *British Medical Journal*, **i,** 767–769.

129. Neerhout, R.C. (1968) Abnormalities of erythrocyte stromal lipids in hepatic disease. *Journal of Laboratory and Clinical Medicine*, **71,** 438–477.

130. Neerhout, R.C. (1968) Erythrocyte stromal lipids in hyperlipemic states. *Journal of Laboratory and Clinical Medicine*, **71,** 448–454.

131. Nunnally, R.M. & Levine, I. (1961) Macronormoblastic hyperplasia of the bone marrow in hepatic cirrhosis. *American Journal of Medicine*, **30,** 972–975.

132. O'Brien, J.R. (1977) The prothrombotic state. In *Recent Advances in Blood Coagulation* (Ed.) Poller, L. pp. 241–266. Edinburgh, London and New York: Churchill Livingstone.

133. Østergaard Kristensen, H.P. (1959) The blood vitamin B_{12} level in liver disease. *Acta Medica Scandinavica*, **163,** 515–523.

134. Outryve, M., van, Baele, G., Weerdi, G.A. de & Barbier, F. (1973) Antihaemophilic factor A (FVIII) and serum fibrin-fibrinogen degradation products in hepatic cirrhosis. *Scandinavian Journal of Haematology*, **11,** 148–152.

135. Pengelly, C.D.R. & Jennings, R.C. (1971) Active chronic hepatitis and haemolytic anaemia associated with Rh-specific antibodies. *Postgraduate Medical Journal*, **47,** 683–686.

136. Pitcher, C.S. & Williams, R. (1963) Reduced red cell survival in jaundice and its relation to abnormal glutathione metabolism. *Clinical Science*, **24,** 239–252.

137. Poller, L. (1977) Coagulation abnormalities in liver disease. In *Recent Advances in Blood Coagulation* (Ed.) Poller, L. pp. 266–292. Edinburgh, London and New York: Churchill Livingstone.

138. Prieto, J., Barry, M. & Sherlock, S. (1975) Serum ferritin in patients with iron overload and with acute and chronic liver diseases. *Gastroenterology*, **68,** 525–533.

139. Rachmilewitz, M., Aronovitch, J. & Grossowicz, N. (1956) Serum concentrates of Vitamin B_{12} in acute and chronic liver disease. *Journal of Laboratory and Clinical Medicine*, **48,** 339.

140. Ratnoff, O.D. (1949) Studies on a proteolytic enzyme in human plasma. *Bulletin of the Johns Hopkins Hospital*, **84,** 29.

141. Ratnoff, O.D. (1977) The haemostatic defects of liver disease. In *Haemostasis: Biochemistry, Physiology and Pathology* (Ed.) Ogston, D. & Bennett, B. pp. 446–466. New York: Wiley.

142. Ratnoff, O.D. & Menzie, C. (1951) A new method for the determination of fibrinogen in small samples of plasma. *Journal of Laboratory and Clinical Medicine*, **37,** 316–320.

143. Retief, F.P., VandenPlas, L. & Visser, H. (1969) Vitamin B_{12} binding proteins in liver disease. *British Journal of Haematology*, **16,** 231–240.

144. Rider, D.M., McDonagh, R.P. & McDonagh, J. (1978) A possible contributory role of the platelet in the formation of plasma factor III. *British Journal of Haematology*, **39,** 579–588.

145. Roberts, H.R. & Cederbaum, A.I. (1972) The liver and blood coagulation: physiology and pathology. *Gastroenterology*, **63,** 297–330.

146. Rubin, M.H., Weston, M.J., Bullock, G., Roberts, J., Langley, P.G., White, Y.S. & Williams, R. (1977) Abnormal platelet function and ultrastructure in fulminant hepatic failure. *Quarterly Journal of Medicine*, **183,** 339–352.

147. Sas, G., Owens, R.E., Smith, J.K., Middleton, S. & Cash, J.D. (1975) In vitro spontaneous thrombin generation in human factor IX concentrates. *British Journal of Haematology*, **31,** 25–35.

148. Scanlon, G.H., Brinkhouse, K.M., Warnerm, E.D., Smith, H.P. & Flynn, J.E. (1939) Plasma prothrombin and the bleeding tendency with special reference to jaundiced patients and vitamin K therapy. *Journal of the American Medical Association*, **112,** 1898–1901.

149. Sears, D.A., George, J.N. & Gold, M.S. (1975) Transient red blood cell aplasia in association with viral hepatitis. Occurrence four years apart in siblings. *Archives of Internal Medicine*, **135,** 1585–1589.

150. Seligsohn, U., Shani, M. & Ramot, B. (1970) Gilbert syndrome and factor VII deficiency. *Lancet*, **i,** 1398.
151. Sharp, A.A., Howie, B., Biggs, R. & Methuen, D.T. (1958) Defibrination syndrome in pregnancy: value of various diagnostic tests. *Lancet*, **ii,** 1309–1312.
152. Sheehy, T.W. & Berman, A. (1960) The anaemia of cirrhosis. *Journal of Laboratory and Clinical Medicine*, **56,** 72–82.
153. Smith, J.A., Lonergan, E.T. & Sterling, K. (1964) Spur cell anaemia. Hemolytic anemia with red cells resembling acanthocytosis in alcoholic cirrhosis. *New England Journal of Medicine*, **271,** 396–398.
154. Soria, J., Coupier, J., Samama, M., Tixier, P. & Bilsk, P.G. (1970) Dysfibrinogenaemia without bleeding tendency with abnormal polymerization of fibrin monomers in a case of severe hepatitis. *XII Congress of the International Society of Haematology, New York*. Abstracts, p. 180.
155. Spector, I. & Corn, M. (1967) Laboratory tests of haemostasis. The relation to haemorrhage in liver disease. *Archives of Internal Medicine*, **119,** 577–582.
156. Starzl, T.E., Marchioro, T.L., Von Kaulla, K.N., Hermann, G., Brittain, R.S. & Waddell, W.R. (1963) Homotransplantation of the liver in humans. *Surgery, Gynecology and Obstetrics*, **117,** 659–676.
157. Stenflo, J. (1974) Vitamin K and the biosynthesis of prothrombin. IV. Isolation of peptides containing prosthetic groups from normal prothrombin and corresponding peptides from dicoumerol-induced prothrombin. *Journal of Biological Chemistry*, **249,** 5527–5535.
158. Subhiyah, B.W. & Al-Hindawi, A.Y. (1967) Red cell survival and splenic accumulation of radio-chromium in liver cirrhosis with splenomegaly. *British Journal of Haematology*, **13,** 773–778.
159. Sullivan, B.H.Jr & Tumen, H.J. (1961) The effect of portacaval shunt on thrombocytopenia associated with portal hypertension. *Annals of Internal Medicine*, **55,** 598–603.
160. Sullivan, L.W. & Herbert, V. (1964) Suppression of haematopoiesis by ethanol. *Journal of Clinical Investigation*, **43,** 2048–2062.
161. Sullivan, L.W., Adams, W.H. & Liu, Y.K. (1977) Induction of thrombocytopaenia by thrombopheresis in man: patterns of recovery in normal subjects during ethanol ingestion and abstinence. *Blood*, **49,** 197–207.
162. Suttie, J.W. (1974) Metabolism and properties of a liver precursor to prothrombin. *Vitamins and Hormones*, **32,** 463–481.
163. Thomas, D.P. (1972) Abnormalities of platelet aggregation in patients with alcoholic cirrhosis. *Annals of the New York Academy of Sciences*, **201,** 243–250.
164. Thomas, D.P., Ream, V.J. & Stuart, R.K. (1967) Platelet aggregation in patients with Laënnec's cirrhosis of the liver. *New England Journal of Medicine*, **276,** 1344–1348.
165. Thomas, D.P., Niewiarowski, S., Myers, A.R., Bloch, K.J. & Colman, R.W. (1970) A comparative study of four methods for detecting fibrinogen degradation products in patients with various diseases. *New England Journal of Medicine*, **283,** 663–668.
166. Thomas, E.D., Buckner, C.D., Clift, R.A., Feter, A., Neiman, P.E. & Storb, R. (1977) Current status of marrow transplantation for leukaemia or aplastic anaemia. In *Recent Advances in Haematology* (Ed.) Hoffbrand, A.V., Brain, M.C. & Hirsh, J. pp. 111–125. Edinburgh, London and New York: Churchill Livingstone.
167. Thorling, E.B. (1972) Paraneoplastic erythrocytosis and inappropriate erythropoietin production. *Scandinavian Journal of Haematology*, (Suppl. 17), **1,** 1–166.
168. Triger, D.R., Alp, M.H. & Wright, R. (1972) Bacterial and dietary antibodies in liver disease. *Lancet*, **i,** 60–63.
169. Tso, S.C. & Hua, A.S.P. (1974) Erythrocytosis in hepatocellular carcinoma – a compensatory phenomenon. *British Journal of Haematology*, **28,** 497–503.
170. Tumen, H.J. (1970) Hypersplenism and portal hypertension. *Annals of the New York Academy of Sciences*, **170,** 332–344.
171. Tytgat, G.M., Collen, D. & Verstraete, M. (1971) Metabolism of fibrinogen in cirrhosis of the liver. *Journal of Clinical Investigation*, **50,** 1690–1701.
172. Vahrman, J. (1971) Viral hepatitis and the ESR. *British Medical Journal*, **ii,** 466–467.
173. Veltkamp, J.J. & Kreuning, J. (1973) Diagnostic value of coagulation studies in chronic liver disease. *Scandinavian Journal of Gastroenterology*, (Suppl. 8), **19,** 93–95.
174. Von Kaulla, E. & Von Kaulla, K.N. (1967) Antithrombin III and diseases. *American Journal of Clinical Pathology*, **48,** 69–80.
175. Von Kaulla, K.N., Kaye, H., Von Kaulla, E., Marchior, T.L. & Starzl, T.E. (1966) Changes in blood coagulation before and after hepatectomy of transplantation in dogs and man. *Archives of Surgery*, **92,** 71–79.
176. Walls, W.D. & Losowsky, M.J. (1971) The hemostatic defect of liver disease. *Gastroenterology*, **60,** 108–119.
177. Werre, J.M., Helleman, P.W., Verloop, M.C. & Degier, J. (1970) Causes of macroplania of erythrocytes in diseases of the liver and biliary tract with special reference to leptocytosis. *British Journal of Haematology*, **19,** 223–235.
178. White, G.C., Roberts, H.R., Kingdon, H.S. & Lundblad, R.L. (1977) Prothrombin complex, concentrates: potentially thrombogenic materials and clues to the mechanisms of thrombosis in vivo. *Blood*, **49,** 159–170.
179. Wiley, J.S., Ellory, J.C., Shuman, M.A., Shaller, C.C. & Cooper, R.A. (1975) Characteristics of the membrane defect in the hereditary stomatocytosis syndrome. *Blood*, **46,** 337–356.
180. Willcox, R.G. & Isselbacher, K.J. (1961) Chronic liver disease in young people. *American Journal of Medicine*, **30,** 185.
181. Williams, R., Williams, H.S., Scheuer, P.J., Pitcher, C.S., Loizeau, E. & Sherlock, S. (1967) Iron absorption and siderosis in chronic liver disease. *Quarterly Journal of Medicine*, **36,** 151–165.
182. Wright, S.G. & Ree, G.H. (1978) Blood in the alcohol stream. *Lancet*, **i,** 49–50.
183. Wu, A., Chanarin, I. & Levi, A.J. (1974) Macrocytosis of chronic alcoholism. *Lancet*, **i,** 829.
184. Yeung, K.Y., Klug, P.P., Brower, M. & Lessin, L.S. (1973) Mechanism of alcohol induced vacuolization in human bone marrow cells. *Blood*, **42,** 998.
185. Zieve, L. (1958) Jaundice, hyperlipemia, hemolytic anemia: a heretofore unrecognized syndrome associated with alcoholic fatty liver and cirrhosis. *Annals of Internal Medicine*, **48,** 471–496.
186. Zieve, L. (1966) Hemolytic anemia in liver disease. *Medicine*, **45,** 497–505.

Chapter 9

Immunological Aspects of Liver Disease

D.R. TRIGER
RALPH WRIGHT

Diseases affecting the liver are notable for the frequency with which immunological phenomena are detectable. Since the liver is a major component of the reticuloendothelial system, such disturbances might be expected, although the mechanism behind many of these abnormalities is poorly understood. The lack of knowledge concerning the aetiology and pathogenesis of liver diseases has prompted investigators to search for an immunological explanation for both the initiation and the perpetuation of many of these disorders. This chapter considers the current status of the liver as a part of the immune system and also reviews the immunological phenomena associated with damage to the liver. The specific immune responses to hepatitis A and B are dealt with in Chapters 28 and 29.

EXPERIMENTAL EVIDENCE FOR THE IMMUNOLOGICAL ROLE OF THE INTACT LIVER

The liver occupies a strategic anatomical position between the gastrointestinal tract and the systemic circulation. Studies in germ-free mice indicate that the intestinal microorganisms provide the major stimulus to gamma globulin production, presumably by the absorption of intact bacteria or their antigenic components into both the lymphatic and portal venous systems.[69]

Supporting experimental evidence has been provided by the ability to demonstrate the presence of radiolabelled type-specific *E. coli* antigen in the liver of coliform-free rabbits following oral feeding.[62] Warshaw, Walker and Isselbacher[90] have studied the absorption of bovine serum albumin (BSA) by the rat small intestine, by cannulating the mesenteric lymphatic duct and portal vein. Following instillation of tritium-labelled BSA into the duodenum, they were able to demonstrate the uptake of ^{3}H-BSA into both lymph and blood and prove that the absorbed BSA was immunologically identical to the instilled protein.

Antigens in the portal venous blood must pass through the hepatic sinusoids before reaching the systemic circulation, and particulate antigens, such as sheep erythrocytes[84] or *Salmonella adelaide*,[75] have been shown to be trapped there in significant quantities. Although the liver is the largest organ in the reticuloendothelial system and is capable of trapping and phagocytosing more antigen than any other component, it may handle antigens differently. Whereas the spleen is able to phagocytose antigens and process them for antibody production, the liver appears to process and degrade antigens much more rapidly and completely without the production of antibody.[36] This may be due to the absence of significant numbers of lymphoid cells from the normal liver, in contrast to other organs in the reticuloendothelial system.

These experimental studies suggest that the liver may act as a filter of exogenous antigens absorbed from the gastrointestinal tract by sequestering part or all of those present in the portal venous system and thereby reducing the amount of antigen available to the antibody-producing components elsewhere (Figure 9.1).

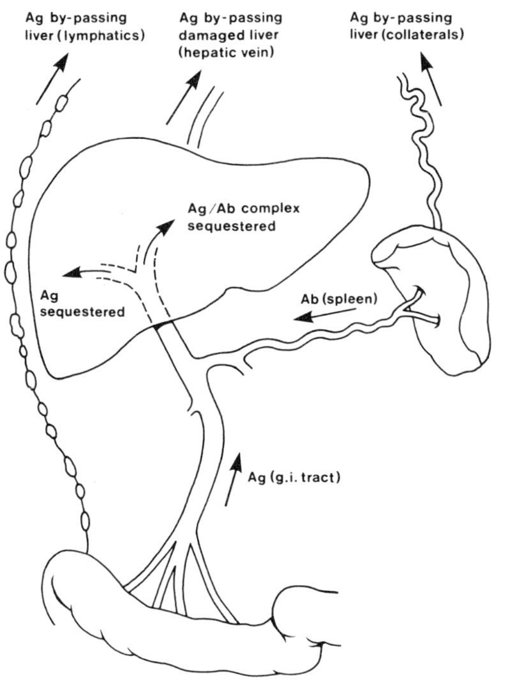

Figure 9.1. The sequestration of exogenous antigen by the liver.

The possibility that this might be a significant in vivo function of the liver was first suggested by Cantor and Dumont.[16] They found that the circulating antibody response in dogs immunized with intramuscular dinitrochlorobenzene (DNCB) was significantly reduced if the animals were fed the hapten prior to the injections, and that this reduction was abolished if the animals were subjected to portacaval shunting before the start of the experiment. They suggested that the liver might help prevent sensitization to antigen absorbed from the gastrointestinal tract into the portal venous system. Subsequent work has emphasized this role of the liver by showing that repeated injection of small amounts of sheep erythrocytes into the portal venous system of rats results in a significantly lower antibody production compared with similar immunization via the inferior vena cava.[84] Supporting evidence has been provided by studies of circulating antibody after the effective phagocytic hepatic function has been altered in various ways, including reticuloendothelial blockade with colloidal carbon,[72] carbon tetrachloride-induced necrosis,[81] portacaval anastomosis[42] and portacaval transposition.[5] All these procedures result in increases in both total and specific antibody production.

Central to this argument is the functional capability of the liver macrophage or Kupffer cell. Traditionally, the cells lining the liver sinusoids are divided into endothelial cells and Kupffer cells. Although the two groups are morphologically distinct,[91] functional differences are often not clear cut. At any given time only about 30 per cent of these cells are phagocytic. Little is known about the kinetics of these macrophages, except that they are sessile under normal conditions and may have a very slow turnover. They are probably derived from cells within the bone marrow, spleen and peripheral blood and are recruited from these sites following liver damage. These cells rarely divide within the liver under normal conditions, although division can be induced experimentally by agents such as zymosan. The macrophages of the reticuloendothelial system have many varied and important immunological functions related chiefly to handling of antigen and participation in T and B cell interaction, as well as playing a vital role in the repair of tissue damage.

Extrapolating these experimental observations to clinical medicine a disturbance of phagocytic function of the liver may be implicated in the mechanism of the hyperglobulinaemia which frequently accompanies liver disease and which is considered later in this chapter. It is also possible that liver macrophages may play a more active role in the disease process, either as cytotoxic cells or by controlling viral replication.

IMMUNOLOGICAL MECHANISMS ASSOCIATED WITH LIVER DISEASE

A wide variety of immunological disturbances has been reported in both acute and chronic liver disease. Disturbances in immunity can be broadly divided into two groups: those involving alterations in B cell function or humoral antibody production and those in which cellular immunity (T cell function) is affected.

Disturbances in B Cell Function

Early studies of serum proteins in chronic liver disease recognized a reversal in albumin : globulin ratio together with an absolute increase in serum globulin. More specifically, it has been shown that this is mainly due to an increase in serum immunoglobulins,[23] with elevations in IgG being most striking in chronic active hepatitis, IgA in alcoholic liver disease and IgM in primary biliary cirrhosis, although there is a considerable overlap. Havens et al[31] showed that the raised serum globulin was due to increased synthesis and this was supported by observations that patients with hepatic cirrhosis had an enhanced capacity to produce circulating antibodies to administered antigens, such as diphtheria toxoid and tetanus antitoxin.[30] Subsequent reports failed to confirm this increased antibody production[12] but interest in the mechanism of hyperglobulinaemia revived following the demonstration of increased anti-salmonella agglutinins in patients with chronic active hepatitis.[60] This was followed by the report of increased antibody titres to intestinal tract organisms (*E. coli* and bacteroides) and dietary proteins in patients with cirrhosis and chronic active hepatitis.[83] Increases in *E. coli* antibody titres were also observed in patients with acute viral hepatitis, these titres returning to normal following resolution of the hepatitis. In contrast, antibody titres to *Haemophilus influenzae* (a non-intestinal tract organism) were normal throughout the acute hepatitis and were not elevated in chronic liver disease, which argues against a non-specific immune response. Simultaneously, Bjørneboe, Prytz and Ørskov[11] confirmed high *E. coli* antibody titres in alcoholic cirrhosis and also observed an increase in *E. coli* antibody titres in patients following portacaval shunt. These observations suggested that Kupffer cells may fail to sequester antigen absorbed from the gut, either because of functional impairment or as a result of shunting of portal blood, an idea which was well supported by the experimental studies cited earlier.

This explanation fails to account for the grossly elevated antibody titres to certain viruses, notably measles, rubella and cytomegalovirus (CMV), which have been reported in patients with chronic active hepatitis.[85] Although elevated titres to CMV are also found in alcoholic cirrhosis, the raised measles and rubella antibody levels seem to occur only in that type of chronic active hepatitis associated with autoantibodies. Cross-reactivity with these autoantibodies was ruled out by absorption experiments.

These apparently unrelated phenomena led us to suggest a number of different mechanisms to account for the hypergammaglobulinaemia of liver disease[82] (Table 9.1). Increased stimulus to antibody production may be provided by the presence of antigens responsible for the liver disease, e.g. the hepatitis virus. Non-specific antigenic stimuli, such as *E. coli*, may also contribute for reasons discussed earlier. Some of the antibody production may be accounted for by the presence of autoantibodies, which will be considered in greater detail in the next section.

Table 9.1. *Hyperglobulinaemia in Liver Disease.*

	Hepatic	Extrahepatic
Stimulus to production	Infective agent e.g. virus ? Autoantigens	? Autoantigens Antigenic stimuli not related to pathogenesis
Mechanism of production	1. Intrahepatic shunting 2. Loss of Kupffer cells	1. Collateral circulation 2. Reduced liver blood flow
	3. Saturation of Kupffer cell phagocytic function	3. Decreased immune surveillance (T/B interaction)
	4. Release of antigens sequestered in the liver 5. Adjuvant effect of liver tissue 6. Loss of normal immuno-suppressive effect of the liver	4. Mitogenic stimulus of endotoxin

There is evidence of increased antibody production in patients with liver disease. The spleen and lymph nodes which are commonly enlarged in patients with chronic liver disease are the sites of increased concentrations of antibody demonstrated by immunofluorescence. Immunoglobulins are not normally detectable in the intact liver although it is capable of synthesizing all other serum proteins.

None of these stimuli is likely to be considerable, but other mechanisms may enhance their ability to induce antibody production. The liver may be unable to sequester antigens because of a functional loss of Kupffer cells, either due to a quantitative loss in the Kupffer cell population or because the cells themselves are committed to other functions, such as handling the products of liver cell breakdown that occurs in acute liver cell necrosis. Alternatively, the antigens may fail to reach the liver because of alterations in liver blood flow which often accompany hepatic disorders, or because of shunting of portal blood past the hepatic sinusoids. Prytz et al,[61] when noting a further increase in serum gamma globulin and *E. coli* antibody titres in patients following portacaval anastomosis, suggested that extrahepatic shunting may play an important role in producing high serum globulin levels, especially of IgG. This has not been confirmed by Simjee et al[70] who favour defective Kupffer cell function or intrahepatic shunting to explain the high bacterial antibody titres. The high viral antibody titres in chronic active hepatitis might be related to release of viral antigens sequestered in the liver, analogous to the measles infection which accompanies subacute sclerosing panencephalitis and which leads to comparably high antibody titres but is confined to measles virus. Endotoxin, which is a potent B cell mitogen, may be found in the circulation of some patients with liver disease, and this may stimulate antibody production. Products of liver cell breakdown, such as nucleic acids, may similarly act as adjuvants to antibody synthesis. T cell function is commonly suppressed in liver disorders (see below) and it has been postulated that a compensatory B cell hyper-reactivity may result from this. In this context, Berger and Bull[8] have reported preliminary data which suggest that circulating lymphocytes in patients with cirrhosis and hyperglobulinaemia show increased immunoglobulin synthesis.

Finally, the observation of Calne et al[15] that simultaneous liver transplantation prolongs the survival of renal allografts raises the possibility that the normal liver might possess an immunosuppressive property, and this has been supported by the isolation of a lymphocyte-inhibiting factor from normal liver.[67]

It seems likely that no single mechanism can account for the elevation in globulins seen in acute and chronic liver disease and their relative importance awaits further elucidation.

Autoantibodies

Gajdusek[27] reported complement-fixing antibodies in the serum of patients with liver disease against an extract of normal human liver, an observation which stimulated much research into the incidence of tissue autoantibodies in hepatic and other disorders. Although most of these have been shown to be neither organ nor species specific, many have proved to be useful clinical markers in the investigation of hepatic disease. Details of the occurrence and importance of some of these antibodies are shown in Table 9.2.

Table 9.2. *Autoantibodies Associated with Liver Disease.*

Autoantibody	Disease	Frequency (%)	Comments
Antinuclear antibody	Chronic active hepatitis	20–50	High titre IgG
	Primary biliary cirrhosis	15–40	
	Drug-associated CAH	10–30	
Anti-DNA antibody	All types of liver disease	30–60	
Anti-smooth muscle antibody	Chronic active hepatitis	20–60	High titre IgG
	Primary biliary cirrhosis	10–30	
	Viral hepatitis	50–80	Low titre IgM – transient
	Alcoholic liver disease	10–15	Low titre IgM
Anti-mitochondrial antibody	Primary biliary cirrhosis	80–95	
	Chronic active hepatitis	10–25	
Bile canalicular antibody	Chronic active hepatitis/ primary biliary cirrhosis	20–40	
Liver membrane antibody	HB_sAg –ve		
	Acute hepatitis	15	
	Chronic active hepatitis	40	
	Cirrhosis	60	

Antinuclear antibody

Haserick, Lewis and Bortz[29] were the first to demonstrate a specific factor in the gamma globulin fraction of patients with systemic lupus erythematosus (SLE) which was responsible for the so-called LE cell phenomenon. This antinuclear factor, subsequently renamed 'antinuclear antibody', can be demonstrated by a variety of immunological techniques, including indirect immunofluorescence, complement fixation, latex precipitation and tanned red cell agglutination. The antibodies are directed against several nuclear constituents, notably deoxyribonucleoprotein, ribonucleic acid and nucleohistones, and they belong to all three major immunoglobulin classes. Because of the heterogeneous nature of the antigen against which they are directed, different immunofluorescent patterns may be produced by antinuclear antibodies and these have been variously described as speckled, diffuse or homogeneous. Initial hopes that these patterns might be of value in clinical diagnosis have not been substantiated. The immunoglobulin class and titre of the antibodies are of some diagnostic value, as will be discussed later.

Although most commonly found in the sera of patients with SLE, antinuclear antibodies are also found in most connective tissue disorders and occasionally in otherwise healthy individuals. An increased frequency is observed in chronic active hepatitis, primary biliary cirrhosis and some drug-associated hepatitis, in contrast to other forms of liver disease.[20] Reports on the frequency of this antibody in the normal population and in certain forms of liver disease (see Table 9.2) are very variable, much of the conflict arising from the difficulty in defining positivity. Low antibody titres of 1 : 10 or less are accepted by most authorities as unimportant, while titres equal to or greater than 1 : 80 are universally considered to be significant. IgG class antibodies are more commonly associated with pathological processes than IgM antibodies.

Anti-DNA antibodies

More specific characterization of the antinuclear antibodies, combined with increasingly sophisticated immunological techniques, led to the development of a radio-immunoassay for double-stranded (native) DNA and the demonstration that it appeared to be specific for SLE.[34] Davis and Read,[18] however, reported that 15 out of 36 patients with chronic active hepatitis exhibited DNA binding of the degree seen in patients with SLE. They reported no abnormalities in 22 patients with other forms of liver disease, but Jain et al[37] found abnormal DNA binding in acute viral hepatitis, alcoholic cirrhosis and primary biliary cirrhosis, as well as in chronic active hepatitis, both HB_sAg positive and HB_sAg negative. We have also detected DNA binding antibodies in a wide variety of liver diseases, including HB_sAg positive carriers, suggesting that DNA antibody levels are unlikely to be of diagnostic help in liver diseases.[43]

It is of interest that Fournié, Lambert and Miescher[24] have shown the induction of anti-DNA antibodies in animals following the injection of bacterial lipopolysaccharides, raising the possibility that the mechanism of anti-DNA antibody production might be related to the elevated *E. coli* antibody titres considered earlier. Alternatively, hepatic- or viral-specific DNA might act as an antigenic stimulus.

Smooth muscle antibody

Although first described by Johnson, Holborow and Glynn[38] in patients with chronic active hepatitis, this autoantibody has been reported in many disorders, both hepatic and non-hepatic. Indirect immunofluorescence remains the sole means of detection and by this technique smooth muscle antibody may stain the actin and myosin of bile canaliculi, renal glomeruli and thyroid epithelial cells. Recent studies have suggested that the antibody is directly produced against actin.[47] The highest antibody titres are usually found in chronic active hepatitis, usually of IgG class, and when present may be of diagnostic value. However, lower antibody titres, mainly IgM, are found transiently in viral infections such as viral hepatitis and infectious mononucleosis. We have observed similar reactions in patients with alcoholic liver disease and the antibodies may also be found in association with malignant disease without any apparent hepatic involvement.

Mitochondrial antibody

This autoantibody is of considerable clinical importance because of its frequent occurrence in primary biliary cirrhosis and rarity in other disorders (see Chapter 31). It is found in over 85 per cent of patients with this disorder, and although some authors report its presence in 10 to 20 per cent of patients with chronic active hepatitis this probably reflects a clinical overlap between these two disorders. Earlier reports of mitochondrial antibodies in halothane-associated hepatitis[65] and prolonged extra-hepatic obstruction[45] have not been confirmed, and although the antibody is occasionally seen in patients with acute hepatitis it is usually transient and present only in low titre. There appears to be an increased incidence in patients with connective tissue disorders and in the relatives of patients with primary biliary cirrhosis.[87] Such patients may have minor histological abnormalities in the liver but there is no evidence that they invariably progress to develop primary biliary cirrhosis and it is thought that the autoantibody may represent a marker of potential autoimmune disease.

The antimitochondrial antibody may be detected by direct immunofluorescence or by complement fixation, and electron microscope studies have shown that it is directed against the inner mitochondrial membrane.[9] The structure of inner mitochondrial membranes resembles the outer coat of certain bacteria, raising the possibility that the antibody might be generated by cross-reacting hitherto unidentified micro-organisms. Recent studies have suggested that there are several different types of mito-chondrial antibodies.[7]

Bile canalicular antibody

This liver-specific antibody has been reported in the serum of some patients with chronic active hepatitis and primary biliary cirrhosis but it has not proved useful as a diagnostic tool. As mentioned earlier, immunofluorescent staining of bile canaliculi may be seen with sera containing strongly positive antibodies to smooth muscle.

Liver cell membrane antibody

Meyer zum Büschenfelde, Kössling and Miescher[51] have purified and characterized a liver-specific protein (LP-2) with which chronic liver disease may be experimentally induced in rabbits. An autoantibody to this liver cell membrane can be detected by immuno-fluorescence using isolated rabbit hepatocytes, and these workers have shown that it is specific for liver disorders, in particular HB_sAg-negative disease.[74] They reported its presence in five out of 31 patients with acute viral hepatitis, 27 out of 72 with chronic active hepatitis and 17 out of 28 with cirrhosis. There was no correlation with the presence of other autoantibodies and no apparent differences between groups with or without the antibody. This important observation requires confirmation from other centres but raises interesting possibilities about the concept of immunological liver injury which will be discussed later. (See also Chapter 29.)

Other liver-specific proteins may also exist. Sugamara and Smith[73] have purified and characterized a human liver protein of molecular weight between 40 000 and 80 000 daltons which has been termed F-antigen. Arakawa et al[1] have induced the antigen by giving rabbits carbon tetrachloride and have shown it to be liver-specific. These workers have also detected it in patients with active liver disease but in only a small minority. It is immunologically distinct from LP-2, but its place in the pathogenesis of chronic liver disease has yet to be established.

Other autoantibodies

Anti-gamma globulin antibodies (rheumatoid factors) may be frequently found in all forms of chronic liver disease. An antibody which appears to react with microsomes has been reported in a number of liver disorders, notably chronic active hepatitis.[64] It does not appear to be specific for this condition, however, and its significance is unknown. Wassermann-type reactions associated with cardiolipin antibodies are occasionally seen in lupoid hepatitis, but they are of no clinical significance. Autoantibodies to thyroid and gastric parietal cells are found with increased frequency in patients with chronic active hepatitis, but the incidence in other types of liver disease is unremarkable. None of the autoantibodies so far described has proved to be a reliable guide to prognosis or to response to therapy in any form of liver disease.

Using immunofluorescent techniques, complement and immunoglobulins can sometimes be detected in the reticuloendothelial system. As mentioned earlier, immunoglobulins are not normally found in the intact liver but in certain types of liver disease they are readily detectable. It is not known whether they are synthesized within the liver or merely deposited there from elsewhere. The type or nature of the immunoglobulin deposition does not appear to correlate with any clinical or histological parameters of liver disease.

Disturbances in T Cell Function

Studies of cellular immunity in liver disease have shown almost uniform depression in this arm of the immune response. In vivo skin-testing to a variety of antigens has shown depressed delayed sensitivity in patients with chronic hepatitis,[79] while Fox, Dudley and Sherlock[25] have demonstrated that induction of cutaneous reactivity, using haemocyanin as antigen, is impaired in primary biliary cirrhosis and cryptogenic cirrhosis. Impaired delayed hypersensitivity is also seen in alcoholic cirrhosis[6] but results in acute hepatitis have been conflicting. In vitro tests have shown that lymphocyte transformation in response to phytohaemagglutinin (PHA) is significantly impaired in chronic active hepatitis,[79] primary biliary cirrhosis,[49] alcoholic liver disease[33] and acute viral hepatitis, both HB_sAg positive and HB_sAg negative.[55]

A major difficulty arises in the interpretation of these results. It is a non-specific finding, since impairment of PHA transformation may be observed in many non-hepatic inflammatory disorders. Recent experimental studies suggest that PHA may stimulate both T and B cells, so its value as an index of T cell function must be questioned. Furthermore, several groups have demonstrated that a serum factor is involved in the impaired lymphocyte transformation, once more raising doubts as to the specificity of the test in relation to T cell function. The nature of this serum factor is unknown, but soluble immune complexes have been implicated.

Leucocyte migration inhibition has replaced lymphocyte transformation as the favoured in vitro test of cell-mediated immunity. This test involves measurement of migration of peripheral leucocytes from a capillary tube into a culture medium containing the antigen under test, usually autologous or heterologous liver tissue. Inhibition of migration is taken as evidence of delayed hypersensitivity, although some workers consider excessive stimulation as evidence of the same phenomenon. Using this test, impairment in cellular immunity has been demonstrated in chronic active hepatitis, primary biliary cirrhosis[2] and alcoholic hepatitis, but not in alcoholic cirrhosis.[53] The results in acute viral hepatitis have been conflicting and difficult to interpret.

One of the major objections to this test is the difficulty in standardizing the test antigen, as normal liver tissue is a heterogeneous assortment of numerous antigens. Preliminary results, using the purified liver-specific protein, suggest that it may be specific for liver disorders but it is unlikely to be of diagnostic value.[52] Other major objections to studies involving the leucocyte migration inhibition test include the variable techniques employed for separation and purification of leucocytes prior to insertion in the capillary tubes and the choice of appropriate control subjects. As with lymphocyte transformation, doubts have been raised as to whether this is a true test of cellular immunity and immune complexes have been shown experimentally to have a significant influence on migration.[44]

Direct studies on the peripheral T cell population show that it is significantly reduced in alcoholic liver disease, chronic active hepatitis and primary biliary cirrhosis.[76] The T cell population is reduced in acute viral hepatitis,[19] although this is also seen in other viral infections and is accompanied by an increase in the population of null cells. The significance of this observation is uncertain, although it may correlate with the impaired cell-mediated immunity. Turnover studies on lymphocyte subpopulations are needed to clarify the position, and since lymphocyte infiltration of the liver is commonly seen in chronic liver disease it is tempting to suggest that the peripheral T cell depletion is related to the cells gathering in the liver. Such a relationship appears to exist in patients with alcoholic liver disease but is less apparent in those with disease of a non-alcoholic aetiology.[35] On the other hand, Sanchez-Tapias, Thomas and Sherlock[66] have demonstrated the presence of 'activated' T cells (defined by the ability to form rosettes with human group O negative erythrocytes) preferentially in the livers of patients with active liver disease but not in those with quiescent disease.

OTHER IMMUNOLOGICAL MECHANISMS

Immune Complex Disorders

Serum complement levels are often low in both acute and chronic liver disease and while impaired synthesis by the liver may be a factor there is good evidence to suggest that the low serum level is partly due to complement consumption which occurs during the formation of antigen–antibody complexes. Experimentally induced complexes are usually cleared from the circulation by the liver and in cirrhotic animals this property is severely impaired.[75]

In situations where the antigen can be defined and quantified (such as hepatitis B surface antigen), good correlation can often be found between the extrahepatic complications of the infection, such as glomerulonephritis or arthritis and the presence of complexes (see Chapter 29). Problems arise when the antigen is unknown. Numerous tests exist for the detection of immune complexes in the serum but they measure complexes of different sizes and it is increasingly recognized that circulating immune complexes may arise in response to any form of inflammation.

Callard et al[14] have shown that immune complexes of an unspecified nature are commonly deposited in the glomerular basement membrane of patients with alcoholic cirrhosis but these are not thought to be of clinical significance. The hypothesis that immune complexes may potentiate liver damage will be discussed later in this chapter.

Cytotoxicity

A recent new development in in vitro immunological techniques has been the demonstration of specific cytotoxicity by lymphocytes against pure cell cultures. Lymphocytes from patients with chronic active hepatitis have been shown to be cytotoxic against a variety of target cells, including Chang liver cells,[89] isolated human hepatocytes[28] and rabbit hepatocytes.[77] Cytotoxicity in the rabbit system can be blocked by liver-specific lipoprotein. Similar phenomena can be shown to occur in patients with alcoholic hepatitis[39] and in various chronic liver disorders as well as uncomplicated acute viral hepatitis.[58] Several different mechanisms have been implicated, including T cells, K cells, antibody-dependent cell-mediated cytotoxicity,[17] suppressor cells[32] and null cells.[41] Cytotoxic systems have also been found in many non-hepatic inflammatory disorders. There are clearly a number of variables in this in vitro system and at present the importance and relevance of this phenomenon to the pathogenesis of liver disease is uncertain.

IMMUNOLOGICAL PHENOMENA ASSOCIATED WITH LIVER DISEASES

Chronic Active Hepatitis (see also Chapter 29)

Much confusion exists in the literature concerning the immunological phenomena associated with chronic active hepatitis, in part at least due to a failure to distinguish between subgroups of the disease. All have the histological picture of mononuclear cell infiltration, erosion of the limiting plate and piecemeal necrosis termed 'chronic aggressive hepatitis' regardless of the aetiology.

The discovery of the hepatitis B antigen has enabled us to divide this group of histologically similar patients into at least two groups according to the presence of markers in the serum and/or liver. Apart from the hepatitis B markers, these two groups show clinical, epidemiological and immunological differences. The HB_sAg negative group commonly show striking abnormalities in B cell parameters. The hyperglobulinaemia associated with this condition is often much higher than is found in any other liver disorder and is largely associated with IgG elevation. Autoantibodies are often found in this group of patients, particularly high titre IgG class antinuclear and anti-smooth muscle antibodies. Some of these patients, both clinically and histologically, resemble patients with primary biliary cirrhosis and this is reflected by the increased incidence of positive antimitochondrial antibodies. Histocompatibility antigens HLA-A1 and HLA-B8 have been reported in association with the presence of high titre autoantibody-positive chronic active hepatitis[48] but not in the HB_sAg positive group. This has been confirmed by others[57] and recently an association with HLA-Dw3 has been described.[56] Extrahepatic manifestations, such as ulcerative colitis, pleurisy, renal tubular acidosis and endocrine disturbances, are also unusually common in the HB_sAg negative group. In contrast, polyarteritis nodosa, arthritis and glomerulonephritis are well recognized in association with HB_sAg positive liver disease, and are thought to be related to the deposition of HB_sAg related antigen–antibody complexes in the tissues.

The mechanism behind the systemic manifestations in the non-hepatitis B group is unknown. Immune complex formation and deposition is possible, but cannot be established without prior identification of the antigen. Cross-reacting antigens, released after damage to hepatocytes, might elicit an immune response on selected target organs, such as the kidney tubule, as has been postulated to account for the renal tubular acidosis.[86]

Increasing knowledge of the aetiology of chronic active hepatitis reveals that the HB_sAg negative group can be further subdivided. Thus, a number of drugs – notably oxyphenisatin and methyldopa – have been implicated in the pathogenesis of chronic active hepatitis, both with and without the production of autoantibodies (see below). Furthermore, some of the autoantibody-negative chronic active hepatitis patients have been shown to suffer from metabolic disturbances, such as alpha-1-antitrypsin deficiency or Wilson's disease. To date, no specific immunological abnormalities have been ascribed to these sub-groups, but further research is needed.

Primary Biliary Cirrhosis (see also Chapter 31)

The most striking serological abnormality associated with this condition is the presence of the antimitochondrial antibody, which is a valuable aid to clinical diagnosis. Although found occasionally in other disorders, the autoantibody has proved valuable in distinguishing this condition from extrahepatic biliary obstruction. The presence and titre of the antibody is in no way related to either the clinical or histological features of the disease and it is unaffected by treatment with immunosuppressive drugs and only transiently by liver transplantation.[71] Antinuclear antibodies and anti-smooth muscle antibodies are also sometimes observed in this condition.

Damage to the bile ducts is a characteristic early histological lesion and although antibodies reacting with bile ductules and bile canaliculi can be demonstrated in the serum by immunofluorescence, they are not specific to primary biliary cirrhosis. All three major immunoglobulins may be raised in this condition, although IgM is the most consistently elevated. The reason for this is unknown. Although modest elevations in total serum globulins are usually found, they are not nearly as high as those seen in lupoid hepatitis. The impairment in cell-mediated immunity by both skin-testing and in vitro tests seems to be more marked in primary biliary cirrhosis. This condition is frequently characterized by the presence of granulomas within the liver and occasionally in other tissues, thus raising the possibility of its association with Crohn's disease or sarcoidosis, which may also be associated with anergic phenomena. The in vitro tests, however, are known to be non-specific in nature and more specific discriminants of these disorders have failed to date to reveal a common aetiology.

Alcoholic Liver Disease (see also Chapter 32)

Autoantibody production is not a noted feature in alcoholic liver disease, although low-titre smooth muscle antibodies are occasionally found. Serum immunoglobulin levels are frequently elevated, particularly IgG and IgA. The IgG levels often reflect the general disease activity, but raised IgA levels, which are more often the most striking abnormality, occur independently of disease activity or severity. Once again, the reason for this selective elevation is unknown. The elevated *E. coli* antibody titres noted in alcoholic liver disease are of IgM and not IgA class,[70] and although immune complexes in the glomeruli of patients with alcoholic cirrhosis are rich in IgA[14] this may well be secondary to the high serum levels. As mentioned earlier, the non-specific in vitro tests of cellular immunity have generally shown impaired T cell function.

Serial observations of alcoholics have shown that alcoholic fatty liver does not predispose to cirrhosis, whereas alcoholic hepatitis is undoubtedly a precirrhotic condition, although the rate of conversion may be very variable. Leevy, Chen and Zetterman[46] have suggested that the conversion to cirrhosis may be the result of alteration in immunological activity to an antigen such as alcoholic hyaline. They have shown that hyaline, when added to lymphocytes from patients with alcoholic hepatitis, causes a significant increase in the stimulation index and production of migration inhibition factor. Similar effects may be produced using ethanol and acetaldehyde. The presence of hyaline may also stimulate antibody production, since circulating antibodies to alcoholic hyaline may be detected in the serum, using a variety of techniques.[40]

Data on histocompatibility antigens in alcoholic liver disease are conflicting. Bailey et al[3] reported an increased incidence of HLA-B8 in this disorder, but this has not been confirmed by Scott, Rajah and Losowsky[68] or by Bell and Nordhagen,[4] although the latter found a significant increase in HLA-Bw40. All these studies have been carried out on small groups and more data are required.

Viral Hepatitis

The specific immunological phenomena related to the viruses of hepatitis A and B are discussed in Chapter 28. There are, in addition, non-specific immunological disturbances in both forms of hepatitis. Serum IgG levels are slightly elevated in both, but IgM levels are said to be higher in HB_sAg negative patients than in hepatitis B,[59] although this has been disputed by other workers. Serum complement is usually low in the early stages of the illness, rising to normal or above later. Anti-smooth muscle antibodies can frequently be detected in serum at some stage of the disease but they are usually of low titre and transient. Antinuclear and antimitochondrial antibodies are only rarely found in acute viral hepatitis and then usually only in low titre. Non-specific elevation of antibody titres to gut-associated bacteria such as *E. coli* may occur transiently during hepatitis. Impairment of T cell function may be demonstrated by in vitro tests during acute hepatitis, with restoration to normal activity on recovery from the hepatitis. To date, however, none of the tests has proved to be of value in predicting which patients will recover uneventfully and which will progress to chronic liver disease.

Drug-Associated Hepatitis (see also Chapter 36)

Many drugs may produce hepatic damage, either as a toxic reaction or on the basis of a hypersensitivity phenomenon. Distinction between the two mechanisms may often be difficult, but certain features tend to support the concept of a hypersensitivity reaction:

1. The liver damage produced by the drug is not dose dependent.
2. Withdrawal of the drug leads to an improvement in liver function, which deteriorates when the patient is subjected to further challenge with small doses of the drug.
3. Extrahepatic manifestations suggestive of an allergic reaction (e.g., rash, arthralgia, eosinophilia) may accompany the liver reaction. The absence of one or more of these phenomena does not, however, exclude the possibility of a hypersensitivity reaction. Diverse histological appearances have been described in association with drug sensitivity, including acute hepatitis, chronic active hepatitis leading to cirrhosis, cholestasis and granulomatous liver disease, although usually only one particular lesion is related to any given drug. Although the list of drugs associated with hypersensitivity reactions involving the liver is large we have selected five for further discussion.

Chlorpromazine

This is recognized as causing a pure cholestatic reaction, with no evidence of a hepatitis-like picture. Cholestasis has been reported to occur after a single tablet and jaundice and pruritus may exist for many months when it may be mistaken for extrahepatic obstruction. Challenge with repeat administration will usually reproduce the clinical features, but is mostly avoided because of the possibility of inducing prolonged symptoms. Despite the deep and prolonged icterus that may develop this condition is benign and usually resolves without any residual damage, although progressive damage may ensue.[50] Eosinophilia is an occasional but unremarkable finding. Immunological tests are generally unrewarding. Disturbances in serum immunoglobulins and appearance of auto-antibodies are not a feature of the disorder. Lymphocyte transformation using chlorpromazine as a mitogen is sometimes positive, but it is not sufficiently reliable to be of diagnostic value.

Alpha-methyldopa

The association of alpha-methyldopa with clinical and histological hepatitis is well documented.[78] Whereas some cases present with an acute hepatitis within the first few months of starting therapy, which resolves on stopping the drug, in other patients the appearance and progression of liver disease may be insidious, such that the diagnosis may not be made until cirrhosis and irreversible liver damage have occurred. Serological abnormalities, including a positive LE cell phenomenon, antinuclear and anti-smooth muscle antibodies, may occur, but are often absent. Immunoglobulin disturbances are similar to those found in chronic active hepatitis of unknown aetiology. A Coombs' positive haemolytic anaemia may be present but this also occurs in patients who take the drug but have no evidence of liver disease. In vitro tests of cell-mediated immunity are not usually helpful in this condition, although this may be due to inappropriate selection of antigen. Torres et al[80] failed to show lymphocyte transformation in response to alpha-methyldopa in any patients with hepatitis related to the drug, but lymphocytes from three of those eight patients did show positive transformation to the oxidized quinone form of the drug. Specific immunological tests are unlikely to be of great value until more is known about the active metabolites of the sensitizing drug.

Oxyphenisatin

Reynolds, Peters and Yamada[63] reported a series of patients with atypical clinical and histological features of chronic active hepatitis who had been taking the purgative oxyphenisatin and whose biochemical abnormalities disappeared on stopping the drug, only to return on subsequent challenge. Out of seven patients, two exhibited a positive LE cell phenomenon, two had positive antinuclear antibodies and three had positive anti-smooth muscle antibodies. Other workers have confirmed the association between this drug and a condition indistinguishable from lupoid hepatitis, although circulating autoantibodies and hyperglobulinaemia are not always present.

Halothane (see also Chapter 47)

Despite much controversy during the past 20 years, it is now generally recognized that a small but significant number of patients develop minor abnormalities in liver function following repeated administration of halothane.[92] These abnormalities are generally minor but occasionally a true hepatitis-like picture, which may even be fulminant, may appear. Repeated exposure using minute quantities of halothane can produce hepatic disturbances, suggesting the sensitivity phenomenon is not dose related. Although the lesion produced is usually an acute hepatitis, repeated exposure may in some cases lead to a chronic aggressive hepatitis with cirrhosis. Unexplained pyrexia is a common finding and skin rashes and eosinophilia occur occasionally. Minor serum immunoglobulin elevations of a non-diagnostic nature may be seen and anti-smooth muscle and antinuclear antibodies are sometimes seen in low titre only. The initial report by Rodriguez et al[65] of positive antimitochondrial antibodies in this condition has not been confirmed but there have been recent reports of microsomal antibodies.[88] Similarly, studies of lymphocyte transformation and leucocyte migration inhibition in response to halothane in these patients have been conflicting[54] but, as in the case of alphamethyldopa, the antigens used may be inappropriate for these in vitro tests.

Isoniazid

The hepatitis-like pattern associated with the antituberculous drug isoniazid provides a good example of the problems of ascribing hypersensitivity phenomena to a drug.[13] The onset of liver damage is variable and often prolonged following exposure to the drug, although rechallenge with isoniazid may produce the clinical biochemical effect usually associated with drug hypersensitivity reactions. Antinuclear antibodies commonly appear in the serum of patients receiving isoniazid but their presence does not relate to liver damage or any other systemic disturbance. Fever, chills, skin rashes and eosinophilia are notably uncommon in association with isoniazid-associated liver damage. Lymphocyte transformation in the presence of isoniazid has produced conflicting results. There is evidence to suggest that genetically determined rapid acetylation of isoniazid might be related to the frequency with which liver damage occurs, raising the possibility that a metabolite of isoniazid may be the provoking substance.[13] Further work should determine whether the hepatitis-like effect is produced by a toxin or by a sensitivity reaction in susceptible individuals.

CONCEPTS OF IMMUNOLOGICAL INJURY

Despite the enormous advances in our understanding of liver disease in recent years, two important questions in relation to immunology remain essentially unanswered:

1. What is the relationship of the disturbances in both T and B cell function that are found in liver diseases to the pathogenesis of the disorders?
2. What factors determine the clinical course following exposure to hepatotoxic agents and are these immunologically mediated?

Two separate mechanisms must be distinguished in the events underlying chronic liver disease. Such disease may arise from a chronic response to a persisting antigen or toxin, such as the hepatitis B virus, and here the defect is due to a failure of the host to eliminate the agent. Alternatively, the damage may result from the production within the host of an autoantigen, thus giving rise to an autoimmune reaction. While it is possible that such a reaction may occur in man and the liver-specific lipoprotein experimental model in the rabbit supports such a mechanism, there is as yet no firm evidence to support it as a clinical entity. The occurrence of serum autoantibodies may reflect the presence of an autoimmune reaction but it cannot be concluded that this is related to the pathogenesis of the liver disease.

Recent theories on the sequence of events leading to the development of chronic liver disease have largely been centred on defective T cell function. Thus Dudley, Fox and Sherlock,[21] using the model of HB_sAg, have suggested that the competence of the cell-mediated immune system determines whether an infection is self-limiting or persists with varying degrees of damage. A wider approach has been taken by Eddleston and Williams[22] who suggest that, in addition to the T cell response to virus antigens on the surface of infected hepatocytes, the elimination of virus is dependent upon a viable B cell response, in the form of the ability to produce appropriate amounts of high-affinity antibody. Autoimmunity itself may result from defective T/B lymphocyte interaction, and they postulate that at least the excessive antibody production might be related to defective suppressor T cell function, although there is no direct evidence to support this. On the basis of earlier work, they suggest that most of the HB_sAg negative chronic liver disease is initiated by the hepatitis B virus, a view which is discussed in Chapter 29.

Other mechanisms are likely to play a role and may interact with the T/B cell system (see Figure 9.2). The association of HLA-A1 and HLA-B8 with HB_sAg negative chronic active hepatitis raises the possibility that this may be a marker of genetic susceptibility to certain infectious or toxic agents. However, attempts to confirm this and to correlate other liver diseases with particular histocompatibility antigens have been disappointing.[68] There is little doubt that circulating immune complexes appear in most if not all forms of liver disease but, as mentioned earlier, their persistence in the circulation is likely to be prolonged in the presence of liver damage. While it seems likely that their presence can be implicated in the pathogenesis of many of the extrahepatic manifestations of liver disease, there is no firm evidence to support the idea that they may contribute to perpetuation or progression of liver damage.

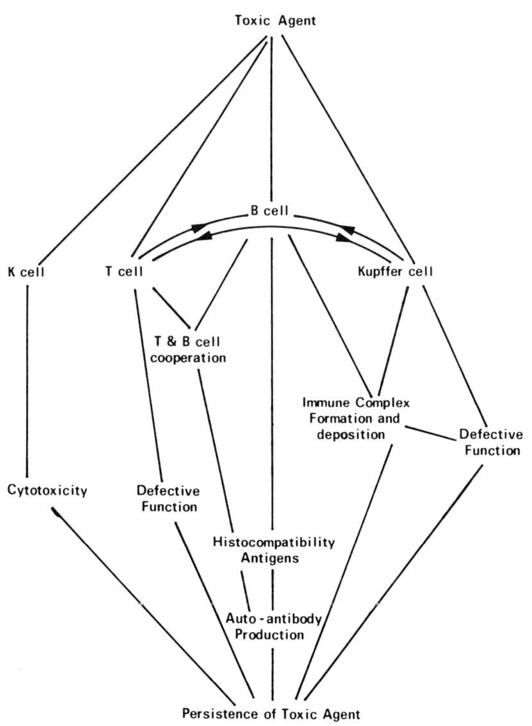

Figure 9.2. Some possible mechanisms involved in the immunological response to liver injury.

A further mechanism which has received scant attention concerns the ability of the Kupffer cell to eliminate viral or other potential toxins. Kupffer cell function appears to be important in acute viral hepatitis in animals and failure of the cells to eliminate virus may lead to replication within the cell and subsequent spill-over with infection of the hepatocyte. Defects in Kupffer cell function in man, due either to an intrinsic defect or to some form of competitive blockade, might lead to a persistence of the provoking agent which could result in chronic liver damage, but such a possibility cannot be tested until adequate methods of assessing Kupffer cell function in vitro become available.

In conclusion, present knowledge suggests that a series of separate but probably related immunological mechanisms are involved in both the initiation and perpetuation of many liver diseases. At present it is impossible to decide whether most of these abnormalities occur as a consequence of the liver damage or whether they are instrumental in producing the destruction. Similarly, the relative importance of different mechanisms cannot be assessed until more sophisticated methods become available for defining individual reactions by reliable in vivo and in vitro tests. Since the liver itself is known to play an important role in the function of the reticuloendothelial system as a whole, this may prove impossible but much further work is required before the role of immune mechanisms in the pathogenesis of liver disease can be defined.

REFERENCES

1. Arakawa, Y., Bull, D.M., Schott, C.F. & Davidson, C.S. (1976) F-antigen: nature, liver specificity and release in experimental liver injury. *Gastroenterology*, **17**, 118–122.

2. Bacon, P.A., Berry, H. & Bown, R. (1972) Cell-mediated immune reactivity in liver disease. *Gut,* **13,** 427–429.
3. Bailey, R.J., Krasner, N., Eddleston, A.L.W.F., Williams, R., Tee, D.E.H., Doniach, D., Kennedy, L.A. & Batchelor, J.R. (1976) Histocompatibility antigens, autoantibodies and immunoglobulins in alcoholic liver disease. *British Medical Journal,* **ii,** 726–728.
4. Bell, H. & Nordhagen, R. (1978) Association between HLA-Bw 40 and alcoholic liver disease with cirrhosis. *British Medical Journal,* **i,** 822.
5. Benjamin, I.S., Ryan, C.J., McLay, A.L.C., Horne, C.H.W. & Blumgart, L.H. (1976) The effects of portacaval shunting and portacaval transposition on serum IgG levels in the rat. *Gastroenterology,* **70,** 661–664.
6. Berenyi, M.R., Straus, B. & Avila, L. (1975) T rosettes in alcoholic cirrhosis of the liver. *Journal of the American Medical Association,* **232,** 44–46.
7. Berg, P.A., Binder, T., Lindner, H., Bannaski, H., Maas, D. & Henning, H. (1975) Heterogenität mitochondrialer Autoantikörper. *Deutsche Medizinische Wochenschrift,* **20,** 1123–1127.
8. Berger, S.R. & Bull, D.M. (1977) Cirrhotic hyperglobulinaemia: increased rates of immunoglobulin synthesis by circulating lymphoid cells. *Clinical Research,* **25,** 307 (abstract).
9. Bianchi, F.B., Penfold, P.L. & Roitt, I.M. (1973) Mitochondrial antibodies in primary biliary cirrhosis. V. Ultrastructural localisation of the antigen to the inner mitochondrial membranes using a direct peroxidase conjugate. *British Journal of Experimental Pathology,* **54,** 652–657.
10. Bjørneboe, M. & Prytz, H. (1976) Mononuclear phagocytic functions of the liver. In *Immunological Aspects of the Liver and Gastrointestinal Tract* (Ed.) Ferguson, A. & MacSween, R.N.M. pp. 7, 251–289. Lancaster, England: Medical and Technical Publishing.
11. Bjørneboe, M., Prytz, H. & Ørskov, F. (1972) Antibodies to intestinal microbes in serum of patients with cirrhosis of the liver. *Lancet,* **i,** 58–60.
12. Bjørneboe, M., Jensen, K.B., Scheibel, I., Thomson, Å. Chr. & Bentzon, M.W. (1970) Tetanus antitoxin production and gamma globulin level in patients with cirrhosis of the liver. *Acta Medica Scandinavica,* **188,** 541–546.
13. Black, M., Mitchell, J.R., Zimmerman, H.J., Ishak, K.G. & Epler, G.R. (1975) Isoniazid-associated hepatitis in 114 patients. *Gastroenterology,* **69,** 289–302.
14. Callard, P., Feldmann, G., Prandi, D., Belair, M.F., Mandet, C., Weiss, Y., Druet, P., Benhamou, J.P. & Bariety, J. (1975) Immune complex type glomerulonephritis in cirrhosis of the liver. *American Journal of Pathology,* **80,** 329–340.
15. Calne, R.Y., Davis, D.R., Hadjiyannakis, D., Sells, R.A., White, D., Herbertson, B.M., Millard, P.R., Joysey, V.C., Davies, D.A.L., Binns, R.M. & Festenstein, H. (1970) Immunosuppressive effects of soluble cell membrane fractions, donor blood and serum on renal allograft survival. *Nature,* **227,** 903–906.
16. Cantor, H.M. & Dumont, A.E. (1967) Hepatic suppression of sensitisation to antigen absorbed into the portal system. *Nature,* **215,** 744–745.
17. Cochrane, A.M.G., Moussouros, A., Thomson, A.D., Eddleston, A.L.W.F. & Williams, R. (1976) Antibody-dependent cell-mediated (K cell) cytotoxicity against isolated hepatocytes in chronic active hepatitis. *Lancet,* **i,** 441–444.
18. Davis, P. & Read, A.E. (1975) Antibodies to double-stranded (native) DNA in active chronic hepatitis. *Gut,* **16,** 413–415.
19. DeHoratius, R.J., Strickland, R.G. & Williams, R.C. Jr (1974) T and B lymphocytes in acute and chronic hepatitis. *Clinical Immunology and Immunopathology,* **2,** 353–360.
20. Doniach, D., Roitt, I.M., Walker, J.G. & Sherlock, S. (1966) Tissue antibodies in primary biliary cirrhosis, active chronic hepatitis, cryptogenic cirrhosis and other liver diseases and their clinical implications. *Clinical and Experimental Immunology,* **1,** 237–262.
21. Dudley, F.J., Fox, R.A. & Sherlock, S. (1972) Cellular immunity and hepatitis-associated Australia antigen liver disease. *Lancet,* **i,** 723–726.
22. Eddleston, A.L.W.F. & Williams, R. (1974) Inadequate antibody response to HB_sAg or suppressor T-cell defect in development of active chronic hepatitis. *Lancet,* **ii,** 1543–1545.
23. Feizi, T. (1968) Serum immunoglobulins in liver disease. *Gut,* **9,** 193–198.
24. Fournié, G.J., Lambert, P.H. & Miescher, P.A. (1974) Release of DNA in circulating blood and induction of anti-DNA antibodies after injection of bacterial lipopolysaccharides. *Journal of Experimental Medicine,* **140,** 1189–1206.
25. Fox, R.A., Dudley, F.J. & Sherlock, S. (1973) The primary immune response to haemocyanin in patients with primary biliary cirrhosis. *Clinical and Experimental Immunology,* **14,** 473–480.
26. Franzl, R.E. (1972) The primary immune response in mice. III. Retention of sheep red blood cell immunogens by the spleen and liver. *Infection and Immunity,* **6,** 469–482.
27. Gajdusek, D.C. (1957) An 'auto-immune' reaction against human tissue antigens in certain chronic diseases. *Nature,* **179,** 666–668.
28. Geubel, A.P., Keller, R.H., Summerskill, W.H.J., Dickson, E.R., Tomasi, T.B. & Shorter, R.G. (1976) Lymphocyte cytotoxicity and inhibition studied with autologous liver cells: observations in chronic active liver disease and the primary biliary cirrhosis syndrome. *Gastroenterology,* **71,** 450–456.
29. Haserick, J.R., Lewis, L.A. & Bortz, D.W. (1950) Blood factor in acute disseminated lupus erythematosus. I. Determination of gamma globulin as specific plasma fraction. *American Journal of Medical Sciences,* **219,** 660–663.
30. Havens, W.P., Meyerson, R.M. & Klatchko, J. (1957) Production of tetanus antitoxin by patients with hepatic cirrhosis. *New England Journal of Medicine,* **257,** 637–643.
31. Havens, W.P., Dickensheets, J., Bierly, J.N. & Eberhard, T.P. (1954) The half-life of I^{131} labelled normal human gamma globulin in patients with hepatic cirrhosis. *Journal of Immunology,* **73,** 256–258.
32. Hodgson, H.J.F., Wands, J.R. & Isselbacher, K.J. (1977) Suppressor lymphocytes: their role in modulating the immune response in acute and chronic active hepatitis. *Gastroenterology,* **72,** 1070.
33. Hsu, C.C.S. & Leevy, C.M. (1971) Inhibition of PHA-stimulated lymphocyte transformation by plasma from patients with advanced alcoholic cirrhosis. *Clinical and Experimental Immunology,* **8,** 749–760.
34. Hughes, G.V.R. (1971) Significance of anti-DNA antibodies in systemic lupus erythematosus. *Lancet,* **ii,** 861–863.

35. Husby, G., Strickland, R.G., Caldwell, J.L. & Williams, R.C. (1975) Localization of T and B cells and alpha fetoprotein in hepatic biopsies from patients with liver disease. *Journal of Clinical Investigation*, **56,** 1198–1209.
36. Inchley, C.J. (1969) The activity of mouse Kupffer cells following intravenous injection of T_4 bacteriophage. *Clinical and Experimental Immunology*, **5,** 173–187.
37. Jain, S., Markham, R., Thomas, H.C. & Sherlock, S. (1976) Double-stranded DNA-binding capacity of serum in acute and chronic liver disease. *Clinical and Experimental Immunology*, **26,** 35–41.
38. Johnson, G.D., Holborow, E.J. & Glynn, L.E. (1965) Antibody to smooth muscle in patients with liver disease. *Lancet*, **ii,** 878–879.
39. Kakumu, S. & Leevy, C.M. (1977) Lymphocyte cytotoxicity in alcoholic hepatitis. *Gastroenterology*, **72,** 594–597.
40. Kanagasundaram, N., Kakumu, S., Chen, T. & Leevy, C.M. (1977) Alcoholic hyalin antigen (AHAg) and antibody (AHAb) in alcoholic hepatitis. *Gastroenterology*, **73,** 1368–1373.
41. Kawanishi, H. & Macdermott, R.P. (1977) Induction of antibody-dependent hepatocyte cytotoxicity by chronic active liver disease serum, mediated by normal null cells. *Gastroenterology*, **72,** 1078.
42. Keraan, M., Meyers, O.L., Engelbrecht, G.H.C., Hickman, R., Saunders, S.J. & Terblanche, J. (1974) Increased serum immunoglobulin levels following portacaval shunt in the rat. *Gut*, **15,** 468–472.
43. Kingham, J.G.C., Rassam, S., Ganguly, N.K., McGuire, M.J., Nasrat, B., Holgate, S.T. & Wright, R. (1978) DNA-binding antibodies and hepatitis B markers in acute and chronic liver disease. *Clinical and Experimental Immunology*, **33,** 204–210.
44. Kotkes, P. & Pick, E. (1975) Studies on the inhibition of macrophage migration induced by soluble antigen–antibody complexes. *Clinical and Experimental Immunology*, **19,** 105–120.
45. Lam, K.C., Mistilis, S.P. & Perrott, N. (1972) Positive tissue antibody tests in patients with prolonged extrahepatic biliary obstruction. *New England Journal of Medicine*, **286,** 1400–1401.
46. Leevy, C.M., Chen, T. & Zetterman, R. (1975) Alcoholic hepatitis, cirrhosis and immunologic reactivity. *Annals of the New York Academy of Sciences*, **252,** 106–115.
47. Lidman, K., Biberfeld, G., Fagraeus, A., Norberg, R., Torstensson, R., Utter, G., Carlsson, L., Luca, J. & Lindberg, U. (1976) Anti-actin specificity of human smooth muscle antibodies in chronic active hepatitis. *Clinical and Experimental Immunology*, **24,** 266–272.
48. MacKay, I.R. & Morris, P.J. (1972) Association of autoimmune active chronic hepatitis with HL-A1, 8. *Lancet*, **ii,** 793–795.
49. MacSween, R.N.M., Galbraith, I., Thomas, M.A., Watkinson, G. & Ludlam, G.B. (1973) Phytohaemagglutinin (PHA) induced lymphocyte transformation and *Toxoplasma gondii* antibody studies in primary biliary cirrhosis. Evidence of impaired cell-mediated immunity. *Clinical and Experimental Immunology*, **15,** 35–42.
50. Maddrey, W.C. & Boitnott, J.K. (1977) Drug-induced chronic liver disease. *Gastroenterology*, **77,** 1348–1353.
51. Meyer zum Büschenfelde, K.H., Kössling, F.K. & Miescher, P.A. (1972) Experimental chronic active hepatitis in rabbits following immunisation with human liver proteins. *Clinical and Experimental Immunology*, **11,** 99–108.
52. Meyer zum Büschenfelde, K.H., Alberti, A., Arnold, W. & Freudenberg, J. (1975) Organ-specificity and diagnostic value of cell-mediated immunity against a liver-specific membrane protein: studies in hepatic and non-hepatic diseases. *Klinische Wochenschrift*, **53,** 1061–1067.
53. Mihas, A.A., Bull, D.M. & Davidson, C.S. (1975) Cell-mediated immunity to liver in patients with alcoholic hepatitis. *Lancet*, **i,** 951–953.
54. Moult, P.J.A., Adjukiewicz, A.B., Gaylarde, P.M., Sarkany, I. & Sherlock, S. (1975) Lymphocyte transformation in halothane-related hepatitis. *British Medical Journal*, **ii,** 69–70.
55. Newble, D.I., Holmes, K.T., Wangel, A.G. & Forbes, I.J. (1975) Immune reactions in acute viral hepatitis. *Clinical and Experimental Immunology*, **20,** 17–28.
56. Opelz, G., Vogten, A.J.M., Summerskill, W.H.J., Schalm, S.W. & Terasaki, P.I. (1977) HLA determinants in chronic active liver disease: possible relation of HLA-Dw3 to prognosis. *Tissue Antigens*, **9,** 36–40.
57. Page, A.R., Sharp, H.L., Greenberg, L.J. & Yunis, E.J. (1975) Genetic analysis of patients with chronic active hepatitis. *Journal of Clinical Investigation*, **56,** 530–535.
58. Paronetto, F. & Vernace, S. (1975) Immunological studies in patients with chronic active hepatitis: cytotoxic activity in lymphocytes to autochthonous liver cells grown in tissue culture. *Clinical and Experimental Immunology*, **19,** 99–104.
59. Peters, C.J. & Johnson, K.M. (1972) Serum immunoglobulin levels in Australia antigen positive and Australia antigen negative hepatitis. *Clinical and Experimental Immunology*, **11,** 381–391.
60. Protell, R.L., Soloway, R.D., Martin, W.J., Schoenfield, L.J. & Summerskill, W.H.J. (1971) Anti-salmonella agglutinins in chronic active liver disease. *Lancet*, **ii,** 330–332.
61. Prytz, H., Bjørneboe, M., Johansen, T.S. & Ørskov, F. (1974) The influence of portosystemic shunt operation on immunoglobulins and *Escherichia coli* antibodies in patients with cirrhosis of the liver. *Acta Medica Scandinavica*, **196,** 109–112.
62. Ravin, H.A., Rowley, D., Jenkins, C. & Fine, J. (1960) On the absorption of bacterial endotoxin from the gastro-intestinal tract of the normal and shocked animal. *Journal of Experimental Medicine*, **112,** 783–792.
63. Reynolds, T.B., Peters, R.L. & Yamada, S. (1971) Chronic active and lupoid hepatitis caused by a laxative, oxyphenisatin. *New England Journal of Medicine*, **285,** 813–820.
64. Rizzetto, M., Swana, G. & Doniach, D. (1973) Microsomal antibodies in active chronic hepatitis and other disorders. *Clinical and Experimental Immunology*, **15,** 331–344.
65. Rodriguez, M., Paronetto, F., Schaffner, F. & Popper, H. (1969) Antimitochondrial antibodies in jaundice following drug administration. *Journal of the American Medical Association*, **208,** 148–150.
66. Sanchez-Tapias, J., Thomas, H.C. & Sherlock, S. (1977) Lymphocyte populations in liver biopsy specimens from patients with chronic liver disease. *Gut*, **18,** 472–475.
67. Schumacher, K., Maerker-Alzer, G. & Wehmer, U. (1974) A lymphocyte-inhibiting factor isolated from normal human liver. *Nature*, **251,** 655–656.
68. Scott, B.B., Rajah, S.M. & Losowsky, M. (1977) Histocompatibility antigens in chronic liver disease. *Gastroenterology*, **72,** 122–125.

69. Sell, S., & Fahey, J.L. (1967) Relationship between gamma-globulin metabolism and low serum gamma-globulin in germ-free mice. *Journal of Immunology,* **93,** 81–87.

70. Simjee, A.E., Hamilton-Miller, J.M.T., Thomas, H.C., Brumfitt, W. & Sherlock, S. (1975) Antibodies to *Escherichia coli* in chronic liver diseases. *Gut,* **16,** 871–875.

71. Smith, M.G.M., Williams, R., Doniach, D. & Calne, R.Y. (1971) Effect of orthoptic liver transplantation on serum auto-antibodies. *Lancet,* **ii,** 1006–1009.

72. Souhami, R.L. (1972) The effect of colloidal carbon on the organ distribution of sheep red cells and the immune response. *Immunology,* **22,** 685–694.

73. Sugamara, K. & Smith, J.B. (1976) Purification and characterisation of human liver specific F antigen. *Clinical and Experimental Immunology,* **26,** 28–34.

74. Tage-Jensen, U., Arnold, W., Dietrichson, O., Hardt, F., Hopf, U., Meyer zum Büschenfelde, K.H. & Nielsen, J.O. (1977) Liver-cell-membrane auto-antibody specific for inflammatory liver diseases. *British Medical Journal,* **i,** 206–208.

75. Thomas, H.C., MacSween, R.N.M. & White, R.G. (1973) Role of the liver in controlling the immunogenicity of commensal bacteria in the gut. *Lancet,* **i,** 1288–1291.

76. Thomas, H.C., Freni, M., Sanchez-Tapias, J., De Villiers, D., Jain, S. & Sherlock, S. (1976) Peripheral blood lymphocyte populations in chronic liver disease. *Clinical and Experimental Immunology,* **26,** 222–227.

77. Thomson, A.D., Cochrane, M.A.G., MacFarlane, I.G., Eddleston, A.L.W.F. & Williams, R. (1974) Lymphocyte cytotoxicity to isolated hepatocytes in chronic active hepatitis. *Nature,* **252,** 721–722.

78. Toghill, P.J., Smith, P.G., Benton, P., Brown, R.C. & Matthews, H.L. (1974) Methyldopa liver damage. *British Medical Journal,* **iii,** 545–548.

79. Toh, B.H., Roberts-Thomson, I.C., Mathews, J.D., Whittingham, S. & MacKay, I.R. (1973) Depression of cell-mediated immunity in old age and the immunopathic diseases, lupus erythematosus, chronic hepatitis and rheumatoid arthritis. *Clinical and Experimental Immunology,* **14,** 193–202.

80. Torres, A.C., Tong, M.J., Chang, K. & Schweitzer, I. (1976) Lymphocyte stimulation in alpha-methyldopa related hepatitis. *Clinical Research,* **24,** 106 (abstract).

81. Triger, D.R. & Wright, R. (1973) Studies on the hepatic uptake of antigen. II. The effect of hepatotoxins on the immune response. *Immunology,* **25,** 951–956.

82. Triger, D.R. & Wright, R. (1973) Hyperglobulinaemia in liver disease. *Lancet,* **i,** 1494–1496.

83. Triger, D.R., Alp, M.H. & Wright, R. (1972) Bacterial and dietary antibodies in liver disease. *Lancet,* **i,** 60–63.

84. Triger, D.R., Cynamon, M.H. & Wright, R. (1973) Studies on the hepatic uptake of antigen. I. Comparison of inferior vena cava and portal vein routes of immunization. *Immunology,* **25,** 941–950.

85. Triger, D.R., Kurtz, J.B. & Wright, R. (1974) Viral antibodies and auto-antibodies in chronic liver disease. *Gut,* **15,** 94–98.

86. Tsantoulas, D.C., McFarlane, I.G., Portmann, B., Eddleston, A.L.W.F. & Williams, R. (1974) Cell-mediated immunity to human Tamm–Horsfall glycoprotein in autoimmune liver disease with renal tubular acidosis. *British Medical Journal,* **iv,** 491–494.

87. Walker, J.G., Bates, D., Doniach, D., Ball, P.A.J. & Sherlock, S. (1972) Chronic liver disease and mitochondrial antibodies. A family study. *British Medical Journal,* **i,** 146–148.

88. Walton, B., Simpson, B.R., Strunin, L., Doniach, D., Perrin, J. & Appleyard, A.J. (1976) Unexplained hepatitis following halothane. *British Medical Journal,* **i,** 1171–1176.

89. Wands, J.R., Perrotto, J.L., Alpert, E. & Isselbacher, K.J. (1975) Cell-mediated immunity in acute and chronic hepatitis. *Journal of Clinical Investigation,* **55,** 921–929.

90. Warshaw, A.L., Walker, W.A. & Isselbacher, K.J. (1974) Protein uptake by the intestine: evidence for absorption of intact macromolecules. *Gastroenterology,* **66,** 987–992.

91. Wisse, E. (1977) Ultrastructure and function of Kupffer *Cells and Other Liver Sinusoidal Cells* (Ed.) Wisse, E. & Knook, D.L. pp. 33–60. Amsterdam: Elsevier/North Holland Biomedical Press.

92. Wright, R., Eade, O.E., Chisholm, M., Hawksley, M., Lloyd, B., Moles, T.M., Edwards, J.C. & Gardner, M.J. (1975) Controlled prospective study of the effect on liver function of multiple exposures to halothane. *Lancet,* **i,** 817–820.

Chapter 10

Regeneration

Part 1: Physical Aspects
STEPHEN KARRAN
CAROL EAGLES

Part 2: Regulatory Mechanisms
NANCY L.R. BUCHER
JOAN A. McGOWAN

Part 1

PHYSICAL ASPECTS

STEPHEN KARRAN
CAROL EAGLES

Extensive resection of normal liver is compatible with survival and return to full health because of the capacity of the remnant to regenerate. Recovery has been reported following 80 to 90 per cent resection (see Chapter 49). Not only is there rapid increase in the size of the liver cells (hypertrophy) but there is also active cell division and multiplication (hyperplasia), with the peak of mitotic activity occurring some 24 to 36 hours after hepatectomy in parenchymal cells and later in littoral and Kupffer cells[69] (Figure 10.1). In both animals and man there is thus an early increase in the mass and

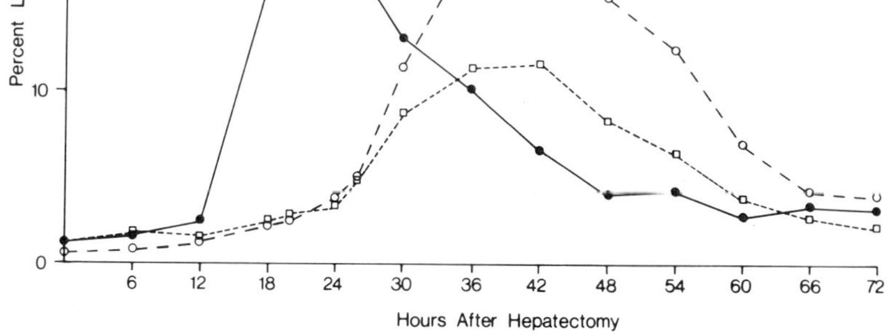

Figure 10.1. Mitotic activity in parenchymal, littoral and Kupffer cells following partial hepatectomy in the rat. From Bucher and Malt,[23] with kind permission of the editor of *New England Journal of Medicine*.

number of cells so that the liver tissue is restored with remarkable rapidity. In addition, repeated hepatectomy is feasible in the same animal following recovery.[157] Liver function also recovers quickly following this restoration of tissue,[17] providing no prior liver damage existed and that complications such as infection or anoxia are avoided. The severity of metabolic abnormality resulting from hepatectomy is directly related to the extent of the resection.[185] The restoration of mass, cell population and function constitutes 'regeneration', which may be contrasted with normal developmental growth and the additive forms of growth seen in pregnancy, lactation and hyperplasia.

SPECIES VARIATIONS

Regeneration of the liver occurs in many species. Man, rodents, dogs, pigs, frogs and birds all exhibit a similar ability to restore lost or damaged tissue. The rate at which the remnant grows varies from species to species. In the rat, for example, following 67 per cent hepatectomy,[77] normal mass and volume are restored within seven to ten days[83] (Figure 10.2). In dogs the process is slower. In children and young adults there is evidence that following hemi-hepatectomy, considerable restoration is detectable within the first 10 days and this progresses considerably within the first few weeks[17] (Figures 10.3 and 10.4). Full restoration of mass has been recognized within six months[6, 64] but the process is probably more rapid than this in previously fit young patients. The gamma camera image in Figure 10.5 was obtained in a girl of nine years three weeks after splenectomy and right hemi-hepatectomy had been performed following a road traffic accident. The heavy lines indicate the costal margins, and it can be seen that not only has the remnant grown to the right to fill most of the space previously occupied by the right lobe of the liver, but also towards the left to occupy the splenic space.

Observations were made on three patients who died from head and chest injuries at one, six and 10 days after right hemi-hepatectomy. Figure 10.6 shows the data obtained at operation and post-mortem. Following operation the weight of the resected lobe was recorded. An estimate of the mass of the remnant was then made after calculating the expected total liver weight for the patient's height and weight using the following formulae:[42, 48]

1. Liver weight (kg) = 1.02 × body surface area (m^2) − 0.22.
2. Surface area (cm^2) = weight $(kg)^{0.425}$ × height $(cm)^{0.725}$ × 71.84.

At post-mortem the mass of the remnant was measured. In the first patient, it was found that the mass of the remnant was approximately

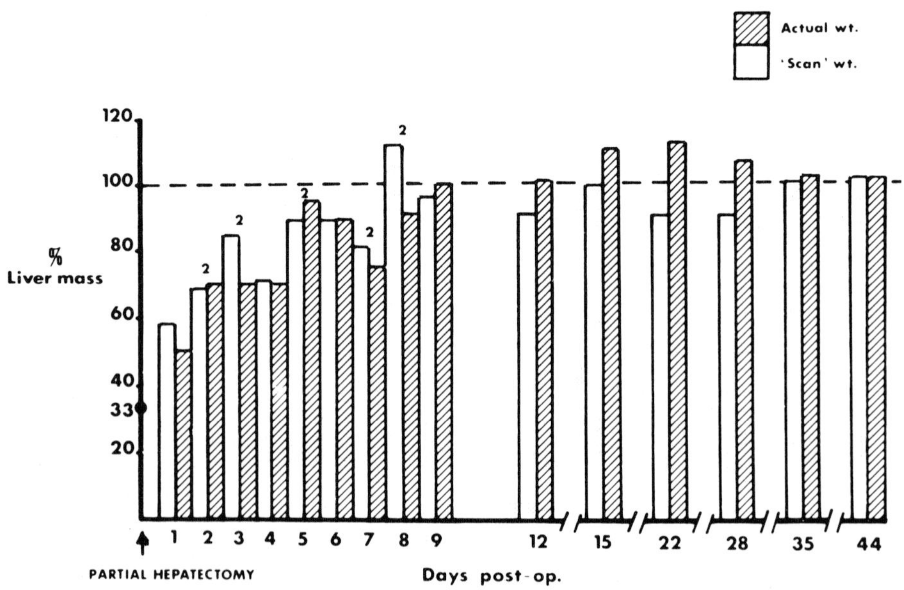

Figure 10.2. Histogram of liver growth in the rat following 67 per cent hepatectomy assessed by in vivo imaging and sacrificial weight measurements. Liver mass is given as percentage of calculated pre-hepatectomy weight. From Karran, Leach and Blumgart,[83] with kind permission of the editor of *Journal of Nuclear Medicine*.

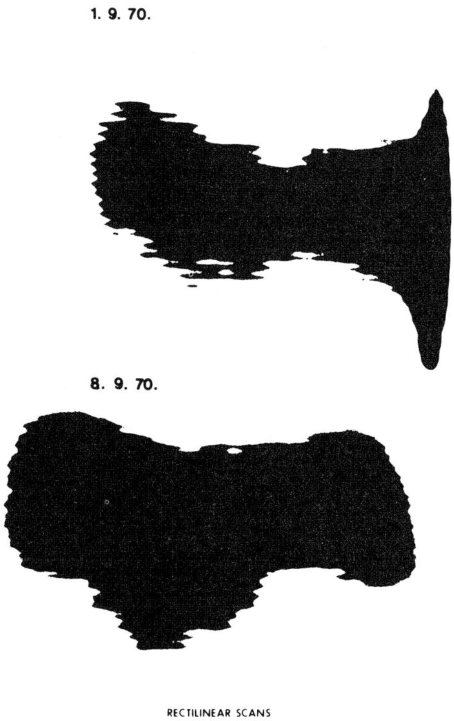

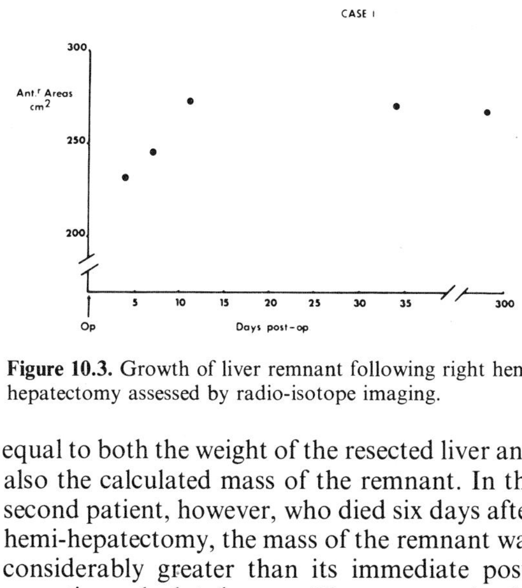

Figure 10.3. Growth of liver remnant following right hemi-hepatectomy assessed by radio-isotope imaging.

equal to both the weight of the resected liver and also the calculated mass of the remnant. In the second patient, however, who died six days after hemi-hepatectomy, the mass of the remnant was considerably greater than its immediate post-operative calculated mass. The remnant in the patient who died 10 days after resection had an increase of some 90 per cent in mass, so that the normal liver weight had been very nearly regained in this short space of time.

From these imaging studies and weight calculations, it therefore appears that the growth of the remnant commences very rapidly after operation, providing complications such as anoxia and sepsis are avoided. Within a few weeks this process is well advanced and liver function returns rapidly to normal.[185] Previous estimates which suggest that four to six months are necessary before full restoration of mass is achieved are therefore almost certainly conservative in fit young patients.[113,114,129]

As the remnant grows its shape is largely determined by external pressure. No new lobes develop although the new liver that is formed is microscopically normal. The residual lobes grow until they are equal in size and volume to the original liver and some small amount of 'overshoot' may be seen. The remnant adapts itself to the available space as it grows. For example, following right hemi-hepatectomy in man the remnant grows in a globular fashion until it becomes moulded within the confines of the diaphragm and abdominal wall (Figure 10.7). Similarly, following splenectomy as well as partial hepatectomy, the remnant grows across to occupy the space previously filled by the spleen as well as growing into the space resulting from removal of the right lobe of the liver (Figure 10.5).

HEPATIC PERFUSION

Controversy has existed for many years about the relevance of alterations in blood flow to the remnant following partial hepatectomy. As a result of the work of Mann and his colleagues,[109] it was postulated that an increase in flow to the remnant was the prime cause of the regenerative response. Increased perfusion results from diversion of all the blood in the portal vein and hepatic artery into the remnant. Associated with this diversion, an increase in portal pressure is found.[135] Following portacaval shunting a decrease in liver size (atrophy) occurs and when partial hepatectomy is performed following portacaval shunting the ability of the remnant to increase in *size* is severely inhibited. However, Weinbren[178] has shown that DNA synthesis and mitotic activity are still increased under these circumstances, indicating the presence of true hyperplasia. Diversion of portal venous blood with possible 'trophic' substances does not, therefore, deprive the remnant of its ability to regenerate. If such 'trophic' substances are responsible for the initiation and control of regeneration (see pages 211–216), these may still reach the remnant through the systemic circulation and ultimately the hepatic artery, even though they may suffer degradation and dilution in the process.

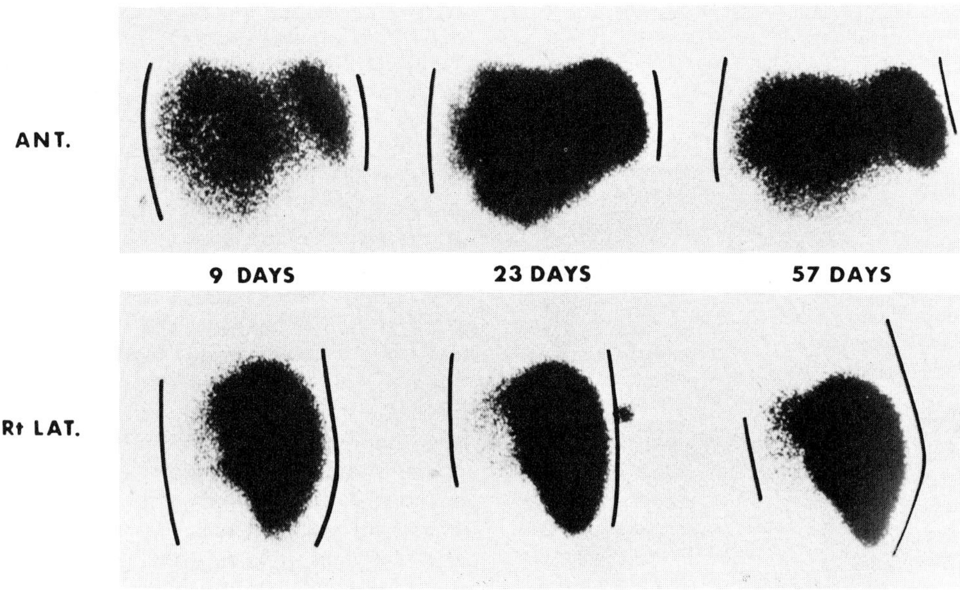

Figure 10.4. Further example of the early growth seen on radio-isotope imaging, with little further increase in size after 23 days.

Perfusion by both portal vein and hepatic artery, however, enables the full regenerative response to occur. It has still to be defined whether this response results from an increased delivery of 'trophic' hormones such as insulin and glucagon, of nutrient substrates such as amino acids, or of both. Following portacaval shunting, partial hepatectomy produces an increased flow in the residual branches of the hepatic artery.[84] Changes in perfusion of the remnant therefore still occur, though the increase is far less than that which occurs in the presence of an intact portal circulation.

Evidence to support this hypothesis has been obtained in an experimental model. Following partial hepatectomy in the rat, a marked increase in 'specific' liver blood flow, i.e. ml/g, to the remnant was shown by both sacrificial uptake studies[15,135] and more recently by in vivo techniques[63,70,85] (Figure 10.8). A similar

Figure 10.5. Gamma camera image in a girl of nine years three weeks after right hemi-hepatectomy and splenectomy. The heavy lines indicate the costal margins. Note that the liver remnant fills both regions previously occupied by the spleen and the right lobe of the liver. From Blumgart, Leach and Karran,[17] with kind permission of the editor of *Gut*.

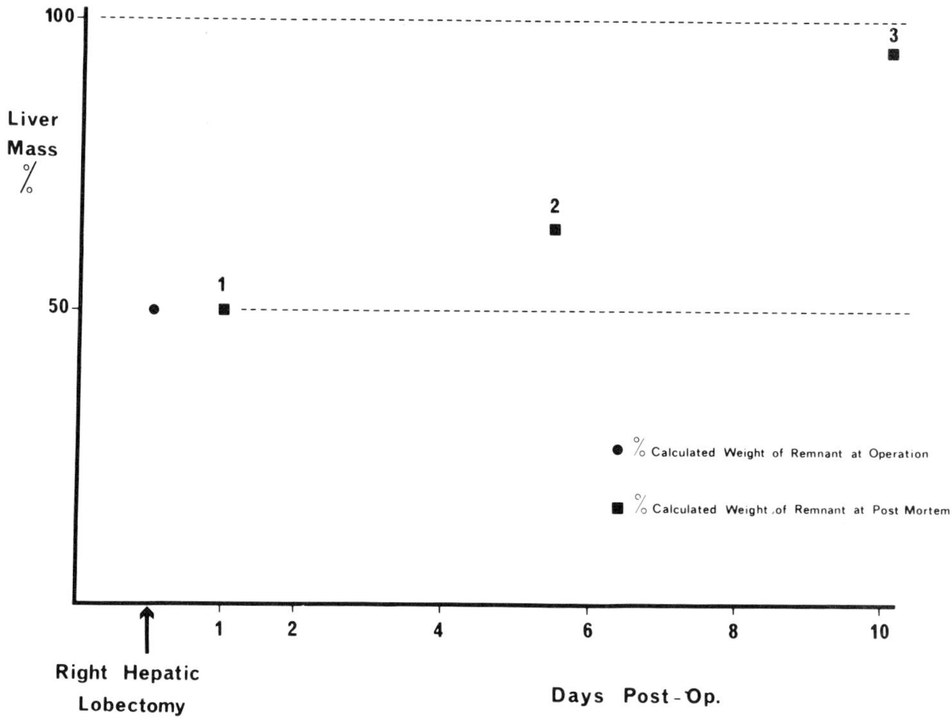

Figure 10.6. Estimations of the growth of the liver remnant in three patients who died at one, six and ten days after right hepatectomy.

pattern is seen in all these studies though there are differences in the extent and timing of the increased perfusion. In both Benacerraf's study and Guest's more recent investigation a delay of 16 and four hours respectively occurred before maximal increases were seen. Both Rabinovici's study and our own recent in vivo dynamic gamma camera study, however, showed that maximal values were obtained *immediately* following hepatectomy. An *immediate* increase in perfusion of the remnant would appear the more probable event following occlusion of inflow to the resected lobes. Colloid uptake studies also show that the maximal increase

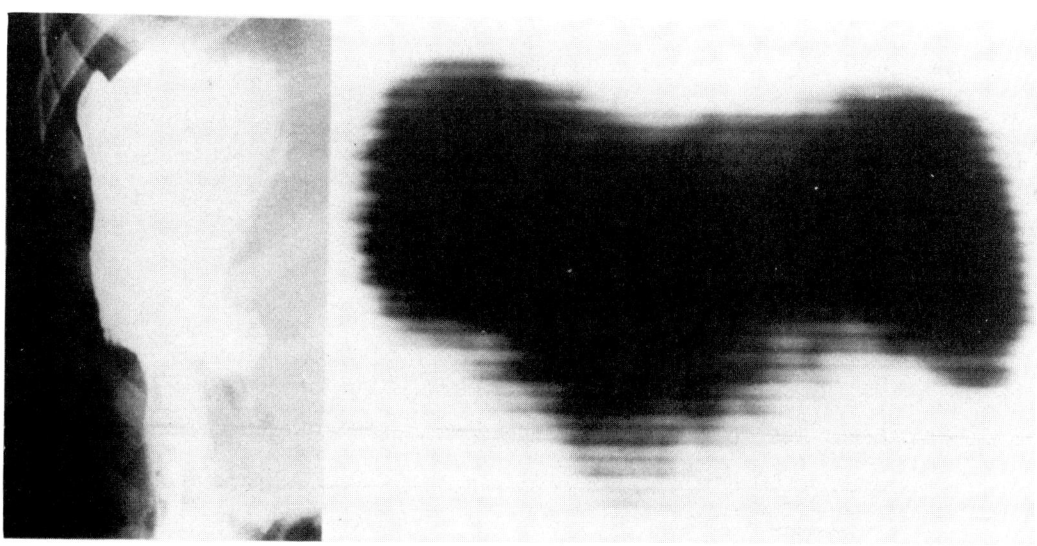

Figure 10.7. Sinogram in a patient who developed a subphrenic abscess following right hemi-hepatectomy, showing the globular enlargement of the remnant which has grown to within 2 cm of the abdominal wall. This was confirmed at laparotomy. From Blumgart, Leach and Karran,[17] with kind permission of the editor of *Gut*.

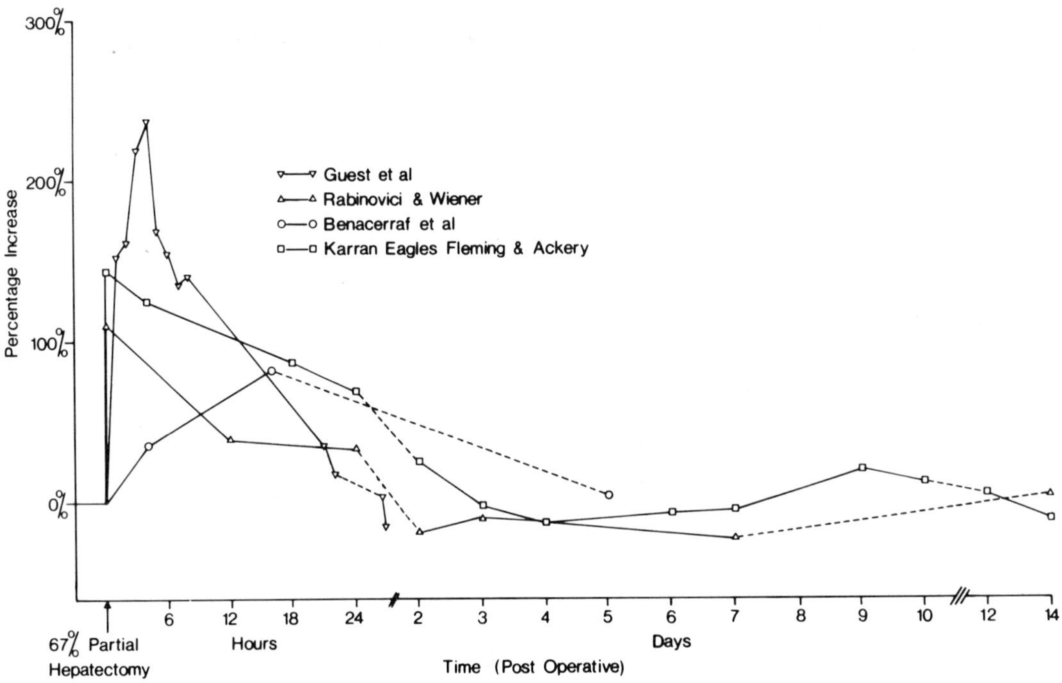

Figure 10.8. Change in 'specific' liver perfusion following 67 per cent hepatectomy in the rat by both sacrificial[15,135] and in vivo techniques.[70,85] From Karran et al[85] with kind permission of the editor of *Journal of Nuclear Medicine*.

occurs immediately following resection[82] (Figure 10.9). Delay in the demonstration of maximal perfusion in the other studies probably results from differences in technique.

The new in vivo method of assessment of hepatic perfusion using the gamma camera and pinhole collimator is relatively simple and allows repeated examinations in the same

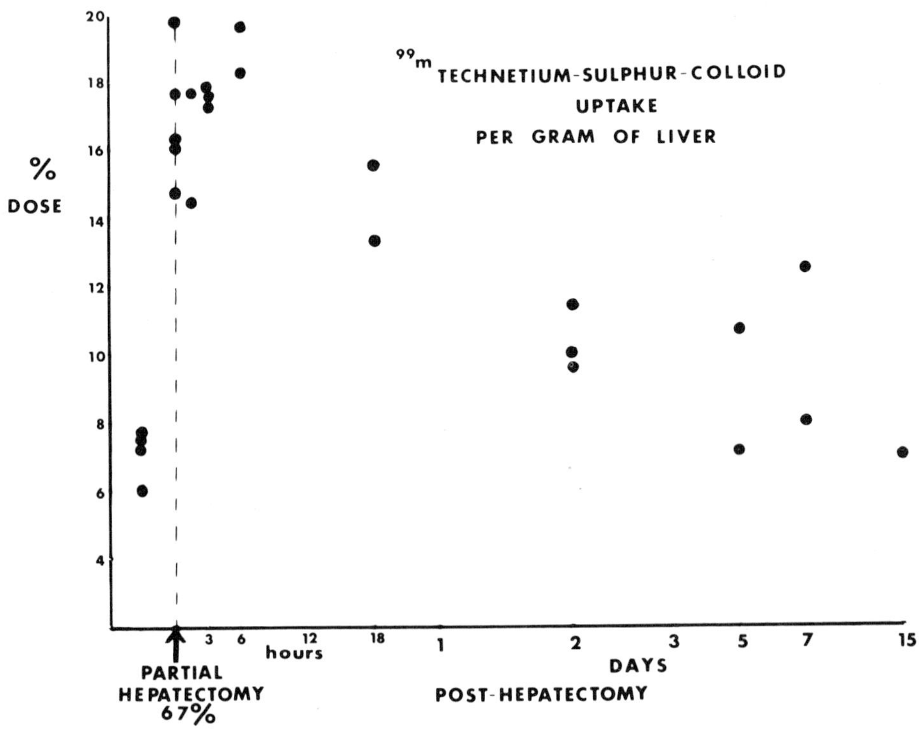

Figure 10.9. Change in hepatic uptake of colloid following 67 per cent hepatectomy in the rat.

animal (Figures 10.10 and 10.11). The isotope used, $^{99}Tc^{m}$, as sulphur colloid, has a half-life of six hours. Residual activity is insignificant 12 hours after previous imaging, and further investigations are therefore possible. Repeated studies (Figure 10.12) are limited only by the ability of the animal to withstand multiple anaesthetics.

A compartmental mathematical model has been developed for the estimation of hepatic perfusion and the technique has been utilized not only for studying the changes produced by partial hepatectomy but also for studying hepatic arterial ligation, portacaval diversion and transposition.[84]

When a colloid is injected into the blood stream it is rapidly taken up by the cells of the reticuloendothelial system, principally the Kupffer cells of the liver and, to a lesser extent, phagocytic cells in the spleen and bone marrow (extrahepatic uptake) (Figure 10.13).

Following intravenous injection of 1 mCi (3.7×10^7 Bq) of $^{99}Tc^{m}$ sulphur colloid the activity within the liver L(t) is detected by the gamma camera fitted with a pinhole collimator and data are stored and then analysed by computer. This activity is given by the formula

$$L(t) = \frac{Bo\,.\,K_1}{K_1 + K_2}\left[1 - \exp^{-}\left(\frac{K_1 + K_2}{V}\right)t\right]$$

where Bo is the injected activity, L(t) the activity in the liver, K_1 the effective hepatic perfusion, K_2 the perfusion of extrahepatic reticuloendothelial tissues and V the blood volume (5.93 ml/100 g).[176]

The rate constant $(K_1 + K_2)/V$ can be measured from this liver uptake curve (Figure 10.14). In addition, the ratio K_1/K_2 can be found, following complete removal of the colloid from the blood, by the measurement of activity within the liver and the rest of the body respectively. From $(K_1 + K_2)/V$ and K_1/K_2, K_1 can then be readily calculated.

Table 10.1 shows the values obtained using the technique and the immediate rise in specific perfusion which occurs following partial hepatectomy can be clearly seen. When partial hepatectomy is performed in a 'shunted' animal, a small rise in 'specific' perfusion occurs through the hepatic artery.[84]

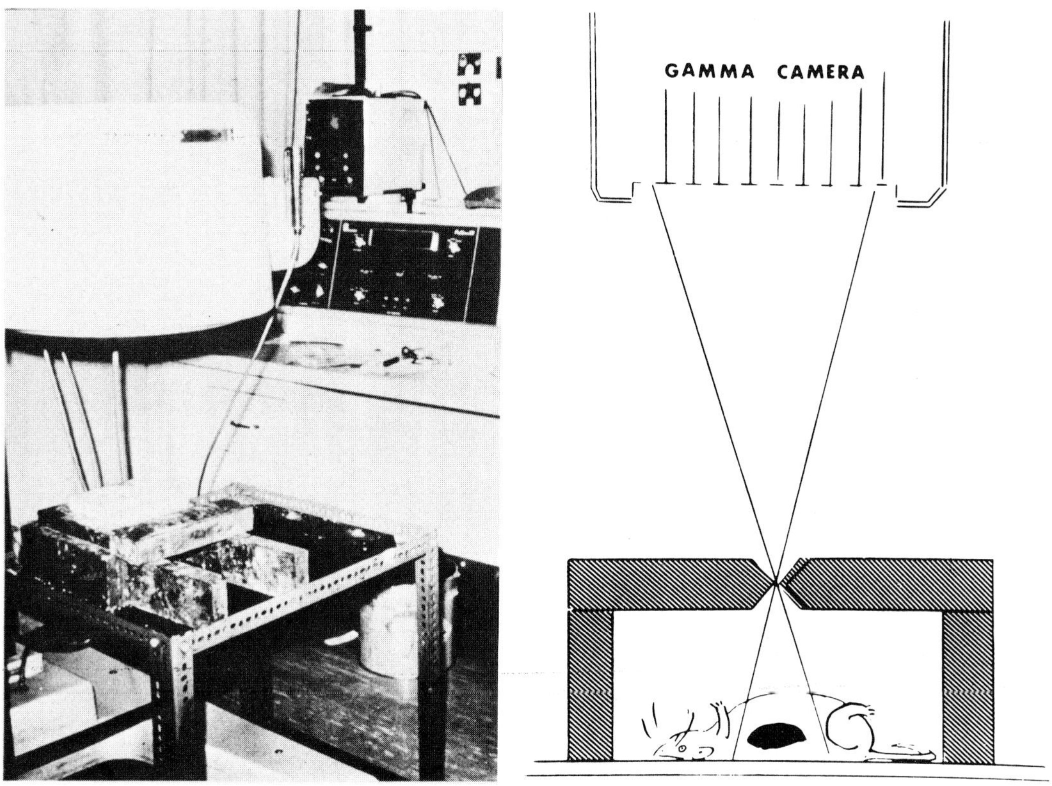

Figure 10.10. Gamma camera with pinhole collimator. Technique for obtaining gamma camera images in small animals using a pinhole collimator to achieve magnification. From Karran, Leach and Blumgart,[83] with kind permission of the editor of *Journal of Nuclear Medicine*.

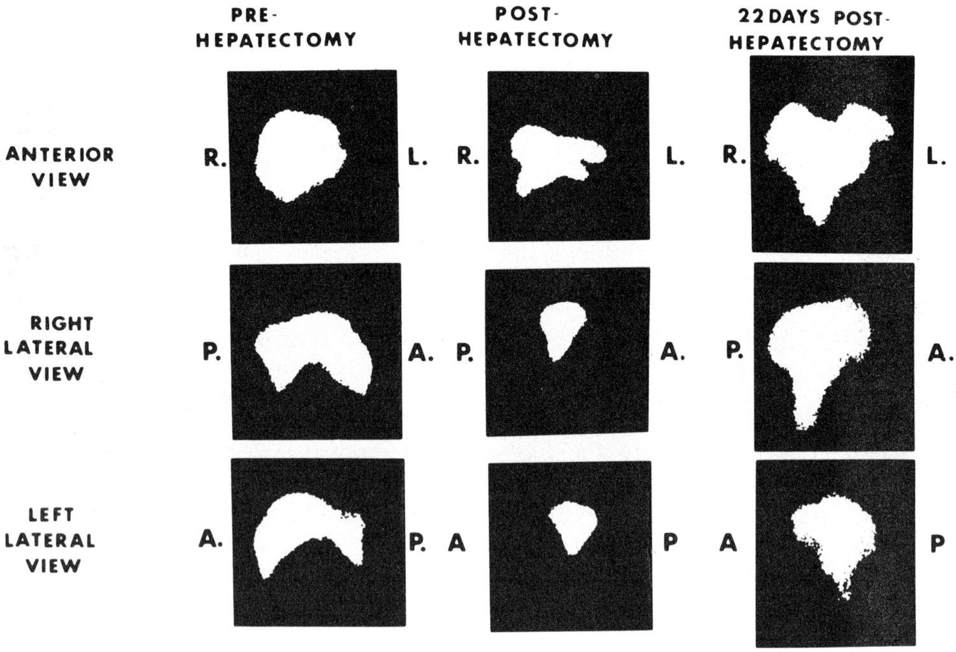

Figure 10.11. Gamma camera images of the liver of the rat. Left-hand column shows anterior and lateral views of normal liver. Middle column shows liver images following 67 per cent hepatectomy. Right-hand column shows liver remnant following regeneration. From Karran, Leach and Blumgart,[83] with kind permission of the editor of *Journal of Nuclear Medicine*.

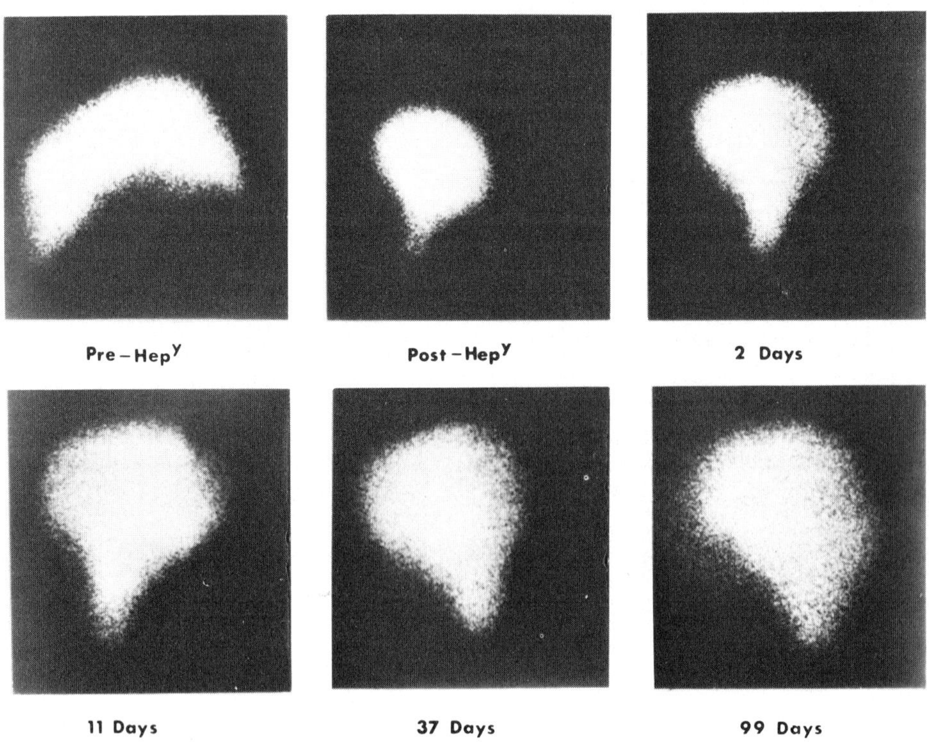

Figure 10.12. Sequential scans obtained following 67 per cent hepatectomy (left lateral views).

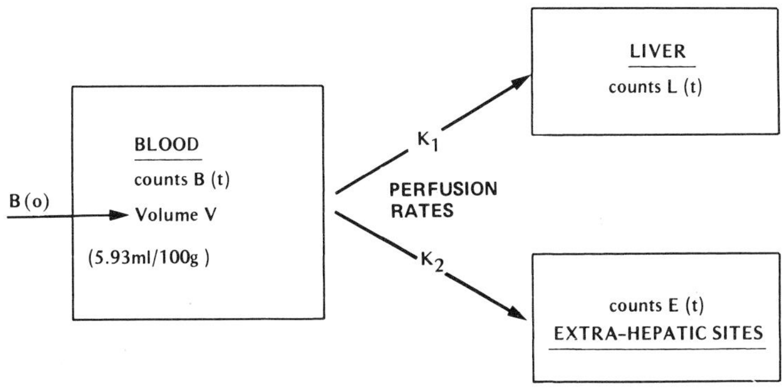

Figure 10.13. Compartmental model for measuring hepatic perfusion. From Karran et al,[85] with kind permission of the editor of *Journal of Nuclear Medicine.*

HISTOLOGICAL CHANGES

Although many of the features previously thought to be characteristic of the regenerative response have been shown by electron microscopy to be artefactual, other features remain undisputed. Following partial hepatectomy, histological changes can be detected in the remnant within a few hours. These changes are first seen in the region surrounding the vascular inflow at the portal triad. Subsequently, they are seen to spread out from the triad until finally they surround the hepatic venous outflow. This sequence of events emphasizes the importance of hepatic perfusion in the initiation and control of this remarkable phenomenon.

Following partial hepatectomy in the rat, the remnant becomes pale during the course of the first day due to fatty infiltration. New constituents of protoplasm are formed and DNA replication commences. By 48 hours the remnant has approximately doubled in size (Figure 10.15). Initially, mitotic activity lags behind the increase in weight, but after this initial delay the increase in cell population proceeds parallel with the increase in mass.[21] Regenerating liver 36 hours after partial hepatectomy in the rat is shown in Figures 10.16 and 10.17.

Synthesis of DNA may be studied by the incorporation of tritiated thymidine. This radioactive precursor is taken up by parenchymal cells at greatly increased rates after 12

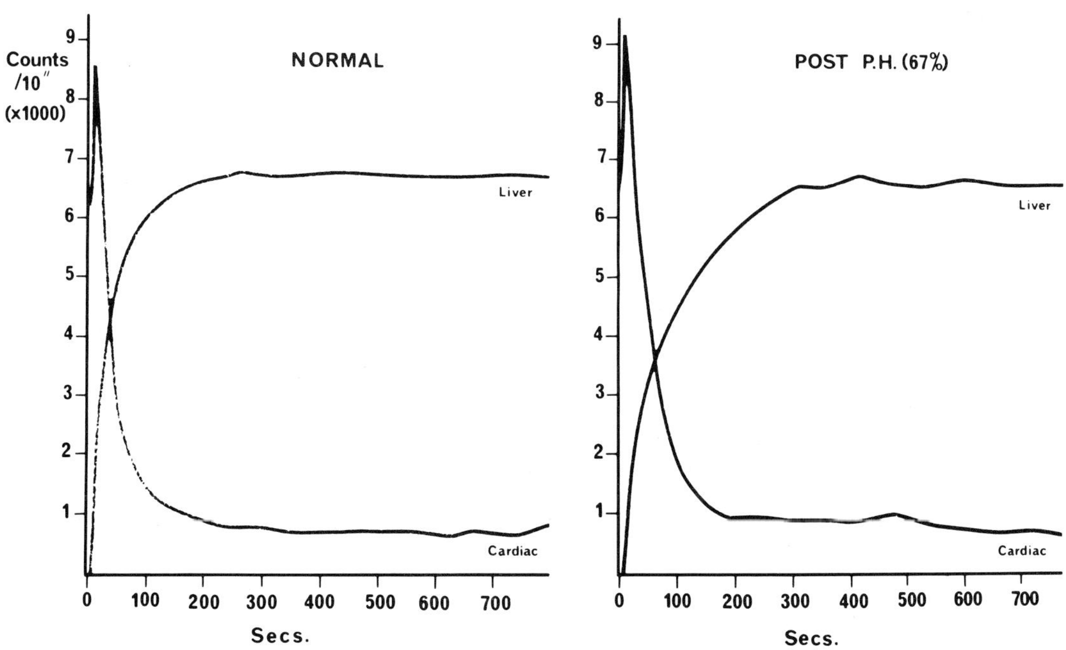

Figure 10.14. Dynamic liver scans using $^{99}Tc^{m}$ sulphur colloid. Liver uptake curves in normal rat (left) and immediately post-hepatectomy (right). From Karran et al,[85] with kind permission of the editor of *Journal of Nuclear Medicine.*

Table 10.1. *Liver Perfusion Following Partial Hepatectomy in the Rat.*

Group	Number of rats	Per cent total counts: Liver (%)	Spleen (%)	Carcass (%)	Efficiency (%)	Total liver perfusion K_1 (ml/min)	Specific liver perfusion K_2 (ml/g/min)
Normal	11	89.71	2.44	7.82	81	25.12	2.15
Post-hepatectomy							
Immediate	8	87.25	2.52	10.27	61	22.46	5.25
4 Hours	6	84.88	4.03	11.03	62.5	23.57	4.83
18 Hours	6	83.90	4.02	12.08	64	23.73	4.02
24 Hours	8	87.77	3.20	9.04	65.5	20.87	3.63
2 Days	10	83.91	3.93	11.57	75.5	17.71	2.69
3 Days	14	87.84	4.09	8.07	79	22.01	2.10
4 Days	6	89.35	4.50	6.15	81	16.88	1.88
6 Days	3	81.00	3.33	15.67		22.00	2.01
7 Days	4	90.75	4.00	5.75		22.36	2.05
9 Days	7	88.48	4.27	7.27		32.52	2.58
10 Days	8	87.57	2.61	9.80		28.11	2.42
12 Days	8	90.82	3.25	5.94		27.64	2.25
14 Days	8	86.95	3.77	9.26		26.91	1.93

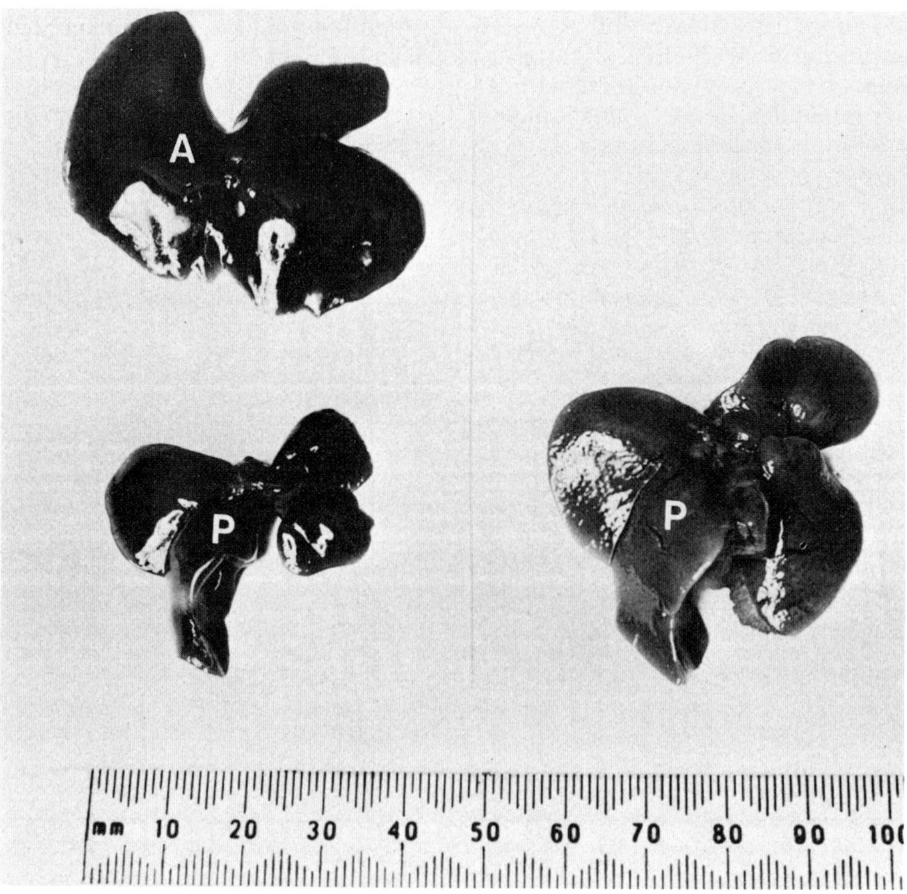

Figure 10.15. Increase in the size of the liver remnant of the rat 48 hours after 67 per cent hepatectomy (A = anterior, P = posterior lobes).

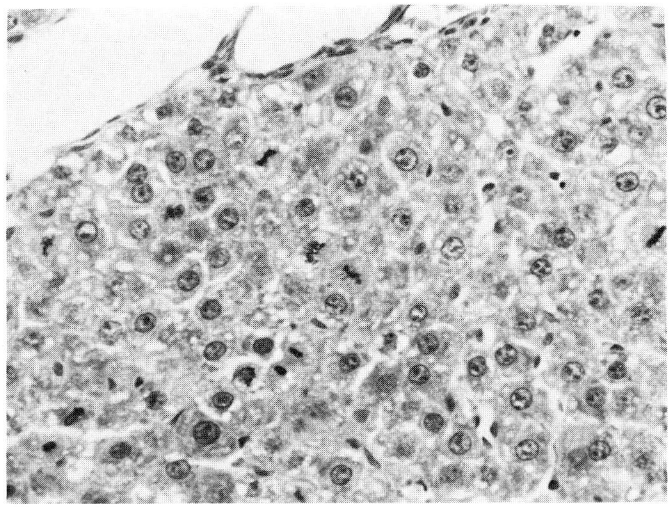

(a)

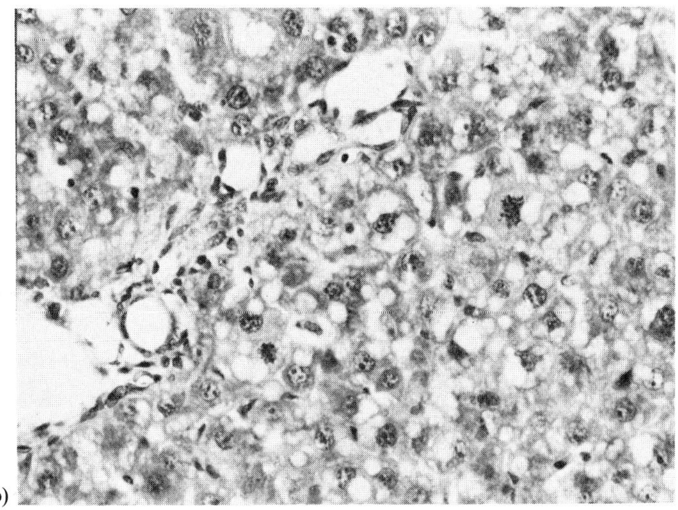

(b)

Figure 10.16. (a) Histological appearances of liver of rat 24 hours after partial hepatectomy. Note the large number of mitoses already visible. A portal tract is seen top left. (b) 66 hours after partial hepatectomy. Mitoses are still visible and there is now prominent cytoplasmic vacuolation due to fatty change.

hours following hepatectomy, and uptake reaches a peak at approximately 18 hours. Doubling of DNA content is a prerequisite for mitosis. There is thus a lag before an increase in mitotic rate is seen and the peak of mitotic activity occurs some 30 hours after resection (Figure 10.18).

In Figure 10.18 the increase in DNA synthesis in parenchymal cells is seen to precede the increase in mitotic activity. A similar sequence of events occurs in ductal and littoral cells except that these changes are delayed with the peak in DNA synthesis occurring in both groups between 36 and 48 hours after hepatectomy.

Although parenchymal cells account for only 60 to 65 per cent of the cell population,[22,163] they account for up to 95 per cent of liver volume. Thus growth of these cells produces immediate changes in the size of the remnant.

Within hours of hepatectomy changes are visible in the parenchymal cells surrounding the portal triad. These changes then involve adjacent cells until eventually central hepatocytes around the hepatic veins are affected. Ductular, littoral and connective tissue cells are relatively unaffected at this time.

The use of improved fixation techniques using glutaraldehyde suggests that many previously reported histological changes are probably artefactual.[56] The stress of hepatectomy possibly alters the susceptibility of tissue to fixation. Hypoxia, various toxins and other stressful conditions may also produce these changes. It has been shown that the endoplasmic reticulum, mitochondria and cell surfaces of hepatocytes are well preserved following hepatectomy, providing the tissues are fixed by this in situ perfusion technique using buffered glutaraldehyde. In these more refined preparations it is difficult to detect features which distinguish regenerating liver at 10 and 20 hours post-hepatectomy from the liver of normal

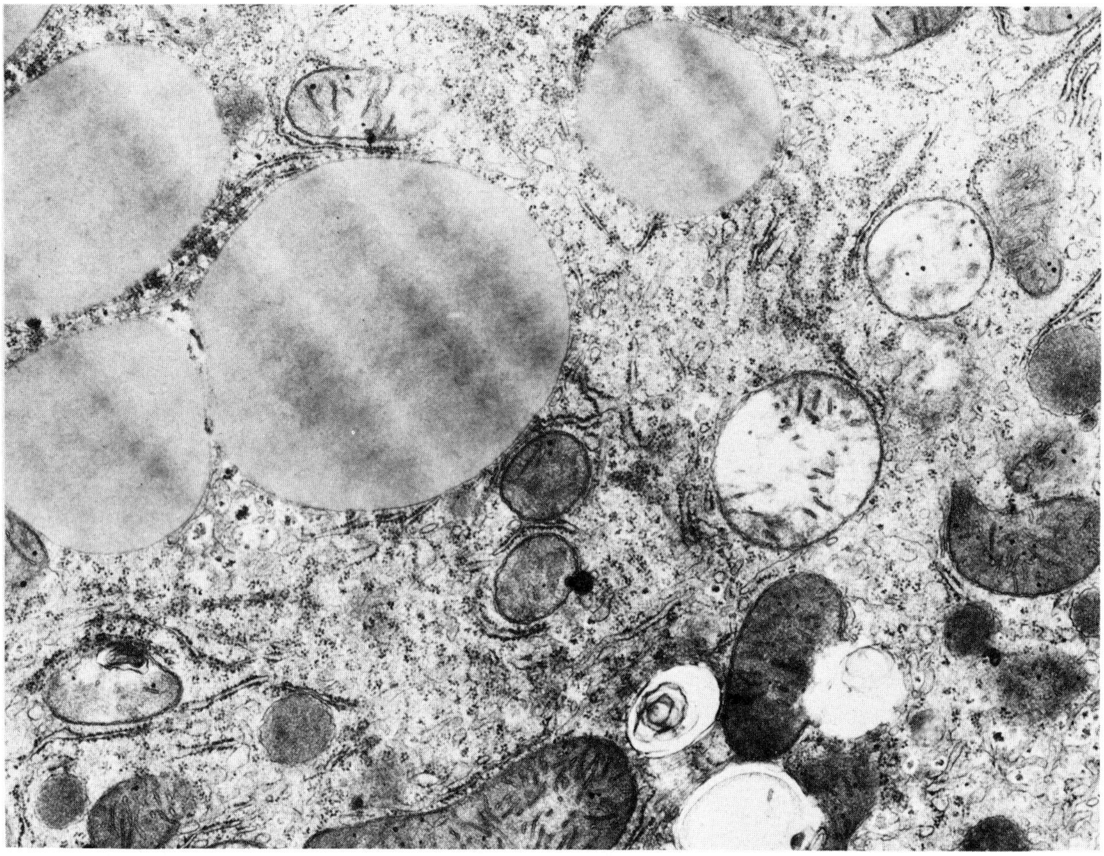

Figure 10.17. Electron microscopy of rat liver 36 hours after partial hepatectomy, showing numerous fat droplets. × 8000.

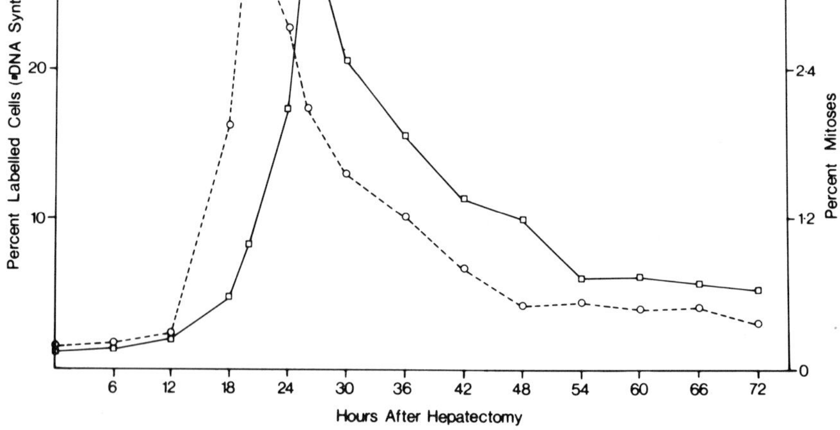

Figure 10.18. The increase in DNA synthesis in parenchymal cells precedes the increase in mitotic activity. Based on Grisham[69].

sham operated animals, apart from the accumulation of large droplets of lipid and a more prominent appearance of the smooth endoplasmic reticulum.

Over the first 10 hours glycogen stores rapidly become depleted but then gradually reappear. Fat globules increase so that at 24 hours the lobular pattern becomes distorted through compression of the sinusoidal spaces by these fat laden hepatocytes. As already mentioned, other cellular structures remain comparatively unchanged at this time.

Non-specific changes, which are common to stressful situations such as hypoxia and biliary obstruction, include vacuolation, appearance of inclusion bodies, activation of lysosomes, loss of microvilli and disorganization of the endoplasmic reticulum.[1,8,12]

At 18 to 20 hours post-hepatectomy, DNA synthesis, as detected by radio-autography with two-hour incorporation of ^{3}H-thymidine, reaches its peak in the periphery of the lobule. Some eight hours later mitosis occurs. Gradually this sequence of events sweeps centrally towards the hepatic venous radicle. It is stressed again that these proliferative events are initiated at that part of the lobule which is perfused with portal blood in the unshunted animal. In animals submitted to portacaval diversion prior to partial hepatectomy, this region still receives nutrients and hormones through the hepatic artery before other parts of the liver.

Mitotic activity proceeds in a relatively asynchronous manner. Though mitosis is completed in individual cells within one hour,[53] the peak of activity in the liver as a whole is spread over 12 hours.[23] Following mitosis, the GI (or 'first gap') phase of growth which precedes the replication of DNA is initially extended from the normal nine-hour period by a further 12 to 15 hours during regeneration. In subsequent cycles, however, this phase lasts only five hours. The period of DNA synthesis (period S), which follows GI, is slightly shortened from nine to eight hours before the GII ('second gap') phase occurs. Following the GII phase, mitosis and division occur (M or D phase). GII and D together remain unchanged during regeneration and occupy a total of 3.5 hours. Thus, in the shortening of the cell life cycle from 21.5 to 16.15 hours, the GI interval is the major variant determining the cell generation time. Control of cell proliferation is probably mediated during this phase.[54] During the early phases of regeneration at least some hepatocytes divide more than once, as demonstrated by double-labelling experiments. This fact is responsible for the production of the maximal initial growth rate which subsequently declines. The regenerative response, as measured by 60-hour ^{3}H-thymidine infusion,[55,155,157,166] occurs diffusely throughout the liver remnant, and there is no evidence, therefore, of a microscopic 'focus' for the initiation of this phenomenon.

Age

The age of the patient or animal is of importance in the regenerative response, not only with regard to recovery following major hepatic resection but also because an inadequate regenerative response in patients more than 40 years old may be responsible for the high incidence of acute hepatic failure following viral hepatitis.[130] Several features of regeneration have been shown to differ with age. The maximal increase in DNA synthesis in rats, for example, is delayed by seven days in old animals.[33] A similar delay in restoration of mass is found, with preoperative values being achieved at three weeks.[124] Differences are also seen in albumin synthesis which occurs at an increased rate in old rats although globulin synthesis is unchanged.[13,143] The increased albumin synthesis which occurs after hepatectomy also occurs later in old rats.[124] Following hepatectomy in old rats the liver ribosomes have a lower specific activity than microsomes from livers of old control rats. In contrast, young rat liver microsomes continue albumin synthesis after hepatectomy at the same rate as young control liver microsomes, with increased synthesis seen 24 hours after operation. This increased synthesis is delayed to 48 hours in old rat liver microsomes.

The ferritin content of liver also differs between young and old rats.[128] The liver of old rats contains four times the amount of ferritin iron/g, and twice the amount of ferritin protein/g of liver tissue. In addition, old rat liver ferritin contains twice as much iron as young rat liver ferritin.

It has also been shown that the proportion of polyploid hepatocytes increases with age[131] so that at two years rat liver contains 10 per cent diploids, 73 per cent tetraploids and 17 per cent octoploids, all of which are active in mitosis. This compares with 20 to 30 per cent of binucleate hepatocytes, 70 to 80 per cent tetraploid and 1 to 2 per cent octaploid nuclei in normal adult rats.[22,122]

It seems probable that functional changes in the liver of old rats do not involve somatic mutations.[124]

The overall decrease in the regenerative response in old age is in harmony with the decrease in metabolic rate in man which falls from 7 MJ/24 hr (1700 kcal/24 hr) in young males to less than 5 MJ/24 hr (1300 kcal/24 hr) with increasing age.[86]

Although the achievement of a 'critical cell mass', as suggested by Johnson,[81] is almost certainly not the means of initiation and control of regeneration (see page 211), changes in hepatic perfusion are still of relevance. Delivery of trophic substances, whether these be hormonal, nutrient or otherwise, is vital for them to exert their effect. It is of interest in portally shunted animals to see the diminished response to hepatectomy in terms of *size*, in the presence of increased mitotic activity indicative of true hyperplasia, particularly as hepatic arterial 'specific' perfusion of the remnant increases thus allowing trophic factors to operate.

Part 2

REGULATORY MECHANISMS

NANCY L.R. BUCHER
JOAN A. McGOWAN

INTRODUCTION

That regeneration of mammalian liver is largely if not entirely controlled by humoral factors now appears to be well established. At the beginning of the present decade it was shown by several groups of investigators that some, but not necessarily all such factors are derived from portal splanchnic organs, and are therefore more concentrated in portal than in peripheral blood.[37,60,92,110,132,160] These substances have been designated portal blood hepatotrophic factors, or simply hepatotrophic factors, and have generally been assigned the dual role of preserving the integrity and promoting the proliferation of hepatocytes. They are the subject of much of the recent research in quest of hepatic growth regulatory mechanisms. There has been new work on non-portal substances as well, however, and we will include investigations dealing with both groups of substances in this brief overview of the most recent advances.

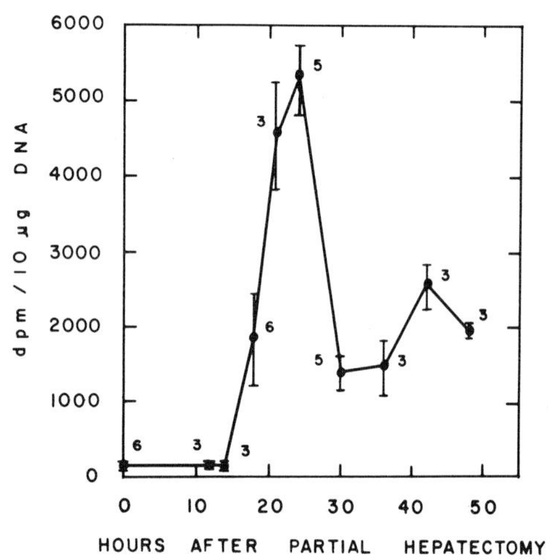

Figure 10.19. One-hour incorporation of ^{3}H-thymidine into hepatic DNA in 200 g male Sprague Dawley rats at intervals after partial hepatectomy. Vertical lines indicate the standard error of the mean, numbers the number of rats per point. From Bucher, Patel and Cohen,[32] with kind permission of Pergamon Press.

Normal adult livers are essentially non-growing, the cells being disengaged from the cell cycle and arrested in the so-called G_0 state. In rats, in which the most recent studies have been conducted, changes in hepatocyte biochemistry start almost immediately after partial hepatectomy, but DNA replication, which signals with certainty that the cells are proliferating, does not get under way for about 14 to 16 hours, as shown in Figure 10.19. The initial peak of DNA synthetic activity occurs at about 22 hours, the timing varying somewhat with age, nutritional status, hormonal balance and other factors. Mitotic activity follows the same course about six to eight hours later.[23] The growth rate gradually diminishes and ceases when the original amount of liver is restored, in one to two weeks. The growth curve in Figure 10.19

provides a frame of reference for the discussion to follow.

For a broader background the reader is referred to reviews by Bucher and Malt,[23] Bresnick,[18] Becker,[14] Hays,[75] Schulte-Hermann,[146] Argyris,[4] Lesch and Reutter[102] and Lewan, Yngner and Engelbrecht.[104]

PORTAL BLOOD HEPATOTROPHIC FACTORS

The momentum gained from the discovery of portal blood hepatotrophic factors has led to two general types of experiments. In the first type the blood supply to all or parts of the liver, or to liver grafts, is altered in ways permitting comparison not only of effects of portal and systemic blood, but also of blood from various sectors of the portal bed. In the second type, various portal splanchnic organs are excised or transplanted, and effects upon liver or liver grafts evaluated with or without replacement of specific hormones and nutrients. The results in most instances point to the pancreas as the major source of hepatotrophic factors, although there are divergencies. This work will be dealt with more fully in the section on insulin and glucagon.

Before discussing the role of pancreatic hormones, however, we would like to emphasize that experimental alterations of hepatic blood supply, mentioned above, often involve deprivation of some or all liver lobes of portal blood, resulting in atrophy. Although the deprived lobes shrink in size, there is little histological evidence of abnormality even over a period of many months.[94,177] Ultrastructural changes also seem relatively minor – mainly depletion of granular endoplasmic reticulum and glycogen granules.[59,112,162] The atrophied hepatocytes retain the ability to proliferate,[94,178] and regenerative capacity following partial hepatectomy shows little or no impairment, although the growth process may be somewhat delayed.[70,184] Indeed, even in the absence of partial hepatectomy, hepatocytes in portacaval-shunted rats are subjected to growth stimulation. Weinbren, Washington and Smith[179] observed concurrent atrophy and hyperplasia in normal livers following short-term portal diversion and thought it quite possible that the liver deficit associated with the atrophy might itself generate the stimulus for cellular proliferation.

The occurrence of active proliferation in hepatocytes that have undergone atrophy is a cogent argument against the critical mass hypothesis,[180] which postulates that cells divide when they reach a critical size, and which has been proposed as a regulatory principle for liver growth.[81] While it is generally the case that cells tend to double in size before undergoing mitosis, and it is well known that certain cells (e.g. amoebae) will not divide if this increase is prevented, many cells, especially in higher organisms, contain variable amounts of storage materials, secretory products and other labile dispensable substances, so that total cell mass is an improbable criterion of preparedness of hepatocytes for division, particularly in vivo. Rather, accumulation of essential substances to requisite levels within the cell is far more likely to be critical, as suggested by recent studies of cells in culture.[66,136] The applicability of the critical mass hypothesis to the liver is also not supported by the work of Stirling, Laughlin and Washington,[165] who showed that the atrophied livers resulting from starvation (instead of portal blood deprivation) could also respond to partial hepatectomy. The hypothesis has recently been evaluated again by Ruhenstroth-Bauer and his associates, with similar conclusions.[169] Hence, atrophy of liver cells, whether from deprivation of portal blood or dietary nutrients, does not seriously interfere with the competence of hepatocytes to undergo division. Further, deviation of portal blood does not prevent growth stimulatory factors from gaining access to the liver. As a result, proliferative activity may be delayed but is not substantially impaired.

Hyperplasia generally refers to an increase in cell number, or to an upward shift in ploidy, such as occurs in developing liver; atrophy and hypertrophy, on the other hand, are defined in terms of cell size or protein content without an increase in genetic substance.[10] In contrast to the process of hyperplasia in the presence of atrophy, discussed in the preceding paragraph, is the more usual combination of hyperplasia and hypertrophy seen following acute loss of liver through injury or surgical resection; in this case the liver remnant receives an actual enrichment of portal blood constituents due to the concomitant reduction in hepatocyte complement and enhancement of portal blood flow.[70,85,135]

Prevention of hepatocyte atrophy and promotion of hypertrophy may be regarded as aspects of the same process, differing in degree, and largely nutrition- and hormone-dependent.

Hyperplasia, however, is a clearly separable process, because it can be associated with either atrophy or hypertrophy. Its regulation seems also to depend upon hormonal, nutritional and possibly other factors, which must therefore differ in some respect from those that promote hypertrophy. 'Hepatotrophic' has been loosely used to designate the factors involved in both hyperplasia and hypertrophy. Some of the divergencies in the literature may be attributable to failure to distinguish between the two processes. In this review growth will be defined as hyperplasia, regardless of associated atrophy or hypertrophy, as hepatic regeneration is basically a hyperplastic process. This definition, however, is not employed universally (e.g. Argyris[4]).

Insulin and Glucagon

More than 10 years ago Steiner and his associates demonstrated a role for insulin in liver growth, using rats made severely diabetic with alloxan.[187] The intact livers in these diabetic animals were already enlarged, reflecting an increase in cell number; they were stimulated to additional growth by treatment with insulin, which caused a further 70 per cent increment in total hepatic DNA. When untreated diabetic rats with already enlarged livers were partially hepatectomized, the rate of DNA synthesis rose to about 60 per cent of that seen in regenerating livers of normal controls. In confirmation, Barra and Hall[11] have shown that regeneration was delayed and prolonged in alloxan diabetic rats, but not inhibited. Thus, although exogenous insulin substantially accelerated hepatocyte proliferation in diabetic rats, active proliferation also occurred in partially resected livers without insulin supplementation. Therefore if liver growth positively requires insulin, the small amounts possibly present in the portal veins of such animals (where indeed it would be maximally effective) must have sufficed.[20] Alternatively, the growth stimulus could be due to substances other than insulin; insulin would then have an enhancing or potentiating role.

In a similar context, DNA synthesis was partially suppressed in the livers of partially hepatectomized rats that were continuously infused with anti-insulin serum; this points to a positive requirement for insulin, at least for maximal expression of proliferative activity.[31]

Employing an entirely different approach, Starzl and his co-workers[160,161,162] have carried out a succession of intricate surgical vascular manipulations in dogs, culminating in a procedure termed 'splanchnic division', in which nutrient-rich venous return from the intestines was directed to the left lobes of the liver, whereas the hormone-rich blood from the pancreas and upper splanchnic organs passed to the right lobes. Both sides of the liver responded to partial hepatectomy, but the regenerative activity was greater on the pancreatic hormone-enriched right side. Either alloxan diabetes or partial hepatectomy deprived the right side of this advantaged state; moreover, treatment of such animals with exogenous insulin, which would go equally to all lobes, shifted the advantage to the nutrient-enriched but previously insulin-deprived left lobes, which then exhibited greater cell renewal than the others. These results were interpreted as showing that insulin was probably the most important specific hepatotrophic factor in portal venous blood, but that additional factors derived from intestinal blood – whether nutrients, hormones or other substances – all contributed to the hepatotrophic effect. In further studies these investigators found that in dogs with portacaval shunts infusion of insulin into the left lobes reduced atrophy, preserved hepatocyte ultrastructure and tripled cell renewal in comparison with the insulin-deprived right lobes. On the other hand, exogenous glucagon had no effect by itself, nor did it potentiate the action of insulin.[161,162] That insulin is hepatotrophic is evident from these studies; it both protects the liver from atrophy and potentiates regeneration. Whether glucagon also has a role was not established; glucagon of gastrointestinal origin is abundant in dogs,[170] and hence this hormone was not eliminated by pancreatectomy. Its possible participation as an additional hepatotrophic factor was therefore not excluded.

Insulin is well known to have anabolic, growth-promoting properties, in keeping with its ability to enhance proliferation of a number of kinds of cells in culture,[74] including hepatocytes.[95,140] Glucagon, on the other hand, is generally thought of as a catabolic hormone, at least with respect to its influence upon hepatic lipid and carbohydrate metabolism, which is generally opposite to that of insulin. For certain functions, however, the actions of the two hormones are complementary; for example, both promote amino acid transport, albeit by different mechanisms, and the effects are additive.[87] Moreover, under certain conditions glucagon also exerts a growth-promoting influence. For example, it is an important constituent of 'TAGH', an empirically devised mixture of tri-iodothyronine (T_3), amino acids, glucagon and heparin that induces a burst of proliferative activity in normal adult rat liver in vivo.[151] In vitro, at least in the presence of other growth factors including insulin, glucagon enhances the growth of adult hepatocytes.[140]

A novel way to study hepatic growth regulation in vivo was introduced by Price and his associates, who partially hepatectomized dogs that were previously deprived of the gastrointestinal tract, pancreas and spleen, and maintained by continuous intravenous infusion of electrolytes, glucose, amino acids and insulin. Modest regenerative activity occurred, as evidenced by ^{3}H-thymidine labelling of hepatic nuclei.[133] Subsequent, more detailed studies in rats showed that the DNA synthetic response was greatly delayed, but could be accelerated considerably by addition of glucagon to the insulin-containing infusion mixture.[184] Bucher and Swaffield[25] meanwhile confirmed in rats the initial findings and, in addition, studied animals eviscerated one day in advance of the partial hepatectomy to permit endogenous pancreatic hormones to decay to negligible levels. In these animals, which were maintained without exogenous insulin and glucagon, and hence largely devoid of these hormones, regenerative activity was significant, although greatly retarded and diminished. Addition of insulin alone (supplemented with glucose) or glucagon alone (supplemented with amino acids) to the saline infusion mixture had little or no effect, but when combined at appropriate dosage levels the two hormones acted synergistically with dramatic effectiveness to abolish the delay and restore the DNA biosynthetic rate in eviscerated rats to the values seen in partially hepatectomized but otherwise normal animals.[25,26] Under these experimental conditions insulin and glucagon, acting in combination but not separately, were seen as striking promoters of hepatocyte proliferation in vivo.

Observations from the several experimental models discussed above – alloxan diabetes, portal deprivation and evisceration – are in general agreement that although liver regeneration does occur it is greatly attenuated when pancreatic hormone levels are minimal or undetectable. Furthermore, it has been observed that when administration of insulin and glucagon to eviscerated rats is delayed for six to seven hours after partial hepatectomy, during which the early steps of the regenerative process are known to be already under way,[23] the effectiveness of the pancreatic hormone treatment is unimpaired.[26,27] On the other hand, infusion of insulin and glucagon into rats with intact livers – either normal or eviscerated, and even when given directly into the portal vein – causes no significant elevation of DNA synthesis,[26,28] although it has been demonstrated repeatedly by cross-circulation experiments between normal and partially hepatectomized partners that the growth stimulus can be transmitted by substances in the blood.[61,105,120] The evidence from the evisceration experiments suggests that the two pancreatic hormones are not primary initiators of the growth process. It also points to the likelihood that at least some of the factors that set the process in motion originate in tissues not drained by the portal venous bed.

Views on the relative significance of the composition of portal blood vis-à-vis the volume of flow are often at variance (see the review by Hays[75]). In the presence of ample provision of exogenous insulin and glucagon, the livers of eviscerated rats were found capable of regenerating at a normal rate even though the hepatic blood supply was reduced to the fractional volume provided by the hepatic artery, the portal vein having been ligated and sectioned at the time of evisceration.[26] This finding, along with earlier studies involving cross-circulation of blood between normal and partially hepatectomized rats which involved no enhancement of hepatic blood flow in the normal partner,[120] underscores the importance of the quality of the blood supplied. A similar view has recently been expressed by Guest et al[70] on the basis of portacaval transposition studies. A recent report by Whittemore, Voorhees and Price,[183] however, indicates that augmentation of hepatic blood flow in eviscerated rats by arterialization of the portal vein increased the DNA synthetic response to partial hepatectomy as well as the sensitivity to glucagon in balancing the effects of insulin. The crux of the matter seems to be the actual quantity of requisite hepatotrophic factors to which the liver cells are exposed, whether they be in low concentrations delivered at a high flow rate, or vice versa.

Further confirmation that the pancreas is an important source of portal blood hepatotrophic factors is provided by the work of Orloff and his collaborators, which is largely dependent upon experiments involving selective ablation and addition of splanchnic organs in association with livers or liver grafts.[19,49,52] Recently, on the basis of replacement studies with insulin and glucagon in pancreatectomized, partially hepatectomized dogs, and in rats with isografts, they concluded, in agreement with the prior studies of eviscerated rats already mentioned, that insulin and glucagon appear to be the major hepatotrophic components of portal blood.[51] There is not universal agreement on this point, however, for Fisher et al,[62] using segmental small intestinal resection or isolation in normal, portacaval-shunted or cross-circulated rats, implicated the intestinal tract as the source, and Chandler,[36] using various diversions of hepatic circulation in rabbits, arrived at a somewhat similar conclusion. Nevertheless, the weight of evidence continues to implicate insulin and glucagon, at least in situations where active hepatocyte proliferation occurs.

A new animal model, recently introduced by Farivar et al,[57] consists of fulminant hepatitis in the mouse, resulting from a 100 per cent lethal dose of A59 murine hepatitis virus. This causes acute massive liver necrosis, thus creating extensive liver insufficiency without surgical intervention. The mean survival time of such mice was unaltered by glucagon administration, and only slightly prolonged by insulin, but it was more than doubled by simultaneous infusion of both hormones; 40 per cent of the mice treated with the insulin–glucagon mixture recovered completely, compared with only six per cent of those treated with insulin, and none of those treated with glucagon. The dual hormone treatment appeared to enhance liver regeneration, and also partially to protect against hepatocellular injury, which progressed more slowly in the hormone-treated animals. Whatever the mechanism of this protection might be, it appeared unrelated to the hepatic regenerative process which occurred many hours later. Very recent observations in a second new animal model, D-galactosamine-induced acute liver cell injury in rats, also suggest an early protective effect of pancreatic hormones.[175] Both new models further emphasize the important hepatotrophic actions of insulin and glucagon.

In normal adult rats, partial hepatectomy causes an abrupt drop in portal venous immunoreactive insulin levels, and a concomitant rise in immunoreactive glucagon.[27,30] Peripheral blood hormone levels also reflect these trends.[50,100] The insulin and glucagon dosages employed in the previously mentioned experiments with eviscerated rats or mice with viral hepatitis were empirical; in both models the optimal doses of glucagon were high, i.e., in the pharmacological range, whereas the insulin doses were more nearly physiological. Although these doses at least follow the trends found in portal blood following partial hepatectomy – high glucagon relative to insulin – the requirement for pharmacological amounts remains puzzling.

Changes not only in hormone levels but also in hormone receptors have been described;[95,99] a 40 to 60 per cent loss of glucagon-binding capacity, but not insulin-binding capacity, was found in plasma membranes from 24-hour regenerating livers, although there was no difference at six to seven hours. The relevance of these findings to liver growth has not yet been clarified.

Although the liver is recognized as a main target of insulin and glucagon action, the evidence cited so far does not prove that the effects upon hepatic growth observed in vivo have resulted from the direct action of these hormones upon the liver. Evidence in support of a direct effect, however, comes from recent work by Richman et al[140] who report that, in monolayer cultures of hepatocytes from partially hepatectomized adult rats, DNA synthesis was stimulated by either insulin or epidermal growth factor (EGF), greatly enhanced by both compounds together and further augmented by glucagon. On the other hand, Leffert et al[101] found that supplementation of their basic medium with glucagon in cultures of normal adult hepatocytes caused no stimulation of growth, although they continue to add glucagon to their multiple-hormone-enriched 'complete medium', presumably because it may be stimulatory in combination with other hormones.

At present the weight of evidence suggests that insulin and glucagon are important potentiators rather than primary initiators of liver growth in vivo, and under at least some experimental conditions they reinforce each other, having an apparent synergistic effect. The extent to which this growth enhancement reflects direct action upon the liver or indirect influence via auxiliary mechanisms is unclear. Hepatic regeneration is generally associated with a rise in endogenous portal vein glucagon concentration and a fall in portal vein insulin; nevertheless, despite the lowered blood levels, there appears to be a positive role for insulin.

Nutritional Factors

The portal blood constituents other than hormones that are of obvious importance are the nutrients. Two general strategies have been employed to assess their effects upon liver growth. The first approach involves starvation or administration of experimental diets to animals for some days prior to partial hepatectomy, to determine consequent effects upon the regenerative process. The second approach, extensively exploited by Lieberman and his colleagues,[152,153,154] involves stimulation of hepatocyte proliferation in intact rats by the sudden shift from a protein-depleted to a high-protein (50 per cent) diet.

Starvation leads to a rapid loss of labile cell constituents – glycogen, protein and RNA – but neither starvation nor protein depletion causes loss of DNA.[3,47,72] Stirling, Laughlin and Washington[165] reported that 48-hour starvation prior to partial hepatectomy delayed the onset of mitosis by at least eight hours, and decreased its intensity in comparison to normally-fed control rats. As mentioned earlier, however, atrophied hepatocytes, whether resulting from starvation or portal diversion, retain the capacity to proliferate.

Animals subjected to nutritionally complete diets containing excessively high fat (45 per cent) or protein (64 per cent) for seven days prior to partial hepatectomy exhibited a delayed mitotic response, which was not attributable to the depression of food intake often associated with unpalatable diets.[167]

The reported effects of protein-free but otherwise complete diets upon the pattern of cell replication after partial hepatectomy are somewhat at variance. Montecuccoli, Novello and Stirpe[119] and Short et al[154] found, respectively, no depression of ^{3}H-thymidine incorporation or per cent of labelled nuclei in 24-hour regenerating livers. On the other hand, decreased ^{3}H-thymidine incorporation at 24 hours was found by both Hilton and Sartorelli[78] and Siimes and Dallman;[156] McGowan and Fausto[115,116] not only agreed that the regenerative response was delayed, but also found that the delay was abolished by administration of a casein hydrolysate to the protein-deprived rats at the time of partial hepatectomy. Stirling, Bourne and Marsh[164] compared protein deprivation and caloric restriction in pair-fed rats; mitotic activity, which is maximal in 29-hour regenerating livers of normally fed animals, was only 40 per cent of the control value at this time in rats fed a calorie-rich but protein-free diet for seven days. The livers of these animals contained substantial amounts of glycogen, in contrast to those of pair-fed controls on a semi-starvation diet whose livers were nearly glycogen-free, and exhibited almost no mitotic activity at 29 hours after the hepatic resection, although a delayed rise was observed at 48 hours. Variable palatability of the food and consequent consumption patterns of rats on different diets may explain some of the diversities reported in these studies.

Barbiroli and Potter[9] have emphasized that the feeding schedule is an important element in the patterning of the normal circadian oscillations in DNA synthesis. A small peak of DNA synthesis occurs about 12 hours after the start of the feeding period in animals fed regularly during a brief, specified interval each day; this periodicity in DNA labelling was abolished when animals were maintained on a protein-free diet.[41] Rats adapted to controlled feeding and lighting schedules were also studied recently by Schulte-Hermann[147] who employed intragastric administration of α-hexachlorocyclohexane (αHCH) as a tool for stimulating liver cell proliferation; DNA synthesis and subsequent mitosis, normally beginning at around 20 hours, were suppressed by fasting or protein deprivation, but were initiated five to eight hours after re-administration of a protein-containing diet. The increase in thymidine uptake failed to occur when the food contained no protein.

That dietary factors – specifically amino acids – can regulate hepatocyte proliferation was shown long ago by the observation of Leduc[91] that liver cells of mice switched from a low to a higher protein diet exhibited a burst of mitotic activity which was proportional to the protein content of the diet after the upshift. Short et al,[152,153] utilizing this model for a series of further studies, found that shifting rats from a protein-free to a 50 per cent protein diet resulted in a rise in DNA synthesis beginning as early as eight hours after the shift – a considerably shorter pre-replicative interval than the 16 to 18 hours required in the case of partial hepatectomy. It was necessary to condition the animals beforehand by deprivation of either protein or particular amino acids for several days for the upshift to be effective. The increases in DNA synthesis and mitosis after the shift were inhibited either by adding specific mixtures of L-amino acids to the initial protein-free diet (especially methionine, phenylalanine, serine and tryptophan), or by deleting particular amino acids from the protein-repleting diet – the lack of lysine, methionine or tryptophan, for example, reduced the DNA synthetic response by 50 per cent, and deletion of isoleucine, threonine or valine was even more inhibitory.

It seems relevant that one of the early pre-replicative changes in the liver remnant following partial hepatectomy is an increase in the free amino acid pools.[58,127] Not only is more amino acid made rather abruptly available per hepatic cell because of the hepatic deficit, but amino acid transport also appears to be enhanced, as shown by Short et al[153] for α-aminoisobutyric acid (AIB), and other amino acids as well, in five-hour regenerating livers. It is noteworthy that both insulin and glucagon increase amino acid transport, although by different mechanisms, as demonstrated by Kletzien et al,[87] insulin effecting an increase in the V_{max} for AIB transport and glucagon lowering the K_m. Whether amino acids are hepatic growth stimulators, or whether they act only in conjunction with hormonal or other factors, is not determined by these in vivo experiments.

To some extent low molecular weight nutrients, including amino acids, seem able to regulate the growth of cells in culture[80] – reminiscent of 'stringent' amino acid control in bacteria – but polypeptide hormones and many other factors are also involved.[79] Although a general increase in the uptake of nutrients may be a necessary precondition for progression through the cell cycle, it is probably not enough by itself to stimulate proliferation particularly in the whole animal where organ size is subservient to the needs of the entire organism.[68,150]

NON-PORTAL FACTORS

In addition to the factors already discussed, numerous 'non-portal' substances have been put forward as regulators of hepatic growth – some as positive or negative effectors, some as promoters or facilitators, or as purveyors of ancillary functions. These putative growth regulators have become incorporated into a number of reviews, some dealing primarily with the liver, others more broadly based.[5,23,38,68,97,102,146] Much of the information is derived from studies of various types of cells in culture, and its applicability to liver growth in the whole animal remains to be firmly established; at present its relevance depends mainly upon inference and analogy. To facilitate the discussion it is convenient to group these numerous substances into the following broad categories.

Hormones and Polypeptide Growth Factors

The liver regenerates to a greater or lesser extent in the absence of the pituitary, thyroid, parathyroid, adrenal, pancreas or gastro-intestinal tract. Conversely, hormones secreted by these organs are often found to influence, in varying degrees, the growth of normal and regenerating livers. The literature has been reviewed frequently,[23,75,146] and we will discuss only the more recent observations.

Growth hormone and somatomedins

Hypophysectomy retards regeneration (DNA synthesis) by about 15 hours, and administration of growth hormone to non-hypophysectomized animals slightly accelerates and enhances it.[146] The growth-promoting effects, of course, extend also to many other tissues. Uthne and Uthne[172] cite evidence suggesting that somatomedins, which are a family of polypeptides (molecular weight around 7000) found in the plasma, are synthesized in the liver following administration or secretion of growth hormone, and appear to be its active principle. They found that, in normal rats, plasma levels of somatomedins were decreased by 75 per cent within four to six hours after partial hepatectomy, and returned slowly to their original values during the next five to six days, in parallel with the rate of restoration of the resected liver tissue. In agreement with previous investigators[134] they conclude that growth hormone is not an absolute necessity for hepatic regeneration, and that mitotic activity can be inaugurated without its participation. The stimulatory influence of somatomedin C upon cultures of fetal rat hepatocytes, noted by Leffert,[95] is in keeping with the previously recognized growth-enhancing effects of growth hormone upon the liver, and many other tissues as well.

Thyroid hormones

In the older literature there are conflicting reports as to whether thyroid hormones and various anti-thyroid drugs enhance or impair hepatic regeneration under a variety of experimental conditions and dosage levels.[22] It is generally agreed, however, that these hormones elicit a hypertrophic and hyperplastic response in the liver;[146] after a single large (pharmacological) dose of tri-iodothyronine (T_3), DNA synthesis and mitosis were significantly stimulated, but after a considerable delay compared to that seen following partial hepatectomy.[93]

Renewed interest in the role of thyroid hormones in liver growth has been aroused by the work of Lieberman and his associates, showing that administration of a mixture designated TAGH, containing T_3, amino acids, glucagon and heparin, could initiate a burst of DNA synthesis in normal adult rat hepatocytes that closely mimicked the DNA synthetic response to partial hepatectomy and was about 60 per cent as effective. Both hormones were present in pharmacological amounts. T_3 was the most important component of the mixture, and was found to cause detectable activity (in combination with the usual large dose of 'AGH') even when reduced to the physiological dose range. It was possible to replace glucagon in the mixture with cyclic AMP with no loss of effectiveness, but cyclic GMP, or 5′-AMP, or high levels of glucose were inactive.[151,154] Malamud and Perrin[108] report that injection of T_3 and glucagon in pharmacological doses modestly stimulated the growth of several mouse tissues, particularly the exocrine pancreas, in which DNA labelling rose four- to sevenfold; this indicates that the effects of T_3 and glucagon are not limited to the liver, although the liver is considerably more responsive.

The TAGH mixture was designed to increase the supply of amino acids and free fatty acids to the liver, the rationale being that serum from partially hepatectomized rats is enriched with these substances; the suggestion is made that the T_3 may alter in some way the metabolism of the excess fatty acids that are brought to the liver by the AGH solution,[151] but this remains speculative.

Leffert and Alexander[96] determined the T_3 and thyroxin content of peripheral blood in normal rats following partial hepatectomy; both substances dropped, the nadir being proportional to the amount of liver excised. Thyroid stimulating hormone (TSH), after an initial fall, increased by 60 to 70 per cent. Metabolic studies suggested that the decreased thyroid hormone levels were due to increased turnover and utilization in the liver remnant, diminished hormone secretion and a slightly reduced concentration of the serum carrier protein for thyroid hormones. In fetal hepatocyte cultures, T_3 had a growth stimulatory effect when combined with insulin, hydrocortisone and other factors,[89] although in adult hepatocyte cultures T_3 was without effect, either alone or in combination with epidermal growth factor (EGF).[140]

Dillman, Schwartz and Oppenheimer[46] have recently noted, in agreement with earlier findings, that the rate of regeneration of the liver remnant in euthyroid and T_4-treated thyroidectomized animals was twice that in thyroidectomized rats. Partial hepatectomy resulted in a fall in plasma T_3, as noted by Leffert and Alexander, and in T_3 bound to hepatic cell nuclei in vivo; T_3-binding capacities of nuclei isolated from euthyroid and thyroidectomized rats, as determined in vitro, were about equally depressed. The authors concluded that although partial hepatectomy causes a significant reduction in the specific T_3 nuclear receptor sites and in the mass of T_3 specifically bound to the nucleus, T_3 is nevertheless necessary for an optimal rate of regeneration.

Short showed that when T_3 was given eight hours in advance of the AGH mixture, DNA synthesis occurred much earlier than when the sequence was reversed. This serves to emphasize the point that the role of T_3 in liver growth is of particular interest because, unlike the other hormones we have been discussing, T_3 can initiate cell proliferation in the normal intact liver.

Adrenal cortical hormones

Both adrenal corticotrophic hormone (ACTH) and glucocorticoids are reported to induce liver growth, but it is a hypertrophic response due almost entirely to cellular enlargement. Indeed these hormones, especially in the pharmacological doses usually employed, actually tend to inhibit or delay the hyperplastic growth of the liver that normally occurs following partial hepatectomy, or carbon tetrachloride intoxication, or during normal development.[146]

Desser-Wiest and her associates recently reexamined the role of the glucocorticoids and report that, in the normal liver, adrenalectomy caused a small increase in DNA synthesis and mitosis. These activities were inhibited by corticosterone, which is the principal glucocorticoid in the rat. They postulate that during the first few hours after partial hepatectomy an observed increase in corticosterone blocked the liver cells at a point in G_1 where they would accumulate, but that the effective hormone activity was then reduced by interaction with serum glucocorticoid-binding proteins which were also increased. This permitted the cells to enter the S phase more or less synchronously.[44] In addition, Desser-Wiest and Desser[45] attribute the increase in hepatic mitosis, well known to occur during pregnancy, to an accompanying rise in progesterone which, they hypothesize, competes with the glucocorticoids for the same receptor sites on the hepatocytes, thereby blocking the inhibitory action of the corticosterone. As these interpretations all rest upon a number of assumptions, further evidence is required. A critical role for adrenal hormones in hepatic regeneration is not supported by results of a recent study in which rates of incorporation of ^{3}H-thymidine into hepatic DNA in rats subjected to adrenalectomy and orchidectomy one week prior to partial hepatectomy did not differ significantly from rates in sham-adrenalectomized, orchidectomized, partially hepatectomized controls (O.T. Terpstra, R.A. Malt and N.L.R. Bucher, unpublished observations).

In fetal hepatocyte cultures, although high concentrations of glucocorticoids are inhibitory, addition of low concentrations potentiate stimulation of DNA synthesis by insulin.[89,95] In adult hepatocyte cultures, addition of hydrocortisone to the basal medium more than doubled the growth rate even without supplementation with other hormones or growth factors;[101] whether this involved macromolecular interactions on the part of the glucocorticoid,[97] or some other function, such as promotion of cellular attachment to the culture dish,[140] is uncertain. The divergence between the in vivo and in vitro actions of glucocorticoids upon the liver cells could perhaps be related to the non-physiological dose levels, but could also be more complex.

Parathyroid hormone and calcium

The role of parathyroid hormone and the related interactions of calcium and cyclic nucleotides, including their participation in hepatic regeneration, have very recently been covered in depth by Whitfield et al,[182] and the role of cyclic nucleotides thoroughly reviewed by Friedman.[67] Rasmussen and Goodman[139] have extensively discussed the relations between calcium and cyclic nucleotides in cell activation, but touch only briefly upon liver growth. In a current series of studies in partially hepatectomized rats, Whitfield, Rixon, MacManus and their associates showed that DNA synthesis, which peaked at about 24 hours, was preceded by two waves of cyclic AMP accumulation with respective maxima at about three and 12 hours after the hepatic resection; infusion of the TAGH mixture (see the section on the thyroid, above) yielded similar results. A delay or lowering of the second cyclic AMP rise, by treatment with certain adrenergic blocking agents, equally delayed or interfered with the initiation of DNA synthesis. Although Thrower and Ord[168] found no such inhibition of DNA synthesis when the cyclic AMP rise was suppressed with a different blocking agent (pindolol), Whitfield et al suggest other mechanisms to explain the discrepancy, which will require additional research for final resolution. Further support for the involvement of cyclic AMP, however, is derived from the demonstration by Short et al[154] that dibutyryl cyclic AMP (but not cyclic GMP) could substitute for glucagon in the TAGH mixture. This is not surprising, for many, if not all, of the effects of glucagon are thought to be mediated by cyclic AMP; the observation by Bucher and Swaffield[26] that glucagon and insulin were not required for the early events of regeneration in eviscerated rats is also in accord with these observations. Overall, the results argue, as noted by Friedman,[67] that cyclic AMP may play a positive role in liver growth, perhaps not early in the conversion of G_0 to the G_+ state, but rather at some point later in G_1.

MacManus, Youdale and Braceland[107] observed a thyroid-dependent hypocalcaemia and hypophosphataemia soon after partial hepatectomy which persisted for at least eight hours; additional data suggested an increased secretion of both calcitonin and parathyroid hormone during the early stages of liver regeneration.

Hepatic regeneration is greatly diminished and delayed in parathyroidectomized or thyroparathyroidectomized rats, despite the occurrence of the two usual bursts of cyclic AMP formation. Either brief elevation of blood calcium (by calcium injection), or treatment with parathyroid hormone, as late as 12 hours after partial hepatectomy, restores the rate of DNA synthesis to control values. Hence hepatocytes appear to be activated even in the hypocalcaemic, parathyroprivic rat, and can reach an advanced pre-DNA synthetic stage of proliferative development, further continuance being calcium dependent. The function of cyclic AMP is thought to be to drive calcium ions from the mitochondria into the cytosol to activate newly synthesized calcium-dependent enzyme assemblies, leading to DNA synthesis, which cannot occur in the calcium-depleted parathyroprivic rats (see Whitfield et al[182] for supporting evidence and a fuller discussion). The investigators conclude that although calcium, cyclic AMP and perhaps cyclic GMP are important intracyclic regulators, they are not involved in the initial proliferative activation of the hepatocytes.

Prostaglandins

MacManus and Braceland[106] recently reported that during the first eight hours after partial hepatectomy the concentration of prostaglandin E (PGE) equivalents in the regenerating liver remnant (but not in peripheral blood) more than doubled. This doubling was attributed to an enhanced rate of prostaglandin synthesis, on the basis of biosynthetic data from liver homogenates. Indomethacin prevented these prostaglandin changes, as well as the subsequent increase in hepatic DNA synthesis. In addition, indomethacin was found to induce a hypocalcaemia, and to block the hypercalcaemic action of parathyroid hormone. The authors suggest that the influence of prostaglandins on DNA synthesis may involve calcium metabolism. Miura and Fukui[117] have also observed an inhibitory effect of indomethacin upon DNA synthesis in the regenerating liver.

Consistent with the above are the findings of Leffert, Koch and Rubalcava[99] that PGE_1 (but not prostaglandins in the A, B and F series) promoted DNA synthesis in fetal hepatocyte cultures, and was elevated two- to threefold in portal venous blood at 12 hours post-hepatectomy.

Although the complex interactions of prostaglandins, parathyroid hormone, cyclic nucleotides and calcium ions cannot yet be fully assessed in relation to liver growth, the emerging patterns provide valuable guidelines for future research.

Epidermal growth factor (EGF)

EGF is a polypeptide, first isolated from the submaxillary glands of male mice, but originating in other tissues, which have not yet been identified, as well. The hormone urogastrone, extracted from human urine, appears to be the human form of EGF, because in amino acid sequence and biological activity it closely resembles mouse EGF. EGF is a potent mitogen for various kinds of cells in culture; it also stimulates epidermal growth in newborn mice, whence its name (for reviews, see Cohen, Carpenter and Lembach[40] and Gospodarowicz and Moran[68]).

The work of Richman et al,[140] mentioned earlier, showed that EGF, especially in combination with pancreatic hormones, was capable of stimulating DNA synthesis when added to adult rat hepatocytes in monolayer cultures. As no mitoses were seen, however, the liver cells apparently did not progress beyond the S phase. In vivo, similarly, continuous intraperitoneal infusion of EGF into normal rats stimulated synthesis of hepatic DNA only slightly, and combination with either insulin or glucagon substantially enhanced its effectiveness, but, in addition, the DNA synthesis was associated with mitosis.[31,32] When glucagon was added to the insulin–EGF mixture, however, contrary to observations in cell cultures, the proliferative activity was considerably diminished. The in vivo EGF model is therefore unlike the earlier models in which insulin and glucagon acted synergistically. The discrepancy could be due to differing experimental conditions, perhaps resolvable by manipulation of hormone dosages, or to more fundamental differences involving the means by which the hormones influence these several model systems. For example, although insulin and glucagon have generally opposite effects upon blood sugar, gluconeogenesis, glycogenolysis and lipolysis, they probably do not act in a plus–minus fashion upon these various functions, but rather operate through quite separate biochemical mechanisms,[103] for they can exert cooperative or counteractive influences, depending upon circumstances. Following a protein meal, for instance, plasma insulin and glucagon levels both rise, promoting gluconeogenesis as well as glycogenolysis, so that blood glucose is maintained in the presence of elevated insulin levels.[35] On the other hand, in isolated hepatocytes, if glycogen stores are high, but not if they are low, insulin stimulates protein synthesis several-fold; the stimulation is abolished by glucagon.[174] Hence insulin and glucagon in enhancing growth stimulation by EGF may operate differently from when promoting hepatocyte proliferation in eviscerated rats or in other models. A combination of EGF and insulin that resulted in a tenfold stimulation of DNA synthesis in livers of normal animals caused negligible or no stimulation in the brain, heart, lung, stomach, spleen, kidney or skin, and thus seems relatively specific for the liver. Although receptors for EGF have been demonstrated in membrane preparations from liver cells, EGF has not yet been shown to have a physiological role in regulating hepatocyte proliferation. This remains an attractive possibility, however.[32]

Continuous infusions of T_3, in either pharmacological or physiological doses, in combination with the same or several-fold higher amounts of glucagon and amino acids that actively potentiated EGF, were without effect, pointing to the possible involvement of different mechanisms in the growth stimulation produced by EGF and by T_3.[31] The necessity for pharmacological doses of pancreatic hormones, particularly glucagon, to augment the growth-stimulating actions of T_3 and EGF, or to promote growth in other animal models discussed earlier, is unexplained; although indirect or ancillary effects merit consideration, perhaps the optimal conditions for effective hormone administration have not yet been found, i.e., the proper combination(s) of hormones and growth factors and prior state of responsiveness of the cells.

Nucleotides

There is an extensive literature on the function of cyclic nucleotides in growth regulation, especially cyclic AMP and to a lesser extent cyclic GMP. The possible role of cyclic AMP in liver growth has been discussed in the section on parathyroid hormone; involvement of cyclic GMP remains inconclusive. Heine, Rapaport and Bucher[76] found no elevation of cyclic CMP or cyclic UMP during the early period of hepatic regeneration, when proliferative activity is high, in contrast to the 50- to 200-fold increase in cyclic CMP reported to occur in the five-day regenerating liver, when proliferative activity is low.[16] The failure of both compounds to incorporate ^{32}Pi (under conditions in which cyclic AMP and cyclic GMP did become labelled) suggested that the cyclic pyrimidine nucleotides are likely to have little if any influence upon hepatocyte proliferation.[76] Whatever the involvement of cyclic nucleotides in liver growth, it is likely that their function may be to serve as mediators of the extracellular regulatory factors that are the primary concern of this review.

A number of other nucleotides and related compounds are also associated with growth and could have regulatory roles. It was found, for example, that purine nucleotides and nucleosides enhanced serum-induced DNA synthesis in quiescent 3T3 cells in culture, whereas pyrimidine compounds were ineffective.[145] Recently Leffert and his associates[89] observed that inosine and hypoxanthine promoted initiation of DNA synthesis in hepatocytes in fetal liver cell cultures, and obtained indirect evidence through use of an inhibitor that hypoxanthine might, in addition, have a potentiating effect in vivo. In other experiments these investigators showed that inosine enhanced proliferation of adult liver cells in culture, both by itself and especially in combination with insulin and hydrocortisone.[101] In addition they isolated from fetal liver cell cultures a 'family' of highly phosphorylated nucleotides which, they postulated, might function in a growth-regulating capacity.[89] Two such substances, which are derivatives of adenine, were previously observed by Rapaport and Bucher[137,138] in regenerating livers; these now appear to occur in similar amounts in normal liver as well[24] and the relevance to liver growth requires re-evaluation. Reports of an association of other unusual nucleotides with proliferative or metabolic activity in other systems suggests that this area merits continuing consideration.

Miscellaneous Liver Growth Inhibitory or Stimulatory Substances

There are several reports that extracts of serum or liver contain substances which inhibit hepatocyte proliferation either in vitro or in vivo during developmental growth or during regeneration following partial hepatectomy. Such inhibitors, if organ- or tissue-specific and operating through a negative feedback system, are termed chalones.[146] Chalones are not cytotoxic, and their effects are reversible. They are generally not species-specific. Some doubts have been expressed concerning their existence in the liver. Recently Verly and his associates have partially purified a protein (40 000 molecular weight) with chalone-like properties from rabbit liver that inhibited DNA synthesis in partially hepatectomized rats.[173] Sekas and Cook[148,149] have obtained a substance with similar activity from rat liver with a molecular weight of less than 10 000, and still different substances are reported by others.[7,126]

Leffert and his associates[98,99] found that the very low density lipoprotein (VLDL) fraction of rat serum inhibited initiation of DNA synthesis in fetal rat hepatocyte cultures; cells already in the 'S' phase were resistant. In vivo, following partial hepatectomy, the serum VLDL levels fell abruptly and remained low for 24 hours or more. In a mutant strain of rats (fatty) which over-produces VLDL, hepatic DNA synthetic rates were only one-quarter of control values, whereas in normal rats stimulation of DNA synthesis by infusion of TAGH at least temporarily depressed the serum VLDL levels. Although there are inconsistencies, this and other evidence suggest that VLDL may function in a chalone-like fashion. It is interesting to note in this connection that glucagon, which tends to be elevated during periods of hepatic growth, is an effective lipolytic agent and would serve to release the liver from the suppressive effects of VLDLs. Heparin acts similarly; its endogenous levels during hepatic regeneration, however, are unknown.[99]

Paralleling the early reports of inhibitory factors in crude serum and liver extracts were a similar number detailing the recovery of stimulatory activities. In some instances both stimulatory and inhibitory factors (generally proteins) were recovered.[22] Along these lines are recent reports by Morley,[121] La Brecque and Pesch,[90] Nadal, Lombard and Zajdela,[123] Marcsek, Merryhart and Grof[111] and others. Frequently the assays employed for these impure preparations lack stringency, and critical evaluation at this stage seems unprofitable.

Stemming from numerous observations that proteases can induce cellular proliferation in vitro, attempts have been made to stimulate liver growth in vivo with these enzymes,[186] or to suppress hepatic regeneration with their inhibitors;[118] the results so far, however, have not provided clear evidence in support of a physiological basis for growth regulation by such means. In a recent evaluation of the plasmin and plasminogen activator proteases of the plasma fibrinolytic system, Rixon, Walker and Whitfield[141] concluded that these substances are unlikely to be blood-borne initiators of hepatocyte proliferation.

Whether it will ultimately be shown that hepatocyte proliferation is controlled by a shifting balance between stimulatory and inhibitory influences still remains speculative.

CONCLUSIONS

From this far from complete survey of the proposed means by which the body exerts its control over the growth of an organ, exemplified here by the liver, it is evident that the operant mechanisms have not yet come clearly into focus.

Unicellular organisms proliferate as a function of the availability of low molecular weight nutrients in the milieu. Mammalian cells in vivo, on the other hand, live in a highly protective environment where fluctuations in temperature, pH, electrolytes and nutrients are maintained within narrow physiological limits. Under these circumstances allocation and utilization of nutrients is at least partially mediated by hormonal agents that regulate the activity of nutrient-specific transport systems, and consequently the availability of nutrients in the intracellular environment. The familiar concept that each cell type has a specific factor that can trigger the cell division programme remains tenable with the proviso that adequate intracellular levels of nutrients are available, these in turn being dependent upon the regulators of the transport systems.[5]

Alternatively, as noted by Holley,[79] cell proliferation may be orchestrated by the interplay of many factors, among which, in addition to a number of hormones and hormone-like substances, are nucleotides, amino acids and peptides, glucose, calcium and phosphate ions and lipopolysaccharides – polypeptide hormones and similar growth-controlling serum factors being considered most important. Holley points out the intriguing possibility that the hormones and growth factors may act by invoking the same intracellular growth-control mechanisms affected by nutrients. In addition to the factors that stimulate growth are chalones and other inhibitory factors which exert a suppressive influence.

In the case of growth regulation by multiple factors, specificity of the stimulus for a single type of cell would presumably be conferred by particular key combinations of factors appropriate for the available receptor sites and metabolic state of those cells.[73] All cells may not be regulated in the same fashion, nor has the possibility been excluded that more than one combination of factors may unlock the interactions that mobilize the programmed progression of a single type of cell through the cell cycle. Heterogeneity has been demonstrated among cells arrested in G_1–G_0,[88,97,142] and there is growing evidence that the responsiveness of cells is dependent upon their prior history.[43,71,97,174] Competence to proliferate, then, is determined by the physiological state of the cell, and the extent of proliferative activity by the availability of regulators appropriate for that state.

ACKNOWLEDGEMENTS

This work was supported by grants from the USPHS No. CA 02146-24 and 5 RO1 AM19435-02. This is Publication No. 1530 of the Cancer Commission of Harvard University.

REFERENCES

1. Abraham, R., Goldbert, L. & Grasso, P. (1967) Hepatic response to lysosomal effects of hypoxia, neutral red and chloroquine. *Nature (London)*, **215,** 194–196.
2. Albano, J.D.M., Ekins, R.P., Maritz, G. & Turner, R.C. (1972) A sensitive, precise radioimmunoassay of serum insulin relying on charcoal separation of bound and free hormone moieties. *Acta Endocrinologica,* **70,** 487–509.
3. Anthony, L.E. & Edozien, J.C. (1975) Experimental protein and energy deficiencies in the rat. *Journal of Nutrition,* **105,** 631–648.
4. Argyris, T.S. (1974) Stimulators, enzyme induction and the control of liver growth. In *Control of Proliferation in Animal Cells* (Ed.) Clarkson, B. & Baserga, R. pp. 49–66. Cold Spring Harbor, New York: Cold Spring Harbor Laboratory.
5. Armelin, H.A. (1975) Hormones and regulation of cell division: mammalian cell cultures as an experimental approach. In *Biochemical Actions of Hormones* (Ed.) Litwack, G. Vol. III, pp. 1–21. New York: Academic Press.
6. Aronsen, K.F., Ericsson, B., Nosslin, B., Nylander, G., Pihl, B. & Waldeskog, B. (1970) Evaluation of hepatic regeneration by scintillation scanning, cholangiography and angiography in man. *Annals of Surgery,* **171,** 567–574.
7. Aujard, C., Chany, E. & Frayssinet, C. (1976) Relation entre la vitesse de croissance du foie de jeune rats et l'action inhibitrice d'extraits de leur foie sur la multiplication de cellules in cultures. *Compte Rendu de l'Académie des Sciences (Paris),* **282,** 1647–1650.
8. Bade, E.G. (1967) In *Control of Cellular Growth in Adult Organisms,* pp. 260–269. New York: Academic Press.
9. Barbiroli, B. & Potter, V. (1971) DNA synthesis and interaction between controlled feeding schedules and partial hepatectomy in rats. *Science,* **172,** 738–740.
10. Barka, T. & Popper, H. (1967) Liver enlargement and drug toxicity. *Medicine,* **46,** 103–117.
11. Barra, R. & Hall, J.C. (1977) Liver regeneration in normal and alloxan-induced diabetic rats. *Journal of Experimental Zoology,* **201,** 93–100.
12. Bassi, M. & Bernelli-Zazzera, A. (1964) Ultrastructural cytoplasmic changes of liver cells after reversible and irreversible ischaemia. *Experimental and Molecular Pathology,* **3,** 332–350.
13. Beauchene, R.E., Roeder, L.M. & Barrows, C.H. (1970) The inter-relationships of age, tissue protein synthesis and proteinaria. *Journal of Gerontology,* **25,** 359.
14. Becker, F.F. (1973) Humoral aspects of liver regeneration. In *Humoral Control of Growth and Differentiation* (Ed.) LoBue, J. & Gordon, E.S. Vol. 1, pp. 249–256. New York: Academic Press.
15. Benacerraf, B., Bilbey, D., Biozzi, G., Halpern, B.N. & Stiffel, G. (1957) The measurement of liver blood flow in partially hepatectomised rats. *Journal of Physiology (London),* **136,** 287–293.
16. Bloch, A. (1975) Isolation of cytidine 3′,5′-monophosphate from mammalian tissues and body fluids and its effects on leukemia L–1210 cell growth in culture. In *Advances in Cyclic Nucleotide Research* (Ed.) Drummond, G.I. & Greengard, P. Vol. **5,** pp. 331–338. New York: Raven Press.
17. Blumgart, L.H., Leach, K.G. & Karran, S.J. (1971) Observations on liver regeneration after right hepatic lobectomy. *Gut,* **12,** 922–928.
18. Bresnick, E. (1971) Regenerating liver: an experimental model for the study of growth. In *Methods in Cancer Research* (Ed.) Busch, H. Vol. VI, pp. 347–397. New York: Academic Press.
19. Broelsch, C.E., Lee, S., Charters, A.C., Chandler, J.G., Grambort, D.E. & Orloff, M.J. (1974) Regeneration of liver isografts transplanted in continuity with splanchnic organs. *Surgical Forum,* **25,** 394–396.
20. Brown, J. Mullen, Y., Molner, I.G. & Clark, W.R. (1976) Importance of hepatic–portal route for control of diabetes. *Diabetes,* **25,** 338.
21. Brues, A.M., Drury, D.R. & Brues, M.C. (1936) A quantitative study of cell growth in regenerating liver. *Archives of Pathology,* **22,** 658–673.
22. Bucher, N.L.R. (1963) Regeneration of mammalian liver. *International Review of Cytology,* **15,** 245–300.
23. Bucher, N.L.R. and Malt, R.A. (1971) Regeneration of the liver and kidney. In *New England Journal of Medicine,* Medical Progress Series, Little, Brown.
24. Bucher, N.L.R. & McGowan, J.A. (1977) Unpublished observations.
25. Bucher, N.L.R. & Swaffield, M.N. (1973) Regeneration of liver in rats in absence of portal splanchnic organs and a portal blood supply. *Cancer Research,* **33,** 3189–3194.
26. Bucher, N.L.R. & Swaffield, M.N. (1975) Regulation of hepatic regeneration in rats by synergistic action of insulin and glucagon. *Proceedings of the National Academy of Sciences of the United States of America,* **72,** 1157–1160.
27. Bucher, N.L.R. & Swaffield, M.N. (1975) Synergistic action of glucagon and insulin in regulation of hepatic regeneration. In *Advances in Enzyme Regulation* (Ed.) Weber, G. Vol. 13, pp. 281–293. New York and Oxford: Pergamon Press.
28. Bucher, N.L.R. & Swaffield, M.N. (1975) Unpublished observations.
29. Bucher, N.L.R. & Wands, J.R. (1977) Hormone cocktails to stimulate hepatocytes. *New England Journal of Medicine,* **296,** 946.
30. Bucher, N.L.R. & Weir, G.C. (1976) Insulin, glucagon, liver regeneration, and DNA synthesis. *Metabolism,* **25,** 1423–1425.
31. Bucher, N.L.R., Patel, U. & Cohen, S. (1978) Hormonal factors concerned with liver regeneration. *Ciba Foundation Symposium No. 55.* (New series) *Hepatotrophic Factors.* pp. 95–107. New York: Elsevier/Excerpta Medica/North Holland.
32. Bucher, N.L.R., Patel, U. & Cohen, S. (1977) Hormonal factors and liver growth. In *Advances in Enzyme Regulation* (Ed.) Weber, G. Vol. 16, pp. 205–213. New York: Pergamon Press.
33. Bucher, N.L.R., Swaffield, M.N. & Di Troia, J.F. (1964) Influence of age upon incorporation of thymidine-2-C^{14} into DNA of regenerating rat liver. *Cancer Research,* **24,** 509–512.
34. Byyny, R.L., Orth, D.N., Cohen, S. & Doyne, E.S. (1974) Epidermal growth factor: effects of androgen and adrenergic agents. *Endocrinology,* **95,** 776–783.
35. Cahill, G.F. (1973) Glucagon. *New England Journal of Medicine,* **288,** 157–158.
36. Chandler, J.G. (1976) Hepatotrophic activity in non-pancreatic non-duodenal portal blood. *Surgical Forum,* **27,** 360–363.
37. Chandler, J.G., Lee, S., Krubel, R., Rosen, H., Nakaji, N.T. & Orloff, M.J. (1971) Inter-liver competition

and portal blood in regeneration of auxiliary liver transplants. *Surgical Forum*, **22**, 341–343.

38. Clarkson, B. & Baserga, R. (Ed.) (1974) *Control of Proliferation in Animal Cells*. pp. 1–1029. Cold Spring Harbor, New York: Cold Spring Harbor Laboratory.
39. Cohen, S. (1972) Epidermal growth factor. *Journal of Investigative Dermatology*, **59**, 13–16.
40. Cohen, S., Carpenter, G. & Lembach, K.J. (1975) Interaction of epidermal growth factor (EGF) with cultured fibroblasts. *Advances in Metabolic Disorders*, **8**, 265–284.
41. Dallman, P.R., Spirito, R.A. & Siimes, M.A. (1974) Diurnal patterns of DNA synthesis in the rat: modification by diet and feeding schedule. *Journal of Nutrition*, **104**, 1234–1241.
42. Deland, F.H. & North, W.A. (1968) Relationship between liver size and body size. *Radiology*, **91**, 1195–1198.
43. DeRubertis, F.R. & Craven, P. (1976) Effect of reduced ATP content on hepatic responses to glucagon. *Metabolism*, **25**, 57–67.
44. Desser-Wiest, L. (1975) Autosynchronization of rat liver cells with endogenous corticosterone after partial hepatectomy. *Cell and Tissue Kinetics*, **8**, 1–9.
45. Desser-Wiest, L. & Desser, H. (1977) Control of liver cell proliferation in pregnant rats. *Journal of Endocrinology*, **72**, 407–408.
46. Dillman, W.H., Schwartz, H.L. & Oppenheimer, J.H. (1977) Specific nuclear T_3 binding sites decrease in the regenerating liver. *Clinical Research*, **25**, A293.
47. Doljanski, F., Rosenthal, J. & Eisenberg, S. (1966) Liver regeneration in starved rats. *Experimental and Molecular Pathology*, **5**, 263–272.
48. Dubois, D. & Dubois, E.F. (1916) A height–weight formula to estimate the surface area of man. *Proceedings of the Society for Experimental Biology (N.Y.)* **13**, 77–78.
49. Duguay, L.R. & Orloff, M.J. (1976) Regulation of liver regeneration by the pancreas in dogs. *Surgical Forum*, **27**, 355–356.
50. Duguay, L.R., Rosenkranz, E. & Orloff, M.J. (1976) Pancreatic hormones in blood during liver regeneration. *Gastroenterology*, **71**, 903.
51. Duguay, L.R., Skivolocki, W.P. & Orloff, M.J. (1977) Regulation of liver regeneration by pancreatic hormones. *Gastroenterology*, **72**, 1053.
52. Duguay, L.R., Charters, A.C., Lee, S., Sviokla, S.C. & Orloff, M.J. (1975) Time course of liver regeneration after splanchnic organ ablation. *Surgical Forum*, **26**, 408–410.
53. Edwards, J.L. & Koch, A. (1964) Parenchymal and littoral cell proliferation during liver regeneration. *Laboratory Investigation*, **13**, 32–43.
54. Fabrikant, J.I. (1968) Kinetics of cellular proliferation in regenerating liver. *Journal of Cell Biology*, **36**, 551–565.
55. Fabrikant, J.I. (1969) Size of proliferating pools in regenerating liver. *Experimental Cell Research*, **55**, 277–279.
56. Fahimi, H.D. (1967) Perfusion and immersion fixation of rat liver with glutaraldehyde. *Laboratory Investigation*, **16**, 736–750.
57. Farivar, M., Wands, J.R., Isselbacher, K.J. & Bucher, N.L.R. (1976) Effect of insulin and glucagon in fulminant murine hepatitis. *New England Journal of Medicine*, **295**, 1517–1519.
58. Ferris, G.M. & Clark, J.B. (1972) Early changes in plasma and hepatic free amino acids in partially hepatectomized rats. *Biochimica et Biophysica Acta*, **273**, 73–79.
59. Fisher, E.R. & Fisher, B. (1963) Ultrastructural hepatic changes following partial hepatectomy and portacaval shunt in the rat. *Laboratory Investigation*, **12**, 929–942.
60. Fisher, B., Szuch, P. & Fisher, E.R. (1971) Evaluation of a humoral factor in liver regeneration utilizing liver transplants. *Cancer Research*, **31**, 322–331.
61. Fisher, B., Szuch, P., Levine, M. & Fisher, E.R. (1971) A portal blood factor as the humoral agent in liver regeneration. *Science*, **171**, 575–577.
62. Fisher, B., Szuch, P., Levine, M., Saffer, E. & Fisher, E.R. (1973) The intestine as a source of a portal blood factor responsible for liver regeneration. *Surgery, Gynecology and Obstetrics*, **137**, 210–214.
63. Fleming, J.S., Karran, S.J., Eagles, C.J. & Ackery, D. (1977) A new in-vivo sequential technique for the measurement of effective liver blood flow in small animals. *Proceedings of the European Society of Surgical Research*, Warsaw.
64. Foster, J.H., Lawler, M.R., Welborn, M.B., Holcom, B.G.W. & Sawyers, J.L. (1968) Recent experience with major hepatic resection. *Annals of Surgery*, **167**, 651–668.
65. Foster, K.J., Alberti, K.G.M.M., Binder, C., Hinks, L., Karran, S., Talbot, S., Turnell, D. & Ørskov, H. (1978) The role of glucocorticoids and glucagon in the metabolic response to moderate injury. *Clinical Science and Molecular Medicine*, **54**, 4–5.
66. Fournier, R.E. & Pardee, A.B. (1975) Cell cycle studies of mononucleate and cytochalasin-B-induced binucleate fibroblasts. *Proceedings of the National Academy of Sciences of the United States of America*, **72**, 869–873.
67. Friedman, D.L. (1976) Role of cyclic nucleotides in cell growth and differentiation. *Physiological Reviews*, **56**, 652–708.
68. Gospodarowicz, D. & Moran, J.S. (1976) Growth factors in mammalian cell culture. *Annual Review of Biochemistry*, **45**, 531–558.
69. Grisham, J.W. (1962) Morphologic study of deoxyribonucleic acid synthesis and cell proliferation in regenerating rat liver; autoradiography with thymidine-H^3. *Cancer Research*, **22**, 842–849.
70. Guest, J., Ryan, C.J., Benjamin, I.S. & Blumgart, L.H. (1977) Portacaval transposition and subsequent partial hepatectomy in the rat: effects on liver atrophy, hypertrophy, and regenerative hyperplasia. *British Journal of Experimental Pathology*, **58**, 140–146.
71. Gunther, G.R., Wang, J.L. & Edelman, G.M. (1974) Kinetics of cellular commitment during stimulation of lymphocytes by lectins. *Journal of Cell Biology*, **62**, 366–377.
72. Harrison, M.F. (1953) Effect of starvation on the composition of the liver cell. .*Biochemical Journal*, **55**, 204–211.
73. Hayashi, I. & Sato, G.H. (1976) Replacement of serum by hormones permits growth of cells in a defined medium. *Nature*, **259**, 132–134.
74. Hayashi, I., Hutchings, S., Mather, J., Larner, J. & Sato, G.H. (1977) Hormonal control of cells in culture. *In Vitro*, **13**, 140.
75. Hays, D.M. (1974) Surgical research aspects of hepatic regeneration. *Surgery, Gynecology and Obstretrics*, **139**, 609–619.
76. Heine, M.C., Rapaport, E. & Bucher, N.L.R. (1977) Unpublished observations. See Foá, P.P., Bajaj,

J.S. & Foá, N.L. (Ed.) *Glucagon: Its Role in Physiology and Clinical Medicine*. pp. 398–399. New York: Springer Verlag.

77. Higgins, G.M. & Anderson, R.M. (1931) Experimental pathology of the liver. I. Restoration of the liver of the white rat following partial surgical removal. *Archives of Pathology*, **12**, 186.

78. Hilton, J. & Sartorelli, A. (1970) Induction of microsomal drug metabolizing enzymes in regenerating liver. In *Advances in Enzyme Regulation* (Ed.) Weber, G. pp. 153–167. New York: Pergamon Press.

79. Holley, R.W. (1975) Control of growth of mammalian cells in cell culture. *Nature*, **258**, 487–490.

80. Holley, R.W. & Kiernan, J.A. (1974) Control of the initiation of DNA synthesis in 3T3 cells: low molecular weight nutrients. *Proceedings of the National Academy of Sciences of the United States of America*, **71**, 2942–2945.

81. Johnson, H.A. (1969) Liver regeneration and the critical mass hypothesis. *American Journal of Pathology*, **57**, 1–15.

82. Karran, S.J., Leach, K.G. & Blumgart, L.H. (1972) Radio-isotope investigation of protein synthesis and reticulo-endothelial activity following partial hepatectomy in the rat. *British Journal of Surgery*, **59**, 907.

83. Karran, S.J., Leach, K.G. & Blumgart, L.H. (1974) Assessment of liver regeneration in the rat using gamma camera. *Journal of Nuclear Medicine*, **15** (1), 10–16.

84. Karran, S.J., Eagles, C.J., Fleming, J. & Ackery, D. (1978) Unpublished data.

85. Karran, S.J., Eagles, C., Fleming, J. & Ackery, D. (1979) In-vivo measurement of liver perfusion in the normal and partially hepatectomised rat using Tc-99m sulfur colloid. *Journal of Nuclear Medicine*, **20**, 26–31.

86. Kinney, J. (1979) Calorie and nitrogen requirements in catabolic states. In *Practical Nutritional Support* (Ed.) Karran, S.J. & Alberti, K.G.M.M. Pitman Medical. In press.

87. Kletzien, R.F., Pariza, M.W., Becker, J.E. & Potter, V.R. (1976) Hormonal regulation of amino acid transport and gluconeogenesis in primary cultures of adult rat liver parenchymal cells. *Journal of Cellular Physiology*, **89**, 641–646.

88. Klevecz, R.R. & Forrest, G.L. (1977) Metabolic regulation in the cell cycle. In *Growth, Nutrition, and Metabolism of Cells in Culture* (Ed.) Rothblat, G.H. & Cristofalo, V.J. Vol. III, pp. 149–196. New York: Academic Press.

89. Koch, K.S., Leffert, H.L. & Moran, T. (1976) Hepatic proliferation control by purines, hormones, and nutrients. In *Oncodevelopmental Gene Expression* (Ed.) Fishman, W.H. & Sell, S. pp. 21–33. New York: Academic Press.

90. La Brecque, D.R. & Pesch, L.A. (1975) Preparation and partial characterization of hepatic regenerative stimulator substances (SS) from rat liver. *Journal of Physiology*, **248**, 273–284.

91. Leduc, E.H. (1949) Mitotic activity in the liver of the mouse during inanition followed by refeeding with different levels of protein. *American Journal of Anatomy*, **84**, 397–421.

92. Lee, S., Edgington, T.S. & Orloff, M.J. (1968) Role of afferent blood supply in regeneration of liver isografts in rats. *Surgical Forum*, **19**, 360.

93. Lee, K.L., Sun, S.-C. & Miller, O.N. (1968) Stimulation of incorporation by triiodothyronine of thymidine-methyl-^{3}H into hepatic DNA of the rat. *Archives of Biochemistry and Biophysics*, **125**, 751–757.

94. Lee, S., Chandler, J.M., Broelsch, C.E., Flamant, Y.M. & Orloff, M.J. (1974) Portal-systemic anastomosis in the rat. *Journal of Surgical Research*, **17**, 53–73.

95. Leffert, H.L. (1974) Growth control of differentiated fetal rat hepatocytes in primary monolayer culture. VII. Hormonal control of DNA synthesis and its possible significance to the problem of liver regeneration. *Journal of Cell Biology*, **62**, 792–801.

96. Leffert, H.L. & Alexander, N.M. (1976) Thyroid hormone metabolism during liver regeneration in rats. *Endocrinology*, **98**, 1205–1211.

97. Leffert, H.L. & Koch, K.S. (1977) In *Growth, Nutrition, and Metabolism of Cells in Culture* (Ed.) Rothblat, G.H. & Cristofalo, V.J. Vol. III, pp. 225–294. New York: Academic Press.

98. Leffert, H.L. & Weinstein, D.B. (1976) Growth control of differentiated fetal rat hepatocytes in primary monolayer cultures. IX. Specific inhibition of DNA synthesis initiation by very low density lipoprotein and possible significance to the problem of liver regeneration. *Journal of Cell Biology*, **70**, 20–32.

99. Leffert, H.L., Koch, K.S. & Rubalcava, B. (1976) Present paradoxes in the environmental control of hepatic regeneration. *Cancer Research*, **36**, 4250–4255.

100. Leffert, H.L., Alexander, N.M., Faloona, G., Rubalcava, B. & Unger, R. (1975) Specific endocrine and hormonal receptor changes associated with liver regeneration in adult rats. *Proceedings of the National Academy of Sciences of the United States of America*, **72**, 4033–4036.

101. Leffert, H.L., Moran, T., Boorstein, R. & Koch, K.S. (1977) Procarcinogen activation and hormonal control of cell proliferation in differentiated primary adult liver cell cultures. *Nature*, **267**, 58–61.

102. Lesch, R. & Reutter, W. (Ed.) (1975) *Liver Regeneration After Experimental Injury. III. Workshop on Experimental Liver Injury*. pp. 1–364. New York: Stratton Intercontinental Medical Book Corporation.

103. Levine, R. (1976) Glucagon and the regulation of blood sugar. *New England Journal of Medicine*, **294**, 494–495.

104. Lewan, L., Yngner, T. & Engelbrecht, C. (1977) The biochemistry of the regenerating liver. *International Journal of Biochemistry*, **8**, 477–487.

105. Lieberman, I. (1969) Studies on control of mammalian deoxyribonucleic acid synthesis. In *Biochemistry of Cell Division* (Ed.) Baserga, R. pp. 119–137. Springfield, Illinois: C.C. Thomas.

106. MacManus, J.P. & Braceland, B.M. (1976) A connection between the production of prostaglandins during liver regeneration and the DNA synthetic responses. *Prostaglandins*, **11**, 609–620.

107. MacManus, J.P., Youdale, T. & Braceland, B.M. (1975) Evidence for the release of calcitonin and parathyroid hormone during liver regeneration in the rat. *Hormone and Metabolic Research*, **7**, 83–87.

108. Malamud, D. & Perrin, L. (1974) Stimulation of DNA synthesis in mouse pancreas by triiodothyronine and glucagon. *Endocrinology*, **94**, 1157–1160.

109. Mann, F.C. (1944) Restoration and pathologic reactions of the liver. *Journal of Mount Sinai Hospital,* **11,** 65–74.
110. Marchioro, T.L., Porter, K.A., Brown, B.I., Otte, J.-B. & Starzl, T.E. (1967) The effect of partial portacaval transposition on the canine liver. *Surgery,* **61,** 723–732.
111. Marczek, Z., Merryhart, J. & Grof, J. (1976) Effects on thymidine incorporation of polypeptides isolated from intact and regenerating liver. *Journal of Cell Biology,* **70,** 187a.
112. Marks, C., Markey, C., Dyer, R. & Vaupel, M.R. (1975) Electron microscopic study of portacaval shunts on ultrastructure of rat livers after partial hepatectomy. *American Journal of Surgery,* **129,** 156–162.
113. McDermott, W.V.Jr (1970) Circulatory changes associated with major hepatic resection. *Annals of the New York Academy of Sciences,* **170,** 246–250.
114. McDermott, W.V.Jr, Greenberger, N.J., Isselbacher, K.J. & Weber, A.L. (1963) Major hepatic resection; diagnostic techniques and metabolic problems. *Surgery,* **54,** 56–66.
115. McGowan, J. (1977) *Liver Regeneration in Protein Deprived Rats.* Ph.D. Thesis, Providence, Rhode Island: Brown University.
116. McGowan, J. & Fausto, N. (1975) Ornithine decarboxylase activity and delayed DNA synthesis in the regenerating liver of protein deprived rats. *Federation Proceedings,* **34** (Abstract), 858.
117. Miura, Y. & Fukui, T. (1976) Pleiotypic responses of regenerating liver. *Advances in Enzyme Regulation,* **14,** 393–405.
118. Miyamoto, M., Terayama, H. & Ohnishi, T. (1973) Effects of protease inhibitors on liver regeneration. *Biochemical and Biophysical Research Communications,* **55,** 84–90.
119. Montecuccoli, G., Novello, F. & Stirpe, F. (1972) Effect of protein deprivation on DNA synthesis in resting and regenerating rat liver. *Journal of Nutrition,* **102,** 507–514.
120. Moolten, F.L. & Bucher, N.L.R. (1967) Regeneration of rat liver: transfer of humoral agent by cross circulation. *Science,* **158,** 272–274.
121. Morley, C.G.D. (1974) Humoral regulation of liver regeneration and tissue growth. *Perspectives in Biology and Medicine,* **17,** 411–428.
122. Nadal, C. & Zajdela, F. (1966) Polyploidie somatique dans le foie de rat. I. Le rôle des cellules binucléées dans la genèse des cellules polyploides. *Experimental Cellular Research,* **42,** 99–116.
123. Nadal, C., Lombard, M.N. & Zajdela, F. (1976) Inhibition of rat hepatocyte multiplication by serum and liver factors. *Virchows Archiv. Abt. B. Cell Pathology,* **20,** 277–285.
124. Obenrader, M., Chen, J., Ove, P. & Lansing, A.I. (1974) Functional regeneration in liver of old rats after partial hepatectomy. *Experimental Gerontology,* **9,** 181–190.
125. Oka, T., Perry, J.W. & Topper, Y. (1974) Changes in insulin responsiveness during development of mammary epithelium. *Journal of Cell Biology,* **62,** 550–556.
126. Onda, H. & Yoshikawa, J. (1974) Studies on the regulatory mechanisms of cell division. α-1-acid glycoprotein as a hepatocyte-specific mitosis inhibitory protein in regenerating rat liver. *Gann,* **66,** 227–235.
127. Ord, M.G. & Stocken, L.A. (1972) Uptake of amino acids and nucleic acid precursors by regenerating rat liver. *Biochemical Journal,* **129,** 175–181.
128. Ove, P., Obenrader, M.L. & Lansing, A.I. (1972) Synthesis and degradation of liver proteins in growing and old rats. *Biochimica et Biophysica Acta,* **277,** 211.
129. Pack, G.T., Islami, A.H., Hubbard, J.C. & Brasfield, R.D. (1962) Regeneration of human liver after major hepatectomy. *Surgery,* **52,** 617–623.
130. Peters, R.L. (1975) Viral hepatitis: a pathologic spectrum. *American Journal of the Medical Sciences,* **270,** 17–32.
131. Post, J. & Hoffman, J. (1972) In *Progress in Liver Diseases* (Ed.) Popper, H. & Schaffner, F. Vol. 2, p. 155. New York: Grune & Stratton.
132. Price, J.B., Voorhees, A.B. & Britton, R.C. (1967) Role of portal blood in regeneration and function of completely revascularized partial hepatic autografts. *Surgery,* **62,** 195–203.
133. Price, J.B.Jr, Takeshige, K., Max, M.H. & Voorhees, A.B.Jr (1972) Glucagon as the portal factor modifying hepatic regeneration. *Surgery,* **72,** 74–82.
134. Rabes, H.M. & Brändle, H. (1969) Synthesis of RNA, protein, and DNA in the liver of normal and hypophysectomized rats after partial hepatectomy. *Cancer Research,* **29,** 817–822.
135. Rabinovici, N. & Wiener, E. (1963) Hemodynamic changes in the hepatectomized liver of the rat and their relationship to regeneration. *Journal of Surgical Research,* **3,** 3–8.
136. Rao, P.N., Sunkara, P.S. & Wilson, B.A. (1977) Regulation of DNA synthesis: age-dependent cooperation among G_1 cells upon fusion. *Proceedings of the National Academy of Sciences of the United States of America,* **74,** 2869–2873.
137. Rapaport, E. & Bucher, N.L.R. (1975) Two new nucleotides in normal and regenerating rat liver. *Journal of Cell Biology,* **67,** 352a.
138. Rapaport, E. & Bucher, N.L.R. (1976) Two new adenine nucleotides in normal and regenerating rat liver. In *Oncodevelopmental Gene Expression* (Ed.) Fishman, W.H. & Sell, S. pp. 13–20. New York: Academic Press.
139. Rasmussen, H. & Goodman, D.B.P. (1977) Relationship between calcium and cyclic nucleotides in cell activation. *Physiological Reviews,* **57,** 421–509.
140. Richman, R.A., Claus, T.H., Pilkis, S.J. & Friedman, D.L. (1976) Hormonal stimulation of DNA synthesis in primary cultures of adult rat hepatocytes. *Proceedings of the National Academy of Sciences of the United States of America,* **73,** 3589–3593.
141. Rixon, R.H., Walker, P.R. & Whitfield, J.F. (1977) Fibrinolysis and liver regeneration. *Journal of Cellular Physiology,* **92,** 13–21.
142. Rossini, M., Lin, J.-C. & Baserga, R. (1976) Effects of prolonged quiescence on nuclei and chromatin of WI–38 fibroblasts. *Journal of Cellular Physiology,* **88,** 1–12.
143. Salatka, K., Kresge, D., Harris, J.L., Edelstein, D. & Ove, P. (1971) Rat serum protein changes with age. *Experimental Gerontology,* **6,** 25.
144. Sander, G. & Pardee, A.B. (1972) Transport changes in synchronously growing CHO and L cells. *Journal of Cellular Physiology,* **78,** 267–272.

145. Schor, S. & Rozengurt, E. (1973) Enhancement by purine nucleosides and nucleotides of serum-induced DNA synthesis in quiescent 3T3 cells. *Journal of Cellular Physiology*, **81,** 339–346.

146. Schulte-Hermann, R. (1974) Induction of liver growth by xenobiotic compounds and other stimuli. *Critical Reviews of Toxicology*, **3,** 79–158.

147. Schulte-Hermann, R. (1977) Two-stage control of cell proliferation induced in rat liver by α-hexachlorocyclohexane. *Cancer Research*, **37,** 166–171.

148. Sekas, G. & Cook, R.T. (1976) Isolation of a low molecular weight inhibitor of [^{3}H]TdR incorporation into hepatic DNA. *Experimental Cell Research*, **102,** 422–425.

149. Sekas, G. & Cook, R.T. (1977) Inhibition of [^{3}H]TdR incorporation into hepatic DNA purification and mode of action. *Federation Proceedings*, **36,** 1078.

150. Shodell, M. & Isselbacher, K.J. (1973) Effect of different media supplements on amino acid uptake and mitotic stimulation in BHK cells. *Nature New Biology*, **242,** 83–85.

151. Short, J., Brown, R.F., Husakova, A., Gilbertson, J.R., Zemel, R. & Lieberman, I. (1972) Induction of DNA synthesis in the liver of the intact animal. *Journal of Biological Chemistry*, **247,** 1757–1766.

152. Short, J., Armstrong, N., Zemel, R. & Lieberman, I. (1973) A role for amino acids in the induction of deoxyribonucleic acid synthesis in liver. *Biochimica et Biophysica Acta*, **50,** 430–437.

153. Short, J., Armstrong, N.B., Kolitsky, M.A., Mitchell, R.A., Zemel, R. & Lieberman, I. (1974) Amino acids and the control of nuclear DNA replication in liver. In *Control of Proliferation in Animal Cells* (Ed.) Clarkson, B. & Baserga, R. pp. 37–48. Cold Spring Harbor, New York: Cold Spring Harbor Laboratory.

154. Short, J., Tsukada, K., Rudert, W.A. & Lieberman, I. (1975) Cyclic adenosine 3′:5′-monophosphate and the induction of deoxyribonucleic acid synthesis in liver. *Journal of Biological Chemistry*, **250,** 3602–3606.

155. Sigel, B., Baldia, L.B., Brightman, S.A., Dunn, M.R. & Price, R.I.M. (1968) Effect of blood flow reversal in liver autotransplants upon the site of hepatocyte regeneration. *Journal of Clinical Investigation*, **47,** 1231–1237.

156. Siimes, M. & Dallman, P. (1974) Nucleic acid and polyamine synthesis in the rat during short term protein deficiency: response of the liver to partial hepatectomy. *Journal of Nutrition*, **104,** 47–58.

157. Simpson, G.E.C. & Finckh, E.S. (1963) Pattern of regeneration of rat liver after repeated partial hepatectomies. *Journal of Pathology and Bacteriology*, **86,** 361–370.

158. Starzl, T.E., Porter, K.A. & Putnam, C.W. (1975) Intraportal insulin protects from the liver injury of portacaval shunt in dogs. *Lancet*, **ii,** 821–825.

159. Starzl, T.E., Porter, K.A. & Putnam, C.W. (1976) Insulin, glucagon, and the control of hepatic structure, function, and capacity for regeneration. *Metabolism*, **25** (No. 11, Supplement 1), 1429–1434.

160. Starzl, T.E., Francavilla, A., Halgrimson, C.G., Francavilla, F.R. & Brown, T.H. (1973) Origin, hormonal nature, and action of hepatotrophic substances in portal venous blood. *Surgery, Gynecology and Obstetrics*, **137,** 179–199.

161. Starzl, T.E., Porter, K.A., Kashiwagi, N., Lee, I.Y., Russell, W.J.I. & Putnam, C.W. (1975) Effect of diabetes mellitus on portal blood hepatotrophic factors in dogs. *Surgery, Gynecology and Obstetrics*, **140,** 549–562.

162. Starzl, T.E., Porter, K.A., Kashiwagi, N. & Putnam, C.W. (1975) Portal hepatrophic factors, diabetes mellitus and acute liver atrophy, hypertrophy and regeneration. *Surgery, Gynecology and Obstetrics*, **141,** 843–858.

163. Steiner, J.W., Perz, Z.M. & Taichman, L.B. (1966) Cell population dynamics in liver: review of quantitative morphological techniques applied to study of physiological and pathological growth. *Experimental and Molecular Pathology*, **5,** 146–181.

164. Stirling, G.A., Bourne, L.D. & Marsh, T. (1975) Effect of protein deprivation and a reduced diet on the regenerating rat liver. *British Journal of Experimental Pathology*, **56,** 502–508.

165. Stirling, G.A., Laughlin, J. & Washington, S.L.A. (1973) Effects of starvation on the proliferative response after partial hepatectomy. *Experimental and Molecular Pathology*, **19,** 44–52.

166. Stöcker, E. (1966) Der Proliferationsmodus in Niere und Leber. *Verhandlungen Deutschen Gesellschaft für Pathologie*, **50,** 53–74.

167. Talarico, K.S., Feller, D.D. & Neville, E.D. (1971) Mitotic response to various dietary conditions in the normal and regenerating rat liver. *Proceedings of the Society for Experimental Biology and Medicine*, **136,** 381–384.

168. Thrower, S. & Ord, M.G. (1974) Hormonal control of liver regeneration. *Biochemical Journal*, **144,** 361–369.

169. Tongendorff, J., Trebin, R. & Ruhenstroth-Bauer, G. (1975) Critique of the 'Critical Mass' hypothesis of the regeneration of liver cells. *American Journal of Pathology*, **80,** 519–524.

170. Unger, R. & Orci, L. (1976) Identification of glucagon-producing cells (A cells) in dog gastric mucosa. *Journal of Cell Biology*, **69,** 455–464.

171. Unger, R.H. & Orci, L. (1976) Physiology and pathophysiology of glucagon. *Physiological Reviews*, **56,** 778–826.

172. Uthne, K. & Uthne, T. (1972) Influence of liver resection and regeneration on somatomedin (sulfation factor) activity in sera from normal and hypophysectomized rats. *Acta Endocrinologica*, **71,** 255–264.

173. Vinet, B. & Verly, W.G. (1976) Purification of a protein inhibitor of DNA synthesis in cells of hepatic origin. *European Journal of Cancer*, **12,** 211–218.

174. Wagle, S.R. & Sampson, L. (1975) Studies on differential response to insulin on the stimulation of amino acid incorporation into protein in isolated hepatocytes containing different levels of glycogen. *Biochemical and Biophysical Research Communications*, **64,** 72–80.

175. Wands, J.R., Storer, R., Patel, U. & Bucher, N.L.R. (1977) Pancreatic hormonal influence on D-galactosamine induced acute liver cell injury. *Gastroenterology*, **73,** 1253.

176. Wang, Louise (1959) Plasma volume, cell volume, total blood volume and F. cells factor in the normal and splenectomised Sherman rat. *American Journal of Physiology*, **196**(1), 188–192.

177. Weinbren, K. & Washington, S.L.A. (1976) Hyperplastic nodules after portacaval anastomosis in rats. *Nature*, **264,** 440–442.

178. Weinbren, K., Stirling, G.A. & Washington, S.L.A. (1972) Development of a proliferative response in

liver parenchyma deprived of portal blood flow. *British Journal of Experimental Pathology,* **53,** 54–58.

179. Weinbren, K., Washington, S.L.A. & Smith, C.Y. (1975) Response of rat liver to alterations in total portal blood flow. *British Journal of Experimental Pathology,* **56,** 148–156.

180. Weinbren, K., Stirling, G.A., Washington, S.L.A., Hooper, S.B. & Laughlin, J. (1971) Critical cytoplasmic mass and the initiation of the proliferative response in the rat liver. *British Journal of Experimental Pathology,* **52,** 583–588.

181. Weir, G.C., Turner, R.C. & Martin, D.B. (1973) Glucagon radioimmunoassay using antiserum 30K: interference by plasma. *Hormone and Metabolic Research,* **5,** 241–244.

182. Whitfield, J.F., MacManus, J.P., Rixon, R.H., Boynton, A.L., Youdale, T. & Swierenga, S. (1976) Positive control of cell proliferation by the interplay of calcium ions and cyclic nucleotides. A review. *In Vitro,* **12,** 1–18.

183. Whittemore, A.D., Voorhees, A.B.Jr & Price, J.B.Jr (1976) Hepatic blood flow and pancreatic hormones as modifiers of hepatic regeneration. *Surgical Forum,* **27,** 363–365.

184. Whittemore, A.D., Kasuya, M., Voorhees, A.B.Jr & Price, J.B.Jr (1975) Hepatic regeneration in the absence of portal viscera. *Surgery,* **77,** 419–426.

185. Wood, C.B., Karran, S.J. & Blumgart, L.H. (1973) Metabolic changes following varying degrees of partial hepatectomy in the rat. *British Journal of Surgery,* **60** (No. 8), 613–617.

186. Yammamoto, K., Omata, S., Ohnishi, T. & Terayama, H. (1973) In vivo effects of proteases on cell surface architecture and cell proliferation in the liver. *Cancer Research,* **33,** 567–572.

187. Younger, L.R., King, J. & Steiner, D.F. (1966) Hepatic proliferative response to insulin in severe alloxan diabetes. *Cancer Research,* **26,** 1408–1414.

Chapter 11

Physiology of the Extrahepatic Biliary Tree

J.A. LYNN

The primary function of the extrahepatic tree is to transport bile from the liver to the duodenum. Its secondary function is to concentrate and modify the composition of bile. This secondary role, which consists of both secretion and absorption by the biliary tree, will be discussed in detail later in this chapter.

In animals with a gallbladder, an organ which concentrates and stores bile, the flow of bile into the duodenum does not parallel its secretion by the liver. Between meals, the ampullary sphincter which lies at the lower end of the common bile duct offers a certain degree of resistance to bile flow. When the gallbladder is relaxed hepatic bile enters it. Elegant studies in a physiological model of gallbladder function in primates have demonstrated that between one-half and one-third of hepatic bile secreted during the fasting of an animal enters the gallbladder. This suggests that between meals there is a leakage of fasting hepatic bile through the ampullary sphincter. This is in part substantiated by the finding of bile in the duodenum in fasting animals. At present, the exact quantity of leakage of bile during fasting through the ampulla is not known.

In animals without a gallbladder (e.g., horse, rat, pigeon) the ampullary sphincter offers little or no resistance to bile flow and the liver secretes large quantities of bile continuously into the duodenum. Experimental studies in man and animals have shown that the secretion pressure of the bile varies, normally from 120 to 250 mm of water. This pressure is the motor of bile flow. At bile duct pressures in excess of 300 mm of water, bile secretion by the liver is totally inhibited. Studies in rhesus monkeys have shown that the pressure in the biliary tree may modify the relative composition of hepatic bile.[15] As the pressure rises in the biliary tree, the secretion of bile salts, phospholipid and cholesterol is reduced. Cholesterol secretion is reduced by a greater extent than either phospholipid or bile salt secretion and as a result the relative composition of hepatic bile is changed so that it becomes less lithogenic. Interestingly, however, when pressure is released it takes several hours for bile salt secretion and phospholipid secretion to return to normal, but there is immediately a tremendous outpouring of cholesterol, resulting in the production of a grossly abnormal hepatic bile supersaturated with cholesterol. The exact significance of these changes in man has yet to be evaluated.

Pressure in the common bile duct must be less than hepatic secretory pressure for bile to flow and it is usually 100 to 150 mm of water. The difference in pressures within the biliary passages and the liver can be considered to be due to three quite separate mechanisms:

1. The activity of the sphincter of Oddi.
2. The filling of the gallbladder.
3. The resorptive activity of the gallbladder.

These mechanisms will now be discussed in detail.

The Physiology of the Sphincter of Oddi

The activity of the sphincter of Oddi may be considered to be the most important factor in pressure regulation within the biliary tree. This activity is not that of a rigid valve. Cine-radiology has clearly demonstrated that the sphincter maintains a brisk peristaltic motion at all times. The basic sphincter rhythm consists of opening and closing. The upper segment relaxes and opens and the ampulla fills and distends. The lower part of the sphincter then opens and bile flows into the duodenum with a final sphincter contraction producing an ejaculatory jet of bile into the duodenum. In the reverse process, the sphincter first closes by contraction of its lowest fibres and this is followed by contraction of its higher fibres. The sphincter is momentarily closed, then the upper part opens once more and the peristaltic cycle is repeated. The basic sphincter rhythm of opening and closing is thus apparent, with contraction taking place from below upwards and relaxation occurring in the opposite direction. It has been demonstrated that one cycle of contraction takes up to three seconds, as does the relaxation phase.[5] As a consequence, approximately 10 contraction cycles occur per minute. This basic rhythm is altered by several factors but in particular by biliary bile duct pressures. A rise in bile duct pressure produces lengthening of both the contraction and the relaxation phases. When the bile duct pressure is artificially raised, the duration of relaxation of the sphincter is different from that of the contraction phase. The opening phase lasts approximately twice as long (six seconds) while the closing phase remains either the same or becomes only a little longer (three to four seconds). This allows more bile to flow into the duodenum. The reverse phenomenon occurs if the bile duct pressure is reduced. The ability of the sphincter to modify its relaxation and contraction phases allows the sphincter to maintain bile duct pressures at a fairly constant level.

For the gallbladder to fill, only a moderate pressure increase (120 to 160 mm of water) is necessary. This pressure increase is achieved by reduction of flow into the duodenum and not by a complete 'shut off' of the sphincter mechanism.

Movements of the duodenum may affect the sphincter. It has been suggested that these movements modify the axis of the sphincter in relation to the rest of the common bile duct. Elevation of the papilla has also been described as producing a balance arm movement which may have a type of pumping action,[5] actively milking bile out of the common bile duct.[19] The role of duodenal musculature on bile flow may not be as important as some workers have suggested. Recent studies simultaneously measuring muscle activity in the duodenal wall and in the sphincter of Oddi have demonstrated that bile flows into the duodenum only when the sphincter shows electrical activity, there being no activity of the duodenal muscle at any time. Further studies are required before the controversy of the effect of the duodenal wall on bile flow can be resolved.

The common bile duct is now known to have no motor role in relation to bile flow. Cholangiography has been claimed to demonstrate peristalsis in the common bile duct.[3,7] These studies have demonstrated three to five waves, lasting one to three seconds each, passing towards the duodenum every minute. Some waves appeared to reach the sphincter while others did not. These early suggestions have not been confirmed by other workers.[1,11,12,16] The depicted waves were almost certainly artefacts produced by shifting and kinking of the biliary passages in association with respiratory movements and vascular movements of nearby structures. True contractile movements are confined to the vaterian segment of the common bile duct. The complete absence of smooth muscle fibres in the wall of the common bile duct, coupled with failure to demonstrate peristalsis in the common bile duct at surgery, suggests that peristalsis in the common bile duct is no more than a radiological illusion.

The Filling and Emptying of the Gallbladder

The gallbladder fills when it has become empty and when its luminal pressure has dropped to 11 to 14 cm of water. The sphincter of Oddi will have adjusted the pressure in the common bile duct to a level higher than the 'empty gallbladder pressure'. Evacuation of the gallbladder occurs with contraction of the gallbladder musculature and a rise in gallbladder pressure up to 200 to 300 mm of water after injection of cholecystokinin (CCK).

The effect of hormones on gallbladder function

Gallbladder contraction is under both nervous and hormonal control. As early as 1928 Ivy and co-workers, using a cross-circulation preparation, showed that contraction of the gallbladder was caused by a hormone, cholecystokinin (CCK), extracted from duodenal mucosa. That the gallbladder is under hormonal control is further emphasized by the fact that an extrinsically denervated gallbladder contracts in response to CCK or to the presence of chyme in the duodenum.

Nervous control of gallbladder function

Before the discovery of CCK in 1917, one suggestion to explain the interplay of the gallbladder and sphincter of Oddi was that of an 'opposing innervation'. It was proposed that contraction of the gallbladder would produce opening of the sphincter through an intramural nervous system, while contraction of the sphincter would produce gallbladder relaxation. This hypothesis of 'antagonistic innervation' is probably incorrect.

There is no doubt that the gallbladder receives an autonomic nerve supply. This nerve supply is predominantly vagal in origin. Animal experiments indicate that vagal fibres stimulate the gallbladder, while sympathetic fibres either inhibit or do not affect gallbladder activity. Recent studies in man, rabbit and cat have confirmed that the gallbladder dilates after vagotomy. The effect of vagotomy on gallbladder function has caused considerable interest following the suggestion that there may be an increased incidence of gallstones following vagotomy. It is not clear whether stasis is the cause of this, or whether some subtle modification of the enterohepatic circulation, due to changes in gallbladder contractility, may produce abnormal hepatic bile. It has been shown that vagotomy does not modify the action of CCK. This suggests that the vagus merely controls gallbladder tone and normally is not very important.

Recent studies of vasoactive intestinal polypeptide (VIP), first thought to be a gut hormone but now localized to a widely distributed system of nerves in the gut wall, have demonstrated the presence of VIP immunoreactive nerve fibres in the human gallbladder wall. This is particularly interesting because the known effects of VIP include relaxation of the gallbladder and inhibition of CCK-induced gallbladder contraction. Demonstration of VIP nerves in the gallbladder wall offers a morphological basis for accepting that the actions of VIP on gallbladder function, which have been shown in isolated preparation, may be physiological.

Pharmacological studies of gallbladder function

Pharmacological studies on strips of healthy gallbladder muscle have demonstrated an inherent slow spontaneous rhythmic activity.[10] Acetylcholine has been shown to produce strong contractions in such a preparation; this effect is potentiated by eserine and is totally abolished by atropine. Histamine, likewise, produces strong contractions. Its effect, however, unlike that of acetylcholine, is not abolished by atropine. Antihistamines abolish all histamine-induced reactions on gallbladder strip contractions.

Cholecystokinin produces powerful contraction of gallbladder strips unaffected either by atropine or hexamethonium. Secretin, however, has a mild effect. Various other substances have been studied for their effect on isolated gallbladder strip preparations. These include 5-HT, morphine, isoprenaline, adrenaline, noradrenaline, nicotine, glyceryl trinitrate, sodium nitrite and gastrin. None of these substances has any effect on muscle contraction in the isolated strip preparation.

The Resorptive Activity of the Gallbladder

The rapid re-absorption of fluid by the gallbladder mucosa stabilizes pressures in the biliary tree. Water and electrolytes are reabsorbed, leaving behind bile salts, bile pigments and cholesterol. Active transport by gallbladder mucosa of Na^+, Cl^- and HCO_3^- from bile to blood is responsible for the concentration of bile. Because ions are transported, water follows in isotonic proportion. K^+ ions diffuse through the gallbladder mucosa so that the final concentration of this electrolyte in bile does not rise as much as that of bile salts. It is now known that the fundamental process responsible for fluid transport is the active pumping of Na^+, Cl^- and HCO_3^- across the apical part of the mucosal cells, where each cell is bound to its neighbour by a tight junction, into lateral channels.

When fluid transport is in a steady state there is a high osmolar pressure at the apex of the lateral channel and a low one at the basal end which is nearly isotonic. At this basal end, fluid crosses the basement membrane, enters the interstitial fluid and is removed by capillaries.

Because Na^+ and Cl^- are already transported into lateral channels at their apices, there is a resultant flow of water into these channels which sweeps solute towards the basement membrane.

BILE DUCT FUNCTION IN BILIARY SECRETION

The estimation of canalicular bile flow, calculated by the biliary clearance of lipid insoluble erythritol, has demonstrated two fractions of bile secreted by hepatocytes into the canaliculus:

1. Canalicular bile salt-dependent bile.
2. Canalicular bile salt-independent bile.

Apart from these two fractions it has been suggested that a third fraction exists, this being ductular ductal bile which is bile salt independent. In addition to secretion into bile ducts, absorption is also thought to occur. The extent and importance of secretion and absorption in the extrahepatic biliary tree have not been fully evaluated.

Secretion into the Extrahepatic Biliary Tree and Ductules

It has been shown that the choloretic effect of secretin results in the addition of an aqueous solution of inorganic electrolytes, specifically chloride and bicarbonate, to basal bile flow without modifying bile salt secretion. Chenderovitch quotes four separate experiments to support the hypothesis that secretion of this electrolytic fluid which is free of bile salts occurs at a ductal or ductular level and not from the hepatocyte.[6]

These experiments are:

1. Infusion of secretin into the hepatic artery results in a 1.5 times greater bile flow than does splenic vein infusion of secretin. This finding suggests that secretin acts primarily on the bile ducts because they are supplied mainly by the hepatic artery.[21]
2. When bromsulphthalein is infused at a constant rate to determine biliary 'washout volumes', secretin infusion results in a smaller 'washout volume' than does a taurocholate choleresis. This finding suggests that secretin increases bile flow by the addition of fluid at a site distal to the site of taurocholate choleresis.[21]
3. Secretin infusion has been shown to have no effect on bromsulphthalein transport maximum, while taurocholate produces a marked increase in this transport maximum.[13]
4. Studies which estimate canalicular bile flow using erythritol or mannitol demonstrate that canalicular bile flow is unaffected in secretin choleresis, suggesting that bile ducts or ductules are the site of action of secretin.[8, 22]

In all of these studies there is no direct evidence of the exact site of action of secretin. The data support Chenderovitch's assumption that bile ducts rather than canaliculi are the structures stimulated by secretin.

The evidence to support the suggestion that bile duct secretion occurs in the absence of secretin is obscure. Chenderovitch has described elegant studies using stop-flow techniques, and has demonstrated secretion of electrolytes in the distal segment of the biliary tree.[6] These studies were performed in the rabbit, a species in which bile flow is unresponsive to secretin stimulation. Isolated canine bile ducts have been shown to secrete a clear alkaline fluid.[14] Studies in rats chronically intoxicated with ethionine or alpha-napthyl-isothiocyanate have demonstrated that, in addition to a proliferation of bile ductules, a hydrocholeresis occurs.[9]

Two quite separate clinical syndromes suggest a role of bile ducts in bile secretion. First, a marked hydrocholeresis occurs in Caroli's disease (congenital cystic dilatation of the intrahepatic bile ducts).[18] Second, the high bile flow in cirrhosis of the liver may be due to proliferation of the bile ductules.[4, 17]

Absorption by the Extrahepatic Biliary Tree and Bile Ductules

The absorption of fluid by the mucosa of the gallbladder is well documented. The role of the extrahepatic bile ducts in the absorption of fluid is unclear.

In an isolated perfused liver preparation of the rat liver, estimated canalicular bile flow is identical to actual bile flow.[2] This suggests that bile ductules and extrahepatic bile ducts do not absorb fluid. The absorption of fluid by bile ductules and the extrahepatic biliary tree, if it does occur, may be species specific because, in the rabbit and rhesus monkey, estimated bile flow exceeds actual bile flow by a significant amount.

In cholecystectomized fasting dogs, the bile stored in the common bile duct is similar in composition to gallbladder bile.[20] In cholecystectomized dogs, estimated canalicular bile flow is less than actual bile flow, indicating a re-absorption of fluid distal to the canaliculus.[22]

The significance of these latter findings is far from clear since they may represent artefacts due to cholecystectomy.

REFERENCES

1. Beneventano, T.C., Hurwitt, E.S., Jacobson, H.G. & Schein, C.J. (1967) Cine-cholangiomanometry: physiologic observations. *American Journal of Roentgenology,* **100,** 673–679.
2. Boyer, J.L. (1971) Canalicular bile formation in the isolated perfused rat liver. *American Journal of Physiology,* **221,** 1156–1163.
3. Burnett, W. & Shields, R. (1958) Movements of common bile duct in man: studies with image intensifier. *Lancet,* **ii,** 387–390.
4. Caroli, J. & Tanasoglu, Y. (1953) Le temps d'apparition de la brome sulfone phtaleine dans la bile. Nouveau test pour le diagnostic des ictères incomplets par retention et les blocages anictériques. *Semaine des Hôpitaux de Paris,* **29,** 591–606.
5. Caroli, J., Porcher, P., Peqvignot, G. & Delatre, M. (1960) Contributions of cineradiography to the study of function of the human biliary tract. *American Journal of Digestive Diseases,* **5,** 677–696.
6. Chenderovitch, J. (1976) Bile duct function in biliary secretion. In *The Hepatobiliary System,* NATO Advanced Study Institutes Series, Series A: Life Sciences, Vol. 7, pp. 267–285. New York: Plenum Press.
7. Daniels, B.T., McGlone, F.B., Job, H. & Sawyer, R.B. (1961) Changing concepts in common bile duct anatomy and embryology. *Journal of the American Medical Association,* **178,** 394–397.
8. Forker, E.L. (1967) Two sites of bile formation as determined by mannitol and erythritol clearance in the guinea pig. *Journal of Clinical Investigation,* **46,** 1189–1195.
9. Goldfarb, S., Singer, E.J. & Popper, H. (1963) Biliary ductules and bile secretion. *Journal of Laboratory and Clinical Medicine,* **62,** 608–615.
10. Mack, A.J. & Todd, J.K. (1968) A study of human gall bladder muscle in vitro. *Gut,* **9,** 546–549.
11. Myers, R.N., Haupt, G.J., Birkhead, N.C. & Deaver, J.M. (1962) Cinefluorographic observations of common bile duct physiology. *Annals of Surgery,* **156,** 442–450.
12. Nebesar, R.A., Pollard, J.J. & Potsaid, M.S. (1966) Cinecholangiography; some physiological observations. *Radiology,* **86,** 475–479.
13. O'Maille, E.R.C., Richards, T.G. & Short, A.H. (1966) Factors determining the maximal rate of organic anion secretion by the liver and further evidence on the hepatic site of action of the hormone secretin. *Journal of Physiology,* **186,** 424–438.
14. Rous, P. & McMaster, P.D. (1921) Physiological causes for the varied character of stasis bile. *Journal of Experimental Medicine,* **34,** 75–96.
15. Strasberg, S.M., Dorne, B.C., Redinger, R.N., Small, D.N. & Egdall, R.H. (1971) Effects of alteration of biliary pressure on bile composition – a method for study: primate biliary physiology, V. *Gastroenterology,* **61,** 357–362.
16. Torsoli, A., Ramorino, M.L. & Alessandrini, A. (1970) Motility of the biliary tract. *Rendiconti Romani di Gastroenterologia,* **2,** 67–80.
17. Turnberg, L.A. & Graham, G. (1970) Bile salt secretion in cirrhosis of the liver. *Gut,* **11,** 126–133.
18. Turnberg, L.A., Jones, C.A. & Sherlock, S. (1968) Biliary secretion in a patient with cystic dilatation of the intra-hepatic biliary tree. *Gastroenterology,* **54,** 1155–1161.
19. Watts, J.McK. & Dunphy, J.E. (1966) The role of the common bile duct in biliary dynamics. *Surgery, Gynecology and Obstetrics,* **122,** 1207–1218.
20. Wheeler, H.O. & Ramos, O.L. (1960) Determinants of flow and composition of bile in the unanesthetized dog during constant infusion of sodium taurocholate. *Journal of Clinical Investigation,* **39,** 161–170.
21. Wheeler, H.O. & Mancusi-Ungaro, P.L. (1966) Role of bile ducts during secretin choleresis in the dog. *American Journal of Physiology,* **210,** 1153–1159.
22. Wheeler, H.O., Ross, E.D. & Bradley, S.E. (1968) Canalicular bile production in dog. *American Journal of Physiology,* **214,** 866–874.

Chapter 12

Bile Salts

K.W. HEATON

The recent explosion of interest and research in bile acids has resulted in a much clearer understanding of their detergent properties, their conservation and recycling mechanisms and their role in certain diarrhoeas. It now seems very likely that disturbed bile acid physiology or metabolism is involved in the pathogenesis of gallstones and the stagnant loop syndrome, probable that it is concerned in the mechanisms of cholestasis and gastric ulcer, and possible that it plays a role in large bowel cancer. Clinical tests of bile acid metabolism are still not widely available, except perhaps for the cholylglycine-^{14}C breath test, but bile acid therapy of gallstones is established as effective in selected cases and as almost certainly safe.

Recent research has been fully documented in a series of symposia[9,101,133] and has been discussed in books, chapters and review articles.[19,59,68,116,117,118,132] Where original references are not given in this chapter they will generally be found in one of these volumes or reviews.

DEFINITIONS AND TERMINOLOGY

Bile acid or bile salt

Under physiological conditions of pH bile acids are mostly ionized and accompanied by plentiful cations, so it is strictly correct to refer to them as bile salts. In the laboratory they are often handled as the pure, protonated acids. Many prefer the term bile acids as less likely to be confused with biliary electrolytes. This chapter uses the terms interchangeably and with no implications regarding the state of conjugation.

Cholyltaurine or taurocholate

Conjugation of a bile acid with taurine or glycine, which always precedes its secretion into bile, involves amidation of its acid radicle (Figure 12.1). The acid radicle on the conjugated compound is that of the amino acid, so it is more correct but less common to refer to 'cholyltaurine' or 'deoxycholylglycine' than to the traditional 'taurocholate' and 'glycodeoxycholate'. Sulphated bile acids follow the same pattern, so that 'sulpholithocholylglycine' is preferred by some to 'glycolithocholate sulphate'. Despite its theoretical inadequacy, the old system is more readily comprehended by most people and will be used here.

With such cumbersome names, the use of abbreviations is inevitable. There is not complete agreement, but a widely used system is shown in Table 12.1.

Chenic or chenodeoxycholic acid

Hofmann has proposed 'chenic' as a more practical name for this famous bile acid. Its acceptance has been limited, possibly because 'chenate' is not euphonious. Logical successors

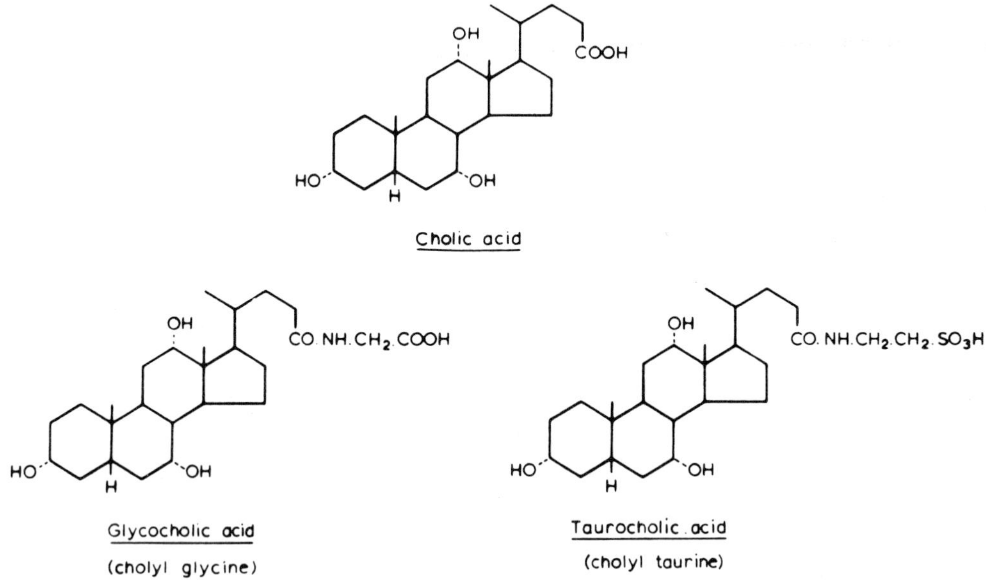

Figure 12.1. Cholic acid and its two conjugates.

Table 12.1. *A System for Abbreviating Bile Acids.*

Cholate/cholic acid	C	Glycocholate	GC
Chenodeoxycholate	CDC	Glycochenodeoxy-cholate	GCDC
Deoxycholate	DC		
Ursodeoxycholate	UDC	Glycodeoxycholate	GDC
Lithocholate	LC		
		Taurocholate	TC, etc.
Glycolithocholate	GLC		
Glycolithocholate sulphate	$GLC\text{-}SO_4$		

might include 'ursic' and 'lithic' acids. Traditional names have the advantage that their inclusion of the ending 'cholate' advertises their biliary nature.

Primary, secondary and tertiary bile acids (Figure 12.2)

Primary bile acids are those which are synthesized by the liver. In man, these are cholate and chenodeoxycholate. Bile acids which are bacterial metabolites are termed secondary. In man, the chief ones are deoxycholate and lithocholate, which arise by 7α-dehydroxylation in the colon of cholate and chenodeoxycholate respectively. Currently, there is interest in a third metabolite found in bile in trace amounts, ursodeoxycholate. The formation of this stereo-isomer of CDC involves a third step, reduction in the liver of a colonic metabolite 7-ketolithocholate which has led to the suggestion that it be called a tertiary bile acid.[69] Sulphated lithocholate may also be considered a tertiary bile acid.

SYNTHESIS AND SECRETION

Bile acid synthesis

The normal human liver converts on average 0.78 to 1.29 mmol (300 to 500 mg) of cholesterol into bile acids daily, the ratio of cholic to chenodeoxycholic acid production being about two to one. The first step in the pathway is the rate-limiting one. It is the insertion of a hydroxyl group into the 7α position of cholesterol under the influence of the enzyme 7α-hydroxylase which is present in the microsomal fraction of the liver cell. The other steps, which have been elucidated mainly in the rat, involve saturation of the double bond, a configurational change of the 3β-hydroxyl group to the 3α position (via the oxo derivative) and, in the case of cholic acid only, 12α-hydroxylation.[19] When all these changes in the steroid nucleus are complete, the side chain is oxidized and shortened in the mitochondria. In this way the 27-carbon cholesterol is converted into 24-carbon bile acids. The overall effect, as with so many hepatic synthetic processes, is to convert a weakly polar, virtually insoluble material into a highly polar, freely soluble one. Alternative pathways have been discovered, but their quantitative importance is uncertain. Probably the most important is oxidation of the side chain (starting with 26-hydroxylation) before any nuclear changes occur in the synthesis of chenodeoxycholate.[6] Another pathway begins with a 25-hydroxylation.[152]

Bile acid synthesis is regulated by feedback inhibition from reabsorbed bile acids reaching

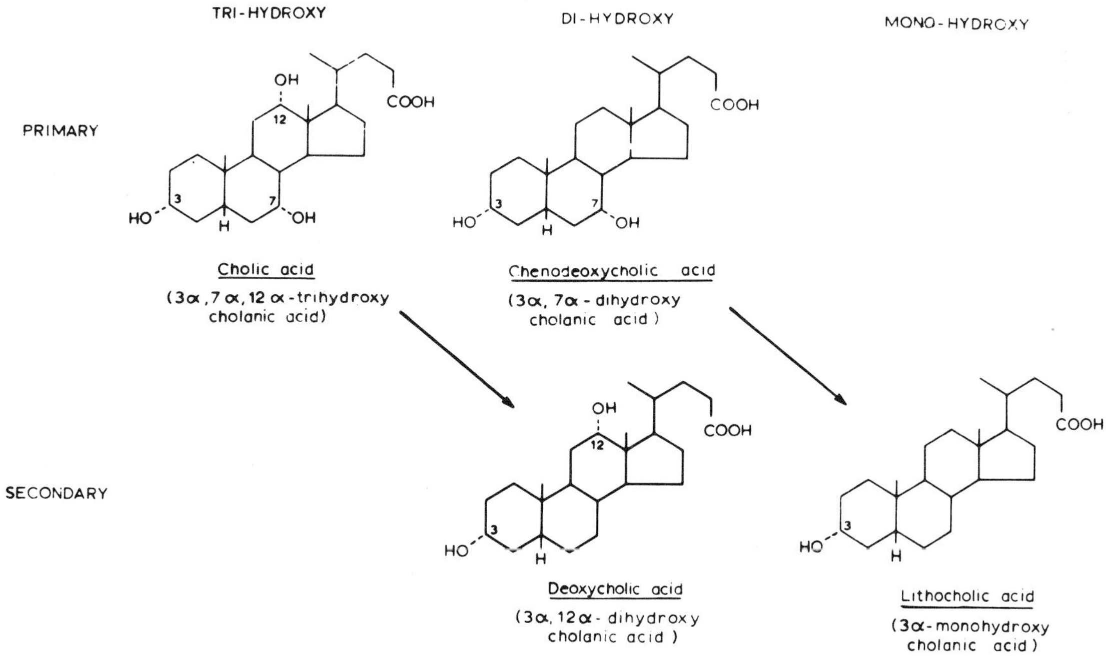

Figure 12.2. The major bile acids of man.

the liver in the portal vein. Procedures which deplete the portal vein of bile acids, such as bile fistula, ileal resection and cholestyramine therapy, cause up to a tenfold increase in synthesis. Feeding bile acids suppresses it. Dihydroxy bile acids suppress overall synthesis more than does cholic acid, at least in the baboon,[143] and there is some evidence that chenodeoxycholate synthesis is more readily inhibited by deoxycholate than is cholate synthesis.[140]

Bile acid synthesis can be measured in various ways. The most direct is the isotope dilution or Lindstedt technique, which also gives information on pool size, but this requires repeated duodenal intubations. Faecal bile acid excretion must, in equilibrium conditions, equal hepatic synthesis and its measurement is more convenient to the subject, but the analytical methods are complex.[72] For reasons which are not clear, faecal measurements tend to give lower figures for daily synthesis than the isotope dilution technique. An indirect assessment of bile acid synthesis is obtained by measuring the activity of cholesterol 7α-hydroxylase in liver tissue. The assumption that the two are correlated is convenient in research but unproven.[146]

Conjugation with glycine and taurine in a ratio of about three to one precedes secretion of bile acids into bile. Conjugation, especially with taurine, increases the solubility of bile acids and also lowers their pK_a, so that they remain ionized at lower pH values. Taurine availability is limited, so that the glycine to taurine conjugation ratio rises whenever there is an increased demand for bile acid synthesis or conjugation, as with ileal dysfunction and small bowel bacterial overgrowth. The ratio tends to fall in cirrhosis.

Hepatic uptake and secretion

Hepatocytes appear to possess a carrier-mediated mechanism for bile acid uptake, which is common to the different bile acids.[1,48] Thanks to this, the liver extracts bile acids from the blood with great avidity and the V_{max} for uptake is far greater than any likely physiological load.[49,145] Hepatic fractional clearance is essentially constant, that is, independent of load. For chenodeoxycholic acid, it has been calculated that 60 per cent of any dose up to 400 mg is cleared at a single passage through the liver.[169] Higher figures are likely for cholic acid and for conjugates; taurocholate is 92 per cent cleared by dog liver.[129] Plasma disappearance curves have been plotted for all the major bile acids after intravenous injection of radiolabelled materials. These curves have two exponentials, whose half-lives are two to three minutes and seven to 16 minutes respectively.[33] Theoretically, measurement of bile acid clearance is a sensitive liver function test but it has proved disappointing in practice (see Chapter 17).

Secretion into the canaliculus rapidly follows uptake, but its mechanisms and kinetics are poorly understood. Certainly, active transport is involved, since the concentration of bile acids rises from 13 to 2700 mmol/l as they travel from portal vein blood to hepatic bile.[89] The rise in osmotic pressure that attends this transport attracts water into the canaliculi and this is believed to be the major driving force in generating canalicular bile flow.[42,77] This bile acid-dependent flow is believed to be essential for the normal excretion of other organic anions, including bilirubin, and its failure is probably the common mechanism in most cases of intrahepatic cholestasis.[77]

An essential characteristic of bile acids, as of all detergents, is the formation of polymolecular aggregates or micelles above a certain concentration in aqueous solution. This critical micellar concentration and the size of the micelles vary with different bile acids, and also with the concentration of counterions such as sodium.[25] Bile acids are normally accompanied by lecithin or monoglyceride. Mixed with water, these and similar polar lipids do not dissolve but swell to form liquid crystals. Mixed with a solution of bile salts, their molecules are incorporated freely into the micelles and efficiently dissolved. As the micelles are expanded by these polar lipids, the critical micellar concentration of bile salts drops dramatically, from say 3 to 0.2 mmol/l. Micellar size is difficult to measure, because most analytical techniques destroy or alter the micelles. By the recently available laser light-scattering technique, sodium glycochenodeoxycholate (molecular weight 472 daltons) was estimated to form micelles weighing 11 400 daltons in pure solution and 27 000 daltons when lecithin was added in the physiological proportion of 3:1 bile acid : lecithin.[74] In bile itself, micelles contain cholesterol as well as lecithin and are presumably larger again. The critical micellar concentration of bile acids in human bile has been estimated as averaging 1.45 mmol/l.[162] This is well below the bile acid concentrations found in hepatic bile and upper small intestinal aspirate, so it can be assumed that the vast majority of bile acid molecules in the body are in micellar solution.

It is not known precisely where in the pathway of bile formation bile acid molecules aggregate into micelles. The possibilities are within the hepatocyte, at the membrane or in the canaliculus. The presence of cholesterol and phospholipid in the micelle suggests closeness of mixed micelle formation to the membrane but does not necessarily imply that it occurs during actual membrane passage.

The well-known choleretic effect of bile acids is reduced by their tendency to form micelles since this reduces the osmolality of canalicular bile (indeed, hepatic bile is always very close to 300 mosmol/l). Bile acids that cannot form micelles, such as the artificial dehydrocholate, cause a relatively greater increase in canalicular bile flow.

ENTEROHEPATIC CIRCULATION

The pivotal fact in the physiology of bile acids is that, after synthesis, they are efficiently conserved and recirculated. The circulating pool provides about 97 per cent of the bile salts entering the biliary tree and duodenum. Hence the availability of detergent in the gallbladder and in the digestive process is governed above all by the size of the pool and the efficiency of its absorption. The composition of the pool, which may be an important variable in the regulation of hepatic cholesterol metabolism, is determined by events in the enterohepatic cycle, especially bacterial metabolism.

The normal bile acid pool is about 5 mmol (2500 mg), and its size is not clearly related to body weight. During the digestion of a meal it is absorbed and re-secreted at least once. The number of circulations per day probably varies with the amount of food eaten.[23] With larger meals, the stomach takes longer to empty and there is more prolonged stimulation of cholecystokinin release. Consequently, the sphincter of Oddi remains relaxed longer and bile acids are kept in circulation instead of being diverted into the gallbladder. Published figures for circulation frequency average about seven per day but these values were derived from subjects given a liquid diet (from methodological necessity) and cannot confidently be extrapolated to normal solid diets. During the overnight fast, the majority of the bile acid pool is sequestered in the gallbladder but according to recent studies it is common for gallbladder emptying to occur during the night[168] and for up to half the pool to be in circulation as breakfast begins.[174] The Mayo Clinic group has demonstrated an inverse relationship between circulation frequency and pool size.[85,125,126] This has been interpreted as meaning that more frequent passage of the pool through the liver leads to increased feedback inhibition of bile acid synthesis and shrinkage of the pool, but another possibility is that small pools are absorbed more rapidly.

The role of the gallbladder

While stored in the gallbladder, bile acids are preserved from the risks of excretion and bacterial attack. Cholecystectomy is followed by greater bacterial degradation of bile acids and an increased proportion of secondary bile acids in the circulating pool,[65,139] and there is more rapid turnover of the primary bile acids.[5] Loss of the reservoir presumably increases cycling frequency and would be expected to cause a reduction in the pool, as indeed happens when the gallbladder is removed in dogs and guinea pigs.[35,56] However, human studies have given conflicting results, a post-cholecystectomy decrease being noted by Pomare and Heaton[139] and Shaffer and Small[151] but not by Almond et al[5] nor by Hepner et al.[65]

The converse situation exists when the gallbladder empties abnormally slowly as it does in coeliac disease.[93] Here, the storage function of the gallbladder is exaggerated and presumably there are fewer enterohepatic cycles. In these patients, the bile acid pool is considerably larger than normal[95] but is turned over abnormally slowly, presumably because it is being sequestered in the gallbladder.[94] In healthy subjects, the rate at which the gallbladder contracts after a meal correlates with the turnover rate of cholic acid, and inversely with its pool size.[57]

Intestinal absorption

This is the key event in the enterohepatic circulation. Theoretically, bile acids can be absorbed by passive diffusion along the entire gut. In practice, diffusion is too slow to cope with the highly polar conjugated bile acids and a special transport system has been developed in the ileum, maximally active in the terminal quarter of the small intestine.[40,177] This system has all the features of a carrier-mediated, energy-requiring, active transport mechanism. It is maximally efficient with the most polar bile acids, namely the taurine conjugates, and the trihydroxy cholate (free or conjugated) is transported six to eight times faster than the dihydroxy bile acids. Unconjugated bile acids cannot compete effectively with the conjugates for active transport because they have relatively low affinity for the transport carriers but, as they can diffuse passively across the mucosa, they are probably conserved equally well.

Overall, the absorption of bile acids is about 96 per cent efficient. This includes the largely unknown factor of colonic absorption. Presented with bile acids in pure solution, the colon can absorb them slowly but almost completely.[113] Absorption is likely to be much slower in the presence of normal colonic contents and is probably limited mainly to the right colon where the contents are liquid. Ileostomy patients do not waste bile acids, but this could mean only that the terminal ileum takes on some of the functions of the colon. The best evidence for a colonic role in the normal enterohepatic circulation is the presence in normal bile of substantial amounts of deoxycholate, since this bile acid is virtually absent after colectomy.[109,114]

Passive absorption across the jejunum is believed by some to be important in the conservation of the glycine-conjugated dihydroxy bile acids, which are the least polar of the conjugates. Certainly, they can be absorbed quite well when the jejunum is perfused with pure solutions, but the existence of such absorption under physiological conditions has not been proved. The crucial question, whether dihydroxy glycine conjugates are the first bile acids to disappear as the pool passes down the jejunum, has received conflicting answers.[7,58]

Bacterial metabolism

The extent to which bile acids are attacked by bacteria depends chiefly on two variables: how distally the pool travels before it is absorbed, and how proximally the anaerobic flora of the intestine extends. Anaerobes, chiefly Bacteroides and bifidobacteria, must be present in concentrations higher than 10^3/ml for significant degradation to occur. Bacterial metabolism of bile acids is of two main types: deconjugation and 7α-dehydroxylation.

Deconjugation begins in the mid-small intestine and may be extensive in the terminal ileum,[127] but it has been calculated from radio-isotope studies that only about 15 per cent of bile acid absorption occurs in unconjugated form.[64] Since unconjugated bile acids are freely absorbed by passive diffusion, deconjugation does not interfere with bile acid conservation.

Indeed, it may even improve it. However, if extensive deconjugation takes place in the upper jejunum, as in the stagnant loop syndrome, there is premature absorption of bile acids and this short circuit leads to bile acid deficiency in the intestinal lumen. This may be aggravated by precipitation of unconjugated bile acids, which are relatively insoluble at acid pH. Glycine liberated by bile acid deconjugation is either absorbed and passed to the general body pool of glycine or metabolized by bacteria with absorption of end products. In any case, about half the carbon in bile acid glycine appears eventually in the breath as carbon dioxide and there is a good correlation between extent of deconjugation and amount of such CO_2 in the breath.[64] This forms the basis of a simple and widely used breath test to detect abnormal deconjugation of bile acids.[46]

Dehydroxylation is limited to the large intestine, and is normally the fate of all cholate or chenodeoxycholate passing into the caecum. Of the deoxycholate so formed, only one-third to one-half is absorbed and recirculated.[64] The rest is precipitated or adsorbed to bacteria. Of newly formed lithocholate only one-fifth is absorbed.[3] Hence dehydroxylation is usually the prelude to excretion. The bile acids which can be extracted from stools are mainly deoxycholate, lithocholate and isolithocholate (3β-hydroxy-5β-cholanoic acid). Keto- or oxo-bile acids are also present due to dehydrogenation of hydroxyl groups. Keto-bile acids are of little general interest except that one (3α-hydroxy-7-keto-5β-cholanoic) is the precursor of ursodeoxycholic acid which is present in normal bile in trace amounts but is abundant in patients being treated with chenodeoxycholic acid for gallstone dissolution. In this case, the absorbed keto bile acid is hydroxylated by the liver to the 7β-epimer of chenodeoxycholic acid.

Return to the liver

Absorbed bile acids in portal blood are largely protein bound, the degree of binding being 96 to 98 per cent with dihydroxy and 83 to 91 per cent with trihydroxy bile acids.[33] The concentration of bile acids in portal serum at laparotomy was found by Lindblad et al[89] to average 12.9 μmol/l, which was two or three times higher than the peripheral serum level. After meals, portal serum levels rose by 50 per cent. The differences between fasting and postprandial levels and between portal and systemic levels are surprisingly small. A possible explanation is absorption of some bile acids via the lymphatics, especially after meals when lymph flow is increased, but data to support this theory are lacking.

Further hepatic metabolism of bile acids

Bile acids which have been deconjugated before absorption are reconjugated before re-entering the bile. Rehydroxylation of dehydroxylated bile acids occurs in some species but not in man.

Sulphation of the 3α-hydroxyl group is an important further step in two circumstances: for the detoxification and excretion of lithocholate, and in cholestasis. The presence of sulphate esters of bile acids in human bile was noted in 1967 by Palmer[130] but their importance has only recently been recognized. After intravenous injection of ^{14}C-labelled lithocholate, 50 to 60 per cent appears in the bile in the form of sulphated glyco- and taurolithocholate, the degree of sulphation being greater with the glycine conjugate.[3,31] Sulphation renders glycolithocholate much more polar and so less easily reabsorbed by passive diffusion.[92] Probably because of this, lithocholate is rapidly excreted from the body and the total circulating pool of 50 to 100 mg is much smaller than might have been expected.[32] Desulphation occurs in the distal intestine, but mostly beyond the point of absorption. Lithocholate and its conjugates are highly toxic materials[28,131] but, in the rat at least, this toxicity is much reduced by sulphation.[45,156] In health, lithocholate is the only bile acid which is sulphated to any extent, but in cholestasis, and to a lesser extent in cirrhosis, there is sulphation of tri- and especially dihydroxy bile acids.

The enterohepatic circulation has been described and analysed in detail by Hofmann.[68,69]

DISEASES INVOLVING BILE ACIDS

Bile acid metabolism is affected when any of the organs involved in the enterohepatic circulation is diseased: liver, biliary tract, upper small intestine, ileum, colon and portal vein.

PARENCHYMAL LIVER DISEASE

Cirrhosis

Synthesis, conjugation, secretion and uptake are all altered in acute and chronic parenchymal liver disease.[50,171] In cirrhosis, even the colonic metabolism of bile acids is altered, though the reason for this is unclear. Cholestasis frequently coexists with hepatocellular disease and contributes its own characteristic abnormalities.

Impaired uptake (and therefore reduced clearance) of bile acids from the blood is due to shunting of blood round the liver as well as to hepatocellular dysfunction. Its most obvious manifestation is a raised serum bile acid concentration. This is often present in the fasting state and is virtually always found two hours after a meal if there is histologically significant liver disease.[12,43,81,165] Indeed, at the present time, the two-hour postprandial serum bile acid concentration seems to be the most sensitive liver function test (Figure 12.3). Presumably this is because after a meal there is maximal absorption of bile acids and, in the presence of portal hypertension, maximal shunting of blood round the liver.

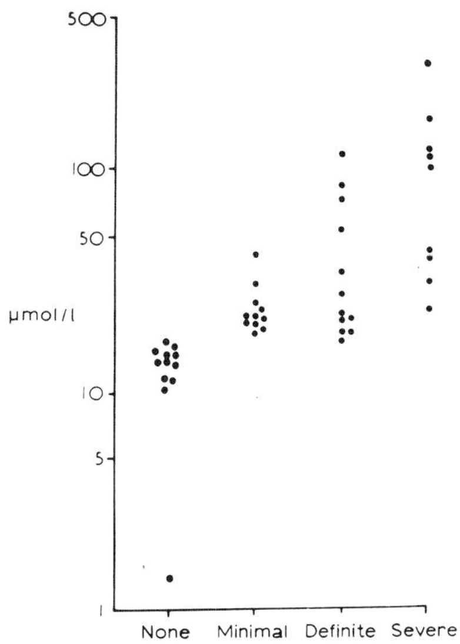

Figure 12.3. Serum total bile acid concentrations two hours after a meal in subjects with various degrees of hepatocellular dysfunction. Modified from Thjodleifsson et al.[165]

The clearance from peripheral blood of intravenously administered bile acid has been measured in many patients with cirrhosis and hepatitis since the pioneer studies of Josephson.[80] The findings of LaRusso et al,[86] using radio-immunoassay to follow the clearance of cholylglycine, raised hopes that a simple, sensitive and specific test of liver function was available. They studied 11 patients who had biopsy-proven chronic active liver disease but whose conventional liver function tests were normal. Cholylglycine clearance was delayed in nine of the 11, although fasting serum cholylglycine was increased in only a few. However, disappointingly, subsequent studies have shown much overlap in bile acid clearance between liver disease and healthy controls[44] and no correlation between clearance rates and the severity of liver disease.[165]

Bile acid synthesis is impaired in cirrhosis.[107] However, this impairment is practically limited to cholic acid and, even in severe liver disease, chenodeoxycholic acid synthesis is normal or virtually so.[171] In a large group of cirrhotics, cholic acid synthesis, measured isotopically, was reduced to less than a third of normal.[171] An inverse correlation was found between the degree of liver failure assessed clinically and the daily synthesis of cholic acid, but even mild cases had significantly reduced synthesis.[102] These findings suggest that cholic acid synthesis is selectively impaired in cirrhosis. This may be due to a specific failure of 12α-hydroxylation, which is the first committed step in the synthetic pathway towards cholic acid. An alternative explanation is that cholic acid synthesis is easily suppressed because there is only one major pathway from cholesterol to cholic acid, whereas chenodeoxycholic acid can be formed by at least two pathways.

The bile acid *pool* is reduced to about half its normal size in cirrhotic patients. This is due mainly to shrinkage of the cholic acid pool (presumably secondary to its poor synthesis), but the pools of the secondary bile acids, deoxycholic and lithocholic, are dramatically reduced as well. That cirrhotics have very low levels of deoxycholate in their bile and blood has long been known, but the mechanism has been obscure. It is now known that, in cirrhotics, the faecal bacteria have markedly reduced dehydroxylating activity, and very little deoxycholate can be found in the faeces.[84] Why faecal bacteria should be inhibited in this way is unknown. Other mechanisms, such as lack of the substrate for dehydroxylation, cholate, and inability to absorb deoxycholate, have been excluded.[103,178]

Individual bile acids in *serum* have been studied many times in the hope of discovering a pattern diagnostic of cirrhosis but there is no consistent picture. The trend is towards a lower trihydroxy to dihydroxy ratio and a lower glycine to taurine conjugation ratio than are found in cholestasis.

Duodenal bile salt concentrations after a test meal were found to be low in English non-alcoholic cirrhotics only if they had steatorrhoea.[11] This may be due not only to the small bile acid pool but also to the copious flow of dilute bile which is characteristic of these patients. Impaired micellar solubilization of dietary fat[11,110] may well contribute to steatorrhoea in non-alcoholic cirrhosis, but in alcoholic patients this is probably less important than pancreatic insufficiency.[100]

Gallbladder bile of cirrhotics is not supersaturated with cholesterol in spite of the small bile salt pool, apparently because cholesterol secretion is also markedly reduced.[171] The increased prevalence of gallstones in cirrhosis is due wholly to pigment stones[122] (and see Chapter 31).

Urinary excretion of bile acids is increased in cirrhosis, but in one study total daily excretion by this route was only 10.2 mg.[157] Urinary excretion is to a great extent preceded by sulphation. The proportion of bile acid sulphated was 100 per cent for lithocholate, 85 per cent for deoxycholate, 76 per cent for chenodeoxycholate and 24 per cent for cholate.[157] Sulphated bile acids have a far greater renal clearance than non-sulphated. This may be because, being more polar, they are less able to diffuse out of the renal tubules.[10] Another possible factor is synthesis of sulphates by the kidney itself. This has been shown to occur quite extensively in the rat,[159] but preliminary data cast doubt on its importance in man.[169]

Portasystemic shunting of blood round the liver is a factor which might be expected to affect bile acid metabolism in cirrhosis. However, in rats with an end-to-side portacaval shunt and consequent hepatic atrophy, there is no reduction in cholate synthesis or pool size.[66] Bile salt secretion is maintained even though the volume of bile flow is reduced.

Acute Hepatitis

Few studies have been reported of bile acid metabolism in hepatitis and it is difficult to separate the effects of liver cell injury from those of cholestasis. In a fully developed case there is markedly delayed clearance of cholic acid from the blood, reduced synthesis and a small pool.[163] Impaired secretion results in low intestinal bile acid concentrations during digestion. This is probably a factor in the steatorrhoea of hepatitis, since intestinal aspirates contain little lipid in the aqueous, micellar phase.[112] Impaired bile acid secretion may also explain why during hepatitis gallbladder bile tends to be supersaturated with cholesterol.[13] Serum bile acid levels are elevated to as much as 100 times normal[120] and their measurement is almost certainly more sensitive than serum bilirubin in detecting hepatitis, especially if postprandial samples are analysed. Of five children inoculated with hepatitis B virus, four remained anicteric, but the onset of hepatitis could be detected in all five by the development of a raised postprandial serum bile acid level.[71]

In *acute hepatic failure* with coma, the plasma disappearance of ^{14}C-cholic acid was more prolonged in patients who died than in those who survived. This might form the basis of a prognostic test.[75]

CHOLESTASIS

Cholestasis may be regarded as the ultimate insult to bile acid metabolism since it deprives bile acids of all access to the enterohepatic circulation. Every aspect of bile acid physiology and biochemistry is disturbed (see Chapter 14).

Synthesis is grossly impaired and perverted. The rate-limiting enzyme for synthesis, 7α-hydroxylase, showed only 22 per cent of its normal activity in the livers of five patients with biliary obstruction,[146] presumably because of intense feedback inhibition from the high serum levels of bile acids. Synthesis matches excretion and in complete biliary obstruction excretion is virtually limited to the urine. Urinary excretion increases markedly but cannot match normal faecal excretion. It amounted to only 33 μmol/24 hr in six obstructed patients studied by Makino et al,[98] and to a maximum of 80 μmol/24 hr in the cases of Stiehl,[156] whereas the normal turnover of bile acids is 600 to 1000 μmol/24 hr. An unknown but probably minor factor is faecal excretion of bile acids which have diffused across the intestinal wall.

Serum bile acid levels are very high in cholestasis. In one series they ranged from 15 to 285 μmol/l, which is four to 60 times the normal level.[120] In the past, a great deal of effort has been spent on analysing the relative amounts of the individual bile acids in the blood of patients with hepatobiliary disease, in the hope of identifying patterns which would be clinically helpful in distinguishing parenchymal liver disease from biliary obstruction.[24,97,120] In fact, there is so much overlap between different groups of patients that these analyses are of little clinical value. However, it is well established that in all cases of cholestasis there is a marked reduction in serum deoxycholate concentrations, presumably because of lack of contact between the cholate pool and intestinal bacteria. When hepatocellular damage is minimal, the ratio of cholate to chenodeoxycholate is greater than one. If cholestasis is prolonged, this ratio tends to fall, possibly because of liver damage. Infants with extrahepatic biliary atresia tend to have a marked preponderance of chenodeoxycholate in their serum, and this has led to the suggestion that the disease is actually a sequel to neonatal hepatitis.[78]

Aberrant bile acids which are produced in cholestasis include sulphates, glucuronides, an unsaturated monohydroxy bile acid (3β-hydroxy-5-cholenic acid), ursodeoxycholic acid, hyocholic acid and a primitive 27-carbon acid normally found in toads and crocodiles, trihydroxycoprostanic acid.[156] Indeed, in one study, 20 different bile acids were found in the urine of a single patient with primary biliary cirrhosis, many being unidentified.[4] The significance of these diversely abnormal pathways is not certain, but some at least can be interpreted as protective mechanisms. Protection may be obtained in two ways. Firstly, the abnormal metabolite may be less toxic and secondly it may be excreted more easily by the kidney. One toxic compound whose formation may be averted is chenodeoxycholic acid (see below). Ursodeoxycholate, the 7β-epimer of chenodeoxycholate, may constitute up to 12 per cent of the bile acids in cholestatic urine.[8] It is probably less hepatotoxic than chenodeoxycholate since it does not share its detergent properties.[29] The aberrant trihydroxy bile acids are also likely to be non-toxic. Sulphates, and probably glucuronides, are not only less toxic but also more efficiently excreted.

Sulphation is an important metabolic step in cholestasis.[156] In normal bile, virtually no sulphates are detectable, but serum bile acids are 9 per cent sulphated and urine bile acids up to 65 per cent sulphated.[98] The concentration of sulphates in the urine is explained, at least in part, by their high renal clearance rates. Radioactive studies have shown that sulphated cholate and chenodeoxycholate are excreted in the urine 10 to 15 times more rapidly than their non-sulphated counterparts.[156] This is probably because sulphated bile acids undergo less reabsorption in the renal tubules. In cholestasis, urinary bile salts are again about 60 per cent sulphated compared with 10 to 20 per cent in serum. Most of these are monosulphates, but disulphates and even trisulphates can be identified. Sulphation probably occurs to some extent in the kidney as well as the liver, and conceivably in the adrenal and the gut which are known to sulphate other steroids.[156]

Bile acid glucuronides have recently been identified in the urine of patients with cholestasis. In one study, patients with intrahepatic cholestasis excreted 7.2 mg glucuronides per 24 hours and those with extrahepatic obstruction 4.7 mg. It is likely that the hepatic glucuronyl transferase responsible for forming these more polar metabolites is inducible by phenobarbitone.[156] Phenobarbitone has been shown to lower serum bile acid concentrations in patients with biliary atresia and primary biliary cirrhosis by promoting the biliary and faecal excretion of bile acids. It may act partly by inducing the formation of bile acid glucuronides.

3β-hydroxy-5-cholenoic acid, an unsaturated monohydroxy bile acid, appears in significant amounts in the urine of both infants and adults with cholestasis.[8,123] Like lithocholate, it is almost wholly sulphated or glucuronidated, so it is not likely to be pathogenic. However, it has attracted interest as a possible intermediate in a minor synthetic pathway from cholesterol to chenodeoxycholic acid which may be increased under the stress of cholestasis.

Pruritus in cholestasis is probably caused by the deposition of bile acids in the skin. Most patients who itch have raised serum bile acid levels, but the correlation is poor. Bile acid concentrations on the skin itself are consistently raised, and Schoenfield[148] showed that, with recovery, skin bile acids return to normal at the same time as pruritus is relieved. Direct evidence that bile acids can cause pruritus was provided by Kirby, Heaton and Burton.[83] Applied to blister bases in a concentration of 1 mmol/l, cholate, chenodeoxycholate and deoxycholate and their conjugates all caused itching, the most active being unconjugated chenodeoxycholate. The most effective treatment for pruritus is cholestyramine, a non-absorbable resin which sequestrates bile acids in the intestine and promotes their excretion. It acts presumably by lowering first serum then skin bile acid concentrations. Phenobarbitone is also effective in intrahepatic cholestasis, relieving pruritus and reducing serum bile acids.[158] Its mode of action is unknown. Two possibilities are stimulation of the bile salt-independent fraction of bile flow[55] and induction of microsomal glucuronidating enzymes.

Role of bile acids in the pathogenesis of intrahepatic cholestasis (see also Chapter 14)

The transport of bile acids into biliary canaliculi is responsible for much or most of the generation of bile flow. The other major organic compounds in bile – phospholipid, cholesterol and bilirubin – are all carried down to the duodenum in bile acid micelles. Failure of bile acid secretion is therefore at least halfway to failure of bile flow or cholestasis. Bilirubin and other organic anions, such as bromsulphthalein, indocyanine green and iopanoic acid, are secreted into bile by an active transport system which is distinct from the bile acid system. However, the secretion of bilirubin conjugates is not accompanied by an increase in bile flow, even when the concentration of bilirubin is increased 100-fold. On the contrary, the secretion of bilirubin seems experimentally to depend on canalicular bile flow, as if such flow is needed to carry bilirubin away from the canalicular membrane. This being so, a marked reduction in canalicular bile flow is bound to decrease the excretion of bilirubin and other organic anions. Thus, even though there is no primary disturbance in bilirubin transport, conjugated hyperbilirubinaemia is bound to occur with severe cholestasis, as indeed occurs with many drug reactions.[77]

Many attempts have been made to prove that intrahepatic cholestasis is caused by failure of bile acid secretion, but the links are still tenuous. The most solid link is the undoubted fact that intravenous administration of lithocholate and other monohydroxy bile acids can induce cholestasis in animals even if given in conjugated form. This was first shown with taurolithocholate by Javitt and Emerman.[79] They found that bile flow was unimpaired if the infusate contained a normal micelle-forming bile salt as well as taurolithocholate. This led originally to the suggestion that monohydroxy bile acids cause cholestasis because, being poorly soluble, they precipitate in the canaliculi unless enough micelles are available to hold them in solution. Later, it was proposed that lithocholate perpetuated cholestasis by damaging the smooth endoplasmic reticulum, which is responsible for the early stages of bile acid synthesis.[147] Currently, however, it is thought that monohydroxy bile acids act by accumulating in and damaging the canalicular membrane. Certainly, the most striking ultrastructural changes which accompany lithocholate cholestasis are those involving the bile canaliculi. These include extensive dilatation, irregular outpouchings and loss of microvilli.[88,111] Similar canalicular changes are seen in human intrahepatic cholestasis and this makes it tempting to blame at least some cases on monohydroxy bile acids, especially as these acids are regularly found in cholestatic urine.

Quite strong arguments are made against a significant role for monohydroxy bile acids in human cholestasis, however. Firstly, when the bile acids present in cholestatic livers were analysed, no more than traces of monohydroxy acids were found.[51] Secondly, these bile acids are present in sulphated form in patients with cholestasis, and experimentally lithocholate sulphate does not cause cholestasis,[88,156] probably because it is quite soluble in water. In addition, there are some forms of cholestasis, notably that induced by oestrogens, in which there is no evidence of canalicular damage.[77] It is unwise to extrapolate directly from animal experiments to human disease. Chenodeoxycholate causes cholestasis in isolated perfused rat livers,[111] but there is no reason to believe it has this effect in man.

The pathogenesis of drug-induced cholestasis is still far from clear.[150] One possible mechanism is precipitation of bile acids by reaction with a positively charged drug. Such precipitation occurs in vitro when chlorpromazine is added to bile[27] and, if this occurred in vivo in the liver cell or the canaliculus, it could help to explain why chlorpromazine is so prone to cause cholestasis. It is easy to imagine that a bile acid–drug precipitate could initiate an immune response and so produce the features of a hypersensitivity reaction.

Bile acids and the hepatocellular damage of cholestasis (see also Chapter 14)

There is persuasive evidence that the liver cell damage which accompanies severe cholestasis is contributed to by high intracellular concentrations of dihydroxy bile acids. Feathery degeneration is the most characteristic histological feature of such damage and, in patients with cholestasis, it is associated with concentrations of chenodeoxycholate which are high enough (68 to 380 nmol/g) to produce detergent effects in vitro.[51] High concentrations of cholate are also found but these are not associated with liver cell damage. In rats, ligation of the common bile duct led to intrahepatic concentrations of dihydroxy bile acids which could be shown to inhibit cytochrome P-450. This implies impairment of a biotransformation system which is concerned with the metabolism of drugs, as well as many natural substances including cholesterol and bile acids.[52]

BILE ACIDS AND CHOLELITHIASIS

The key role of bile acids in cholelithiasis (see also Chapter 53) is emphasized by the fact that, in selected patients, gallstones can be dissolved in situ by the long-term oral administration of chenodeoxycholic or ursodeoxycholic acid. The only gallstones which are suitable for this treatment, and the only ones in whose pathogenesis bile acids are known to be concerned, are those which are rich in cholesterol. Cholesterol-rich stones in the gallbladder in fact constitute the majority of biliary calculi occurring in economically developed countries. In Philadelphia, USA, cholesterol stones were found in 73 per cent of 92 consecutive cholecystectomies.[167] In an x-ray powder analysis of the crystalline material in 331 gallstones from several different countries, cholesterol comprised 58 per cent of the average stone in England, 74 per cent in the USA, 80 per cent in Australia, 82 per cent in Germany and 89 per cent in Sweden.[160] Thus, the major problem in the pathogenesis of gallstones is the precipitation of cholesterol crystals out of micellar solution in the gallbladder, and the growth of these crystals into macroscopic stones. The key step, precipitation of cholesterol, can take place (though it does not necessarily do so) only if gallbladder bile is supersaturated with cholesterol. This discussion will focus largely on the problem of supersaturated or lithogenic bile. Other factors which may be important in the pathogenesis of cholesterol gallstones, but are outside the scope of this chapter, are stasis and stratification of bile, inhibitors of crystal growth, bacterial infection and excess of glycoprotein or mucus.[22]

Cholesterol in bile

Cholesterol is virtually insoluble in water. In body fluids it is transported by incorporation into negatively charged particles – lipoproteins in plasma, micelles in bile. The efficient dispersal of cholesterol in bile requires not only a detergent to provide micelles, but also a polar lipid to swell the micelles into two molecule-thick discs.[153] In bile the polar lipid is a phospholipid, lecithin, which does not itself dissolve in water but is swollen by it into a liquid crystalline phase which is efficiently dispersed into bile salt micelles. Hence, lecithin is termed a swelling amphipath whereas bile acids are soluble amphipaths. Addition of lecithin to a mixture of bile salts as found in human bile reduces the number of bile salt molecules required to solubilize one cholesterol molecule from about 35 to 10.[62] There are probably no important differences between the cholesterol-solubilizing capacities of the different bile salts. With pure bile salt solutions, dihydroxy glycine conjugates are the most effective but this difference is minimized by the presence of lecithin.[36,62]

The degree to which bile is saturated with cholesterol depends chiefly on the relative proportions of bile acid, phospholipid and cholesterol. Under physiological conditions the amount of water present makes little difference but, paradoxically, more concentrated biles tend to have a greater cholesterol-holding capacity.[26]

The source and function of cholesterol in bile are surprisingly little understood. There is no doubt that secretion into bile is a major pathway of cholesterol loss from the body, accounting for around 30 mg/hr, or 700 mg/24 hr.[54,151] Radioactive studies have suggested that the majority of bile cholesterol is derived from plasma,[149] which fits with the concept of bile cholesterol as the end product of effete plasma lipoproteins.[155] However, newly synthesized cholesterol seems to be the preferred substrate for bile acid synthesis in rats.[124] In any case, there seems to be a correlation between the synthesis of cholesterol and its secretion into bile.

Supersaturated bile

Bile is supersaturated when it contains more cholesterol than can be held in micellar solution. The capacity of bile to dissolve cholesterol has been studied extensively on the assumption that it depends entirely on the availability of bile acid phospholipid micelles. Admirand and Small[2] examined the physical state of all possible combinations of bile acids, lecithin and cholesterol and determined the limits of a micellar zone. To depict this zone it was necessary to use triangular co-ordinates (Figure 12.4). This physicochemical approach to bile

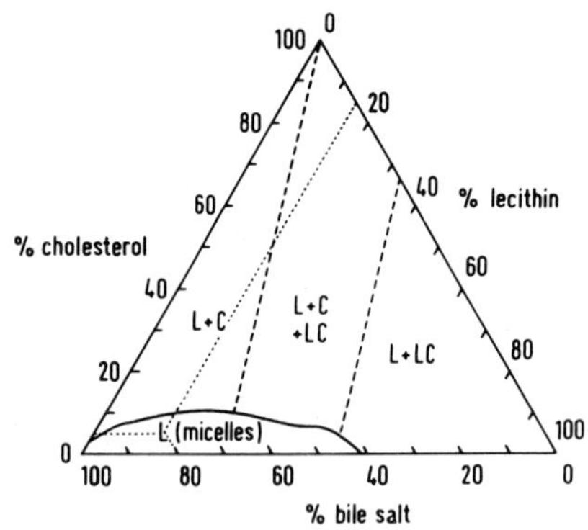

Figure 12.4. Triangular co-ordinates used to plot the composition of bile in terms of its content of cholesterol, lecithin (phospholipid) and bile salts. The point joined by the dotted lines represents a mixture of 5 per cent cholesterol, 15 per cent lecithin and 80 per cent bile salts. A bile sample with this composition lies in the micellar zone and is undersaturated with cholesterol. Bile samples above the curved line are supersaturated and contain crystals or liquid crystals according to the zone they fall into. This diagram is appropriate only for bile samples with a total solute concentration of 5 to 20 per cent. (Modified from Admirand and Small.[2]) Later studies have indicated that the zone of true cholesterol solubility is somewhat smaller than shown.[73]

was validated by the fact that, in patients with cholesterol stones, the composition of gallbladder bile was nearly always outside the micellar zone whereas in normal subjects it was always within the micellar zone. Later workers found that supersaturated bile is often present in normal subjects, indicating that stone formation requires other factors as well, perhaps nucleating agents.[73]

A disadvantage of using triangular co-ordinates to represent bile lipid composition is that a single numeral cannot be read from it to indicate the degree of cholesterol saturation. Because of this, various formulae have been devised to allow the calculation of a lithogenic or saturation index or of percentage cholesterol saturation. The most popular formula is that of Thomas and Hofmann.[166] This method ignores the total concentration of biliary lipids, but to take these into account requires complicated tables.[26]

Determinants of the cholesterol saturation of bile

As bile appears in the canaliculus its saturation with cholesterol depends on the relative secretion rates of bile acids, phospholipid and cholesterol. These are closely related in that the secretion of both the other lipids stops if the secretion of bile acids stops. However, as the secretion of bile acids increases that of phospholipid increases proportionately more than that of cholesterol, so that at higher bile acid secretion rates the saturation of bile decreases.[144] In fact, there seems to be a cut-off point at a bile acid secretion rate of about 12 μmol/min, or 10 μmol/kg/hr, below which bile becomes supersaturated with cholesterol.[175] During fasting, when the bile salt pool is largely sequestered in the gallbladder, there is naturally a low bile salt secretion rate. Hence, even in normal subjects, fasting hepatic bile is supersaturated with cholesterol. During digestion, when the bile salt pool is in circulation, the secretion rate is higher and hepatic bile is undersaturated, at least in normal subjects.[105]

These considerations have led some to the erroneous conclusion that the key factor in gallstone formation is a low total daily bile salt secretion. Others have measured the hours per day in which bile secreted into the duodenum is supersaturated and have tried to relate this to gallstone risk. However, both viewpoints fail to recognize the crucial fact that cholesterol gallstones form in the gallbladder and not in the bile ducts. Furthermore, it is highly probable that stone formation occurs mainly in the resting, relaxed gallbladder, namely during the overnight fast.

The saturation of bile in the gallbladder is determined above all by the size of the bile acid pool. This can be deduced from the fact that, as the gallbladder relaxes and the sphincter of Oddi contracts at the end of digestion, the circulating bile acid pool is diverted into the gallbladder, priming it with detergent. As the fast continues, water is extracted from the gallbladder contents and replaced with freshly secreted supersaturated bile. The ability of the gallbladder contents to remain unsaturated will depend chiefly on two factors: the original priming dose of bile salts, that is the size of the pool, and the cholesterol content of later incoming bile, that is the cholesterol secretion rate. These theoretical considerations are borne out by the finding of Swell, Gregory and Vlahcevic[161] that there is a strong negative correlation between the size of the bile acid pool and the cholesterol saturation of bile (Figure 12.5). The small size of the bile acid pool in cholesterol gallstone patients was first shown by Vlahcevic et al[172] and has since been abundantly confirmed.[65,134,138,151] The smallness

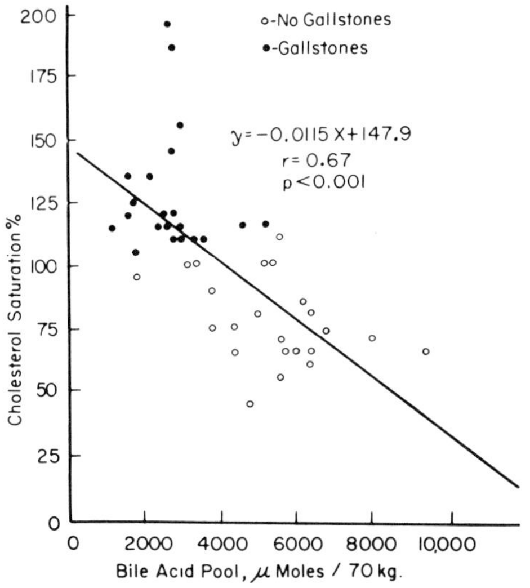

Figure 12.5. Relation between the size of the bile acid pool and the cholesterol saturation of gallbladder bile. From Swell et al[161] with kind permission of the authors and the editor of *Medical Clinics of North America*.

of the bile acid pool could be partly due to the gallstones encroaching on the gallbladder lumen or otherwise interfering with its storage capacity,[138] but this is certainly not the whole explanation since a small pool is also found in American Indians with a high probability of developing gallstones later but without actual calculi.[16,173] Furthermore, the pool is of normal size in patients with pigment stones.[151]

Determinants of bile acid pool size

When the bile acid pool is depleted, for example by bile diversion or cholestyramine therapy, there is a compensatory increase in bile acid synthesis by the liver. In gallstone patients daily synthesis is normal even though the pool is chronically depleted.[16] This suggests that hepatic synthesis is in fact inhibited, and this is supported by the finding that, in the livers of gallstone patients, there is reduced activity of the rate-limiting enzyme in bile acid synthesis, cholesterol 7α-hydroxylase.[146] The obvious interpretation is that reduced hepatic synthesis leads to a small bile acid pool. Northfield and Hofmann[125] have suggested that the primary event is more frequent circulation of the pool which intensifies the feedback inhibition of bile acid synthesis, and have shown a negative correlation between the size of the pool and the frequency of its circulation. A negative correlation has also been found between the rate of gallbladder emptying and the size of the cholate pool.[57] However, gallstone patients probably do not empty their gallbladders unusually fast[168] and it is hard to understand why they should. Furthermore, it is possible that a small pool circulates more frequently simply because it is small and requires less time for intestinal absorption.

Impaired hepatic synthesis of bile acids implies reduced cholesterol catabolism. Evidence that some patients with gallstones have defective cholesterol catabolism has been provided by Hepner and Quarfordt,[63] using isotopically labelled cholesterol. The cause of this hepatic defect is quite unknown. Dietary factors could be important. Certainly, in a variety of mammals, feeding a semi-synthetic diet rich in refined, fibre-depleted carbohydrate results in reduced bile acid synthesis and pool size. Similar diets, with or without added cholesterol, induce gallstones in monkeys, dogs, prairie dogs, rabbits, hamsters and mice.[60]

Composition of the bile acid pool in gallstone patients

The bile of patients with gallstones tends to have an increased proportion of dihydroxy bile acids[170] and this is due to increased amounts of deoxycholate. It is uncertain whether increased deoxycholate precedes gallstone formation or is the result of it. It can reasonably be attributed to interference by the gallstones with the storage function of the gallbladder, such that the bile acid pool circulates more often and so is more degraded by intestinal bacteria.[138] When a patient's gallbladder ceases to function to the extent that it does not opacify on oral cholecystography, there is a further increase in biliary deoxycholate.[142] Physiologically, the patient has performed autocholecystectomy, and his bile now resembles that of a cholecystectomy patient.[65,139] On the other hand, increased deoxycholate could be due to altered colonic function and could constitute a risk factor for gallstones by allowing greater secretion of cholesterol.[91]

Cholesterol synthesis and secretion in gallstone disease

Many patients with cholesterol gallstones are obese. In such patients an important factor in the production of supersaturated bile is excessive secretion of cholesterol. This was first shown in young Arizona Indian women, who are extraordinarily prone to gallstones,[53] but was soon demonstrated also in fat white women with stones.[54] Later, it became apparent that, even if they do not have gallstones, very obese people secrete twice the normal amount of cholesterol and, because of this rather than lack of bile salts, their bile is normally supersaturated.[17,151] In these studies the cholesterol secretion rate correlated with excess body weight, which suggests that adiposity of any degree may be a risk factor for the secretion of lithogenic bile. Weight reduction reverses the abnormality but cholesterol secretion remains high during the period of weight loss, perhaps because of mobilization of cholesterol from adipose tissue.[17]

Excessive cholesterol secretion is presumably the end-result of excessive synthesis. It is well established that obesity increases body synthesis of cholesterol. Indeed, cholesterol production is related directly to the weight of body fat.[106,121] It has not so far been possible to show increased cholesterol synthesis in non-obese gallstone patients,[136] but in their livers there is increased activity of the rate-limiting hormone for cholesterol synthesis, HMG-CoA reductase,[146] and there is a correlation between the activity of this enzyme and the rate of cholesterol secretion.[82] Patients with gallstones tend to have high fasting plasma triglyceride levels[15] and plasma triglyceride levels closely reflect cholesterol production rates.[155]

Effects of Bile Acid Feeding on Bile

The discovery by the Mayo Clinic group that feeding chenodeoxycholic acid reduces the saturation of bile and can lead to the dissolution of gallstones[37] prompted intensive study of the effects of feeding different bile acids on bile. Favourable changes are obtained only with chenodeoxycholic acid itself and its 7β-epimer ursodeoxycholic acid.[99] When either bile acid is fed, it becomes the predominant bile acid in bile, but there is also a marked increase in its epimer because the two bile acids are metabolically interchangeable. Ursodeoxycholate desaturates bile in doses as low as 150 mg/24 hr,[119] whereas with chenodeoxycholate it is usually necessary to give 750 to 1000 mg/24 hr.[76] This raises the possibility that chenodeoxycholate operates by being transformed to ursodeoxycholate.

Feeding chenodeoxycholate expands the total bile salt pool in most cases and originally this was thought to be its mode of action. However, it can desaturate the bile without expanding the pool[38] and it is now believed to act by decreasing the secretion of cholesterol. In fact, there is a change in the coupling between bile salt secretion and cholesterol secretion such that for a given rise in bile acid output there is only half the expected rise in cholesterol secretion.[128] This is probably not due to an effect on the actual process of canalicular bile secretion since, in acute experiments in the cat, chenodeoxycholate favours the secretion of more, not less, cholesterol than does cholate.[154] The theory currently favoured is that chenodeoxycholate acts by suppressing cholesterol synthesis. Certainly, feeding chenodeoxycholate reduces the activity of HMG-CoA reductase in the liver[34] and total body production of cholesterol is probably lowered.[135] Bile acid synthesis is suppressed as well, but the size of the circulating pool is maintained by absorption of exogenous bile acid.

Feeding cholic acid expands the bile acid pool but has no favourable effect on cholesterol secretion or the saturation of bile.[87] The composition of the pool is changed, with marked increases in cholate and its metabolite deoxycholate at the expense of chenodeoxycholate.

Deoxycholate feeding studies have given discordant results, possibly due to the different dosages used. When the dosage was 100 to 150 mg/24 hr, which should merely double or treble the normal deoxycholate input, there was a striking difference in the effects on cholate and chenodeoxycholate metabolism.[140] Chenodeoxycholate synthesis and pool size were reduced but there was no effect on cholate synthesis or pool size. This specific inhibitory effect on the synthesis of chenodeoxycholate was accompanied by increased cholesterol saturation of the bile, which led to the speculation that excess secondary bile acids in bile could be a risk factor for gallstone formation.[91] This speculation was rendered more plausible by the simultaneous discovery that feeding wheat bran made bile less saturated with cholesterol and had effects on bile acid metabolism which were exactly opposite to those of deoxycholate feeding, namely a fall in the deoxycholate pool, an increase in the chenodeoxycholate pool and synthesis rate, and no change in cholate synthesis.[141] When the dosage of deoxycholate was 750 mg/24hr, there was a decrease in the synthesis of cholate as well as of chenodeoxycholate.[85] This could be explained as the result of a supra-physiological dose of deoxycholate, but it is puzzling that in the latter study there was no increase in biliary saturation. One intriguing and unexplained finding common to both deoxycholate feeding studies was a 12 to 15 per cent fall in serum cholesterol.

Clinical application of bile acid treatment

Medical treatment of gallstones is now a reality. Chenodeoxycholic acid is available for prescription by doctors in several European countries. In the USA, a large multicentred trial is in progress (1977). The efficacy of treatment is not in doubt. If the gallbladder opacifies on cholecystography, if the stones are wholly radiolucent (which makes them 80 per cent probable cholesterol-rich stones) and if they are less than 15 mm in diameter, there is an 80 per cent chance that they will dissolve with an adequate dose of chenodeoxycholate.[164] An adequate dose probably means 15 mg/kg body weight/24 hr[76] but obese subjects may need more.[41] Success, which can be assessed only by repeated cholecystograms, comes in less than six months with some small stones but can be delayed for two to three years with large ones. If treatment is then stopped, stones recur within a year or two in up to 50 per cent of patients.[41]

Side effects of chenodeoxycholate treatment are few. The only proven one is diarrhoea, but this is seldom troublesome and settles when the dose is reduced. It is probably due to the secretory effects of dihydroxy bile acids on the colonic mucosa.[104] Fears of hepatotoxicity have delayed the introduction of this therapy in Britain, the USA and other countries. These fears spring from the fact that feeding chenodeoxycholate causes liver damage in many mammalian species, including baboons and rhesus monkeys.[115,176] However, there is no good evidence that chenodeoxycholate causes significant damage to the human liver. Histological examination of liver biopsies from over a hundred patients has shown no more than the trivial abnormalities which are found in untreated gallstone patients.[41,70] Elevations in the serum levels of 'liver enzymes' such as aspartate aminotransferase occur in about 30 per cent of patients, but these are transient and usually moderate. A few follow episodes of biliary colic and may be caused by the passage of a stone but most are unexplained and probably represent a non-injurious leak of enzymes from the liver cells. All other tests of liver function, including the clearance of bromsulphthalein, are normal.[14] The lack of hepatotoxicity in man is probably due to the fact that the toxic metabolite, lithocholate, is efficiently detoxicated by sulphation. Certainly, sulphation of intravenously administered lithocholate occurs much more rapidly in man than in the rhesus monkey, a species which does develop liver damage with chenodeoxycholate.[47]

The limitations of bile acid treatment of gallstones are considerable. To be suitable, patients must have mild or infrequent symptoms, their gallbladders must opacify and the stones must be radiolucent and not too large. This probably excludes up to 80 per cent of patients complaining of gallstone-induced symptoms. Therapy is prolonged and expensive and requires numerous hospital visits and x-ray films. It may make the patient dependent on hospital treatment for the rest of his life. In spite of this, it is at best 80 per cent effective, and eventual recurrence is likely in most cases. The most pressing problem is how to manage patients once their stones have dissolved. Lifetime treatment, even with small doses, is unattractive. The logical approach is the removal of the cause. According to current evidence, the major causes are obesity and the consumption of refined, fibre-depleted foods such as sugar and white flour.[60] Trials are needed to show that gallstone recurrence can be prevented by maintenance of a slim physique and avoidance of refined foods. Other agents which should be avoided are drugs which are known to cause gallstones, especially clofibrate and oestrogens, including the contraceptive pill.

Oestrogens, Bile and Gallstones

Cholesterol gallstones are commoner in women than in men and are associated with pregnancy. They are also increased in frequency in women who take oral contraceptives and in those who are treated with oestrogens after the menopause.[20,21,30] During oral contraceptive therapy gallbladder bile is more saturated with cholesterol, indeed it is usually supersaturated.[18] The mechanisms for this unfavourable change in bile are probably twofold: increased secretion of cholesterol and reduced synthesis of bile acids leading to a reduced bile acid pool.[137] A decrease in the proportion of chenodeoxycholate has been described during oral contraceptive therapy and also in pregnant baboons[18,39] but it is not established that this results in increased cholesterol saturation of bile. During the normal menstrual cycle bile becomes more saturated after ovulation has occurred, but there is no change in bile salt composition.[96]

BILE ACID MALABSORPTION AND CHOLEGENIC DIARRHOEA

Conservation of bile acids depends on a normally functioning terminal ileum. Resection of as little as 40 cm of terminal ileum can cause significant bile acid malabsorption. This has numerous effects. The most striking is diarrhoea, which can be intense and disabling, especially if the right colon has been resected as well. This diarrhoea is caused by the laxative action of dihydroxy bile acids, which not only inhibit the absorption of water and electrolytes, but actually promote secretion of an isotonic sodium chloride solution by the colonic mucosa. These secretory actions resemble those of cholera toxin on the small intestine in being mediated by stimulation of the enzyme adenyl cyclase, which catalyses the production of cyclic AMP in the intestinal mucosa. Bile acids also increase colonic motility. Cholegenic diarrhoea is sometimes not relieved by ordinary anti-diarrhoeal drugs. In this case, it usually responds to bile acid inactivating agents such as the anion exchange resin cholestyramine or aluminium hydroxide gel. With extensive ileal resections diarrhoea is partly due to unabsorbed fatty acids, which also have secretory effects on the colonic mucosa, and cholestyramine is less effective than reduction of dietary fat.

Bile acid malabsorption provokes a compensatory increase in the catabolism of cholesterol, and bile acid synthesis increases up to tenfold. During an overnight fast, when most secreted bile acids are sequestered in the gallbladder, a near-normal bile acid pool may be collected and the absorption of breakfast lipids may be nearly normal. Failure of the pool to recirculate, however, means that there is a marked deficiency of bile acids for the digestion of later meals. This is probably a major factor in the steatorrhoea of intestinal resection and helps to explain why steatorrhoea and malabsorption of fat-soluble vitamins are worse after distal than proximal resections. Another consequence of bile acid deficiency is supersaturated bile, and this is probably the reason for the three- to fivefold increase in the incidence of gallstones in ileectomized patients.

Other secondary effects of bile acid malabsorption are a raised glycine to taurine conjugation ratio in the bile, due to relative unavailability of taurine, and absence of secondary bile acids in the faeces (with all but large resections), due probably to inhibition of bacterial dehydroxylases by high colonic bile acid concentrations. Hyperoxaluria and oxalate urinary stones are common. The likely mechanism is increased absorption of dietary oxalate in the colon due to bile acid-induced permeability of the mucosa.

Bile acid malabsorption and cholegenic diarrhoea also occur, for reasons which are quite obscure, in patients with severe post-vagotomy diarrhoea. They are also found in a few patients with idiopathic diarrhoea who have till then been regarded as having the irritable bowel syndrome. Bile acid malabsorption has been described in children, but not adults, with cystic fibrosis.

The diagnostic test for cholegenic diarrhoea is a successful trial of cholestyramine therapy. The ^{14}C-glycocholate breath test is positive in some but not all patients, but faecal radioactivity is consistently increased.

Unresected Crohn's disease leads to bile acid malabsorption only if it is extensive in the ileum. It is more likely to disturb bile acid metabolism by causing bacterial overgrowth in the small bowel.

This topic has recently been reviewed in detail.[61]

BILE ACIDS AND THE STAGNANT LOOP SYNDROME

Malabsorption of fat, vitamin B_{12} and sometimes other nutrients is prone to occur whenever the upper small intestine contains faecal-type anaerobic bacteria in counts greater than 10^3/ml. In these circumstances, there is almost always extensive deconjugation of bile acids in the upper small intestine. There are two ways in which such deconjugation could lead to steatorrhoea. The abnormally high concentration of deconjugated dihydroxy bile acids could damage the mucosal cells and interfere with their absorptive functions. Alternatively, there could be precipitation of unconjugated bile acids, which are poorly soluble at alkaline pH. Together with rapid absorption of unconjugated bile acids by passive diffusion across the jejunal mucosa this would lead to intraluminal bile acid deficiency and lack of lipid-dissolving micelles. In fact, evidence exists for both these mechanisms, though latterly more emphasis has been laid on mucosal damage. There is no doubt that unconjugated dihydroxy bile acids can interfere with the active transport mechanisms of the brush border as well as with the enzymatic activities of the enterocyte. The toxicity of dihydroxy bile acids is reduced by incorporation into mixed micelles, and in any contaminated small bowel the pathogenic factors are likely to be constantly changing, depending on the supply of conjugated bile acids, the number and activity of bacteria, the pH and the rate of absorption of unconjugated bile acids.

The ^{14}C-glycocholate breath test provides a simple and reliable screening test for significant bacterial overgrowth.

These topics have been reviewed recently and in detail.[61,67]

REFERENCES

1. Accatino, L. & Simon, F.R. (1976) Identification and characterisation of a bile acid receptor in isolated liver surface membranes. *Journal of Clinical Investigation,* **57,** 496–508.
2. Admirand, W.H. & Small, D.M. (1968) The physico-chemical basis of cholesterol gallstone formation in man. *Journal of Clinical Investigation,* **47,** 1043–1052.
3. Allan, R.N., Thistle, J.L. & Hofmann, A.F. (1976) Lithocholate metabolism during chenotherapy for gallstone dissolution. 2. Absorption and sulphation. *Gut,* **17,** 413–419.
4. Almé, B., Bremmelgaard, A., Sjövall, J. & Thomassen, P. (1975) Complexity of the bile acid mixture in human urine. In *Advances in Bile Acid Research* (Ed.) Matern, S., Hackenschmidt, J., Back, P. & Gerok, W. pp. 145–147. Stuttgart: Schattauer Verlag.
5. Almond, H.R., Vlahcevic, Z.R., Bell, C.C., Gregory, D.H. & Swell, L. (1973) Bile acid pools, kinetics and biliary lipid composition before and after cholecystectomy. *New England Journal of Medicine,* **289,** 1213–1216.
6. Anderson, K.E., Kok, E. & Javitt, N.B. (1972) Bile acid synthesis in man: metabolism of 7α-hydroxy cholesterol-^{14}C and 26-hydroxycholesterol-^{3}H. *Journal of Clinical Investigation,* **51,** 112–117.
7. Angelin, B., Einarsson, K. & Hellström, K. (1976) Evidence for the absorption of bile acids in the proximal small intestine of normo- and hyper-lipidaemic subjects. *Gut,* **17,** 420–425.
8. Back, P. (1973) Identification and quantitative determination of urinary bile acids excreted in cholestasis. *Clinica Chimica Acta,* **4,** 199–207.
9. Back, P. & Gerok, W. (1972) (Eds.) *Bile Acids in Human Diseases.* Stuttgart: Schattauer Verlag.
10. Back, P. & Gerok, W. (1977) Differences in renal excretion between glyco-, tauroconjugates, sulfo-conjugates and glucuronoconjugates of bile acids in cholestasis. In *Bile Acid Metabolism in Health and Disease* (Ed.) Paumgartner, G. & Stiehl, A., pp. 93–100. Lancaster: Medical and Technical Publishers.
11. Badley, B.W.D., Murphy, G.M., Bouchier, I.A.D. & Sherlock, S. (1970) Diminished micellar phase lipid in patients with chronic non-alcoholic liver disease and steatorrhea. *Gastroenterology,* **58,** 781–789.
12. Barnes, S., Gallo, G.A., Trash, D.B. & Morris, J.S. (1975) Diagnostic value of serum bile acid estimations in liver disease. *Journal of Clinical Pathology,* **28,** 506–509.
13. Begemann, F. & Herget, H.J. (1975) Lithogenic bile in acute hepatitis. In *Advances in Bile Acid Research* (Ed.) Matern, S., Hackenschmidt, J., Back, P. & Gerok, W., pp. 335–338. Stuttgart: Schattauer Verlag.
14. Bell, G.D. (1974) The present position concerning gallstone dissolution. *Gut,* **15,** 913–929.
15. Bell, G.D., Lewis, B., Petrie, A. & Dowling, R.H. (1973) Serum lipids in cholelithiasis: effect of chenodeoxycholic acid therapy. *British Medical Journal,* **iii,** 520–523.
16. Bell, C.C., McCormick, W.C., Gregory, D.H., Law, D.H., Vlahcevic, Z.R. & Swell, L. (1972) Relationship of bile acid pool size to the formation of lithogenous bile in male Indians of the Southwest. *Surgery, Gynecology and Obstetrics,* **134,** 473–478.
17. Bennion, L.J. & Grundy, S.M. (1975) Effects of obesity and caloric intake on biliary lipid metabolism in man. *Journal of Clinical Investigation,* **56,** 996–1011.
18. Bennion, L.J., Ginsberg, R.L., Garnick, M.B. & Bennett, P.H. (1976) Effects of oral contraceptives on the gallbladder bile of normal women. *New England Journal of Medicine,* **294,** 189–192.
19. Björkhem, I. & Danielsson, H. (1976) Biosynthesis and metabolism of bile acids in man. In *Progress in Liver Disease. V* (Ed.) Popper, H. & Schaffner, F. New York: Grune & Stratton.
20. Boston Collaborative Drug Surveillance Programme (1973) Oral contraceptives and venous thromboembolic disease, surgically confirmed gallbladder disease, and breast tumours. *Lancet,* **i,** 1399–1403.
21. Boston Collaborative Drug Surveillance Program (1974) Surgically confirmed gallbladder disease, venous thromboembolism, and breast tumors in relation to postmenopausal estrogen therapy. *New England Journal of Medicine,* **290,** 15–19.
22. Bouchier, I.A.D. (1975) Gallstones. In *Modern Trends in Gastroenterology – 5* (Ed.) Read, A.E., London: Butterworths.
23. Brunner, H., Northfield, T.C., Hofmann, A.F., Go, V.L.W. & Summerskill, W.H.J. (1974) Gastric emptying and secretion of bile acids, cholesterol, and pancreatic enzymes during digestion. Duodenal perfusion studies in healthy subjects. *Mayo Clinic Proceedings,* **49,** 851–860.
24. Carey, J.B. (1970) Bile salts and hepatobiliary disease. In *Diseases of the Liver,* 3rd ed. (Ed.) Schiff, L. pp. 103–146. Philadelphia: Lippincott.
25. Carey, M.C. & Small, D.M. (1970) The characteristics of mixed micellar solutions with particular reference to bile. *American Journal of Medicine,* **49,** 590–608.

26. Carey, M.C. & Small, D.M. (1978) The physical chemistry of cholesterol solubility in bile: relationship to gallstone formation and dissolution in man. *Journal of Clinical Investigation*, **61,** 998–1026.
27. Carey, M.C., Hirom, P.C. & Small, D.M. (1974) Precipitation of bile salts by chlorpromazine (CPZ); the protective effect of lecithin (LEC). *Gastroenterology*, **66,** 671.
28. Carey, J.B., Wilson, I.D., Zaki, F.G. & Hanson, R.F. (1966) The metabolism of bile acids with special reference to liver injury. *Medicine (Baltimore)*, **45,** 461–470.
29. Chadwick, V.S., Gaginella, T.S., Debongnie, J.C., Phillips, S.F. & Hofmann, A.F. (1976) Different effects of chenodeoxycholic and ursodeoxycholic acids on colonic secretion, permeability and morphology. *Gastroenterology*, **71,** 900.
30. Coronary Drug Project Research Group (1977) Gallbladder disease as a side effect of drugs influencing lipid metabolism. *New England Journal of Medicine*, **296,** 1185–1190.
31. Cowen, A.E., Korman, M.G., Hofmann, A.F. & Cass, O.W. (1975a) Metabolism of lithocholate in healthy man. I. Biotransformation and biliary excretion of intravenously administered lithocholate, lithocholylglycine, and their sulfates. *Gastroenterology*, **69,** 59–66.
32. Cowen, A.E., Korman, M.G., Hofmann, A.F. & Coffin, S.B. (1975b) Metabolism of lithocholate in healthy man. II. Enterohepatic circulation. *Gastroenterology*, **69,** 67–76.
33. Cowen, A.E., Korman, M.G., Hofmann, A.F. & Thomas, P.J. (1975c) Plasma disappearance of radioactivity after intravenous injection of labelled bile acids in man. *Gastroenterology*, **68,** 1567–1573.
34. Coyne, M.J., Bonorris, G.G., Goldstein, L.I. & Schoenfield, L.J. (1976) Effect of chenodeoxycholic acid and phenobarbital on the rate-limiting enzymes of hepatic cholesterol and bile acid synthesis in patients with gallstones. *Journal of Laboratory and Clinical Medicine*, **87,** 281–291.
35. Crook, D.N., Smith, D.C., McAllister, R.A. & Mackay, C. (1971) The effect of cholecystectomy on the size of the bile-salt pool in the dog. *British Journal of Surgery*, **58,** 867.
36. Dam, H. (1971) Determinants of cholesterol cholelithiasis in man and animals. *American Journal of Medicine*, **51,** 596–613.
37. Danzinger, R.G., Hofmann, A.F., Schoenfield, L.J. & Thistle, J.L. (1972) Dissolution of cholesterol gallstones by chenodeoxycholic acid. *New England Journal of Medicine*, **286,** 1–8.
38. Danzinger, R.G., Hofmann, A.F., Thistle, J.L. & Schoenfield, L.J. (1973) Effect of oral chenodeoxycholic acid on bile acid kinetics and biliary lipid composition in women with cholelithiasis. *Journal of Clinical Investigation*, **52,** 2809–2821.
39. Deitrick, J.E., McSherry, C.K., Javitt, N.B. & Glenn, F. (1973) Bile salt kinetics in the pregnant baboon: a new model for the study of gallbladder function. *Gastroenterology*, **65,** 536.
40. Dietschy, J.M. (1968) Mechanisms for the intestinal absorption of bile acids. *Journal of Lipid Research*, **9,** 297–309.
41. Dowling, R.H. (1977) Chenodeoxycholic acid therapy of gallstones. *Clinics in Gastroenterology*, **6,** 141–163.
42. Erlinger, S. & Dhumeaux, D. (1974) Mechanisms and control of secretion of bile water and electrolytes. *Gastroenterology*, **66,** 281–304.
43. Fausa, O. & Gjone, F. (1976) Serum bile acid concentrations in patients with liver disease. *Scandinavian Journal of Gastroenterology*, **11,** 537–543.
44. Ferguson, D.R., Calcraft, B.J., Hofmann, A.F. & Belobaba, D.T.A. (1976) Lack of sensitivity of a bile acid clearance test in the detection of liver disease. *Gastroenterology*, **71,** 905.
45. Fisher, M.M. & Miyai, K. (1971) Lithocholic acid induced intrahepatic cholestasis. *Gastroenterology*, **60,** 193.
46. Fromm, H. & Hofmann, A.F. (1971) Breath test for altered bile-acid metabolism. *Lancet*, **ii,** 621–625.
47. Gadacz, T.R., Allan, R.N., Mack, E. & Hofmann, A.F. (1976) Impaired lithocholate sulfation in the rhesus monkey: a possible mechanism for chenodeoxycholate toxicity. *Gastroenterology*, **70,** 1125–1129.
48. Glasinovic, J.-C., Dumont, M., Duval, M. & Erlinger, S. (1975a) Hepatocellular uptake of bile acids in the dog: evidence for a common carrier-mediated transport system. *Gastroenterology*, **69,** 973–981.
49. Glasinovic, J.-C., Dumont, M., Duval, M. & Erlinger, S. (1975b) Hepatocellular uptake of taurocholate in the dog. *Journal of Clinical Investigation*, **55,** 419–426.
50. Greim, H. (1976) Bile acids in hepato-biliary diseases. In *The Bile Acids*, Vol. 3, (Ed.) Nair, P.P. & Kritchevsky, D. pp. 53–80. New York: Plenum.
51. Greim, H., Trülzsch, D., Czygan, P., Rudick, J., Hutterer, F., Schaffner, F. & Popper, H. (1972a) Mechanism of cholestasis. 6. Bile acids in human livers with or without biliary obstruction. *Gastroenterology*, **63,** 846–850.
52. Greim, H., Trülzsch, D., Roboz, J., Dressler, K., Czygan, P., Hutterer, F., Schaffner, F. & Popper, H. (1972b) Mechanism of cholestasis. 5. Bile acids in normal rat livers and in those after bile duct ligation. *Gastroenterology*, **63,** 837–845.
53. Grundy, S.M., Metzger, A.L. & Adler, R.D. (1972) Mechanisms of lithogenic bile formation in American Indian women with cholesterol gallstones. *Journal of Clinical Investigation*, **51,** 3026–3043.
54. Grundy, S.M., Duane, W.C., Adler, R.D., Aron, J.M. & Metzger, A.L. (1974) Biliary lipid outputs in young women with cholesterol gallstones. *Metabolism*, **23,** 67–73.
55. Gumucio, J.J., Accatino, L., Macho, A.M. & Contreras, A. (1973) Effect of phenobarbital on the ethynyl estradiol-induced cholestasis in the rat. *Gastroenterology*, **65,** 651–657.
56. Hammerman, K., Thiel, M. & Admirand, W.H. (1976) Effects of increased bile salt enterohepatic cycling on bile composition and bile salt kinetics. *Gastroenterology*, **70,** A-35.
57. Hanson, K.C. & Duane, W.C. (1976) Role of the gallbladder in regulation of bile acid metabolism in man. *Gastroenterology*, **71,** A-17.
58. Hardison, W.G., Grundy, S.M. & von Bergmann, K. (1976) Small bowel absorption of endogenous conjugated bile acid in man. *Gastroenterology*, **71,** A-18.
59. Heaton, K.W. (1972) *Bile Salts in Health and Disease.* Edinburgh: Churchill Livingstone.
60. Heaton, K.W. (1975) Gallstones and cholecystitis. In *Refined Carbohydrate Foods and Disease. Some*

Implications of Dietary Fibre (Ed.) Burkitt, D.P. & Trowell, H.C. pp. 173–194. London: Academic Press.

61. Heaton, K.W. (1977) Disturbances of bile acid metabolism in intestinal disease. *Clinics in Gastroenterology*, **6,** 69–89.
62. Hegardt, F.G. & Dam, H. (1971) The solubility of cholesterol in aqueous solutions of bile salts and lecithin. *Zeitschrift für Ernährungswissenschaft*, **10,** 223–233.
63. Hepner, G.W. & Quarfordt, S.H. (1975) Kinetics of cholesterol and bile acids in patients with cholesterol cholelithiasis. *Gastroenterology*, **69,** 318–325.
64. Hepner, G.W., Hofmann, A.F. & Thomas, P.J. (1972) Metabolism of steroid and amino acid moieties of conjugated bile acids in man. I. Cholylglycine. *Journal of Clinical Investigation*, **51,** 1889–1897.
65. Hepner, G.W., Hofmann, A.F., Malagelada, J.R., Szczepanik, P.A. & Klein, P.D. (1974) Increased bacterial degradation of bile acids in cholecystectomised patients. *Gastroenterology*, **66,** 556–564.
66. Herz, R., Paumgartner, G. & Preisig, R. (1974) Bile salt metabolism and bile formation in the rat with a portacaval shunt. *European Journal of Clinical Investigation*, **4,** 223–228.
67. Hess Thaysen, E. (1977) Diagnostic value of the ^{14}C-cholylglycine breath test. *Clinics in Gastroenterology*, **6,** 227–245.
68. Hofmann, A.F. (1976) The enterohepatic circulation of bile acids in man. *Advances in Internal Medicine*, **21,** 501–534.
69. Hofmann, A.F. (1977) The enterohepatic circulation of bile acids in man. *Clinical Gastroenterology*, **6,** 3–24.
70. Hofmann, A.F. & Paumgartner, G. (1975) *Chenodeoxycholic Acid Therapy of Gallstones. Progress Report, 1975.* Stuttgart: Schattauer Verlag.
71. Hofmann, A.F., Korman, M.G. & Krugman, S. (1974) Sensitivity of serum bile acid assay for detection of liver damage in viral hepatitis type B. *American Journal of Digestive Diseases*, **19,** 908–910.
72. Hofmann, A.F., Schoenfield, L.J., Kottke, B.A. & Poley, J.R. (1970) Methods for the description of bile acid kinetics in man. In *Methods in Medical Research*, Vol. 12 (Ed.) Olson, R.E. pp. 149–180. Chicago: Year Book Medical Publishers.
73. Holzbach, R.T., Marsh, M., Olszewski, M. & Holan, K. (1973) Cholesterol solubility in bile. Evidence that supersaturated bile is frequent in healthy man. *Journal of Clinical Investigation*, **52,** 1467–1479.
74. Holzbach, R.T., Oh, S.Y., McDonnel, M.E. & Jamieson, A.M. (1977) Quasielastic laser spectrometry studies of pure bile salt and bile-salt-mixed lipid micellar systems. In *Proceedings of the Symposium on Micellization, Solubilization and Microemulsions* (Ed.) Mittal, K.L. pp. 403–418. New York: Plenum.
75. Horak, W., Waldram, R., Murray-Lyon, I.M., Schuster, E. & Williams, R. (1976) Kinetics of (^{14}C) cholic acid in fulminant hepatic failure: a prognostic test. *Gastroenterology*, **71,** 809–813.
76. Iser, J.H., Dowling, R.H., Mok, H.Y.I. & Bell, G.D. (1975) Chenodeoxycholic acid treatment of gallstones. A follow-up report and analysis of factors influencing response to therapy. *New England Journal of Medicine*, **293,** 378–383.
77. Javitt, N.B. (1976a) Hepatic bile formation. *New England Journal of Medicine*, **295,** 1464–1469 and 1511–1516.
78. Javitt, N.B. (1976b) Cholestasis in infancy. *Gastroenterology*, **70,** 1172–1181.
79. Javitt, N.B. & Emerman, S. (1968) Effect of sodium taurolithocholate on bile flow and bile acid excretion. *Journal of Clinical Investigation*, **47,** 1002–1014.
80. Josephson, B. (1941) The circulation of the bile acids in connection with their production, conjugation and excretion. *Physiological Reviews*, **21,** 463–486.
81. Kaplowitz, N., Kok, E. & Javitt, N.B. (1973) Postprandial serum bile acid for the detection of hepatobiliary disease. *Journal of the American Medical Association*, **225,** 292–293.
82. Key, P.H., Bonorris, G.G., Coyne, M.J., Taub, M. & Schoenfield, L.J. (1977) Hepatic cholesterol synthesis: a determinant of cholesterol secretion in gallstone patients. *Gastroenterology*, **72,** A-159.
83. Kirby, J., Heaton, K.W. & Burton, J.L. (1974) Pruritic effect of bile salts. *British Medical Journal*, **iv,** 693–695.
84. Knodell, R.G., Kinsey, M.D., Boedeker, E.C. & Collin, D.P. (1976) Deoxycholate metabolism in alcoholic cirrhosis. *Gastroenterology*, **71,** 196–201.
85. LaRusso, N.F., Szczepanik, P.A. & Hofmann, A.F. (1977) Effect of deoxycholic acid ingestion on bile acid metabolism and biliary lipid secretion in normal subjects. *Gastroenterology*, **72,** 132–140.
86. LaRusso, N.F., Hoffman, N.E., Hofmann, A.F. & Korman, M.G. (1975) Validity and sensitivity of an intravenous bile acid tolerance test in patients with liver disease. *New England Journal of Medicine*, **292,** 1209–1214.
87. LaRusso, N.F., Hoffman, N.E., Hofmann, A.F., Northfield, T.C. & Thistle, J.L. (1975) Effect of primary bile acid ingestion on bile acid metabolism and biliary lipid secretion in gallstone patients. *Gastroenterology*, **69,** 1301–1314.
88. Layden, T.J., Schwarz, J. & Boyer, J.L. (1975) Scanning electron microscopy of the liver. Studies of the effect of taurolithocholate and other models of cholestasis. *Gastroenterology*, **69,** 724–738.
89. Lindblad, L., Lundholm, K. & Scherstén, T. (1977) Bile acid concentrations in systemic and portal serum in presumably normal man and in cholestatic and cirrhotic conditions. *Scandinavian Journal of Gastroenterology*, **12,** 395–400.
90. Losowsky, M.S. & Walker, B.E. (1969) Liver disease and malabsorption. *Gastroenterology*, **56,** 589–600.
91. Low-Beer, T.S. & Pomare, E.W. (1975) Can colonic bacterial metabolites predispose to cholesterol gallstones? *British Medical Journal*, **i,** 438–440.
92. Low-Beer, T.S., Tyor, M.P. & Lack, L. (1969) Effect of sulfation of taurolithocholic and glycolithocholic acids on their intestinal transport. *Gastroenterology*, **56,** 721–726.
93. Low-Beer, T.S., Harvey, R.F., Davies, E.R. & Read, A.E. (1975) Abnormalities of serum cholecystokinin and gallbladder-emptying in celiac disease. *New England Journal of Medicine*, **292,** 961–963.
94. Low-Beer, T.S., Heaton, K.W., Heaton, S.T. & Read, A.E. (1971) Gallbladder inertia and sluggish enterohepatic circulation of bile-salts in coeliac disease. *Lancet*, **i,** 991–994.
95. Low-Beer, T.S., Heaton, K.W., Pomare, E.W. & Read, A.E. (1973) The effect of coeliac disease upon bile salts. *Gut*, **14,** 204–208.
96. Low-Beer, T.S., Wicks, A.C.B., Heaton, K.W., Durrington, P. & Yeates, J. (1977) Fluctuations of serum and bile lipid concentrations during the

menstrual cycle. *British Medical Journal*, **i**, 1568–1570.

97. Makino, I., Nakagawa, S. & Mashimo, K. (1969) Conjugated and unconjugated serum bile acid levels in patients with hepatobiliary diseases. *Gastroenterology*, **56**, 1033–1039.
98. Makino, I., Hashimoto, H., Shinozaki, K., Yoshino, K. & Nakayawa, S. (1975a) Sulfated and non-sulfated bile acids in urine, serum, and bile of patients with hepatobiliary diseases. *Gastroenterology*, **68**, 545–553.
99. Makino, I., Shinozaki, K., Yoshino, K. & Nakagawa, S. (1975b) Dissolution of cholesterol gallstones by ursodeoxycholic acid. *Japanese Journal of Gastroenterology*, **72**, 690–702.
100. Marin, G.A., Clark, M.L. & Senior, J.R. (1969) Studies of malabsorption occurring in patients with Laennec's cirrhosis. *Gastroenterology*, **56**, 727–736.
101. Matern, S., Hackenschmidt, J., Back, P. & Gerok, W. (1975) *Advances in Bile Acid Research*. Stuttgart: Schattauer Verlag.
102. McCormick, W.C., Bell, C.C., Swell, L. & Vlahcevic, Z.R. (1973) Cholic acid synthesis as an index of the severity of liver disease in man. *Gut*, **14**, 895–902.
103. Mehta, S.J., Struthers, J.E., Kaye, M.D. & Naylor, J.L. (1974) Biliary deoxycholate in patients with alcoholic cirrhosis. *Gastroenterology*, **67**, 674–679.
104. Mekhjian, H.S., Phillips, S.F. & Hofmann, A.F. (1971) Colonic secretion of water and electrolytes induced by bile acids: perfusion studies in man. *Journal of Clinical Investigation*, **50**, 1569–1577.
105. Metzger, A.L., Adler, R., Heymsfield, S. & Grundy, S.M. (1973) Diurnal variation in biliary lipid composition. Possible role in cholesterol gallstone formation. *New England Journal of Medicine*, **288**, 333–336.
106. Miettinen, T.A. (1971) Cholesterol production in obesity. *Circulation*, **44**, 842–850.
107. Miettinen, T.A. (1972) Lipid absorption, bile acids and cholesterol metabolism in patients with chronic liver disease. *Gut*, **13**, 682–689.
108. Miettinen, T.A. (1975) Bile acid metabolism. In *Handbook of Experimental Physiology* (Ed.) Kritchevsky, D. pp. 109–150. Berlin: Springer.
109. Miettinen, T.A. & Peltokallio, P. (1971) Bile salt, fat, water and vitamin B_{12} excretion after ileostomy. *Scandinavian Journal of Gastroenterology*, **6**, 543–552.
110. Miettinen, T.A. & Siurala, M. (1971) Micellar solubilisation of intestinal lipids and sterols in gluten enteropathy and liver cirrhosis. *Scandinavian Journal of Gastroenterology*, **6**, 527–535.
111. Miyai, K., Price, V.M. & Fisher, M.M. (1971) Bile acid metabolism in mammals. Ultrastructural studies on the intrahepatic cholestasis induced by lithocholic and chenodeoxycholic acids in the rat. *Laboratory Investigation*, **24**, 292–302.
112. Modai, M. & Theodor, E. (1970) Intestinal contents in patients with viral hepatitis after a lipid meal. *Gastroenterology*, **58**, 379–387.
113. Morris, J.S. & Heaton, K.W. (1974) The fate of labelled bile salts introduced into the colon. *Scandinavian Journal of Gastroenterology*, **9**, 33–39.
114. Morris, J.S., Low-Beer, T.S. & Heaton, K.W. (1973) Bile salt metabolism and the colon. *Scandinavian Journal of Gastroenterology*, **8**, 425–431.
115. Morrissey, K.P., McSherry, C.K., Swarm, R.L., Nieman, W.H. & Deitrick, J.E. (1975) Toxicity of chenodeoxycholic acid in the non-human primate. *Surgery*, **77**, 851–860.
116. Nair, P.P. & Kritchevsky, D. (1971) *The Bile Acids, Volume 1. Chemistry*. New York: Plenum.
117. Nair, P.P. & Kritchevsky, D. (1973) *The Bile Acids, Volume 2. Physiology and Metabolism*. New York: Plenum.
118. Nair, P.P. & Kritchevsky, D. (1976) *The Bile Acids, Volume 3. Pathophysiology*. New York: Plenum.
119. Nakagawa, S., Makino, I., Ishizaki, T. & Dohi, I. (1977) Dissolution of cholesterol gallstones by ursodeoxycholic acid. *Lancet*, **ii**, 367–370.
120. Neale, G., Lewis, B., Weaver, V. & Panveliwalla, D. (1971) Serum bile acids in liver disease. *Gut*, **12**, 145–152.
121. Nestel, P.J., Schreibman, P.H. & Ahrens, E.H. (1973) Cholesterol metabolism in human obesity. *Journal of Clinical Investigation*, **52**, 2389–2397.
122. Nicholas, P., Rinaudo, P.A. & Conn, H.O. (1972) Increased incidence of cholelithiasis in Laennec's cirrhosis. A postmortem evaluation of pathogenesis. *Gastroenterology*, **63**, 112–121.
123. Norman, A. & Strandvik, B. (1973) Excretion of bile acids in extrahepatic biliary atresia and intrahepatic cholestasis of infancy. *Acta Pediatrica Scandinavica*, **62**, 253–263.
124. Normann, P.T. & Norum, K.R. (1976) Newly synthesised hepatic cholesterol as precursor for cholesterol and bile acids in rat bile. *Scandinavian Journal of Gastroenterology*, **11**, 427–432.
125. Northfield, T.C. & Hofmann, A.F. (1973) Biliary lipid secretion in gallstone patients. *Lancet*, **i**, 747.
126. Northfield, T.C. & Hofmann, A.F. (1975) Biliary lipid output during three meals and an overnight fast. I. Relationship to bile acid pool size and cholesterol saturation of bile in gallstone and control subjects. *Gut*, **16**, 1–11.
127. Northfield, T.C. & McColl, I. (1973) Postprandial concentrations of free and conjugated bile acids down the length of the normal human small intestine. *Gut*, **14**, 513–518.
128. Northfield, T.C., LaRusso, N.F., Hofmann, A.F. & Thistle, J.L. (1975) Biliary lipid output during three meals and an overnight fast. II. Effect of chenodeoxycholic acid treatment in gallstone subjects. *Gut*, **16**, 12–17.
129. O'Maille, E.R.L., Richards, T.G. & Short, A.H. (1967) The influence of conjugation of cholic acid on its uptake and secretion: hepatic extraction of taurocholate and cholate in the dog. *Journal of Physiology*, **189**, 337–350.
130. Palmer, R.H. (1967) Formation of bile acid sulfates: a new pathway of bile acid metabolism in humans. *Proceedings of the National Academy of Sciences*, **58**, 1047–1050.
131. Palmer, R.H., Glickman, P.B. & Kappas, A. (1962) Pyrogenic and inflammatory properties of certain bile acids in man. *Journal of Clinical Investigation*, **41**, 1573–1577.
132. Paumgartner, G. (1977) Bile acids. *Clinics in Gastroenterology*, **6**, 1–250.
133. Paumgartner, G. & Stiehl, A. (1977) *Bile Acid Metabolism in Health and Disease*. Lancaster: Medical and Technical Publishing.
134. Pedersen, L. & Arnfred, T. (1975) Kinetics and pool size of chenodeoxycholic acid in cholesterol gallstone patients. *Scandinavian Journal of Gastroenterology*, **10**, 557–560.
135. Pedersen, L., Arnfred, T. & Hess Thaysen, E. (1974) Cholesterol kinetics in patients with cholesterol gallstones before and during chenodeoxycholic acid

treatment. *Scandinavian Journal of Gastroenterology*, **9**, 787–791.
136. Pedersen, L., Arnfred, T. & Hess Thaysen, E. (1975) Turnover of plasma cholesterol in patients with cholesterol gallstones. *Acta Medica Scandinavica*, **197**, 421–425.
137. Pertsemlidis, D., Panveliwalla, D. & Ahrens, E.H. (1974) Effects of clofibrate and of an estrogen-progestin combination on fasting biliary lipids and cholic acid kinetics in man. *Gastroenterology*, **66**, 565–573.
138. Pomare, E.W. & Heaton, K.W. (1973a) Bile salt metabolism in patients with gallstones in functioning gallbladders. *Gut*, **14**, 885–890.
139. Pomare, E.W. & Heaton, K.W. (1973b) The effect of cholecystectomy on bile salt metabolism. *Gut*, **14**, 753–762.
140. Pomare, E.W. & Low-Beer, T.S. (1975) The selective inhibition of chenodeoxycholate synthesis by cholate metabolites in man. *Clinical Science and Molecular Medicine*, **48**, 315–321.
141. Pomare, E.W., Heaton, K.W., Low-Beer, T.S. & Espiner, H.J. (1976) The effect of wheat bran upon bile salt metabolism and upon the lipid composition of bile in gallstone patients. *American Journal of Digestive Diseases*, **21**, 521–526.
142. Redinger, R.N. (1976) The effect of loss of gallbladder function on biliary lipid composition in subjects with cholesterol gallstones. *Gastroenterology*, **71**, 470–474.
143. Redinger, R.N. & Grace, D.M. (1977) Specificity and interrelation of bile acids on bile acid synthesis in the baboon. *Gastroenterology*, **72**, A-141.
144. Redinger, R.N. & Small, D.M. (1972) Bile composition, bile salt metabolism and gallstones. *Archives of Internal Medicine*, **130**, 618–630.
145. Reichen, J. & Paumgartner, G. (1975) Kinetics of taurocholate uptake by the perfused rat liver. *Gastroenterology*, **68**, 132–136.
146. Salen, G., Nicolau, G., Shefer, S. & Mosbach, E.H. (1975) Hepatic cholesterol metabolism in patients with gallstones. *Gastroenterology*, **69**, 676–684.
147. Schaffner, F. & Popper, H. (1969) Cholestasis is the result of hypoactive hypertrophic smooth endoplasmic reticulum in the hepatocyte. *Lancet*, **ii**, 355–359.
148. Schoenfield, L.J. (1969) The relationship of bile acids to pruritus in hepatobiliary disease. In *Bile Salt Metabolism* (Ed.) Schiff, L., Carey, J.B. & Dietschy, J.M. pp. 257–265. Springfield: Thomas.
149. Schwartz, C.C., Vlahcevic, Z.R., Berman, M., Halloran, L.G., Gregory, D.H. & Swell, L. (1976) Kinetic analysis of the metabolic pathways of cholesterol for bile acid (BA) synthesis and biliary cholesterol (BC) secretion in man. *Gastroenterology*, **70**, 992.
150. Schwarz, L.R., Schwenk, M. & Greim, H. (1977) Current concepts in intrahepatic cholestasis. *Acta Hepato-gastroenterologica*, **24**, 210–215.
151. Shaffer, E.A. & Small, D.M. (1977) Biliary lipid secretion in cholesterol gallstone disease. The effect of cholecystectomy and obesity. *Journal of Clinical Investigation*, **59**, 828–840.
152. Shefer, S., Cheng, F.W., Dayal, B., Hauser, S., Tint, G.S., Salen, G. & Mosbach, E.H. (1976) A 25-hydroxylation pathway of cholic acid biosynthesis in man and rat. *Journal of Clinical Investigation*, **57**, 897–903.
153. Small, D.M. (1970) The formation of gallstones. *Advances in Internal Medicine*, **16**, 243–264.
154. Smallwood, R.A. & Hoffman, N.E. (1976) Bile acid structure and biliary secretion of cholesterol and phospholipid in the cat. *Gastroenterology*, **71**, 1064–1066.
155. Sodhi, H.S. & Kudchodkar, B.J. (1973) Correlating metabolism of plasma and tissue cholesterol with that of plasma-lipoproteins. *Lancet*, **i**, 513–519.
156. Stiehl, A. (1977) Disturbances of bile acid metabolism in cholestasis. *Clinics in Gastroenterology*, **6**, 45–68.
157. Stiehl, A., Earnest, D.L. & Admirand, W.H. (1975) Sulfation and renal excretion of bile salts in patients with cirrhosis of the liver. *Gastroenterology*, **68**, 534–544.
158. Stiehl, A., Thaler, M.M. & Admirand, W.H. (1972) The effects of phenobarbital on bile salts and bilirubin in patients with intrahepatic and extrahepatic cholestasis. *New England Journal of Medicine*, **286**, 858–861.
159. Summerfield, J.A., Gollan, J.L. & Billing, B.H. (1976) Synthesis of bile acid monosulphates by the isolated perfused rat kidney. *Biochemical Journal*, **156**, 339–345.
160. Sutor, D.J. & Wooley, S.E. (1971) A statistical survey of the composition of gallstones in eight countries. *Gut*, **12**, 55–64.
161. Swell, L., Gregory, D.H. & Vlahcevic, Z.R. (1974) Current concepts of the pathogenesis of cholesterol gallstones. *Medical Clinics of North America*, **58**, 1449–1471.
162. Tamesue, N. & Juniper, K. (1967) Concentration of bile salts at the critical micellar concentration of human gallbladder bile. *Gastroenterology*, **52**, 473–479.
163. Theodor, E., Spritz, N. & Sleisenger, M.H. (1968) Metabolism of intravenously injected isotopic cholic acid in viral hepatitis. *Gastroenterology*, **55**, 183–190.
164. Thistle, J.L., Hofmann, A.F., Ott, B.J. & Yu, P.Y.S. (1976) Gallstone dissolution with chenodeoxycholic acid, 1969–1976: the Mayo Clinic studies. *Gastroenterology*, **70**, 943.
165. Thjodleifsson, B., Barnes, S., Chitranukroh, A., Billing, B.H. & Sherlock, S. (1977) Assessment of the plasma disappearance of cholyl-1 ^{14}C-glycine as a test of hepatocellular disease. *Gut*, **18**, 697–702.
166. Thomas, P.J. & Hofmann, A.F. (1973) A simple calculation of the lithogenic index of bile: expressing biliary lipid composition on rectangular coordinates. *Gastroenterology*, **65**, 698–700.
167. Trotman, B.W. & Soloway, R.D. (1975) Pigment vs. cholesterol cholelithiasis: clinical and epidemiological aspects. *American Journal of Digestive Diseases*, **20**, 735–740.
168. van Berge Henegouwen, G.P. & Hofmann, A.F. (1976) Measurement of gallbladder storage and emptying in man: method and preliminary application. *Gastroenterology*, **71**, A-39.
169. van Berge-Henegouwen, G.P. & Hofmann, A.F. (1977) Pharmacology of chenodeoxycholic acid. II. Absorption and metabolism. *Gastroenterology*, **73**, 300–309.
170. Van der Linden, W. (1971) Bile acid pattern of patients with and without gallstones. *Gastroenterology*, **60**, 1144–1145.
171. Vlahcevic, Z.R., Prugh, M.F., Gregory, D.H. and Swell, L. (1977) Disturbances of bile acid metabolism in parenchymal liver cell disease. *Clinics in Gastroenterology*, **6**, 25–43.
172. Vlahcevic, Z.R., Bell, C.C., Buhac, I., Farrar, J.T. & Swell, L. (1970) Diminished bile acid pool size in

patients with gallstones. *Gastroenterology,* **59,** 165–173.

173. Vlahcevic, Z.R., Bell, C.C., Gregory, D.H., Buker, G., Juttijudata, P. & Swell, L. (1972) Relationship of bile acid pool size to the formation of lithogenic bile in female Indians of the South-West. *Gastroenterology,* **62,** 73–83.

174. von Bergmann, K., Mok, H.Y.I. & Grundy, S.M. (1976) Distribution of the bile acid pool in the fasting state in man. *Gastroenterology,* **71,** A-41.

175. Wagner, C.I., Trotman, B.W. & Soloway, R.D. (1976) Kinetic analysis of biliary lipid excretion in man and dog. *Journal of Clinical Investigation,* **57,** 473–477.

176. Webster, K.H., Lancaster, M.C., Hofmann, A.F., Wease, D.F. & Baggenstoss, A.H. (1975) Influence of primary bile acid feeding on cholesterol metabolism and hepatic function in the Rhesus monkey. *Mayo Clinic Proceedings,* **50,** 134–138.

177. Weiner, I.M. & Lack, L. (1968) Bile salt absorption; enterohepatic circulation. In *Handbook of Physiology, Section 6: Alimentary Canal, Vol. III: Intestinal Absorption* (Ed.) Code, C.F. pp. 1439–1455. Washington: American Physiological Society.

178. Yoshida, T., McCormick, W.C., Swell, L. & Vlahcevic, Z.R. (1975) Bile acid metabolism in cirrhosis. IV. Characterisation of the abnormality in deoxycholate metabolism. *Gastroenterology,* **68,** 335–341.

Chapter 13

Bilirubin Metabolism and Hyperbilirubinaemic Disorders

JOHN GOLLAN
RUDI SCHMID

Bilirubin is the principal waste product resulting from the degradation of haem in mammals. Its formation reflects the continuing turnover of haem and essential haemoproteins such as haemoglobin, myoglobin and cytochromes; under physiological conditions the overall rate of bilirubin formation is equalled by a comparable rate of haem synthesis. In humans, the relatively low plasma bilirubin concentration observed under physiological conditions, 5.1 to 17.1 μmol/l (0.3 to 1.0 mg/dl),[80] represents a balance between the rate of production and the hepatic clearance of bilirubin. Consequently, enhanced production of bilirubin or its impaired handling in the liver, caused by abnormalities of uptake, conjugation, or secretion of the pigment into bile, are manifested by hyperbilirubinaemia. Jaundice (icterus) is usually apparent by clinically yellow colouration of the sclerae, mucous membranes and skin when the plasma bilirubin concentration has reached values in excess of 50 μmol/l (3 mg/dl). When hyperbilirubinaemia develops abruptly, the appearance of jaundice may lag one to two days behind the rise in plasma bilirubin concentration. Although hyperbilirubinaemia per se only rarely results in secondary tissue damage, in the form of encephalopathy, haemolysis or renal tubular dysfunction, it is of considerable clinical and pathophysiological interest as a manifestation of a variety of inherited and acquired disease processes. In addition, a basic understanding of bilirubin metabolism has direct application for the hepatic transport of other organic anions or xenobiotics which share similar pathways of metabolism and excretion.

In this chapter, consideration will be given primarily to the recent developments in bilirubin metabolism, to the pathophysiology of jaundice, and to the various clinical disorders of bilirubin metabolism, with emphasis on the hereditary syndromes. Several recent reviews contain comprehensive discussions of various aspects of bilirubin metabolism and hyperbilirubinaemia.[22, 40, 42, 45, 58, 63, 89, 142, 174, 336, 339, 340, 341]

BILIRUBIN METABOLISM

Physicochemical Properties of Bilirubin

Bilirubin consists of a chain of four pyrrole rings linked by three carbon bridges (a central $—CH_2—$ and two outer $—CH=$ groups). In the vast majority of naturally occurring mammalian bile pigments, the sequence of the four methyl, two vinyl, and two propionic acid side chains is the same, since they are formed by cleavage of the cyclic tetrapyrrole ferroprotoporphyrin IX (haem) at the α-methene bridge position (i.e. between the pyrrole rings bearing the vinyl groups). Recent spectroscopic and x-ray crystallographic studies have demonstrated that crystalline bilirubin IX–α has the involuted structure shown in Figure 13.1.[86] The double bonds adjacent to the two outer rings are constrained to a Z-Z (or trans-) configuration, and the hydrophilic —COOH and —NH groups are linked by strong intramolecular hydrogen bonds, both in the solid state and probably in solution. This leaves no sites for attachment of water and hence the naturally occurring bilirubin IX-α (Z-Z) is virtually insoluble in water (approximately 0.1 μmol/l at pH 7.4)[91] but surprisingly lipid soluble and soluble in non-polar organic solvents such as chloroform and dimethylsulphoxide.[266] In alkaline solution the hydrogen bonds are opened and several hydrophilic sites are exposed, forming the divalent anion, the consequence of which is greatly enhanced solubility in polar solvents.

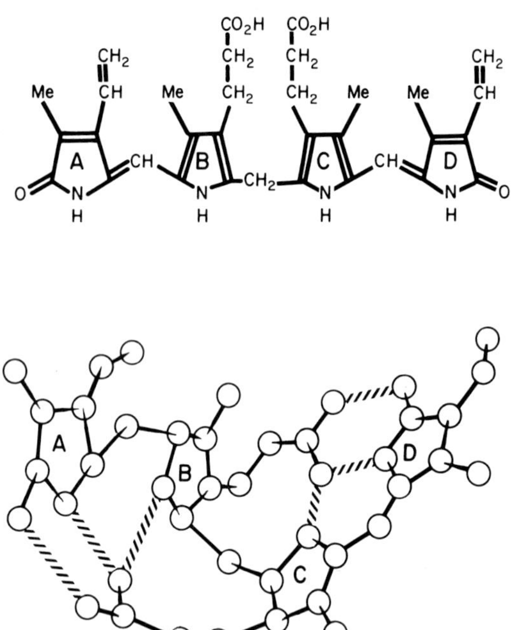

Figure 13.1. Structure of bilirubin IX-α: conventionally written structure (top panel) and involuted hydrogen-bonded structure (bottom panel). In the latter, the propionic acid groups of pyrrole rings B and C are linked to the nitrogens of the opposite pyrrole rings (interrupted lines). From Schmid,[336] with kind permission of Williams & Wilkins.

In aqueous solution, the bilirubin IX-α anion may be cleaved at the central —CH_2— bridge and the non-identical left and right halves may then spontaneously reunite at random (dipyrrole exchange). This leads to formation in vitro of III-α and XIII-α isomers,[267] both of which are found as minor constituents in commercial bilirubin preparations. In mammals, very small amounts of haem may be cleaved at the non-α carbon bridge positions, giving rise to β-, γ- and δ-isomers of bilirubin IX, which appear in trace amounts in the bile.[73, 85] Characterization of these isomeric pigments has shown that in contrast to bilirubin IX-α they are unable to form intramolecular hydrogen bonds and, as a result of their increased polarity, are excreted in the bile of rats largely as unconjugated pigments.[72] It has been postulated that rotation of either of the outer pyrrole rings of bilirubin IX-α at the double bonds may give rise to geometric isomers which differ physically from the normal Z-Z configuration. [265] Indeed, it appears likely that the E-E, Z-E, or E-Z forms may be produced by photo-isomerization,[249] and since intramolecular hydrogen bonding is absent in these geometric isomers this may be the mechanism whereby bilirubin IX-α (unconjugated) is excreted in the bile of hyperbilirubinaemic infants[256] and Gunn rats during phototherapy.[298, 407]

Although bilirubin IX-α (Z-Z) accounts for most of the excreted bile pigments in mammals, it cannot be secreted into bile in its native form. This problem has been circumvented by the development of a series of conjugating mechanisms in the liver, which enzymatically convert the lipid-soluble internally hydrogen-bonded pigment to more polar and readily excreted carbohydrate esters, particularly glucuronides. The esterification of bilirubin IX-α occurs on the propionic side chains and disrupts the intramolecular hydrogen bonds of the —COOH groups so that the central —CH_2— bridge is exposed, rendering the pigment less stable and more susceptible to autoxidation.[146] Physiological properties of the bilirubin IX-α conjugates and presumably of the soluble bilirubin isomers (e.g. IX-β, IX-γ, IX-δ and IX-α (E-E)), which do not form intramolecular hydrogen bonds, are strikingly different from those of bilirubin IX-α (Z-Z). In contrast to the water-soluble conjugates which are excreted as such in bile or urine, unconjugated bilirubin IX-α diffuses freely across most biological membranes such as the blood–brain barrier,[123] placenta[332] and intestinal and gallbladder epithelium.[239, 297] Thus, conjugation confers on the pigment the properties that inhibit its intestinal reabsorption and permit its elimination from the body. Moreover, bilirubin encephalopathy is never seen in conjugated hyperbilirubinaemia, regardless of the plasma level.

Sources of Bilirubin

Daily bilirubin production in adults measured by endogenous CO production,[108,234] or in turnover studies with radiolabelled bilirubin[46] averages 250 to 350 mg or 3.8 ± 0.6 (mean ± s.e.) mg/kg. Since haem is degraded in vivo to yield equimolar amounts of bilirubin and CO, the measurement of CO production reflects the total body haem turnover, whereas plasma bilirubin turnover measures only that pigment fraction which enters the plasma compartment prior to excretion (and hence fails to account for the bilirubin fraction formed in the liver from turnover of intrinsic haem compounds, which is excreted directly into the bile[223]). Plasma bilirubin turnover studies yield values, therefore, which are slightly lower than those calculated from the rate of CO production.[48]

The prosthetic haem moiety of haemoglobin is the major source of bilirubin and in humans accounts for about 70 per cent of the excreted pigment. All mammalian cells contain varying amounts of haem, in the form of haemoproteins (e.g. mitochondrial and microsomal cytochromes) which are essential for aerobic metabolism. With the notable exception of the liver, however, the tissue concentrations of these haemoproteins are so low, or their rates of turnover so slow (e.g. myoglobin) that their contribution to total bilirubin production is insignificant. Evidence for non-erythroid sources of bilirubin was first provided by injection of the haem precursor glycine, isotopically labelled, into humans.[178,253] The label was recovered in faecal stercobilin and, as expected, the major peak of labelled stercobilin excretion corresponded to the destruction of senescent erythrocytes (100 to 140 days), but between 10 and 20 per cent of the labelled pigment appeared within the first few days after administration of the glycine. Further studies established that production of this 'early-labelled bilirubin' (ELB) begins within minutes of administration of the labelled precursor, achieves maximum levels in one to three hours, and subsequently declines asymptotically over a period of several days.[340] Using isotopically labelled δ-amino laevulinic acid (ALA), which is preferentially incorporated into the haem of liver cells rather than into haemoglobin of maturing erythroid cells in bone marrow, the existence of two or more ELB components has been demonstrated.[319,399] The initial component appears to be derived largely from haemoproteins and haem in the liver, and the second component predominantly from the premature destruction of newly formed erythrocytes, either in the marrow or soon after their release into the circulation. The latter fraction appears to be responsible for only a minor fraction of the ELB in normal rats or humans.[316]

Initial estimates of the hepatic contribution to total bilirubin production in normal subjects ranged from 10 to 20 per cent,[316] but recent observations suggest that this fraction may be greater than had previously been assumed, ranging between 23 and 37 per cent.[50,216,223] Although it appears that the initial ELB component itself may comprise several phases, it has not yet been possible to equate these with specific haem or haemoprotein compounds in the liver. It is assumed, however, that hepatic bilirubin is formed primarily from turnover of the microsomal cytochromes P-450 and b_5, catalase, tryptophan pyrrolase, and mitochondrial cytochrome-*b*. A priori, cytochrome P-450 which mediates the oxidative biotransformation of many lipophilic compounds[159] would be expected to provide a major contribution, as it has been estimated in the rat that this haemoprotein requires at least 70 per cent of the total haem synthesized in the liver.[263] Moreover, when hepatic cytochrome P-450 synthesis is accelerated by treatment with xenobiotics, the shape and size of the ELB peak is significantly altered.[247,342] Catalase is the only other hepatic haemoprotein which is likely to provide a major contribution to ELB formation, since the molecule has a relatively short biological half-life, and is a tetramer containing four haem groups.[237] Analysis of the early phase of the ELB peak indicates that the liver[247] and developing erythroid cells[400,401] contain small pools of 'free' haem, which exhibit rapid turnover rates (60 to 90 min), exceeding those of any known haemoproteins.[64,65] It has been postulated that in the liver this pool represents haem, newly formed in the mitochondria, in transit to the subcellular sites of haemoprotein synthesis.[334]

Although the latter component(s) of ELB are also derived largely from turnover of hepatic haem, the normally small erythropoietic fraction may increase in magnitude and distort the shape of the ELB peak when erythropoiesis is accelerated or abnormal. In clinical disorders associated with premature destruction of developing or young erythroid cells ('ineffective erythropoiesis'),[191,317] such as the megaloblastic anaemias, iron deficiency anaemia, sideroblastic anaemia, thalassaemia minor, congenital erythropoietic porphyria and lead poisoning,[299] between 30 and 80 per cent of the faecal bile pigments may originate from this source. As could be expected, a decreased erythropoietic contribution to the ELB peak is observed in patients with aplastic anaemia.[30]

Formation of Bilirubin

In humans most normal erythrocytes are sequestered from the circulation after approximately 120 days by the reticuloendothelial cells ('mononuclear phagocytic cells') of the spleen, liver, or bone marrow.[190] Intracellular (extravascular) lysis follows within minutes and the degradation of haemoglobin then proceeds within the phagocytic cells. In haemolytic states or after splenectomy, the role of the hepatic sinusoidal cells in erythrocyte removal is enhanced.[66, 208]

In contrast to intact altered red cells which are sequestered and catabolized by the reticuloendothelial system, free haemoglobin, whether released into the plasma by intravascular haemolysis or administered intravenously, is taken up predominantly by hepatic parenchymal cells and converted to bile pigment.[66, 197] The hepatic parenchymal cells are also largely responsible for uptake of the haem moiety of haptoglobin-bound haemoglobin, methaemoglobin, methaemalbumin, haemin, and haem-haemopexin.[63, 281] It is not known whether bilirubin formed in the parenchymal cells, following the removal of haem from the circulation, is directly secreted into bile or first refluxes back into the plasma bilirubin pool, as occurs for the initial component of ELB[38, 223] or following the infusion of biliverdin.[165] In the presence of severe intravascular haemolysis, when the plasma haptoglobin-binding capacity is exceeded, free haemoglobin is filtered by the glomeruli and then partially re-absorbed and degraded by the proximal tubule cells of the kidney.[98] Thus, the parenchymal cells of both the liver and kidney assume importance as sites of bilirubin formation in the presence of intravascular haemolysis.[307] The observation that significant haemoglobinaemia or methaemalbuminaemia is unusual in haemolytic states, whereas unconjugated hyperbilirubinaemia is relatively common, indicates that the rate of haem degradation generally exceeds the rate of haemoglobin release and probably also exceeds the maximum rate of bilirubin removal by the liver.[340]

When haemoglobin is catabolized the globin moiety is degraded and the products returned to the amino acid pool. The remaining ferroprotoporphyrin ring is cleaved by oxidative cleavage of the α-meso-bridge carbon atom which is eliminated as CO (Figure 13.2). The haem iron is transferred to iron-carrying proteins (e.g. ferritin) and partially re-utilized for haem synthesis. A specific haem-cleaving enzyme, microsomal haem oxygenase,[365] has been identified and found to be most active in those tissues which are normally concerned with the

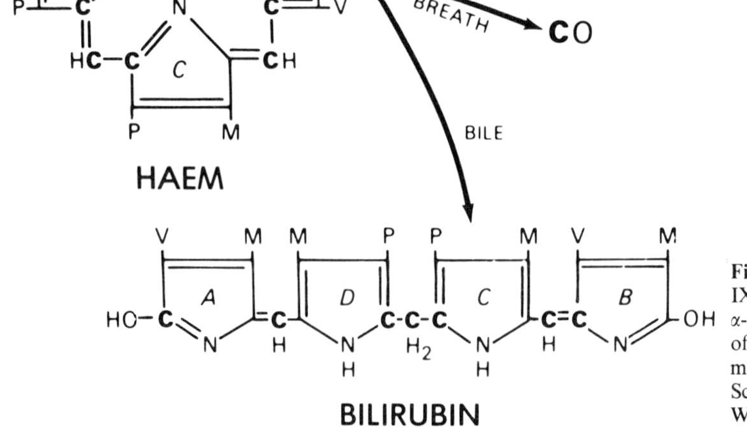

Figure 13.2. Conversion of protohaem IX to bilirubin IX-α. Cleavage of the α-methene bridge results in formation of equimolar amounts of iron, carbon monoxide and bilirubin IX-α. From Schmid,[335] with kind permission of William J. Dornan, Inc.

degradation of haem. Haem oxygenase activity in the liver, spleen, bone marrow, macrophages, renal tubules and brain (choroid plexus) can be stimulated three- to fivefold by haem or haemoglobin, presumably as a result of substrate-mediated enzyme induction.[340, 367] This adaptive response provides an efficient mechanism to catabolize the increased amounts of haemoglobin released in haemolytic disorders or internal haemorrhage (e.g. subcutaneous, pleural, or subarachnoid). Haem oxygenase has recently been purified to apparent homogeneity from pig spleen[403] and partially purified from rat liver,[258] and the enzyme appears to be distinct from cytochrome P-450, even though both are terminal oxidases of the microsomal electron-transport system. The finding of an inverse relationship between the level of cytochrome P-450 and haem oxygenase activity in a variety of experimental systems suggests, however, that the former may be indirectly involved in haem catabolism. Activity of haem oxygenase, which is rate limiting in the overall conversion of haem to bilirubin, is dependent on molecular oxygen (3 mol of O_2 are consumed per mol of haem degraded) and NADPH, with the latter being regenerated by microsomal NADPH-cytochrome-*c* reductase.[366] Although some details of the haem oxygenase reaction remain uncertain, evidence obtained from in vitro model systems[339] and recent animal studies using $^{18}O_2$ combined with mass spectrometric analysis[96, 97] are consistent with the following concepts. Cleavage of the protoporphyrin ring requires the presence of a central iron[95] or cobalt atom,[257] since free porphyrins do not yield linear tetrapyrroles and are excreted unchanged. Microsomal haem oxygenase exhibits a high degree of substrate specificity and is most active with free haem or haem loosely associated with protein (e.g. methaemalbumin). It is postulated that in the enzymatic degradation of haemoproteins, including haemoglobin, haem is dissociated from its parent apoprotein and bound to haem oxygenase in the membrane of the endoplasmic reticulum in such a manner that oxidation at the β-, γ-, and δ-carbon bridges is prevented.[94] The enzyme-bound haem, reduced to its ferrous form by NADPH, binds a molecule of molecular oxygen, which then probably is activated by the reduced haem-iron. The activated oxygen attacks the α-methene carbon bridge of the haem to form α-hydroxyhaem. This unstable intermediate reacts spontaneously with additional molecular oxygen at the hydroxylated α-bridge to produce a biliverdin–iron complex, which is hydrolysed to biliverdin IX-α and CO. In the presence of molecular oxygen and a reducing system haem thus mediates its own destruction. In many non-mammalian vertebrates (e.g. birds and amphibia) haem degradation terminates at this step and consequently the green tetrapyrrole biliverdin is excreted in bile, probably in the unconjugated form. In mammals biliverdin is hydrogenated to bilirubin (Figure 13.3) by the cytosolic NADPH-dependent enzyme biliverdin reductase,[368] which has a stereochemical preference for the IX-α isomer of biliverdin.[110] Since this enzyme is most abundant in tissues with high haem oxygenase activities and always appears to be in excess, biliverdin is rarely detected in human plasma or bile. Recent in vivo studies have indicated that the total time required for the chemical transformations involved in the formation of biliverdin, its reduction to bilirubin, and the conjugation and excretion of bilirubin is of the order of one to two minutes.[97, 165]

Plasma Bilirubin Transport

Unconjugated bilirubin is only sparingly soluble in aqueous solutions at physiologic pH. In plasma, it is bound reversibly to albumin by one high affinity site, which has a reported binding constant at 37°C of 3×10^7 $(\text{mol/l})^{-1}$.[204] The histidine residues of albumin are essential for the binding of bilirubin at this locus, and arginine and tyrosine may also be involved.[206] Since this primary binding site is relatively hydrophobic, low concentrations of water-soluble organic anions that also bind to albumin do not readily displace bilirubin;[292] in addition, pH changes within the physiological range do not significantly alter the dissociation of bilirubin from this site.[291] Beyond a molar ratio of 1 : 1, bilirubin binds to albumin on at least two lower affinity sites. Bilirubin can be displaced from these secondary sites by other organic anions, and small reductions in pH also result in an increased dissociation of the pigment from albumin.[287] The unbound or free bilirubin fraction in plasma, although exceedingly small, is of great physiological significance because only unbound bilirubin is available for transit across cell membranes, such as the blood–brain barrier. Direct analytical methods for the determination of free bilirubin in plasma are not yet available;[89] binding studies performed with crystalline human albumin preparations do not necessarily reflect the in vivo binding of bilirubin in hyperbilirubinaemic

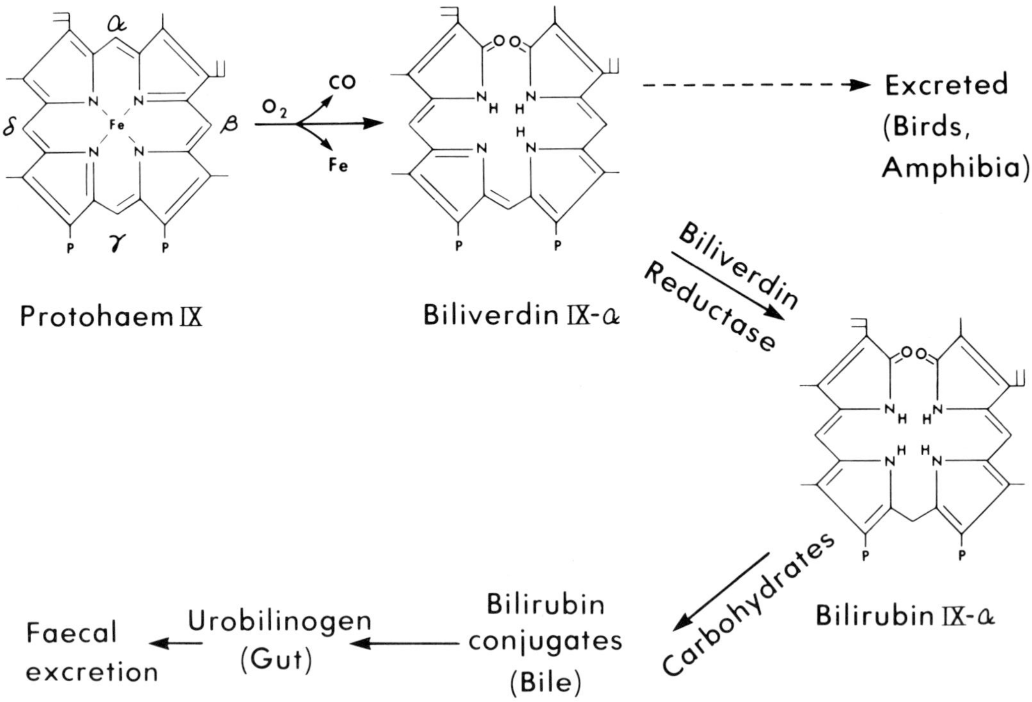

Figure 13.3. The metabolic degradation of protohaem IX to bile pigments in mammals and other vertebrates. From Schmid,[335] modified and reproduced with kind permission of William J. Dornan, Inc.

plasma.[207] Brodersen[89] has calculated that the plasma concentration of free bilirubin in normal adults is of the order of 0.12 nmol/l (7 pg/dl), and from the peroxidase technique described by Jacobsen and Wennberg[207] the safe upper limit of free bilirubin in neonates, beyond which kernicterus may occur, is shown to be about 50 nmol/l (2.9 ng/dl). This level of free bilirubin is achieved when approximately 80 per cent of the high-affinity binding sites of albumin are saturated with bilirubin.

The long-chain fatty acids are amongst those compounds that compete with bilirubin for common binding sites on the albumin molecule. Although fatty acids are normally transported bound to albumin without interfering with bilirubin binding, increasing the molar ratio of fatty acids to albumin up to 4:1 progressively blocks the binding of bilirubin at the primary site and forces its transport at secondary sites, making it susceptible to displacement by water-soluble organic anions. At higher molar ratios of fatty acid to albumin (⊳5 : 1), there is also direct competition for binding between fatty acid and bilirubin at the secondary sites.[295] Since human breast milk contains high concentrations of fatty acids, the elevated levels of free fatty acids present in the plasma of breast-fed infants may result in the displacement of bilirubin from albumin.[402] A large number of drugs can competitively displace bilirubin from its binding site on albumin and potentially increase the risk of kernicterus in jaundiced newborn infants. These have been reviewed by Brodersen[89] and include certain sulphonamides (e.g. sulphisoxazole), antibiotics (e.g. penicillin derivatives), analgesics (e.g. salicylate and phenylbutazone), food additives (e.g. parabenes), x-ray contrast media for cholangiography, and diuretics (e.g. furosemide).[351, 387] Other compounds, including the benzodiazepines, are bound strongly to albumin but do not displace bilirubin as they presumably bind to different molecular sites.[92] It is thus important that all drugs used in newborns or in pregnant or lactating women should be considered with regard to their ability to displace bilirubin from albumin.

Conjugated bilirubin also is transported in the plasma bound to albumin[205] but its affinity for the protein appears to be less than that of the unconjugated pigment. This may explain the observation that the non-protein-bound fraction of conjugated bilirubin (which accounts for <1 per cent of total plasma conjugated bilirubin in jaundiced patients), but not unconjugated bilirubin,[153] is freely filtered by the glomeruli; this filtered fraction is largely reabsorbed by the renal tubules[163] with the residual non-reabsorbed component giving rise to the bilirubinuria which is characteristic in hepatocellular and cholestatic jaundice.

Hepatic Uptake of Bilirubin

Under normal circumstances unconjugated bilirubin entering the plasma is rapidly cleared by the liver. It is generally assumed that bilirubin is separated from the carrier albumin prior to its uptake by the liver cell.[66, 172] The sinusoidal surface of the cell membrane may initiate the uptake process by interacting with the albumin molecule on receptor sites which bind bilirubin and detach it from its carrier protein.[82] The uptake mechanism appears to be a carrier-mediated, saturable process that obeys Michaelis–Mentin kinetics, and is shared by a variety of other organic anions (e.g. bromsulphthalein and indocyanine green) which exhibit mutually competitive inhibition.[173, 330] Bile acids on the other hand do not compete with bilirubin for hepatic uptake.[303] The finding in a mutant strain of Southdown sheep of impaired hepatic uptake of a variety of organic anions, including bilirubin,[112, 276] lends support to the existence of a common carrier-mediated system, which may involve integral proteins of the sinusoidal plasma membrane.[314, 392] The hepatic uptake system operates far below saturation at normal plasma bilirubin concentrations, and in experimental animals the maximal initial uptake rate has been shown to exceed greatly the steady-state excretory transport maximum; thus, the uptake of bilirubin does not appear to be the rate-limiting step in its excretion.[303]

Direct experimental evidence obtained in animals has established that the flux of bilirubin and other organic anions across the plasma membrane is bidirectional.[173, 188, 330] Compartmental analysis of radiobilirubin plasma disappearance curves suggests that, in normal individuals, about 40 per cent of the bilirubin taken up by the hepatocytes in a single pass through the liver refluxes unchanged to the plasma.[46] In Gilbert's syndrome,[47, 223] congenital non-haemolytic jaundice[80] and Gunn rats,[330] despite the presence of unconjugated hyperbilirubinaemia, the rate of hepatic bilirubin uptake is reported to be normal although there is a corresponding increase in reflux to the plasma. Hence the initial hepatic uptake of bilirubin appears to be independent of its cytoplasmic binding and subsequent metabolism but, due to the bidirectional flux, *net* uptake reflects the irreversible removal of pigment by intracellular metabolic pathways. Conjugated bilirubin is taken up by the liver even more rapidly than unconjugated bilirubin and the two compounds compete with one another and other organic anions for hepatic uptake, suggesting that the uptake mechanism for conjugated bilirubin may be the same as that for unconjugated bilirubin.[354]

Significant amounts of bilirubin have been shown to accumulate in the normal liver, i.e. storage,[313, 396] but the low polarity of the pigment argues against its existence in the free form. Two protein fractions have been demonstrated in the hepatic cytosol and these exhibit a high affinity for bilirubin and, together with albumin, bind most of the intrahepatic pigment.[244] Ligandin,[251] which is also known as aminoazodye-binding protein B,[222] or Y protein,[244] is identical with glutathione *S*-transferase B.[184] In addition to bilirubin, it binds a variety of ligands including carcinogens, haem, synthetic dyes, cholecystographic agents and hormones.[12] Z protein,[244] which is probably identical with aminoazodye-binding protein A and fatty acid-binding protein,[290] has a lesser affinity but a greater capacity than ligandin for bilirubin; binding to Z protein occurs only after ligandin has become saturated. It appears likely that Z protein is involved principally with fatty acid transport since it has a high affinity for long-chain fatty acids and is found in intestinal mucosa, liver, myocardium, and other tissues which take up and metabolize fatty acids. Ligandin constitutes 6 per cent of the cytoplasmic protein in rat liver and is also found to a lesser extent in kidney and small intestine. The protein consists of two non-identical monomeric subunits which may be responsible for different catalytic and binding functions.[57]

It has been proposed that ligandin influences the net hepatic uptake of bilirubin specifically by reducing bilirubin efflux from the cell back into the plasma.[12] The evidence in support of this hypothesis remains circumstantial and it has yet to be demonstrated directly at a cellular level that hepatic bilirubin uptake depends critically on the presence of ligandin. Phylogenetic studies suggest that ligandin evolved with terrestrial reptiles, birds and mammals and that its presence correlated with the appearance of selective hepatic organic anion uptake.[246] In newborn monkeys and humans the 'maturation' of hepatic ligandin to adult levels during the first five to 10 days of life coincides with maturation of the hepatic uptake mechanism(s) for organic anions.[245] Drugs such as phenobarbitone which induce ligandin have been shown to accelerate the hepatic uptake of organic anions.[315] However, phenobarbitone treatment has many additional effects on the liver, including stimulation of hepatic blood flow and bile secretion, which may be responsible for this effect. Nevertheless, recent studies with the isolated perfused liver pre-treated with phenobarbitone[269] and in vivo in thyroidectomized rats, in which hepatic ligandin concentration is increased but hepatic blood flow reduced,[395] support the concept that ligandin may be involved in the regulation of bilirubin efflux from the liver. Opposing this view is the report that some inducers of ligandin (e.g. 3-methylcholanthrene) do not influence the hepatic uptake of organic anions.[264] Indeed, until recently it has been difficult to reconcile the suggestion that ligandin is involved in hepatic bilirubin uptake with the observations that purified ligandin has a lower binding affinity than plasma albumin for bilirubin,[217] and that bilirubin migrates with albumin rather than ligandin on gel chromatography.[82] It is now established, however, that the binding affinity of ligandin for bilirubin diminishes rapidly on fractionation of the isolated cytosol; thus ligandin prepared by moving boundary sedimentation (in which lower molecular weight molecules remain associated with the protein) exhibits a much higher binding activity than that obtained by zonal centrifugation.[274] Further studies have shown that in native cytosol most ligandin is bound to reduced glutathione. In this complexed form the cytosolic protein binds bilirubin more strongly than does albumin[275] and hence may serve to limit organic anion efflux from the liver. Very little is known about bilirubin transport within the hepatocytes, although it appears to be highly compartmentalized since bilirubin produced from hepatic haem turnover within the liver cell seems to utilize hepatic transport channels that differ from those carrying the pigment from plasma to bile.[223]

Bilirubin Conjugation

In the process of conjugation, bilirubin is esterified with polar endogenous molecules which greatly enhance the water solubility of the pigment and facilitate its excretion. In mammalian bile most of the excreted bilirubin is conjugated and, with the exception of Gunn rats or patients with unconjugated hyperbilirubinaemia undergoing phototherapy,[249,298] only trace amounts of the unconjugated pigment are present.

Esterification occurs on the carboxyl groups of one or both of the propionic acid side chains with a variety of carbohydrate moieties, forming mono- or diesters. The conjugates are unstable, since the two dipyrrolic halves of the molecule are able to rotate about the central methene bridge. Therefore, most analytical studies on the structure and formation of conjugates have utilized the more stable red azopigments which may readily be separated by thin-layer chromatography.[194] In this reaction bile pigments are coupled with diazotized anthranilate and the central —CH_2— bridge is cleaved to form two dipyrrolic azopigments with the ester linkages remaining unaffected. Using this approach together with recently developed quantitative methods for the direct separation of native tetrapyrroles[170, 370] it has been established that bilirubin β-D-diglucuronide (Figure 13.4) constitutes the major pigment

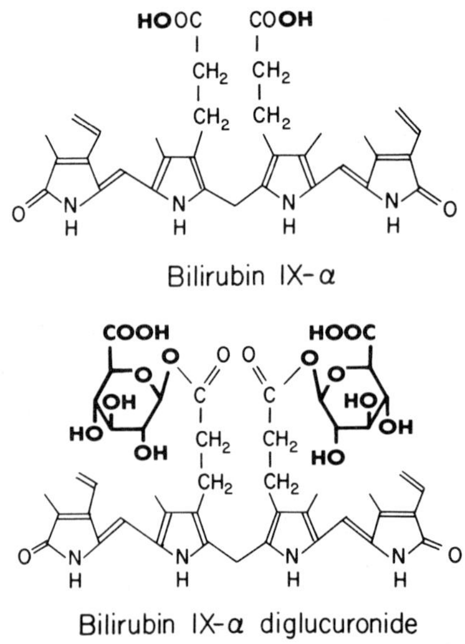

Figure 13.4. Structure of bilirubin IX-α and bilirubin IX-α diglucuronide. In the diglucuronide, the two molecules of glucuronic acid attached to the propionic acid groups prevent intramolecular hydrogen bonding between the latter groups and the pyrrole ring nitrogens. From Schmid,[336] with kind permission of Williams & Wilkins.

fraction in normal human bile[141, 169] and that monoglucuronides represent only a minor fraction. Trace amounts of other conjugates (e.g. glucosides and xylosides) have also been demonstrated[141] but they are of minor physiological significance. Although bilirubin glucuronide is the predominant bile pigment in mammals, significant species differences exist in the nature and relative distribution of other conjugates.[144] In contrast to humans, in whom the excretion of neutral glycosides is unimportant, the cat, mouse, rabbit and dog eliminate considerable amounts of bilirubin as glucoside and xyloside conjugates. In dogs, an extremely complex pattern of bilirubin conjugates, mostly acylglycosides, has been identified, including heterogeneous diconjugates containing two different carbohydrate moieties.[196] It is controversial whether bilirubin sulphate occurs in human and rat bile.[203,231,288]

Esterification of the propionic acid side chains of bilirubin with glucuronic acid forms the 1-*o*-acylglucuronides found in fresh normal bile. However, following cholestasis and during storage of bile in vitro, chromatographic analysis reveals additional azopigment bands[141] which result from isomerization to the non-*C*-1-glucuronides by sequential migration of the bilirubin acyl group from position 1 to positions 2, 3 and 4 of the sugar moiety (yielding 2-, 3-, and 4-*o*-acylglucuronides), particularly at slightly alkaline pH.[74] It is possible that such intramolecular rearrangement may also account for the complex bilirubin conjugates (e.g. aldobiouronides) which Kuenzle[231] has isolated in small amounts from pooled human T-tube bile.

Formation of bilirubin monoglucuronide is mediated by uridine diphosphate glucuronate glucuronyltransferase (UDP-glucuronyltransferase) which is located in the membranes of smooth and rough endoplasmic reticulum. The enzyme transfers the glucuronyl group from the co-substrate UDP-glucuronic acid to bilirubin or other acceptor molecules (e.g. *p*-nitrophenol).[127] The UDP-glucuronic acid itself is synthesized from glucose-1-phosphate through the formation of UDP-glucose, which is oxidized by a soluble dehydrogenase. Although glucuronyltransferase has been extensively studied,[404] its purification and characterization has been only partially successful.[99,177] As with other membrane-bound enzymes, interaction of the glucuronyltransferase with the phospholipid components of the microsomal membrane profoundly influences its activity, so that solubilization usually results in inactivation. The in vitro activity of hepatic microsomal preparations is greatly enhanced or 'activated' by a variety of agents which perturb membrane integrity (e.g. detergents). The use of digitonin 'activated' microsomes has been widely adopted as a means of determining bilirubin glucuronyltransferase activity with greater sensitivity than can be achieved for the 'native' enzyme activity.[193] Following digitonin treatment the enzyme exhibits altered kinetics, and although it has not been established that the assay accurately reflects the rate of hepatic bilirubin glucuronidation in vivo, the relative differences in activity measured in needle biopsy specimens obtained from both normal and hyperbilirubinaemic individuals (e.g. Gilbert's syndrome) appear to be retained.[67]

Hepatic glucuronyltransferase activity is enhanced by treatment with phenobarbitone, glutethimide and other drugs which apparently cause substrate-mediated enzyme induction.[75,406] From observations that the K_m for UDP-glucuronic acid in the in vitro assay of the enzyme is much higher than the UDP-glucuronic acid concentration in the liver in vivo,[380] and that the liver contains a considerable excess of glucuronyltransferase activity relative to that required for the elimination of bilirubin in the basal state,[235] it has been suggested that the availability of hepatic UDP-glucuronic acid, rather than the amount of enzyme present (except in Crigler–Najjar syndrome and Gunn rats in which glucuronyltransferase activity is congenitally absent), may control the rate of bilirubin conjugation in vivo, particularly in neonates.[235]

The measurement of glucuronyltransferase activity using non-bilirubin aglycones (e.g. *p*-nitrophenol) yields results which differ from those obtained when bilirubin is used as the substrate.[404] Indeed, it appears that the liver contains several glucuronyltransferases with overlapping substrate specificity for a variety of endogenous compounds and xenobiotics.[127,186,235,405] It is evident, however, that a specific conjugating form of the enzyme exists for bilirubin, since in patients with Crigler–Najjar syndrome and Gunn rats, bilirubin conjugation is not detectable, in vivo or in vitro, but glucuronide synthesis of numerous other substrates is unimpaired or only slightly reduced.[299,340]

Bilirubin glucuronyltransferase activity has been demonstrated also in the renal cortex and gastrointestinal mucosa,[127] and studies in hepatectomized animals confirmed that these tissues are the main sites of extrahepatic bilirubin formation.[151,324] Under physiological conditions it is unlikely that extrahepatic conjugation of bilirubin is of importance, but it has been shown that grafting of normal rat kidneys into Gunn rats results in the conjugation and subsequent biliary excretion of a considerable portion of the plasma bilirubin pool.[147] Extrahepatic conjugation results largely in formation of bilirubin monoglucuronide.[151] Moreover, the in vitro assay of hepatic UDP-glucuronyltransferase in rats measures predominantly or exclusively formation of the mono-, rather than the diglucuronide,[193] although recent studies in human and dog liver indicate some diglucuronide formation.[144] There is experimental evidence that synthesis of bilirubin diglucuronide from bilirubin may involve two enzymatic steps which have different pH optima.[209] Indeed, conversion of mono- to diglucuronide may be catalysed by a separate enzyme which is located in the hepatocyte at a site different from that of glucuronyltransferase.[187] The observation that bilirubin mono-, but not diglucuronide, normally accumulates within the liver cell is consistent with this concept.[396] This further supports the postulate by Jansen et al[210] that conversion of mono- to diglucuronide reflects transglucuronidation of monoglucuronides (resulting in equimolar formation of diglucuronide and unconjugated bilirubin), and that the enzyme catalysing this reaction is located in the liver plasma membrane (Figure 13.5). Several technical and conceptual questions have been raised with regard to this hypothesis,[336] including the apparent metabolic inefficiency of this postulated mechanism which necessitates deconjugation of one-half of the bilirubin monoglucuronide formed in order to produce diglucuronide. In addition, recent studies in intact rats infused with purified bilirubin monoglucuronide isotopically labelled in the glucuronyl group indicated that bilirubin diglucuronide is not formed in vivo by transglucuronidation of monoglucuronide.[71] Finally, considering the fact that monoglucuronide is readily excreted in the bile of patients with Crigler–Najjar and Gilbert's syndrome[143, 166, 168] and in normal individuals, it might reasonably be asked why bilirubin diglucuronide should be formed at all. Further investigation is necessary in order to resolve these questions and apparent ambiguities, and to clarify the mechanism and subcellular site of conversion of bilirubin monoglucuronide to diglucuronide.

Biliary Secretion of Bilirubin

Unlike the natural bilirubin IX-α (Z-Z), other isomers including the artificial isomers IX-β, -γ, and -δ[72] and probably the geometric E-isomers of bilirubin IX-α produced by photo-isomerization,[249] all of which lack intramolecular hydrogen bonding, are excreted directly into bile without conjugation with carbohydrate moieties. Normal human bile contains only very small amounts of unconjugated bilirubin IX-α (less than 1.2 per cent of total bilirubin in gallbladder bile), which appears to be excreted as such rather than to represent conjugated bilirubin that has been hydrolysed by β-glucuronidase.[87] Small amounts of unconjugated bilirubin are also found in the bile of patients with Gilbert's and Crigler–Najjar syndromes.[143, 338] Studies in a patient with sickle cell disease and pigment gallstones demonstrated that unconjugated bilirubin output is hyperbolically related to bile salt output, although maximum excretion of unconjugated pigment represented only 3 per cent of the total bilirubin output.[393] From the fact that a similar hyperbolic relationship exists for biliary lipids, cholesterol and phospholipids, this has been taken as indirect evidence that unconjugated

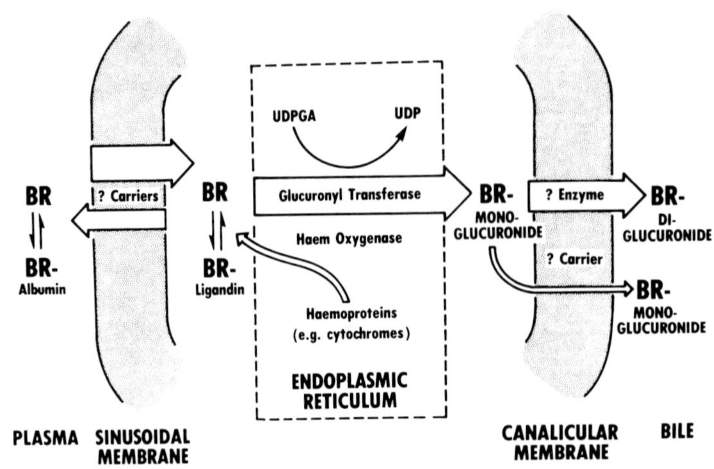

Figure 13.5. Bilirubin transport and conjugation in the hepatocyte. Bilirubin that has been transferred across the sinusoidal membrane into the hepatocyte is converted by microsomal glucuronyltransferase to bilirubin monoglucuronide. The monoconjugate is either excreted directly into bile or converted to diglucuronide (possibly by an enzyme located in the canalicular membrane) and then excreted. From Schmid,[336] modified and reproduced by kind permission of Williams & Wilkins.

bilirubin is transported into bile in the form of mixed micelles. This concept is supported by studies in Gunn rats, which have shown that the excretion of unconjugated bilirubin may be greatly enhanced by infusing either bile acids or conjugated bilirubin.[61, 102]

The mode of conjugated bilirubin transport within the hepatocytes and the potential role of the Golgi apparatus and microtubular system in the secretory process have not been defined. Furthermore, the determinants involved in the process of pigment secretion at the canalicular membrane level remain largely unknown. It is apparent, however, that secretion proceeds against a considerable concentration gradient and that the mechanism displays saturation kinetics, and operates with a lower capacity than either pigment uptake or conjugation.[149] It may therefore be assumed that secretion is rate limiting in the overall transport of bilirubin from plasma to bile.[173] The process probably involves a membrane carrier system which appears to be shared by a variety of endogenous and exogenous organic anions (e.g. bromsulphthalein [BSP], rose bengal, indocyanine green [ICG] and cholecystographic dyes) but is functionally distinct from that for bile acids.[4, 131, 148] It is not clear whether there is a single membrane carrier which serves to concentrate a variety of structurally unrelated anions or whether there are multiple systems which are subject to allosteric interaction.[148] These hypothetical carrier(s) may be genetically absent or defective in patients with the Dubin–Johnson syndrome and in mutant Corriedale sheep, in whom the secretion of conjugated bilirubin and BSP is markedly defective, whereas bile acid transport is unimpaired.[4, 182] In contrast to conjugated BSP, the excretion of unconjugated BSP is almost normal in the mutant Corriedale[25] and in Dubin–Johnson patients,[1] suggesting that at least two different canalicular carriers are involved in organic anion secretion.[25]

Despite the presence of separate secretory mechanisms for bile acids and for organic anions, these are not functionally independent of each other, since infusion of taurocholate substantially increases the maximum secretory rate (Tm) of bilirubin, BSP, ICG and iopanoic acid.[149, 175] This effect on Tm is specific for bile acids and is not produced by stimulants of bile salt-independent bile flow such as theophylline.[24, 155] From these observations Goresky[173] has proposed that, in addition to the canalicular membrane transport processes, the formation of mixed micelles at the canalicular surface or within the canalicular lumen may be an important determinant of net hepatic bilirubin transport. It is postulated that the passive binding to micelles creates a 'sink' which reduces the luminal concentration of conjugated bilirubin in the non-micellar phase of bile, decreasing its availability for back diffusion across the canalicular membrane. This association may thus create a net concentration gradient that favours flux of pigment into bile, thereby effectively reducing the energy barrier required for transport. Although the functional importance of micellar sequestration of bilirubin and other organic anions within the canalicular lumen has yet to be established, the concept is supported by the finding that conjugated bilirubin and BSP are present in bile almost entirely in the form of mixed micelles.[329, 382] A second hypothesis which has emerged from the observation that bilirubin Tm is increased by taurocholate infusion is that of a lobular gradient in the liver.[173, 175] This is based on the concept that a concentration gradient for bile acids exists in the sinusoidal blood from the portal to the central zone of the hepatic lobule, so that ordinarily only the more peripheral (periportal) hepatocytes are involved in the extraction and secretion of bile acids. During bile acid infusion centrilobular hepatocytes are progressively recruited for bile acid transport (which results in a flattened lobular profile for bile acid secretion). This postulated mechanism, which is supported by preliminary functional and morphological findings,[180, 215, 236] would readily explain the observed increase in bilirubin Tm associated with taurocholate infusion.

Fate of Bilirubin in the Gastrointestinal Tract

The absorption of conjugated bilirubin in both the gallbladder[297] and intestine[239, 240] is negligible because of its polar nature and molecular size. In healthy adults the conjugates probably remain largely intact during transit through the small intestine, so that there is no appreciable enterohepatic circulation of bilirubin. However, in the presence of intestinal stasis or obstruction and in newborns there is increased formation and absorption of unconjugated bilirubin; in the latter, this may contribute to neonatal hyperbilirubinaemia.[90, 308]

Bilirubin glucuronides are hydrolysed to the unconjugated pigment predominantly in the terminal ileum and colon by bacterial β-glucuronidase. Bilirubin is reduced by the action of intestinal bacteria to a complex series of colourless tetrapyrroles, collectively termed 'urobilinogen'.[129,384] It is not known whether deconjugation precedes reduction in the in vivo formation of urobilinogen. Urobilinogen can be formed from bilirubin in vitro by anaerobic cultures of *Clostridia*, *Bacteroides*, or mixed faecal flora[134,386] and the reaction appears to be mediated by enzymes bound to bacterial membranes.[372] Oral administration of broad-spectrum antibiotics greatly diminishes the formation of urobilinogen[384] and, in infants, lack of appropriate colonic flora during the first two to six months of life results in greatly reduced faecal urobilinogen excretion.[299] Normal adult faeces contain a mixture of urobilinogens and their corresponding orange coloured oxidation products, urobilins.[385] The ultimate composition of faecal pigments is probably dependent primarily on the nature of the bacterial flora of the colon. In normal subjects only about 50 per cent of the daily bilirubin turnover can be recovered as faecal urobilinogen (measured by Ehrlich's aldehyde reaction). There is, therefore, a poor correlation between bilirubin production and faecal urobilinogen excretion, so that measurement of faecal urobilinogen is of limited diagnostic value.[78]

Urobilinogen undergoes an enterohepatic circulation, although less than 20 per cent of the amount produced daily is re-absorbed since it is formed mostly in the colon where the absorption rate is low; about 90 per cent of this is promptly re-excreted by the liver into bile by the anionic transport system.[241,243] The remaining 10 per cent reaching the systemic circulation is excreted in the urine (approximately 2 per cent of daily urobilinogen production). Urinary urobilinogen is increased in haemolytic disorders and in patients with hepatocellular disease and/or portasystemic shunts.[54] The mechanism of renal excretion involves glomerular filtration of the non-protein-bound plasma fraction (approximately 20 per cent of total plasma urobilinogen) followed by tubular re-absorption and secretion.[88,248] Urinary urobilinogen excretion is related to urine pH, higher values being recorded in alkaline than in acid urine, and a diurnal variation has also been demonstrated.[385]

DISORDERS OF BILIRUBIN METABOLISM

Laboratory Methods

The routine determination of plasma bilirubin concentration is most commonly achieved by one of several modifications of the diazo reaction or by direct spectrophotometry.[60] Although bilirubin has a characteristic absorption spectrum, with a maximum at 460 nm when bound to albumin (or 453 nm in chloroform, dimethyl sulphoxide or common organic solvents), the presence of turbidity, haemoglobin and dietary lipochromes in plasma may interfere with direct spectrophotometric readings. Despite these limitations this method may be useful for the rapid and approximate estimation of total bilirubin concentration. In the more widely used diazo reaction, stable red-violet dipyrrolic azoderivatives are formed by the reaction of bilirubin with diazonium salts of aromatic amines, such as sulphanilic acid (van den Bergh reaction),[374] and the products formed are measured spectrophotometrically. The overall reaction is a multistep process[266] which leads to disruption of the bilirubin molecule into formaldehyde and two diazotized dipyrroles (azopigments). Since bilirubin IX-α is asymmetrically substituted, it forms non-identical pairs of azopigments, which are sometimes referred to as 'vinyl' and 'isovinyl' azoderivatives.

In plasma, bilirubin IX-α reacts very slowly with diazotized sulphanilic acid, but the reaction is greatly accelerated by addition of solvents such as methanol, ethanol, diphylline or caffeine benzoate ('indirect-reacting bilirubin'). These accelerators disrupt the intramolecular hydrogen-bonded structure of the unconjugated pigment, thereby facilitating reaction with the diazo reagent. In contrast, conjugated bilirubin in plasma reacts almost immediately without the addition of accelerators ('direct-reacting bilirubin'). In the method of Malloy and Evelyn[259] and its many modifications, methanol is employed as accelerator. Although the sensitivity of this method is reduced by the required dilution of plasma (which is necessary to prevent protein precipitation), and the presence of lipaemia and haemolysis may cause errors,[60] it is widely used in clinical practice. The most satisfactory procedure currently available for the determination of unconjugated bilirubin in plasma appears to be that of Michaelsson, Nosslin and Sjölin[278] which is based on the method of Jendrassik and Gróf,[211] and uses diphylline or caffeine benzoate as accelerator. The sensitivity of this method is enhanced by converting the azopigments from red to blue by the addition of alkali. Estimation of conjugated bilirubin is generally less accurate than that for the unconjugated pigment. Thus, in predominantly conjugated hyperbilirubinaemia only an approximate value is obtained for both the conjugated and total bilirubin levels. However, the estimates obtained are adequate for most clinical purposes, since it is generally sufficient to ascertain the relative degree to which conjugated or unconjugated bilirubin predominates in the plasma. More accurate determination of individual pigment concentrations does not provide additional diagnostic information.

A variety of other procedures has been advocated for the measurement of plasma bilirubin level,[189, 250] and different accelerating agents have been proposed, [252] but these do not appear to represent a significant advance over existing methods. Finally, methods have been developed using diazotized ethyl anthranilate or *p*-iodoaniline[194, 195, 376] which yield azopigments that can readily be extracted into organic solvents for chromatographic separation and quantification. These methods are more sensitive than the classical diazo procedure and have been applied successfully in the analysis of individual bilirubin conjugates, but have not been widely adopted for routine clinical assays.

Pathophysiology of Hyperbilirubinaemia

The plasma bilirubin in normal subjects is virtually all in the unconjugated form[39] and values obtained for conjugated bilirubin are probably largely spurious, representing artefacts inherent in the method employed. The normal plasma bilirubin concentration (5.1 to 17.1 μmol/l [0.3 to 1.0 mg/dl]) varies directly with bilirubin turnover and inversely with hepatic bilirubin clearance.[81] Whether estimated by means of this relationship or determined directly[311] the normal distribution is skewed, and slightly higher values have been observed in males than females. Individuals with a plasma unconjugated bilirubin level between 17 and 68 μmol/l (1 and 4 mg/dl) may have haemolysis, abnormal hepatic function, or both. The finding of concentrations persistently in excess of 68 μmol/l (4 mg/dl) implies reduced hepatic function, irrespective of the presence of haemolysis, since the maximum achievable rate of bilirubin production (eight times normal under steady-state conditions) seems to elevate plasma unconjugated bilirubin no higher than 60 to 68 μmol/l (3.5 to 4 mg/dl).[39] During acute haemolytic crises, such as occur in sickle cell disease or paroxysmal nocturnal haemoglobinuria, bilirubin production and plasma bilirubin may transiently exceed these levels.

Unconjugated hyperbilirubinaemia may be caused by accelerated pigment formation associated with haemolysis or 'ineffective erythropoiesis', by impaired hepatic blood flow or by defective hepatic uptake or conjugation of the pigment. Cholestasis due to impaired bile flow either at the canalicular or bile duct level results in accumulation of conjugated bilirubin in plasma. Despite recent progress in understanding of the nature of bile secretion, the mechanisms underlying defective canalicular bile flow have not yet been established. Nor is it known whether in cholestasis conjugated bilirubin refluxes to the sinusoidal plasma by reverse pinocytosis from the liver cell, or from damaged canaliculi either directly or via the intercellular space, or a combination of these postulated defects. With the exception of the familial hyperbilirubinaemias, the clinically important causes of jaundice attributable to primary liver disease probably involve more than one defect in hepatic transport and may also be associated with over-production of bilirubin. Hence, in diffuse hepatocellular injury (e.g., hepatitis or cirrhosis), the plasma concentrations of both conjugated and unconjugated bilirubin are increased, with the former usually predominating, although the relative proportion of the two pigments is variable and of little diagnostic significance. Since the specific abnormalities in bilirubin metabolism that lead to jaundice in diffuse liver disease are unclear, the subsequent discussion will consider only those causes of hyperbilirubinaemia which are attributable to identified and recognizable defects.

Unconjugated Hyperbilirubinaemia due to Increased Bilirubin Formation

Haemolysis per se generally gives rise to a mild degree of hyperbilirubinaemia as discussed in the previous section. Although the plasma bilirubin level increases linearly in relation to bilirubin production, the plasma bilirubin concentration may still be normal in patients with a 50 per cent reduction in red cell survival, provided that hepatic bilirubin clearance is normal. Although the unconjugated fraction predominates in haemolytic jaundice, increased plasma levels of conjugated bilirubin (>15 per cent of the total plasma bilirubin) may be present in association with hepatic dysfunction,[371] and in occasional patients with acute haemolytic crises, in whom the amount of bilirubin generated and conjugated may exceed the biliary secretory transport maximum for conjugated bilirubin.[327,357] Increased bilirubin production results in elevated excretion of faecal and urinary urobilinogen, but these parameters are of little value in the diagnostic evaluation of jaundice. Haemolysis due to hereditary abnormalities of erythrocytes (e.g., hereditary spherocytosis, pyruvate kinase deficiency, sickle cell disease) generally produces only a mild degree of jaundice which may present within a few days of birth or as recurrent episodes during later life, frequently in association with febrile illnesses. Cholelithiasis, reflecting precipitation of bilirubin, is the major complication of long-standing excessive bilirubin production.

Ineffective erythropoiesis is associated with the premature destruction of defective red cells in the bone marrow and consequent augmentation of the erythropoietic component of 'early-labelled bilirubin'. Diagnosis of the various disorders of haem, haemoglobin or erythroid cell formation which give rise to ineffective erythropoiesis (detailed under 'Sources of bilirubin', above) usually presents no difficulties. Jaundice is of a mild degree and the reticulocyte count is normal or only moderately increased, but elevated levels of faecal and urinary urobilinogen in the absence of a marked reduction in the survival of circulating red cells are characteristic of this condition.

Markedly increased ineffective erythropoiesis is the basis of a rare disorder known as 'primary shunt hyperbilirubinaemia'[201] or *'idiopathic dyserythropoietic jaundice'*.[37] Since the former name incorrectly implies that bilirubin is formed directly from the pyrrolic precursors of haem and not via the breakdown of haem, the latter title is more appropriate. This heterogeneous group of disorders is frequently familial and characterized by the onset of asymptomatic jaundice in the second or third decades of life, in the presence of a marked increase in faecal urobilinogen excretion and a normal or near normal red cell life span.[9, 202, 224, 379] Israels[200] reviewed 11 such cases in which about half had splenomegaly, but hepatomegaly was absent and liver function tests were uniformly normal, apart from an elevated plasma unconjugated bilirubin concentration (20 to 136 μmol/l [1.2 to 8 mg/dl]). The presence of values exceeding 68 μmol/l (4 mg/dl) in some patients suggested the coexistence of defective hepatic bilirubin clearance. In the majority of patients, the disorder was further characterized by a reticulocytosis, normoblastic erythroid hyperplasia of bone marrow and increased iron turnover with diminished red cell incorporation, reflecting the state of ineffective erythropoiesis. The underlying defect responsible for the high rate of haem turnover within the marrow remains unknown. In addition, some cases exhibit an increased serum iron concentration and haemosiderosis of hepatic parenchymal and Kupffer cells. A mild haemolytic anaemia with spherocytosis and increased osmotic fragility has also been described but, unlike congenital spherocytic anaemia, autohaemolysis and mechanical fragility tests were normal. Splenectomy resulted in a prolongation of red cell survival and a partial reduction in plasma bilirubin level, but marrow erythroid hyperplasia persisted and faecal urobilinogen excretion remained high. Although the prognosis of this rare, idiopathic form of ineffective erythropoiesis appears to be excellent, like other causes of enhanced bilirubin production, it predisposes to cholelithiasis.

Unconjugated Hyperbilirubinaemia due to Reduced Hepatic Clearance of Bilirubin

The major aspects of the pathogenesis and diagnosis of non-haemolytic unconjugated hyperbilirubinaemia in the neonatal period have been reviewed recently by Johnson,[213] Seligman,[345] Thaler,[369] and Schmid and McDonagh.[340] So-called *'physiologic jaundice'*, a transient elevation of plasma unconjugated bilirubin during the first week of life, is the most common form. The cause of this condition is multifactorial, reflecting accelerated erythrocyte breakdown, impaired hepatic uptake, conjugation and excretion of bilirubin by the newborn liver, and enhanced enterohepatic circulation of bilirubin. However, the quantitative contributions of these various factors have not been established.

Impaired hepatic bilirubin clearance due specifically to reduced hepatic uptake or competition for binding to Z protein or ligandin is associated with the administration of *drugs* such as rifampicin (and other rifamycin antibiotics),[2, 103, 221] bunamiodyl,[56] flavaspidic acid[188] and probenecid.[220] Plasma bilirubin concentration reverts rapidly to normal following discontinuation of the offending drug. Hepatic uptake of bilirubin and a variety of other organic anions is impaired in *mutant Southdown sheep*.[112] This condition is inherited as an autosomal recessive trait, and the animals exhibit chronic facial eczema due to phylloerythrin-mediated photosensitivity, a mild unconjugated hyperbilirubinaemia, and abnormal renal function.[340]

A mutant strain of Wistar rat described by Gunn[181] and subsequently by Malloy and Lowenstein[260] has provided a unique experimental model for investigation of the underlying metabolic defect in type I Crigler–Najjar syndrome (which it closely resembles), and for study of bilirubin metabolism in the newborn, and the mechanism and efficacy of phototherapy. The major characteristics of the *Gunn rat* have been considered in detail by Schmid and McDonagh.[340] The disorder is inherited as an autosomal recessive trait,[181] and the absence of hepatic bilirubin UDP-glucuronyltransferase activity gives rise to a severe unconjugated hyperbilirubinaemia (usually >120 μmol/l [>7 mg/dl]), which leads to tissue deposition of bilirubin and functional impairment of the central nervous system,[214] kidneys[101, 293] and thyroid.[167] Recent attempts to replace glucuronyltransferase in these mutant Gunn rats have been of interest because replacement of the enzyme in patients with Crigler–Najjar type I syndrome would represent a significant therapeutic advance. However, such experiments have met with only limited success. When rat hepatoma cells[325] or normal rat kidney[147] were grafted into homozygous Gunn rats, the recipients acquired the ability to conjugate endogenous bilirubin and excrete it in bile. Similarly, it has been claimed that the level of hyperbilirubinaemia was reduced in Gunn rats following infusion of enzyme-replete hepatocytes into the portal vein[179, 362] but the results of this series of experiments were less convincing because they lacked some essential controls. Grafting normal liver tissue on to the liver of enzyme-deficient rats has produced conflicting results[280, 375] and further studies, including the demonstration of bilirubin glucuronide in the bile of grafted animals, are necessary in order to assess the potential of this form of enzyme replacement.[229]

Chronic non-haemolytic unconjugated hyperbilirubinaemia is a feature of several genetically transmitted syndromes in humans. This spectrum of disorders is distinguished primarily on the basis of the plasma bilirubin level, the response to phenobarbitone administration, and the presence or absence of bilirubin glucuronide in bile. While most patients can readily be categorized as having one of the three syndromes listed in Table 13.1, occasional patients manifest features which make precise classification difficult. The three syndromes may be defined as follows: Crigler–Najjar type I syndrome,[116] an extremely rare and almost invariably fatal form of severe unconjugated hyperbilirubinaemia, which is caused by a genetic defect in bilirubin conjugation similar to that found in homozygous Gunn rats; Gilbert's syndrome,[157] a relatively common, benign, and possibly heterogeneous condition presenting with a mild, fluctuating and often subclinical hyperbilirubinaemia; and a third condition characterized by an intermediate degree of hyperbilirubinaemia, arbitrarily defined as greater than 103 μmol/l (6 mg/dl), and clinical and biochemical features which merge with those of the other two syndromes. This last disorder is considered to be due to a partial defect in bilirubin conjugation and is commonly referred to as Crigler–Najjar type II syndrome.[15]

Crigler–Najjar Type I Syndrome (Congenital Non-haemolytic Jaundice with Glucuronyltransferase Deficiency)

Clinicopathological features

In 1952 Crigler and Najjar[116] reported a familial form of severe non-haemolytic jaundice associated with neurological dysfunction. Six infants from three interrelated families were observed with markedly elevated plasma bilirubin concentration (445 to 770 μmol/l [26 to 45 mg/dl]) which appeared between the first and third post-natal days and persisted throughout life. The plasma bilirubin was virtually all unconjugated, bilirubinuria was absent and there was no evidence of haemolysis. Hepatosplenomegaly was absent and hepatic histology and conventional liver function tests, including BSP clearance, were normal. Five of these icteric infants developed a neurological syndrome resembling kernicterus, which resulted in rapid deterioration and death by the age of 15 months. Autopsy examination of the brain in a 17-day-old infant revealed intense staining of the cerebral cortex and basal ganglia with bilirubin. The sixth affected child in this family group initially escaped overt neurological damage[105] and developed normally into the teens despite persistent hyperbilirubinaemia. Approaching the age of 15 and in the absence of an apparent precipitating event, this boy developed symptoms and signs closely resembling those of kernicterus which led to his death within six months.[84] In contrast to the autopsy findings in infants, pigment staining was not evident in the brain and the cerebral cortex was

Table 13.1. *Comparison of the Chronic Non-haemolytic Unconjugated Hyperbilirubinaemic Syndromes.*

	Type I Crigler–Najjar syndrome	Type II Crigler–Najjar syndrome	Gilbert's syndrome
Incidence	Rare M : F 1 : 1	Uncommon M : F 1 : 1	≤ 7% of population M : F 4 : 1
Mode of inheritance	Autosomal recessive	? Autosomal dominant with variable penetrance	? Autosomal dominant
Bilirubin UDP-glucuronyl-transferase activity	Absent	Markedly decreased or absent	Decreased
Associated defects	None	? Decreased hepatic bilirubin uptake	(a) Decreased hepatic uptake of bilirubin, BSP (≤ 40%) and ICG (≤ 20%); (b) mild haemolysis (≤ 50%)
Plasma bilirubin concentration (μmol/l [mg/dl])	308–855 (18–50), usually > 340 (> 20)	103–376 (6–22), usually < 340 (< 20)	≤ 103 (≤ 6), usually < 50 (< 3)
Age hyperbilirubinaemia recognized	1–3 days after birth	Usually 1st year of life; occasionally not until adulthood	Usually early adulthood; may be associated with fasting
Clinical features	Jaundice and kernicterus in infants; occasionally bilirubin encephalopathy in young adults	Usually asymptomatic jaundice, kernicterus rare	Asymptomatic or non-specific symptoms; occasional mild jaundice
Routine liver function tests, cholecystography, and liver histology	Normal	Normal	Normal
Bile	Usually pale yellow; contains a trace of unconjugated bilirubin and monoconjugates	Yellow; contains mostly bilirubin monoglucuronide	Normal colour; relative increase in monoglucuronide and decrease in diglucuronide
Effect of phenobarbitone on plasma bilirubin	None	Marked reduction	Reduction
Prognosis	Usually fatal in infancy, or later onset of neurological damage	Usually good; neurological damage rare	Good

normal, but neuronal loss and gliosis of the thalamus and basal ganglia were evident.[154] In addition, bilirubin deposits were found in the renal papillae, intestinal mucosa, endocardium, connective tissue and perivascular adventitia. In a further patient born in the same kindred,[105] and jaundiced since the second day of life, neuropsychiatric manifestations appeared at the age of 18 years in association with a rise in plasma bilirubin concentration to around 680 μmol/l (40 mg/dl).[77] Despite the development of severe extrapyramidal abnormalities and grand mal seizures her condition appeared to stabilize for about 12 months following a temporary reduction in plasma bilirubin level produced by exchange plasmapheresis.[49] Subsequently her neurological status fluctuated somewhat and tended to correlate with plasma bilirubin levels (340 to 600 μmol/l); overall her condition deteriorated inexorably and she died aged 23 years.[328] Sporadic cases have also been recorded from other kindreds in whom neurological damage was absent during early childhood.[160, 322] Since the original description of this syndrome, more than 60 additional patients have been reported from many different countries in association with a further 30 or so probable cases among family members of the propositi.[340] In the vast majority of affected individuals kernicteric brain damage and death ensued within 18 months of birth, although rarely patients survived beyond puberty before the development of bilirubin encephalopathy.

Mode of inheritance

The familial nature of this syndrome has been widely established in kindreds other than that reported by Crigler and Najjar,[116] and a history of consanguinity is frequently obtained.[15, 32] The available evidence indicates that the disorder is inherited as an autosomal recessive trait. This mode of inheritance is supported by excretion studies of compounds which form glucuronides such as salicylates[106] and menthol[15, 363] in non-icteric parents and siblings of patients. Despite the observation that formation of the glucuronides of these aglycones was uniformly reduced in the heterozygous carriers of the gene, none of these individuals exhibited an elevated plasma bilirubin concentration. Although it appears that the enzymatic defect in carriers is usually not severe enough to interfere with pigment excretion, family studies using bilirubin as the test substrate have not been performed. Moreover, menthol excretion was normal in both parents of a negro patient, but the mother was shown to have impaired hepatic clearance of radiobilirubin.[80] Although mild unconjugated hyperbilirubinaemia has been reported occasionally in relatives of patients,[238, 338] this is observed far more frequently in association with the Crigler–Najjar type II syndrome (see below).

Laboratory findings

The evidence accumulated from many case studies indicates that bilirubin production is consistently normal. Hence haemoglobin concentration, reticulocyte count, red cell survival,[80, 390] magnitude and kinetics of the early-labelled bilirubin fraction,[319] plasma bilirubin turnover rate[51, 80, 338] and bone marrow structure are normal. Light microscopic examination of the liver has generally revealed a normal appearance, although the presence of occasional and unexplained bile thrombi was observed by Crigler and Najjar.[116] On electron microscopy, subcellular structure also appears normal apart from prominence of the smooth endoplasmic reticulum[120, 279] and minor non-specific changes at the sinusoidal pole of the hepatocytes.[198]

Except for the elevated plasma bilirubin concentration, conventional liver function tests (including clearance of BSP) and cholangiography are uniformly normal. In the majority of cases plasma bilirubin levels exceed 340 μmol/l (20 mg/dl), with all of the pigment in the unconjugated form.[338] The small amounts of direct-reacting bilirubin reported were probably artefactual and reflected the inadequacy of the methodology (see 'Laboratory methods', above). Plasma bilirubin concentration may fluctuate, with a tendency to higher values in winter or during intercurrent illnesses.[338] Predictably, the urine contains no bilirubin, but a chloroform-soluble pigment has been found which may be similar to a presumed photoderivative of bilirubin, obtained on ultrafiltration of plasma.[218] The faeces are normal in colour and the concentration of faecal urobilinogen is usually markedly reduced in both children[15, 338] and adults.[360] Bile obtained from the gallbladder or following duodenal intubation is pale lemon-yellow. In a detailed examination of bile from patients, Fevery et al[143] have confirmed that biliary excretion of bilirubin is markedly reduced (<68 μmol/l [<4 mg/dl]). It was shown also that the proportion of unconjugated bilirubin IX-α was increased to 30 to 57 per cent of the total excreted bile pigment (<1 per cent in control subjects), although the actual amount of unconjugated bilirubin in bile was only one to seven times that observed in normal adults or patients with Gilbert's syndrome and constituted only a minor fraction of total bilirubin production. In addition, trace amounts of conjugated bilirubin were present in bile, predominantly in the form of bilirubin monoglucuronide. Glucose and xylose conjugates were also detectable.

Radiobilirubin kinetic studies in this syndrome showed a normal bilirubin production rate, greatly diminished hepatic bilirubin clearance (1 to 2 per cent of normal) and a biological half-life of the pigment in excess of 156 hours.[51, 80, 115, 338] The fractional transfer rate of bilirubin from plasma to liver was reduced to approximately half that of normal individuals. This finding may reflect saturation of either the hepatic uptake process or intracellular binding sites as a result of the high plasma bilirubin levels. Isotopic studies also suggested that little more than half of the calculated extrahepatic bilirubin pool was present in extravascular tissues.[80, 338] However, removal by plasmapheresis of an amount of pigment equal to the total exchangeable bilirubin pool produced only a moderate and transient reduction in plasma bilirubin concentration,[49] suggesting that some tissues contain additional pigment deposits which do not readily exchange with bilirubin in the plasma. The tissue storage site of this excess pigment has not been determined. Only a small portion of the computed daily bile pigment turnover is eliminated in the form of bilirubin in the bile or as urobilinogen in the faeces. The major fraction of the bilirubin appears to be converted to polar diazo-negative derivatives that are excreted mainly in bile and to a lesser extent in urine.[49, 338] These pigment catabolites probably resemble those excreted by the Gunn rat [298, 338] and, at least in part, may represent dihydroxyl derivatives of bilirubin.[55]

The primary metabolic defect in Crigler–Najjar type I syndrome which leads to the markedly diminished hepatic bilirubin clearance involves the conjugation of bilirubin. In vitro assay of bilirubin UDP-glucuronyltransferase activity in liver biopsy specimens revealed complete absence of bilirubin glucuronide formation.[15, 77, 296, 364] Glucuronide formation in vivo was also found to be reduced, but not absent, after administration of the following compounds that are normally excreted as glucuronides: *N*-acetyl-*p*-aminophenol,[19] tetrahydrocortisol,[306] menthol,[363] chloral hydrate, trichloroethanol and salicylates,[106] *o*-aminophenol and 4-methyl-umbelliferone.[15] Thus, the genetic defect in hepatic glucuronide synthesis appears to be virtually complete for bilirubin, although trace amounts of bilirubin conjugates have been identified in the bile of some patients.[143] For several other aglycones the defect seems to be less severe in that glucuronide formation and excretion are only partially reduced. Since the glucuronyltransferase system probably consists of a series of distinct but related enzymes with overlapping substrate specificity, the genetic defect may not simply involve lack of the specific enzyme for bilirubin conjugation but rather reflect a more generalized abnormality possibly in the microenvironment of the endoplasmic reticulum.[283]

Treatment

Various therapeutic modalities have been tried in an attempt to produce a sustained reduction of plasma bilirubin concentration, in the hope of preventing bilirubin encephalopathy, particularly in patients who survived the neonatal period. However, no form of treatment has been found to be consistently effective. As in the homozygous Gunn rat, phenobarbitone and other microsomal enzyme-inducing agents fail to stimulate bilirubin glucuronide formation or to reduce plasma bilirubin concentration in patients with Crigler–Najjar type I syndrome.[15, 16, 49, 84] Failure to respond to phenobarbitone therapy has been advocated as a useful means of distinguishing patients with an absolute defect in bilirubin glucuronide formation from those considered to have a partial enzyme defect,[15] but this distinction does not appear to hold true in all instances.[115, 143] Several experimental manoeuvres, such as exchange transfusion, or plasmapheresis,[49, 84, 154] have been attempted in order to remove bilirubin from the body. Although these procedures remove substantial amounts of bilirubin and result in a transient reduction in plasma level, the rapid rebound in plasma bilirubin and inherent practical problems limit the usefulness of this approach. Similarly, continuous extracorporeal perfusion through an affinity chromatography column containing albumin-covered agarose beads has proved successful in Gunn rats,[331] but major problems relating to the sterility, rheology and biocompatibility of such a system need to be overcome before it can be applied to humans. From the observation that in normal individuals and patients with Gilbert's syndrome, hepatic bilirubin clearance is independent of pigment turnover, Berk et al[50] subjected a patient with Crigler–Najjar type I syndrome (and Gunn rats) to repeated phlebotomy to reduce plasma bilirubin turnover. However, plasma bilirubin concentration remained essentially unchanged and this was found to be caused by an unexpected and unexplained reduction in plasma bilirubin clearance accompanying the fall in plasma bilirubin turnover. To prevent re-absorption and enterohepatic circulation of the small amount of unconjugated bilirubin which may be excreted in the bile, the potential value of orally administered binding agents such as agar or cholestyramine has been investigated. Although this approach has proved successful in neonatal jaundice[308] and in Gunn rats [242, 294] it has not consistently been beneficial in the treatment of Crigler–Najjar patients.[16, 77, 296]

The efficacy of phototherapy in the management of neonatal jaundice is well established,[254] and this therapeutic modality also has been successful in reducing plasma bilirubin levels to below 170 µmol/l (10 mg/dl) in some infants with Crigler–Najjar type I syndrome.[5, 176, 219] However, at least 12 hours per day of exposure to an artificial light source (425 to 475 nm region of the visible spectrum) are necessary to maintain an adequate response and little is known about possible long-term effects of such extensive illumination. It has recently been suggested that in hyperbilirubinaemic infants the duration of daily phototherapy may be reduced by oral administration of cholestyramine,[16] making treatment at home a possibility.[296] Nevertheless, since this approach has proved ineffective in at least one reported adult case[77] and its long-term efficacy has not been evaluated, it hardly appears to be a practical measure for life-long management of this condition.

Crigler–Najjar Type II Syndrome (Congenital Non-haemolytic Jaundice with a Partial Defect in Bilirubin Conjugation)

Clinicopathological features

This condition was described in detail by Arias,[9] who reported a group of eight patients aged 14 to 52 years. In half of these patients jaundice was noted within the first year of life, and in the remaining four cases between the ages of two and 34 years. Jaundice was the only abnormal physical sign and, apart from the social problems imposed by chronic jaundice, most individuals led a relatively normal life. Although plasma bilirubin concentration ranged from 110 to 340 μmol/l (6.4 to 20 mg/dl), and virtually all of the pigment was in the unconjugated form, neurological manifestations presumably due to bilirubin encephalopathy were evident in only one patient.[212] This patient died at the age of 44, having been confined to a psychiatric institution for the last 20 years of her life; during this time her neurological signs and plasma bilirubin level (270 to 375 μmol/l [15.8 to 22 mg/dl]) had remained relatively stable. At autopsy, the brain was reduced in weight and on histological examination showed degenerative changes consistent with kernicterus.[212] Subsequently, many additional patients with this syndrome have been described.[43, 340] Evidence of bilirubin encephalopathy was encountered much less frequently than in the more severe Crigler–Najjar type I syndrome, and the great majority of patients developed normally without signs of intellectual or extrapyramidal impairment.[15] Indeed, two of three icteric brothers, all over 50 years of age, with plasma bilirubin concentrations consistently in excess of 340 μmol/l (20 mg/dl) exhibited no neurological dysfunction, and the third had only minor and non-specific electroencephalographic changes.[166] However, presumably transient and reversible bilirubin encephalopathy has been observed in association with an increase in plasma bilirubin level related to prolonged fasting or an intercurrent illness.[168] Light microscopic examination of the liver has not revealed morphological abnormalities, but on electron microscopy hypertrophy and hyperplasia of smooth endoplasmic reticulum and prominence of the Golgi apparatus have been noted, particularly in the region of bile canaliculi.[166, 389]

Mode of inheritance

The frequent occurrence of Crigler–Najjar type II syndrome in families suggested that it is genetically determined but, unlike the type I syndrome, consanguinity appeared to be infrequent. Although jaundice may occur in successive generations, the exact pattern of inheritance has not been established. Some hold that the syndrome is transmitted as an autosomal dominant with incomplete penetrance.[9, 59, 355] This view is supported by the occurrence of significant hyperbilirubinaemia in three or four successive generations, and by the results of the menthol glucuronide test used as a screening procedure to identify carriers of the trait without hyperbilirubinaemia. For example, in a study of five families, reduced menthol glucuronide excretion was noted consistently on only one side of the family, and in no instance were abnormal test results found in both parents of a jaundiced patient.[15] However, mild unconjugated hyperbilirubinaemia was present on the other side of the pedigree in two families, in whom menthol glucuronide excretion was normal. This finding, together with the abnormal menthol glucuronide excretion noted in anicteric individuals presumed to be heterozygous for the type I syndrome,[363] indicates that the menthol excretion test fails to identify all carriers of the abnormal gene and hence its predictive value is limited. Since individuals with mild unconjugated hyperbilirubinaemia (Gilbert's syndrome) appear quite frequently in the families of patients with Crigler–Najjar type II syndrome,[166, 199] others have postulated that the disorder is transmitted as a recessive trait. Crigler–Najjar type II syndrome is a very rare condition, however, whereas Gilbert's syndrome occurs in up to 7 per cent of the population, so that this genetic interpretation may be an over-simplification. It has therefore been suggested that two allelic genes may be involved, each being transmitted by a different parent, and that Gilbert's syndrome results when one or the other gene is present in a single dose.[199] It is evident that identification of the defect at a molecular level is required in order to establish the precise mode of inheritance of this syndrome.

Laboratory findings

Plasma unconjugated bilirubin levels usually range between 103 and 428 μmol/l (6 to 25 mg/dl), but values approaching 700 μmol/l (41 mg/dl) have been recorded in association with fasting or an intercurrent illness.[166, 168] The plasma conjugated bilirubin fraction is normal and bilirubinuria is absent. Red cell survival and bilirubin production are normal, but hepatic bilirubin clearance is markedly diminished[70] and faecal urobilinogen excretion is moderately reduced. Bile obtained by duodenal aspiration or at laparotomy contains a considerable amount of bilirubin, but the bilirubin secretion rate is reduced in relation to the calculated pigment production rate.[168] Bilirubin monoglucuronide is the major bile pigment, with bilirubin diglucuronide and unconjugated bilirubin representing only minor fractions.[143, 166, 168] Bilirubin glucosides and xylosides are usually present in slightly higher proportion than in the bile of normal individuals. However, formation of these conjugates far from compensates for the deficient glucuronide conjugation.[143] Although bilirubin monoglucuronide is the major bile pigment fraction in bile, bilirubin glucuronyltransferase activity in liver biopsy specimens is either not detectable[9, 15, 199, 230] or greatly reduced.[166] With other aglycones, including *o*-aminophenol and *p*-nitrophenol, hepatic glucuronide formation was also found to be reduced.[9, 15] In addition, glucuronide formation in vivo, measured by the menthol or salicylamide test, was diminished in most[9, 199, 230] but not in all cases.[15, 389]

Treatment

It is now widely recognized that phenobarbitone and related drugs produce a dramatic fall in the plasma bilirubin concentration in this syndrome (in contrast to patients with Crigler–Najjar type I syndrome).[15, 356, 398] Although in most instances phenobarbitone treatment is merely desirable, but not essential, for the management of this condition, many patients benefit cosmetically and in terms of their social adjustment. Depending on the age of the patient, daily administration of 60 to 180 mg phenobarbitone in divided doses usually brings about a progressive reduction in plasma bilirubin concentration over a period of two to three weeks, frequently to levels at which clinical jaundice is no longer recognizable. Therapy is effective regardless of when it is initiated in relation to the course of the disorder[166] and, on withdrawal of the drug, the pigment level gradually returns to pretreatment values.[115] Results comparable to those with phenobarbitone have been obtained with oral administration of other microsomal enzyme-inducing agents, such as dicophane, glutethimide, antipyrine, bucolone or the nonhypnotic barbiturate phetharbital.[58]

It has been widely assumed that the response to phenobarbitone and related compounds is due to drug-mediated induction of hepatic microsomal glucuronyltransferase, particularly in view of the observation that hepatic enzyme activity and bilirubin transport capacity in heterozygous Gunn rats are substantially enhanced by phenobarbitone.[318] Similarly, in patients with acute hepatitis[137] or undergoing surgery,[69] activity of the enzyme was increased during phenobarbitone therapy. In patients with Crigler–Najjar type II syndrome, phenobarbitone has been shown to enhance significantly the hepatic clearance of bilirubin,[70] but with one possible exception no corresponding increase in bilirubin glucuronyltransferase activity could be demonstrated in the liver.[166] Furthermore, it has been shown that in patients with Gilbert's syndrome phenobarbitone does not cause an increase in hepatic enzyme activity despite the demonstrated reduction in plasma bilirubin level.[137] Thus the weight of evidence indicates that Crigler–Najjar type II syndrome is due to a partial deficiency of hepatic bilirubin glucuronyltransferase activity, but the dramatic reduction of hyperbilirubinaemia in response to phenobarbitone cannot be ascribed solely or largely to induction of the enzyme.[166, 230, 389] The finding that bilirubin monoglucuronide is the predominant pigment in bile, and that this pattern is unchanged by phenobarbitone therapy,[166] remains at present unexplained, but may require reassessment of the postulated enzymatic defect in this condition.[168]

Gilbert's Syndrome (Low-grade Chronic Hyperbilirubinaemia)

Clinicopathological features

In 1901 Gilbert and Lereboullet[157] described a syndrome of chronic benign, intermittent jaundice, characterized by mild hyperbilirubinaemia in the absence of bilirubinuria or symptoms and signs of liver disease. The disorder was later shown to be distinct from haemolytic disease.[158] Although some of the original cases described by Gilbert probably had a state of compensated haemolysis, the term 'Gilbert's syndrome' has gained popular acceptance in the face of a variety of alternative proposals, which include constitutional hepatic dysfunction,[111] familial non-haemolytic jaundice,[117] hereditary non-haemolytic bilirubinaemia[6] and constitutional hyperbilirubinaemia.[21]

Since the introduction of routine biochemical screening, it has become apparent that mild elevation of plasma unconjugated bilirubin is not uncommon. The actual incidence is difficult to estimate and obviously depends on the value selected as the upper limit for normal plasma bilirubin concentration. Population studies have shown that, in general, men exhibit a higher plasma bilirubin level than women[21,300] and that a clear bimodal distribution is frequently,[300,311] but not invariably, present.[21,377] On the basis of these and other investigations[45,227] the incidence of Gilbert's syndrome appears to be approximately 3 to 7 per cent of the population, with males predominating over females by ratios of 2 to 7 : 1.[7,150,273,311]

The presence of hyperbilirubinaemia is recognized most often during the second and third decades of life, although many older persons may be unaware of the abnormality until it is detected by incidental laboratory examination[150] or in the course of family studies.[311] Jaundice or scleral icterus is the only presenting symptom or abnormal physical finding in approximately 30 per cent of patients. In some series, hyperbilirubinaemia was commonly an incidental finding in asymptomatic individuals,[45] whereas in others the disorder was associated with a variety of non-specific and protean symptoms, most frequently abdominal discomfort, fatigue or malaise.[311] In general, these symptoms do not correlate with the plasma bilirubin level, and it has been suggested that they are, in fact, related to anxiety rather than to the underlying disorder in pigment metabolism. Since an increase in the level of plasma bilirubin in Gilbert's syndrome usually results from fasting[138] (see below), hyperbilirubinaemia in previously subclinical individuals may first be detected in association with caloric withdrawal due to an intercurrent febrile illness, 'morning sickness' of pregnancy, achalasia,[140] or postoperatively, especially following oral surgery.[312] Many patients with Gilbert's syndrome are initially misdiagnosed as having acute or persistent hepatitis or cholelithiasis.[311] Consequently, the major importance of diagnosing this benign disorder is to distinguish it from more serious causes of hepatic dysfunction.

An essential component of the syndrome is that on light microscopy no significant abnormalities of liver structure are detectable. Although in a few individual cases a variety of minor and generally unimpressive histological abnormalities have been reported, the only finding noted by several investigators was accumulation of a lipofuscin-like pigment, predominantly in the centrilobular zones.[31,289,326] The histochemistry and ultrastructure of this pigment appear to differ from that found in the Dubin–Johnson syndrome. Electron microscopic studies have shown a variety of minor abnormalities,[93] but the only consistent and notable finding in a series of patients was gross hypertrophy of the smooth endoplasmic reticulum.[268] This observation is reminiscent of that in Crigler–Najjar type II syndrome.[166]

Mode of inheritance

The occurrence of more than one case of mild unconjugated hyperbilirubinaemia within a given family has been recognized since the report of Gilbert and Lereboullet.[157] However, the heterogeneity of the disorder, as demonstrated by reduced red cell survival and mild abnormalities of hepatic clearance of BSP and/or ICG in some individuals (see below), has complicated family studies so that the mode of inheritance has not been clearly defined. In addition, many seemingly sporadic cases have been reported. Hence, the reported familial incidence of Gilbert's syndrome varies considerably in different series. A positive family history of hyperbilirubinaemia was obtained from only eight of 58 patients studied by Foulk et al,[150] whereas icterus was noted in three successive generations of a family reported by

Baroody and Shugart.[27] In another series of 15 patients with Gilbert's syndrome, 55 per cent of the siblings and 26 per cent of parents of the index cases had mild unconjugated hyperbilirubinaemia,[7] and in a further study of 122 first-degree relatives of 42 patients, 27 per cent of the siblings and 16 per cent of the parents were found to have elevated bilirubin levels.[311] No affected relatives were observed in the kindred of 25 of the 42 patients. A higher incidence of hyperbilirubinaemia among relatives could be anticipated if plasma bilirubin levels were determined on repeated occasions or after fasting for 48 hours. The accumulated evidence suggests that, in many cases, Gilbert's syndrome is probably inherited as an autosomal dominant, and the patients are heterozygous for a single abnormal gene. Furthermore, the observation that cases of Gilbert's syndrome are occasionally found in families of Crigler–Najjar type II patients suggests that the two disorders may be genetically related.

Laboratory findings

Although, by definition, in Gilbert's syndrome the hyperbilirubinaemia is less than 103 µmol/l (6 mg/dl),[58] the majority of patients exhibit a level below 50 µmol/l (3 mg/dl) and there is considerable daily and seasonal fluctuation. In a series of 58 patients reported by Foulk et al,[150] and in another 55 observed by Powell et al,[311] normal plasma bilirubin concentration was observed in 22 per cent and 33 per cent, respectively, of the patients at least once during the period of observation. In other series the mean value obtained during the initial evaluation of patients ranged from 27 to 34 µmol/l (1.6 to 2 mg/dl).[45,162]

A variety of factors has been shown to produce fluctuations in plasma bilirubin concentration. Gilbert and Herscher[156] noted that in normal individuals *fasting* resulted in a slight rise of plasma bilirubin. In subjects with Gilbert's syndrome, a two- to threefold increase in plasma bilirubin concentration is observed within 48 hours of reducing the daily intake to 400 cal (1.6 MJ).[28,29,138,162] Twelve to 24 hours after resuming a regular diet, plasma bilirubin returns to baseline level. Although fasting has also been shown to increase plasma unconjugated bilirubin levels in patients with liver disease or haemolysis, the magnitude of this rise is considerably less than that observed in Gilbert's syndrome.[135,301] Recent findings in Gunn rats[164] and in patients with Crigler–Najjar type II syndrome and Gilbert's syndrome[29,162,166] indicate that the degree of unconjugated hyperbilirubinaemia may be influenced by dietary composition as well as total caloric intake. A normocaloric but lipid-free diet or intravenous infusion of glucose or amino acids increases hyperbilirubinaemia to an extent similar to that produced by fasting. Since addition of a small amount of lipid rapidly reverses the effect of these dietary manipulations and of fasting, it appears likely that in both situations the enhanced hyperbilirubinaemia is attributable, at least in part, to lipid withdrawal. It is not known, however, whether the mechanism responsible for the hyperbilirubinaemia is the same in fasting per se and in dietary lipid withdrawal. Since similar dietary effects are observed in Gunn rats, it must be concluded that they are unrelated to hepatic bilirubin glucuronyltransferase activity because the enzyme is deficient in these animals. Kinetic studies have demonstrated a reduction in hepatic clearance of bilirubin both in fasting Gunn rats and in patients with Gilbert's syndrome,[79,223] and in Gunn rats fed a lipid-free diet.[161] Fasting does not appear to affect hepatic uptake of bilirubin significantly,[330] although the hepatic content of ligandin and Z protein is reduced.[359] With regard to changes in bilirubin production in fasting the evidence is contradictory; enhanced catabolism of haem has been suggested by the finding of increased hepatic haem oxygenase activity[23] and carbon monoxide production,[232,255,270] but other investigators using kinetic methods have failed to find an increase in bilirubin production.[36,79,223] From the observation that plasma-free fatty acid levels correlate with the rise in plasma bilirubin concentration both in fasting normal subjects[114] and in Gunn rats,[62,320] it has been postulated that fasting hyperbilirubinaemia may be due to lipolytic increase of bilirubin sequestered in adipose tissues. It is evident that further investigation is necessary to clarify the complex mechanism(s) of dietary-induced hyperbilirubinaemia.

Intravenous administration of *nicotinic acid* (50 mg) to patients with Gilbert's syndrome has been shown to cause a two- to threefold increase in plasma unconjugated bilirubin concentration within three hours of administration, whereas in normal individuals or in patients with haemolysis or liver disease the rise is less impressive.[119,152] The underlying mechanism is unknown, but the observation that this response is largely prevented by prior splenectomy[152,183] suggests that nicotinic acid may enhance erythrocyte breakdown and haem catabolism in the spleen, either by a direct effect on the red cell or by inducing reticuloendothelial hyperactivity. Alternatively, Rosental and Thaler[321] have shown that nicotinic acid produces a transient inhibition of hepatic bilirubin glucuronyltransferase activity in heterozygous (anicteric) Gunn rats, which may explain the enhanced hyperbilirubinaemic response observed in Gilbert's syndrome. Administration of *phenobarbitone* or glutethimide for one to two weeks reduces plasma unconjugated bilirubin concentration in patients with Gilbert's syndrome, frequently to normal levels.[68] Kinetic studies have shown that the reduction in plasma bilirubin is due both to accelerated hepatic bilirubin clearance and to reduced plasma bilirubin turnover.[70, 76]

Since virtually all plasma bilirubin is in the unconjugated form, bilirubinuria is absent. The faecal excretion of urobilinogen is usually normal, but it may be slightly decreased.[9, 117] Hepatosplenomegaly is absent and conventional liver function tests are normal.

In about one-third of patients with Gilbert's syndrome, minor abnormalities of plasma BSP[44] and/or ICG disappearance[262] have been observed, reflecting a defect in hepatic anion transport. These abnormalities are probably due to defects in different stages of the hepatic uptake process. Similarly, it has been shown that in patients with Gilbert's syndrome the plasma half-life of tolbutamide is prolonged and its metabolic clearance is reduced.[104] Since tolbutamide is bound to ligandin, but does not undergo glucuronidation, and clearance of the drug is generally enhanced by phenobarbitone administration, it would appear that hepatic uptake of this compound is defective in Gilbert's syndrome.

Although the pathogenesis of Gilbert's syndrome is unresolved, kinetic studies with radiobilirubin have established that the mild unconjugated hyperbilirubinaemia is due to a reduction in hepatic bilirubin clearance to approximately 30 per cent of normal,[47] resulting in increased retention of the pigment in the plasma. In addition to this hepatic defect in pigment clearance it has been found that up to 60 per cent of patients in several reported series have a mild and fully compensated haemolytic state.[41, 49, 83, 310] In this group of patients bilirubin turnover is increased in proportion to the rate of haemolysis. Reduced hepatic bilirubin clearance indicative of Gilbert's syndrome has been observed in association with hereditary spherocytosis, glucose-6-phosphate dehydrogenase deficiency and a variety of non-spherocytic haemolytic anaemias.[41] In these instances, the coexistence of the two conditions is believed to be incidental rather than causal. The apparent prevalence of the combined appearance of the two abnormalities may simply reflect enhanced detection of Gilbert's syndrome due to the higher plasma bilirubin levels that result from the haemolysis-related pigment overload.

The mechanism underlying the reduction of bilirubin clearance in Gilbert's syndrome is not clear and is a subject of considerable controversy. Measurement of ligandin concentration indicated that this intracellular binding protein is not reduced in the liver[145] or plasma.[373] From the analysis of kinetic studies with radiobilirubin it has been suggested that defects exist in both the hepatic uptake and the microsomal conjugation of the pigment.[47, 70] Whereas direct evidence for an uptake defect has not yet been obtained, hepatic bilirubin UDP-glucuronyltransferase activity measured in biopsy material is almost always reduced.[13, 18, 33, 67, 137] With aglycones other than bilirubin, glucuronide formation in vitro or in vivo has been found to be unimpaired or reduced depending on the substrate examined. Thus, in vitro glucuronidation of methyl umbelliferone has been reported as normal[9, 381] whereas that of *p*-nitrophenol may be reduced significantly.[18] Similarly, in vivo conjugation of menthol,[150] salicylamide[26] and *N*-acetyl-*p*-aminophenol[337] is unimpaired, but urinary excretion of clofibrate glucuronide has been found to be diminished.[233]

The pathogenic significance of this partial and seemingly selective reduction in glucuronide formation and particularly of the reduced hepatic bilirubin UDP-glucuronyltransferase activity is unclear. Several observations are difficult to reconcile with the concept that reduced bilirubin glucuronyltransferase activity alone is responsible for the impaired hepatic clearance of the pigment in Gilbert's syndrome.[340] *First*, even the reduced hepatic enzyme activity is greatly in excess of the calculated enzyme activity in the whole liver required to conjugate all of the bilirubin produced in vivo. *Second*, since enzyme activity in vitro is generally measured after digitonin activation, it is difficult to determine to what extent this artificially perturbed enzyme level reflects the physiological situation. *Third*, the limitations of the in vitro enzyme assay may also be responsible for the repeated observation that treatment with phenobarbitone or related drugs fails to increase measurably hepatic bilirubin glucuronyltransferase activity[68,70,137] despite a drug-mediated reduction of plasma bilirubin concentration and improved hepatic pigment clearance. *Fourth*, the finding that hepatic bilirubin glucuronyltransferase activity may be reduced in chronic persistent hepatitis,[136] end-stage cirrhosis,[139] a variety of haemolytic disorders,[17] and in several anicteric disorders such as non-cirrhotic portal fibrosis, extrahepatic portal vein obstruction or granulomatous involvement of the liver,[118] suggests that the reduced enzyme activity in Gilbert's syndrome may not represent the primary defect. *Fifth*, the striking changes in the pattern of bilirubin glucuronides in the bile of patients with Gilbert's syndrome (reduction in diglucuronide with a relative increase in monoglucuronides)[143,171] are consistent with the hypothesis that there is an abnormality in the second enzymatic step which is presumed to add the second glucuronic acid moiety to form the diglucuronide. *Sixth*, as mentioned above, all patients with Gilbert's syndrome have a moderately reduced rate of hepatic bilirubin uptake,[47] in contrast to patients with Crigler–Najjar syndrome type I[51] and homozygous Gunn rats,[330] where initial hepatic uptake of bilirubin appears normal despite a lack of bilirubin glucuronyltransferase activity. This does not necessarily imply, however, that the moderate reduction in uptake rate is the cause of the syndrome, since the intrinsic capacity of the hepatic uptake system enormously exceeds the normal net transport rate of bilirubin from blood to bile.[303,330] *Lastly*, a significant proportion of patients with Gilbert's syndrome exhibit abnormalities in hepatic transport of BSP, ICG, tolbutamide and/or oestrogens.[3] Since BSP is conjugated by a soluble hepatic enzyme and ICG is not conjugated prior to excretion, it is apparent that the reduction in glucuronyltransferase activity cannot account for these findings. It is thus evident that hepatic uptake of organic anions is defective, at least in this sub-group of patients with Gilbert's syndrome,[272] and that this abnormality is of variable selectivity. Considering the multiplicity of associated hepatic transport anomalies, the frequency of occult haemolysis and the apparent problems in ascribing the primary defect solely to reduced bilirubin glucuronyltransferase activity, it appears likely that Gilbert's syndrome represents a heterogeneous group of pathogenetic defects.

The diagnosis of Gilbert's syndrome is established primarily by exclusion of overt haemolysis and acquired liver disease. Further ascertainment of the diagnosis may be achieved by determining the effect of dietary restriction[162,301] or intravenous nicotinic acid administration[119,152] on the plasma bilirubin concentration. Either manipulation generally results in a two- to threefold rise in plasma bilirubin concentration although negative results are observed occasionally. Other diagnostic manoeuvres which have been advocated are measurement of the effect of phenobarbitone on plasma bilirubin concentration[68] and administration of a tracer dose of radiobilirubin for estimation of the percentage of the dose remaining in the plasma after four hours.[47] Percutaneous liver biopsy for both histological examination and determination of bilirubin glucuronyltransferase activity[67] is warranted if the diagnosis remains in any doubt.

Treatment

Once the diagnosis is established it is important to reassure the patient with regard to the benign and inconsequential nature of the disorder and the excellent prognosis. Although phenobarbitone, glutethimide and related drugs have been employed experimentally to reduce the hyperbilirubinaemia, there is little justification for the long-term use of these agents.

Conjugated Hyperbilirubinaemia

Dubin–Johnson syndrome (chronic idiopathic jaundice)

In 1954, Dubin and Johnson[126] and Sprinz and Nelson[358] independently described a benign disorder characterized by chronic or intermittent jaundice and a grossly pigmented liver (Table 13.2). Many additional cases have subsequently been reported in both sexes and in a wide variety of ethnic groups, including caucasians, negroes, Indians and Japanese.[52,100,125,226,361] The highest incidence of the disorder, about one per 1300, occurs in Persian Jews.[350]

Dubin[125] noted that jaundice was evident at birth or by the time of puberty in about half, and by the age of 20 in about two-thirds of all afflicted individuals. Apart from chronic or recurrent jaundice of fluctuating intensity, most patients are asymptomatic, although some complain of vague right upper quadrant abdominal pain, weakness, nausea or vomiting.

Table 13.2. *Comparison of the Hereditary Conjugated Hyperbilirubinaemias.*

	Dubin–Johnson syndrome	Rotor's syndrome
Incidence	Uncommon (1 : 1300 in Iranian Jews)	Rare
Mode of inheritance	Autosomal recessive	Autosomal recessive
Defect in bilirubin metabolism	Impaired biliary excretion	Impaired biliary excretion
Plasma bilirubin concentration (μmol/l [mg/dl])	17–430 (1–25), usually 35–85 (2–5) (average of 60% conjugated); increased by oestrogens and pregnancy	17–340 (1–20), usually 35–85 (2–5) (average of 60% conjugated)
Age hyperbilirubinaemia recognized	Usually early adulthood (variable)	Usually childhood (variable)
Clinical features	Asymptomatic or non-specific symptoms; jaundice, occasional hepatosplenomegaly	Asymptomatic or non-specific symptoms; jaundice
Routine liver function tests	Usually normal	Normal
Plasma BSP disappearance	Slow initial disappearance (45 min retention ≤ 20%); secondary rise at 90 min usual	Markedly slow initial disappearance (45 min retention 30–50%); no secondary rise
Oral cholecystography	Gallbladder usually not visualized	Usually normal
Gross appearance and histology of liver	Black-brown colour; pigment granules (melanin) in centrilobular areas	Normal
Urinary coproporphyrin excretion	Normal total, > 80% coproporphyrin I (c.f. normal, 75% coproporphyrin III)	Increased total, proportion of coproporphyrin I elevated but < 80%
Prognosis	Good	Good

Many patients are anicteric at the time of diagnosis and their inherited abnormality is detected during the course of family studies for evaluation of a jaundiced relative. In women, subclinical hyperbilirubinaemia is often unmasked by pregnancy or the use of oral contraceptives.[109] Physical examination is frequently normal except for slight icterus. In about 50 per cent of cases the urine is darker than normal and the liver is moderately enlarged and/or tender.[125] On visual examination, the liver is darkly pigmented; it has been described variously as green, slate blue, dark grey, or even black in appearance. Indeed, gross black discolouration of liver biopsy tissue is characteristic of this disorder. Although pigment may be observed occasionally in phagocytic cells of lymph nodes and bone marrow, there is usually no generalized pigmentation of other tissues. The liver is histologically normal except for a conspicuous coarse-granular intracellular brown pigment which is most often limited to the centrilobular areas (Figure 13.6). The pigment tends to be confined to parenchymal cells[358] but small amounts may be present also in Kupffer cells.[125, 391] On electron microscopy, apart from inconstant evidence of mitochondrial damage,[130] the predominant finding is the aforementioned granular pigment which is present as dense membrane-enclosed bodies located primarily in the pericanalicular region.[289] It has been suggested that these are pigment-laden lysosomes.[282, 347] Subcellular fractionation of liver tissue has shown increased activity of some lysosomal acid hydrolases, but the structural integrity of subcellular organelles seems generally preserved and the accumulation of pigment appears to represent a benign type of secondary lysosomal storage.[347] The observation that pigment disappears from the liver during the convalescent phase of acute viral hepatitis, whereas the hepatic excretory defect

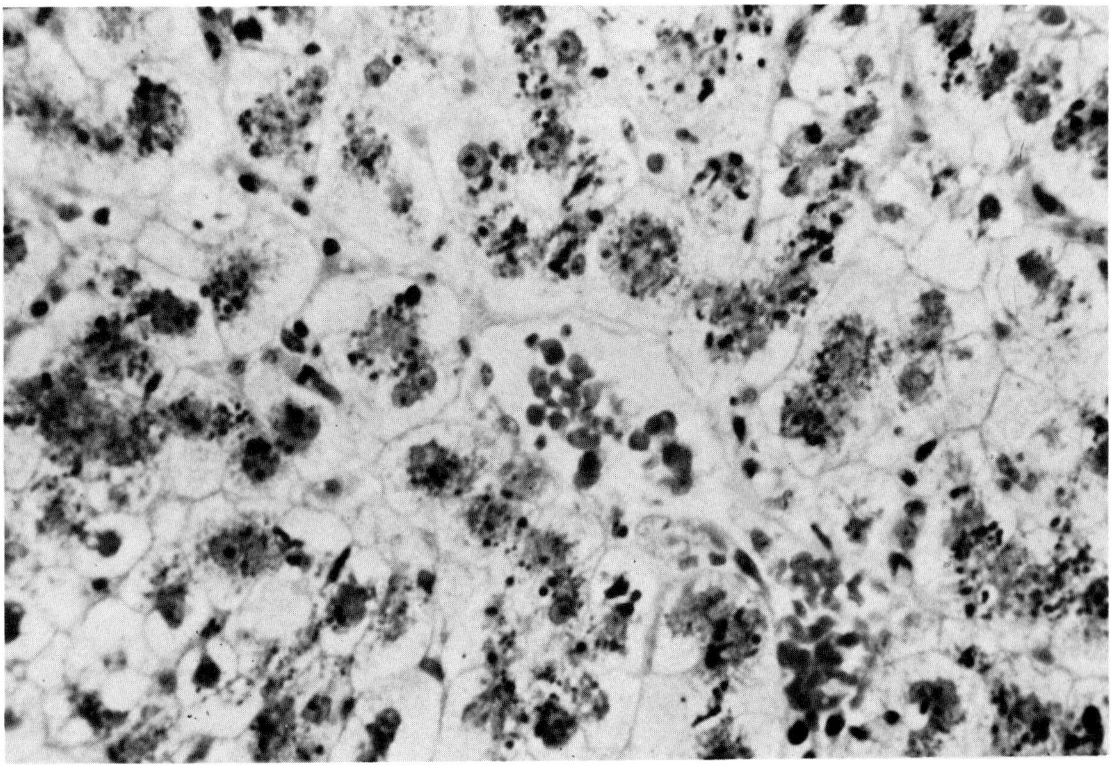

Figure 13.6. Hepatic histology in Dubin–Johnson syndrome (chronic idiopathic jaundice). Dark pigment granules are located predominantly in hepatocytes around the central vein.

for organic anions (see below) persists, further supports the concept that the accumulation of pigment is the result, rather than the cause, of the primary hepatic defect.[383] Furthermore, the degree of hepatic pigmentation is highly variable and is poorly correlated with plasma bilirubin concentration.[8,391] The chemical nature of the pigment remains unclear. Earlier investigators had assumed that the pigment belonged to the ill-defined group of lipofuscins,[125,126] but histochemical, spectroscopic and physiochemical analyses suggest that it is closely related to melanin.[11,133]

Hyperbilirubinaemia is usually slight to moderate and exhibits considerable fluctuation.[125,350,358] Although values as high as 400 μmol/l (23 mg/dl) have been reported, most of the patients have plasma bilirubin levels of less than 86 μmol/l (5 mg/dl). Characteristically the plasma contains a significant fraction of 'direct-reacting' bilirubin (mean 60 per cent). Both conjugated bilirubin and urobilinogen are detectable in the urine of most patients.[125] Red cell survival and conventional liver function tests are generally normal. Hepatic uptake of BSP and other organic dyes is normal or only mildy impaired, and the relative hepatic storage capacity of BSP is preserved.[286,350,388] However, the biliary excretion of both bilirubin[8] and BSP is markedly impaired, and the maximal hepatic secretory rate (Tm) for BSP approaches zero.[348,349] This results in prolonged hepatic storage of the dye.[226] Consequently, plasma BSP levels 45 minutes after a 5 mg/kg intravenous dose may be normal or only slightly increased but, because of the hepatic excretory defect, conjugated BSP refluxes from the liver into the plasma producing a secondary rise in plasma concentration 60 to 90 minutes after injection. This peculiarity is demonstrable in more than 90 per cent of all cases and is virtually pathognomonic for Dubin–Johnson syndrome.[261,344,349] Recent studies in humans[1] and in the mutant Corriedale sheep,[25] which represents the ovine counterpart of the Dubin–Johnson syndrome (see below), indicated that whereas the biliary excretion of conjugated BSP is profoundly depressed, unconjugated BSP excretion is impaired to a much lesser degree. With dibromsulphthalein, ICG and rose bengal, which do not require conjugation for excretion in bile, a secondary rise in plasma concentration is not observed.[132] Treatment with phenobarbitone frequently reduces the plasma level of conjugated bilirubin and increases the hepatic transport maximum of BSP, but this effect is inconstant.[271, 348] Hepatic transport of conjugated oestrogens is defective[3] but the biliary excretion of bile acids is unaffected.[107, 109, 182] In the majority of patients, oral cholecystography fails to outline the gallbladder or results in only faint visualization,[125] but intravenous administration of contrast medium may improve visualization. An isolated deficiency of factor VII has been described in a significant proportion of patients with Dubin–Johnson syndrome reported from Israel,[346] but in family studies the two defects were found to segregate independently, suggesting that they are unrelated.

Metabolic defects in the *mutant Corriedale sheep* appear to be remarkably similar to those of the Dubin–Johnson syndrome.[113, 340] The disorder is transmitted as an autosomal dominant trait and affected sheep have a mild conjugated hyperbilirubinaemia with greatly reduced biliary secretion of conjugated bilirubin, BSP, ICG, rose bengal, and iodopanoic acid, but unimpaired hepatic transport of bile acids.[4, 11, 14, 277] About six months after birth, brown-black pigment becomes apparent in the lysosomes of the centrilobular hepatic parenchymal cells. The physicochemical properties of the pigment resemble those of melanin and it has been suggested that its formation may be related to defective biliary excretion of catecholamines.[11] Facial photosensitivity, which is an additional feature of this ovine disorder, results from the accumulation in plasma of phylloerythrin, a cyclic tetrapyrrole formed by bacterial degradation of chlorophyll in the gut.

Patients with Dubin–Johnson syndrome have a unique and diagnostic abnormality of urinary coproporphyrin excretion. The urine of healthy individuals contains coproporphyrin isomers I and III, with about 75 per cent in the isomer III form, reflecting the fact that porphyrins of the isomer III series are precursors in haem biosynthesis. In Dubin–Johnson syndrome, although total urinary coproporphyrin excretion is normal, or only slightly increased, 84 to 90 per cent of the total urinary coproporphyrin is the type I isomer.[34, 225, 228, 393] In heterozygous carriers of the trait, who are phenotypically normal, an intermediate urinary coproporphyrin isomer ratio is present (approximately 35 per cent coproporphyrin I).[35, 225, 393] However, in presumed heterozygotes, the range and overlap of values are too great for the isomer ratio to serve as an accurate diagnostic tool for detection of individual cases. The recent finding that uroporphyrinogen III cosynthetase activity is normal in both erythrocytes and liver of patients with Dubin–Johnson syndrome[352] suggests that the altered urinary coproporphyrin excretion is not related to an abnormality in the relative production rates of porphyrinogen isomers I and III, but rather to the defect in biliary excretion.

Family studies based on detection of presumptive carriers by determination of the urinary coproporphyrin isomer ratio indicated that Dubin–Johnson syndrome is inherited as an autosomal recessive trait.[35, 128, 393] This mode of inheritance is further supported by the high frequency of consanguinity noted in parents of affected individuals.[226] The primary defect appears to involve impaired biliary canalicular transport of organic anions, possibly due to an abnormality in the membrane carrier system.[25] Impaired biliary secretion has been demonstrated for conjugated bilirubin[125] and BSP,[1, 261] ICG,[344] rose bengal[391] and cholecystographic contrast media.[125] Since this benign disorder has a good prognosis with a normal life expectancy, no specific therapy is necessary other than reassurance. Female patients should be warned about the aggravating effect of oestrogen-containing preparations or pregnancy on the intensity of jaundice.

Rotor's Syndrome

In 1948, Rotor, Manahan and Florentin[323] described a benign disorder of familial non-haemolytic jaundice with direct-reacting bilirubin in a Philippino family. Some of these patients have been studied further by other investigators[302, 394, 397] and additional cases of the syndrome have been reported in both sexes and in other ethnic groups.[192, 285, 304, 305, 309, 333, 378, 394] This disorder is seen much less commonly than the Dubin–Johnson syndrome from which it appears to differ pathophysiologically (Table 13.2).

Rotor's syndrome is characterized by chronic, relatively mild jaundice which fluctuates in intensity and is usually apparent before the age of 20 years. Although patients are usually asymptomatic, mild epigastric discomfort and weakness have been described, with occasional frank abdominal pain and fever. Hepatosplenomegaly is unusual, jaundice being the only abnormal physical finding. Both the gross and microscopic appearance of the liver are normal;

pigmentation of the liver is conspicuously absent, but this is not a reliable feature by which to distinguish it from Dubin–Johnson syndrome since the amount of hepatic pigmentation is highly variable in the latter condition.[8] With the exception of one reported family, evidence of haemolysis was lacking.[124] Conventional liver function tests are normal, apart from a predominantly conjugated hyperbilirubinaemia; plasma bilirubin concentration is usually elevated in the range of 34 to 86 μmol/l (2 to 5 mg/dl), with occasional values up to 400 μmol/l (23 mg/dl) being recorded. Bilirubinuria is evident, provided that the plasma level of conjugated bilirubin is sufficiently high. In contrast to Dubin–Johnson syndrome, the gallbladder is usually, although not invariably, visualized on oral cholecystography.

After intravenous injection of a single loading dose of bilirubin, plasma clearance of both bilirubin and conjugated bilirubin is reduced.[333] In addition, plasma clearance of BSP is markedly delayed in Rotor's syndrome, so that between 30 and 50 per cent of the dye is usually retained in plasma 45 minutes after administration of a 5 mg/kg dose. However, in contrast to Dubin–Johnson syndrome there is no reflux of conjugated BSP from the liver into the circulation and hence no secondary rise in plasma BSP occurs after 90 minutes. Moreover, the computed hepatic storage capacity for BSP is only 10 per cent of normal, whereas Tm is only modestly reduced.[397] Reduced plasma disappearance, Tm, and relative hepatic storage capacity of ICG have also been observed in Rotor's syndrome.[284] The abnormalities in BSP and ICG transport in Rotor's syndrome differ from those in the Dubin–Johnson syndrome and suggest that Rotor's syndrome represents a defect in hepatic uptake and/or storage of organic anions. Furthermore, the derangement in BSP transport resembles that of other hepatobiliary disorders[343, 388] so that it is not diagnostic for Rotor's syndrome. Analysis of urinary coproporphyrin excretion is a further means of differentiating this disorder from Dubin–Johnson syndrome.[394] Patients with Rotor's syndrome exhibit markedly increased (i.e. sixfold) total urinary coproporphyrin excretion. Although more than 60 per cent is excreted as the type I isomer, there is an absolute increase in coproporphyrin III excretion, in sharp contrast to the findings in Dubin–Johnson syndrome. A similar pattern of coproporphyrin isomer excretion is found in many cholestatic disorders[20] and this may simply reflect impaired hepatic porphyrin excretion.

Pedigree analyses of families with Rotor's syndrome suggest an autosomal recessive mode of inheritance.[302] This is consistent with the more recent observations that phenotypically normal heterozygous carriers of the trait have a mildly elevated plasma retention of BSP at 45 minutes,[397] and a total urinary coproporphyrin excretion intermediate between that of normal subjects and of patients with the syndrome.[394]

Hepatic Storage Disease

A third type of congenital conjugated hyperbilirubinaemia associated with hepatic uptake and storage impairment has been described by Dhumeaux and Berthelot.[122] Other presumed cases of this so-called 'hepatic storage disease' have been reported also by De Groote et al[121] and by Hadchouel et al.[185] In this disorder, jaundice appeared early in childhood and the plasma bilirubin concentration fluctuated between 50 and 70 μmol/l (3 and 4.1 mg/dl), comprising around 50 per cent conjugated bilirubin. Conventional liver function tests, plasma bile acid concentration, and hepatic bilirubin UDP-glucuronyltransferase activity were all normal. Hepatic histology was normal and intrahepatocytic pigment was lacking. The gallbladder was visualized on oral cholecystography, but only after a delay of 20 hours. The plasma disappearance of BSP, dibromsulphthalein, ICG and rose bengal were all significantly reduced. The most striking finding was, however, a marked impairment of the relative hepatic storage capacity of BSP, and this defect was associated with a decrease in the biliary Tm. Although conjugated BSP was demonstrable in the plasma and urine, no distinct secondary rise of conjugated dye was evident in the plasma. These findings suggest that the primary defect is an impairment of hepatic uptake and/or storage of bilirubin and other organic anions. These hepatic transport abnormalities appear to be similar to those which have been described in the mutant Southdown sheep.[112] Since ligandin and Z protein content of hepatocytes in the mutant Southdown sheep is normal,[244] and phenobarbitone administration modifies neither plasma bilirubin level nor BSP clearance in hepatic storage disease (although phenobarbitone increases hepatic ligandin concentration), a deficiency of these intracellular binding proteins appears unlikely. There are distinct similarities between hepatic storage disease and Rotor's syndrome, and on the basis of the available evidence a clear separation of the two syndromes may be difficult. Except for reduced Tm and storage capacity of ICG,[284] details of dye transport and hepatic storage capacity have not been reported in Rotor's syndrome. It is possible that the tentative distinction between the two syndromes may prove to be artificial or that some of the patients previously believed to have Rotor's syndrome actually may have hepatic storage disease.

REFERENCES

1. Abe, H. & Okuda, K. (1975) Biliary excretion of conjugated sulfobromophthalein (BSP) in constitutional conjugated hyperbilirubinaemias. *Digestion,* **13,** 272–283.
2. Acocella, G. & Billing, B.H. (1965) The effect of rifamycin SV on bile pigment excretion in rats. *Gastroenterology,* **49,** 526–530.
3. Adlercreutz, H. & Tikkanen, M.J. (1973) Defects in hepatic uptake and transport and biliary excretion of estrogens. *Médecine et Chirurgie Digestives,* **2,** 59–65.
4. Alpert, S., Mosher, M., Shanske, A. & Arias, I.M. (1969) Multiplicity of hepatic excretory mechanisms for organic anions. *Journal of General Physiology,* **53,** 238–247.
5. Altay, C. & Say, B. (1973) Phototherapy in nonobstructive nonhemolytic jaundice. *Pediatrics,* **51,** 124–126.
6. Alwall, N. (1946) On hereditary nonhemolytic bilirubinemia. *Acta Medica Scandinavica,* **123,** 560–595.
7. Alwall, N., Laurell, C.B. & Nilsby, I. (1946) Studies on heredity in cases of 'non-haemolytic hyperbilirubinaemia without direct van den Bergh reaction' (hereditary non-haemolytic bilirubinaemia). *Acta Medica Scandinavica,* **124,** 114–125.
8. Arias, I.M. (1961) Studies of chronic familial nonhemolytic jaundice with conjugated bilirubin in the serum with and without an unidentified pigment in the liver cells. *American Journal of Medicine,* **31,** 510–518.
9. Arias, I.M. (1962) Chronic unconjugated hyperbilirubinemia without overt signs of hemolysis in adolescents and adults. *Journal of Clinical Investigation,* **41,** 2233–2245.
10. Arias, I.M. (1962) Chronic unconjugated hyperbilirubinemia (CUH) with increased production of bile pigment not derived from the hemoglobin of mature, circulating erythrocytes. *Journal of Clinical Investigation,* **41,** 1341–1342.
11. Arias, I.M. (1968) Chronic idiopathic jaundice. In *Ikterus* (Ed.) Beck, K. pp. 65–71. Stuttgart: F.K. Schattauer Verlag.
12. Arias, I.M. & Jansen, P. (1975) Protein binding and conjugation of bilirubin in the liver cell. In *Jaundice* (Ed.) Goresky, C.A. & Fisher, M.M. pp. 175–188. New York: Plenum.
13. Arias, I.M. & London, I.M. (1957) Bilirubin glucuronide formation in vitro; demonstration of a defect in Gilbert's disease. *Science,* **126,** 563–564.
14. Arias, I., Bernstein, L., Toffler, R., Cornelius, C., Novikoff, A.B. & Essner, E. (1964) Black liver disease in Corriedale sheep: a new mutation affecting hepatic excretory function. *Journal of Clinical Investigation,* **43,** 1249–1250.
15. Arias, I.M., Gartner, L.M., Cohen, M., Ben-Ezzer, J. & Levi, A.J. (1969) Chronic nonhemolytic unconjugated hyperbilirubinemia with glucuronyl transferase deficiency. Clinical, biochemical, pharmacologic and genetic evidence for heterogeneity. *American Journal of Medicine,* **47,** 395–409.
16. Arrowsmith, W.A., Payne, R.B. & Littlewood, J.M. (1975) Comparison of treatments for congenital nonobstructive nonhemolytic hyperbilirubinemia. *Archives of Diseases in Childhood,* **50,** 197–201.
17. Auclair, C., Feldman, G., Hakim, J., Boivin, P., Boucherot, J. & Troube, H. (1976) Bilirubin and paranitrophenol glucuronyl transferase activities and ultrastructural aspect of the liver in patients with chronic hemolytic anemias. *Biomedicine,* **25,** 61–65.
18. Auclair, C., Hakim, J., Boivin, P., Troube, H. & Boucherot, J. (1976) Bilirubin and paranitrophenol glucuronyl transferase activities of the liver in patients with Gilbert's syndrome. *Enzyme,* **21,** 97–107.
19. Axelrod, J., Schmid, R. & Hammaker, L. (1957) A biochemical lesion in congenital, non-obstructive, non-haemolytic jaundice. *Nature (London),* **180,** 1426–1427.
20. Aziz, M.A., Schwartz, S. & Watson, C.J. (1964) Studies of coproporphyrin. VIII. Reinvestigation of the isomer distribution in jaundice and liver diseases. *Journal of Laboratory and Clinical Medicine,* **63,** 596–604.
21. Bailey, A., Robinson, D. & Dawson, A.M. (1977) Does Gilbert's disease exist? *Lancet,* **i,** 931–933.
22. Bakken, A.F. & Fog, J. (1975) *Metabolism and Chemistry of Bilirubin and Related Tetrapyrroles.* Oslo: Rikshospitalet.
23. Bakken, A.F., Thaler, M.M. & Schmid, R. (1972) Metabolic regulation of heme catabolism and bilirubin production. 1. Hormonal control of hepatic heme oxygenase activity. *Journal of Clinical Investigation,* **51,** 530–536.
24. Barnhart, J.L. & Combes, B. (1974) The effect of theophylline on hepatic excretory function. *American Journal of Physiology,* **227,** 194–199.
25. Barnhart, J.L., Gronwall, R.R. & Combes, B. (1977) Selective defect in biliary excretion of conjugated BSP compounds in mutant Corriedale sheep. Evidence for a second canalicular carrier. *Gastroenterology,* **73,** A-59/1257.
26. Barniville, H.T.F. & Misk, R. (1959) Urinary glucuronic acid excretion in liver disease and the effect of a salicylamide load. *British Medical Journal,* **i,** 337–340.
27. Baroody, W.G. & Shugart, R.T. (1956) Familial nonhemolytic icterus. *American Journal of Medicine,* **20,** 314–316.
28. Barrett, P.V.D. (1971) Hyperbilirubinemia of fasting. *Journal of the American Medical Association,* **217,** 1349–1353.
29. Barrett, P.V.D. (1975) Effects of caloric and noncaloric materials in fasting hyperbilirubinemia. *Gastroenterology,* **68,** 361–369.

30. Barrett, P.V.D., Cline, M.J. & Berlin, N.I. (1966) The association of the urobilin 'early peak' and erythropoiesis in man. *Journal of Clinical Investigation.* **45,** 1657–1665.
31. Barth, R.F., Grimley, P.M., Berk, P.D., Bloomer, J.R. & Howe, R.B. (1971) Excess lipofuscin accumulation in constitutional hepatic dysfunction (Gilbert's syndrome). *Archives of Pathology,* **91,** 41–47.
32. Bartolozzi, G., Ciampolini, M.,Salti, R. & Verrotti, M. (1969) La Malattia di Crigler–Najjar: presentazione di un caso. *Minerva Pediatrica,* **21,** 2393–2406.
33. Bellet, H. & Raynaud, A. (1974) An assay of bilirubin UDP-glucuronyl transferase on needle-biopsies applied to Gilbert's syndrome. *Clinica Chimica Acta,* **53,** 51–55.
34. Ben-Ezzer, J., Rimington, C., Shani, M., Seligsohn, U., Sheba, Ch. & Szeinberg, A. (1971) Abnormal excretion of the isomers of urinary coproporphyrin by patients with Dubin–Johnson syndrome in Israel. *Clinical Science,* **40,** 17–30.
35. Ben-Ezzer, J., Blonder, J., Shani, M., Seligsohn, U., Post, C.A., Adam, A. & Szeinberg, A. (1973) Dubin–Johnson syndrome. Abnormal excretion of the isomers of urinary coproporphyrin by clinically unaffected family members. *Israel Journal of Medical Sciences,* **9,** 1431–1436.
36. Bensinger, T.A., Maisels, M.J., Carlson, D.E. & Conrad, M.E. (1973) Effect of low calorie diet on endogenous carbon monoxide production: normal adults and Gilbert's syndrome. *Proceedings of the Society for Experimental Biology and Medicine,* **144,** 417–419.
37. Berendsohn, S., Lowman, J., Sundberg, D. & Watson, C.J. (1964) Idiopathic dyserythropoietic jaundice. *Blood,* **24,** 1–18.
38. Bergan, A., Östrem, T. & Gjelstad, N. (1973) Conjugation of non-erythroid bilirubin in chronic experimental cholestasis in the dog. *Scandinavian Journal of Gastroenterology,* **10,** 565–569.
39. Berk, P.D. (1975) Total body handling of bilirubin. In *Jaundice* (Ed.) Goresky, C.A. & Fisher, M.M. pp. 135–157. New York: Plenum.
40. Berk, P.D. & Berlin, N.I. (1977) *Chemistry and Physiology of Bile Pigments.* Washington, D.C.: U.S. Government Printing Office.
41. Berk, P.D. & Blaschke, T.F. (1972) Detection of Gilbert's syndrome in patients with hemolysis. A method using radioactive chromium. *Annals of Internal Medicine,* **77,** 527–531.
42. Berk, P.D. & Javitt, N.B. (1978) Hyperbilirubinemia and cholestasis. *American Journal of Medicine,* **64,** 311–326.
43. Berk, P.D., Berlin, N.I. & Howe, R.B. (1974) Disorders of bilirubin metabolism. In *Duncan's Diseases of Metabolism* (Ed.) Bondy, P.K. & Rosenberg, L. pp. 825–880A. Philadelphia: W.B. Saunders.
44. Berk, P.D., Blaschke, T.F. & Waggoner, J.G. (1972) Defective bromosulfophthalein clearance in patients with constitutional hepatic dysfunction (Gilbert's syndrome). *Gastroenterology,* **63,** 472–481.
45. Berk, P.D., Wolkoff, A.W. & Berlin, N.I. (1975) Inborn errors of bilirubin metabolism. *Medical Clinics of North America,* **59,** 803–816.
46. Berk, P.D., Howe, R.B., Bloomer, J.R. & Berlin, N.I. (1969) Studies of bilirubin kinetics in normal adults. *Journal of Clinical Investigation,* **48,** 2176–2190.
47. Berk, P.D., Bloomer, J.R., Howe, R.B. & Berlin, N.I. (1970) Constitutional hepatic dysfunction (Gilbert's syndrome). A new definition based on kinetic studies with unconjugated radiobilirubin. *American Journal of Medicine,* **49,** 296–305.
48. Berk, P.D., Rodkey, F.L., Blaschke, T.F., Collison, H.A. & Waggoner, J.G. (1974) Comparison of plasma bilirubin turnover and carbon monoxide production in man. *Journal of Laboratory and Clinical Medicine,* **83,** 29–37.
49. Berk, P.D., Martin, J.F., Blaschke, T.F., Scharschmidt, B.F. & Plotz, P.H. (1975) Unconjugated hyperbilirubinemia. Physiologic evaluation and experimental approaches to therapy. *Annals of Internal Medicine,* **82,** 552–570.
50. Berk, P.D., Blaschke, T.F., Scharschmidt, B.F., Waggoner, J.G. & Berlin, N.I. (1976) A new approach to quantitation of the various sources of bilirubin in man. *Journal of Laboratory and Clinical Medicine,* **87,** 767–780.
51. Berk, P.D., Scharschmidt, B.F., Waggoner, J.G. & White, S.C. (1976) The effect of repeated phlebotomy on bilirubin turnover, bilirubin clearance and unconjugated hyperbilirubinemia in the Crigler–Najjar syndrome and the jaundiced Gunn rat: application of computers to experimental design. *Clinical Science and Molecular Medicine,* **50,** 333–348.
52. Berkowitz, D., Entine, J. & Chunn, L. (1960) Dubin–Johnson syndrome: report of a case occurring in a Negro male. *New England Journal of Medicine,* **262,** 1028–1029.
53. Bernstein, L.H., Ben-Ezzer, J., Gartner, L. & Arias, I.M. (1966) Hepatic intracellular distribution of tritium-labeled unconjugated and conjugated bilirubin in normal and Gunn rats. *Journal of Clinical Investigation,* **45,** 1194–1201.
54. Bernstein, R.B., Troxler, R.F. & Lester, R. (1968) The effect of hepatobiliary disease on urobilinogen excretion. *Gastroenterology,* **54,** 150.
55. Berry, C.S., Zarembo, J.E. & Ostrow, J.D. (1972) Evidence for conversion of bilirubin to dihydroxyl derivatives in the Gunn rat. *Biochemical and Biophysical Research Communications,* **49,** 1366–1375.
56. Berthelot, P. & Billing, B.H. (1966) Effect of bunamiodyl on hepatic uptake of sulfobromophthalein in the rat. *American Journal of Physiology,* **211,** 395–399.
57. Bhargava, M., Listowsky, I. & Arias, I.M. (1977) Ligandin: subunits and function. *Gastroenterology,* **73,** A-15/1213.
58. Billing, B.H. (1975) Bilirubin metabolism. In *Diseases of the Liver* (Ed.) Schiff, L. pp. 287–313. Philadelphia: J.B. Lippincott.
59. Billing, B.H. (1975) Genetics of unconjugated hyperbilirubinaemia. In *Metabolism and Chemistry of Bilirubin and Related Tetrapyrroles* (Ed.) Bakken, A.F. & Fog, J. pp. 96–100. Oslo: Rikshospitalet.
60. Billing, B., Haslam, R. & Wald, N. (1971) Bilirubin standards and the determination of bilirubin by manual and technicon auto-analyzer methods. *Annals of Clinical Biochemistry,* **8,** 21–30.
61. Billing, B.H., Jansen, F.H. & Bilton, E. (1973) The effect of bile depletion on the biliary excretion of unconjugated bilirubin and bilirubin conjugates. In *The Liver. Quantitative Aspects of Structure and Function* (Ed.) Paumgartner, G. & Preisig, R. pp. 386–391. Basel: Karger.
62. Billing, B.H., Hole, D.R., Tickner, T.R. & Gollan, J.L. (1977) The role of lipids in the dietary regulation

of plasma bilirubin concentration in Gunn rats. *Gastroenterology*, **73**, A-15/1213.

63. Bissell, D.M. (1975) Formation and elimination of bilirubin. *Gastroenterology*, **69**, 519–538.
64. Bissell, D.M. & Hammaker, L.E. (1976) Cytochrome P-450 heme and the regulation of δ-aminolevulinic acid synthetase in the liver. *Archives of Biochemistry and Biophysics*, **176**, 103–112.
65. Bissell, D.M. & Hammaker, L.E. (1977) Effect of endotoxin on tryptophan pyrrolase and δ-aminolaevulinate synthetase: evidence for an endogenous regulatory haem fraction in rat liver. *Biochemical Journal*, **166**, 301–304.
66. Bissell, D.M., Hammaker, L. & Schmid, R. (1972) Hemoglobin and erythrocyte catabolism in rat liver: the separate roles of parenchymal and sinusoidal cells. *Blood*, **40**, 812–822.
67. Black, M. & Billing, B.H. (1969) Hepatic bilirubin UDP-glucuronyl transferase activity in liver disease and Gilbert's syndrome. *New England Journal of Medicine*, **280**, 1266–1271.
68. Black, M. & Sherlock, S. (1970) Treatment of Gilbert's syndrome with phenobarbitone. *Lancet*, **i**, 1359–1362.
69. Black, M., Perrett, R.D. & Carter, A.E. (1973) Hepatic bilirubin UDP-glucuronyl transferase activity and cytochrome P450 content in a surgical population, and the effects of pre-operative drug therapy. *Journal of Laboratory and Clinical Medicine*, **81**, 704–712.
70. Black, M., Fevery, J., Parker, D., Jacobson, J., Billing, B.H. & Carson, E.R. (1974) Effect of phenobarbitone on plasma [^{14}C]bilirubin clearance in patients with unconjugated hyperbilirubinaemia. *Clinical Science and Molecular Medicine*, **46**, 1–17.
71. Blanckaert, N., Gollan, J.L. & Schmid, R. (1978) Is bilirubin diglucuronide formed in vivo by transglucuronidation of bilirubin monoglucuronide? *Gastroenterology*, **74**, 1166.
72. Blanckaert, N., Heirwegh, K.P.M. & Zaman, Z. (1977) Comparison of the biliary excretion of the four isomers of bilirubin-IX in Wistar and homozygous Gunn rats. *Biochemical Journal*, **164**, 229–236.
73. Blanckaert, N., Fevery, J., Heirwegh, K.P.M. & Compernolle, F. (1977) Characterization of the major diazo-positive pigments in bile of homozygous Gunn rats. *Biochemical Journal*, **164**, 237–249.
74. Blanckaert, N., Compernolle, F., Leroy, P., Van Houtte, R., Fevery, J. & Heirwegh, K.P.M. (1978) The fate of bilirubin-IXα glucuronide in cholestasis and during storage in vitro: intramolecular rearrangement to positional isomers of glucuronic acid. *Biochemical Journal*, **171**, 203–214.
75. Blaschke, T.F. & Berk, P.D. (1972) Augmentation of bilirubin UDP-glucuronyltransferase activity in rat liver homogenates by glutethimide. *Proceedings of the Society for Experimental Biology and Medicine*, **140**, 1315–1318.
76. Blaschke, T.F., Berk, P.D., Rodkey, F.L., Scharschmidt, B.F., Collison, H.A. & Waggoner, J.G. (1974) Effects of glutethimide and phenobarbital on hepatic bilirubin clearance, plasma bilirubin turnover and carbon monoxide production in man. *Biochemical Pharmacology*, **23**, 2795–2806.
77. Blaschke, T.F., Berk, P.D., Scharschmidt, B.F., Guyther, J.R., Vergalla, J.M. & Waggoner, J.G. (1974) Crigler–Najjar syndrome: an unusual course with development of neurologic damage at age eighteen. *Pediatric Research*, **8**, 573–590.
78. Bloomer, J.R., Berk, P.D., Howe, W.B., Waggoner, J.G. & Berlin, N.I. (1970) Comparison of faecal urobilinogen excretion with bilirubin production in normal volunteers and patients with increased bilirubin production. *Clinica Chemica Acta*, **29**, 463–471.
79. Bloomer, J.R., Barrett, P.V., Rodkey, F.L. & Berlin, N.I. (1971) Studies on the mechanism of fasting hyperbilirubinemia. *Gastroenterology*, **61**, 479–487.
80. Bloomer, J.R., Berk, P.D., Howe, R.B. & Berlin, J.I. (1971) Bilirubin metabolism in congenital nonhemolytic jaundice. *Pediatric Research*, **5**, 256–264.
81. Bloomer, J.R., Berk, P.D., Howe, R.B. & Berlin, N.I. (1971) Interpretation of plasma bilirubin levels based on studies with radioactive bilirubin. *Journal of the American Medical Association*, **218**, 216–220.
82. Bloomer, J.R., Berk, P.D., Vergalla, J. & Berlin, N.I. (1973) Influence of albumin on the hepatic uptake of unconjugated bilirubin. *Clinical Science and Molecular Medicine*, **45**, 505–516.
83. Blueger, A.F., Krupnikova, E.Z., Sondore, V. Yu & Semushina, E.P. (1977) Study of the etiology and pathogenesis of low grade non-hemolytic unconjugated hyperbilirubinemia (Gilbert's disease). *Acta Hepato-Gastroenterologica*, **24**, 140–147.
84. Blumenschein, S.D., Kallen, R.J., Storey, B., Natzschka, C., Odell, G.B. & Childs, B. (1968) Familial nonhemolytic jaundice with late onset of neurological damage. *Pediatrics*, **42**, 786–792.
85. Blumenthal, S.G., Taggart, D.B., Ikeda, R.M., Ruebner, B.H. & Bergstrom, D.E. (1977) Conjugated and unconjugated bilirubins in bile of humans and Rhesus monkeys. Structure of adult human and Rhesus monkey bilirubins compared with dog bilirubins. *Biochemical Journal*, **167**, 535–548.
86. Bonnett, R., Davies, J.E. & Hursthouse, M.B. (1976) Structure of bilirubin. *Nature (London)*, **262**, 326–328.
87. Boonyapisit, S.T., Trotman, B.W. & Ostrow, J.D. (1978) Unconjugated bilirubin, and the hydrolysis of conjugated bilirubin, in gallbladder bile of patients with cholelithiasis. *Gastroenterology*, **74**, 70–74.
88. Bourke, E., Milne, M.D. & Stokes, G.S. (1965) Mechanisms of renal excretion of urobilinogen. *British Medical Journal*, **ii**, 1510–1514.
89. Brodersen, R. (1977) Prevention of kernicterus, based on recent progress in bilirubin chemistry. *Acta Paediatrica Scandinavica*, **66**, 625–634.
90. Brodersen, R. & Hermann, L.S. (1963) Intestinal reabsorption of unconjugated bilirubin. A possible contributing factor in neonatal jaundice. *Lancet*, **i**, 1242.
91. Brodersen, R. & Theilgaard, J. (1969) Bilirubin colloid formation in neutral aqueous solution. *Scandinavian Journal of Clinical and Laboratory Medicine*, **24**, 395–398.
92. Brodersen, R., Sjödin, T. & Sjöholm, J. (1977) Independent binding of ligands to human serum albumin. *Journal of Biological Chemistry*, **252**, 5067–5072.
93. Brown, N.K. & Smuckler, E.A. (1970) Alkaptonuria and Gilbert's syndrome. Report of two affected siblings and hepatic ultrastructure in one sibling. *American Journal of Medicine*, **48**, 759–765.

94. Brown, S.B. (1976) Stereospecific haem cleavage. A model for the formation of bile-pigment isomers in vivo and in vitro. *Biochemical Journal,* **159,** 23–27.

95. Brown, S.B. & Grundy, M.S. (1977) The role of iron in haem degradation. *Biochemical Society Transactions,* **5,** 1017–1020.

96. Brown, S.B. & King, R.F. (1975) An ^{18}O double-labelling study of haemoglobin catabolism in the rat. *Biochemical Journal,* **150,** 565–567.

97. Brown, S.B. & King, R.F. (1978) The mechanism of haem catabolism. Bilirubin formation in living rats by [^{18}O]oxygen labelling. *Biochemical Journal,* **170,** 297–311.

98. Bunn, H.F. & Jandl, J.H. (1969) The renal handling of hemoglobin. II. Catabolism. *Journal of Experimental Medicine,* **129,** 925–934.

99. Burchell, B. (1977) Studies on the purification of rat liver uridine diphosphate glucuronyltransferase. *Biochemical Journal,* **161,** 543–550.

100. Butt, H.R., Anderson, V.E., Foulk, W.T., Baggenstoss, A.H., Schoenfield, L.J. & Dickson, E.R. (1966) Studies of chronic idiopathic jaundice (Dubin–Johnson syndrome). II. Evaluation of a large family with the trait. *Gastroenterology,* **51,** 619–630.

101. Call, N.B. & Tisher, C.C. (1975) The urinary concentrating defect in the Gunn strain of rat. Role of bilirubin. *Journal of Clinical Investigation,* **55,** 319–329.

102. Callahan, E.W. & Schmid, R. (1969) Excretion of unconjugated bilirubin in the bile of Gunn rats. *Gastroenterology,* **57,** 134–137.

103. Capelle, P., Dhumeaux, D., Mora, M., Feldmann, G. & Berthelot, P. (1972) Effect of rifampicin on liver function in man. *Gut,* **13,** 366–371.

104. Carulli, N., Ponz de Leon, M., Mauro, E., Manenti, F. & Ferrari, A. (1976) Alteration of drug metabolism in Gilbert's syndrome. *Gut,* **17,** 581–587.

105. Childs, B. & Najjar, V.A. (1956) Familial nonhemolytic jaundice with kernicterus: report of two cases without neurologic disease. *Pediatrics,* **18,** 369–377.

106. Childs, B., Sidbury, J.B. & Migeon, C.J. (1959) Glucuronic acid conjugation by patients with familial nonhemolytic jaundice and their relatives. *Pediatrics,* **23,** 903–913.

107. Clarenburg, R. & Kao, C.-C. (1973) Shared and separate pathways for biliary excretion of bilirubin and BSP in rats. *American Journal of Physiology,* **225,** 192–200.

108. Coburn, R.F., Williams, W.J. & Forster, R.E. (1964) Effect of erythrocyte destruction on carbon monoxide production in man. *Journal of Clinical Investigation,* **43,** 1098–1103.

109. Cohen, L., Lewis, C. & Arias, I.M. (1972) Pregnancy, oral contraceptives, and chronic familial jaundice with predominantly conjugated hyperbilirubinemia (Dubin–Johnson syndrome). *Gastroenterology,* **62,** 1182–1190.

110. Colleran, E. & O'Carra, P. (1977) Enzymology and comparative physiology of biliverdin reduction. In *Chemistry and Physiology of Bile Pigments* (Ed.) Berk, P.D. & Berlin, N.I. pp. 69–80. Washington, D.C.: U.S. Government Printing Office.

111. Comfort, M.W. (1935) Constitutional hepatic dysfunction. *Proceedings of the Staff Meetings of the Mayo Clinic,* **10,** 57–61.

112. Cornelius, C.E. & Gronwall, R.R. (1968) Congenital photosensitivity and hyperbilirubinemia in Southdown sheep in the United States. *American Journal of Veterinary Research,* **29,** 291–295.

113. Cornelius, C.E., Arias, I.M. & Osburn, B.I. (1965) Hepatic pigmentation with photosensitivity: a syndrome in Corriedale sheep resembling Dubin–Johnson syndrome in man. *Journal of the American Veterinary Medical Association,* **146,** 709–713.

114. Cowan, R.E., Thompson, R.P.H., Kaye, J.P. & Clark, G.M. (1977) The association between fasting hyperbilirubinaemia and serum non-esterified fatty acids in man. *Clinical Science and Molecular Medicine,* **53,** 155–163.

115. Crigler, J.F. & Gold, N.I. (1969) Effect of sodium phenobarbital on bilirubin metabolism in an infant with congenital, nonhemolytic, unconjugated hyperbilirubinemia, and kernicterus. *Journal of Clinical Investigation,* **48,** 42–55.

116. Crigler, J.F. & Najjar, V.A. (1952) Congenital familial nonhemolytic jaundice with kernicterus. *Pediatrics,* **10,** 169–180.

117. Dameshek, W. & Singer, K. (1941) Familial nonhemolytic jaundice: constitutional hepatic dysfunction with indirect van den Bergh reaction. *Archives of Internal Medicine,* **67,** 259–285.

118. Datta, D.V., Nair, R. & Nair, C.R. (1975) Estimation of hepatic bilirubin UDP-glucuronyl transferase in patients with noncirrhotic portal fibrosis and liver disease: significance and limitations. *Digestive Diseases,* **20,** 961–967.

119. Davidson, A.R., Rojas-Bueno, A., Thompson, R.P.H. & Williams, R. (1975) Reduced caloric intake and nicotinic acid provocation tests in the diagnosis of Gilbert's syndrome. *British Medical Journal,* **i,** 480.

120. De Brito, T., Borges, M.A. & Da Silva, L.C. (1966) Electron microscopy of the liver in nonhemolytic acholuric jaundice with kernicterus (Crigler–Najjar) and in idiopathic conjugated hyperbilirubinemia (Rotor). *Gastroenterologia,* **106,** 325–335.

121. De Groote, J., Ramboer, C., Versieck, J. & Barbier, F. (1968) Pathologie isolée de la B.S.P. Étude chez quatre malades. *Revue Internationale d'Hématologie,* **18,** 833–844.

122. Dhumeaux, D. & Berthelot, P. (1975) Chronic hyperbilirubinemia associated with hepatic uptake and storage impairment. *Gastroenterology,* **69,** 988–993.

123. Diamond, I. & Schmid, R. (1966) Experimental bilirubin encephalopathy: the mode of entry of bilirubin-^{14}C into the central nervous system. *Journal of Clinical Investigation,* **45,** 678–689.

124. Dollinger, M.R., Brandborg, L.L., Sartor, V.E. & Bernstein, J.M. (1967) Chronic familial hyperbilirubinemia. Hepatic defect(s) associated with occult hemolysis. *Gastroenterology,* **52,** 875–881.

125. Dubin, I.N. (1958) Chronic idiopathic jaundice. A review of fifty cases. *American Journal of Medicine,* **24,** 268–292.

126. Dubin, I.N. & Johnson, F.B. (1954) Chronic idiopathic jaundice with unidentified pigment in liver cells. A new clinicopathologic entity with a report of 12 cases. *Medicine,* **33,** 155–197.

127. Dutton, G.J. (1966) The biosynthesis of glucuronides. In *Glucuronic Acid, Free and Combined* (Ed.) Dutton, G.J. pp. 185–299. New York: Academic.

128. Edwards, R.H. (1975) Inheritance of the Dubin–Johnson–Sprinz syndrome. *Gastroenterology,* **68,** 734–749.

129. Elder, G., Gray, C.H. & Nicholson, D.G. (1972) Bile pigment fate in gastrointestinal tract. *Seminars in Hematology,* **9,** 71–90.

130. Enat, R. & Barzilai, D. (1977) Mitochondrial pathology in the liver in a patient with the Dubin–Johnson syndrome. *Israel Journal of Medical Sciences,* **13,** 1197–1205.

131. Erlinger, S. & Dhumeaux, D. (1974) Mechanisms and control of secretion of bile water and electrolytes. *Gastroenterology,* **66,** 281–304.

132. Erlinger, S., Dhumeaux, D., Desjeux, J.F. & Benhamou, J.P. (1973) Hepatic handling of unconjugated dyes in the Dubin–Johnson syndrome. *Gastroenterology,* **64,** 106–110.

133. Essner, E. & Novikoff, A.B. (1960) Human hepatocellular pigments and lysosomes. *Journal of Ultrastructural Research,* **3,** 374–391.

134. Fahmy, K., Gray, C.H. & Nicholson, D.C. (1972) The reduction of bile pigments by faecal and intestinal bacteria. *Biochimica et Biophysica Acta,* **264,** 85–97.

135. Felsher, B.F. & Carpio, N.M. (1975) Caloric intake and unconjugated hyperbilirubinemia. *Gastroenterology,* **69,** 42–47.

136. Felsher, B.F. & Carpio, N.M. (1977) Non-familial unconjugated hyperbilirubinemia and reduced hepatic bilirubin UDP-glucuronyl transferase activity in patients with chronic persistent hepatitis. *Gastroenterology,* **73,** A-22/1220.

137. Felsher, B.F., Craig, J.R. & Carpio, N. (1973) Hepatic bilirubin glucuronidation in Gilbert's syndrome. *Journal of Laboratory and Clinical Medicine,* **81,** 829–837.

138. Felsher, B.F., Rickard, D. & Redeker, A.G. (1970) The reciprocal relation between caloric intake and the degree of hyperbilirubinemia in Gilbert's syndrome. *New England Journal of Medicine,* **283,** 170–172.

139. Fevery, J., De Groote, J. & Heirwegh, K.P.M. (1973) Quantitation of hepatic bilirubin conjugation. In *The Liver. Quantitative Aspects of Structure and Function* (Ed.) Paumgartner, G. & Preisig, R. pp. 203–209. Basel: Karger.

140. Fevery, J., Heirwegh, K.P.M. & De Groote, J. (1974) Unconjugated hyperbilirubinaemia in achalasia. *Gut,* **15,** 121–124.

141. Fevery, J., Van Damme, B., Michiels, R., De Groote, J. & Heirwegh, K.P.M. (1972) Bilirubin conjugates in bile of man and rat in the normal state and in liver disease. *Journal of Clinical Investigation,* **51,** 2482–2492.

142. Fevery, J., Blanckaert, N., Heirwegh, K.P.M. & De Groote, J. (1976) Bilirubin conjugates: formation and detection. In *Progress in Liver Diseases* (Ed.) Popper, H. & Schaffner, F. pp. 183–214. New York: Grune & Stratton.

143. Fevery, J., Blanckaert, N., Heirwegh, K.P.M., Préaux, A.-M. & Berthelot, P. (1977) Unconjugated bilirubin and an increased proportion of bilirubin monoconjugates in the bile of patients with Gilbert's syndrome and Crigler–Najjar disease. *Journal of Clinical Investigation,* **60,** 970–979.

144. Fevery, J., Van De Vijver, M., Michiels, R. & Heirwegh, K.P.M. (1977) Comparison in different species of biliary bilirubin-IXα conjugates with the activities of hepatic and renal bilirubin-IXα-uridine diphosphate glycosyltransferases. *Biochemical Journal,* **164,** 737–746.

145. Fleischner, G., Kamisaka, K., Habig, W., Jacoby, W. & Arias, I.M. (1975) Human ligandin: characterization and quantitation. *Gastroenterology,* **69,** A-21/821.

146. Fog, J. & Jellum, E. (1963) Structure of bilirubin. *Nature (London),* **198,** 88–89.

147. Foliot, A., Christoforov, B., Petite, J.P., Etienne, J.P., Housset, E. & Dubois, M. (1975) Bilirubin UDP-glucuronyltransferase activity of Wistar rat kidney. *American Journal of Physiology,* **229,** 340–343.

148. Forker, E.L. (1975) Canalicular anion transport, pathogenetic mechanisms, and a steady-state distributed model for measuring kinetics. In *Jaundice* (Ed.) Goresky, C.A. & Fisher, M.M. pp. 229–240. New York: Plenum.

149. Forker, E.L. (1977) Mechanisms of hepatic bile formation. *Annual Review of Physiology,* **39,** 323–347.

150. Foulk, W.T., Butt, H.R., Owen, C.A., Whitcomb, F.F. & Mason, H.L. (1959) Constitutional hepatic dysfunction (Gilbert's syndrome): its natural history and related syndromes. *Medicine,* **38,** 25–46.

151. Franco, D., Préaux, A.-M., Bismuth, H. & Berthelot, P. (1972) Extra hepatic formation of bilirubin glucuronides in the rat. *Biochimica et Biophysica Acta,* **286,** 55–61.

152. Fromke, V.L. & Miller, D. (1972) Constitutional hepatic dysfunction (CHD; Gilbert's disease); a review with special reference to a characteristic increase and prolongation of the hyperbilirubinemic response to nicotinic acid. *Medicine,* **51,** 451–464.

153. Fulop, M., Sandson, J. & Brazeau, P. (1965) Dialyzability, protein binding and renal excretion of plasma conjugated bilirubin. *Journal of Clinical Investigation,* **44,** 666–680.

154. Gardner, W.A. & Konigsmark, B. (1969) Familial non-hemolytic jaundice: bilirubinosis and encephalopathy. *Pediatrics,* **43,** 365–376.

155. Gibson, G.E. & Forker, E.L. (1974) Canalicular bile flow and bromosulfophthalein transport maximum: the effect of a bile salt-independent choleretic, SC-2644. *Gastroenterology,* **66,** 1046–1053.

156. Gilbert, A. & Herscher, M. (1906) Sur les variations de la cholémie physiologique. *Presse Médicale,* **14,** 209–211.

157. Gilbert, A. & Lereboullet, P. (1901) La cholémie simple familiale, *Semaine Medicale (Paris),* **21,** 241–245.

158. Gilbert, A., Lereboullet, P. & Herscher, M. (1907) Les trois cholémies congénitales. *Bulletins et Mémoires de la Société Médicale des Hôpitaux de Paris,* **24,** 1203–1210.

159. Gillette, J.R., Davis, D.C. & Sasame, H.A. (1972) Cytochrome P-450 and its role in drug metabolism. *Annual Review of Pharmacology,* **12,** 57–84.

160. Girotti, F., Finocchi, G., Sartori, L. & Boscherini, B. (1969) Congenital non-haemolytic jaundice in a four-years-old girl without disease of the central nervous system. *Helvetica Paediatrica Acta,* **24,** 399–403.

161. Gollan, J.L., Bateman, E.C. & Billing, B.H. (1975) Effects of carbohydrate and lipid feeding on the plasma bilirubin concentration in Gilbert's syndrome. *Digestion,* **12,** 256.

162. Gollan, J.L., Bateman, E.C. & Billing, B.H. (1976) Effect of dietary composition on the unconjugated hyperbilirubinaemia of Gilbert's syndrome. *Gut,* **17,** 335–340.

163. Gollan, J.L., Dallinger, K.J. & Billing, B.H. (1978) Factors influencing excretion of conjugated bilirubin in the isolated kidney. *Clinical Science and Molecular Medicine*, **54**, 381–389.

164. Gollan, J.L., Hatt, K.J. & Billing, B.H. (1975) The influence of diet on unconjugated hyperbilirubinaemia in the Gunn rat. *Clinical Science and Molecular Medicine*, **49**, 229–235.

165. Gollan, J.L., McDonagh, A.F. & Schmid, R. (1977) Biliverdin IXα: a new probe of hepatic bilirubin metabolism. *Gastroenterology*, **72**, A-163/1186.

166. Gollan, J.L., Huang, S.N., Billing, B.H. & Sherlock, S. (1975) Prolonged survival in three brothers with severe type 2 Crigler–Najjar syndrome. Ultrastructural and metabolic studies. *Gastroenterology*, **68**, 1543–1555.

167. Gomba, Sz., Gautier, A., Lemarchand-Béraud, Th. & Gardiol, D. (1976) Pigmentation and dysfunction of Gunn rat thyroid. Correlation between morphological and biochemical data. *Virchows Archiv; B: Cell Pathology*, **20**, 41–54.

168. Gordon, E.R., Shaffer, E.A. & Sass-Kortsak, A. (1976) Bilirubin secretion and conjugation in the Crigler–Najjar syndrome type II. *Gastroenterology*, **70**, 761–765.

169. Gordon, E.R., Goresky, C.A., Chang, T.-H. & Perlin, A.S. (1976) The isolation and characterization of bilirubin diglucuronide, the major bilirubin conjugate in dog and human bile. *Biochemical Journal*, **155**, 477–486.

170. Gordon, E.R., Chan, T.-H., Samodai, K. & Goresky, C.A. (1977) The isolation and further characterization of the bilirubin tetrapyrroles in bile-containing human duodenal juice and dog gall-bladder bile. *Biochemical Journal*, **167**, 1–8.

171. Gordon, E.R., Shaffer, E.A., Paré, P. & Goresky, C.A. (1977) Gilbert's syndrome: the qualitative basis of the disorder. *Gastroenterology*, **73**, A-24/1222.

172. Goresky, C.A. (1971) Bilirubin and sulfobromophthalein uptake by liver. *Gastroenterology*, **60**, 194.

173. Goresky, C.A. (1975) The hepatic uptake process: its implications for bilirubin transport. In *Jaundice* (Ed.) Goresky, C.A. & Fisher, M.M. pp. 159–174. New York: Plenum.

174. Goresky, C.A. & Fisher, M.M. (1975) *Jaundice*. New York: Plenum.

175. Goresky, C.A., Haddad, H.H., Kluger, W.S., Nadeau, B.E. & Bach, G.G. (1974) The enhancement of maximal bilirubin excretion with taurocholate-induced increments in bile flow. *Canadian Journal of Physiology and Pharmacology*, **52**, 389–403.

176. Gorodischer, R., Levy, G., Krasner, J. & Yaffe, S.J. (1970) Congenital nonobstructive, nonhemolytic jaundice: effect of phototherapy. *New England Journal of Medicine*, **282**, 375–377.

177. Gorski, J.P. & Kasper, C.B. (1977) Purification and properties of microsomal UDP-glucuronyltransferase from rat liver. *Journal of Biological Chemistry*, **252**, 1336–1343.

178. Gray, C.H., Neuberger, A. & Sneath, P.H. (1950) Studies in congenital porphyria. 2. Incorporation of ^{15}N in the stercobilin in the normal and in the porphyric. *Biochemical Journal*, **47**, 87–92.

179. Groth, C.G., Arborgh, B., Björkén, C., Sundberg, B. & Lundgren, G. (1977) Correction of hyperbilirubinemia in the glucuronyltransferase-deficient rat by intraportal hepatocyte transplantation. *Transplantation Proceedings*, **9**, 313–316.

180. Gumucio, J.J., Balabaud, C., Miller, D.L., De Mason, L.J., Appelman, H.D., Stoecker, T.J. & Franzblau, D.R. (1978) Bile secretion and liver cell heterogeneity in the rat. *Journal of Laboratory and Clinical Medicine*, **91**, 350–362.

181. Gunn, C.H. (1938) Hereditary acholuric jaundice in a new mutant strain of rats. *Journal of Heredity*, **29**, 137–139.

182. Gutstein, S., Alpert, S. & Arias, I.M. (1968) Studies of hepatic excretory function. IV. Biliary excretion of sulfobromophthalein sodium in a patient with the Dubin–Johnson syndrome and a biliary fistula. *Israel Journal of Medical Sciences*, **4**, 36–40.

183. Gydell, K. (1959) Nicotinic acid induced hyperbilirubinemia and hypersideremia. *Acta Medica Scandinavica*, **164**, 305–320.

184. Habig, W.H., Pabst, M.J., Fleischner, G., Gatmaitan, Z., Arias, I.M. & Jacoby, W.B. (1974) The identity of glutathione S-transferase B with ligandin, a major binding protein of liver. *Proceedings of the National Academy of Sciences of the United States of America*, **71**, 3879–3882.

185. Hadchouel, P., Charbonnier, A., Lageron, A., Lemonnier, F., Rautureau, M., Scotto, J. & Caroli, J. (1971) A propos d'une nouvelle forme d'ictère chronique idiopathique. Hypothèse physiopathologique. *Revue Médico-Chirurgicale des Maladies du Foie*, **46**, 61–68.

186. Halac, E. & Reff, A. (1967) Studies on bilirubin UDP-glucuronyltransferase. *Biochimica et Biophysica Acta*, **139**, 328–343.

187. Halac, E., Dipiazza, M. & Detwiler, P. (1972) The formation of bilirubin mono- and diglucuronide by rat liver microsomal fractions. *Biochimica et Biophysica Acta*, **279**, 544–553.

188. Hammaker, L. & Schmid, R. (1967) Interference with bile pigment uptake in the liver by flavaspidic acid. *Gastroenterology*, **53**, 31–37.

189. Hargreaves, T. (1969) Neonatal serum bilirubin estimation. *Clinica Chimica Acta* **26**, 331–337.

190. Harris, J.W. & Kellermeyer, R.W. (1970) *The Red Cell. Production, Metabolism, Destruction: Normal and Abnormal.* Cambridge, Massachusetts: Harvard University.

191. Haurani, F.I. & Tocantins, L.M. (1961) Ineffective erythropoiesis. *American Journal of Medicine*, **31**, 519–531.

192. Haverback, B.J. & Wirtschafter, S.K. (1960) Familial non-hemolytic jaundice with normal liver histology and conjugated bilirubin. *New England Journal of Medicine*, **262**, 113–117.

193. Heirwegh, K.P.M., Van de Vijver, M. & Fevery, J. (1972) Assay and properties of digitonin-activated bilirubin uridine diphosphate glucuronyltransferase from rat liver. *Biochemical Journal*, **129**, 605–618.

194. Heirwegh, K.P.M., Van Hees, G.P., Leroy, P., Van Roy, F.P. & Jansen, F.H. (1970) Heterogeneity of bile pigment conjugates as revealed by chromatography of their ethyl anthranilate azopigments. *Biochemical Journal*, **120**, 877–890.

195. Heirwegh, K.P.M., Fevery, J., Meuwissen, J.A.T.P., Compernolle, F., Desmet, V. & Van Roy, F.P. (1974) Recent advances in the separation and analysis of diazo-positive bile pigments. *Methods of Biochemical Analysis*, **22**, 205–250.

196. Heirwegh, K.P.M., Fevery, J., Michiels, R., Van Hees, G.P. & Compernolle, F. (1975) Separation by thin-layer chromatography and structure elucidation

of bilirubin conjugates isolated from dog bile. *Biochemical Journal*, **145**, 185–199.

197. Hershko, C., Cook, J.D. & Finch, C.A. (1972) Storage iron kinetics. II. The uptake of hemoglobin iron by hepatic parenchymal cells. *Journal of Laboratory and Clinical Medicine*, **80**, 624–634.
198. Huang, P.W.H., Rozdilsky, B., Gerrard, J.W., Goluboff, N. & Holman, G.H. (1970) Crigler–Najjar syndrome in four of five siblings with postmortem findings in one. *Archives of Pathology*, **90**, 536–542.
199. Hunter, J.O., Thompson, R.P.H., Dunn, P.M. & Williams, R. (1973) Inheritance of type 2 Crigler–Najjar hyperbilirubinaemia. *Gut*, **14**, 46–49.
200. Israels, L.G. (1970) The bilirubin shunt and shunt hyperbilirubinemia. In *Progress in Liver Diseases* (Ed.) Popper, H. & Schaffner, F. pp. 1–12. New York: Grune & Stratton.
201. Israels, L.G. & Zipursky, A. (1962) Primary shunt hyperbilirubinaemia. *Nature (London)*, **193**, 73–74.
202. Israels, L.G., Suderman, H.J. & Ritzmann, S.E. (1959) Hyperbilirubinemia due to an alternate path of bilirubin production. *American Journal of Medicine*, **27**, 693–702.
203. Isselbacher, K.J. & McCarthy, E.A. (1959) Studies on bilirubin sulphate and other nonglucuronide conjugates of bilirubin. *Journal of Clinical Investigation*, **38**, 645–651.
204. Jacobsen, J. (1969) Binding of bilirubin to human serum albumin. Determination of the dissociation constants. *FEBS Letters*, **5**, 112–114.
205. Jacobsen, J. (1970) Dimerisation of bilirubin diglucuronide and formation of a complex of bilirubin and the diglucuronide. *Scandinavian Journal of Clinical and Laboratory Investigation*, **26**, 395–398.
206. Jacobsen, J. (1972) Chemical modification of the high-affinity bilirubin-binding site of human serum albumin. *European Journal of Biochemistry*, **27**, 513–519.
207. Jacobsen, J. & Wennberg, R.P. (1974) Determination of unbound bilirubin in the serum of newborns. *Clinical Chemistry*, **20**, 783–789.
208. Jandl, J.H., Jones, A.R. & Castle, W.B. (1957) The destruction of red cells by antibodies in man. 1. Observations on the sequestration and lysis of red cells altered by immune mechanism. *Journal of Clinical Investigation*, **36**, 1428–1459.
209. Jansen, P.L.M. (1974) The enzyme-catalyzed formation of bilirubin diglucuronide by a solubilized preparation from cat liver microsomes. *Biochimica et Biophysica Acta*, **338**, 170–182.
210. Jansen, P.L.M., Chowdhury, J.R., Fischberg, E.B. & Arias, I.M. (1977) Enzymatic conversion of bilirubin monoglucuronide to diglucuronide by rat liver plasma membranes. *Journal of Biological Chemistry*, **252**, 2710–2716.
211. Jendrassik, L. & Gróf, P. (1938) Vereinfachte photometrische Methoden zur Bestimmung des Blutbilirubins. *Biochemische Zeitschrift*, **297**, 81–89.
212. Jervis, G.A. (1959) Constitutional nonhemolytic hyperbilirubinemia with findings resembling kernicterus. *American Medical Association Archives of Neurology and Psychiatry*, **81**, 55–64.
213. Johnson, J.D. (1975) Neonatal nonhemolytic jaundice. *New England Journal of Medicine*, **292**, 194–197.
214. Johnson, L., Sarmiento, F., Blanc, W.A. & Day, R. (1959) Kernicterus in rats with an inherited deficiency of glucuronyl transferase. *American Medical Association Journal of Diseases of Children*, **97**, 591–608.
215. Jones, A.L., Schmucker, D.L., Mooney, J.S., Adler, R.D. & Ockner, R.K. (1976) Morphometric analysis of rat hepatocytes after total biliary obstruction. *Gastroenterology*, **71**, 1050–1060.
216. Jones, E.A., Shrager, R., Bloomer, J.R., Berk, P.D., Howe, R.B. & Berlin, N.I. (1972) Quantitative studies of the delivery of hepatic-synthesized bilirubin to plasma utilizing δ-aminolevulinic acid-4-^{14}C and bilirubin-^{3}H in man. *Journal of Clinical Investigation*, **51**, 2450–2458.
217. Kamisaka, K., Listowsky, I. & Arias, I.M. (1973) Circular dichroism studies of Y protein (Ligandin), a major organic anion binding protein in liver, kidney, and small intestine. *Annals of the New York Academy of Sciences*, **226**, 148–153.
218. Kapitulnik, J., Kaufmann, N.A., Goitein, K., Cividalli, G. & Blondheim, S.H. (1974) A pigment found in Crigler–Najjar syndrome and its similarity to an ultrafiltrable photoderivative of bilirubin. *Clinica Chimica Acta*, **57**, 231–237.
219. Karon, M., Imach, D. & Schwartz, A. (1970) Effective phototherapy in congenital nonobstructive, nonhemolytic jaundice. *New England Journal of Medicine*, **282**, 377–380.
220. Kenwright, S. & Levi, A.J. (1973) Impairment of hepatic uptake of rifamycin antibiotics by probenecid, and its therapeutic implications. *Lancet*, **ii**, 1401–1405.
221. Kenwright, S. & Levi, A.J. (1974) Sites of competition in the selective hepatic uptake of rifamycin-SV, flavaspidic acid, bilirubin, and bromsulphthalein. *Gut*, **15**, 220–226.
222. Ketterer, B., Ross-Mansell, P. & Whitehead, J.K. (1967) The isolation of carcinogen-binding protein from livers of rats given 4-di-methylamino-azobenzene. *Biochemical Journal*, **103**, 316–324.
223. Kirshenbaum, G., Shames, D.M. & Schmid, R. (1976) An expanded model of bilirubin kinetics: effect of feeding, fasting, and phenobarbital in Gilbert's syndrome. *Journal of Pharmacokinetics and Biopharmaceutics*, **4**, 115–155.
224. Klaus, D. & Feine, U. (1965) Primary shunt hyperbilirubinaemia. *German Medical Monthly*, **10**, 89–93.
225. Kondo, T., Kuchiba, K. & Shimizu, Y. (1976) Coproporphyrin isomers in Dubin-Johnson syndrome. *Gastroenterology*, **70**, 1117–1120.
226. Kondo, T., Kuchiba, K., Ohtsuka, Y., Yanagisawa, W., Shiomura, T. & Taminato, T. (1974) Clinical and genetic studies on Dubin–Johnson syndrome in a cluster area in Japan. *Japanese Journal of Human Genetics*, **18**, 378–392.
227. Kornberg, A. (1942) Latent liver disease in persons recovered from catarrhal jaundice and in otherwise normal medical students as revealed by the bilirubin excretion test. *Journal of Clinical Investigation*, **21**, 299–308.
228. Koskelo, P., Toivonen, I. & Adlercreutz, H. (1967) Urinary coproporphyrin isomer distribution in the Dubin–Johnson syndrome. *Clinical Chemistry*, **13**, 1006–1009.
229. Krasner, J. & Mukherjee, A.B. (1978) Letter to the editor: Importance of technique in the induction of glucuronyl transferase in Gunn rats. *Pediatric Research*, **12**, 58–59.
230. Kreek, M.J. & Sleisenger, M.H. (1968) Reduction of serum unconjugated bilirubin with phenobarbitone

in adult congenital nonhaemolytic unconjugated hyperbilirubinaemia. *Lancet*, **ii**, 73–78.

231. Kuenzle, C.C. (1970) Bilirubin conjugates of human bile: the excretion of bilirubin as the acyl glycosides of aldobiouronic acid, with a branched-chain hexuronic acid as one of the components of the hexuronosylhexuronide. *Biochemical Journal*, **119**, 411–435.
232. Kutz, K., Egger, G., Bachofen, H. & Preisig, R. (1977) Effect of fasting on endogenous carbon monoxide production in normal subjects and those with constitutional hepatic dysfunction (Gilbert's syndrome). In *Chemistry and Physiology of Bile Pigments* (Ed.) Berk, P.D. & Berlin, N.I. pp. 156–167. Washington, D.C.: U.S. Government Printing Office.
233. Kutz, K., Schulte, A., Jensen, C. & Gugler, R. (1977) Impaired drug conjugation in subjects with Gilbert's syndrome. *Gastroenterology*, **73**, A-31/1229.
234. Landaw, S.A. (1975) Carbon monoxide production as a measurement of heme catabolism. In *Jaundice* (Ed.) Goresky, C.A. & Fisher, M.M. pp. 103–107. New York: Plenum.
235. Lathe, G.H. (1972) The degradation of haem by mammals and its excretion as conjugated bilirubin. *Essays in Biochemistry*, **8**, 107–148.
236. Layden, T.J. & Boyer, J.L. (1977) Evidence that bile acids are a determinant of the lobular gradient for canalicular bile secretion. *Gastroenterology*, **73**, A-33/1231.
237. Lazarow, P.B. & de Duve, C. (1973) The synthesis and turnover of rat liver peroxisomes. Biochemical pathway of catalase synthesis. *Journal of Cell Biology*, **59**, 491–506.
238. Lelong, M., Colin, J., Alagille, D., Gentil, C., Bretagne, J. & Houllemare, L. (1961) Ictère familial non-hémolytique avec ictère nucléaire (maladie de Crigler–Najjar). *Archives Françaises de Pédiatrie*, **18**, 272–275.
239. Lester, R. & Schmid, R. (1963) Intestinal absorption of bile pigments. II. Bilirubin absorption in man. *New England Journal of Medicine*, **269**, 178–182.
240. Lester, R. & Schmid, R. (1963) Intestinal absorption of bile pigments. I. The enterohepatic circulation of bilirubin in the rat. *Journal of Clinical Investigation*, **42**, 736–746.
241. Lester, R. & Schmid, R. (1965) Intestinal absorption of bile pigments. III. The enterohepatic circulation of urobilinogen in the rat. *Journal of Clinical Investigation*, **44**, 722–730.
242. Lester, R., Hammaker, L. & Schmid, R. (1962) A new therapeutic approach to unconjugated hyperbilirubinaemia. *Lancet*, **ii**, 1257.
243. Lester, R., Schumer, W. & Schmid, R. (1965) Intestinal absorption of bile pigments. IV. Urobilinogen absorption in man. *New England Journal of Medicine*, **272**, 939–943.
244. Levi, A.J., Gatmaitan, Z. & Arias, I.M. (1969) Two hepatic cytoplasmic protein fractions, Y and Z, and their possible role in the hepatic uptake of bilirubin, sulfobromophthalein, and other anions. *Journal of Clinical Investigation*, **48**, 2156–2167.
245. Levi, A.J., Gatmaitan, Z. & Arias, I.M. (1970) Deficiency of hepatic organic anion binding protein, impaired organic anion uptake by liver and 'physiologic' jaundice in newborn monkeys. *New England Journal of Medicine*, **284**, 1136–1139.
246. Levine, R.I., Reyes, H., Levi, A.J., Gatmaitan, Z. & Arias, I.M. (1971) Phylogenetic study of organic anion transfer from plasma into the liver. *Nature (New Biology)*, **231**, 277–279.
247. Levitt, M., Schacter, B.A., Zipursky, A. & Israels, L.G. (1968) The nonerythropoietic component of early bilirubin. *Journal of Clinical Investigation*, **47**, 1281–1294.
248. Levy, M., Lester, R. & Levinsky, N.G. (1968) Renal excretion of urobilinogen in the dog. *Journal of Clinical Investigation*, **47**, 2117–2124.
249. Lightner, D.A. (1977) The photoreactivity of bilirubin and related pyrroles. *Photochemistry and Photobiology*, **26**, 427–436.
250. Lipsitz, P.J. & London, M. (1973) A rapid total bilirubin test using sodium hypochlorite. *Journal of Laboratory and Clinical Medicine*, **81**, 625–631.
251. Litwack, G., Ketterer, B. & Arias, I.M. (1971) Ligandin: an abundant hepatic protein which binds steroids, bilirubin, carcinogens, and a number of exogenous organic anions. *Nature (London)*, **234**, 466–467.
252. Lolekha, P.H. & Limpavithayakul, K. (1977) Promoting ability of 5 accelerating agents for diazotization of several types of bilirubin samples. *Clinical Chemistry*, **23**, 778–779.
253. London, I.M., West, R., Shemin, D. & Rittenberg, D. (1950) On the origin of bile pigment in normal man. *Journal of Biological Chemistry*, **184**, 351–358.
254. Lucey, J.F., Ferreiro, M. & Hewitt, J. (1968) Prevention of hyperbilirubinemia of prematurity by phototherapy. *Pediatrics*, **41**, 1047–1054.
255. Lundh, B., Johansson, M.-B., Mercke, C. & Cavallin-Ståhl, E. (1972) Enhancement of heme catabolism by caloric restriction in man. *Scandinavian Journal of Clinical and Laboratory Investigation*, **30**, 421–427.
256. Lundh, H.T. & Jacobsen, J. (1972) Influence of phototherapy on unconjugated bilirubin in duodenal bile of newborn infants with hyperbilirubinaemia. *Acta Paediatrica Scandinavica*, **61**, 693–696.
257. Maines, M.D. & Kappas, A. (1977) Enzymatic oxidation of cobalt protoporphyrin IX: observations on the mechanism of heme oxygenase action. *Biochemistry*, **16**, 419–423.
258. Maines, M.D., Ibrahim, N.G. & Kappas, A. (1977) Solubilization and partial purification of heme oxygenase from rat liver. *Journal of Biological Chemistry*, **252**, 5900–5903.
259. Malloy, H. & Evelyn, K. (1937) The determination of bilirubin with the photoelectric colorimeter. *Journal of Biological Chemistry*, **119**, 481–490.
260. Malloy, H. & Lowenstein, L. (1940) Hereditary jaundice in the rat. *Canadian Medical Association Journal*, **42**, 122–125.
261. Mandema, E., de Fraiture, W.H., Nieweg, H.O. & Arends, A. (1960) Familial chronic idiopathic jaundice (Dubin–Sprinz disease), with a note on bromsulphalein metabolism in this disease. *American Journal of Medicine*, **28**, 42–50.
262. Martin, J.F., Vierling, J.M., Wolkoff, A.W., Scharschmidt, B.F., Vergalla, J., Waggoner, B.A. & Berk, P.D. (1976) Abnormal hepatic transport of indocyanine green in Gilbert's syndrome. *Gastroenterology*, **70**, 385–391.
263. Marver, H.S. & Schmid, R. (1972) The porphyrias. In *The Metabolic Basis of Inherited Disease* (Ed.) Stanbury, J.B., Wyngaarden, J.B. & Fredrickson, D.S. pp. 1087–1140. New York: McGraw-Hill.

264. McDevitt, D.G., Nies, A.S. & Wilkinson, G.R. (1977) Influence of phenobarbital on factors responsible for hepatic clearance of indocyanine green in the rat: relative contributions of induction and altered blood flow. *Biochemical Pharmacology,* **26,** 1247–1250.

265. McDonagh, A.F. (1976) Photochemistry and photometabolism of bilirubin IXα. In *Bilirubin Metabolism in the Newborn* (II) (Ed.) Bergsma, D. & Blondheim, S.H. pp. 30–40. New York: American Elsevier.

266. McDonagh, A.F. (1978) Bile pigments. Bilatrienes and 5,15-biladienes. In *The Porphyrins* (Ed.) Dolphin, D. New York: Academic Press.

267. McDonagh, A.F. & Assisi, F. (1972) The ready isomerization of bilirubin IX-α in aqueous solution. *Biochemical Journal,* **129,** 797–800.

268. McGee, J. O'D., Allan, J.G., Russell, R.I. & Patrick, R.S. (1975) Liver ultrastructure in Gilbert's syndrome. *Gut,* **16,** 220–224.

269. Meijer, D.K.F., Vonk, R.J., Keulemans, K. & Weitering, J.G. (1977) Hepatic uptake and biliary excretion of dibromosulphthalein. Albumin dependence, influence of phenobarbital and nafenopin pretreatment and the role of Y and Z protein. *The Journal of Pharmacology and Experimental Therapeutics,* **202,** 8–21.

270. Mercke, C., Cavallin-Ståhl, E. & Lundh, B. (1975) Diurnal variation in endogenous production of CO. Effect of caloric restriction. *Acta Medica Scandinavica,* **198,** 161–164.

271. Merdler, C., Burke, M., Shani, M., Felner, S. & Lurie, I. (1976) The effect of phenobarbital on patients with Dubin–Johnson syndrome. *Digestion,* **14,** 394–399.

272. Metreau, J.-M., Dhumeaux, D., Gisselbrecht, C., Préaux, A.-M. & Berthelot, P. (1977) Constitutional unconjugated hyperbilirubinaemia. *Lancet,* **i,** 318.

273. Meulengracht, E. (1947) A review of chronic intermittent juvenile jaundice. *Quarterly Journal of Medicine,* **16,** 83–98.

274. Meuwissen, J.A.T.P., Ketterer, B. & Heirwegh, K.P.M. (1977) Role of soluble binding proteins in overall hepatic transport of bilirubin. In *Chemistry and Physiology of Bile Pigments* (Ed.) Berk, P.D. & Berlin, N.I. pp. 323–337. Washington, D.C.: U.S. Government Printing Office.

275. Meuwissen, J.A.T.P., Zeegers, M., Srai, K.S. & Ketterer, B. (1977) Effect of glutathione on the activity of bilirubin-binding proteins from rat liver cytosol. *Biochemical Society Transactions,* **5,** 1404–1407.

276. Mia, A.S., Gronwall, R.R. & Cornelius, C.E. (1970) Bilirubin-^{14}C turnover studies in normal and mutant Southdown sheep with congenital hyperbilirubinemia. *Proceedings of the Society for Experimental Biology and Medicine,* **133,** 955–959.

277. Mia, A.S., Gronwall, R.R. & Cornelius, C.E. (1970) Unconjugated and conjugated bilirubin transport in normal and mutant Corriedale sheep with Dubin–Johnson syndrome. *Proceedings of the Society for Experimental Biology and Medicine,* **135,** 33–37.

278. Michaelsson, M., Nosslin, B. & Sjölin, S. (1965) Plasma bilirubin determination in the newborn infant. *Pediatrics,* **35,** 925–931.

279. Minio-Paluello, F., Gautier, A. & Magnenat, P. (1968) L'ultrastructure du foie humain dans un cas de Crigler–Najjar. *Acta Hepato-Splenologica,* **15,** 65–71.

280. Mukherjee, B. & Krasner, J. (1973) Induction of an enzyme in genetically deficient rats after grafting of normal liver. *Science,* **182,** 68–70.

281. Muller-Eberhard, U. & Liem, H.H. (1974) Hemopexin, the heme-binding serum β-glycoprotein. In *Structure and Function of Plasma Proteins* (Ed.) Allison, A.C. Vol. 1, pp. 35–53. London: Plenum.

282. Muscatello, U., Mussini, I. & Agnolucci, M.T. (1967) The Dubin–Johnson syndrome: an electron microscopic study of the liver cell. *Acta Hepato-Splenologica,* **14,** 162–170.

283. Nakata, D., Zakim, D. & Vessey, D.A. (1976) Defective function of a microsomal UDP-glucuronyltransferase in Gunn rats. *Proceedings of the National Academy of Sciences of the United States of America,* **73,** 289–292.

284. Namihisa, T. & Nambu, M. (1977) Rotor's and Dubin–Johnson syndromes. *New England Journal of Medicine,* **297,** 560.

285. Namihisa, T. & Yamaguchi, K. (1973) The constitutional hyperbilirubinemia in Japan: studies on 139 cases reported during the period from 1963 to 1969. *Gastroenterologia Japonica,* **8,** 311–321.

286. Namihisa, T., Yamaguchi, K. & Nambu, M. (1973) The constitutional conjugated hyperbilirubinemia. *Gastroenterologia Japonica,* **8,** 217–223.

287. Nelson, J., Jacobsen, J. & Wennberg, R.P. (1974) Effect of pH on the interaction of bilirubin with albumin and tissue culture cells. *Pediatric Research,* **8,** 963–967.

288. Noir, B.A. & Nanet, H. (1974) A study of the ethyl anthranilate azo derivatives of bilirubin sulphate. Confirmation of the existence of bilirubin sulphate conjugates in bile. *Biochimica et Biophysica Acta,* **372,** 230–236.

289. Novikoff, A.B. & Essner, E. (1960) The liver cell. *American Journal of Medicine,* **29,** 102–131.

290. Ockner, R.K., Manning, J.A., Poppenhausen, R.B. & Ho, W.K. (1972) A binding protein for fatty acids in cytosol of intestinal mucosa, liver, myocardium, and other tissues. *Science,* **177,** 56–58.

291. Odell, G.B. (1965) Influence of pH on the distribution of bilirubin between albumin and mitochondria. *Proceedings of the Society for Experimental Biology and Medicine,* **120,** 352–354.

292. Odell, G.B. (1966) The distribution of bilirubin between albumin and mitochondria. *Journal of Pediatrics,* **68,** 164–180.

293. Odell, G.B., Natzschke, J.C. & Storey, G.N. (1967) Bilirubin nephropathy in the Gunn strain of rat. *American Journal of Physiology,* **212,** 931–938.

294. Odell, G.B., Bolen, J.L., Poland, R.L., Seungdamrong, S. & Cukier, J.O. (1974) Protection from bilirubin nephropathy in jaundiced Gunn rats. *Gastroenterology,* **66,** 1218–1224.

295. Odell, G.B., Cukier, J.O., Ostrea, E.M., Maglalang, A.C. & Poland, R.L. (1977) The influence of fatty acids on the binding of bilirubin to albumin. *Journal of Laboratory and Clinical Medicine,* **89,** 295–307.

296. Odièvre, M., Trivin, F., Eliot, N. & Alagille, D. (1978) Case of congenital nonobstructive, nonhaemolytic jaundice. Successful long-term phototherapy at home. *Archives of Diseases in Childhood,* **53,** 81–82.

297. Ostrow, J.D. (1967) Absorption of bile pigments by the gallbladder. *Journal of Clinical Investigation,* **46,** 2035–2052.

298. Ostrow, J.D. (1971) Photocatabolism of labeled bilirubin in the congenitally jaundiced (Gunn) rat. *Journal of Clinical Investigation,* **50,** 707–718.

299. Ostrow, J.D. (1974) Bilirubin and jaundice. In *The Liver. Normal and Abnormal Functions* (Ed.) Becker, F.F. pp. 303–369. New York: Marcell Dekker.

300. Owens, D. & Evans, J. (1975) Population studies in Gilbert's syndrome. *Journal of Medical Genetics,* **12,** 152–156.

301. Owens, D. & Sherlock, S. (1973) Diagnosis of Gilbert's syndrome: role of reduced caloric intake test. *British Medical Journal,* **iii,** 559–563.

302. Pascasio, F.M. & de la Fuente, D. (1969) Rotor–Manahan–Floretin syndrome: clinical and genetic studies. *Philippine Journal of Internal Medicine,* **7,** 151–157.

303. Paumgartner, G. & Reichen, J. (1976) Kinetics of hepatic uptake of unconjugated bilirubin. *Clinical Science and Molecular Medicine,* **51,** 169–176.

304. Peck, O.C., Rey, D.F. & Snell, A.M. (1960) Familial jaundice with free and conjugated bilirubin in the serum and without liver pigmentation. *Gastroenterology,* **39,** 625–627.

305. Pereira Lima, J.E., Utz, E. & Roisenberg, I. (1966) Hereditary non-hemolytic conjugated hyperbilirubinemia without abnormal liver cell pigmentation. A family study. *American Journal of Medicine,* **40,** 628–633.

306. Peterson, R.E. & Schmid, R. (1957) A clinical syndrome associated with a defect in steroid glucuronide conjugation. *Journal of Clinical Endocrinology and Metabolism,* **17,** 1485–1488.

307. Pimstone, N.R., Engel, P., Tenhunen, R., Seitz, P., Marver, H.S. & Schmid, R. (1971) Inducible heme oxygenase in the kidney: a model for the homeostatic control of hemoglobin catabolism. *Journal of Clinical Investigation,* **50,** 2042–2050.

308. Poland, R.L. & Odell, G.B. (1971) Physiologic jaundice: the enterohepatic circulation of bilirubin. *New England Journal of Medicine,* **284,** 1–6.

309. Porush, J.G., Delman, A.J. & Feuer, M.M. (1962) Chronic idiopathic jaundice with normal liver histology. *Archives of Internal Medicine,* **109,** 102–109.

310. Powell, L.W., Billing, B.H. & Williams, H.S. (1967) The assessment of red cell survival in idiopathic unconjugated hyperbilirubinaemia (Gilbert's syndrome) by the use of radioactive diisopropylfluorophosphate and chromium. *Australasian Annals of Medicine,* **16,** 221–225.

311. Powell, L.W., Hemingway, E., Billing, B.H. & Sherlock, S. (1967) Idiopathic unconjugated hyperbilirubinemia (Gilbert's syndrome). A study of 42 families. *New England Journal of Medicine,* **277,** 1108–1112.

312. Quinn, N.W. & Gollan, J.L. (1975) Jaundice following oral surgery: Gilbert's syndrome. *British Journal of Oral Surgery,* **12,** 285–288.

313. Raymond, G.D. & Galambos, J.T. (1971) Hepatic storage and excretion of bilirubin in man. *American Journal of Gastroenterology,* **55,** 135–144.

314. Reichen, J. & Berk, P.D. (1977) Isolation of an organic anionic dye binding protein from rat liver plasma membrane. *Gastroenterology,* **73,** A-44/1242.

315. Reyes, H., Levi, A.J. & Arias, I.M. (1971) Studies of Y and Z, two hepatic cytoplasmic organic anion-binding proteins: effect of drugs, chemicals, hormones and cholestasis. *Journal of Clinical Investigation,* **50,** 2242–2252.

316. Robinson, S.H. (1968) The origins of bilirubin. *New England Journal of Medicine,* **279,** 143–149.

317. Robinson, S.H. & Tsong, M. (1970) Hemolysis of 'stress' reticulocytes: a source of erythropoietic bilirubin formation. *Journal of Clinical Investigation,* **49,** 1025–1034.

318. Robinson, S.H., Yannoni, C. & Nagawawa, S. (1971) Bilirubin excretion in rats with normal and impaired bilirubin conjugation: effect of phenobarbital. *Journal of Clinical Investigation,* **50,** 2606–2613.

319. Robinson, S.H., Lester, R., Crigler, J.F. & Tsong, M. (1967) Early-labeled peak of bile pigment in man. Studies with glycine-^{14}C and δ-aminolevulinic acid-^{3}H. *New England Journal of Medicine,* **277,** 1323–1329.

320. Rosental, E. & Thaler, M.M. (1977) Inhibition of lipolysis prevents fasting hyperbilirubinemia in Gunn rats. *Gastroenterology,* **72,** A-99/1122.

321. Rosental, E. & Thaler, M.M. (1977) Inhibition of bilirubin conjugation and induction of hyperbilirubinemia by nicotinic acid. *Gastroenterology,* **73,** A-46/1244.

322. Rosenthal, I.M., Zimmerman, H.J. & Hardy, N. (1956) Congenital nonhemolytic jaundice with disease of the central nervous system. *Pediatrics,* **18,** 378–386.

323. Rotor, A.B., Manahan, L. & Florentin, A. (1948) Familial non-hemolytic jaundice with direct van den Bergh reaction. *Acta Medica Philippina,* **5,** 37–48.

324. Royer, M., Noir, B.A., Sfarcich, D. & Nanet, H. (1974) Extrahepatic bilirubin formation and conjugation in the dog. *Digestion,* **10,** 423–434.

325. Rugstad, H.E., Robinson, S.H., Yannoni, C. & Tashjian, A.H. (1970) Transfer of bilirubin uridine disphosphate-glucuronyltransferase to enzyme-deficient rats. *Science,* **170,** 553–555.

326. Sagild, U., Dalgaard, O.Z. & Tygstrup, N. (1962) Constitutional hyperbilirubinemia with unconjugated bilirubin in the serum and lipochrome-like pigment granules in the liver. *Annals of Internal Medicine,* **56,** 308–314.

327. Schalm, L. & Weber, A.P. (1964) Jaundice with conjugated bilirubin in hyperhaemolysis. *Acta Medica Scandinavica,* **176,** 549–553.

328. Scharschmidt, B.F. (1978) Personal communication.

329. Scharschmidt, B.F. & Schmid, R. (1979) The micellar sink: a quantitative assessment of the association of organic anions with mixed micelles and other macromolecular aggregates in rat bile. *Journal of Clinical Investigation,* **62.** In press.

330. Scharschmidt, B.F., Waggoner, J.G. & Berk, P.D. (1975) Hepatic organic anion uptake in the rat. *Journal of Clinical Investigation,* **56,** 1280–1292.

331. Scharschmidt, B.F., Plotz, P.H., Berk, P.D., Waggoner, J.G. & Vergalla, J. (1974) Removing substances from blood by affinity chromatography. II. Removing bilirubin from the blood of jaundiced rats by hemoperfusion over albumin-conjugated agarose beads. *Journal of Clinical Investigation,* **53,** 786–795.

332. Schenker, S., Dawber, N.H. & Schmid, R. (1964) Bilirubin metabolism in the fetus. *Journal of Clinical Investigation,* **43,** 32–39.

333. Schiff, L., Billing, B.H. & Oikawa, Y. (1959) Familial nonhemolytic jaundice with conjugated bilirubin in the serum. A case study. *New England Journal of Medicine,* **260,** 1315–1318.

334. Schmid, R. (1973) Synthesis and degradation of microsomal hemoproteins. *Drug Metabolism and Disposition*, **1**, 256–258.

335. Schmid, R. (1976) Pyrrolic victories. *Transactions of the Association of American Physicians*, **84**, 64–76.

336. Schmid, R. (1978) Bilirubin metabolism: state of the art. *Gastroenterology*, **74**, 1307–1312.

337. Schmid, R. & Hammaker, L. (1959) Glucuronide formation in patients with constitutional hepatic dysfunction (Gilbert's syndrome). *New England Journal of Medicine*, **260**, 1310–1314.

338. Schmid, R. & Hammaker, L. (1963) Metabolism and disposition of C^{14}-bilirubin in congenital non-hemolytic jaundice. *Journal of Clinical Investigation*, **42**, 1720–1734.

339. Schmid, R. & McDonagh, A.F. (1975) The enzymatic formation of bilirubin. *Annals of the New York Academy of Sciences*, **244**, 533–552.

340. Schmid, R. & McDonagh, A.F. (1978) Hyperbilirubinemia. In *The Metabolic Basis of Inherited Disease* (Ed.) Stanbury, J.B., Wyngaarden, J.B. & Frederickson, D.S. pp. 1221–1257. New York: McGraw-Hill.

341. Schmid, R. & McDonagh, A.F. (1978) Formation and metabolism of bile pigments in vivo. In *The Porphyrins* (Ed.) Dolphin, D. New York: Academic Press.

342. Schmid, R., Marver, H.S. & Hammaker, L. (1966) Enhanced formation of rapidly labeled bilirubin by phenobarbital: hepatic microsomal cytochromes as a possible source. *Biochemical and Biophysical Research Communications*, **24**, 319–328.

343. Schoenfield, L.J., Foulk, W.T. & Butt, H.R. (1964) Studies of sulfobromophthalein sodium (BSP) metabolism in man. I. In normal subjects and patients with hepatic disease. *Journal of Clinical Investigation*, **43**, 1409–1418.

344. Schoenfield, L.J., McGill, D.B., Hunton, D.B., Foulk, W.T. & Butt, H.R. (1963) Studies of chronic idiopathic jaundice (Dubin–Johnson syndrome). I. Demonstration of hepatic excretory defect. *Gastroenterology*, **44**, 101–111.

345. Seligman, J.W. (1977) Recent and changing concepts of hyperbilirubinemia and its management in newborn. *Pediatric Clinics of North America*, **24**, 509–528.

346. Seligsohn, U., Shani, M., Ramot, B., Adam, A. & Sheba, C. (1970) Dubin–Johnson syndrome in Israel. II. Association with factor-VII deficiency. *Quarterly Journal of Medicine*, **39**, 569–584.

347. Seymour, C.A., Neale, G. & Peters, T.J. (1977) Lysosomal changes in liver tissue from patients with the Dubin–Johnson–Sprinz syndrome. *Clinical Science and Molecular Medicine*, **52**, 241–248.

348. Shani, M., Seligsohn, U. & Ben-Ezzer, J. (1974) Effect of phenobarbital on liver functions in patients with Dubin–Johnson syndrome. *Gastroenterology*, **67**, 303–308.

349. Shani, M., Gilon, E., Ben-Ezzer, J. & Sheba, C. (1970) Sulfobromophthalein tolerance test in patients with Dubin–Johnson syndrome and their relatives. *Gastroenterology*, **59**, 842–847.

350. Shani, M., Seligsohn, U., Gilon, E., Sheba, C. & Adam, A. (1970) Dubin–Johnson syndrome in Israel. I. Clinical, laboratory, and genetic aspects of 101 cases. *Quarterly Journal of Medicine*, **39**, 549–567.

351. Shankaran, S. & Poland, R.L. (1977) Displacement of bilirubin from albumin by furosemide. *Journal of Pediatrics*, **90**, 642–646.

352. Shimizu, Y., Kondo, T., Kuchiba, K. & Urata, G. (1977) Uroporphyrinogen III cosynthetase in liver and blood in the Dubin–Johnson syndrome. *Journal of Laboratory and Clinical Medicine*, **89**, 517–523.

353. Shull, S.D., Wagner, C.I., Trotman, B.W. & Soloway, R.D. (1977) Factors affecting bilirubin excretion in patients with cholesterol or pigment gallstones. *Gastroenterology*, **72**, 625–629.

354. Shupeck, M. (1977) Studies of the hepatic uptake of conjugated bilirubin in the rat. *Gastroenterology*, **72**, A-166/1189.

355. Sleisenger, M.H., Kahn, I., Barniville, H., Rubin, W., Ben-Ezzer, J. & Arias, I.M. (1967) Nonhemolytic unconjugated hyperbilirubinemia with hepatic glucuronyl transferase deficiency: a genetic study in four generations. *Transactions of the Association of American Physicians*, **80**, 259–266.

356. Smith, P.M., Middleton, J.E. & Williams, R. (1967) Studies on the familial incidence and clinical history of patients with chronic unconjugated hyperbilirubinaemia. *Gut*, **8**, 449–453.

357. Snyder, A.L., Satterlee, W., Robinson, S.H. & Schmid, R. (1967) Conjugated plasma bilirubin in jaundice caused by pigment overload. *Nature (London)*, **213**, 93.

358. Sprinz, H. & Nelson, R.S. (1954) Persistent non-hemolytic hyperbilirubinemia associated with lipochrome-like pigment in liver cells: report of 4 cases. *Annals of Internal Medicine*, **41**, 952–962.

359. Stein, L.B., Mishkin, S., Fleischner, G., Gatmaitan, Z. & Arias, I.M. (1976) Effect of fasting on hepatic ligandin, Z protein, and organic anion transfer from plasma in rats. *American Journal of Physiology*, **231**, 1371–1376.

360. Sugar, P. (1961) Familial nonhemolytic jaundice. Congenital, with kernicterus. *Archives of Internal Medicine*, **108**, 189–195.

361. Suri, V.P., Chatterjee, T. & Sagaraya, K. (1966) Dubin–Johnson syndrome. *Journal of the Indian Medical Association*, **47**, 32–34.

362. Sutherland, D.E.R., Matas, A.J., Steffes, M.W., Simmons, R.L. & Najarian, J.S. (1977) Transplantation of liver cells in an animal model of congenital enzyme deficiency disease: the Gunn rat. *Transplantation Proceedings*, **9**, 317–320.

363. Szabó, L. & Ebrey, P. (1963) Studies on the inheritance of Crigler–Najjar syndrome by the menthol test. *Acta Paediatrica Hungarica*, **4**, 153–158.

364. Szabó, L., Kovács, Z. & Ebrey, P.B. (1962) Crigler–Najjar's syndrome. *Acta Paediatrica Hungarica*, **3**, 49–70.

365. Tenhunen, R., Marver, H.S. & Schmid, R. (1968) The enzymatic conversion of heme to bilirubin by microsomal heme oxygenase. *Proceedings of the National Academy of Sciences of the United States of America*, **61**, 748–755.

366. Tenhunen, R., Marver, H.S. & Schmid, R. (1969) Microsomal heme oxygenase. Characterization of the enzyme. *Journal of Biological Chemistry*, **244**, 6388–6394.

367. Tenhunen, R., Marver, H.S. & Schmid, R. (1970) The enzymatic catabolism of hemoglobin: stimulation of microsomal heme oxygenase by hemin. *Journal of Laboratory and Clinical Medicine*, **75**, 410–421.

368. Tenhunen, R., Ross, M.E., Marver, H.S. & Schmid, R. (1970) Reduced nicotinamide-adenine dinucleotide phosphate dependent biliverdin reductase: partial purification and characterization. *Biochemistry*, **9**, 298–303.

369. Thaler, M.M. (1977) Jaundice in the newborn. Algorithmic diagnosis of conjugated and unconjugated hyperbilirubinemia. *Journal of the American Medical Association,* **237,** 58–62.

370. Thompson, R.P.H. & Hofmann, A.F. (1973) Free and conjugated bile pigments of body fluids: qualitative analysis by thin-layer chromatography. *Journal of Laboratory and Clinical Medicine,* **82,** 483–488.

371. Tisdale, W.A., Klatskin, G. & Kinsella, E.D. (1959) The significance of the direct-reacting fraction of serum bilirubin in hemolytic jaundice. *American Journal of Medicine,* **26,** 214–227.

372. Troxler, R.F., Dawber, N.H. & Lester, R. (1968) Synthesis of urobilinogen by broken cell preparations of intestinal bacteria. *Gastroenterology,* **54,** 568–574.

373. Tsuru, M., Kamisaka, K., Hirano, M. & Kameda, H. (1978) Quantification of human serum ligandin by radioimmunoassay. *Clinica Chimica Acta,* **84,** 251–253.

374. van den Bergh, H.A.A. & Müller, P. (1916) Über eine direkte und indirekte Diazoreaktion auf Bilirubin. *Biochemische Zeitschrift,* **77,** 93–103.

375. Van Houwelingen, C.A.J. & Arias, I.M. (1976) Attempts to induce hepatic uridine diphosphate glucuronyl transferase in genetically deficient Gunn rats by grafting of normal liver tissue. *Pediatric Research,* **10,** 830–832.

376. Van Roy, F.P., Meuwissen, J.A.T.P., De Meuter, F. & Heirwegh, K.P.M. (1971) Determination of bilirubin in liver homogenates and serum with diazotized p-iodoaniline. *Clinica Chimica Acta,* **31,** 109–118.

377. Vaughan, J.M. & Haslewood, G.A.D. (1938) The normal level of plasma bilirubin. *Lancet,* **i,** 133–135.

378. Vaughan, J.P., Marubbio, A.T., Maddocks, I. & Cooke, R.A. (1970) Chronic idiopathic jaundice in Papua and New Guinea: a report of nine patients with Dubin–Johnson's or Rotor's syndrome. *Transactions of the Royal Society of Tropical Medicine and Hygiene,* **64,** 287–292.

379. Verwilghen, R., Verhaegen, H., Waumans, P. & Beert, J. (1969) Ineffective erythropoiesis with morphologically abnormal erythroblasts and unconjugated hyperbilirubinaemia. *British Journal of Haematology,* **17,** 27–33.

380. Vessey, D.A., Goldenberg, J. & Zakim, D. (1973) Kinetic properties of microsomal UDP-glucuronyltransferase: evidence for cooperative kinetics and activation by UDP-N-acetylglucosamine. *Biochimica et Biophysica Acta,* **309,** 58–66.

381. Wakisaka, G., Ichida, F., Kuge, T., Yamamoto, T., Sasaki, H., Yamamoto, Y., Imai, Y., Okawa, S., Harada, T., Taguchi, Y. & Nakagawa, T. (1961) Clinical and enzymological observation on cases with Gilbert's disease. *Japanese Archives of Internal Medicine,* **8,** 634–648.

382. Ware, A.J., Carey, M.C. & Combes, B. (1976) Solution properties of sulfobromophthalein sodium (BSP) compounds alone and in association with sodium taurocholate (TC). *Journal of Laboratory and Clinical Medicine,* **87,** 443–456.

383. Ware, A.J., Eigenbrodt, E.H., Shorey, J. & Combes, B. (1972) Viral hepatitis complicating the Dubin–Johnson syndrome. *Gastroenterology,* **63,** 337–339.

384. Watson, C.J. (1969) Gold from dross: the first century of urobilinoids. *Annals of Internal Medicine,* **70,** 839–851.

385. Watson, C.J. & Weimer, M. (1959) Composition of the urobilin group in urine, bile, and feces and the significance of variations in health and disease. *Journal of Laboratory and Clinical Medicine,* **54,** 1–25.

386. Watson, C.J., Campbell, M. & Lowry, P.T. (1958) Preferential reduction of conjugated bilirubin to urobilinogen by normal fecal flora. *Proceedings of the Society for Experimental Biology and Medicine,* **98,** 707–711.

387. Wennberg, R.P., Rasmussen, L.F. & Ahlfors, C.E. (1977) Displacement of bilirubin from human albumin by 3 diuretics. *Journal of Pediatrics,* **90,** 647–650.

388. Wheeler, H.O., Meltzer, J.I. & Bradley, S.E. (1960) Biliary transport and hepatic storage of sulfobromophthalein sodium in the unanaesthetized dog, in normal man, and in patients with hepatic disease. *Journal of Clinical Investigation,* **39,** 1131–1141.

389. Whelton, M.J., Krustev, L.P. & Billing, B.H. (1968) Reduction in serum bilirubin by phenobarbital in adult unconjugated hyperbilirubinemia: is enzyme induction responsible? *American Journal of Medicine,* **45,** 160–164.

390. Whitington, G.L. (1960) Congenital nonhemolytic icterus with damage to the central nervous system. Report of a case in a negro child. *Pediatrics,* **25,** 437–440.

391. Wolf, R.L., Pizette, M., Richman, A., Dreiling, D.A., Jacobs, W., Fernandez, O. & Popper, H. (1960) Chronic idiopathic jaundice: a study of two afflicted families. *American Journal of Medicine,* **28,** 32–41.

392. Wolkoff, A.W. & Arias, I.M. (1977) ^{35}S-BSP binding by purified rat liver cell plasma membrane subfractions. *Gastroenterology,* **73,** A-57/1255.

393. Wolkoff, A.W., Cohen, L.E. & Arias, I.M. (1973) The inheritance of the Dubin–Johnson syndrome. *New England Journal of Medicine,* **288,** 113–117.

394. Wolkoff, A.W., Wolpert, E., Pascasio, F.N. & Arias, I.M. (1976) Rotor's syndrome. A distinct inheritable pathophysiologic entity. *America Journal of Medicine,* **60,** 173–179.

395. Wolkoff, A.W., Sellin, J., Gatmaitan, Z., Goresky, C.A. & Arias, I.M. (1977) Role of ligandin in the transfer of bilirubin from plasma into the liver. *Gastroenterology,* **73,** A-57/1255.

396. Wolkoff, A.W., Ketley, J.N., Waggoner, J.G., Berk, P.D. & Jakoby, W.B. (1978) Hepatic accumulation and intracellular binding of conjugated bilirubin. *Journal of Clinical Investigation,* **61,** 142–149.

397. Wolpert, E., Pascasio, F.M., Wolkoff, A.W. & Arias, I.M. (1977) Abnormal sulfobromophthalein metabolism in Rotor's syndrome and obligate heterozygotes. *New England Journal of Medicine,* **296,** 1099–1101.

398. Yaffe, S.J., Levy, G., Matsuzawa, T. & Baliah, T. (1966) Enhancement of glucuronide-conjugating capacity in a hyperbilirubinemic infant due to apparent enzyme induction by phenobarbital. *New England Journal of Medicine,* **275,** 1461–1466.

399. Yamamoto, T., Skanderbeg, J., Zipursky, A. & Israels, L.G. (1965) The early appearing bilirubin: evidence for two components. *Journal of Clinical Investigation,* **44,** 31–41.

400. Yannoni, C.Z. & Robinson, S.H. (1975) Early-labelled haem in erythroid and hepatic cells. *Nature (London),* **258,** 330–331.

401. Yannoni, C.Z. & Robinson, S.H. (1976) Early labeled heme synthesis in normal rats and rats with iron

deficiency anemia. *Biochimica et Biophysica Acta,* **428,** 533–549.

402. Yong, F.-C. & Cheah, S.-S. (1977) Breast milk jaundice: an *in vitro* study of the effect of free fatty acids on the bilirubin-serum albumin complex. *Research Communications in Chemical Pathology and Pharmacology,* **17,** 679–688.
403. Yoshida, T. & Kikuchi, G. (1977) Heme oxygenase purified to apparent homogeneity from pig spleen microsomes. *Journal of Biochemistry,* **81,** 265–268.
404. Zakim, D. & Vessey, D.A. (1973) Techniques for the characterization of UDP-glucuronyltransferase, glucose-6-phosphatase, and other tightly-bound microsomal enzymes. *Methods of Biochemical Analysis,* **21,** 1–37.
405. Zakim, D., Goldenberg, J. & Vessey, D.A. (1973) Differentiation of homologous forms of hepatic microsomal UDP-glucuronyltransferase. 1. Evidence for the glucuronidation of o-aminophenol and p-nitrophenol by separate enzymes. *Biochimica et Biophysica Acta,* **309,** 67–74.
406. Zeidenberg, P., Orrenius, S. & Ernster, L. (1967) Increase in levels of glucuronylating enzymes and associated rise in activities of mitochondrial oxidative enzymes upon phenobarbital administration in the rat. *Journal of Cell Biology,* **32,** 528–531.
407. Zenone, E.A., Stoll, M.S. & Ostrow, J.D. (1977) Mechanism of excretion of unconjugated bilirubin (UCB) during phototherapy. *Gastroenterology,* **72,** A-157/1180.

Chapter 14

Classification and Mechanism of Cholestasis

FENTON SCHAFFNER
HANS POPPER

Cholestasis is an important component of many liver and biliary tract diseases, and discussion of it concerns and overlaps with the description of disease entities in many parts of this book. Here, the emphasis is placed on the definition and features of cholestasis. The diseases involved are listed primarily from the point of view of differential diagnosis, and the problem of mechanism is put into focus. More detailed descriptions are provided of jaundice in pregnancy and of benign recurrent jaundice because these conditions are not covered elsewhere. The concept of mechanism is referred to, despite the prevailing ignorance about the molecular basis of this phenomenon, with the intention of offering assistance in the understanding of the pathogenesis, diagnosis and management of clinical disorders. The consequences of cholestasis, as well as its prognosis, are discussed. A short review of the diagnosis and therapy of cholestasis, partly overlapping and supplementing presentations in other parts of the book, concludes the chapter.

DEFINITION OF CHOLESTASIS

'Cholestasis', literally translated, is 'stagnation of bile',[169] but the application of this term depends on the viewpoint of the user.[159] The morphologist considers cholestasis to be the visualization of bile in the tissue which, on histological examination, implies bile pigment in hepatocytes, bile thrombi in bile canaliculi, and bile in the Kupffer cells and other macrophages. However, visualization of bile depends upon the technique applied; in reality, some bile is always in transit in normal hepatocytes and biliary passages and cholestasis really means an excess of morphologically demonstrable bile. Electron microscopically, cholestasis is associated with characteristic alterations of the hepatocytes; specifically, lesions of the bile canaliculi and the hepatocytic organelles surrounding them.[158,171,181,210] This can therefore be applied as the morphological characteristic of milder cholestasis. It is particularly important in experimental rodents, in which bile thrombi do not form even in severe cholestasis except in neonatal rats or after overload with bilirubin.[52] The clinician considers cholestasis to be piling up in the serum of all biliary substances, although the increase in serum bilirubin may be less conspicuous than that of the others. Jaundice is not a necessary requirement, but bilirubinuria occurs at some time in almost all instances. The radiologist demonstrates cholestasis by the visualization of an obstacle in the biliary passages. The physiologist characterizes cholestasis as disturbed secretion into canaliculi of whole bile by the hepatocytes, and this represents the best functional identification of the disorder. It excludes conditions in which the secretory defect does not involve all biliary substances; for instance, the selective inability to secrete organic anions, such as bilirubin or injected dyes, which is characteristic of the conjugated bilirubinopathies like Dubin–Johnson or Rotor's syndrome.[9] The latter conditions do not represent cholestasis, nor are they associated with elevation of serum bile acids or with the characteristic electron microscopic findings. The exclusion of the early stages of primary biliary cirrhosis is less well accepted (see Chapter 31). Bile presumably regurgitates through the altered bile ducts in the early stage of chronic destructive non-suppurative cholangitis to raise the level of all biliary substances in blood, with electron microscopic[108] or functional evidence of disturbed secretion of bile by the hepatocytes.[124]

CLASSIFICATION OF CHOLESTASIS

Cholestasis produced by demonstrable obstruction of the extrahepatic and large intrahepatic bile ducts is separated from the form in which such an obstruction cannot be demonstrated anatomically or by cholangiography. The mechanism of the cholestasis in the forms without demonstrable obstruction, discussed below, is not fully established, and the noncommittal designation 'intrahepatic cholestasis' is most widely applied to describe a phenomenon that is a common feature of liver disease.[156,159] Ambiguity arises in that intrahepatic cholestasis may be the result of obstruction within the liver, but in practice this ambiguity interferes but little, and no substitute for the term 'intrahepatic cholestasis' has been accepted.

Extrahepatic Biliary Obstruction

Any obstacle to bile flow in the common hepatic duct or common bile duct between the papilla of Vater and the bifurcation within the liver may produce cholestasis, resulting in a dilatation of the ducts above the obstacle. When the obstruction lasts long enough, the intrahepatic bile duct system dilates, a feature designated as hydrohepatosis.[169] Although jaundice is common in this form it may be absent or inconspicuous, while the activities of enzymes such as alkaline phosphatase, which are considered as markers for cholestasis, are greatly increased. Aminotransferase activity rises before that of alkaline phosphatase, but it falls within several days to normal, or nearly so, despite deepening jaundice. Itching may occur with any form of prolonged cholestasis, as may hypercholesterolaemia, although the latter occurs less regularly. Bacterial infection with cholangitis and, later, abscess formation accompanied by chills, fever and septicaemia are common complications explained by interference with drainage of the bile. There are four common and many uncommon causes of this obstruction.

Gallstones

Stones in the common bile duct lead the list of causes of obstruction. Initially, they may be impacted anywhere in the course of the duct system, including at the papilla of Vater. Relaxation of the initially contracted duct and subsidence of the oedema of the duct wall usually loosen the impaction; and, if the stone is not delivered into the duodenum, an incomplete obstruction, sometimes without jaundice, may result, recognizable only by other laboratory abnormalities referable to cholestasis. A ball-valve effect of the stone produces fluctuation in the degree of cholestasis. A stone in the cystic duct does not produce cholestasis except when located near the junction with the common duct and bulging into the lumen of the latter. Stones in the common hepatic duct and its branches are uncommon and, as a rule, develop only after cholecystectomy.

Tumours

Carcinoma at the papilla of Vater may produce varying degrees of cholestasis because of temporary relief of the obstruction of the bile flow by sloughing of carcinomatous tissue, usually associated with bleeding. Tumours in and around the extrahepatic biliary ducts produce cholestasis. Intrinsic benign tumours, like papillomas, often cause cholestasis which varies in intensity when the tumour changes position. This also includes benign papillomatous tumours on the papilla of Vater. Malignant tumours, primarily carcinomas of the duct, consistently create increasing cholestasis, with obstruction becoming complete without fluctuation, except after manipulative intervention. Extrinsic malignant tumours originating from organs around the liver, particularly from the head of the pancreas but also from the stomach, also cause relentlessly progressing cholestasis when they grow towards the bile duct and invade its wall, preventing the lateral movement of the duct in the loose, delicate connective tissue of the lesser omentum. Enlarged lymph nodes without fixation of the duct do not produce cholestasis even if they form large clusters.[87] Most forms of cholestasis in leukaemia and many lymphomas have an intrahepatic basis. The exceptions are chloroma, histiocytic non-Hodgkin's lymphomas, and occasionally Hodgkin's disease when the process extends into and thus fixes the duct. Metastatic carcinomas in the hilar lymph nodes only exceptionally produce cholestasis, again because they do not fix the duct. However, metastases to the hilar connective tissue of the liver from distant sites do produce cholestasis.

Inflammatory lesions of the bile ducts

These lesions, usually associated with strictures, are a frequent cause of extrahepatic mechanical obstruction. Previously, emphasis was laid on sequelae of surgical intervention on the ducts as a common cause of these strictures, with infection a frequent complication and the degree of obstruction varying but being mostly incomplete. Primary or idiopathic sclerosing cholangitis is diagnosed more frequently now than in previous years.[42,174,230] It is not clear whether this indicates increased incidence or better delineation of the disease. Sclerosing cholangitis is most frequently associated with ulcerative colitis and less often with retroperitoneal fibrosis. A relation to the use of methysergide (Sansert) is substantiated in rare instances. As this disorder may involve the gallbladder sometimes without involving the extrahepatic bile ducts, the disease probably represents some of the cases previously designated as acalculous cholecystitis. The intrahepatic bile ducts may be involved in association with extrahepatic sclerosing cholangitis or, rarely, alone. Sclerosing cholangitis may be a transient or relapsing disease. Extrahepatic biliary atresia with or without involvement of the intrahepatic duct system is a disease of infancy and childhood (see Chapter 41).

Pancreatic diseases

Diseases of the pancreas, particularly cancer[57, 134] (see Chapter 55), but also pancreatitis, may cause extrahepatic biliary obstruction. The importance of the latter is more frequently emphasized on the basis of endoscopic retrograde cholangiography, by which tapering of the common duct is demonstrated.[190] Jaundice is reported in 15 to 25 per cent of cases of acute pancreatitis. While other causes of the jaundice can be incriminated, in over 40 per cent mechanical obstruction of the pars pancreatica of the common bile duct was responsible.[119] Similarly, in chronic pancreatitis both inflammation and fibrosis distort and kink the common duct,[189,204] as can acute pancreatitis and pseudocysts of the pancreas.[190] Retention cysts may also produce obstructive jaundice.[122]

Unusual causes

A series of rare conditions produces mechanical extrahepatic biliary obstruction. This includes choledochal cysts, strategically located amoebic abscesses, diverticula of the duodenum, parasitic infections such as fascioliasis and ascariasis, and haemobilia.[17] Two conditions have been incriminated repeatedly as producing extrahepatic mechanical obstruction, but these findings have just as frequently been challenged. One condition is the so-called inspissated bile syndrome diagnosed in infants, particularly when the cause of the accompanying jaundice is not established.[98,113,219] Inspissated bile in the biliary passages in this syndrome is the result of an underlying disease usually associated with increased red-cell breakdown. The hepatic alterations, including morphological evidence of cholestasis, are also expressions of the underlying disease and are not produced mechanically. Similarly, it is not established that dyskinesia or spasm of the bile ducts and at the sphincter of Oddi causes cholestasis. Fibrotic lesions secondary to inflammation at the sphincter may produce cholestasis, as suggested by the reported beneficial effects of sphincterotomy.[76] Fibrosis of the sphincter of Oddi may also be a variant of sclerosing cholangitis.

Intrahepatic Mechanical Obstruction

Distortion with associated narrowing of intrahepatic bile ducts is produced by several processes which may result in focal cholestasis in the parenchyma drained by this bile duct. However, only exceptionally is jaundice produced by such focal obstruction since the remaining part of the liver is able to compensate for the local biliary obstruction. Depending on the extent of the obstructed part of the parenchyma, however, biochemical evidence of obstruction may be recognized; for instance, by elevated activities of the alkaline phosphatase. The characteristic example is obstruction of one main bile duct at the bifurcation of the common hepatic duct within the liver by either ligation or tumour or other space-occupying process. This obstruction is not associated with jaundice or significant hyperbilirubinaemia as long as the liver is otherwise normal, but is accompanied by itching and a rise in the activities of alkaline phosphatase or other enzymes and even by hypercholesterolaemia. Minor stresses of the liver, however, cause jaundice. The spectrum of conditions producing focal alterations with or without biochemical evidence of cholestasis includes any fibrosing lesion, particularly cirrhosis, abscesses and granulomas. In all of these jaundice may result from the minor contribution of other factors to the obstructive features.

Cystic fibrosis of the pancreas is associated with steatosis and plugging of bile ducts and bile ductules by inspissated mucus, proliferation of ductules and periductular fibrosis. PAS stains of the mucous material are diagnostic. Focal biliary cirrhosis develops in 25 per cent of the survivors of the disease but only in less than 3 per cent does this lead to end-stage liver disease with portal hypertension and oesophageal varices. Jaundice is not part of the disease except in infancy and, unusually, in the end stage.[34]

The less common conditions in which intrahepatic mechanical biliary obstruction is extensive enough to produce jaundice include:

1. Carcinoma of the bifurcation of the common hepatic duct. Although technically intrahepatic, this obstruction has all the features of a tumour of the extrahepatic biliary tract (see Chapter 55). The different degree of involvement in both branches accounts for variations in the clinical picture as well as for the different morphological changes in both lobes of the liver.
2. Infantile obstructive cholangiopathy (extrahepatic atresia). This lesion may or may not have an intrahepatic atretic component and giant cell hepatitis. While it may be associated with trisomy 18, its frequent occurrence after viral infections like rubella in pregnancy suggests an acquired condition during intrauterine life. Recently, the presence of dilated small bile ducts at the hilum of the liver in early infancy and their obliteration later in childhood[7] have been listed as an indication for early surgical intervention in the form of a portoenterostomy of Kasai.[104,118,225] The changing manifestations of the disease during life and the late appearance of cirrhotic transformation all point to the dynamic character of the disease. Cholestasis occurs in children with congenital pyloric stenosis, possibly due to associated bile duct atresia or hypoplasia.[115]
3. Intrahepatic cholangitis. Both intrahepatic suppurative and sclerosing cholangitis are potential causes of cholestasis. While much emphasis had been placed on intrahepatic suppurative cholangitis as a cause of jaundice, sometimes without involvement of the extrahepatic ducts (cholangitis lenta), little attention is now paid to this possibility, particularly because antibiotic therapy has largely eliminated the clinical entity. Reference was made to intrahepatic sclerosing cholangitis which may be associated with ulcerative colitis. Pericholangitis in later stages of this disease should also be listed.[105]
4. Mechanical intrahepatic interference with the bile flow by periductal and periductular fibrosis. This phenomenon occurs late in primary biliary cirrhosis and in many forms of prolonged cholestasis, particularly in extrahepatic biliary obstruction lasting for more than a year. The lesion is seldom uniform throughout the liver, but it is uniform around a given portal tract. It may become severe enough to cause jaundice and functional sequelae (see 'Consequences of Cholestasis' below). The clinically most important aspect is mechanical intrahepatic cholestasis from periportal scarring in long-lasting extrahepatic biliary obstruction, particularly from strictures. Surgical restoration of the extrahepatic bile ducts results, slowly if at all, in normal bile flow from the liver. This obstruction may become the cause of sustained morbidity even after mechanically successful reconstructive surgery of the biliary tract.
5. Metastatic carcinoma. Jaundice, largely cholestatic, is frequent in terminal stages of metastatic disease of the liver. Occasionally, however, it is the first symptom of a cancer.

Hepatocellular carcinoma is responsible in a few instances.[142] The extent and location of the tumour, early or late, primary or metastatic, may explain jaundice, at least in part, by a mechanical effect on intrahepatic bile ducts. More frequently, however, this explanation is inadequate, and a metabolic reason has to be assumed as in other instances of pure intrahepatic cholestasis.

6. Rarely, polycystic liver disease causes mechanical cholestasis.

Intrahepatic Cholestasis (Without Demonstrable Biliary Obstruction)

Jaundice, with conjugated hyperbilirubinaemia and the histological manifestations of cholestasis, has been one of the most difficult diagnostic problems in liver disease. While the aetiology is known in most instances, the mechanism of the cholestasis, discussed below, remains problematical. Cholestasis may be a component of a hepatitis or cirrhosis of different aetiologies in which other manifestations of lesions of the hepatocytes are present to a variable degree. Organelles, other than those around the bile canaliculi and the bile canalicular membrane itself, are altered by the responsible agent. Less frequently, the structural, functional and clinical manifestations of cholestasis predominate or are present alone. Organelles concerned with bile secretion, mainly around the bile canaliculus, are primarily involved, although secondary injury of the other organelles may eventually develop. The separation of primary and pure cholestasis from the combined forms becomes difficult in advanced stages. Nevertheless, such separation may be desirable in diagnosis and management. A role of metabolic factors is postulated to be responsible for producing cholestasis, although not to a degree to justify the term 'metabolic cholestasis', particularly since microphysical factors cannot be fully excluded.

Pure intrahepatic cholestasis

This diagnosis is made, where possible, on an aetiological basis and, where not, on a descriptive basis. Many cases primarily affect infants and children.[100] Moreover, multiple factors often prevail, complicating or triggering the cholestatic phenomenon.

Cholestasis in infection. Pure cholestasis complicating lobar pneumonia was common[244] but is now a rare phenomenon;[221] it conveyed a grave prognosis at a time when effective antibacterial therapy did not exist. γ-Glutamyl transpeptidase (γ-GTP) activity is often increased in lobar pneumonia. One cause of cholestasis in children is urinary tract infection.[14,153] It occurs less frequently in gram-negative infections of adults.[130] The demonstration of the cholestatic potential of endotoxin in cell cultures [224] and in vivo[117] provides an explanation, although this form of cholestasis may also be associated with disseminated intravascular coagulation as another aetiological factor.[112]

Alpha-1-antitrypsin deficiency (see Chapter 35). This is considered a frequent cause of neonatal cholestasis by a mechanism not understood[82] and not necessarily associated with hepatitis.[161] The cholestasis spontaneously disappears in most babies, and only a few show the cirrhotic manifestations associated with alpha-1-antitrypsin deficiency later in childhood or as adults.[194]

Hyperalimentation. In children,[138,167] and also in adults, hyperalimentation may be accompanied by a cholestasis related hypothetically to an alteration of the bile acid metabolism.[165,220]

Cholestasis in haemolytic conditions (see Chapter 8). Bile plugs, usually rather slender, can be demonstrated by light microscopy in many forms of moderate or severe haemolysis. The characteristic pericanalicular changes of cholestasis can be seen by electron microscopy. The conjugated hyperbilirubinaemia in more severe haemolysis probably has a cholestatic component. Since biliary secretion is the rate-limiting step in bilirubin removal from the liver cell, minor interference with this step causes retention of bilirubin. Indeed, the highest bilirubin levels recorded with a large contribution of the direct reacting form occur in the presence of haemolysis.[71,109] Whether hyperbilirubinaemia by itself produces cholestasis is conjectural, but bilirubin has been proven to be cholestatic in experimental animals.[237] Severe cholestasis can occur in patients with sickle cell crisis; histologically, bile stasis is most impressive.[109] Urinary bilirubin excretion, impaired because of renal failure, may contribute to the extreme hyperbilirubinaemia in all haemolytic conditions.[71]

Postoperative cholestasis. This condition (see Chapter 47) is the result of many cooperative factors including spontaneous haemolysis, blood transfusions, bilirubin shifts, anoxia and shock.[187,214]

Congestive cholestasis. Acute, as well as chronic, cardiac failure may be associated with cholestasis not clearly related to the degree of congestion; nor is the degree of cholestatic jaundice related to the extent of hepatocellular necrosis which is often present. The previous assumption that increased venous pressure may mechanically interfere with bile flow[62] cannot be maintained. Congestive cholestasis may be due to reduced oxygen tension, suggesting a specific effect on the cholestatic phenomenon. However, pressure on the hepatocytes cannot be excluded as an important phenomenon. This is suggested by the severity of cholestasis in tricuspid insufficiency as well as in the Budd–Chiari syndrome.[32] Pulmonary infarcts are frequently associated with jaundice, and a haemolytic component may be a contributory factor. That it is not the only factor is suggested by experiments in which injection into tissue of blood equivalent to the amount likely to accumulate in pulmonary infarcts does not produce jaundice or cholestasis.[198] Cholestasis in shock can be explained by similar factors: a combination of haemolytic with cholestatic factors including oxygen deficiency, a presumed effect of tissue breakdown products and possible endotoxinaemia.[234] The histological manifestations are characteristic of cholestasis, while hyperbilirubinaemia is particularly prominent due to the associated renal failure.

Amyloidosis. Enzyme activity referable to cholestasis is frequently elevated in diffuse or parenchymal amyloidosis, in contrast to the portal or perivascular form. Hyperbilirubinaemia with jaundice is the exception and may be explained both by interference with microcirculation as well as by compression of the hepatocytes by amyloid deposition.

Malignancies including lymphomas. While carcinoma metastases or lymphomas may mechanically interfere with bile drainage sufficiently to cause cholestasis, this hydrodynamic explanation usually does not suffice except in terminal stages. Therefore, a metabolic component is postulated to be contributing in varying degrees. Its nature is entirely hypothetical. An example is Hodgkin's disease and, less frequently, diffuse histiocytic or mixed non-Hodgkin's lymphomas. While jaundice is frequent in terminal stages, it may also occur in earlier stages by a mechanism presumed to be metabolic and not clearly understood, with the incidence of jaundice varying between 10 and 13 per cent. Pruritus frequently occurs in Hodgkin's disease and may in part be explained by cholestasis. Patients with Hodgkin's disease may develop jaundice after taking oestrogenic preparations. Diffuse destruction of bile ducts is rare but is seen in rapidly progressing cholestatic Hodgkin's disease of the liver. Cholestatic jaundice is an early phenomenon in histiocytic medullary reticulosis to which severe haemolysis contributes, as it may in any other lymphoma (see Chapters 8 and 39).

Viral cholestasis. Cholestasis may be the only alteration in rare instances of liver disease presumably caused by one of the hepatitis viruses,[7,25,28,58,73] including hepatitis B virus.[6] The differential diagnosis in these instances is difficult and the aetiology seldom established beyond any doubt.

Drug-induced cholestasis (Chapter 36). Administration of a series of drugs, with phenothiazines and anabolic steroids as examples, may be followed by pure cholestasis without any other clinical, laboratory or histological manifestations[149,152] (see Chapter 36). Other drugs, including even halothane, exceptionally cause pure cholestasis.

Cholestasis of pregnancy. In uncomplicated pregnancy, particularly in the last trimester, pruritus and biochemical manifestations referable to cholestasis are present despite a histologically normal liver. The activities of serum alkaline phosphatase and leucine aminopeptidase are elevated. Bromsulphthalein (BSP) retention is moderately increased with reduction of BSP secretory activity (Tm) but with a slight increase of storage capacity. Occasionally, serum bilirubin is mildly increased, and bilirubin may appear in the urine. Moderate elevation of serum triglycerides and total cholesterol are also found. By contrast, the activities of the serum aminotransferases, 5′-nucleotidase and particularly γ-GTP are always normal, as is hepatic blood flow. The abnormal findings are variable and sometimes associated histologically with non-specific reactive hepatitis. These irregular abnormalities are probably explained by elevated oestrogen levels, which also may be reflected in palmar erythema and spider naevi. All these manifestations rapidly return to normal after delivery.

Cholestatic jaundice in pregnancy can be subdivided into jaundice in pregnancy and jaundice from pregnancy; the former is more frequent, with viral hepatitis being the leading cause.[116] An incidence has been calculated from the literature of one case per 1500 pregnancies, of which 41 per cent were considered to be viral hepatitis.[84,85] This latter figure is determined by the prevalence of hepatitis in the population. Pregnancy usually does not significantly influence the course of viral hepatitis which is not considered an indication for interruption of the pregnancy; however, this statement may not be true for all parts of the world. Choledocholithiasis is the second, but far less frequent, cause of cholestasis in pregnancy, while chronic or alcoholic hepatitis is rare, presumably because of infrequent conception. Cholestasis from drugs or urinary infection, as well as haemolysis, must be listed for completeness.

Recurrent cholestasis of pregnancy. The most frequent cause of cholestasis induced by pregnancy is recurrent jaundice of pregnancy. The first manifestation is pruritus, particularly at bedtime, followed often but not invariably after one or two weeks by jaundice.[84] The onset is usually early in the third trimester, but it occasionally begins earlier. Clinically, severe pruritus is the predominant symptom, sometimes becoming unbearable. Otherwise, however, no manifestations of liver disease are noted, and prodromal symptoms are absent. The liver and spleen are not enlarged. Itching and jaundice persist up to delivery, after which both subside within about a week. As a rule, delivery is not premature or delayed by the condition. Serum bilirubin rises to 103 to 171 μmol/l (6 to 10 mg/dl) and remains constant until delivery. Most is direct reacting. Alkaline phosphatase and 5′-nucleotidase activities rise moderately, hardly ever exceeding five times the upper limit of normal, whereas γ-GTP characteristically remains normal. Activities of aminotransferases are moderately elevated, SGOT more so than SGPT. Serum bile acids are significantly elevated, but the relative amounts of individual bile acids are the same as in other cholestatic conditions. Bromsulphthalein retention is increased, and is mainly explained by reduced transport maxima. Serum cholesterol is elevated, and there is an increased tendency to gallstone formation. Serum protein partition is normal except for reported high levels of cryoglobulin. Prothrombin time is occasionally prolonged, with decrease in vitamin K-dependent factors II, VII, IX and X. Otherwise, haematological findings are essentially normal.

Histologically, centrilobular cholestasis is the predominant finding, with the bile thrombi being rather delicate and inflammation in portal tracts subdued or absent. Electron microscopy reveals the typical features of cholestasis.[3] The disease is self-limiting, and permanent sequelae are not reported. In several women, features of primary biliary cirrhosis developed following cholestasis of pregnancy.[8] This is probably best explained by unmasking of pre-existing primary biliary cirrhosis during pregnancy, similar to that reported for other cholestatic agents like chlorpromazine.

The major problem is that of pathogenesis, a clue to which may lie in several observations:

1. The disease seems to be an accentuation of the mild tendency to cholestasis in normal pregnancy.
2. It usually recurs in subsequent pregnancies, as a rule, with increasing severity. Sometimes it is milder, and exceptionally it will not recur.
3. Familial occurrence involving mothers and daughters, sisters or other relatives has been repeatedly reported.[197]
4. The disease has a distinct geographical predominance, with a high incidence in Chile and Scandinavia, a predominance shared with jaundice following administration of contraceptive drugs.[3,144]
5. Cholestatic jaundice following contraceptive steroids and recurrent jaundice of pregnancy may be manifestations of the same condition. Repeatedly, women with cholestasis following contraceptive steroids subsequently had cholestatic jaundice of pregnancy and vice versa. Contraceptive steroid cholestasis may precede jaundice in pregnancy and subsequently develop again on intake of contraceptives. All these factors point to increased sensitivity to oestrogen.[110] Hyperoestrogenaemia in the last trimester of pregnancy produces some cholestasis, and there are also a few reports of similar cholestasis in premenopausal women. Administration of high doses of oestrogen produces BSP retention, and thus a genetically determined sensitivity can be assumed. There is no evidence for increased oestrogen synthesis but rather for reduced biliary excretion. Whether this is the cause or effect of cholestasis is difficult to distinguish since urinary oestrogen excretion is altered in all forms of cholestasis. According to Adlercreutz and Tenhunen,[2] plasma 20-OH steroids and 3-alpha-5-alpha and 3-alpha-5-

beta C-21 steroids are increased while 3-beta-5-alpha C-21 steroids are decreased. Moreover, steroids not found normally have been detected.

Pruritus of pregnancy is probably a milder form of the same condition in which biochemical but no clinical parameters of cholestasis prevail.

Fatty liver of pregnancy. A rarer form of jaundice produced by pregnancy is pernicious steatosis, also called acute fatty metamorphosis of pregnancy or obstetrical acute yellow atrophy.[195] It is an acute condition involving mainly young obese primiparas with toxaemia of pregnancy. Dramatic symptoms develop in the later portion of the last trimester, occasionally even at birth, with abdominal pain, vomiting, severe headache, tachycardia and some jaundice, but without fever.[26,89] Rapidly increasing somnolence and haematemesis present an alarming picture. Muscle pain and renal failure are frequent, as is stillbirth. Few mothers and children survive with renal failure. Death may occur days after delivery. The white blood count is greatly elevated. Serum bilirubin, by contrast, is only mildly elevated and rarely reaches 171 μmol/l (10 mg/dl). Aminotransferase and alkaline phosphatase activities are only mildly raised, uric acid and blood urea nitrogen (BUN) are usually high, and hypoglycaemia is common and difficult to correct. Blood coagulation is severely impaired.

Morphological findings, observed mainly at autopsy, include a liver usually slightly smaller than normal, despite severe steatosis which involves almost the whole lobule and leaves only a small portion of the periportal hepatocytes fat-free.[111] The steatosis is characterized by small fat droplets crowding the cell but not dislocating the nucleus to one side. They accentuate the thickness of the cell membrane to give the cell a plant-cell-like appearance. Centrilobular cholestasis is moderate. Inflammation indicating hepatocellular necrosis is subdued in some instances, while in others it is prominent and loss of hepatocytes probably explains the lack of enlargement of the steatotic liver. The sinusoidal lining cells are loaded with lipofuscin. The portal tracts are entirely normal, indicating the acuity of the process.

The clinical separation from massive necrotic hepatitis may be difficult, while pathologically the two conditions differ greatly. The same anatomical lesion has been observed after the intravenous administration of large doses of tetracycline, particularly if given for pyelonephritis in pregnant women.[35] However, the occurrence of this lesion in non-pregnant persons treated with tetracycline and in pregnant women not receiving this therapy suggests independent disease entities with a higher susceptibility in pregnancy.[111] The pathogenesis, however, remains a riddle. It is probably metabolic in nature. The analogy with the tetracycline lesion suggests inhibition with hepatocytic lipoprotein secretion as part of the pathogenesis but cannot explain necrosis. The toxic effects of free fatty acids have been implicated.[61]

Brief reference should be made to cholestatic phenomena in toxaemia of pregnancy, although these are not in the foreground. Activities of serum alkaline phosphatase and aminotransferases are usually elevated, but jaundice is exceptional. Even in fully developed fatal eclampsia, jaundice is primarily haemolytic and is associated with the characteristic intravascular coagulopathy and the deposition of fibrin thrombi.[124]

Idiopathic recurrent intrahepatic cholestasis. This is a rare hereditary disorder, autosomal recessive in character with poor penetrance. It expresses itself in repeated attacks of intrahepatic cholestasis. First described in 1958 by Summerskill and Walshe[217] in England, and by Tygstrup[222] in siblings and in five male patients from the Faroe Islands, the condition is often called by the name of the describers. It is best designated by the descriptive form used above.[216] A familial basis has been claimed for idiopathic recurrent cholestasis, cholestasis of pregnancy and contraceptive steroid cholestasis.[51] After prodromal symptoms of anorexia, pruritus and weight loss without pain or severe fever, episodes of jaundice develop which last up to three months and are associated with more or less severe itching but not with hepatosplenomegaly.[216] The evidence of jaundice is absent in the intervals which sometimes last for years. The attacks, up to 25 in one patient, start in childhood or in adult life. Serum bilirubin may rise to 342 μmol/l (20 mg/dl), mostly conjugated. The activity of serum alkaline phosphatase is greatly elevated, that of aminotransferases only slightly so. BSP retention is conspicuous, with impaired storage and transport maxima. Serum bile acids are very high, as are beta globulins. Other serum proteins are not significantly altered.

Histologically, conspicuous centrilobular cholestasis is seen during attacks without significant alterations of the hepatocytes. On electron microscopy these show only non-specific alterations as seen in any other type of cholestasis.[16] Mild portal inflammatory reactions, disappearing during the jaundice-free interval in which only portal fibrosis has been reported, indicate the minor lasting effect of the cholestasis. Electron-microscopically detected alterations of bile ductules have been incriminated in the pathogenesis of the jaundice in the patients from the Faroe Islands.[223] Abnormal metabolism of bile acids has been considered the key pathogenetic factor. Cholestyramine is recommended as therapy during the attack, primarily to relieve itching. Children have been treated with phenobarbital without uniform results, and corticosteroids, which may reduce the serum bilirubin level, have been recommended but are probably without effect on the underlying disorder.

Cholestasis in children. Besides recurrent benign cholestasis which may start in infancy,[170] three types of familial cholestasis have been described but, in contrast to benign cholestasis, they are progressive, not intermittent, and are not explained by atresia. The description of all of them is based on relatively few case reports, and their separation may not be final. Byler's disease was described in children of several related families descended from a man named Byler.[33,119] They initially show intermittent and non-progressive cholestatic jaundice with pruritus and hepatosplenomegaly. Bile acids in the serum are high in the cases examined, and a defect in bile acid secretion is postulated. Initially, no significant histological changes by light microscopy are noted except for cholestasis. At least in one instance cirrhosis developed. A non-specific picture is found in most instances by electron microscopy,[147] but in one instance a characteristic lesion was seen.[53] The second syndrome, in a non-Byler kindred, was marked by prolonged survival but complicated by mental retardation, ataxia and facial or digital abnormalities.[5] An available biopsy, obtained late, showed reduction of intralobular bile ducts. A third syndrome begins with severe pruritus and dermal changes before cholestatic jaundice with steatorrhoea develops.[232] Histologically, only cholestasis is seen. Years later, cirrhosis ensues, leading to hepatic failure. All these cases are characterized by early integrity of the hepatocytes and bile ducts and by the absence of hyperlipidaemia or xanthomatosis characteristic of biliary atresia. Evidence suggests congenital alterations of bile acid metabolism and a subsequent toxic effect of retained bile acids, possibly a monohydroxylated one such as lithocholate. These syndromes possibly share this defect with other genetic types of intrahepatic cholestasis; for instance, idiopathic recurrent cholestasis in which the disturbance of bile acid metabolism may be intermittent.

Adult forms of cholestasis of unknown aetiology. The classification presented does not cover a group of rare instances of unexplained cholestasis in adults. Some of them are progressive and terminate in cirrhosis. They defy any pathogenetic or aetiological classification, apparently being not familial and not related to the various factors mentioned.

Multifactorial cholestasis. In many conditions cholestasis is the result of a variety of contributing factors, such as infection, interference with microcirculation, intravascular haemolysis, intravascular coagulation and multiple blood transfusions. Since renal blood flow is reduced, usually on a functional basis, urinary excretion of bilirubin is decreased. The serum bilirubin levels in these instances are elevated far more than the raised activity of alkaline phosphatase.

Cholestasis as the predominant sign in various forms of hepatitis

Manifestations of cholestasis are occasionally in the foreground of the clinical and laboratory picture in almost all forms of hepatitis. This raises the differential diagnostic possibility of extrahepatic mechanical obstruction. Liver biopsy rapidly establishes the underlying hepatitis in almost all these instances, with the possible exception of drug-induced hepatitis. However, cholangiography performed endoscopically or percutaneously should be obtained first.

Viral hepatitis. Characteristically, in the initial stages of viral hepatitis morphological cholestasis reflected in bile thrombi is absent or minimal and, also, the activity of alkaline phosphatase is only moderately raised even if the serum bilirubin level is high. Cholestasis, both morphologically and biochemically, may become prominent in later stages, often when the other manifestations of hepatitis regress. This form of delayed cholestatic viral hepatitis, occurring both in hepatitis B and in non-A non-B hepatitis, has a delay in full recovery. Steroid therapy, which may reduce the bilirubin level somewhat, does not otherwise influence the course of the disease. This evolution seldom represents a diagnostic problem. Viral hepatitis, apparently not hepatitis A, with cholestatic manifestations including hypercholesterolaemia and pruritus has also been described in uncommon epidemics.[60] These cases vary in clinical intensity and have the usual histological manifestations of hepatitis. They also have a good long-term prognosis.

Alcoholic hepatitis. As in viral hepatitis, uncommon cases of alcoholic liver disease show laboratory findings pointing to cholestasis, sometimes prompting unjustified and dangerous abdominal exploration,[12,150,157] particularly since fever, abdominal pain, and leucocytosis are usually present. The characteristic histology of alcoholic liver injury readily establishes the prognosis. However, pancreatitis, choledocholithiasis and tumours interfering with biliary drainage also occur in patients with alcoholic liver disease. The complication may be recognized by cholangiography. Histological appearances of mechanical obstruction may be recognized despite the sometimes prominent alcoholic hepatitis. Zieve's syndrome with hyperlipidaemia and haemolysis in alcoholics may be associated with high direct-reacting bilirubin, hyperlipidaemia, centrilobular cholestasis, and often mild steatosis.[243] The haemolytic component aggravates cholestasis, but elevation of the alkaline phosphatase activity is less conspicuous than the bilirubin level would suggest. Jaundice may be particularly severe in alcoholic liver disease with haemolysis when numerous burr or spur forms of erythrocytes are present.[39,40]

Drug hepatitis. The most frequent hepatic drug reaction with jaundice is cholestatic hepatitis in which the cholestasis is frequently prominent but, histologically, intralobular and particularly portal inflammation distinguishes it from pure cholestasis. However, in this respect, liver biopsy need not be as diagnostic as in the other instances listed. The hepatitic component can be recognized clinically by fever, anorexia, malaise and hepatic tenderness, and functionally by raised aminotransferase activities. Usually, the hepatitic component is of shorter duration than the cholestatic one, and late in the course only pure cholestasis remains.

Combination of hepatitis with cholestasis

Diffuse hepatocellular alterations with disturbed liver function are conveniently called hepatitis in a generic sense, although the hepatocyte lesions are functionally more important in most instances than the inflammatory reaction. This necro-inflammatory component is combined with a cholestatic component in many acute and chronic liver diseases, that is, with failure of hepatocytic bile secretion. Most of the agents causing hepatitis produce both components in a spectrum from anicteric to cholestatic hepatitis. Thus cholestasis is an important component in almost all acute and chronic liver diseases, as already mentioned for viral, alcoholic and drug-induced hepatitis. The same holds true for cirrhosis of every variety, not only primary biliary and obstructive cirrhosis. Histologically, the degree of cholestasis may vary throughout the cirrhotic liver and may involve some nodules preferentially and sometimes part of the nodule, in which plump bile thrombi are conspicuous. Focal cholestasis may lead to destruction of nodules in cirrhosis of any type. This is frequently associated with Mallory's hyalin, with no relation to alcohol intake.[77] Intrahepatic cholestasis may complicate any stage and aetiological form of cirrhosis; it is more frequent in cryptogenic macronodular cirrhosis for unknown reasons.[38,45] It does not necessarily imply a poor diagnosis, since the cholestasis may suddenly disappear.[157,196] Cholestasis is also a complicating component in some cases of metabolic liver diseases like Wilson's disease in adults and children and, primarily in children, Niemann–Pick disease, galactosaemia, late stages of glycogen storage disease type IV, Wolman's disease, tyrosinosis, and familial hepatosteatosis due to a presumed enzyme defect so far not established.[153]

MECHANISM OF CHOLESTASIS

Descriptions of the mechanism and consequences of cholestasis can be largely based on light and ultrastructural studies of the morphological alterations. Therefore, the histological characteristics of cholestasis are interwoven with these descriptions.

Morphological Features of Acute Cholestasis

These histological changes can be divided into the primary or essential manifestations and secondary or accompanying features of cholestasis. The secondary features are of greater significance in the aetiological differential diagnosis than the essential features, which are identical in virtually all forms of cholestasis. The essential features result from alteration of what has been designated as the bile-secretory apparatus of the hepatocytes.[154] This includes the modified portion of the hepatocytic plasma membrane of the hepatocytes lining the bile canaliculus. The canalicular membrane is normally about 13 per cent of the total plasma membrane. Histologically, early cholestasis is characterized by dilatation of centrilobular bile canaliculi, the lumens of which contain bile thrombi. Since each centrilobular region is formed by several zones 3 of the Rappaport acinus and the degree of cholestasis may vary in these acini, cholestasis is frequently not concentric around the hepatic vein tributaries, but rather paracentral. Bile pigment granules in the cytoplasm of the hepatocytes may be noted in addition to the bile thrombi, as well as bile pigment granules in Kupffer cells after somewhat prolonged cholestasis. Macrophages may also contain engulfed bile thrombi. The hepatocytes in the cholestatic area may have an eosinophilic ground-glass appearance in the cytoplasm because of increased smooth endoplasmic reticulum, or they may exhibit hyperplasia or hypertrophy reflected also in numerous binucleated hepatocytes.

On transmission electron microscopy, the earliest lesion involves dilatation of the bile canaliculus and changes of the microvilli.[158] Normally, microvilli are regular finger-like extensions almost filling the bile canaliculus, which is formed by two and sometimes three hepatocytes (Chapter 2). The microvilli in cholestasis become distorted, either bleb-like and swollen, or shortened and deformed, and sometimes they are even missing. However, the few microvilli at the tight junction, which seals the canaliculus, remain intact, at least for a long time, as seen on scanning electron microscopy.[36,114,136,226] Even in normal individuals, however, portions of bile canaliculi may show irregularities or absence of microvilli, suggesting variations in function. The dilated lumen may contain a bile thrombus which is usually variegated in appearance, in that portions are fibrillar, granular, homogeneous, or crystalline, and even lamellar progressing to whorls. The differences are due to variations in age and the contribution of bile and of phospholipid components of the canalicular membranes. Bile thrombi, sometimes together with swollen oedematous microvilli, have been said to form a mechanical obstacle to bile flow. Actual obstruction, however, is doubtful because the bile canaliculi form an extensive communicating network. Dilated bile canaliculi have diverticular outpouchings into the cytoplasm of the hepatocytes. Since this appearance resembles the developmental stages of the bile canaliculi in the neonatal liver, cholestasis may be associated with new formation of canaliculi.[54,55] Although bile thrombi are predominantly in zone 3, bile-canalicular dilatation usually extends through the entire acinus or lobule. However, the degree of dilatation varies greatly even in the same canaliculus. This often depends on the hepatocyte forming its wall, suggesting variation in degree of cholestasis in neighbouring hepatocytes even in the centrilobular zone. Canaliculi with an almost normal lumen can be noted even in severe cholestasis. These cellular variations also involve features within the hepatocytes. The cytoplasm bordering the microvilli, the pericanalicular ectoplasm, is widened. It is homogeneous and contains a few cytoplasmic vacuoles similar to the terminal web of the intestinal epithelium. The vesicles and cisternae of the Golgi zone, located between the nucleus and the canaliculus, are large, and the vesicles contain electron-opaque granules. The smooth endoplasmic reticulum appears to be increased.[185,205] Several morphometric studies have been carried out in rats with ligated bile ducts, with conflicting results.[47,102,156,240] The volume of both the rough and the smooth endoplasmic reticulum is unchanged, while the surface area of both doubles. This is reflected chemically in an increase of the microsomal fraction in the total liver without alterations in the protein phospholipid ratio, but with significant reduction in cytochrome P-450.[93,102,166,185] Activities of some but not all drug-handling enzymes and of glucose-6-phosphatase are reduced, while conjugating enzymes remain normal.[102] The cytoplasm contains increased lysosomes, also reflected in PAS-positive diastase-resistant granules. Moreover, lamellated whorl-like electron-opaque material, presumably phospholipid components of bile, are surrounded by membranes.[15,158] Less dense fibrillar and usually non-membrane-bound material may represent bilirubin. The tight junction between neighbouring hepatocytes[133] remains intact even in severe cholestasis and appears disrupted only after hepatocellular necrosis. As seen particularly by scanning electron microscopy, the intercellular space, an extension between hepatocytes of the perisinusoidal space, and also endowed with microvilli, is lengthened; it may almost reach to the tight junction, thus reducing the size of the gap junction.[114,226]

Morphological observations indicate that early stages of cholestasis are characterized by alterations of organelles around the biliary pole of the hepatocyte and by dilatation of the bile canaliculi, the latter suggesting a possible local micromechanical component. This picture is seen in intrahepatic as well as obstructive cholestasis. The localization of bile thrombi as far as possible from the site of obstruction, that is, in the centrilobular zone, can be explained in several ways.[77,155] Some bile probably continues to be secreted by hepatocytes. The rate of flow in the lobule is slowest in the central zone and most rapid near the entry of the canalicular system into the bile duct. The slower central flow allows for greater absorption of water and is more likely to lead to inspissation. Bile thrombi also form on the lobular periphery when bile flow is obstructed because of bile duct obstruction or portal fibrosis. Under these circumstances, flow is slowest immediately behind the obstruction. Hepatocellular alterations may also play a role in centrilobular cholestasis. This zone is more vulnerable to injury because it has the lowest oxygen tension. The centrilobular hepatocytes also have more smooth endoplasmic reticulum responsible for microsomal biotransformation.

Cholestasis is therefore a hepatocytic alteration caused by pressure in the mechanical form and by metabolic processes in intrahepatic cholestasis. The identity of the morphological features by conventional, histochemical, and ultrastructural techniques in all forms suggests the same basic process and explains why morphological analysis of the essential cholestatic process does not assist in aetiological differential diagnosis. The same holds true for biochemical parameters reflecting cholestasis and explains their relative lack of usefulness in differential diagnosis, although biochemical parameters do reflect the intensity and duration of cholestasis just as the morphological changes do.

Pathogenesis of Centrilobular Cholestasis

Bile entering the intestines is the net result of five different fluid currents (Figures 14.1 and 14.2): (1) canalicular bile salt-independent secretion; (2) canalicular bile salt-dependent secretion; (3) fluid transfer through tight junctions; (4) ductular and ductal (including gallbladder) absorption and secretion; and (5) glycoprotein-rich mucus release from adnexal glands.[155,159,183] Of these, in cholestasis, (1) and (2) are regularly altered, (3) and (4) potentially changed, while (5), about 20 ml/day, is only secondarily, if at all, affected.

Bile salt-independent flow

The fluid current forming this flow has been determined in animals and man by extrapolation to zero bile salt secretion, the linear relationship between bile flow and bile salt secretion.[63] This line intercepts with the vertical

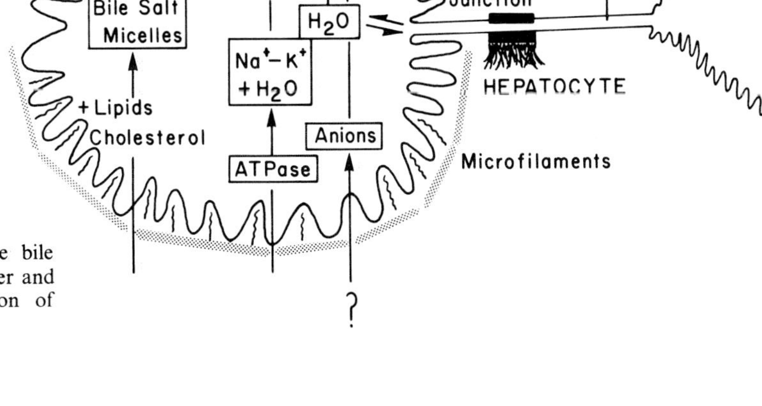

Figure 14.1. Transport site at the bile canaliculus. From Popper, Schaffner and Denk[159] with the kind permission of Plenum Press.

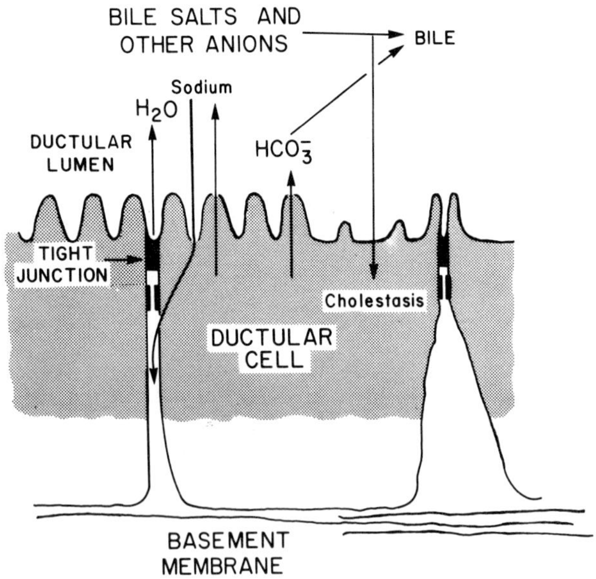

Figure 14.2. Transport sites in the ductule. From Popper, Schaffner and Denk[159] with the kind permission of Plenum Press.

ordinate, above the zero point indicating that a varying amount of bile is secreted without relation to bile salts. This bile salt-independent flow is greater in rodents and rabbits than in man, where it approximates 0.16 ml/min. In general, it represents 30 to 60 per cent of the basal bile flow not stimulated by food. It is increased by phenobarbital and by theophylline, in contrast to the bile salt-dependent flow. It is inhibited by ouabain and ethacrynic acid. The main process is sodium transport which is dependent on Na^+-K^+-ATPase activity (Figure 14.1).[20,55,107] This ion pump is presumably located in the microvilli of bile canaliculi. The relation of bile salt-independent flow to erythritol clearance indicates a canalicular origin. It is questionable whether bile acid-independent bile flow carries bilirubin, dyes, or other organic anions. Stimulated increase of the bile salt-independent bile flow does not alter secretion of bile salts but decreases that of cholesterol and phospholipids.

Bile salt-dependent secretion

The flow represents the portion of canalicular bile secretion which rises on postprandial nutritional stimulation of bile flow. It is driven by the secretory flow of the bile salts[63,207,231] but, presumably, sodium delivery has to precede that of bile salts to initiate water flow into the canaliculus (Figure 14.1). Thus, both the osmotic force derived from the delivery of sodium as well as bile salts provide the energy for the active transport of the bulk of water, electrolytes and other solutes into the bile canaliculus. Hydromechanical factors including arterial blood flow are less important than metabolic processes, in contrast to renal glomerular filtration.

Bile salt-dependent flow depends on the availability of bile salts for transport. It is determined by (1) the blood level of bile salts which depends on enterohepatic circulation and much less so on hepatocellular bile acid synthesis, and (2) the uptake of bile salts by hepatocytes, which depends on an active saturable transport system.[120] Uptake is sodium-dependent and more efficient for trihydroxy than for dihydroxy bile salts and for conjugated salts than unconjugated ones. Under normal circumstances it is far more efficient than biliary secretion by the hepatocytes; (3) the transport of bile salts in hepatocytes in part related to specific transport proteins, and (4) the ability of hepatocytes to secrete bile salts, which, in turn, is related to the amount of fluid and other solutes obligated during bile salt secretion.

Bile ductular flow

The bile ductules under normal circumstances both reabsorb electrolyte-containing fluid and secrete one which is rich in bicarbonate (Figure 14.2).[81,177] The secretion is stimulated by secretin and exceeds reabsorption to provide, normally, an increment of about 150 ml/day, yielding a total average bile flow of 600 ml/day.

The role of bile salt metabolism in initiation of cholestasis

Both the bile salt-independent and salt-dependent flow may be inhibited in cholestasis. Many agents, such as lithocholate and sex steroids, diminish both. However, there is no evidence that the inhibition of the bile salt-independent fraction, for instance by ethinyloestradiol, causes the characteristic morphological alteration of cholestasis or jaundice. Nonetheless, inhibition of bile salt-independent flow secondarily reduces bile salt-dependent flow by inhibition of sodium secretion. Depression of this flow by various agents results in morphological features characteristic of cholestasis. That cholestasis reflects impaired bile salt secretion was first illustrated by lithocholate administration to hamsters which produced the functional and electron microscopic features of cholestasis.[99,180] Two mechanisms were implicated. Polyionic aggregates consisting of micelles composed of bile salts, phospholipids and cholesterol are essential in the transport of cholesterol and phospholipids in bile (see Chapter 12). Micelles may also play a role in the biliary secretion of these substances. Since lithocholate is a poor micelle former, this transport could be inhibited. Recent evidence, however, incriminates another mechanism. Lithocholate is deposited within the microvilli, causing them to become deformed and increasing the cholesterol content of the canalicular membrane while inhibiting secretion of phospholipids and cholesterol into the bile.[132] While the study of lithocholate cholestasis had major heuristic value in emphasizing the role of bile salts in cholestasis, the theory that primary alterations of the bile salt metabolism cause cholestasis[97,182] now has little support.[152,155,159] Bile acids are formed from cholesterol by the microsomal biotransformation system in the smooth endoplasmic reticulum.[18] This organelle is altered in that morphometry indicates excess formation of seemingly inactive membranes and at least some cytochrome P-450-dependent drug metabolism is reduced in rats.[47,159] Contradictory observations were made in uncomplicated human cholestasis.[29,88] It appeared reasonable to apply the concept of hypoactive hypertrophic endoplasmic reticulum[94] to cholestasis[91] and to assume impaired ring hydroxylation of bile acids with synthesis of cholestatic monohydroxy bile salts. In addition, preferential formation of dihydroxy bile salts was assumed, which under some experimental circumstances also produce cholestasis by membrane alterations different from those induced by monohydroxy bile salts. Monohydroxy bile salts have been found in the urine in neonatal cholestasis.[11,101,127] However, the enzyme in the rate-limiting 7-alpha-hydroxylation of cholesterol differs from that of drug-handling enzymes by being not inducible by phenobarbital. If it therefore depends on cytochrome P-450, this must be a different form of the haem protein. Moreover, in cholestasis, the alterations of microsomal transformation occur later, and the haemoproteins show normal degradation in turnover studies but, if anything, reduced synthesis.[50,126] Thus, the alterations of the endoplasmic reticulum are probably a consequence of cholestasis rather than its cause.

More important than quantitative alterations of bile salt metabolism in initiation of cholestasis is a reduced amount of bile salts available to the hepatocytes in hepatocellular injury. A lesion of the perisinusoidal and intercellular plasma membrane of the hepatocytes, which is endowed with specific bile salt receptors, may impair the uptake of bile salts from the blood in hepatocellular injury. This may interrupt the intrahepatic circulation, not only by impaired canalicular secretion but also because of impaired uptake, as demonstrated in isolated hepatocytes.[79] Moreover, the availability of carrier proteins within the hepatocytes may be decreased. Primary bile salts are significantly elevated in the serum in cholestasis. In addition to reduced hepatocellular uptake, however, this elevation can be accounted for by leakage of bile salts from the hepatocytes into the blood. Excretion of excess serum bile salts by the kidney, some involving renal sulphation, results.[128,145,212,215] The net reduction in uptake of bile salts by the hepatocytes, complicated by reduced transformation of cholesterol to bile acid, may be a key factor in the cholestasis-associated hepatocellular injury in a non-specific fashion.

Sites of Initiation of Cholestasis

Lesions of several hepatocellular sites have to be considered in pure cholestasis; namely, the canalicular plasma membrane, the cytoskeleton and the tight junction (Figure 14.3). Changes in the portal tracts also deserve consideration.

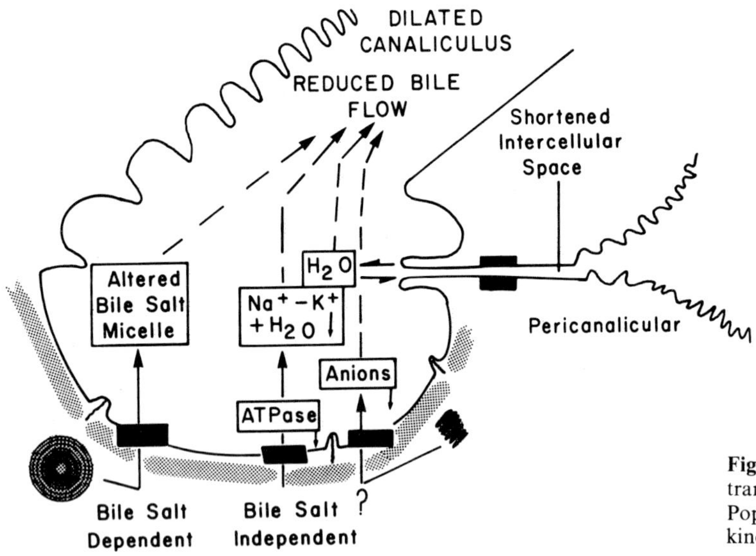

Figure 14.3. Blocks in canalicular transport sites in cholestasis. From Popper, Schaffner and Denk[159] with the kind permission of Plenum Press.

Alterations of the canalicular plasma membrane

The plasma membrane is characterized by carrier proteins, receptors for bile acids,[1] Na^+-K^+-ATPase-dependent ion pumps which may be stimulated by phenobarbital[103] and by the ability to convert bilirubin monoglucuronide to diglucuronide.[96] The canalicular membrane, by lacking many of these features, differs from the rest of the plasma membrane. Changes of the canalicular membrane in cholestasis have been demonstrated by histochemical studies and by chemical analysis of plasma membrane fractions. Histochemically, canalicular membrane-associated ectoenzymes, like magnesium-dependent ATPase and 5′-nucleotidase, are reduced[139,159,233] while alkaline phosphatase is increased.[73] They are located in the deeper portion of the thin glycocalix, which is rich in carbohydrate and covers the outer aspect of the microvilli. Moreover, γ-glutamyl transpeptidase supposedly appears earlier in metabolically induced cholestasis than in obstructive jaundice. In the latter, it is visualized in the hepatocytes after it has been demonstrated in the ductules.[168] Chemical analysis depends on the lack of contamination of the canalicular membrane fraction.[65,66,163,206,235] The Na^+-K^+-ATPase activity was found reduced in cholestasis. The sialic acid content increased[202] and the amount of phospholipids and cholesterol altered in the membrane.[137,241] Increased cholesterol is one of the main alterations, although different cholestatic agents, such as monohydroxy or dihydroxy bile acids or steroids, have varying effects. There is some evidence that the effectiveness of the ion pump depends on the lipid constitution of the membrane.[3] The combination of all these observations suggests reduced permeability of the membrane in cholestasis. However, Forker[67] demonstrated increased permeability at least to sucrose, which might be interpreted as reduced viscosity.

Changes in the microfilaments

The cytoskeleton below the cell membrane consists of rigid microtubules and contractile myosin-associated actin filaments.[1,78,140] The cytoskeleton not only maintains the tone of the membrane but also favours biliary secretion. Available evidence suggests that microfilaments are more important in the canalicular membrane, in contrast to the rest of the plasma membrane, although microtubules have been related to lipid secretion at the canalicular membrane also.[162] Cytochalasin B, which specifically alters actin microfilaments, produces cholestasis.[151] Cholestatic sex steroids are supposed to inhibit microfilament action.[69]

Leaky tight junction[56]

Cytoskeleton fibres condense at the tight junction which also has an adjacent mitochondrion, suggesting a local energy-dependent process.[211] Phalloidin increases the visibility of actin filaments around the tight junction.[4,72] It weakens the hepatocyte cell membrane, producing invaginations in hepatocytes in situ and local protrusions in isolated cells, depending on hydrostatic pressure.[10] Phalloidin may influence the tight junction, through which an electrolyte-containing fluid enters the bile canaliculus from the perisinusoidal space.[71] Functionally, this fluid contribution seems to be increased in cholestasis.[22] This may be the specific site of the increased permeability,[22,68,186] which would be in keeping with morphological preservation of microvilli at the tight junction and shortening of the intercellular space.[36]

Portal and bile duct changes

Bile ducts and ductules are potentially altered in cholestasis which may also involve the portal tracts. Changes occur in this location in prolonged cholestasis; ductules appear disfigured and have vacuolated and bile-pigmented cytoplasm.[30,177] This suggests reabsorption of bile through the ductules even with complete obstruction, creating a hepatoductular circulation (Figure 14.2). This fluid flush in the peripheral zone of the lobule may be a reason, already mentioned, for the preferential stagnation of bile in the centrilobular zone. Bile ducts and ductules appear to be increased in prolonged cholestasis, either from proliferation of ductules by sprouting as a reaction to inflammation, or by lengthening, producing tortuosity also involving the small bile ducts, in response to increased intraluminal pressure. The proliferated ductules are flattened cylinders on three-dimensional reconstruction.[103] Proliferated ductules are surrounded initially by inflammatory exudate and eventually by increased collagen bundles.[24,209] The stimulus for ductular proliferation and alteration is not understood. Lithocholate on injection produces ultrastructural changes in the ductules at the time when the canalicular changes are subsiding.[180] Ductular proliferation and alterations, as well as periductular inflammation and fibrosis, develop on prolonged feeding of lithocholate.[90,146] The microcirculation in the portal tracts may be altered. Arterial flow may exceed venous blood flow, and oedema may develop. Both may add a mechanical obstructive component.

Causes of Bile Canalicular Dilatation

Four factors can be postulated to explain dilatation of the bile canaliculi, the basic feature of cholestasis. The most important seems to be reduced membrane tone, from cytoskeleton failure, overcoming intracellular hydrostatic pressure. The second is slowing of bile flow, where bile thrombi and oedematous microvilli may be a contributing factor. The third is increased bile flow, in some forms of cholestasis at least, as illustrated by the effects of administration of dehydrocholate. The fourth is obstruction by lesions in the portal tracts. The last is hard to evaluate but probably quite effective.

Intrahepatic mechanical factors in cholestasis therefore include (1) a hydromechanical effect from portal changes including oedema, (2) the complexity of the proliferated bile ductular system, (3) portal fibrosis potentially leading to compression and even disappearance of ducts, and (4) bile duct lesion in various forms of hepatitis. The combination of all these factors creates a microphysical element in addition to the chemical one even in intrahepatic cholestasis.

Cholestasis and Drugs

The following mechanisms can be implicated in cholestatic drug reactions:[152,155,159,183] anabolic and oestrogenic steroids (a) compete for organic ion secretion, (b) inhibit the Na^+-K^+-ATPase pump, (c) stimulate biotransformation and (d) depending on steric configuration, may be deposited in the canalicular membrane. Chlorpromazine and related drugs, and particularly their metabolites, also reduce ATPase activity[21,176] and complex with bile salts, disturbing micelle formation.[27] Phenobarbital increases bile salt-independent flow by influencing the ATPase pump and increasing blood flow but has little effect on bile salt formation and excretion.

CONSEQUENCES OF CHOLESTASIS

While the mechanism of cholestasis remains shrouded in mystery, the consequences are far better understood. Of major significance is retention of two substances in the hepatocytes, namely, bile salts and unconjugated bilirubin. Phospholipid retention leads to whorl-shaped deposits but probably is more a morphological marker than injurious to the cytoplasm, and the same holds true for cholesterol deposits.

Bilirubin, in concentrations found in cholestasis, decreases oxygen uptake by hepatic mitochondria and uncouples oxidative phosphorylation.[208] Moreover, mitochondrial cytochromes are decreased, and this may be related to altered carbohydrate metabolism.[239] Cholate[236] and lithocholate excesses[131,180] cause curling of mitochondrial cristae before jaundice develops.

Bile acid retention is the most important consequence of cholestasis. Reference has been made to the effects of lithocholate and other monohydroxy bile acids. Competitive binding of dihydroxy and trihydroxy bile acids to microsomes as shown in experimental animals inhibits biotransformation of drugs in cholestasis. This has not been confirmed in man,[88] but physiological regulation of the cytochrome P-450-dependent microsomal biotransformation by bile salts has been postulated. Greater concentrations of the bile salts lead to a dose-dependent detergent action on microsomes.[92] Dihydroxy bile salts are more effective than trihydroxy ones and unconjugated ones more than conjugated ones. Exposure of microsomes to bile salts in vitro results in their gradual disintegration, with reduction of cytochrome P-450, inhibition of its reductase, destruction of its lipoprotein-binding site, and transformation into inactive cytochrome P-420. This may account for the observed alterations of the smooth endoplasmic reticulum in all species studied, as well as for the lesions in rat livers perfused with chenodeoxycholate. Since determination of bile salts in liver tissue does not reflect the relative distribution in cytoplasm, blood and bile, the observation in rats with ligated bile ducts that the hepatic bile salt concentration reaches only levels causing competitive binding is not necessarily convincing, as is the similar observation that, after prolonged biliary obstruction in man, detergent levels of dihydroxy bile salts are found.[80]

Cholestasis also affects the rough endoplasmic reticulum in addition to the smooth form. Synthesis of proteins, particularly of lipoproteins, is increased in rats. This accounts also for the presence of the abnormal low density lipoprotein-X (LPX)[192] which is rich in cholesterol, the microsomal synthesis of which is raised in cholestasis.[191] Excess bile salts, moreover, solubilize canalicular membrane components, particularly phospholipids,[65,242] leading to the appearance in blood of abnormal membranous components.

The cytoplasmic change characteristic for cholestasis is rarefaction of the cytoplasm with brown remaining strands. The rarefactions correspond electron microscopically to electron-opaque myelin-like whorls. This lesion, which involves single cells in centrilobular cholestasis, is explained by the detergent action of bile salts since its intensity parallels the tissue content of dihydroxy bile salts.[80] The identical lesion is seen in renal tubules with bile salt retention. Another effect, representing hydration more than feathery degeneration, is caused by alteration of hepatocytic tubulin. The appearance of such hepatocytes is similar to those in alcoholic liver injury, where such an antitubulin effect has been demonstrated, resulting in retention of proteins secreted by the hepatocyte.[13] Moreover, cytoplasmic deposits of Mallory's hyalin are noted in prolonged cholestasis.[77] Hyalin has been produced in mice by griseofulvin,[48] which causes cholestasis[31] and has an antitubulin effect. It also alters the activities of some microsomal enzymes.[49]

Feathery degeneration proceeds to single cell necrosis associated with focal reactive inflammation.[158] This hepatitic reaction caused by cholestasis has to be differentiated from an unrelated hepatitis by its restrictions to the cholestatic zone. Intralobular inflammation is accompanied by reactive portal inflammation which, in turn, leads to ductular alterations with proliferation as well as fibrosis.[199] The portal reaction persists after subsidence of cholestasis of any aetiology and is the lesion seen between episodes of recurrent benign cholestasis. This 'cholangiolitis'[169] is the result of the cholestasis, and not its cause, in almost all situations.

Eventually, portal and periportal fibrosis can develop in any form of cholestasis. The first type of collagen to appear in both man and experimental animals is the more pliable type III, or reticulin, soon followed by the formation of hard, doubly refractile type I collagen. It causes scarring fibrosis around bile ducts and ductules secondary to the intralobular cholestasis. If severe enough, it interferes mechanically with ductular and ductal bile flow and produces a mechanical intrahepatic obstructive component secondary to any cholestasis. It is reflected in periportal or zone 1 cholestasis which characteristically varies in intensity throughout the liver but is more uniform around a given portal tract than in centrilobular cholestasis. Destruction of the layer of hepatocytes around the portal tracts with relatively little but often leucocytic inflammation (biliary piecemeal necrosis) leads to apparent enlargement of the portal tracts, similar to chronic active hepatitis, although, histologically, vacuolated cells predominate. The lesion need not be associated with conspicuous bile pigment accumulation, although it otherwise shows 'feathery degeneration' and is presumably 'cholate stasis'. Copper and copper-binding protein, demonstrable by orcein staining, accumulates in the periportal cells.[166] Periportal cholestasis associated with portal and periportal scarring is the lesion seen in later stages of primary biliary cirrhosis[172] and other conditions associated with bile duct lesions,[199] such as sarcoidosis.[173] It may account for residual impairment of biliary secretion following successful surgical correction of extrahepatic mechanical obstruction. It probably represents the end stage of prolonged cholestasis, which is initially free of liver cell injury or obstruction, for instance, in hereditary infantile cholestasis. In all these conditions, including uncorrected or infected biliary obstruction, strictures, sclerosing cholangitis and atresia, unremitting fibrosis with septa formation eventually terminates in biliary cirrhosis in which the original aetiology cannot be ascertained. Moreover, the deposition of hard type I collagen favours development of portal hypertension.

Peripheral cholestasis must be distinguished from ductal cholestasis, often associated with dense bile deposits or microliths in ductules. This results from dehydration, usually in liver disease, but does not necessarily reflect jaundice.[158]

INTERACTION OF CAUSES AND EFFECTS

The considerations presented for mechanisms and consequences can best be integrated if cholestasis is regarded as a result of multifactorial processes with variable initial targets. Wherever the latter is, the processes reinforce each other to produce two vicious circles (Figure 14.4).[159,183] One is on a molecular or organelle level within the hepatocyte, and the other is on a ductular or lobular level and is obviously hydromechanical. The two reinforcing vicious circles are connected by the retention of both bilirubin and bile salts. Both bile acid-independent and -dependent flow diminish regardless of where the process is initiated. Similarly, on the lobular level, hepatocellular changes interact with ductular and ductal lesions.

DIAGNOSIS

Clinical

Cholestasis by itself does not produce the usual clinical manifestations of acute and chronic liver disease such as malaise and fatigability. The

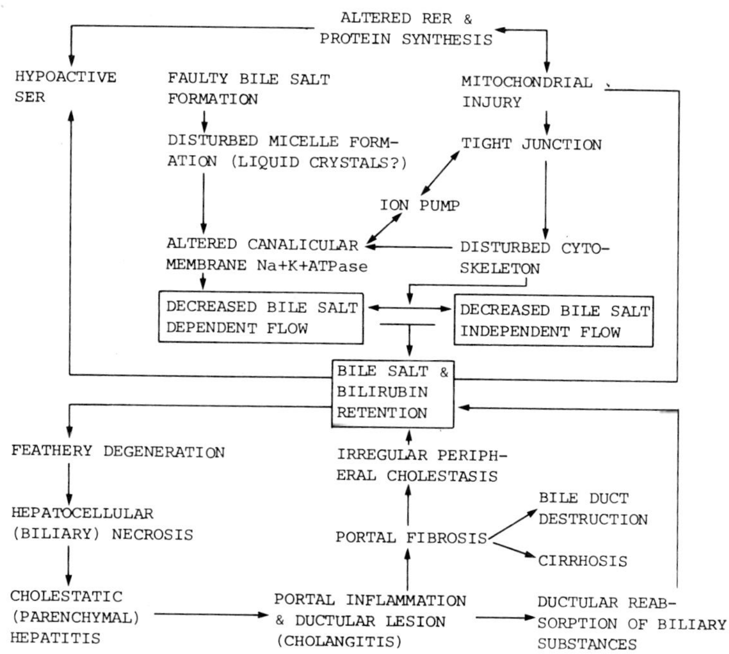

Figure 14.4. Vicious circles operative in cholestasis; the one in the upper half is at the molecular-organelle level while the one in the lower portion is at the lobular-hydromechanical level. From Popper, Schaffner and Denk[159] with the kind permission of Plenum Press.

only specific systemic manifestation in cholestasis is pruritus due to intradermal disposition of bile salts. Trihydroxy bile salts were held responsible[188] but now dihydroxy ones are felt to be responsible.[106] The history in the jaundiced patient is of great help in ascertaining factors pointing to viral hepatitis, alcohol intake, and exposure to drugs or chemicals. Chills and fever, anorexia and loss of taste for cigarettes are not diagnostic. A family history of gallstones or anaemia speaks for gallstone disease. Cutaneous stigmata of liver disease favour but do not prove intrahepatic disease. Right upper quadrant pain and also back pain suggest an obstructive disorder. A grossly enlarged and very tender liver is seldom seen in extrahepatic obstruction, while a mass or an enlarged gallbladder is the most significant feature pointing to either obstruction or tumour.

Laboratory

Since the basic lesion in cholestasis is the same in the mechanical form and in the metabolic form, there is little hope of developing a biochemical laboratory test to separate the two. Most test results reflect the intensity and degree of cholestasis rather than its aetiology. Accompanying features help and may make themselves felt in the use of statistical and computer methods integrating various parameters. The most reliable laboratory parameter of cholestasis is increased activity of alkaline phosphatase, particularly if this is related to hyperbilirubinaemia and refined by specific isoenzyme determinations including those referable to the liver and the intestine. Elevation of the latter suggests an intrahepatic cause.[229] Alkaline phosphatase activity is not always significantly elevated in malignant obstruction. Elevation out of proportion to that of bilirubin speaks for primary biliary cirrhosis, granulomatosis, or space-occupying lesions, obstruction of one main bile duct or a stone in the common duct. Elevation of bilirubin without appropriately increased alkaline phosphatase activity suggests an increased supply of bilirubin from haemolysis; Dubin–Johnson's or Rotor's syndrome; or the early stage of viral hepatitis. γ-Glutamyl transpeptidase (γ-GTP) parallels alkaline phosphatase except in alcoholics, where γ-GTP may be more elevated, while in sex steroid or pregnancy jaundice it tends to be normal. The activities of leucine aminopeptidase and 5′-nucleotidase usually parallel that of alkaline phosphatase except that the former is elevated in pancreatic diseases even without cholestasis. When measured in rat serum and liver after bile duct ligation, the activities of alkaline phosphatase, γ-GTP, and 5′-nucleotidase do not parallel each other.[238] Simultaneous elevation of liver and bone enzyme alkaline phosphatase raises the suspicion of a malignant lesion with bone metastases. The activities of aminotransferases, more that of SGOT than of SGPT, are elevated in pure cholestasis, although far less than alkaline phosphatase. Relatively high levels of aminotransferase activity are found in early cholestasis and stone obstruction and then decline rapidly. Serum protein partition is not significantly altered in pure cholestasis. Gamma globulin need not be elevated but, in prolonged cholestasis, beta globulins rise. There is also considerable hyperlipidaemia with total cholesterol being high, while cholesterol esters are not reduced. Many other biochemical tests have been recommended, but most of them, like determination of LPX,[164] have little value in the separation of aetiological factors. Some hints may be obtained from older tests. For instance, the sedimentation rate is low in viral hepatitis but normal or high in other liver and biliary tract diseases. Very high levels suggest malignancies or bacterial infections. Leucocytosis characterizes infected biliary obstruction, alcoholic hepatitis, and massive hepatic necrosis. Hyperglycaemia suggests pancreatic carcinoma in the absence of long-standing diabetes.

Histology

Large bile duct obstruction is suggested by oedema of the portal tracts, tortuosity of bile ducts and ductules, location of ductules close to the margin of the portal tracts, and prominent fibroblasts and segmented leucocytes in the portal tracts.[74,135,158,199] None of these findings is pathognomonic.

The following features are of little diagnostic significance in cholestasis: central or peripheral feathery degeneration, ductular proliferation and alteration, vacuolization of peripheral hepatocytes, intraparenchymal foam cells and any type of inflammation. More reliable are features developing after prolonged obstruction. These include extravasation of bile from bile ducts, often with granuloma formation, and biliary necrotic foci or bile infarcts near the portal tracts. Extravasations of bile in the parenchyma, as well as bile infarcts remote from portal tracts, also occur in various forms of intrahepatic cholestasis, particularly in late primary biliary cirrhosis. Segmented leucocytes intermixed with mononuclear inflammatory cells around proliferated bile ductules do not point to any specific aetiology, like bacterial infection; they speak for the latter only if they are the prominent infiltrating cells. If segmented leucocytes are absent, the intensity of the portal inflammation serves as a preliminary indicator. A conspicuous reaction in the first three weeks of jaundice speaks for intrahepatic cholestasis; it is absent only in the form induced by sex steroids. By contrast, intense portal inflammation after three weeks of cholestasis suggests large bile duct obstruction, since hepatitis, both viral and drug-induced, has usually subsided. However, errors in the histological evaluation are common, and there is a risk with biopsy in large bile duct obstruction. Therefore, enthusiasm for histological differential diagnosis of cholestasis is waning, especially with the development of more decisive physical techniques like cholangiography.

Two specific problems deserve mention. First, with direct reacting hyperbilirubinaemia without histological cholestasis and with normal hepatic structure, an early stage of primary biliary cirrhosis or Rotor's syndrome should be considered. Secondly, cholestasis in the biopsy specimen in the absence of jaundice suggests a focal space-occupying lesion.

Physical Methods

Cholestasis established by clinical and laboratory examinations without recognized aetiology calls for a series of procedures, depending on availability of equipment and skill of the examiner. This includes cholangiography, either endoscopic retrograde cholangio-pancreatography (ERCP)[41,141,245] or percutaneous transhepatic (or transjugular)[125] cholangiography using the thin flexible Chiba needle.[143,148] The latter localizes the upper end of the obstruction, and this is important for surgical relief. Ultrasonography, an inexpensive non-invasive and risk-free procedure, is increasingly being used as an initial study.[95,218,227] Scanning[86] with biopsy into a cold area, computerized tomography and selected coeliac angiography are useful. Peritoneoscopy is recommended by those with experience in the procedure.[121] Radiological studies with barium should be deferred until the newer techniques are applied, since the barium may interfere with results. Exploratory laparotomy can no longer be justified.

Liver Biopsy

A high percentage of biopsy differential diagnoses of cholestasis are correct when made by experienced pathologists, but there is a risk of biliary peritonitis in the presence of extrahepatic biliary obstruction. While this risk is small,[135] the greater accuracy with greater safety of the physical procedures mentioned in the previous paragraph makes liver biopsy a procedure that should be conducted only if mechanical obstruction has been ruled out.

A Simple Algorithm for Approaching the Problem of Cholestasis[179]

1. Check urine for bilirubin and serum for direct or indirect reacting bilirubin.
2. If bilirubin is mainly indirect reacting (unconjugated) and the urine is free of bilirubin, work up for haemolysis (reticulocytes, haptoglobin, haemoglobin electrophoresis). If no haemolysis is found, further investigation is unnecessary and a diagnosis of a variant of Gilbert's disease can be made.
3. If the urine contains bilirubin and the serum bilirubin is mainly direct reacting, check SGOT, SGPT, alkaline phosphatase, γ-GTP, serum protein electrophoresis, hepatitis B surface antigen, and mitochondrial, smooth muscle and antinuclear antibodies.
   (a) If everything but bilirubin is normal, undertake a liver biopsy to look for the pigment of the Dubin–Johnson syndrome.
   (b) If activities of aminotransferases are greater than five times normal after a week but that of alkaline phosphatase is less than three times normal and gamma globulin is normal with all negative immunological studies, it is viral, chemical (drug), or alcoholic hepatitis. A liver biopsy facilitates recognition of alcoholic hepatitis. If gamma globulin level is high, especially IgG, a liver biopsy should be carried out to diagnose chronic hepatitis with or without cirrhosis.
   (c) If activities of aminotransferases are less than five times normal after a week but that of alkaline phosphatase (and γ-GTP) are more than three times normal, a variant of intrahepatic cholestasis should be distinguished from large bile duct obstruction.

Pruritus is a usual complaint, and serum cholesterol is elevated. Sonography, scanning, and endoscopic and thin-needle cholangiography should be used, in that order, until an obstruction is found or the biliary tree is seen to be normal. Computerized tomography should be used only if an abnormality found by sonography cannot be clearly defined. An upper gastrointestinal radiological study with barium is less likely to be helpful, and in most cases need not be ordered. Under any circumstances, barium studies should be delayed until the studies first listed are complete. If no obstruction is found, the diagnosis is intrahepatic cholestasis. A liver biopsy should be performed to see if alcoholic or viral hepatitis is present, and the drug history should be reinvestigated.

(d) If the diagnostic features in the preceding paragraph are present with a normal biliary tree and mitochondrial antibody is found, IgM should be determined, and a liver biopsy should be obtained to diagnose primary biliary cirrhosis.

(e) Scanning or sonographic areas suggestive of a space-occupying lesion, in addition to the features described in paragraph 3 above, should lead to a liver biopsy to detect metastases.

THERAPY

There is no rational therapy for intrahepatic cholestasis. Phenobarbital reduces the bilirubin level in some forms of jaundice,[19,23] especially in infants.[193,213] Corticosteroids do not influence the course of the disease but often reduce the bilirubin level in any variety of jaundice without influencing the basic process. They may alter bilirubin metabolism by increasing production of non-pigmented metabolites and by increasing shortened red cell survival. Cholestyramine relieves pruritus by binding bile salts in the gut, but it is not recommended when the serum bilirubin level is above 171 μmol/l (10 mg/dl).[44,45,184] Hypolipidaemic drugs are contraindicated in liver disease; in primary biliary cirrhosis they have a paradoxical hyperlipidaemic effect.[178] Anabolic steroids, although they relieve itching, accentuate jaundice. Fat-soluble vitamins can be given orally in a water-soluble form. The preferred preparation of vitamin D is 25-hydroxycholecalciferol or 1,25-dihydroxycholecalciferol. The liver is responsible for the 25-hydroxylation of vitamin D, a function depressed in liver diseases[228] in addition to malabsorption.[37,46] Absorption of vitamins A and K may also be impaired, and parenteral administration may be needed.

REFERENCES

1. Accatino, L. & Simon, F.R. (1976) Identification and characterization of a bile acid receptor in isolated liver surface membranes. *Journal of Clinical Investigation,* **57,** 496–508.
2. Adlercreutz, H. & Tenhunen, R. (1970) Some aspects of the interaction between natural and synthetic female sex hormones and the liver. *American Journal of Medicine,* **49,** 630–648.
3. Adlercreutz, H., Svanborg, A. & Ånberg, Å. (1967) Recurrent jaundice in pregnancy. I. A clinical and ultrastructural study. *American Journal of Medicine,* **42,** 335–340.
4. Agostini, B., Govindan, V.M. & Hofmann, W. (1975) Morphological changes induced by phalloidin in the rat liver. In *Pathogenesis and Mechanism of Liver Cell Necrosis* (Ed.) Keppler, D. pp. 175–197. Baltimore: University Park Press.
5. Alagille, D., Odievre, M., Gautier, M. & Dommerques, J.P. (1975) Hepatic ductular hypoplasia associated with characteristic facies, vertebral malformations, retarded physical, mental and sexual development and cardiac murmur. *Journal of Pediatrics,* **86,** 63–71.
6. Albot, G. & Toulet, J. (1974) De la cholostase au cours des ictères viraux. *Semaine des Hôpitaux de Paris,* **50,** 2853–2865.
7. Albot, G., Jezequel, A.M. & Lunel, J. (1962) Les épisodes cholostatiques au cours des ictères par hépatites virales. *Acta Hepato-Splenologica,* **9,** 140–154.
8. Albot, G., Zerolo, J., Camilleri, J.P., Kapandji, I.A. & Lafon, J. (1972) Ictère récidivant de la grossesse et cholangiolite chronique isolée ou maladie de Hanot et MacMahon. *Semaine des Hôpitaux de Paris,* **48,** 3425–3441.
9. Alpert, S., Mosher, M., Shanske, A. & Arias, I.M. (1969) Multiplicity of hepatic excretory mechanisms for organic anions. *Journal of General Physiology,* **53,** 238–247.
10. Baccino, F.M., Cantino, D. & Zuretti, M.F. (1976) Studies on the hepatotoxicity of *Amanita phalloides* in the rat. 1. Liver cell vacuolation. *Experimental and Molecular Pathology,* **24,** 159–175.
11. Back, P. (1973) Identification and quantitative determination of urinary bile acids excreted in cholestasis. *Clinica Chimica Acta,* **44,** 199–207.
12. Ballard, H., Bernstein, M. & Farrar, J.T. (1961) Fatty liver presenting as obstructive jaundice. *American Journal of Medicine,* **30,** 196–201.
13. Barona, E., Leo, M.A., Borowsky, S.A. & Lieber, C.S. (1975) Alcoholic hepatomegaly: accumulation of protein in the liver. *Science,* **190,** 794–796.
14. Bernstein, J. & Brown, A.K. (1962) Sepsis and jaundice in early infancy. *Pediatrics,* **29,** 873–882.

15. Biava, C. (1964) Studies on cholestasis. The fine structure and morphogenesis of hepatocellular and canalicular bile pigment. *Laboratory Investigation,* **13,** 1099–1123.
16. Biempica, L., Gutstein, S. & Arias, I.M. (1967) Morphological and biochemical studies of benign recurrent cholestasis. *Gastroenterology,* **52,** 521–535.
17. Bismuth, H. (1973) Hemobilia. *New England Journal of Medicine,* **288,** 617–619.
18. Björkhem, I. & Danielsson, H. (1974) Hydroxylations in biosynthesis and metabolism of bile acids. *Molecular and Cellular Biochemistry,* **4,** 79–95.
19. Bloomer, J.R. & Boyer, J.L. (1975) Phenobarbital effects in cholestatic liver disease. *Annals of Internal Medicine,* **82,** 310–317.
20. Boyer, J.L. (1971) Canalicular bile formation in the isolated perfused rat liver. *American Journal of Physiology,* **221,** 1156–1163.
21. Boyer, J.L. & Root, M. (1976) Chlorpromazine metabolites – inhibitors of Na^+-K^+-ATPase in liver plasma membranes (LPM) enriched in bile canaliculi. *Clinical Research,* **14,** 281a.
22. Bradley, S., Morris, A. & Baker, K.J. (1974) Mechanism of proteobilia. *Clinical Research,* **22,** 558a.
23. Braun, W., Wöckel, W., Giertler, U. & Vollmar, F. (1972) Phenobarbitalbehandlung der benignen rezidivierenden intrahepatischen cholestase. *Schweizerische Medizinische Wochenschrift,* **102,** 1769–1772.
24. Brooks, S.E.H., Reynolds, P., Audretsch, J.J. & Haggio, G. (1975) Scanning electron microscopy of proliferating bile ductules. *Laboratory Investigation,* **33,** 311–315.
25. Burke, J.A. (1974) The cholestatic form of viral hepatitis. *Clinical Pediatrics,* **13,** 636–639.
26. Cano, R., Delman, R., Pitchemoni, C.S., Lev, R. & Rosenthal, W.S. (1975) Acute fatty liver of pregnancy. *Journal of the American Medical Association,* **231,** 159–161.
27. Carey, M.C., Hirom, P.C. & Small, D.M. (1976) A study of the physicochemical interactions between biliary lipids and chlorpromazine hydrochloride. Bile salt precipitation as a mechanism of phenothiazine-induced bile secretory failure. *Biochemical Journal,* **153,** 519–531.
28. Caroli, J., Thiery, J.P. & Andre, S. (1962) Les hépatites hypercholostatiques. Étude clinique, histologique (microscope optique et électronique), physiopathologique. *Semaine des Hôpitaux de Paris,* **38,** 1294–1328.
29. Carulli, N., Manenti, F., Ponz de Leon, M., Ferrari, A., Salvioli, G. & Gallo, M. (1975) Alteration of drug metabolism during cholestasis in man. *European Journal of Clinical Investigation,* **5,** 455–462.
30. Chedid, A., Spellberg, M.A. & DeBeer, R.A. (1974) Ultrastructural aspects of primary biliary cirrhosis and other types of cholestatic liver disease. *Gastroenterology,* **67,** 858–869.
31. Chiprut, R.O., Viteri, A., Jamroz, C. & Dyck, W.P. (1976) Intrahepatic cholestasis after griseofulvin administration. *Gastroenterology,* **70,** 1141–1143.
32. Clain, D., Freston, J., Krell, L. & Sherlock, S. (1967) Clinical diagnosis of the Budd–Chiari syndrome. *American Journal of Medicine,* **43,** 544–554.
33. Clayton, R.J., Iber, F.L., Ruebner, B.H. & McKusick, V.A. (1969) Byler disease: fatal familial intrahepatic cholestasis in an Amish kindred. *American Journal of Diseases of Childhood,* **117,** 112–124.
34. Cohn, D. (1977) Multilobular biliary cirrhosis of the liver associated with cystic fibrosis (mucoviscidosis). *Medical Journal of Australia,* **i,** 101–104.
35. Combes, B., Whalley, P.J. & Adams, R.H. (1972) Tetracycline and the liver. In *Progress in Liver Diseases,* Vol. 4 (Ed.) Popper, H. & Schaffner, F. pp. 589–596. New York: Grune & Stratton.
36. Compagno, J. & Grisham, J.W. (1974) Scanning electronmicroscopy of extrahepatic biliary obstruction. *Archives of Pathology,* **97,** 348–351.
37. Compston, J.E. & Thompson, R.P.H. (1977) Intestinal absorption of 25-hydroxy-vitamin D and osteomalacia in primary biliary cirrhosis. *Lancet,* **i,** 721–724.
38. Cooksley, W.G., Powell, L.W., Kerr, J.F. & Bhathal, P.S. (1972) Cholestasis in active chronic hepatitis. *American Journal of Digestive Diseases,* **17,** 495–504.
39. Cooper, R.A. (1977) Abnormalities in cell-membrane fluidity in the pathogenesis of disease. *New England Journal of Medicine,* **297,** 371–377.
40. Cooper, R.A., Kimball, D.B. & Durocher, J.R. (1974) Role of the spleen in membrane conditioning and hemolysis of spur cells in liver disease. *New England Journal of Medicine,* **290,** 1279–1284.
41. Cotton, P.B. (1977) Progress report: ERCP. *Gut,* **18,** 316–341.
42. Danzi, J.T., Makipour, H. & Farmer, R.G. (1976) Primary sclerosing cholangitis, a report of nine cases and clinical review. *American Journal of Gastroenterology,* **65,** 109–116.
43. Datta, D.V. & Sherlock, S. (1963) Treatment of pruritus of obstructive jaundice with cholestyramine. *British Medical Journal,* **i,** 216–219.
44. Datta, D.V. & Sherlock, S. (1966) Cholestyramine for long term relief of the pruritus complicating intrahepatic cholestasis. *Gastroenterology,* **50,** 323–332.
45. Datta, D.V., Sherlock, S. & Scheuer, P.D. (1963) Postnecrotic cirrhosis with chronic cholestasis. *Gut,* **4,** 223–230.
46. Daum, F., Rosen, J.F., Roginsky, M., Cohen, M.I. & Finberg, L. (1976) 25-hydroxycholecalciferol in the management of rickets associated with extrahepatic biliary atresia. *Pediatrics,* **88,** 1041–1043.
47. Denk, H., Eckerstorfer, R. & Rohr, H.P. (1977) The endoplasmic reticulum of rat liver cell in experimental mechanical biochemical and ultrastructural–morphometric studies on structure and enzyme composition. *Experimental and Molecular Pathology,* **26,** 193–203.
48. Denk, H., Gschnait, F. & Wolff, K. (1975) Hepatocellular hyalin (Mallory bodies) in long-term griseofulvin-treated mice. A new experimental model for the study of hyalin formation. *Laboratory Investigation,* **32,** 773–776.
49. Denk, H., Eckerstorfer, R., Talcott, R.E. & Schenkman, J.B. (1977) Alteration of hepatic microsomal enzymes by griseofulvin treatment of mice. *Biochemical Pharmacology,* **26,** 1125–1130.
50. Denk, H., Greim, H., Hutterer, F., Schaffner, F. & Popper, H. (1973) Turnover of hepatic cytochrome P-450 in experimental cholestases. *Experimental and Molecular Pathology,* **19,** 241–247.
51. De Pagter, A.G.F., van Berge Henegouwen, G.P., Ten Bokkel Huinink, J.A. & Brandt, K.H. (1976) Familial benign recurrent intrahepatic cholestasis. Interrelation with intrahepatic cholestasis of pregnancy and from oral contraceptives. *Gastroenterology,* **71,** 202.

52. Desmet, V.J. (1972) Morphologic and histochemical aspects of cholestasis. In *Progress in Liver Diseases*, Vol. 4 (Ed.) Popper, H. & Schaffner, F. pp. 97–132. New York and London: Grune & Stratton.
53. De Vos, R., De Wolf-Peeters, C., Desmet, V., Eggermont, E. & Van Acker, K. (1975) Progressive intrahepatic cholestasis (Byler's disease): case report. *Gut*, **16**, 943–950.
54. De Wolf-Peeters, C., De Vos, R. & Desmet, V. (1971) Histochemical evidence of a cholestatic period in neonatal rats. *Pediatric Research*, **5**, 704–709.
55. De Wolf-Peeters, C., De Vos, R., Desmet, V., Bianchi, L. & Rohr, R.P. (1974) Electron microscopy and morphometry of canalicular differentiation in fetal and neonatal rat liver. *Experimental and Molecular Pathology*, **21**, 339–350.
56. Diamond, J.M. (1974) Tight and leaky junctions of epithelia; a perspective on kisses in the dark. *Federation Proceedings*, **33**, 2220–2224.
57. Douglass, H.O. Jr & Holyoke, E.D. (1974) Pancreatic cancer, initial treatment as the determinant of survival. *Journal of the American Medical Association*, **229**, 793–797.
58. Dubin, I.N. (1959) Intrahepatic bile stasis in acute non-fatal viral hepatitis; its incidence, pathogenesis and correlation with jaundice. *Gastroenterology*, **36**, 645–660.
59. Dubin, I.N. & Peterson, L.H. (1958) An explanation for the centrolobular localization of intrahepatic bile stasis in acute liver diseases. *American Journal of Medical Sciences*, **236**, 45–52.
60. Dubin, I.N., Sullivan, B.H. Jr, Le Golvan, P.C. & Murphy, L.C. (1960) The cholestatic form of viral hepatitis, experiences with viral hepatitis at Brooke Army Hospital during the years 1951 to 1953. *American Journal of Medical Sciences*, **29**, 55–72.
61. Eisele, J.W., Barker, E.A. & Smuckler, E.A. (1975) Lipid content in the liver of fatty metamorphosis of pregnancy. *American Journal of Pathology*, **81**, 545–560.
62. Eppinger, H. (1937) *Die Leberkrankheiten. Allgemeine und spezielle Pathologie und Therapie der Leber.* Vienna: Springer.
63. Erlinger, S. & Dhumeaux, D. (1974) Mechanisms and control of secretion of bile water and electrolytes. *Gastroenterology*, **66**, 281–304.
64. Erlinger, S., Dhumeaux, D., Berthelot, P. & Dumont, M. (1970) Effect of inhibitors of sodium transport on bile formation in the rabbit. *American Journal of Physiology*, **219**, 416–422.
65. Evans, W.H., Kremmer, T. & Culvenor, J.B. (1976) Role of membranes in bile formation. Comparison of the composition of bile and a liver bile-canalicular plasma-membrane subfraction. *Biochemical Journal*, **154**, 589–595.
66. Fisher, M.M., Bloxam, D.L., Oda, M., Phillips, M.J. & Yousef, I.M. (1975) Characterization of rat liver cell plasma membranes. *Proceedings of the Society for Experimental Biology and Medicine*, **150**, 177–184.
67. Forker, E.L. (1970) Hepatocellular uptake of inulin, sucrose and mannitol in rats. *American Journal of Physiology*, **219**, 1568–1573.
68. Forker, E.L. (1975) Canalicular anion transport, pathogenetic mechanisms and a steady state distributed model for measuring kinetics. In *Hepatology – Research and Clinical Issues, Vol. 2. Jaundice.* (Ed.) Goresky, C.A. & Fisher, M.M. pp. 229–240. New York and London: Plenum Press.
69. French, S. (1976) Is cholestasis due to microfilament failure? *Human Pathology*, **7**, 243–244.
70. Frimmer, M. (1975) Phalloidin, a membrane specific toxin. In *Pathogenesis and Mechanisms of Liver Cell Necrosis* (Ed.) Kepler, D. pp. 163–173. Baltimore: University Park Press.
71. Fulop, M., Katz, S. & Lawrence, C. (1971) Extreme hyperbilirubinemia. *Archives of Internal Medicine*, **127**, 254–258.
72. Gabbiani, G., Montesano, R., Tuchweber, B., Salas, M. & Orci, L. (1975) Phalloidin-induced hyperplasia of actin filaments in rat hepatocytes. *Laboratory Investigation*, **33**, 562–569.
73. Gall, E.A. & Braunstein, H. (1955) Hepatitis with manifestations simulating bile duct obstruction (so-called cholangiolitic hepatitis). *American Journal of Clinical Pathology*, **25**, 1113–1127.
74. Gardiol, D. & Loup, P. (1971) Critères histologiques de la cholostase extrahépatique. *Acta Hepato-Splenologica*, **18**, 253–261.
75. Gautier, M., Jehan, P. & Odievre, M. (1976) Histologic study of biliary fibrous remnants in 48 cases of extrahepatic biliary atresia: correlation with postoperative bile flow restoration. *Journal of Pediatrics*, **89**, 704–709.
76. Geenen, J.E., Hogan, W.J., Shaffer, R.D., Stewart, E.T., Dodds, W.J. & Arndorfer, R.C. (1977) Endoscopic electrosurgical papillotomy and manometry in biliary tract disease. *Journal of the American Medical Association*, **237**, 2075–2078.
77. Gerber, M.A., Orr, W., Denk, H., Schaffner, F. & Popper, H. (1973) Hepatocellular hyalin in cholestasis and cirrhosis: its diagnostic significance. *Gastroenterology*, **64**, 89–98.
78. Graf, J. (1976) Possible role of a microtubular microfilamentous system in bile formation (Abstract). *Digestion*, **12**, 306.
79. Greim, H., Schwartz, L., Czygan, P. & Popper, H. (1975) Mechanism of necrosis induced by hepatotoxic bile acids. In *Pathogenesis and Mechanisms of Cell Necrosis* (Ed.) Keppler, D. pp. 199–208. Baltimore: University Park Press.
80. Greim, H., Trülzsch, D., Czygan, P., Rudick, J., Hutterer, F., Schaffner, F. & Popper, H. (1972) Mechanism of cholestasis: 6. Bile acids in human livers with or without biliary obstruction. *Gastroenterology*, **63**, 846–850.
81. Guzelian, P. & Boyer, J.L. (1974) Glucose reabsorption from bile. Evidence for a biliohepatic circulation. *Journal of Clinical Investigation*, **53**, 526–534.
82. Hadchouel, M. & Gautier, M. (1976) Histopathological study of the liver in the early cholestatic phase of alpha-1-antitrypsin deficiency. *Journal of Pediatrics*, **89**, 211–215.
83. Hägerstrand, I. (1976) Bile canalicular alkaline phosphatase and disease. *Acta Pathologica et Microbiologica Scandinavica*, Section A, **84**, 217–277.
84. Haemmerli, U.P. (1966) Jaundice during pregnancy, with special emphasis on recurrent jaundice during pregnancy and its differential diagnosis. *Acta Medica Scandinavica* (Suppl.) **444**, 1–111.
85. Haemmerli, U.P. (1975) Jaundice during pregnancy. In *Diseases of the Liver* (Ed.) Schiff, L. pp. 1336–1353. Philadelphia: Lippincott.
86. Handmaker, H. (1975) Nuclear medicine in the evaluation of the patient with jaundice. *Journal of the American Medical Association*, **231**, 1172–1176.
87. Hardy, K.J., Wheatley, I.C., Anderson, A.I.E. & Bond, R.J. (1976) The lymph nodes of the porta

hepatis. *Surgery, Gynecology and Obstetrics,* **143,** 225–228.

88. Hepner, G.W. (1975) Hepatic microsomal function is not severely impaired by cholestasis. *Gastroenterology,* **70,** A-16.
89. Holzbach, R.T. (1974) Acute fatty liver of pregnancy with disseminated intravascular coagulation. *Obstetrics and Gynecology,* **43,** 740–744.
90. Hunt, R., Leveille, G. & Sauberlich, H. (1964) Dietary bile acids and lipid metabolism. Effects of lithocholic acid in mammalian species. *Proceedings of the Society for Experimental Biology and Medicine,* **115,** 277–280.
91. Hutterer, F., Bacchin, P.G., Raisfeld, I.H., Schenkman, J.B., Schaffner, F. & Popper, H. (1970a) Alteration of microsomal biotransformation in the liver in cholestasis. *Proceedings of the Society for Experimental Biology and Medicine,* **133,** 702–706.
92. Hutterer, F., Denk, H., Bacchin, P.G., Schenkman, J.B., Schaffner, F. & Popper, H. (1970b) Mechanism of cholestasis. 1. Effect of bile acids on microsomal cytochrome P-450 dependent biotransformation system *in vitro*. *Life Sciences,* **9,** 877–887.
93. Hutterer, F., Greim, H., Trülzsch, D., Czygan, P. & Schenkman, J.B. (1972) Microsomal biotransformation system in cholestases. In *Progress in Liver Diseases,* Vol. 4 (Ed.) Popper, H. & Schaffner, F. pp. 151–171. New York: Grune & Stratton.
94. Hutterer, F., Klion, F.M., Wengraf, A., Schaffner, F. & Popper, H. (1969) Hepatocellular adaptation and injury. Structural and biochemical changes following dieldrin and methyl butter yellow. *Laboratory Investigation,* **20,** 455–464.
95. Isikoff, M.B. & Diaconis, J.N. (1977) Ultrasound; a new diagnostic approach to the jaundiced patient. *Journal of the American Medical Association,* **238,** 221–223.
96. Jansen, P.L.M., Chowdhury, J.R., Fischberg, E.B. & Arias, I.M. (1977) Enzymatic conversion of bilirubin monoglucuronide to diglucuronide by rat liver plasma membranes. *Journal of Biological Chemistry,* **252,** 2710–2716.
97. Javitt, N.B. (1975) Current status of cholestasis induced by monohydroxy bile acids. In *Hepatology – Research and Clinical Issues,* Vol. 2. Jaundice (Ed.) Goresky, C.A. & Fisher, M.M. pp. 401–409. New York and London: Plenum Press.
98. Javitt, N.B. (1976) Cholestasis in infancy. Status report and conceptual approach. *Gastroenterology,* **70,** 1172–1181.
99. Javitt, N.B. & Emerman, S. (1968) Effect of sodium taurolithocholate on bile flow and bile acid excretion. *Laboratory Investigation,* **47,** 1002–1014.
100. Javitt, N.B., Morrissey, K.P., Siegel, E., Goldberg, H., Gartner, L.M., Hollander, M. & Kok, E. (1973) Cholestatic syndromes in infancy: diagnostic value of serum bile acid pattern and cholestyramine administration. *Pediatric Research,* **7,** 119–125.
101. Jenner, R.E. & Howard, E.R. (1975) Unsaturated monohydroxy bile acids as a cause of idiopathic obstructive cholangiopathy. *Lancet,* **ii,** 1073–1074.
102. Jones, A.L., Schmucker, D.L., Mooney, J.S., Adler, R.D. & Ockner, R.K. (1976) Morphometric analysis of rat hepatocytes after total biliary obstruction. *Gastroenterology,* **71,** 1050–1060.
103. Jørgenson, M. (1973) A stereological study of intrahepatic bile duct. 2. Bile duct proliferation in some pathologic conditions. *Acta Pathologica et Microbiologica Scandinavica,* Section A, **81,** 663–669.
104. Kasai, M. (1974) Treatment of biliary atresia with special reference to hepatic porto-enterostomy and its modifications. *Progress in Pediatric Surgery,* **6,** 5–50.
105. Kern, F. Jr (1976) Hepatobiliary disorders in inflammatory bowel disease. In *Progress in Liver Diseases,* Vol. 5 (Ed.) Popper, H. & Schaffner, F. pp. 575–589. New York: Grune & Stratton.
106. Kirby, J., Heaton, K.W. & Burton, J.L. (1974) Pruritic effect of bile salts. *British Medical Journal,* **iv,** 693–695.
107. Klaasen, C. (1971) Does bile acid secretion determine canalicular bile production in rats? *American Journal of Physiology,* **220,** 667–673.
108. Klion, F.M. & Schaffner, F. (1966) Electron microscopic observations in primary biliary cirrhosis. *Archives of Pathology,* **81,** 152–161.
109. Klion, F.M., Weiner, M.J. & Schaffner, F. (1964) Cholestasis in sickle cell anemia. *American Journal of Medicine,* **37,** 829–832.
110. Kreek, M.J. & Sleisinger, M.H. (1970) Estrogen induced cholestasis due to endogenous and exogenous hormones. *Scandinavian Journal of Gastroenterology,* **5,** 123–131.
111. Kunelis, C.T., Peter, J.L. & Edmonson, H.A. (1965) Fatty liver of pregnancy and its relationship to tetracycline therapy. *American Journal of Medicine,* **38,** 359–377.
112. Künzer, W., Sutor, A.H., Niederhoff, H. & Küzer, W. Jr (1975) Cholestatischer Ikterus nach disseminierter intravascular Gerinnung ('Schockleber'). *Klinische Wochenschrift,* **53,** 441–443.
113. Landing, B.H. (1975) Protracted obstructive jaundice in infancy with emphasis on neonatal hepatitis, biliary atresia, and choledochal cyst. In *The Liver. Normal and Abnormal Functions, Part B* (Ed.) Becker, F.F. pp. 821–849. New York: Marcel Dekker, Inc.
114. Layden, T.J., Schwarz, J. & Boyer, J.L. (1975) Scanning electron microscopy of the rat liver; studies of the effect of taurolithocholate and other models of cholestasis. *Gastroenterology,* **69,** 724–738.
115. Levine, G., Favara, B.E., Mierau, G. & Bailey, W.G. (1973) Jaundice, liver ultrastructure, and congenital pyloric stenosis. *Archives of Pathology,* **95,** 267–270.
116. Levy, V.G., Chevrel, B. & Caroli, J. (1977) Les ictères au cours de la grossesse. *Médecine et Chirurgie Digestives,* **6,** 111–116.
117. Levy, E., Slusser, R.J. & Ruebner, B.H. (1968) Hepatic changes produced by a single dose of endotoxin in the mouse. *American Journal of Pathology,* **52,** 477–502.
118. Lilly, J.R. & Altman, R.P. (1975) Hepatic portoenterostomy (the Kasai operation) for biliary atresia. *Surgery,* **78,** 76–86.
119. Linarelli, L.G., Williams, C.N. & Phillips, M.J. (1972) Byler's disease: fatal intrahepatic cholestasis. *Journal of Pediatrics,* **81,** 484–492.
120. Lindblad, L., Lundholm, K. & Schersten, T. (1977) Bile and concentrations in systemic and portal serum in presumably normal man and in cholestatic and cirrhotic conditions. *Scandinavian Journal of Gastroenterology,* **12,** 395–400.
121. Lindner, H. & Laulenschlager, H.J. (1974) Die laparoskopische Differentialdiagnose des intra- und extrahepatischen Verschlusssyndroms. *Leber Magen Darm,* **4,** 319–329.

122. LoIudice, T.A., Jarmolych, J. & Buhac, I. (1977) Pancreatic retention cyst; a cause of obstructive jaundice. *Journal of the American Medical Association,* **238,** 889–890.

123. Long, R.G., Scheuer, P.J. & Sherlock, S. (1977a) Pre-eclampsia presenting with deep jaundice. *Journal of Clinical Pathology,* **30,** 212–215.

124. Long, R.G., Scheuer, P.J. & Sherlock, S. (1977b) Presentation and course of asymptomatic primary biliary cirrhosis. *Gastroenterology,* **72,** 1204–1207.

125. Luska, G., Freyschmidt, J. & Huchzermeyer, H. (1977) Perkutane transjugulare Cholangiographie. *Roentgen-Berichte,* **6,** 13–19.

126. Mackinnon, A.M. & Simon, F.R. (1974) Reduced synthesis of hepatic microsomal cytochome P_{450} in the bile duct ligated rat. *Biochemical and Biophysical Research Communications,* **56,** 437–443.

127. Makino, I., Sjövall, J., Norman, A. & Strandvik, B. (1971) Excretion of 3β-hydroxy-5-cholenoic and 3α-hydroxy-5α-cholenoic acids in urine of infants with biliary atresia. *FEBS Letters,* **15,** 161–164.

128. Makino, I., Hashimoti, H., Shinozaki, K., Yoshino, K. & Nakagawa, S. (1975) Sulfated and nonsulfated bile acids in urine, serum and bile of patients with hepatobiliary diseases. *Gastroenterology,* **68,** 545–553.

129. McCollum, W.B. & Jordan, P.H. Jr (1975) Obstructive jaundice in patients with pancreatitis without associated biliary tract disease. *Annals of Surgery,* **182,** 116–120.

130. Miller, D.J., Keeton, G.R., Webber, B.L. & Saunders, S.J. (1976) Jaundice in severe bacterial infection. *Gastroenterology,* **71,** 94–97.

131. Miyai, K., Mayr, W.E. & Richardson, A.L. (1975) Acute cholestasis induced by lithocholic acid in the rat. A freeze-fracture replica and thin section study. *Laboratory Investigation,* **32,** 527–535.

132. Miyai, K., Richardson, A.L., Mayr, W. & Javitt, N.B. (1977) Subcellular pathology in rat liver in cholestasis and choleresis induced by bile salts. 1. Effects of lithocholic, 3β-hydroxy-5-cholenoic, cholic, and dehydrocholic acids. *Laboratory Investigation,* **36,** 249–258.

133. Montesano, R., Friend, D.S., Perret, A. & Orci, L. (1975) *In vivo* assembly of tight junctions in fetal rat liver. *Journal of Cell Biology,* **67,** 310–319.

134. Morgan, R.G.H. & Wormsley, K.G. (1977) Cancer of the pancreas. *Gut,* **18,** 580–596.

135. Morris, J.S., Gallo, G.A., Scheuer, P.J. & Sherlock, S. (1975) Percutaneous liver biopsy in patients with large bile duct obstruction. *Gastroenterology,* **68,** 750–754.

136. Motta, P. & Fumagalli, G. (1975) Structure of rat bile canaliculi as revealed by scanning electron microscopy. *Anatomical Record,* **182,** 499–514.

137. Nemchausky, B.A., Boyer, J.L., Layden, T.J. & Schwartz, J. (1976) *In vivo* effects of bile acids on canalicular membrane enzyme, lipid composition and three dimensional structure. *Gastroenterology,* **70,** A-131.

138. Obling, H., Engels, A.-M. & Dönges, K.G. (1969) Hepatocellular jaundice after multiple infusions of fat emulsions in two children with extensive jejunal resection. *Deutsche Medizinische Wochenschrift,* **94,** 1825–1827.

139. Oda, M. & Phillips, M.J. (1975) Electron microscopic cytochemical characterization of bile canaliculi and bile ducts *in vitro. Virchows Archiv B. Cellular Pathology,* **18,** 109–118.

140. Oda, M., Price, V.M., Fisher, M.M. & Phillips, M.J. (1974) Ultrastructure of bile canaliculi, with special reference to the surface coat and pericanalicular web. *Laboratory Investigation,* **31,** 314–323.

141. Oi, L., Kobayashi, S. & Kondo, T. (1970) Endoscopic pancreatocholangiography. *Endoscopy,* **2,** 103–106.

142. Okuda, K. & Peters, R.L. (1976) *Hepatocellular Carcinoma.* New York: John Wiley.

143. Okuda, K., Tanikawa, K., Emura, T., Kuratomi, S., Jinnouchi, S., Urabe, K., Sumikoshi, T., Kanda, Y., Fukuyama, Y., Musha, H., Mori, H., Shimokawa, Y., Yakushiji, F. & Matsuura, Y. (1974) Nonsurgical, percutaneous transhepatic cholangiography – diagnostic significance in medical problems of the liver. *American Journal of Digestive Diseases,* **19,** 21–36.

144. Orellana-Alcalde, J.M. & Dominguez, J.P. (1966) Jaundice and oral contraceptive drugs. *Lancet,* **i,** 1278–1280.

145. Palmer, R.H. & Bolt, M.G. (1971) Bile and sulfates. 1. Synthesis of lithocholic acid sulfates and their identification in human bile. *Journal of Lipid Research,* **12,** 671–679.

146. Palmer, R.H. & Hruban, Z. (1966) Production of bile duct hyperplasia and gallstones by lithocholic acid. *Journal of Clinical Investigation,* **45,** 1255–1267.

147. Partin, J.S., Schubert, W.K. & Partin, J.C. (1975) Unique ultrastructural abnormality of hepatic mitochondria in a patient with Byler like cholestatic syndrome. *Gastroenterology,* **69,** A-52.

148. Pereiras, R. Jr, Chiprut, R.O., Greenwald, R.A. & Schiff, E.R. (1977) Percutaneous transhepatic cholangiography with the 'skinny' needle. A rapid, simple and accurate method in the diagnosis of cholestasis. *Annals of Internal Medicine,* **86,** 562–568.

149. Perez, V., Schaffner, F. & Popper, H. (1972) Hepatic drug reactions. In *Progress in Liver Diseases,* Vol. 4 (Ed.) Popper, H. & Schaffner, F. pp. 597–625. New York: Grune & Stratton.

150. Phillips, G.B. & Davidson, C.S. (1954) Acute hepatic insufficiency in the chronic alcoholic and pathological study. *Archives of Internal Medicine,* **94,** 585–603.

151. Phillips, M.J., Oda, M., Mak, E., Fisher, M.M. & Jeejeebhoy, K.N. (1975) Microfilament dysfunction as a possible cause of intrahepatic cholestasis. *Gastroenterology,* **69,** 48–58.

152. Plaa, G.L. & Priestly, B.G. (1977) Intrahepatic cholestasis induced by drugs and chemicals. *Pharmacological Reviews,* **28,** 207–273.

153. Poley, J.R. & Magnani, H.N. (1976) Cholestatic jaundice in infancy; diagnosis, differential diagnosis and treatment. *Australian Paediatric Journal,* **12,** 134–153.

154. Popper, H. (1968) Cholestasis. *Annual Review of Medicine,* **19,** 39–56.

155. Popper, H. (1977) The mechanism of cholestasis. In *The Liver and Bile* (Ed.) Bianchi, L., Gerok, W. & Sickinger, K. pp. 187–199. Baltimore: University Park Press.

156. Popper, H. & Schaffner, F. (1952) Laboratory diagnosis of liver disease. Coordinated use of histological and biochemical observations. *Journal of the American Medical Association,* **150,** 1367–1372.

157. Popper, H. & Schaffner, F. (1970) Alcoholic hepatitis in the spectrum of ethanol-induced liver injury. *Scandinavian Journal of Gastroenterology* (Suppl.) **7,** 69–78.

158. Popper, H. & Schaffner, F. (1970) Pathophysiology of cholestasis. *Human Pathology,* **1,** 1–24.

159. Popper, H., Schaffner, F. & Denk, H. (1976) Molecular pathology of cholestasis. In *The Hepatobiliary System, Fundamental and Pathological Mechanisms* (Ed.) Taylor, W. pp. 605–629. New York: Plenum Press.

160. Porter, C.A., Mowat, A.P. & Cook, P.J.L. (1972) α_1-antitrypsin deficiency and neonatal hepatitis. *British Medical Journal,* **iii,** 435–439.

161. Prandi, D., Erlinger, S., Glasinovic, J.-C. & Dumont, M. (1975) Canalicular bile production in man. *European Journal of Clinical Investigation,* **5,** 1–6.

162. Prugh, M.F., Gregory, D.H., Vlahcevic, Z.R. & Swell, L. (1976) Role of the 'microtubular-golgi' network in the hepatocellular transport of biliary lipids. *Gastroenterology,* **70,** A-132.

163. Reichen, J. & Paumgartner, G. (1977) Relationship between bile flow and Na^+,K^+-adenosinetriphosphatase in liver plasma membranes enriched in bile canaliculi. *Journal of Clinical Investigation,* **60,** 429–434.

164. Ritland, S. (1975) The abnormal 'lipoprotein of cholestasis,' lipoprotein-X. *Scandinavian Journal of Gastroenterology,* **10,** 785–789.

165. Rodgers, B.M., Hallenbeck, J.I., Donnelly, W.H. & Talbert, J.L. (1976) Intrahepatic cholestasis with parenteral alimentation. *American Journal of Surgery,* **131,** 149–155.

166. Roessner, A., Uchida, Y., Van Husen, N., Gerlach, U., Witting, U. & Themann, H. (1976) Vergleichende feinstrukturell-morphometrische und biochemische Befunde an der Rattenleber nach Gallengangsligatur. *Research in Experimental Medicine,* **169,** 9–20.

167. Roger, R. & Finegold, M.J. (1974) Cholestasis in low birth weight prematures: is parenteral alimentation the cause? *American Journal of Pathology,* **74,** 6a–7a.

168. Ronchi, G. & Desmet, V. (1973) Histochemical studies of so-called 'marker enzymes of cholestasis' during extrahepatic bile duct obstruction in the rat. *Beiträge für Pathologie,* **149,** 213–226.

169. Rössle, R. (1930) Die cholangiolitische Zirrhose. In *Entzundungen der Leber,* Vol. **5,** No. 1 of *Handbuch der Speziellen Pathologischen Anatomie und Histologie* (Ed.) Henke, F. & Lubarsch, O. pp. 448–452. Berlin: Springer.

170. Rotthauwe, H.W. & Rotthauwe, I. (1971) Familiäre rekurrierende intrahepatische Cholestase seit dem frühen Kindesalter. *Zeitschrift für Kinderheilkunde,* **110,** 292–316.

171. Rouiller, C. (1956) Les canalicules biliares. Étude au microscope électronique. *Acta Anatomica (Basel),* **26,** 94–109.

172. Rubin, E., Schaffner, F. & Popper, H. (1965) Primary biliary cirrhosis. Chronic non-suppurative destructive cholangitis. *American Journal of Pathology,* **46,** 387–407.

173. Rudzki, C., Ishak, K.G. & Zimmerman, H.J. (1975) Chronic intrahepatic cholestasis of sarcoidosis. *American Journal of Medicine,* **59,** 373–387.

174. Ruskin, R.B., Katon, R.M., Bilbao, M.K. & Smith, F. (1976) Evaluation of sclerosing cholangitis by endoscopic retrograde cholangiopancreatography. *Archives of Internal Medicine,* **136,** 232–235.

175. Salaspuro, M. & Sipponen, P. (1976) Demonstration of an intracellular copper-binding protein by orcein in long-standing cholestatic liver diseases. *Gut,* **17,** 787–790.

176. Samuels, A.M. & Carey, M.C. (1976) Effects of chlorpromazine (CPZ) and its metabolites on Na^+-K^+-ATPase activity of canalicular enriched liver plasma membranes. *Gastroenterology,* **70,** A-75.

177. Sasaki, H., Schaffner, F. & Popper, H. (1967) Bile ductules in cholestasis: morphologic evidence for secretion and absorption in man. *Laboratory Investigation,* **96,** 84–95.

178. Schaffner, F. (1969) Paradoxical elevation of serum cholesterol by clofibrate in patients with primary biliary cirrhosis. *Gastroenterology,* **57,** 253–255.

179. Schaffner, F. (1977) The jaundiced patient. In *Current Diagnosis 5* (Ed.) Conn, H.F. & Conn, R.B. pp. 32–36. Philadelphia: Saunders.

180. Schaffner, F. & Javitt, N.B. (1966) Morphologic changes in hamster liver during intrahepatic cholestasis induced by taurolithocholate. *Laboratory Investigation,* **15,** 1783–1792.

181. Schaffner, F. & Popper, H. (1959) Morphologic studies of cholestasis. *Gastroenterology,* **37,** 565–573.

182. Schaffner, F. & Popper, H. (1969) Hypothesis: cholestasis is the result of hypoactive hypertrophic smooth endoplasmic reticulum in the hepatocyte. *Lancet,* **ii,** 355–359.

183. Schaffner, F. & Popper, H. (1975) Causation and consequences of cholestasis. In *Hepatology: Research and Clinical Issues,* Vol. 2. Jaundice (Ed.) Goresky, C.A. & Fisher, M.M. pp. 329–349. New York: Plenum Press.

184. Schaffner, F., Klion, F.M. & Latuff, A.J. (1965) Long term use of cholestyramine in the treatment of primary biliary cirrhosis. *Gastroenterology,* **48,** 293–298.

185. Schaffner, F., Bacchin, P.G., Hutterer, F., Scharnbeck, H.H., Sarkozi, L.L., Denk, H. & Popper, H. (1971) Mechanism of cholestasis. 4. Structural and biochemical changes in the liver and serum in rats after bile duct ligation. *Gastroenterology,* **60,** 888–897.

186. Schatzki, P.F. (1969) Bile canaliculus and space of Disse: electron microscopic relationships as delineated by lanthanum. *Laboratory Investigation,* **20,** 87–93.

187. Schmid, M., Hefti, M.L., Gattiker, R. & Kistler, H.J. (1965) Benign postoperative intrahepatic cholestasis. *New England Journal of Medicine,* **272,** 545–550.

188. Schoenfield, L.J., Sjövall, J. & Perman, E. (1967) Bile acids on skin of patients with pruritic hepatobiliary disease. *Nature (London),* **213,** 93–94.

189. Scott, J., Summerfield, J.A., Elias, E., Dick, R. & Sherlock, S. (1976) Chronic pancreatitis: a cause of cholestasis. *Gastroenterology,* **70,** A-135.

190. Seeff, L.B. & Zimmerman, H.J. (1976) Relationship between hepatic and pancreatic disease. In *Progress in Liver Diseases,* Vol. 5 (Ed.) Popper, H. & Schaffner, F. pp. 590–608. New York: Grune & Stratton.

191. Seidel, D., Buff, H.U., Fauser, U. & Bleyl, U. (1976) On the metabolism of lipoprotein-X (LP-X). *Clinica Chimica Acta,* **66,** 195–207.

192. Seidel, D., Alaupovic, P., Furman, R.H. & McConathy, W.J. (1970) A lipoprotein characterizing obstructive jaundice. II. Isolation and partial characterization of the protein moieties of low density lipoproteins. *Journal of Clinical Investigation,* **49,** 2396–2407.

193. Sharp, H.L. & Mirkin, B.L. (1972) Effect of phenobarbital on hyperbilirubinemia, bile acid

metabolism and microsomal enzyme activity in chronic intrahepatic cholestasis of childhood. *Journal of Pediatrics,* **81,** 116–126.

194. Sharp, H.L., Bridges, R.A. & Krivit, W. (1969) Cirrhosis associated with alpha-1-antitrypsin deficiency: a previously unrecognized inherited disorder. *Journal of Laboratory and Clinical Medicine,* **73,** 934–939.
195. Sheehan, H.L. (1961) Jaundice in pregnancy. *American Journal of Obstetrics and Gynecology,* **81,** 427–440.
196. Sherlock, S. (1966) Biliary secretory failure in man. *Annals of Internal Medicine,* **65,** 397–408.
197. Sherlock, S. (1968) Jaundice in pregnancy. *British Medical Bulletin,* **24,** 39–43.
198. Sherlock, S. (1975) The liver in circulatory failure. In *Diseases of the Liver,* 4th ed. (Ed.) Schiff, L. pp. 1033–1050. Philadelphia: Lippincott.
199. Shorter, R.G. & Baggenstoss, A.H. (1959) Extrahepatic cholestasis. I. Histologic changes in hepatic interlobular bile ducts and ductules in extrahepatic cholestasis. *American Journal of Clinical Pathology,* **32,** 1–4.
200. Shorter, R.G. & Baggenstoss, A.H. (1959) Extrahepatic cholestasis. II. Histologic features of diagnostic importance. *American Journal of Clinical Pathology,* **32,** 5–9.
201. Shorter, R.G. & Baggenstoss, A.H. (1959) Extrahepatic cholestasis. III. Chronology of histologic changes in the liver. *American Journal of Clinical Pathology,* **32,** 10–17.
202. Simon, F.R. & Arias, I.M. (1973) Alteration of bile canalicular enzymes in cholestasis. A possible cause of bile secretory failure. *Journal of Clinical Investigation,* **52,** 765–775.
203. Simon, F.R., Sutherland, E. & Accatino, L. (1977) Stimulation of hepatic sodium and potassium-activated adenosine triphosphatase activity by phenobarbital; its possible role in regulation of bile flow. *Journal of Clinical Investigation,* **59,** 849–861.
204. Snape, W.J. Jr, Long, W.B., Trotman, B.W., Marin, G.A. & Czaja, A.J. (1976) Marked alkaline phosphatase elevation with partial common bile duct obstruction due to calcific pancreatitis. *Gastroenterology,* **70,** 70–73.
205. Solymoss, B. & Zsigmond, G. (1974) Effect of microsomal enzyme inducers on the liver changes produced by common bile-duct ligature. *Proceedings of the Society of Experimental Biology and Medicine,* **147,** 430–433.
206. Song, C.S., Rubin, W., Rifkind, A.B. & Kappas, A. (1969) Plasma membranes of rat liver. Isolation and enzymatic characterization of a fraction rich in bile canaliculi. *Journal of Cell Biology,* **41,** 124–132.
207. Sperber, I. (1965) Biliary secretion of organic anions and its influence on bile flow. In *The Biliary System. A Symposium of the NATO Advanced Study Institute* (Ed.) Taylor, W. pp. 457–467. Philadelphia: Davis.
208. Stakeberg, H., Lundborg, H. & Schersten, T. (1974) Rate of *in vitro* incorporation of precursors into hepatic lipids and proteins in patients with extrahepatic cholestasis. *European Journal of Clinical Investigation,* **4,** 399–403.
209. Steiner, J.W., Carruthers, J.S. & Kalifat, S.R. (1962) The ductular cell reaction of rat liver in extrahepatic cholestasis. I. Proliferated biliary epithelial cells. *Experimental and Molecular Pathology,* **1,** 162–185.
210. Steiner, J.W., Jezequel, A.M., Phillips, M.J., Miyai, K. & Arakawa, K. (1965) Some aspects of the ultrastructural pathology of the liver. In *Progress in Liver Diseases,* Vol. 2 (Ed.) Popper, H. & Schaffner, F. pp. 303–372. New York: Grune & Stratton.
211. Sternlieb, I. (1969) Mitochondrion–desmosome complexes in human hepatocytes. *Zeitschrift für Zellforschung,* **93,** 249–253.
212. Stiehl, A., Earnest, D.L. & Admirand, W.H. (1975) Sulfation and renal excretion of bile salts in patients with cirrhosis of the liver. *Gastroenterology,* **68,** 534–544.
213. Stiehl, A., Thaler, M.M. & Admirand, W.H. (1973) Effects of phenobarbital on bile salt metabolism in cholestasis due to bile duct hypoplasia. *Pediatrics,* **51,** 992–997.
214. Strohmeyer, G. & Berges, W. (1976) Der postoperative Ikterus. *Internist,* **17,** 313–319.
215. Summerfield, J.A., Cullen, J., Barnes, S. & Billing, B.H. (1977) Evidence for renal control of urinary excretion of bile acids and bile acid sulphates in the cholestatic syndrome. *Clinical Science and Molecular Medicine,* **52,** 51–65.
216. Summerskill, W.H.J. (1965) The syndrome of benign recurrent cholestasis. *American Journal of Medicine,* **38,** 298–305.
217. Summerskill, W.H.J. & Walshe, J.M. (1959) Benign recurrent intrahepatic 'obstructive' jaundice. *Lancet,* **ii,** 686–690.
218. Taylor, K.J.W. & Rosenfield, A.T. (1977) Grey-scale ultrasonography in differential diagnosis of jaundice. *Archives of Surgery,* **112,** 820–825.
219. Thaler, M.M. (1976) Cryptogenic liver disease in young infants. In *Progress in Liver Diseases,* Vol. **5** (Ed.) Popper, H. & Schaffner, F. pp. 476–493. New York: Grune & Stratton.
220. Touloukian, R.J. & Downing, S.E. (1973) Cholestasis associated with long-term parenteral hyperalimentation. *Archives of Surgery,* **106,** 58–62.
221. Tugwell, P. & Williams, A.O. (1977) Jaundice associated with lobar pneumonia. A clinical laboratory and histological study. *Quarterly Journal of Medicine, n.s.* **46,** 97–118.
222. Tygstrup, N. (1960) Intermittent possibly familial intrahepatic cholestatic jaundice. *Lancet,* **i,** 1171.
223. Tygstrup, N. (1977) Personal communication.
224. Utili, R., Abernathy, C.O. & Zimmerman, H.J. (1976) Cholestatic effects of *Escherichia coli* endotoxin on the isolated perfused rat liver. *Gastroenterology,* **70,** 248–253.
225. Valayer, J. (1976) Hepatic porto-enterostomy. Surgical problems and results. In *Liver Diseases in Infancy and Childhood* (Ed.) Berenberg, S.R. pp. 84–96. The Hague: Martinus Nijhoff.
226. Vial, J.D., Simon, F.R. & Mackinnon, A.M. (1976) Effect of bile duct ligation on the ultrastructural morphology of hepatocytes. *Gastroenterology,* **70,** 85–92.
227. Vicary, F.R., Cusick, G., Shirley, I.M. & Blackwell, R.J. (1977) Ultrasound and jaundice. *Gut,* **18,** 161–164.
228. Wagonfeld, J.B., Nemchausky, B.A., Bolt, M., Vander Horst, J., Boyer, J.L. & Rosenberg, I.H. (1976) Comparison of vitamin D and 25-hydroxy-vitamin-D in the therapy of primary biliary cirrhosis. *Lancet,* **ii,** 391–394.
229. Warnes, T.W., Hine, P. & Kay, G. (1977) Intestinal alkaline phosphatase in the diagnosis of liver disease. *Gut,* **18,** 274–278.
230. Warren, K.W., Athassiades, S. & Monge, J.I. (1966) Primary sclerosing cholangitis, a study of forty-two cases. *American Journal of Surgery,* **111,** 23–38.

231. Wheeler, H.O. (1972) Secretion of bile acids by the liver and their role in the formation of hepatic bile. *Archives of Internal Medicine,* **130,** 533–541.
232. Williams, C.N., Kaye, R., Baker, L., Hurwitz, R. & Senior, J.R. (1972) Progressive familial cholestatic cirrhosis and bile acid metabolism. *Journal of Pediatrics,* **81,** 493–500.
233. Wills, E.J. & Epstein, M.E. (1966) Subcellular changes in surface adenosine triphosphatase activity of human liver in extrahepatic obstructive jaundice. *American Journal of Pathology,* **49,** 605–635.
234. Wilkinson, S.P., Moodie, H., Stamatakis, J.D., Kakkar, V.V. & Williams, R. (1976) Endotoxaemia and renal failure in cirrhosis and obstructive jaundice. *British Medical Journal,* **ii,** 1415–1418.
235. Wisher, M.H. & Evans, W.H. (1977) Preparation of plasma-membrane subfractions from isolated rat hepatocytes. *Biochemical Journal,* **164,** 415–422.
236. Witzleben, C.L. (1972) Hepatic ultrastructural effects of cholic acid overload. *Experimental and Molecular Pathology,* **16,** 47–53.
237. Witzleben, C.L. & Boyce, W.H. (1975) Bilirubin as a cholestatic agent. III. Prevention of bilirubin-related cholestasis by sulfobromophthalein. *Archives of Pathology,* **99,** 492–495.
238. Wootton, A.M., Neale, G. & Moss, D.W. (1977) Enzyme activities of cells of different types isolated from livers of normal and cholestatic rats. *Clinical Science and Molecular Medicine,* **52,** 585–590.
239. Yamada, T., Ida, T., Yamaoka, Y., Ozawa, K., Takasan, H. & Honjo, I. (1975) Two distinct patterns of glucose intolerance in icteric rats and rabbits. Relationship to impaired liver mitochondria functions. *Journal of Laboratory and Clinical Medicine,* **86,** 38–45.
240. Yamauchi, H., Koyama, K., Otawa, T., Ouchi, K., Anezaki, T. & Sato, T. (1976) Morphometric studies on the rat liver in biliary obstruction. *Tohoku Journal of Experimental Medicine,* **119,** 9–25.
241. Yousef, I.M., Kakis, G. & Fisher, M.M. (1976) Lithocholate-induced intrahepatic cholestasis. *Gastroenterology,* **70,** A-138.
242. Yousef, I.M., Bloxam, D.L., Phillips, M.J. & Fisher, M.M. (1975) Liver cell plasma membrane lipids and the origin of biliary phospholipids. *Canadian Journal of Biochemistry,* **53,** 989–997.
243. Zieve, L. (1966) Hemolytic anemia in liver disease. *Medicine,* **45,** 497–505.
244. Zimmerman, H.J. & Thomas, L.J. (1950) The liver in pneumococcal pneumonia: observations in 94 cases on liver function and jaundice in pneumonia. *Annals of Internal Medicine,* **35,** 556–567.
245. Zimmon, D.S., Breslaw, J. & Kessler, R.E. (1975) Endoscopy with endoscopic cholangiopancreatography; the combination as a primary diagnostic procedure. *Journal of the American Medical Association,* **233,** 447–449.

Chapter 15

Haem Metabolism and the Porphyrias

D.M. BISSELL

BACKGROUND

Porphyrins are planar molecules with four pyrrole rings joined by carbon bridges to form a macrocycle, the centre of which readily binds transition metals (Figure 15.1). As complexes with iron, magnesium or cobalt they act as the prosthetic group for molecules essential to oxidative respiration (haem), photosynthesis (chlorophyll) and are found also as vitamin B_{12} (Figure 15.1). The presence of these structurally closely related compounds in both the plant and animal kingdoms suggests that they must have arisen early in evolution. Indeed, phylogenetic studies as well as biosynthetic considerations indicate that uroporphyrinogen III was a common precursor to all three in evolution.[54]

In mammals, porphyrins function exclusively as metal complexes, primarily with iron as haem, and with cobalt as vitamin B_{12}. Free porphyrins serve no biologically useful function in humans. They are produced only in minute amounts and then only as accidental side products of haem synthesis. The pathway of haem synthesis normally operates at high efficiency; intermediates are utilized nearly quantitatively so that less than 1 per cent escape from the biosynthetic route to appear in blood and undergo excretion. The appearance of increased amounts of porphyrins or porphyrin precursors in urine or faeces implies a disturbance in haem synthesis. Collectively, these disturbances are termed *porphyria.* Individually, they represent several discrete genetic or acquired defects in haem synthesis, which vary in their clinical expression, depending on the nature and biochemical localization of the defect. These distinctions form the basis for classifying the porphyrias, as will be discussed below.

The first published cases of porphyria were recognized as having more than a single aetiology. Günther's patient, Petry, exhibited a congenital (and presumably hereditary) form; in other instances, the condition clearly was toxin-related, as in the numerous cases following introduction (in 1888) of the hypnotic, sulphomethane (Sulphonal). In the latter cases, there was no evidence for a hereditary sensitivity to the drug. The spectrum of the porphyrias was enlarged still further in the 1930s with the description of a type that involved excretion of a compound that was colourless in urine but gave a red reaction with Ehrlich's reagent. Waldenström suggested correctly that the compound was a pyrrole precursor of haem, and it was later identified as porphobilinogen.[83] Patients with pyrroluria exhibited severe abdominal pains, often associated with a peripheral neuropathy and psychological disturbances, and these symptoms were frequently elicited or markedly exacerbated by administration of barbiturates. The unique sensitivity to barbiturates in these patients was recognized as hereditary. This condition is known today as acute intermittent porphyria, a misnomer in view of the fact that the characteristic

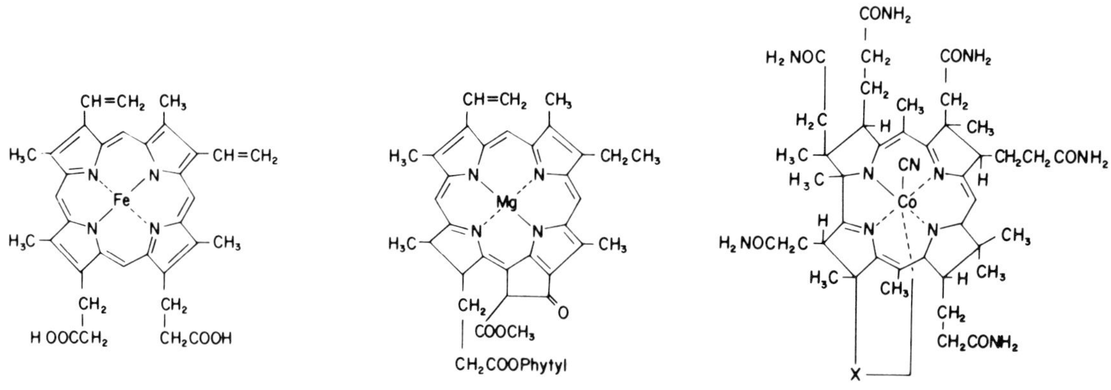

Ferriprotoporphyrin IX (heme) — Chlorophyll a — Vitamin B_{12}

Figure 15.1. Biologically important metalloporphyrins.

abnormality is increased excretion of a pyrrole, not a porphyrin. Nonetheless, the designation is widely accepted and serves to group this disease correctly with the closely related 'true' porphyrias.

In addition to the above forms of porphyria, types were described which were discrete in some respects but to an extent appeared to overlap with those previously described. This situation led to some confusion in the classification and nomenclature of the porphyrias. However, important developments over the past 30 years have provided a secure basis for delineating most, if not all, of these diseases. These include elucidation of the pathway of haem biosynthesis, studies of the regulation of haem biosynthesis and measurement of the enzymes catalysing specific steps in the pathway of haem synthesis. Model systems – particularly animals with congenital or chemically-induced porphyria – have provided much of the insight in these areas. Such work has been reviewed recently and will not be described in detail here.[57,81] However, a summary of current concepts will be given below, inasmuch as an understanding of haem biosynthesis and its regulation is essential to a coherent view of the porphyrias.

HAEM BIOSYNTHESIS

Formation of δ-Aminolaevulinic Acid (ALA)

As shown in Figure 15.2, glycine and succinic acid provide the constituent carbons for haem. One mol glycine and one mol succinyl CoA, derived from the tricarboxylic acid cycle, combine in the presence of pyridoxal phosphate to form ALA. The reaction is catalysed by the mitochondrial enzyme, ALA synthetase, and the product, ALA, is considered to be the first compound of the pathway committed to haem synthesis although its metabolism by minor alternate routes occurs.[57] The reaction is rate-limiting for the formation of haem in the liver and possibly in other tissues; therefore, ALA synthetase plays a key role in regulating the pathway, as will be discussed below.

Formation of Porphobilinogen

Porphobilinogen, the pyrrole subunit of the porphyrin ring, is formed by condensation of 2 mol ALA, with elimination of water, in a reaction catalysed by the cytosolic enzyme, porphobilinogen synthetase (ALA dehydrase). The enzyme appears to contain sulphydryl groups, is activated in vitro by sulphydryl-reducing agents and is particularly sensitive to inhibition by lead. A requirement for zinc also has been suggested by recent studies.[33]

Examination of rates of product formation in vitro by ALA synthetase and porphobilinogen synthetase suggests that the latter enzyme is present in relative abundance and therefore is unlikely to be involved significantly in regulation of the rate of haem synthesis. Both ALA and porphobilinogen are soluble in aqueous solution at physiological pH, are colourless and non-fluorescent and, therefore, impart no unusual hue to urine.

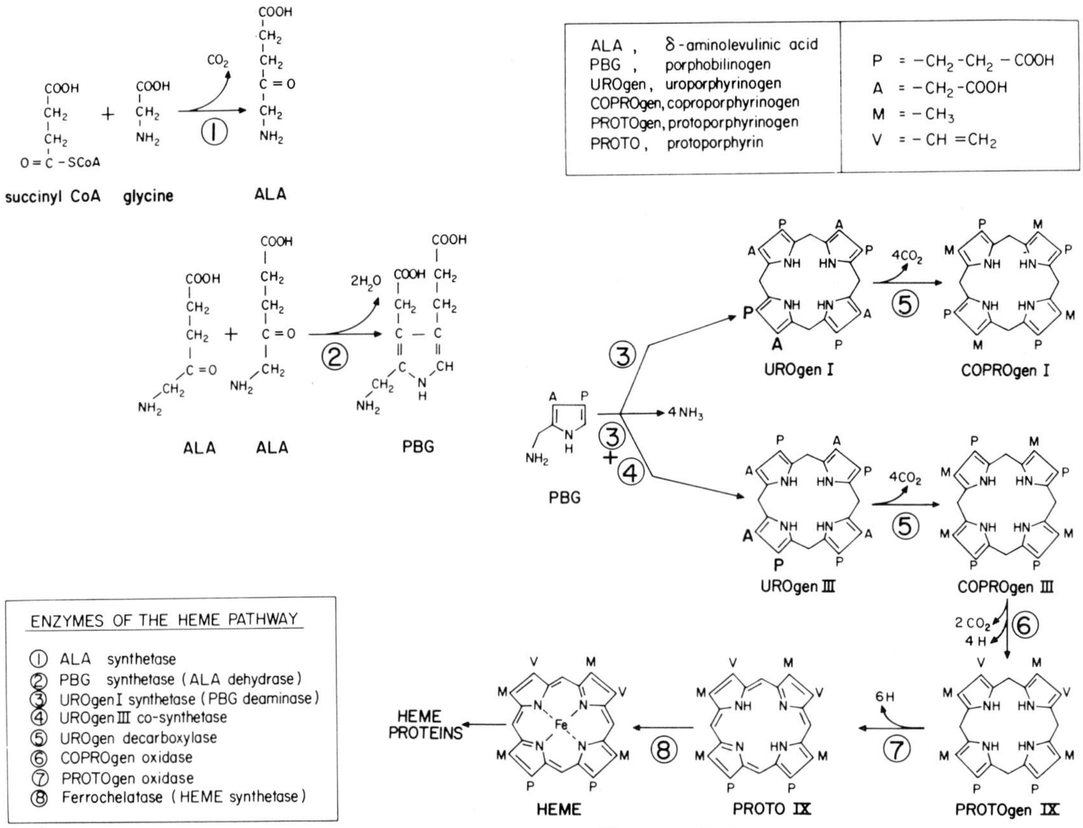

Figure 15.2. The pathway of haem synthesis.

Formation of Uroporphyrinogen

Condensation of 4 mol porphobilinogen and ring closure yields the first porphyrin-like compound of the haem pathway, uroporphyrinogen. As depicted in Figure 15.3, the true intermediates in haem synthesis (up to protoporphyrin) are *porphyrinogens*, reduced porphyrins containing six additional hydrogen atoms. They are colourless, non-fluorescent compounds which are readily converted in the presence of light and air to the corresponding porphyrin by an irreversible oxidation (Figure 15.3). The resulting porphyrins, with the exception of protoporphyrin, cannot be reincorporated into the pathway and undergo elimination from the organism. A feature of porphobilinogen with important biological consequences is its asymmetry, conferred by two different side chains, one an acetic and the other a propionic group (Figure 15.2). Because of the asymmetry, condensation of 4 mol porphobilinogen in theory may yield four possible isomeric forms: a regular (head-to-tail) arrangement, with strictly alternating acetic and propionic acid groups (type I), an arrangement in which two opposite pyrrole substituents are reversed (type II), a single pyrrole is reversed (type III) or two adjacent pyrroles are reversed (type IV). Of these, only types I and III are found in nature (Figure 15.2), and only the isomer III series serve as intermediates in haem synthesis.

This striking isomeric specificity for uroporphyrinogen is achieved in a reaction of intriguing complexity. The principal enzyme of the reaction is uroporphyrinogen-I synthetase, which, as its name implies, catalyses the conversion of 4 mol porphobilinogen to uroporphyrinogen I. Formation of the physiologically 'correct' uroporphyrinogen III requires, in addition to this enzyme, a second protein known as uroporphyrinogen-III cosynthetase. Although by itself inactive in mediating porphyrin formation, the cosynthetase acts in concert with uroporphyrinogen-I synthetase to form the III isomer. Recent studies suggest that the two proteins act as a complex (rather than sequentially), directing formation of either the I or III isomer from the start of the reaction, and that free intermediates do not occur. The precise manner in which the cosynthetase catalyses a 'reversal' (head-to-head condensation) of one of the pyrrole units is a subject of current investigation in several laboratories.[3, 34, 35]

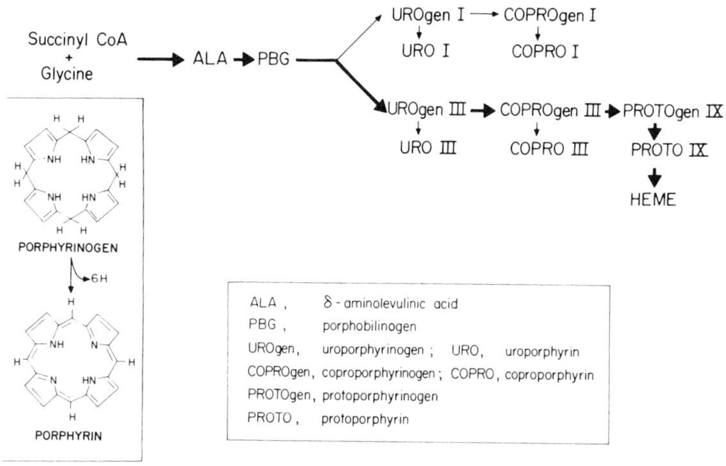

Figure 15.3. The relationship of porphyrinogens and porphyrins to the haem synthetic pathway.

Separation and assay of the synthetase and cosynthetase in vitro suggest that in normal liver the latter activity is present in relative excess. This may ensure that porphobilinogen is carried through to uroporphyrinogen III, with minimal formation of the biologically useless I-isomer series.

Formation of Coproporphyrinogen

Uroporphyrinogen is converted to coproporphyrinogen by sequential decarboxylation of the four acetyl side chains of the molecule. Intermediate porphyrins containing seven, six or five carboxyl groups are found in small amounts in normal urine. Present evidence suggests that a single enzyme, uroporphyrinogen decarboxylase, mediates all four decarboxylations of both the isomer-III and -I compounds.[43]

Formation of Protoporphyrinogen

Conversion of coproporphyrinogen-III to protoporphyrinogen IX (coproporphyrinogen I is not further metabolized) involves decarboxylation and dehydrogenation of two of the propionic side chains on adjacent pyrrole units, yielding vinyl groups. The latter modification, mediated by coproporphyrinogen oxidase, confers additional asymmetry on the molecule. The number of possible isomers increases to 15, and these were arbitrarily designated as I to XV by Fischer, without regard to the biosynthetic precursors of specific isomers. Isomer IX of protoporphyrinogen belongs to the III series of uro- and coproporphyrin and is the only naturally occurring isomer of protoporphyrinogen.

Formation of Haem

Finally, protoporphyrinogen is oxidized to protoporphyrin and iron is inserted to form ferriprotoporphyrin IX, or haem. The oxidation of protoporphyrinogen was believed formerly to be non-enzymatic, because this occurs readily in vitro in the presence of air. However, in the reducing atmosphere of cells, spontaneous oxidation may be prevented, and recent studies suggest that the process is enzymatically mediated.[64] The insertion of iron is catalysed by a mitochondrial enzyme activity termed ferrochelatase. Although this process can also occur non-enzymatically in vitro, the evidence for an enzymatically mediated catalysis under physiological conditions is convincing.[19]

SUBCELLULAR AND EXTRACELLULAR TRANSPORT OF HAEM AND HAEM PRECURSORS

The pathway of haem synthesis takes in both the mitochondrial and cytosolic portions of the cell, and the final product, haem, undergoes distribution to multiple subcellular compartments and, at least in the case of hepatic parenchymal cells, transport out of the cell. The initial enzyme of the pathway, ALA synthetase, is formed on the rough endoplasmic reticulum, subsequently passing to mitochondria where it catalyses the formation of ALA. Thus, potential points of regulation of this key enzyme exist at the level of transcription of specific messenger RNA, translation on the rough endoplasmic reticulum, post-translocational modification, its transport into mitochondria, and direct negative feedback of its activity in mitochondria. With formation of ALA, the haem pathway leaves the mitochondrion as the next three enzymes – porphobilinogen synthetase, uroporphyrinogen synthetase-cosynthetase and uroporphyrinogen decarboxylase – are located in the extra-mitochondrial cytosol. The product of the latter reaction, coproporphyrinogen, re-enters the mitochondrion where coproporphyrinogen oxidase, protoporphyrinogen oxidase and ferrochelatase catalyse the formation of haem.

A substantial portion of newly synthesized haem passes from the mitochondrion to combine with protein acceptors on the endoplasmic reticulum. Presumably, haem proteins in other sites (microbodies or cytosol) similarly draw on mitochondrial haem. In addition, haem may undergo transfer out of the cell, either into plasma or directly into bile.[9]

An unsolved, and largely unexplored, problem in haem metabolism concerns the manner in which constituents and intermediates of the pathway are translocated within the cell. The presence of haem-carrying proteins in liver cytosol has been postulated;[40] specific transport mechanisms for haem precursors similarly may reasonably be inferred although these lack direct confirmation. Their significance lies in the fact that they represent potential points of regulation of haem synthesis in addition to the specific enzymes of the pathway.

In plasma, ALA and porphobilinogen appear to be only loosely associated with protein, so that they undergo efficient elimination by the kidneys. Haem is transported on albumin or on the beta-glycoprotein, haemopexin.[59] In most species, the affinity of haem for haemopexin is measurably greater than for albumin, although in plasma albumin is present in 30 to 40 fold greater concentration than is haemopexin and therefore may be quantitatively the more important carrier. Porphyrins are associated with the same serum proteins but with less affinity than is haem. Whether the association between these proteins and haem or porphyrins serves a specific function in the metabolism of the compounds is not known.

PHYSIOLOGICAL EFFECTS OF HAEM PRECURSORS

Although haem synthesis is highly efficient, small amounts of intermediates escape the pathway and enter the circulation. In porphyria, these amounts are substantially increased. Their distribution in body tissues or excreta (hence their detection) reflects to a large extent their physical properties. In general, the intermediates of haem synthesis, viewed in their biosynthetic sequence, comprise increasingly lipophilic compounds. Up to and including uroporphyrin, the intermediates of the pathway contain sufficient ionizable groups to be relatively water soluble at physiological pH, be filtered by renal glomeruli and appear in urine. The decarboxylation of uroporphyrinogen, however, and formation of subsequent intermediates involve progressive removal of ionizable groups, with a parallel increase in lipophilicity. As a result, coproporphyrin is excreted preferentially into bile, and hence appears in faeces, although substantial amounts appear also in urine. Protoporphyrin is excreted solely by the faecal route.

Porphyrins are red-purple in colour and are fluorescent, in contrast to ALA and porphobilinogen which are colourless and non-fluorescent. The fluorescence reflects the fact that porphyrins undergo excitation by light, the effect being maximal with light of wavelength of about 400 nm, which corresponds to the absorption maximum for porphyrins. Relaxation of 'excited-state' porphyrins back to ground state occurs spontaneously. The released energy appears in vitro as a fluorescent emission with a peak intensity at about 600 nm (the precise wavelength varies for the different porphyrins and can be used for their quantification). Porphyrins exposed to light in vivo (in skin or epidermal capillaries) undergo a similar excitation; in vivo, however, relaxation of the molecule gives rise to active intermediates (possibly singlet oxygen) which cause pathological change in contiguous tissues, e.g., erythrocytes or capillary endothelial cells. The nature of the light-induced damage varies with the type of porphyrin, probably because of differences in the subcutaneous distribution of uro-, copro- or protoporphyrin. Accordingly, the clinical manifestations of photosensitivity differ among the various porphyrias but include urticaria, oedema, bullae or ulceration and may include haemolysis.[76] By contrast, those porphyrias associated with over-production of only ALA or porphobilinogen exhibit no photosensitivity.

REGULATION OF HEPATIC HAEM SYNTHESIS

Role of ALA Synthetase

Studies in animals and in cell culture have established that in normal liver the rate-determining step in haem synthesis is the formation of ALA which directly reflects the activity of the enzyme, ALA synthetase, catalysing this reaction. Numerous findings point also to the fact that ALA synthetase is subject to regulation by haem, thereby establishing a homeostatic mechanism for adjusting the level of haem synthesis to the needs of the organism. Based on cogent, albeit circumstantial, evidence, a haem 'pool' serving this regulatory function has been postulated, as indicated in Figure 15.4. This pool appears to consist of haem-in-transit and is fed by endogenous synthesis as well as being in equilibrium with cytochrome-associated haem.[72] In addition, exogenously administered haem, in part, may enter the pool, effecting a reduction in the activity of ALA synthetase, as shown in experimental animals given haem intraperitoneally or intravenously.[52] Conversely, a manipulation that results in withdrawal of haem from the regulatory pool, e.g., new synthesis of apocytochrome, results in stimulation of ALA synthetase activity. Administration of barbiturate to experimental animals constitutes a model for the latter sequence of events. Recent studies have provided evidence that the initial event after administration of phenobarbital to rats is formation of apocytochrome P-450 followed by stimulation of the haem synthetic pathway.[21,65]

In addition to serving the biosynthesis of tissue haem proteins, haem in the regulatory pool presumably also undergoes degradation to bile pigment. Haem degradation involves irreversible oxidative cleavage of the porphyrin ring, and the alpha-methene bridge carbon is released as CO (Figure 15.4). In liver, the process appears to be mediated by a microsomal enzyme, haem oxygenase, which is present in the parenchymal cell fraction of the liver as well as in sinusoidal lining cells.[8] After administration of a haem load to experimental animals, hepatic haem oxygenase activity increases, apparently serving to eliminate excess intracellular haem.[80] It is not known whether haem oxygenase may be stimulated in the absence of an increased haem load and thereby deplete intracellular hepatic haem. Although the activity increases after administration of a variety of non-haem substances, this response may reflect shifts in intracellular haem and presentation of an 'endogenous' haem load to the enzyme.[6] Experimental porphyria in rats is associated with subnormal activity of hepatic haem oxygenase.[67]

The precise way in which haem alters the activity of ALA synthetase is uncertain. Evidence has been obtained for a decrease in enzyme synthesis (haem acting as a co-repressor), direct (feedback) inhibition of the enzyme itself or post-transitional interaction of haem and ALA synthetase, which prevents transfer of the enzyme from cytosol to mitochondria. Any one or a combination of these mechanisms could be operative in vivo.[36]

Role of Cytochrome P-450

All tissues, other than erythrocytes, exhibit aerobic metabolism and therefore require mitochondrial cytochromes. Presumably all such cells synthesize haem to meet the need for cytochrome formation. Requirements for haem synthesis vary widely among individual tissues, reflecting the type of haem protein present in a tissue, its concentration and its half-life. Haem formation in bone marrow is active because of the relatively large amounts required for haemoglobin synthesis, although the turnover of haemoglobin is slow (the red cell life span in humans is 120 days; in the rat, 57 days). In the liver, 50 per cent of newly synthesized haem is utilized in the formation of cytochrome P-450. Although the amount of cytochrome P-450 in liver is only a very small fraction of the haemoglobin in the organism, the half-life of cytochrome P-450 is short (in the rat its decay is biphasic, with an average half-life of about 16 hours). The haem requirement for hepatic cytochrome P-450 in the rat can be estimated at approximately 10 per cent of that for haemoglobin. Therefore, synthesis of cytochrome P-450

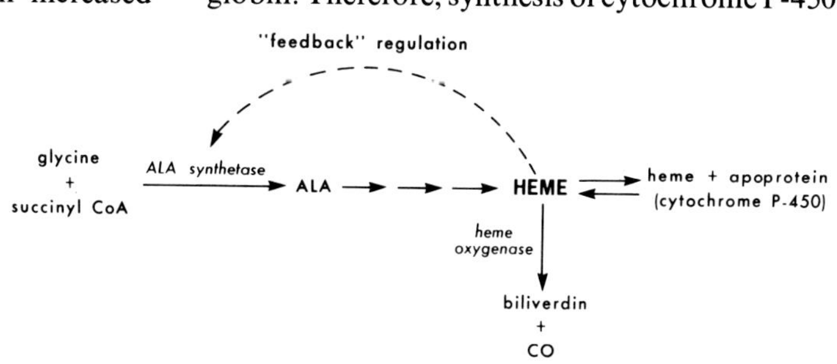

Figure 15.4. A postulated model for end-product regulation of haem synthesis in the liver. From Bissell and Hammaker,[7] with kind permission of the authors and Academic Press, Inc.

appears to account for the high rate of haem synthesis in the liver, and changes in the production of cytochrome P-450 would be expected to exert major changes in the rate of hepatic haem synthesis. The liver contains a number of haem proteins, in addition to cytochrome P-450, which collectively undoubtedly affect the rate of haem synthesis. Individually, however, none of these is comparable either in concentration or rate of turnover to cytochrome P-450.

An important characteristic of cytochrome P-450 is its inducibility by a substrate (administered drug or lipophilic endogenous substances such as gonadal steroids). Ultimately, induction brings about accelerated removal (and/or inactivation) of the substrate from the organism. This response requires new synthesis of cytochrome P-450, a process which in turn requires increased haem synthesis. Normal liver meets this demand with increased activity of ALA synthetase and new production of haem precursors. In porphyric individuals, the flow of precursors may be partially blocked (a complete block presumably would be lethal) by a defective or deficient enzyme, thus limiting the capacity for increasing haem synthesis. In such an individual, depletion of the haem pool may occur, so that ALA synthetase is derepressed and the defective enzymatic step becomes rate-determining for haem synthesis. Under these conditions, the intermediates prior to the block accumulate, spilling over into the circulation and appearing in urine or faeces. This type of porphyria may be regarded as a *haem-deficient* condition; characteristically, it is exacerbated by the administration of inducers of cytochrome P-450 (of which barbiturates are the archetype). The haem-deficient porphyrias may be contrasted with porphyrias with a normal capacity for haem synthesis which are unaffected by inducers of cytochrome P-450: these may be termed *haem-compensated*. This distinction is important in the diagnosis and management of the various porphyrias.

CLASSIFICATION OF THE PORPHYRIAS

The porphyrias may be classified according to pathogenesis (hereditary or acquired) and to tissue localization (bone marrow or liver) (Table 15.1). With regard to the latter, presumably all cells in the body synthesize haem, as noted above, and thus all potentially may be affected by a genetic defect in the haem pathway. However, because the liver and marrow are the major sites of haem synthesis, they are also the most important sources of porphyrin. The possibility remains that the porphyric state has important consequences in tissues not contributing quantitatively to the overproduction of porphyrins or porphyrin precursors. Indeed, neural dysfunction is prominent in acute intermittent porphyria and may be an expression of the genetic defect in this tissue (see below). A phenomenon that remains unexplained is why porphyria involves predominantly either bone marrow or liver but not both.

The specific enzyme defect associated with each porphyria is listed in Table 15.1. In the case of the hepatic porphyrias, the position of the defect in the haem pathway is shown in Figure 15.5, as well as the individual pattern of excretion of precursors associated with each type. Of the three porphyrias that comprise the haem-deficient group (Table 15.1), the pattern of precursor excretion provides the principal means for their differentiation, their main clinical features being essentially identical, as will be discussed.

ERYTHROPOIETIC PORPHYRIA

Extensive discussion of erythropoietic porphyria is beyond the scope of this chapter; the reader is referred to a recent detailed review.[57] In brief, *congenital erythropoietic porphyria* is a rare, recessively inherited disease, with less than 100 cases in the world literature. Affected individuals display markedly porphyric urine (mainly uroporphyrin I) from infancy and usually are severely photosensitive from an early age. Haemolytic anaemia and disfiguring cutaneous changes (hypertrichosis and scar formation) are common. The neurological symptoms of the haem-deficient hepatic porphyrias (see below) do not occur in this condition.

ERYTHROHEPATIC PROTOPORPHYRIA

Erythrohepatic protoporphyria is a relatively common disorder, characterized by a variable

Table 15.1. *Classification of the Porphyrias.*

	Synonym	Inheritance	Enzyme defect	Haem status
Hereditary erythropoietic				
Congenital	Günther's disease	Recessive	Uroporphyrinogen-III cosynthetase or Uroporphyrinogen-I synthetase	Compensated (?)
Hereditary erythrohepatic				
Protoporphyria	Erythropoietic protoporphyria	Dominant	Ferrochelatase	Compensated
Hereditary hepatic				
Acute intermittent	Swedish porphyria Pyrroloporphyria	Dominant	Uroporphyrinogen-I synthetase	Deficient
Coproporphyria		Dominant	Coproporphyrinogen oxidase	Deficient
Variegate	South African porphyria	Dominant	Undetermined (Protoporphyrinogen oxidase?)	Deficient
Cutanea tarda	Symptomatic porphyria	Dominant	Uroporphyrinogen decarboxylase	Compensated
Acquired				
Intoxications (heavy metals, hexachlorobenzene, etc.)		–	Variable	Variable
Nutritional deficiencies (iron, pyridoxine)		–	Variable	Variable
Liver disease		–	Variable	Variable

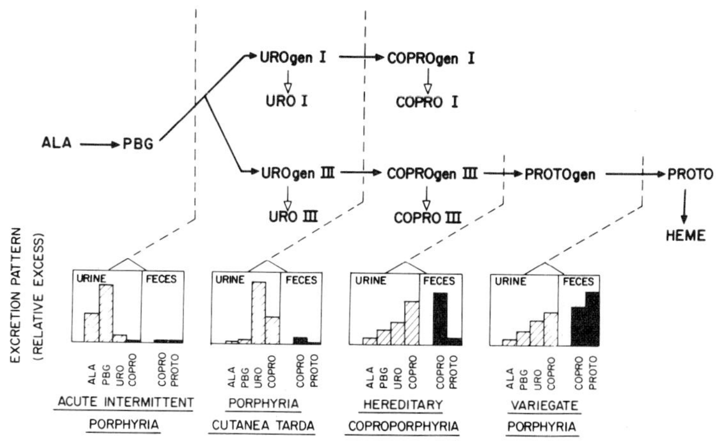

Figure 15.5. Patterns of precursor excretion in the hereditary hepatic porphyrias. The vertical dashed line for each type of porphyria indicates the point in the haem pathway at which defective enzymatic activity has been identified or is presumed to exist (see also Table 15.1). The abbreviations used are the same as in Figure 15.3.

(usually mild) cutaneous photosensitivity. Patients exhibit moderately to markedly elevated plasma and faecal protoporphyrin, with a lesser increase in coproporphyrin. The cutaneous reaction consists acutely of oedema (solar urticaria) which may progress to chronic eczema after repeated light-induced injury.[49] Betacarotene is effective in increasing tolerance to sunlight, apparently by blocking the active intermediate (singlet oxygen?) in porphyrin-induced tissue damage[76] and, apart from the rare patients in whom hepatic complications develop, the prognosis of the disease is good. Recent studies of bone marrow[17] and cultured skin fibroblasts[15] indicate that ferrochelatase activity is strikingly decreased in persons with this disorder.

The relative contribution of erythroid tissue and liver to the overproduction of protoporphyrin apparently varies among individual patients. In some studies, leakage of protoporphyrin from erythrocytes appears to be entirely responsible for the excess excretion of porphyrin,[63] while other studies document a significant contribution by the liver.[74] Whether these divergent findings reflect an underlying heterogeneity of this type of porphyria or only variation in its biochemical expression is unclear at the present time.

While it is typically only a dermatological disorder, hepatic deposition of protoporphyrin has been documented in many patients with this disease; protoporphyrin-containing gallstones also occur.[11] A few individuals with strikingly elevated blood porphyrin concentrations present with jaundice, which initially may occur in the absence of other manifestations of hepatic disease but leads relatively rapidly to portal hypertension, hepatic failure and death. Liver biopsy demonstrates massive deposition of protoporphyrin in bile canaliculi, hepatocytes and sinusoidal cells, as well as inflammatory exudate and fibrosis. The seriousness of this complication suggests that persons with symptomatic protoporphyria – particularly those with circulating porphyrin in excess of 1000 μg/dl red cells – should be observed closely and subjected to liver biopsy if signs of hepatic dysfunction are present.[10] Bromsulphthalein retention is the most sensitive test of liver function in this setting, and liver biopsy may reveal histological changes of unexpected severity. Preliminary reports suggest that cholestyramine therapy is associated with reduction of hepatic protoporphyrin and amelioration of pathological changes in the liver.[22,41]

HEPATIC PORPHYRIAS WITH HAEM DEFICIENCY: ACUTE INTERMITTENT PORPHYRIA, HEREDITARY COPROPORPHYRIA AND VARIEGATE PORPHYRIA

Although these porphyrias are distinct genetic entities, they will be described as a group because they are indistinguishable in terms of their main clinical features. Each involves an enzyme defect that results in a potential – or actual – deficiency of hepatic haem synthesis, which may account for their many clinical characteristics in common. These porphyrias differ primarily with regard to their respective patterns of haem precursor excretion, which are of importance for screening of carriers and account also for the presence of cutaneous symptoms in hereditary coproporphyria and variegate porphyria.

Clinical Presentation

Acute attacks are accompanied by the manifestations listed in Table 15.2. Abdominal pain, often colicky and severe, is a frequent symptom and mimics acute inflammation of a hollow viscus. Many patients complain of severe constipation for a considerable period of time, beginning in some cases in puberty.

Table 15.2. *Clinical Presentation of Acute Attacks of Haem-deficient Porphyria.*

Percentage of patients presenting with symptom or sign			
Symptoms		Physical findings	
Abdominal pain	90	Tachycardia	83
Vomiting	80	Hypertension	55
Constipation	80	Motor neuropathy	53
Pain in limbs	51	Pyrexia	38
Pain in back	50	Leucocytosis (12 000)	20
Confused state	32	Bulbar involvement	18
Urinary frequency	30	Sensory loss	15
Dysuria	28	Cranial nerve involvement	9
Abnormal behaviour	23	Proteinuria	8
Seizures	12	Hepatomegaly	5
Diarrhoea	8		
Stupor	7		
Coma	6		

The data are taken from Eales,[27] a study of 80 patients with variegate porphyria. The presentation of acute intermittent porphyria[77,83] and of hereditary coproporphyria[18] is entirely similar.

Nausea and vomiting are frequent. Neurological symptoms are protean, ranging from headache and psychiatric disturbances to paraesthesias and paralysis. A family history may elicit information concerning relatives who succumbed to an obscure 'neurological' disease that, in retrospect, was probably porphyria.

Physical examination may reveal abdominal tenderness and diminished bowel sounds, although the findings are characteristically less impressive than the symptoms; rebound tenderness is distinctly unusual. Attacks are accompanied almost invariably by sinus tachycardia, which parallels disease activity in many patients. Approximately one-third of patients present with altered mental status and a minor proportion of these with seizures. Motor and sensory neurological abnormalities may develop rapidly during the early phase of an attack. These begin with distal motor deficits, progressing in severe cases to quadriplegia and respiratory failure. Death is usually due to respiratory failure and the complications associated with its management.

Laboratory studies may be useful in differentiating acute porphyric attacks from other intra-abdominal crises (Table 15.3). The total leucocyte count is usually within normal limits and, even when elevated, the differential cell count is normal. An abdominal radiograph may reveal distended bowel loops. Liver function studies are typically within normal limits, except for transient increases in bromsulphthalein retention.[77] Dark urine, when it is present, should suggest the diagnosis (see below:

Table 15.3. *Normal Values for the Laboratory Determination of Porphyrins and Porphyrin Precursors.*

	Urine 24 h	Faeces dry wt	Erythrocytes
ALA	<57 μmol (<7.5 mg)	–	–
Porphobilinogen	<9 μmol (<2.0 mg)	–	–
Uroporphyrin	12–60 nmol (0.01–0.05 mg)	trace	–
Coproporphyrin	76–382 nmol (0.05–0.25 mg)	<76 nmol/g (<50 μg/g)	<23 nmol/l (<1.5 μg/dl)
Protoporphyrin	–	<215 nmol/g (<120 μg/g)	<1.3 μmol/l (<75 μg/dl)

The ranges for δ-aminolaevulinic acid and porphobilinogen are those for the procedure of Davis and Andelman,[23] which is available in kit form (Bio-Rad Laboratories, Richmond, California). The measurement includes both ALA and aminoacetone, the latter normally being present in only small amounts.[53] Porphyrin analyses were carried out according to Schwartz et al[75]; the normal ranges are those utilized by the author and are similar to those of Meyer and Schmid[57] and Elder, Gray and Nicholson.[30]

'Differentiation of the haem-deficient porphyrias'). Hyponatraemia may also occur, possibly due to inappropriate secretion of antidiuretic hormone; it may develop rapidly in patients receiving large volumes of dextrose-in-water as part of their therapy and be responsible for acute mental changes unrelated to porphyria per se. Total serum thyroxine is elevated in many patients, and this, with other manifestations, suggests a hyperthyroid state. However, the increase reflects elevation only of thyroid-binding globulin and other parameters of thyroid function are normal; this appears to occur more often in females than in males with porphyria.[77]

Pathogenesis

The enzyme defects in acute intermittent porphyria, hereditary coproporphyria and variegate porphyria (Table 15.1)

The defect in acute intermittent porphyria has been studied in several laboratories and consists of a 50 per cent reduction in uroporphyrinogen-I synthetase activity.[78] In hereditary coproporphyria (Figure 15.5), relatively few individuals have been studied, in part because coproporphyrinogen oxidase is mitochondrial and therefore requires blood leucocytes or skin fibroblasts for its assay. In these cells, decreases of 50 per cent or more in enzyme activity have been recorded in affected individuals.[31] Comparable information in variegate porphyria is lacking although a defect in the conversion of protoporphyrinogen to haem can be postulated from the precursor excretion pattern typical of the disease (Figure 15.5).

The net result of any one of these defects is to limit the capacity for haem synthesis. This may be inferred from the fact that all three conditions exhibit stimulation of ALA synthetase activity (presumably secondary to derepression of the enzyme) and all are markedly sensitive to agents that increase the need for haem synthesis (i.e., inducers of hepatic cytochrome P-450).

Drug sensitivity

In known carriers of these defects the biochemical manifestations of disease vary from minimal to marked, undoubtedly reflecting the importance of secondary factors in the clinical disease. A fixed capacity for haem synthesis will be of little consequence if the demand for haem remains within that capacity. Many patients with porphyria, in fact, appear to enjoy a haem-compensated state, are asymptomatic and exhibit minimally increased excretion of haem precursors. However, an endogenous or exogenous challenge to the haem synthetic system may rapidly induce a haem-deficient state. Many acute attacks follow the unwitting administration of drug inducers of cytochrome P-450. 'Spontaneous' attacks occur also (more frequently, it appears, in acute intermittent porphyria than in the other two), reflecting the importance of endogenous factors. Acute attacks are more frequent in women than in men, and first attacks are rare before puberty. Pregnancy may exacerbate the condition in some women, and cyclical attacks associated with menstruation have been described.[88] These findings emphasize the importance of hormonal changes in the pathogenesis of acute attacks, possibly related to the fact that gonadal steroids are metabolized in part by cytochrome P-450 and may stimulate endogenously the rate of hepatic haem synthesis. Exogenous progesterone induces cytochrome P-450 in experimental animals, and exogenous hormones (oral contraceptives) have provoked acute attacks in some porphyrics.

Neurological dysfunction

Most, if not all, of the symptoms and findings of acute attacks suggest neurological dysfunction, including abdominal pain, which may result from a neurogenic motility disorder of the bowel. Hyperactivity of the sympathetic nervous system may account for tachycardia and constipation which are seen frequently. Increased excretion of catecholamines has been documented in persons during attacks of acute intermittent porphyria, as have abnormalities in the uptake of norepinephrine (noradrenaline) by platelets from individuals with this disorder.[4] The aetiology of neurological dysfunction in these types of porphyria remains a major unresolved problem. To date, attention has centred on ways in which elevated circulating levels of porphyrins or porphyrin precursors might affect the nervous system. While the haem-deficient porphyrias differ with respect to the pattern of precursor over-production, they exhibit in common excess excretion of ALA and porphobilinogen, and these compounds characteristically undergo striking increases during acute attacks in all three types of porphyria. In addition, in two diseases unrelated to porphyria – heavy metal intoxication and hereditary tyrosinaemia – acute abdominal manifestations occur in association with increased urinary excretion of ALA and are similar to those in porphyrics.[47] Furthermore, 'neurological' symptoms are absent in those porphyrias involving over-production of porphyrins but not ALA or porphobilinogen, i.e., the haem-compensated porphyrias (Table 15.1). While these findings suggest that increased plasma ALA may alter neural function, correlation between the plasma level of ALA or porphobilinogen and the severity of symptoms is poor. Moreover, attempts to demonstrate direct toxicity of ALA to neural tissues, either in vivo or in vitro, have produced results that are either negative or inconclusive, despite the use of pharmacological concentrations of ALA. An alternative possibility is that neurological dysfunction reflects intrinsic haem deficiency at the cellular level, either because cells of the nervous system, like the liver, are sensitive to inducers of cytochrome P-450 or because they require exogenous haem. The latter might normally be supplied by the liver (see above, 'Subcellular and extracellular transport of haem and haem precursors') but decrease during an acute attack associated with intrahepatic haem depletion (see below). The recently demonstrated efficacy of haem administration in acute attacks is consistent with either hypothesis, since the administered haem may supply the nervous system directly, or it may inhibit hepatic ALA synthetase, thereby reducing over-production and circulating concentrations of ALA and porphobilinogen.

Diagnosis

Acute porphyric attacks

An initial attack of porphyria in which 'classic' manifestations readily suggest the diagnosis is a rare event. Commonly, only a part of the symptom complex is present, and many patients suffer intermittent and sub-acute attacks of pain, in which symptoms may be unaccompanied by abnormal physical findings. Such patients are often told that their complaints are psychosomatic; the less fortunate are those deemed to have a surgically correctable abdominal process. While the diagnosis may be suggested by history and physical examination, definitive evaluation virtually always requires appropriate laboratory investigation. Decisions as to the laboratory tests to be ordered depend on the type of porphyria under consideration, since the principal precursor excess (as well as its route of excretion) differs among the three haem-deficient porphyrias (Figure 15.5). Elevation of urinary porphobilinogen is characteristic of acute intermittent porphyria, faecal coproporphyrin of hereditary coproporphyria and faecal protoporphyrin of variegate porphyria. During an acute attack of any of the three, urinary porphobilinogen will be elevated, and this can be assessed qualitatively by means of the Watson–Schwartz test in which porphobilinogen forms a pink complex with Ehrlich's reagent.[84] The test is positive in virtually all patients suffering acute attacks, although its sensitivity is insufficient for screening carriers. It is also specific, when performed properly. In this regard, it should be emphasized that extraction of the pink complex with chloroform or butanol is essential to a correct interpretation of the colour reaction. The porphobilinogen complex will remain in the aqueous phase after extraction with organic solvents, whereas a number of other substances in urine (notably, urobilinogen, indoles and Pyridium), which also yield a red reaction with Ehrlich's reagent, are extractable with organic solvents. Other causes of false-positive tests have been noted but are relatively infrequent.[30] A modification of the

Ehrlich's procedure (the Hoesch test) has recently been re-evaluated.[46] It eliminates the necessity for extraction of the pink reaction product and may prove superior to the Watson–Schwartz test in its ease of handling.

Tests for the carrier state

In screening for carriers of acute intermittent porphyria, urinary porphobilinogen is measured by a column chromatographic procedure originally introduced by Mauzerall and Granick.[55] The column method is both quantitative and, with few exceptions, specific. Urine from persons taking large amounts of phenothiazines may contain chromogens which are eluted from the column together with porphobilinogen and interfere with the analysis.[66] The sensitivity of the column procedure permits measurement of urinary porphobilinogen in normal individuals. Porphobilinogen excretion exceeds the normal range in at least 80 per cent of persons with acute intermittent porphyria, regardless of the presence or absence of symptoms of the disease. In a small proportion of affected individuals, and in most prepubertal carriers, the urinary findings are normal. For this reason, negative results based on urine analysis alone carry a definite measure of uncertainty. In acute intermittent porphyria, this difficulty can be circumvented by assay of the hereditary enzyme defect, decreased activity of uroporphyrinogen-I synthetase. The enzyme, being cytosolic, is present in mature erythrocytes and therefore may be measured in red cell haemolysates. The genetically determined decrease in activity is expressed regardless of age or clinical state of the individual. The original assay method has undergone recent modifications,[58] and the determination is suitable for routine clinical use.[50, 60] Cultured skin fibroblasts and amniotic cells from affected individuals also display diminished activity of uroporphyrinogen-I synthetase.[16, 56, 70] While porphyric individuals exhibit, on the average, 50 per cent of normal activity, occasional determinations with erythrocytes from affected individuals fall into the low-normal range. In persons with a reticulocytosis, enzyme activity may be elevated. The activity is highest in young red cells and progressively declines as erythrocytes age in the circulation. In other instances, relatively high enzyme activity in porphyrics may be genetically determined, and unaffected family members display approximately twice the activity of porphyric members.[68]

Deficient activity of coproporphyrinogen oxidase in hereditary coproporphyria has been documented.[18, 31] The assay is relatively demanding and at the present time is a research procedure only. However, elevated faecal coproporphyrin excretion appears to be a constant finding in all affected individuals, so that estimation of coproporphyrinogen oxidase activity may be unnecessary as a screening procedure. In variegate porphyria, the enzyme defect remains to be determined. Measurement of faecal protoporphyrin is the appropriate test for carriers.

Management

Prevention of attacks

In the management of the haem-deficient porphyrias, prevention of attacks is of paramount importance. This requires screening of families with a known case and education of affected family members as to circumstances that may precipitate acute attacks. Information concerning hazardous drugs should be provided, and Table 15.4 lists compounds that have been implicated in acute attacks of porphyria. Barbiturates are the most frequent offenders, reflecting in part their widespread use. Also in Table 15.4 is a short list of agents that have been administered without ill effects

Table 15.4. *Drug Usage in Persons with Haem-deficient Porphyria (Acute Intermittent Porphyria, Hereditary Coproporphyria, Variegate Porphyria).*[a]

May precipitate acute attacks[b]	Believed to be safe
Barbiturates	Aspirin
Griseofulvin	Bromides
Sulphonamides	Chlorpromazine
Glutethimide	Chloral hydrate
Hydantoins	Corticosteroids
Meprobamate	Diazepam
Oestrogens	Dicoumarol
Ergot preparations	Digoxin
Methyldopa	Diphenhydramine
Chloroquine	Ether
Chlorpropamide	Guanethidine
Chlordiazepoxide	Meperidine
Tolbutamide	Morphine
Ethanol	Neostigmine
Halothane	Nitrous oxide
Chloramphenicol	Penicillins
Pyrazinamide	Propranolol
	Tetracyclines

[a] The data are taken, in part, from Wetterberg.[86]
[b] Listed in decreasing order of importance as precipitants of acute attacks.

to persons with haem-deficient porphyria. Although these should not provoke acute attacks, porphyrics may be unusually sensitive to 'usual' doses. For example, propranolol appears to be efficacious in some patients, alleviating tachycardia and hypertension[5] but even in small doses may cause profound hypotension in others.[13] Also, hepatic metabolism of drugs may be significantly protracted in persons with acute intermittent porphyria.[1]

Fasting has been implicated in producing acute attacks in a number of individuals. The basis for the effect is unclear. Fasting in experimental animals increases the activity of ALA synthetase and produces an exaggerated response to inducers of haem synthesis.[52] Carriers of porphyria should be advised that stringent dieting is dangerous and that caloric intake should be maintained, if possible, during periods of anorexia due to viral illness or other cause. Surgical operations pose a hazard because of the routinely imposed preoperative fast; if the fast cannot be modified, caloric intake should be maintained with intravenous solutions. On the other hand, caloric intake in excess of normal needs is discouraged: there is no evidence that a high carbohydrate diet prevents acute attacks, and weight-control problems are frequent.

Acute attacks

The management of acute porphyric attacks includes supportive care, judicious use of analgesics, administration of carbohydrate and intravenous haematin. (In the context of this discussion, 'haem', 'haematin' and 'haemin' should be regarded as equivalent terms. Haematin and haemin are the hydroxide and chloride salts, respectively, of haem. Since only the hydroxide is soluble in aqueous solution, haem is prepared as haematin (at pH 8.0) for intravenous injection. In plasma, the compound undoubtedly exists as haem, bound to plasma protein and the hydroxyl replaced by a protein ligand.) Pain symptoms in some patients are controlled with chlorpromazine; other patients will require meperidine. The latter, because of its addicting potential, should be used for short periods only; indeed, given the remitting nature of acute attacks, chronic administration of meperidine should not only be unnecessary but should suggest that the pain symptoms are due to causes other than porphyria. When seizures are a feature of the acute presentation, they usually remit early in the course of therapy and may be controlled with diazepam. Chronic seizure disorders in porphyrics may respond with bromides;[51] barbiturates, hydantoins and related compounds are contraindicated. Glucose is given by whatever route is most convenient, although it usually is necessary to use the intravenous route, with the aim of giving at least 2.2 mol/24 hr (400 g/24 hr). The rationale for glucose therapy is the fact that the effect of fasting on ALA synthetase in animals (described above) is reversed promptly after administration of glucose,[14,82] and the efficacy of glucose infusions has been documented in individual clinical reports.[77]

Intravenous haematin

Administration of haematin should be undertaken in those patients with acute attacks showing progressive deterioration despite the above regimen. The mortality of acute porphyric attacks was formerly placed as high as 25 per cent. Modern techniques of intensive care undoubtedly have brought about a reduction in that figure, and haematin therapy promises to reduce it still further. The fact that acute intermittent porphyria, hereditary coproporphyria and variegate porphyria represent haem-deficient conditions has been recognized for several years. Only recently, however, has it been demonstrated that haematin may be administered safely to patients and in amounts large enough to suppress endogenous hepatic haem synthesis (most of the administered haem is degraded rapidly and irreversibly to bile pigment, leaving only a small fraction of the dose to mix with the intracellular haem 'pool', where it exerts a regulatory effect). The initial studies of haematin therapy were carried out in patients with respiratory failure and little chance of survival. Nonetheless, striking successes with this group occurred, encouraging more extensive trials. Watson and his colleagues[85] have reviewed 20 patients treated with haematin, virtually all of whom responded both biochemically and clinically to the therapy. Moreover, haematin appears to be remarkably safe, provided that the published guidelines with regard to maximal dose are adhered to.[25] In one case of transient renal failure, the patient had received an unusually large dose. The available data suggest that intravenous haematin should be offered not just to the desperately ill but to all patients failing to respond to conventional measures, so that the severe neurological complications of the disease hopefully may be avoided.

A haematin solution is not yet available commercially, and the stability of the compound in alkaline salt solution is uncertain. At the present time, it is prepared fresh daily. It also should be noted that, while haematin will promptly (within 24 to 48 hr) abort acute attacks, its effect on the biochemical manifestations of the disease is transient. Suppression of ALA levels is achieved only as long as plasma haem is elevated. For this reason, and also because it requires intravenous administration, haematin is unsuited for chronic therapy. Fortunately, the clinical remission induced by haematin usually persists despite the return of porphobilinogen excretion to elevated values.

Prognosis

Neurological deficits comprise the most important residue of acute attacks of porphyria of the haem-deficient type. While these are highly variable in extent and severity, a large measure of recovery can be expected in nearly all patients. Repeated acute attacks are uncommon, particularly if a precipitating agent has been identified. It should be stressed that, while mental aberrations are a component of acute attacks, these uniformly resolve in survivors, and there is no evidence that progressive mental deterioration occurs in these forms of porphyria; longevity also appears to be unimpaired.[24] A number of patients who have suffered acute attacks (and indeed many carriers who have not) complain of chronic sub-acute symptoms, typically without physical findings and often unassociated with any predictable change in the excretion of haem precursors. It may be impossible to establish whether or not such complaints are due to porphyria, and the symptoms should be treated empirically, with due regard for the precautions concerning drug therapy outlined above. It is noteworthy that, although these disorders involve the liver, there is no clinically significant impairment of liver function.

Differentiation of the Haem-deficient Porphyrias

Cutaneous manifestations

The over-production of precursors in acute intermittent porphyria, hereditary coproporphyria or variegate porphyria reflects the site in the haem pathway at which the flow of intermediates has been partially blocked (Figure 15.5); haem precursors prior to the block in each case spill over into plasma. The presence of excess *porphyrins* in hereditary coproporphyria and variegate porphyria – but not in acute intermittent porphyria – is responsible for differences in the clinical presentation of the three conditions. In about 80 per cent of patients with variegate porphyria and 25 per cent of those with hereditary coproporphyria, circulating porphyrins cause cutaneous photosensitivity and/or increased fragility of exposed skin areas. The skin lesions consist of a bullous eruption, leading eventually to ulceration and chronic scarring, typically involving the extensor surface of the hands and also the face. By contrast, persons with acute intermittent porphyria experience no photosensitivity whatsoever. Over-production of porphyrins also gives the urine an abnormal colour, which varies from wine-red to brownish. Because porphyrins are not usually elevated in acute intermittent porphyria, the colour of the urine is often unaltered. Urine that has been standing (particularly if exposed to sunlight) may darken noticeably, however, reflecting non-enzymatic conversion of porphobilinogen to uroporphyrin-like compounds of undetermined structure.

Geographical and racial distribution

These three porphyrias have distinctive geographical and racial associations, which may be useful in their differential diagnosis. The prevalence of acute intermittent porphyria appears to be less than one case per 10 000 persons, except in isolated, in-bred groups,[83] both in Europe and in the white population of the United States; the disease appears to be unusual in non-white populations. Variegate porphyria is extremely common in the Cape area of South Africa, but it is less common than acute intermittent porphyria in Europe and the United States. The prevalence of variegate porphyria has been estimated at 0.3 per cent of the Afrikaner population of South Africa, where the disease was introduced in 1688 by a Dutch immigrant to the Cape.[24] Hereditary coproporphyria appears to be distributed in a pattern similar to that of acute intermittent porphyria. However, large numbers of cases have not been reported, possibly because it appears to be more often latent and clinically less severe when symptomatic than is acute intermittent porphyria.[37] The differentiation of these types by laboratory diagnosis (virtually always required) has been described in a preceding section (see 'Diagnosis' above).

HAEM-COMPENSATED PORPHYRIA: PORPHYRIA CUTANEA TARDA

Clinical Presentation

The sole clinical manifestations of this form of porphyria are dark urine and cutaneous photosensitivity. The skin lesions resemble those of variegate porphyria (see above) and their severity is roughly proportional to the degree of porphyrin over-production (as reflected in urinary porphyrin content). The porphyria is classified as a haem-compensated type because it is associated with normal excretion of ALA and porphobilinogen and is unaffected by barbiturates or other inducers of cytochrome P-450. Indeed, hepatic concentrations of cytochrome P-450 may be elevated in this condition.[61] The urine contains markedly elevated concentrations of uroporphyrin I and also coproporphyrin I, the excretion of uroporphyrin typically exceeding 960 nmol/24 hr (800 μg/24 hr) (cf. Table 15.3 for normal values) when cutaneous symptoms are present. The cutaneous symptoms of the disease are due to increased circulating concentrations of uroporphyrin, by the mechanisms discussed above (see 'Physiological effects of haem precursors').

In Europe and the United States porphyria cutanea tarda is probably seen more frequently than any other form of porphyria. For this reason, its differentiation from the haem-deficient porphyrias is important, given the very different management of these conditions. Unlike the haem-deficient porphyrias, porphyria cutanea tarda carries no associations with a neurological syndrome, with attacks of abdominal pain or psychosis. The condition arises most often in persons with underlying liver disease, which is usually related to excessive ethanol intake. Patients may complain of acute photosensitivity (bulla formation) or may notice only that exposed skin (in particular, the back of the hands) is unusually fragile. Seemingly trivial trauma to these skin areas produces ulceration and scar formation. Similar cutaneous symptoms are absent in acute intermittent porphyria and, in variegate porphyria or hereditary coproporphyria, are secondary in importance to the 'neurological' symptom complex. Examination of haem precursors in urine and faeces conclusively differentiates these porphyrias from each other (see Figure 15.5).

Pathogenesis

Because of its occurrence in persons with liver disease, porphyria cutanea tarda was viewed formerly as an acquired porphyria. While familial clustering of cases has been reported, this has been an infrequent occurrence and could be explained on an environmental basis. Increased hepatic iron deposition is present in most patients, and an inhibitory effect of iron on uroporphyrinogen-III cosynthetase could be demonstrated in vitro. A defect at this enzymatic step appeared to account for the characteristic over-production of isomer-I porphyrins.[44] Finally, it has been shown that serial phlebotomy results in amelioration of the porphyria in virtually all cases, presumably because it diminishes hepatic iron stores.

These findings, in aggregate, provide cogent evidence for a role of iron in the pathogenesis of porphyria cutanea tarda. However, it remains unexplained that many persons with hepatic siderosis and fibrosis exhibit no abnormality of porphyrin metabolism; moreover, in cases of porphyria cutanea tarda, the degree of hepatic siderosis (as well as the liver disease, per se) is often relatively minor. Finally, partial inhibition by iron of uroporphyrinogen-III cosynthetase fails to account for a constant feature of the excretion pattern in porphyria cutanea tarda, namely, that the amount of uroporphyrin in urine markedly exceeds that of coproporphyrin (Figure 15.5). The latter finding suggests that a partial block to the flow of haem precursors exists at the level of uroporphyrinogen decarboxylase, and recent studies indicate that this activity is reduced in persons with porphyria cutanea tarda. Moreover, this enzyme defect has been detected in family members of patients with porphyria cutanea tarda; several apparent 'carriers' displayed subclinical abnormalities of porphyrin metabolism.[43]

These studies provide a basis for regarding porphyria cutanea tarda as a genetic disease, one in which the hereditary enzyme abnormality is a necessary, but probably not the sole, determinant of clinically apparent disease.[28] In ways that remain poorly understood, the defect in uroporphyrinogen decarboxylase activity, in concert with an inhibitory effect of iron and possibly of alcohol, partially blocks the formation of uroporphyrinogen III, resulting in shunting of porphobilinogen to the isomer-I pathway. Despite the over-production of porphyrins, sufficient haem is synthesized to maintain homeostasis, and the activity of ALA synthetase is either normal or minimally elevated in hepatic tissue of patients with porphyria cutanea tarda. In addition to alcohol, drugs and other chemicals may also exert a direct toxic effect on enzymes of the haem pathway, precipitating or aggravating porphyria cutanea tarda. Administration of oestrogen has been implicated in several cases.[28]

Management

Patients should discontinue drugs which may be aggravating the condition and also alcohol.[38] While improvement may result from this manipulation alone, serial phlebotomy is usually necessary and is virtually always effective.[39] Provided that the patient maintains a satisfactory haemoglobin level, one unit of blood (500 cc) may be removed bi-weekly until a response occurs, as judged by decreasing urinary porphyrin excretion. The cutaneous manifestations of the disease resolve as urinary uroporphyrin excretion drops below 1200 nmol/24 hr (1000 μg/24 hr). The time between initiation of phlebotomy therapy and response varies widely among individual patients but averages several months.[32] The duration of the response is similarly unpredictable; uroporphyrin excretion may remain low for years, without further phlebotomy, particularly if factors aggravating the condition have been identified and eliminated. For patients unable to tolerate phlebotomy and significantly disabled by cutaneous symptoms, therapy with chloroquine may be undertaken. Although serious hepatotoxic reactions to chloroquine have been described in patients with porphyria cutanea tarda, a recent report suggests that 'low-dose' treatment is relatively safe.[79] Chloroquine administration results in depletion of hepatic stores of uroporphyrin, apparently by complexing in situ with the porphyrin.[73]

Prognosis

The prognosis of porphyria cutanea tarda is that of the underlying liver disease. The role of screening procedures in families with an affected person is not clear at the present time. Recent studies suggest that detection of carriers will require assay of uroporphyrinogen decarboxylase activity.[43] While the enzyme is present in erythrocytes and therefore readily accessible, its determination presents methodological difficulties that prevent its routine clinical use. However, recognition that porphyria cutanea tarda is a genetic condition is recent, and developments in this area may be anticipated.

ACQUIRED PORPHYRIA

Toxins

Chlorinated phenols

The most severe of the acquired porphyrias result from toxins such as hexachlorobenzene, as documented in a widespread poisoning in Turkey.[71] These substances also cause porphyria in experimental animals, probably directly inhibiting one or more enzymes of the haem synthetic pathway.[29] The biochemical and clinical abnormalities resemble those of porphyria cutanea tarda. Exposure to such toxins should be a rare event under current health and safety regulations but may arise unwittingly, as after casual mixing of commonly used cleaning agents.[48]

Lead

Intoxication with lead results in increased urinary excretion of ALA, together with lesser increases in coproporphyrin. This pattern reflects inhibition of porphobilinogen synthetase by lead, which may react with sulphydryl groups on the enzyme or displace zinc, which appears to be essential for normal enzyme activity. Presumably, partial inhibition of coproporphyrinogen oxidase also occurs, accounting for the increased excretion of urinary coproporphyrin. In erythrocytes of lead-poisoned individuals, decreased activity of porphobilinogen synthetase correlates well with blood lead concentrations.[68] Although abdominal pain and neurological deficits occur with lead intoxication, the disorder can be distinguished readily from acute intermittent porphyria by the absence of increased urinary porphobilinogen.

In addition to porphobilinogen synthetase, ferrochelatase activity in erythroid cells appears to be inhibited in lead intoxication. As a result, protoporphyrin in circulating erythrocytes is substantially increased.[62] In both lead intoxication and iron deficiency (see below), the porphyrin appears to be trapped within the cell as a metal chelate (zinc protoporphyrin), so that it fails to diffuse into plasma and does not, therefore, cause symptoms of cutaneous photosensitivity.[45] Also, faecal excretion of protoporphyrin in these disorders is normal. In these respects, the porphyria of iron deficiency or lead intoxication differs strikingly from that of protoporphyria (see above).

Iron Deficiency

Lack of iron would be expected to impair the conversion of protoporphyrin to haem, and in persons with iron deficiency, erythrocytes contain increased amounts of protoporphyrin. As in lead intoxication the increased protoporphyrin serves as a convenient parameter of iron deficiency but is otherwise of no clinical significance. It can be quantitated by a simple one-step extraction procedure which lends itself to rapid and sensitive clinical screening.[12,20,62]

Liver Disease

The porphyrin abnormalities of acute liver disease are generally mild, being most notable in cholestasis and in resolving acute viral hepatitis.[2] The urine exhibits modest increases of uro- and coproporphyrin without elevation of ALA or porphobilinogen. The main clinical significance of this benign porphyrinuria is that it may be misconstrued as evidence for a hereditary condition.

In persons with hereditary conjugated hyperbilirubinaemia (Rotor Syndrome), urinary coproporphyrin is moderately elevated.[87] In the closely related Dubin–Johnson syndrome, total coproporphyrin in urine is normal, although the ratio of isomer I/III (normally 1/9) is reversed.[42] These conditions involve impaired biliary excretion of a variety of organic compounds, including coproporphyrin. They are unaccompanied by clinical manifestations of porphyria.

CONCLUSION

The porphyrias are abnormalities of haem synthesis, in which haem precursors – ALA, porphobilinogen or porphyrins – are over-produced and appear in increased amounts in blood, urine or faeces. Several types of porphyria occur, differing in pathogenesis (hereditary or acquired), organ involvement (bone marrow or liver) and the presence or absence of a relative haem deficiency in affected tissues. These distinctions form the basis for classifying the various porphyrias, as well as providing a rationale for the clinical and laboratory characteristics of the individual types.

Congenital erythropoietic porphyria is a rare disease which appears to involve only the bone marrow and is characterized by severe photosensitivity from early childhood.

Erythrohepatic protoporphyria involves over-production of protoporphyrin predominantly by erythroid cells but also by liver. In the vast majority of cases, the clinical manifestations are dermatological only. However, in persons in whom over-production is striking, massive deposition of protoporphyrin in the liver has occurred, followed by rapidly progressive hepatic failure.

Acute intermittent porphyria, hereditary coproporphyria and *variegate porphyria* comprise the hepatic *haem-deficient porphyrias.* While each type is associated with a distinct, inherited enzymatic defect, the abnormality in all cases potentially compromises the haem-synthetic capacity of the liver. This fact may account for the similar clinical manifestations of these diseases. The major symptom complex consists of neuropsychiatric abnormalities and is commonly precipitated by drug inducers of hepatic haem synthesis, notably barbiturates. Cutaneous photosensitivity is present in variegate porphyria and, to a lesser extent, in hereditary coproporphyria; it is absent in acute intermittent porphyria. Treatment with haematin infusions represents a major therapeutic advance which promises to reduce substantially the mortality of acute attacks.

Porphyria cutanea tarda is a *haem-compensated porphyria* characterized by cutaneous photosensitivity and excessive excretion of urinary uroporphyrin, without increased ALA or porphobilinogen and without neurological symptoms. An inherited abnormality appears to act in concert with environmental factors (typically, excess ethanol ingestion) to produce clinical manifestations. Effective treatment is provided by serial phlebotomy, which reduces the burden of iron in the liver.

Acquired porphyrias can result from specific intoxications (e.g. hexachlorobenzene, lead), from iron deficiency or from liver injury of diverse aetiology. Attention should be directed to the underlying cause; the porphyrinuria per se is seldom of clinical importance.

REFERENCES

1. Anderson, K.E., Alvares, A.P., Sassa, S. & Kappas, A. (1976) Studies in porphyria. V. Drug oxidation rates in hereditary hepatic porphyria. *Clinical Pharmacology and Therapeutics,* **19,** 47–54.
2. Aziz, M.A., Schwartz, S. & Watson, C.J. (1964) Studies of coproporphyrin. VIII. Reinvestigation of the isomer distribution in jaundice and liver diseases. *Journal of Laboratory and Clinical Medicine,* **63,** 596–604.
3. Battersby, A.R., Buckley, D.G., McDonald, E. & Williams, D.C. (1977) Enzymic formation of the type-III porphyrin macrocycle from unrearranged AP-AP pyromethane. *Journal of the Chemical Society, Chemical Communications,* 115–117.
4. Beal, M.F., Atuk, N.O., Westfall, T.C. & Turner, S.M. (1977) Catecholamine uptake, accumulation, and release in acute porphyria. *Journal of Clinical Investigation,* **60,** 1141–1148.
5. Beattie, A.D., Moore, M.R., Goldberg, A. & Ward, R.L. (1973) Acute intermittent porphyria: response of tachycardia and hypertension to propranolol. *British Medical Journal,* **iii,** 257–260.
6. Bissell, D.M. & Hammaker, L.E. (1976) Cytochrome P-450 heme and the regulation of hepatic heme oxygenase activity. *Archives of Biochemistry and Biophysics,* **176,** 91–102.
7. Bissell, D.M. & Hammaker, L.E. (1976) Cytochrome P-450 heme and the regulation of δ-aminolevulinic acid synthetase in the liver. *Archives of Biochemistry and Biophysics,* **176,** 103–112.
8. Bissell, D.M., Hammaker, L. & Schmid, R. (1972) Hemoglobin and erythrocyte catabolism in rat liver: the separate roles of parenchymal and sinusoidal cells. *Blood,* **40,** 812–822.
9. Bissell, D.M., Liem, H.H. & Muller-Eberhard, U. (1977) Heme secretion by the liver. *Clinical Research,* **25,** 307A.
10. Bloomer, J.R., Bonkowsky, H.L. & Klatskin, G. (1975) The liver in protoporphyria. *Gastroenterology,* **69,** 810.
11. Bloomer, J.R., Phillips, M.J., Davidson, D.L. & Klatskin, G. (1975) Hepatic disease in erythropoietic protoporphyria. *American Journal of Medicine,* **58,** 869–882.
12. Blumberg, W.E., Eisinger, J., Lamola, A.A. & Zuckerman, D.M. (1977) The hematofluorometer. *Clinical Chemistry,* **23,** 270–274.
13. Bonkowsky, H.L. & Tschudy, D.P. (1974) Hazard of propranolol in treatment of acute porphyria. *British Medical Journal,* **iv,** 47–48.
14. Bonkowsky, H.L., Collins, A., Doherty, J.M. & Tschudy, D.P. (1973) The glucose effect in rat liver: studies of δ-aminolevulinate synthase and tyrosine amino-transferase. *Biochimica et Biophysica Acta,* **320,** 561–576.
15. Bonkowsky, H.L., Bloomer, J.R., Ebert, P.S. & Mahoney, M.J. (1975) Heme synthetase deficiency in human protoporphyria. Demonstration of the defect in liver and cultured skin fibroblasts. *Journal of Clinical Investigation,* **56,** 1139–1148.
16. Bonkowsky, H.L., Tschudy, D.P., Weinbach, E.C., Ebert, P.S. & Doherty, J.M. (1975) Porphyrin synthesis and mitochondrial respiration in acute intermittent porphyria: studies using cultured human fibroblasts. *Journal of Laboratory and Clinical Medicine,* **85,** 93–102.
17. Bottomley, S.S., Tanaka, M. & Everett, M.A. (1975) Diminished erythroid ferrochelatase activity in protoporphyria. *Journal of Laboratory and Clinical Medicine,* **86,** 126–131.
18. Brodie, M.J., Thompson, G.G., Moore, M.R., Beattie, A.D. & Goldberg, A. (1977) Hereditary coproporphyria. Demonstration of the abnormalities in haem biosynthesis in peripheral blood. *Quarterly Journal of Medicine,* **46,** 229–241.
19. Burnham, B.F. (1969) Metabolism of porphyrins and corrinoids. In *Metabolic Pathways* (Ed.) Greenberg, D.M. Vol. 3, Ch. 18. New York: Academic Press.
20. Chisolm, J.J., Mellits, E.D., Keil, J.E. & Barrett, M.B. (1974) A simple protoporphyrin assay-microhematocrit procedure as a screening technique for increased lead absorption in young children. *Journal of Pediatrics,* **84,** 490–496.
21. Correia, M.A. & Meyer, U.A. (1975) Apocytochrome P-450: reconstitution of functional cytochrome with hemin in vitro. *Proceedings of the National Academy of Sciences,* **72,** 400–404.
22. Davidson, D.L., Bloomer, J.R. & Klatskin, G. (1973) Therapy of hepatic disease in erythropoietic protoporphyria. *Gastroenterology,* **65,** 535.
23. Davis, J.R. & Andelman, S.L. (1967) Urinary delta-aminolevulinic acid (ALA) levels in lead poisoning. I. A modified method for the rapid determination of urinary delta-aminolevulinic acid using disposable ion-exchange chromatography columns. *Archives of Environmental Health,* **15,** 53–59.
24. Dean, G. (1971) *The Porphyrias. A Story of Heredity and Environment.* 2nd ed. London: Pitman Medical.
25. Dhar, G.J., Bossenmaier, I., Petryka, Z.J., Cardinal, R. & Watson, C.J. (1975) Effects of hematin in hepatic porphyria. Further studies. *Annals of Internal Medicine,* **83,** 20–30.
26. Donaldson, E.M., McCall, A.J., Magnus, I.A., Simpson, J.R., Caldwell, R.A. & Hargreaves, T. (1970) Erythropoietic protoporphyria: two deaths from hepatic cirrhosis. *British Journal of Dermatology,* **84,** 14–24.
27. Eales, M. (1963) Porphyria as seen in Cape Town: a survey of 250 patients and some recent studies. *South African Journal of Laboratory and Clinical Medicine,* **9,** 151–162.
28. Elder, G.H. (1977) Porphyrin metabolism in porphyria cutanea tarda. *Seminars in Hematology,* **14,** 227–242.
29. Elder, G.H., Evans, J.O. & Matlin, S.A. (1976) The effect of the porphyrogenic compound, hexachlorobenzene, on the activity of hepatic uroporphyrinogen decarboxylase in the rat. *Clinical Science and Molecular Medicine,* **51,** 71–80.
30. Elder, G.H., Gray, C.H. & Nicholson, D.C. (1972) The porphyrias: a review. *Journal of Clinical Pathology,* **25,** 1013–1033.
31. Elder, G.H., Evans, J.O., Thomas, N., Cox, R., Brodie, M.J., Moore, M.R., Goldberg, A. & Nicholson, D.C. (1976) The primary enzyme defect in hereditary coproporphyria. *Lancet,* **ii,** 1217–1219.
32. Epstein, J.H. & Redeker, A.G. (1968) Porphyria cutanea tarda. A study of the effect of phlebotomy. *New England Journal of Medicine,* **279,** 1301–1304.
33. Finelli, V.N., Murthy, L., Peirano, W.B. & Petering, H.G. (1974) δ-Aminolevulinate dehydratase, a zinc

dependent enzyme. *Biochemical and Biophysical Research Communications*, **60,** 1418–1424.
34. Franck, B., Fels, G. & Ufer, G. (1977) Heme biosynthesis from [^{14}C]- and [^{3}H]-labeled tripyrroles. *Angewandte Chemie*, **16,** 652–653.
35. Frydman, B. & Frydman, R.B. (1975) Biosynthesis of uroporphyrinogens from porphobilinogen. Mechanism and nature of the process. *Accounts of Chemical Research*, **8,** 201–208.
36. Gidari, A.S. & Levere, R.D. (1977) Enzymatic formation and cellular regulation of heme synthesis. *Seminars in Hematology*, **14,** 145–168.
37. Goldberg, A., Rimington, C. & Lochhead, A. (1967) Hereditary coproporphyria. *Lancet*, **i,** 632–636.
38. Haberman, H.F., Rosenberg, F. & Menon, I.A. (1975) Porphyria cutanea tarda: comparison of cases precipitated by alcohol and estrogens. *Journal of the Canadian Medical Association*, **113,** 653–655.
39. Ippen, H. (1961) Allgemeinsymptome der späten Hautporphyrie (Porphyria cutanea tarda) als Hinweise für deren Behandlung. *Deutsche Medizinische Wochenschrift*, **86,** 127–133.
40. Ketterer, B., Srai, K.S. & Christodoulides, L. (1976) Haem-binding proteins of the rat liver cytosol. *Biochimica et Biophysica Acta*, **428,** 683–689.
41. Kniffen, J.C. (1970) Porphyrin removal in intrahepatic porphyrastasis. *Gastroenterology*, **58,** 1027.
42. Koskelo, P., Toivonen, I. & Adlercreutz, H. (1967) Urinary coproporphyrin isomer distribution in the Dubin–Johnson syndrome. *Clinical Chemistry*, **13,** 1006–1009.
43. Kushner, J.P., Barbuto, A.J. & Lee, G.R. (1976) An inherited enzymatic defect in porphyria cutanea tarda. Decreased uroporphyrinogen decarboxylase activity. *Journal of Clinical Investigation*, **58,** 1089–1097.
44. Kushner, J.P., Lee, G.R. & Nacht, S. (1972) The role of iron in the pathogenesis of porphyria cutanea tarda. An in vitro model. *Journal of Clinical Investigation*, **51,** 3044–3051.
45. Lamola, A.A., Piomelli, S., Poh-Fitzpatrick, M.B., Yamane, T. & Harber, L.C. (1975) Erythropoietic protoporphyria and lead intoxication: the molecular basis for difference in cutaneous photosensitivity. II. Different binding of erythrocyte protoporphyrin in hemoglobin. *Journal of Clinical Investigation*, **56,** 1528–1535.
46. Lamon, J., With, T.K. & Redeker, A.G. (1974) The Hoesch test: bedside screening for urinary porphobilinogen in patients with suspected porphyria. *Clinical Chemistry*, **20,** 1438–1440.
47. Lindblad, B., Lindstedt, S. & Steen, G. (1977) On the enzymic defects in hereditary tyrosinemia. *Proceedings of the National Academy of Sciences*, **74,** 4641–4645.
48. Lynch, R.E., Lee, G.R. & Kushner, J.P. (1975) Porphyria cutanea tarda associated with disinfectant misuse. *Archives of Internal Medicine*, **135,** 549–552.
49. Magnus, I.A., Jarret, A., Prankerd, T.A.J. & Rimington, C. (1961) Erythropoietic protoporphyria — a new porphyria syndrome with solar urticaria due to protoporphyrinaemia. *Lancet*, **ii,** 448–451.
50. Magnussen, C.R., Levine, J.B., Doherty, J.M., Cheesman, J.O. & Tschudy, D.P. (1974) A red cell enzyme method for the diagnosis of acute intermittent porphyria. *Blood*, **44,** 857–868.
51. Magnussen, C.R., Doherty, J.M., Hess, R.A. & Tschudy, D.P. (1975) Grand mal seizures and acute intermittent porphyria. The problem of differential diagnosis and treatment. *Neurology*, **25,** 1121–1125.
52. Marver, H.S. (1969) The role of heme in the synthesis and repression of microsomal protein. In *Microsomes and Drug Oxidations* (Ed.) Gillette, J.R., Conney, A.H., Cosmides, G.J., Estabrook, R.W., Fouts, J.R. & Mannering, G.J. pp. 495–515. New York: Academic Press.
53. Marver, H.S., Tschudy, D.P., Perlroth, M.G., Collins, A. & Hunter, G. Jr (1966) The determination of aminoketones in biological fluids. *Analytical Biochemistry*, **14,** 53–60.
54. Mauzerall, D. (1976) Chlorophyll and photosynthesis. *Philosophical Transactions of the Royal Society, London*, **B 273,** 287–294.
55. Mauzerall, D. & Granick, S. (1956) The occurrence and determination of delta-aminolevulinic acid and porphobilinogen in urine. *Journal of Biological Chemistry*, **219,** 435–446.
56. Meyer, U.A. (1973) Intermittent acute porphyria. Clinical and biochemical studies of disordered heme biosynthesis. *Enzyme*, **16,** 334–342.
57. Meyer, U.A. & Schmid, R. (1978) The porphyrias. In *The Metabolic Basis of Inherited Disease* (Ed.) Stanbury, J.B., Wyngaarden, J.B. & Frederickson, D.S. pp. 1166–1220. New York: McGraw-Hill.
58. Meyer, U.A., Strand, L.J., Doss, M., Rees, A.C. & Marver, H.S. (1972) Intermittent acute porphyria – demonstration of a genetic defect in porphobilinogen metabolism. *New England Journal of Medicine*, **286,** 1277–1282.
59. Muller-Eberhard, U. & Liem, H.H. (1974) Hemopexin, the heme-binding serum β-glycoprotein. In *Structure and Function of Plasma Proteins* (Ed.) Allison, A.C. Ch. 2, pp. 35–53. London: Plenum Press.
60. Peterson, L.R., Hamernyik, P., Bird, T.D. & Labbe, R.F. (1976) Erythrocyte uroporphyrinogen I synthase activity in diagosis of acute intermittent porphyria. *Clinical Chemistry*, **22,** 1835–1840.
61. Pimstone, N.R., Biekkenhorst, G. & Eales, L. (1973) Enzymatic defects in hepatic porphyria. Preliminary observations in patients with porphyria cutanea tarda and variegate porphyria. *Enzyme*, **16,** 354–366.
62. Piomelli, S. (1973) A micromethod for free erythrocyte porphyrins: the FEP test. *Journal of Laboratory and Clinical Medicine*, **81,** 932–940.
63. Piomelli, S., Lamola, A.A., Poh-Fitzpatrick, M.B., Seaman, C. & Harber, L.C. (1975) Erythropoietic protoporphyria and lead intoxication: the molecular basis for difference in cutaneous photosensitivity. I. Different rates of disappearance of protoporphyrin from the erythrocytes, both in vivo and in vitro. *Journal of Clinical Investigation*, **56,** 1519–1527.
64. Poulson, R. (1976) The enzymic conversion of protoporphyrinogen IX to protoporphyrin IX in mammalian mitochondria. *Journal of Biological Chemistry*, **251,** 3730–3733.
65. Rajamanickman, C., Satyanarayana Rao, M.R. & Padmanaban, G. (1975) On the sequence of reactions leading to cytochrome P-450 synthesis-effect of drugs. *Journal of Biological Chemistry*, **250,** 2305–2310.
66. Reio, L. & Wetterberg, L. (1969) False porphobilinogen reactions in the urine of mental patients. *Journal of the American Medical Association*, **207,** 148–150.
67. Rothwell, J.D., LaCroix, S. & Sweeney, G.D. (1973) Evidence against a regulatory role for heme oxygenase in hepatic heme synthesis. *Biochimica et Biophysica Acta*, **304,** 871–874.
68. Sassa, S., Granick, S. & Kappas, A. (1975) Effect of lead and genetic factors on heme biosynthesis in the human red cell. *Annals of the New York Academy of Sciences*, **244,** 419–440.

69. Sassa, S., Granick, S., Bickers, D.R., Bradlow, H.L. & Kappas, A. (1974) A microassay for uroporphyrinogen I synthase, one of three abnormal enzyme activities in acute intermittent porphyria, and its application to the study of the genetics of this disease. *Proceedings of the National Academy of Sciences*, **71**, 732–736.
70. Sassa, S., Solish, G., Levere, R.D. & Kappas, A. (1975) Studies in porphyria IV. Expression of the gene defect of acute intermittent porphyria in cultured human skin fibroblasts and amniotic cells: prenatal diagnosis of the porphyric trait. *Journal of Experimental Medicine*, **142**, 722–731.
71. Schmid, R. (1960) Cutaneous porphyria in Turkey. *New England Journal of Medicine*, **263**, 397–398.
72. Schmid, R. (1973) Synthes and degradation of microsomal hemoproteins. *Drug Metabolism and Disposition*, **1**, 256–258.
73. Scholnick, P.L., Marver, H.S. & Epstein, J. (1973) The molecular basis of the action of chloroquine in porphyria cutanea tarda. *Journal of Investigative Dermatology*, **61**, 226–232.
74. Scholnick, P., Marver, H.S. & Schmid, R. (1971) Erythropoietic protoporphyria: evidence for multiple sites of excess protoporphyrin formation. *Journal of Clinical Investigation*, **50**, 203–207.
75. Schwartz, S., Berg, M.H., Bossenmaier, I. & Dinsmore, H. (1960) Determination of porphyrins in biological materials. *Methods of Biochemical Analysis*, **8**, 221–293.
76. Spikes, J.D. (1975) Porphyrins and related compounds as photodynamic sensitizers. *Annals of the New York Academy of Sciences*, **244**, 496–508.
77. Stein, J.A. & Tschudy, D.P. (1970) Acute intermittent porphyria, a clinical and biochemical study of 46 patients. *Medicine*, **49**, 1–16.
78. Strand, L.J., Felsher, B.W., Redeker, A.G. & Marver, H.S. (1970) Enzymatic abnormalities in heme biosynthesis in intermittent acute porphyria: decreased hepatic conversion of porphobilinogen to porphyrins and increased δ-aminolevulinic acid synthetase activity. *Proceedings of the National Academy of Sciences of the United States of America*, **67**, 1315–1320.
79. Taljaard, J.F.F., Shanley, B.C., Stewart-Wynne, E.G., Deppe, W.M. & Joubert, S.M. (1972) Studies on low dose chloroquine therapy and the action of chloroquine in symptomatic porphyria. *British Journal of Dermatology*, **87**, 261–269.
80. Tenhunen, R., Marver, H.S. & Schmid, R. (1970) The enzymatic catabolism of hemoglobin: stimulation of microsomal heme oxygenase by hemin. *Journal of Laboratory and Clinical Medicine*, **75**, 410–421.
81. Tschudy, D.P. & Bonkowsky, H.L. (1972) Experimental porphyria. *Federation Proceedings*, **31**, 147–159.
82. Tschudy, D.P., Welland, F.H., Collins, A. & Hunter, G. (1964) The effect of carbohydrate feedings on the induction of δ-aminolevulinic acid synthetase. *Metabolism*, **13**, 396–405.
83. Waldenström, J. (1957) The porphyrias as inborn errors of metabolism. *American Journal of Medicine*, **22**, 758–773.
84. Watson, C.J. & Schwartz, S. (1941) A simple test for urinary porphobilinogen. *Proceedings of the Society for Experimental Biology and Medicine*, **47**, 393–394.
85. Watson, C.J., Pierach, C.A., Bossenmaier, I. & Cardinal, R. (1977) Postulated deficiency of hepatic heme and repair by hematin infusions in the 'inducible' hepatic porphyrias. *Proceedings of the National Academy of Sciences of the United States of America*, **74**, 2118–2120.
86. Wetterberg, L. (1975) Report on an international survey of safe and unsafe drugs in acute intermittent porphyria. *Supplement to the Proceedings of the First International Porphyrin Meeting, 'Porphyrias in Human Disease'*, Freiburg, pp. 191–202. Freiburg, Germany: Falk.
87. Wolkoff, A.W., Wolpert, E., Pascasio, F.N. & Arias, I.M. (1976) Rotor's syndrome: a distinct inheritable pathophysiologic entity. *American Journal of Medicine*, **60**, 173–179.
88. Zimmerman, T.S., McMillin, J.M. & Watson, C.J. (1966) Onset of manifestations of hepatic porphyria in relation to the influence of female sex hormones. *Archives of Internal Medicine*, **118**, 229–240.

Chapter 16

The Liver and Response to Drugs

CHARLES F. GEORGE
PETER J. WATT

INTRODUCTION: FACTORS INFLUENCING THE RESPONSE TO DRUGS

Drugs may exert their pharmacological and therapeutic effects in one of several ways.[75] Firstly, they may mimic or block the effects of endogenous hormones and neurotransmitter substances including acetylcholine, noradrenaline and enkephalins through an interaction with specific drug receptors. Secondly, they can affect the activity of certain enzymes, monoamine oxidase for example, in a more or less specific manner. Alternatively, they may have a non-specific action on cellular function in cell membranes and affect ionic fluxes, a property which is shared by anaesthetic agents.

Whatever the precise mechanism and locus of action, the magnitude of a drug's operation is related to its free concentration in extracellular fluid[10,15,28,29,98,123] and the latter is in equilibrium with the concentration of drug free in plasma water. The most important factors affecting drug action are the dose, the proportion of this which reaches the systemic circulation, its distribution volume in the body, protein binding and the rate of elimination,[64] all of which may be influenced by hepatic function.

Pharmacokinetic Factors

Absorption

Whatever the route of administration the major factors which govern drug absorption are the formulation, its physicochemical characteristics and the surface area available. For injected drugs, the local blood supply is also important in determining the rate and amount absorbed. In contrast, with orally administered treatment gastric and intestinal motility have similar consequences.

Bioavailability of orally administered drugs

With the exception of a few whose molecular size is sufficiently small to allow them to pass between intercellular gaps, and others, like levodopa, which are absorbed by active transport, drugs are absorbed by passive diffusion across mucosal barriers. Most lipid-soluble drugs that are non-ionized at intestinal pH are well absorbed.[89] Despite this, the proportion of the dose which reaches the systemic circulation unchanged (bioavailability) may be low. Figure 16.1 shows the sites which limit the bioavailability of drugs and hence their effectiveness. For many the liver (site 6) is the most important of these. For example, the anti-anginal, antihypertensive, β-adrenoceptor antagonist, propranolol, is almost completely absorbed after oral administration[136,163] but its bioavailability is low.

This phenomenon has been extensively studied[59,67,160,164] and the explanation resides

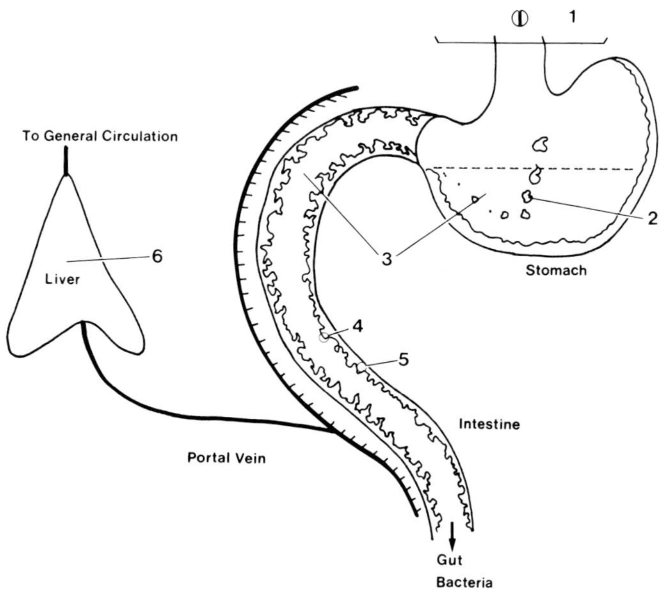

Figure 16.1. Sites at which the bioavailability of orally administered drugs may be reduced. Site 1 – compliance. Site 2 – disintegration and dissolution. Site 3 – gastric and intestinal motility. Site 4 – physicochemical characteristics of the drug. Site 5 – metabolism by intestinal enzymes. Site 6 – hepatic metabolism at the first pass.

in the liver which extracts and biotransforms this and other drugs as they pass through it on their way to the systemic circulation. This phenomenon, which is frequently referred to as a 'first-pass effect', is lacking after the creation of a portacaval anastomosis.[79, 160]

An example of this occurrence for propranolol after intravenous dosing is shown in Figure 16.2. The hepatic extraction of propranolol (E) was derived from the equation

$$E = \frac{(A - H)}{A} \times 100$$

where A was the concentration in arterial blood, and H the concentration in hepatic venous blood and amounted to over 80 per cent. Thus, when given orally (Figure 16.3), a substantial proportion of the dose is removed by the liver before it reaches the systemic circulation (Figure 16.4).

Other drugs which exhibit a large hepatic first-pass effect include the β-adrenoceptor antagonists, alprenolol[1] and oxprenolol,[119] the analgesics, paracetamol[126] and pentazocine,[19] lignocaine[69, 79, 170] and tricyclic antidepressants such as nortriptyline.[77]

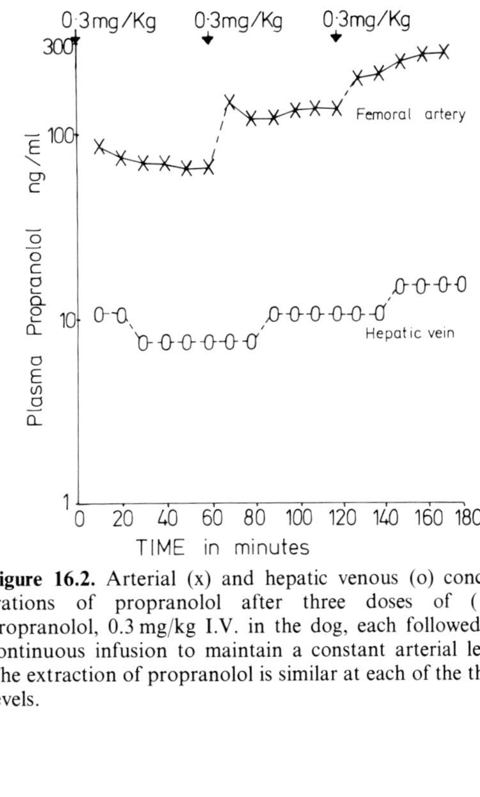

Figure 16.2. Arterial (x) and hepatic venous (o) concentrations of propranolol after three doses of (−)-propranolol, 0.3 mg/kg I.V. in the dog, each followed by continuous infusion to maintain a constant arterial level. The extraction of propranolol is similar at each of the three levels.

Distribution volume

After reaching the systemic circulation, drugs become distributed to the tissues according to their physicochemical characteristics, binding to plasma proteins (see below) and blood flow. The volume of distribution of a drug is a theoretical measurement based upon an assumption that instantaneous mixing occurs throughout the body. Thus, volume of distribution (V_d) is calculated from the dose divided by the concentration in blood and can be obtained in two ways. Firstly, a concentration–time curve for drug in the blood can be constructed and the concentration at zero time estimated by

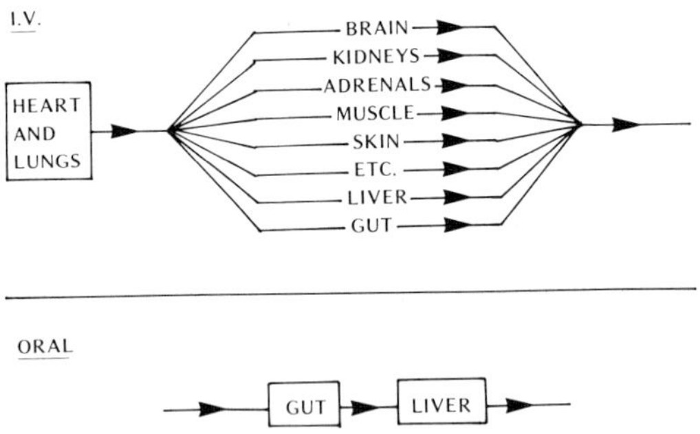

Figure 16.3. The effects of dosing by two different routes with a drug which undergoes extensive metabolism at the first pass in the liver. For intravenously administered drugs the liver is in parallel with other organs and the rate of removal of drugs from the circulation is dependent upon liver blood flow. In contrast, when given orally, virtually all of the drug is presented to the liver, and intrinsic metabolism will determine the bioavailability.

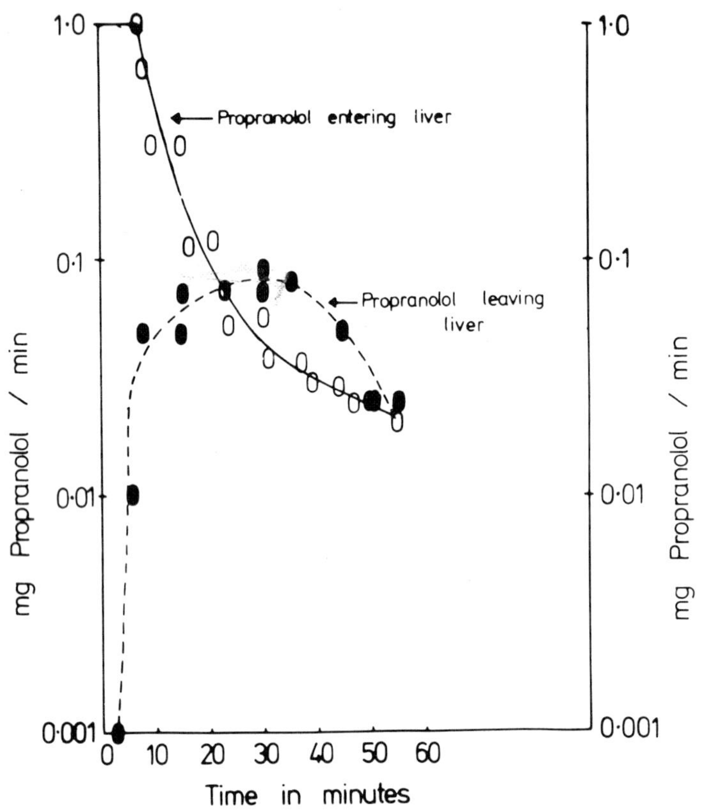

Figure 16.4. Kinetics of propranolol administered via the portal vein of a dog. ○ represents the amount of propranolol entering the liver and ● that leaving the liver. During the first five minutes of the experiment, extraction was almost 100 per cent and the total systemic availability was approximately 30 per cent.

extrapolating the second exponential (Figure 16.5) to obtain the apparent volume of distribution (V_d(a)). This parameter is useful in calculating loading doses of drugs as well as infusion rates. It is also of fundamental importance in determining the rate of drug elimination (see below). Alternatively, the volume of distribution can be calculated at steady-state (V_d(ss)). This can be regarded as the volume of distribution that would be attained if the drug were infused intravenously until a steady concentration in blood were attained.[138] V_d(ss) is a better measurement than V_d(a) because the former is dependent only on the distribution volume and the distribution rate constant, whereas the latter is affected also by the elimination process itself.[94,151]

Drug distribution volumes vary widely: some, such as heparin, are confined in plasma water because of their high molecular weight and ionization; others, like antipyrine, are distributed throughout body water,[38] whereas lipid-soluble drugs like propanolol have a V_d of several litres/kg[163] because they are widely distributed and concentrated in the tissues, especially those of brain, liver and lung.[83]

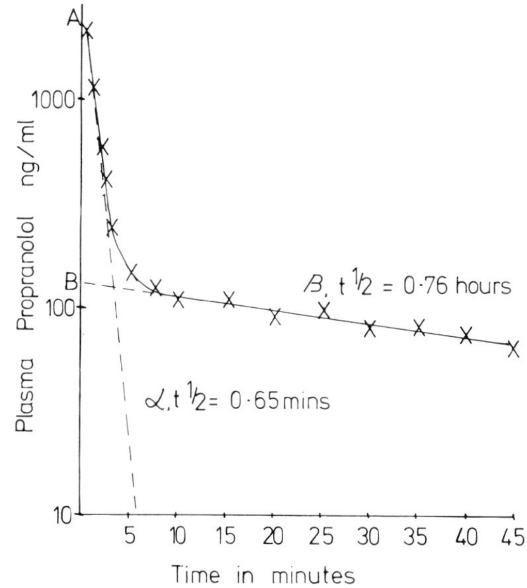

Figure 16.5. Concentration–time curve for intravenously administered propranolol. The log-linear plot can be resolved into two exponentials, and extrapolation back of the second exponential or β-phase to zero time allows calculation of the volume of distribution.

Protein binding

Many drugs are carried in the blood bound to non-specific sites on plasma proteins. Albumin is the most important protein for the majority of drugs, but for some, tubocurarine for example, binding to globulin is more relevant.[15] Drug bound to protein is in equilibrium with that free in plasma water, but only the latter exerts a pharmacological and therapeutic effect (see above). The amount of drug bound to protein is determined by the number of binding sites available, which varies for different drugs, their affinity for the drug and its concentration.[101] Plasma protein binding is an important factor in determining drug distribution and the rate of elimination. Only the unbound fraction is available for distribution: thus, the higher the degree of binding of sulphonamides to albumin, the greater is the proportion that remains in the blood and the lower the concentration which enters cerebrospinal fluid.[63] Similarly, the distribution of most antibiotics into the tissues is closely related to their binding on plasma proteins.[17] Drugs and drug metabolites can displace one another from binding to plasma proteins and the resultant increase in free concentration will lead to a temporary increase in their effects.[37, 101]

For most drugs, except those which show a high hepatic extraction,[58] only free drug can be eliminated. Because of this, protein binding will lessen the removal of drugs and delay their elimination.[12, 112, 129] Details of the extent to which large numbers of drugs are bound to plasma proteins can be found in the review by Koch-Weser and Sellers.[101]

Rates of elimination

The rate of elimination of a drug from the body will determine its duration of action.[108] In addition, together with the frequency of administration, the rate of elimination determines the concentration in blood during regular dosing, which is frequently known as the steady-state concentration (Figure 16.6). For many water-soluble drugs, including digoxin,[49] chlorpropamide,[152] aminoglycosides[80, 103] and practolol,[27] the kidney is the most important route of elimination. However, others which are largely non-ionized at physiological pH are extensively reabsorbed from the kidney. Thus, for the majority of drugs the duration and intensity of action are largely determined by the speed at which they are metabolized in the body by the enzymes in the liver microsomes.[45]

Drug metabolism in the liver

Although metabolism can occur at several sites in the liver, including mitochondria and the cytosol, for the majority of drugs the smooth endoplasmic reticulum (Figure 16.7) is the most important. In the endoplasmic reticulum, enzymes attached to lipid layers of the membranes catalyse the metabolism of drugs to more water-soluble compounds which are subsequently eliminated either in bile or urine (see below). Experimentally, separation of the smooth endoplasmic reticulum can be achieved by ultracentrifugation at 1×10^5 *g*. This produces a pellet of membranes known as the microsomal fraction. Metabolism of drugs by this fraction is usually referred to as 'microsomal enzyme metabolism'.

Among the enzymes located in the endoplasmic reticulum are cytochrome P-450, so called because of its striking absorption peak at 450 nm in the presence of carbon monoxide,[57] flavin enzymes, responsible for reduction of azo and nitro groups, esterases and transferases. Pathways of drug metabolism in the microsomal system can broadly be categorized into two

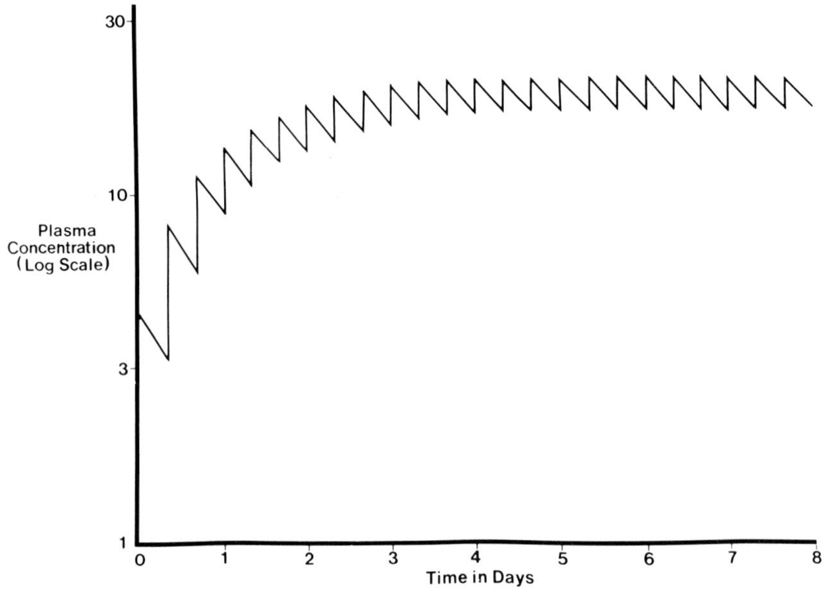

Figure 16.6. Concentration–time profile for a drug during repetitive dosing. A 'steady-state' is achieved after approximately five half-lives have elapsed. At this time fluctuations from one day to the next in concentrations do not differ.

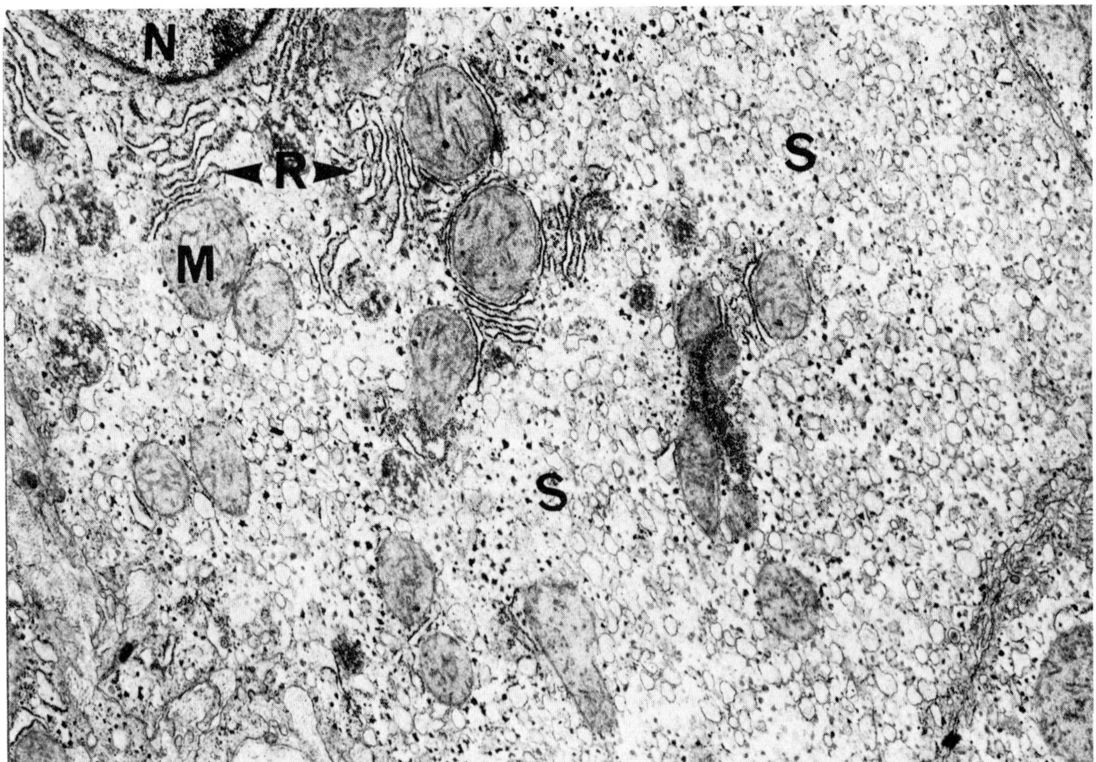

Figure 16.7. Electron micrograph of an hepatocyte showing smooth endoplasmic reticulum. M, mitochondrion; N, nucleus; R, ribosomes; S, smooth endoplasmic reticulum.

main types: firstly, pre-conjugation or phase I reactions which serve to append or reveal suitable chemical groups such as OH, NH_2 and COOH within the drug; and secondly, conjugation, synthetic, or phase II reactions in which groupings revealed by phase I reactions are coupled to endogenous compounds such as glucuronic acid and sulphate (Table 16.1). Phase II reactions may occur without prior oxidation, reduction or hydrolysis if suitable groupings already exist.

Most phase I metabolites are generated by a common hydroxylating enzyme system, cytochrome P-450. This system was first described by Estabrook, Cooper and Rosenthal[57] and further elucidated by the same group initially in the adrenal cortex.[132] Later, however, the same enzyme system was found to be present and more active in the liver.[56, 147]

This enzyme system has the capacity to transport electrons to a cytochromal acceptor and in the process an oxygen atom is donated to the drug:

$$X + 2e^- + 2H^+ + O_2 \rightarrow X{:}O + H_2O$$

Thus, one of the two electrons is used for the reduction of one atom of oxygen to water and the second oxygen atom is incorporated into the substrate. The electron donor is reduced NADP and the electrons are picked up by a flavoprotein known as cytochrome *c* reductase.[95] Thereafter, the electrons flow from the reduced flavin enzymes to cytochrome P-450 (Figure 16.8). The activity of the cytochrome P-450 system is in part genetically determined[6, 181, 184] but is also under the influence of environmental factors including substances present in the diet and various medicines.[45] Drugs may affect the activity of the P-450 cytochrome system in one of two ways. Firstly, the amount and activity of the enzyme may be increased by drugs which are referred to as

Table 16.1. *Pathways of Drug Elimination in Man.*

Phase	Reaction	Enzyme	Example(s)
I	Oxidation of aliphatic and aromatic groups, etc.	Cytochrome P-450	Barbiturates Meprobamate Phenytoin Phenothiazines Chlordiazepoxide Antihistamines Phenacetin Antipyrine Mefenamic acid Steroids Diazoxide, etc.
	Reduction of azo and nitro groups, etc.	Flavin enzymes	Prontosil Chloramphenicol Chloralhydrate
	Hydrolyses	Esterases Amidases	Esters Procaine Lignocaine Indomethacin Atropine substitutes
II	Glucuronide synthesis	Glucuronyl transferase	Paracetamol Chloramphenicol
	Glycine conjugation	Transacylase	Salicylate
	Ethereal sulphate synthesis	Sulphokinase	Isoprenaline
	Methylation	Catechol-o-methyl transferase	Isoprenaline
	Acetylation	N-acetyl transferase	Isoniazid Sulphomethazine
	Mercapturic acid synthesis	Glutathione transferases	Paracetamol

Other phase II reactions include glutamine synthesis and thiocyanate formation

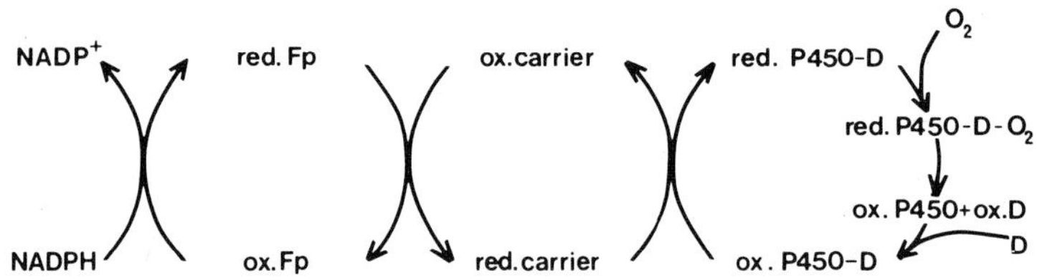

Figure 16.8. The cytochrome P-450 hydroxylating system.

inducers of microsomal oxidation.[56,147] They include barbiturates, glutethimide, dichloralphenazone, haloperidol, alcohol and griseofulvin.[50] When an inducer of microsomal oxidation is introduced into the treatment of a patient stabilized on another drug which is metabolized by hepatic microsomal enzymes the effect is to increase gradually the rate of inactivation of the latter. Thus, to maintain the previous pharmacological and therapeutic effects it may be necessary to increase the dose several fold.[35] Secondly, drugs may inhibit the action of hepatic microsomal enzymes: these include methylphenidate, chloramphenicol, disulfiram, allopurinol, alcohol and dextropropoxyphene.[50]

Generally, phase I reactions lead to a diminution of the pharmacological activity but there are important exceptions to this rule. They include the red dye, Prontosil, and the antidepressant, imipramine, which are converted to the active metabolites, sulphanilamide and desipramine respectively.[47] Toxic metabolites of phenacetin and paracetamol may also be generated by this system.[126]

Synthetic, conjugation or phase II reactions. These are listed in Table 16.1. Glucuronic acid conjugation is probably the most widespread and versatile synthetic reaction in the liver: glucuronic acid can be transferred to many chemical groupings including hydroxyls (alcoholic, phenolic and hydroxyl amino), carboxyl, amino and sulphydryl.[168] In contrast, sulphate conjugation occurs only on hydroxyl groupings, usually phenolic. Methylation can occur on hydroxyl (OH), sulphydryl (SH) and amino (NH_2) groupings. Conjugation with amino acids may also be important; aspirin, for example, is normally conjugated with glycine.

A few phase II reactions take place in the cytosol; among the enzymes located therein, *N*-acetyl transferase is responsible for the acetylation of isoniazid, hydrallazine, sulphonamides and procainamide. The activity of this enzyme is genetically determined in an autosomal recessive manner and patients are either fast or slow acetylators.[135] The proportion of the genotypes varies among ethnic groups; about 95 per cent of Eskimos are fast acetylators whereas among caucasians the proportion is less than half.

Metabolism outside the liver

Finally, hydrolysis of some drugs takes place in the blood where non-specific esterases exist in plasma. These are responsible for the hydrolysis of drugs which include succinylcholine, procaine and procainamide. The activity of this plasma esterase (pseudocholinesterase) is genetically determined and the trimodal distribution of activity suggests an autosomal, autonomous inheritance.[135] Pseudocholinesterase is synthesized within the liver which is, therefore, important in terminating the action of some neuromuscular blocking drugs.

Fate of metabolites formed within the liver

After the formation of polar metabolites within the liver these are excreted either in bile or urine.

Biliary excretion of drugs has been the subject of an extensive review by Smith.[167] Most of our understanding of the basic mechanisms involved stems from animal experiments. In man, ethical considerations have precluded the widespread use of radiolabelled drugs for metabolic studies so that reliance has been placed on bile collections made from patients with T-tube drainage after surgery on the biliary tree. Such data do not provide an accurate quantitative guide to normal biliary excretion of drugs because of the underlying disease, which may induce variable degrees of hepatic damage and obstruction to bile flow. Furthermore, the collection of bile may be incomplete and most studies have been based on single doses of drugs.

Normal bile contains bile salts, lecithin and cholesterol as stable ionic mixed micelles. For drugs to be excreted in this manner they must have a molecular structure which possesses affinities for both the aqueous and lipid domains of the micelle. This conclusion is based on the very slow elimination of non-polar compounds such as dieldrin which cannot be metabolized by the liver[167] and the fact that highly polar compounds, for example, the aminoglycoside antibiotics such as gentamicin (which have large numbers of amino and hydroxyl groups), are not excreted in the bile. However, trapping of some drugs can occur in mixed micelles and may, in part, explain the secretion of compounds into the bile against an apparent concentration gradient.

Another important determinant of whether or not a drug is eliminated in bile is its molecular weight. There are significant species differences in the patterns and pathways of drug elimination. Biliary excretion tends to be relatively unimportant in man because the threshold for elimination by this route lies at a molecular weight of the drug by 176 which may facilitate which the threshold occurs at 325.[86] Thus, glucuronidation has two important effects: firstly, since glucuronides are strong acids such metabolites are highly water soluble (at physiological pH the carboxyl group of the conjugate is almost completely ionized and readily inserts into water by attracting dipoles in the vicinity); and secondly, addition of the glucuronide grouping increases the molecular weight of the drug by 176 which may facilitate excretion into the bile.

Among the drugs which undergo biliary excretion in man are fusidic acid, a tetracyclic turpene which is extensively metabolized by the liver so that less than 1 per cent appears in the bile as unchanged drug.[72] Although the fusidic acid molecule already possesses polar groups in the form of hydroxyl groups in the 3 and 11 positions and a carboxyl at C21, the oxidated metabolites (Figure 16.9) show enhanced polarity. These have comparable micellar properties to sodium taurocholate and are capable of solubilizing lecithins.[41] Rifampicin is also excreted in the bile after undergoing partial O-dealkylation in the liver; the metabolite, 25-desacetyl rifampicin, is more polar and largely excreted in the faeces via the bile.[173]

Other compounds which are eliminated in bile include digitoxin[40] and practolol.[154] However, a proportion of these drugs is reabsorbed from the small intestine, a process referred to as enterohepatic recirculation.

Methods of estimating the rate of drug elimination in man

With the exception of alcohol, phenytoin in high doses[149] and phenylbutazone,[48] the majority of drugs are removed in an exponential fashion which implies that a fixed proportion of the dose is removed in unit time: this type of removal is said to obey first order kinetics. It contrasts with that of alcohol of which a fixed amount is removed in unit time, about 10 mg/hr,[76] and which thus exhibits zero order kinetics. For the majority of drugs, if the logarithm of the blood concentration is plotted against time (by the method of least squares), a straight-line relationship will be obtained: from this, the time taken to fall from a concentration of 2X to X units can be calculated (Figure 16.5). In practice, the usual way of estimating the half-life ($t\frac{1}{2}$) is from the slope of the regression which is equal to:

$$\frac{-k_{el}}{2.3}$$

where k_{el} is the overall first-order elimination rate constant and has the dimensions of either per min or per hr, and 2.3 represents $\log_e 10$.

$t\frac{1}{2}$ is then equal to

$$\frac{0.693}{k_{el}}$$

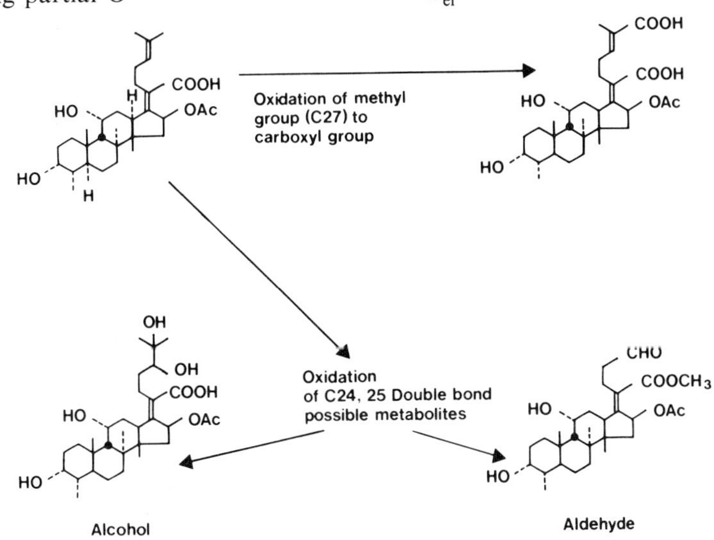

Figure 16.9. Metabolism of fusidic acid.

$t_{\frac{1}{2}}$ has been by far the most widely-used estimate of drug elimination but is subject to numerous errors since it assumes that the β-phase of the concentration-time curve (see Figure 16.5) represents only drug elimination. This is, however, frequently not the case since $t_{\frac{1}{2}}$ calculated in this way may lengthen on successive doses,[51] which suggests that distribution to the tissues (where access is slow) may contribute to the β-phase and the overall k_{el}. *Clearance* (Cl) represents a more precise estimate of the body's efficiency to remove a drug since it refers to the total volume of blood or plasma from which a drug is irreversibly removed in unit time. This is particularly important when trying to estimate changes produced by liver disease, where changes in protein binding, blood flow and capacity for metabolism may not necessarily be reflected in the $t_{\frac{1}{2}}$.

$$Cl = V_d \frac{0.693}{t_{\frac{1}{2}}}$$

Alternatively, clearance can be estimated from the ratio of the injected dose to the area under the concentration–time curve from the zero time to infinity.

Estimation of P-450 activity

There are comparatively few situations where it is possible to estimate drug metabolism directly in man and the indirect measurements described above will usually have to suffice. There have been a few studies undertaken, however, in which the activity of hepatic cytochrome P-450 has been estimated in samples of liver either biopsied with a needle[165] or by wedge biopsy at surgical operation.[48]

Pharmacodynamics

Strictly speaking, pharmacodynamics refers to studies of the response to a given concentration of drug at the target organ or effector tissue, but since it is not usually possible to measure the concentration in the tissue itself, pharmacodynamics will be defined in this chapter as 'a study of the response to a given concentration of a drug in the blood'.

Surprisingly few well-conducted pharmacodynamic studies have been undertaken either in health or disease. Furthermore, relatively little is known about individual differences in response to the same concentration of drug in the blood.[65,169] There is, however, evidence for individual differences in receptor sensitivity and increasing information on alterations in response to drugs with ageing. Despite this paucity of information, pharmacodynamic factors should be remembered when considering the potential response of an individual to drugs. Changes relating to hepatic disease are discussed in the following section.

LIVER DISEASE AND THE RESPONSE TO DRUGS

Introduction

Despite the obvious importance of the liver in the handling of drugs, there have been few well-controlled studies on the effects of hepatic disease. However, from the foregoing discussion it should be apparent that liver disease could affect the response to drugs in a number of ways: firstly, by changing the bioavailability, half-life or clearance of a drug; secondly, the unbound fraction may increase, thereby altering the pharmacological effects; and finally, the response of the end organ may vary.

Much of the work done previously has assumed that patients with liver disease represent a homogeneous group. This is clearly erroneous and in the present review liver disease will be subdivided into (a) acute liver disease due to toxins, e.g. paracetamol overdosage and acute viral hepatitis (AVH), and (b) chronic liver disease, that is chronic hepatitis and cirrhosis. The severity of chronic liver disease varies from one patient to another, but whether the illness is compensated or not is among the more important factors which will determine the response to drugs. Thus, patients who are jaundiced, hypoproteinaemic or show evidence of encephalopathy will tend to respond differently from others who are well compensated. Finally, most hospital patients and a high proportion of those in general practice will be receiving drug treatment. Inevitably, some of these will have an effect on drug protein binding and on the activity of the microsomal enzyme oxidizing system. Concurrent or recent drug therapy may, therefore, mask the effects of liver disease[109] or possibly aggravate it.[143]

Bioavailability and Liver Disease

Absorption

There are no reliable data on drug absorption in hepatic disease. It might, however, be anticipated that absorption of some drugs would be reduced in patients with obstructive jaundice. Furthermore, interruption of the enterohepatic circulation could alter the half-life of digitoxin and some antibiotics. The ion exchange resin, cholestyramine, which has been used to treat pruritus associated with biliary obstruction,[46] can also reduce the reabsorption of drugs which undergo an enterohepatic recirculation, thereby reducing their half-lives.[40]

Metabolism at the first pass

The best evidence for an alteration in the bioavailability produced by hepatic disease exists for propranolol[160] and lignocaine[79] and relates to subjects or dogs in whom a portacaval anastomosis has been created. Similar changes should be expected in patients with cirrhosis and oesophageal varices or other portasystemic anastomoses.

More recently, attention has been focused on the plasma concentration–time profile for propranolol in patients with coeliac and Crohn's disease. The higher plasma concentrations seen in these diseases[134,155] do not relate to altered gastrointestinal transit[81] but are due in all probability to complicating hepatic disease.[66]

Altered volumes of distribution

Extensive data are now available on the volumes of distribution of analgesics,[9,30,98,124] anticonvulsants,[25] anticoagulants,[191] minor tranquillizers,[33,99,166] cardioactive drugs including lignocaine,[62,175,176,190] propranolol[31] and barbiturates.[36,120] See tables for individual drug data. From these it would appear that there is no alteration in the volume of distribution of drugs in acute viral hepatitis. In contrast, the volume of distribution is usually increased in patients with cirrhosis, particularly in those whose serum albumin concentrations are depressed. The most prominent changes are seen with lignocaine[176] and propranolol.[31]

Protein binding

Protein binding may be significantly reduced, particularly where a drug is heavily bound to plasma proteins; for example, phenylbutazone,[183] phenytoin,[5] diazepam[99] and tolbuamide.[174] There is usually a good correlation between the serum albumin concentration and the degree of protein binding which will, therefore, be reduced in the presence of hypoalbuminaemia. In addition, an elevated serum bilirubin in jaundiced patients may displace drugs from their binding to sites on plasma proteins. Finally, binding may be particularly lowered in patients who, in addition to being jaundiced and having a lowered serum albumin concentration, are uraemic – the hepatorenal syndrome[131] (see Chapter 46).

Elimination half-life

This is by far the most widely studied parameter in liver disease. Little change has been demonstrated in the half-life of most drugs during acute viral hepatitis, except in patients who are severely ill. However, diazepam is an exception and shows a prolonged half-life in this situation,[99] as does pethidine.[124] In contrast, the half-life of many drugs is prolonged in patients with cirrhosis or chronic active hepatitis, particularly those who are hypoalbuminaemic, jaundiced and show a diminished clearance of indocyanine green.[30,32] Data relating to individual drugs can be found in the tables.

Clearance

This parameter has been measured only comparatively recently in patients with liver disease but is probably the most sensitive index of overall dysfunction. Thus, the clearance of antipyrine,[8] pethidine[124] and lignocaine,[190] is depressed during attacks of acute viral hepatitis but increases during recovery. However, clearance tends to be disturbed to a greater degree in patients with chronic liver disease, the extent varying according to the serum albumin, bilirubin and indocyanine green clearance.[30,32] Data relating to individual drugs can be found in the tables.

Individual Drugs

Anti-inflammatory analgesics

Antipyrine. Although not widely used as an anti-inflammatory analgesic, antipyrine has been widely studied as a 'model drug' because of its distribution throughout body water, total dependence on liver metabolism for elimination and uniformly low degree of protein binding. Data relating to studies published to date are detailed in Table 16.2.

Paracetamol. The half-life of paracetamol is unchanged in the great majority of patients with liver disease, including those with cirrhosis[62] in whom the half-life averages 2.9 ± 0.3 hr compared with the normal 2.0 ± 0.4 hr. Only in patients with severe liver damage due to paracetamol overdosage is there a clinically significant prolongation of the half-life[142] (see Table 16.2).

Phenylbutazone. The protein binding of phenylbutazone is diminished in patients with hepatic disease.[183] This may, in part, account for the failure of Brodie, Burns and Weiner[39] and Hvidberg, Andreasen and Ranck[91] to demonstrate prolongation of the half-life in patients with cirrhosis. However, a prolongation of the

Table 16.2. *Drug Class: Anti-inflammatory Analgesics.*

Type of patient	No.	Dose	Route	Protein binding %	V_d(1/kg)	$t_{\frac{1}{2}}$(hr)	Cl/ml/min/kg	Reference
Antipyrine								
Controls	20	1 g	I.V.	—	—	11.9 (5.3–13.9)	—	Brodie, Burns & Weiner[39]
Cirrhotics	9	1 g	I.V.	—	—	9.0 (3.3–11.9)	—	
Controls	6	1.2 g	o	—	33.3±2.8	—	38.4±4.4	Branch, Herbert & Read[30]
Chronic liver disease								
Albumin > 3 g/100 ml	5	1.2 g	o	—	33.6±2.4	—	27.1±2.1	
Albumin < 3 g/100 ml	9	1.2 g	o	—	41.3±3.2	—	10.3±1.6	
Chronic active hepatitis	1	18 mg/kg	o	—	—	137	—	Adjepon-Yamoah, Nimmo & Prescott[4]
Controls	9	15 mg/kg	I.V.	—	36.9±9.3	7.9±1.7	58.6±16.6	Andreasen et al[9]
Cirrhotics	11 }							
Halothane hepatitis	1 }	15 mg/kg	I.V.	—	38.5±7.3	31.8±19.5	18.5±11.8	
Biliary obstruction	1 }							
Cirrhotics	5	15 mg/kg	I.V.	—	—	—	9.6±1.9	Andreasen & Ranek[8]
Cirrhotics with encephalopathy	13	15 mg/kg	I.V.	—	—	—	4.6±1.4	
AVH	1	15 mg/kg	I.V.	—	—	—	5.9	
5/12 later							54.5	
Cirrhotics (17)+2 others	19	18 mg/kg	o	—	—	30.3±6.8	—	Forrest et al[62]
Paracetamol								
Paracetamol overdosage	17	N.K.	o	—	—	7.6±0.8	—	Prescott et al[143]
Healthy normals	17	—	—	—	—	2.0±0.4	—	
Cirrhotics (15)+2 others	17	1.5 g	o	—	—	2.9±0.3	—	Forrest et al[62]
Phenylbutazone								
Controls	10	800 mg	o	—	—	72 (44–114)	—	Brodie, Burns & Weiner[39]
Cirrhotics	11	800 mg	o	—	—	51 (32–122)	—	
Normals	36	400–600 mg	o	—	—	78.1±14.6	—	Levi, Sherlock & Walker[109]
Liver disease (no inducing drugs)	34	400–600 mg	o	—	—	100±29	—	
Liver disease (on inducing drugs)	61	400–600 mg	o	—	—	54.3±18.4	—	
Normals (on inducing drugs)	19	400–600 mg	o	—	—	57.2±17.4	—	
Controls	8	—	—	94±1.1	—	—	—	Wallace & Brodie[183]
Chronic hepatic disease	6	—	—	90±2.0	—	—	—	
Salicylic acid								
Controls	6	1.3 g	I.V.	—	—	6.1 (4.7–9.0)	—	Brodie, Burns & Weiner[39]
Cirrhotics	8	1.3 g	I.V.	—	—	6.6 (3.3–10.3)	—	

V_d = volume of distribution; $t_{\frac{1}{2}}$ = half-life in blood or plasma; Cl = clearance; I.V. = intravenous; o = oral; AVH = acute viral hepatitis; N.K. = not known. Range shown in parentheses.

half-life was encountered by Levi, Sherlock and Walker[109] but only in patients who were not receiving drugs known to induce microsomal enzyme oxidation (see Table 16.2).

Salicyclic acid (see Table 16.2).

Narcotic analgesics

Morphine. Although there is some evidence for an increased sensitivity to morphine in patients with cirrhosis[107] there are no data on its pharmacokinetics in liver disease. However, protein binding is significantly depressed in hepatic failure[131] (see Table 16.3).

Pethidine. The half-life of pethidine is more than doubled in patients with cirrhosis[98] and during acute viral hepatitis.[124] This drug is best avoided in patients with hepatic disease. Pharmacokinetic details are shown in Table 16.3.

Anticonvulsants

Phenobarbitone (see Table 16.4). Phenobarbitone is only partially metabolized in the liver, and renal excretion can therefore compensate to some degree for alterations in hepatic metabolism. Nevertheless, the half-life is prolonged in patients with cirrhosis and to a lesser degree in patients with acute viral hepatitis.[7]

Phenytoin (see Table 16.4). The unbound fraction is increased in patients with hepatic disease.[5,25,131] Since the pharmacological and therapeutic effects relate to the free concentration, patients with hepatic disease tend to have their epilepsy controlled at lower total plasma phenytoin concentrations than usual. Furthermore, intoxication is particularly likely to occur in patients with liver disease.[97,106] There are, however, few data on the half-life of phenytoin in liver disease.

Anticoagulants (see Chapter 8)

The half-life of dicoumarol is prolonged in patients with cirrhosis[39] and an accentuation of its hypoprothrombinaemic effects has been seen following exposure to carbon tetrachloride,[14] a hepatotoxin which is known to impair oxidative enzymes in liver microsomes by decreasing the amount of cytochrome P-450.[153] However, the half-life of phenprocoumon (Marcumar) is unchanged in cirrhotics[84] and the pharmacokinetics of warfarin are unchanged in patients with acute viral hepatitis[191] (see Table 16.5).

Anti-asthma drugs

Theophylline. The half-life of theophylline is substantially prolonged in patients with cirrhosis[139,144] (see Table 16.6).

Corticosteroids (see Chapter 29; Table 16.6). The half-life of prednisolone is slightly prolonged in patients with chronic liver disease[142] but total serum concentrations of prednisolone are depressed following oral administration of prednisone due, presumably, to decreased 11β-hydroxy-dehydrogenase activity. Nevertheless, the activity of corticosteroids is increased in patients with hepatic disease due to lowered serum protein concentrations:[111] the frequency of prednisone side-effects is doubled when serum albumin concentrations are less than 2.5 g/100 ml.

Minor tranquillizers: benzodiazepines

Unwanted CNS effects of diazepam are considerably more frequent in patients with reduced serum albumin concentrations.[78] In patients with normal serum albumin concentrations 2.9 per cent have unwanted CNS depression compared with 9.3 per cent in those with severe hypoalbuminaemia (<3 g/100 ml). (Similar effects were reported for chlordiazepoxide.)[78] This finding accords with reduced binding of diazepam recorded by Klotz et al[99] and Thiessen et al.[174] Furthermore, only 17.9 ± 5.8 mg of intravenous diazepam was required as a premedication for endoscopy in patients with liver disease compared with 27 ± 12.1 mg in normals,[33] and individual doses showed a strong correlation with the serum albumin concentration. Thus, diazepam, which is known to produce substantial reductions in arterial blood-gas tensions during upper gastrointestinal endoscopy,[185] should be used with caution in patients with hepatic disease. In contrast, oxazepam does not show an appreciable alteration in its pharmacokinetics in patients with hepatic disease[166] (see Table 16.7).

Major tranquillizers

Few data are available on phenothiazines and butyrophenones in hepatic disease. There is, however, no evidence for prolongation of the chlorpromazine half-life in patients with cirrhosis[121] (see Table 16.8).

Table 16.3. *Drug Class: Narcotic Analgesics.*

Type of patient	No.	Dose	Route	Protein binding %	V_d(1/kg)	$t\frac{1}{2}$(hr)	Cl/ml/min/kg	Reference
Morphine								
Normals	—	—	—	35.1	—	—	—	Olsen, Bennett & Porter[131]
Hepatic failure	2	—	—	25.0 (21.2–28.8)	—	—	—	
Pethidine								
Normals	8	0.8 mg/kg	I.V.	64.3±13.5	4.17±1.33	3.21±0.80	1316±383	Klotz et al[98]
Cirrhotics	10	0.8 mg/kg	I.V.	64.9±5.8	5.76±2.55	7.04±0.92	664±293	
Normals	15	—	—	58.3±8.2	5.94±2.65	3.37±0.82	1261±527	McHorse et al[124]
AVH	14	—	—	56.0±11.8	5.56±1.8	6.99±2.74	649±278	
In recovery	(5)	—	—	—	—	3.25±0.8	—	

V_d = volume of distribution; $t\frac{1}{2}$ = half-life in blood or plasma; Cl = clearance; I.V. = intravenous; AVH = acute viral hepatitis.

Table 16.4. *Drug Class: Anticonvulsants.*

Type of patient	No.	Dose	Route	Protein binding %	V_d(l/kg)	$t\frac{1}{2}$(hr)	Cl/ml/min/kg	Reference
Phenobarbitone								
Normals	8	0.85–2.55 mg/kg	o	—	—	86±3	—	Alvin et al[7]
Cirrhotics	9			—	—	130±15	—	
AVH	8			—	—	104 (60–177)	—	
Phenytoin								
Normals	—	—	—	10.6±1.3 (free)	—	—	—	Hooper et al[90]
Hepatic disease	—	—	—	15.9±6.0 (free)	—	—	—	
Normals	—	—	—	8.3±0.8% (free)	—	—	—	Affrime & Reidenberg[5]
Cirrhotics	8	—	—	11.7±6.2% (free)	—	—	—	
AVH								
Acute	5	250 mg	I.V.	12.6% (free)	0.68	13.2	2.55	Blaschke et al[25]
Recovery	—	—	—	9.9% (free)	0.63	13.5	2.22	
Hepatic failure	2	—	—	76.3 (63–89.6)	—	—	—	Olsen, Bennett & Porter[131]
Hepatorenal syndrome	3	—	—	77.5±2.2	—	—	—	

V_d = volume of distribution; $t\frac{1}{2}$ = half-life in blood or plasma; Cl = clearance; AVH = acute viral hepatitis; o = oral; I.V. = intravenous.

Table 16.5. *Drug Class: Anticoagulants.*

Type of patient	No.	Dose	Route	Protein binding %	V_d(l/kg)	$t\frac{1}{2}$(hr)	Cl/ml/min/kg	Reference
Dicoumarol								
Controls	19	0.3 g	I.V.	—	—	30.7 (7.2–100)	—	Brodie, Burns & Weiner[39]
Cirrhotics	6	0.3 g	I.V.	—	—	50.6 (15.4–100)	—	
Phenprocoumon								
Cirrhotics	3	20 mg	I.V.	—	—	139 (103–160)	—	Heni, Lehnhardt & Glogner[84]
	2	10 mg	I.V.	—	—	132 (128–136)	—	
Normals						150		
Warfarin								
AVH	5	15 mg	o	—	0.19 ± 0.04	23 ± 5	6.1 ± 0.9	Williams et al[191]
Acute recovery	—	15 mg	o	—	0.21 ± 0.02	25 ± 3	61 ± 0.7	

V_d = volume of distribution; $t\frac{1}{2}$ = half-life in blood or plasma; Cl = clearance; I.V. = intravenous; AVH = acute viral hepatitis; o = oral.

Table 16.6. *Drug Class: Anti-asthma Compounds.*

Type of patient	No.	Dose	Route	Protein binding %	V_d(1/kg)	t½(hr)	Cl/ml/min/kg	Reference
Theophylline								
Normals	5	2.8 mg/kg	I.V.	—	—	9.2±1.5	—	Piafsky et al[139]
Cirrhotics	4	2.8 mg/kg	I.V.	—	No change	30.0±17.8	—	
Normals	—	5.6 mg/kg	I.V.	—	—	6.7 (2.8–12.4)	—	Rangno et al[144]
Cirrhotics	—	5.6 mg/kg	—	—	—	30.8 (11.5–55.8)	—	
Corticosteroids								
Prednisolone								
Controls	3	—	—	—	—	2.92 (2.5–3.25)	—	Powell & Axelsen[142]
Chronic liver disease	3	—	—	—	—	3.69 (3.25–4.16)	—	
Normals	8	—	—	53.5±5.2	—	—	—	
Active chronic hepatitis	9	—	—	46.6±5.8	—	—	—	
Inactive chronic hepatitis	7	—	—	54.3±4.1	—	—	—	
AVH	6	—	—	50.4±7.0	—	—	—	

V_d = volume of distribution; t½ = half-life in blood or plasma; Cl = clearance; I.V. = intravenous; AVH = acute viral hepatitis.

Table 16.7. *Drug Class: Tranquillizers (Benzodiazepines).*

Type of patient	No.	Dose	Route	Protein binding %	V_d(l/kg)	$t\frac{1}{2}$(hr)	Cl/ml/min/kg	Reference
Diazepam								
Normals	5	0.1 mg/kg	I.V.	97.8 ± 1.0	1.13 ± 0.28	46.6 ± 14.2	44.8 ± 9.1	Klotz et al[99]
Cirrhotics	9	0.1 mg/kg	I.V.	95.3 ± 1.8	1.74 ± 0.21	105.6 ± 15.2	24.8 ± 12.7	
AVH	8	10 mg	o	—	—	74.5 ± 27.5	—	
CAH	4	10 mg	o	—	—	59.7 ± 23.0	—	
Controls	5	27 ± 5.4 mg	I.V.	—	0.98 ± 0.41	43 ± 7.2	15.1 ± 6.9	Branch et al[33]
Chronic liver disease								
No ascites	10	17.9 ± 1.5 mg	I.V.	—	0.69 ± 0.44	48.7 ± 38.3	10.6 ± 6.2	
With ascites	7	17.9 ± 1.5 mg	I.V.	—	0.59 ± 0.29	77.4 ± 11.4	6.0 ± 3.9	
Normals	21	—	—	98.5 ± 0.4	—	—	—	Thiessen et al[174]
Alcoholics	14	—	—	97.8 ± 1.2	—	—	—	
Oxazepam								
Young normals	8	45 mg[a]	o	86.7 ± 4.7	52.5 ± 15.6	5.1 ± 1.4	112.5 ± 32.8	Shull et al[166]
AVH	7	45 mg	o	86.0 ± 3.8	62.0 ± 22.0	5.3 ± 0.8	137.4 ± 55.6	
Middle-aged normals	8	45 mg[a]	o	89.6 ± 4.5	70.6 ± 13.6	5.6 ± 0.8	136.0 ± 49.5	
Cirrhotics	6	45 mg	o	87.6 ± 3.5	76.5 ± 29.9	5.8 ± 1.2	155.5 ± 52.7	

[a] Except 2 who received 15 mg o.
V_d = volume of distribution; $t\frac{1}{2}$ = half-life in blood or plasma; Cl = clearance; I.V. = intravenous; AVH = acute viral hepatitis; o = oral; CAV = chronic active hepatitis.

Table 16.8. *Drug Class: Tranquillizers (Phenothiazines).*

Type of patient	No.	Dose	Route	Protein binding %	V_d(l/kg)	$t\frac{1}{2}$(hr)	k_{el}/hr	Reference
Chlorpromazine								
Normals	13	25 mg	I.V.	—	—	31	0.053	Maxwell et al[121]
Cirrhotics	24 }							
On inducing drugs	7 }	25 mg	I.V.	—	—	7	0.078	
No drugs	14 }			—	—	14	0.078	

V_d = volume of distribution; $t\frac{1}{2}$ = half-life in blood or plasma; k_{el}/hr = overall first-order elimination rate constant (see text); I.V. = intravenous.

Oral hypoglycaemic agents

Data are confined to tolbutamide (see Table 16.9) and they are conflicting. Ueda et al[179] have claimed that the half-life of tolbutamide was prolonged in five of ten cirrhotic patients whom they studied. These findings were challenged by Nelson[127] because of a failure to take account of the normal range of variability. However, it seems likely that the pharmacological effect may be slightly increased due to a reduction in protein binding.[179]

Cardioactive drugs (see also George[194])

Digoxin. There is no evidence of an alteration in half-life of this drug.[17,193] It is possible, however, that its distribution volume may be altered, but there are no data on this point.

Lignocaine. Data showing that the handling of this drug is abnormal in patients with acute viral hepatitis and markedly altered in those with chronic hepatic disease are extensive (see Table 16.10). This drug must therefore be used with extreme caution in patients with liver disease.

Propranolol. Similarly, the pharmacokinetics of propranolol are highly abnormal in liver disease. The bioavailability is increased,[160] the clearance reduced and the half-life prolonged,[31] due in part to diminished protein binding[58] and, in all probability, to a diminution of hepatic blood flow as there is a close correlation between the clearance of propranolol and that of indocyanine green.[31] Liver blood flow is known to determine the half-life of propranolol.[58,67] Furthermore, the intrinsic clearance rate by metabolism is important[162,188] (see Table 16.10). Finally, since the pharmacological effect depends upon the free concentration[123] and the latter may be increased when the serum albumin concentration is reduced, the effects of propranolol may be accentuated in liver disease.

Quinidine. The protein binding of quinidine is considerably reduced in patients with alcoholic liver disease and this necessitates reduction in the dosage.[5]

Barbiturates

The effects of liver disease on the pharmacokinetics of individual barbiturate drugs are summarized in Tables 16.4 and 16.11. The half-life of amylobarbitone is prolonged and its clearance diminished, particularly in patients with reduced serum albumin concentrations;[120] similar findings have been reported for hexobarbitone in acute viral hepatitis.[36] However, the removal of pentobarbitone appears to be 'more rapid' in patients with cirrhosis.[159] The anaesthetic induction agent, thiopentone, has a prolonged duration of action in patients with hepatic disease (mean 489 sec compared with 152 sec) after 4 mg/kg I.V.[165] Thus, the dose required to produce anaesthesia for 60 min was 0.54 g in patients with severe liver damage compared with 1.04 g in normal subjects.[53] This is probably due to diminished protein binding in patients with hepatic disease.[68]

Neuromuscular blocking drugs

The requirements for *d*-tubocurarine are also reduced in patients with hepatic disease,[53] due to diminished hydrolysis.[61,122,182] Similarly, the rate of procaine hydrolysis is reduced from 0.66 ± 0.14 min to 2.3 ± 0.9 min.[146]

Data relating to these and a few other drugs, published mainly in abstract form, are summarized by Closson.[42]

Antibiotics

Penicillins and cephalosporins (see Table 16.12). Penicillins are significantly metabolized by the liver,[43] 10 to 20 per cent of an oral dose being excreted as penicilloic acids and other derivatives. Nevertheless, the rapid urinary excretion of unmetabolized penicillins permits normal therapeutic dosage in patients with liver disease. Most penicillins are secreted in an active form into the bile but this becomes a significant route for excretion only in patients with severe renal failure. Thus, Hoffman, Cestero and Bullock[88] found that in five oliguric patients with severe hepatic dysfunction the mean half-life of carbenicillin was 23.2 ± 2.9 hr, some 7.5 hr longer than in those with oliguric renal failure alone. Clearly care must be taken in order to prevent toxicity from penicillins occurring in patients with hepatorenal failure. Two penicillins should be avoided in patients with liver disease: talampicillin, which is hydrolysed in part by the liver to ampicillin and an ester moiety,[100] and nafcillin, which is largely excreted via the bile.[130]

Table 16.9. *Drug Class: Oral Hypoglycaemics.*

Type of patient	No.	Dose	Route	Protein binding %	V_d(l/kg)	$t\frac{1}{2}$(hr)	Cl/ml/min/kg	Reference
Tolbutamide								
Normals	7	20 mg/kg	I.V.	—	—	4.4±0.7	—	Ueda et al[179]
Cirrhotics	10	20 mg/kg	I.V.	—	—	normal in 5; 9.3 in 5 (7.8±11.2)	—	
Unspecified liver disease	10	0.56	o	—	—	6.0 (3.2–10.0)	—	Nelson[127]
Normals	21	50 μg/ml[a]	—	97.9±0.3	—	—	—	Thiessen et al[174]
		300 μg/ml	—	95.2±0.6	—	—	—	
Alcoholics	14	50 μg/ml	—	96.3±2.6	—	—	—	
		300 μg/ml	—	88.1±8.5	—	—	—	

V_d = volume of distribution; $t\frac{1}{2}$ = half-life in blood or plasma; Cl = clearance; I.V. = intravenous; o = oral.
[a]Concentration per ml plasma.

Table 16.10. *Drug Class: Cardioactive Drugs.*

Type of patient	No.	Dose	Route	Protein binding %	V_d(l/kg)	$t\frac{1}{2}$(hr)	Cl/ml/min/kg	Reference
Digoxin								
Cirrhotics	3	1 mg	I.V.	—	—	33.6 ± 38.4 (normal 30–40)	—	Marcus & Kapadia[117]
AVH	5	0.375–0.75 mg	I.V.	—	—	0.78 ± 0.23 ng/ml at 24 hr (normal 1.06 ± 0.32)	—	Zilly, Richter & Rietbrock[193]
Lignocaine								
Normals	10	50 mg	I.V.	—	1.70 ± 0.21	1.80 ± 0.17	701 ± 41	Thomson, Rowland & Melmon[175]
Liver disease (alcoholic)	8	50 mg	—	—	2.22 ± 0.94	5.72 ± 3.90	368 ± 180	
Normals	10	50 mg	—	—	1.32	1.8	10.0	Thomson et al[176]
Liver disease (alcoholic)	8	50 mg	—	—	2.31	4.9	6.0	
Normals	4	400 mg	o	—	—	1.40 ± 0.26	—	Adjepon-Yamoah, Nimmo & Prescott[4]
CAH	1	400 mg	—	—	—	19.1	—	
AVH	6	1 mg/kg	I.V.	56 ± 8 (free)	3.1 ± 1.8	2.67 (1.1–7.2)	13.0 ± 3.9/kg	Williams et al[190]
AVH in recovery	—	—	—	49 ± 12 (free)	2.0 ± 0.5	1.5 (1.2–3.5)	20.0 ± 3.9/kg	
Cirrhotics 16, CAH 3, Others 2	21	400 mg	o	—	—	6.6 ± 1.1	—	Forrest et al[62]
Propranolol (+)–isomer					V_d(l)			
Normals	6	40 mg	I.V.	—	221.5 (121–286)	2.9 (2.1–3.8)	919 (512–1326)	Branch, James & Read[31]
Cirrhotics 12, CAH 6, Others 2	20	40 mg	I.V.	—	460.1 (183–787)	15.6 (2.8–35.4)	463 (137–1086)	
Quinidine								
Normals	7	5 μg/ml[a]		14.1 ± 4.6 (free)	—	—	—	Affrime & Reidenberg[5]
Alcoholics	10			51.5 ± 16.0 (free)	—	—	—	

V_d = volume of distribution; $t\frac{1}{2}$ = half-life in blood or plasma; Cl = clearance; I.V. = intravenous; AVH = acute viral hepatitis; o = oral; CAH = chronic active hepatitis.
[a]Concentration per ml plasma.

Table 16.11. *Drug Class: Barbiturates.*

Type of patient	No.	Dose	Route	Protein binding %	V_d(l)	$t\frac{1}{2}$(hr)	Cl/ml/min	Reference
Amylobarbitone								
Normals	10	3.23 mg/kg	I.V.	60.7±5.3	91.3±32.3	21.1±3.9	92.0±22.1	Mawer, Miller & Turnberg[120]
Mixed liver disease								
Normal albumin	5	3.23 mg/kg	I.V.	60.5±2.4	114±43.4	17.7±4.1	118.9±28.0	
Low albumin	5	3.23 mg/kg	I.V.	31.0±13.8	79.5±40.0	39.4±14.8	41.0±11.4	
Hexobarbitone								
Normals	14	2.97–	I.V.	—	1.1±0.12/kg	4.35±1.15	3.57±0.83/kg	Breimer, Zilly & Richter[36]
AVH	13	7.32 mg/kg	—	—	1.1±0.40/kg	8.17±3.09	1.94±0.85/kg	
Pentobarbitone								
Controls	35	—	—	—	—	—	—	Sessions et al[159]
Liver disease (17 cirrhotics)	21	—	—	—	—	'more rapid'	—	
Thiopentone								
Normals	10	—	—	72 (28±0.9% free)	—	—	—	Ghoneim & Pandya[68]
Cirrhotics	10	—	—	47 (53±2.1% free)	—	—	—	

V_d = volume of distribution; $t\frac{1}{2}$ = half-life in blood or plasma; Cl = clearance; I.V. = intravenous; AVH = acute viral hepatitis.

Table 16.12. *Drug Class: Antibiotics (Penicillins and Cephalosporins).*

Type of patient	No.	Dose	Route	Protein binding %	$t\frac{1}{2}$(hr)	Renal excretion (% dose given)	Common duct bile concentration (mg/l)	References
Ampicillin[a]								
Normals	—	500 mg	o	20	0.8–1.0	92 I.V.	22.3 (10–36)	Acocella et al[3]
Amoxycillin[a]								
Normals	—	500 mg	o	25	1.0–1.3	50–64 (o)	9.5 (1–53)	Barza & Weinstein[16]
Cloxacillin[a]								
Normals	—	500 mg	o	93	0.5	41 (o)	—	Giusti[70]
Carbenicillin								
Normals	5	2 g	I.V.	50	1.0 ± 0.25	85	14–33	Hoffman, Cestero & Bullock[88]
Hepatic dysfunction	9	2 g	I.V.	—	1.9 ± 0.6	—	—	Jackson & McLeod[93]
Penicillin G[a]								
Normals	—	3 MU	I.V.	60	0.7	58–85 I.V.	10–20	Kosmidis et al[102]
Cephradine								
Normals	15	0.5 g	I.V.	28	0.48	88.4	14 mg/l (2.2–41)	Renzini et al[148]
Cephazolin								
Normals	15	0.5 g	I.V.	70	0.49	91.5	—	Paradelis[133]
Cephaloridine								
Normals	15	0.5 g	I.V.	41	0.49	88.9	—	

[a] Data calculated from more than one source.
$t\frac{1}{2}$ = half life in blood or plasma; o = oral; I.V. = intravenous.

Hepatic metabolism of cephalosporins is insignificant and biliary concentrations of the derivatives are low. Even after intravenous cephradine, a drug which is concentrated in the bile with peak concentrations occurring between one and two hours,[118] the elimination half-life is 0.49 hr and 61.4 per cent of the dose appears in the urine within two hours.[133] Thus, in the absence of concomitant renal failure cephalosporins may be used without special precautions in patients with hepatocellular damage.

Aminoglycosides. The aminoglycosides are excreted unchanged as a function of the glomerular filtration rate; no adjustment of the dosage is required in liver disease without concomitant renal failure.

Chloramphenicol (see Table 16.13). In patients with severely impaired liver function the rate of conjugation of chloramphenicol with glucuronic acid is reduced, resulting in prolongation of the serum half-life of unmetabolized drug.[14,104] Suhrland and Weisberger[172] showed definite erythropoietic depression in 8 of 16 patients with hepatic insufficiency who received chloramphenicol 2 g daily for 10 to 28 days. The suggestion was that only unmetabolized chloramphenicol is toxic to the marrow; certainly the mean free drug levels of 19 mg/l in cirrhotics with impaired red cell production was significantly higher than the mean level of 3 to 9 mg/l in patients with normal erythropoiesis. The relationship of direct toxicity to chloramphenicol-induced marrow aplasia is not clear. Nevertheless, with the availability of alternative treatments for meningitis (ampicillin) and salmonellosis (cotrimoxazole; mecillinam) there can be few indications for the use of chloramphenicol in patients with liver disease.

Tetracyclines (see Table 16.13). The fact that only 31 per cent of minocycline and 70 per cent of doxycycline can be recovered from faeces and urine in an active form[115] is suggestive of significant hepatic metabolism of these drugs. Hepatic metabolism is enhanced by induction of microsomal enzymes with anticonvulsants, as shown by the reduced half-life of doxycycline from 15.1 hr in normals to 7.4 hr in patients receiving drugs.[137] Despite reports by Bernard, Yin and Simons[20] that serum levels of minocycline are unaffected by hepatic disease, special care must be taken to avoid their accumulation in severe hepatocellular failure because tetracyclines are potent antimetabolites and are potentially hepatotoxic.[113] Erythromycin seems a safer choice for the treatment of chlamydial and rickettsial infections in patients with liver disease.

Clindamycin, lincomycin and erythromycin (see Tables 16.14 and 16.15). Excretion of clindamycin is significantly impaired in patients with liver disease; in hepatitis the half-life may be prolonged to 14 hr compared to the normal 3 hr.[34]

Accumulation of clindamycin may be hepatotoxic, resulting in raised serum alkaline phosphatase, glutamic oxaloacetic and glutamic pyruvic transaminases.[60,189] Single case studies suggest that clindamycin may be a cause of drug hepatitis.[55] Although other workers have not experienced problems using clindamycin in patients with liver disease,[85] caution is clearly indicated. The simplest approach is to use alternative antibiotics for the treatment of staphylococcal and anaerobic infections. If used in severe liver disease dosage reduction of clindamycin is required and should be monitored by serial blood assays.

The use of lincomycin in patients with liver disease is less well documented; nevertheless, the evidence indicates impaired excretion.[18]

Little unchanged erythromycin is excreted by the kidney. This suggests extensive secretion by the liver, some as the des-*N*-methyl derivative.[116] Hepatotoxicity appears to be confined to erythromycins substituted at the 2 'position' since Tolman, Sannella and Feston[177] found no cross-sensitivity between the toxic erythromycin estolate and erythromycin base, stearate, gluceptate or the ethylsuccinate. Given precautions to avoid overdosage erythromycin is potentially valuable for the treatment of chlamydial and rickettsial infections in patients with liver disease.

Fusidic acid. Less than 1 per cent of fusidic acid is excreted unchanged in the urine, indicating extensive metabolism by the liver.[71] Although fusidic acid is remarkably non-toxic, some impairment of bromsulphthalein excretion occurs[192] and there are anecdotal reports of jaundice: the drug should therefore be used with extreme caution in patients with hepatic failure.

Cotrimoxazole (see Table 16.16). Chemical assays have shown that although the sulphamethoxazole component is excreted normally in patients with liver disease, the half-life of trimethoprim may be prolonged to twice normal in patients with severe hepatic damage.[15]

Table 16.13. *Drug Class: Antibiotics (Chloramphenicol and Tetracyclines).*

Type of patient	No.	Dose	Route	Protein binding %	$t_{\frac{1}{2}}$(hr)	Renal excretion (% dose given)	Common duct bile concentration (mg/l)	References
Chloramphenicol								
Normals	4	10 mg/kg	I.V.	60	2.29 (1.72–2.82)	Total 75–90	—	Azzollini et al[14]
	18	500 mg	I.V.	—	2.9 (1.3–4.2)	Active 5–15	—	
Cirrhosis	8	10 mg/kg	I.V.	—	4.05 (2.19–6.42)	—	—	
Cirrhosis	11	500 mg	I.V.	—	5 (2–12)	Total 73 Active 11.9	—	Kunin, Glasko & Finland[104]
Tetracycline	10	1 g	o	65	10.8	60	0.5–4	Acocella et al[3]
Doxycycline	10	200 mg	o	90	16.7	33	—	Doluisio & Dittert[51]
Minocycline	10	600 mg	o	75	14.3	6	—	Macdonald et al[115]

$t_{\frac{1}{2}}$ = half-life in blood or plasma; I.V. = intravenous; o = oral.

Table 16.14. *Drug Class: Antibiotics (Clindamycin and Lincomycin).*

Type of patient	No.	Dose	Route	Protein binding %	$t\frac{1}{2}$(hr)	Renal excretion (% dose given)	Common duct bile concentration (mg/l)	References
Clindamycin								
Normals	6	300 mg	I.M.	—	3 (2.4–4.2)	15	—	Brandl et al[34]
	7	300 mg	I.V.	—	3.42±0.45	—	—	Avant, Schenker & Alford[13]
Acute hepatitis	6	300 mg	I.M.	—	7.3 (3.0–14.2)	—	—	
Hepatic dysfunction	—	varied	—	—	—	33	50	Williams et al[189]
Lincomycin								
Normals	6	600 mg	I.M.	72	4.9 (4.4–5.7)	6–15	—	Bellamy, Bates & Reinarz[18]
Hepatic insufficiency	9	600 mg	I.M.	—	9.0 (6.1–11.8)	—	—	Medina et al[125]

$t\frac{1}{2}$ = half-life in blood or plasma; I.M. = intramuscular; I.V. = intravenous.

Table 16.15. *Drug Class: Antibiotics (Erythromycin and Fusidic Acid).*

Type of patient	No.	Dose	Route	Protein binding %	$t\frac{1}{2}$(hr)	Renal excretion (% dose given)	Common duct bile concentration (mg/l)	References
Erythromycin								
Normals	14	125 to 500 mg	o	90	1.2	6–7 (parenteral)	200–500	Wiegand & Chun[186] Twiss et al[178]
Fusidic acid								
Normals	10	500 mg	o	95	8	<1	—	Godtfredsen, Roholt & Tybring[73] Godtfredsen[71]

$t\frac{1}{2}$ = half-life in blood or plasma; o = oral.

Table 16.16. *Drug Class: Antibiotics (Cotrimoxazole).*

Type of patient	No.	Dose	Route	Protein binding %	$t\frac{1}{2}$(hr)	Renal excretion (% dose given)	Common duct bile concentration (mg/l)	References
Cotrimoxazole								
Normals	6	2 tabs	o	—	—	—	161 (128–200)	Neuman, Kazmierczak & Cachin[128]
Hepatic dysfunction	6	2 tabs	o	—	—	—	50 (15–150)	
Trimethoprim								
Normals	13	320 mg	o	42–46	11.5 (8.4–13.5)	40.7 (24 hr)	—	Rieder & Schwartz[150]
Hepatic dysfunction	7	320 mg	o	—	14.3 (6.6–23.7)	25.3 (24 hr)	—	
Sulphamethoxazole								
Normals	13	1800 mg	o	62	12.1 (7.9–17.4)	57 (24 hr)	—	
Hepatic dysfunction	7	1800 mg	o	—	12.3 (9.3–15.1)	47.7 (24 hr)	—	

$t\frac{1}{2}$ = half-life in blood or plasma; o = oral.

However, the same workers found that following a single oral dose of cotrimoxazole the maximum plasma levels of both sulphamethoxazole and trimethoprim were lower by an average factor of 1.6 to 2.0 in patients with liver disease compared to normal controls. The suggested explanation was impaired absorption secondary to changes in the bile. The alternative possibility, that the lower plasma levels reflect an increased distribution volume, is untenable if the findings by Hitzenberger et al[87] of a reduced volume of distribution of trimethoprim in patients with cirrhosis (1.0 versus 1.71/kg) are correct. Lower than normal maintenance doses should be given in order to prevent accumulation of trimethoprim when cotrimoxazole is being used parenterally in patients with severe parenchymal damage. There is no reliable information on patients receiving oral therapy but similar precautions would seem sensible.

Metronidazole. Metronidazole is partially metabolized in the liver by oxidation of the hydroxy group on the side chain or by conjugation with glucuronic acid.[92] Significant amounts are excreted into the bile, mean levels of 28 mg/l being reported.[140] However, this drug may be reabsorbed since urinary excretion accounted for all of a 4.2 g course of therapy given over seven days.[96] Although there are no data on the use of metronidazole in patients with liver disease the fact that it is excreted by the kidneys together with its bactericidal action and ability to penetrate tissues suggest that it is the drug of choice for the treatment of anaerobic infections in patients with hepatic dysfunction.

Antifungal agents (see Table 16.17)

5-fluorocytosine. There is no evidence of metabolism of this drug by the liver; 90 per cent of the drug is recovered unchanged in the urine within 48 hours. A report of the administration of the drug to a single patient with cirrhosis showed serum levels of 5-fluorocytosine to be unchanged.[26] Hepatic dysfunction is not, therefore, a contraindication to the use of 5-fluorocytosine.

Amphotericin B. The metabolic fate of this drug is uncertain. The long half-life with continued detection in the urine up to seven days after administration suggests that metabolism is not an important means of disposal but that it is bound within the body and slowly released from this site.[22] There is no reason, on present evidence, to avoid this drug on grounds of liver disease.

Miconazole. Little information is available concerning the extent of this drug's metabolism by the liver. Although the drug appears to be generally safe, in the absence of such data it would be wise to treat patients who have hepatic dysfunction with antifungal agents whose pharmacokinetics have been defined.

Antituberculous drugs (see Chapter 36; Table 16.18)

Rifampicin. Rifampicin is extensively metabolized by the liver and can cause mild hepatotoxicity which may subside with continuation of treatment. Patients with pre-existing liver disease are at greater risk of developing other toxic manifestations.[21] Alternative drugs should be used in such subjects.

Isoniazid. Isoniazid is occasionally hepatotoxic but chronic liver disease in itself does not appear to predispose to further damage by this drug[23] and is not a contraindication to the use of this drug.

Ethambutol. Of the ethambutol which is absorbed from the gut, approximately 75 per cent is excreted unchanged in the urine; the remainder is excreted in urine as the aldehyde and dicarboxylic acid metabolites. No data are available on the handling of the drug in the presence of hepatic dysfunction, but in view of the small proportion of the drug which is metabolized it seems unlikely that liver disease would significantly increase the risk of toxicity from ethambutol.

Pyrazinamide. The principal toxicity of pyrazinamide is hepatic and fatal instances have been recorded. Although there are no studies of its metabolism in patients with pre-existing liver disease its use can be justified only in a desperate situation where no alternative drug is available.

Drugs not studied to date

Several attempts have been made to devise pharmacokinetic models for the effects of liver disease on drug handling: these have been summarized by Wilkinson and Shand,[188] Wilkinson and Schenker[187] and Blaschke.[24] Although the models produced by these authors

Table 16.17. *Drug Class: Antibiotics (Antifungal Agents).*

Type of patient	No.	Dose	Route	Protein binding %	$t_{\frac{1}{2}}$(hr)	Renal excretion (% dose given)	Common duct bile concentration (mg/l)	References
5-Fluorocytosine								
Normal	10	2 g	o	—	2.89	87	—	Schonebeck et al[157]
Miconazole								
Normal	18	522–3000 mg/day	I.V.	81–93	0.75	—	—	Lewi et al[110] Stevens, Levine & Deresinski[171]
Amphotericin B								
Normal	15	45 mg/day	I.V.	91–95	24	2–5	—	Bindschadler & Bennett[22] Block[26]

$t_{\frac{1}{2}}$ = half-life in blood or plasma; o = oral; I.V. = intravenous.

Table 16.18. *Drug Class: Antibiotics (Antituberculars).*

Type of pateint	No.	Dose	Route	Protein binding %	$t_{\frac{1}{2}}$(hr)	Renal excretion (% dose given)	Common duct bile concentration (mg/l)	References
Ethambutol								
Normal	10	25 mg/kg	o	—	6	70	—	Place & Thomas[141]
Isoniazid								
Normal	12	600 mg	o	None	3.24±0.14 6.74±0.33	5–25	—	Acocella et al[3]
Chronic liver disease	13	600 mg	o	—	—	—	—	Jackson & McLeod[93]
Pyrazinamide								
Normal	27	1.5 g/day	o	—	6.1	34	—	Ellard[54]
Rifampicin								
Normal	12	600 mg	o	75	2.8±0.22	5–24	—	Acocella et al[3]
Chronic liver disease	13	600 mg	o	—	6.74±0.33	—	—	Binda et al[21] Jackson & McLeod[93]

$t_{\frac{1}{2}}$ = half life in blood or plasma; o = oral.

have some value they are no substitute for studies of individual drug pharmacokinetics in various disease states.[47] Nevertheless, the following conclusions may be drawn. Hepatic disease may lead to increased bioavailability of orally administered drugs if they undergo a high clearance at the first pass. The distribution volume tends to be increased in patients with chronic hepatic disease, particularly those with reduced serum albumin concentrations. Protein binding is also reduced in patients who are hypoalbuminaemic, jaundiced and/or uraemic, leading to increased pharmacological and therapeutic effects. The elimination half-lives of drugs which are metabolized by the microsomal enzymes as well as metabolic clearances are usually unchanged in acute viral hepatitis, but considerable alterations can occur in patients with decompensated chronic liver disease. These changes are accompanied by a reduction in serum albumin and reduced clearance of indocyanine green or portasystemic encephalopathy. Smaller than normal doses of most drugs should be used in such patients.

Cytochrome P-450 activity in liver disease

Studies of this and other enzyme activity in hepatic disease are comparatively few. Three studies have been published. The first, by Doshi, Luisada-Opper and Leevy concerned microsomal pentobarbital hydroxylate activity in acute viral hepatitis.[52] In the second, cytochrome P-450 content has been studied in patients with severe hepatitis and cirrhosis.[156] Finally, *N*-oxidation of dimethyl aniline and oxidative demethylation of aminopyrine has been studied by Gold and Ziegler.[74] All three studies confirmed that enzymic activity is preserved in hepatitis, except in the most severe cases, and the P-450 content may fall to 50 per cent of normal values. Similar changes can occur in cirrhosis. However, NADPH-cytochrome-*c*-reductase activity remains unimpaired even in severe liver damage. Furthermore, P-450 activity may be increased in areas of regenerating tissue.

Pharmacodynamics

Altered pharmacodynamic responses have been clearly demonstrated for three groups of drugs in hepatic diseases: anticoagulants, sedatives and diuretics.

Anticoagulants

The ability to synthesis the vitamin K_1-dependent clotting factors II, VII, IX and X in patients with severe liver disease is reduced. Thus, their sensitivity to oral anticoagulants of either the coumarin or indanedione series is increased.[180]

Sedatives

Morphine tolerance is diminished in patients with hepatic cirrhosis, particularly those who have previously had episodes of portasystemic encephalopathy.[107] These authors attributed the changes to an increased sensitivity of the CNS to morphine but it is equally possible that they reflect the diminished protein binding demonstrated by Olsen, Bennett and Porter.[131] However, patients with cirrhosis are more susceptible to the effects of chlorpromazine[145] and this is almost certainly due to an altered end organ response.[121] The increased sensitivity to diazepam[33] may be explained by pharmacokinetic changes.

Diuretics

Whilst there is no doubt of the usefulness of these agents in the treatment of patients with oedema due to hepatic disease, they are extremely hazardous.[44] Encephalopathy is likely to develop in up to 20 per cent of patients treated with frusemide and great care must be taken to give adequate potassium replacement therapy.

ACKNOWLEDGEMENTS

Figures 16.2 and 16.4 are reproduced from *Journal of Pharmacokinetics and Biopharmaceutics* (1976) with the kind permission of the Plenum Publishing Corporation. Figure 16.5 is reproduced from George[65] with the kind permission of the publishers, Kimpton.

Finally, we wish to thank Mrs F.D. Lowman who typed the original manuscript.

REFERENCES

1. Ablad, B., Ervik, M., Hallgren, J., Johnsson, G. & Solvell, L. (1972) Pharmacological effects and serum levels of orally administered alprenolol in man. *European Journal of Clinical Pharmacology*, **5**, 44–52.

2. Acocella, G., Mattiussi, R., Nicolis, F.B., Pallanza, R. & Tenconi, L.T. (1968) Biliary excretion of antibiotics in man. *Gut*, **9**, 536–545.
3. Acocella, G., Bonollo, L., Garimoldi, M., Mainardi, M., Tenconi, L.T. & Nicolis, F.B. (1972) Kinetics of rifampicin and isoniazid administered alone and in combination to normal subjects and patients with liver disease. *Gut*, **13**, 47–53.
4. Adjepon-Yamoah, K.K., Nimmo, J. & Prescott, L.F. (1974) Gross impairment of hepatic drug metabolism in a patient with chronic liver disease. *British Medical Journal*, **iv**, 387–388.
5. Affrime, M. & Reidenberg, M.M. (1975) The protein binding of some drugs in plasma from patients with alcoholic liver disease. *European Journal of Clinical Pharmacology*, **8**, 267–269.
6. Alexanderson, B., Price Evans, D.A. & Sjoqvist, F. (1969) Steady-state levels of nortripyline in twins: influence of genetic factors and drug therapy. *British Medical Journal*, **iv**, 764–768.
7. Alvin, J., McHorse, T., Hoyumpa, A., Bush, M.T. & Schenker, S. (1975) The effect of liver disease in man on the disposition of phenobarbital. *Journal of Pharmacology and Experimental Therapeutics*, **192**, 224–235.
8. Andreasen, P.B. & Ranek, L. (1975) Liver failure and drug metabolism. *Scandinavian Journal of Gastroenterology*, **10**, 293–297.
9. Andreasen, P.B., Ranek, L., Statland, B.E. & Tygstrup, N. (1974) Clearance of antipyrine-dependence on quantitative liver function. *European Journal of Clinical Investigation*, **4**, 129–134.
10. Anton, A.H. (1960) The relation between the binding of sulfonamides to albumin and their antibacterial efficacy. *Journal of Pharmacology and Experimental Therapeutics*, **129**, 282–290.
11. Anton, A.H. (1973) Increasing activity of sulfonamides with displacing agents: a review. *Annals of the New York Academy of Sciences*, **226**, 273–292.
12. Anton, A.H. & Boyle, J.J. (1964) Alteration of the acetylation of sulphonamides by protein binding, sulphinpyrazone and suramin. *Canadian Journal of Physiology and Pharmacology*, **42**, 809–817.
13. Avant, G.R., Schenker, S., Alford, R.H. (1975) The effect of cirrhosis on the disposition and elimination of clindamycin. *American Journal of Digestive Diseases*, **20**, 223–230.
14. Azzollini, F., Gazzaniga, A., Lodola, E. & Natangelo, R. (1972) Elimination of chloramphenicol and thiamphenicol in subjects with cirrhosis of the liver. *International Journal of Clinical Pharmacology, Therapy and Toxicology*, **6**, 130–134.
15. Baraka, A. & Gabali, F. (1968) Correlation between tubocurarine requirements and plasma protein pattern. *British Journal of Anaesthetics*, **40**, 89–93.
16. Barza, M. & Weinstein, L. (1976) Pharmacokinetics of the penicillins in man. *Clinical Pharmacokinetics*, **1**, 297–308.
17. Barza, M., Samuelson, T. & Weinstein, L. (1974) Penetration of antibiotics into fibrin loci in vivo. II. Comparison of nine antibiotics: effect of dose and degree of protein binding. *Journal of Infectious Diseases*, **129**, 66–72.
18. Bellamy, H. Jr, Bates, B.B. & Reinarz, J.A. (1966) Lincomycin metabolism in patients with hepatic insufficiency: effect of liver disease on lincomycin serum concentration. In *Antimicrobial Agents and Chemotherapy*. (Ed.) Hobby, G.L. pp. 36–41. Michigan: The American Society for Microbiology.
19. Berkowitz, B.A., Asling, J.H., Shnider, S.M. & Way, E.L. (1969) Relationship of pentazocine plasma levels to pharmacologic activity in man. *Clinical Pharmacology and Therapeutics*, **10**, 320–328.
20. Bernard, B., Yin, E.J. & Simon, H.J. (1971) Clinical pharmacological studies with minocycline. *Journal of Clinical Pharmacology*, **11**, 332–348.
21. Binda, G., Domenichini, E., Gottardi, A., Orlandi, B., Orrelli, E., Paeini, B. & Fowst, G. (1971) Rifampicin, a general review. *Arzneimittel Forschung*, **21**, 1907–1978.
22. Bindschadler, D.D. & Bennett, J.E. (1969) A pharmacologic guide to the clinical use of amphotericin B. *Journal of Infectious Diseases*, **120**, 427–436.
23. Black, M. (1974) Isoniazid and the liver. *American Review of Respiratory Diseases*, **110**, 1–3.
24. Blaschke, T.F. (1977) Protein binding and kinetics of drugs in liver diseases. *Clinical Pharmacokinetics*, **2**, 32–44.
25. Blaschke, T.F., Meffin, P.J., Melmon, K.L. & Rowland, M. (1975) Influence of acute viral hepatitis on phenytoin kinetics and protein binding. *Clinical Pharmacology and Therapeutics*, **17**, 685–691.
26. Block, E.R. (1973) Effect of hepatic insufficiency on 5-fluorocytosine concentrations in serum. *Antimicrobial Agents and Chemotherapy*, **3**, 141–142.
27. Bodem, G. & Chidsey, C.A. (1973) Pharmacokinetic studies of practolol, a beta adrenergic antagonist, in man. *Clinical Pharmacology and Therapeutics*, **14**, 26–29.
28. Booker, H.E. & Darcey, B. (1973) Serum concentrations of free diphenylhydantoin and their relationship to clinical intoxication. *Epilepsia*, **14**, 177–184.
29. Borgå, O., Hamberger, B., Malmfors, T. & Sjoqvist, F. (1970) The role of plasma protein binding in the inhibitory effect of nortriptyline on the neuronal uptake of norepinephrine. *Clinical Pharmacology and Therapeutics*, **11**, 581–588.
30. Branch, R.A., Herbert, C.M. & Read, A.E. (1973) Determinants of serum antipyrine half-lives in patients with liver disease. *Gut*, **14**, 569–573.
31. Branch, R.A., James, J. & Read, E.A. (1976a) A study of factors influencing drug disposition in chronic liver disease, using the model drug (+)-propranolol. *British Journal of Clinical Pharmacology*, **3**, 243–249.
32. Branch, R.A., James, J.A. & Read, A.E. (1976b) The clearance of antipyrine and indocyanine green in normal subjects and in patients with chronic liver disease. *Clinical Pharmacology and Therapeutics*, **20**, 81–89.
33. Branch, R.A., Morgan, M.H., James, J. & Read, A.E. (1976) Intravenous administration of diazepam in patients with chronic liver disease. *Gut*, **17**, 975–983.
34. Brandl, R., Arkenau, C., Simon, C., Malerczyk, V. & Eidelloth, G. (1972) The pharmacokinetics of clindamycin in the presence of impaired liver and kidney function. *Deutsche Medizuische Wochey Schimtt*, **91**, 1051–1059.
35. Breckenridge, A., Orme, M. L'E., Davies, L., Thorgeirsson, S.S. & Davies, D.S. (1973) Dose-dependent enzyme induction. *Clinical Pharmacology and Therapeutics*, **14**, 514–520.

36. Breimer, D.D., Zilly, W. & Richter, E. (1975) Pharmacokinetics of hexobarbital in acute hepatitis and after apparent recovery. *Clinical Pharmacology and Therapeutics*, **18**, 433–440.
37. Brodie, B.B. (1967) Idiosyncrasy and intolerance. In *Drug Responses in Man* (Ed) Wolstenholme, G.E.W. & Porter, R. pp. 188–213. London: J. & A. Churchill.
38. Brodie, B.B. & Axelrod, J. (1950) The fate of antipyrine in man. *Journal of Pharmacology and Experimental Therapeutics*, **98**, 97–104.
39. Brodie, B.B., Burns, J.J. & Weiner, M. (1959) Metabolism of drugs in subjects with Laennec's cirrhosis. *Medicina Experimentalis*, **1**, 290–292.
40. Caldwell, J.H. & Greenberger, N.J. (1970) Cholestyramine enhances digitalis excretion and protects against lethal intoxication. *Journal of Clinical Investigation*, **49**, 16a.
41. Carey, M.C. & Small, D.M. (1971) Micellar properties of sodium fusidate, a steroid antibiotic structurally resembling the bile salts. *Journal of Lipid Research*, **12**, 604–613.
42. Closson, R.G. (1977) Terminal half-lives of drugs studied in patients with hepatic diseases. *American Journal of Hospital Pharmacy*, **34**, 520–524.
43. Cole, M., Kenig, M.D. & Hewitt, V.A. (1973) Metabolism of penicillins to penicilloic acids and 6-aminopenicillanic acid in man and its significance in assessing penicillin absorption. *Antimicrobial Agents and Chemotherapy*, **3**, 463–468.
44. Conn, H.O. (1972) The rational management of ascites. *Progress in Liver Disease*, **4**, 269–288.
45. Conney, A.H. (1967) Pharmacological implications of microsomal enzyme induction. *Pharmacology Reviews*, **19**, 317–366.
46. Datta, D.V. & Sherlock, S. (1963) Treatment of pruritus of obstructive jaundice with cholestyramine. *British Medical Journal*, **i**, 216–219.
47. Davies, D.S. (1972) Drug metabolism and poisoning. *Medicine*, **4**, 287–293.
48. Davies, D.S. & Thorgeirsson, S.S. (1971) Mechanism of hepatic drug oxidation and its relationship to individual differences in rates of oxidation in man. *Annals of the New York Academy of Sciences*, **179**, 411–420.
49. Doherty, J.E., Flanigan, W.J., Patterson, R.M. & Dalrymple, G.V. (1969) The excretion of tritiated digoxin in normal human volunteers before and after unilateral nephrectomy. *Circulation*, **40**, 555–561.
50. Dollery, C.T., George, C.F. & Orme, M. L'E. (1974) Drug interactions affecting cardiovascular therapy. In *Clinical Effects of Interaction Between Drugs* (Ed.) Cluff, L.E. & Petrie, J.C. Amsterdam: Excerpta Medica.
51. Doluisio, J.T. & Dittert, L.W. (1969) Influence of repetitive dosing of tetracycline on biologic half-life in serum. *Clinical Pharmacology and Therapeutics*, **10**, 690–701.
52. Doshi, J., Luisada-Opper, A. & Leevy, C.M. (1972) Microsomal pentobarbital hydroxylase activity in acute viral hepatitis. *Proceedings of the Society for Experimental Biology in Medicine*, **140**, 492–495.
53. Dundee, J.W. (1952) Thiopentone narcosis in the presence of hepatic dysfunction. *British Journal of Anaesthetics*, **24**, 81–100.
54. Ellard, G.A. (1969) Absorption, metabolism and excretion of pyrazinamide in man. *Tubercle*, **50**, 144–158.
55. Elmore, M., Rissing, J.P., Rink, L. & Brooks, G.F. (1974) Clindamycin-associated hepatotoxicity. *American Journal of Medicine*, **57**, 627–630.
56. Ernster, L. & Orrenius, S. (1965) Substrate induced synthesis of the hydroxylating enzyme system of liver microsomes. *Federation Proceedings*, **24**, 1190–1199.
57. Estabrook, R.W., Cooper, D.Y. & Rosenthal, O. (1963) The light reversible carbon monoxide inhibition of the steroid C21-hydroxylase system of the adrenal cortex. *Biochemische zeitschrift*, **338**, 741–755.
58. Evans, G.H., Nies, A.S. & Shand, D.G. (1973) The disposition of propranolol, III: Decreased half-life and volume of distribution as a result of plasma binding in man, monkey, dog and rat. *Journal of Pharmacology and Experimental Therapeutics*, **186**, 114–122.
59. Evans, G.H., Wilkinson, G.R. & Shand, D.G. (1973) The disposition of propranolol. IV. A dominant role for tissue uptake in the dose-dependent extraction of propranolol by the perfused rat liver. *Journal of Pharmacology and Experimental Therapeutics*, **186**, 447–454.
60. Fass, R.J., Scholand, J.F., Hodges, G.R. & Saslaw, S. (1973) Clindamycin in the treatment of serious anaerobic infections. *Annals of Internal Medicine*, **78**, 853–859.
61. Foldes, F.F., Swerdlow, M., Lipschitz, E., van Hees, G.R. & Shanor, S.P. (1956) Comparison of the respiratory effects of suxamethonium and suxethonium in man. *Anesthesiology*, **17**, 559–568.
62. Forrest, J.A.H., Finlayson, N.D.C., Adjepon-Yamoah, K.K. & Prescott, L.F. (1977) Antipyrine, paracetamol and lignocaine elimination in chronic liver disease. *British Medical Journal*, **i**, 1384–1387.
63. Garrod, L.P. & O'Grady, F.W. (1971) *Antibiotic and Chemotherapy*. Edinburgh and London: Churchill Livingstone.
64. George, C.F. (1976) Diseases of the alimentary system: absorption, distribution and metabolism of drugs; effects of disease of the gut. *British Medical Journal*, **ii**, 742–744.
65. George, C.F. (1978) *Topics in Clinical Pharmacology*. London: Kimpton.
66. George, C.F. & Castleden, C.M. (1977) Propranolol absorption. *British Medical Journal*, **i**, 47.
67. George, C.F., Orme, M. L'E., Buranapong, P., MacErlean, D., Breckenridge, A.M. & Dollery, C.T. (1976) Contribution of the liver to overall elimination of propranolol. *Journal of Pharmacokinetics and Biopharmaceutics*, **4**, 17–27.
68. Ghoneim, M.M. & Pandya, H. (1975) Plasma protein binding of thiopental in patients with impaired renal or hepatic function. *Anesthesiology*, **42**, 545–549.
69. Gibaldi, M., Boyes, R.W. & Feldman, S. (1971) Influence of first-pass effect on availability of drugs on oral administration. *Journal of Pharmaceutical Sciences*, **60**, 1338–1340.
70. Giusti, D.L. (1973) A review of the clinical use of antimicrobial agents in patients with renal and hepatic insufficiency. I. The penicillins. *Drug Intelligence and Clinical Pharmacy*, **7**, 62–74.
71. Godtfredsen, W.O. (1967) *Fusidic Acid and Some Related Antibiotics*. Copenhagen: Leo Pharmaceutical Products.
72. Godtfredsen, W.O. & Vangedal, S. (1966) On the metabolism of fusidic acid in man. *Acta Chemica Scandinavica*, **20**, 1599–1607.

73. Godtfredsen, W.O., Roholt, K. & Tybring, L. (1962) Fucidin, a new orally active antibiotic. *Lancet*, **i**, 928–931.
74. Gold, M.S. & Ziegler, D.M. (1973) Dimethylaniline N-oxidase and aminopyrine N-demethylase activities of human liver tissue. *Xenobiotica*, **3**, 179–189.
75. Goldstein, A., Aranow, L. & Kaplan, S.M. (1974) *Principles of Drug Action*. 2nd ed. New York, Evanston and London: Harper & Row.
76. Goodman, L.S. & Gilman, A. (1975) *The Pharmacological Basis of Therapeutics*. 5th ed. New York: Macmillan.
77. Gram, L.F. & Overo, K.F. (1975) First pass metabolism of nortriptyline in man. *Clinical Pharmacology and Therapeutics*, **18**, 305–314.
78. Greenblatt, D.J. & Koch-Weser, J. (1974) Clinical toxicity of chlordiazepoxide and diazepam in relation to serum albumin concentration: a report from the Boston Collaborative Drug Surveillance Program. *European Journal of Clinical Pharmacology*, **7**, 259–262.
79. Gugler, R., Lain, P. & Azarnoff, D.L. (1975) Effect of portacaval shunt on the disposition of drugs with and without first pass effect. *Journal of Pharmacology and Experimental Therapeutics*, **195**, 416–423.
80. Gyselnyck, A.M., Forrey, A. & Cutler, R. (1971) Pharmacokinetics of gentamicin: distribution and plasma and renal clearance. *Journal of Infectious Diseases*, **124** (Suppl. 124), 70–76.
81. Hamlyn, A.N., McKenna, K. & Douglas, A. (1977) Gastric emptying in coeliac disease. *British Medical Journal*, **i**, 1257–1258.
82. Hammer, W. & Sjoqvist, F. (1967) Plasma levels of monomethylated tricyclic antidepressants during treatment with imipramine-like compounds. *Life Sciences*, **6**, 1895–1903.
83. Hayes, A. & Cooper, R.G. (1971) Studies on the absorption, distribution and excretion of propranolol in rat, dog and monkey. *Journal of Pharmacology and Experimental Therapeutics*, **176**, 302–311.
84. Heni, N., Lehnhardt, G. & Glogner, P. (1976) Elimination kinetics of phenprocoumon (Marcoumar) in liver cirrhosis and after premedication with phenobarbital. *International Journal of Clinical Pharmacology and Biopharmaceutics*, **13**, 253–261.
85. Hinthorn, D.R., Baker, L.H., Romig, D.A., Hassanein, K. & Liu, C. (1976) Use of clindamycin in patients with liver disease. *Antimicrobial Agents and Chemotherapy*, **9**, 498–501.
86. Hirom, P.C., Millburn, P., Smith, R.L. & Williams, R.T. (1972) Species variations in the threshold molecular-weight factor for the biliary excretion of organic amines. *Biochemical Journal*, **129**, 1071–1077.
87. Hitzenberger, G., Bonelli, J., Korn, A. & Pesendorfer, F. (1974) Pharmacokinetics of cotrimoxazole in patients with impaired liver function. *Proceedings of the 8th International Congress of Chemotherapy*, **1**, 692–695.
88. Hoffman, T.A., Cestero, R. & Bullock, W.E. (1970) Pharmacodynamics of carbenicillin in hepatic and renal failure. *Annals of Internal Medicine*, **73**, 173–178.
89. Hogben, C.A.M., Tocco, D.J., Brodie, B.B. & Schanker, L.S. (1959) On the mechanism of intestinal absorption of drugs. *Journal of Pharmacology and Experimental Therapeutics*, **125**, 275–282.
90. Hooper, W.D., Bochner, F., Eadie, M.J. & Tyrer, J.H. (1974) Plasma protein binding of diphenylhydandoin. Effects of sex hormones, renal and hepatic disease. *Clinical Pharmacology and Therapeutics*, **15**, 276–282.
91. Hvidberg, E.F., Andreasen, P.B. & Ranek, L. (1974) Plasma half-life of phenylbutazone in patients with impaired liver function. *Clinical Pharmacology and Therapeutics*, **15**, 171–177.
92. Ings, R.M.J., Law, G.L. & Parnell, E.W. (1966) The metabolism of metronidazole. *Biochemical Pharmacology*, **15**, 515–519.
93. Jackson, E.A. & McLeod, D.C. (1974) Pharmacokinetics and dosing of antimicrobial agents in renal impairment, part I. *American Journal of Hospital Pharmacy*, **31**, 36–52.
94. Jusko, W.J. & Gibaldi, M. (1972) Effects of change in elimination on various parameters of the two-compartment open model. *Journal of Pharmaceutical Sciences*, **61**, 1270–1273.
95. Kamin, H., Siler Masters, B.S., Gibson, Q.H. & Williams, C.H. (1965) Microsomal TPNH-cytochrome-C-reductase. *Federation Proceedings*, **24**, 1164–1171.
96. Kane, P.O., McFadzean, J.A. & Squires, S. (1961) Absorption and excretion of metronidazole. Part II. Studies on primary failures. *British Journal of Venereal Diseases*, **37**, 276–277.
97. Karlin, J.M. & Kutt, H. (1970) Acute diphenylhydantoin intoxication following halothane anesthesia. *Journal of Pediatrics*, **76**, 941–944.
98. Klotz, U., McHorse, T.S., Wilkinson, G.R. & Schenker, S. (1974) The effect of cirrhosis on the disposition and elimination of meperidine in man. *Clinical Pharmacology and Therapeutics*, **16**, 667–675.
99. Klotz, U., Avant, G.R., Hoyumpa, A., Schenker, S. & Wilkinson, G.R. (1975) The effects of age and liver disease on the disposition and elimination of diazepam in adult man. *Journal of Clinical Investigation*, **55**, 347–359.
100. Knudsen, E.T. & Harding, J.W. (1975) A multicentre comparative trial of talampicillin and ampicillin in general practice. *British Journal of Clinical Practice*, **29**, 255–266.
101. Koch-Weser, J. & Sellers, E.M. (1976) Binding of drugs to serum albumin. *New England Journal of Medicine*, **294**, 311–316.
102. Kosmidis, J., Williams, J.D., Andrews, J., Goodall, J.A.D. & Geddes, A.M. (1972) Amoxycillin – pharmacology, bacteriology and clinical studies. *British Journal of Clinical Practice*, **26**, 341–346.
103. Kunin, C.M. (1967) A guide to use of antibiotics in patients with renal disease. *Annals of Internal Medicine*, **67**, 151–158.
104. Kunin, C., Glazko, A.J. & Finland, M. (1959) Persistence of antibiotics in blood of patients with acute renal failure. II. Chloramphenicol and its metabolic products in the blood of patients with severe renal disease or hepatic cirrhosis. *Journal of Clinical Investigation*, **38**, 1498–1508.
105. Kunin, C.M., Craig, W.A., Kornguth, M. & Monson, R. (1973) Influence of binding on the pharmacologic activity of antibiotics. *Annals of the New York Academy of Sciences*, **226**, 214–224.

106. Kutt, H., Winters, W., Scherman, R. & McDowell, F. (1964) Diphenylhydantoin and phenobarbital toxicity; the role of liver disease. *Archives of Neurology*, **11**, 649–656.
107. Laidlaw, J., Read, A.E. & Sherlock, S. (1961) Morphine tolerance in hepatic cirrhosis. *Gastroenterology*, **40**, 389–396.
108. Levy, G. (1966) Kinetics of pharmacologic effects. *Clinical Pharmacology and Therapeutics*, **7**, 362–372.
109. Levi, A.J., Sherlock, S. & Walker, D. (1968) Phenylbutazone and isoniazid metabolism in patients with chronic liver disease in relation to previous drug therapy. *Lancet*, **i**, 1275–1279.
110. Lewi, P.J., Boelaert, J., Daneels, R., De Meyere, R., Van Landuyt, H., Heykants, J.J.P., Symonens, J. & Wynants, J. (1976) Pharmacokinetic profile of intravenous miconazole in man. *European Journal of Clinical Pharmacology*, **10**, 49–54.
111. Lewis, G.P., Jick, H., Slone, D. & Shapiro, S. (1971) The role of genetic factors and serum protein binding in determining drug response as revealed by comprehensive drug surveillance. *Annals of the New York Academy of Sciences*, **179**, 729–738.
112. Letteri, J.M., Mellk, H., Louis, S., Kutt, H., Durante, P. & Glazko, A. (1971) Diphenylhydantoin metabolism in uraemia. *New England Journal of Medicine*, **285**, 648–652.
113. Lloyd-Still, J.D., Grand, R.J. & Vawter, G.F. (1974) Tetracycline hepatotoxicity in the differential diagnosis of postoperative jaundice. *Journal of Pediatrics*, **84**, 366–370.
114. Luton, E. (1965) Carbon tetrachloride exposure during anticoagulant therapy. *Journal of the American Medical Association*, **964**, 1386–1387.
115. Macdonald, H., Kelly, R.G., Allen, S.E., Nobel, J.F. & Kanegis, L.A. (1973) Pharmacokinetic studies on minocycline in man. *Clinical Pharmacology and Therapeutics*, **14**, 852–861.
116. Mao, J.C.H. & Tardrew, P.L. (1965) Demethylation of erythromycins by rabbit tissues in vitro. *Biochemical Pharmacology*, **14**, 1049–1058.
117. Marcus, F.I. & Kapadia, G.G. (1964) The metabolism of tritiated digoxin in cirrhotic patients. *Gastroenterology*, **47**, 517–524.
118. Maroske, D., Knothe, H. & Rox, A. (1976) Die Lebergewebekonzentration von Cephradin und Cephacetril sowie deren Gallenausscheidung. *Journal for the Clinical Study and Treatment of Infections*, **4**, 159–165.
119. Mason, W.D. & Winer, N. (1976) Pharmacokinetics of oxprenolol in normal subjects. *Clinical Pharmacology and Therapeutics*, **20**, 401–412.
120. Mawer, G.E., Miller, N.E. & Turnberg, L.A. (1972) Metabolism of amylobarbitone in patients with chronic liver disease. *British Journal of Pharmacology*, **44**, 549–560.
121. Maxwell, J.D., Carrella, M., Parkes, J.D., Williams, R., Mould, G.P. & Curry, S.H. (1972) Plasma disappearance and cerebral effects of chlorpromazine in cirrhosis. *Clinical Science*, **43**, 143–151.
122. McArdle, B. (1940) The serum choline esterase in jaundice and diseases of the liver. *Quarterly Journal of Medicine*, **9**, 107–119.
123. McDevitt, D.G., Frisk-Holmberg, M., Hollifield, J.W. & Shand, D.G. (1976) Plasma binding and the affinity of propranolol for a beta-receptor in man. *Clinical Pharmacology and Therapeutics*, **20**, 152–157.
124. McHorse, T.S., Wilkinson, G.R., Johnson, R.F. & Schenker, S. (1975) Effect of acute viral hepatitis on the disposition and elimination of meperidine. *Gastroenterology*, **68**, 775–780.
125. Medina, A., Fiske, N., Hjelt-Harvey, I., Brown, C.D. & Prigot, A. (1963) Absorption, diffusion, excretion of a new antibiotic, lincomycin. *Antimicrobial Agents Chemotherapy*, **4**, 189–196.
126. Mitchell, J.R., Jollow, D.J., Potter, W.Z., Davis, D.C., Gillette, J.R. & Brodie, B.B. (1973) Acetaminophen-induced hepatic necrosis. I. Role of drug metabolism. *Journal of Pharmacology and Experimental Therapeutics*, **187**, 211–217.
127. Nelson, E. (1964) Rate of metabolism of tolbutamide in test subjects with liver disease or with impaired renal function. *American Journal of Medical Sciences*, **248**, 657–659.
128. Neuman, M., Kazmierczak, A. & Cachin, M. (1971) The serum biliary and urinary antibacterial levels of trimethoprim-sulfamethoxazole in relation to the liver function. *Proceedings of the 7th International Congress of Chemotherapy*, **1**, 85–87.
129. Newbould, B.B. & Kilpatrick, R. (1960) Long-acting sulphonamides and protein-binding. *Lancet*, **i**, 887–891.
130. Nunes, H.L., Pecoro, C.C., Judy, K., Rosenman, S.B., Warren, G.H. & Martin, C.M. (1964) Turnover and distribution of nafcillin in tissues and body fluids of surgical patients. In *Antimicrobial Agents and Chemotherapy* (Ed.) Sylvester, J.C. pp. 237–249. Michigan: The American Society for Microbiology.
131. Olsen, G.D., Bennett, W.M. & Porter, G.A. (1975) Morphine and phenytoin binding to plasma proteins in renal and hepatic failure. *Clinical Pharmacology and Therapeutics*, **7**, 677–684.
132. Omura, T., Sato, R., Cooper, D.Y., Rosenthal, O. & Estabrook, R.W. (1965) Function of cytochrome P-450 of microsomes. *Federation Proceedings*, **24**, 1181–1189.
133. Paradelis, S.G. (1975) Absorption and excretion studies of cephalosporins in human subjects. *Chemotherapy (Penicillins and Cephalosporins)* (Ed.) Williams, J.D. & Geddes, A.M. pp. 5, 283–292. London: Plenum Press.
134. Parsons, R.L., Kaye, C.M., Raymond, K., Trounce, J.R. & Turner, P. (1976) Absorption of propranolol and practolol in coeliac disease. *Gut*, **17**, 139–143.
135. Paterson, J.W. (1972) Pharmacogenetics in relation to poisoning. *Medicine* (1st series), **4**, 294–300.
136. Paterson, J.W., Conolly, M.E., Dollery, C.T., Hayes, A. & Cooper, R.G. (1970) The pharmacodynamics and metabolism of propranolol in man. *European Journal of Clinical Pharmacology*, **2**, 127–133.
137. Pentilla, O., Neuvonen, P.J., Aho, K. & Lehtovaara, R. (1974) Interaction between doxycycline and some antiepileptic drugs. *British Medical Journal*, **ii**, 470–472.
138. Perrier, D. & Gibaldi, M. (1973) Relationship between plasma or serum drug concentration and amount of drug in the body at steady state upon multiple dosing. *Journal of Pharmacokinetics and Biopharmaceutics*, **1**, 17–22.
139. Piafsky, K.M., Sitar, D., Rango, R.E. & Ogilvie, R.I. (1975) Disposition of theophylline in chronic liver disease. *Clinical Pharmacology and Therapeutics*, **17**, 241.

140. Pieri, F., Andre, L.J. & Abed, L. (1969) Étude du métabolisme du métronidazole chez l'homme: demonstration de la présence de cet amoebicide dans la bile. *Médecine Tropicale,* **29,** 375–376.
141. Place, V.A. & Thomas, J.P. (1963) Clinical pharmacology of ethambutol. *American Review of Respiratory Disease,* **87,** 901–904.
142. Powell, L.W. & Axelsen, E. (1972) Corticosteroids in liver disease: studies on the biological conversion of prednisone to prednisolone and plasma protein binding. *Gut,* **14,** 690–696.
143. Prescott, L.F., Wright, N., Roscoe, P. & Brown, S.S. (1971) Plasma-paracetamol half-life and hepatic necrosis in patients with paracetamol overdosage. *Lancet,* **i,** 519–522.
144. Rango, R.E., Piafsky, K.M., Sitar, D. & Ogilvie, R.I. (1976) The clinical pharmacology of theophylline and its pharmacokinetics in pulmonary edema and cirrhosis. *Arzneimittel Forschung,* **26,** 1268–1269.
145. Read, A.E., Laidlaw, J. & McCarthy, C.F. (1969) Effects of chlorpromazine in patients with hepatic disease. *British Medical Journal,* **ii,** 497–499.
146. Reidenberg, M.M., James, M. & Dring, L.G. (1972) The rate of procaine hydrolysis in serum of normal subjects and diseased patients. *Clinical Pharmacology and Therapeutics,* **13,** 279–284.
147. Remmer, H. & Merker, H.J. (1965) Effect of drugs on the formation of smooth endoplasmic reticulum and drug-metabolizing enzymes. *Annals of the New York Academy of Sciences,* **123,** 79–97.
148. Renzini, G., Ravagnan, G., Oliva, B. & Salvetti, E. (1974) Cephradine microbiological activity in vitro and in vivo serum and tissue levels. *Medicamentos de Actualidad,* **10,** 75–83.
149. Richens, A. & Houghton, G.W. (1975) Effect of drug therapy on the metabolism of phenytoin. In *Clinical Pharmacology of Anti-epileptic Drugs* (Ed.) Schneider, H., Janz, D., Gardner-Thorpe, G., Meinardi, H. & Sherwin, A.L. pp. 87–110. Berlin: Springer-Verlag.
150. Rieder, J. & Schwartz, D.E. (1975) Pharmakokinetik der Wirkstoffkombination Trimethoprim + Sulfamethoxazol bei Leberkranken im Vergleich zu Gesunden. *Arzneimittel Forschung Drug Research,* **25,** 656–666.
151. Riegelman, S., Loo, J. & Rowland, M. (1968) Concept of a volume of distribution and possible errors in evaluation of this parameter. *Journal of Pharmaceutical Sciences,* **57,** 128–133.
152. Rothfeld, E.L., Crews, A.H., Ribot, S. & Bernstein, A. (1965) Severe hypoglycaemia. Result of renal retention of chlorpropamide. *Archives of Internal Medicine,* **115,** 468–469.
153. Sasame, H.A., Castro, J.A. & Gillette, J.R. (1968) Studies on the destruction of liver microsomal cytochrome P-450 by carbon tetrachloride administration. *Biochemical Pharmacology,* **17,** 1759–1768.
154. Scales, B. & Cosgrove, M.B. (1970) The metabolism and distribution of the selective adrenergic blocking agent, practolol. *Journal of Pharmacology and Experimental Therapeutics,* **175,** 338–347.
155. Schneider, R.E., Babb, J., Bishop, H., Mitchard, M., Hoare, A.M. & Hawkins, C.F. (1976) Plasma levels of propranolol in treated patients with coeliac disease and patients with Crohn's disease. *British Medical Journal,* **ii,** 794–795.
156. Schoene, B., Fleischmann, R.A., Remmer, H. & Oldershausen, H.F.V. (1972) Determination of drug metabolizing enzymes in needle biopsies of human liver. *European Journal of Clinical Pharmacology,* **4,** 65–73.
157. Schonebeck, J., Polak, A., Fernex, M. & Scholer, H.J. (1973) Pharmacokinetic studies on the oral antimycotic agent 5-fluorocytosine in individuals with normal and impaired kidney function. *Chemotherapy,* **18,** 321–336.
158. Seltzer, H.S. (1972) Drug-induced hypoglycaemia. A review based on 473 cases. *Diabetes,* **21,** 955–966.
159. Sessions, J.T., Minkel, H.P., Bullard, J.C. & Ingelfinger, F.J. (1954) The effect of barbiturates in patients with liver disease. *Journal of Clinical Investigation,* **33,** 1116–1127.
160. Shand, D.G. & Rangno, R.E. (1972) The disposition of propranolol. 1. Elimination during oral absorption in man. *Pharmacology,* **7,** 159–168.
161. Shand, D.G., Evans, G.H. & Nies, A.S. (1971) The almost complete hepatic extraction of propranolol during intravenous administration in the dog. *Life Sciences,* **10,** 1417–1421.
162. Shand, D.G., Kornhauser, D.M. & Wilkinson, G.R. (1975) Effects of route of administration and blood flow on hepatic drug elimination. *Journal of Pharmacology and Experimental Therapeutics,* **195,** 424–432.
163. Shand, D.G., Nuckolls, E.M. & Oates, J.A. (1970) Plasma propranolol levels in adults with observations in four children. *Clinical Pharmacology and Therapeutics,* **11,** 112–120.
164. Shand, D.G., Rangno, R.E. & Evans, G.H. (1972) The disposition of propranolol. II. Hepatic elimination in the rat. *Pharmacology,* **8,** 344–352.
165. Shideman, F.E., Kelly, A.R., Lee, L.E., Lowell, V.F. & Adams, B.J. (1949) The role of the liver in the detoxication of thiopental (Pentothal) in man. *Anesthesiology,* **10,** 421.
166. Shull, H.J., Wilkinson, G.R., Johnson, R. & Schenker, S. (1976) Normal disposition of oxazepam in acute viral hepatitis and cirrhosis. *Annals of Internal Medicine,* **84,** 420–425.
167. Smith, R.L. (1973) *The Excretory Function of Bile.* London: Chapman & Hall.
168. Smith, R.L. & Caldwell, J. (1977) Drug metabolism in non-human primates. In *Drug Metabolism from Microbe to Man* (Ed.) Parke, D.V. & Smith, R.L. pp. 331–356. London: Taylor & Francis.
169. Smith, S.E. & Rawlins, M.D. (1973) *Variability in Human Drug Response.* London: Butterworth.
170. Stenson, R.E., Constantino, R.T. & Harrison, D.C. (1971) Interrelationships of hepatic blood flow, cardiac output and blood levels of lidocaine in man. *Circulation,* **43,** 205–211.
171. Stevens, D.A., Levine, H.B. & Deresinski, S.C. (1976) Miconazole in coccidioidomycosis. *The American Journal of Medicine,* **60,** 191–202.
172. Suhrland, L.G. & Weisberger, A. (1963) Chloramphenicol toxicity in liver and renal disease. *Archives of Internal Medicine,* **112,** 747–753.
173. Sunahara, S. & Nakagawa, H. (1972) Metabolic study and controlled clinical trials of rifampin. *Chest,* **61,** 526–532.
174. Thiessen, J.J., Sellers, E.M., Denbeigh, P. & Dolman, L. (1976) Plasma protein binding of diazepam and tolbutamide in chronic alcoholics. *Journal of Clinical Pharmacology,* **16,** 345–351.
175. Thomson, P.D., Rowland, M. & Melmon, K.L. (1971) The influence of heart failure, liver disease and renal failure on the disposition of lidocaine in man. *American Heart Journal,* **82,** 417–421.

176. Thomson, P.D., Melmon, K.L., Richardson, J.A., Cohn, K., Steinbrunn, W., Cudihie, R. & Rowland, M. (1973) Lidocaine pharmacokinetics in advanced heart failure, liver disease, and renal failure in humans. *Annals of Internal Medicine,* **78,** 499–508.
177. Tolman, K.G., Sannella, J.J. & Feston, J.W. (1974) Chemical structure of erythromycin and hepatotoxicity. *Annals of Internal Medicine,* **81,** 58–60.
178. Twiss, J.R., Berger, W.V., Gillette, L., Aronson, A.R. & Siegel, L. (1956) The biliary excretion of erythromycin (Ilotycin). *Surgery, Gynecology and Obstetrics,* **102,** 355–357.
179. Ueda, H., Sakurai, T., Ota, M., Nakajima, A., Kamii, K. & Maezawa, H. (1963) Disappearance rate of tolbutamide in normal subjects and in diabetes mellitus, liver cirrhosis and renal disease. *Diabetes,* **12,** 414–419.
180. Verstraete, M. & Verwilghen, R. (1976) Haematological disorders. In *Principles and Practice of Clinical Pharmacology and Therapeutics* (Ed.) Avery, G.S., Ch. XXII, pp. 661–716. Edinburgh and London: Churchill Livingstone.
181. Vesell, E.S., Passananti, G.T., Greene, F.E. & Page, J.G. (1971) Genetic control of drug levels and of the induction of drug-metabolizing enzymes in man: individual variability in the extent of allopurinol and nortriptyline inhibition of drug metabolism. *Annals of the New York Academy of Sciences,* **179,** 752–773.
182. Vorhaus, L.J. & Kark, R.M. (1953) Serum cholinesterase in health and disease. *American Journal of Medicine,* **14,** 707–719.
183. Wallace, S. & Brodie, M.J. (1976) Decreased drug binding in serum from patients with chronic hepatic disease. *European Journal of Clinical Pharmacology,* **9,** 429–432.
184. Whittaker, J.A. & Price-Evans, D.A. (1970) Genetic control of phenylbutazone metabolism in man. *British Medical Journal,* **iv,** 323–328.
185. Whorwell, P.J., Smith, C.L. & Foster, K.J. (1976) Arterial blood gas tensions during upper gastrointestinal endoscopy. *Gut,* **17,** 797–800.
186. Wiegand, R.G. & Chun, A.H.C. (1972) Serum protein binding of erythromycin and erythromycin 2′-propionate ester. *Journal of Pharmaceutical Sciences,* **61,** 425–428.
187. Wilkinson, G.R. & Schenker, S. (1976) Effects of liver disease on drug disposition in man. *Biochemical Pharmacology,* **25,** 2675–2681.
188. Wilkinson, G.R. & Shand, D.G. (1975) A physiological approach to hepatic drug clearance. *Clinical Pharmacology and Therapeutics,* **18,** 377–390.
189. Williams, D.N., Crossley, K., Hoffman, F. & Sabath, L.D. (1975) Parenteral clindamycin phosphate: pharmacology with normal and abnormal liver function and effect on nasal staphylococci. *Antimicrobial Agents and Chemotherapy,* **7,** 153–158.
190. Williams, R.L., Blaschke, T.F., Meffin, P.J., Melmon, K.L. & Rowland, M. (1976) Influence of viral hepatitis on the disposition of two compounds with high hepatic clearance: lignocaine and indocyanine green. *Clinical Pharmacology and Therapeutics,* **20,** 290–299.
191. Williams, R.L., Schary, W.L., Blaschke, T.F., Meffin, P.J., Melmon, K.L. & Rowland, M. (1976) Influence of acute viral hepatitis on disposition and pharmacologic effect of warfarin. *Clinical Pharmacology and Therapeutics,* **20,** 90–97.
192. Wynn, V. (1965) Metabolic effects of steroid antibiotic fusidic acid. *British Medical Journal,* **i,** 1400–1404.
193. Zilly, W., Richter, E. & Rietbrock, N. (1975) Pharmacokinetics and metabolism of digoxin- and β-methyl-digoxin-12a-^{3}H in acute hepatitis. *Clinical Pharmacology and Therapeutics,* **17,** 302–309.
194. George, C.F. (1979) Drug kinetics and hepatic blood flow. *Clinical Pharmacokinetics,* **4,** 433–448.

PART TWO

Diagnosis and Management

Chapter 17

Biochemical Assessment of Liver Function

C.P. PRICE
K.G.M.M. ALBERTI

The concept of 'liver function tests' came into being with the development and growth of clinical chemistry laboratories where large numbers of samples could be analysed by automated techniques. These tests have tended to become stereotyped due to usage and may not reflect the best means available for testing hepatic integrity. The liver has arguably more biochemical functions than any other organ in the body and there are many possible ways, both in practice and theoretically, for testing these functions (Table 17.1). It should also be emphasized that many so-called liver 'function' tests are not tests of function at all, but are tests of hepatocellular damage or bile duct patency. Such tests are enumerated in Table 17.2. One of the major problems in biochemical diagnosis is that nearly all commonly available tests are indirect, relying on measurements in blood, urine and faeces. This strains the specificity of many of these tests. In the future it is hoped that more tests will become available which are based on chemical analysis of biopsy specimens. This will necessitate refinement of microanalytical techniques, but this should be possible with modern technology.

Distinction must also be drawn between tests which inform the clinician that there is *some* disease or damage of the liver, tests which indicate the *extent* of damage or the disease process, and tests which are designed to differentiate between, and help in, the diagnosis of *specific* diseases of the liver. These distinctions will be drawn in the ensuing chapters when relevant tests are discussed.

In the rest of this chapter we shall consider first each of the functions of the liver, discussing tests of these functions. Certain sections will be brief where the topics have been covered in other chapters. A discussion of tests reflecting morphological change will follow, together with sections on the use of computers in the diagnosis of liver disease and a discussion on the selection of the best available tests of function or damage.

TESTS OF LIVER FUNCTION

Carbohydrate Metabolism (see also Chapters 3 and 32)

One of the major roles of the liver is that of maintaining glucose homeostasis. Apart from a minor contribution by the kidney, the liver alone is responsible for meeting the demands of other tissues for glucose, and, placed as it is astride the portal system, it is of prime importance in disposing of the ingested carbohydrate, in particular glucose and fructose. It has the capacity to store glucose as glycogen and vice versa, to convert the excess glucose into lipid, and to convert precursors such as lactate, pyruvate, alanine, other glucogenic amino acids and glycerol into new glucose.

In spite of this, it is of interest that none of the commonly used liver function or damage tests involves carbohydrate metabolism. Part of the reason for this lies in the large functional reserve of the liver. It might be considered that fasting blood glucose concentration would reflect hepatic integrity, but this has proved a poor discriminant and only shows a significant fall in severe acute liver disease and then only

Table 17.1 *Liver Functions and Related Biochemical Tests.*

Function	Biochemical tests related to function	Refer to chapter
Carbohydrate metabolism		
Glucose homeostasis Galactose metabolism Glycogen metabolism Fructose metabolism Alcohol metabolism	Fasting blood glucose, oral/I.V. glucose tolerance tests, fasting and postprandial blood lactate, I.V. glycerol and lactate tolerance tests, galactose tolerance test, I.V. or I.M. glucagon test, fructose tolerance test	3, 32
Lipid metabolism		
Ketogenesis Fatty acid turnover Triglyceride metabolism Lipoprotein production Cholesterol synthesis Phospholipid metabolism	Serum free fatty acids, fasting triglycerides, serum cholesterol and cholesterol esters, serum lipoprotein fractions, serum total lipids and total phospholipids, serum lecithin cholesterol acyl transferase, lipoprotein-X, fasting blood ketone body concentrations	4
Protein metabolism		
Amino acid turnover Urea synthesis, ammonia synthesis/clearance Albumin turnover Globulin synthesis	Plasma ammonia, urea and amino acids, serum octopamine, serum albumin and protein electrophoresis, turbidity and flocculation tests, acute phase and other specific proteins, serum pseudocholinesterase	5, 42
Hormone metabolism		
Polypeptide hormone action and degradation, steroid conjugation	Serum insulin and C-peptide, serum growth hormone, glucagon, insulin clearance, plasma sex hormone levels	7
Digestion		
Bile acid production and	Serum two-hour postprandial total bile acids, chenodeoxycholate:cholate ratio, bile acid tolerance tests, ^{14}C-cholylglycine breath test	12
Detoxification and excretion		
Bilirubin Steroids Microsomal enzyme induction Drug metabolism Alcohol	Serum total bilirubin and fractions, urine bilirubin and urobilinogen, faecal stercobilinogen; bromsulphthalein and indocyanine green excretion tests, rose bengal elimination, ^{14}C-aminopyrine breath test, antipyrine half-life, urine glucaric acid, urine 6β-hydroxycortisol, serum γ-glutamyl transferase	13, 32
Storage function		
Iron and trace metals Lipids Glycogen Vitamins	Serum iron, iron binding capacity, ferritin, serum copper and caeruloplasmin, 24 hour urine copper; specific tissue enzyme assays on liver, muscle, leucocytes and cultured skin fibroblasts; red cell galactose-1-phosphate uridyl transferase	33, 34, 37, 40
Haematological functions		
Coagulation factor production Vitamin B_{12} and folate status Iron status	Measurement of clotting factors, fibrinogen factor VII, serum vitamin B_{12} and folate levels, serum iron and transferrin	8
Immunological functions		
Complement metabolism Kupffer cell function	Serum complement levels, complement turnover, uptake of ^{131}I-albumin	9

inconstantly. The reasons for this are detailed in Chapter 3. Similarly glucose tolerance tests are abnormal in so many different disease states that their discriminant function is negligible. The combination of glucose intolerance with hyperinsulinism (see Chapter 7) in the non-obese individual gives some clue to parenchymal damage, but insulin assays are relatively costly and time-consuming, so that this type of test is comparatively unhelpful.

It is possible to test hepatic glycogen reserve by administering glucagon (1 mg I.V. or I.M.). The consequent rise in blood glucose concentration gives an index of hepatic glycogen content,[46] but again the test lacks specificity. Any decrease in nutritional input over the days preceding the test will decrease hepatic glycogen reserves. In addition it is not known to what extent glucagon receptors in the liver are damaged or lost in different hepatic diseases, so that an abnormal response may reflect merely receptor changes and not genuine changes in glycogen. Tests such as this were used initially to identify glycogen storage diseases, but have been largely replaced by direct tissue studies either of cultured cells, such as fibroblasts, or using liver biopsies (see below under 'Storage').

Tests of gluconeogenic capacity have proved to be more sensitive to date than measurements of glucose or glucose disposal. As related in Chapter 3, blood levels of the gluconeogenic precursors, particularly lactate and glycerol, are abnormal in many patients with liver disease both in the fasting and postprandial states. Blood lactate concentration correlates closely with other tests of liver function such as serum albumin and plasma bilirubin levels. It is of interest that in chronic liver disease the most marked changes occur in liver cirrhosis, and indeed it is rare to find a patient with moderate or severe cirrhosis who has a normal blood lactate concentration. There appears to be little advantage, however, in measuring lactate and, in view of the special precautions required in taking blood for this assay (no muscle movement, immediate deproteinization), there is little likelihood of its coming into common usage. There is one situation in which measurement of lactate may be useful in subjects with liver disease. This is in acute liver failure or fulminant liver disease, when parenteral nutritional support is being considered. Such patients are in danger of developing lactic acidosis due to the impaired ability of the diseased liver to remove lactate. If intravenous nutrients such as fructose, ethanol and sorbitol are used, lactate may accumulate rapidly in the blood. In such situations monitoring of lactate directly may be of use, although similar information can be gained by monitoring acid–base status. Infusions of lactate and glycerol with measurement of disappearance rates from the circulation also afford tests of hepatic gluconeogenic capacity. However, again these are time-consuming, complicated and costly, and are probably unnecessary unless a special investigation of carbohydrate metabolism is intended.

In certain inherited disorders (see Chapters 3, 37 and 40) it may be useful to perform fructose or galactose loading tests.[116] The fructose tolerance test is used in the diagnosis of hereditary fructose intolerance. The fructose (0.25 g/kg body weight in adults; 3 g/m^2 surface area in children) must be given intravenously as oral administration can result in profound gastrointestinal symptoms. In affected individuals administration of fructose is followed by symptomatic hypoglycaemia and a prolonged fall in serum inorganic phosphate concentration. The galactose tolerance test has been used in the past as a liver function test, but now is used primarily in the diagnosis of hereditary galactokinase deficiency and congenital galactosaemia. The subject is given 40 g galactose P.O.; a rise of greater than 3 mmol/l (54 mg/dl) in blood galactose level signifies either liver disease or galactokinase deficiency. It should be noted that such tests can be dangerous in patients with galactosaemia.

Lipid Metabolism (see also Chapter 4)

Many abnormalities in circulating lipid concentrations have been described in liver disease including elevated concentrations of free fatty acids and triglycerides.[142] These are, however, totally non-specific and uninformative. It might also be expected that ketogenesis would be defective. Blood ketone body levels are low, however, in normal man and provocation such as prolonged fasting, unjustifiable in patients with liver disease, would be required to prove this.

Abnormalities in circulating lipoproteins have long been known to exist in liver disease, with serum triglyceride concentrations often markedly elevated. In contrast, an early fall in the ability to synthesize apolipoproteins is said to be one of the predetermining factors in the development of fatty liver. This inability to synthesize carrier proteins is opposite to the effects of liver disease on enzyme induction, as shown by the frequently elevated levels of serum γ-glutamyl transferase. There is indeed a close correlation between raised serum triglycerides and γ-glutamyl transferase.[36, 117] Thus whilst a fall in alpha-lipoprotein may be present, elevation in pre beta-lipoprotein will also be observed.

It has been pointed out by Agorastos et al[2] that there are many similarities in the lipoprotein patterns of patients with liver disease and those with lecithin cholesterol acyl-transferase (LCAT) deficiency. Changes in the enzyme level can lead to an increase in free cholesterol and phospholipids in the circulation. It would appear that there is also a change in the lipoprotein pattern with the triglyceride rich fraction moving in the beta-lipoprotein position. In general, however, the changes in normal lipoproteins are relatively non-specific for liver disease, unless detailed time-consuming ultracentrifugation studies are undertaken.

The most striking abnormality of lipoprotein pattern is seen in patients with biliary obstruction where an abnormal lipoprotein, lipoprotein-X, is found in the serum. The presence of lipoprotein-X does not appear to be related to LCAT deficiency despite the fact that the abnormal lipoprotein contains mainly free cholesterol and phosphatidylcholine.[154] In a study of over 600 patients with jaundice Magnani and Alaupovic[113] found that lipoprotein-X was present in serum in 98 per cent of patients with extrahepatic biliary obstruction. Only 26.5 per cent of patients with intrahepatic cholestasis showed lipoprotein-X in the serum. The point was made by the authors that measurement of lipoprotein-X gave a better differentiation than alkaline phosphatase and other standard liver function tests, between jaundice requiring medical treatment and that needing surgical intervention.

In a smaller study Miller and Johnson[125] showed a lesser ability to discriminate using lipoprotein-X levels. In an attempt to improve the discrimination the lipoprotein-X measurement was undertaken together with measurement of LCAT activity in serum. This second parameter failed, however, to add any further information. Similar conclusions were reached by Ritland et al[155] despite the earlier claims of Wengeler, Greten and Seidel.[199] Further studies are required to establish whether measurement of lipoprotein-X and/or LCAT add significantly to our diagnostic armamentarium.

Alcoholic liver disease brings marked changes in lipoprotein fractions as might be expected. A significant increase in free fatty acids is observed, in excess of that seen in other types of liver disease; increases in the pre beta-lipoprotein fraction are also quite marked. Factors influencing this condition include increased peripheral lipolysis, reduced hepatic lipoprotein lipase and enzyme induction.[117] The problems of alcoholic hyperlipidaemia are discussed fully in Chapter 32.

It is apparent that, as with carbohydrate metabolism, measurement of lipid functions of the liver, again due to lack of specificity rather than of sensitivity, offers little in diagnostic terms, apart from a possible contribution from lipoprotein-X measurement. Further details are given in Chapter 4.

Protein Metabolism

The role of the liver in protein metabolism is reviewed in Chapter 5.

Amino acids

Removal of 90 per cent of the functional capacity of the liver is necessary before significant alterations in amino acid metabolism are found. Because of this large reserve the amino acid content of blood and urine may be within normal limits in patients with chronic liver disease. However, elevated levels of amino acids will be found where there is gross liver cell breakdown and this is seen in acute hepatic necrosis, viral hepatitis, and portal cirrhosis. The increase probably represents a combination of tissue breakdown and inability to metabolize incoming amino acids. Increasing tyrosinuria is thought to indicate a rapidly progressive degenerative process of the hepatic parenchyma and is of prognostic significance, although the opposite finding should not provide an optimistic outlook.

Many studies of circulating amino acid levels have been performed in patients with hepatic encephalopathy, but these are of more interest from a pathophysiological, than from a diagnostic or prognostic standpoint (see Chapter 42).

Urea

Urea is formed in the liver from amino groups derived from the deamination of amino acids and from ammonia derived from bacterial metabolism in the large intestine. A fall in urea concentration is associated with decreased deamination of amino acids and is associated with either increased levels of amino acids in hepatic disease,[172] or low amino acid levels in severe nutritional disorders. Changes in blood urea are not usually extreme except when the hepatic condition is associated with renal failure. The blood urea may fall toward zero and this is a poor prognostic sign.[173] In general, however, measurement of urea is of little use in liver disease.

Ammonia

Ammonia arises from the metabolism of intestinal bacteria and to a lesser extent from the deamination of amino acids in extrahepatic tissues or in the liver itself. Whilst most is removed from the body in the form of urea, a minute amount may escape in the expired air.

The level of ammonia in the blood may increase in cases of severe hepatic functional impairment, particularly in portal cirrhosis with shunting of blood across the liver.[161] The increase in circulating ammonia was implicated early in the development of hepatic encephalopathy (see Chapter 42), although it is now considered to be a minor factor. Increases in ammonia concentration in these conditions will be exacerbated by any increase in protein content of the diet. Therefore care must be taken in balancing the protein intake against the depressed circulating albumin level and the effects of circulating ammonia levels. Monitoring of blood ammonia levels may be of therapeutic aid in such cases.[168]

Ammonium chloride tolerance test. Ammonium chloride tolerance tests have been used in the past to demonstrate abnormalities of ammonia metabolism in cases where the resting blood ammonia levels are within normal limits.[179] In one procedure blood is taken before and 45 minutes after oral administration of three grams of ammonium chloride. Normal tolerance, which represents a return to normal ammonium levels within 45 minutes, is usually found in patients with jaundice caused by biliary obstruction, metastatic carcinoma and uncomplicated cirrhosis.[31]

Elevated levels are found in patients with significant portasystemic shunting, the extent of the abnormality probably being related to the degree of shunting.[121] This test is little used nowadays, probably as a result of greater understanding of the biochemical aspects of hepatic encephalopathy.

Octopamines

Fischer and Baldessarini[47] proposed that features of hepatic encephalopathy were related to an accumulation of β-hydroxylated phenylethylamines, octopamine and β-phenylethanolamine (see Chapter 42). These substances are weak neurochemical transmitters and may replace physiological transmitters at nerve endings in the peripheral and central nervous system. Increased levels of octopamine have been demonstrated in the serum and urine of patients with hepatic encephalopathy and in the brains and other tissues of animals with experimentally induced liver damage.[48]

In a study of the patients with proven liver disease, Manghani et al[115] found statistically significant increases in urine and serum octopamine levels between patients with and without encephalopathy, and between grade 0 and grade 1 encephalopathy. Levels of urinary octopamine excretion overlapped for the different grades of encephalopathy. There appeared to be no prognostic value in the measurement of either serum or urine octopamine levels. In another study, plasma levels of octopamine and ammonia were compared in 65 patients with chronic liver disease.[28] There was a significant correlation between venous ammonia and octopamine levels, but no correlation was found with arterial blood samples, probably reflecting the number of patients with portasystemic shunts. Patients with portasystemic anastomosis displayed low octopamine and high ammonia levels and this was evident in 10 of 31 shunted cirrhotics without signs of hepatic encephalopathy and 6 of 16 with grade 1 or 2 encephalopathy. The authors concluded that there may be other biogenic amines which may also be responsible for hepatic encephalopathy, which is supported by the observation of inhibition of the transmethylation reaction in the octopamine assay. Measurement of octopamine has found little use in the diagnosis or assessment of patients with liver disease.

Serum proteins

The liver is the major site for synthesis of many of the proteins circulating in the body. The liver cells are the sole sites of formation of alpha and beta globulins. The gamma globulins are synthesized in cells of the reticuloendothelial system and thus most of these proteins are extrahepatic in origin.

Changes in serum proteins in liver disease will reflect a multifactorial reaction which includes a response to foreign agents and the effects of decreased protein synthesis. The simple concept of diminished synthesis, however, may not be a true reflection of protein turnover status.

Changes in protein levels may frequently be due to alteration in distribution or catabolism of plasma proteins, sometimes due to factors similar to those present in a variety of other types of tissue injury. Furthermore a change in the synthesis of a plasma protein in the liver may reflect variations in the *regulation* of synthesis rather than a change in *capacity* for this function.

Albumin (see Chapter 5). Albumin is quantitatively the most important plasma protein synthesized by the liver. The average adult contains approximately 300 g albumin with some 12 g produced daily; a reduction in synthetic rate of 50 per cent would result in only a 20 per cent fall in the serum albumin value. This may explain why only minimal changes in the serum albumin value are found in patients with typical acute viral hepatitis.[123] More marked changes in serum albumin are seen when there is gross tissue necrosis, as, for example, in solvent poisoning. Albumin has a fairly long half-life in the circulation (approximately 20 days) and thus it is not a particularly useful marker of protein synthesis in acute situations.[177]

Hypoalbuminaemia may occur in chronic liver diseases such as portal cirrhosis and hepatic malignancy. It may be quite marked in cirrhosis, contributing to the development of the ascites and generalized oedema that may be associated with the condition. In advanced stages of the disease the hypoalbuminaemia may in part be due to the progressively increased shunting of blood in the liver as a result of a raised portal pressure.[212]

Hypoalbuminaemia may also result from inadequate nutrition. This is thought to contribute to the hypoalbuminaemia that may be found in patients with extrahepatic biliary obstruction; hepatocellular damage may be a further contributory factor. Protein malnutrition will also produce hypoalbuminaemia as seen in 'kwashiorkor', a form of hepatic disease seen in children in tropical countries resulting from a low protein intake.

Measurement of albumin provides a reasonable guide to the severity of chronic liver disease, although yielding no aetiological clues. Albumin levels correlate well with other measurements of liver function in cirrhosis such as bilirubin and lactate concentration. In that it is a reasonably easy measurement it will doubtless continue to be useful as a long-term guide to hepatic synthetic function in chronic liver disease, providing that care is taken to rule out other hypoalbuminaemic states such as severe renal disease, malnutrition, protein losing gastroenteropathy, severe catabolic states (e.g. burns), and dilutional states.

Globulins. The changes in the globulins, and indeed basic globulin fractions, may mask considerable changes occurring with individual proteins within these fractions. It is useful, however, to consider the globulins together, although more attempts are now being made to identify specific proteins rather than determine changes in whole groups of proteins.

The long half-life of albumin means that only minimal changes will be seen in serum albumin levels in acute conditions; however, more marked changes will be seen in proteins with shorter half-lives. Proteins with rapid turnover rates include pre-albumin and the alpha-lipoproteins (half-lives of less than two days and four days respectively).[177] Several of the coagulation factors also have short half-lives. In acute viral hepatitis, and also fluctuating chronic active hepatitis, the serum albumin may remain within normal limits, whilst the pre-albumin value will be much reduced.[177] In quiescent chronic liver disease, the correlation between albumin and pre-albumin is good. When proteins of similar turnover rates are compared, the correlation is good whatever the course of the disorder, as for example with pre-albumin and alpha-lipoprotein levels.[177]

The changes in alpha-lipoprotein are mirrored in the changes of the globulins as a group, with decreases seen in acute viral hepatitis.[123] Changes seen in the globulins may reflect the changes seen in flocculation tests described later.

Changes in the beta globulin fraction are encountered more consistently than those in the alpha globulin fraction. Increases may be seen in viral hepatitis, extrahepatic biliary obstruction and biliary cirrhosis;[74] these changes are frequently related to changes in lipoproteins.

Most changes are, however, seen in the gamma globulin fraction (see Chapter 9). This must be due to a variety of factors including the production of antibodies and the leakage of cellular contents when damage occurs. In acute viral hepatitis the gamma globulin fraction increases soon after exposure to the infectious agent and may remain elevated for up to five months. Progression to chronic liver disease may be indicated if elevation of the gamma globulin fraction persists.

A variety of techniques has been employed in the assessment of changes in serum proteins.

Early tests dependent on changes in serum protein fractions included the cephalin–cholesterol flocculation test, the thymol turbidity and flocculation tests, and the zinc sulphate turbidity test. The flocculation and turbidity tests do not necessarily depend on changes in the concentration of one protein or protein fraction, but on the relationship that exists between several protein fractions.

Cephalin–cholesterol flocculation test. This test is said to respond to an increase in serum globulins and a decrease in albumin.[22] It has been claimed that the test is extremely sensitive to changes in serum albumin with a rapid response in acute viral hepatitis; the lack of change in serum albumin concentrations would dispute this claim in the absence of evidence to support qualitative changes in the albumin molecule. It has also been claimed that the reaction seen early in acute viral hepatitis is due to a fall in the alpha globulin concentration.[151] The conditions for production of a positive reaction are met in a large proportion of cases of hepatocellular damage and a lesser incidence of reaction is seen in obstructive liver disease.[70] The specificity of the test is slight, and it adds little to measurement of albumin together with quantitative serum protein electrophoresis.

Thymol turbidity and flocculation tests. These tests are influenced by a decrease in serum albumin and an increase in globulin fractions, but are mainly affected by increases in the lipoprotein and beta globulin fractions.[105] Therefore one may see positive results associated with hyperlipidaemia, e.g. in diabetes, and in normal subjects after a fatty meal. The test does not respond as rapidly as the cephalin–cholesterol flocculation test to the onset of viral hepatitis, but an abnormal response is maintained over a longer period.

Zinc sulphate turbidity test. This test is more affected by changes in gamma globulins alone than the other two tests. The high levels of gamma globulin characteristic of chronic hepatitis and cirrhosis are readily detected by the zinc sulphate turbidity test.[105] Therefore, whilst results for this test may parallel changes seen with the other turbidity tests, the parallelism is not consistent because the zinc sulphate test is not so affected by changes in albumin and lipid concentrations. The main claim for this test is its ability to distinguish between hepatocellular damage and extra-hepatic obstruction.[105]

In a comparison of several biochemical liver function tests with the protein-dependent turbidity and flocculation tests, Weinrib, Schaefer and Oikawa[198] found that no added information could be obtained from the inclusion of turbidity tests with a group of tests that included serum bilirubin, alkaline phosphatase and the aminotransferases. It has been suggested that these tests are now outdated and should be replaced by more specific tests, namely protein electrophoresis and immunological measurement of specific proteins. Countering this argument is the point that flocculation tests are simple, quick and inexpensive to perform – but with the use of automated immunoprecipitation measurement techniques, it is reasonable to expect an increasing use of specific protein assays. The full value of specific protein measurement will, however, only be achieved with understanding of the underlying pathophysiological changes.

Serum protein electrophoresis. It is possible to recognize electrophoresis patterns associated with certain hepatic diseases (Figure 17.1). Thus, in acute viral hepatitis there may be a fall in the alpha-1-globulin with an increase in beta globulin.[123] A gradual increase in the gamma globulin fraction over a period of months after the onset of hepatitis is a prognostic index of the transition from acute to chronic hepatitis. In cases of cirrhosis the albumin is reduced with a generalized increase in the gamma globulin fraction. This may be accompanied by a merging of the beta and gamma globulin bands, due to an increase in the IgA immunoglobulin.[74] In cholestasis, on the other hand, the increases in the gamma globulin fraction are smaller but with significant increases in alpha and beta globulin, due in part to the increased concentrations of lipoproteins.

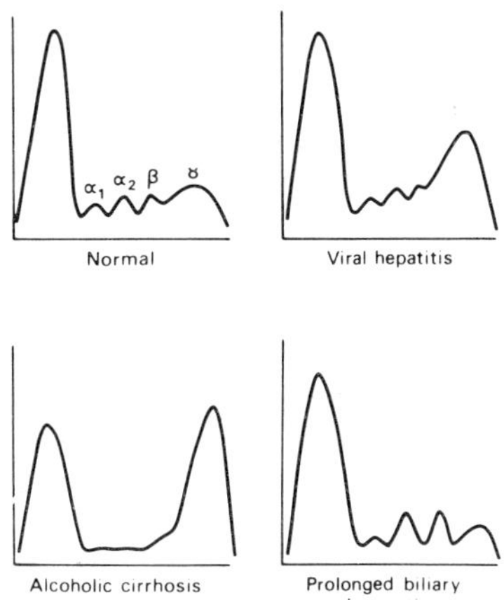

Figure 17.1. Serum protein electrophoresis patterns in various types of liver disease.

Measurement of specific proteins

Fibrinogen. The hepatic cells are the sole site of formation of fibrinogen. Mild liver damage is usually associated with normal or slightly elevated levels of fibrinogen in the circulation.[196] Severe cellular damage will, however, cause the fibrinogen level to fall to as low as 1.5 μmol/l (500 mg/l).[149] The measurement of fibrinogen is of little value in the diagnosis of hepatic dysfunction, but low values do indicate extensive liver damage.

Acute phase proteins. In diseases associated with tissue necrosis, changes can be seen in a number of serum proteins; these proteins are called the 'acute phase reacting proteins'.[201] In liver disease associated with tissue injury there may be an increase in some of the serum proteins (positive acute phase reactants), a decrease in concentration of other serum proteins (negative acute phase reactants) and unchanged concentration in other proteins, e.g. alpha-2-macroglobulin.

Changes in the acute phase reactants, including alpha-1-antitrypsin, alpha-1-acid glycoprotein, haptoglobin, fibrinogen and C-reactive protein, are not always easy to interpret. The concentration of haptoglobin may fall in acute viral hepatitis,[177] yet an increase is generally found in other types of acute infection. It is unlikely that defective synthesis is responsible for the decrease as haptoglobin levels are generally normal in cirrhotic patients who have impaired albumin synthesis. It is possible that haptoglobin has been consumed in this situation due to increased erythrocyte breakdown. The levels of transferrin have also been shown to be increased in acute viral hepatitis.

By measurement of acute phase proteins in patients with myocardial infarction, Smith et al[178] were able to show a quantitative relationship between the acute phase protein pattern and the extent of tissue injury. This supports the theory of Darcy[38] that humoral factors released from the site of tissue damage give rise to a change in the rate of protein synthesis in the liver. Certainly cortisol and catecholamines have been shown to influence the rate of protein synthesis in the liver.[193]

There appears to be little value in measuring the acute phase proteins in patients with liver disease in that they add little to prognosis or diagnosis. At present there is insufficient knowledge of the factors affecting the rate of synthesis of these proteins in the liver.

There is one particular acute phase protein, however, which has attracted attention in recent years. This is alpha-1-antitrypsin. It is a protein synthesized solely in the liver and levels in the serum are known to increase in many inflammatory states. In many types of liver disease the alpha-1-antitrypsin levels are either normal or increased. It is now thought that alpha-1-antitrypsin deficiency may be an important cause of liver disease (see Chapter 35).[24]

Pseudocholinesterase. The use of enzymes in diagnosis is generally related to the assessment of tissue damage, and enzyme measurement is not often utilized in the assessment of protein synthesis, although γ-glutamyl transferase is sometimes used in this way as a measure of the activity of the microsomal enzyme system.

The level of pseudocholinesterase in patients with liver disease has been found to follow the pattern of protein metabolism, falling in catabolism and rising in anabolism.[26] The level of enzyme in the serum falls in response to trauma and in response to marked infection. Evidence suggests that its synthesis parallels that of serum albumin. It is generally considered that if the enzyme level falls to a low level it is indicative of serious disease. It has been found to be of value in predicting whether liver function will deteriorate after a shunt operation in any given patient.[79]

Coagulation factors. The use of coagulation factors in relation to the assessment of protein metabolism is discussed in Chapter 8. Early studies involved a broad spectrum of tests of blood clotting but more recently the measurement of specific factors has been used. Good correlation has been shown between Factor VII levels, prothrombin time and serum albumin in patients with liver disease.[62] However, it would appear that the prothrombin time technique employed by these workers favoured the assessment of Factor VII and therefore the correlation may not be as good if other techniques are used. The haematological techniques may be of greater value than the estimation of serum albumin because the latter is affected by other non-hepatic factors.

Hormone Metabolism

The liver is intimately involved in the actions and metabolism of many hormones. Polypeptide hormones are degraded by proteolytic enzymes after interaction with specific cell surface receptors, although much remains to be learned about the specific sites at which degradation takes place. The evidence to date suggests that receptor binding precedes degradation. Failure to degrade these hormones has important implications for whole body metabolic homeostasis in that increased concentrations of these hormones may reach peripheral tissues. Non-protein hormones also act on and are degraded by the liver, by oxidation and conjugation. As yet no liver function tests have been based on altered hormone metabolism (for further details see Chapter 7).

Digestion

The liver plays an important role in the function of the alimentary tract through the provision of bile acids. The metabolism and function of bile acids are described in detail in Chapter 12.

There are very few commonly performed tests of bile acid metabolism, although there has been a great deal of recent interest in measurement of bile acids in the serum. It is generally accepted that the measurement of serum bile acids two hours after a meal is of more value than measurement in the fasting state.[89] The question is what function is being assessed? Clearly measurement in the postprandial state reflects the ability of the liver not only to synthesize the bile acids, but also to clear them from the portal blood stream. The value of the measurement of serum bile acids may be that they provide a single test which depends on several liver functions giving a very sensitive index of overall hepatic dysfunction.[8, 87]

The most commonly performed test of bile acid metabolism is the cholylglycine or bile acid tolerance test. This involves giving cholylglycine and measuring the plasma disappearance using a radioimmunoassay technique.[103] The tolerance test was compared with the measurement of fasting conjugated cholic acid in the serum and it was found that the tolerance test was a more sensitive index of liver dysfunction. One could in fact consider the single measurement of postprandial bile acid as a bile acid tolerance test using endogenous bile acid. Evidence suggests that the postprandial bile acid measurement is both sensitive and reliable and little is to be gained from the more complicated bile acid tolerance test.[87]

The ^{14}C-cholylglycine breath test has also been described recently.[189] This test does not appear to have many advantages in the assessment of hepatic function, although it does assess the state of the bile acid pool. It reflects more the level of bile acid deconjugation and metabolism in the bowel than hepatic bile acid metabolism and finds its main use as a gastrointestinal function test.

Detoxification and Excretory Function

The liver plays an important part in removing potentially harmful substances from the body. Many of the detoxifying functions involve the processing of substances by oxidation, generally through the microsomal system, and conjugation into relatively non-toxic substances which are excreted in the bile and urine. The term detoxification is not necessarily a correct description of the process taking place, as it implies that the substance being transformed is harmful; this may not always be the case.

Steroid metabolism

The liver plays a major role in the metabolism of many steroids; thus the liver is involved in the conversion of progesterone to pregnanediol which has no biological activity and is excreted in the bile and the urine.[12] The androgen, testosterone, produced in the testes is metabolized in the liver to several unknown compounds, although one of the commonest metabolites is androsterone. Some of the androsterone is secreted into the bile but most is conjugated with sulphate and eventually excreted in the urine.

Changes in androgen metabolism have been demonstrated in patients with liver disease including viral hepatitis, chronic active hepatitis, and cirrhosis. A fall is seen in the level of urinary 17-oxosteroid (one-third of this group of steroid metabolites being androsterone). There is also a decrease in the conjugation of the steroid and reduced removal of steroid from the circulation. It would appear that there may also be an increase in urine oestrogen and fall in gonadotrophins which suggests that the change in androgen status and possibly also testicular atrophy may be secondary to an increase in circulating oestrogens.

The possible involvement of oestrogens in androgenic steroid metabolism changes in liver disease suggests that the liver may play a part in oestrogen metabolism. The liver is known to contain enzyme systems that convert oestradiol to less active oestrogens. Conjugation takes place in the liver and there is evidence to suggest an enterohepatic circulation of free oestrogens, free oestrogen often being found in the bile.[4]

The liver is also responsible for the modification of adrenocortical hormones to inactive metabolites. The biologically inactive metabolites are conjugated and eventually excreted in the urine. The adrenocorticoids undergo reduction and conjugation to form sulphates and glucuronides. No liver function tests are based on steroid metabolism or measurement. The pathophysiological aspects of the subject are dealt with in detail in Chapter 7.

Bilirubin metabolism

The subject of bilirubin metabolism is dealt with extensively in Chapter 13. There are essentially five stages at which changes in the metabolism may occur. These can be identified as: (a) increased load presented to the liver cell; (b) reduced uptake and intracellular transport by the liver cell; (c) reduction in conjugating ability; (d) reduced excretion at the canulicular surface; and (e) reduced biliary flow. Derangement of hepatic architecture may involve all stages.

Haemolysis, increasing the production of bilirubin, will lead to a situation of 'overload jaundice' where the ability of the liver to remove the pigment is saturated. The maximum handling capacity of the liver is approximately 770 μmol (450 mg) bilirubin per day, which represents a doubling of the erythrocyte destruction rate. Overload jaundice may also be produced in the absence of haemolysis; it is thought that in this case the bilirubin arises from unwanted haem produced in the bone marrow. Both situations are demonstrated by an increase in the unconjugated bilirubin fraction in the blood.

A reduction in the removal of bilirubin from the circulation has been observed after administration of flavaspidic acid and various cholecystographic agents.[170] Flavaspidic acid displaces bilirubin and BSP from intracellular binding sites. *Gilbert's* syndrome may also represent defective bilirubin removal, although some workers have demonstrated a conjugation defect.[15]

Gilbert's syndrome presents as an asymptomatic unconjugated bilirubinaemia with serum bilirubin levels ranging from normal to 90 μmol/l (5.3 mg/dl). Conventional bromsulphthalein (BSP) excretion tests are normal, although abnormalities of dye excretion kinetics have been demonstrated in some cases. The condition is often detected accidentally either as a sequel to viral hepatitis or when a person undergoes routine biochemical profiling. The picture presents as a moderate unconjugated bilirubinaemia with absence of conjugated bilirubinaemia and no other abnormalities of liver function. An increase in unconjugated bilirubin is observed following a 400 kcal diet for 24 hours or after the administration of nicotinic acid.[138]

Recently it has been suggested that Gilbert's disease may reflect a 'statistical phenomenon'. Bailey, Robinson and Dawson[7] studied biochemical profiles on almost 24 000 people attending a screening centre. Both sexes showed a skewed distribution for bilirubin concentration, but analysis of the data showed no evidence of bimodality for either sex. The term 'constitutional hyperbilirubinaemia' was suggested as a name for a condition that reflects an unusual statistical distribution, rather than a disease state.

There is a genetically determined deficiency of bilirubin glucuronyl transferase in the *Crigler–Najjar* syndrome. Levels of bilirubin in the circulation may rise to over 1000 μmol/l (58 mg/dl). The BSP excretion is normal in this condition.

This deficiency of the conjugating enzyme is distinct from other conditions, such as the *Lucey–Driscoll* syndrome, in which it is thought there are circulating steroid-like substances in the serum of pregnant women that inhibit the activity of the conjugating enzymes.[104] In some cases breast milk has also been shown to contain an inhibitor of bilirubin conjugation.[67]

The increase of conjugated bilirubin in the serum is the result of reduced excretion of bile, either at the canalicular junction or in the biliary tree. The *Dubin–Johnson* syndrome is a chronic intermittent conjugated hyperbilirubinaemia with bilirubin present in the urine. Other biochemical liver function tests are normal except for a reduced BSP excretion rate. Another condition, *Rotor's* syndrome, shows many similar features, but lacks the presence of a black pigment in the liver tissue, which is seen in Dubin–Johnson syndrome.[169] The BSP excretion pattern is similar in both conditions with a BSP level at 120 minutes that exceeds the level at 45 minutes (Figure 17.2).

The post-canalicular reduction in bilirubin excretion may result from varying levels of obstruction to the flow of bile in the biliary tree; these are discussed in greater detail in Chapter 13.

Drugs may interfere with the metabolism of bilirubin at most levels, from its production to its excretion. Thus the sulphonamides can cause haemolysis due to a hypersensitivity which results in decreased hepatocellular function. The effects of drugs on bilirubin excretion are discussed in Chapters 16 and 36, and show that effects can occur at the level of bilirubin uptake, conjugation and canalicular excretion. There are also drugs that will reduce the ability of the liver to excrete bilirubin by virtue of their effects on hepatic architecture, e.g. solvents like carbon tetrachloride.

The value of serum bilirubin measurement lies in the quantitative assessment of jaundice: it is not a particularly sensitive index of parenchymal damage, levels being higher with cholestasis.

Bromsulphthalein excretion

The dye bromsulphthalein (BSP) is taken up by the liver cell, conjugated with glutathione and excreted in the bile. Thus bilirubin and bromsulphthalein are treated similarly by the liver cell. The use of this dye and other similar dyes in tests of liver function or functional capacity requires that a dose be given that approaches the normal maximal handling capacity of the liver.

The standard test involves the infusion of a known amount of dye into an arm vein over a five-minute period, with removal of blood samples from the other arm at 5, 25 and 45 minute intervals, after the commencement of the infusion.[85] There is a variety of factors that can affect the determination of the dye in serum and it is important, in view of the low levels of dye retained in normal subjects, that the test is carefully controlled.[50] The dye is given in relation to body weight and the concentration of dye in the serum of the five minute blood sample is regarded as equivalent to 100 per cent retention.

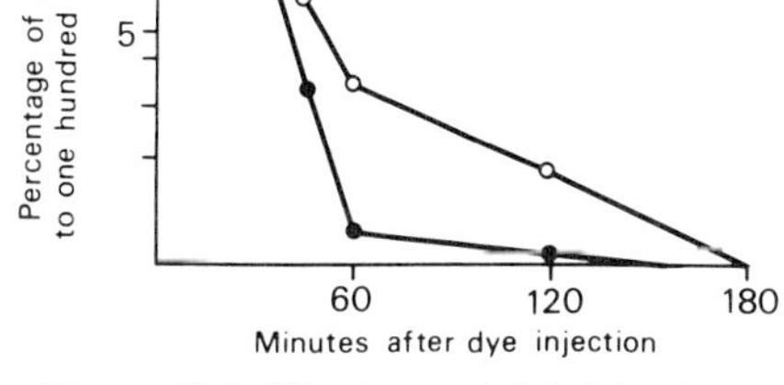

Figure 17.2. The bromsulphthalein dye retention curve over a period of three hours in a normal subject (●---●), in a patient with metastatic carcinoma (○——○), and in a patient with Dubin–Johnson syndrome (□——□).

It is generally considered that normal dye excretion results in only 5 per cent being retained at 45 minutes. However, Zieve and Hill[211] performed bromsulphthalein excretion tests on 718 normal subjects and noted that 50 per cent had retentions of less than 4 per cent, 90 per cent of subjects less than 8 per cent, and 99 per cent of subjects less than 14 per cent retention in 45 minutes, suggesting a wider reference range. Furthermore, it is known that increased dye retention is seen in obesity, old age, fever, prolonged fasting, pregnancy and prior administration of drugs, for example cholecystographic agents.[85] The reasons for these differences are not clear, although differing compartmental distribution is likely in obese patients. In these situations it is difficult to predict the possible importance of competition between the dye and endogenous materials for protein transport and uptake by the liver. There is little point in undertaking a dye excretion test when a raised serum bilirubin has been noted, or in the patient already known to have liver disease.

The BSP test is said to be useful in detecting minor or early changes in liver function, although this is not universally accepted.[87] The test is said to be more sensitive and reliable if the initial removal capacity is assessed by obtaining blood specimens at five-minute intervals for up to half an hour.[85] In patients suspected of having Dubin–Johnson syndrome, additional samples should be taken for up to two hours (Figure 17.2). An estimation of the hepatic storage capacity and transport maximum (Tm) requires continuous infusion of dye and serial blood sampling. The BSP_{Tm} is reported to be the best single determinant of hepatic dysfunction and is valuable in assessing the response to therapy in chronic active hepatitis.[60]

Indocyanine green excretion

The reporting of side-effects such as thrombophlebitis and anaphylactic reactions with BSP has led to the search for other tests. Indocyanine green is said to be free from side-effects and is rapidly excreted by the liver in an unconjugated form.[23, 107] The dye has the further advantage that it can be assayed directly and has been accurately and continuously monitored by dichromatic ear densitometry. The rate of disappearance of the dye is thought to be related to hepatic blood flow and significant alteration in dye excretion has been noted in experimental myocardial infarction, myocardial infarction in man and in obstructive airways disease.[44] The indocyanine green clearance test is performed by injecting first 0.5 mg/kg I.V. with blood samples taken at two, four, six and eight minutes. If the percentage disappearance rate is normal (28 ± 3%/min) then 5 mg/kg are given, which approaches V_{max} for the normal liver, and the test is repeated. Normal percentage disappearance rate is 23 ± 2%/min for the bigger dose.[108] This is probably the dye excretion test of choice at the present time.[106]

Rose bengal excretion

The use of rose bengal excretion as an index of hepatic dysfunction is discussed in Chapter 20 together with the use of other isotopically labelled compounds employed in a similar way.

Microsomal Enzyme Induction

The effect of phenobarbitone in increasing the conjugation of bilirubin by inducing the synthesis of the conjugating enzyme has been mentioned earlier. This observation represents an aspect of alteration in hepatic function that is ill-understood in terms of the breadth of its involvement in hepatic dysfunction. It has been known for some years that the enzyme composition of cells can be altered by nutritional factors, hormonal factors and the administration of foreign chemical agents.[98] The evidence for alteration in the synthesis of enzymes is based first on an inability to demonstrate activation of pre-existing enzymes and secondly on the fact that agents that abolish de novo protein synthesis suppress the effects of 'enzyme-inducing agents'.[33]

There are two groups of enzyme-inducing agents. The first group acts in a rather non-specific way, increasing a variety of metabolic processes associated with drug metabolism. The agents themselves are not necessarily related and include phenobarbitone and phenytoin. The second group of agents has more specific effects and often acts in a different way from the first group. Thus an agent from the second group can further enhance enzyme activity already stimulated by an agent from the first group.[133]

The most appropriate technique for demonstrating enzyme induction is the direct demonstration of enhanced specific activities in the tissue. Obviously this has limited possibilities in man, although it has been applied to liver biopsy specimens.[16] Usually, therefore, enzyme induction is assessed indirectly.

The effects of enzyme-inducing agents on drug metabolism may be determined by measuring the changes produced in the duration of action of a standard drug. Alternatively, changes in the rate of metabolism of a drug can be determined by measurement of drug metabolites in blood or urine. Phenylbutazone and antipyrine are two drugs that have been used in this context, primarily because their concentrations can be measured easily.

Antipyrine

Since the liver is the major site of drug metabolism, one might expect alteration in drug metabolism in the presence of liver disease. Several investigations of antipyrine half-life in blood have been undertaken in patients with liver disease, using determination of antipyrine half-life after a single dose of drug (1200 mg). Branch, Herbert and Read[20] showed that in patients with liver disease, the metabolism of the antipyrine was impaired. The abnormality was less in patients with acute forms of liver disease, viral hepatitis and obstructive jaundice, compared with patients with chronic forms of liver disease. The greatest prolongation of antipyrine half-life was seen in patients with evidence of reduced hepatic protein synthesizing ability (reduced serum albumin and prolonged prothrombin time not responding to vitamin K). Prolonged antipyrine half-life did not, however, correlate with other biochemical liver function or damage tests. Administration of phenobarbitone over three days produced a significant reduction in antipyrine half-life, as did prednisone when given over a longer period. In studies of this type the effect of variation in hepatic blood flow should not be overlooked as the rate at which drugs are presented to the liver cell will also have an effect on the clearance from the circulation.[21]

Aminopyrine breath test. Assessment of the kinetics of drug disappearance depends in part on the ability to measure the drug in the blood, and is not always straightforward. Attempts have been made to overcome this problem by measuring labelled carbon dioxide in the breath derived from a small dose of radioactively labelled aminopyrine. The test is based on the fact that the ^{14}C-labelled methyl groups of aminopyrine are metabolized to $^{14}CO_2$; elimination in the breath is related to the rate of aminopyrine metabolism.[14] An oral dose of 1.5 μCi (5.55×10^4 Bq) ^{14}C(-dimethylamine)-aminopyrine is given; two hours later the breath is collected by blowing through hyamine-hydroxide in ethanol, until an indicator changes colour (equivalent to the collection of 2 mmol CO_2). After addition of scintillation fluid the radioactively labelled carbon dioxide is determined. The percentage of the dose excreted is then calculated. In a series of patients with alcoholic liver disease it was shown that the $^{14}CO_2$ excretion was decreased in patients with cirrhosis (Figure 17.3).[109] Widely scattered and generally higher values were found in patients without cirrhosis. Four patients with cirrhosis showed excretion in the high normal range and these cases were known to be taking enzyme-inducing drugs. It may also be of note that patients with the lowest values showed a very poor prognosis. In alcoholic liver disease there would appear to be a progression from a state where the microsomal enzyme system may be activated with reduced half-life of some drugs, to a state where there is an overall reduction in microsomal enzyme activity due to diminished protein synthesis. Further progress in this direction has a poor prognostic outlook.[109]

A further evaluation of the aminopyrine breath test by Galizzi et al[56] confirmed the view that reduced excretion of $^{14}CO_2$ was related to the degree of hepatocellular failure. In assessing its value as a liver function test it was thought to be more sensitive for detecting hepatocellular disease than serum albumin, serum bilirubin and prothrombin, as might be expected. However, it was no more sensitive than serum aspartate aminotransferase and a serum two-hour postprandial bile acid level. It has been shown to correlate well with bromsulphthalein excretion index and galactose elimination capacity.[14] Its main value would appear to be in relation to the status of the microsomal enzyme system, and the full value of assessment of this functional aspect has yet to be determined.

Other methods of assessing microsomal enzyme induction

The level of activity of the microsomal enzyme system may be of importance in its own right, as distinct from being part of a multifactorial problem as is likely in patients with liver disease. Measurement of the plasma antipyrine half-life in patients with chronic renal failure suggests that the microsomal enzyme system is activated in these patients;[112] the plasma antipyrine half-life was half that found in normal subjects. The clinical significance of these findings is yet to be appreciated, but clearly activation of drug metabolizing enzymes may have an effect on vitamin D metabolism and so contribute to the osteomalacia seen in some of these patients.

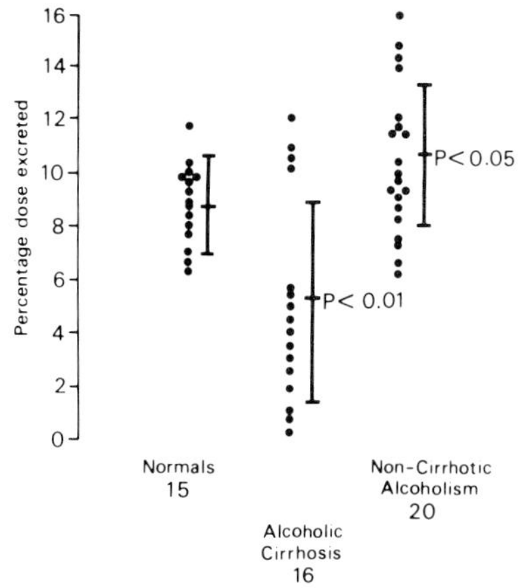

Figure 17.3. Aminopyrine breath test. Two hour $^{14}CO_2$ excretion as a percentage of the oral dose in normal subjects and in alcoholic liver disease (mean ± 1 SD). From Lewis et al,[109] with kind permission of the authors and the editor of *Journal of Clinical Pathology*.

Two metabolic pathways of endogenous compounds have been used as indices of enzyme induction. The behaviour of the microsomal hydroxylating system for steroids appears to be identical to that for drugs.[188] The excretion of 6β-hydroxycortisol, a polar metabolite of cortisol, in relation to the total excretion of 17-hydroxycorticosteroids (which are not changed by inducing agents), has been used as an index of microsomal enzyme induction.[102] However, there may be disadvantages to this approach as 6β-hydroxycortisol may be formed outside the liver and indeed increased urinary levels have been observed with no other evidence of altered drug metabolism or enzyme induction.[27]

The ratio of 6β-hydroxycortisol to 17-hydroxycorticosteroids was studied in patients with liver disease by Eade et al.[43] They found that the mean ratio was increased in the urine in all groups of patients studied, and was even elevated in some patients in the recovery phase of viral hepatitis in whom traditional liver function tests were normal. The results showed a wide overlap between patients reflecting acute and chronic liver disease groups. The ratio was significantly increased in patients with secondary carcinoma compared with patients having a single carcinoma. It is obvious from these findings that the test has little discriminatory use, and in general is an unnecessary part of the hepatologist's diagnostic armamentarium.

The second metabolic pathway which may be enhanced by enzyme-inducing agents involves the conversion of hexoses to glucuronic acid.[76] It has been shown that aminopyrine will increase the urinary excretion of xylulose, an end product of glucuronic acid metabolism. In human beings D-glucaric acid is one of the major metabolites of D-glucuronic acid and it has been shown that D-glucaric acid excretion is increased in patients given enzyme-inducing drugs;[1] the urine levels of D-glucaric acid correlate well with the concentration of microsomal enzyme cytochrome P-450.[80] Again, however, measurement of D-glucaric acid must remain in the field of special investigations.

γ-Glutamyl transferase

Levels of the enzyme γ-glutamyl transferase are raised in the blood of patients taking enzyme-inducing drugs.[160] Evidence has been produced that supports the idea that this elevation is due to enzyme induction. The change in serum γ-glutamyl transferase activity in patients on enzyme-inducing drugs is not great, although it is possible to show a good correlation with the concomitant effects of such agents on warfarin metabolism. Results are, however, somewhat erratic.[203]

Elevated levels of serum γ-glutamyl transferase have been found in over 80 per cent of heavy drinkers and alcoholics, this incidence being much higher than changes in other biochemical liver function tests.[156] Increases in γ-glutamyl transferase activity may be present without any other clinical evidence of liver disease being present. Whilst the levels of serum γ-glutamyl transferase may reflect various alterations of hepatic function beyond just microsomal enzyme induction, they are of value in monitoring the progress of alcoholics and checking for abstention from alcohol. When drinking stops, the serum γ-glutamyl transferase falls by as much as 50 per cent within ten days.[156]

There would appear to be little value in the use of serum γ-glutamyl transferase levels in the differential diagnosis of liver disease, because of its varied distribution within the liver. It is further complicated by the fact that in many instances we do not know the extent of enzyme induction or de novo protein synthesis that takes place in any type of liver disease. The main value of serum γ-glutamyl transferase measurement therefore probably lies in its sensitivity as a broad index of hepatic dysfunction, and as a means of monitoring truthfulness in alcoholic patients.

Storage Functions

The liver plays an important role in the storage of many constituents of the body. Alteration in the metabolism of any one constituent whilst affecting the respective metabolic pathway may also grossly alter other functions of the liver.

Iron storage

There have in the past been attempts to differentiate two conditions, representing excess iron in the liver with or without tissue damage. The subject of iron storage disease is discussed in Chapter 34.

The biochemical liver function tests will depend in part on the severity of the condition and most often reflect a cirrhotic pattern. The serum iron concentration is often raised and serum transferrin may be saturated to as much as 95 per cent. The assay of serum ferritin has proved of diagnostic value with increased levels seen in haemochromatosis, with the advent of radio-immunoassay techniques for its measurement.[148]

Copper storage

The subject of Wilson's disease is discussed in detail in Chapter 33. Patients with this condition present with a picture of cirrhosis; a wide pattern of change in routine biochemical liver function tests will be observed, reflecting the effects of the copper deposition on other aspects of liver function. The serum caeruloplasmin and copper levels will be decreased. An increased twenty-four hour urine copper level will be found, but care must be taken in the collection of the specimen to avoid contamination of collection vessels.

Lipid storage

The lipoidoses are disorders in which abnormal amounts of lipids are stored in the cells of the reticuloendothelial system (see Chapter 37).

There is a very rare inherited disease known as cholesteryl ester storage disease which involves the liver. The defect appears to relate to two lysosomal enzymes, cholesteryl ester hydrolase and triglyceride lipase.[52]

Gaucher's disease is a rare condition in which

a glucocerebroside, containing sphingosine, fatty acid and glucose, is deposited in the reticuloendothelial system, because it cannot be cleared due to a deficiency of the enzyme glucocerebrosidase.[139] The biochemical changes are very variable. The serum cholesterol is normal. A persistently elevated tartrate-stable acid phosphatase may suggest Gaucher's disease. Diagnosis of Gaucher's disease may be confirmed by measurement of tissue enzyme levels in cultured skin fibroblasts or leucocytes. A method has recently been described for the detection of individual heterozygotes and homozygotes for Gaucher's disease employing a fluorogenic substrate for the estimation of leucocyte glucocerebroside: β-glucocerebrosidase.[140]

Niemann–Pick disease is a condition in which sphingomyelin is deposited in the reticuloendothelial system.[51] Biochemical tests in blood are of no value in the diagnosis and management of this condition. Diagnosis of this condition may be made with the aid of tissue enzyme levels in cultured skin fibroblasts. A chromogenic substrate has recently been synthesized whereby sphingomyelinase can be estimated in liver tissue, blood leucocytes, cultured skin fibroblasts and cultured amniotic cells.[54, 213] The results agree with earlier techniques employing isotopically labelled lipids and the method is able to detect heterozygous carriers in utero.[54]

The term histiocytosis X has been used to describe a group of conditions involving some unknown lipid storage defect.[175] Alteration in liver function may be quite profound with evidence of hepatocellular damage or biliary obstruction, whilst in some cases no change will be seen.

Amyloid

Amyloidosis is a condition characterized by the extracellular deposition of amyloid, a fibrous protein of the connective tissue (see Chapter 37). Biochemical changes in the blood are very variable with evidence of reduced BSP excretion, increased serum alkaline phosphatase and raised serum cholesterol.[186] The picture is most typical of intrahepatic cholestasis. There is no satisfactory biochemical test in the diagnosis of this condition.

Glycogen

The subject of the glycogen storage diseases is discussed in Chapter 40. The biochemical findings reflect the altered relationship between glycogen and circulating blood glucose. Hypoglycaemia, ketosis, hyperlactataemia and hyperlipidaemia are quite common. Alterations in routine biochemical liver function tests are not often found, although the more sensitive tests may show abnormalities.

Glucagon tolerance tests (1 mg given I.V., I.M. or S.C.) give some indication of the amount of glycogen which can be mobilized as glucose, but are now little used.

Modern diagnosis of the various conditions is accomplished by direct enzyme assays using liver or cultured skin fibroblasts. The enzyme deficiencies and techniques for demonstrating the abnormality are summarized in Table 40.4, Chapter 40. Two recent reviews are recommended for more detailed information on the classification and diagnostic procedures for glycogen storage disease.[77, 114]

Haematological Function

The reader is referred to Chapter 8 for details of the assessment of the haematological functions of the liver.

Immunological Function

The reader is referred to Chapter 9 for details of the assessment of the immunological functions of the liver.

TESTS OF MORPHOLOGICAL CHANGE

The point has already been made that hepatic function may be altered either by abnormalities within the liver cell or by changes that take place outside the cell. These two factors often coexist, which can make interpretation of functional disturbances difficult. Whilst it is not easy to identify the contribution that any one factor makes, it can be useful both diagnostically and prognostically to assess the morphological changes that take place. The biochemical tests of morphological change are employed first to determine the presence of damage or structural alteration, and secondly to assess progress of changes.

Tests involved in the biochemical assessment of morphological change are given in Table 17.2.

Tests of Hepatocellular Damage

The majority of tests used to detect and assess the presence of cellular injury involve the measurement of enzymes in the serum or plasma (Table 17.2). The presence of hepatic enzymes in the circulation is taken as a measure of the damage to the cell. There are three main variables that will affect the level of the enzyme in the circulation: (a) activity in the liver cell; (b) amount of leakage from the cell; and (c) rate of disappearance of the enzyme from the circulation. The choice of enzymes as markers is because smaller molecules, for example metabolites, are more labile, influenced by many more factors and less specific, while other proteins have either not yet been identified or are more difficult to measure.

Transferases

Aminotransferases. The commonest enzymes employed as indicators of hepatocellular damage are aspartate (AST) and alanine (ALT) aminotransferases. These enzymes are both present in high concentrations in the liver. Aspartate aminotransferase is found in the cell cytoplasm and the mitochondria, differing isoenzyme forms being present in each, whilst alanine aminotransferase is found solely in the cytoplasm.[19] Both enzymes are also found in the bile, but this is not considered a major excretory route.[130] Details of distribution of the aminotransferases in other tissues together with other characteristics are given in Table 17.3.

The aminotransferases are released from the hepatic cell when damage occurs or when there is an increase in cell membrane permeability. Serum levels are particularly high in acute hepatocellular damage, and are also increased in chronic hepatocellular disease and in cholestatic conditions. It is generally thought that alanine aminotransferase is the more sensitive and specific test of acute hepatocellular damage,[34] whereas increases in aspartate aminotransferase are more marked in chronic liver cell damage. Hence in the presence of an inflammatory condition where there is simply leakage of cytoplasmic enzymes into the circulation, ALT will rise more than AST. In contrast, when there is gross cellular necrosis, as in carbon tetrachloride or paracetamol poisoning, the level of AST may rise above the ALT level. As will be seen from Table 17.3, the half-life of AST is less than that of ALT, thus the AST levels will decay at a faster rate than that of ALT, which will influence interpretation of the results.

A feature of the use of serum enzymes in the assessment of morphological change is the effect of variation in the distribution of the particular enzymes within the liver. This may explain apparent anomalies as far as the aminotransferases are concerned. Thus, it is common to find an elevated serum AST with normal ALT level in patients with hepatic malignancy, although gross cellular necrosis would not be expected.

Acute liver disease. Elevated serum aminotransferase levels may be found in the preicteric phase of acute viral hepatitis, as much as four weeks before the clinical onset of type A viral hepatitis and even longer in type B[157] (see Chapter 28). The peak enzyme levels are commonly seen about seven to ten days before maximum bilirubin levels are observed. Serum enzyme values are often between 20 and 50 times the upper limit of the reference range;[30,123] when using opti-

Table 17.2. *Morphological Changes in the Liver and Biliary Tract and Related Biochemical Tests.*

Morphological change	Biochemical tests[a]
Hepatocellular damage	
Enzymes	Aspartate and alanine aminotransferases, ornithine carbamyl transferase, lactate dehydrogenase, isocitrate dehydrogenase, sorbitol dehydrogenase, glutamate dehydrogenase
Other	Iron and ferritin
Bile duct patency	
Enzymes	Alkaline phosphatase, 5′-nucleotidase, leucine aminopeptidase, γ-glutamyl transferase
Bile contents	Bilirubin, bile acids, cholesterol, lipoprotein-X, urine urobilinogen
Hepatic fibrosis	Galactosamine, prolyl hydroxylase, free proline, and hydroxyproline, monoamine oxidase
Hepatic blood flow	Xenon elimination, ICG excretion index
Malignancy	α-fetoprotein, carcino embryonic antigen

[a] Serum or plasma unless otherwise stated.

Table 17.3. *Characteristics of Serum Enzymes Employed in the Assessment of Liver Function.*

Enzyme	Enzyme commission number	Molecular weight (approx.)	Blood half-life (hours)	Tissues of origin	Disease specificity
Aspartate aminotransferase	2.6.1.1	100 000	17 ± 5	Heart, liver, skeletal muscle, kidney, brain	Myocardial damage, hepatocellular damage skeletal muscle damage
Alanine aminotransferase	2.6.1.2	110 000	47 ± 10	Liver	Hepatocellular damage
Lactate dehydrogenase	1.1.1.27	135 000	113 ± 60 (LD1) 10 ± 2 (LD5)	Heart, liver, skeletal muscle, kidney, red cells, pancreas, lung	Skeletal muscle damage, myocardial damage, hepatocellular damage, anaemia
Isocitrate dehydrogenase	1.1.1.42	64 000	–	Liver	Hepatocellular damage
Sorbitol dehydrogenase	1.1.1.14	115 000	–	Liver	Hepatocellular damage
Glutamate dehydrogenase	1.4.1.3	1 000 000	18 ± 1	Liver	Hepatocellular damage
Ornithine carbamyl transferase	2.1.3.3	260 000	–	Liver	Hepatocellular damage
Alkaline phosphatase	3.1.3.1	120 000	41 ± 2 (bone)	Bone, intestinal mucosa, liver, placenta, kidney	Biliary obstruction, osteoblastic activity, pregnancy
5′-Nucleotidase	3.1.3.5	120 000	–	Hepatobiliary tract, thyroid, aorta, pancreas	Biliary obstruction
Leucine aminopeptidase	3.4.11.1	80 000	–	Liver, intestine, pancreas, kidney	Biliary obstruction
γ-Glutamyl transferase	2.3.2.2	$80–150 \times 10^3$	–	Hepatobiliary tract, pancreas, kidney, spleen, intestine	Biliary obstruction, hepatocellular damage, microsomal enzyme induction
Pseudocholinesterase	3.1.3.1	$2–12 \times 10^6$	–	Red cell, liver	Chronic liver disease, untreated deficiency

mized methodology the level of alanine aminotransferase exceeds that of aspartate aminotransferase. The correlation with symptoms in the individual patient is not particularly good, but the enzyme measurements complement clinical assessment.

Both of the aminotransferases fall rapidly within a few days of onset of jaundice, paralleling clinical improvement (Figure 17.4). Normal serum enzyme levels are achieved within two to five weeks of the onset of the jaundice. If the aminotransferase levels remain elevated and continue to rise, massive hepatic cell necrosis and hepatic failure are indicated. In this situation, when the AST level exceeds that of ALT, widespread cell necrosis is present with poor prognosis. Persistent mild aminotransferase elevations, with values up to twice the upper limit of the reference range, may indicate the onset of chronic hepatitis or cirrhosis.[35] However, this is not diagnostic, as up to one-quarter of patients may still show enzyme elevations at six months, returning to normal by one year without other clinical or biochemical indications of liver disease.

In other acute conditions, elevations of serum aminotransferases may also be demonstrated. Thus, in infectious mononucleosis elevations of ALT and AST are seen in about 80 per cent of cases. Increased levels are found early in the disease, but maximal levels are not seen until the second or third week, returning to normal by the fifteenth week. Peak levels are up to three times the upper limit of the reference range.[131,159]

Drugs and toxins. Aminotransferase elevations are also frequently the first finding in hepatocellular reactions to drugs and toxic agents. The extent of the changes is related to the nature and dose of the toxic agent. The increases in the aminotransferases are generally more striking with drugs and chemicals producing acute cellular necrosis. The ingestion of carbon tetrachloride is a classic illustration of the situation where small amounts of the toxin produce rapid onset of jaundice and widespread hepatocellular necrosis, resulting in huge elevations of the aminotransferases with AST being greater than ALT due to liberation of both cytoplasmic and mitochondrial enzyme.[207] In survivors, recovery is rapid with enzyme levels falling to normal within two weeks. Dose-dependent changes are also seen during tetracycline, cytotoxic drug and salicylate therapy.[81]

There is a second type of drug reaction, mimicking a hepatitic reaction, which is independent of drug dosage or duration of therapy. It is more frequent with multiple drug exposure and is thought to be a hypersensitivity reaction. The condition may occur in a subclinical, anicteric form or as a florid condition indistinguishable from acute viral hepatitis. During antituberculous therapy, raised aminotransferase levels are common during the first six months of treatment, although this may be due to direct toxicity.[167] If the increases in aminotransferase levels are small it is generally considered safe to continue therapy with monitoring of enzyme levels from time to time. The more classic example of this type of drug reaction is that seen following frequent exposure to halothane (see Chapter 16).

Chronic liver disease. In chronic liver disease, the picture of hepatocellular damage is often complicated by the presence of cholestasis which in itself may increase the leakage of cellular enzymes into the circulation. Aminotransferase levels are increased in the majority of patients with chronic active hepatitis and levels correlate with the activity and progression of the disease.[128] In cases with gradual onset, enzyme levels average five times normal, but with an acute presentation more marked elevations are seen. If there is a rapid rise with the AST levels higher than that of ALT then the prognosis is poor with the likelihood of hepatic coma.[171]

Cirrhosis may result from several types of hepatocellular damage and cholestatic conditions. In most forms of cirrhosis the aminotransferase levels show marked increases during active phases (Figure 17.5). In primary biliary cirrhosis the AST level may exceed that of ALT.[61] Elevation of enzyme levels is often

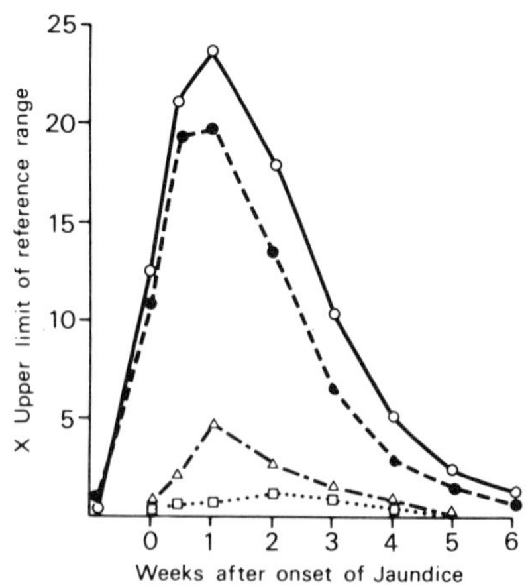

Figure 17.4. Serial estimations of serum aminotransferase activities, alkaline phosphatase activity and bilirubin in a patient with acute viral hepatitis. ○——○ alanine aminotransferase, ●---● aspartate aminotransferase, □ . . . □ alkaline phosphatase, △-·-·△ bilirubin.

independent of the presence of jaundice and presumably this reflects the presence of reserve detoxifying capacity despite the hepatocellular damage in an already cirrhotic liver.

Cholestatic liver disease. In cholestatic liver disease moderate elevations of both aminotransferases are found with ALT invariably higher than AST.[208] Occasionally high levels of the enzymes may be encountered with cell necrosis as a result of sudden bile stasis.[42] Increases of aminotransferases may also be due to complicating ascending cholangitis. Higher levels of enzymes are found in the presence of complete obstruction due to the ensuing hepatocellular damage. The possible contribution of regurgitation of biliary aminotransferases in biliary obstruction has yet to be proven.

Infiltrations. Hepatic infiltration can lead to elevations of the serum aminotransferase levels.[174, 187] An increase in these enzymes may be the first clue to hepatic involvement, but normal levels do not exclude hepatic malignancy. Primary hepatic carcinoma is invariably associated with elevated serum aminotransferase levels.[165]

Clinical uses. In recent years many laboratories have chosen to estimate only one of the aminotransferases, the choice being dependent in part upon the cost, type of equipment and availability of other tests. No clear favourite has emerged between the two aminotransferases and the evidence for the choice of either one of the enzymes is not entirely convincing. De Ritis, Coltorti and Giusti[41] proposed the measurement of both aminotransferases together with the calculation of the ratio, but this idea did not find favour because of wide methodological variations. The conclusion of De Ritis[40] when reviewing his ideas in the light of improved, more uniform methodologies, was that serum alanine aminotransferase offered better discriminatory power for the diagnosis of viral hepatitis. Measurement of the ratio added to the assessment, in that it provided additional information on the course of the hepatitis and its prognosis.

The use of the ratio of AST to ALT gives a rough indication of the presence of minimal and gross cell necrosis, roughly paralleling changes that might be expected if one were to study mitochondrial and cytoplasmic isoenzymes. Indeed Ideo et al[82] have shown that the mitochondrial isoenzyme of AST appears in the circulation in large amounts only when gross cellular damage is present.

In recent years increasing attention has been paid to the reactivation of the AST with pyridoxal phosphate. It would be expected that

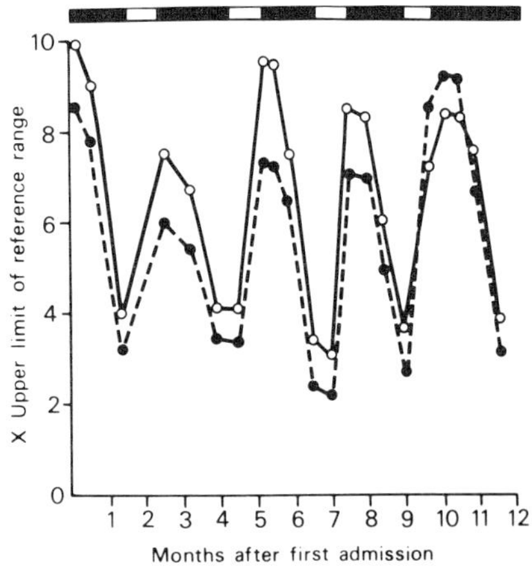

Figure 17.5. Serial estimations of serum aminotransferase activities in a patient admitted to hospital on several occasions over a period of two years with evidence of alcoholic liver damage. ○——○ alanine aminotransferase, ●---● aspartate aminotransferase, ■ inpatient, □ outpatient.

enhancement of AST by pyridoxal phosphate would be particularly prominent in such patients because of the high known incidence of nutritional vitamin deficiency in certain patients with liver disease. However, Rosalki and Bayoumi,[158] in studying patients with chronic alcoholic liver disease, showed that preincubation with pyridoxal phosphate did not increase the AST activity. There was significant activation in isolated cases, but the findings were not correlated with any known factors or disease group.

In general the aminotransferases continue to be amongst the more useful biochemical tests in diagnosis and in the assessment of liver disease, although as with many of the other tests, their discriminatory ability is increased markedly by using them in conjunction with other tests rather than in isolation. In addition other enzymes may be more specific for the liver per se.

Ornithine carbamyl transferase. This enzyme is not often used in the routine laboratory because of the relatively complicated methodology involved. However, it is an enzyme which is elevated only in the blood of patients with liver disease.[150] Very high levels are found in patients with hepatocellular damage, paralleling changes in the aminotransferases.[150] Very high levels may also be found in the active phases of cirrhosis, but only moderate changes will be found in patients with biliary obstruction. It has been used as a sensitive indicator of hepatotoxicity following the administration of drugs or after ingestion of excessive amounts of alcohol.[101]

Dehydrogenases

The aminotransferases have proved to be the most popular 'hepatocellular enzymes' over the years. Despite this, there are other enzymes which offer a greater degree of organ specificity. This may not, however, be as important as finding tests which are specific to individual liver diseases.

Lactate dehydrogenase. The measurement of serum lactate dehydrogenase has little to offer in the assessment of hepatic function. The presence of lactate dehydrogenase in the cytoplasm of cells of many organs of the body gives it poor diagnostic specificity. There are, however, five major isoenzymes of lactate dehydrogenase of which the slowest migrating band on electrophoresis (LD5) predominates in hepatic tissue.[206] This isoenzyme is often increased in hepatitis and other conditions involving hepatocellular damage.[119] Elevations in lactate dehydrogenase levels may also be seen in hepatic malignancy but the isoenzyme pattern will depend on the activity of the malignant process.[83, 205] The specificity of the enzyme as a diagnostic test can be improved in a negative sense by the use of the substrate 2-hydroxybutyric acid; hydroxybutyrate dehydrogenase activity is a property of the heart isoenzymes LD1 and LD2. Measurement of the isoenzymes has not, however, proved useful when compared with other more easily performed enzyme assays.

Isocitrate dehydrogenase. This enzyme is present in the cytoplasm of the liver cell. The enzyme is also present in significant amounts in heart, kidney, and skeletal muscle.[157] Despite this wide tissue distribution, increases in the activity of this enzyme in the serum are almost totally confined to patients with liver disease.[137] The highest isocitrate dehydrogenase levels are found in acute viral hepatitis, infectious mononucleosis and toxic hepatitis.[11, 137]

In viral hepatitis serum levels of the enzyme are almost always raised with values maximal in the first week of illness, returning to normal by the third or fourth week.[181] The increases average up to about seven times the upper limit of the reference range, and whilst levels parallel changes in the aminotransferases, it is less sensitive and is thus not recommended. In chronic liver disease the isocitrate dehydrogenase shows similar changes to those seen in the aminotransferases.[11] In cases of hepatic malignancy the enzyme levels are elevated in more than half of the cases, but it is worth noting that increased levels have been reported in disseminated malignancy without any apparent hepatic involvement.[202] Isocitrate dehydrogenase therefore does not appear to offer any significant diagnostic advantage and is not common in routine laboratory practice.

Sorbitol dehydrogenase. Sorbitol dehydrogenase is found almost exclusively in the liver with only small amounts present in the prostate and kidney.[157] Very little activity is found in the serum of normal people. Elevated levels of the enzyme are found in patients with hepatocellular damage, but its diagnostic usefulness is impaired by its relative instability in serum. In acute viral hepatitis changes in the serum enzyme level parallel changes in the aminotransferases.[42] In cirrhosis and other chronic forms of liver disease, levels may remain within the normal range unless hepatocellular damage is present. Very high activities may be encountered in congestive cardiac failure when secondary liver damage occurs as a result of hypoxia.[143] Changes appear to parallel those of alanine aminotransferase and again it appears to offer little diagnostic improvement.

Glutamate dehydrogenase. This enzyme differs slightly from those mentioned above in that it is located solely in mitochondria. It is found mainly in liver, heart, muscle and kidneys. The enzyme has a very high molecular weight and is present in normal serum in very small amounts. Its intracellular location suggests that elevations of glutamate dehydrogenase would parallel the changes seen with aspartate aminotransferase. However, a comparison of serum levels of glutamate dehydrogenase and aspartate aminotransferase in alcoholics suggests that the former enzyme is a more sensitive index of hepatic cell damage in these patients (see also Chapter 32).[192]

The difference between aspartate aminotransferase and glutamate dehydrogenase, whilst being partly explained by the presence of the former enzyme in the cytoplasm in addition to mitochondria, may lie in the distribution of the enzymes in the liver as a whole, that is their relative intercellular differences. It has been known for some time that a feature of enzyme changes after acute right-sided cardiac failure is a relatively high serum glutamate dehydrogenase activity exceeding that found in acute viral hepatitis. This led Guder et al[63] to investigate the intercellular distribution of glutamate dehydrogenase and other enzymes within the liver, and they showed a high concentration of glutamate dehydrogenase in the centrilobular region, while, in contrast, larger amounts of alanine aminotransferase were found in the peripheral cells, showing an inverse correlation to glutamate dehydrogenase. Thus not only intracellular distribution but also intercellular distribution of enzymes must be considered in the choice of enzyme tests.

Van Waes and Lieber[192] chose to use glutamate dehydrogenase as a marker of liver cell damage that is known to be concentrated mainly in the centrilobular region. These authors found that in the management of patients with alcoholic liver disease, the aminotransferases did not reflect adequately the extent of cell necrosis. It was argued that the major effects of alcoholic liver injury were seen in the centrilobular part of the liver; furthermore mitochondrial damage is known to occur. The intracellular location and intercellular distribution in the liver of glutamate dehydrogenase suggested its possible use as a marker of alcoholic cellular injury. The results of Van Waes and Lieber's study[192] showed the superiority of glutamate dehydrogenase over the aminotransferases and γ-glutamyl transferase as a marker of liver cell necrosis in the alcoholic.

Use of enzyme tests in hepatocellular damage

In reviewing the data available on the use of enzymes as indicators of hepatic cell injury, it is clear that the two aminotransferases, either separately or in combination, are probably the most popular diagnostic tests. Other enzymes in general do not offer greater sensitivity and even where they may this cannot be further explored until detailed knowledge of the morphological changes in relation to the distribution of enzymes has been considered. The work of Van Waes and Lieber[192] reflects this approach to the selection of a diagnostic test. This point is further support for De Ritis[40] who argued that the main problem is not the need for organ-specific markers but for disease-specific markers.

Non-enzymatic markers

Enzymes have been employed as markers of cellular damage because they represent proteins present in the hepatic cell and have certain properties that can be measured, and therefore the amount of protein can be quantified. It would be possible to consider the measurement of other cellular protein constituents but quantification could prove tedious and expensive to undertake.

There is a paucity of literature on the use of constituents of hepatic cells other than enzymes as indicators of cellular damage. Some data are available on the levels of ferritin and the mathematical product of the serum aspartate aminotransferase and liver iron concentration in patients with hepatocellular damage.[148] There is strong evidence that the ferritinaemia of liver disease is largely derived from damaged hepatic cells, the circulating level depending on the activity of the cellular damage and the parenchymal iron stores. Increased levels of serum iron are also found in a large proportion of patients with viral hepatitis. An elevation of the serum iron is only usually observed in cirrhosis if there is evidence of cell necrosis. Levels of serum iron are usually normal in obstructive liver disease.[166]

Tests of Bile Duct Patency

Just as hepatocellular damage is, to some degree, a feature of most types of liver disease, so also is obstruction to the passage of bile. There is considerable evidence to suggest that obstruction to the flow of bile can lead to the appearance of biliary contents in the blood. It is useful, therefore, to view the assessment of bile duct patency in the light of this. Whilst it is easy to consider the level of bilirubin as reflecting diminished clearance in the bile, there are many factors that can affect the excretion of bilirubin. Not only can the elimination of bilirubin be affected at several stages, but there is also a large reserve excretory capacity of the liver. Furthermore the presence of a low molecular weight water soluble waste product in the circulation means that it can be eliminated in the urine.

The assessment of bile duct patency requires some understanding of the conditions that comprise this functional abnormality. The term cholestasis is used to describe the stagnation of bile in the biliary passages as visualized using the light microscope. The functional aspect of this problem relates to the defect in the secretion of bile, whilst the biochemical result is the accumulation of all components of bile in the blood. Cholestasis may occur at different levels of the biliary tree, thereby possibly affecting only one part of the liver; in this situation jaundice may be absent, although other biochemical indications of cholestasis may be present.

Alkaline phosphatase

Several enzymes have been employed as indicators of abnormality of bile duct patency. Alkaline phosphatase is probably the most popular test used in this context. The enzyme is found in the liver and in the bile, whilst also being present in other parts of the body (bone, intestine, kidney, placenta). The liver enzyme is found predominantly at the microvilli of the bile canaliculi located in the plasma membrane.[65]

Isoenzymes. In patients with biliary obstruction an increase is seen in the serum alkaline phosphatase activity with highest levels in cases of complete biliary obstruction.[147] This activity has been shown to comprise two major isoenzyme fractions. One fraction is derived from the liver cell, having properties identical to the liver isoenzyme. The other isoenzyme fraction only appears when there is obstruction to the flow of bile and study of its properties suggests that it is derived from the bile.[146] It has been shown in experimental animals that ligature of the bile ducts in rats leads to an increase in alkaline phosphatase activity in the liver at the canalicular membrane.[88] It has been proposed that the elevation seen in patients with obstructive liver disease represents overspill of the enzyme from the liver cell, whose content is increased, together with regurgitation of the biliary isoenzyme into the circulation.[146]

This idea led the authors to propose that the 'biliary isoenzyme' may represent a better index of bile duct patency than the total enzyme activity. This has been demonstrated in patients with liver disease where biliary obstruction has been fairly well defined. Price and Sammons[147] showed that quantitation of the 'biliary isoenzyme', rather than total activity, allowed better differentiation of patients with complete extrahepatic, partial intrahepatic and minimal obstruction (Figure 17.6). Isolation of the abnormal alkaline phosphate isoenzyme by gel filtration from serum of patients with biliary obstruction led to the observation that the enzyme activity was associated with vesicular structures.[39] The authors suggested that fragments of liver cell membranes appear and continue to circulate in the blood of patients with cholestasis. Another biliary enzyme, γ-glutamyl transferase, was also noted in the vesicular structures.

Extrahepatic obstruction. In the case of extrahepatic biliary obstruction due to neoplasm, biliary obstruction is usually complete and prolonged. There is an early marked elevation of the serum alkaline phosphatase which continues to increase as the obstruction persists, up to ten times the upper reference range limit. The absence of a marked early rise in the serum alkaline phosphatase with jaundice is against complete biliary obstruction. Biliary obstruction due to stone or stricture is more often incomplete. In consequence the increases in serum alkaline phosphatase are less marked. However, values may still rise to $2\frac{1}{2}$ times the upper limit of the reference range (Figure 17.7). The serum alkaline phosphatase activity may rise still further if the situation is complicated by ascending cholangitis.

Intrahepatic obstruction. Intrahepatic cholestasis due to mechanical obstruction, biliary cirrhosis or drug reaction cannot be clearly differentiated from extrahepatic obstruction on the basis of serum total alkaline phosphatase levels.[64] The values may rise up to ten times the upper reference limit as in extrahepatic obstruction.

In patients with hepatic malignancy the greatest incidence of elevation and highest level of alkaline phosphatase are found in patients with the most extensive liver involvement.[6] In the absence of jaundice or hepatic enlargement the incidence of increased serum alkaline phosphatase activity is about 50 per cent, with levels up to three times the upper reference limit. In many cases the raised serum alkaline phosphatase may be the only abnormal finding, although increases in serum AST may also be seen. The explanation for the raised alkaline phosphatase may be that whilst any regurgitated bilirubin can be excreted by the kidney, any enzyme released into the circulation has to be catabolized by the usual mechanisms.[68] This dissociation of serum bilirubin and alkaline phosphatase levels has been noted in other types of liver diseases producing mild intrahepatic cholestasis, mainly chronic liver diseases including alcoholic cirrhosis.[13]

Whilst the correlation between degree of hepatic malignant infiltration and elevation of serum alkaline phosphatase is understandable, the situation in other forms of intrahepatic cholestasis is less clear. In cirrhosis resulting from longstanding hepatocellular damage, the levels of serum alkaline phosphatase may be only marginally increased as a result of minimal biliary tract involvement. In primary and secondary biliary cirrhosis there is more marked cholestasis and significant elevations in serum alkaline phosphatase levels are seen.[61]

In conditions with predominantly hepatocellular damage the increases in serum alkaline phosphatase are less marked.[147] Patients with

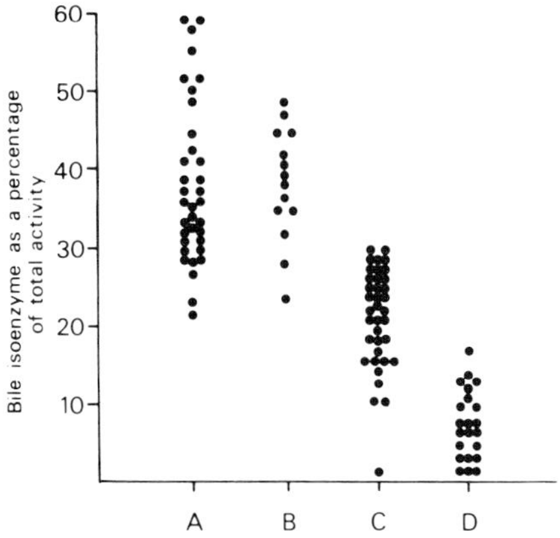

Figure 17.6. Variation of the abnormal serum alkaline phosphatase isoenzyme activity as a percentage of the total activity in patients with certain hepatobiliary diseases: (A) extrahepatic obstruction; (B) metastatic carcinoma with jaundice; (C) metastatic carcinoma without jaundice; (D) viral hepatitis. From Price and Sammons,[147] with kind permission of the authors and the editor of *Journal of Clinical Pathology*.

acute viral hepatitis may develop evidence of minimal cholestasis in the second or third week of the illness with small increases in the serum alkaline phosphatase. In chronic active hepatitis, with the appearance of significant cholestasis on histological examination of the liver, marked elevations of serum alkaline phosphatase may be seen.

Increases in the serum alkaline phosphatase may be due to isoenzymes other than those arising from liver and bone. The intestinal isoenzyme may be elevated in patients with cirrhosis.[49] It has recently been suggested that the intestinal isoenzyme may offer a means of differentiating intra- and extrahepatic cholestasis.[197] Whilst this is a somewhat unusual observation, it is pointed out by the authors that bile affects the release of intestinal alkaline phosphatase into lymph and this might explain the absence of intestinal alkaline phosphatase in the serum of patients with extrahepatic biliary obstruction.

Alkaline phosphatase measurement is thus a useful guide to obstruction, particularly if the isoenzymes are measured. It is, however, a poor discriminant between different causes of obstruction and, because of its distribution in other tissues, can occasionally give misleading information (Table 17.4).

5′-Nucleotidase

The presence of alkaline phosphatase in the blood arising from the skeleton has led to the search for other enzymes to offer greater specificity for diseases of the hepatobiliary system. The enzyme 5′-nucleotidase is widely distributed in the body, but elevations in the serum are confined to liver disease.[17] Serum 5′-nucleotidase activity may be elevated in all types of liver disease, but is more frequently and markedly elevated in the presence of cholestasis of intra- or extrahepatic origin.[57] In extrahepatic obstruction, enzyme levels generally parallel those of alkaline phosphatase, but may fall more rapidly when the obstruction is relieved.[210] Such a correlation is associated with histological evidence of bile duct proliferation, rather than bile stasis as is the case with alkaline phosphatase.[75]

The similarity between the behaviour of alkaline phosphatase and 5′-nucleotidase is seen in uncomplicated acute obstructive liver disease.[141] Greater elevations in serum 5′-nucleotidase may, however, be found in chronic forms of liver disease, primary and secondary biliary cirrhosis and chronic active hepatitis. It is claimed by several workers that 5′-nucleotidase is a more sensitive index of malignant liver disease and may be superior in monitoring antitumour therapy.[191]

One of the somewhat misguided uses of the estimation of serum 5′-nucleotidase has been as an alternative to alkaline phosphatase isoenzyme fractionation. This stems from the fact

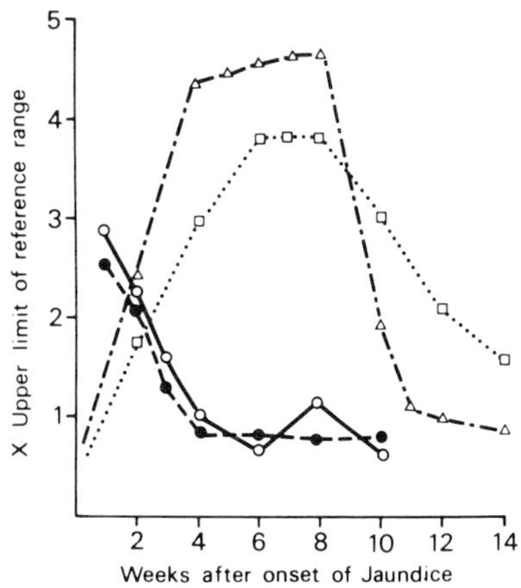

Figure 17.7. Serial estimations of serum aminotransferase activities, alkaline phosphatase activity and bilirubin in a patient with a history of biliary colic. Surgical exploration of the patient's bile ducts revealed a stone in the common bile duct. ○——○ alanine aminotransferase, ●---● aspartate aminotransferase, □...□ alkaline phosphatase, △-·-·△ bilirubin.

that serum 5′-nucleotidase levels are not elevated in serum in patients with diseases of the bone. However, the differing sensitivities of the two enzymes in different types of liver disease have led to a situation where a normal serum 5′-nucleotidase in the presence of a raised alkaline phosphatase does not necessarily signify the presence of bone disease.[32] The main value of serum 5′-nucleotidase may be in the confirmation of liver disease in childhood.[69, 209]

Leucine aminopeptidase

Serum concentrations of this enzyme are elevated significantly only in diseases of the pancreas and hepatobiliary system, although its tissue distribution is much more widespread.[132] Its distribution in the liver is similar to alkaline phosphatase with weak activity also present in the microsomal fraction of liver cells.[195] Serum leucine aminopeptidase levels are particularly elevated in cholestatic liver disease with the highest levels seen in complete biliary obstruction due to carcinoma of the pancreas.[164] Surprisingly, enzyme levels are not elevated in cases of carcinoma of the pancreas, where there is no hepatobiliary involvement.

In most varieties of liver disease serum leucine aminopeptidase shows a similar incidence and sensitivity to alkaline phosphatase with parallel enzyme changes. However, it is not so useful for differentiating between hepatocellular and cholestatic jaundice, since there is a considerable overlap between values in these conditions.[124, 126] Furthermore, it is less sensitive in cholestatic jaundice compared with 5′-nucleotidase, and more frequently elevated in hepatocellular jaundice.

γ-Glutamyl transferase

In recent years the enzyme γ-glutamyl transferase has been used to complement the measurement of alkaline phosphatase in the assessment of hepatobiliary disease.[110] Elevated serum levels of the enzyme are confined to diseases of the pancreas and hepatobiliary system and to a lesser extent the kidney.[59] The serum enzyme level is raised in all types of liver disease, with an incidence of about 90 per cent, with greatest elevations being seen in obstructive liver disease.[110]

In acute viral hepatitis the enzyme level is almost invariably raised; elevation is present in the first week and is maximal in the second or third weeks. Levels may be elevated for more than six weeks after the peak.[156] There is little correlation with severity and other biochemical

Table 17.4. *Laboratory Data from a Patient with a History of Epilepsy, Biliary Colic and Skeletal Pain.*[a]

Hospital visit	Biochemical parameters					
	Bilirubin µmol/l ref. range 2–17 µmol/l (0.12–1.00 mg/dl)	Aspartate aminotransferase I.U./l at 37°C[b] ref. range 5–42 I.U./l	Alkaline phosphatase I.U./l at 37°C[b] ref. range 50–275 I.U./l	γ-Glutamyl transferase I.U./l at 37°C ref. range 6–48 I.U./l	Calcium mmol/l	Albumin g/l
First visit – epilepsy diagnosed	12 (0.70 mg/dl)	24	195	–	–	–
One year later – routine	14 (0.82 mg/dl)	26	220	–	–	–
Four years later – routine	10 (0.58 mg/dl)	19	220	–	–	–
Eight years later – biliary colic	30 (1.75 mg/dl)	65	290	–	2.52 (10.1 mg/dl)	41
Eleven years later – routine	10 (0.58 mg/dl)	20	480	195	2.20 (8.82 mg/dl)	40
Twelve years later – routine	10 (0.58 mg/dl)	25	580	250	2.08 (8.35 mg/dl)	40

[a] Male, 32 years old. *1966* – diagnosed as suffering from epilepsy. *1974* – admitted with biliary colic. *1978* – he complained of pains in his legs. Alkaline phosphatase isoenzyme analysis at last visit indicated that the activity was due to the presence of the bone isoenzyme.

[b] These methods have changed over the years that this patient has attended the hospital; results have been converted to current method ranges.

parameters; this, and the presence of increased activity at a time of clinical recovery, has led to the suggestion that the enzyme elevation results from increased enzyme synthesis as an inflammatory response.[185] In more longstanding hepatocellular damage, higher levels of serum-γ-glutamyl transferase levels are found, presumably reflecting hepatocellular and cholestatic components.

There is no doubt that the highest levels are found in patients with obstructive liver disease. This presumably reflects the contribution of the biliary enzyme. Recent work indicates the presence of a biliary enzyme in the serum of patients with extrahepatic biliary obstruction.[200] The high levels seen in biliary obstruction are, however, not sufficient for satisfactory discrimination between so called medical and surgical jaundice.[90,110]

There is also a high incidence of raised levels of serum γ-glutamyl transferase in the presence of hepatic metastases.[204] However, the lack of disease specificity of the enzymes makes it of little value in the diagnosis of hepatic malignancy. Furthermore it has been noted recently that the serum γ-glutamyl transferase may be raised in the absence of hepatic metastases.[96] These latter findings are supported by Beck et al,[10] who pointed to the limited use of γ-glutamyl transferase levels in preoperative detection of liver metastases.

In cirrhosis the levels of serum γ-glutamyl transferase are extremely variable and an increase in the enzyme level may be the only abnormal finding.[86] It is noteworthy that there is a tendency for a serum γ-glutamyl transferase level to fall, sometimes to below normal, in the terminal stages of the illness, presumably reflecting reduced synthesis.[37,136,194]

The absence of serum γ-glutamyl transferase elevation in bone disease combined with its greater sensitivity for liver disease, compared with other cholestatic enzymes, has led to its use as a means of confirming the hepatic origin of a raised alkaline phosphatase.[110] However, as more experience is gained in this field, especially with regard to the involvement of the so-called enzyme-inducing agents, this strategy has to be questioned (see page 397). The ideal means for differentiating hepatic alkaline phosphatase has to be on 'biliary tract specific' parameters that behave similarly, and γ-glutamyl transferase does not meet this requirement and thus there is no real substitute for alkaline phosphatase isoenzyme fractionation (Table 17.3).

Serum γ-glutamyl transferase activity therefore does not offer much in the differential diagnosis of diseases of the hepatobiliary system. In fact one of its main values may be in its use as a screening test for liver disease.

Serum γ-glutamyl transferase determination has been shown to be a valuable test for the detection of liver involvement in the suspected alcoholic and heavy drinker. It has been found to be more sensitive and specific than the aminotransferase determinations and far more sensitive than alkaline phosphatase.[156] This is no doubt due to the effect of alcohol as an enzyme-inducing agent as discussed earlier.

Biliary pigments

There are many other constituents of bile that appear in the circulation of patients with biliary obstruction. Some of these are large molecular weight materials such as the enzymes already described whilst others are small molecular weight materials which may be removed by the kidney. Several of the constituents are dealt with in other sections of this chapter and will therefore only be mentioned briefly here.

Serum. The fact that the bilirubin in its conjugated form can be eliminated by the kidney and, furthermore, excreted by the liver if there is sufficient remaining viable tissue, contributes to the disparity that often exists between serum bilirubin and other markers of biliary obstruction.

The serum bilirubin level is not a good indication of bile duct patency. The level will be increased in complete biliary obstruction, but with incomplete or intermittent biliary obstruction the serum bilirubin level may be normal, whilst there are increases in serum alkaline phosphatase and γ-glutamyl transferase. This situation is sometimes seen in patients with hepatic metastases where only a portion of the biliary tree is obstructed.[68]

Urine. The presence of bilirubin in the urine has often been considered an early clue to the presence of liver disease.[134] In acute viral hepatitis the appearance of bilirubin in the urine precedes that of urobilinogen, or jaundice. The presence of bilirubin in the urine also offers an early indication that hepatotoxic agents are having an adverse effect on the liver. Urobilinogen may disappear from the urine completely with complete biliary obstruction, while if the obstruction is incomplete the picture is one of intermittent increases in urine urobilinogen. The urine urobilinogen may be increased in cases where there is increased red cell destruction.[22] This is thought to be due to the fact that the liver cannot handle the urobilinogen load because of the large amounts of bilirubin entering the intestine. Sudden increases in urine urobilinogen may be seen in patients who suffer pulmonary infarction with congestive cardiac failure presumably as a result of localized haemolysis.

Urobilinogenuria is seen in patients with hepatocellular damage as long as adequate quantities of bilirubin reach the intestine. Therefore one sees increases in urine urobilinogen in the early stages of hepatitis and also in the late stages.[173] When little bile pigment is secreted into the bile duct the urine urobilinogen levels fall to zero. The urine urobilinogen level may be increased in cases of portal cirrhosis even when serum bilirubin levels are normal. In this situation a part of the portal blood supply reaches the general circulation without passing through the liver.

The chief value of tests for urobilinogen in the urine lies in the demonstration that some bile pigment is entering the intestine. It can further be used to differentiate between complete and incomplete biliary obstruction.

Faeces. The presence of bile pigment in the faeces is an indication of the fact that pigment is entering the intestine from the bile. In general, if the pigment is completely absent from the faeces then there is a complete obstruction to the flow of bile, as for example with a neoplasm. If the obstruction is only intermittent then pigment will be found in the faeces. Antibiotic therapy may affect the production of urobilinogen in the intestine and in these circumstances bilirubin may appear in the faeces.[173] The colour of the faeces may also be markedly affected by the presence of excessive amounts of fat.

Bile acids

Marked changes in bile acid metabolism take place in biliary obstruction. These are considered in greater detail in Chapter 12. It is thought that the changes in bile acid metabolism may be responsible for some of the changes seen in the blood lipids in patients with biliary obstruction. Hypercholesterolaemia is found in the majority of patients with extrahepatic biliary obstruction, whether it be complete or incomplete, and there is usually an increase in the proportion of free cholesterol. The release of the biliary obstruction is usually followed by a return to normal of the serum cholesterol level. In contrast there is little rise in the serum cholesterol in conditions associated with predominantly hepatocellular damage.

Cholestasis is characterized by the appearance of an abnormal low density lipoprotein, lipoprotein-X.[162] Apart from increases in patients with lecithin cholesterol acyltransferase deficiency the appearance of the abnormal lipoprotein is thought to be specific for cholestatic liver disease. The use of lipoprotein-X in the diagnosis of liver disease is discussed in Chapter 4.

Tests of Hepatic Fibrosis

The liver depends for its basic framework on the presence of a small amount of connective tissue. In hepatic injury, the metabolism of hepatic connective tissue is changed, depending on the severity and duration of the injury. This results in reversible or irreversible hepatic fibrosis. An increase in the hepatic connective tissue results when more connective tissue is formed than is broken down. The increase in hepatic connective tissue is one of the major factors in the development of chronic liver disease.

Hepatic fibrosis occurs in three locations: (a) in the portal tracts; (b) around the parenchymal cell; and (c) around proliferating bile ductules which are located in the portal tract but extend into the parenchyma. Portal fibrosis is similar to that of connective tissue in general, but the parenchymal fibrosis is thought to result from mesenchymal/epithelial interactions and is one of the significant changes seen in chronic liver disease and important in the development of cirrhosis.[145]

Collagen

The development of fibrosis is thought to be due in part to increased fibrogenesis which can be demonstrated biochemically by an increase in collagen during the development of cirrhosis.[92] Evidence is based mostly on the determination of hydroxyproline. The hydroxyproline is formed from the proline present in the peptide chain by the action of the enzyme peptidylproline hydroxylase. In cirrhosis, the collagen content of the liver may increase as much as fivefold, there being good correlation with the amount of reticulum and collagen fibres demonstrated histologically.[71] The activity of prolyl hydroxylase has been shown to increase in patients who develop chronic liver disease.[180,190] In the livers of patients with cirrhosis, the pool of free proline is increased in proportion to the extent of liver fibrosis.[93] This has led to the suggestion that in conditions of increased fibrogenesis the pool of free proline or the amount of prolyl tRNA may play an important role in the regulation of collagen synthesis. Mata et al,[120] in studying the serum free proline and free hydroxyproline in patients with chronic liver disease, showed that levels of the free amino acids were significantly elevated in alcoholic cirrhotics. Furthermore, the levels fell when the patients stopped drinking. There is therefore little doubt that these imino acids are implicated in the fibrotic changes, but at present there is insufficient evidence to suggest any diagnostic significance for the measurement of the compounds.

There has been considerable interest in changes of the collagen of basement membrane.[91] Attempts have been made to measure the enzymes involved in basement membrane synthesis. The enzyme lysine hydroxylase is responsible for the production of hydroxylysine from lysine, this amino acid acting as the acceptor for galactose in the production of dissaccharide residues.[78] A galactosyl transferase has been measured in serum (not employing hydroxylysine as an acceptor) and it was shown that increases in enzyme activity occurred in hepatocellular damage and the levels appeared to correlate with the severity of the condition.[95]

Biochemical studies on collagen have also suggested that a monoamine oxidase may catalyse the maturation of connective tissue fibres, specifically the cross-linking of both collagen and elastin.[18] Changes in the level of serum monoamine oxidase have been reported in chronic congestive cardiac failure, cirrhosis, diabetes mellitus and thyrotoxicosis.[122,135] Ito et al[84] studied serum monoamine oxidase levels in patients with various diseases and showed that about 80 per cent of patients in their study with hepatic cirrhosis, and 60 per cent with chronic active hepatitis, had elevated enzyme activities. The levels were also found to increase with the progress of hepatic fibrosis. Levels were also elevated in other conditions involving increased collagen turnover. These changes in monoamine oxidase are, however, too nonspecific to warrant its use as a liver damage/fibrosis test.

Mucopolysaccharides

The mucopolysaccharides, particularly the acid types, are important components of the fibrous matrix. There is an increase in the acid mucopolysaccharide content of the liver with hepatic injury.[99] Furthermore galactosamine containing glycoprotein is increased in liver injury.[72] These alterations in the liver are not generally thought to occur in other organs. In the serum there may be an increase in the hexosamine level in liver injury.[53] The increased hexosamine is mainly galactosamine and its elevation is claimed to be diagnostic of hepatic fibrosis. In a study of 30 patients with liver disease, Hirayama, Yoshikawa and Tada[73] showed a strong correlation between the serum galactosamine level and the degree of hepatic fibrosis. The urine in hepatic fibrosis is said to contain excess mucopolysaccharide derivatives and also excess hydroxyproline.[45,55]

The degree of hepatic fibrosis, as well as its reversibility, depends on either continued increase in synthesis or reduced breakdown of connective tissue. Increased levels of enzymes involved in the degradation of mucopolysaccharides have been noted in the liver with reversible hepatic fibrosis. Studies of β-glucuronidase and *N*-acetyl glucosaminidase levels in serum of patients with cirrhosis have demonstrated changes in enzyme levels that are correlated with the activity of the disease.[71]

Clearly at present a reliable biochemical method for the assessment of hepatic fibrosis has not been finally established. The results obtained to date in patients with liver disease have indicated that despite their apparent lack of specificity, many of the tests described do reflect altered connective tissue metabolism. The activity in the serum of various enzymes which are involved in collagen metabolism such as prolyl hydroxylase and amine oxidase are increased in cirrhosis and other types of liver diseases.[152,153] In addition, the activities of hyaluronidase, β-glucuronidase and β-glucosaminidase, enzymes which metabolize acid mucopolysaccharides, are increased in hepatocellular injury and also in chronic liver disease.[100,144] The activity of amine oxidase among these enzyme systems roughly correlates with the degree of hepatic fibrosis. Undoubtedly this is a developing area and useful tests should be available within the next few years.

Tests of Hepatic Blood Flow

The important physiological functions of the liver and the central role that it plays in the metabolism of the body means that an adequate circulation is essential. Evaluation of the functional status of the hepatic circulation is important in patients with chronic liver disease, because of the problems of portal hypertension and its complications (see Chapter 43). Assessment of the hepatic circulation identifies the portal blood flow component and total hepatic flow.

Xenon

The use of radioactive xenon (^{133}Xe) has been reported for the estimation of portal blood flow.[183] The xenon is introduced into the gastrointestinal tract and then monitored using combined hepatic and umbilical vein catheterization. In a preliminary study of patients with alcoholic liver disease there was a reduction in extraction of xenon from the circulation in patients with portal hypertension.

Indocyanine green excretion

Excretion of this dye is regarded as a good indirect indication of changes in total hepatic blood flow. Indocyanine green excretion has been used to evaluate hepatic function (see earlier). It is a dye that does not require conjugation for its extraction and the rate of its disappearance from the circulation is related to liver blood flow. Edwards, Saunders and Thomas[44] compared indocyanine green excretion with galactose tolerance in patients with pulmonary disease. They showed that in a large proportion of patients there was impaired dye excretion, the conventional liver function tests being normal. Changes were also seen in galactose tolerance and it was suggested that alterations in hepatic blood flow were responsible for both observations.

Tests for Primary Hepatic Malignancy

Hepatic malignancy can be due either to a primary cancer of the hepatic tissue or to infiltration with the growth of secondary metastatic deposits. The subject of primary tumours of the liver is dealt with extensively in Chapter 38. The results of various tests in secondary malignancy have been discussed earlier. As far as primary cancer is concerned the assessment of liver function can be considered in two stages. Firstly the recognition and evaluation of the tumour and secondly the effects, metabolic and morphological, due to the presence of the lesion.

Alpha-fetoprotein

The most useful diagnostic test in primary hepatic cancer is the detection of alpha-fetoprotein in the circulation.[5] It is a glycoprotein with an electrophoretic mobility between albumin and alpha-1-globulin. It has a molecular weight of approximately 70000. Fetal and cancer alpha-fetoprotein have similar properties and give a reaction of immunological identity, although the cancer-associated protein has been split into four bands on starch gel electrophoresis.

The use of sensitive radio-immunoassay techniques has led to the recognition of alpha-fetoprotein in approximately 90 per cent of patients with primary hepatoma.[94] There does appear to be considerable ethnic and geographical variations, however, in the frequency of positive determinations. Early workers using insensitive techniques found a large incidence of false-negative results which was much reduced by employing the sensitive radio-immunoassay. Indeed the employment of sensitive radio-immunoassay techniques, whilst enhancing the sensitivity of the test for primary hepatoma, has reduced the specificity of the test.[29]

The use of a sensitive radio-immunoassay has led to the recognition of alpha-fetoprotein in the circulation of patients with other types of liver disease including viral hepatitis, toxic hepatitis, chronic active hepatitis and cirrhosis.[163] Liver cell damage and regeneration are common to all of these conditions, although the source of the protein has not been clearly identified. There is a great deal of work on alpha-fetoprotein in viral hepatitis showing that maximum levels are attained during the recovery phase;[3] this is consistent with the idea of alpha-fetoprotein production being associated with regeneration. The observation that alpha-fetoprotein levels run in parallel with aminotransferase levels suggests an acute phase response.[94]

It is now generally considered that the measurement of serum alpha-fetoprotein is useful not only as an indicator of the presence of hepatocellular cancer but also as a marker of disease activity.[94] As might be expected the serum alpha-fetoprotein levels fall following resection of tumour tissue.[118] Results with chemotherapy are not spectacular, but more effective drugs are required before this point can be clarified further.

Carcinoembryonic antigen

Carcinoembryonic antigen is another oncofetal

marker that can be detected in the circulation by various immunoassay techniques.[129] Its value in the diagnosis of hepatic malignancy may be that a negative finding makes it highly unlikely that there is widespread metastatic cancer. The carcinoembryonic antigen levels may also be of value in monitoring the results of resection and chemotherapy treatment in patients with cancer, especially colonic cancer.[176] A progressive rise in the level of carcinoembryonic antigen may indicate the development of hepatic metastases long before their presence is detected by other tests.[111]

In a recent study of carcinoembryonic antigen in patients with liver disease it was shown that the antigen was present in the serum of 90 per cent of patients with chronic liver disease and 50 per cent of patients with acute liver damage.[25] The levels of antigen increased with increasing chronicity and with the severity of damage, and in individual patients the antigen level fluctuated with the clinical condition. Although the source of the carcinoembryonic antigen is unknown, it may be associated with cellular regeneration.

THE USE OF COMPUTERS IN THE ASSESSMENT OF LIVER FUNCTION

The wide variety of biochemical tests of liver function has led to many approaches to the ultimate choice of tests employed. The bulk of data produced has encouraged many clinical and laboratory staff to look to the computer as a means of data handling and interpretation. The majority of applications for computers have been in the area of differential diagnosis. Various mathematical models have been used to study clinical and laboratory data from patients with hepatobiliary disease. Baron[9] tried to identify the problems facing the clinician with regard to the presence of liver disease, the type of liver disease and the severity. The available tests were specified in relation to functional criteria; however, other tests were then employed for the statistical analysis.

The technique of canonical variate analysis (a type of discriminant function analysis) was used to distinguish various types of liver disease. On achieving this, the degree of differentiation of disease groups could be broadly identified with three 'functions': (a) assessment of bile duct patency; (b) degree of hepatocellular damage; and (c) the ability of the liver to synthesize proteins. A similar study was undertaken by Miloszewski et al[127] who prepared a correlation matrix between eight biochemical liver function tests. Factorial analysis was applied to the correlation matrix using the method of principal components and this showed that the correlation between the eight tests could be interpreted in terms of no more than four factors and possibly only three. The eight tests were serum bilirubin, alanine aminotransferase, albumin, globulin, alkaline phosphatase, zinc sulphate and thymol turbidity and prothrombin time. The first factor with a high loading comprised the alanine aminotransferase and tubidity tests. The second factor identified prothrombin time and albumin; the third factor identified alkaline phosphatase, and the fourth, serum globulin. The conclusions drawn supported the view of Baron,[9] arguing that the tests assessed hepatocellular damage, bile duct patency and hepatocellular synthetic ability.

Another approach using computer assisted pattern recognition was employed by Strandjord, Clayson and Roby.[184] The system employed an interactive graphical scheme where three dimensional relationships of several tests and the time parameter were selected according to available clinical data, and an attempt made to identify relationships with disease clusters based on the previously documented experience of that hospital or clinical team.

The availability of data on previously diagnosed patients gives a data bank whereby the probability of any test being abnormal in a particular disease can be calculated. This approach is the basis for the use of a sequential Bayesian model which has been used in the diagnosis of jaundice.[97] To the probability of a certain result being found in a particular disease was added the refinement of a sequential approach, whereby pieces of information were obtained in a sequence to give the greatest amount of information as quickly as possible. The employment of this technique with a base of information on 300 patients resulted in an accuracy of 80 per cent in a medical versus surgical decision with an accuracy of just over 60 per cent in the distinguishing among 11 causes of jaundice.[182] The data from each patient comprised 72 pieces of information from clinical and laboratory findings available within 48 hours of admission, and it was considered valuable to have a rapid feedback to the clinician using this technique.

The subject of the use of computer in diagnosis of liver disease is fascinating in that it demands that the investigator returns to basic principles in the application of science. The topic demands separate consideration which is not possible in this chapter. The reader is referred to a recent review by Goldberg and Ellis[58] where consideration is given to the potential use of mathematical and computer assisted procedures in the diagnosis of liver disease.

The main problem with this type of mathematical approach is that the final result depends entirely on the validity of the component tests. Efforts must continue to be made to improve the primary tests used. This multiple approach does, however, have the advantage of taking assessment of tests out of the sphere of 'clinical impression' and gives an objective assessment of the usefulness of individual tests and groups of tests. It is also worth noting that recent advances in physical techniques, such as ultrasound (Chapter 21), improved biopsy methods (Chapter 18), and peritoneoscopy (Chapter 25) have lessened the need for such precision in the biochemical tests.

THE CHOICE OF TESTS OF LIVER FUNCTION AND INTEGRITY

Many reviews have been published about the biochemical assessment of liver function. There are, however, very few discussions which identify the problems to which the clinicians apply biochemical tests. The most common introduction to a discussion of liver function tests usually begins with a comment on the number of tests available. The failure of these discussions lies in the fact that this observation does not lead to an identification of the problems that the hepatologist faces *before* the various tests are evaluated. It is necessary therefore to identify the problems that face the clinician in the diagnosis and management of patients with liver disease.

The first consideration must be the recognition of the presence of liver disease. This can call for what might loosely be termed a 'screening test'. In the jaundiced patient the screening tests have been completed at the clinical examination and a biochemical test will confirm only the clinical observation of jaundice. In non-jaundiced patients tests have been developed that challenge the idea previously held, that the BSP excretion test is the most sensitive test of liver dysfunction. It has been claimed that the serum two-hour postprandial bile acid level is more sensitive than the dye excretion test.[87] In view of the many factors known to influence serum γ-glutamyl transferase, this enzyme may also be a sensitive index of liver disease, but one must be aware of the possibility of false-positive results.

Establishing the presence of liver disease is followed by the differential diagnosis which is immediately considered in the context of subsequent medical or surgical management. The main application of computers has been in the sphere of differential diagnosis. It has been quite clearly shown by Stern, Knill-Jones and Williams[182] that as more questions are asked of the system, efficiency falls. Hence a computer can accurately answer the medical versus surgical question, but cannot differentiate between several disease categories with the same degree of accuracy. It is interesting to note the conclusion of several groups who have employed computers in differential diagnosis, because the impression is that there are a core of investigations beyond which the yield, resulting from introducing further tests, is small. Thus, Miloszewski et al[127] and Baron[9] identified four tests that they related to four basic functions. Hamilton[66] produced a discriminant function based on four tests for the assessment of hepatic function; it was further claimed that assessment of severity could be made. The four tests chosen, total bilirubin, alanine aminotransferase, zinc turbidity and alkaline phosphatase, are known to result from different pathological processes and, whilst it may be possible to use this combination in differential diagnosis, it is hard to see its application in the assessment of the severity of the disease.

The third role of the biochemical liver function test is in the assessment of severity of the condition and its subsequent management. It is not necessary for this role to be undertaken by tests that are employed in differential diagnosis. Therefore Van Waes and Lieber[192] chose to use serum glutamate dehydrogenase activity in the assessment of hepatocellular damage in patients with alcoholic hepatitis. The value of this enzyme in differential diagnosis is generally considered to be limited, but in a situation where a diagnosis has been achieved and a specific pathological change has to be monitored, then a different test is used.

CONCLUSION

There are many functions of the liver and there are many tests both of function and of integrity. The future of the biochemical assessment of liver function lies in two fundamental areas. First, that we seek to establish the nature of the pathological change in relation to tests available or tests being developed. Secondly we must establish the true nature of the problem to which the tests are to be applied.

REFERENCES

1. Aarts, E.M. (1965) Evidence for the function of D-glucaric acid as an indicator for drug induced enhanced metabolism through the glucuronic acid pathway in man. *Biochemical Pharmacology*, **14**, 359–363.
2. Agorastos, J., Boswell, C., Harry, D.S. & McIntyre, N. (1976) Plasma lipoproteins in liver disease. *Biochemical Society Transactions*, **4**, 593–596.
3. Akeyama, T., Koyama, T. & Kamada, T. (1972) Alpha-fetoprotein in acute viral hepatitis. *New England Journal of Medicine*, **287**, 989.
4. Aldercrueuta, H. (1974) Hepatic metabolism of estrogen in health and disease. *New England Journal of Medicine*, **290**, 1081–1083.
5. Alpert, E., Hershberg, R., Schur, P.H. & Isselbacher, K.J. (1971) Alpha-fetoprotein in human hepatoma: improved detection in serum, and quantitative studies using a new sensitive technique. *Gastroenterology*, **61**, 137–143.
6. Baden, H., Anderson, H., Augustenborg, G. & Hanel, H.K. (1971) Diagnostic value of gamma-glutamyl transpeptidase and alkaline phosphatase in liver metastases. *Surgery, Gynecology and Obstetrics*, **133**, 769–773.
7. Bailey, A., Robinson, D. & Dawson, A.M. (1977) Does Gilbert's disease exist? *Lancet*, **i**, 931–933.
8. Barnes, S., Gallo, G.A., Trash, D.B. & Morris, J.S. (1975) Diagnostic value of serum bile acid estimations in liver disease. *Journal of Clinical Pathology*, **28**, 506–509.
9. Baron, D.N. (1970) A critical look at the value of biochemical liver function tests with special reference to discriminant function analysis. *Annals of Clinical Biochemistry*, **7**, 100–103.
10. Beck, P.R., Belfield, A., Spooner, R.J., Blumgart, L.H. & Wood, C.B. (1978) Serum enzymes in the diagnosis of hepatic metastatic carcinoma. *Clinical Chemistry*, **24**, 839.
11. Bell, J.L., Shaldon, S. & Baron, D.N. (1962) Serum isocitrate dehydrogenase in liver disease and some other conditions. *Clinical Science*, **23**, 57–66.
12. Berliner, D.L. & Dougherty, T.F. (1961) Hepatic and extrahepatic regulation of corticosteroids. *Pharmacological Review*, **13**, 329–359.
13. Betro, M.G., Oon, R.C.S. & Edwards, J.B. (1972) Gamma-glutamyl transpeptidase in diseases of the liver and bone. *American Journal of Clinical Pathology*, **60**, 672–678.
14. Bircher, J., Platzer, R., Gikalov, I., Kupfer, A. & Preisig, R. (1976) Aminopyrine breath test for evaluation of liver function. How to analyse the $^{14}CO_2$ data. *Radioaktive Isotopen in Klinik und Forschung*, **12**, 347–352.
15. Black, M. & Billing, B.H. (1969) Hepatic bilirubin UDP-glucuronyl transferase activity in liver disease and Gilbert's syndrome. *New England Journal of Medicine*, **280**, 1266–1271.
16. Black, M. & Sherlock, S. (1970) Treatment of Gilbert's syndrome with phenobarbitone. *Lancet*, **i**, 1359–1361.
17. Bodansky, O. & Schwartz, M.K. (1968) 5′-nucleotidase. *Advances in Clinical Chemistry*, **11**, 277–328.
18. Bornstein, P., Kang, A.H. & Piez, K.A. (1966) The nature and location of intramolecular cross links in collagen. *Proceedings of the National Academy of Science (Washington)*, **55**, 417–424.
19. Boyde, T.R.C. & Latner, A.L. (1961) Starch gel electrophoresis of transaminase in human tissue extracts and serum. *Biochemical Journal*, **82**, 52 p.
20. Branch, R.A., Herbert, C.M. & Read, A.E. (1973) Determinants of serum antipyrine half-lives in patients with liver disease. *Gut*, **14**, 569–573.
21. Branch, R.A., James, J.A. & Read, A.E. (1976) The clearance of antipyrine and indocyanine green in normal subjects and in patients with chronic liver disease. *Clinical Pharmacology and Therapeutics*, **20**, 81–89.
22. Breen, K.J. & Schenker, S. (1971) Liver function tests. *CRC Criticial Reviews in Clinical Laboratory Sciences*, **2**, 573–593.
23. Brugmann, E. & Towe, J. (1974) Indocyanine green clearance in a liver function test. *Materia Medica Polona*, **6**, 123–126.
24. Brunt, P.W. (1975) Alpha-1-antitrypsin deficiency and liver disease. In *Modern Trends in Gastroenterology* (Ed.) Read, A.G., Vol. 5, pp. 134–148. London: Butterworth.
25. Bullen, A.W., Losowsky, M.S., Carter, S., Patel, S. & Munro Neville, A. (1977) Diagnostic usefulness of plasma carcinoembryonic antigen levels in acute and chronic liver disease. *Gastroenterology*, **73**, 673–678.
26. Burnett, W. (1960) An assessment of the value of serum cholinesterase as a liver function test and in the diagnosis of jaundice. *Gut*, **1**, 294–302.
27. Burstein, S., Kimball, H.L. & Klaiber, E.L. (1967) Metabolism of 2α- and 6β hydroxycortisol in man: determination of production rates of 6β hydroxycortisol with and without phenobarbital administration. *Journal of Clinical Endocrinology and Metabolism*, **27**, 491–499.
28. Capocaccia, L., Cangiano, C., Attili, A.F., Angelico, M., Cascino, A. & Rossi Fanelli, F. (1977) Octopamine and ammonia plasma levels in hepatic encephalopathy. *Clinica Chimica Acta*, **75**, 99–105.
29. Chayvialle, J.A.P., Touillon, C., Crozier, C. & Lambert, R. (1974) Radioimmunoassay of α-fetoprotein in human serum. *Digestive Diseases*, **19**, 1102–1110.
30. Clermont, R.J. & Chalmers, T.C. (1967) The transaminase tests in liver disease. *Medicine*, **46**, 197–207.
31. Conn, H.O. (1961) Ammonia tolerance as an index of portal systemic collateral circulation in cirrhosis. *Gastroenterology*, **41**, 97–106.
32. Connell, M.D. & Dinwoodie, A.J. (1970) Diagnostic use of serum alkaline phosphatase isoenzymes and 5′-nucleotidase. *Clinica Chimica Acta*, **30**, 235–241.
33. Conney, A.H., Miller, E.C. & Miller, J.A. (1958) Metabolism of methylated aminoazo dyes; evidence for induction of enzyme synthesis in rat by 3-methylchloranthrene. *Cancer Research*, **16**, 450–459.
34. Coodley, E.L. (1971) Enzyme diagnosis in hepatic disease. *American Journal of Gastroenterology*, **56**, 413–419.
35. Cooper, W.C., Gershon, R.K., Sun, S.G. & Fresh, J.W. (1966) Anicteric viral hepatitis: a clinico-pathological follow-up study in Taiwan. *New England Journal of Medicine*, **274**, 585–595.
36. Cucuianu, M., Zdrenghea, D., Pop, M. & Opincaru, A. (1976) Increased serum γ-glutamyl transferase in hypertriglyceridemia: comparison with serum pseudocholinesterase. *Clinica Chimica Acta*, **71**, 419–427.

37. Cuschieri, A. & Baker, P.R. (1974) γ-Glutamyl transpeptidase in hepatobiliary disease – values as an enzymatic liver function test. *British Journal of Experimental Pathology*, **55**, 110–115.
38. Darcy, D.A. (1964) Response of a serum glycoprotein to tissue injury and necrosis. I. The response to necrosis, hyperplasia and tumour growth. *British Journal of Experimental Pathology*, **45**, 281–293.
39. DeBroe, M.E., Borgers, M. & Wieme, R.J. (1975) The separation and characterisation of liver plasma membrane fragments circulating in the blood of patients with cholestasis. *Clinica Chimica Acta*, **59**, 369–372.
40. DeRitis, F. (1970) Diagnostic enzymology in diseases of the liver and biliary tract. *Polskie Archiwum Medycyny Wewnetrznej (Warszawa)*, **4**, 509–523.
41. DeRitis, F., Coltorti, M. & Giusti, G. (1956) Ulteriore contributo al valore diagnostico ed al significato patogenetico delle modificazioni delle attivita transaminasiche del siero nella epatite virale. *Minnesota Medicine*, **47**, i, 167–172.
42. DeRitis, F., Giusti, G., Piccinino, F. & Cacciatore, L. (1965) Biochemical laboratory tests in viral hepatitis and other hepatic diseases. *Bulletin of the World Health Organization*, **32**, 59–72.
43. Eade, O.E., Maddison, A., Leonard, P.J. & Wright, R. (1977) Ratio of urinary β-hydroxycortisol to 17-hydroxycorticosteroids in patients with liver disease. *Digestion*, **16**, 169–174.
44. Edwards, M., Saunders, R.A. & Thomas, A.J. (1972) The indocyanine green extraction test of liver function in pulmonary disease. *Annals of Clinical Biochemistry*, **9**, 26–28.
45. Emmrich, R., Haentschel, H.J. & Haentschel, H. (1967) Die klinische bedeutung der hydroxyprolineanscheidung in Harn. *Zeitschrift für die Gesamte Innere Medizin und Ihre Grenzgebiete*, **22**, 193–199.
46. Felig, P., Brown, W.V., Levine, R.A. & Klatskin, G. (1970) Glucose homeostasis in viral hepatitis. *New England Journal of Medicine*, **283**, 1436–1440.
47. Fischer, J.E. & Baldessarini, R.J. (1971) False neurotransmitters and hepatic failure, *Lancet*, **ii**, 75–80.
48. Fischer, J.E. & James, J.H. (1972) Treatment of hepatic coma and hepatorenal syndrome. Mechanism of action of L-dopa and aramine. *American Journal of Surgery*, **123**, 222–230.
49. Fishman, W.H., Inglis, N.I. & Krant, M.J. (1965) Serum alkaline phosphatase of intestinal origin in patients with cancer and with cirrhosis of the liver. *Clinica Chimica Acta*, **12**, 298–303.
50. Fleck, A. & Morrison, B.A. (1970) The determination of bromsulphthalein in serum. *Clinica Chimica Acta*, **30**, 751–759.
51. Fredrickson, D.S. & Sloan, H.R. (1972) Sphingomyelin lipidoses: Niemann–Pick disease. In *The Metabolic Basis of Inherited Disease* (Ed.) Stanbury, J.B., Wyngaarden, J.B. & Fredrickson, D.S. pp. 783–807. New York: McGraw Hill.
52. Fredrickson, D.S., Sloan, H.R., Ferrans, V.J. & Demosky, S.J. (1972) Cholesteryl ester storage disease: a most unusual manifestation of deficiency of two lysosomal enzyme activities. *Transactions of the Association of American Physicians*, **85**, 109–119.
53. Froehlich, A.L. (1967) Les glycoproteines du serum dans la cirrhose alcoolique. *Revue Internationale d'Hepatologie*, **7**, 565–571.
54. Gal, A.E., Brady, R.O., Hibbert, S.R. & Pentchen, P.G. (1975) A practical chromogenic procedure for the detection of homozygotes and heterozygous carriers of Niemann Pick disease. *New England Journal of Medicine*, **293**, 632–636.
55. Galambos, J.T. (1967) The effect of acute and chronic liver disease on sulfate metabolism in man. *American Journal of Gastroenterology*, **47**, 105–112.
56. Galizzi, J., Long, R.G., Billing, B.H. & Sherlock, S. (1978) Assessment of the (^{14}C) aminopyrine breath test in liver disease. *Gut*, **19**, 40–45.
57. Goldberg, D.M. (1973) 5′-nucleotidase: recent advances in cell biology, methodology and clinical significance. *Digestion*, **8**, 87–99.
58. Goldberg, D.M. & Ellis, G. (1978) Mathematical and computer assisted procedures in the diagnosis of liver and biliary tract disorders. *Advances in Clinical Chemistry*, **20**, 50–128.
59. Goldberg, D.M. & Martin, J.V. (1976) Role of γ-glutamyl transpeptidase activity in the diagnosis of hepatobiliary disease. *Digestion*, **12**, 232–246.
60. Goldstein, G. & Mistilis, S.P. (1972) Active chronic hepatitis: use of bromosulphthalein TM and S in estimating disease activity. *Scandinavian Journal of Gastroenterology*, **7**, 737–742.
61. Goudie, R.B., MacSween, R.N.M. & Goldberg, D.M. (1966) Serological and histological diagnosis of primary biliary cirrhosis. *Journal of Clinical Pathology*, **19**, 527–538.
62. Green, G., Poller, L., Thomson, J.M. & Dymock, I.W. (1976) Factor VII as a marker of hepatocellular synthetic function in liver disease. *Journal of Clinical Pathology*, **29**, 971–975.
63. Guder, W.G., Habicht, A., Kleissl, J., Schmidt, U. & Wieland, O.H. (1975) The diagnostic significance of liver cell inhomogeneity: serum enzymes in patients with central liver necrosis and the distribution of glutamate dehydrogenase in normal human liver. *Zeitschrift für Klinische Chemie und Klinische Biochemie*, **13**, 311–318.
64. Gutman, A.B. (1959) Serum alkaline phosphatase activity in diseases of the skeletal and hepatobiliary systems. A consideration of the current status. *American Journal of Medicine*, **27**, 875–901.
65. Hägerstrand, I. (1975) On histochemical enzyme changes in association with canalicular activity of alkaline phosphatase in human liver. *Acta Pathologica et Microbiologica Scandinavica, Section A*, **83**, 527–533.
66. Hamilton, M. (1977) A simple discriminant function for hepatic disease. *Journal of Clinical Pathology*, **30**, 454–459.
67. Hargreaves, T. & Piper, R.F. (1971) Breast milk jaundice. Effects of inhibitory breast milk and 3α20β pregnanediol on glucuronyl transferase. *Archives of the Diseases of Childhood*, **46**, 195–198.
68. Hill, P.G. & Sammons, H.G. (1967) An interpretation of the elevation of serum alkaline phosphatase in disease. *Journal of Clinical Pathology*, **20**, 654–659.
69. Hill, P.G. & Sammons, H.G. (1967) An assessment of 5′-nucleotidase as a liver function test. *Quarterly Journal of Medicine*, **36**, 457–468.
70. Hill, E. & Zieve, L. (1957) Discrimination between obstructive and hepatocellular jaundice by means of the commonly used serum tests. *American Journal of Clinical Pathology*, **27**, 6–12.
71. Hirayama, C. (1974) Hepatic fibrosis: biochemical considerations. In *The Liver and its Diseases* (Ed.) Schaffner, F., Sherlock, S. & Leevy, C.M. pp. 273–282. New York: Stratton Intercontinental.
72. Hirayama, C. & Hartman, F. (1961) Zur Biochemie des Leberbindegewebes während der Entincklung einer durch Thioacetamid bei Ratten induzierten

Leberfibrose. *Acta Hepato-Splenologica (Stuttgart)*, **8,** 102–109.

73. Hirayama, C., Yoshikawa, T. & Tada, H. (1961) Serum galactosamine. A diagnostic index of liver fibrosis in liver disease. *Lancet*, **i,** 532–533.
74. Hobbs, J.R. (1967) Serum proteins in liver disease. *Proceedings of the Royal Society of Medicine*, **60,** 1250–1254.
75. Hobbs, J.R., Campbell, D.M. & Scheuer, P.J. (1968) The clinical value of serum 5′-nucleotidase assay. In *6th International Congress of Clinical Chemistry, Munich, 1966. Clinical Enzymology*, Vol. 2, p. 106. Basle and New York: Karger.
76. Hollman, J. & Touster, D. (1962) Alteration in tissue levels of uridine diphosphate glucose dehydrogenase, uridine diphosphate glucuronic acid pyrophosphatase and glucuronyl transferase induced by substances influencing the production of ascorbic acid. *Biochimica et Biophysica Acta*, **62,** 338–352.
77. Howell, R.R. (1972) The glycogen storage diseases. In *The Metabolic Basis of Inherited Disease* (Ed.) Stanbury, J.B., Wyngaarden, J.B. & Fredrickson, D.S. pp. 149–173. New York: McGraw Hill.
78. Hudgin, R.L. & Schachter, H. (1971) Porcine sugar nucleotide: glycoprotein glycosyl transferase. II. Blood serum and liver galactosyl transferase. *Canadian Journal of Biochemistry*, **49,** 838–846.
79. Hunt, A.H. & Lehmann, H. (1960) Serum albumin, pseudocholinesterase and transaminases in the assessment of liver function before and after venous shunt operations. *Gut*, **1,** 303–311.
80. Hunter, J., Maxwell, J.D., Carella, M., Stewart, D.A. & Williams, R. (1971) Urinary D-glucaric acid excretion as a test of hepatic enzyme induction in man. *Lancet*, **i,** 572–575.
81. Iancu, T. (1972) Serum transaminases and salicylate therapy. *British Medical Journal*, **ii,** 167.
82. Ideo, G., De Franchis, R., Bellobuono, A., Sforzini, S. & Dioguardi, N. (1972) Serum cytosolic/mitochondrial enzyme ratio: a tool for the estimation of the severity of acute hepatitis. *Zeitschrift für Klinische Chemie und Klinische Biochemie*, **10,** 74–76.
83. Ishibe, T. (1976) Prognostic usefulness of serum lactic dehydrogenase and its fifth isoenzyme level in carcinoma of the prostate. *International Urology and Nephrology*, **8,** 221–225.
84. Ito, K., Nakagawa, J., Minakuchi, C. & Fukase, M. (1971) A clinical evaluation of serum monoamine oxidase, with special reference to hepatic fibrosis. *Digestion*, **4,** 49–58.
85. Jablonski, P. & Owen, J.A. (1969) The clinical chemistry of bromsulfophthalein and other cholephilic dyes. *Advances in Clinical Chemistry*, **12,** 310–386.
86. Jacobs, W.L.W. (1972) γ Glutamyl transpeptidase in diseases of the liver, cardiovascular system and diabetes mellitus. *Clinica Chimica Acta*, **38,** 419–434.
87. Javitt, N.B. (1977) Diagnostic value of serum bile acids. *Clinics in Gastroenterology*, **6,** 219–226.
88. Kaplan, M.M. & Righetti, A. (1970) Induction of rat liver alkaline phosphatase: the mechanism of the serum elevation in bile duct obstruction. *Journal of Clinical Investigations*, **49,** 508–516.
89. Kaplowitz, N., Kok, E. & Javitt, N.B. (1973) Post prandial serum bile acid for the detection of hepatobiliary diseases. *Journal of the American Medical Association*, **225,** 292–293.
90. Keane, P.M., Garcia, L., Gupta, R.N. & Walker, W.H.C. (1973) Serum γ glutamyl transpeptidase in liver disorders. *Clinical Biochemistry*, **6,** 41–45.
91. Kefalides, N.A. (1970) Comparative biochemistry of mammalian basement membranes. In *Chemistry and Molecular Biology of the Intercellular Matrix* (Ed.) Balazs, E.A. Vol. 1, pp. 535–573. New York: Academic Press.
92. Kent, G., Fels, I.G., Dubin, A. & Popper, H. (1959) Collagen content based on hydroxyproline determinations in human and rat livers. Its relation to morphologically demonstrable reticulum and collagen fibres. *Laboratory Investigation*, **8,** 48–56.
93. Kershenobich, D., Fierro, F.J. & Rojkind, M. (1970) The relationship between the free pool of proline and collagen content in human liver cirrhosis. *Journal of Clinical Investigation*, **49,** 2246–2249.
94. Kew, M.C. (1975) Alpha-fetoprotein. In *Modern Trends in Gastroenterology* (Ed.) Read, A.E. Vol. 5, pp. 91–114. London and Boston: Butterworth.
95. Kim, Y.S., Perdomo, J., Whitehead, J.S. & Curtis, K.J. (1972) Glycosyltransferases in human blood. II. Study of serum galactosyltransferase and N-acetylgalactosyl-aminyltransferase in patients with liver disease. *Journal of Clinical Investigation*, **51,** 2033–2039.
96. Kim, N.K., Yasmineh, W.G., Freier, E.F., Goldman, A.J. & Theologides, A. (1977) Value of alkaline phosphatase, 5′-nucleotidase, γ glutamyl transferase and glutamate dehydrogenase activity measurements (single and combined) in serum in diagnosis of metastases to the liver. *Clinical Chemistry*, **23,** 2034–2038.
97. Knill-Jones, R.P., Stern, R.B., Girmes, D.H., Maxwell, J.D., Thompson, R.P.H. & Williams, R. (1973) Use of sequential Bayesian model in diagnosis of jaundice by computer. *British Medical Journal*, **i,** 530–533.
98. Knox, W.E. (1954) Metabolic adaptation in animals. In *Cellular Metabolism and Infections* (Ed.) Racker, E. pp. 45–60. New York: Academic Press.
99. Koizumi, T., Nakamura, N. & Abe, H. (1967) Changes in acid mucopolysaccharide in the liver in hepatic fibrosis. *Biochimica et Biophysica Acta*, **148,** 749–756.
100. Koizumi, T., Suematsu, T., Iwabozi, N. & Abe, H. (1968) Changes in N-acetyl βglucosaminidase activity in hepatic damage. *Biochimica et Biophysica Acta*, **151,** 628–636.
101. Konttinen, A., Hartel, G. & Louhija, A. (1970) Multiple serum enzyme analysis in chronic alcoholics. *Acta Medica Scandinavica*, **188,** 257–264.
102. Kuntzman, R., Jacobson, M., Schneidman, K. & Conney, A.H. (1964) Similarities between oxidative drug-metabolizing enzymes and steroid hydroxylases in liver microsomes. *Journal of Pharmacology and Experimental Therapeutics*, **146,** 280–285.
103. LaRusso, N.E., Hoffman, N.E., Hoffman, A.F. & Korman, M.G. (1975) Validity and sensitivity of an intravenous bile acid tolerance test in patients with liver disease. *New England Journal of Medicine*, **292,** 1209–1214.
104. Lathe, G.H. & Walker, M. (1958) Inhibition of bilirubin conjugation in rat liver by human pregnancy and neonatal serum and steroids. *Quarterly Journal of Experimental Physiology*, **43,** 257–265.
105. Latner, A.L. (1975) Hepatic function. In *Clinical Biochemistry* (Ed.) Cantarow, A.T. & Trumper, M. pp. 610–683. Philadelphia, London, Toronto: W.B.

Saunders.

106. Leevy, C.M., Popper, H. & Sherlock, S. (1977) Standardisation of nomenclature, diagnostic criteria, and diagnostic methodology. In *Diseases of the Liver and Biliary Tract*. Chicago, London: Year Book Medical Publishers.

107. Leevy, C.M., Bender, J., Silverberg, M. & Naylor, J. (1963) Physiology of dye extraction by the liver: comparative studies of sulfobromphthalein and indocyanine green. *Annals of the New York Academy of Sciences*, **111**, 161–175.

108. Leevy, C.M., Smith, F., Longueville, J., Paumgartner, G. & Howard, M.M. (1967) Indocyanine green clearance as a test of hepatic function. *Journal of the American Medical Association*, **200**, 236–240.

109. Lewis, K.O., Nicholson, G., Lance, P. & Paton, A. (1977) Aminopyrine breath test in alcoholic liver disease and in patients on enzyme inducing drugs. *Journal of Clinical Pathology*, **30**, 1040–1043.

110. Lum, G. & Gambino, S.R. (1972) Serum gamma-glutamyl transpeptidase activity as an indicator of disease of liver, pancreas or bone. *Clinical Chemistry*, **18**, 358–362.

111. Mach, J.P., Jaeger, P., Bertholet, M.M., Ruegsegger, O.H., Loosli, R.M. & Pettavel, J. (1974) Detection of recurrence of large bowel carcinoma by radioimmunoassay of circulating carcinoembryonic antigen (CEA). *Lancet*, **ii**, 535–540.

112. Maddocks, J.L., Wake, C.J. & Harber, M.J. (1975) The plasma half life of antipyrine in chronic uraemic and normal subjects. *British Journal of Clinical Pharmacology*, **2**, 339–343.

113. Magnani, H.N. & Alaupovic, P. (1976) Utilization of the quantitative assay of lipoprotein X in the differential diagnosis of extrahepatic obstructive jaundice and intrahepatic diseases. *Gastroenterology*, **71**, 87–93.

114. Mahler, R.F. (1976) Disorders of carbohydrate metabolism excluding diabetes. *Clinics in Endocrinology and Metabolism*, **5**, 579–598.

115. Manghani, K.K., Lunzer, M.R., Billing, B. & Sherlock, S. (1975) Urinary and serum octopamine in patients with portal systemic encephalopathy. *Lancet*, **ii**, 943–946.

116. Marks, V. & Alberti, K.G.M.M. (1976) Selected tests of carbohydrate metabolism. *Clinics in Endocrinology and Metabolism*, **5**, 805–820.

117. Martin, P.J., Martin, J.V. & Goldberg, D.M. (1975) γ-glutamyl transpeptidase, triglycerides and enzyme induction. *British Medical Journal*, **i**, 17–18.

118. Masopust, J., Kithier, K., Radl, J., Koutecky, J. & Kotal, L. (1968) Occurrence of fetoprotein in patients with neoplasms and non-neoplastic diseases. *International Journal of Cancer*, **3**, 364–373.

119. Massey, W.H., Dennis, D.L., Fletcher, W.S. & Wood, D.C. (1971) Lactic dehydrogenase isoenzyme alterations in malignant disease of the liver. *American Journal of Surgery*, **122**, 209–216.

120. Mata, J.M., Kershenobich, D., Villarreal, E. & Rojkind, M. (1975) Serum free proline and free hydroxyproline in patients with chronic liver disease. *Gastroenterology*, **68**, 1265–1269.

121. McDermott, W.V. (1960) The ammonium tolerance test in the diagnosis of disease of the liver and portal hypertension. *Surgical Forum*, **10**, 282–286.

122. McEwen, C.M. & Harrison, D.C. (1965) Abnormalities of serum monoamine oxidase in chronic congestive heart failure. *Journal of Laboratory and Clinical Medicine*, **65**, 546–559.

123. McIntyre, N. & Heathcote, J. (1974) The laboratory in the diagnosis and management of viral hepatitis. *Clinics in Gastroenterology*, **3**, 317–336.

124. Mericas, G., Anagostau, E., Hadziyannis, St. & Kakar, S. (1964) The diagnostic value of serum leucine aminopeptidase. *Journal of Clinical Pathology*, **17**, 52–55.

125. Miller, J.P. & Johnson, K. (1976) A critical examination of the value of combined determinations of lecithin: cholesterol acyl transferase and lipoprotein-X in the differential diagnosis of liver disease. *Clinica Chimica Acta*, **69**, 81–84.

126. Miller, A.L. & Worsley, L. (1960) Serum leucine aminopeptidase in carcinoma of the pancreas and other diseases. *British Medical Journal*, **ii**, 1419–1422.

127. Miloszewski, K., Walker, B.E., Hamilton, M. & Losowsky, M.S. (1970) A new look at biochemical tests of liver function. *European Journal of Clinical and Biochemical Research*, **15**, 878–881.

128. Mistilis, S.P. & Blackburn, C.R.R. (1970) Active chronic hepatitis. *American Journal of Medicine*, **48**, 484–495.

129. Moore, T.L., Kupchik, H.Z., Marcon, N. & Zamcheck, N. (1971) Carcinoembryonic antigen assay in cancer of the colon and pancreas and other digestive tract disorders. *American Journal of Digestive Diseases*, **16**, 1–7.

130. Mossberg, S.M. & Ross, G. (1963) High serum transaminase activity associated with extrahepatic biliary disease. *Gastroenterology*, **45**, 345–353.

131. Mygind, N. (1976) Serial enzyme studies in infectious mononucleosis. *Scandinavian Journal of Infectious Diseases*, **8**, 139–142.

132. Nachlas, M.M., Crawford, D.T. & Seligman, A.M. (1957) Histochemical demonstration of leucine aminopeptidase. *Journal of Histochemistry and Cytochemistry*, **5**, 264–278.

133. Neale, G. (1975) The effects of agents which induce hepatic microsomal enzymes. In *Modern Trends in Gastroenterology* (Ed.) Read, A.E. pp. 262–288. London, New York: Butterworth.

134. Neefe, J.R. & Reinhold, J.G. (1964) Laboratory aids in diagnosis and management of infectious (epidemic) hepatitis. Analysis of results obtained on 34 volunteers during the early and convalescent stages of induced hepatitis. *Gastroenterology*, **7**, 393–407.

135. Nillson, S.E., Tryding, N. & Tufvesson, G. (1968) Serum monoamine oxidase in diabetes mellitus and some other internal diseases. *Acta Medica Scandinavica*, **184**, 105–108.

136. Nosslin, B., Aronsen, K.F. & Hanson, A. (1966) The value of glutamyl transpeptidase in liver diagnosis. *Scandinavian Journal of Clinical and Laboratory Investigation*, **18**, (Suppl. 92), 178–180.

137. Okumura, M. & Spellberg, M.A. (1960) Serum isocitric dehydrogenase activity in the differential diagnosis of liver disease. *Gastroenterology*, **39**, 305–311.

138. Owens, D. & Sherlock, S. (1973) The diagnosis of Gilbert's syndrome: role of the reduced caloric intake test. *British Medical Journal*, **iii**, 559–563.

139. Patrick, A.D. (1965) A deficiency of glucocerebrosidase in Gaucher's disease. *Biochemical Journal*, **97**, 17c–18c.

140. Peters, S.P., Lee, R.E. & Glew, R.H. (1975) A microassay for Gaucher's disease. *Clinica Chimica Acta*, **60**, 391–396.

141. Phelan, M.B., Neale, G. & Moss, D.W. (1971) Serial studies of serum alkaline phosphatase and 5′-nucleotidase levels in hepatobiliary disease. *Clinica*

Chimica Acta, **32,** 95–102.

142. Phillips, G.B. (1960) The lipid composition of serum in patients with liver disease. *Journal of Clinical Investigation,* **39,** 1639–1650.
143. Pitkanen, E. & Servo, C. (1971) Polyol oxidoreductase activity in human blood serum during acute hepatitis. *Clinica Chimica Acta,* **33,** 273–278.
144. Platt, D. & Leinweber, B. (1969) Untersuchungen zum katabole mukopolysaccharidstoffwechsel bei lebererkrankunggen. *Acta Hepato-splenologica (Stuttgart),* **16,** 324–330.
145. Popper, H. & Udenfriend, S. (1970) Hepatic fibrosis. Correlation of biochemical and morphological investigations. *American Journal of Medicine,* **49,** 707–721.
146. Price, C.P. & Sammons, H.G. (1974) The nature of the serum alkaline phosphatases in liver disease. *Journal of Clinical Pathology,* **27,** 392–398.
147. Price, C.P. & Sammons, H.G. (1976) An interpretation of the serum alkaline phosphatase isoenzyme patterns in patients with obstructive liver disease. *Journal of Clinical Pathology,* **29,** 976–980.
148. Prieto, J., Barry, M. & Sherlock, S. (1975) Serum ferritin in patients with iron overload and with acute and chronic liver disease. *Gastroenterology,* **68,** 525–533.
149. Ratnoff, O.D. (1975) Disordered hemostasis in hepatic disease. In *Diseases of the Liver* (Ed.) Schiff, L. pp. 183–203. Philadelphia: Lippincott.
150. Reichard, H. (1961) Ornithine carbamyl transferase activity in human serum in diseases of the liver and biliary system. *Journal of Laboratory and Clinical Medicine,* **57,** 78–87.
151. Reinhold, J.G. (1960) Flocculation tests and their application to the study of liver disease. *Advances in Clinical Chemistry,* **3,** 84–156.
152. Ristteli, J. & Kivirikko, K.I. (1974) Activities of polyl hydroxylase, lysyl hydroxylase, collagen galactosyl transferase and collagen glucosyl transferase in the liver of rats with hepatic injury. *Biochemical Journal,* **144,** 115–122.
153. Ristteli, J. & Kivirikko, K.I. (1976) Intracellular enzymes of collagen biosynthesis in rat liver as a function of age and in hepatic injury induced by dimethylnitrosamine. *Biochemical Journal,* **158,** 361–367.
154. Ritland, S., Blomhoff, J.P. & Gjone, E. (1973) Lecithin: cholesterol acyl-transferase and lipoprotein-X in liver disease. *Clinica Chimica Acta,* **49,** 251–259.
155. Ritland, S., Blomhoff, J.P., Elgjo, K. & Gjone, E. (1973) Lipoprotein X (LP-X) in liver disease. *Scandinavian Journal of Gastroenterology,* **8,** 155–160.
156. Rosalki, S.B. (1975) Gamma glutamyl transpeptidase. *Advances in Clinical Chemistry,* **17,** 53–107.
157. Rosalki, S.B. (1976) Enzyme tests in diseases of the liver and hepatobiliary tract. In *The Principles and Practice of Diagnostic Enzymology* (Ed.) Wilkinson, J.H. pp. 303–360. London: Edward Arnold.
158. Rosalki, S.B. & Bayoumi, R.A. (1975) Activation by pyridoxal 5-phosphate of aspartate aminotransferase in serum of patients with heart and liver disease. *Clinica Chimica Acta,* **59,** 357–360.
159. Rosalki, S.B., Jones, T.G. & Verney, A.F. (1960) Transaminase and liver function studies in infectious mononucleosis. *British Medical Journal,* **i,** 929–933.
160. Rosalki, S.B., Tarlow, D. & Rau, D. (1971) Plasma gamma glutamyl transpeptidase elevation in patients receiving enzyme-inducing drugs. *Lancet,* **ii,** 376–377.
161. Rosoff, L. & Rosoff, L. (1977) Biochemical tests for hepatobiliary disease. *Surgical Clinics of North America,* **57,** 257–273.
162. Ross, A., Murphy, G.M., Wilkinson, P.A., Mills, G.L. & Sherlock, S. (1970) Occurrence of an abnormal lipoprotein in patients with liver disease. *Gut,* **11,** 1035–1037.
163. Ruoslahti, E. & Seppälä, M. (1972) Normal and increased alpha-feto-protein in neoplastic and non-neoplastic liver disease. *Lancet,* **ii,** 278–279.
164. Rutenberg, A.M., Goldbarg, J.A. & Pineda, E.P. (1958) Leucine aminopeptidase activity. Observations in patients with cancer of the pancreas and other diseases. *New England Journal of Medicine,* **259,** 469–472.
165. San Jose, D., Cady, A., West, M., Chomet, B. & Zimmerman, H.J. (1965) Primary carcinoma of the liver. Analysis of clinical and biochemical features of 80 cases. *American Journal of Digestive Diseases,* **10,** 657–674.
166. Schamroth, L., Edelstein, W., Politzer, W.M. & Stevens, N. (1956) Serum iron in the diagnosis of hepatobiliary disease. *British Medical Journal,* **i,** 960–964.
167. Scharer, L. & Smith, J.P. (1969) Serum transaminase elevations and other hepatic abnormalities in patients receiving isoniazid. *Annals of Internal Medicine,* **71,** 1113–1120.
168. Schenker, S., Breen, K.J. & Hoyumpa, A.M. (1974) Hepatic encephalopathy: current status. *Gastroenterology,* **66,** 121–154.
169. Schiff, L., Billing, B.H. & Oikawa, Y. (1959) Familial non-haemolytic jaundice with conjugated bilirubin in the serum. A case study. *New England Journal of Medicine,* **260,** 1315–1318.
170. Schmid, R. (1972) Bilirubin metabolism in man. *New England Journal of Medicine,* **287,** 703–709.
171. Schmidt, E. & Schmidt, F.W. (1967) *Guide to Practical Enzyme Diagnosis.* Mannheim: Boehringer.
172. Shambaugh, G.E. (1978) Urea biosynthesis. II. Normal and abnormal regulation. *American Journal of Clinical Nutrition,* **31,** 126–133.
173. Sherlock, S. (1975) *Diseases of the Liver and Biliary System,* 5th edition. Oxford, London, Edinburgh and Melbourne: Blackwell Scientific Publications.
174. Shimokawa, Y., Okuda, K., Kubo, Y., Kaneko, A., Arishima, T., Nagata, E., Hashimoto, M., Sawa, Y., Nagasaki, Y., Kojiro, M., Sakamoto, K. & Nakashima, T. (1977) Serum glutamic oxaloacetic transaminase/glutamic pyruvic transaminase ratio in hepatocellular carcinoma. *Cancer,* **40,** 319–324.
175. Silverstein, M.N., Ellefson, R.D. & Ahern, E.J. (1970) The syndrome of the sea-blue histiocyte. *New England Journal of Medicine,* **282,** 1–4.
176. Skarin, A.T., Delwiche, R., Zamcheck, N., Lokich, J.J. & Frei, E. (1974) Carcinoembryonic antigen; clinical correlation with chemotherapy for metastatic gastrointestinal cancer. *Cancer (Philadelphia),* **33,** 1239–1245.
177. Skrede, S., Blomhoff, J.P., Elgjo, K. & Gjone, E. (1973) Biochemical tests in evaluation of liver function. *Scandinavian Journal of Gastroenterology,* **8** (Suppl. 19), 37–46.
178. Smith, S.J., Bos, G., Esseveld, M.R., van Eijk, H.G. & Gerbrandy, J. (1977) Acute-phase proteins from the liver and enzymes from myocardial infarction: a quantitative relationship. *Clinica Chimica Acta,* **81,** 75–85.

179. Steigman, F. & Clowdus, B.F. (1971) *Hepatic Encephalopathy*. p. 104. Springfield: Charles C. Thomas.
180. Stein, H.D., Keiser, H.R. & Sjoerdsma, A. (1970) Proline hydroxylase activity in human blood. *Lancet*, **i**, 106–109.
181. Sterkel, R.L., Spencer, J.A., Wolfson, S.K. & Williams-Ashman, H.G. (1958) Serum isocitric dehydrogenase activity with particular reference to liver disease. *Journal of Laboratory and Clinical Medicine*, **52**, 176–184.
182. Stern, R.B., Knill-Jones, R.P. & Williams, R. (1975) Use of computer programme for diagnosing jaundice in district hospitals and specialized liver units. *British Medical Journal*, **ii**, 659–662.
183. Stones, R.M., ten Hove, W., Effros, R. & Leevy, C.M. (1972) Portal venous blood flow; its estimation and significance. *Gastroenterology*, **62**, 186–187.
184. Strandjord, P.E., Clayson, K.J. & Roby, R.J. (1973) Computer assisted pattern recognition and the diagnosis of liver disease. *Human Pathology*, **4**, 67–77.
185. Szczeklik, E., Orlowski, M. & Szewczuk, A. (1961) Serum γ-glutamyl transpeptidase activity in liver disease. *Gastroenterology*, **41**, 353–359.
186. Tachdjian, V. (1976) Metabolic disorders and the liver. In *Gastroenterology* (Ed.) Bockus, H.L. Vol. 3, pp. 576–600. Philadelphia, London, Toronto: W.B. Saunders.
187. Tan, C.O., Cohen, J., West, M. & Zimmerman, H.J. (1963) Serum enzymes in disease. XIV. Abnormality of levels of transaminases and glycolytic and oxidative enzymes and of liver function as related to the extent of metastatic carcinoma of the liver. *Cancer*, **16**, 1373–1387.
188. Tephly, T.R. & Mannering, G.J. (1964) Inhibition of microsomal drug metabolism by steroid hormone. *Pharmacologist*, **6**, 186 (Abstract).
189. Thaysen, E.H. (1977) Diagnostic value of the ^{14}C-cholylglycine breath test. *Clinics in Gastroenterology*, **6**, 227–245.
190. Tsujii, T., Kimura, K. & Fukuhara, M. (1977) Liver protocollagen proline hydroxylase in human liver disease and experimental liver fibrosis. *Gastroenterology (Japan)*, **12**, 21–27.
191. Van der Slik, W., Persijn, J.P., Engelsman, E. & Riethorst, A. (1970) Serum 5′-nucleotidase. *Clinical Biochemistry*, **3**, 59–80.
192. Van Waes, L. & Lieber, C.S. (1977) Glutamate dehydrogenase: a reliable marker of liver cell necrosis in the alcoholic. *British Medical Journal*, **ii**, 1508–1510.
193. Vetter, N.J., Strange, R.C., Adams, W. & Oliver, M.F. (1974) Initial metabolic and hormonal response to acute myocardial infarction. *Lancet*, **i**, 284–288.
194. Villa, L., Dioguardi, N., Agostini, A., Ideo, G. & Stabilini, R. (1966) Prognostic value of serum γ-glutamyl transpeptidase activity in liver disease. *Enzymologia Biologica et Clinica*, **7**, 109–114.
195. Wachstein, M. (1959) Enzymatic histochemistry of the liver. *Gastroenterology*, **37**, 525–537.
196. Wardle, E.N. (1974) Fibrinogen in liver disease. *Archives of Surgery*, **109**, 741–746.
197. Warnes, T.W., Hine, P. & Kay, G. (1977) Intestinal alkaline phosphatase in the diagnosis of liver diseases. *Gut*, **18**, 274–278.
198. Weinrib, M., Schaefer, J.W. & Oikawa, Y. (1971) An evaluation of liver function tests in the differential diagnosis of jaundice. *Journal of the Medical Association of the State of Alabama*, **40**, 641–643.
199. Wengeler, H., Greten, H. & Seidel, D. (1972) Serum cholesterol esterification in liver disease. Combined determinations of lecithin:cholesterol acyltransferase and lipoprotein X. *European Journal of Clinical Investigation*, **2**, 372–378.
200. Wenham, P.R., Price, C.P. & Sammons, H.G. (1978) The γ-glutamyl transferase isoenzymes of human bile. *Journal of Clinical Pathology*, **31**, 666–670.
201. Werner, M. (1969) Serum protein changes during the acute phase reaction. *Clinica Chimica Acta*, **25**, 299–305.
202. West, M., Schwartz, M.A., Cohen, J. & Zimmerman, H.J. (1964) XV Glycolytic and oxidative enzymes and transaminases in patients with carcinoma of the kidney, prostate and urinary bladder. *Cancer*, **17**, 432–437.
203. Whitfield, J.B., Pounder, R.E., Neale, G. & Moss, D.W. (1972) Serum γ-glutamyl transpeptidase activity in liver disease. *Gut*, **13**, 702–708.
204. Wieme, R.J. & Demeulenaire, L. (1970) Enzyme assays in liver disease. *Journal of Clinical Pathology*, **24** (Suppl. 4), 51–59.
205. Wieme, R.J., Van Hove, W.Z. & Van Der Straeten, M.E. (1968) The influence of cytostatic treatment on serum LDH patterns of patients with bronchial carcinoma and its relation to tumour regression. *Annals of the New York Academy of Sciences*, **151**, 213–221.
206. Wilkinson, J.H. (1976) *The Principles and Practice of Diagnostic Enzymology*. pp. 43–79. London: Edward Arnold.
207. Wroblewski, F. (1959) The clinical significance of transaminase activities of serum. *American Journal of Medicine*, **27**, 911–923.
208. Wroblewski, F. & Ladue, J.S. (1956) SGPT in hepatic disease: a preliminary report. *Annals of Internal Medicine*, **45**, 801–811.
209. Yeung, C.Y. (1972) Serum 5′-nucleotidase in neonatal hepatitis and biliary atresia: preliminary observations. *Pediatrics*, **50**, 872–914.
210. Young, I.I. (1958) Serum 5′-nucleotidase: characterization and evaluation in disease states. *Annals of the New York Academy of Sciences*, **75**, 357–362.
211. Zieve, L. & Hill, E. (1955) An evaluation of factors influencing the discriminative effectiveness of a group of liver function tests. IV. Nature of the interrelationships among hepatic tests in cirrhosis. *Gastroenterology*, **28**, 914–923.
212. Zimmon, D.S., Oratz, M., Kessler, R., Schreiber, S.S. & Rothschild, M.A. (1969) Albumin to ascites: demonstration of a direct pathway bypassing the systemic circulation. *Journal of Clinical Investigation*, **48**, 2074–2078.
213. Zitman, D., Chazan, S. & Klibansky, C. (1978) Sphingomyelinase activity levels in human peripheral blood leukocytes, using (^{3}H) sphingomyelin as substrate: study of heterozygotes and homozygotes for Niemann–Pick's disease variants. *Clinica Chimica Acta*, **86**, 37–43.

Chapter 18

Liver Biopsy: Methods, Diagnostic Value and Interpretation

G.H. MILLWARD-SADLER
P.J. WHORWELL

Although first used before the turn of the century, the technique of liver biopsy did not become firmly established in clinical practice until the 1940s.[23] Refinements in techniques have led to its being widely accepted as a routine part of the investigation of a patient with liver disease in any general hospital. This wide use must not, however, detract from the fact that it remains a potentially hazardous procedure that should not be lightly undertaken.

INDICATIONS

1. Diagnosis of primary liver disease.
2. Assessment of progression of disease and response to therapy.
3. Confirmation of malignant disease.
4. Staging and diagnosis of lymphomas.
5. Diagnosis of metabolic disease, such as glycogen storage disease.
6. Diagnosis of multisystem disease, such as sarcoidosis, amyloidosis or haemochromatosis.
7. Diagnosis of pyrexia of unknown origin and uncommon infections. In addition to histology, the biopsy may be cultured and stained for specific organisms such as tubercle bacilli.
8. Assessment of advisability on the use of potentially hepatotoxic drugs such as methotrexate in psoriasis.

PRECAUTIONS AND CONTRAINDICATIONS

A skilled operator is required, as not only is this more likely to result in an adequate biopsy specimen but the patient's cooperation is considerably enhanced by a confident, assured attendant.

A clotting profile, which should at least include the prothrombin ratio and platelet count, must be obtained shortly before biopsy. If any abnormality is detected, biopsy should be delayed until it has been corrected by the appropriate use of vitamin K or clotting factor concentrates. It should be borne in mind that dysproteinaemias and some drugs can lead to platelet dysfunction, despite a normal count. We are prepared to biopsy a patient with a platelet count greater than 80 000 000/l and a prothrombin ratio of 1.3 or below. It is usual to group and cross-match two units of blood beforehand.

In any situation where a space-occupying lesion of the liver is suspected, previous ultrasound and a colloid liver scan may indicate the nature of the lesion and its location, thus enabling a specific area to be aimed for. Suspicion of a hydatid cyst or haemangioma are absolute contraindications to biopsy.

Biopsy in the presence of biliary obstruction is not often indicated, and has an increased risk of biliary peritonitis. However, when indicated, the risks are not unacceptable.[46, 67] Our practice is to refrain from biopsy in anybody who is shown, either by ultrasound or retrograde cholangiography, to have dilated ducts. We are also reluctant to biopsy patients who have had previous biliary surgery, particularly if it was in any way complicated.

Passive congestion of the liver is associated with an increased risk of haemorrhage, and the congestion should be minimized before biopsy. A series of biopsies without complication in this situation has been reported.[63]

Fine needle liver biopsy

Liver biopsy using a fine 0.7 mm external diameter needle has been advocated for cytodiagnosis[34] or where repeat biopsies are needed for such purposes as enzyme estimations. It is claimed to have a greater safety than any of the other techniques. This method is unlikely to become acceptable for routine use, due to the inadequate size of the biopsy, but it may find a place as a research tool.

Types of Needles

The original needles consisted of a trocar and cannula with a bore of up to 3 mm.[23] It soon became apparent that the incidence of haemorrhage could be reduced by decreasing the size of the bore.[28] Safety was also adversely affected by the slow speed of the manoeuvre, which was revolutionized by the introduction of the 'one-second' technique by Menghini.[42] He designed a needle with an oblique tip, slightly convex towards the outside, which has an internal nail to prevent the biopsy being drawn up into the syringe. The needles come in sizes of 1.0, 1.5 and 2.00 mm in diameter, the 1.5 mm version being the most commonly used. There have been several modifications of the Menghini needle, and we use the one introduced by Klatskin, in which the whole circumference of the tip is sharpened. We also prefer to use the needle without the nail, as otherwise this may lead to crushing artefact when the biopsy impacts on it. In addition, there is immediate confirmation that a biopsy has been obtained, and undue fragmentation does not occur.

The other needle in common use is the Vim-Silverman or its disposable derivative, the Trucut.[55] In the former, a trocar and cannula are introduced into the liver, the trocar is removed and a split cannula with a tendency to spring open is advanced through the other cannula into the liver. The split cannula is then closed by advancing the outside one over it, and after rotation of the two they are withdrawn. No suction is required, but distortion can be considerable. The main advantage in this technique is that it is usually possible to obtain biopsies from fibrotic livers in which the Menghini needle has failed. Today the Trucut modification, in which the inside cannula has a 2 cm notch cut out of one side and the sliding cannula has a cutting edge, is more often used.

PROCEDURE

Preparation

Although there have been recent reports of outpatient liver biopsy,[27, 51] we prefer the patient to be admitted to hospital for biopsy. Premedication is not usually necessary, although an intramuscular injection of diazepam will calm the unduly anxious patient. Sedation should never be so extensive that patient cooperation is lost. The patient should lie flat on the edge of the bed with one head-pillow and the right hand placed behind the head. Except when it is necessary to biopsy a specific area, the intercostal route should be used. The site for biopsy is selected by percussing out the borders of the liver and then choosing the area of maximum dullness on expiration in the mid-axillary line. This usually involves traversing either the eighth, ninth or tenth intercostal space.

Technique

After cleansing the skin with a suitable antiseptic, local anaesthetic is introduced at the biopsy site and infiltrated down to and including the liver capsule. A small incision is made in the skin to facilitate entry of the biopsy needle. At this point the bleeding time should be noted and, if unacceptable, the procedure should be abandoned despite a normal clotting screen. The forthcoming events should then be explained and rehearsed with the patient, with particular emphasis given to the importance of breath-holding. He should also be warned that there may be some local and perhaps shoulder-tip pain. The needle should be placed on a 10 ml syringe, which is filled with 6 ml of sterile normal saline. With the patient breathing quietly, the needle is advanced until it is felt to give into the space overlying the liver. Two ml of saline is injected to clear any debris from the needle. The patient is told to breathe out and then stop breathing. Two ml of suction is applied to the syringe and the Klatskin needle can then be rapidly advanced in and out of the liver in one movement. The appearance of blood in the syringe at the time of the biopsy should not cause alarm and is not indicative of subsequent haemorrhage. On withdrawal, the biopsy appears in the barrel of the syringe and is easily removed by withdrawing the plunger and pouring the contents into a suitable container which should have a small piece of gauze in the bottom. In situations where malignant disease is suspected, a second pass of the needle in a different direction is justified, particularly if the first biopsy appears macroscopically normal (see Chapter 38). After the biopsy the patient is asked to lie on his right side for two hours and remain in bed for 24 hours. Regular recordings of pulse and blood pressure should be made for the first few hours.

The Specimen

Most of the specimen should be fixed in 10 per cent formalin for routine histology, but small portions may be fixed in 2 to 4 per cent glutaraldehyde for electron microscopy and snap-frozen for storage in liquid nitrogen. If there is a suspicion of infection, a piece may be sent for culture.

Complications

Pain

Some pain may be experienced at the site of biopsy, and there is occasionally shoulder-tip pain secondary to diaphragmatic irritation. If there is any bleeding into the pleural cavity, there may be some pleuritic-type pain with an associated friction rub.

Perforation of other abdominal organs

This is rare, with the colon being the most commonly punctured viscus. Pancreatic and renal tissue is occasionally found in the biopsy specimen, usually from inexperienced operators. Perforation of a distended gallbladder occasionally complicates the abdominal approach, but has also been recorded with the intercostal technique.[38] Pneumothorax may also occur.

Biliary peritonitis

Biliary leakage may complicate a biopsy in patients with obstructed, dilated intrahepatic ducts. This complication is potentially lethal, and if suspected is an indication for early laparotomy and decompression.

Needle fracture

Purow, Grosberg and Wapnick[53] recently reported fracture of the biopsy needle during the procedure with retention of the broken end. They were able to obtain information on three similar incidents. The fracture site was approximately level with the tip of nail when in situ and may be of significance if metal fatigue were responsible in any way.

Intrahepatic haematoma

Raines et al,[54] in a prospective study of 40 patients undergoing needle biopsy of the liver, found three (7 per cent) to have a solitary filling defect on a post-biopsy liver scan. Except for a fall in haematocrit and in one case some transitory pain, none of the patients experienced any other effects. There has subsequently been a report of an intrahepatic haematoma causing biliary obstruction.[6]

Haemorrhage

This is the commonest complication and cause of death. Provided the precautions previously described are taken, the risk can be minimized but is occasionally unavoidable, particularly if a deep breath is taken at the moment of biopsy or some major vessel is punctured. Terry[68] estimated that significant bleeding complicated 0.2 per cent of biopsies. Strict observations should give an early indication of bleeding, and if blood transfusion fails to stabilize the situation, laparotomy has to be considered.

Mortality

Haemorrhage and peritonitis account for the majority of deaths complicating liver biopsy. One of the highest figures of 1 per cent was given by Snapper in 1951,[66] although at about the same time Gallison and Skinner[13] suggested the figure was 0.35 per cent. Two large reviews of 10 600 and 20 016 patients gave figures of 0.12

per cent and 0.17 per cent respectively.[68, 74] More recently, a review of 79 381 biopsies has given a figure of 0.015 per cent.[33] It seems likely that the current rate of mortality lies somewhere between 0.1 and 0.01 per cent.

LIVER BIOPSY IN CHILDREN

This is increasingly used and is safe, provided the child is appropriately sedated and properly restrained.[20] A general anaesthetic may be required if a biopsy is particularly necessary in a very uncooperative child. The subcostal or intercostal route is used, depending on the liver size, and the Menghini needle is usually employed. Movement of the liver may be minimized by an assistant who pushes it upwards from below the costal margin.

THE LIVER BIOPSY

Macroscopic Features

A limited amount of information is available from macroscopic appearances.

Architecture

A normal architecture can be identified in a cylinder of liver when a regular dark brown/pale brown mottling is seen. This results from the centrilobular distribution of lipofuscin.

Abnormal fibrosis is seen as a grey-white tissue that is usually narrower than the rest of the biopsy. In a micronodular cirrhosis this fibrous tissue may predominate and a few tiny nodules of pale brown parenchyma may be embedded within it. A macronodular cirrhosis may not be identified grossly but a fragmented biopsy is suggestive of a cirrhosis.

Pigments

Lipofuscin has been mentioned; as a 'wear and tear' pigment it shows zonal emphasis around the central vein and its presence indicates lack of regeneration. Other pigments may also be seen and these include bile, haemosiderin and the Dubin–Johnson pigments. Bile will produce a green to dark green colour in the biopsy which with any zonal accentuation will be reflected as a mottled green pattern. In haemochromatosis the iron is present in such excess that the biopsy may be a uniform dark brown but lesser degrees of iron retention may show a dark brown/light brown mottling that is very similar to lipofuscin deposition. By light microscopy the iron pigmentation is distinguished by its periportal distribution and staining reactions. Dubin–Johnson pigment may be suspected in a very dark brown or almost black liver.

Miscellaneous

The most frequently identified abnormality is fatty liver which is seen as a very pale cream cylinder of liver. Tumour may closely resemble fibrosis in gross appearance and indeed many tumours are desmoplastic but a glistening, slightly mucoid and pearly-grey appearance suggests carcinoma. The presence of flecks of yellowing necrosis may be seen grossly within areas of tumour and sometimes there is a cylinder of liver with which to contrast the abnormal appearances. Primary tumours of the liver may have these gross appearances on biopsy but hepatocellular carcinoma may be tan, yellow or yellow-green and fragmented. These appearances may mimic a cirrhosis with multiple fragmented tiny nodules.

Handling

The specimen must be handled with great care, especially for light microscopy and ultrastructural examination. Squeezing by forceps should be avoided: instead, the biopsy should be gently lifted out on the paper or gauze from the container and transferred to fixative.

Fixation

The properties of the various fixatives have been reviewed by Hopwood[21] and Glauert.[15]

A perfect fixative does not exist but a 10 per cent solution of neutral buffered formol-saline has fewest disadvantages and several advantages. Carnoy's, Helly's and Zenker's fixatives are excellent for histological and especially nuclear detail but unfortunately are unsatisfactory for the orcein or immunoperoxidase techniques and are preferably avoided[43] (Table 18.1). Fixation in formalin requires at least four hours for small biopsies at ambient temperatures but is quicker at higher (37°C) temperatures. For formalin fixation it should be appreciated that

1. fixation is progressive and not complete for several days;
2. penetration of the fixative is limited;
3. the process involves interaction of aldehyde with the amino groups in tissue proteins and requires a great excess by volume (×20) of fixative.

These are minor points for a small needle biopsy but become of increasing importance for wedge biopsies of liver, hepatic (lobar) resections and the occasional liver removed during transplantation.

Table 18.1. *Effect of Fixative on Demonstration of HB_sAg.*

Fixative	Orcein	Immunoperoxidase[a]
Formalin pH 7	++++	++++
Bouin	+++	++
Carnoy	−	+
Zenker	++	+
Helly	+	−

[a] Peroxidase antiperoxidase (PAP) technique standardized for our laboratory at rabbit anti-HBs 1/10, swine anti-rabbit 1gG 1/20, and rabbit PAP at 1/200.

Electron microscopy

For ultrastructural studies glutaraldehyde (electron microscopy grades) remains the fixative of choice but good detail is preserved after fixation in buffered paraformaldehyde of adequate osmolarity, and this has been recommended as an appropriate general fixative for combined light microscopy with transmission and scanning electron microscopic studies.[17] We use a 4.5 per cent solution of glutaraldehyde with a cacodylate buffer (at pH 7.4) and keep the solution at 4° centigrade for up to four weeks. Phosphate buffer may be substituted for cacodylate.

Intrinsic enzyme activity is normally demonstrated on frozen sections which are then processed for electron microscopy, but some can also be demonstrated after fixation. There is great variation in the effect of a fixative on various enzymes and in the effect of various fixatives on a particular enzyme.[56]

Processing

After fixation, routine histopathology processing schedules are adequate. These will dehydrate the specimen in a series of graded alcohols, clear in chloroform or toluene, and impregnate with hot paraffin wax. Thin epoxy resin sections may also be prepared from thick sections of paraffin-embedded material[5] or, alternatively, if facilities are available a methacrylate embedding procedure may be employed by which sections 1 to 2 μm thick may be cut.[30]

Other Techniques

Diagnostic techniques apart from those required for standard light and electron microscopy can be used but usually require fresh or snap-frozen liver. Culture of the specimen for bacteria or viruses,[75] assays of enzymes,[32,61,62,71] metals,[3,12] or other hepatocellular constituents,[29] and frozen sections of liver for histochemistry,[11] for fluorescence of porphyrins,[35] immunofluorescence or, very rarely, for a rapid histopathological diagnosis may all be employed as indicated by clinical circumstances.

Immunofluorescence has been widely employed in liver for the demonstration of virus antigens such as hepatitis A and B (see Chapters 28 and 29), serum immunoglobulins and products of the hepatocyte such as albumin and alpha-1-antitrypsin.[69] With the advent of the immunoperoxidase technique some, and probably many, of these fluorescent demonstrations will be superseded. The disadvantages of fluorescence are the requirements of fresh and therefore potentially infected and infective material, the use of specialized fluorescence microscopy, the lack of a permanent record unless photographs are taken, and poor correlation with diagnostic histopathology. The use of an immunoperoxidase technique overcomes these handicaps but is limited by the stability of the antigen in the fixative and in the processing to paraffin blocks. This limitation may not be as considerable as first feared. By using proteolytic enzymes, particularly trypsin, for pre-digestion of sections we have recently been able to restore antigenicity of HB_sAg lost after formalin fixation[45] while both extracellular immunoglobulin and components of complement have been demonstrated in renal glomeruli.[37]

Application of immunoperoxidase techniques

will revolutionize diagnostic histopathology in all areas including liver biopsies. As they will identify a specific feature rather than produce a variable pattern for diagnostic interpretation they must supplement general biopsy interpretation rather than replace it.

MICROSCOPY: STAINING

We prefer not to section our liver biopsies serially. Rather, a small series of 10 to 15 consecutive sections 3 to 4 µm thick are cut and stained with haematoxylin and eosin (H & E), silver impregnation,[16] periodic acid-Schiff after diastase digestion (DPAS), orcein[64] and Perl's Prussian blue. A series of sections at different levels is then cut if the clinical information or the biopsy features suggest a focal lesion which is not apparent on these sections.

The additional stains routinely employed demonstrate extra detail not seen or only poorly seen in routine H & E sections. Trichrome preparations of varying hues (Masson, Goldner, Mallory, Picro-Mallory, M.S.B. etc.) are popular, aesthetically attractive and photogenic but rarely provide any information that cannot be identified with advantage on either an H & E, or on a non-gold-toned reticulin preparation. We use them only to search for fibrin thrombi.

Reticulin Preparations

Omission of gold toning from the reticulin preparation results in collagen in portal tracts and in the wall of the central vein staining a dark golden brown while sinusoid reticulin is grey black. Collapsed reticulin remains black but collagen that forms within the lobule stains as the portal tracts. A counterstain such as neutral red may be employed but is not necessary. Alcian blue has also been used in combination with non-toned preparations to demonstrate connective tissue mucins.[36]

Iron

The Perl's Prussian blue technique is a reliable histochemical stain for iron and often demonstrates it in scanty amounts in periportal hepatocytes. A grading system of 0 to 4 can be employed[60] which reliably identifies symptomatic and latent haemochromatosis.[12] This stain is also useful in that other pigments, such as lipofuscin and bile, are not obscured unless there is gross excess of iron. A light counterstain such as neutral red is usually employed.

Periodic Acid-Schiff (PAS)

Glycogen

Glycogen can be demonstrated histochemically in formalin-fixed paraffin-processed liver by the PAS technique. This is unreliable because of its solubility in aqueous media. For a definitive demonstration alcohol-based reagents must be used either on frozen sections or on tissue fixed and processed in non-aqueous media. Specificity of the reaction for glycogen is confirmed by prior diastase (or amylase) digestion of the section but quantitation of the glycogen present is suspect unless these precautions are taken. Even then any reduction in glycogen has to be gross before it is detectable. The generalized intense staining of glycogen also obscures other positively-stained non-glycogen structures in the biopsy. Consequently, a section stained by the PAS technique after diastase digestion is the more valuable preparation as then ceroid pigment, globules and basement membranes can be identified when present.

Ceroid

Phagocytosed granular material within Kupffer cells is frequently intensely PAS positive and then is termed 'ceroid pigment'. It is closely allied to the lipofuscins, having similar light microscopic appearances and staining reactions. The main distinction is that lipofuscin is positive in Schmorl's reaction and ceroid is negative. This pigment is a consequence of death of hepatocytes and occurs in both viral hepatitis and a focus of non-specific necrosis. During the evolution of extrahepatic bile duct obstruction, bile is found in Kupffer cells and is accompanied by PAS positive pigment. With relief of the obstruction the bile rapidly disappears, but this pigment may persist.

Globules

Apart from lipofuscin, PAS positive diastase resistant material may be present in hepatocytes. When present as globules in periportal

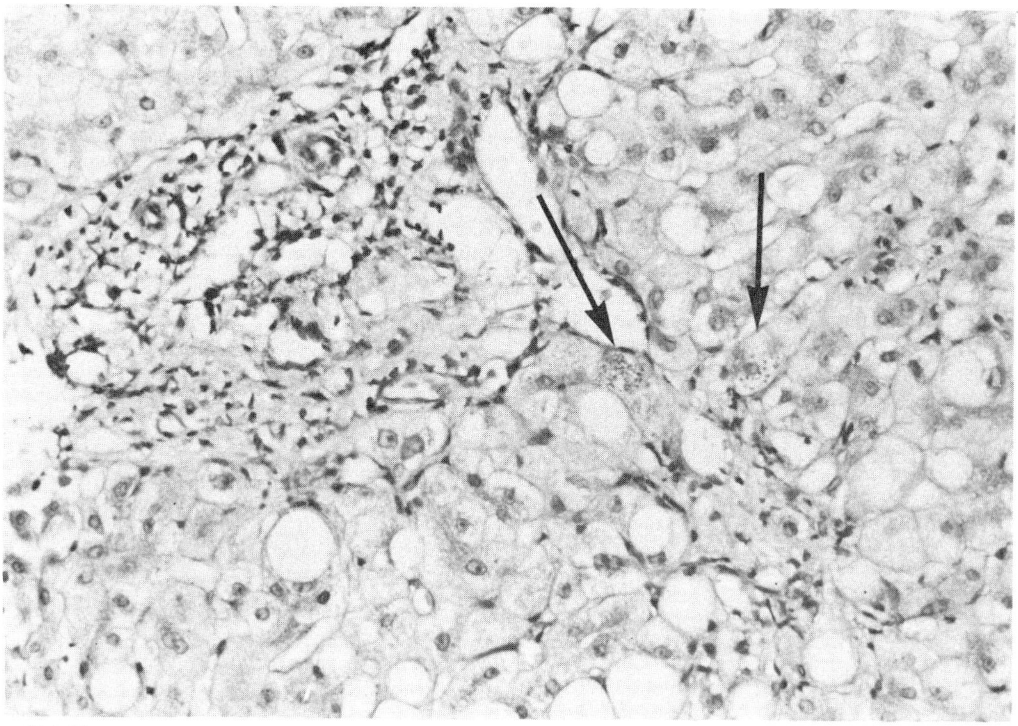

Figure 18.1. Heterozygous MZ alpha-l-antitrypsin deficiency: globules (arrows) are tiny and only present in two hepatocytes adjacent to this portal tract. Not all portal tracts were involved. Incidental finding in patient with acute alcoholic hepatitis. DPAS × 500.

hepatocytes they are regarded as diagnostic of alpha-1-antitrypsin deficiency until proved otherwise (see Chapter 35). In this respect it must be indicated that these globules may be very small and appear more as a coarse granularity, particularly in association with the heterozygous deficiency state (Figure 18.1). On other occasions palely stained globules may be seen in hepatocytes adjacent to zones of necrosis. Immunocytochemical techniques demonstrate that these are also globules of alpha-1-antitrypsin. They do not have the same genetic implication as periportal globules and disappear with resolution of the hepatocellular damage.

Nuclei

Nuclei of hepatocytes may be vacuolated as a result of cytoplasmic invagination. This occurs in normal liver and in many conditions associated with non-specific changes in the liver such as diabetes mellitus and psoriasis. Glycogen may occur in these but occasionally some of the vacuoles are intensely PAS positive after diastase digestion. The significance of this is not known.

Basement membranes

Within portal tracts, basement membranes, particularly around bile ducts and ductules, can be demonstrated. No disorders of the bile duct basement membrane equivalent to those of the renal glomerulus are described.

Others

Infiltrations within the liver such as amyloid may be positive and the mucin in adenocarcinomas can be identified.

Orcein

The orcein technique also provides specific diagnostic information. It is one of several stains which can demonstrate hepatocytes containing hepatitis B surface antigen (HB_sAg).[64] The most frequently used alternative to orcein for this demonstration is aldehyde fuchsin. Recently a trichrome modification for HB_sAg has been described.[18] In addition, orcein will demonstrate a copper-

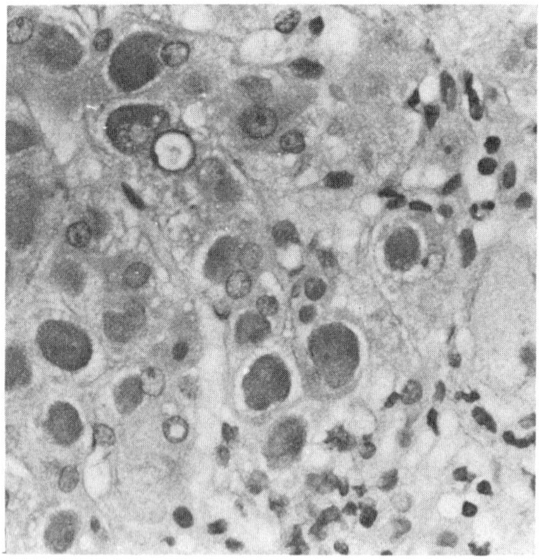

Figure 18.2. Positive cytoplasmic staining for HB_sAg by orcein. Note the clear rim of cytoplasm under the plasma membrane. Patient with cirrhosis and HB_sAg positive chronic active hepatitis. Orcein × 800.

binding protein in periportal hepatocytes (see below) and the elastic fibres in portal tracts.

HB_sAg

We have found that batches of orcein vary tremendously in both the staining of HB_sAg positive hepatocytes and their general background staining. New batches are therefore carefully checked against known positive control tissue and the staining carefully adjusted. Positive hepatocytes (Figure 18.2) contain a discrete area of evenly stained but finely honeycombed brown to brown-black cytoplasm. The smallest positive areas are simply a perinuclear rim of stained cytoplasm but even when large they rarely reach the plasma membrane. Care must be taken as acidophil degenerate cells take up the stain non-specifically and various other positively stained features must be distinguished (see below).

Granules

Ceroid pigments are stained brown but are readily identified by their granularity and position in Kupffer cells. Their identity can be confirmed if necessary by their other staining reactions.[50]

Copper-binding protein is demonstrated as blue-black granules within periportal hepatocytes (Figure 18.3). Evidence has been presented that these are copper binding proteins within hepatocytes and that they are increased in conditions of chronic cholestasis such as biliary atresia and the later stages of primary biliary cirrhosis.[57, 65] There is good correlation between the orcein demonstration of copper binding protein and the demonstration of copper by the rhodanine technique.[22]

Elastic

The elastic fibres in the connective tissue of the portal tracts are still demonstrated by this modified orcein technique. Demonstration of these fibres identifies the original portal tracts and consequently the extent of any new fibrous tissue which lacks these fibres can be more accurately assessed. In normal portal tracts there is often a narrow peripheral zone lacking in elastic but this should rarely cause confusion. In some biopsies, particularly in alcoholic liver disease, fine fibrils may stain as elastic fibres but differ from the more coarse serpiginous elastic fibres of the portal tract, being finer, straighter and more aligned so that distinction is not usually a problem.

MICROSCOPIC FEATURES

Despite the helpful and sometimes diagnostic features provided by these additional stains, most biopsy interpretation relies on sections stained with H & E. The main objectives of a liver biopsy are to provide or confirm a

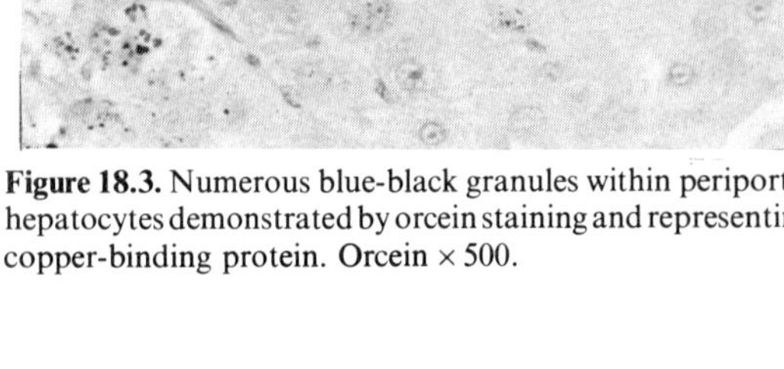

Figure 18.3. Numerous blue-black granules within periportal hepatocytes demonstrated by orcein staining and representing copper-binding protein. Orcein × 500.

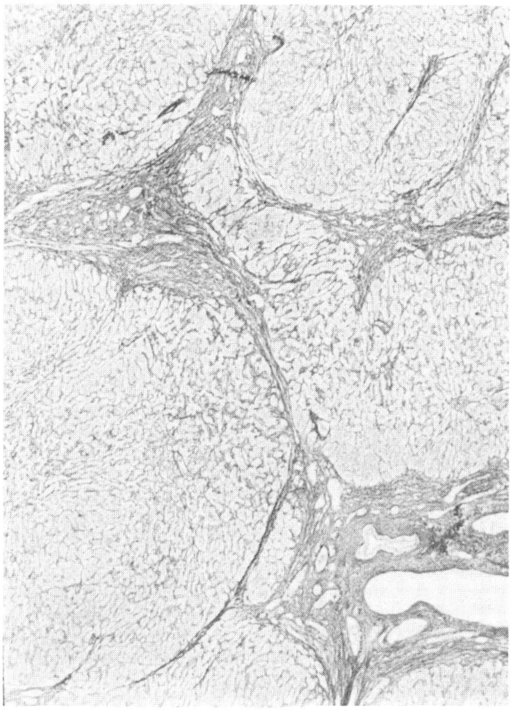

Figure 18.4. Macronodular cirrhosis with portal tract bottom right, slender bands of abnormal fibrous tissue and abnormal cell plate patterns. A needle biopsy demonstrating only the right half of the figure may show mild fibrosis only. Wedge biopsy, reticulin × 20.

diagnosis, to offer a prognosis and to study the effects of treatment. Furthermore, the biopsy should be critically evaluated initially without clinical details and a presumptive diagnosis with differential diagnosis made. Only then should comparison and correlation with clinical details and investigations be made. Meaningful discussion often results. In all instances it is essential to examine the biopsy in a systematic and logical manner.

Architecture

Firstly the architecture of the biopsy should be established. This is usually obvious either with a regular arrangement of portal tracts to central veins or alternatively with abnormal fibrous bands and regenerative nodules of cirrhosis but occasionally difficulty may be encountered. Sometimes this is because the portal tracts on the edge of the biopsy have been torn out of the specimen by a blunt biopsy needle. On other occasions part of a large macronodule may have been biopsied. Features which may then help when present are slender abnormal bands of fibrous tissue (Figure 18.4), an abnormal cell plate pattern (Figures 18.5 and 18.6), an excess of 'central' efferent veins in the biopsy frequently with an abnormal approximation to fibrous bands, and absence of lipofuscin in hepatocytes. In difficult cases careful examination of the individual components of the acinus (or lobule) are required.

Portal Tracts

Large portal tracts present no problem with identification but smaller ones may be difficult to separate from bands of fibrous tissue containing a few bile ductules. Even in obvious portal tracts the individual structures should be identified and any abnormalities noted. The relative size and calibre of the bile duct, artery and vein should be studied: portal vein thrombosis may be reflected in the biopsy only by branches of smaller calibre relative to their accompanying bile ducts and arteries. Bile ducts may be hypoplastic[1] as well as atretic or, in acquired large duct obstruction, dilated. Characteristic changes also occur in primary biliary cirrhosis (sec Chapter 31) and chronic hepatitis (see Chapter 29). The nature of the stroma should be noted: the collagen becomes more dense and hyaline with increasing age and becomes oedematous in bile duct obstruction.

The quality and location of any inflammatory infiltrate should be identified. Neutrophils around peripheral proliferating bile ductules indicate obstruction to bile ducts but when present in the lumen of the bile duct indicate a cholangitis. Likewise an inflammatory infiltrate within the artery or vein wall indicates a corresponding arteritis or endophlebitis. Both are relatively rare events: branches of the hepatic artery can be involved by polyarteritis nodosa and are claimed to be more frequently involved in acute rather than subacute bacterial endocarditis; portal endophlebitis usually indicates portal pyaemia due to sepsis within the portal venous drainage. A mixed lymphocytic and macrophage infiltrate is a common reactive component in portal tracts and distinction between this, chronic persistent hepatitis and pericholangitis can be extremely difficult if not impossible. Indeed, sometimes no clear histological distinction can be made between the pericholangitis and non-specific reactive inflammatory infiltrate. The presence of plasma cells in more than scanty numbers is suggestive of significant liver disease or a complication.

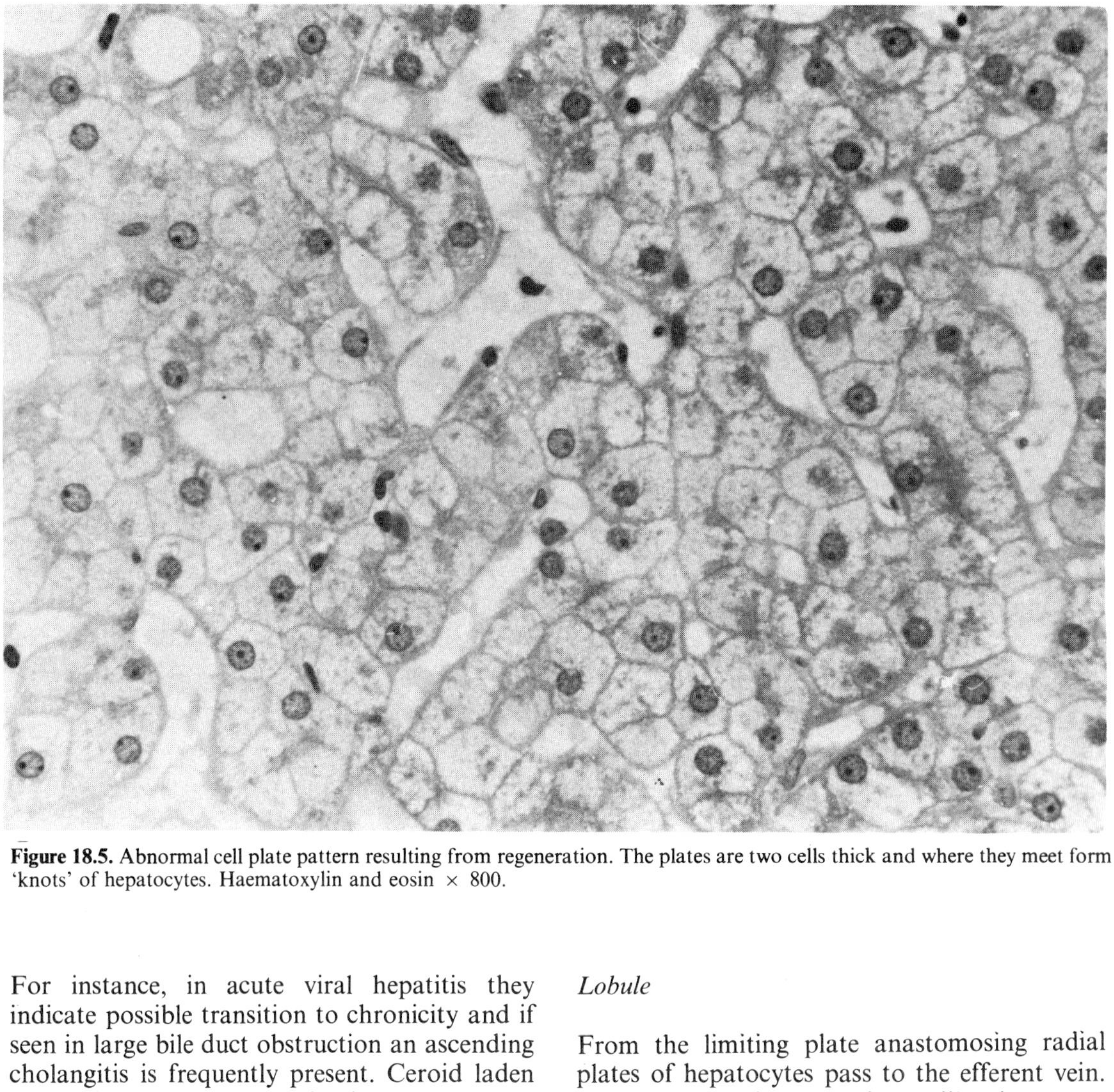

Figure 18.5. Abnormal cell plate pattern resulting from regeneration. The plates are two cells thick and where they meet form 'knots' of hepatocytes. Haematoxylin and eosin × 800.

For instance, in acute viral hepatitis they indicate possible transition to chronicity and if seen in large bile duct obstruction an ascending cholangitis is frequently present. Ceroid laden macrophages usually persist in portal tracts after resolution elsewhere and rarely can be demonstrated up to 4 to 6 months after the clinical onset of an acute viral hepatitis.

Parenchyma

The limiting plate

Examination of the lobule begins with the limiting plate which is simply the concentric layer of hepatocytes opposed to the connective tissue of the tracts. This plate is obviously interrupted by the entry of vessels into the sinusoids but is comprehensively distorted in many liver diseases ranging from piecemeal necrosis in chronic hepatitis (Figure 18.7) to portal tract expansion and bile ductule proliferation in large bile duct obstruction.

Lobule

From the limiting plate anastomosing radial plates of hepatocytes pass to the efferent vein. This pattern is altered readily in many conditions ranging from focal necroses to regeneration and is most reliably identified in reticulin preparations. The anatomical location of such lesions is important and particular attention should be paid to the hepatocytes around the efferent vein. Damage is emphasized here in acute viral hepatitis, alcoholic liver disease and some cases of drug-induced hepatitis but is minor in bile duct obstruction and pure drug-induced cholestasis.

Hepatocytes

These should be carefully examined and types of degeneration identified. These are rarely specific for one disease and it is usually a combination of the types of degeneration present and their distribution that indicate different diagnoses.

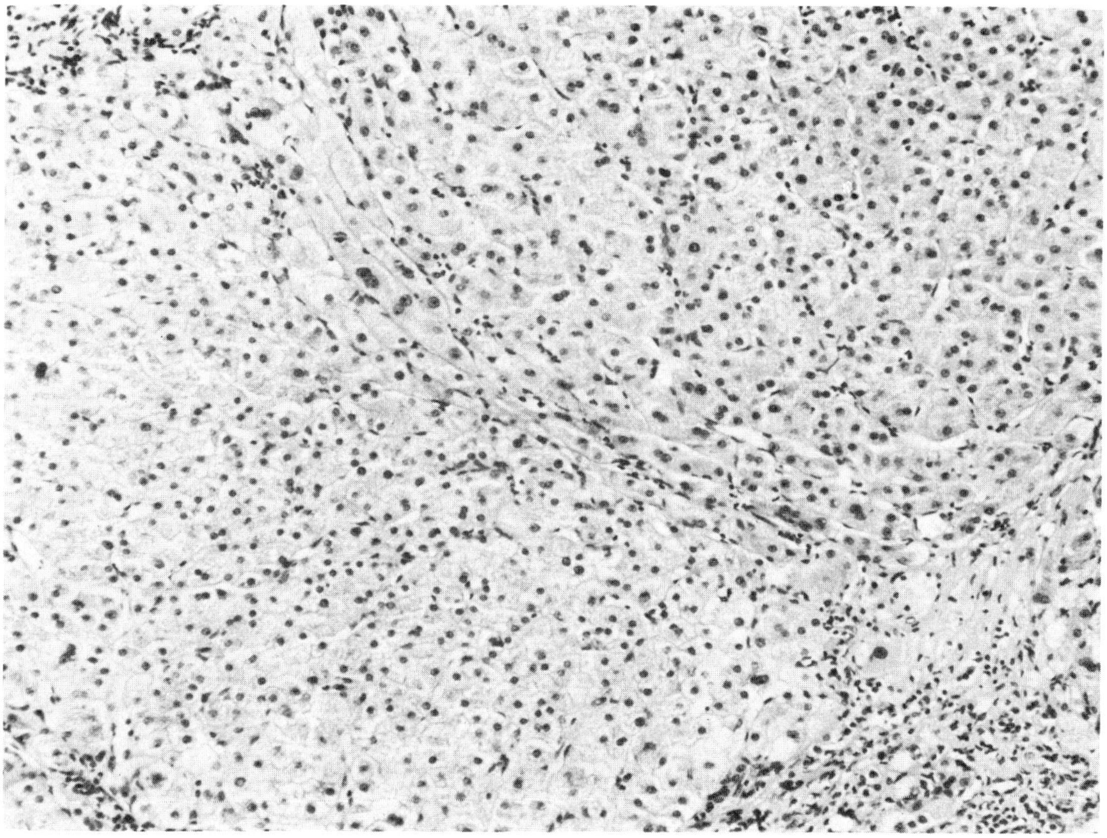

Figure 18.6. Abnormal cell plate pattern from regeneration. Asynchronous growth between two areas of parenchyma has resulted in a line of compression. This pattern most commonly occurs in cirrhosis. Haematoxylin and eosin × 400.

Thus Mallory's alcoholic hyalin (Figure 18.8) may be found in any established cirrhosis, in chronic cholestasis,[14] in primary biliary cirrhosis, in Wilson's disease,[58] in Indian childhood cirrhosis[48] and following intestinal by-pass operations for obesity,[40] as well as in alcoholic liver disease. When combined with fatty change and ballooning degeneration of hepatocytes and concentrated in hepatocytes around the efferent vein the pattern is virtually pathognomonic for alcohol (see Chapter 32). Fatty change itself is a very common finding, particularly in small amounts and around the efferent vein, but a periportal distribution indicates malnutrition and cachexia or rarely phosphorus poisoning (see Chapters 6 and 37).

Even less florid changes such as the number of binucleate hepatocytes, variation in nuclear size and staining, and the presence and distribution of intracellular pigments should be systematically sought. Increased numbers of binucleate and trinucleate hepatocytes and increased variation in nuclear pleomorphism are found with increasing age. These changes also occur during regeneration following hepatocellular damage and then persist after other signs of regeneration have disappeared. An increased variation in size and number of hepatocyte nuclei for the age of the patient may therefore give an indication of previous disease within the liver.

Pigments. Pigments within hepatocytes are most commonly iron, lipofuscin and bile. Iron is easily identified by its periportal location and specific staining reactions but bile and lipofuscin are more difficult. Both are usually found in hepatocytes around the efferent vein. Lipofuscin has fairly uniform golden brown granules which are refractile and has characteristic staining reactions[50] and electron microscopic appearances (see 'Lysosomes' in Chapter 2). It is a 'wear and tear' pigment and is noted for its absence in regenerating liver. It has significance therefore in suggesting that cirrhosis is not present in biopsies where identification of the architecture is equivocal. Bile, by contrast, is more variable in appearance and may range

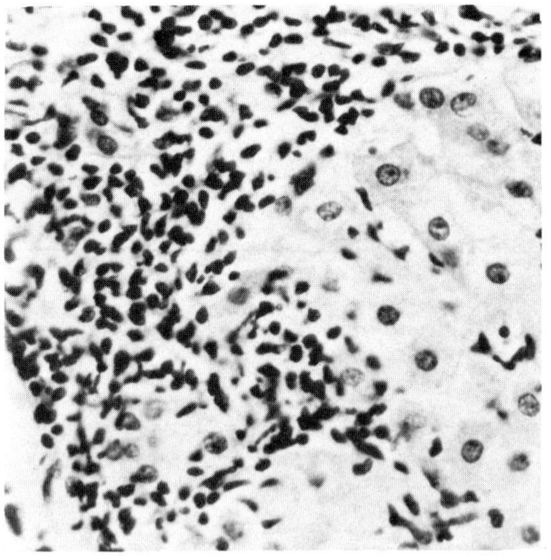

Figure 18.7. Piecemeal necrosis: mononuclear cells are isolating small groups of hepatocytes at an interface. The limiting plate has been destroyed. Haematoxylin and eosin × 500.

from brown through yellow to green in colour. Definitive identification of bile is made by finding it within the canaliculi.

Copper is also found on occasions and can be specifically demonstrated by the very sensitive rubeanic acid technique, the sensitive and more reliable rhodanine technique,[22] or by orcein which stains copper-binding protein.[57]

Sinusoids

These narrow channels are usually less than half the width of a hepatocyte. Identification of relative width is helpful as apparent occlusion of the sinusoids indicates pathological change in the liver. This may be damage to hepatocytes such as fatty change or ballooning degeneration, or focal proliferation of sinusoidal cells as occurs in viral hepatitis (Figure 18.9), or twinning of cell plates as in regeneration (Figure 18.6). The first two are usually obvious so that bland obliteration of the sinusoidal space should result in a careful search for regenerative activity. Unfortunately, over-enthusiastic aspiration using a nail within the Menghini needle, or subsequent forceful expulsion with the stilette, can produce a similar artefact.

Conversely, dilatation of sinusoids may be associated with loss of hepatocytes, passive venous congestion, infarcts of Zahn,[73] metastases within the liver (see Chapter 38), and drugs.[72] Passive venous congestion produces centrilobular dilatation while portal vein occlusion (infarct of Zahn) will be multiacinar and affect all zones of an acinus. The sinusoidal ectasia associated with the 'pill' and with metastases is usually random in the acinus but a periportal pattern has been associated with the 'pill'.[72]

Congested sinusoids are rarely identified in a biopsy as the blood readily escapes from such small fragments of tissue. Persistence of many red cells in sinusoids, particularly dilated ones, is unusual. Two possible causes are erythrophagocytosis by Kupffer cells as occurs in some haemolytic anaemias, and engorgement of the space of Disse. Originally described as pathognomonic for veno-occlusive disease of the liver[31] this has also been identified in left ventricular failure without right heart failure.[8]

Cells within the sinusoids should be noted. Malignant cells ranging from carcinoma to hairy cell leukaemia, reactive (or infected) cells as in infectious mononucleosis and aberrant normal or hyperplastic tissue as in extramedullary haemopoiesis may all occur. Endothelial cells and Kupffer cells are usually inconspicuous

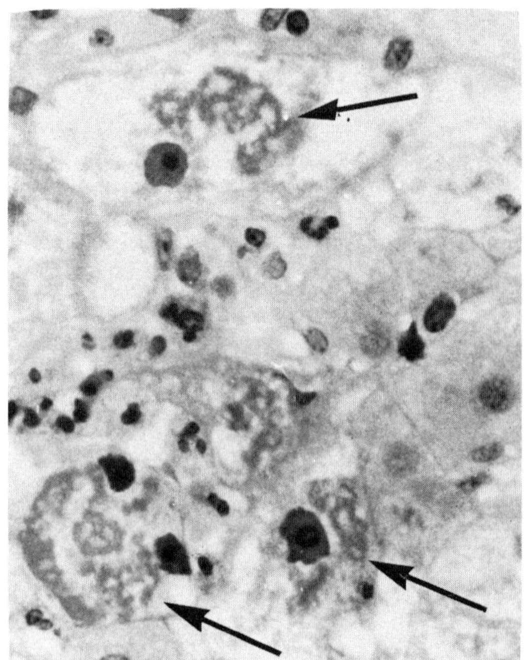

Figure 18.8. Mallory bodies (arrows) are best seen in swollen ballooned hepatocytes and are characterized by their denseness and irregular form. Haematoxylin and eosin × 1200.

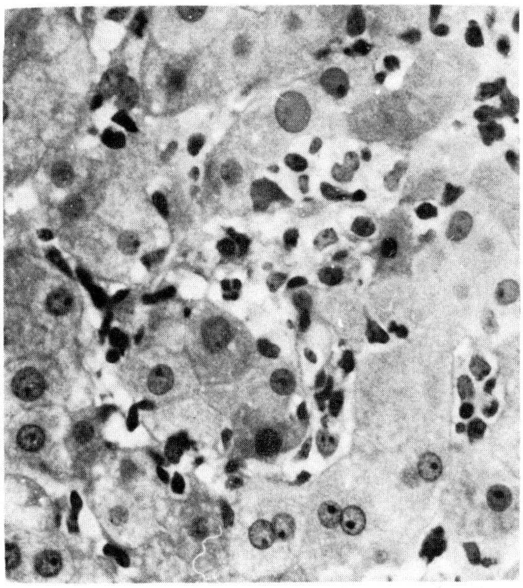

Figure 18.9. Sinusoids filled with inflammatory cells and proliferating Kupffer cells. Haematoxylin and eosin × 1000.

but the latter especially may show hyperplasia and phagocytic activity in response to hepatocellular damage and death (Figure 18.9) or may contain extraneous pigment such as Thorotrast[10] or malarial pigment.

The space of Disse is also a common site for deposition of amyloid (see Chapter 37) which can be seen as an acellular eosinophilic zone between the hepatocyte and sinusoidal lumen. With increasing degrees of amyloidosis hepatocytes become atrophic but in the earliest stages special techniques such as Congo red staining may be required to demonstrate it.

Central Vein

Last, but not least, the central vein should be identified. It has already been noted that an excess of apparent 'central' veins may be found in a macronodular cirrhosis, but important diagnostic information is provided in differentiating acute liver disease. This is the area involved in minor degrees of cholestasis, hepatocellular damage in viral hepatitis and commonly fibrosis in alcoholic liver disease. 'Prolapse' of hepatocytes through the wall of the central vein has been described in association with prolonged androgenic steroid therapy.[49]

DIAGNOSIS

Diagnosis in liver biopsies varies between primary and secondary liver lesions and the presence of focal or diffuse changes in the liver. Of these the most important distinction is between focal and diffuse liver disease as the latter is more reliably present and sampling error may be considerable with focal lesions. A normal or 'non-specific' biopsy therefore does not contradict the clinical diagnosis.

Diffuse Lesions

In this group are some of the major indications for liver biopsy. These include the differential diagnosis of jaundice (see Chapter 26) and the confirmation and differential diagnosis of cirrhosis (see Chapter 30).

Jaundice

There are many causes of jaundice but the common differential diagnosis in *acute* liver disease includes viral hepatitis, drug-induced jaundice, and large bile duct obstruction. Congenital disorders of bilirubin metabolism affecting children or young adults can usually be readily separated by their clinical and biochemical features, sometimes in association with a biopsy (see Chapter 13). Cholestasis is considered in more detail in Chapter 14.

The emphasis in acute viral hepatitis (see also Chapter 28) is on panlobular hepatocellular damage including ballooning and acidophil degeneration with accentuation of the cell damage around centrilobular veins (Figure 18.10). Cholestasis is present as bile within hepatocytes and canaliculi but usually does not reflect the degree of hyperbilirubinaemia. Portal tracts may be expanded but the emphasis is on a mononuclear cell inflammatory infiltrate and there is rarely any significant bile ductule proliferation. There is generalized hyperplasia of Kupffer cells, particularly around central veins where they are also hypertrophied and laden with phagocytosed debris. These cells may fill a sinusoid and the features are associated with hepatocellular damage and death.

In obstruction to the biliary tree cholestasis is the earliest feature and correlates with the degree of hyperbilirubinaemia.[7,46,47,52] Again, it is identified within hepatocytes and canaliculi around the centrilobular vein but there is no

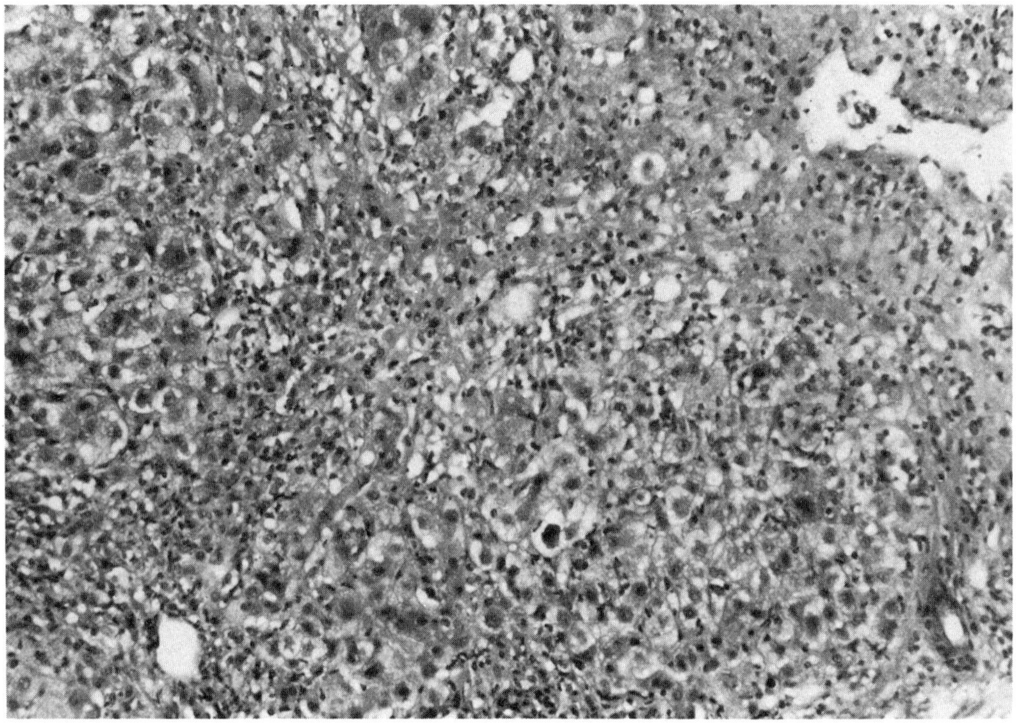

Figure 18.10. Lobular disarray in acute viral hepatitis. Central vein top right and portal tract bottom left. Haematoxylin and eosin × 250.

significant hepatocellular damage (Figure 18.11). Any that is present is consequent upon the cholestasis and therefore occurs as a relatively late event. Bile damaged hepatocytes show feathery degeneration – a term which denotes enlargement of the cell with cytoplasm arranged in fine strands irregularly traversing between plasma membranes and containing bile.

Within the first week cholestasis may be the only notable feature so that for any accurate biopsy interpretation the duration of jaundice is critical clinical information.

After the first week changes also occur in portal tracts. These initially become rounded in cross-section and the cells and fibres of the stroma more widely separated as a result of oedema. The bile duct is distended and later the epithelium shows considerable distortion as a result of focal degeneration and regeneration (Figure 18.12). A multilayered epithelium may thus form while at the same time parts of the duct wall are degenerate and lined by epithelial cells with flattened contours and pyknotic nuclei (Figure 18.13).

An inflammatory reaction initially is scanty and confined to a few neutrophils which may be easily overlooked. As the numbers of neutrophils increase they concentrate along the margins of the portal tracts and characteristically around the bile ductules. Lymphocytes and macrophages appear but remain central within the tract. Plasma cells, if present, indicate a complication, particularly a cholangitis: otherwise an alternative diagnosis should be sought.

As the obstruction progresses so the portal tracts expand by the formation of new fibrous tissue. This occurs irregularly around the portal tract edge so that the spur-like projections are eventually formed. Prominent in this fibrosis

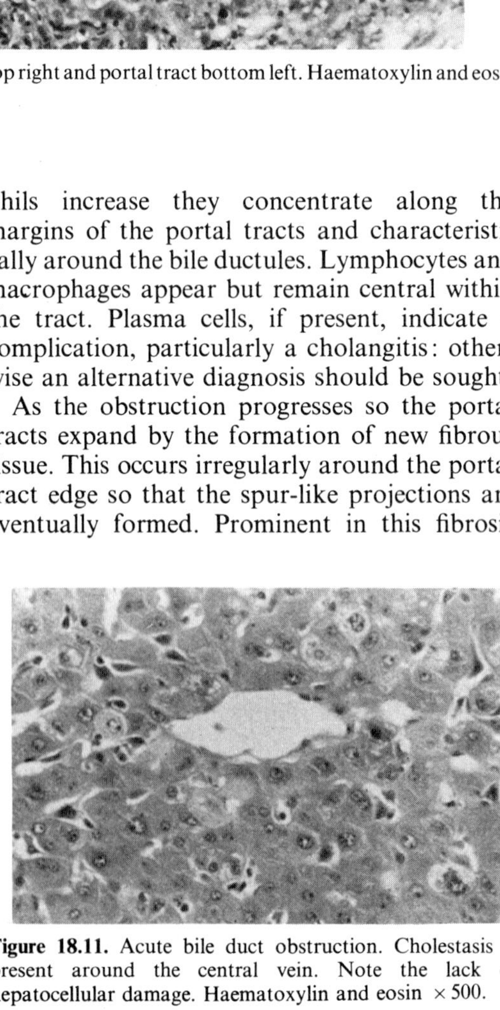

Figure 18.11. Acute bile duct obstruction. Cholestasis is present around the central vein. Note the lack of hepatocellular damage. Haematoxylin and eosin × 500.

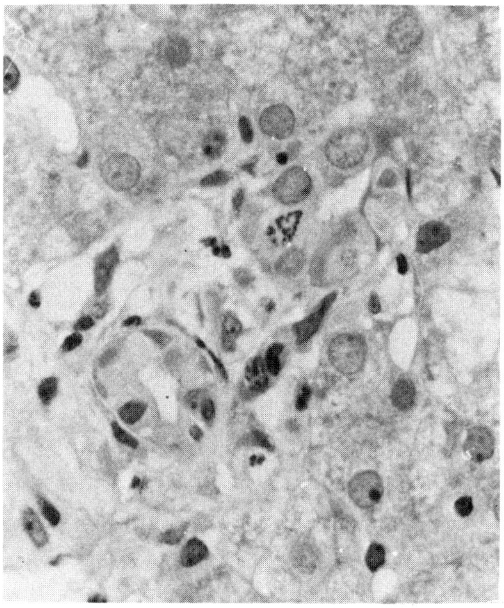

Figure 18.12. Mitotic activity in bile ductule on edge of portal tract: early acute bile duct obstruction. Haematoxylin and eosin × 1000.

and most consistently found are the proliferating bile ductules at the edge of the tract[52] (Figure 18.14). These are in columns of low cuboidal biliary epithelial cells usually around a small but definite lumen which may be filled with bile in severe obstruction. They are frequently angulate and may be perpendicular to the parenchymal interface.

Occasionally bile infarcts within the lobule and bile granulomas within the portal tracts may be found. These are attributed to the escape of bile into the tissues and are virtually pathognomonic for obstruction. The bile infarct is an area of extracellular bile within the lobule surrounded by the ghost outlines of hepatocytes admixed with some foamy and bile laden macrophages (Figure 18.15). In long-standing cases the bile disappears and a network of reticulin fibres and macrophages remains. Within the portal tract escape of bile from bile duct results in a foreign body giant cell granulomatous reaction usually positioned against the bile duct. This should not be confused with the granuloma associated with primary biliary cirrhosis. Epithelioid cells are characteristic of the granulomas in primary biliary cirrhosis and are not a feature of the reaction to bile. Very rarely bile does escape from the bile duct in primary biliary cirrhosis and incite a foreign body giant cell reaction. These extravasations of bile may rarely occur in the first week of obstruction but most frequently are seen in long-standing cases of obstruction.

Ancillary stains assist by the negative information they provide. The normality of the central zone in obstruction is clearly demonstrated in the reticulin preparations while the absence of focal Kupffer cell proliferation can be seen on diastase PAS preparations. These latter preparations do demonstrate positively-stained pigment within the Kupffer cells but the distribution of such cells is uniform around the central vein and numbers diminish drastically in the mid-zone and even more in the periportal areas. Focal clusters of Kupffer cells reflect a response to hepatocyte death and are usually a late event in obstruction. These features are particularly important in distinguishing between

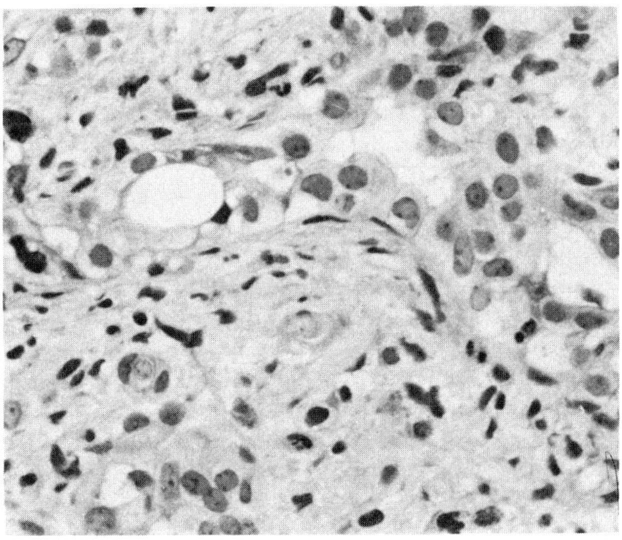

Figure 18.13. Bile duct in duct obstruction showing distension with focal hyperplasia and atrophy of the epithelium. Haematoxylin and eosin × 1000.

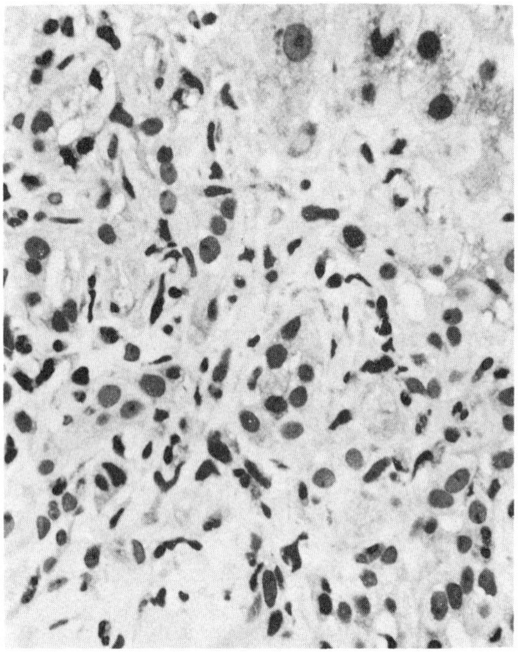

Figure 18.14. Hepatocytes (top) with proliferating bile ductules in the edge of the expanded portal tract. Haematoxylin and eosin × 800.

obstruction and the cholestatic variety of viral hepatitis (see Chapter 28).

It should be emphasized that these are the classical features in a liver biopsy following total large bile duct obstruction. They are now rarely seen because, with the advent of ERCP, percutaneous transhepatic cholangiography and ultrasound, biopsy is relatively contraindicated in bile duct obstruction. Biopsies are much more likely to be taken in 'odd' cases or those showing complications.

When obstruction to the major ducts is intermittent the degree of bile retention may be minimal and overshadowed by the portal tract changes of fibrosis with bile ductule proliferation and surrounding neutrophils. A similar lack of cholestasis may be seen with focal intrahepatic obstruction. Then not only may the portal tract changes be relatively emphasized but there may be considerable variation between portal tracts. Some tracts may show prominent enlargement with fibrosis, bile ductules and neutrophils while others are apparently unaffected or only mildly affected. The changes of active obstruction should not be confused with those that may be found non-specifically in liver biopsies from patients with cholelithiasis and chronic cholecystitis. Mild portal tract fibrosis may be found and there may be bile ductule proliferation but neutrophils are not a feature and there is no readily visible lumen to the ductules. Also the ductules often lie parallel to the limiting plate whereas in obstruction they appear more irregularly orientated.

The evolution of the changes is difficult to time because the onset of obstruction is rarely known accurately in a patient. Experimentally, ligation of the common bile duct in rats results in mitotic activity in bile duct epithelium detectable by autoradiography within 48 hours. By the eighth day the proportion of bile ductules by volume has approximately doubled and gradually increases thereafter. New fibrous tissue is formed after the bile ductule proliferation and apparently in response to it.[24]

The morphology of drug-induced jaundice is varied and complex (see Chapter 36) but very few drugs mimic the portal tract changes of biliary obstruction. When there is only cholestasis with minimal or no inflammation or hepatocellular damage, distinction between drug-induced jaundice and large bile duct obstruction can be impossible without knowledge of the duration of jaundice. Clinical or biochemical features of jaundice of more than two weeks' duration without portal tract changes are unlikely to be due to obstruction. Drugs most likely to create diagnostic confusion are the anabolic and 17α-substituted steroids and those drugs producing a cholestatic hepatitis: chief among these are the phenothiazines.

Distinction between viral hepatitis and drug hepatitis can be extremely difficult and sometimes impossible.[4] Points in favour of a drug-induced hepatitis are the more sharply circumscribed focal or even zonal distribution of the hepatocellular degenerative changes, fatty change in hepatocytes and minimal reactive mesenchymal and inflammatory changes away from the degenerate hepatocytes.

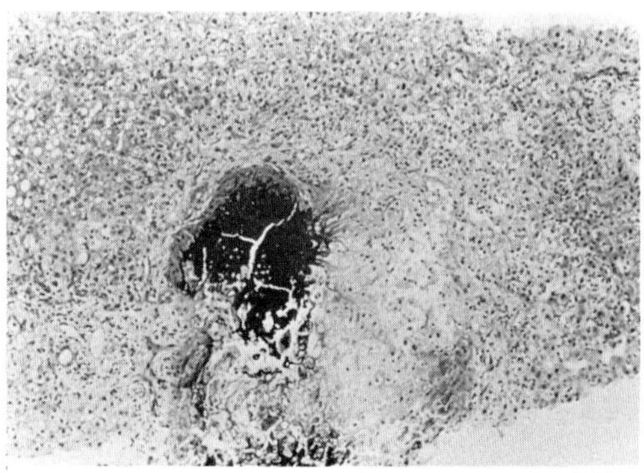

Figure 18.15. Bile infarct: a lake of extracellular bile within the lobule surrounded by a pale zone of histiocytes and degenerate hepatocytes. Haematoxylin and eosin ×20.

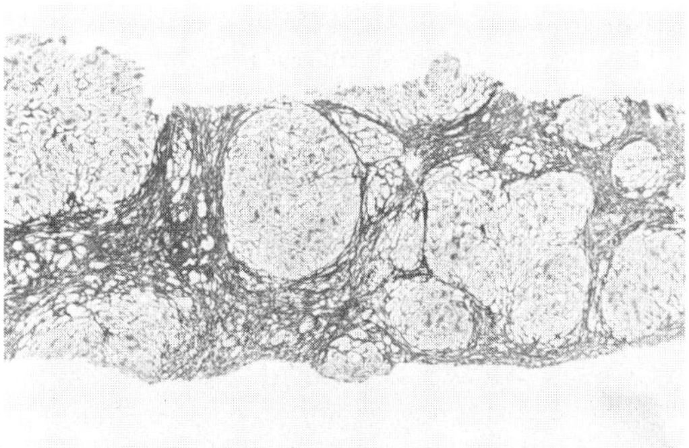

Figure 18.16. Micronodular cirrhosis. Numerous tiny nodules are identified within a needle biopsy × 10.

Cirrhosis

This is considered in Chapter 30. The value of needle biopsy varies with the type of needle and the technique employed. Cutting needles such as Vim-Silverman and Trucut are not deflected by the connective tissue and so are more accurate. Blunt needles such as the Menghini needle core out the softer parenchyma and slide along connective tissue bands. Cirrhosis may then be underdiagnosed.[59]

Generally a micronodular cirrhosis (Figure 18.16) shows uniformity throughout the liver and is not affected by sampling. The most difficult problem is to establish when, for instance, severe central hyaline sclerosis in an alcoholic is or is not an early micronodular cirrhosis. In a macronodular multilobular cirrhosis (Figures 18.4 and 18.17) with areas of apparently normal architecture, sampling error can be considerable and in the absence of obvious regenerative nodules diagnosis is difficult. The presence of slender bands of fibrous tissue (Figure 18.4), the abnormal cell plate patterns (Figure 18.6) and the excess of efferent veins are important features in these cases. In such cases there should also be an absence of lipofuscin around these efferent veins. Conversely, its presence suggests a lack of regeneration, infers an 'ageing' hepatocyte and indicates that the efferent vein is an anatomical central vein.

Focal Lesions

A significant proportion of the liver biopsies performed in routine clinical practice is for a tissue diagnosis in non-hepatic diseases that involve the liver. There may be diffuse involvement of the liver as in amyloidosis and malaria but focal lesions are more common. Consequently, considerable sampling error occurs and examination of multiple levels of the biopsy may be necessary. There is thus a conflict

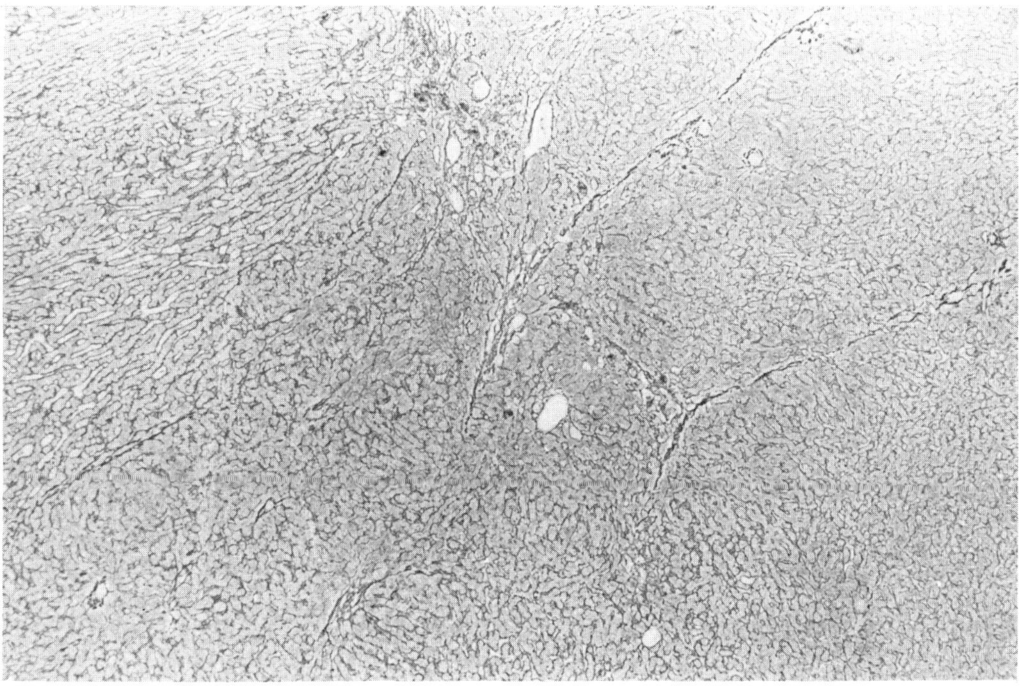

Figure 18.17. A macronodular multilobular cirrhosis showing very slender bands of fibrous tissue, an excess of efferent veins and an abnormal cell plate pattern × 20.

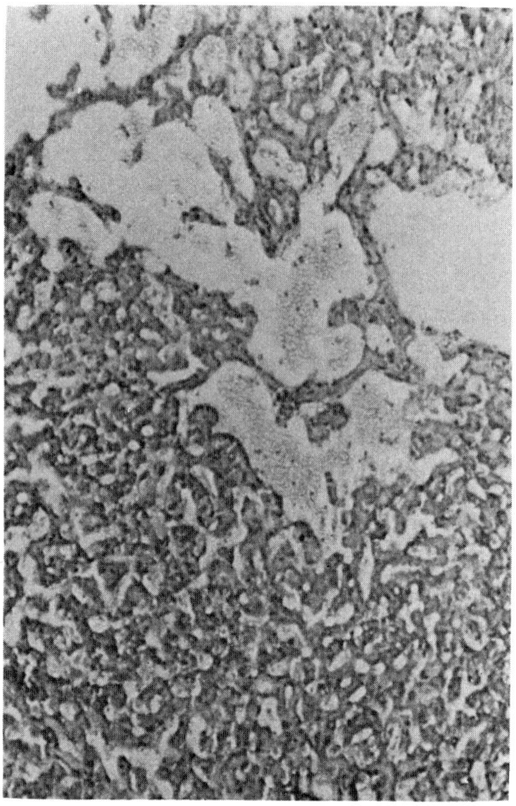

Figure 18.18. Focal sinusoidal ectasia: sudden widening of the sinusoids with associated atrophy of hepatocytes. Haematoxylin and eosin ×250.

between the examination of biopsies for focal lesions and the need for retention of tissue for additional diagnostic techniques such as the search for organisms in tuberculosis or the immunoperoxidase method for viruses, proteins or other antigens.

The accurate identification of focal lesions when present is usually simple: metastatic liver disease rarely presents diagnostic problems except for identification of its origin and most difficulty arises with the leukaemic and lymphomatous infiltrates (see Chapter 39). Likewise, epithelioid granulomas are not difficult to identify but their aetiology can rarely be determined from the morphology. Many causes have been described (see Chapter 37) but the most common in the UK are sarcoidosis, sarcoidal reaction to tumour, tuberculosis, drug reactions and primary biliary cirrhosis. Despite this a significant proportion remains undiagnosed.

Sometimes secondary changes related to a focal lesion may be identified. The presence of neutrophils around proliferating bile ductules in some but not all portal tracts suggests a focal intrahepatic lesion involving a branch of the biliary tree. Focal sinusoidal ectasia may be identified where sinusoids in one area are dilated and hepatocytes are small and atrophic (Figure 18.18). This feature has various associations such as severe wasting illness, drugs, cirrhosis and vascular disturbances but is also seen sometimes around metastases. Its architectural localization may indicate a particular association, such as the periportal ectasia described with the contraceptive pill.[72] The centrilobular sinusoidal dilatation from heart failure is similar but identified by its regular distribution and even appearance. When focal sinusoidal ectasia is the only abnormality in a biopsy, particularly when metastatic liver disease is suspected clinically, multiple levels through the specimen must be examined for microscopic deposits of tumour in portal tract or sinusoids.

Focal lesions may also be primary within the liver. Apart from hepatoma, adenoma and focal nodular hyperplasia, small microhamartomas of the biliary tree (von Meyenburg complexes) may also be found. They are most commonly an incidental finding and bear no relationship to other hepatic changes but they may be associated with congenital hepatic fibrosis,[26] even in adults,[9, 39] and polycystic liver.[41]

PROGNOSTIC FEATURES

Making a specific diagnosis inevitably implies a prognosis for the patient but occasionally additional features in the biopsy may indicate the further natural history of the disease more clearly. This has been most intensively investigated and debated in acute viral hepatitis where such features as bridging hepatic necrosis (Figure 18.19), excessive numbers of plasma cells, bile duct lesions, piecemeal necrosis, impaired hepatocyte regeneration and the presence of complement in hepatocytes have all been incriminated (see Chapter 28).

Similarly prognostic features may be found in other conditions. In alcoholics the presence of centrilobular fibrosis is a bad prognostic sign indicating inevitable progression to cirrhosis if drinking continues[70] (Figure 18.20), and in alpha-1-antitrypsin deficiency the absence of bile ducts within a child's liver biopsy may be a favourable feature.[19]

A slightly different use is to predict the outcome of a portoenterostomy performed for extrahepatic biliary atresia. Here a core of tissue

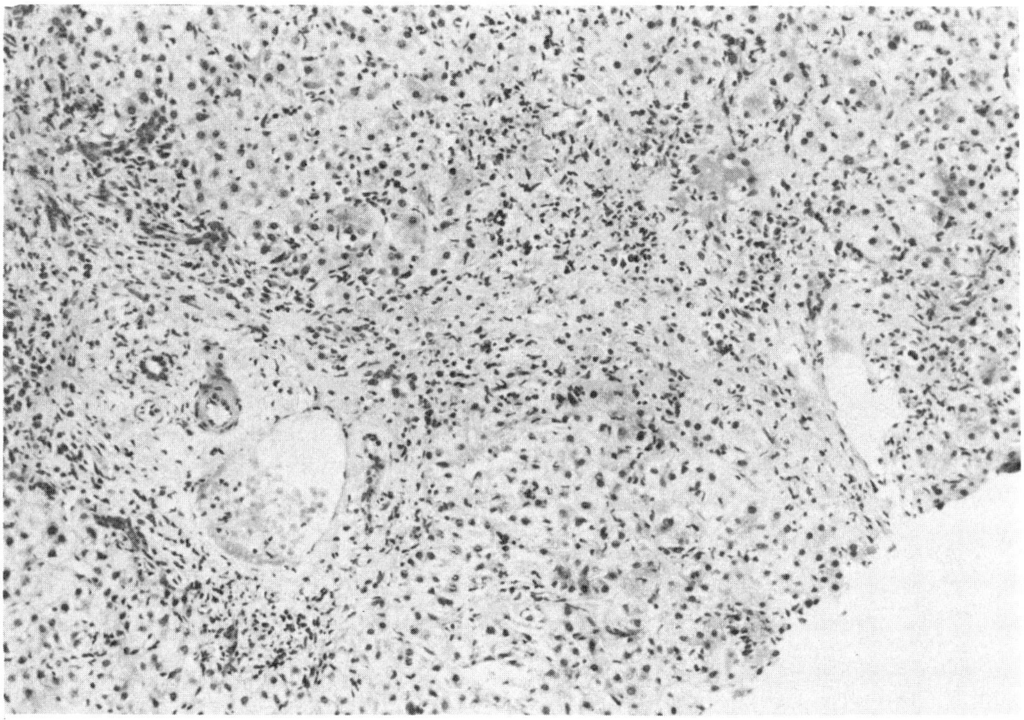

Figure 18.19. Bridging hepatic necrosis in acute viral hepatitis. The portal tract (left) and central vein (right) are bridged by a zone of collapsed reticulin. Haematoxylin and eosin × 250.

is removed from the porta hepatis and a loop of bowel anastomosed to the raw surface of the liver. The presence of tiny bile ductules within this excised core indicates an increased chance of successful bile drainage.[25]

RESPONSE TO THERAPY

The restricted use of liver biopsy for assessing the results of therapy reflects as much the limited range of therapeutic manoeuvres available in liver disease as the sampling error and consequent variation that occur in biopsy material. The most obvious use is to assess the reduction in iron (or copper) overload in response to venesection or chelation therapy. Iron in particular can be assessed in a semi-quantitative fashion by histochemical techniques and shows a reasonable correlation with liver iron measured biochemically.[12] The effects of venesection can then be accurately followed and treatment suspended when demonstrable iron is grade I or less, although continual reassessment may be necessary (see Chapter 34).

The biopsy is also used to assess the effects of steroid therapy in chronic active hepatitis. Piecemeal necrosis, particularly its lymphocytic component, sometimes subsides dramatically on steroid therapy. Unfortunately, any reduction in activity may simply reflect the geographical variation of activity within the liver that is a feature of this disease and consequently a misleading impression of therapeutic response may be obtained. Nevertheless, by so employing liver biopsy, workers at the Mayo Clinic assessed the relative merits of steroids and azathioprine and found a combination of the two to be most effective.[2]

It can be used to follow the consequences of a portoenterostomy performed for extrahepatic biliary atresia. In such a patient recently there was initial clinical improvement. A follow-up liver biopsy three months later demonstrated continuing bile duct obstruction and at subsequent re-exploration a mass of clot and mucin within the enterostomy was removed. A further biopsy has demonstrated a dramatic decrease in activity although considerable scarring is now present.

Liver biopsy is used to anticipate the complications of methotrexate therapy for

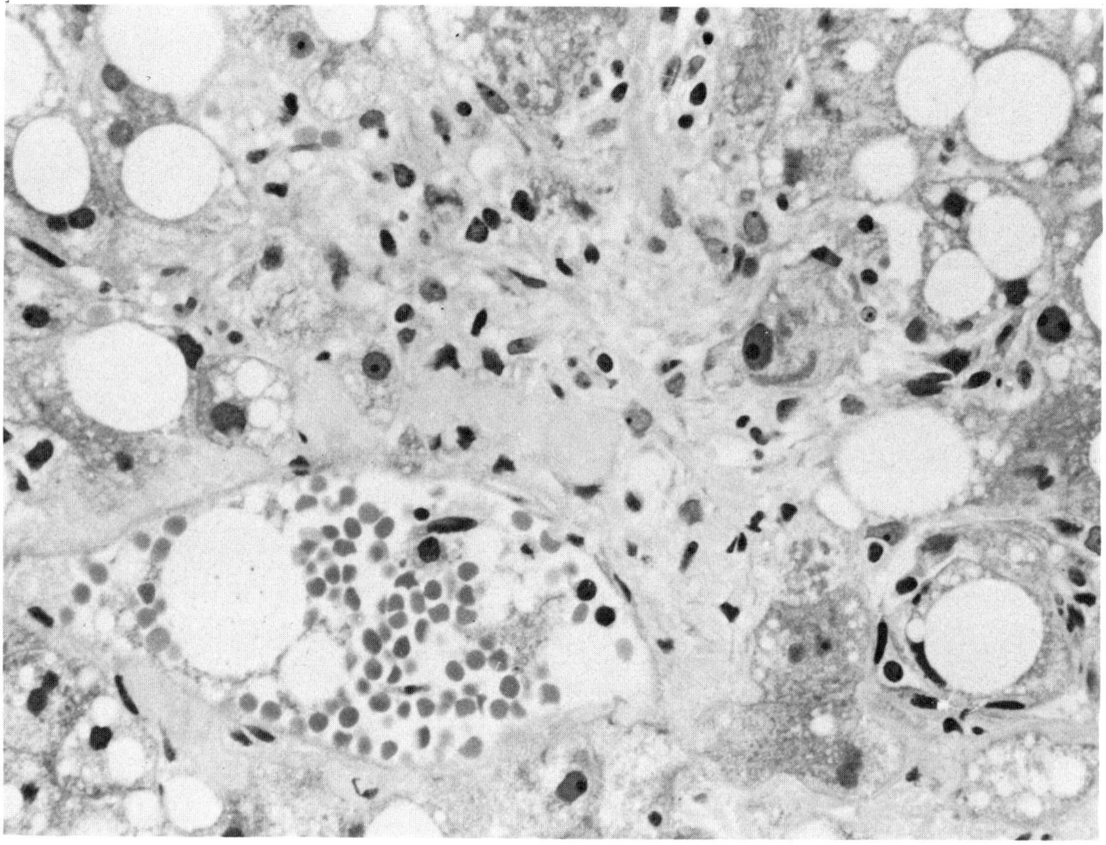

Figure 18.20. Alcoholic liver disease. The central vein is surrounded by dense fibrous tissue which is also extending into adjacent sinusoids. Hepatocytes show fatty change and some also contain Mallory bodies. Haematoxylin and eosin × 1200.

psoriasis. Prolonged administration of methotrexate, particularly orally, can result in cirrhosis.[44] The development of the cirrhosis cannot be predicted by clinical features or liver function tests. Consequently, if this therapy is employed regular liver biopsy is mandatory.

REFERENCES

1. Alagille, D., Odièvre, M., Gautier, M. & Domergues, J.P. (1975) Hepatic ductular hypoplasia associated with characteristic facies, vertebral malformations, retarded physical, mental and skeletal development and cardiac murmur. *Journal of Pediatrics*, **86**, 63–71.
2. Baggenstoss, A.H., Soloway, R.D., Summerskill, W.H.J., Elveback, L.R. & Schoenfield, L.J. (1972) Chronic active liver disease. The range of histologic lesions, their response to treatment and evolution. *Human Pathology*, **3**, 183–198.
3. Barry, M. & Sherlock, S. (1971) Measurement of liver-iron concentration in needle biopsy specimens. *Lancet*, **i**, 100–103.
4. Bianchi, L., De Groote, J., Desmet, V.J., Gedigk, P., Korb, G., Popper, H., Poulsen, H., Scheuer, P.J., Schmid, M., Thaler, H. & Wepler, W. (1974) Guidelines for diagnosis of therapeutic drug induced liver injury in liver biopsies. Review by an international group. *Lancet*, **i**, 854–857.
5. Burns, J. (1970) Preparation of thin epoxy resin sections from thick sections of paraffin-embedded material. *Journal of Clinical Pathology*, **23**, 643–645.
6. Chiprut, R.O., Greenwald, R.A., Morris, S.J., Zeppa, R. & Schiff, E.R. (1978) Intrahepatic hematoma resulting in obstructive jaundice. *Gastroenterology*, **74**, 124–127.
7. Christoffersen, P. & Poulsen, H. (1970) Histological changes in human liver biopsies following extrahepatic biliary obstruction. *Acta Pathologica et Microbiologica Scandinavica* (Suppl.) **212**, 150–157.
8. Cohen, J.A. & Kaplan, M.M. (1978) Left-sided heart failure presenting as hepatitis. *Gastroenterology*, **74**, 583–587.
9. Daroca, P.J., Tuthill, R. & Reed, R.J. (1975) Cholangiocarcinoma arising in congenital hepatic fibrosis. *Archives of Pathology*, **99**, 592–595.
10. da Silva Horta, J., Abbatt, J.D., da Motta, L.C. & Roriz, M.L. (1965) Malignancy and other late effects following administration of Thoratrast. *Lancet*, **ii**, 201–205.

11. Desmet, V.J., Bullens, A.M., De Groote, J. & Heirwegh, K.P.M. (1968) A new diazo reagent for specific staining of conjugated bilirubin in tissue sections. *Journal of Histochemistry and Cytochemistry*, **16,** 419–427.
12. Edwards, C.Q., Carroll, M., Bray, P. & Cartwright, G.E. (1977) Hereditary haemochromatosis. Diagnosis in siblings and children. *New England Journal of Medicine*, **297,** 7–13.
13. Gallison, D.T.Jr & Skinner, D. (1950) Bile peritonitis complicating needle biopsy of liver. *New England Journal of Medicine*, **243,** 47–50.
14. Gerber, A.M., Orr, W., Denk, H., Schaffner, F. & Popper, H. (1973) Hepatocellular hyalin in cholestasis and cirrhosis: its diagnostic significance. *Gastroenterology*, **64,** 89–98.
15. Glauert, A.M. (1975) *Fixation Dehydration and Embedding of Biological Specimens.* Amsterdam: North-Holland Publishing Co.
16. Gordon, H. & Sweets, H.H.Jr (1936) Simple method for silver impregnation of reticulum. *American Journal of Pathology*, **12,** 545–552.
17. Grisham, J.W., Nopanitaya, W. & Compagno, J. (1976) Scanning electron microscopy of the liver: a review of methods and results. In *Progress in Liver Diseases* (Ed.) Popper, H. & Schaffner, F. Vol. V, pp. 1–23. New York: Grune & Stratton.
18. Gubetta, L., Rizzetto, M., Crivelli, O., Verme, G. & Aricò, S. (1977) A trichrome stain for the intrahepatic localisation of the hepatitis B surface antigen (HB_sAg). *Histopathology*, **1,** 277–288.
19. Hadchouel, M. & Gautier, M. (1976) Histopathologic study of the liver in the early cholestatic phase of αIAT deficiency. *Journal of Pediatrics*, **89,** 211–215.
20. Hong, R. & Schubert, W.K. (1960) Menghini needle biopsy of the liver. *American Journal of Diseases of Children*, **100,** 42–46.
21. Hopwood, D. (1969) Fixatives and fixation: a review. *Histochemical Journal*, **1,** 323–360.
22. Irons, R.D., Schenk, E.A. & Lee, J.C.K. (1977) Cytochemical methods for copper. Semiquantitative screening procedure for identification of abnormal copper levels in liver. *Archives of Pathology and Laboratory Medicine*, **101,** 298–301.
23. Iversen, P. & Roholm, K. (1939) On aspiration biopsy of the liver, with remarks on its diagnostic significance. *Acta Medica Scandinavica*, **102,** 1–16.
24. Johnstone, J.M. & Lee, E.G. (1976) A quantitative assessment of the structural changes in the rat's liver following obstruction of the common bile duct. *British Journal of Experimental Pathology*, **57,** 85–94.
25. Kasai, M., Watanabe, I. & Ohi, R. (1975) Follow-up studies of long-term survivors after portoenterostomy for 'non-correctable' biliary atresia. *Journal of Pediatric Surgery*, **10,** 173–182.
26. Kerr, D.N.S., Harrison, C.V., Sherlock, S. & Milnes-Walker, R. (1961) Congenital hepatic fibrosis. *Quarterly Journal of Medicine*, **30,** 91–117.
27. Knauer, C.M. (1978) Percutaneous biopsy of the liver as a procedure for outpatients. *Gastroenterology*, **74,** 101–102.
28. Krarup, N.B. (1949) Aspiration biopsy of the liver with special reference to the method of Iversen-Roholm. *Acta Medica Scandinavica* (Suppl.), **234,** 199–209.
29. Laurell, S. & Lundquist, A. (1971) Lipid composition of human liver biopsy specimens. *Acta Medica Scandinavica*, **189,** 65–68.
30. Lee, R.L. (1977) 2-hydroxyethyl methacrylate embedded tissue – a method complementary to routine paraffin embedding. *Medical Laboratory Sciences*, **34,** 231–239.
31. Leopold, J.G., Parry, T.E. & Storring, F.K. (1970) A change in the sinusoid trabecular structure of the liver with hepatic venous outflow block. *Journal of Pathology*, **100,** 87–98.
32. Levin, B., Dobbs, R.H., Burgess, A. & Palmer, T. (1969) Hyperammonaemia. A variant type of deficiency of liver ornithine transcarbamylase. *Archives of Disease in Childhood*, **44,** 162–169.
33. Lindner, H. (1967) Grenzen und Gefahren der perkutanen Leberbiopsie mit der Menghi-Ninadel. *Deutsch Medizinische Wochenschrift*, **92,** 1751–1757.
34. Lundquist, A. (1970) Liver biopsy with a needle of 0.7 mm outer diameter. *Acta Medica Scandinavica*, **188,** 471–474.
35. Lundvall, O. & Enerbäck, L. (1969) Hepatic fluorescence in porphyria cutanea tarda studied in fine needle aspiration biopsy smears. *Journal of Clinical Pathology*, **22,** 704–709.
36. Lyon, H. & Prento, P. (1973) Alcian blue-silver impregnation. A method differentiating between acid carbohydrates, reticulin fibres and collagen fibres. *Acta Pathologica et Microbiologica Scandinavica*, Section A, **81,** 6–8.
37. MacIver, A.G., Giddings, J., Mepham, B.L. (1979) Demonstration of extracellular immunoglobulins, complement components and fibrinogen/fibrin in formalin fixed paraffin sections of renal tissue using the trypsin-immunoperoxidase (PAP) technique. In preparation.
38. Madden, R.E. (1961) Complications of needle biopsy of the liver. *Archives of Surgery*, **83,** 788–781.
39. Manes, J.L., Kissane, J.M. & Valdes, A.J. (1977) Congenital hepatic fibrosis, liver cell carcinoma and adult polycystic kidneys. *Cancer*, **39,** 2619–2623.
40. McGill, D.B., Humphreys, S.R., Baggenstoss, A.H. & Dickson, E.R. (1972) Cirrhosis and death after jejunoileal shunt. *Gastroenterology*, **63,** 872–877.
41. Melnick, P.J. (1955) Polycystic liver. Analysis of seventy cases. *Archives of Pathology*, **59,** 162–172.
42. Menghini, G. (1958) One-second needle biopsy of the liver. *Gastroenterology*, **35,** (2), 190–199.
43. Millward-Sadler, G.H. & Giddings, J. (1978) Unpublished observations.
44. Millward-Sadler, G.H. & Ryan, T.J. (1974) Methotrexate induced liver disease in psoriasis. *British Journal of Dermatology*, **90,** 661–667.
45. Millward-Sadler, G.H., Giddings, J. & Mepham, B.L. (1979). In preparation.
46. Morris, J.S., Gallo, G.A., Scheuer, P.J. & Sherlock, S. (1975) Percutaneous liver biopsy in patients with large bile duct obstruction. *Gastroenterology*, **68,** 750–754.
47. Movitt, E.R. & Davis, A.E. (1954) Extrahepatic biliary obstruction: experience with needle biopsy of the liver. *Annals of Internal Medicine*, **40,** 952–962.
48. Nayak, N.C., Sagreiya, K. & Ramalingaswami, V. (1969) The nature and significance of cytoplasmic hyalin of hepatocytes. *Archives of Pathology*, **88,** 631–637.
49. Paradinas, F.J., Bull, T.B., Westaby, D. & Murray-Lyon, I.M. (1977) Hyperplasia and prolapse of hepatocytes into hepatic veins during long-term methyltestosterone therapy: possible relationships of these changes to the development of peliosis hepatis and liver tumours. *Histopathology*, **1,** 225–246.

50. Pearse, A.G.E. (1972) *Histochemistry*, 3rd ed. Edinburgh: Churchill Livingstone.
51. Perrault, J., McGill, D.B., Ott, B.J. & Taylor, W.F. (1978) Liver biopsy: complications in 1000 inpatients and outpatients. *Gastroenterology*, **74**, 103–106.
52. Poulsen, H. & Christoffersen, P. (1970) Histological changes in liver biopsies from patients with surgical bile duct disorders. *Acta Pathologica et Microbiologica Scandinavica*, Section A, **78**, 571–579.
53. Purow, E., Grosberg, S.J. & Wapnick, S. (1977) Menghini needle fracture after attempted liver biopsy. *Gastroenterology*, **73**, 1404–1405.
54. Raines, D.R., van Heertum, R.L. & Johnson, L.F. (1974) Intrahepatic hematoma: a complication of percutaneous liver biopsy. *Gastroenterology*, **67**, 284–289.
55. Rake, M.O., Murray-Lyon, I.M., Ansell, I.D. & Williams, R. (1969) Improved liver-biopsy needle. *Lancet*, **ii**, 1283.
56. Sabatini, D.D., Bensch, K. & Barrnett, R.J. (1963) Cytochemistry and electron microscopy. The preservation of cellular ultrastructure and enzymatic activity by aldehyde fixation. *Journal of Cell Biology*, **17**, 19–58.
57. Salaspuro, M. & Sipponen, P. (1976) Demonstration of an intracellular copper binding protein by orcein staining in long-standing cholestatic liver disease. *Gut*, **17**, 787–790.
58. Schaffner, F., Sternlieb, I., Barka, T. & Popper, H. (1962) Hepatocellular changes in Wilson's disease. Histochemical and electron microscopic studies. *American Journal of Pathology*, **41**, 315–328.
59. Scheuer, P.J. (1970) Liver biopsy in the diagnosis of cirrhosis. *Gut*, **11**, 275–278.
60. Scheuer, P.J., Williams, R. & Muir, A.R. (1962) Hepatic pathology in relatives of patients with haemochromatosis. *Journal of Pathology and Bacteriology*, **84**, 53–64.
61. Seymour, C.A. & Peters, T.J. (1977) Enzyme activities in human liver biopsies: assay methods and activities of some lysosomal and membrane-bound enzymes in control tissue and serum. *Clinical Science and Molecular Medicine*, **52**, 229–239.
62. Seymour, C., Neale, G. & Peters, T.J. (1977) Lysosomal changes in liver tissue from patients with the Dubin–Johnson–Sprinz syndrome. *Clinical Science and Molecular Medicine*, **52**, 241–248.
63. Sherlock, S. (1951) The liver in heart failure: relation of anatomical, functional and circulatory changes. *British Heart Journal*, **13**, 273–293.
64. Shikata, T., Uzawa, T., Yoshiwara, N., Akatsuka, T. & Yamazaki, S. (1974) Staining methods of Australia antigen in paraffin section. *Japanese Journal of Experimental Medicine*, **44**, 25–36.
65. Sipponen, P. (1976) Orcein positive hepatocellular material in long-standing biliary diseases. I. Histochemical characteristics. *Scandinavian Journal of Gastroenterology*, **11**, 545–552.
66. Snapper, I. (1951) In (Ed.) Rappaport, E.M. Liver biopsy, *Review of Gastroenterology*, **18**, 649–650.
67. Spellberg, M.A. & Bermudez, F. (1977) Value and safety of percutaneous liver biopsy in obstructive jaundice. *American Journal of Gastroenterology*, **67**, 444–448.
68. Terry, R. (1952) Risks of needle biopsy of the liver. *British Medical Journal*, **i**, 1102–1105.
69. Triger, D.R., Millward-Sadler, G.H., Czaykowski, A.A., Trowell, T. & Wright, R. (1976) Alpha-1-antitrypsin deficiency and liver disease in adults. *Quarterly Journal of Medicine*, **45**, 51–72.
70. Van Waes, L. & Lieber, C.S. (1977) Early perivenular sclerosis in alcoholic fatty liver: an index of progressive liver injury. *Gastroenterology*, **73**, 646–650.
71. Wagner, R., Huijing, F. & Porter, E. (1971) Hepatic gluconeogenesis due to phosphorylase deficiency. Limitations of enzyme studies on liver biopsy specimens. *American Journal of Medicine*, **51**, 685–691.
72. Winkler, K. & Poulsen, H. (1975) Liver disease with periportal sinusoidal dilatation. A possible complication to contraceptive steroids. *Scandinavian Journal of Gastroenterology*, **10**, 699–704.
73. Woolling, K.R., Baggenstoss, A.H. & Weir, J.F. (1951) Infarcts of liver. *Gastroenterology*, **17**, 479–493.
74. Zamcheck, N. & Klausenstock, O. (1953) Liver biopsy (concluded). II. The risk of needle biopsy. *New England Journal of Medicine*, **249**, 1062–1069.
75. Zuckerman, A.J. (1970) In *Virus Diseases of the Liver*. London: Butterworths.

Chapter 19

Some Aspects of Ultrastructural Pathology

A.M. JEZEQUEL

In the past 15 years much has been learned about the liver response to injury and the significance of some elementary alterations has begun to emerge. A great part of our information comes from experimental studies but a body of knowledge has also been obtained through studies on human material. This chapter will cover mainly the latter and will focus on some areas which have aroused a special interest in recent years. Specific pathological situations are considered in other chapters. For more extensive reviews, the reader is referred to the papers by Jezequel and Orlandi,[36] Trump, Dees and Shelburne,[85] Schaffner[72] and Schaffner and Popper.[73]

The most conspicuous alteration of the single hepatocyte is the shrinkage necrosis, in which the cell loses all relationship with the neighbouring hepatocytes and tends to become round in shape, with smooth contours and disappearance of microvilli. The cytoplasm is electron dense, deprived of glycogen, and the usual organization of cytoplasmic organelles is lost. However, stacks of rough endoplasmic reticulum, mitochondria and lysosomes retain their structural features. The nucleus becomes pyknotic with increased density of the chromatin and is later expelled from the cellular body. The denaturation of cytoplasmic proteins with an increased affinity for eosin leads to the formation of 'acidophilic' or 'eosinophilic' bodies seen under the light microscope. Such cell remnants can be seen free in the parenchyma, or engulfed in the cytoplasm of fixed or circulating macrophages. They are a usual feature during acute hepatitis, viral or drug-induced, and are known as Councilman-like bodies.[43] (Figure 19.1.) Other forms of necrosis can be observed, such as the necrosis following ischaemia associated with prominent mitochondrial swelling and formation of intracytoplasmic vacuoles[2] or the feathery degeneration observed during cholestasis.[20,62] These represent gross alterations of the liver cell and are usually accompanied by the presence of an inflammatory reaction or an infiltration of the portal tracts, with or without collagen proliferation. But electron microscopic studies have shown that cellular alterations do not need to involve the whole hepatocyte. Although hepatic response to injury rarely produces specific structural changes, a pattern of response involving groups of organelles can be expected in a number of circumstances.

NUCLEUS

Except for gross alterations occurring in pyknosis and during the formation of Councilman-like bodies, ultrastructural alterations in liver cell nuclei are rarely observed in human pathology. Modifications in size and shape, with occasional cytoplasmic invaginations occur in tumour cells or in regenerating nodules but do not present characteristic features. Nuclear abnormalities, with enlarged nucleoli associated with proliferation of rough endoplasmic reticulum and formation of cytolysomes, are frequent in hereditary tyrosinaemia; the alterations are similar to those observed in experimental intoxication with ethionine.[74] Inclusions of viral origin are rarely observed in human liver. However, eosinophilic inclusions which

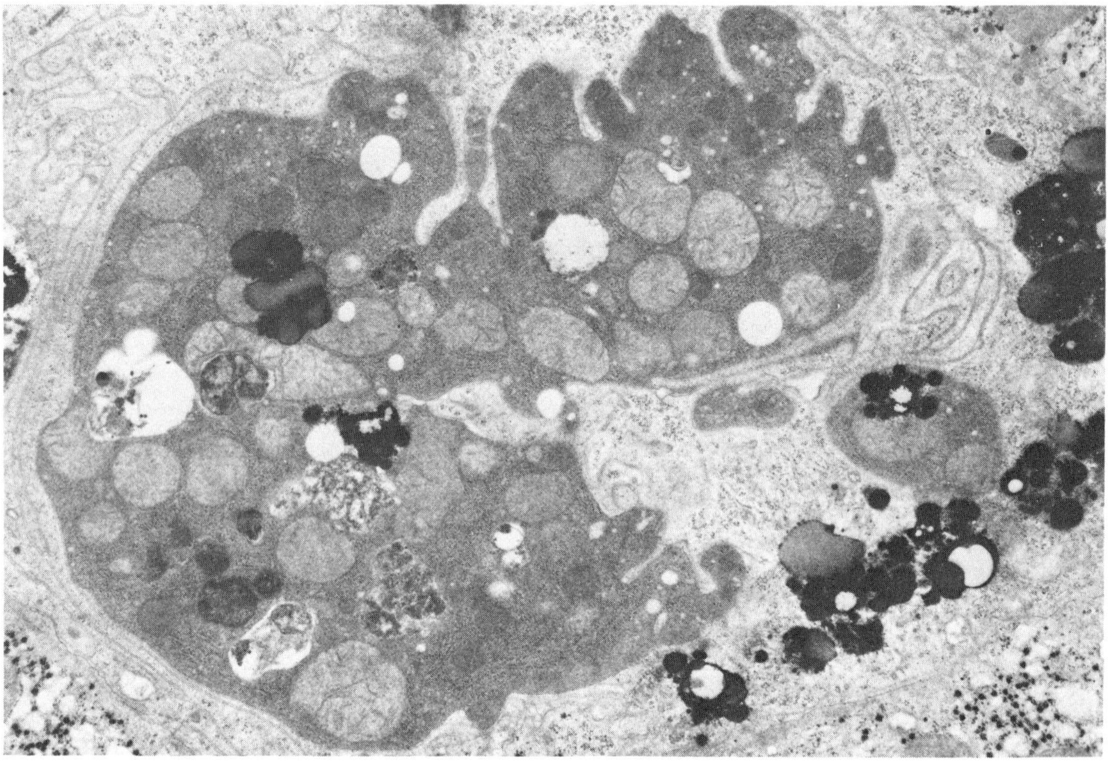

Figure 19.1. Councilman-like body in drug-induced hepatitis (chloramphenicol). Some components of hepatocytes, rough ER, mitochondria and lipofuscin granules, can be identified in the dense cytoplasm. No nucleus is visible in the plane of section. The cell remnants appear engulfed in a macrophage. × 9000.

give a 'sanded' appearance to the nuclei may be seen in chronic hepatitis B and are due to the presence of excess viral core material in the nucleoplasm.[5, 28, 29]

ENDOPLASMIC RETICULUM

Changes of the configuration of the endoplasmic reticulum are among the most prominent cytoplasmic alterations and are often the earliest changes observed in various experimental situations in animals[40, 79] or after administration of a number of drugs in man.[35, 36] As mentioned previously (see Chapter 2) the endoplasmic reticulum is the site of synthesis and action of some enzymes of the drug-metabolizing system. These enzymes are responsible for the transformation of some compounds into inactive or active metabolites. Among the mechanisms leading to cell necrosis, a great importance has been given to the covalent, irreversible binding of metabolites with cytoplasmic proteins.[54] However, covalent binding may occur during the metabolism of various substances and is not necessarily a harmful process.[64] At the moment the 'point of no return' of cellular alterations remains unknown.

A conspicuous increase of the smooth endoplasmic reticulum in hepatocytes may follow the administration of some drugs and has been extensively studied especially after administration of phenobarbitone in animals. The increase of smooth membranes is accompanied by an increase of drug-metabolizing enzymes[65] and morphometric studies show that in the rat there is an early and short-lived increase of the membranes of the rough endoplasmic reticulum which returns to normal values by the fifth day of treatment, whereas the smooth membranes continue to increase. The increase of the smooth endoplasmic reticulum is positively correlated with the increase of drug-metabolizing enzymes such as cytochrome P-450.[76] However, an increase of smooth membranes is not specifically correlated with enzyme induction. Several substances produce the same response as phenobarbitone;[11] others stimulate a more limited number of pathways and like

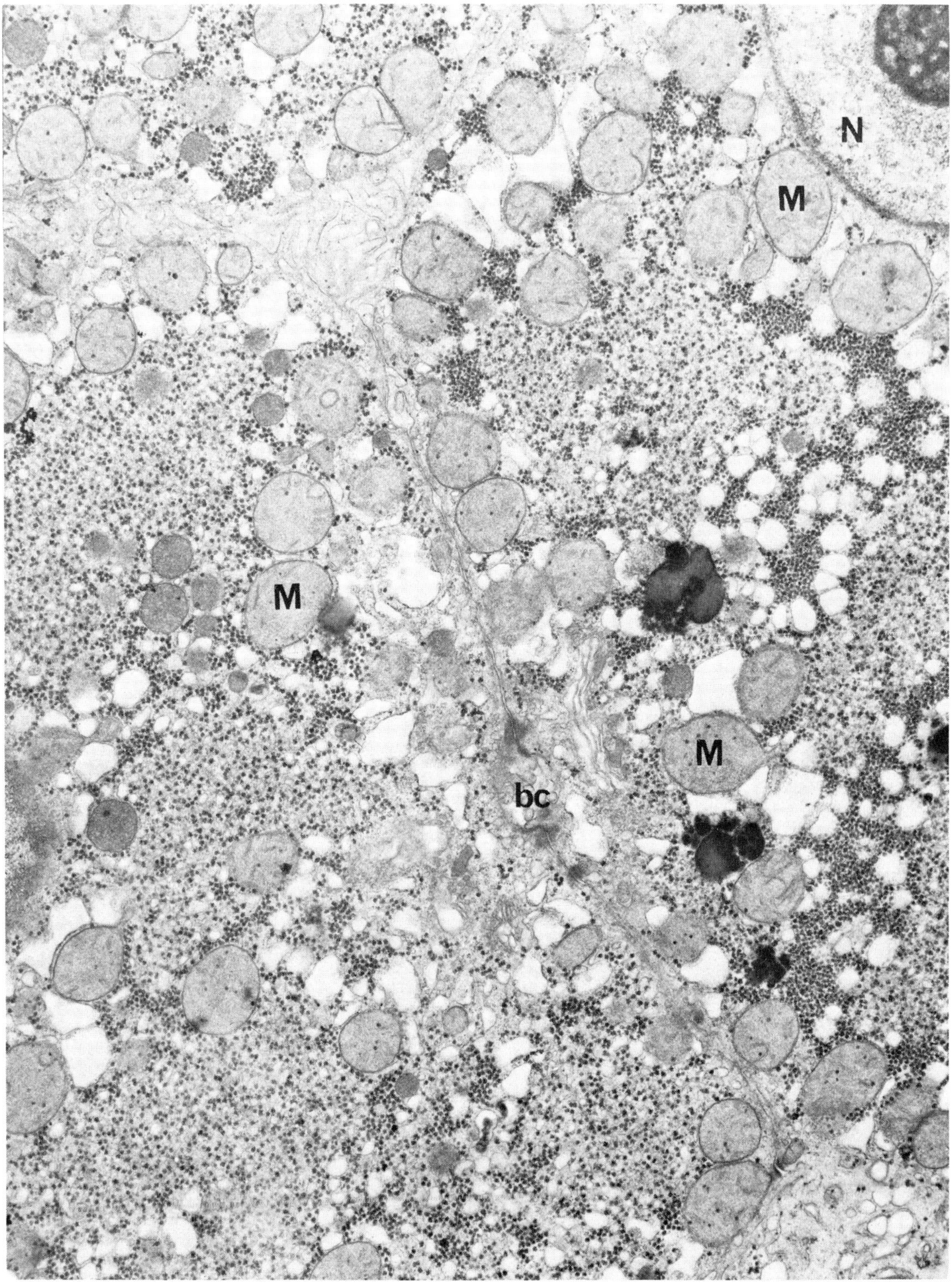

Figure 19.2. Low-power view of hepatic parenchyma in a patient under long-term anticonvulsant therapy. In the three hepatocytes present in the field, the smooth endoplasmic reticulum is prominent and the other cell components appear normal. N = nucleus; bc = bile canaliculus; M = mitochondria. × 11 250.

3-methylcholanthrene may lead to an increase of a variant of cytochrome P-450 (P-448) without quantitative changes of smooth membranes.[16] On the other hand, an increase of smooth membranes may not be accompanied by changes in microsomal enzyme activity, as observed in D-galactosamine-induced hepatitis.[49]

In man, changes in the distribution or amount of the endoplasmic reticulum have often been described, but the evaluation of such changes has often been hampered by the lack of baseline data. As previously mentioned (see Chapter 2) the human hepatocytes contain a relatively large amount of smooth endoplasmic reticulum which makes it likely that some images of 'increased' smooth membranes in humans should be interpreted with caution. Quantitative studies have shown, for instance, that an increase in smooth membranes does occur in the hepatocytes of patients under treatment with drugs inducing microsomal drug-metabolizing enzymes. This was especially evident in patients undergoing long-term anticonvulsant therapy (Figures 19.2 and 19.3) where an eightfold increase of smooth endoplasmic reticulum was measured.[39] A discrete increase also occurred in a patient with Crigler–Najjar type II syndrome treated with phenytoin.[47] The pattern of proliferation of the smooth endoplasmic reticulum in man is somewhat different from the pattern observed in rat and at low magnification it assumes the 'pepper and salt' appearance first described in patients under therapy with rifampicin[38] and due to the formation of scattered foci of densely packed smooth membranes.

A proliferation of the smooth endoplasmic reticulum has been described following the administration of ethanol in rat and in man, together with an increase of various drug-metabolizing enzymes,[52, 70] but this aspect remains controversial. Quantitative studies have suggested that a degranulation of the rough endoplasmic reticulum may occur.[57] Others have found an inconstant increase[48] or even a true decrease of the smooth reticulum.[14] The discrepancies may lie in the experimental procedure itself, inter-species variations, lack of a standardized diet or difficulties in recognizing intralobular variations.

An increase of the endoplasmic reticulum

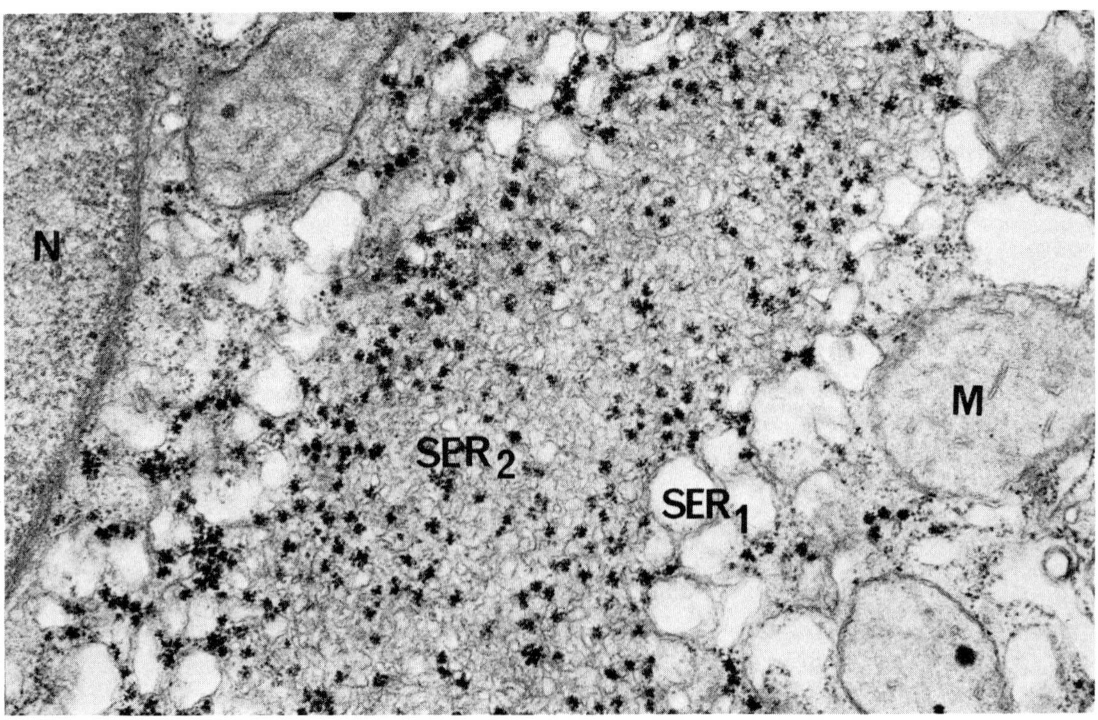

Figure 19.3. Same patient as in Figure 19.1. Part of a hepatocyte shows large clumps of densely packed smooth membranes (SER_2) next to vesicles with a wide lumen (SER_1). The respective increase of each component was eightfold and threefold as measured by quantitative morphometry.[39] M = mitochondria. × 30 000.

may also be related to an altered turnover of membranous components, due to interactions with a drug or its metabolites. Many examples have been reported in experimental conditions. In man, a similar phenomenon may occur in drug-induced phospholipidosis,[12, 33] or in the alcoholic hepatitis-like reaction following therapy with perhexiline maleate.[4] According to a hypothesis recently suggested by studies on perfused rat liver, the cholestasis induced by chlorpromazine (CPZ) could also be due to a binding of CPZ to membrane phospholipids with consequent widespread alterations of membrane properties.[27]

A peculiar alteration of the endoplasmic reticulum may be observed in the hepatocytes of subjects with HB_sAg positive hepatitis (Figure 19.4), giving rise to the 'ground-glass' appearance of liver cells under the light microscope. This aspect is due to the formation of a rich network of cisternae of the smooth reticulum which contain rod-like structures showing in cross-section as tubules about 35nm in diameter, and occasionally containing a small core. These elements are thought to represent excess formation of viral protein coat.[28,29,30,60,77] This structural change can be estimated at the level of the light microscope with special staining[75] but the incidence of altered hepatocytes is highly variable and has not been correlated with any feature of the disease. Hepatocytes showing eosinophilic cytoplasm with a rim of basophilic material may be observed after steroid administration (Figure 19.5), due to the increased amount of smooth endoplasmic reticulum and the crowding of mitochondria and rough endoplasmic reticulum along the nuclear and the peripheral cell membrane.[56] 'Ground-glass' hepatocytes may be seen in other situations where an increase of the smooth reticulum occurs, such as following the administration of barbiturates or other microsomal enzyme inducers. In these cases, intracisternal rods are not present and special staining is negative.[60,84,91]

Changes of the endoplasmic reticulum are a prominent feature in subjects with alpha-1-antitrypsin deficiency whether they are homozygotes or heterozygotes. In these patients, hepatocytes contain globules of PAS-positive, diastase-resistant material, which is moderately electron dense, shows a finely granular structure and is contained within enlarged cisternae. The inclusion bodies have been localized both in the rough and in the smooth endoplasmic reticulum[15,93] and have been shown to contain asialo α-1-antitrypsin.[34] Despite prominent morphological alterations of the endoplasmic reticulum in these patients, the hepatic microsomal enzymes involved in aminopyrine demethylation are not impaired.[51]

MITOCHONDRIA

Apparent swelling of mitochondria or 'bizarre' shapes are not necessarily evidence of degenerative changes but may reflect an adaptive phenomenon as suggested after administration of cortisone.[88] In these conditions the increase in volume density of mitochondria is accompanied by a numerical decrease so that the total volume per cell remains constant. In man, megamitochondria, often containing crystalloid material, occur in a number of circumstances[78] and appear especially prominent in alcoholics.[50, 69] It is well established that megamitochondria and alcoholic hyalin are distinct entities.[32] Enlarged mitochondria with an expanded matrix are present in nearly all hepatocytes in Reyes's syndrome at the onset of the illness and return to normal during recovery[31, 58] but no changes are 'characteristic' as claimed by some workers. Swelling and pleomorphism of mitochondria also occur when thyroid function is altered.[45] Although various hypotheses have been proposed, the nature of these alterations is not understood at the moment. In intra- or extrahepatic cholestasis, changes in the conformation of cristae with images of 'curling' are frequently observed.[13,61] (Figure 19.6.) Morphometric studies have shown that this configurational change is associated with an increase in the surface density of mitochondrial cristae.[9] The significance of this alteration is not known but it is of interest that similar qualitative and quantitative changes have been observed in patients with uncomplicated cholelithiasis, i.e. in the absence of jaundice.[46] This suggests that disturbances in bile salts and cholesterol metabolism may be responsible for changes in the molecular structure and consequently in enzymatic properties of mitochondrial membranes.

Much emphasis has been placed on mitochondrial changes during halothane hepatitis, with variations in size and shape of mitochondria or breaks in the outer envelope,[44, 86] which could help in differentiating between acute viral hepatitis and unexplained postoperative hepatitis. However, the presence of specific features has not been confirmed by a recent survey on a large number of patients.[90] By a mechanism which appears to apply to a large

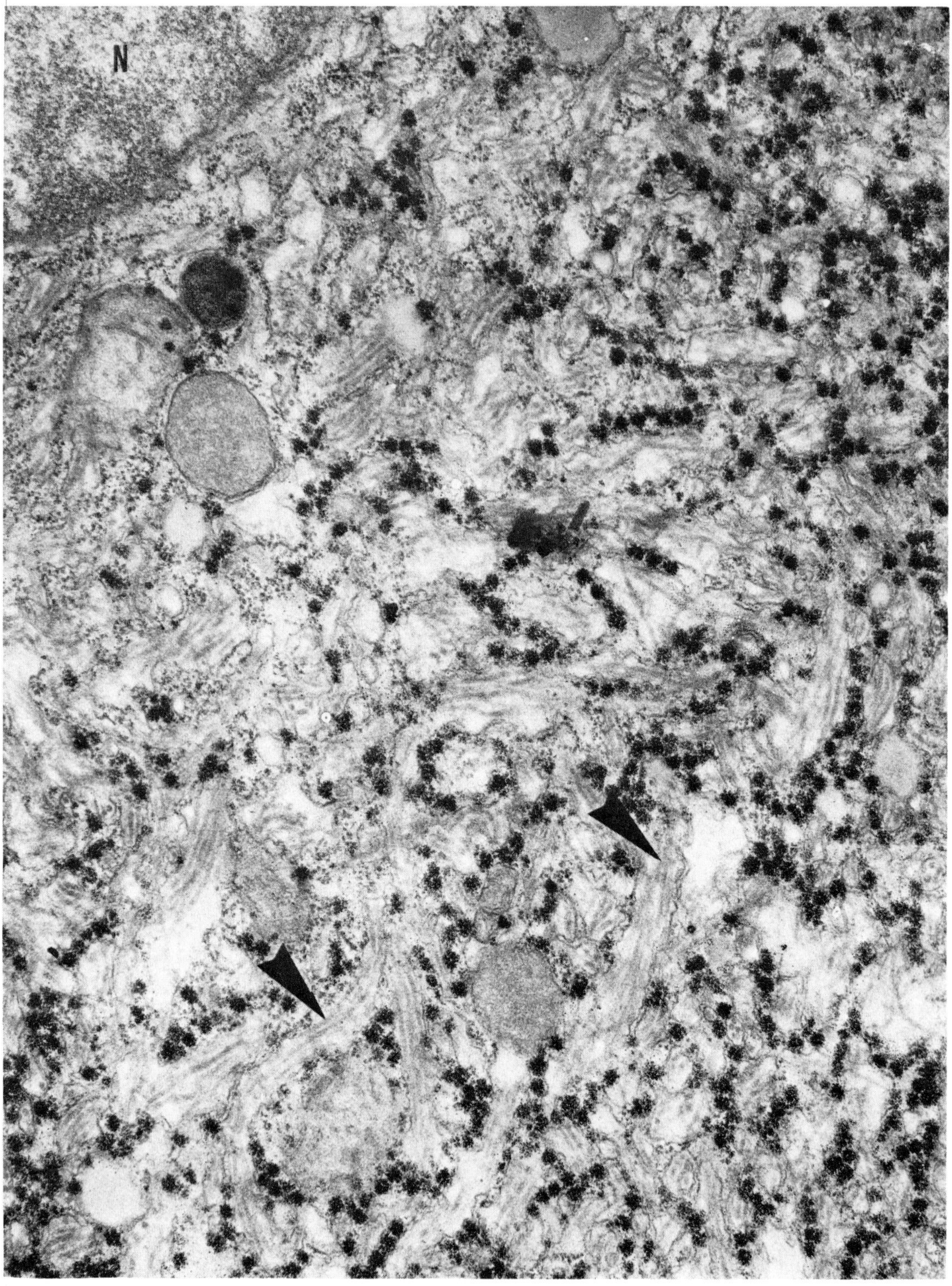

Figure 19.4. Part of the cytoplasm of a hepatocyte showing a disruption of the normal architecture of the cytoplasm. Numerous filamentous structures 35 nm in diameter (arrowheads) fill the cisternae of the endoplasmic reticulum and are seen in longitudinal, oblique or cross-sections. These filaments represent excess production of hepatitis B virus protein coat (HB_sAg). × 35 000.

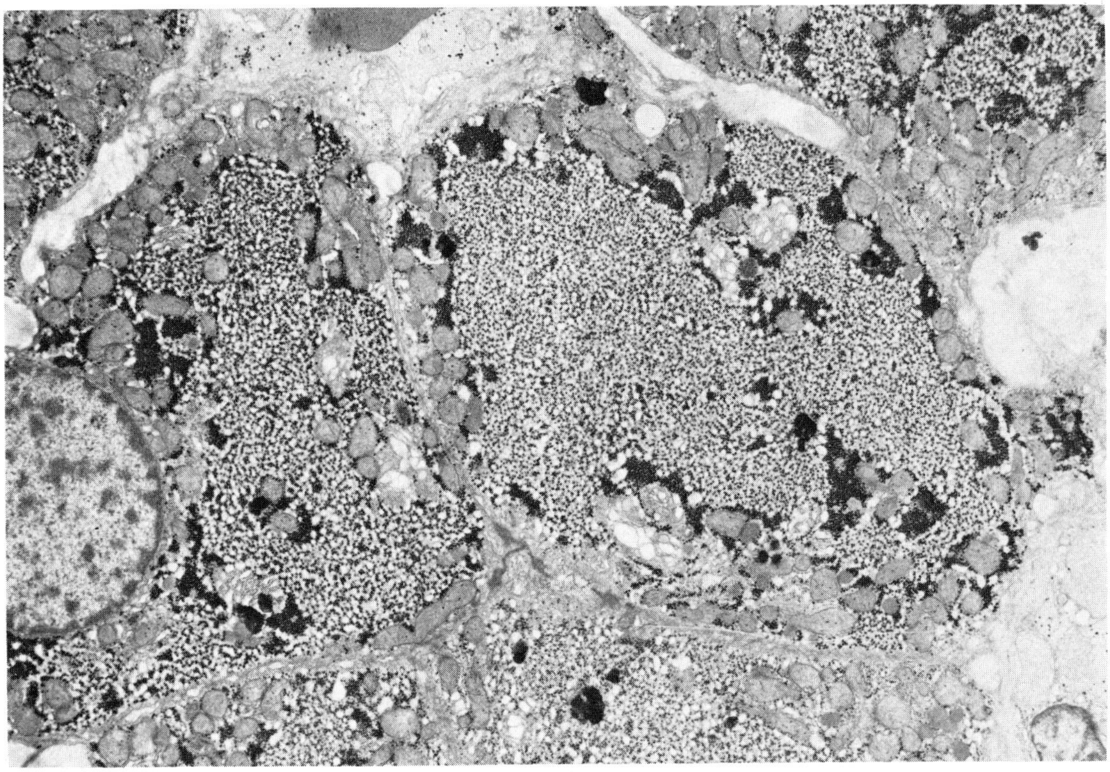

Figure 19.5. The picture illustrates the 'margination' of mitochondria in a group of hepatocytes of a patient receiving anabolic steroids. The smooth membranes occupy most of the cytoplasm while the mitochondria and rough endoplasmic reticulum are concentrated along the cell membrane and around the nucleus. × 6000.

number of compounds, it has been suggested that the toxic effects of halothane would be mediated through the binding of its metabolites with microsomal phospholipids, which could in turn trigger the formation of antigenic complexes.[10, 25]

Mitochondrial abnormalities, together with a variety of cytoplasmic alterations, are frequently observed in patients with Wilson's disease[80] and are being dealt with in Chapter 33.

PEROXISOMES

Changes in the number or structure of peroxisomes have been observed especially in experimental conditions. Until now, the proliferation of peroxisomes which occurs following administration of hypolipidaemic agents or unrelated substances to animals[24, 26, 63, 81] has not been reported in man. Only in patients under immunosuppressive therapy with

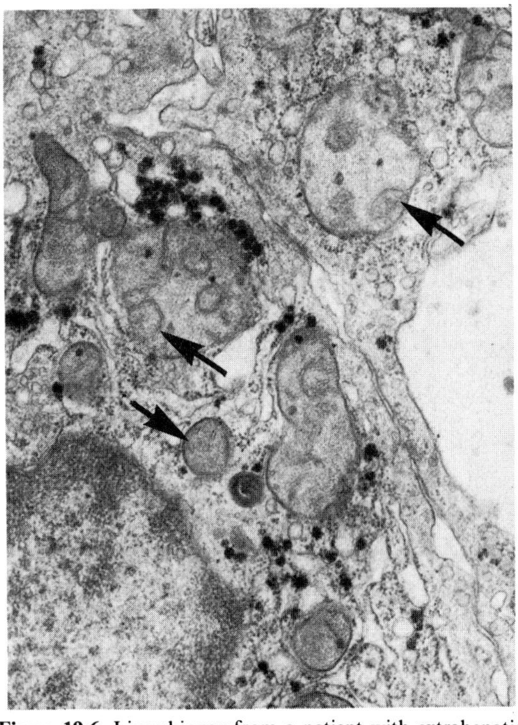

Figure 19.6. Liver biopsy from a patient with extrahepatic cholestasis showing curled or circular cristae in numerous mitochondria (arrows). × 17 500.

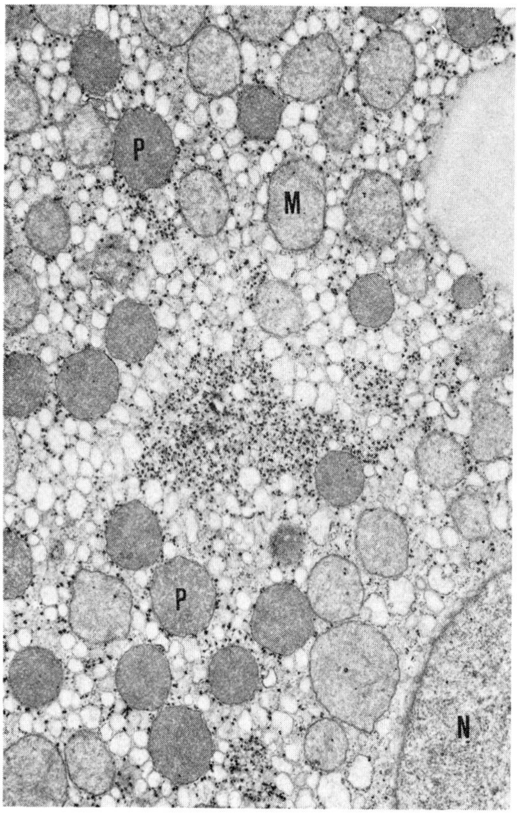

Figure 19.7. Increased number of peroxisomes (P) in a patient under therapy with 6-mercaptopurine. The ratio of peroxisomes to mitochondria is about 1:1. M = mitochondria; N = nucleus. × 10 500. From Jezequel,[35] with kind permission of Plenum Press.

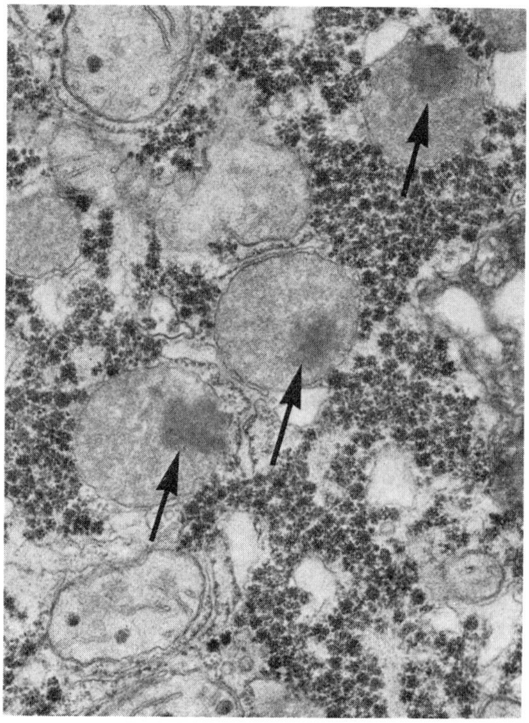

Figure 19.8. Part of a hepatocyte in a patient with extrahepatic cholestasis, showing numerous peroxisomes with an amorphous, core-like material (arrows). × 30 000.

6-mercaptopurine does there seem to be a numerical increase of peroxisomes.[35] (Figure 19.7.) The presence of an electron dense material in peroxisomes has been reported in cholestasis by various authors[13] and has also been observed in patients with cholelithiasis.[46] This core-like material is amorphous in appearance (Figure 19.8) and lacks the crystalloid configuration described in one case of benign recurrent cholestasis.[7] A variety of inclusions is occasionally observed in the peroxisomes in normal individuals (see Chapter 2).

LYSOSOMES AND RESIDUAL BODIES

As previously mentioned, cellular lysis does not need to involve the whole hepatocyte and the occurrence of focal cytoplasmic degradation (FCD) is not an uncommon phenomenon. In FCD, only a segment of the cell is affected, so that a defined area of the cytoplasm, containing a variety of organelles, becomes progressively surrounded by a membranous system arising from the endoplasmic reticulum, and is later entrapped into autophagic vacuoles or 'cytolysomes' (Figure 19.9). The products of complete or incomplete lysis will become part of the various 'residual bodies'. This may be part of a pathological or physiological process.[1,22,36,82] Apart from the process of autophagocytosis and the formation of cytolysomes, storage of various substances may occur at the level of lysosomes by temporary or permanent impairment of lysosomal enzymatic activity. Evidence of genetic alterations in the synthesis or activation of lysosomal enzymes has led to the concept of 'inborn lysosomal disease' which has been applied to some storage diseases, especially polysaccharidoses and lipidoses. In type II glycogenosis (Pompe's disease) glycogen in excess in the liver is deposited mainly as monoparticulate elements

(*Text continues on p. 449*)

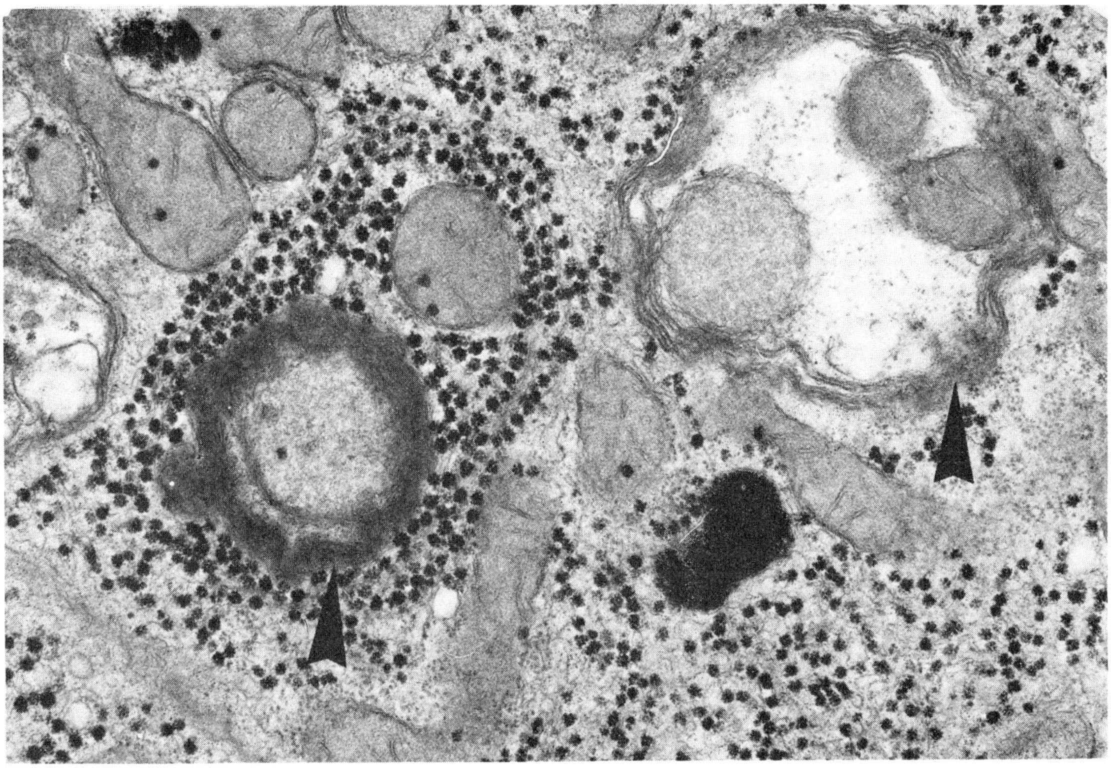

Figure 19.9. Part of a hepatocyte in a patient under treatment with 6-mercaptopurine. Cytolysosomes (arrowheads) are present and contain various cytoplasmic components surrounded by a multi-layered envelope. From Jezequel and Orlandi,[36] with kind permission of Academic Press, London. × 17 500.

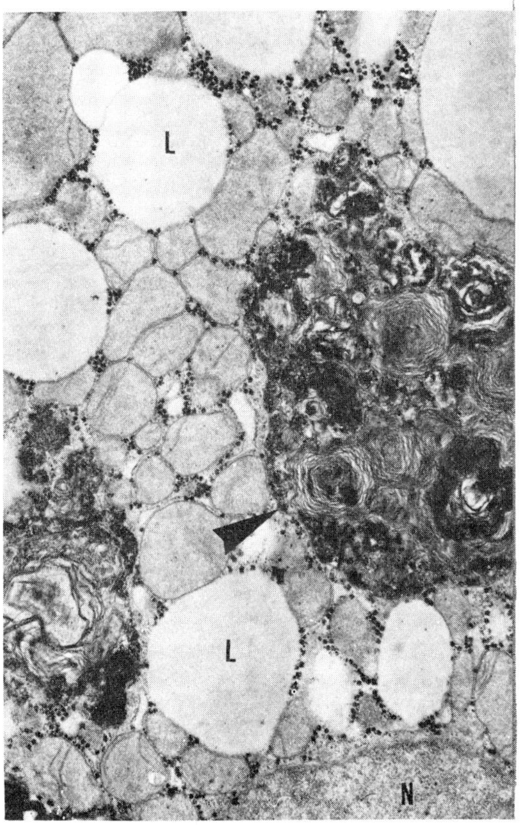

Figure 19.10. (Left) Part of a hepatocyte in a child with lipid storage disease. The cytoplasm contains numerous lipid droplets (L) of various sizes and large electron-dense bodies with a complex lamellar structure (arrowheads) presumably of lysosomal origin. N = nucleus. × 10 500.

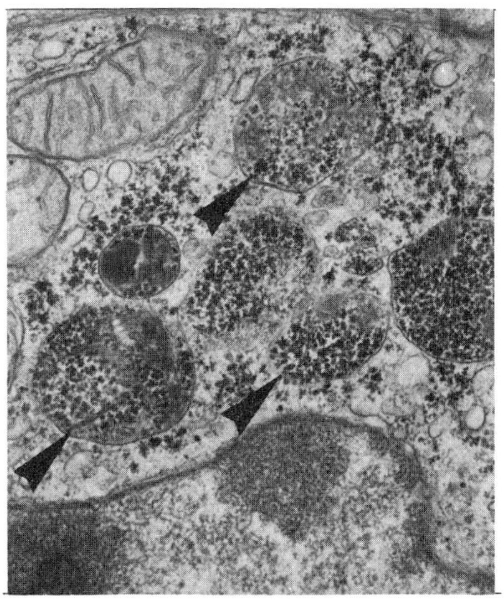

Figure 19.11. (Above) Part of a hepatocyte showing residual bodies (arrowheads) loaded with glycogen, as observed in type II glycogenosis. × 16 000. Courtesy of Dr Benhamou.

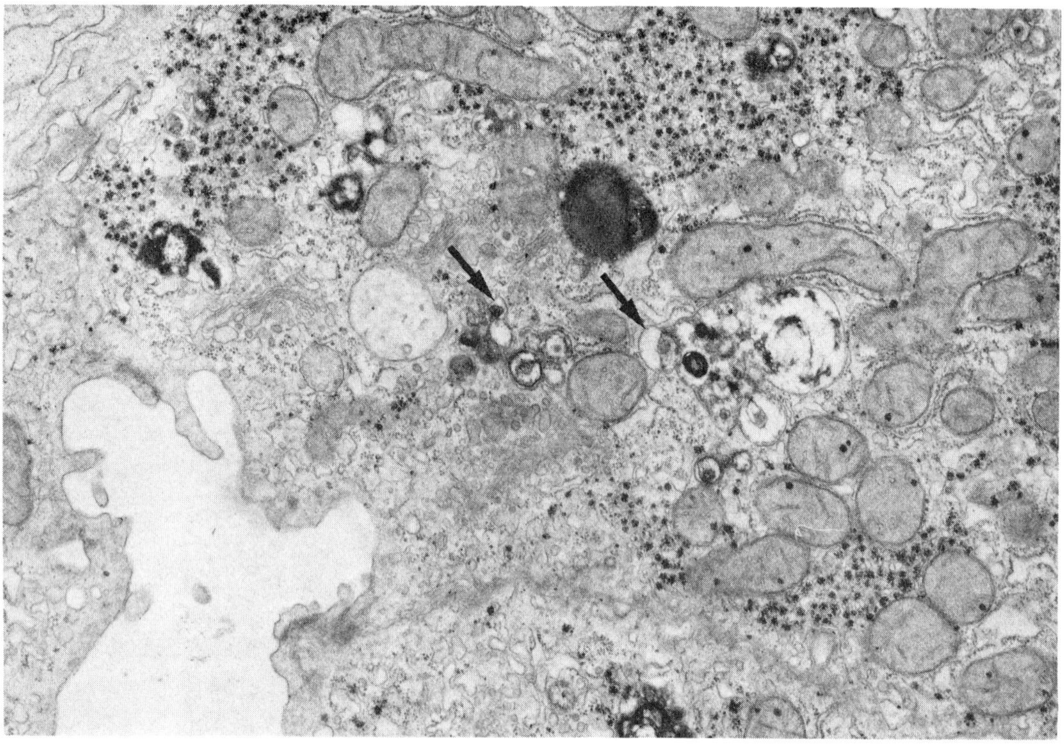

Figure 19.12. Part of a hepatocyte in a patient under treatment with 6-mercaptopurine. Numerous multilobulated dense bodies are evident. They contain heterogeneous ring-shaped osmiophilic material associated with bile retention (arrows). The lumen of the bile canaliculus is distended and lacks microvilli. From Jezequel and Orlandi,[36] with kind permission of Academic Press, London. × 17 500.

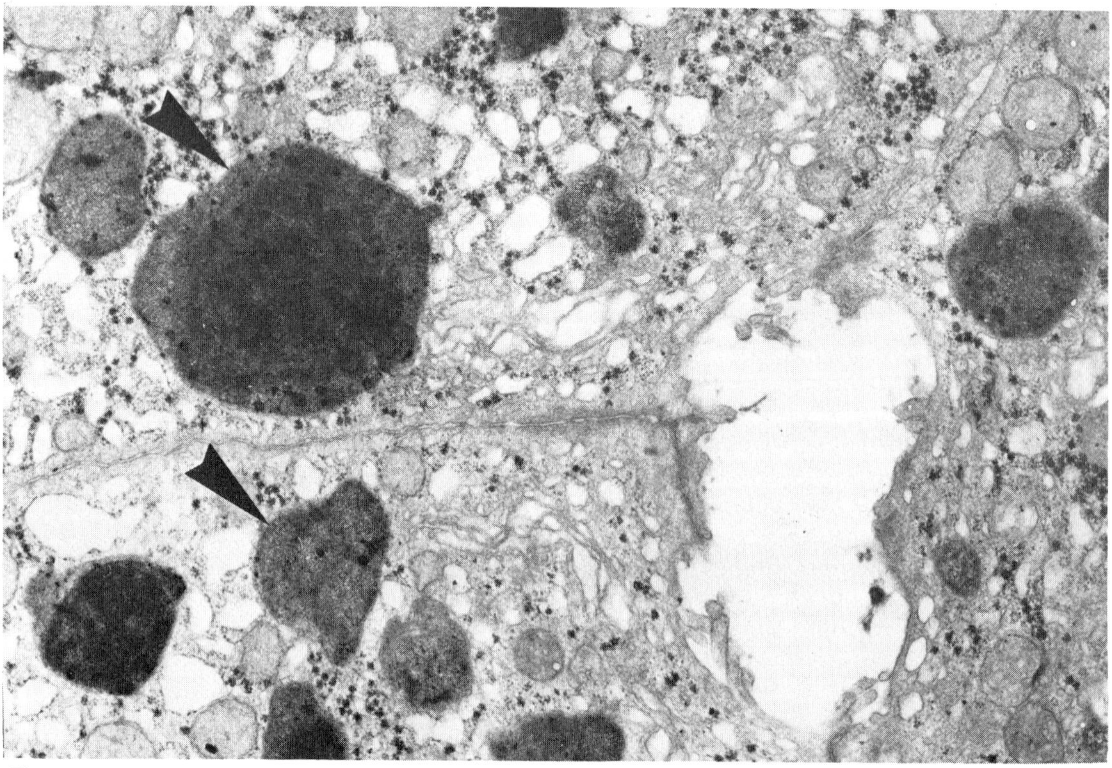

Figure 19.13. Large heterogeneous granules, limited by a single membrane (arrowheads), are present in the juxta-canalicular areas of hepatocytes in a patient with Dubin–Johnson syndrome. The lumen of the bile canaliculus is distended and microvilli are rare. The junctional complexes around the canalicular lumen are normal. × 18 200.

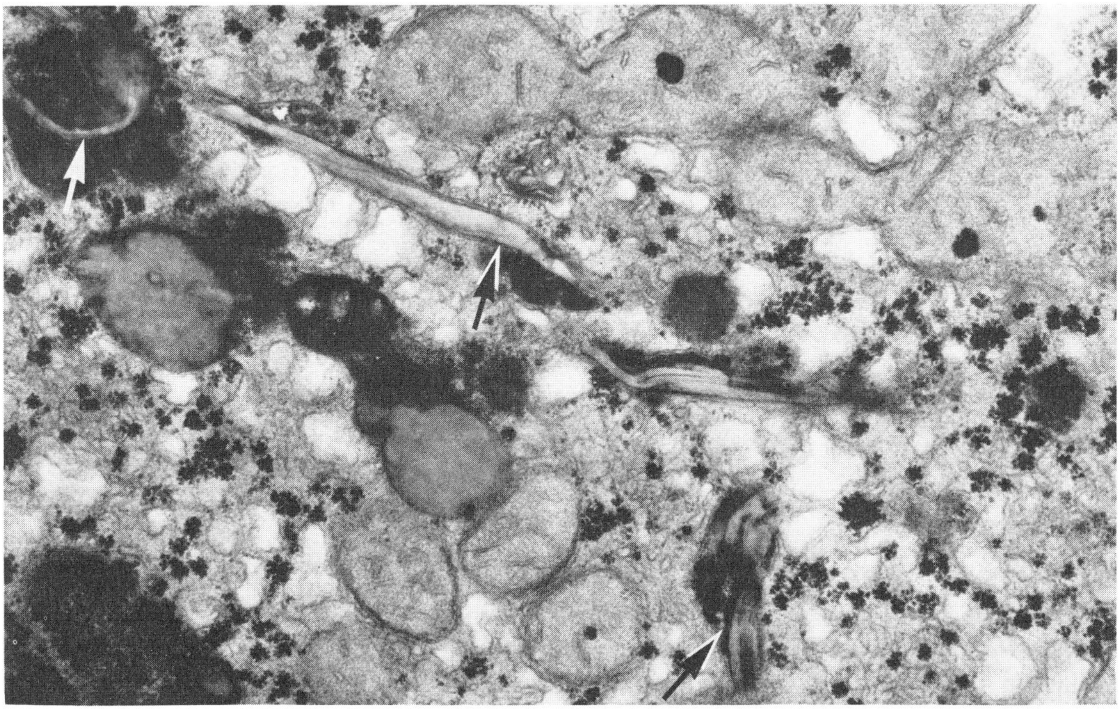

Figure 19.14. Part of the cytoplasm of a hepatocyte in a patient under long-term anticonvulsant therapy. Numerous ribbon-like formations (arrows) extending into the cytoplasm are associated with the lipofuscin granules. They are variable in width and in length, and show a dense limiting membrane surrounding an electron-lucent core. × 30 000.

inside lysosomes and is accumulated by an autophagic process.[3,23,53] In mucopolysaccharidoses such as Hurler and pseudo-Hurler diseases, enlarged lysosomes in the hepatocytes contain fluffy, electron lucent material, different from the features observed in the brain.[23] In fucosidosis, features similar to those present in Hurler's disease have been observed together with numerous intralysosomal dense lamellar deposits.[23] Pericanalicular dense bodies containing dense laminated material have also been described in some hepatocytes of children with Tay–Sachs disease[87] or in Fabry's disease,[23] whereas in Niemann–Pick disease numerous inclusions filled with dense membranous material are distributed throughout the hepatocytes.[87] All these alterations have in common an inherited defect of one or more lysosomal enzymes with consequent accumulation of undigested products (Figures 19.10 and 19.11). Similar changes may be produced by temporary overload or inefficiency of lysosomal enzymes in some pathological situations (Figures 19.12 and 19.13). This may explain the unusual, lysosome-associated formations observed in hepatocytes of subjects under long-term anticonvulsant therapy[37] and in patients with untreated cholelithiasis.[46] (Figure 19.14.) In these situations an alteration in cholesterol metabolism and formation of abnormal membranous components have been hypothesized. A similar mechanism could explain the changes observed in 'phospholipidosis'[33] or following therapy with perhexiline maleate.[4]

Lysosomal overload is also involved in the formation of 'siderosomes' or iron-laden lysosomes. Ferritin particles, sometimes in crystalline arrays, non-ferritin iron, carbohydrates, lipids and protein components have been identified in haemochromatosis and systemic iron overload.[41,42,66,67] This localization is not specific since excess storage iron also occurs in the cytoplasmic matrix and in lysosomes of phagocytic cells throughout the body.[67]

MALLORY BODIES

The term 'alcoholic hyalin' often used to describe Mallory bodies implies some specificity of this alteration. However, hyalin has been observed in a variety of conditions, in cirrhosis of various aetiologies – including primary

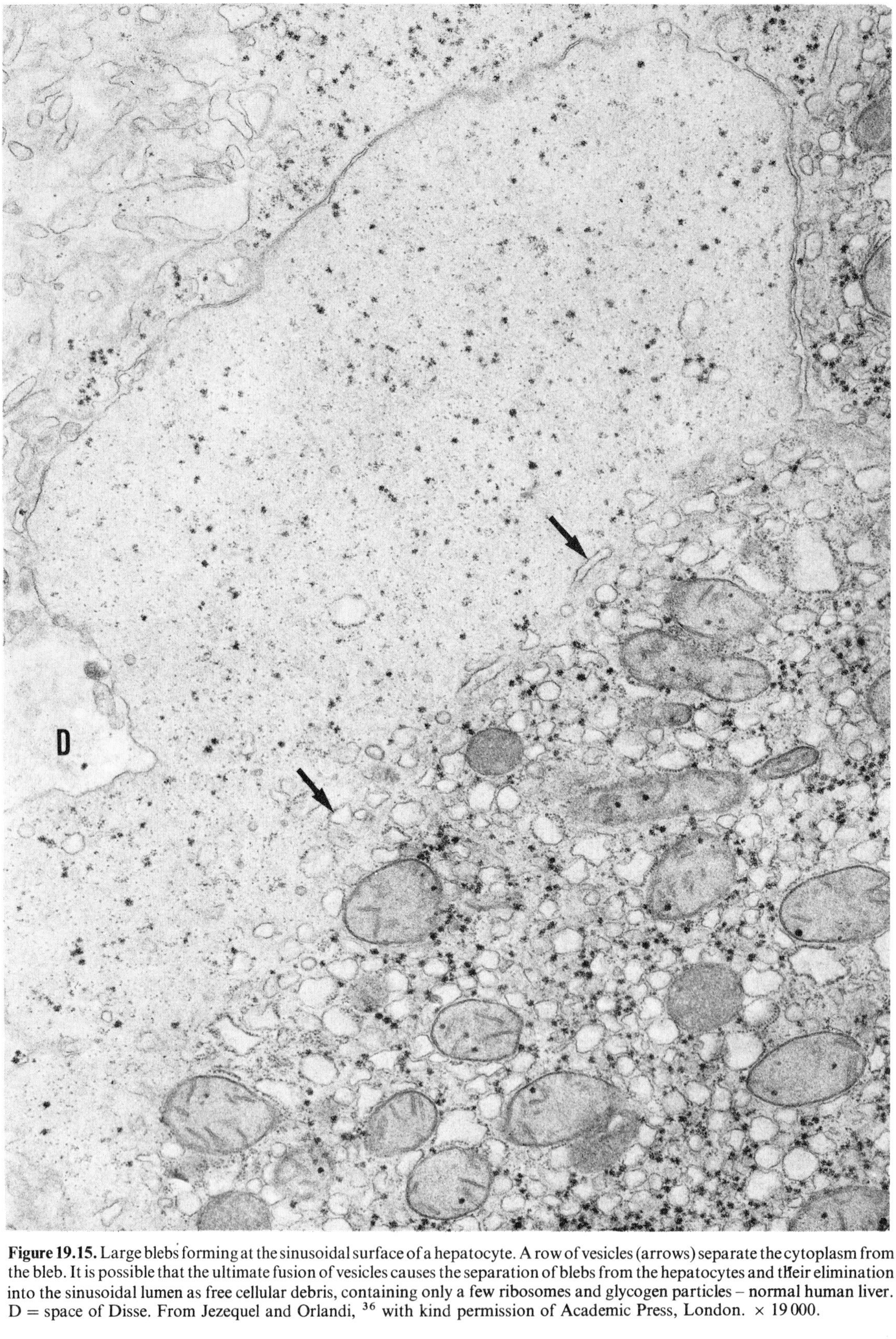

Figure 19.15. Large blebs forming at the sinusoidal surface of a hepatocyte. A row of vesicles (arrows) separate the cytoplasm from the bleb. It is possible that the ultimate fusion of vesicles causes the separation of blebs from the hepatocytes and their elimination into the sinusoidal lumen as free cellular debris, containing only a few ribosomes and glycogen particles – normal human liver. D = space of Disse. From Jezequel and Orlandi, [36] with kind permission of Academic Press, London. × 19 000.

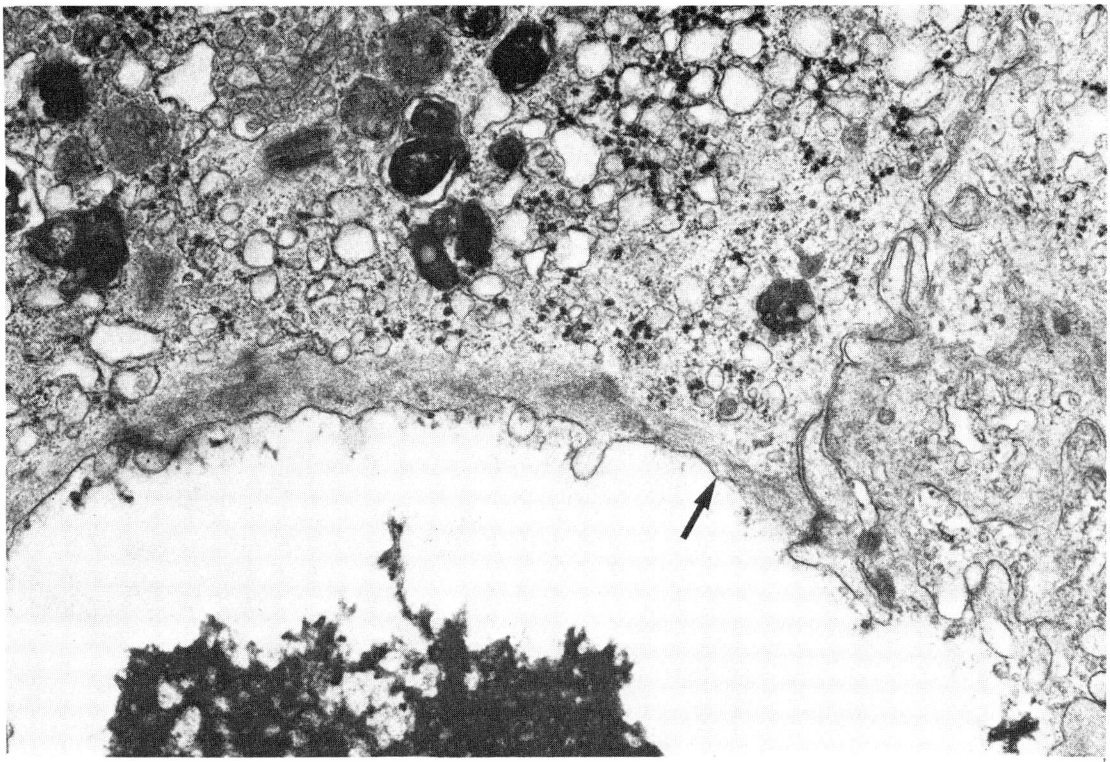

Figure 19.16. Alterations of the canalicular membrane in a patient with cholestasis; microvilli are rare and microfilaments can be seen in the pericanalicular area (arrow). The bile canaliculus (lower margin) contains a large thrombus and there is evidence of intracytoplasmic bile retention. × 20 000.

biliary cirrhosis – as well as in unrelated pathological situations.[21, 89, 92] It seems that the presence of centrilobular hyalin together with intact lobular architecture is pathognomonic of alcoholic liver injury.[21]

The first extensive ultrastructural study of Mallory bodies was published in 1964[6] and has been enlarged recently with the description of three types of 'alcoholic hyalin',[92] i.e. bundles of filaments in parallel arrays, clusters of randomly oriented fibrils and granular or amorphous substance. It has been suggested that Mallory bodies are made up of actin-like filaments capable of binding antiactin antibodies.[55] However, a comparative study of griseofulvin-induced Mallory bodies in mice and hyperplastic microfilaments induced by phalloidin has not confirmed this hypothesis, but tends to demonstrate that Mallory bodies are made up of intermediate (10 nm) filaments. Their formation might result from an antitubulin action of griseofulvin (in mice) or of alcohol (in man).[19]

PLASMA MEMBRANE

Alterations of the plasma membrane have often been invoked in the pathogenesis of various diseases, especially in cholestasis. However, evidence of structural changes rests on biochemical or immunological rather than on morphological data. The formation of blebs or localized swelling of microvilli, with occasional shedding of parts of the cytoplasm at the sinusoidal or at the canalicular pole of the hepatocytes, is often observed in cholestasis[13,61,62] but is not a specific change (Figure 19.15). Large pinocytic vacuoles may form from deep invaginations of the cell surface, especially in hypoxic conditions.[71] Invaginations of the cell membrane at the level of the space of Disse seem also to occur in peliosis[68,83] and may be secondary to the profound changes occurring in the vascular bed. More meaningful may be the modifications observed in membrane-associated cytoplasmic components from the 'cytoskeleton', such as actin-like microfilaments, which may play a role in membrane flow, transport and bile secretion into the canaliculus (Figure 19.16). Such modifications have been implicated in the pathogenesis of cholestasis,[17,18,59] but it has been suggested that these could be secondary rather than primary events, due to a toxic action of bile salts on the canalicular membrane.[8]

In summary, abnormal features of hepatocytes involving single organelles or groups of organelles, and not appreciable with the light microscope, may be recognized by electron microscopy. Although this may add little to the diagnosis and management of liver diseases at present, it increases our understanding of the structure and function of the liver cell, and helps to elucidate the mechanisms of some pathological processes.

REFERENCES

1. Arstila, A.U. & Trump, B.F. (1968) Studies on cellular autophagocytosis. The formation of autophagic vacuoles in the liver after glucagon administration. *American Journal of Pathology*, **53,** 687–733.
2. Bassi, M. & Bernelli-Zazzera, A. (1964) Ultrastructural cytoplasmic changes of liver cells after reversible and irreversible ischemia. *Experimental and Molecular Pathology*, **3,** 332–350.
3. Baudhuin, P., Hers, H.G. & Loeb, H. (1964) An electron microscopic and biochemical study of type II glycogenosis. *Laboratory Investigation*, **13,** 1139–1152.
4. Beaugrand, M., Chousterman, M., Callard, P., Camilieri, J.P., Petite, J.P. & Ferrier, J.P. (1977) Hépatites au maléate de perhexiline (Pexid) évoluant vers la cirrhose malgré l'arrêt du traitment (2 cas). *Gastroenterologie Clinique et Biologique*, **1,** 745–750.
5. Bianchi, L. & Gudat, F. (1976) Sanded nuclei in hepatitis B. Eosinophilic inclusions in liver cell nuclei due to excess in hepatitis B core antigen formation. *Laboratory Investigation*, **35,** 1–5.
6. Biava, C. (1964) Mallory alcoholic hyalin: a heretofore unique lesion of hepatocellular ergastoplasm. *Laboratory Investigation*, **13,** 301–320.
7. Biempica, L., Gutstein, S. & Arias, I.M. (1967) Morphological and biochemical studies of benign recurrent cholestasis. *Gastroenterology*, **52,** 521–535.
8. Boyer, J.L., Layden, T.J. & Hruban, Z. (1977) Mechanisms of cholestasis. Taurolithocholate alters canalicular membrane composition, structure and permeability. In *Membrane Alterations as Basis of Liver Injury* (Ed.) Popper, H., Bianchi, L., & Reutter, W. pp. 353–369. Lancaster: MTP Press.
9. Capurso, L., Koch, M.M., Freddara, U., Lorenzini, I., Jezequel, A.M. & Orlandi, F. (1975) Contribution of morphometry to the study of cholestasis in man. *Digestion*, **12,** 294.
10. Carney, F.M. & Van Dyke, R.A. (1972) Halothane hepatitis. A critical review. *Anesthesia and Analgesia (Cleveland)*, **51,** 135–160.
11. Conney, A.H. (1967) Pharmacological implications of microsomal enzyme induction. *Pharmacological Reviews*, **19,** 317–366.
12. de la Iglesia, F., Feuer, G., Takada, A. & Matsuda, Y. (1974) Morphological studies on secondary phospholipidosis in human liver. *Laboratory Investigation*, **30,** 539–549.
13. Desmet, V.J. (1972) Morphological and histochemical aspects of cholestasis. In *Progress in Liver Diseases* (Ed.) Popper, H. & Schaffner, F. Vol. 3, pp. 97–132. New York: Grune & Stratton.
14. Dobbins, W.O.III, Rollins, E.L., Brooks, S.G. & Fallon, M.J. (1972) A quantitative morphological analysis of ethanol effect upon rat liver. *Gastroenterology*, **62,** 1020–1033.
15. Feldman, G., Bignon, J., Chahinian, P., Degott, C. & Benhamou, J.P. (1974) Hepatocyte ultrastructural changes in α_1-antitrypsin deficiency. *Gastroenterology*, **67,** 1214–1224.
16. Fouts, J.R. & Rogers, L.A. (1965) Morphological changes in the liver accompanying stimulation of drug metabolizing enzyme activity by phenobarbital, chlordane, benzpyrene or methylcholanthrene in rats. *Journal of Pharmacology and Experimental Therapeutics*, **147,** 112–119.
17. French, S.W. (1976) Is cholestasis due to microfilament failure? *Human Pathology*, **7,** 243–244.
18. French, S.W. & Davis, P.L. (1975) Ultrastructural localization of actin-like filaments in rat hepatocytes. *Gastroenterology*, **68,** 765–774.
19. French, S.W., Sim, J.S. & Caldwell, M.G. (1977) Thick microfilaments (intermediate filaments) and chronic alcohol ingestion. In *Membrane Alterations as Basis of Liver Injury* (Ed.) Popper, H., Bianchi, L. & Reutter, W. pp. 311–325. Lancaster: MTP Press.
20. Gall, E.A. & Dabrogorki, O. (1964) Hepatic alterations in obstructive jaundice. *American Journal of Clinical Pathology*, **41,** 126–139.
21. Gerber, M.A., Orr, W., Denk, H., Schaffner, F. & Popper, H. (1973) Hepatocellular hyalin in cholestasis and cirrhosis: its diagnostic significance. *Gastroenterology*, **64,** 89–98.
22. Goldfischer, S., Novikoff, A.B., Albala, A. & Biempica, L. (1970) Hemoglobin uptake by rat hepatocytes and its breakdown within lysosomes. *Journal of Cell Biology*, **44,** 513–530.
23. Hers, H.G. & Van Hoof, F. (1970) The genetic pathology of lysosomes. In *Progress in Liver Diseases* (Ed.) Popper, H. & Schaffner, F. Vol. 3, pp. 185–205. New York: Grune & Stratton.
24. Hess, R., Staubli, W. & Reiss, W. (1965) Nature of the hepatomegalic effect produced by ethyl chlorophenoxy-isobutyrate in the rat. *Nature*, **208,** 856–858.
25. Howard, L.C.Jr, Brown, D.R. & Blake, D.A. (1973) Sub-cellular binding of halothane 1-^{14}C- in mouse liver and brain. *Journal of Pharmaceutical Sciences*, **62,** 1021–1023.
26. Hruban, Z., Gotoh, M., Slesers, A. & Chou, S. (1974) Structure of hepatic microbodies in rats treated with acetylsalicylic acid, clofibrate and dimethrin. *Laboratory Investigation*, **30,** 64–75.
27. Hruban, Z., Tavoloni, N., Reed, J.S. & Boyer, J.L. (1978) Ultrastructural changes during cholestasis induced by chloropromazine in the isolated perfused rat liver. *Virchows Archiv. Abt.* B, **26,** 289–306.
28. Huang, S.N. & Groh, V. (1973) Immunoagglutination electron microscopic study on virus-like particles and Australia antigen in liver tissue. *Laboratory Investigation*, **4,** 353–366.

29. Huang, S.N., Millman, I., O'Connell, A., Aronoff, A., Gault, H. & Blumberg, B.S. (1972) Virus-like particles in Australia-antigen-associated hepatitis: an immunoelectronmicroscopic study of human liver. *American Journal of Pathology,* **67,** 453–470.
30. Huang, S.N., Groh, V., Beaudoin, J.G., Dauphinee, W.D., Guttmann, R.D., Morehouse, D.D., Aronoff, A. & Gault, H. (1974) A study of the relationship of virus-like particles and Australia antigen in the liver. *Human Pathology,* **5,** 209–222.
31. Iancu, T.C., Mason, W.H. & Neustein, H.B. (1977) Ultrastructural abnormalities of liver cells in Reye's syndrome. *Human Pathology,* **8,** 421–431.
32. Iseri, O.A. & Gottlieb, L.S. (1971) Alcoholic hyalin and megamitochondria as separate and distinct entities in liver disease associated with alcoholism. *Gastroenterology,* **60,** 1027–1035.
33. Ito, S. & Tsukada, Y. (1973) Clinico-pathological and electron microscopical studies on a coronary dilating agent: 4-4′ diethyl-amino-ethoxyexestrol-induced liver injuries. *Acta Hepato-Gastroenterologica,* **20,** 204–215.
34. Jeppsson, J.O., Larsson, C. & Eriksson, S. (1975) Characterization of alpha-1-antitrypsin in the inclusion bodies from the liver in alpha-1-antitrypsin deficiency. *New England Journal of Medicine,* **293,** 576–580.
35. Jezequel, A.M. (1976) Ultrastructural changes induced by drugs in the liver. In *The Hepatobiliary System* (Ed.) Taylor, W. pp. 179–203. London: Plenum Press.
36. Jezequel, A.M. & Orlandi, F. (1972) Fine morphology of the human liver as a tool in clinical pharmacology. In *Liver and Drugs* (Ed.) Orlandi, F. & Jezequel, A.M. pp. 145–192. London: Academic Press.
37. Jezequel, A.M. & Orlandi, F. (1976) Unusual residual bodies in human liver cells. *Journal of Ultrastructure Research,* **57,** 87–93.
38. Jezequel, A.M., Orlandi, F. & Tenconi, L.T. (1971) Changes of the smooth endoplasmic reticulum induced by rifampicin in human and guinea-pig hepatocytes. *Gut,* **12,** 984–987.
39. Jezequel, A.M., Koch, M.M., Galeazzi, R., Lorenzini, I. & Orlandi, F. (1976) Liver response to drugs in man. A correlated morphometric and functional study. In *Diseases of the Liver and Biliary Tract* (Ed.) Leevy, C.M. pp. 153–157. Basel: S. Karger.
40. Jones, A.L. & Schmucker, D.L. (1977) Current concepts of structure as related to function. *Gastroenterology,* **73,** 833–851.
41. Kent, G. (1965) Iron storage diseases and the liver. In *Progress in Liver Diseases* (Ed.) Popper, H. & Schaffner, F. Vol. 2, pp. 253–271. New York: Grune & Stratton.
42. Kerr, D.N.S. & Muir, A.R. (1960) A demonstration of the structure and deposition of ferritin in the human liver cell. *Journal of Ultrastructure Research,* **3,** 313–319.
43. Klion, F.M. & Schaffner, F. (1966) The ultrastructure of acidophilic 'Councilman-like' bodies in the liver. *American Journal of Pathology,* **48,** 755–767.
44. Klion, F.M., Schaffner, F. & Popper, H. (1969) Hepatitis after exposure to halothane. *Annals of Internal Medicine,* **71,** 467–477.
45. Klion, F.M., Segal, R. & Schaffner, F. (1971) The effect of altered thyroid function on the ultrastructure of the human liver. *American Journal of Medicine,* **50,** 317–324.
46. Koch, M.M., Freddara, U., Lorenzini, I., Giampieri, M.P., Jezequel, A.M. & Orlandi, F. (1978) A stereological and biochemical study of the human liver in uncomplicated cholelithiasis. *Digestion.* In press.
47. Koch, M.M., Lorenzini, I., Freddara, U., Jezequel, A.M. & Orlandi, F. (1978) Type 2 Crigler–Najjar syndrome. Quantitation of ultrastructural data and evolution under therapy with phenytoin. *Gastroenterologie Clinique et Biologique.* In press.
48. Koff, S., Carter, E.A., Lui, S. & Isselbacher, K.L. (1970) Prevention of the ethanol-induced fatty liver in the rat by phenobarbital. *Gastroenterology,* **59,** 50–61.
49. Koff, R.S., Davidson, L.J., Gordon, G. & Sabesin, S. (1973) D-galactosamine hepatotoxicity. III. Normoactive smooth endoplasmic reticulum and modification by phenobarbital. *Experimental and Molecular Pathology,* **19,** 168–177.
50. Lane, B.P. & Lieber, C.S. (1966) Ultrastructural alterations in human hepatocytes following ingestion of ethanol with adequate diets. *American Journal of Pathology,* **49,** 593–603.
51. Larsson, C. & Eriksson, S. (1977) Liver function in asymptomatic adult individuals with severe α_1-antitrypsin deficiency. *Scandinavian Journal of Gastroenterology,* **12,** 543–546.
52. Lieber, C.S. (1973) Hepatic and metabolic effects of alcohol. *Gastroenterology,* **65,** 821–846.
53. McAdams, A.J. & Wilson, H.E. (1966) The liver in generalized glycogen storage disease. *American Journal of Pathology,* **49,** 99–111.
54. Mitchell, J.R. & Jollows, D.J. (1975) Metabolic activation of drugs to toxic substances. *Gastroenterology,* **68,** 390–410.
55. Nenci, I. (1975) Identification of actin-like protein in alcoholic hyalin by immunofluorescence. *Laboratory Investigation,* **32,** 257–260.
56. Orlandi, F. & Jezequel, A.M. (1962) Electron microscopy of the human liver after methandrostenolone administration. In *Aktuelle Probleme der Hepatologie* (Ed.) Martini, G.A. pp. 41–47. Stuttgart: G. Thieme Verlag.
57. Oudea, M.C., Collette, M. & Oudea, P. (1973) Morphometric study of ultrastructural changes induced in rat liver by chronic alcohol intake. *American Journal of Digestive Diseases,* **18,** 398–402.
58. Partin, J.C., Schubert, W.K. & Partin, J.S. (1971) Mitochondrial structure in Reye's syndrome (encephalopathy and fatty degeneration of the viscera). *New England Journal of Medicine,* **285,** 1339–1343.
59. Phillips, M.J., Oda, M., Mak, E., Fisher, M.M. & Jeejebhoy, K.N. (1975) Microfilament dysfunction as a possible cause of intrahepatic cholestasis. *Gastroenterology,* **69,** 48–58.
60. Popper, H. (1975) The ground-glass hepatocyte as a diagnostic hint. *Human Pathology,* **6,** 517–520.
61. Popper, H. & Schaffner, F. (1970) Pathophysiology of cholestasis. *Human Pathology,* **1,** 1–24.
62. Popper, H., Schaffner, F. & Denk, H. (1976) Molecular pathology of cholestasis. In *The Hepatobiliary System* (Ed.) Taylor, W. pp. 605–629. London: Plenum Press.
63. Reddy, J.K., Azarnoff, D.L., Svoboda, D.H. & Prasad, J.D. (1974) Nafenopin-induced hepatic microbody (peroxisomes) proliferation and catalase synthesis in rats and mice. Absence of sex difference in response. *Journal of Cell Biology,* **61,** 344–358.

64. Remmer, H. & Bock, K.W. (1974) The role of the liver in drug metabolism. In *The Liver and its Diseases* (Ed.) Schaffner, F., Sherlock, S. & Leevy, C.M. pp. 34–42. New York: Intercontinental Medical Book Co.
65. Remmer, H. & Merker, H.J. (1963) Drug-induced changes in the endoplasmic reticulum; association with drug-metabolizing enzymes. *Science,* **142,** 1657–1658.
66. Richter, G.W. (1960) The nature of storage iron in idiopathic hemochromatosis and in hemosiderosis. *Journal of Experimental Medicine,* **112,** 551–570.
67. Richter, G.W. (1978) The iron-loaded cell. The cytopathology of iron storage. A review. *American Journal of Pathology,* **91,** 361–404.
68. Ross, R.C., Kovacks, K. & Horvath, E. (1972) Ultrastructure of peliosis hepatis in a percutaneous biopsy. *Pathologia Europaea,* **7,** 273–282.
69. Rubin, E. & Lieber, C.S. (1967) Early fine structural changes in the human liver induced by alcohol. *Gastroenterology,* **52,** 1–13.
70. Rubin, E., Hutterer, F. & Lieber, C.S. (1968) Ethanol increases smooth endoplasmic reticulum and drug metabolizing enzymes. *Science,* **159,** 1469–1471.
71. Schaffner, F. (1970) Oxygen supply and the hepatocyte. *Annals of the New York Academy of Sciences,* **170,** 67–77.
72. Schaffner, F. (1974) Some unresolved ultrastructural problems encountered in the study of the liver and its diseases. In *The Liver and its Diseases* (Ed.) Schaffner, F., Sherlock, S. & Leevy, C.M. pp. 7–18. New York: Intercontinental Medical Book Co.
73. Schaffner, F. & Popper, H. (1975) Electron microscopy of the liver. In *Diseases of the Liver* (Ed.) Schiff, L. 4th ed., pp. 51–85. Philadelphia: Lippincott.
74. Scotto, J.M., Stralin, H.G. & Landrieu, P. (1977) Étude ultrastructurale du foie dans deux cas de tyrosienémie héréditaire. *Gastroenterologie Clinique et Biologique,* **1,** 139–149.
75. Shikata, T., Uzawa, T., Yoshiwara, N., Akatsuka, T. & Yamazaki, S. (1974) Staining methods of Australia antigen in paraffin section. Detection of cytoplasmic inclusion bodies. *Japanese Journal of Experimental Medicine,* **44,** 25–36.
76. Staubli, W., Hess, R. & Weibel, E.R. (1969) Correlated morphometric and biochemical studies on the liver cell. II. Effect of phenobarbital on rat hepatocytes. *Journal of Cell Biology,* **42,** 92–112.
77. Stein, O., Fainaru, M. & Stein, Y. (1972) Visualization of virus-like particles in endoplasmic reticulum of hepatocytes of Australia antigen carriers. *Laboratory Investigation,* **26,** 262–269.
78. Steiner, J.W., Jezequel, A.M., Phillips, M.J., Miyai, K. & Arakawa, K. (1965) Some aspects of the ultrastructural pathology of the liver. In *Progress in Liver Diseases* (Ed.) Popper, H. & Schaffner, F. Vol. 2, pp. 303–372. New York: Grune & Stratton.
79. Stenger, R.J. (1970) Organelle pathology of the liver. The endoplasmic reticulum. *Gastroenterology,* **58,** 554–574.
80. Sternlieb, I. & Scheinberg, I.H. (1974) Wilson's disease. In *The Liver and its Diseases* (Ed.) Schaffner, F., Sherlock, S. & Leevy, C.M. pp. 328–336. New York: Intercontinental Medical Book Co.
81. Svoboda, D.J. & Azarnoff, D.L. (1966) Response of hepatic microbodies to a hypolipidemic agent, ethylchlorophenoxyisobutyrate (CPIB). *Journal of Cell Biology,* **30,** 442–450.
82. Swift, H. & Hruban, Z. (1964) Focal degradation as a biological process. *Federal Proceedings,* **23,** 1026–1037.
83. Taxy, J.B. (1978) Peliosis: a morphological curiosity becomes an iatrogenic problem. *Human Pathology,* **9,** 331–340.
84. Thomsen, P., Poulsen, H. & Petersen, P. (1977) Different types of ground glass hepatocytes in human liver biopsies. Morphology, occurrence and diagnostic significance. *Scandinavian Journal of Gastroenterology,* **11,** 113–119.
85. Trump, B.F., Dees, J.H. & Shelburne, J.D. (1973) The ultrastructure of the human liver cell and its common patterns of reaction to injury. In *The Liver* (Ed.) Gall, E.A. & Mostofi, F.K. pp. 80–120. Baltimore: Williams & Wilkins.
86. Uzunalimoglu, B., Yardley, J.H. & Boitnott, J.K. (1970) The liver in mild halothane hepatitis. *American Journal of Pathology,* **61,** 457–478.
87. Volk, B.W., Wellmann, K.F. & Wallace, B.J. (1970) Hepatic changes in various lipidoses: electron microscopic and histochemical studies. In *Progress in Liver Diseases* (Ed.) Popper, H. & Schaffner, F., Vol. 3, pp. 206–221. New York: Grune & Stratton.
88. Wiener, J., Loud, A.V., Kimberg, D.V. & Spiro, D. (1968) A quantitative description of cortisone-induced alterations in the ultrastructure of rat liver parenchymal cells. *Journal of Cell Biology,* **37,** 47–61.
89. Wiggers, K.D., French, S.W., French, B.A. & Carr, B.N. (1973) The ultrastructure of Mallory bodies filaments. *Laboratory Investigation,* **29,** 652–658.
90. Wills, E.J. & Walton, B. (1978) A morphological study of unexplained hepatitis following halothane anesthesia. *American Journal of Pathology,* **91,** 11–32.
91. Winkler, K., Junge, U. & Creutzfeldt, W. (1977) Ground-glass hepatocytes in unselected liver biopsies. Ultrastructure and relationship to Hepatitis B antigen. *Scandinavian Journal of Gastroenterology,* **11,** 167–170.
92. Yokoo, H., Minick, O.T., Batti, F. & Kent, G. (1972) Morphologic variants of alcoholic hyalin. *American Journal of Pathology,* **69,** 25–40.
93. Yunis, E.J., Agostini, R.M. & Glew, R.H. (1976) Fine structural observations on the liver in α_1-antitrypsin deficiency. *American Journal of Pathology,* **82,** 265–286.

Chapter 20

Radio-isotope Imaging

D.M. ACKERY

Radio-isotope studies of the morphology and function of the liver and its related structures are firmly established in the investigation of patients with hepatobiliary disease.[16] The investigation usually involves the intravenous administration of a radioactive pharmaceutical followed by measurement of gamma radiation emitted from the body. The procedure is simple for the patient, with minimal risk, and is now used widely in the initial investigation of hepatic disorders, particularly if focal disease is suspected. Physiological mechanisms play an essential part in the uptake of radioactivity by the liver. Since these functions may be impaired by a variety of causes, the radio-isotope image is usually unspecific for pathogenesis; but it can provide a sensitive indication of early disease, and point the direction for subsequent investigation.

INSTRUMENTATION

Distribution of radioactivity is measured by a scintillation detector placed close to the surface of the patient. The detector consists of a sodium iodide crystal which converts the energy of interacting gamma photons into voltage pulses and, by means of suitable electronics, displays these events on an oscilloscope or a film. Lead shielding (collimation) enables analysis of the photon spatial distribution.

The simplest type of detector is a scintillation probe, which has coarse collimation and measures photons arising from a large region of an organ. Finer collimation permits concentration on a small volume of tissue, and a profile of activity can be obtained when the detector is driven mechanically across the surface of the body.

The *rectilinear scanner* constructs a two-dimensional representation of activity. The detector passes to and fro across the patient measuring the activity profile in each plane, and moves laterally by a small incremental distance at the end of each traverse. The scan thus obtained is displayed either on photographic film or on paper, the activity variation being shown as relative optical density or as a colour contour print.

Rectilinear scanners are reasonably stable and reliable instruments, and have been used successfully for several years to give images of hepatic distribution of radioactivity. Their principal limitation is that they are rather slow; a typical hepatic image requires a period of 10 to 15 minutes for completion. This means that they can be used only for 'static' images of activity distribution, and cannot make rapid sequential measurements of changing activity with time.

The imaging time can be reduced by using two detector heads which scan two sides of the patient simultaneously.

The *gamma camera* is now increasingly used for hepatic radio-isotope imaging. It has a static detector consisting of a large single sodium iodide crystal manufactured as a disc. On the patient surface of the crystal is fitted a multihole lead collimator, which limits entry into the crystal to those gamma photons which are emitted perpendicular to the crystal face. The spatial distribution of gamma interactions within the sodium iodide crystal is analysed electronically, and this gives an image which can be displayed on photographic or polaroid film, or by a printer. Since scanning is not required, the image is obtained more rapidly than by a rectilinear scanner, typically in under five minutes.

Most gamma cameras do not give a direct digital output, and for image quantification an analogue to a digital converter must be used. This transposes the image into a digital matrix in which each intercept point is characterized by an X and Y value. The counts at each XY location are given by a Z value. These values of X, Y and Z are stored in a digital memory, usually magnetic tape or disc. A matrix of 64 by 64 lines has a total of 4096 XY intercept points each with its Z value for the counts at that position.

This digital system enables serial images to be stored during an investigation in order to show temporal changes in liver activity during a 'dynamic' study. By analysis of stored data a histogram of changes in count-rate with time for each hepatic region can be constructed. The final result is analogous to a quantitative contrast angiographic investigation. An on-line mini computer allows mathematical treatment of data which are used for correction of non-uniformity of detection across the field of the gamma camera, for statistical smoothing and for the analysis of activity–time relationships.

TECHNIQUES AND PHARMACOLOGY

For high-quality gamma camera images intravenously administered radioactivity should be localized in the liver. For this, two types of radioactive pharmaceutical are used: colloid preparations, which are phagocytosed by the Kupffer cells of hepatic vascular sinuses; and dyes or chemicals, which are actively transported by hepatic parenchymal cells. The final liver concentration of both types of pharmaceutical will depend upon the hepatic blood flow and the functional capacity of the liver to clear the pharmaceutical from the blood (the extraction efficiency). The product of these factors gives the effective hepatic blood flow.

Several different radio-isotopes have been used as labels for these pharmaceuticals. The physical requirements of an ideal radio-isotope are that its gamma photon energy should be optimal for detection by a gamma camera or rectilinear scanner (approximately between 100 and 500 keV), and that radioactive decay takes place with a short half-life (preferably a few hours) and with no beta emission. The patient radiation dose is thereby minimized, enabling greater initial administrations of activity. This gives images of good statistical quality.

At present most routine hepatic gamma imaging is done with colloid labelled with $^{99}Tc^{m}$. $^{99}Tc^{m}$ is available from a ^{99}Mo generator. It has a half-life of six hours, a monochromatic gamma emission of 140 keV, and no beta emission. Pharmaceutical grade preparations of colloid are available commercially, and these are easily labelled with $^{99}Tc^{m}$. 4 to 5 mCi (1.5 to 1.9×10^8 Bq) of $^{99}Tc^{m}$-colloid give good images of reticulo-endothelial function 10 to 15 minutes after intravenous administration. Alternative colloid preparations, such as ^{198}Au-colloid, have been used but they usually give higher patient radiation doses.

Hepatocyte cell function and biliary excretion are usually assessed with ^{131}I-labelled rose bengal. This has a dose limitation due to the long half-life (eight days) and beta emission of ^{131}I. Interest is now being shown in a number of compounds which are concentrated by the hepatobiliary system and can be labelled with $^{99}Tc^{m}$. Of these, pyridoxyline glutamate and iminodiacetic acid and its derivatives show the greatest promise and several millicuries can be administered, enabling good visualization of the gallbladder and biliary ducts.[42]

Radiation Dosimetry

Before radio-isotopes are administered to patients careful consideration has to be given to the potential risks resulting from absorbed radiation doses to tissues. The dose delivered by any radio-isotope will depend on its physical half-life and its residence time in the body. A further factor is beta particle emission, which greatly increases the radiation dose to surrounding tissue but plays no useful part in the imaging process. Detailed calculation of radiation doses is usually unnecessary since these are published for adult routine procedures.[20,48] Those for paediatric investigation are given by Treves and Spencer.[55]

Positioning

As a routine procedure images should be taken in the anterior, posterior and right and left lateral positions. This allows comprehensive examination of both liver and spleen, since the gamma camera and rectilinear scanner preferentially detect radiation from tissue which lies closest to the detector.

The anterior image gives the best overall view of hepatic morphology and its relationship to the costal edge, and to clinical examination. It provides optimal detection of the anterior surface of the liver, including the left lobe and porta hepatis. The posterior view shows the posterior aspect of the right lobe and its relationship to the right kidney, and also is the view used for judging splenic enlargement. The left lobe of the liver is seen less well in this view since it lies anteriorly and much of its photon emission is attenuated by the spine. The right lateral image is of particular value in guiding needle biopsy of a focal lesion within the right lobe. The left lateral image shows the lateral shape of the spleen, and also displays the left hepatic lobe 'end-on' which can enhance the detection of focal lesions which may be seen poorly in the anterior view. Images should be accompanied in all cases by appropriate anatomical landmarks. In order to avoid variations in image quality, sufficient counts (usually more than 200 000 per image) should be collected to minimize errors due to statistical factors. Typical normal liver images are shown in Figure 20.1.

INTERPRETATION OF THE HEPATIC RADIONUCLIDE STATIC IMAGE

The $^{99}Tc^{m}$ colloid image is judged firstly for its technical quality. This is necessary in order to avoid pitfalls due to faulty performance of the detector or electronics, and secondly to assess that the pharmaceutical is properly labelled. If significant amounts of free $^{99}Tc^{m}$ are administered, activity will be seen to concentrate in the kidneys, bladder, thyroid and gastric mucosa. With good colloid labelling, most of the activity in a normal individual is concentrated in the liver and spleen.

Interpretation of hepatic and splenic images is based upon four criteria: organ size; morphological shape; uniformity of uptake; and the relative uptake in liver, spleen and bone marrow.

Hepatic enlargement

Clinical estimation of liver size by palpation of the lower border, and percussion over the thorax, may be misleading, even in the non-obese subject.[14,49] Generally, the radionuclide image gives a better impression of true liver size, and this can be assessed subjectively with reasonable accuracy. There appears to be little additional value in attempting to calculate liver volume by fitting mathematical models to the images.[41] The radiocolloid image also gives a reliable assessment of splenic size. This is usually obtained from the posterior image, when a length in the adult of greater than 13 cm indicates enlargement.[35]

True hepatic enlargement is usually a consequence of significant focal or diffuse liver disease, but the liver image may be generally enlarged without obvious pathological abnormality, or may show a Riedel's extension to the right lobe. On the other hand, the liver may be of normal size but still contains an abscess cavity or metastases. The hepatic image may appear unusually small in advanced cirrhosis.

Hepatic morphology

A wide variation has been reported for the shapes of normal livers.[33] These may give a clinical impression of focal intrahepatic disease or pressure from extrahepatic lesions.[9] The gallbladder fossa, the porta hepatis, thinning of the left lobe as it passes over the spine, lower costal margin indentation and impression on the medial superior aspect of the right lobe due to confluence of the hepatic veins are among the normal variations which require careful consideration. Change in hepatic shape may also follow splenectomy, with migration of the left lobe into the left upper quadrant.[4] Care must be exercised to avoid reporting these normal variations as hepatic lesions.

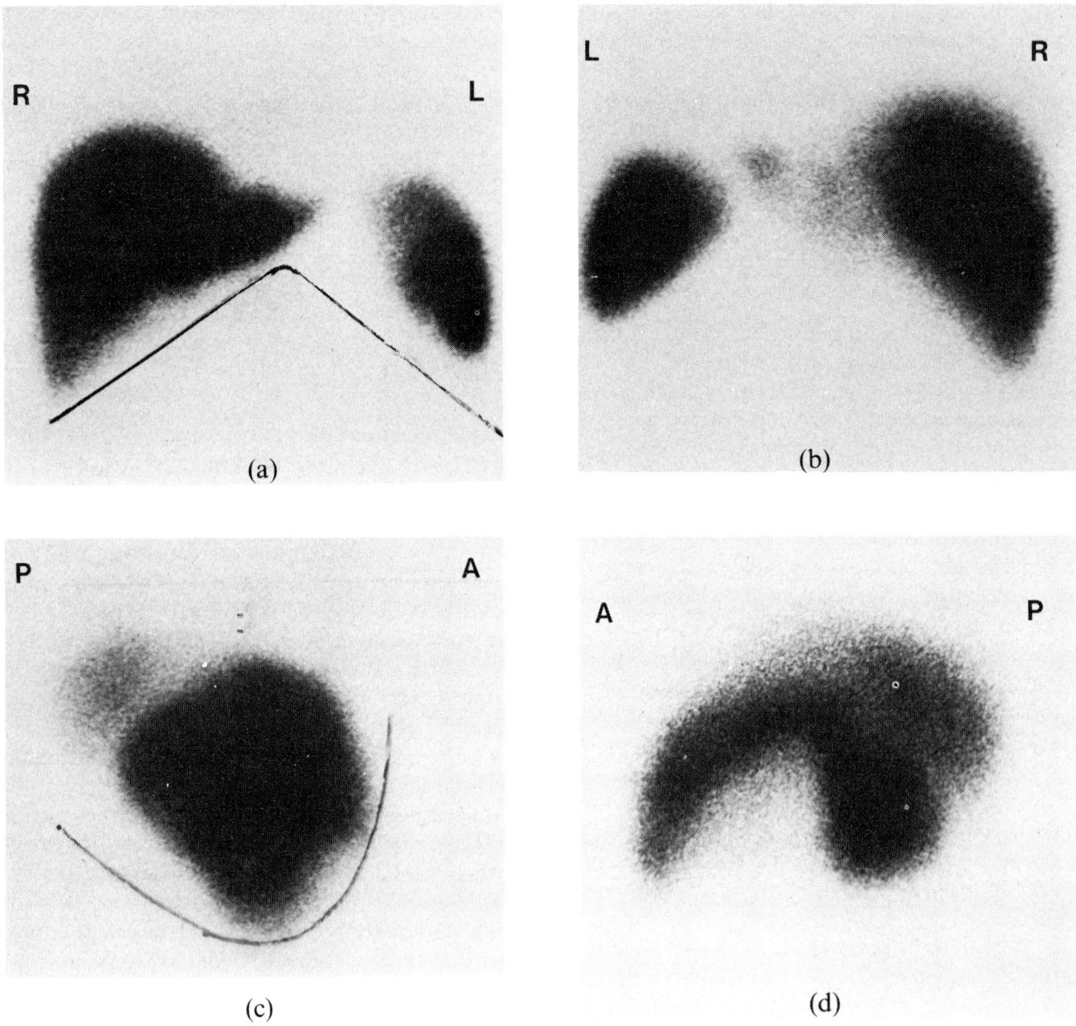

Figure 20.1. Gamma camera images of the normal liver and spleen: (a) Anterior, showing normal hepatic and splenic morphology and position; (b) Posterior, activity from the left lobe is attenuated by the spine; (c) Right lateral, right hepatic lobe activity is seen predominantly; (d) Left lateral, the spleen is seen best, with the left hepatic lobe arching anteriorly, and the right hepatic lobe seen above and posterior to the spleen.

Liver shape may also be a useful sign in congenital or post-traumatic eventration of the right diaphragm.[47, 61]

Uniformity of uptake

Apart from the exceptions given above, the normal liver shows homogeneous uptake of radiocolloid, and any departure from this pattern indicates potential liver disease. The right hepatic lobe usually shows a higher count-rate than the left due to its larger volume and the incisura between the two lobes may be marked. Minor inhomogeneity can be caused by statistical fluctuations, but this should be avoided by good technique. Well-defined focal lesions in the image are almost always pathological, once the possibility of an artefact has been excluded.

Relative uptake of colloid by the liver, spleen and bone marrow

Generalized disease affecting the reticulo-endothelial function of the liver will lead to poor hepatic accumulation of colloid. Preferential uptake of activity is then seen in the spleen which may be enlarged, and in the bone marrow which in the healthy subject shows relatively little concentration of activity.

Focal Hepatic Disease

Radio-isotope imaging has been shown to be a particularly effective procedure for identifying space-occupying lesions within the liver.[33, 34, 38] It compares favourably with other diagnostic imaging techniques such as angiography, at least for the detection of lesions down to about 2 cm in diameter, but it lacks diagnostic specificity.[29] Due to difficulties in interpretation arising from variations in the normal hepatic appearances, the frequency of false positive reporting may be high, and this will lead to an over-diagnosis of focal liver disease.[36] Table 20.1 gives the causes for a single area of decreased uptake in a radiocolloid image. This classification serves as a useful guide to the expected frequency of different conditions in an average hospital, although this will of course vary with the types of patient referred and the geographical region.

The radio-isotope colloid image is most frequently used as a non-invasive method for determining the presence of *liver metastases*.[15] The accuracy of the technique compared with needle biopsy or laparotomy, with histological confirmation, varies from between 75 and 85 per cent.[32] False positive lesions commonly result when the patient has severe obstructive jaundice, or marked hepatic dysfunction. A frequent reason for false negative interpretation of the image is the small size of some metastases which go undetected by the limited resolution of the gamma imaging technique. Recent advances in radiopharmaceuticals and detector technology do not seem to have resulted in an improvement in the diagnostic accuracy of the investigation. For this reason it is questionable if the procedure is of value for the routine screening of cancer patients to detect early spread to the liver, or as a guide to surgical management.[8, 37, 45]

The combination of either angiography[27] or computed axial tomography[13] has little to offer in increasing the diagnostic accuracy of the radio-isotope investigation, but the addition of grey-scale ultrasound does add further definition to an equivocal radio-isotope result.[53]

The colloid image is of direct value in confirming the presence of metastases in many patients and may make exploratory laparotomy unnecessary. It often provides guidance for needle biopsy since 'blind' biopsy alone has a large sampling error.[2] The radio-isotope image can be virtually diagnostic when multiple hepatic metastases are present (Figures 20.2 and 20.3), and even if the result is equivocal at first examination it is readily repeated after some weeks.

Other tumours of the liver may also be detected by radio-isotope imaging, but generally show no distinctive features. *Primary hepatomas* may present a difficult diagnostic problem since they normally arise in a liver which already shows uneven uptake of activity due to impaired reticuloendothelial function.[26, 54] For instance, in alcoholic cirrhosis poor uptake of colloid in regions of fibrosis and regeneration leads to patchiness in the image which may be difficult to distinguish from tumour. Sequential imaging can assist in the differentiation since the persistence over a long period of a large focal lesion is greatly indicative of hepatoma. Radio-isotope methods have been used for the selection of patients for hepatic lobectomy in this condition.[10] *Haemangioma* of the liver may appear as a large space-occupying lesion often producing a concave defect on the surface of the liver. Since needle biopsy of these tumours is best avoided, further assistance to

Table 20.1. *Causes for a Single Area of Decreased Uptake in the Radiocolloid Hepatic Image.*

Common	Less common	Rare
Metastatic neoplasm	Cirrhosis	Haemangioma
Pyogenic abscess	Primary hepatic neoplasm	Focal nodular hyperplasia
False positive causes	Trauma	Hamartoma
	Lymphoma	Hepatic vein thrombosis
	Post-radiotherapy	Amyloidosis
	Cysts (a) Simple	Viral hepatitis
	(b) Hydatid	Gumma
	Abscess (a) Amoebic	
	(b) Tuberculous	
	(c) Actinomycotic	
	Arteriovenous malformations	

Modified from Holder et al.[17]

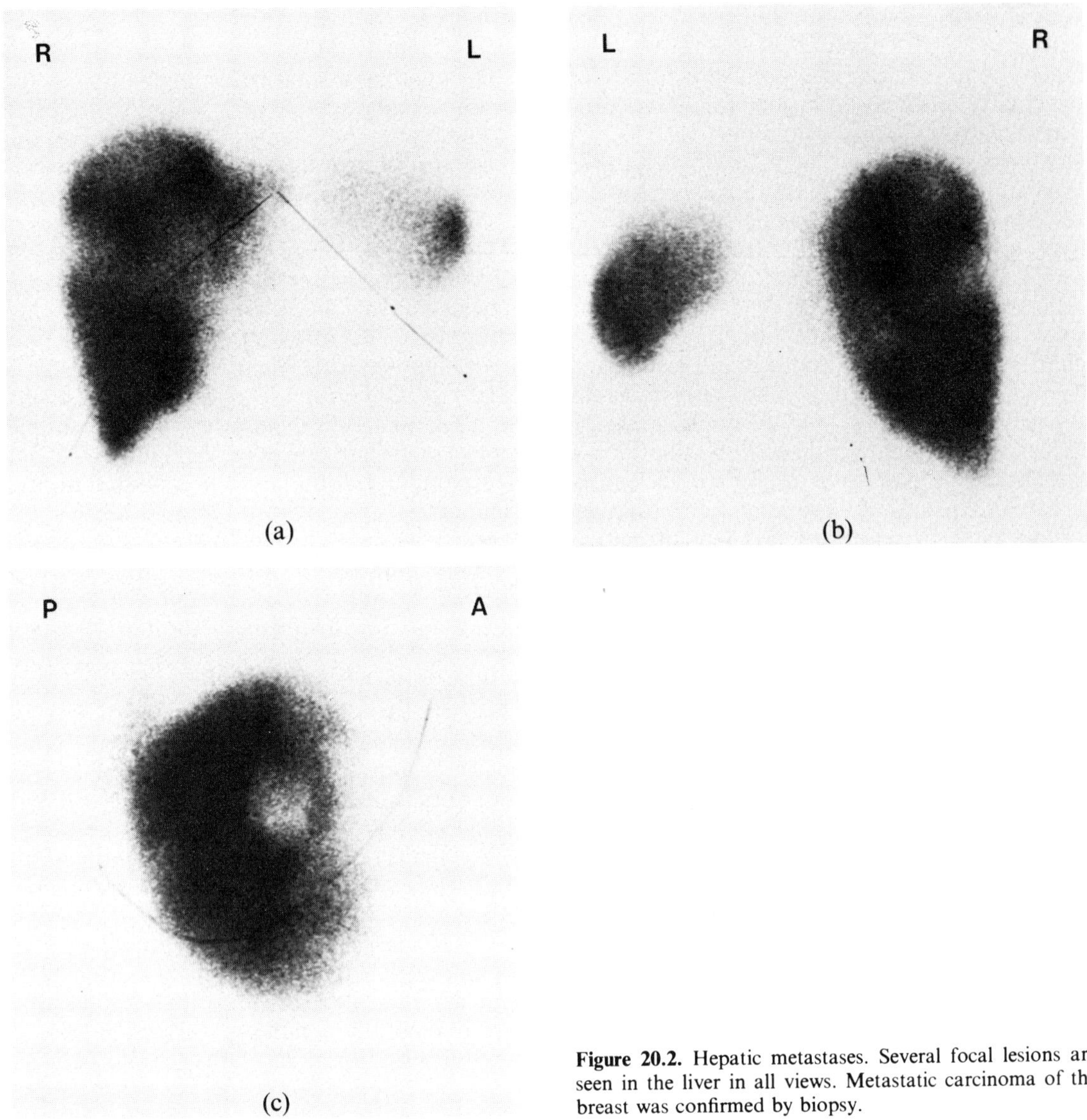

Figure 20.2. Hepatic metastases. Several focal lesions are seen in the liver in all views. Metastatic carcinoma of the breast was confirmed by biopsy.

the diagnosis can be given by completion of a 'blood-pool' image with $^{99}Tc^{m}$-labelled red cells, or with a radio-isotope of indium, usually $^{113}In^{m}$ or ^{111}In, which remains in the circulation bound to transferrin. Because of its greater vascularity a haemangioma usually shows a higher level of activity than normal liver parenchyma.[52] Regions of *focal nodular hyperplasia* may show radiocolloid concentration to be either absent or normal.[57]

Radio-isotope colloid imaging has a useful localizing role to play in those patients who have clinical evidence of an abscess. The image may show either a focal lesion due to intrahepatic *pyogenic abscess*[40,44] or evidence of an extrinsic lesion above the right lobe due to a subdiaphragmatic abscess. An intrahepatic abscess cavity may not be large, and may need careful examination in all views to show its presence. The size and extent of loculation seen in the image give guidance on drainage procedures, and follow-up images show the results of treatment. The diagnosis of *amoebic abscess* (Figure 20.4) is also facilitated by liver imaging.[3] In regions where amoebiasis is uncommon, this diagnosis should be considered in patients with unexplained fever who have travelled abroad, even when the liver is not enlarged. Often the radio-isotope image may give the first evidence of amoebic abscess within the liver.

Cysts of the liver may be single or multiple (Figures 20.5 and 20.6). An identical appearance will be seen in the liver image with congenital

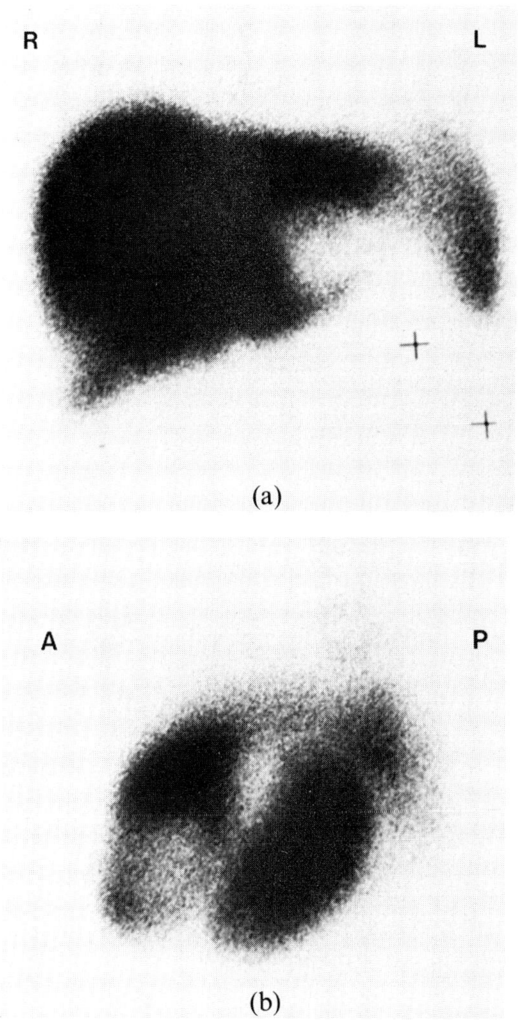

Figure 20.3. Hepatic metastases. Large metastases from colonic carcinoma seen particularly well in the anterior and left lateral images.

and parasitic cysts. In polycystic disease hepatic cysts of widely different sizes may occur and the image appearance is therefore indistinguishable from that of a metastatic liver.[34] If no diagnostic clues are available from the history or from the presence of cysts in other organs, the problem can normally be resolved by ultrasonic examination. This should also always be carried out if parasitic cysts are suspected, to avoid the risk of hepatic needle biopsy.

During the interpretation of liver images for focal disease, care must be taken to avoid pitfalls due to artefacts. Articles external to the patient will attenuate the emitted photon radiation, so that coins, buckles and jewellery will be clearly seen as apparent defects within the liver. The effect of a large right breast, or breast prosthesis, can often be discerned as a region of reduced count-rate over the upper right lobe (Figure 20.7). A faulty gamma camera photomultiplier can produce the appearance of a circumscribed 'lesion' within the liver (Figure 20.8). Certain pathological lesions can also confuse the search for focal liver disease: an enlarged or intrahepatic gallbladder (Figure 20.9), dilated biliary ducts at the porta hepatis,[1] focal impairment of function in cirrhosis[23] or hepatitis [59] can all lead to misinterpretation. In addition, space-occupying lesions of the right kidney can displace the liver so that a concavity is seen on the posterior surface in the right lateral image (Figure 20.10).

Special techniques

A search for focal disease within the liver relies upon the detection of regions of absent radiocolloid accumulation. As the changes seen in the image are usually unrelated to pathogenesis, attempts have been made to use different techniques and radiopharmaceuticals in order to add more specific information to the radiocolloid image.

An assessment of vascularity can be obtained by comparing the count-rate of the lesion with that of surrounding liver tissue during early arrival of the radiocolloid in the hepatic arterial perfusion soon after bolus intravenous administration.[58] This technique has some similarity with contrast angiography and may show an early 'flush' of activity in vascular lesions. Alternatively, radioactivity which does not easily diffuse out of the circulation can be administered, and the vascularity of the lesion is assessed after radiopharmaceutical equilibration within the blood.[31] Radio-isotopes of indium which label transferrin, labelled human serum albumin, or $^{99}Tc^{m}$-labelled red cells are used.

The second approach is to use a radiopharmaceutical which is actively concentrated in tumour or inflammatory tissue. ^{75}Se-selenomethionine has been used since it might be expected to be taken up by actively metabolizing tumour tissue. Uptake is seen in some metastatic tumours, and also in some hepatomas, but this is variable and may require digital subtraction of the colloid image to show the lesion.[24]

A better agent for tumour localization, which is also concentrated in inflammatory lesions, is ^{67}Ga citrate.[21,28] Although ^{67}Ga may be concentrated well in some tumour tissue, its reliability is variable. Unfortunately, it is

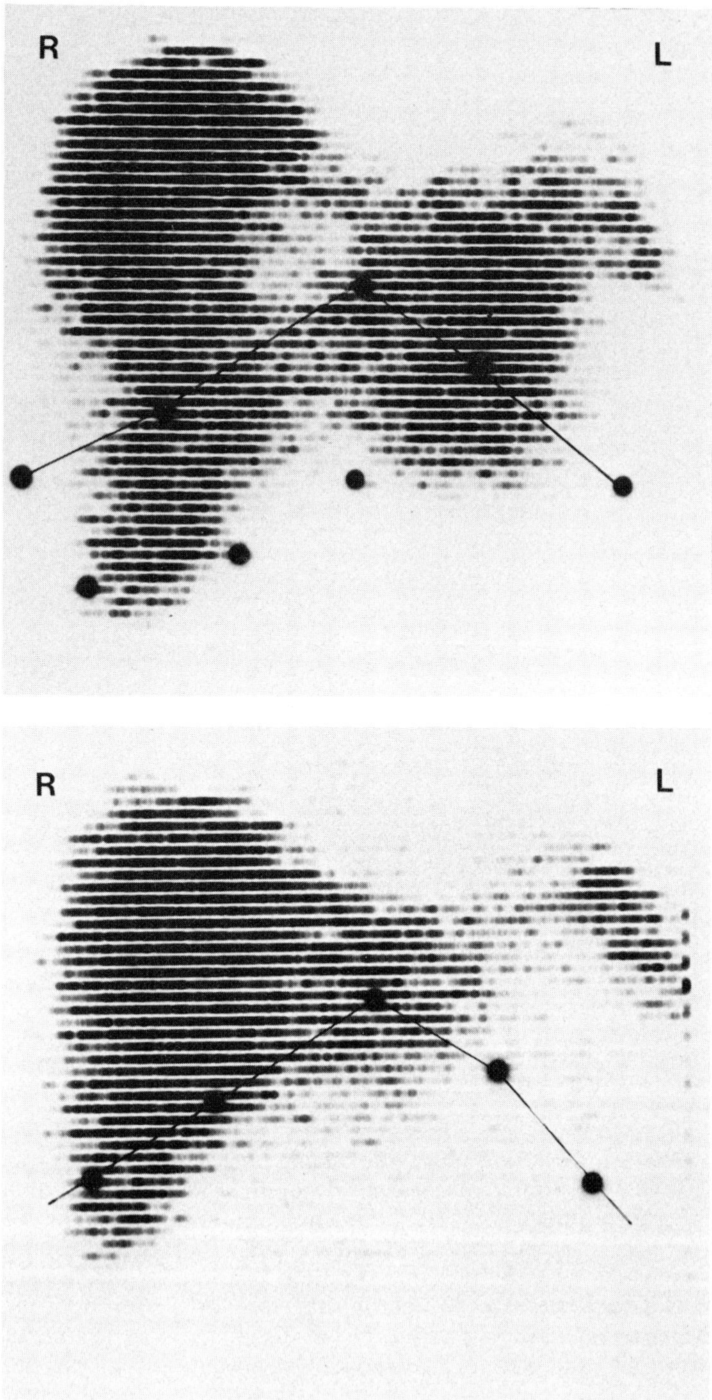

Figure 20.4. Amoebic abscess. (a) Hepatomegaly and amoebic abscess cavity in a Goanese patient with pyrexia, abdominal pain and jaundice; (b) same patient after treatment for three weeks.

concentrated to some extent in the normal liver, and also in the colon, so that colonic cleansing is essential to avoid false positive interpretation.[39] Imaging is usually performed at 48 hours following administration. In spite of the drawbacks of ^{67}Ga, including its cost, it has been used more extensively than other radiopharmaceuticals for the identification of hepatic malignancy, and for the localization of both intrahepatic and extrahepatic abscess cavities.[5]

Although these techniques go some way towards adding specificity to the routine hepatic image, and in some cases have shown a high degree of accuracy, they can seldom alone give the correct diagnosis. For most patients ^{99}Tc^{m}-colloid imaging, followed by liver ultra-

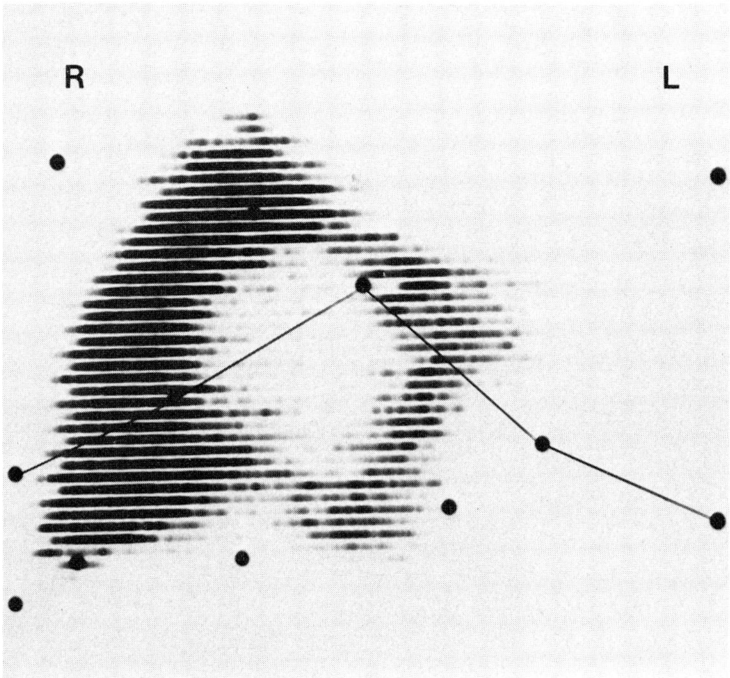

Figure 20.5. Large solitary cyst of the liver, giving obstructive jaundice.

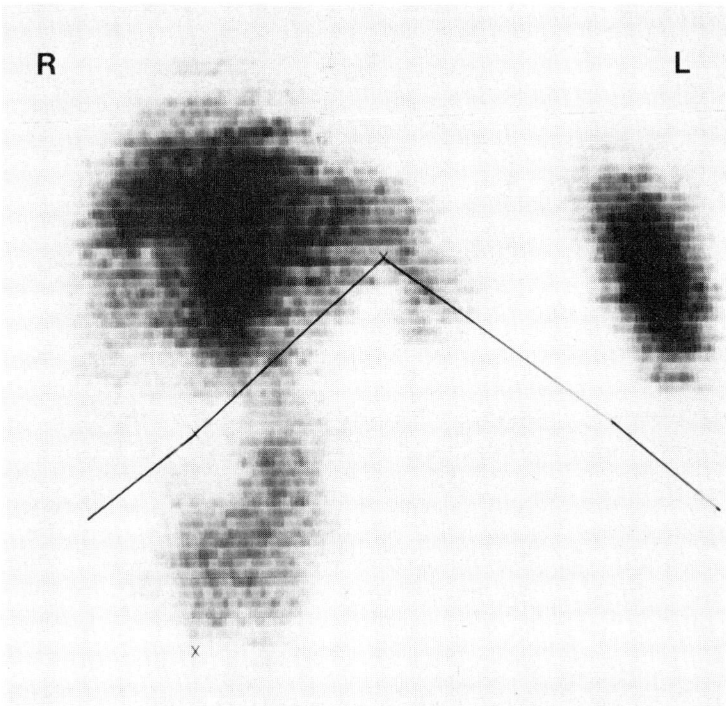

Figure 20.6. Polycystic liver disease. Focal lesions are seen in the right and left lobes of the enlarged liver.

sonography, gives sufficiently reliable information to enable direct intervention to be made for histological confirmation or drainage. Specialized radio-isotope techniques should be reserved for those patients for whom biopsy, or surgery, is contraindicated.

Trauma

The ease with which liver radio-isotope imaging can be carried out as an emergency procedure makes it particularly useful in the investigation of the localization and extent of hepatic

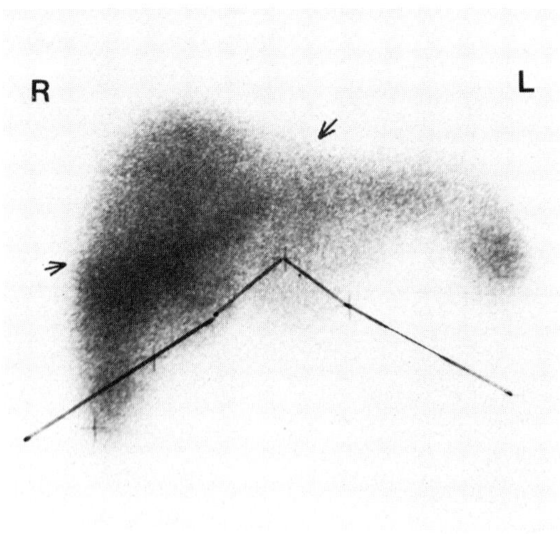

Figure 20.7. (Left.) Breast attenuation. Reduced count-rate from the upper part of the right hepatic lobe due to overlying breast.

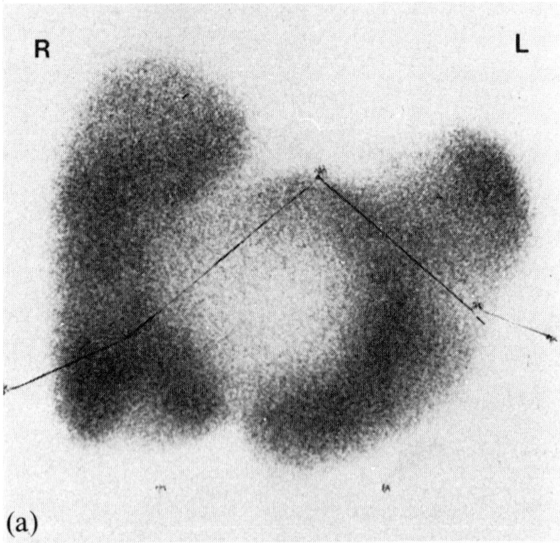

(a)

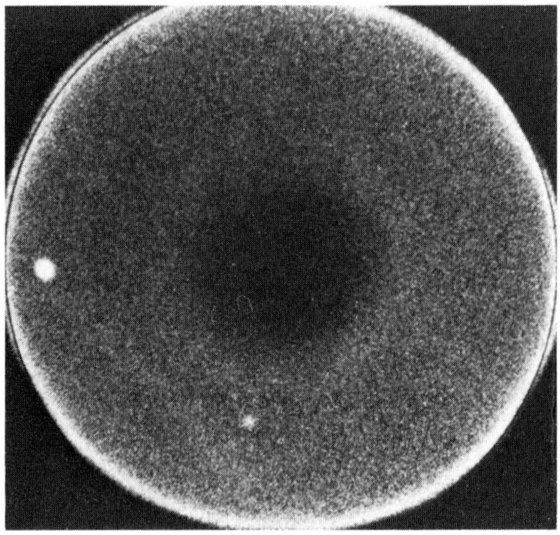

(b)

Figure 20.8. Photomultiplier fault. Apparent large focal lesion in enlarged liver (a) due to a central photomultiplier defect detected in the uniformity source image (b).

injury.[7,12] A subcapsular or parenchymal haematoma can usually be demonstrated, and this information can guide the surgical or medical management of the patient. In addition, serial radio-isotope images can show the resolution of a haematoma, which may take several months, or can show the rate of regeneration following surgery.[6,25]

Diffuse Parenchymal Disease

Irregular and patchy hepatic uptake of radiocolloid is observed in many disorders which alter the normal hepatic function and anatomical architecture. The mechanisms for these appearances include impairment of normal hepatic macrophage function, alterations in blood flow and replacement of liver parenchyma by fibrous tissue. When hepatic function is impaired, the macrophage systems of spleen, bone marrow and lung, which comprise 35 per cent of the total reticuloendothelial system, clear a larger proportion of radiocolloid from the circulation. The appearances seen in the radio-isotope image are an enlarged liver, usually with irregular distribution of activity, splenomegaly with high splenic uptake, and increased uptake of activity in the skeleton (bone marrow), which is seen particularly in the vertebrae, sacroiliac regions and ribs. Rarely, activity may also be seen in the lungs. There are many causes for these appearances and the changes are typically seen in fatty liver, extensive metastatic infiltration, cirrhosis of all types, portal fibrosis and acute and chronic hepatitis.

With fatty infiltration alone, the hepatic image is normally enlarged with little or no

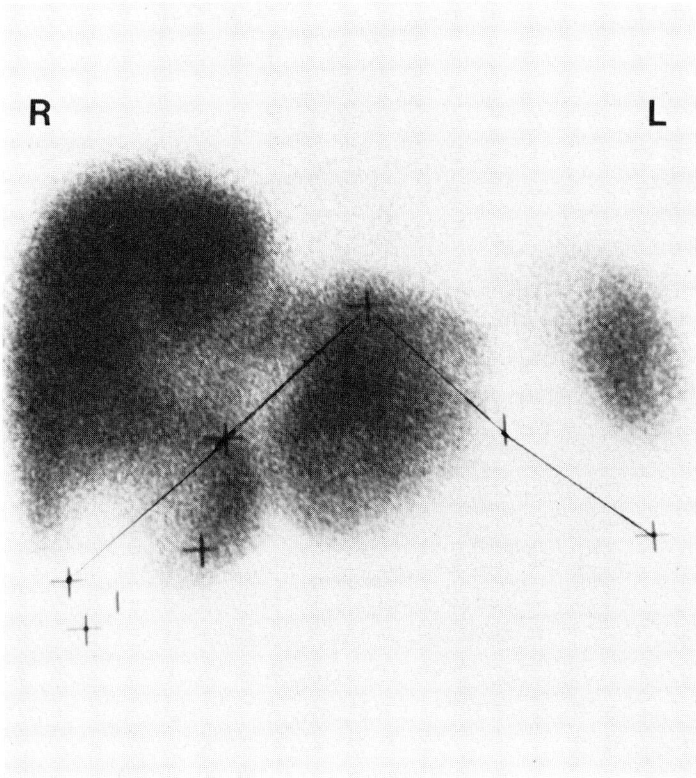

Figure 20.9. Obstructive jaundice. Focal lesion in the lower right hepatic lobe due to enlarged gallbladder; in addition, activity is reduced at the porta hepatis due to biliary dilatation.

increase in splenic activity. Further impairment of hepatic function typical of cirrhosis gives a characteristic pattern of hepatomegaly with patchy colloid distribution, and clear evidence of increased splenic and marrow uptake (Figure 20.11). These findings usually correlate reasonably well with the extent of the disease shown by histological examination[11] although the image appearances alone give little clue as to the aetiology. The relative uptake of activity in the spleen and liver, particularly when expressed as a quantitative ratio, may be used in follow-up studies to show progression of the disease or its response to therapy.

The wide variety of appearances which are seen in many generalized disorders of the liver limit the diagnostic contribution of the radiocolloid image. In Hodgkin's disease, as with other lymphomas, the liver and spleen may show general enlargement, which does not correlate with histological evidence of infiltration (Figure 20.12). The use of radio-isotope imaging for classifying the stage of these diseases has been disappointing.[30] Obstructive jaundice may cause secondary impairment of Kupffer cell function, with patchy uptake of colloid, but more usually a focal loss is seen at the porta hepatis due to distension and dilatation of the hepatic bile ducts. The liver may be small in advanced cirrhosis and in portal vein obstruction, but usually portal vein occlusion does not lead to the high splenic activity expected in cirrhosis. The size of the liver can also be decreased with hepatic infestation in schistosomiasis. In this condition atrophy of the right hepatic lobe may be seen, although in general the appearances are variable, and patients do not necessarily show splenic enlargement with increased activity.[19] A more characteristic appearance may be seen in the Budd–Chiari syndrome. Often the hepatic images of these patients show high uptake of activity centrally in the anterior image, and posteriorly in the right lateral image.[51] This activity probably is in the caudate lobe, which is spared the effects of venous occlusion by its separate venous drainage direct into the inferior vena cava. A similar image appearance is seen with superior vena caval occlusion, when intravenous colloid is administered in the arm. The collateral circulation diverts the active colloid via the umbilical vein into small segments of the liver.[18] Unlike the appearance of the Budd–Chiari syndrome, thrombosis of smaller hepatic veins usually gives a generalized heterogenous uptake of activity which may be confused with metastatic infiltration. In the same way, many other generalized liver disorders may severely affect

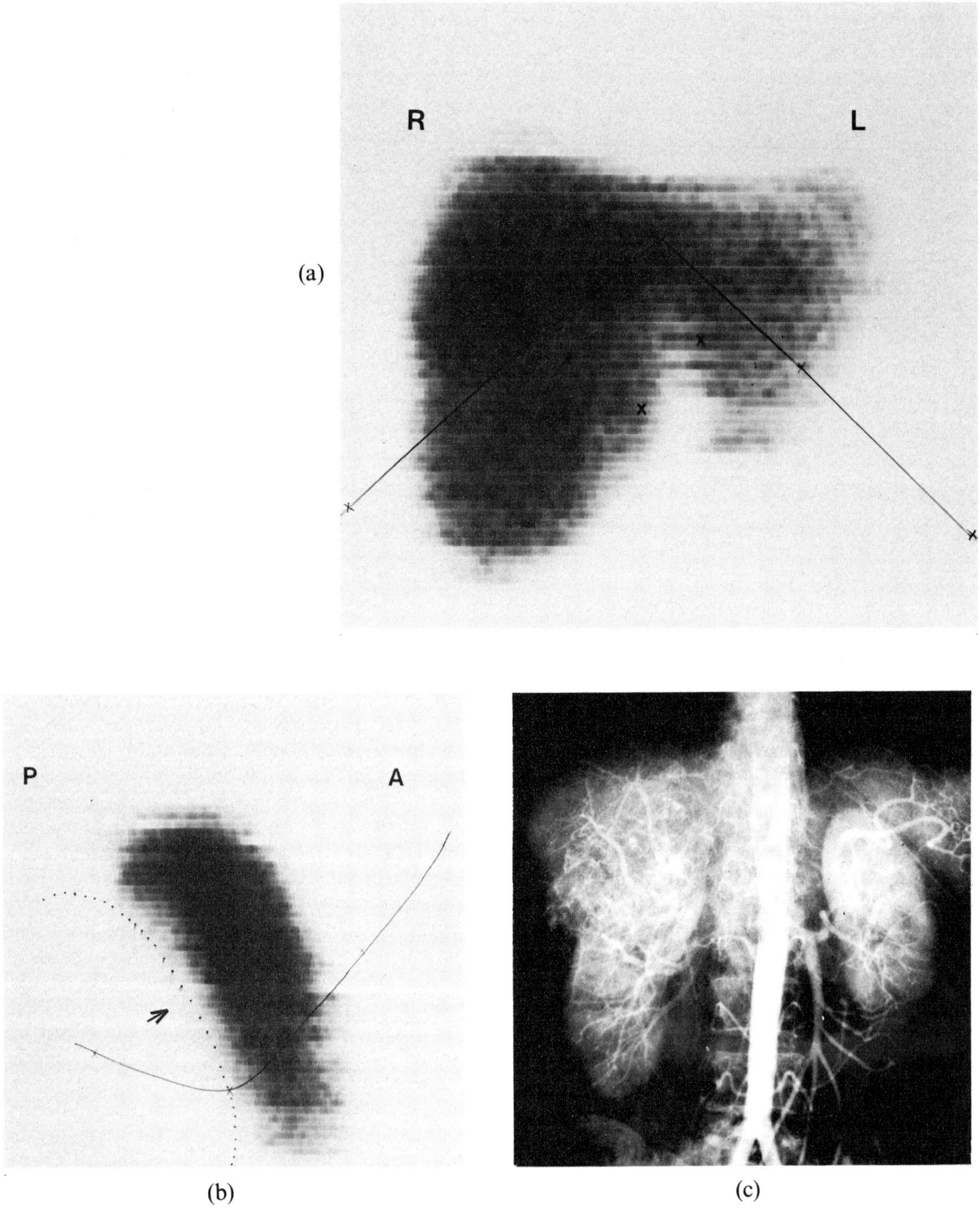

Figure 20.10. Hypernephroma of the right kidney. (a) Anterior hepatic image shows enlargement only; (b) Right lateral image shows concave impression on posterior surface of right hepatic lobe; (c) Abnormal circulation in tumour in upper pole of right kidney displayed by renal arteriography.

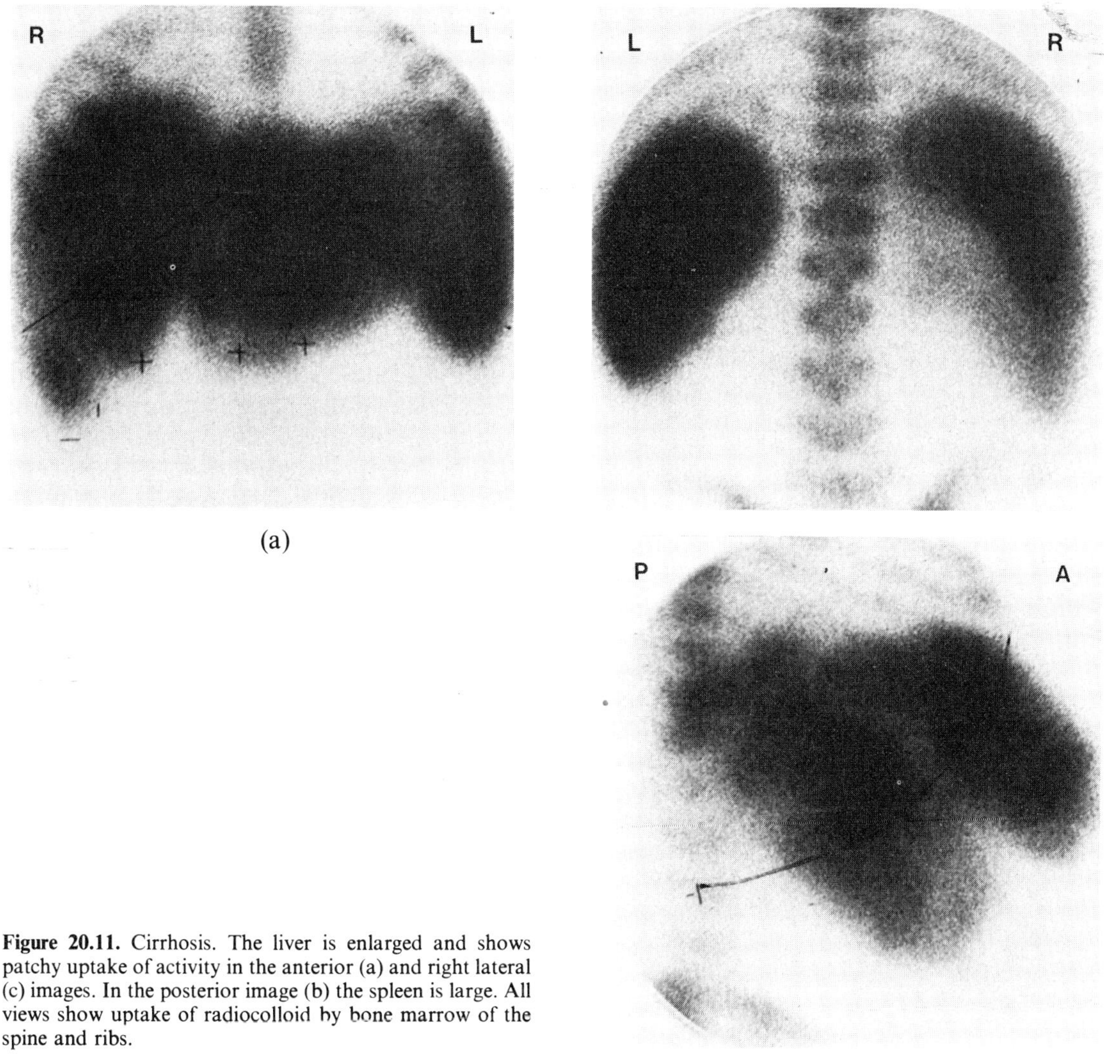

(a) (b) (c)

Figure 20.11. Cirrhosis. The liver is enlarged and shows patchy uptake of activity in the anterior (a) and right lateral (c) images. In the posterior image (b) the spleen is large. All views show uptake of radiocolloid by bone marrow of the spine and ribs.

hepatic function in discrete regions and thus give the appearance of focal disease. These 'pseudo-tumours' are particularly common in cirrhosis, in which they may be mistaken for neoplastic change.

DYNAMIC STUDIES

This term refers to the sequential measurement of changing radioactivity in the liver and other organs. Relative activity levels can be examined as a series of images, or the data contained in the images may be quantified to give a plot of activity levels against time. These studies can be used to give an expression of the functional capacity of the liver to handle labelled compounds, and to show the degree of impairment following pathological change. They have been used mostly to study liver blood flow and the mechanisms of jaundice.

Blood Flow Studies

It was hoped initially that a radio-isotope technique might replace the classical but difficult methods of measuring blood flow using arterial and venous blood sampling.[50] This hope was based on the premise that the liver is the primary site of clearance of activity from the blood, and activity entering it would be cleared in the 'first pass' so that concentration in the venous drainage would be negligible. For many radiopharmaceuticals the first condition is true; radiocolloids and certain radioactive labelled dyes, e.g. rose bengal, are largely cleared from the perfusing arterial or portal blood when the

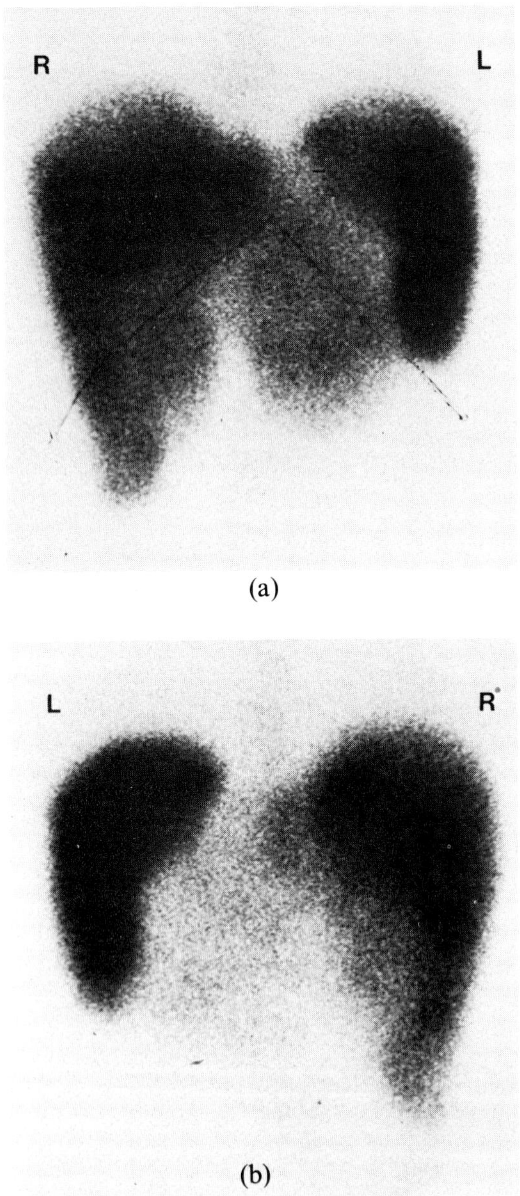

Figure 20.12. Hodgkin's disease. Generalized enlargement of the liver and spleen, with no clear focal lesions and no significant increase in bone marrow uptake.

liver is healthy, although some difference is observed between agents, e.g. between different colloid preparations. But in disease the extraction efficiency for these agents is decreased. In cirrhosis the blood flow to the liver is reduced with intrahepatic shunting, and at the same time the ability to extract colloid is diminished, so that a simple clinical measurement of hepatic clearance of intravenously administered radiocolloid does not by itself give the degree of reduction in hepatic blood flow. Attempts to overcome the problem of extraction efficiency have not been successful since no radiopharmaceutical has yet been found which is cleared totally by either the liver macrophages or polygonal cells under pathological conditions. Intrasplenic injection of larger particles of labelled macro-aggregated albumin has been used to show the relative quantity of portal blood which is shunted past the liver in disease. The size of these particles does not permit passage through the capillary bed so that they become trapped and, under normal circumstances, remain in the liver, showing the distribution of portal perfusion. However, when shunting of the portal circulation takes place particles bypass the liver and are eventually trapped in the pulmonary capillaries. Measurement of the partition of activity between liver and lung gives the degree of portal shunting.[56]

Clinical Studies

For a number of years labelled rose bengal has been used clinically for the study of hepatocyte function and biliary patency. Most studies have concentrated on distinguishing extrahepatic biliary obstruction from jaundice of intrahepatic origin. The degree of success of these studies has varied, but on the whole it has been limited, and the procedure has not been adopted widely for routine investigation of jaundiced patients. Rose bengal can be successfully labelled only with ^{131}I, and this limits the amount that can be administered to patients, due to the relatively high radiation dose delivered by ^{131}I. As a result, the radio-isotope images are of poor quality with inadequate definition of the biliary system. In the last few years a number of new compounds has been developed, all of which can be labelled with $^{99}Tc^{m}$.[60] Of these, the iminodiacetic acid derived compounds, for example HIDA, appear best, since they are rapidly extracted from the blood and excreted through the hepatocytes, giving early and high concentration in bile. Labelling with $^{99}Tc^{m}$ prior to administration is an easy procedure. It is hoped that these radiopharmaceuticals will have a useful role to play in the investigation of jaundice.[42] Demonstration of the major biliary ducts should be of value in defining the level and degree of extrahepatic biliary obstruction (Figures 20.13 and 20.14; and see Chapter 26).

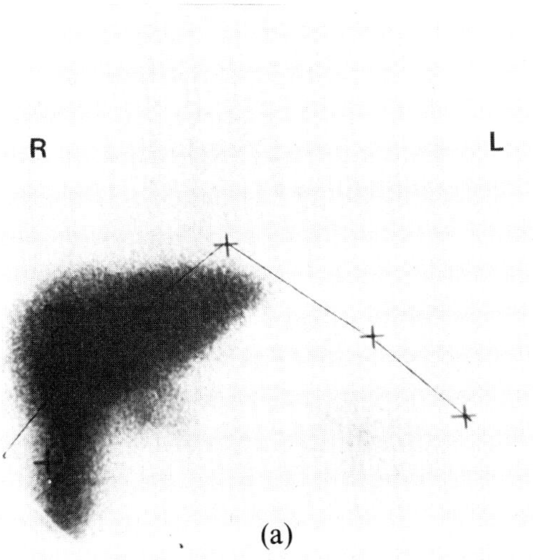

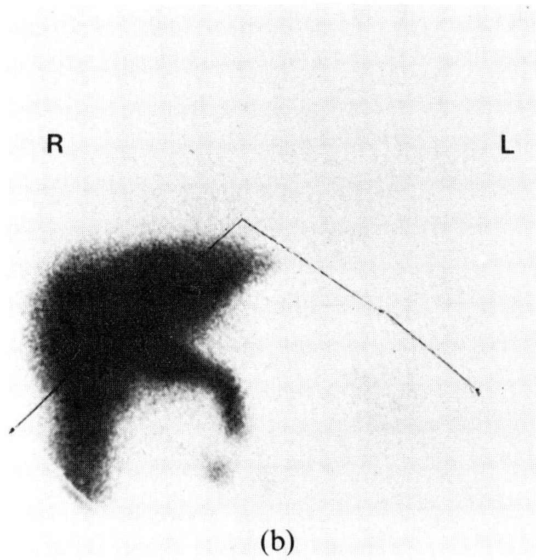

(c)

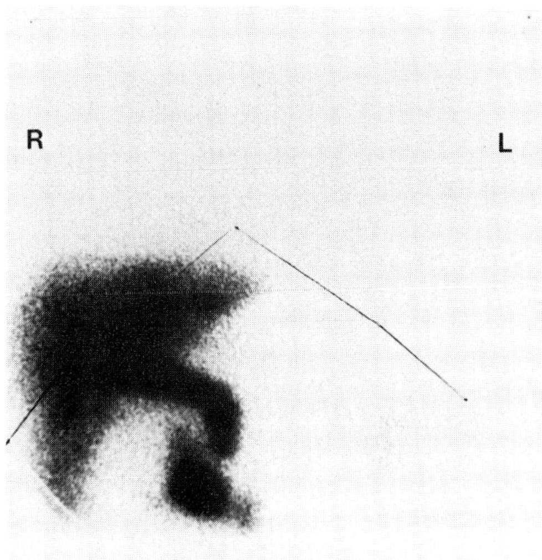

Figure 20.13. Normal hepatobiliary images ($^{99}Tc^m$-HIDA). (a) Normal concentration of activity by the liver at 10 minutes; (b) Activity in biliary ducts at 30 minutes, but no concentration is present in the gallbladder (previous cholecystectomy); (c) At 45 minutes, activity has passed into the intestine.

PAEDIATRIC INVESTIGATIONS

The non-invasive nature of radio-isotope investigations makes them particularly suited for the investigation of children. With reassurance and mild sedation the child can be persuaded to lie quietly under a gamma camera, and a good-quality image can be obtained with the administered dose of radiopharmaceutical kept to a minimum. A converging collimator, which gives magnification of the image size and enhanced spatial resolution, can be used for smaller children.

The indications for paediatric study include investigation of hepatosplenomegaly, diagnosis of a space-occupying lesion, assessment of congenital abnormalities, and detection of extrahepatic lesions, e.g. renal masses, which cause extrinsic pressure on the liver. $^{99}Tc^m$ sulphur colloid is used, and the technique is very similar to that for adults.[55]

Radio-isotopes have been used particularly in the investigation of neonatal cholestasis. Sequential imaging by a gamma camera with data acquisition following intravenous administration of ^{131}I rose bengal can help to distinguish between neonatal hepatitis and biliary atresia. Infants who have a patent biliary system show prompt, or at least only moderately delayed, arrival of activity in the intestinal region; failure to excrete activity over a period of up to one week strongly suggests a diagnosis of biliary atresia. Silverberg, Rosenthal and Freeman[46] emphasize the importance of extending the investigation over several

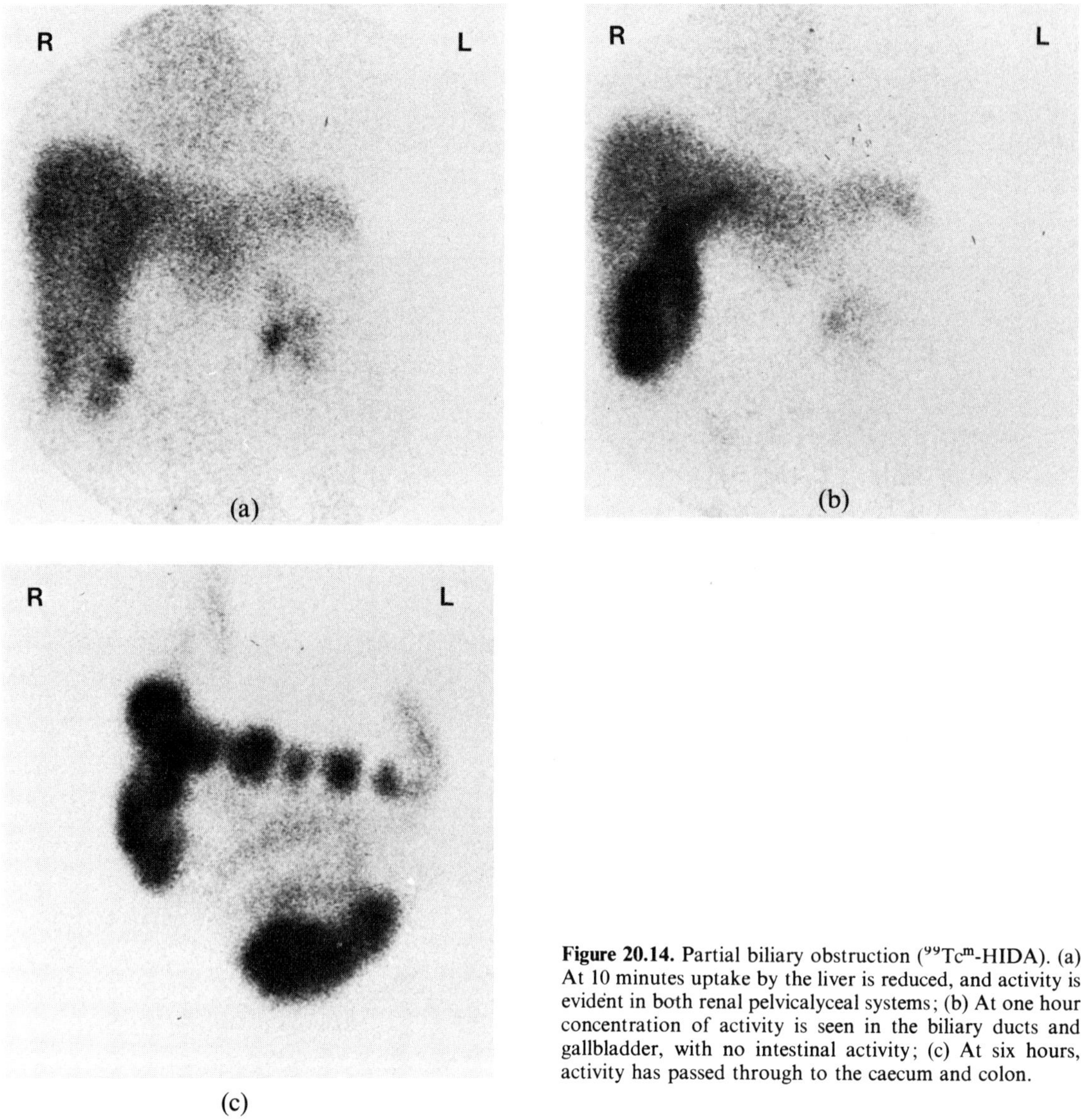

Figure 20.14. Partial biliary obstruction ($^{99}Tc^m$-HIDA). (a) At 10 minutes uptake by the liver is reduced, and activity is evident in both renal pelvicalyceal systems; (b) At one hour concentration of activity is seen in the biliary ducts and gallbladder, with no intestinal activity; (c) At six hours, activity has passed through to the caecum and colon.

days in order not to miss delayed excretion of activity through a partially patent biliary system, and they also point out the risk of mistaking intestinal activity for that accumulated in the kidneys due to increased renal clearance of rose bengal in severe jaundice. Radio-isotope imaging procedures have advantages over measurements of faecal activity, when it may be difficult to avoid contamination of specimens by radioactivity excreted in the urine (Figure 20.15). Studies in young pigs suggest that the new $^{99}Tc^m$ hepatobiliary agents may be able to detect extrahepatic biliary obstruction in early life, and assist in the diagnosis of biliary atresia.[22] It has yet to be shown if this will be successful in humans.

SUMMARY

The rapid and extensive advances which have taken place in organ imaging in recent years make it necessary to define precisely the validity of radio-isotope liver and biliary imaging, so that it takes its proper place in the diagnostic assessment of patients with hepatic disorders. Its accuracy in the detection of focal intrahepatic lesions is good – about 80 per cent, which is better than that reported for blind hepatic biopsy or biochemical evaluation.[43]

Its interrelationship to grey-scale ultrasound imaging and computerized axial tomography is still not established with certainty. Both these techniques have the advantage of better

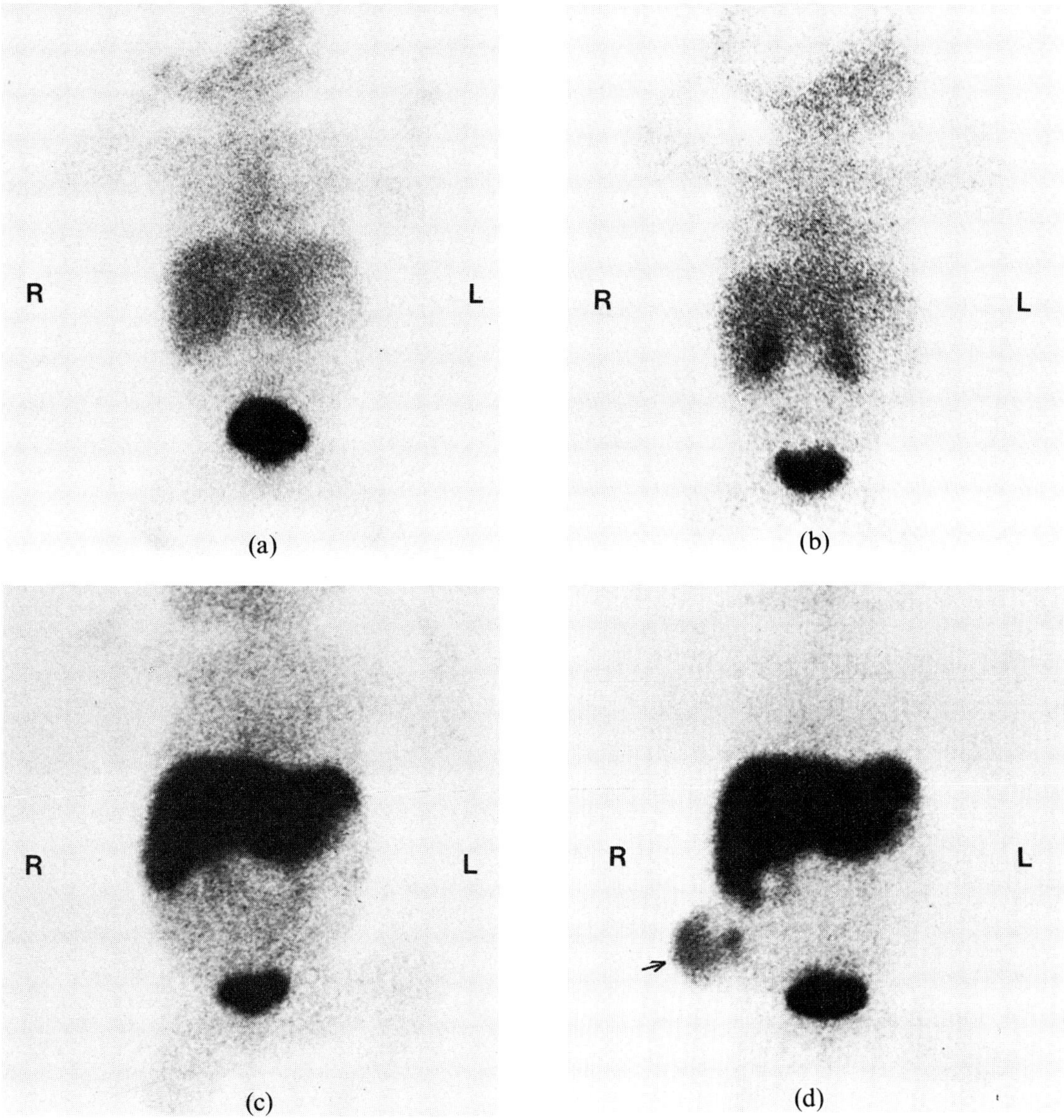

Figure 20.15. Biliary atresia ($^{99}Tc^{m}$-HIDA). Investigation at age of three months showed poor hepatic uptake and increased renal clearance at 10 minutes (a) and 45 minutes (b). After surgical porto-enterostomy hepatic uptake is improved at 10 minutes (c) and activity is concentrated in biliary drainage bag (arrowed) at 30 minutes (d).

diagnostic specificity for hepatic lesions and are able to show other abdominal viscera. This is of value in the recognition of disease in organs related to the liver, such as the biliary system, pancreas and kidneys. Grey-scale ultrasound is already being used in many centres for routine evaluation of the liver, but it requires careful attention to technique and interpretation for successful diagnosis. Even if these conditions are satisfied, focal lesions which are seen in the radio-isotope image may be missed. It seems likely that both techniques will play a complementary role in the future.

The place of radio-isotopes in diffuse hepatic disease is less certain. Imaging gives a quantitative measurement of overall hepatic function, but is unlikely ever to replace histology and biochemistry for the diagnosis and classification of acute and chronic liver disease. It may be used to add morphological and functional information to the total picture of hepatic pathology and has a potential role as a non-invasive method of assessing the progression or regression of hepatic disorders.

REFERENCES

1. Agnew, J.E., James, O. & Bouchier, I.A.D. (1975) Liver and pancreas scanning in extrahepatic obstructive jaundice (with special reference to tumours of the bile and hepatic ducts). *British Journal of Radiology*, **48,** 190–199.
2. Conn, H.O. (1972) Rational use of liver biopsy in the diagnosis of hepatic cancer. *Gastroenterology*, **62,** 142–146.
3. Cuaron, A., Sepulveda, B. & Landa, L. (1965) Topographic distribution of amoebic abscesses studied by liver scanning. *International Journal of Applied Radiation and Isotopes*, **16,** 603–609.
4. Custer, J.R. & Shafer, R.B. (1975) Changes in liver scan following splenectomy. *Journal of Nuclear Medicine*, **16,** 194–195.
5. Damron, J.R., Beihn, R.M., Selby, J.B. & Rosenbaum, H.D. (1974) Gallium–technetium subtraction scanning for the localisation of subphrenic abscess. *Radiology*, **113,** 117–122.
6. Deland, F.H. & Wagner, N.H. (1968) Regeneration of the liver after hepatectomy. *Journal of Nuclear Medicine*, **9,** 587–589.
7. Evans, G.W., Curtin, F.G., McCarthy, H.F. & Kiernan, J.H. (1972) Scintigraphy in traumatic lesions of liver and spleen. *Journal of the American Medical Association*, **6,** 665–667.
8. Fee, H.J., Prokop, E.K., Cameron, J.L. & Wagner, H.N. (1974) Liver scanning in patients with suspected abdominal tumour. *Journal of the American Medical Association*, **230,** 1675–1677.
9. Freeman, L.M., Meng, C.H., Johnson, P.M., Berstein, R.G. & Bosniak, M.A. (1969) False positive liver scans caused by disease processes in adjacent organs and structures. *British Journal of Radiology*, **42,** 651–656.
10. Gammill, S.L., Takahashi, M., Jingu, K., Stumpe, W. & Font, R. (1975) A comparison of scans and angiograms in selecting patients with hepatomas for hepatic lobectomy. *American Journal of Roentgenology, Radium Therapy and Nuclear Medicine*, **123,** 522–530.
11. Geslien, G.E., Pinsky, S.M., Poth, R.K. & Johnson, M.C. (1976) The sensitivity and specificity of 99mTc-sulphur colloid liver imaging in diffuse hepatocellular disease. *Radiology*, **118,** 115–119.
12. Gilday, D.L. & Alderson, P.O. (1974) Scintigraphic evaluation of liver and spleen injury. *Seminars in Nuclear Medicine*, **4,** 357–370.
13. Grossman, Z.D., Wistow, B.W., Bryan, P.J., Dinn, W.M., McAfee, J.G. & Kieffer, S.A. (1977) Radionuclide imaging, computed tomography and grey-scale ultrasonography of the liver: a comparative study. *Journal of Nuclear Medicine*, **18,** 327–332.
14. Halpern, S., Coel, M., Ashburn, W., Alazraki, N., Littenberg, R., Hurwitz, S. & Green, J. (1974) Correlation of the liver and spleen size. *Archives of Internal Medicine*, **134,** 123–124.
15. Hatfield, P.M. (1975) Role of liver scanning in the diagnosis of hepatic metastases. *Medical Clinics of North America*, **59,** 247–276.
16. Holder, L.E. & Saenger, E.L. (1975) The use of nuclear medicine in evaluating liver disease. *Seminars in Roentgenology*, **10,** 215–222.
17. Holder, L.E., Ashare, A.B., Tomsick, T., Colley, D.P., Fernandez, M., Catz, S. & Saenger, E.L. (1975) The gamut approach to scintigram interpretation – diagnostic aid and teaching method. *Journal of Nuclear Medicine*, **16,** 1121–1124.
18. Holmquest, D.L. & Burdine, J.A. (1973) Caval-portal shunting as a cause of a focal increase in radiocolloid uptake in normal livers. *Journal of Nuclear Medicine*, **14,** 348–351.
19. Iio, M., Iuchi, M., Kitani, K., Yamada, H., Ishiwa, M., Kameda, H. & Chiba, K. (1971) Scintigraphic evaluation of the liver with schistosomiasis japonica. *Journal of Nuclear Medicine*, **12,** 655–659.
20. ICRP Publication 17 (1969) Protection of the patient in radionuclide investigations. *Report prepared for the International Commission on Radiological Protection 1969*. Oxford, New York: Pergamon Press.
21. James, O., Wood, E.J. & Sherlock, S. (1974) ^{67}Ga scanning in the diagnosis of liver disease. *Gut*, **15,** 404–410.
22. Jenner, R.E., Clarke, M.B. & Howard, E.R. (1976) Liver and gall-bladder imaging with technetium-99m dihydrothiotic acid and technetium-99m pyridoxoline glutamate – a study in the young pig. *British Journal of Radiology*, **49,** 852–857.
23. Johnson, P.M. & Sweeney, W.A. (1967) The false-positive hepatic scan. *Journal of Nuclear Medicine*, **8,** 451–460.
24. Kaplan, E. & Domingo, M. (1972) ^{75}Se-selenomethionine in hepatic focal lesions. *Seminars in Nuclear Medicine*, **2,** 139–149.
25. Karran, S.J., Leach, K.G. & Blumgart, L.H. (1974) Assessment of liver regeneration in the rat using the gamma camera. *Journal of Nuclear Medicine*, **15,** 10–16.
26. Kido, C. (1975) Primary liver cancer (angiography and scintigraphy). *Australasian Radiology*, **19,** 129–139.
27. Kim, D.K., McSweeney, S.D. & Yeh, J. (1975) Tumours of liver as demonstrated by scan and laparotomy. *Surgery, Gynecology and Obstetrics*, **141,** 409–410.
28. Lavender, J.P., Lowe, J., Barker, J.R., Burn, J.I. & Chaudhri, M.A. (1971) Gallium 67 citrate scanning in neoplastic and inflammatory lesions. *British Journal of Radiology*, **44,** 361–366.
29. Lerona, P.T., Go, R.T. & Cornell, S.H. (1974) Limitations of angiography and scanning in diagnosis of liver masses. *Radiology*, **112,** 139–145.
30. Lipton, M.J., Denardo, G.L., Silverman, S. & Glatstein, E. (1972) Evaluation of the liver and spleen in Hodgkin's disease. 1. The value of hepatic scintigraphy. *American Journal of Medicine*, **52,** 356–361.
31. Lubin, E. & Lewitus, Z. (1972) Blood pool scanning in investigating hepatic mass lesions. *Seminars in Nuclear Medicine*, **2,** 128–132.
32. Lunia, S., Parthasarathy, S., Bakshi, S. & Bender, M.A. (1975) An evaluation of 99mTc-sulfur colloid liver scintiscans and their usefulness in metastatic work-up: a review of 1,424 studies. *Journal of Nuclear Medicine*, **16,** 62–65.
33. McAfee, J.G., Ause, R.G. & Wagner, H.N. (1965) Diagnostic value of scintillation scanning of the liver. *Archives of Internal Medicine*, **116,** 95–110.
34. McCready, V.R. (1972) Scintigraphic studies of space-occupying liver disease. *Seminars in Nuclear Medicine*, **2,** 108–127.
35. McIntyre, P.A. (1972) Diagnostic significance of the spleen scan. *Seminars in Nuclear Medicine*, **2,** 278–287.
36. Nishiyama, H., Lewis, J.T., Ashare, A.B. & Saenger, E.L. (1975) Interpretation of radionuclide liver images: do training and experience make a difference? *Journal of Nuclear Medicine*, **16,** 11–16.

37. Operchal, J.A., Bowen, R.D. & Grove, R.B. (1976) Efficacy of radionuclide procedures in staging bronchogenic carcinoma. *Journal of Nuclear Medicine,* **17,** 530.
38. Oster, Z.H., Larson, S.M., Strauss, H.W. & Wagner, H.N. (1975) Analysis of liver scanning in a general hospital. *Journal of Nuclear Medicine,* **16,** 450–453.
39. Pinsky, S.M. & Henkin, R.E. (1976) Gallium-67 tumour scanning. *Seminars in Nuclear Medicine,* **6,** 397–409.
40. Ranson, J.H., Madayag, M.A., Localio, S.A. & Spencer, F.C. (1975) New diagnostic and therapeutic techniques in the management of pyogenic liver abscesses. *Annals of Surgery,* **181,** 508–518.
41. Rollo, F.D. & Deland, F.H. (1968) The determination of liver mass from radionuclide images. *Radiology,* **91,** 1191–1194.
42. Ronai, P.M. (1977) Hepatobiliary radiopharmaceuticals: defining their clinical role will be a galling experience. *Journal of Nuclear Medicine,* **18,** 488–490.
43. Rothschild, M.A. (1976) Hepatic radionuclide imaging: an effective diagnostic procedure! *American Journal of Digestive Diseases,* **21,** 655–659.
44. Schraibman, I.G. (1974) Non-parasitic liver abscess. *British Journal of Surgery,* **61,** 709–712.
45. Sears, H.F., Gerber, F.H., Sturtz, D.L. & Fouty, W.J. (1975) Liver scan and carcinoma of the breast. *Surgery, Gynecology and Obstetrics,* **140,** 409–411.
46. Silverberg, M., Rosenthal, L. & Freeman, L.M. (1973) Rose bengal excretion studies as an aid in the differential diagnosis of neonatal jaundice. *Seminars in Nuclear Medicine,* **3,** 69–80.
47. Soucek, C.D. (1975) Foramen of Morgagni hernia diagnosed by liver scan. *Journal of Nuclear Medicine,* **16,** 261–263.
48. Spencer, R.P., Hosian, F. & Spitznagle, L.A. (1976) Kinetics and dosimetry of radiopharmaceuticals in evaluating liver, gall bladder and spleen. In *Radiopharmaceutical Dosimetry Symposium. Proceedings of conference held at Oak Ridge, Tennessee, April 26–29* (Ed.) Cloutier, R.J. pp. 256–266. Department of Health, Education and Welfare.
49. Sullivan, S., Krasner, N. & Williams, R. (1976) The clinical estimation of liver size: a comparison of techniques and an analysis of the source of error. *British Medical Journal,* **ii,** 1042–1043.
50. Taplin, G.V. (1971) Review paper: Dynamic studies of liver function with radioisotopes. In *Dynamic Studies with Radioisotopes in Medicine: Proceedings.* pp. 373–392. Rotterdam: International Atomic Energy Agency.
51. Tavill, A.S., Wood, E.J., Kreel, L., Jones, E.A., Gregory, M. & Sherlock, S. (1975) The Budd-Chiari syndrome: correlation between hepatic scintigraphy and the clinical, radiological and pathological findings in nineteen cases of hepatic venous outflow obstruction. *Gastroenterology,* **68,** 509–518.
52. Taylor, R.D., Anderson, P.M., Winston, M.A. & Blahd, W.H. (1976) Diagnosis of hepatic hemangioma using multiple radionuclide and ultrasound techniques. *Journal of Nuclear Medicine,* **17,** 362–364.
53. Taylor, K.J., Sullivan, D.C., Rosenfield, A.T. & Gottschalk, A. (1977) Grayscale ultrasound and isotope scanning: complementary techniques for imaging the liver. *American Journal of Roentgenology,* **128,** 277–281.
54. Tonami, N., Aburano, T. & Hisada, K. (1975) Comparison of alpha 1 fetoprotein radioimmunoassay method and liver scanning for detecting primary hepatic cell carcinoma. *Cancer,* **36,** 466–470.
55. Treves, S. & Spencer, R.P. (1973) Liver and spleen scintigraphy in children. *Seminars in Nuclear Medicine,* **3,** 55–68.
56. Ueda, H., Kitani, K., Kameda, H., Yamada, H. & Iio, M. (1967) Detection of hepatic shunts by the use of ^{131}I-macroaggregated albumin. *Gastroenterology,* **52,** 480–487.
57. Uszler, J.M. & Swanson, L.A. (1975) Focal nodular hyperplasia of the liver: case report. *Journal of Nuclear Medicine,* **16,** 831–832.
58. Waxman, A.D., Finck, E.J. & Siemsen, J.K. (1974) Combined contrast and radionuclide angiography of the liver. *Radiology,* **113,** 123–129.
59. Winston, M.A. & Shapiro, M. (1974) Pseudotumours in acute hepatitis. *Journal of Nuclear Medicine,* **15,** 1039–1040.
60. Wistow, B.W., Subramanian, G., van Heertum, R.L., Henderson, R.W., Gagne, G.M., Hall, R.C. & McAfee, J.G. (1977) An evaluation of 99mTc-labelled hepatobiliary agents. *Journal of Nuclear Medicine,* **18,** 455–461.
61. Yeung, W.C., Haines, J.E. & Larson, S.M. (1976) Diagnosis of posterolateral congenital diaphragmatic (Bochdalek) hernia by liver scintigram: case report. *Journal of Nuclear Medicine,* **17,** 110–112.

Chapter 21

Ultrasound Imaging and Computed Tomography

K.C. DEWBURY
H.B. MEIRE
J.E. HUSBAND

ULTRASOUND: INTRODUCTION

Diagnostic procedures using ultrasound are painless, harmless, relatively inexpensive and have no contraindications at the intensities used. The liver is perhaps the one organ in which ultrasound can offer more diagnostic information than it can for any other organ, and in this chapter its main diagnostic uses and some indication as to its current limitations are included.

PRINCIPLES OF ULTRASOUND

In order to understand the value and limitations of ultrasound it is helpful to have at least some knowledge of the basic principles involved in production of the images.

Diagnostic ultrasound scanners utilize very short pulses (about one-millionth of a second) of high frequency sound, usually two to five million cycles per second. At this very high frequency sound can be focused into a fine beam a few millimetres in diameter, and when this beam impinges on the junction between two substances of different density and elasticity a proportion of it is reflected, as in marine echo sounding. Diagnostic scanners employ a transducer which acts both as transmitter and receiver of the sound. When scanning a patient this is held in contact with the skin and moved over the region of interest. To ensure good acoustic contact between transducer and skin, the skin is coated with oil or another suitable coupling medium. Electronic devices record the position of the transducer and also calculate the precise position of any tissue discontinuities (interfaces) from which echoes are received. The received echoes are displayed as dots on the screen, the position of each dot corresponding to the locus of the interface which gave rise to that echo. In general, there are more echoes from heterogeneous tissues than from homogeneous tissues. Higher level or bright echoes are received from interfaces between tissues with large differences in acoustic impedence. More homogeneous tissues cause lower amplitude echoes which are displayed as grey dots; the lower the amplitude the darker the grey. Fluid-filled spaces generate no echoes and so appear black. As the transducer is moved over the patient an image is therefore built up of all the interfaces contained within the thin slice of the patient over which the transducer has been moved.

The limitations of the system result from total reflection of sound at gas/soft tissue or bone/soft tissue interfaces. In practice, therefore, ultrasound cannot see through gas or bone and, when the liver is examined, the interposition of ribs or bowel gas between liver and transducer has to be avoided. This is possible in over 80 per cent of patients, failures occurring in patients with high diaphragms, low ribs or excessive upper abdominal bowel gas.

SCANNING TECHNIQUE

It is preferable to examine the liver with the patient maintaining suspended deep inspiration. Since each scan takes only about one second to perform this is generally possible. If the patient has pulmonary emphysema or hepatomegaly, inspiration may be unnecessary. No patient preparation is necessary except for attempts at reducing bowel gas in patients who have had a failed examination from this cause.

Since each scan examines only a thin slice of liver it is essential to perform many adjacent scans to image the whole volume of the organ. Most operators employ a series of longitudinal scans initially, each of these corresponding to the lateral view of a parasagittal section. It is generally advisable to perform transverse scans also, to facilitate imaging of the extreme lateral portion of the right lobe and to verify the nature of structures seen on the longitudinal scans. By convention, the transverse scans are displayed as if the section is viewed from the foot of the bed, perhaps because the apparatus was developed by a gynaecologist!

NORMAL ULTRASOUND APPEARANCES

An appreciation of the normal ultrasound appearances in the upper abdomen is essential to the understanding of the pathological variations discussed in the following sections. The best assessment of the liver parenchyma is made in the longitudinal scan. The liver parenchyma produces a soft, even, low-level echo pattern, which is interspersed with higher-level echoes from the portal vein walls (Figure 21.1). These vascular echoes form rings or parallel lines depending on the plane in which the vessel is cut by the ultrasound beam. Hepatic veins within the liver are seen as echo-free rings or tubular structures with no surrounding bright echoes.[6] In addition to the left and right lobes of the liver, the caudate lobe is also often seen lying cephalad and posterior to the portal vein and anterior to the inferior vena cava. In our experience this lobe may rarely show an echo pattern which differs from that of the remainder of the liver. The superior and posterior surface of the liver is clearly defined by the diaphragm, identified as a thin, bright bow. The posterior surface is usually also partly defined by the right kidney, well seen through the ultrasound 'window' of the liver. The inferior surface forms a smooth concave border under which the gallbladder is usually found. This surface of the liver may be partially obscured by colonic gas. The normal gallbladder is a smooth, pear-shaped, echo-free sac.

On technically good scans it is always possible to identify a large number of vascular structures in the upper abdomen, both intra- and extrahepatic. The extrahepatic portal system is best seen on the transverse scan. At the level of the first lumbar vertebra the inferior vena cava and aorta lie anteriorly to right and left of the spine. Just anterior to the aorta a small echo-free ring surrounded by a bright cuff of echoes represents the superior mesenteric artery. Anterior to these vessels the splenic and then portal veins are seen passing across the midline to enter the liver anterior to the inferior vena cava. At this point the right portal vein usually extends onwards into the hepatic parenchyma. On a longitudinal scan just to the right of the aorta the superior mesenteric vein is seen running up to join the splenic vein, so forming the portal vein.

The body of the pancreas lies parallel to the splenic vein and a little below and anterior to it. The superior mesenteric artery and superior mesenteric vein pass through the head of the pancreas, the majority of the head lying above and anterior to these vessels (Figure 21.2). Identification of these landmarks on longitudinal and transverse scans aids in the accurate localization of the pancreas, allowing its visualization in some 80 per cent of normal patients.[27] For visualization of head, body and tail on a single section an oblique scan may be more suitable than a transverse scan.

The normal intrahepatic biliary tree is not visualized, although very occasionally the main hepatic ducts and the common bile duct may be traced in some patients.

DIAGNOSIS OF LIVER DISEASE

Patients are generally referred for liver ultrasound examination for one of the following main reasons:

1. Confirmation of hepatomegaly and determination of its cause.

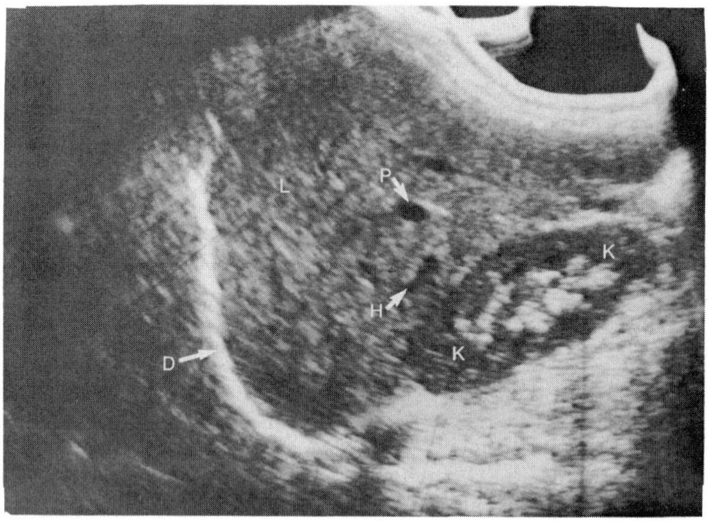

Figure 21.1. Longitudinal scan of right lobe of normal liver. L – liver. K – kidney. H – hepatic vein. P – portal vein branch. D – diaphragm.

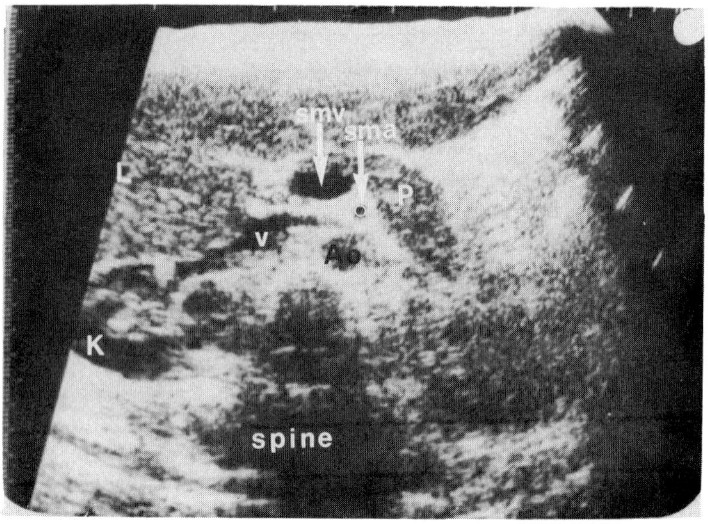

Figure 21.2. Transverse scan of upper abdomen showing pancreas and adjacent vessels. L – liver. K – kidney. Ao – aorta. V – vena cava. SMA – superior mesenteric artery. SMV – superior mesenteric vein. P – pancreas.

2. Further investigation of an abnormal isotope image.
3. Confirmation or exclusion of hepatic metastases after diagnosis of primary malignancy.
4. Investigation of jaundice.

Hepatomegaly may, of course, also be present in patients in group 2 or be caused by metastatic disease. These categories are therefore somewhat artificial, but are perhaps helpful from the clinical viewpoint.

Hepatomegaly

When examining a patient with suspected hepatomegaly one must firstly exclude non-hepatic causes for this clinical finding. The common cause is a low, flat diaphragm secondary to pulmonary emphysema and this is very easily seen at ultrasound examination. Non-hepatic masses inferior to the liver may also be detected and can generally be shown to be extrahepatic. Lesions arising in the upper pole of the right kidney displace the liver anteriorly and inferiorly and may be clinically indistinguishable from genuine hepatomegaly. A Riedel's lobe is easily identified by ultrasound and is shown to be of the same echo consistency as the remainder of the liver.

Clinical assessment of liver size is rather subjective whilst ultrasound images yield objective measurements. However, the shape of the liver varies considerably from one patient to another and its volume will depend on the patient's build. It is therefore difficult to confirm or exclude hepatomegaly with absolute confidence in any one case without making liver volume measurements. In practice, however, an adequate assessment of liver size can be made by eye, based on a series of longitudinal scans. If necessary, an accurate measurement of liver volume can be made by taking serial longitudinal scans at known intervals, measuring the area of liver seen on each and adding all the areas together after allowing for slice thickness (scan spacing).[7] This technique is useful for monitoring changes in liver volume during therapy but is seldom necessary for the actual diagnosis of hepatomegaly.

Whilst we have so far discussed liver enlargement, the disease processes which may cause this may also be present in normal- or small-sized livers and we will therefore now discuss the different forms of liver disease which can be demonstrated or diagnosed by ultrasound.

Focal Disease

This may be unifocal or multifocal, benign or malignant and may have been previously diagnosed by other techniques or initially diagnosed at the time of the ultrasound examination.

Isotope scanning detects focal disease as 'cold' areas, but can usually give no further differential diagnosis. Ultrasound imaging, however, will reliably differentiate many forms of focal disease and we shall now consider each in turn, dealing with benign conditions first.

Benign

The commonest abnormality in this group seen in our patients has been simple cyst. These are usually single, though occasionally three or four may be present. They are seen as clearly-defined, echo-free spaces with thin walls and accentuation of the echoes from distal structures (Figure 21.3). Their size can be accurately measured and followed by serial scans if required. When these cysts are seen, especially if they are multiple, one should also examine the kidneys and pancreas for cysts. The polycystic liver is unlikely to be diagnosed initially by ultrasound but we have seen localized areas of this disease in patients with polycystic kidneys.

Hydatid cysts are not often seen in the UK but nevertheless will occasionally present. These may be multiple, usually have thicker walls which may be laminated, and frequently daughter cysts can be seen within the main cyst. Not uncommonly, a hydatid cyst will present as a single, simple, thin-walled cyst and thus this diagnosis can never be ruled out by ultrasound when a cyst is detected.

Rarely, metastases may become cystic but these will be discussed in the following section. Liver abscesses are also readily demonstrated by ultrasound.[23] Since the centre of these abscesses contains fluid, they appear as thick-walled cysts, the inner margin being very irregular (Figure 21.4). The quantity of fluid present and the wall thickness will depend on the stage in the natural history of the disorder when the scan is performed. A rim of rather dense liver tissue may occasionally be seen around an abscess and the echoes from distal structures may also be accentuated. No reliable differences have been noted between amoebic abscesses and those caused by other organisms. Hepatic metastases may occasionally cavitate and produce a similar appearance but the clinical history is usually helpful in differentiating these two conditions.

A rare abnormality that may have a rather characteristic ultrasound appearance is a vascular malformation of the liver. This appears as several echo-free spaces adjacent to one another; the feeding vessels may also be visualized. If real time imaging is available, the pulsation from the vascular walls can be imaged.

Malignant

Primary hepatoma is a rare disorder in the United Kingdom and the United States and its vascularity at angiography is very variable. The ultrasound appearances of this tumour are also variable, ranging from dense high-amplitude echoes in the vascular lesions to almost completely cystic appearances in others. There are therefore no ultrasound criteria specific for this disorder but, when clinical suspicion exists, ultrasound is useful to confirm or exclude a focal mass lesion.

Metastatic malignant disease of the liver is common and the precise role of ultrasound in the diagnosis and management of this disease remains incompletely resolved at the present time.

To date, experience has proved that it is possible to detect metastases of about 2 cm in diameter.[11]

Smaller lesions may be detected if they are multiple, whereas in obese patients lesions of 4 cm can be overlooked. Despite these limitations, ultrasound has been shown to be at least

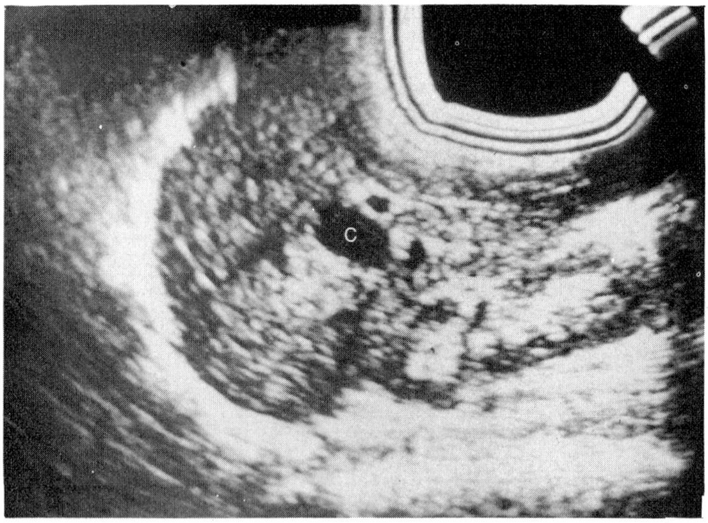

Figure 21.3. Longitudinal scan of right lobe of liver. C – simple liver cyst.

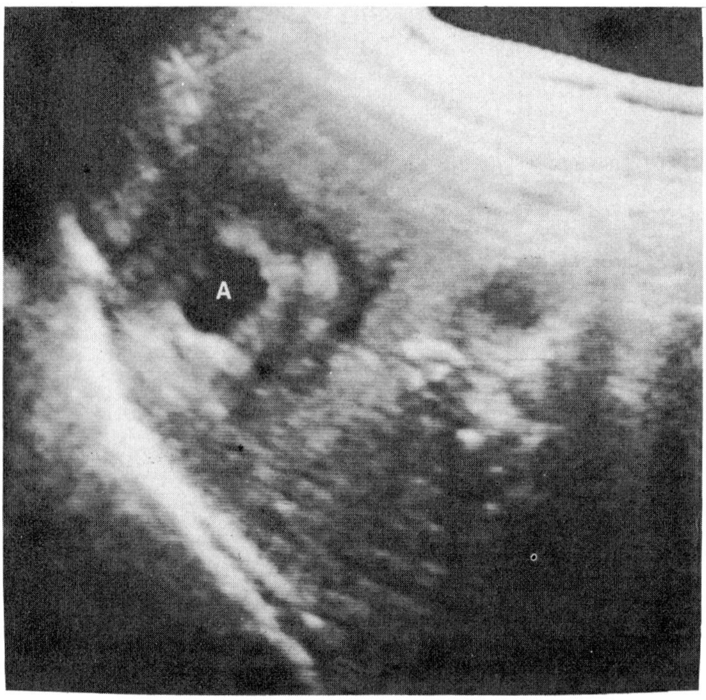

Figure 21.4. Longitudinal scan of right lobe of liver. A – abscess.

as accurate as isotope scanning in the diagnosis of metastases. The different patterns of lesion detected by ultrasound may give some clue as to the primary site where this is not known.[38]

The appearances of metastases described in the published literature vary enormously,[4,33] but this probably reflects differences in patient population from centre to centre. Basically, six different patterns have been described and, although none of these correlate precisely with a given tumour type, there are certain loose correlations which will be mentioned as we describe each pattern:[28]

1. Most centres report that the majority of hepatic metastases exhibit echo amplitudes below those of normal liver (Figure 21.5). In practice, most of these are from breast, bronchus and lymphoma, but many other tumours may produce identical metastases.
2. Carcinoma of the colon and many other intra-abdominal adenocarcinomas have metastases producing high-amplitude echoes which make them readily visible on ultrasound images (Figure 21.6). Whilst this appearance is not specific for any one condition, when it is seen in a patient with an

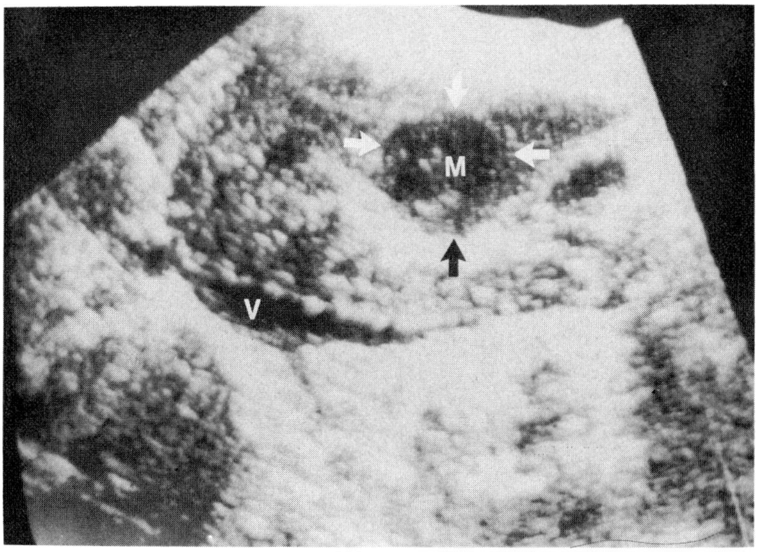

Figure 21.5. Longitudinal scan of liver over the spine. M – low-amplitude metastases. V – inferior vena cava.

unknown primary lesion we normally recommend barium studies as the next investigation.

3. The large majority of malignancies produce liver deposits with one or other of the above appearances. However, as metastases may exhibit echo amplitudes both above and below normal liver, it is not surprising that some return echoes that are similar to those from liver. The proportion of lesions exhibiting this characteristic is small (probably about 3 per cent) but, when encountered, this form of metastasis may be undetectable by ultrasound scanning. Occasionally, the presence of such lesions may be inferred from distortion of the normal vascular architecture of the liver.
4. Although most primary tumours produce hepatic metastases of only one type, we have also seen both high- and low-amplitude lesions present in the same liver. The reasons for this remain uncertain but it may well be that differences in vascularity may be responsible. The presence of necrosis or haemorrhage in some deposits may also be expected to alter their echo pattern.
5. Several complex patterns have been reported, particularly by workers using early ultrasound equipment without grey scale display.[25] In general, these patterns are rings or 'targets' in which the echo amplitudes in the centre of the lesions are the reverse of those in the periphery (Figure 21.7). Such appearances are relatively uncommon but occur in the larger solitary metastases from various sites and no specific significance can be attached to them. The explanation for these patterns probably lies once again in differences in vascularity, and the presence or absence of central necrosis.
6. The sixth pattern seen is that of cystic metastases. Cystic change may be apparent in some or all metastases present. The walls are usually thick and irregular and may have nodules of tissue on them (Figure 21.8). When thin-walled cystic metastases are encountered it may be impossible to be certain that they represent malignant disease. The clinical situation might be helpful, but benign liver cysts can occur in a patient with carcinoma of the breast! In cases when doubt exists serial scans may be useful, since cystic metastases generally enlarge rapidly while benign cysts remain unchanged for years. Cystic metastases are very rare but may be seen from ovary, kidney, gastric sarcoma and primary hepatoma.

Aspiration and biopsy

Whilst discussing focal liver disease, the value of ultrasound in guiding an aspiration or biopsy needle must be mentioned. This technique was originally used for renal puncture,[9] but has been extended to amniocentesis, pericardiocentesis, the aspiration of fluid in many other sites and the biopsy of kidneys, pancreas and masses. Special sterilizable transducers with a central hole are now available and the aspiration/biopsy needle can be passed down through the hole whilst the transducer is 'aimed' at the mass lesion seen on the ultrasound image. The technique is said to aid more accurate placement

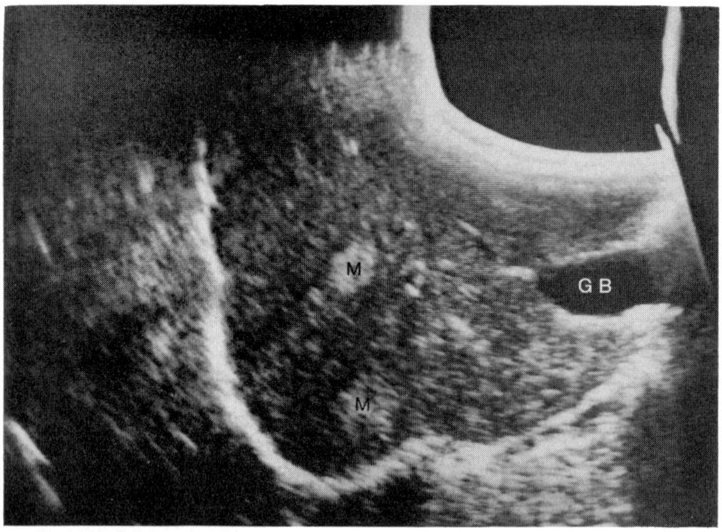

Figure 21.6. Longitudinal scan of right lobe of liver. M – high-amplitude metastases. GB – gallbladder.

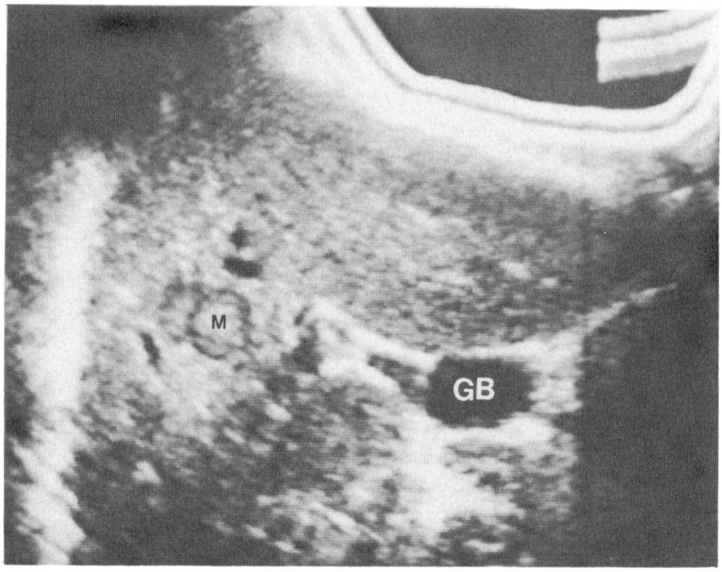

Figure 21.7. Longitudinal scan of right lobe of liver. M – 'target' metastasis. GB – gallbladder.

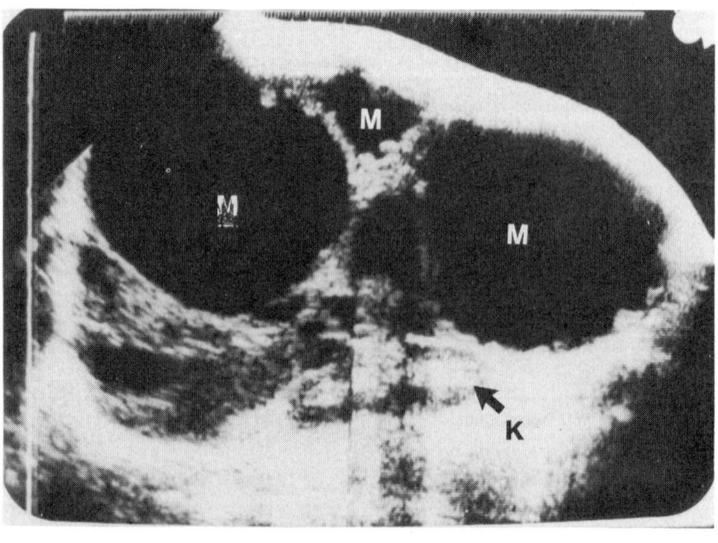

Figure 21.8. Longitudinal scan of right lobe of liver showing cystic metastases. M – cystic metastases. K – kidney.

of the needle than can be achieved by conventional techniques.[14]

Jaundice

There are numerous causes of jaundice. It is of considerable importance in the further management of the patient that obstructive jaundice is differentiated from hepatocellular jaundice. There can be no doubt nowadays that, where ultrasound is available, this should be performed early in the further investigation of jaundice (see Chapter 22).

Although the normal non-dilated biliary tree is not usually visualized, the intrahepatic radicles become readily visible when dilated (Figure 21.9). The accuracy of diagnosis of moderate to severe obstruction approaches 100 per cent. False negative examinations may occur in early acute obstruction when the bilirubin level is below 100 μmol/l (6 mg/dl).[24] The criterion for the diagnosis of biliary duct dilatation is the recognition of tubular, branching, fluid-filled structures radiating out from the porta hepatis. It is possible to confuse portal radicles with enlarged bile ducts. There are, however, a number of differentiating features. The distended biliary tree is usually best seen in the longitudinal scan where the dilated ducts have rather short straight courses. Multiple branch points may be seen and the directional changes may be rather sharp and angular. Acoustic enhancement beyond the dilated ducts occurs commonly. The dilated (and normal) portal venous system is best seen in transverse scans. The vessels form smooth curves and acoustic enhancement does not usually occur beyond the individual veins; indeed, acoustic shadowing may be seen beyond larger vessels. Finally, of course, a particular tubular structure should, if possible, be traced back in sequential scans to either common bile duct (CBD) or portal vein. Biliary radicles measuring 4 mm and more and a CBD measuring 10 mm or more indicate unequivocal dilatation.

A diagnosis of obstruction is made on the identification of dilated biliary radicles in a jaundiced patient. The next step is to define the level of obstruction. In practice, this entails identification of the CBD. Transverse or oblique scans usually show the dilated upper CBD lying nearly parallel and anterolateral to the portal vein.[29] Scans closer to the longitudinal plane may show the lower CBD lying anterior to the inferior vena cava. The site of obstruction is most conveniently classified into two groups:

1. At the level of the porta hepatis.
2. Lower CBD or pancreas.

In our experience, the accuracy of identifying the level of obstruction into these two groups is over 70 per cent, the main limiting factor being the presence of gas in the duodenal bulb and pyloric antrum, which may obscure much of the CBD.

If the level of obstruction is clearly shown, ultrasound will indicate the cause in approximately 50 per cent. In a majority of cases this will fall into the category of stone, tumour or stricture (Figure 21.10).

Biliary calculi are visualized as bright echoes since they strongly reflect the ultrasound beam. As a consequence, little energy is left to pass beyond the stone, which gives rise to the characteristic shadow distal to the stone. This acoustic shadow is sometimes more obvious

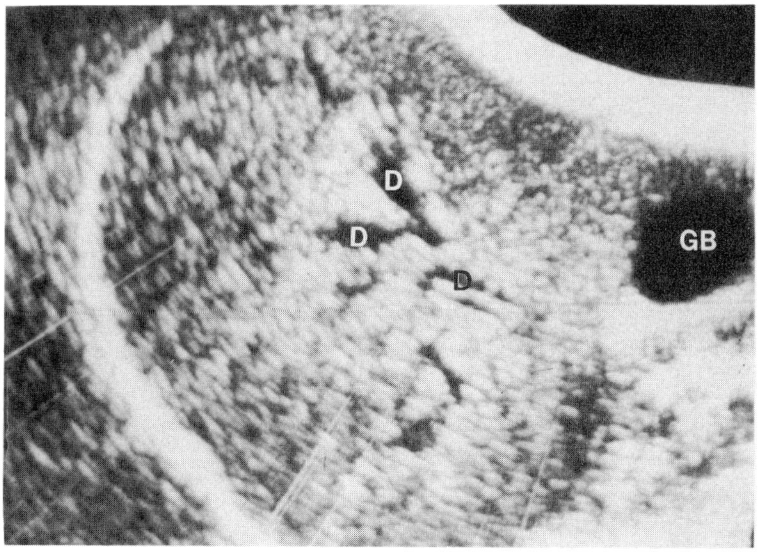

Figure 21.9. Transverse scan of liver showing minimal dilatation of bile ducts. D – dilated ducts. GB – gallbladder.

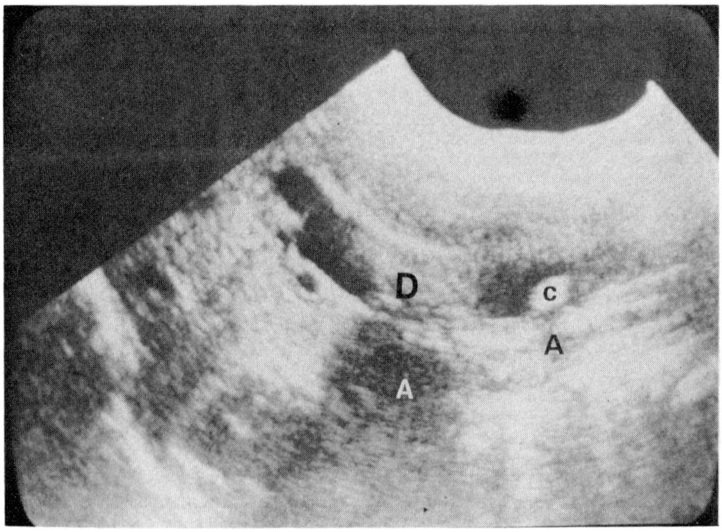

Figure 21.10. Scan along the long axis of dilated common bile duct. C – calculus at lower end of CBD. D – debris. A – acoustic shadow.

than the calculus itself. Calculi may be found at any level in the biliary tree. In general, the higher they are lodged the easier they are to see. In practice, the majority of stones causing obstruction lodge in the region of the ampulla. In this difficult region a stone may best be seen in the transverse scan as a dense spot in the head of the pancreas – the so-called 'target sign'. Differentiation from a small ampullary carcinoma in this instance may not be possible.

Numerous tumours may cause biliary obstruction. Pancreatic carcinoma is undoubtedly the commonest, where small tumours may cause low obstruction and larger tumours extend up to the porta hepatis (Figure 21.11). Ampullary carcinomas are usually small and difficult to identify. Cholangiocarcinomas most commonly infiltrate around the ducts at the level of the porta hepatis. Metastatic deposits in the liver and portal nodes cause high obstruction due to compression.

The identification of the pancreas has already been described, and tumours of the pancreatic head larger than 4 cm in diameter can usually be recognized. However, it may be difficult to distinguish tumour from chronic pancreatitis, particularly if the latter is localized. The normal pancreas is homogeneous and has an even echo pattern. Tumours are shown as an irregular heterogeneous mass, with areas of high and low echo amplitudes. When a tumour causes obstruction the CBD is seen to end abruptly at the upper end of the mass. In addition to pancreatic tumours, a pseudocyst in the head of the pancreas may also cause biliary obstruction. Pseudocysts almost always occur in association with generalized acute pancreatitis. The pancreas is enlarged and, being oedematous, returns lower level echoes than normal. The pseudocyst is identified as a localized cystic area (Figure 21.12). This is most commonly rounded but may have a more bizarre shape. Debris is commonly seen within the pseudocyst. The detection of pseudocysts by ultrasound approaches 100 per cent.[32] Serial scans will show the progress of the cyst which may abruptly change in size if it discharges spontaneously into a neighbouring viscus.

The positive identification of cholangiocarcinoma is difficult, and one may often only identify obstruction at the porta hepatis. However, these tumours may be shown as an ill-defined infiltrating mass around the bile ducts, more often returning rather higher level echoes than does normal liver tissue. Nodal deposits at the porta hepatis have the non-specific appearance of an irregular lobulated mass at this site (Figure 21.13). The appearance of liver metastases has been fully described in the preceding section.

At its best, ultrasound may be expected to show the presence of biliary obstruction, define its level and suggest its cause, thus obviating the need for any further investigation prior to laparotomy. With technically satisfactory scans, ultrasound will at least distinguish obstructive from other causes of jaundice.

A significant proportion of patients with cirrhosis may be jaundiced, and ultrasound may be of value in suggesting this as a positive diagnosis in the undiagnosed case. The echo pattern is characteristic, with bright large-amplitude echoes returned from the liver (Figure 21.14). In addition to being bright, the echoes are tightly packed to give a mesh appearance.

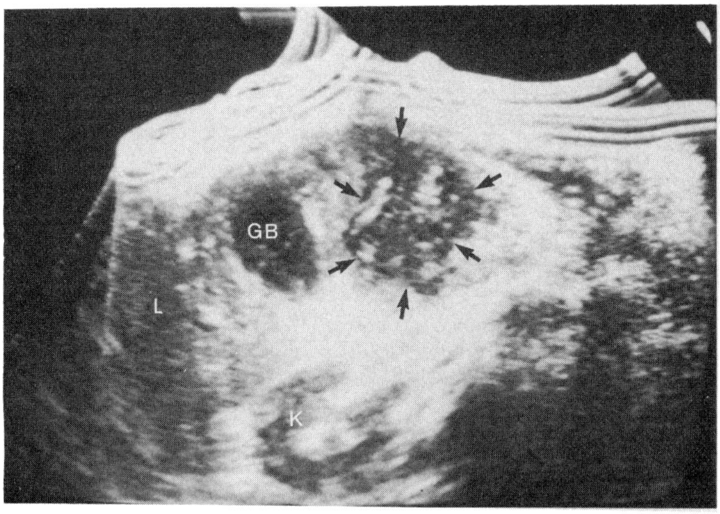

Figure 21.11. Transverse scan of upper abdomen showing carcinoma in head of pancreas. Carcinoma arrowed. GB – dilated gallbladder. L – liver. K – right kidney.

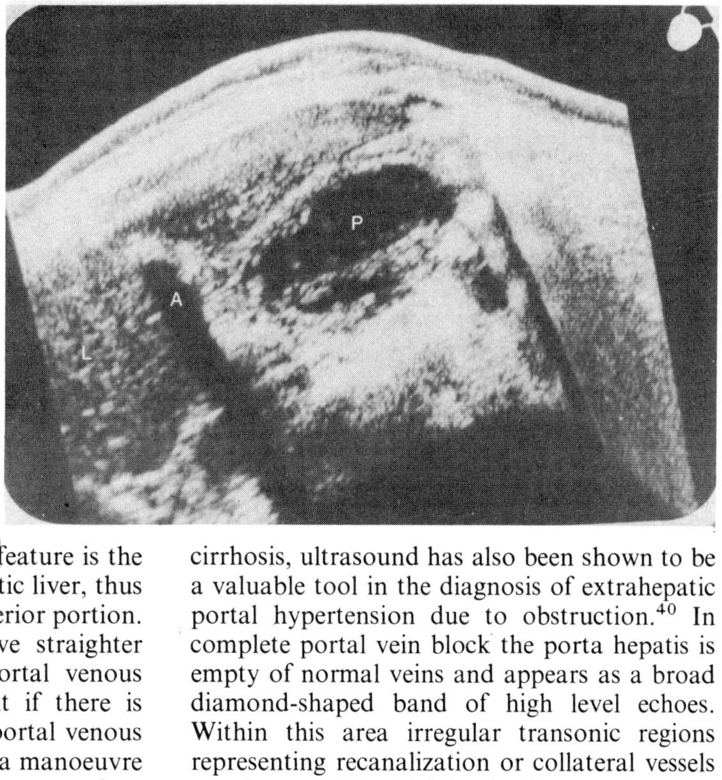

Figure 21.12. Transverse scan of upper abdomen showing pseudocyst in pancreas. P – pseudocyst. L – liver. A – acoustic shadow from biliary calculus.

Perhaps the most characteristic feature is the attenuation of sound by the cirrhotic liver, thus preventing visualization of its posterior portion. Venous structures appear to have straighter courses than normal, and the portal venous system shows central enlargement if there is portal hypertension. The normal portal venous system enlarges during the Valsalva manoeuvre but this does not occur in portal hypertension. The portal vein is detected in nearly 100 per cent of patients with technically satisfactory scans. When it was measured just to the right of its origin in suspended inspiration, Doust and Pearce[8] found that the average AP diameter was 10.3 mm and the maximum AP diameter 15 mm. Webb, Berger and Sherlock[40] reported a mean diameter of 6.3 ± 2.3 mm and a maximum AP diameter of 10 mm. In addition to aiding the diagnosis of intrahepatic portal hypertension in cirrhosis, ultrasound has also been shown to be a valuable tool in the diagnosis of extrahepatic portal hypertension due to obstruction.[40] In complete portal vein block the porta hepatis is empty of normal veins and appears as a broad diamond-shaped band of high level echoes. Within this area irregular transonic regions representing recanalization or collateral vessels may be seen. The high level echoes at the porta are most probably associated with surrounding fibrosis. Portal venography gives a more exact picture of the portal venous system than does ultrasound and is necessary where surgery is contemplated. However, in a small proportion of patients with cirrhosis the portal vein is not displayed by venography because contrast medium has passed into massive portasystemic collaterals. Ultrasound can then determine whether the portal vein is patent.

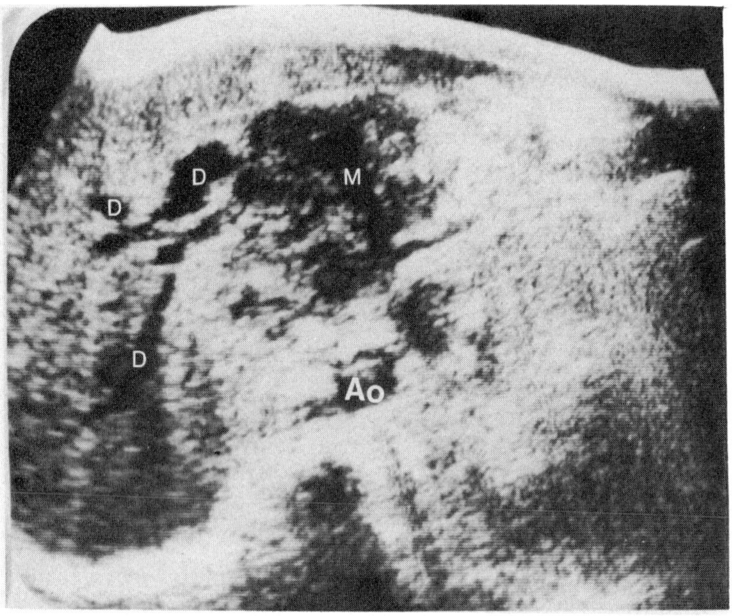

Figure 21.13. Transverse scan of upper abdomen showing lobulated mass in the porta hepatis. M – mass. D – dilated bile ducts within the liver. Ao – aorta.

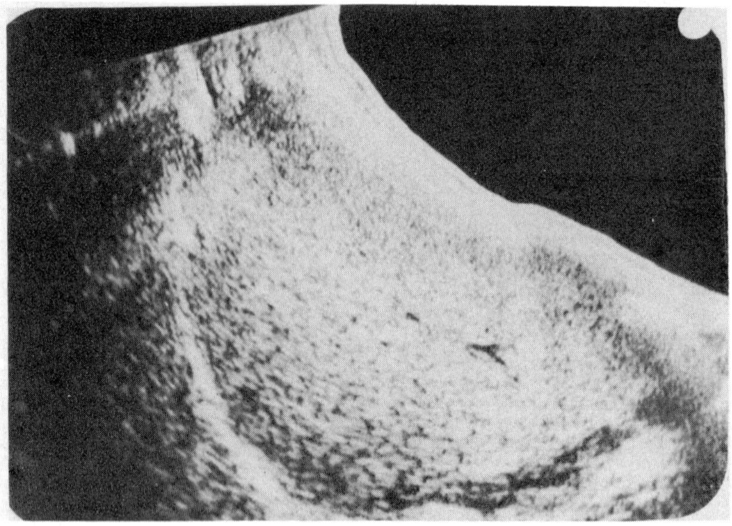

Figure 21.14. Longitudinal scan of right lobe of cirrhotic liver. Compare echo amplitudes with Figure 21.1.

A common accompaniment of cirrhosis is ascites, and ultrasound sensitively detects even small amounts of ascitic fluid, often first seen in the hepatorenal angle. Unfortunately, whilst the bright liver echo pattern is characteristic, it does not identify aetiological groups except for severe congestive cardiac failure (cardiac cirrhosis). In the latter instance diagnosis is easy as the distended hepatic veins are readily demonstrated and, in addition, the posterior attenuation is minimal or absent.[41]

GALLBLADDER

The primary imaging examination of the gallbladder is the oral cholecystogram. This examination has a high degree of accuracy in diagnosing gallbladder disease. Ultrasound imaging at this time does not compete with, or replace, this examination as a screening procedure. The major role of ultrasound is for the further investigation of patients with a failed oral cholecystogram and in the jaundiced patient.

The gallbladder is most frequently located under the inferior surface of the liver between the right and quadrate lobe. However, its position varies considerably in relationship to external landmarks. A rapid series of longitudinal scans about the mid-clavicular line will usually show the position of the gallbladder. Once located, oblique scans may optimally demonstrate the entire length of the organ. The gallbladder can be satisfactorily outlined in about 95 per cent of normal fasting subjects and there is a considerable variation in its size and shape. The contractile response of the normal gallbladder to a fatty meal may be recorded by ultrasound as by other techniques (Figure 21.15).

The typical appearance of gallstones has already been described (Figure 21.16). Gallstones as small as 2 to 3 mm may be detected and their presence may be confirmed by a repeat scan in the erect position. This will demonstrate the gravitational change in the position of the stones. Small single calculi may be missed unless meticulous sequential scans along both axes of the gallbladder are performed. The accuracy of ultrasound in the detection of stones is in the order of 80 per cent, as compared with 90 per cent for oral cholecystography.[10] Stones may be demonstrated in the cystic duct as well as in the common bile duct and gallbladder. In acute cholecystitis, a halo of oedema around the gallbladder wall may be identified. Following repeated episodes of acute or sub-acute cholecystitis, the gallbladder may become fibrotic and contracted. Gallbladders measuring less than 2.5 cm in diameter tend to lose their normal echo-free characteristics and may be impossible to identify accurately. However, if, as is common, they contain stones, these may still be demonstrated by ultrasound (Figure 21.17). In this instance, the bright echoes from the stone and the accompanying acoustic shadow may be seen in the anticipated position of the gallbladder. Care must be taken to differentiate this appearance from shadowing due to gas in the hepatic flexure of the colon.

Tumours of the gallbladder are uncommon and their diagnosis by any technique is difficult.

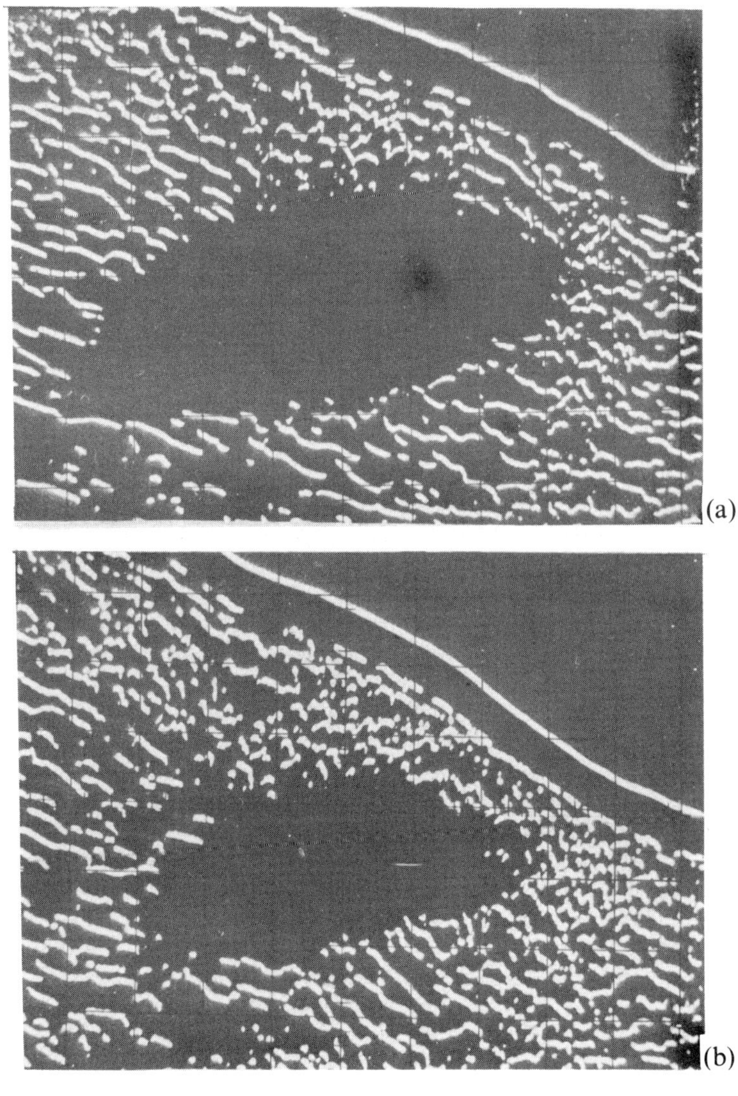

Figure 21.15. (a) Non-grey scale image of gallbladder in fasted patient. (b) Repeat scan after fatty meal. Note reduction in the size of the gallbladder.

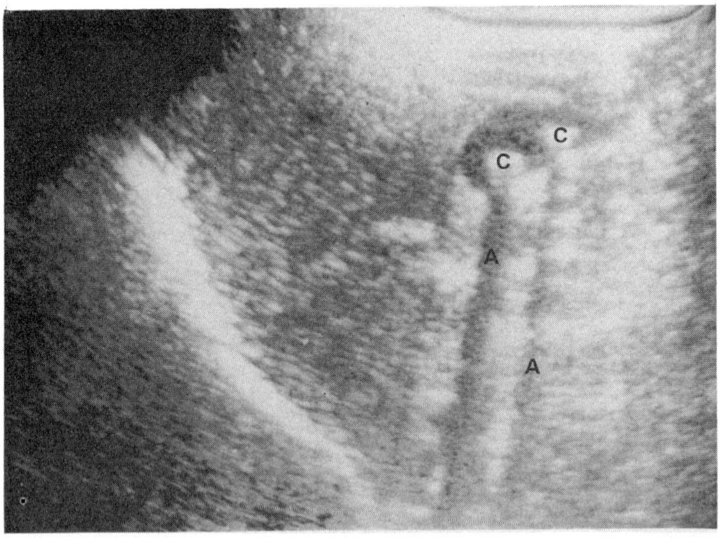

Figure 21.16. Longitudinal scan of right lobe of liver and gallbladder. C – calculi within gallbladder. A – acoustic shadow beyond calculi.

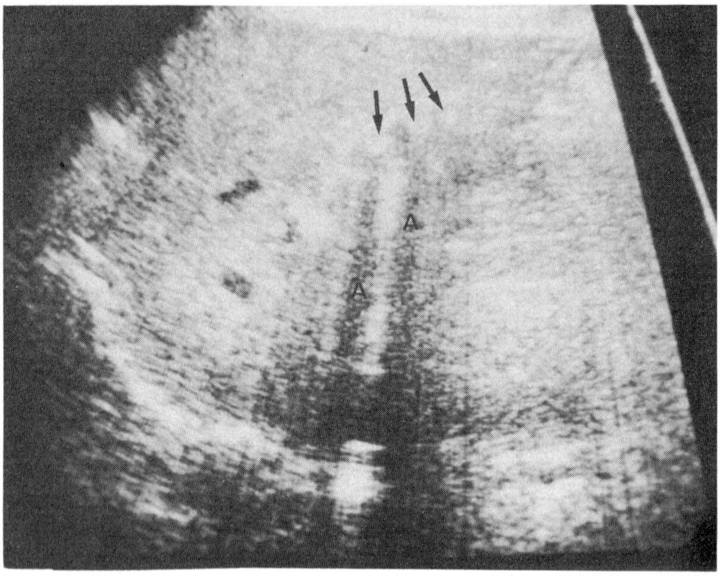

Figure 21.17. Longitudinal scan of right lobe of liver and gallbladder. Gallbladder is contracted and fibrotic and contains three calculi; calculi are arrowed. A – acoustic shadowing.

This is true of ultrasound, since such tumours most commonly occur in contracted gallbladders. However, polyps are occasionally demonstrated.

In the young child or infant, the diagnosis of choledochal cyst is easily made.[5] As one might anticipate, this is seen as an echo-free lesion in the right upper quadrant, separate from the gallbladder. The cyst usually involves the common bile duct and may also involve the intrahepatic ducts. Following decompression of the choledochal cyst, ultrasound is a convenient way to follow resolution.

Although there is a wide variation in the size of the normal gallbladder, marked distension is readily recognized. The most distended gallbladders are seen in patients with longstanding obstruction secondary to pancreatic or ampullary carcinoma. The intrahepatic biliary ducts and the CBD will also be distended, but recognition of the distended gallbladder may help one arrive at the correct diagnosis. It is important in this context to remember that a significant proportion of patients with obstructive jaundice, secondary to a tumour, may also have gallstones in the gallbladder. The demonstration of gallstones in a distended gallbladder should not limit the search for a definitive cause for the obstruction.

Frequently, very thick bile (biliary sludge) is present in the chronically obstructed gallbladder. This layers out in the dependent position, and is demonstrated as a layer of low-amplitude echoes situated posteriorly in the supine position. This thick bile produces no acoustic shadow, in contrast to multiple tiny stones. On changing the patient's position, this sludge will slowly slide to the most dependent portion of the gallbladder (Figure 21.18).

Ultrasound and radiography should be regarded as complementary techniques for investigating the gallbladder. At the present time, the failure rate for both techniques is somewhat similar. By combining the two techniques as described, the overall accuracy may be increased to over 95 per cent.

FUTURE DEVELOPMENTS IN ULTRASOUND IMAGING

There are three main fronts on which future progress will be made. The first, and probably the most important, is to make the image

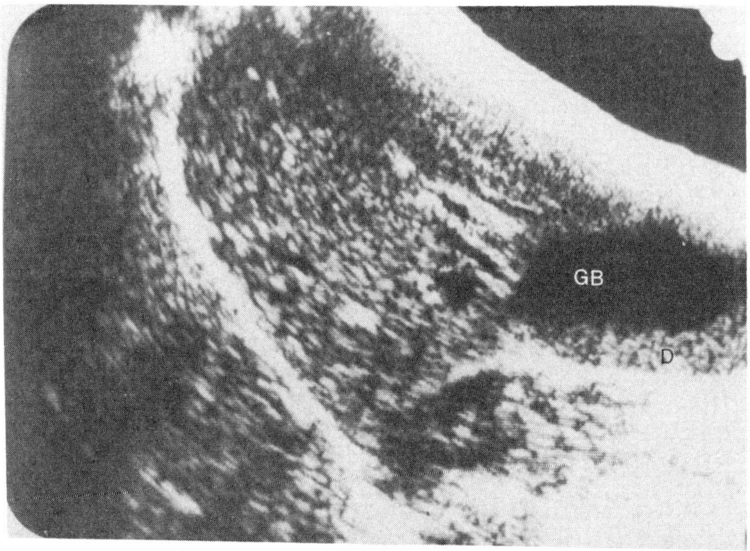

(a)

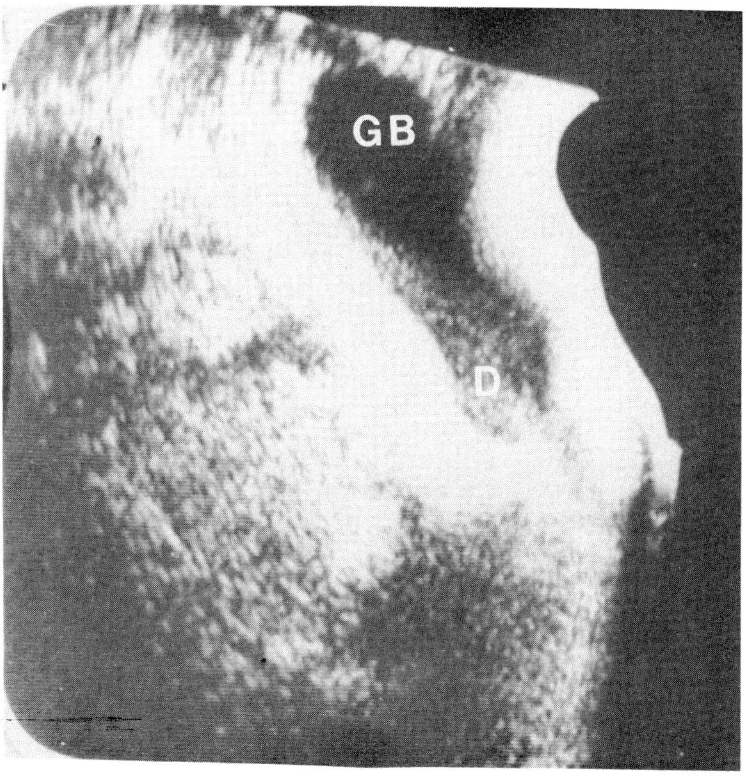

(b)

Figure 21.18a. Longitudinal scan of gallbladder in a patient with long-standing obstructive jaundice. Debris is present in the dependent portion of the gallbladder. GB – gallbladder. D – debris.

Figure 21.18b. Repeat scan with patient in erect position. The debris has moved under the influence of gravity. GB – gallbladder. D – debris.

quality less dependent on the expertise of the operator. This will presumably require a degree of automation which may involve some sacrifice of the versatility and operator interaction which current machines permit. Secondly, the ability of the apparatus to detect smaller structures will continue to improve. Over the past five years resolution has improved from 2 cm to nearer 2 mm today.

Lastly, greater use will be made of the specific nature of the returning echo so that 'tissue signatures' will be determined and this will permit non-invasive 'biopsy' of certain tissues.[39]

COMPUTED TOMOGRAPHY: INTRODUCTION

Whole body computed tomography (CT) is an important advance in diagnostic imaging, but experience of its use in the investigation of liver disease remains limited. The precise role of CT in clinical management and its relationship to ultrasound and isotope techniques cannot yet be defined with any certainty.

BASIC PRINCIPLES

Computed tomography utilizes x-radiation to produce an anatomical display of the body in cross-section. The main advantage of the system is the ability to detect very small differences in attenuation of x-radiation so that structures not visible on conventional radiographs are clearly identified. The basic principles of CT have been described.[16,17] The EMI Whole Body Scanner (CT 5005), with which our experience has been gained, uses a tightly collimated fan beam of x-rays from a single source. The x-ray tube and an array of detectors are mounted on a frame which moves across the patient then rotates through 10°. The process is repeated until the total rotation is 180°. The whole process takes 20 seconds. The detector array, which is mounted diametrically opposite to the x-ray source, records the attenuation of the x-ray beam during the scan. This information is converted into electrical signals which are then digitized for storage and processing. The information is reconstructed as a grey scale image with a matrix of 320 by 320 on a television monitor. Scans are carried out at 140 kV and 28 mA. Each slice is 13 mm thick. Using the standard settings indicated above, with a 13-inch field size, the absorbed skin dose for an examination of 10 slices is approximately 3.5 rad.

Since absorption values are directly related to tissue density, measurements have been established on an arbitrary scale, with water equal to 0, air approximately equal to −500 and bone extending to +500. Soft tissues have a density of 20 to 30, whereas fat has a density of −40 to −50. It is clearly impossible to display this wide range of absorption values on a single image. The system provides controls which allow interrogation of the data at a particular window level and window width. The wider the window width, the lower the contrast between the different tissues, and conversely a narrow window width increases contrast. The window level is appropriately set for the type of tissue being examined, and measurements of density can be fairly accurately assessed by reducing the window width to a minimum (001). By variation of the window settings, it is possible to distinguish cystic from solid lesions and indeed to detect lesions at a narrow window setting which are not obvious when a wide window is used.[37]

FACTORS INFLUENCING IMAGE QUALITY

Liver CT scans may be degraded by certain artefacts. These are caused by moving structures of very high or very low density.[26] The ribs can cause streaks across the liver, making detection of the lesion difficult. Surgical metal clips and high density contrast media also cause streaking across the scans. Since the liver is closely related to the heart, cardiac movement frequently causes artefacts near the dome of the diaphragm. Respiratory movement also degrades the CT image,[1] but these artefacts can be eliminated by performing all scans during arrested respiration. Gas in moving bowel frequently causes problems unless an anticholinergic agent is given. The advent of scanners with scan times of a few seconds should significantly reduce these artefacts.[15]

An important factor which influences CT liver scans is the partial volume effect. If a lesion occupies the whole thickness of a slice, its recorded attenuation value corresponds directly to the lesion. However, if the lesion is only partially contained within the slice, the attenuation values recorded represent the attenuation values of the lesion and a contribution from normal liver tissue. Hence the overall attenuation of the lesion may be significantly different from its true reading, and may be subsequently misinterpreted or the lesion may even remain completely undetected.

Both spatial and density resolution influence the quality of the CT image. These two factors are closely interrelated: the higher the density difference between the lesion and the normal liver, the smaller the lesion that can be identified. For example, tiny specks of calcification can be identified, whereas tumours cannot be seen unless they are approximately 1 to 2 cm in size.

TECHNIQUE

Examination of the liver using CT requires supervision by an experienced radiologist if optimal results are to be obtained. Prior to the examination, a long film of the chest and abdomen is taken using a slit beam of x-rays to overcome distortion. This is known as the scanogram.[19] Metal markers are placed on the suprasternal notch, the iliac crests and upper border of the symphysis pubis. It is then possible to relate the level of the proposed tomographic slices to the anatomical vertebral level. This is not only useful in planning the precise location of CT slices, but provides a reasonably accurate method of reproducing the same slice at a later examination. For investigation of the liver, slices are taken at 1.5 cm intervals from the dome of the diaphragm to the tip of the right lobe. An anticholinergic agent is given five to ten minutes before the procedure in order to minimize artefacts from gas in moving bowel. We currently use Buscopan (hyoscine-*N*-butyl bromide) 20 mg intramuscular injection. It is essential that the scans are carried out during suspended respiration. This is particularly important when examining the liver because of its close proximity to the diaphragm.

Iodinated contrast agents, given intravenously, may be helpful in detecting a space-occupying lesion of the liver, which is only suspected on initial scans, by increasing the density of the normal liver. A urographic contrast agent, for example 60 ml sodium iothalamate (70 per cent w/v), may be given as an infusion or as a bolus injection. Since the majority of space-occupying lesions have a lower density than normal liver parenchyma, the administration of contrast medium increases this density difference. Occasionally, however, the space-occupying lesion is enhanced after intravenous contrast and detection becomes more difficult. This is probably related to the vascularity of the lesion.[37]

THE NORMAL LIVER

The CT scan demonstrates the detailed anatomy across the whole abdomen at the level of the slice (Figure 21.19). It is therefore possible not only to identify the individual lobes of the liver but also to assess the relationship of the liver to other organs and structures. All CT scans are viewed as though from the foot of the patient.

The left lobe varies considerably in size and shape. It may be flattened, triangular or large and rounded. The right lobe is more constant in shape, occupying the greater part of the right half of the abdomen. The caudate lobe is clearly identified, in the majority of patients, lying anterior to the inferior vena cava, posterolateral to the fissure for the ligamentum venosum. The quadrate lobe lies anteriorly between the gallbladder and the fissure for the ligamentum teres. Both the fissures containing the falciform ligament and ligamentum teres, and the fissure containing the gastrohepatic ligament and ligamentum venosum can be clearly identified in most patients. Fat lying in these fissures has a low density which makes them easy to identify.

The liver parenchyma has a homogeneous density which is usually greater than other intra-abdominal organs such as the kidneys, pancreas and spleen. The density values range from 20 to 40 EMI units.

Within the normal liver are areas of diminished density due to the major vascular channels. The inferior vena cava is clearly shown in the posteromedial aspect of the right lobe. Anterior to this it is usually possible to identify the major portal veins. These may be seen as small round areas of low density and must not be mistaken for space-occupying lesions or dilated intrahepatic bile ducts. Examination of serial slices will usually reveal their branching nature and convergence towards the porta hepatis. If there is doubt regarding their nature, intravenous urographic contrast medium will opacify the vessels, whereas the majority of space-occupying lesions and dilated

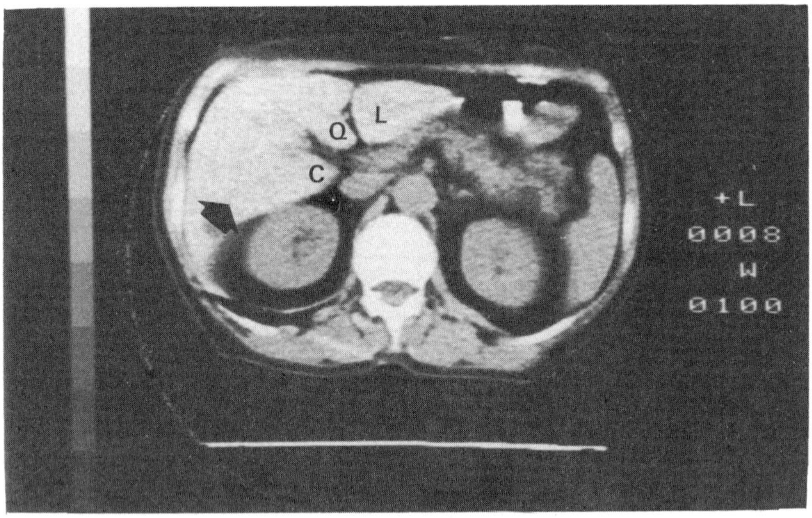

Figure 21.19. The normal liver. Right lobe (arrowhead). Left lobe (L). Caudate lobe (C) and quadrate lobe (Q).

bile ducts remain unaffected.[22] As with ultrasound, normal sized intrahepatic bile ducts are not shown on the CT scan.[2] However, it is occasionally possible to identify the common bile duct and hepatic artery within the porta hepatis.

The gallbladder lies on the anterior surface of the liver and is almost invariably seen on a normal liver scan.

Occasionally, a caudal extension of the right lobe of the liver, Riedel's lobe, is noted. This is more common in females than males.

THE ABNORMAL LIVER

The main indications for computed tomography in liver disease are likely to be in the detection of space-occupying lesions and in the evaluation of obstructive jaundice.

Space-occupying Lesions

Space-occupying lesions in the liver are recognized by CT if the attenuation values are significantly different from normal liver parenchyma. The vast majority of lesions have a lower attenuation value and are therefore seen as areas of diminished density.[30] Density measurements of the lesion also provide information regarding its composition. If the abnormal area contains calcium or extravasated blood, the density of the lesion will be higher than that of normal liver.[37] With CT it is therefore possible to detect tumours, both primary and secondary, benign and malignant, and to distinguish these from cysts and abscesses.

Malignant tumours

Since primary hepatoma is an extremely rare condition, there are as yet few reports of the CT appearances in the world literature. Sheedy et al[34] report one patient with a large hepatoma, the only abnormal sign of which on the CT scan was massive liver enlargement. In retrospect, minimal alteration in tissue density was shown. Figure 21.20 shows a primary hepatoma originating in the left lobe, with metastases in the right lobe. The density of the tumour is lower than that of normal liver, confirming the findings of other investigators.[2] Para-aortic lymph node involvement was also demonstrated. These findings indicated that the tumour was inoperable. The value of computed tomography in primary malignant liver tumours is therefore not only to establish the diagnosis, but to define the extent of disease if surgery is considered, or to monitor response to chemotherapy.

Metastatic disease in the liver is extremely common. Practically all liver metastases appear as areas of diminished density on the CT scan

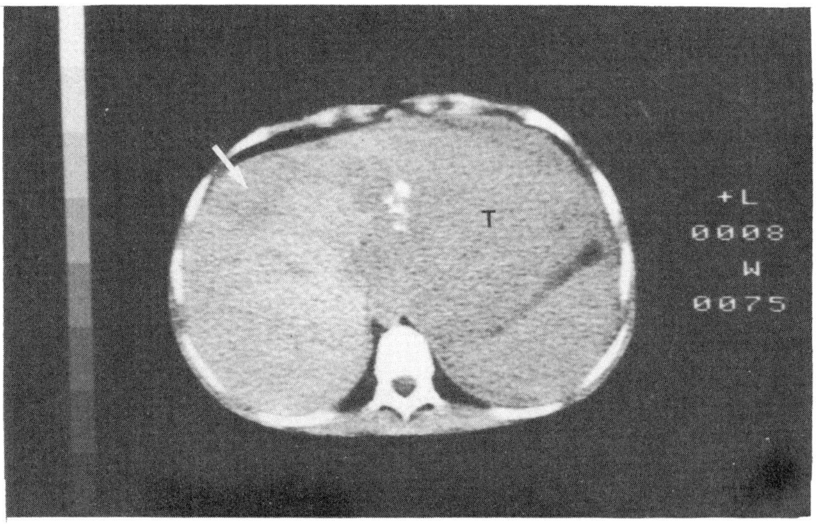

Figure 21.20. Primary hepatoma involving the left lobe (T). Metastases are also present in the right lobe (arrowed).

(EMI units approximately 10 to 20). It is impossible to determine the site of origin of the primary tumour on the CT scan appearances. However, metastases occasionally contain calcium, suggesting that the primary tumour is either an osteogenic sarcoma, an ovarian tumour or colloid carcinoma of the colon.[20] An unusual appearance is an area of extremely low density in the centre of the metastasis; this probably represents central necrosis (Figure 21.21).

It has already been emphasized that lesions are demonstrated only if there is sufficient contrast between the normal liver and a lesion. It is therefore possible for metastases to remain undetected, particularly if these are small (less than 2 cm). Even in retrospect, we were unable to identify multiple metastases 2 to 4 mm in size throughout the liver in a patient with a pancreatic carcinoma. Intravenous urographic contrast medium may be helpful in confirming the presence of a suspected lesion by increasing the contrast between normal liver and the suspected deposit.

Benign tumours

Benign tumours are rare and our own experience is therefore limited. Figure 21.22 shows a large benign hepatic adenoma. It has a lower density than normal liver and was not enhanced after administration of intravenous contrast medium. Stephens, Hattery and Sheedy[36] have reported the appearances of a cavernous haemangioma which became denser after contrast infusion.

Cysts

Cysts can usually be identified with little difficulty because they have a very low density (EMI units approximately 0 to 10) (Figure 21.23). They are well demarcated from the normal liver parenchyma because their density is so low and can be detected when they are as small as 1 cm in diameter.

Hydatid cysts may contain calcification in the wall and, occasionally, septa are visible traversing the cyst. However, it is not always possible to distinguish an hydatid from a simple cyst.

Abscesses

The density of a liver abscess usually lies between that of a cyst and a solid tumour. However, the diagnosis is usually made in the light of the clinical history rather than on the basis of the CT scan alone. A subphrenic abscess can be identified as a collection of fluid adjacent to the liver margin. CT may be used for needle guidance for aspiration.[13,20] This must be distinguished from ascites, which surrounds not only the liver but also the spleen.

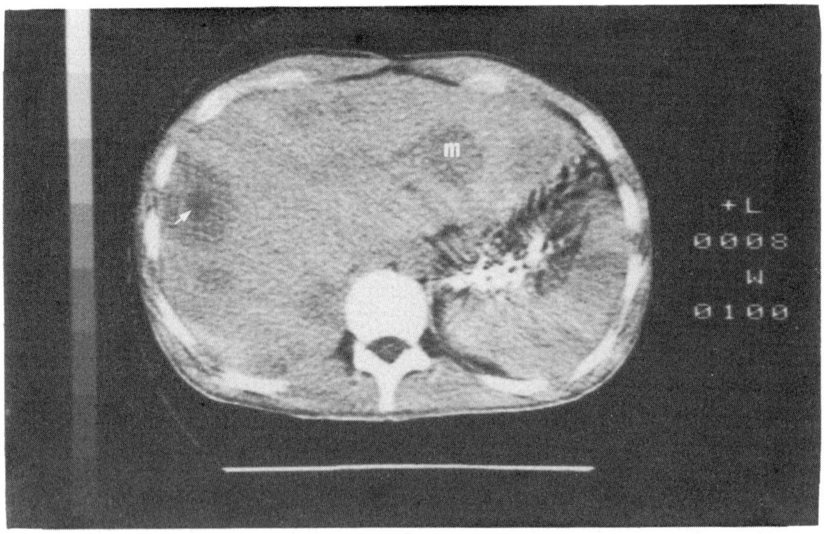

Figure 21.21. Multiple metastases. One metastasis shows a central area of low density (arrowed).

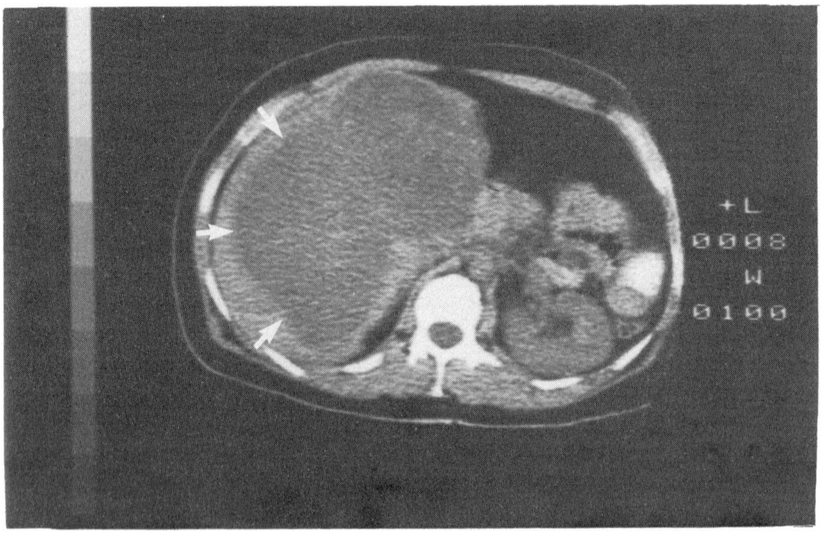

Figure 21.22. Benign hepatic adenoma. The tumour (arrowed) has a lower density than normal liver but did not enhance after administration of intravenous contrast. Courtesy of the BUPA Medical Centre.

Differential diagnosis

There is little difficulty in making the diagnosis of multiple metastases. The solitary space-occupying lesion, however, can present a diagnostic problem, particularly if it is small. In this instance, the differential diagnosis of a cyst from a solid tumour depends entirely upon the density values obtained. Since the standard deviation of a given attenuation value is high, it is not always possible to reach a definitive diagnosis.

CT may be helpful in demonstrating the site of origin of a lesion considered to be situated in the liver by other imaging techniques, such as isotope scanning or ultrasound (Figure 21.24).

Obstructive Jaundice

Normal intrahepatic bile ducts are not shown with computed tomography but can be clearly identified as multiple rounded or tubular structures of low density if dilated.[2,18,35] These

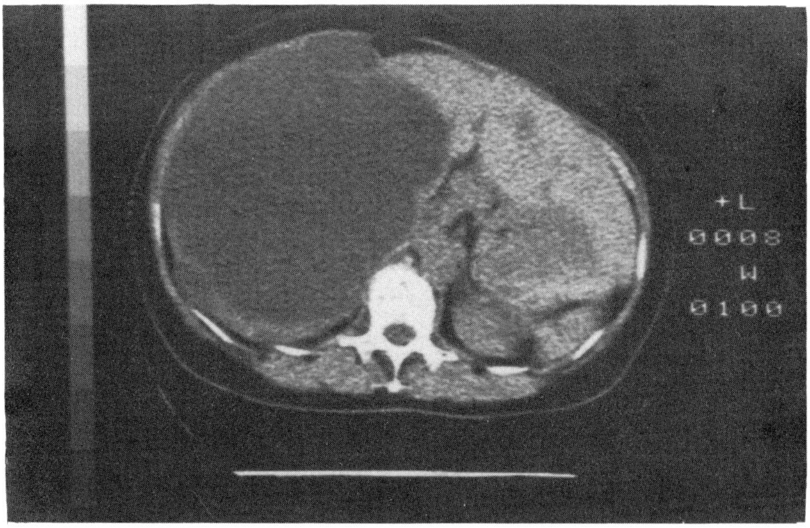

Figure 21.23. Benign liver cyst.

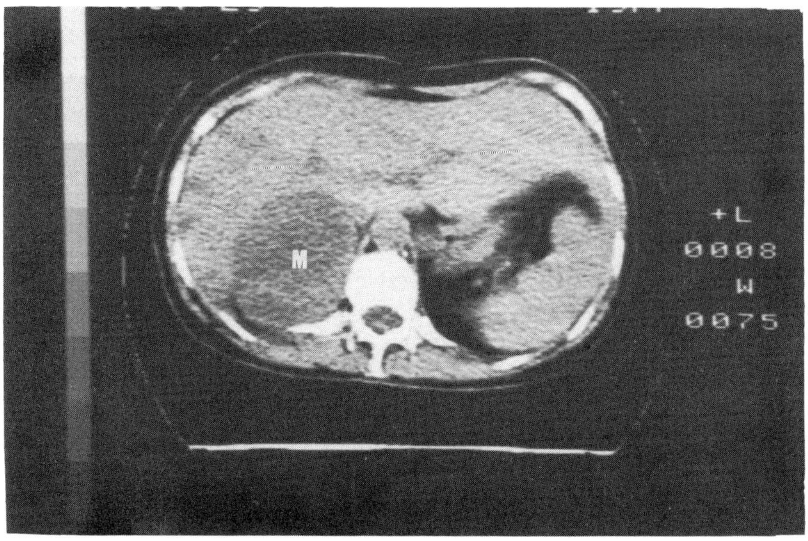

Figure 21.24. Metastasis (M) in right suprarenal gland from malignant melanoma, interpreted on ultrasound as metastasis in right lobe of liver.

can be distinguished from normal vascular channels after administration of contrast medium since the vessels become opacified. It may also be possible to demonstrate the obstructing lesion, for example a carcinoma in the head of the pancreas. Stephens et al[37] found a mass in the head of the pancreas or porta hepatis in seven of 13 patients with dilated ducts.

Intrahepatic bile ducts are also visualized if they contain air. Since ultrasound is completely reflected by air, assessment of the liver in these patients is extremely difficult. We have demonstrated multiple metastases in a patient with air in the intrahepatic bile ducts which was interpreted as normal by ultrasound.

Diffuse Liver Disease

There is probably little place for computed tomography in the diagnosis of diffuse liver disease. There is no change in density of the liver in patients with cirrhosis, although an unusually high density has been reported in patients with haemochromatosis.[2] Fatty liver has a characteristic appearance; as the whole parenchyma is replaced by tissue of very low density, the normal vessels appear as areas of high density.[31]

The Gallbladder

Although gallstones can be identified on the CT scan, there is little place for computed tomography as a method of choice in the investigation of gallbladder disease. Occasionally, however, large malignant tumours of the gallbladder may be shown on the CT scan. The precise location of the mass and its relation to normal structures is helpful in radiotherapy treatment planning.

RELATIONSHIP OF ULTRASOUND, COMPUTED TOMOGRAPHY AND ISOTOPE TECHNIQUES

The precise relationship of ultrasound to computed tomography for the diagnosis of liver disease will depend on the ultimate accuracy of both systems and their alternatives.[21] The development of ultrasound scanners is advancing rapidly and it is now possible to detect metastases of 1 cm in diameter under ideal circumstances. It is also possible to demonstrate vascular structures a few millimetres in diameter. Computed tomography (CT) has caught the imagination of many workers recently, but its application to the liver is still in its infancy and its precise clinical role remains uncertain. Both ultrasound and CT produce images of a thin slice of the patient but since CT uses ionizing radiation it measures a totally different characteristic of tissues than does ultrasound. The advantages and limitations of CT might therefore be expected to be different from ultrasound. Certainly the resolution of CT images is limited at present by patient movement during scanning and it is probable that ultrasound has a greater ability not only to identify normal vessels but also to detect and differentiate metastases. It must be emphasized that the results of ultrasound are highly dependent upon the skill of the operator. However, as instrumentation in both fields improves, the relative roles of each modality may well alter. The gap which is less likely to close is the cost differential which is currently about 20:1 in favour of ultrasound.

Isotope techniques in liver imaging include the use of colloidal agents for static imaging, hepatocellular agents, and vascular agents for dynamic studies. Whilst isotope studies may detect space-occupying lesions of 1 to 2 cm in diameter, all show as reduced areas of uptake. Dynamic imaging may resolve the nature of some of these lesions, but ultrasound studies more readily add specificity to the lesion. Newer hepatocellular agents such as pyridoxylidene glutamate and iminodiacetic acid derivatives show great promise in outlining the gallbladder and biliary ducts. In particular, the entire length of the common bile duct may be outlined, which is not always possible with ultrasound due to overlying gas. These agents may be a valuable addition to assist in the differential diagnosis of jaundice. However, the resolution is not adequate to indicate the cause.

Whilst there is a considerable overlap of information gained from computed tomography, ultrasound imaging and isotope imaging, there can be no doubt that the techniques are best regarded as complementary. The diagnostic accuracy is considerable when they are used together.[12]

At present, it seems reasonable to utilize the cheaper, painless, harmless ultrasound as the first imaging procedure and to reserve the more expensive, time-consuming and possibly hazardous procedures for those cases where ultrasound is inconclusive or supporting evidence is required.

REFERENCES

1. Alfidi, R.J., MacIntyre, W.J. & Haaga, R.J. (1976) The effects of biological motion on CT resolution. *American Journal of Roentgenology,* **127,** 11–15.
2. Alfidi, R.J., Haaga, J.R., Meaney, T.F., MacIntyre, W.J., Gonzales, L., Tarar, R., Zelch, M.G., Boller, M., Cook, S.A. & Jelden, G. (1975) Computed tomography of the thorax and abdomen: a preliminary report. *Radiology,* **117,** 257–264.
3. Alfidi, R.J., Haaga, J.R., Havrilla, T.R., Pepe, R.G. & Cook, S.A. (1976) Computed tomography of the liver. *American Journal of Roentgenology,* **127,** 69–74.
4. Bree, R.L., Stanley, C.T., Goldstein, H.M. & Green, B. (1977) The spectrum of grey scale sonographic findings in hepatic neoplasms. *Ultrasound in Medicine,* **3A,** 467–468.
5. Carlsen, E. (1975) Liver, gallbladder and spleen. *Radiologic Clinics of North America,* **13,** 543–556.
6. Carlsen, E.N. & Filly, R.A. (1976 Newer ultrasonographic anatomy of the upper abdomen: I. The portal and hepatic venous anatomy. *Journal of Clinical Ultrasound,* **4,** 85–90.

7. Carr, D., Duncan, J.G., Railton, R. & Smith, C.B. (1976) Liver volume determination by ultrasound: a feasibility study. *British Journal of Radiology,* **49,** 776–778.
8. Doust, B.D. & Pearce, J.D. (1976) Grey scale ultrasonic properties of the normal and inflamed pancreas. *Radiology,* **120,** 653–657.
9. Goldberg, B.B. & Pollack, H.M. (1973) Ultrasonically guided renal cyst aspiration. *Journal of Urology,* **109,** 5–7.
10. Goldberg, B., Harris, K. & Brooker, W. (1974) Ultrasonic and radiographic cholecystography. *Radiology,* **111,** 405–409.
11. Green, B., Bree, R.L., Goldstein, H.M. & Stanley, C. (1977) Grey scale ultrasound evaluation of hepatic neoplasms: patterns and correlations. *Radiology,* **124,** 203–208.
12. Grossman, Z.D., Wistow, B.W., Bryan, P.J., Dinn, W.M., McAfee, J.G. & Kieffer, S.A. (1977) Radionuclide imaging, computed tomography, and gray-scale ultrasonography of the liver: a comparative study. *Journal of Nuclear Medicine,* **18,** 327–332.
13. Haaga, J.R. & Alfidi, R.J. (1976) Precise biopsy localization by computed tomography. *Radiology,* **118,** 603–607.
14. Hancke, S., Holm, H.H. & Koch, F. (1975) Ultrasonically guided percutaneous fine needle biopsy of the pancreas. *Surgery, Gynecology and Obstetrics,* **140,** 361–364.
15. Harell, G.S., Marshall, W.H., Brieman, R.S. & Seppi, E.J. (1977) Early experience with the varian six second body scanner in the diagnosis of hepatobiliary tract disease. *Radiology,* **123,** 335–360.
16. Hill, K.R. (1974) The EMI scanner: technical aspects. *British Journal of Hospital Medicine – Equipment* (Suppl.), **11,** 5–14.
17. Hounsfield, G.N. (1973) Computerized transverse axial scanning (tomography): (1) description of system. *British Journal of Radiology,* **46,** 1016–1022.
18. Husband, J.E., Meire, H.B. & Kreel, L. (1977) Comparison of ultrasound and computer-assisted tomography in pancreatic diagnosis. *British Journal of Radiology,* **50,** 855–862.
19. Kreel, L. (1977) Computerized tomography using the EMI general purpose scanner. *British Journal of Radiology,* **50,** 2–14.
20. Kreel, L. (1977) Computerized tomography of the liver. *Clinical Radiology,* **28,** 571–581.
21. Kreel, L. & Meire, H.B. (1977) The diagnostic process – a comparison of scanning techniques. *British Medical Journal,* **ii,** 809–811.
22. Kressel, H.Y., Korobkin, M., Goldberg, H.I. & Moss, A.A. (1977) The portal venous tree simulating dilated biliary ducts on computed tomography of the liver. *Journal of Computer Assisted Tomography,* **1** (2), 169–175.
23. Lawson, T.L. (1977) Hepatic abscess: ultrasound as an aid to diagnosis. *Digestive Diseases,* **22,** 33–37.
24. Malini, S. & Sabel, J. (1977) Ultrasonography in obstructive jaundice. *Radiology,* **123,** 429–433.
25. McCarthy, C.F., Wells, P.N.T., Ross, F.G.M. & Read, E.A. (1969) The use of ultrasound in the diagnosis of cystic lesions of the liver and upper abdomen and in the detection of ascites. *Gut,* **10,** 904.
26. McCullough, E.C., Payne, J.T., Baker, H.L. Jr, Hattery, R.R., Sheedy, P.F., Stephens, D.H. & Gedgaudus, E. (1976) Performance evaluation and quality assurance of computed tomography scanners, with illustrations from the EMI, ACTA and Delta scanners. *Radiology,* **120,** 173–188.
27. Meire, H.B. (1977) Upper abdominal vascular anatomy demonstrated by grey scale ultrasound. *Ultrasound in Medicine,* **3A,** 357–361.
28. Meire, H.B. (1977) Grey scale echographic appearances of liver metastases. *Ultrasound in Medicine,* **3A,** 315–319.
29. Perlmutter, G. & Goldberg, B. (1976) Ultrasonic evaluation of the common bile duct. *Journal of Clinical Ultrasound,* **4,** 107–111.
30. Petasnick, J.P. & Clark, J.W. (1976) Computed tomography of the abdomen: initial experience. *Gastrointestinal Radiology,* **1,** 201–208.
31. Sagel, S.S., Stanley, R.J. & Evens, R.G. (1976) Early clinical experience with motionless whole-body computed tomography. *Radiology,* **119,** 321–330.
32. Sanders, A. & Sanders, R. (1977) Complementary use of B-scan ultrasound and radionuclide imaging techniques. *Journal of Nuclear Medicine,* **18,** 205–219.
33. Scheible, W., Gosink, B.B. & Leopold, G.R. (1977) Echographic patterns of hepatic metastatic disease. *Ultrasound in Medicine,* **3A,** 463–464.
34. Sheedy, P.S., Stephens, D.H., Hattery, R.R., Muhm, J.R. & Hartman, G.W. (1976) Computed tomography of the body; initial clinical trial with the EMI prototype. *American Journal of Roentgenology,* **127,** 23–51.
35. Stanley, R., Sagel, S.S. & Levitt, R. (1976) Computed tomography of the body: early trends in application and accuracy of the method. *American Journal of Roentgenology,* **127,** 53–67.
36. Stephens, D.H., Hattery, R.R. & Sheedy, P.F. II (1976) Computed tomography of the abdomen: early experience with the EMI body scanner. *Radiology,* **119,** 331–335.
37. Stephens, D.H., Sheedy, P.F.II, Hattery, R. & MacCarty, R. (1977) Computed tomography of the liver. *American Journal of Roentgenology,* **128,** 579–590.
38. Taylor, K.J.W. (1977) Investigation of the hepatobiliary system and spleen. In *Ultrasonics in Clinical Diagnosis* (Ed.) Wells, P.N.T. London: Churchill Livingstone.
39. Waag, R.C., Gramiak, R., Lerner, R.M., Lee, P.P.K., Hunter, L.P. & Schenk, E. (1977) Tissue characterisation by ultrasonic diffraction. *Ultrasound in Medicine,* **3B,** 1815.
40. Webb, L.J., Berger, L.A. & Sherlock, S. (1977) Grey scale ultrasonography of portal vein. *Lancet,* **ii,** 675–677.
41. Weill, F. & Maurat, P. (1974) The sign of the vena cava: echotomographic illustration of right cardiac insufficiency. *Journal of Clinical Ultrasound,* **2,** 27.

Chapter 22

Angiography

R. DICK

Newer imaging techniques for the liver and biliary tract, including some which do not involve ionizing irradiation or patient discomfort, have led to more careful selection for angiography. Though it is an 'intrusive' investigation, it provides, in properly selected patients, diagnostic information which outweighs the risks of the necessary irradiation and of the iodinated media used. Angiography is certain to retain its place in the diagnostic work-up, though the future will see increasing use of it in an 'interventional'[24] or 'therapeutic'[4] role.

As with ultrasonography, angiography provides an anatomical or pathological display, yet has the advantage of providing the additional haemodynamic information so important in liver disease. In the investigation of the biliary tract, especially that of the patient with obstructive jaundice, angiography is much less important in the diagnostic work-up than cholangiography and ultrasonography,[22] as most biliary tract tumours are avascular. It may nevertheless provide important information if curative surgery is being planned.

Each patient requires an individual rather than a collective approach. It is essential that clinician, radiologist and physicist establish the correct order of investigation. For example, in a patient with acute or continuing gastrointestinal bleeding, angiography is the prime investigation, whereas in suspected cystic liver disease ultrasonography is prime. Wherever possible, non-invasive tests should be performed before invasive investigations. In some patients, ultrasonography, radio-isotope scanning, computed tomography and angiography will all be justified and will give cumulative information. Wherever the process of investigation ceases, it should be rare for the surgeon to be surprised at the pathology found at elective laparotomy.

EQUIPMENT, TECHNIQUE AND RISKS

To achieve the best angiograms, sophisticated equipment is essential. Basic requirements are a high output generator, x-ray tubes with standard and small (0.3 mm) focal spot for routine and magnification radiography respectively, biplane fluoroscopy, videotape recording, electrically-operated flow-rate injector, rapid film changers and automatic film processing. The present cost of such a unit exceeds £200 000.

Angiography requires meticulous care of the patient both during and after the procedure. Use of guided catheters and deflector assemblies allows users with reasonable manual dexterity to become proficient at main trunk and branch catheterization in both the arterial and venous systems. It is important to avoid long examinations, and to use the smallest diameter catheter possible with as few catheter changes as necessary. The aim is selective, or if necessary superselective, catheterization of vessels to give maximum opacification of the territories supplied by the coeliac and superior mesenteric arteries, and of the portal and hepatic venous systems, keeping total contrast injected to below 1 g iodine per kg body weight. Provided that bleeding tendencies are corrected and the risk of further hepatic and/or renal insufficiency is minimized, complications are rare in careful hands.

LIVER AND BILIARY TUMOURS

Many liver neoplasms have characteristic arteriographic features[12] that differ widely from the normal hepatic arterial pattern (Figure 22.1). If the neoplasm is vascular, it is often possible to distinguish haemangioma, liver cell adenoma and primary liver cancer (hepatoma). Haemangioma develops a 'mimosa' blush which persists beyond 12 seconds, and the tumour may be circumscribed (Figure 22.2). Liver cell adenomas (Figure 22.3), hepatomas and the rare angiosarcoma are mostly highly vascular.

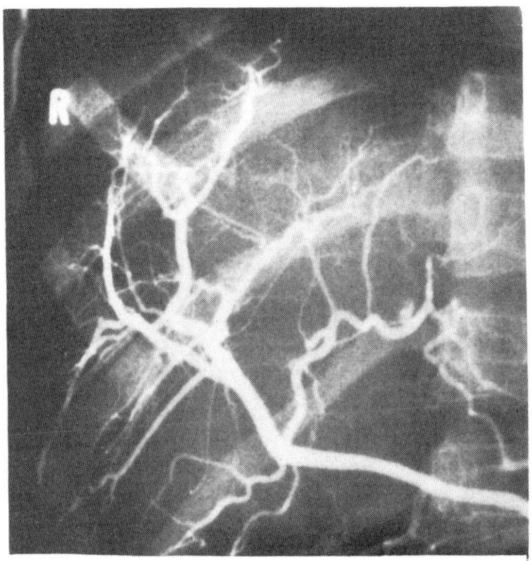

Figure 22.1. Hepatic arteriogram. Normal arterial/arteriolar pattern.

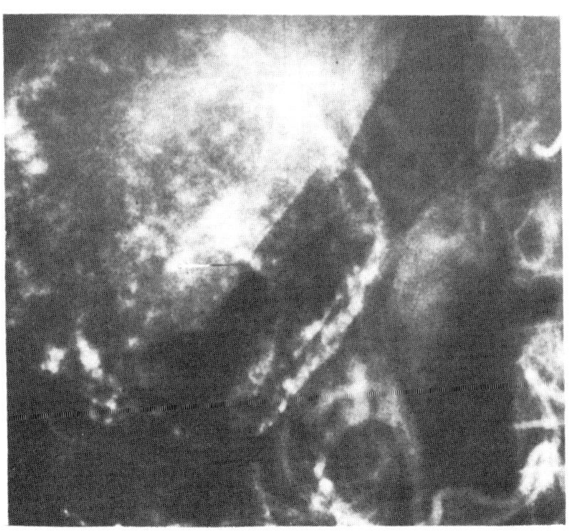

Figure 22.2. Palpable liver mass, 60-year-old male. Discrete blush at 20 s typical of haemangioma. Operative proof. Cure.

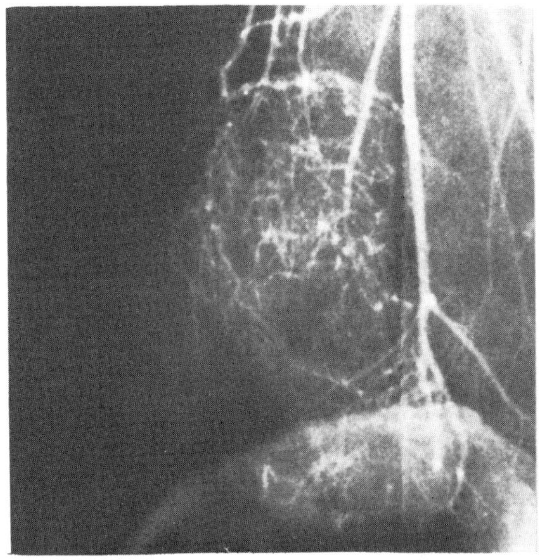

Figure 22.3. Selective hepatic arteriogram. Defined vascular tumour lower right lobe. Liver cell adenoma. Female on contraceptive pill.

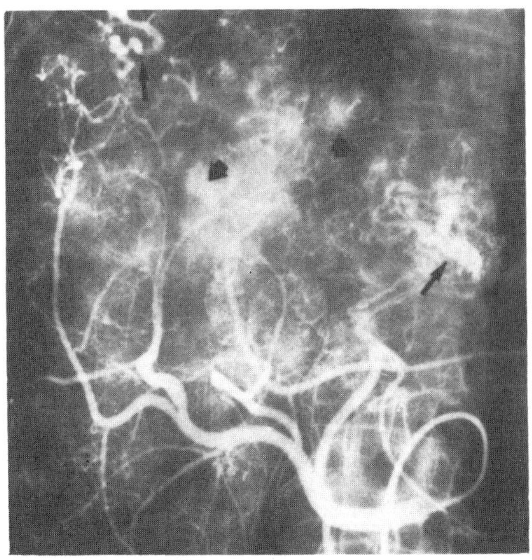

Figure 22.4. Superselective hepatic arteriogram. Diffuse malignant circulation. Tumour stains (short fat arrows) and abnormal veins (long thin arrows). Biopsy = primary liver cell cancer.

The diagnosis of primary liver cancer by angiography is usually straightforward, and this is undoubtedly the best method of all for indicating operability.[6] The angiographic extent correlates well with the surgical findings in 80 per cent of cases.[18] Liver cell cancer has a bizarre vascularity, with dilated tumour arterioles and irregular veins (Figure 22.4).

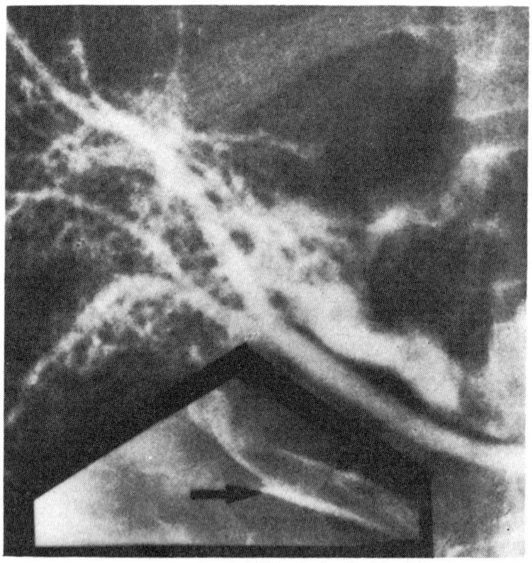

Figure 22.5. Selective hepatic arteriogram. Tumour circulation liver hilum with shunt to portal vein containing tumour thrombus. Primary liver cancer. Embolized (inset).

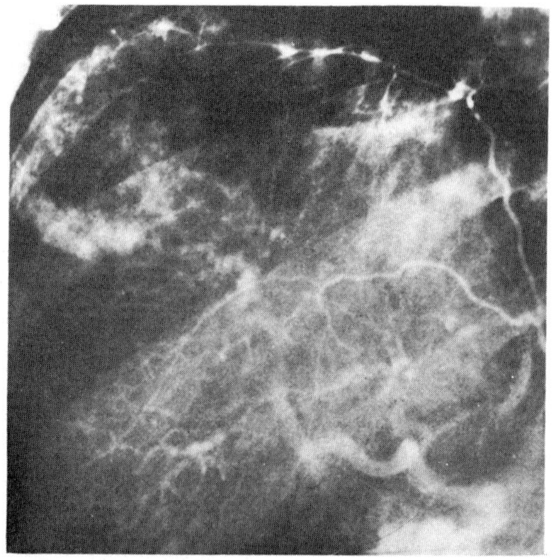

Figure 22.7. Coeliac arteriogram. Peripheral necrotic primary liver cancer. Phrenic artery supply superiorly suggests tumour involves hemidiaphragm (inoperable).

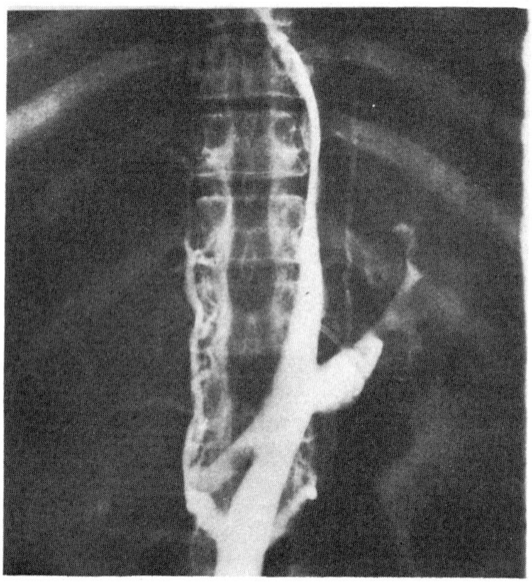

Figure 22.6. Inferior venacavogram. Hepatic cava displaced and invaded by liver cancer right lobe. Vertebral venous plexus fills.

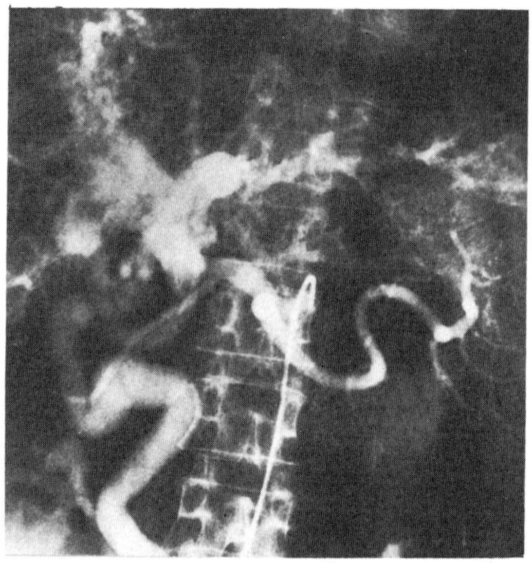

Figure 22.8. Selective coeliac arteriogram. Primary liver cancer right lobe liver, massive portal venous shunt. (Large umbilical vein.) Splenomegaly. (Published by courtesy of Dr D. Irving.)

Extrahepatic or intrahepatic arteriovenous shunting may occur. Such early portal venous filling may rarely be a feature of cirrhosis or follow liver biopsy, but if widespread is virtually diagnostic of primary liver cancer (Figure 22.5). It sometimes occurs locally in regenerative nodules and other neoplasms.[26] Angiograms may show the primary cancer spreading to hepatic veins, inferior vena cava (Figure 22.6) or extrahepatic structures (Figure 22.7), as well as the presence of associated cirrhosis (Figure 22.8). Hopefully, one may demonstrate an uninvolved lobe, making hemihepatectomy worth while (Figure 22.9a and b). In inoperable malignancy, an arterial catheter may be left in the hepatic artery for cytotoxic drug perfusion. The possibility of embolizing large tumour fistulae at the time of arteriography should be considered.

Metastases are much commoner than any

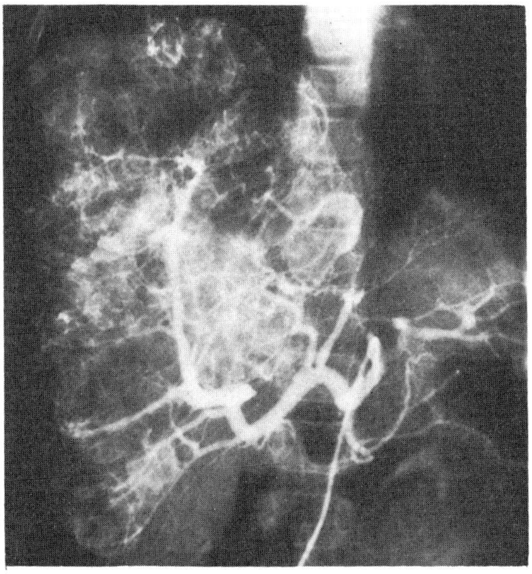

(a)

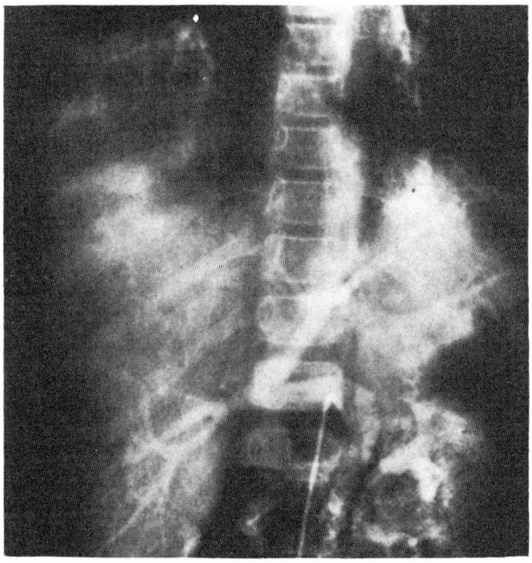

(b)

Figure 22.9. (a) Coeliac arteriogram. Female aged seven years. Very vascular tumour right lobe, normal left lobe. Biopsy = multifocal primary liver cell cancer. (b) Superior mesenteric arteriogram. Venous phase. Tumour displaces portal vein branches. Normal left lobe veins. Extended right hemihepatectomy performed. (Portal vein may contribute to blood supply of liver cell adenoma and carcinoma.)

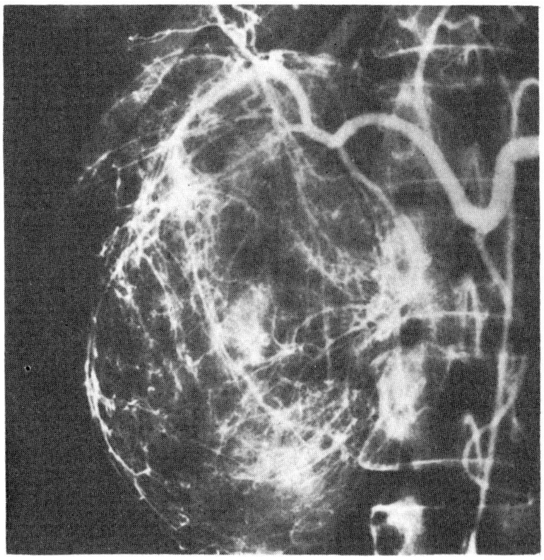

Figure 22.10. Common hepatic arteriogram. Highly vascular tumour right lobe. Carcinoid origin suggested by study. Ileal primary at operation.

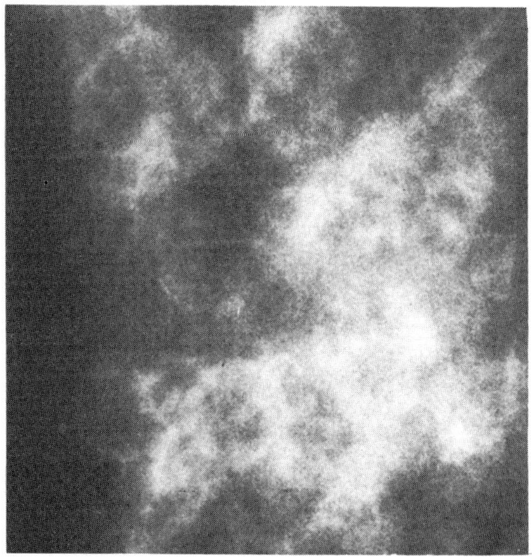

Figure 22.11. Superselective hepatic arteriogram. Capillary phase. Multiple round defects with vascular periphery = metastases. Malignant gastrinomas.

other liver neoplasm. They may be highly vascular, especially those from endocrinomas poorly opacified but may have a diagnostic dense peripheral ring of contrast (Figure 22.11). Some metastases, such as the mucoid-secreting colonic variety, are totally avascular. If minimal neovascularity is suspected, it can be highlighted with the use of pharmacoangiography (Figure 22.12a and b), namely the use of intra-arterial drugs prior to repeat injection of contrast. Vasoconstrictors (adrenaline 20 μg) or, alternatively, vasodilators (Tolazoline 25 to 50 mg) have been advocated for injection into the hepatic artery to enhance tumour circulation and are without added risk to the patient.[7] However, a generous volume of contrast agent is the most important factor in opacifying normal or abnormal tissues.

Arteriography is disappointing in the diagnosis of the occasional avascular primary liver cell cancer and with avascular metastases. Very small (1 to 2 cm) avascular intrahepatic lesions

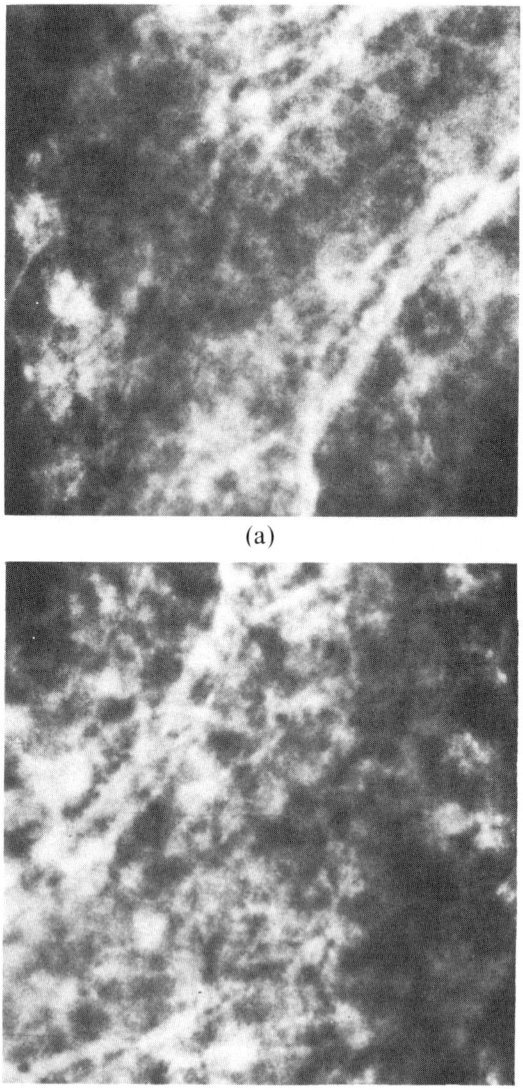

(a)

(b)

Figure 22.12. (a) Enhanced hepatic contrast with pharmacoangiography. Initial study without drugs. (b) Improved contrast following Tolazoline 50 mg injected into catheter prior to contrast. Multifocal primary liver cancer.

sometimes cause filling defects on a well-filled portal venogram long before they are detected on arteriography.[19] Hepatic lymphoma is always hypovascular, with an absence of arteriovenous shunting.[3]

Cholangiocarcinomas are avascular tumours, causing invasion and fixity of nearby arteries and veins. Dilated bile ducts causing lucencies in the hepatogram phase are distinguished from metastases because of their linear shape.[25] The size of the gallbladder can be assessed (Figure 22.13) and the venous phase of the coeliac arteriogram provides important information about the calibre and patency of the splenic, portal and intrahepatic veins. Nevertheless, unless resection is contemplated, angiography is not routinely indicated if cholangiography or ultrasonography have indicated the site and probable nature of the biliary pathology.

PORTAL HYPERTENSION

The patient deserves an integrated approach, the team consisting of a physician, a surgeon and a radiologist. Timing, both of investigations and treatment, is important. Most patients will require angiography. This should be performed promptly to allow maximum time to plan management. Early in the course of a bleed, a slow infusion of Pitressin (0.1 u/min) into the superior mesenteric artery will lower portal venous pressure and may stop variceal bleeding. However, not only may bleeding recommence when the drug is discontinued, but Pitressin experimentally is as effective if given by the more simple intravenous route.[10]

Angiography is the best imaging technique to demonstrate the precise portal venous anatomy, including the number and direction of venous collaterals. Vital haemodynamic information, including flow rates and pressures, is concurrently obtained. The normal portal venous

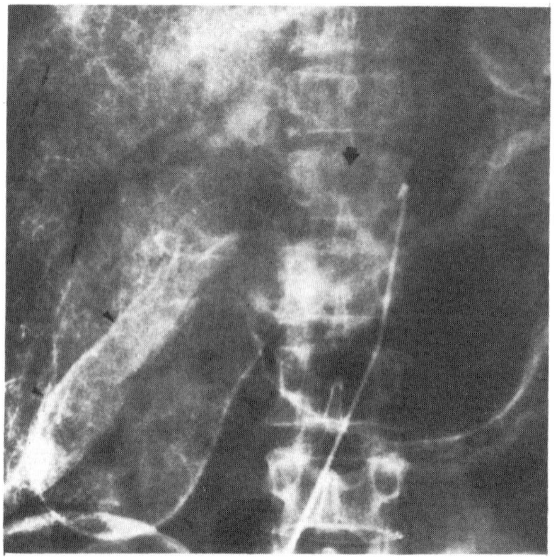

Figure 22.13. Selective coeliac arteriogram. Late hepatogram/portal venous phase. 60-year-old male, carcinoma pancreatic head. Tumour pressure on portal vein (large arrow). Enlarged gallbladder (arrow heads). Multiple small negative defects in liver due to dilated bile ducts (small arrows). Autopsy proof.

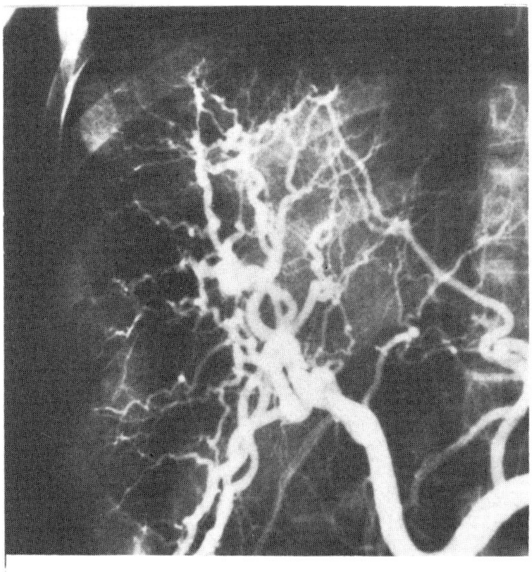

Figure 22.14. Selective hepatic arteriogram. Corkscrewing of arteries and arterioles. Advanced cirrhosis. (c.f. Figure 22.1.)

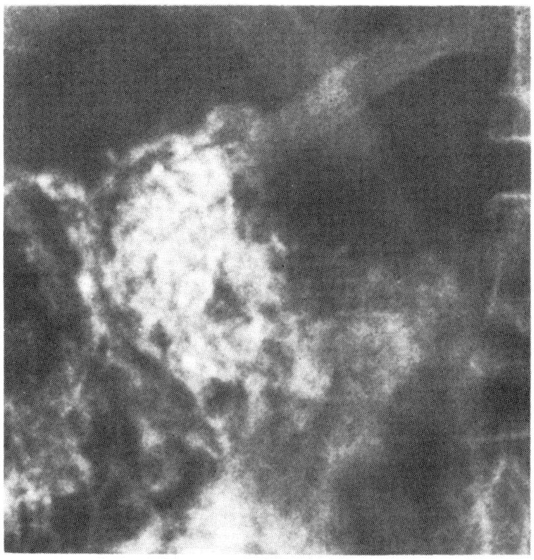

Figure 22.16. Patient with cirrhosis/portal hypertension. Superior mesenteric arteriogram. Capillary haemangioma duodenal wall (found at endoscopy).

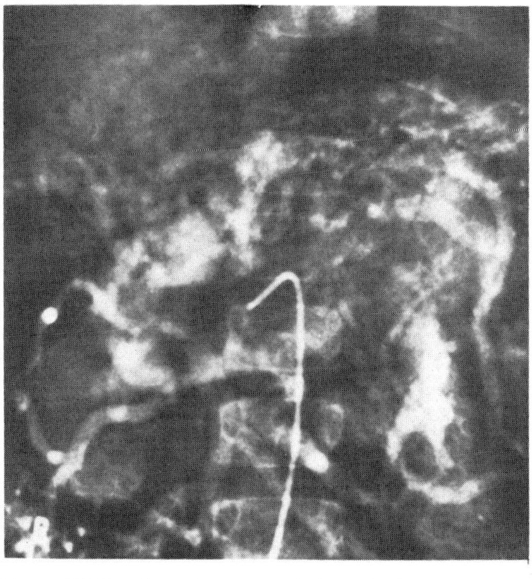

Figure 22.15. Superior mesenteric arteriogram, venous phase. Thrombosed portal vein. Many periportal and gastric collaterals. Past umbilical sepsis.

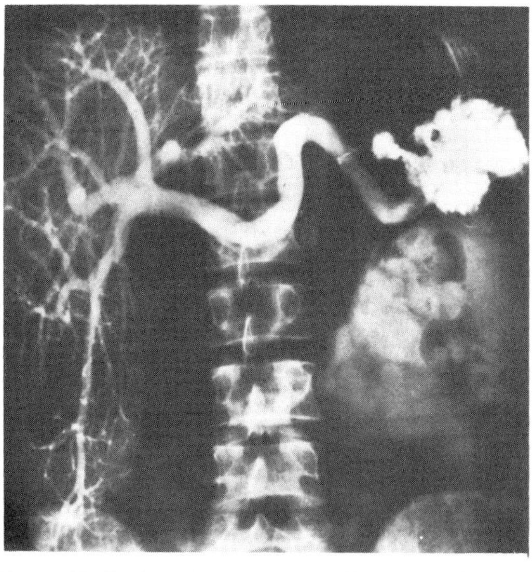

Figure 22.17. Splenic portogram. Normal study. Note Riedel's lobe.

pressure does not exceed 11 mmHg. A pressure in the portal vein of 30 mmHg in a patient with a normal wedge hepatic venous pressure indicates a presinusoidal cause of portal hypertension. Thus a diagnosis may be made even before angiography has commenced.

High-dose arterioportography (50 to 70 ml Urografin 370 successively into coeliac axis and superior mesenteric artery) is advantageous in outlining *both* the arterial and venous systems at the same examination (Figures 22.14 and 22.15). Despite the addition of vasodilators such as bradykinin[2] or prostaglandins,[13] dense variceal filling is not always achieved, and in some patients selective left gastric pharmacoarteriography should follow.[14] Arteriography in portal hypertension may show associated non-variceal causes of bleeding, namely arteriovenous

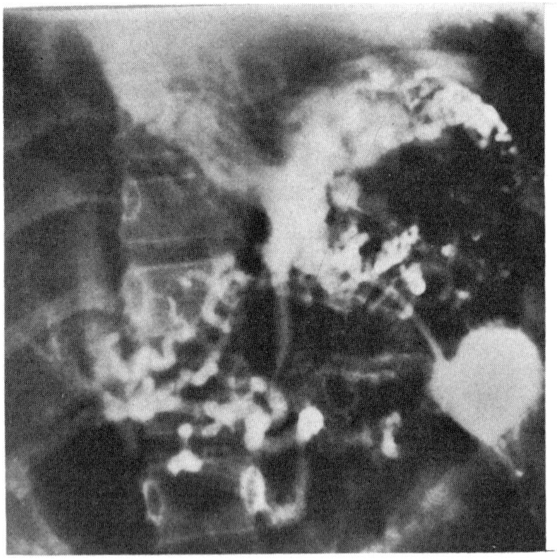

Figure 22.18. Splenic portogram. Child with past portal pyaemia. Splenic and portal vein thrombosis. Oesophageal, gastric and renocaval collaterals.

fistulae, haemangiomas (Figure 22.16), and gastric or duodenal ulcers. In the poor-risk patient, the vessel feeding a bleeding ulcer should be embolized forthwith.[1]

Unquestionably, a *direct* injection of contrast into the portal venous system will show collaterals most fully, including those in unusual sites.[8] Splenic pulp injection is quick, and even in inexperienced (though careful) hands is technically straightforward and free of serious complications.[5] The pattern of collateral venous filling depends upon the site of obstruction,[11] the appearance deviating markedly from the normal (Figures 22.17 and 22.18). Percutaneous transhepatic portography[15] is possible provided that the portal vein is patent. It gives superb venograms and has the advantage of allowing subsequent selective catheterization and thus thrombosis of gastro-oesophageal collaterals (Figure 22.19a, b and c). Access to the portal vein via the umbilical vein has not been universally adopted.

Armed with a good portal venogram, the medical team can choose between sclerotherapy and a decompressing surgical shunt for the individual patient. Successful sclerosis of varices either by the oesophagoscope or the trans-

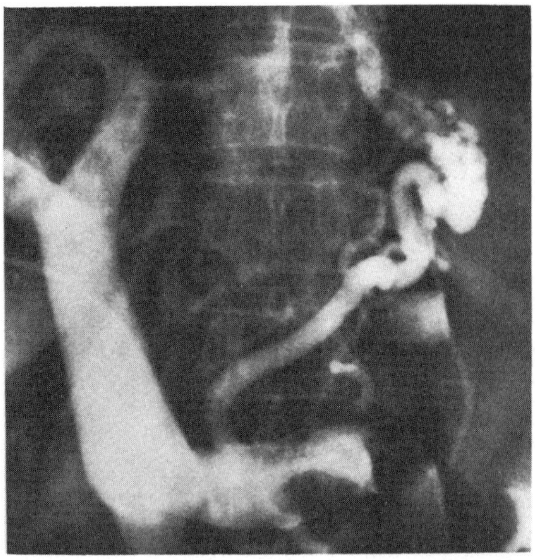

(a)

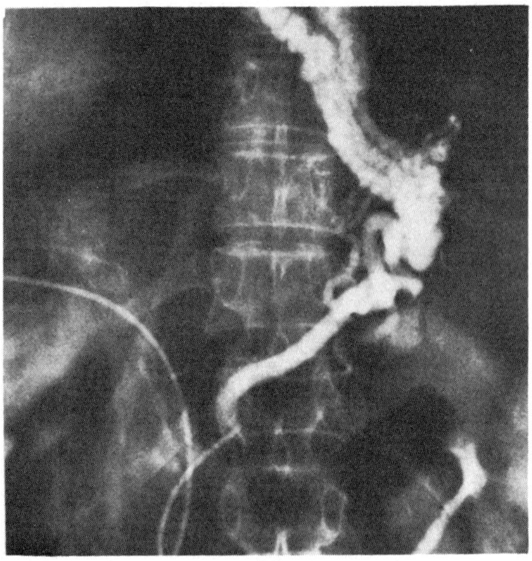

(b)

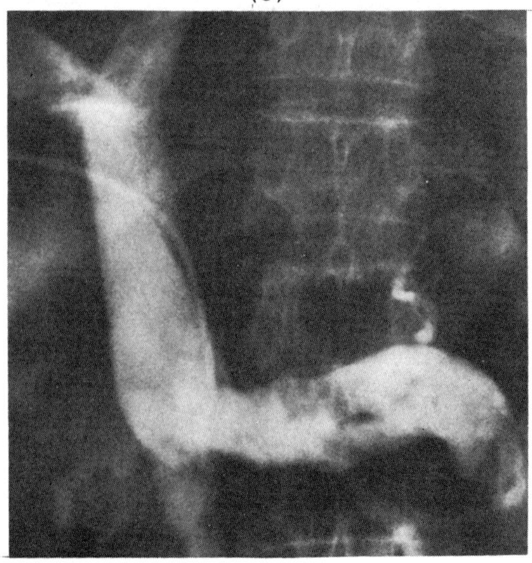

(c)

Figure 22.19. (a) Transhepatic portogram. Left gastric, superior and inferior mesenteric collaterals. (b) Selective left gastric venogram. Gastric and oesophageal varices. (c) Final portogram shows left gastric vein occluded. A thin short gastric vein remains to be obliterated.

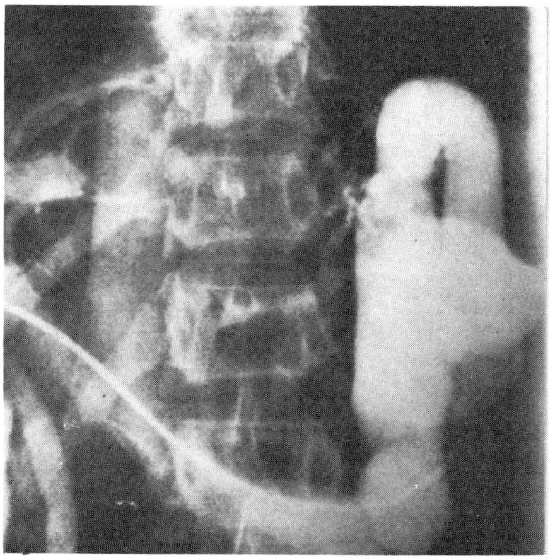

Figure 22.20. Transhepatic portogram. Large retroperitoneal shunt to left renal vein and inferior vena cava.

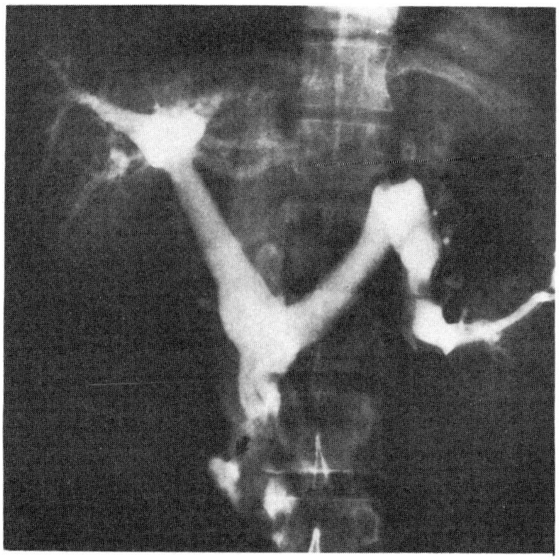

Figure 22.21. Splenic portogram showing patent mesocaval shunt (arrowed). Flow preserved to small cirrhotic liver.

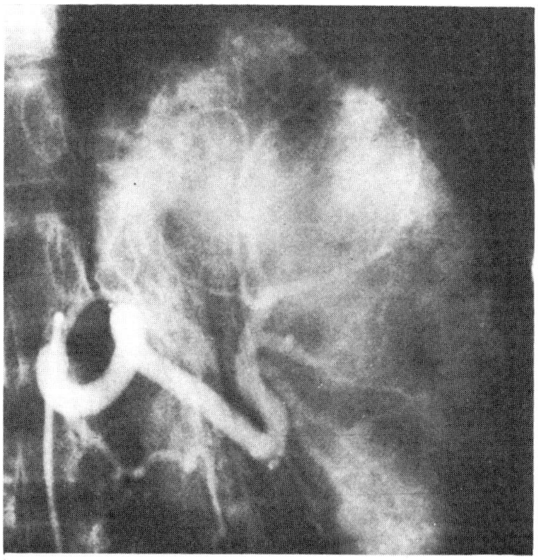

Figure 22.22. Selective splenic arteriogram. Multiple defects in enlarged spleen were due to sarcoid granuloma. Note lymphogram.

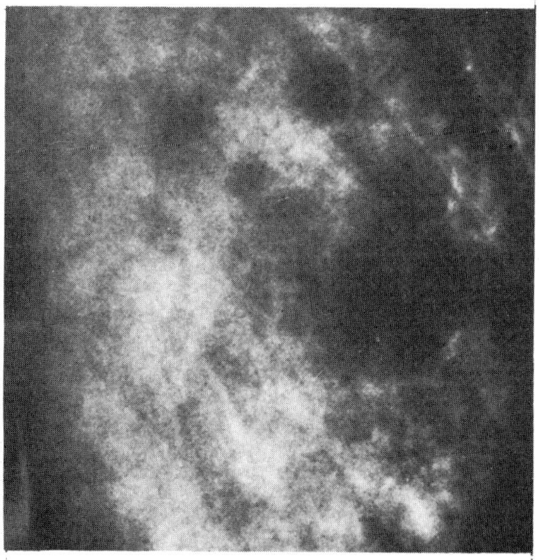

Figure 22.23. Selective left hepatic arteriogram. Multiple abscess cavities left lobe, confirmed by retrograde cholangiogram.

hepatic portal approach stops bleeding instantly and dramatically. Results of transhepatic sclerosis are encouraging.[16,21,23] The average results of these three groups show a portal vein catheterization rate of 92 per cent and initial variceal sclerosis in 66 per cent. The technique is challenging and initially time-consuming. Useful retroperitoneal shunting veins must be carefully distinguished from large gastric collaterals (Figure 22.20). Thrombin, Gelfoam and Sotradecol combinations and the monomer, isobucrylate, are four of the common agents used. The perfect occluding agent should be both easy to handle and cause guaranteed permanent occlusion but it is not yet available. Follow-up studies up to two years indicate recanalization of some veins in over 50 per cent of patients. The message is clear. Following successful sclerotherapy the patient with fair liver function ought, within four months, to have elective shunt surgery to decompress the portal system. Unfortunately, many patients

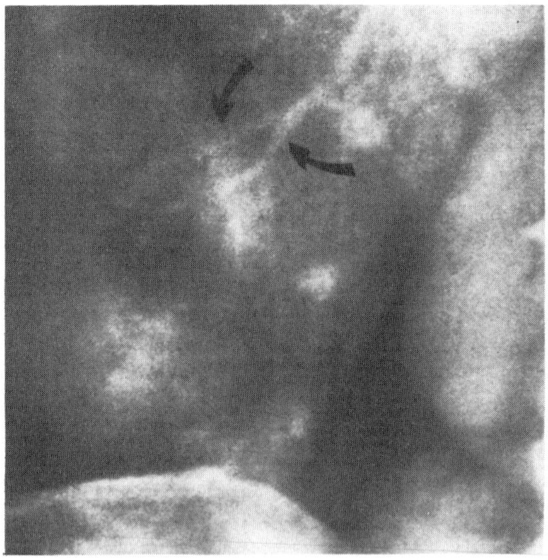

Figure 22.24. Budd–Chiari syndrome. Arteriogram–hepatogram phase. Slow sinusoidal clearance. Note portal vein radicles (arrows).

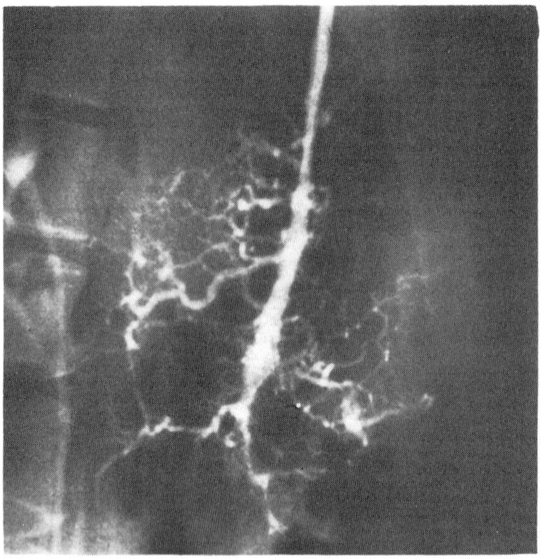

Figure 22.25. Budd–Chiari syndrome. Wedge hepatic venogram, lateral view. Intrahepatic spider's web venous pattern is diagnostic.

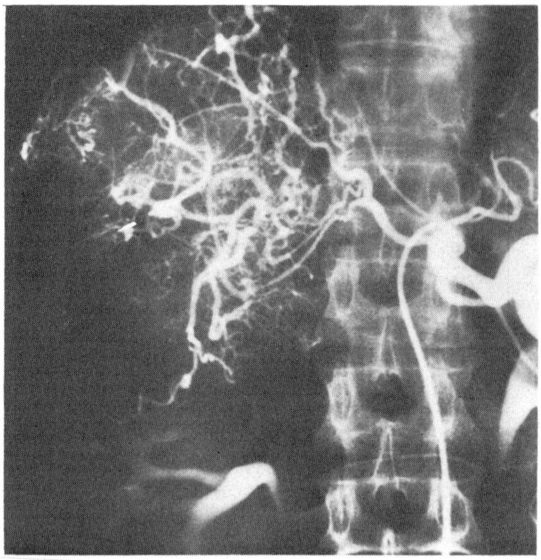

Figure 22.26. Selective coeliac arteriogram. Blood supply of vascular tumour in right hypochondrium is by inferior phrenic arteries, not hepatic. Lesion distorts upper right kidney. Adrenal adenoma.

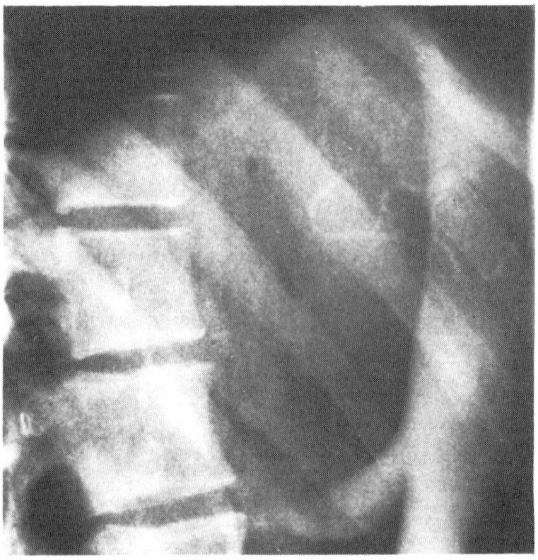

Figure 22.27. Inferior venacavogram. Forward displacement of upper cava due to retroperitoneal tumour.

offered for initial and later repeat sclerotherapy are surgically rejected end-stage cirrhotics with gross ascites and coagulopathy. Complications of the procedure are low in all centres and no subsequent pulmonary emboli have been diagnosed clinically or radiologically.

In the preparation of a patient for definitive shunt surgery, angiography should demonstrate patency of vessels to be used for the particular portasystemic shunt. The presence and position of the left kidney must be shown prior to any type of splenorenal shunt. It cannot be assumed that anatomy, as demonstrated on a study made weeks or months previously, will remain unaltered. Timely use of ultrasound will prevent some repeat angiograms. Following shunt surgery, patency may be proven by arteriography, venacavography, or splenic pulp injections should the spleen remain (Figure 22.21). If the approach is via the venous system (either portal or systemic), pressures may be recorded and should show a significant fall from preoperative readings.

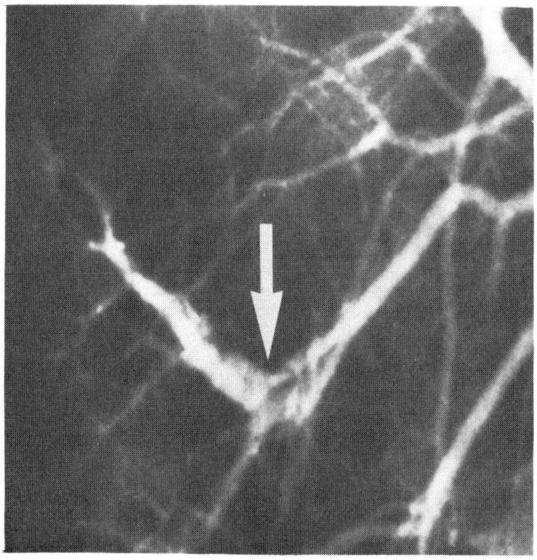

(a)

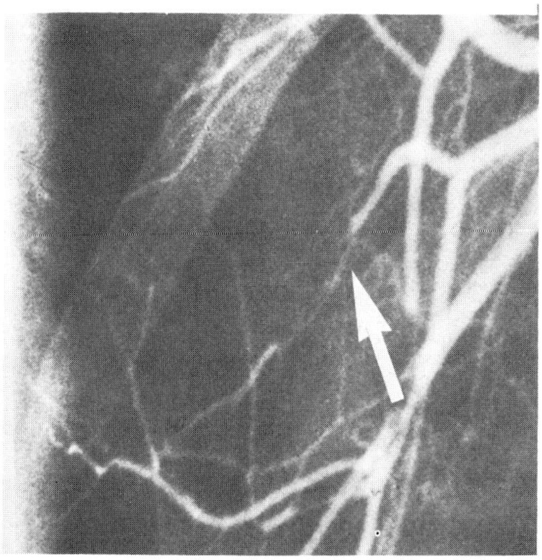

(b)

Figure 22.28. (a) Selective hepatic arteriogram. Patient has traumatic hepatic arterioportal venous shunt (arrow) and haemobilia. (b) Shunt has closed (arrow) following Gelfoam embolization. Immediate cessation of blood loss.

FURTHER APPLICATIONS

Granulomas in liver or spleen appear as well-defined avascular defects (Figure 22.22), whereas abscesses show the minimal vascularity of a shaggy wall surrounding a necrotic centre (Figure 22.23). Small areas of increased vascularity ('pseudo-tumours') are sometimes seen in the liver in the Budd–Chiari syndrome.[9] *Slowly*-fading adjacent portal vein radicles may confirm the radiologist's suspicion (Figure 22.24). Other patients with occluded hepatic veins will show on wedged hepatic venography a diagnostic plexiform web pattern (Figure 22.25). These have been proven to be due to veno-venous connections between hepatic veins.[17]

ANGIOGRAPHIC PITFALLS

Both regenerative nodules and focal nodular hyperplasia may be highly vascular with hepatic arterioportal venous shunting, and resemble liver cell cancer.[26] The radio-isotope scan can prove the presence of a nodule because of increased rather than decreased isotope uptake by the vascular lesion.[20] Some retroperitoneal tumours may mimic vascular liver tumours closely unless their major vascular supply is carefully studied (Figure 22.26). Inferior vena-cavography is usually decisive (Figure 22.27).

THERAPEUTIC ARTERIAL EMBOLIZATION

In certain patients this should be considered *at the time of angiography*. Patients with sites of active bleeding, highly vascular neoplasms and arteriovenous fistulae (some iatrogenic in origin) should benefit from timely successful embolization (Figure 22.28a and b).

REFERENCES

1. Allison, D.J. (1977) Haematemesis and melaena. *British Medical Journal,* **i,** 1279.
2. Aspelin, P., Nylander, G. & Pettersson, H. (1976) Bradykinin-induced changes in calibre of portal vein during splanchnic angiography. *Investigative Radiography,* **11,** 10–13.
3. Chuang, V.P., Bree, R.L. & Bookstein, J.J. (1974) Angiographic features of focal lymphoma of the liver. *Radiology,* **111,** 53–55.
4. Dick, R. (1977) Therapeutic angiographic embolization. *British Journal of Radiology,* **50,** 241–242.
5. Frimann-Dahl, J. (1970) Percutaneous splenoportography. In *Modern Trends in Diagnostic Radiology – 4* (Ed.) McLaren, J.W. pp. 175–189. London: Butterworths.
6. Gammill, S.L., Takahashi, M., Jingu, K., Stumpe, W. & Font, R. (1975) A comparison of scans and angiograms in selecting patients with hepatomas for hepatic lobectomy. *American Journal of Roentgenology,* **123,** 522–530.
7. Goldstein, H.M., Thaggard, A., Wallace, S. & Neiman, H.L. (1976) Priscoline-augmented hepatic angiography. *Radiology,* **119,** 275–279.

8. Hamlyn, A.N., Morris, J.S., Dick, R., Lunzer, M.R. & Puritz, H. (1974) Portal hypertension with varices in unusual sites. *Lancet,* **ii,** 1531–1534.
9. Hungerford, G.D., Lunzer, M.R., Dick, R., Hamlyn, A.N. & Sherlock, S. (1976) Pseudo-metastases in the liver: a presentation of the Budd–Chiari syndrome. *Radiology,* **120,** 627–628.
10. Kaufmann, S.L., Harrington, D.P., Barth, K.H., Maddrey, W.C. & White, R.I. Jr (1977) Control of variceal bleeding by superior mesenteric artery vasopressin infusion. *American Journal of Roentgenology,* **128,** 567–570.
11. Laws, J.W. (1964) The liver, spleen, gall bladder and pancreas. In *Recent Advances in Radiology,* 4th ed. (Ed.) Lodge, T. pp. 125–155. London: J. & A. Churchill.
12. Lea Thomas, M. & Carty, H. (1974) Hereditary haemorrhagic telangiectasia of the liver demonstrated angiographically. *Acta Radiologica Diagnosis,* **15,** 433–438.
13. Legge, D.A. (1977) The use of prostaglandin F_2 alpha in selective visceral angiography. *British Journal of Radiology,* **50,** 251–255.
14. Lunderquist, A. (1974) Pharmacoangiography of the left gastric artery in oesophageal varices. *Acta Radiologica Diagnosis,* **15,** 157–160.
15. Lunderquist, A. & Vang, J. (1974) Transhepatic catheterization and obliteration of the coronary vein in patients with portal hypertension and oesophageal varices. *New England Journal of Medicine,* **291,** 646–649.
16. Lunderquist, A., Simert, G., Tylen, U. & Vang, J. (1977) Follow up of patients with portal hypertension and oesophageal varices treated with percutaneous obliteration of gastric coronary vein. *Radiology,* **122,** 59–63.
17. Maguire, R. & Doppman, J.L. (1977) Angiographic abnormalities in partial Budd–Chiari syndrome. *Radiology,* **122,** 629–635.
18. Okuda, K., Obata, H., Jinnouchi, S., Kubo, Y., Nagasaki, Y., Shimokawa, Y., Motoike, Y., Muto, H., Nakajima, Y., Musha, H., Yamazaki, T., Sakamoto, K., Kojiro, M. & Nakashima, T. (1977) Angiographic assessment of gross anatomy of hepatocellular carcinoma: comparison of coeliac angiograms and liver pathology in 100 cases. *Radiology,* **123,** 21–29.
19. Pinet, F., Amiel, M., Bourgoin, J., Clermont, A., Pierluca, P. & Dargent, M. (1972) Microangiographie des tumeurs malignes du foie. *Annals Radiologie,* **15,** 437–443.
20. Reuter, S.R., Redman, H.C. & Siders, D.B. (1970) The spectrum of angiographic findings in hepatoma. *Radiology,* **94,** 89–94.
21. Scott, J., Dick, R., Long, R.G. & Sherlock, S. (1976) Percutaneous transhepatic obliteration of gastro-oesophageal varices. *Lancet,* **ii,** 53–56.
22. Viamonte, M. Jr & Schiff, E. (1977) Diagnostic approach to hepatic malignant neoplasms. *Journal of the American Medical Association,* **238,** 2191–2193.
23. Viamonte, M. Jr, Pereiras, R., Russell, E., Le Page, J. & Hutson, D. (1977) Transhepatic obliteration of oesophageal varices: results in acute and non-acute bleeders. *American Journal of Roentgenology,* **129,** 237–241.
24. Wallace, S. (1976) Interventional radiology. *Cancer,* **37** (Suppl.), 517–531.
25. Walter, J.F., Bookstein, J.J. & Bouffard, E.V. (1976) Newer angiographic observations in cholangiocarcinoma. *Radiology,* **118,** 19–23.
26. Winograd, J. & Palubinskas, A.J. (1977) Arterial-portal venous shunting in cavernous haemangioma of the liver. *Radiology,* **122,** 331–332.

Chapter 23

Endoscopic–Radiological Examination and Therapy in Biliary Tract Disease

F.W. OSSENBERG
M. CLASSEN

After the first endoscopic cannulation of the papilla of Vater by McCune, Shorb and Moscovitz[66] its widespread introduction followed the development of new fibreoptic duodenoscopes in 1970. The rapid development of suitable endoscopic–radiological techniques for diagnostic and therapeutic procedures in the area of the pancreatic and biliary tract system resulted in a deluge of mainly enthusiastic reports (see the detailed survey by Cotton.[17,18])

For the first time direct access was made possible to the papilla of Vater, the key point of a functional system comprising the duodenum, biliary tract, liver and pancreas. By means of retrograde cannulation the pancreatic and biliary tract system can be visualized independently of hepatic function and extrahepatic obstruction can be exactly assessed radiologically. In addition, this technique enables manometric examination of the two ducts and permits the collection of pure pancreatic juice bile for cytological, serological and biochemical examinations. A new chapter in the treatment of gallstone disease has been started with electropapillotomy and stone extraction from the common bile duct. The latest development is direct endoscopic inspection of the biliary tree by peroral transpapillary choledochoscopy.

ENDOSCOPIC–RADIOLOGICAL DIAGNOSTIC TECHNIQUES OF THE BILIARY TRACT

Technical Aspects of Endoscopic–Radiological Retrograde Cholangiopancreatography (ERCP)

Indications and contraindications

Because of their close topography and functional relationship the biliary tract and the pancreatic duct system are usually visualized under the same procedure of ERCP. This provides an excellent diagnostic method for distinguishing medical and surgical jaundice[7,8] and can be used in early stages of the illness. Since, even in the absence of jaundice, intravenous cholangiograms often fail to provide diagnostic information, ERCP is indicated for all patients suspected of biliary tract disease who have negative conventional x-rays. Furthermore, ERCP is indicated on suspicion of pancreatic disease. It permits definite documentation of chronic pancreatitis, demonstrating duct abnormalities such as strictures and stones, and thus provides a basis for surgical drainage. ERCP permits the diagnosis of pancreatic cancer at the stage at which it usually presents for specialist investigation. In patients with obscure epigastric pain, a normal pancreatogram cannot exclude relapsing pancreatitis although advanced chronic pancreatitis can be excluded.

Like other endoscopic examinations, ERCP is contraindicated in severe cardiorespiratory insufficiency or after recent cardiovascular attacks. Following acute pancreatitis, pancreatography should not be performed for at least three to four weeks. In patients with recurrent pancreatitis or continuing pain and hyperamylasaemia, ultrasonographic exclusion of pseudocysts is obligatory prior to ERCP. If pseudocysts can be demonstrated, pancreatography is rarely indicated and should be performed only as an immediate preoperative examination. In view of the difficulty in disinfecting fibrescopes and the possibility of transmitting viral hepatitis, the presence of hepatitis B antigen in the serum should be excluded in all jaundiced patients prior to the performance of the ERCP. Many endoscopists decline to examine hepatitis B-antigen carriers[7,11,19,68] although transmission is rare.[65]

Complications

Serious complications of upper gastrointestinal tract endoscopy related to premedication and instrument manipulation are rare. Specific risks are incurred by cannulation and injection of contrast into the pancreatic and bile duct systems.[19] Respiratory and circulatory reactions to the premedication, aspiration of gastric juice and perforation of the alimentary tract with the fibrescope occur extremely rarely. However, diminution of arterial oxygen saturation following the procedure is common.[98] Perforation of the pancreatic and common bile ducts with the plastic catheter are very rare complications.

Sepsis and pancreatitis are the two main hazards. They are particularly to be expected after the filling with contrast of an abnormal and poorly draining duct system. In the majority of patients a transient rise in serum amylase and lipase in the absence of pancreatic symptoms is observed after pancreatography, especially if pancreatic parenchymal opacification is present.[91] In 25 per cent of cases an increase in serum amylase is observed even after selective retrograde cholangiography. Acute pancreatitis following retrograde pancreatography results from an excessive injection of the contrast material; this risk can be diminished by careful fluoroscopic monitoring of the injection of contrast by means of a powerful television image-intensifier system. A comprehensive collection of the results of many workers indicates that the risk of pancreatitis is 1 to 1.3 per cent.[5,70] Sepsis is the principal cause of mortality following ERCP. It occurs almost exclusively in patients with poor drainage of the pancreatic and biliary systems.[18] In pancreatic lesions such as malignant stenosis and pseudocysts poor drainage presumably results from the introduction of infection by the procedure. Patients with biliary stasis invariably have infected bile and cholangitis and septicaemia may occur as a result of dissemination of bacteria already present. A sudden pressure increase in the biliary tree can cause bacteraemia by cholangiovenous reflux.[44,46]

Instruments

The equipment for duodenoscopy with cannulation of the papilla of Vater consists of a polydirectional, flexible, small-sized fibrescope with a high-quality lateral-viewing optical system and a channel large enough for the passage of tubes, Dormia baskets or biopsy forceps. These requirements are met by the majority of endoscope manufacturers (ACMI, Machida, Fuji, Wolf). We most frequently use the JFB2 duodenoscope (Olympus Optical Co.). Standard forward-viewing panendoscopes are suitable only in patients with Billroth II (Polya) partial gastrectomy, when the papilla is approached from below via the afferent loop.

Graduated catheters of polyvinyl chloride or teflon, with an outer diameter of 1.5 to 1.7mm, are used for the cannulation. Metal tip inserts may facilitate cannulation of the minor papilla or of a smooth or indurated major papilla.

Premedication: cannulation technique

Prior to the examination the fasting patient receives 0.5 mg atropine and an individually 'titrated' dose of diazepam. The mouth and throat are swabbed or sprayed with a suitable local anaesthetic. Because of the altered pharmacodynamics of drugs in patients with liver disease[75] (see Chapter 16), the dosage of diazepam must be tailored to avoid respiratory depression or hepatic precoma in susceptible patients. The presence of duodenal ileus is helpful in locating the papilla, and intermittent intravenous injections of hyoscine-*N*-butyl bromide (Buscopan) (20 to 40 mg) or glucagon 0.5mg) are effective in achieving this.[18,27]

The patient is examined in the prone position on the x-ray table. The duodenoscope is first introduced into the antrum of the stomach; to avoid strong peristalsis little air should be insufflated. After locating the pylorus the tip of the instrument is advanced as near as possible to it by a slight dorsal flexion. The tip is then squared off ventrally in the direction of the lesser curvature and is simultaneously pushed forward until it enters the duodenal bulb with a slight jerk. By turning the instrument through 180° further introduction is performed with slight air insufflation. The lumen of the descending part of the duodenum then becomes visible.

For cannulation we prefer the endoscope to be straight. This position can be achieved by hooking the tip of the instrument in the second part of the duodenum and then withdrawing it with the lens facing the patient's left side. Further withdrawal brings the lens up the medial wall of the duodenum to the longitudinal fold and the papilla. The control of the distal tip is thus enhanced and less of the shaft is exposed to radiation. The longitudinal fold is the guide to the papilla, which is located proximally partly directly on it and partly adjacent to it (Plate 23.1; see page 548). The orifice is located in the centre of the papillary area; it is either slit-like or rounded and of variable size. The minor papilla, the end of the duct of Santorini, is located 2 cm above the major papilla towards the posterior wall. The positioning of the catheter tip is crucial for successful cannulation. The tip of the instrument is adjusted so that the extended catheter lies at a right angle with the papillary orifice.[26] After cannulation of the papillary orifice the contrast medium, Urografin (diatrizoate sodium 60 per cent) or Angiografin (diatrizoate meglumine 65 per cent) is injected under careful fluoroscopic monitoring. Usually the pancreatic duct is visualized first; cholangiography may then be achieved by placing the catheter tip a short distance inside the papillary orifice and then angling it upwards in a craniodorsal direction.

The technique of cannulation of the papilla is difficult to learn and requires good manual skill by the endoscopist.[5, 67] Both the cannulation success rate and the complication rate depend largely on the skill and experience of the operator. A recent survey demonstrated that in expert hands there was a 15 per cent failure rate for cannulation and a 3.5 per cent complication rate. In less experienced hands the failure rate was 62 per cent and the complication rate 15 per cent. With a perfect examination technique the pancreatic duct is visualized in 92 per cent of cases and the common bile duct in 87 per cent.[18] Failure may be due to lack of cooperation by the patient or abnormal anatomy, as with pyloric or duodenal stenosis, following Billroth II partial gastrectomy, with inflammatory or neoplastic stenosis of the papilla or in the presence of peripapillary duodenal diverticula where the papilla is hidden in the diverticulum.

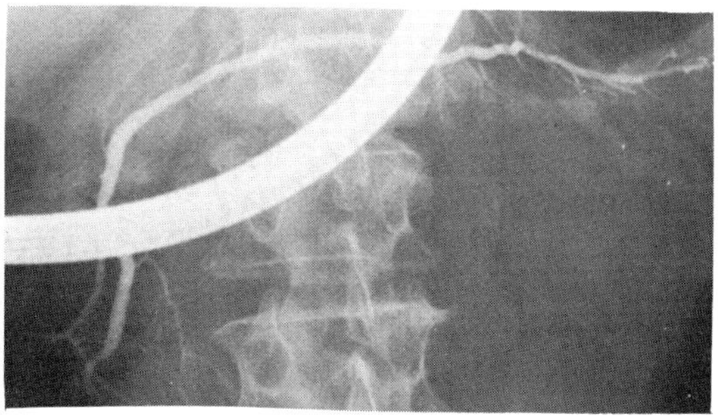

Figure 23.1. Normal pancreatography. Opacification of the main pancreatic duct, Santorini's duct and their primary and secondary duct branches.

Technical features of cholangiography

After cannulation of the papilla, contrast medium should be injected until there is adequate filling of the intrahepatic ducts and the gallbladder. However, in the presence of bile duct stenosis contrast injection should be kept to the minimum consistent with making a diagnosis to reduce the risk of producing acute suppurative cholangitis. There is no evidence that incorporation of an antibiotic into the injected contrast material is beneficial, but antibiotics should be administered immediately after the procedure if contrast medium has entered poorly drained ducts. Prophylactic antibiotic therapy (see Chapter 53) may be indicated if 'high risk' factors are present.

Changing the position of the patient is often more effective than increasing the volume of contrast material. Cystic duct obstruction can be diagnosed if the gallbladder fails to fill after suitable positioning and adequate filling of the intrahepatic tree with contrast has occurred. Filling of the biliary tree commonly provides high-quality retrograde cholangiograms which are easy to interpret. Difficulties in interpretation may result from layering or streaming effects caused by incomplete mixing of contrast material and bile. Air bubbles which are injected together with the contrast material may be confused with common bile duct stones. If this is suspected, rotation of the patient on his body axis with radiographs taken in different positions and projections may prove helpful.

Diagnostic Findings at the Papilla of Vater, the Pancreatic Duct and the Biliary Tract System

Papilla of Vater: ampullary and periampullary diseases

At endoscopy, hemispherical, papillary and flat-form variants of the papilla are found. Above it the intraduodenal part of the common bile duct penetrates the duodenal wall into the lumen and, together with the major duodenal fold, covers the papilla like a roof.[26] The commonest site for the occurrence of duodenal diverticula is the concave side of the duodenal loop, mainly in the papillary region (Plate 23.1). Diverticula vary from the size of a pea to that of a tennis ball and occur singly or in groups. The papilla is often located in the border or in the cavity of a diverticulum. Endoscopically the orifice of the diverticulum can be easily recognized by the radial mucosal folds. When manipulating the endoscope near diverticula the endoscopist must consider the risk of perforation of the thin wall. According to Hoffmann and Weiss[43] there is a significant relationship between juxtapapillary duodenal diverticula and gallstones: 74 per cent of patients with duodenal diverticula who are examined suffer from gallstones.

Periampullary carcinoma arising from the distal common bile duct, the head of the pancreas, the duodenum or the papilla of Vater itself can be diagnosed duodenoscopically.[16, 85]

Ulcerated tumours in the area of the papilla are almost exclusively malignant; the histological and cytological proof of malignancy is easily obtained by biopsy and brush cytology.[30] The diagnosis of non-ulcerated tumours is difficult. The endoscopic appearance of a coarsely enlarged papilla with a smooth, villous or nodular surface can resemble a carcinoma of the papilla, papillitis or adenomyomatosis of the papilla. The results of histological examination may prove falsely negative because only the upper epithelial layers are seized by the biopsy forceps. For reliable histological diagnosis it is necessary in these cases to split the papilla with the electropapillotome and to cut away a larger piece of tissue with the diathermy loop. Furthermore, an enlarged and swollen papilla may be caused by impaction of a gallstone within the papilla. A discharge from the papillary orifice may indicate a suppurative cholangitis, whilst the discharge of blood may indicate a tumour located higher in the biliary tree. A reddened, dilated and irregularly shaped orifice in the presence of upper abdominal pain and transient jaundice may indicate the recent passage of a gallstone through the papilla.

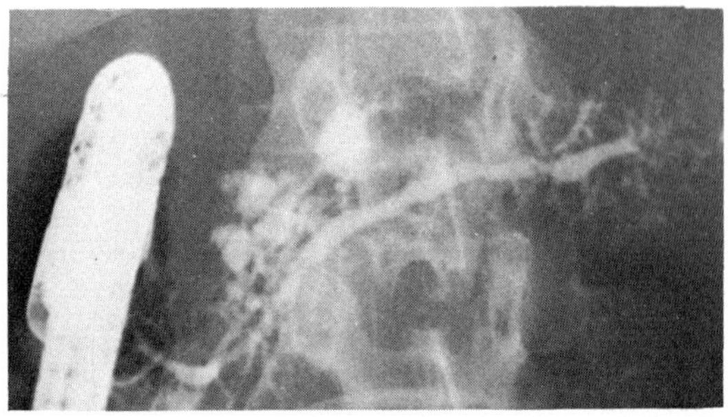

Figure 23.2. Pancreatography in chronic pancreatitis. Enlargement and variation in the calibre of the main pancreatic duct and its branches. Opacification of some small pseudocysts.

The importance of pancreatography in diagnosis

The course of the main pancreatic duct (MPD) is subject to considerable variation, the ascending type being the most frequent variant[49, 84] (Figure 23.1). The average diameter of the duct is 4 mm in the area of the head, 3 mm in the body and 2 mm in the tail of the pancreas. The normal contour of the wall is smooth. Injection of increasing volumes of contrast material results in opacification of the duct branches (primary, secondary and tertiary), the fine pancreatic ducts and, finally, the acini. Because greater degrees of opacification are associated with an increased incidence of pancreatitis, only the main pancreatic duct and the primary duct branches should be filled.

Inflammatory pancreatic processes are seen in the pancreatogram as deformations of the duct system or pseudocysts.[50, 78, 84, 87, 102] These cysts connect with the duct system in about 60 per cent of cases. Filling defects in the area of the duct branches, complete obstruction of the MPD and displacement or narrowing of the common bile duct are indirect signs of pseudocysts.[88] In chronic pancreatitis the earliest changes are minor variations in the calibre of the fine branches. In advanced chronic pancreatitis marked enlargement and variation in calibre of the MPD and its branches, strictures, obstructions, calculi or coarse acinar opacification are seen in the pancreatogram (Figures 23.2 and 23.3). The radiological differentiation between chronic pancreatitis and

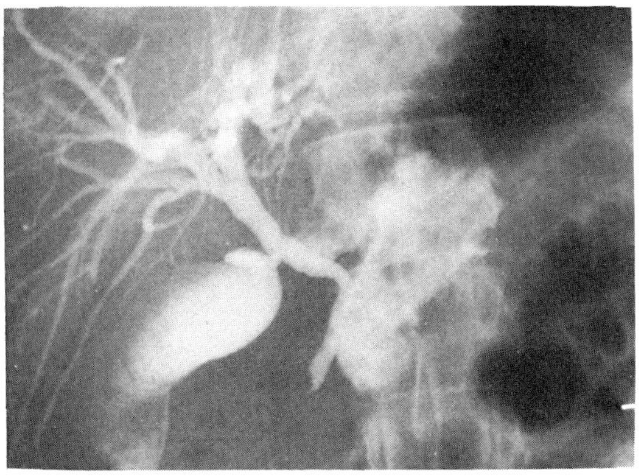

Figure 23.3. Retrograde cholangiopancreatography with opacification of a large pseudocyst. Early obstruction of bile flow, as suggested by a slight enlargement of the intrahepatic bile ducts and the gallbladder.

carcinoma is difficult and these conditions may coexist.[84,93]

Pancreatic cancer, arising almost exclusively from duct tissue, is seen most commonly on the pancreatogram as complete duct obstruction or stenosis with distal dilatation. Rarely, it may appear as a tapering stricture, ectasia or coarse acinar opacification[16,35,50,93] (Figure 23.4).

Special problems arise with cancer involving the head of the pancreas when the pancreatic duct is blocked close to the papilla and pancreatography fails,[93] or when, in spite of the tumour's progressing, the pancreatogram appears normal. In these cases retrograde cholangiography will sometimes demonstrate a lesion.[59,63,90] Mistakes in the interpretation of the pancreatogram result from injection of insufficient contrast material, the introduction of air bubbles, or faulty positioning causing inadequate filling with contrast material, giving the appearance of complete duct obstruction. Due to difficulty in distinguishing cancer and pancreatitis by radiographs alone, additional information is required. Positive results have been obtained in 50 to 80 per cent of cases by cytological examination of pure pancreatic juice aspirated following secretin stimulation from the intubated main pancreatic duct.[41,61] However, the results are poor in early cancer, in exocrine pancreatic insufficiency and in tumours located in the body or the tail.[30] Brush cytology from the pancreatic and common bile ducts has also been recommended.[74,97] In an attempt to provide better diagnosis, the measurement of carcino-embryonic antigen (CEA) in pure pancreatic juice is being investigated. Pure bile can be aspirated for cytological examination by means of a balloon catheter.[89]

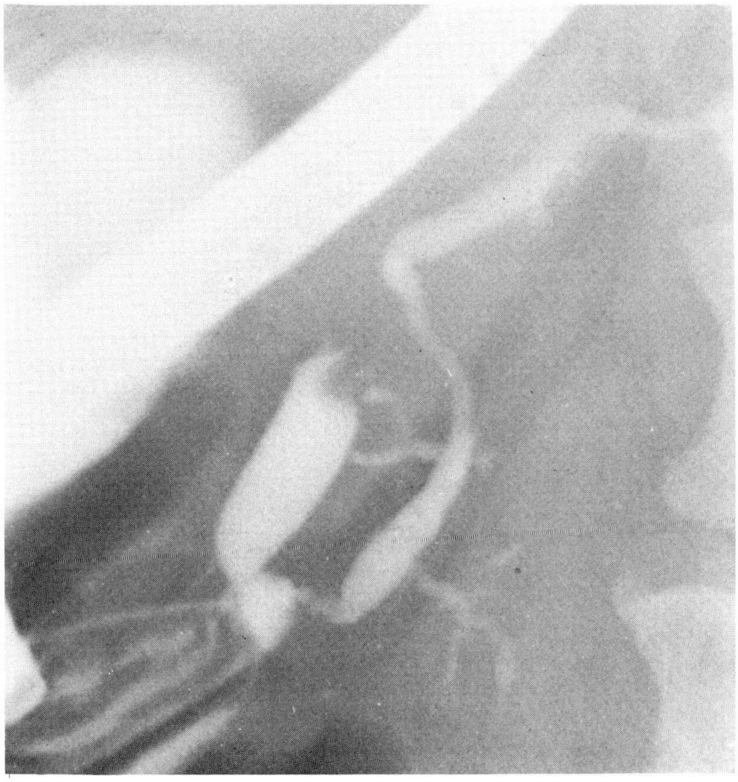

Figure 23.4. Retrograde cholangiopancreatography in a patient with cancer of the head of the pancreas. Radiography demonstrates a complete obstruction of the distal common bile duct and a tubular narrowing of the main pancreatic duct.

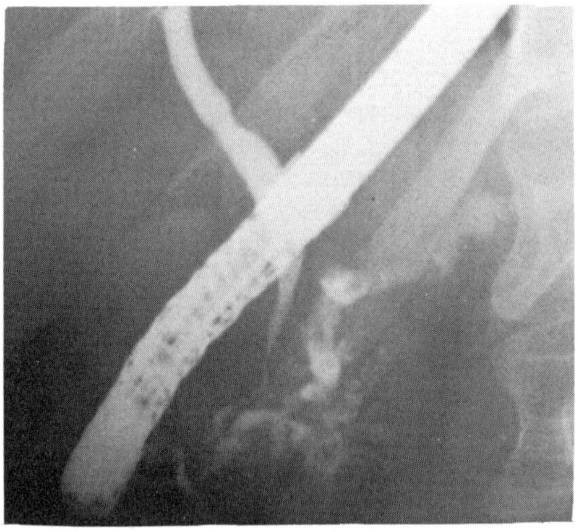

Figure 23.5. Retrograde cholangiopancreatography in chronic pancreatitis. Enlargement and calibre variations of the pancreatic duct with coarse parenchymal opacification. Thread-like stenosis of the distal common bile duct.

Alterations of the common bile duct in pancreatic disease

Both chronic pancreatitis and cancer are located predominantly in the head of the pancreas. By constriction of the intrapancreatic portion of the common bile duct they often cause extrahepatic obstructive jaundice (Figures 23.5 and 23.6). Koch, Classen and Demling[59] found involvement of the common bile duct in approximately 50 per cent of patients with chronic pancreatitis, but stenosis of the bile duct was not sufficiently severe to cause significant obstruction. Knowledge of biliary tract involvement is of great importance in considering pancreatectomy for patients with chronic pancreatitis. In 75 per cent of patients with cancer of the head of the pancreas a tight stenosis of the common bile duct with obstruction was observed. Three to five cm tubular waist-like or thread-like stenoses of the distal common bile duct with distal dilatation are seen on the cholangiogram. It must be

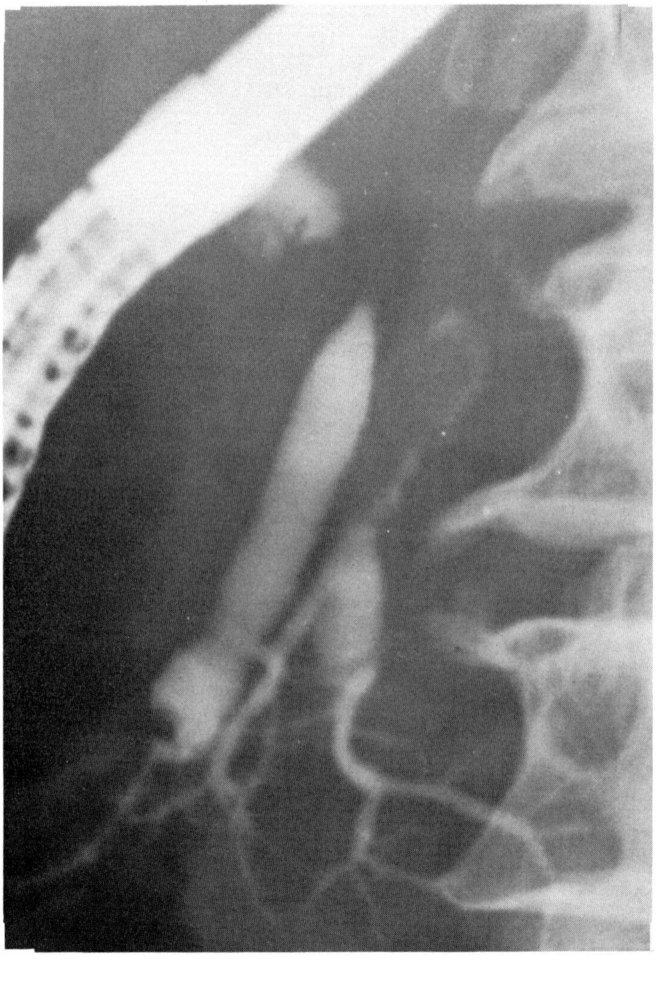

Figure 23.6. Retrograde cholangiopancreatography in a patient with cancer of the head of the pancreas. Obstruction of the common bile duct and the main pancreatic duct is nearly complete.

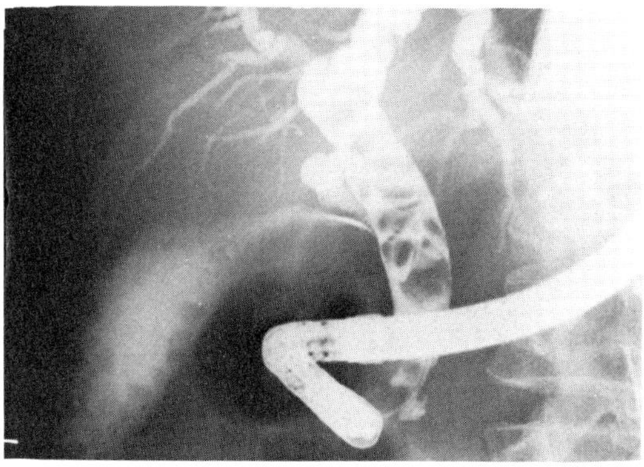

Figure 23.7. Retrograde cholangiography. Multiple gallstones in the gallbladder and the common bile duct. Deep cannulation of the common bile duct with the teflon catheter.

stressed that, in patients with cancer of the head of the pancreas when the pancreatic ducts either appear normal or fail to opacify, partial stenosis of the common bile duct is often the abnormality leading to the detection of the pancreatic disease.[59, 63]

Common bile duct stones

Radiographs of the biliary tree containing gallstones are familiar to clinicians and radiologists and most radiographs are easy to interpret (Figure 23.7). Calculi usually float up the duct during injection of contrast and only rarely produce complete obstruction. With impaction of a stone in the papilla of Vater the papilla appears swollen, and on tapping it with the probe it feels hard. In such cases, as well as with impaction of a stone in the lower common bile duct, cannulation of the papilla and injection of contrast may not be possible. Large stones occluding the lumen appear radiologically as convex obstructions in the bile duct or as ring-like lesions. Very small gallstones may easily be overlooked if the volume of contrast medium injected is excessive. In such cases detection may be facilitated by late radiographs in the outflow phase or by the use of diluted contrast solution. In patients with common bile duct stones a fine indentation of the distal wall contour of the bile duct seems to indicate secondary cholangitis. Considering the risk of infection by cholangiography in partial duct obstruction, endoscopic papillotomy should, if indicated, follow immediately.

Cholangiocarcinoma

Seifert et al[88] distinguish three types of bile duct tumour by means of retrograde cholangiography: (a) stenosis of the duct system with dilatation of the upper duct system and its branches, (b) complete obstruction of the common bile duct and (c) complete obstruction of one of the hepatic ducts without filling of its branches (Figure 23.8). Spot films demonstrate the irregular contour and sometimes an exophytic border of the constriction.[90] The localization of the cholangiocarcinoma is equally frequent in the areas of the right and left and common hepatic ducts as well as in the triple junction of the common hepatic, cystic and common bile ducts. Carcinomas in the area of the distal common bile duct and the diffuse spreading types are rarely observed. Isolated stenoses found in bile ducts free of gallstones and in the absence of a history of previous surgery to the ducts are indicative of carcinoma. Differentiation from tumours arising in surrounding tissues, namely the head of the pancreas, from postoperative strictures and from inflammatory stenosis is usually simple.

Primary sclerosing cholangitis

Primary sclerosing cholangitis is a chronically progressive inflammation of the biliary tree involving the extrahepatic as well as the intrahepatic bile ducts. Twenty to forty per cent of patients suffer simultaneously from ulcerative colitis.[1] In the presence of jaundice or with involvement of the intrahepatic bile ducts conventional cholangiography is often unsuccessful. Elias, Summerfield and Sherlock[28] stress the importance of retrograde cholangiography which will demonstrate the characteristic radiological appearance of the disease. The hazards of laparotomy and exploration of the biliary tree may thus be avoided in most cases. The typical radiological appearances of sclerosing cholangitis are multiple strictures with 'beading' of ducts between the narrowed segments and involvement of both intrahepatic and extrahepatic duct systems.[3, 29] Diffuse alterations of the entire bile duct system are not exceptional but the gallbladder is typically not involved. Located short stenoses, in contrast, favour the diagnosis of cholangiocarcinoma rather than sclerosing cholangitis and their presence is a clear indication for surgery (Figure 23.9).

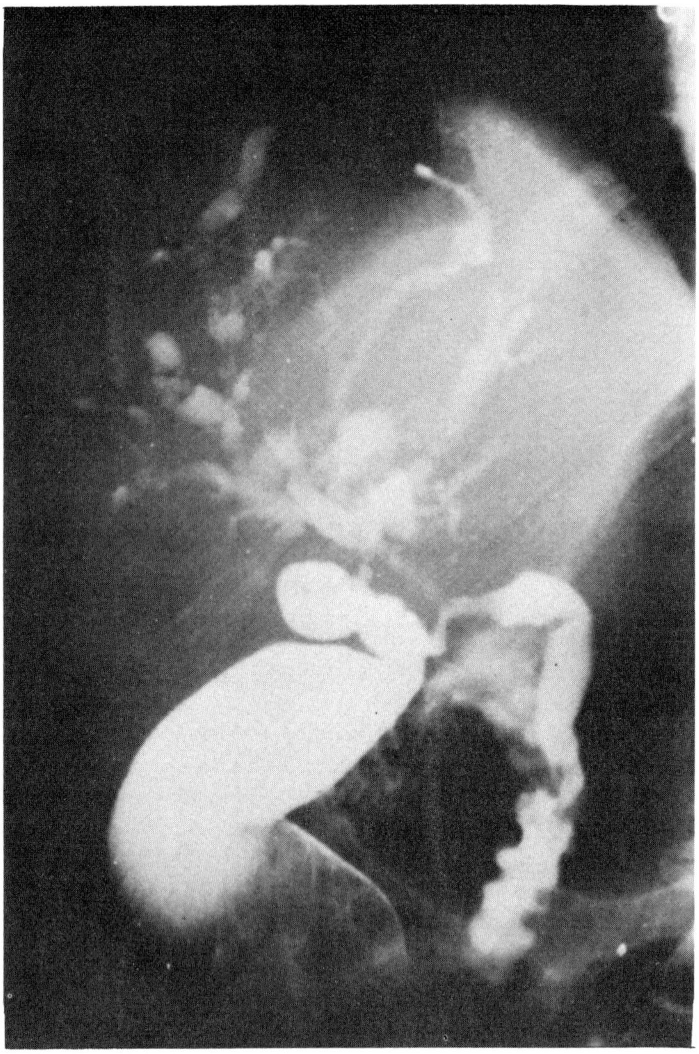

Figure 23.8. Retrograde cholangiography in common hepatic duct carcinoma. Marked enlargement of the intrahepatic bile ducts and the gallbladder.

Common bile duct cysts

Cystic dilatation of the common bile duct is very rarely observed. It may be suspected in patients presenting with intermittent jaundice, upper abdominal pain and an upper abdominal mass. Conventional cholangiography is usually unsuccessful. Since any volume of contrast material may be instilled into the dilated common bile duct by retrograde cholangiography, the diagnosis of even large cysts is possible without difficulty[71] (Figure 23.10).

Choledochoduodenal fistula and biliary–digestive anastomosis

Before the introduction of duodenal fibreoscopy the diagnosis of choledochoduodenal fistula was difficult if not impossible. Choledochoduodenal fistulae are commonly situated on or around the longitudinal fold of the duodenum and are usually caused by the spontaneous passage of gallstones. Ikeda and Okada[47] describe two types of choledochoduodenal fistulae. Type I is usually present on the longitudinal fold just proximal to the papilla. It is small and arises from the intramural portion of the common bile duct. Type II is found in the duodenal mucosa, adjacent to the longitudinal fold. It is large and arises from the extramural portion of the common bile duct. Type II fistulae are probably caused by stones which are too big to enter the narrow intramural portion of the common bile duct. The diagnosis of choledochoduodenal fistulae is made by direct observation of the fistula orifice with outflow of bile or contrast medium injected through the papilla. Successful cholangiography performed through the papilla

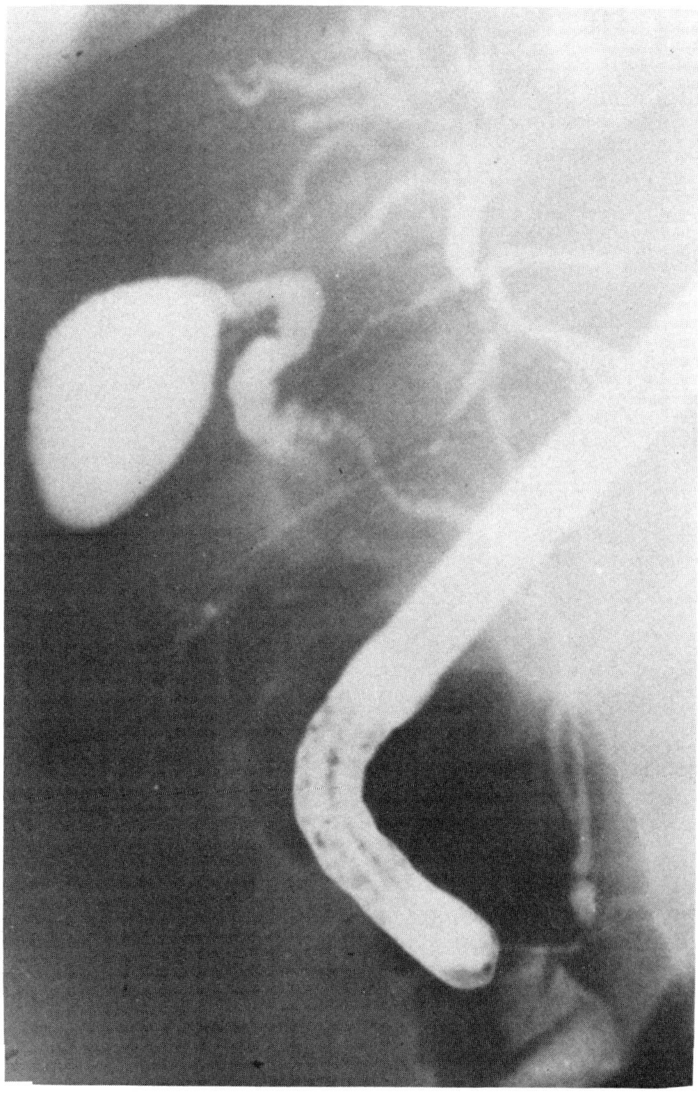

Figure 23.9. Retrograde cholangiography in a patient with ulcerative colitis and primary sclerosing cholangitis, mainly involving the extrahepatic bile ducts. Consequent dilatation of the intrahepatic bile ducts. As is typical of sclerosing cholangitis, the gallbladder appears normal.

in addition to visualization of the fistula orifice confirms the diagnosis.

Formerly the most frequently employed form of biliary–digestive anastomosis was the external supraduodenal choledochoduodenostomy, where the common bile duct is anastomosed to the anterior wall of the bulb or to the postbulbar duodenum. The anastomosis can be located and cannulated by means of both lateral-viewing duodenoscopes and forward-viewing panendoscopes.[32] The most frequent findings in patients with postoperative complaints are shrinkage of the anastomosis and retention of gallstones or food particles, particularly in the common duct stump below the anastomosis[15,32] (Figure 23.11). The stenosed anastomosis can be enlarged by incision using the papillotome of Demling and Classen. Retained gallstones and food remnants in the common duct stump can be extracted with the Dormia basket after endoscopic papillotomy. Following choledochojejunostomy, a more frequently performed anastomosis, retrograde cholangiography cannot be performed.

Alterations of the intrahepatic bile ducts

Retrograde cholangiography should always include an attempt to fill the biliary system beyond the bifurcation in order to avoid overlooking abnormalities of the intrahepatic ducts. Primary alterations of the intrahepatic ducts, such as cystic ectasia in the Caroli

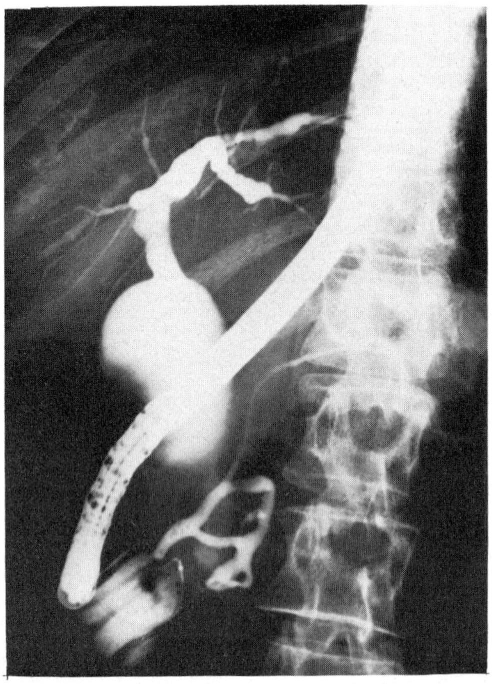

Figure 23.10. Retrograde opacification of a large common bile duct cyst. Abnormal junction between the main pancreatic duct and Santorini's duct. (By courtesy of Dr N. Soehendra, Hamburg.)

syndrome (Figure 23.12), intrahepatic gallstones or primary sclerosing cholangitis, are infrequent findings but can be readily demonstrated by retrograde cholangiography. Secondary alterations of the intrahepatic bile ducts, as in cirrhosis or metastatic liver disease, are observed more often. Ayoola et al[3] describe the characteristic changes in cirrhosis as 'pruning' of intrahepatic ducts, with the presence of segments of ductular stenosis, tortuosity, ductular displacement and an absence of dilatation. The stenosis and displacement are due to compression by regenerative nodules; 'pruning' may reflect a severe degree of portal fibrosis. While small metastatic tumour nodules may easily give findings similar to cirrhosis, progressive metastatic liver disease is distinguishable by the presence of irregular dilatation, abrupt obstruction of branches and marked ductular displacement giving rise to 'mass effects'. These findings are probably due to compression of ducts by tumour nodules. In seven of 23 patients with primary biliary cirrhosis, irregularities in calibre and a tortuous course of the small intrahepatic ducts have been described;[94] it is supposed that these changes are probably related to the distorted hepatic architecture due to cirrhosis and they may be interpreted as signs that cirrhosis has supervened (Figure 23.13).

Papillary stenosis

Duodenoscopic assessment of papillary abnormalities in papillitis, adenomyomatosis and ampullary carcinoma has already been mentioned. In such cases deep cannulation of the papilla may be difficult if not impossible. However, visualization of the biliary tree is generally possible. Common findings in papillary stenosis are dilatation of the extra- and intrahepatic bile ducts as well as the absence of motility of the sphincter of Oddi with consequent delay in emptying of the duct. However, it must be stressed that the retrogradely filled duct may appear to be larger than when visualized by intravenous cholangiography. Spot films of the papillary region may demonstrate abnormalities of the distal common bile duct, such as a thread-like stenosis of the ampullary segment or gross dilatation and irregularity of the contour of the wall. Using fluoroscopy or, preferably, radiocinematography it can be seen that the discharge of the contrast medium is delayed; also, a papillary movement is not detectable (Figure 23.14). In border-line cases the duodenobiliary pressure gradient should, if possible, be measured by manometry to substantiate the diagnosis (see below).

Supplementary Procedures during Retrograde Cholangiography

Choledochal manometry

Microsensor catheters[96] and perfused teflon catheter systems[38, 69, 79] are available to measure the duodenobiliary pressure gradient. Microsensor catheters do not readily fit the normal channel of the duodenoscope so that the sensitive tip is easily damaged. We therefore now use an open-tip perfused catheter system.

Technique. Premedication, duodenoscopy and cannulation of the papilla are performed in the usual way. Pressure transmission is made via an open-tip teflon catheter (300 cm long; inner diameter 1.2 mm) which is advanced through the instrument channel of the duodenoscope to the papilla. After cannulation it is pushed forward 2.5 cm into the common bile duct. The correct position of the catheter tip is verified endoscopically by the graduated scale at the

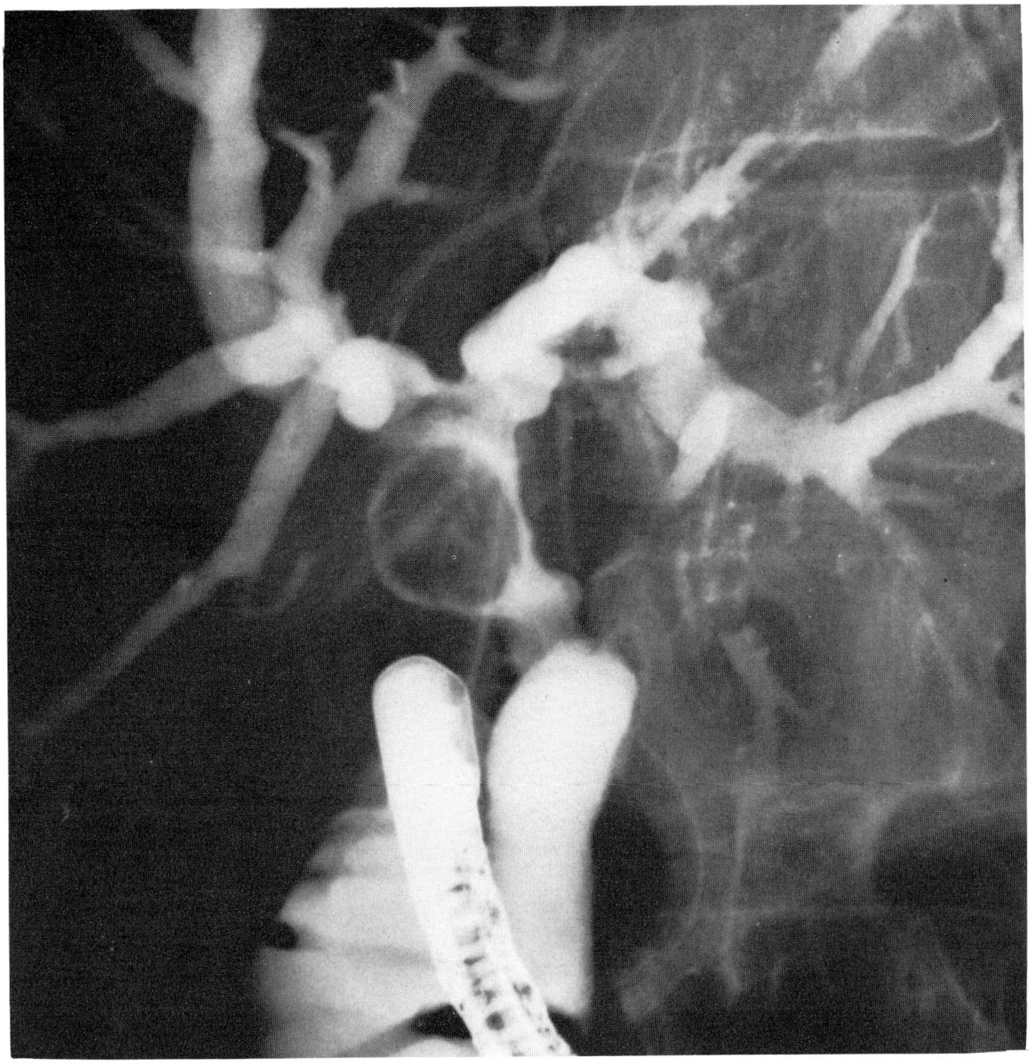

Figure 23.11. Retrograde cholangiography through a choledochoduodenostomy. Obstructing gallstone in the common hepatic duct with consequent enlargement of the intrahepatic bile ducts. Wall irregularities and calibre variations of the left hepatic duct and its branches suggest cholangitis. Prepapillary obstructing gallstone with consequent enlargement of the common bile duct stump distal to the anastomosis.

distal end of the catheter and by observing bile entering the catheter under aspiration. A second catheter of the same size is attached to the outside of the duodenoscope for measuring the duodenal intraluminal pressure as the zero reference point. Both catheters are perfused with saline at a rate of 0.5 ml/min. The intraluminal pressures of the duodenum and the common bile duct are transmitted simultaneously via these catheters to an external transducer (Statham element PB 23) and are recorded continuously by a two-channel direct writing recorder (Helcoscriptor HE 17; Hellige, Freiburg). The results are given in cm H_2O. The duodenobiliary pressure gradient is calculated from the difference between common bile duct and duodenal pressures.

The disadvantages of this measuring system are its inertia, caused by the length and small diameter of the manometric catheter, artefacts resulting from duodenal peristalsis, angulation of the catheter end and contact of the catheter tip with the wall, as well as difficulties encountered in achieving deep cannulation in patients with papillary stenosis.

According to our experience the normal duodenobiliary pressure gradient is 6.3 ± 3.8 cm H_2O. Values above 15 cm H_2O suggest papillary stenosis. After endoscopic papillotomy the pressure gradient is significantly lower than

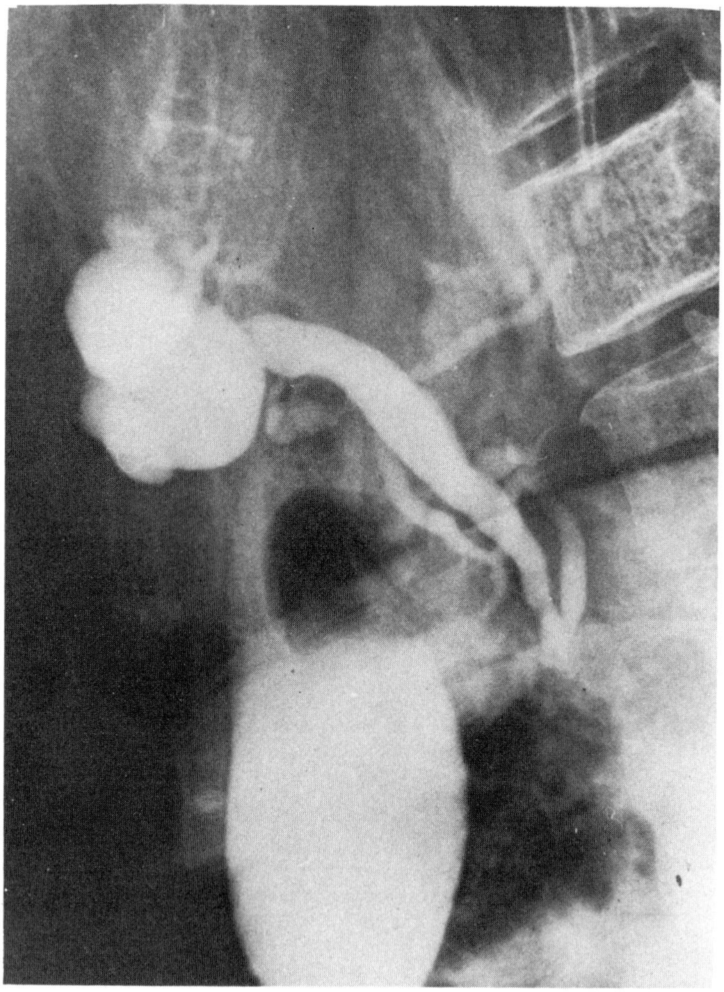

Figure 23.12. Circumscribed cystic dilatation of an intrahepatic bile duct in Caroli's disease. (By courtesy of Dr N. Soehendra, Hamburg.)

normal; in half of our patients there was no measurable pressure gradient.

Measurement of the pressure in the sphincter of Oddi by means of water perfused through side-hole catheters and catheter tip transducers has also been proposed for manometric evaluation of papillary function.[79, 96] However, Rösch, Koch and Demling[79] were unable to obtain reproducible results with either procedure and are convinced that the pressures recorded hitherto were artefacts originating from intermittent occlusion of the catheter by respiratory movements.

Peroral transpapillary cholangioscopy

Peroral cholangiopancreatoscopy opens a new field in fibre-endoscopic inspection of small hollow organs in the human body. The prototypes of various cholangioscopes are at present being tested in some centres.[18,54,79]

Technique. A long side-viewing duodenoscope ('motherscope') is used for the location of the papilla. A second, very thin endoscope ('babyscope') with a diameter of 2.3 mm is passed through the instrument channel and advanced through the papilla of Vater (Figure 23.15). So far this procedure has been used only following endoscopic papillotomy. Following this procedure the 'babyscope', which is difficult to manipulate because of its rigidity, is easily introduced. Rinsing facilities allow a good view within the ductal system. The disadvantages of the present instruments are that they are not steerable, they have no instrument channel for biopsy and they cannot be sterilized. Furthermore, these small fibrescopes are fragile and provide images of poor quality. In the future,

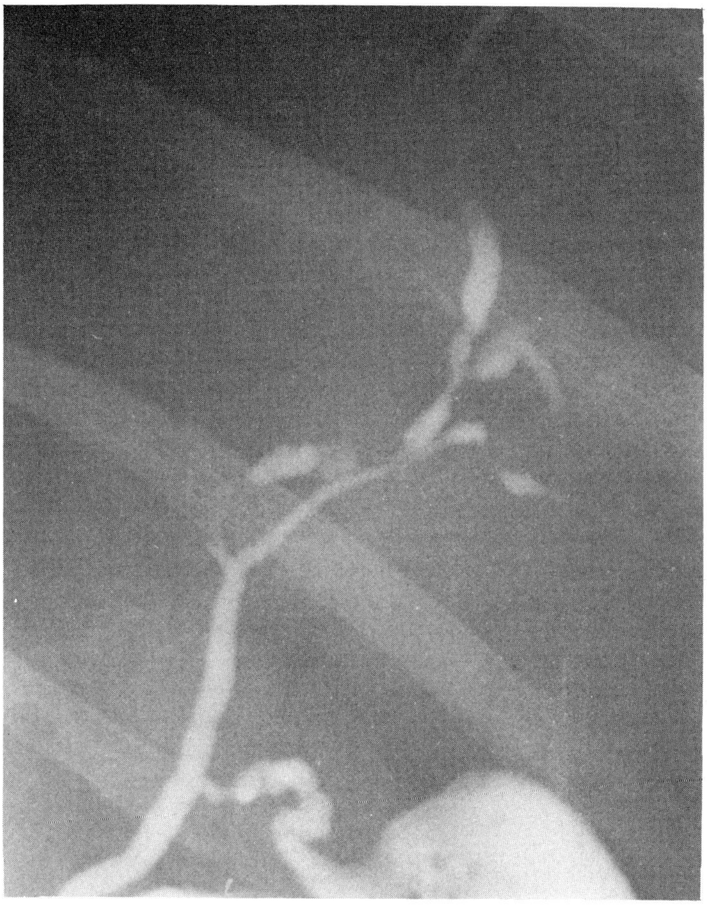

Figure 23.13. Narrowing and irregularities of the intrahepatic bile ducts simulating the characteristic findings in primary sclerosing cholangitis.

improved instruments will probably have a limited application in a few complex cases.

Cholangiography – Which is the Technique of Choice?

The precise role of ERCP alongside other developing techniques is still being clarified. For a non-icteric patient conventional excretion cholangiography following oral or intravenous administration of the contrast medium will continue to be the method of choice. Comparative studies of conventional and retrograde cholangiography have demonstrated, however, the limited diagnostic yield of conventional methods of opacification.[37] In 27 per cent of 103 patients with biliary disease identical findings were obtained with both techniques. In 20 per cent of cases conventional cholangiography gave falsely-negative results and in 55 per cent of the examinations no satisfactory opacification of the bile ducts could be achieved. Therefore, in patients strongly suspected of having biliary tract disease and with no pathological findings demonstrated by conventional cholangiography, performance of ERCP is indicated.

Differentiation between intrahepatic or 'medical' and extrahepatic or 'surgical' jaundice is nowadays facilitated by the development of several techniques which permit direct cholangiography when the intravenous method is inadequate. Since 1937, percutaneous transhepatic cholangiography (PTC) has been the most commonly used procedure in the demonstration of biliary obstruction. The danger from haemorrhage, bile leakage and septicaemia which may complicate this procedure has restricted its use to the immediate preoperative period. More sophisticated modifications of this original procedure which minimize the risk of complication by laparoscopic or transjugular hepatic venous access to the liver for the transhepatic injection of contrast have not gained wide acceptance.[39] The current vogue is to employ the technique used at Chiba University and described by Okuda et al.[73] In

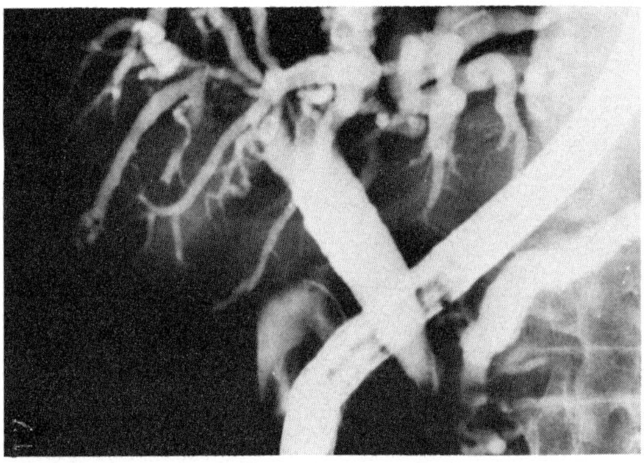

Figure 23.14. Retrograde cholangiopancreatography in papillary stenosis following surgical sphincterotomy. Marked dilatation of the intra- and extrahepatic bile ducts and of the main pancreatic duct.

this modification of PTC the 'skinny' needle is used. This is made of stainless steel with an outer diameter of 0.7 mm and is extremely flexible so that the patient may breathe normally while it lies in situ. The advantages of the Chiba technique are convincing: it is simple and cheap; complications are few and even non-obstructed ducts may be opacified in most cases. Comparisons between the Chiba modification of PTC and ERCP have more or less demonstrated that these are complementary rather than competitive procedures.[28, 33, 34, 45] Both procedures have their advantages and disadvantages and each clinician must select the procedure which he regards as most suitable with regard to the facilities and resources available as well as his own personal experience.

In common with other authors it is our practice to start with retrograde cholangiography. If retrograde opacification of the bile

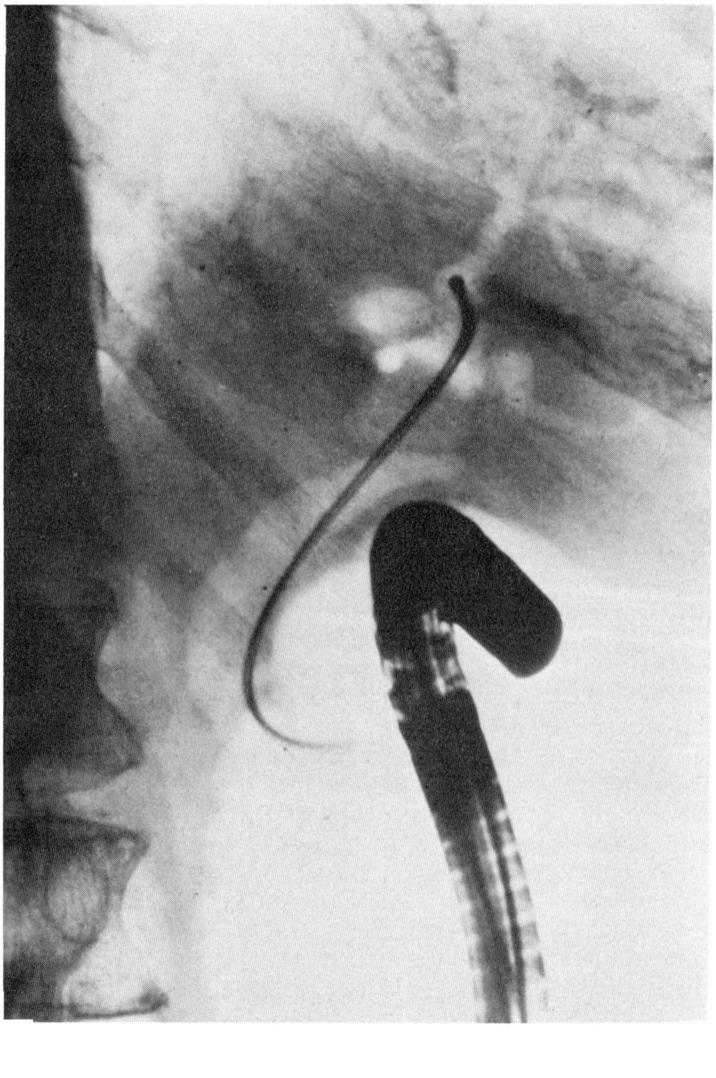

Figure 23.15. Transduodenal cholangioscopy. Via the 'motherscope', the 'babyscope' is introduced in the common bile duct.

ducts is unsuccessful, PTC using the Chiba needle follows immediately. Even if complete common bile duct obstruction is demonstrated by ERCP, subsequent performance of PTC is required to locate with reliability the proximal demarcation of the obstructing process which is decisive for planning the surgical procedure (see Chapter 26 for further discussion).

ENDOSCOPIC THERAPY OF COMMON BILE DUCT STONES AND PAPILLARY STENOSIS

The technique of retrograde cannulation of the papilla of Vater serves as the basis for endoscopic papillotomy in the treatment of papillary stenosis and for the removal of stones from the common bile duct. This therapeutic adaptation was developed simultaneously by Demling and Classen[10] in Germany and by Kawai et al[52] in Japan. At present this method is finding increasing application in western Europe,[10,12,20,22,57,64] in Japan[53,54] and in the United States.[36,101]

Technique of Endoscopic Papillotomy (EPT)

Instruments

We use the same instruments as for diagnostic ERCP: duodenoscope JFB2 (Olympus Optical Co.), duodenoscope TX6 (ACMI) or duodenoscope FDS (Machida). For patients following a Billroth II partial gastrectomy, forward-viewing panendoscopes such as the GIFD3 (Olympus Optical Co.) are used. Two papillotomes have been developed: the bridged pulsed papillotome by the Japanese, Soma, and the arched tracted papillotome by Demling and Classen. The great majority of procedures carried out to date have been performed with the papillotome developed by Demling and Classen. This papillotome comprises a plastic catheter containing a wire snare. The wire passes out of the lumen of the catheter 3cm short of the tip and is reintroduced through the wall into the lumen 5 mm from the tip. The wire is drawn taut by the application of tension on the proximal end of the catheter. By passing a high-frequency diathermy current along the wire, it can be used as an electrical knife (manufacturer: Storz, Tuttlingen). The diathermy source used is the Wappler Pneumotome which supplies a mixed current for cutting and coagulation, or the Olympus PSD source or the Erbotom FR-2 (Erbe, Tübingen) with separate currents. We prefer to use a mixture of cutting and coagulation current at a ratio of 2:3. Stone retrieval from the common bile duct is made by means of Dormia basket catheters (Storz, Tuttlingen; Olympus Optical Co., Tokyo) or modified Fogarty catheters (Edwards Co., Los Angeles) which can be passed down the instrument channel of the duodenoscope into the bile duct.

Technique

Premedication, duodenoscopy and filling of the common bile duct with contrast are the same as in diagnostic ERC. Subsequently the papillotome designed by Demling and Classen is advanced selectively into the common bile duct under radiological and endoscopic control[12] (Figure 23.16). After applying tension to the wire and intermittently passing a mixed cutting and coagulation current, the roof of the papilla is slit in the direction between 11 and 12 o'clock for a length of approximately 1.5 cm. The sudden emptying of contrast medium tinged with bile and the successful achieving of the endoscopic

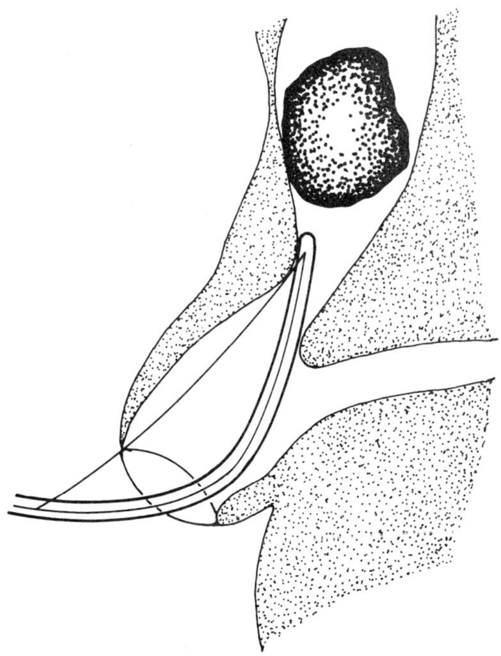

Figure 23.16. Sketch of endoscopic papillotomy by means of the papillotome described by Demling and Classen. The papillotome is introduced selectively into the distal common bile duct. The wire snare is directed to the roof of the papilla for incision.

view into the lumen of the bile duct indicate that the newly created opening is adequately large (Plate 23.2; see page 548). The entire operation takes 30 to 60 minutes. When the introduction of the papillotome into the bile duct is impossible a minicut is performed:[22] when the tip of the catheter of the papillotome is fixed in the papillary orifice, a subpapillary mucous section is realized by upward movement of the wire. This precutting then permits the deep introduction of the papillotome into the common bile duct and allows a classical anterograde section by retracted movement of the papillotome.[22]

One week after endoscopic papillotomy, the duodenum, papilla of Vater and the duct systems are examined with diagnostic ERC. If stones still persist in the bile duct the inadequately large papillary stoma is extended. If extension of the incision appears either to hold no promise of success or to be dangerous, persistent stones can be removed with extraction instruments under radiological control (Figure 23.17).

Results of Endoscopic Papillotomy for Removal of Common Bile Duct Stones

So far more than 2000 endoscopic papillotomies have been performed, mainly in western Europe, for the removal of stones from the common bile duct (Table 23.1). In 63 per cent of patients the stones disappeared spontaneously some days after EPT. In a further 30 per cent of patients stones could be extracted by means of a Dormia basket. In 93 per cent of cases, therefore, EPT was successful in removing common bile duct stones.

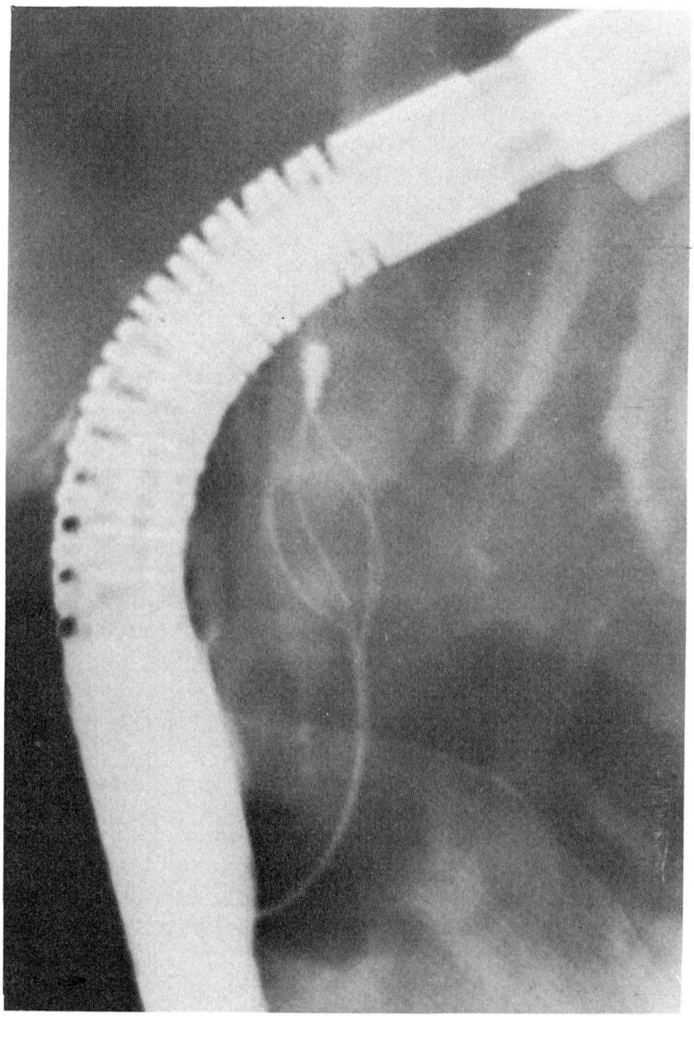

Figure 23.17. A Dormia basket advanced in the common bile duct for stone extraction.

Table 23.1. *Results of Endoscopic Papillotomy (EPT) for Removal of Common Duct Stones.*

Centre	EPT	Spontaneous stone disappearance	Extraction	Residual stones	Failed attempts
Classen, M. Ossenberg, F.W. (Hamburg) Wurbs, D.	248	196	18		14
Cotton, P.B. (London)	84	68	10		6
Cremer, M. (Brussels)	220	203	26	14	3
Demling, L. Koch, H. (Erlangen) Rösch, W.	247	117	102	16	16
Geenen, J.E. (Milwaukee)	65	44	16		5
Kawai, K. Nakajima, M. (Kyoto)	56	33	17		6
Liguory, C. (Paris)	202	168	28		13
Manegold, B.C. (Mannheim)	138	79	49		10
Safrany, L. (Wilhelmshaven)	498	180	290	28	23
Salmon, P.R. (Bristol)	34	30	1		3
Soehendra, M. (Hamburg)	112	57	29	21	5
Zimmon, D.S. (New York)	85	78	23		15
Totals	1989	1253 (63%)	609 (31%)		119 (6%)

Data from personal communications.

Complications of Endoscopic Papillotomy

As with every invasive therapy, EPT is not without risk of serious complications (Table 23.2).[62, 76] In 150 patients (7.5 per cent) who underwent papillotomy for common bile duct stone removal complications such as pancreatitis, perforation, bleeding and septic cholangitis were observed. The EPT-related mortality in these patients was 1.2 per cent. In our experience acute pancreatitis and retroperitoneal perforation are rare and benign complications. By contrast, septic cholangitis is a serious hazard, often necessitating urgent surgical intervention. Septic cholangitis results from stagnation of bile flow caused by common duct obstruction and simultaneous ascending infection facilitated by papillotomy. Thus the risk of septic cholangitis increases with the size and eventual impaction of the common duct stones. The use of a prophylactic antibiotic regimen (see Chapter 53) may be effective in reducing this complication.

Besides cholangitis, bleeding is a relatively frequent and most serious complication of EPT. In our experience bleeding resulted in nearly every case from a repeated second or third large incision for the removal of big stones. The risk of bleeding thus seems to correlate with the length of the incision and with the size of the stones to be removed. Anatomical studies of the arterial blood supply to the papilla of Vater and the distal common bile duct by Spängler[92] stressed the importance of the retroduodenal artery, an anastomotic vessel between the gastroduodenal and the superior mesenteric artery. This vessel crosses the terminal common bile duct from the dorsal aspect. From this crossing, branches ramify to lead on to the ventral and dorsal aspects of the common bile duct to the papilla. Arterial bleeding after EPT may originate from the retroduodenal artery itself, from one of its branches in the area of the distal common bile duct or from another branch which supplies the duodenal wall above the papilla of Vater.

Treatment of Septic Cholangitis

Acute suppurative cholangitis, presenting clinically as Charcot's triad of symptoms, with chills and fever, upper abdominal pain and jaundice, results from biliary obstruction by common bile duct stones in more than 90 per cent of cases.[2, 83] In its advanced form acute sup-

Table 23.2. *Complications of Endoscopic Papillotomy (EPT) for Removal of Common Duct Stones.*

Centre	EPT	Bleeding	Perforation	Cholangitis	Pancreatitis	Mortality
Classen, M. Ossenberg, F.W. (Hamburg) Wurbs, D.	248	7 (4)	1	14 (4)	2	5
Cotton, P.B. (London)	84	3 (2)		2 (2)		0
Cremer, M. (Brussels)	220	9 (4)	1 (1)	2	2	4
Demling, L. Koch, H. (Erlangen) Rösch, W.	247	7 (5)	2 (2)	6 (3)	9	3
Geenen, J.E. (Milwaukee)	65	1			2	1
Kawai, K. Nakajima, M. (Kyoto)	56	1	0	0	1	0
Liguory, C. (Paris)	202	13 (2)	5 (2)	5 (1)	1	2
Manegold, B.C. (Mannheim)	138	2 (1)	3 (1)	2	3 (1)	3
Safrany, L. (Wilhelmshaven)	498	9 (1)	8 (1)	8 (6)	3	5
Salmon, P.R. (Bristol)	34	1	0	1	0	0
Soehendra, M. (Hamburg)	112	3	2 (2)	1	2	0
Zimmon, D.S. (New York)	85	1	0	2	3	1
Totals	1989	57 (19)	22 (9)	43 (16)	28(1)	24 (=1.2%)

Data from personal communications.
Numbers in parentheses indicate the number of patients subjected to surgical treatment of their complications.

purative cholangitis is characterized by hypotension and endotoxic shock, lethargy and mental confusion, and acute renal failure or liver abscess. It is commonly accepted that most of these patients will die in the absence of surgical decompression of the biliary tree. The reported surgical mortality varies from 13 to 60 per cent.[42] The following order of priorities for the management of acute suppurative cholangitis, based on newly developed endoscopic diagnostic and therapeutic procedures, is proposed: (a) retrograde cholangiography should be performed as an emergency procedure within 12 hours; (b) if cholangiography demonstrates the presence of common bile duct stones or papillary stenosis, endoscopic papillotomy should be performed subsequently during the same session.

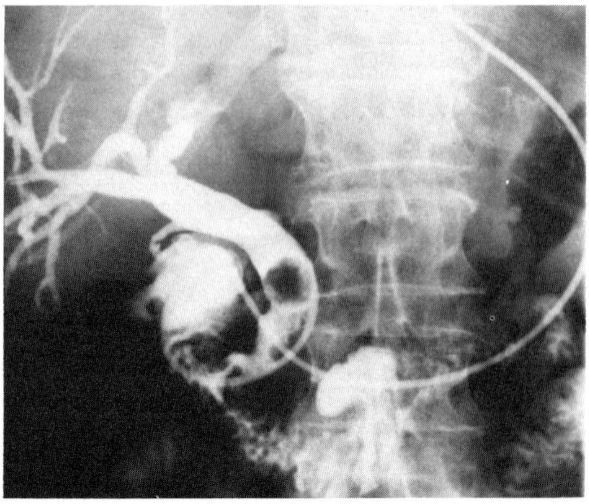

Figure 23.18. Transduodenal biliary drainage for common bile duct stones. The Oedmann catheter is advanced in the common bile duct proximal to the obstructing stone.

Endoscopic papillotomy is often sufficient to achieve an initial adequate drainage of the common bile duct. If an obvious discrepancy between the size of the gallstone and the diameter of the newly created opening suggests difficulty in spontaneous passage of the stone, biliary drainage is indicated.

Technique of duodenoscopic biliary drainage

A preformed green Oedmann catheter is advanced via the large instrument channel of the duodenoscope GFB2 (Olympus Optical Co.), retrogradely in the common bile duct proximally beyond the obstructing stone (Figure 23.18). Leaving the catheter in place, the instrument is withdrawn and the oral catheter end is fed out through the nose of the patient. This biliary drainage permits continuous bile aspiration for some days, with intermittent rinsing using heparin and infusion of cholate (for a detailed survey, see Classen and Ossenberg[14]), in an attempt to dissolve the stones. In addition, it permits the local application of antibiotics. Following this drain-

Table 23.3. *Indications for Endoscopic Papillotomy.*

Current established indications	Residual common bile duct stones following cholecystectomy. Common bile duct stones in poor-risk patients, particularly in obstructive jaundice. Benign papillary stenosis.
Exceptional indications	Peripapillary carcinoma with obstructive jaundice: (a) palliative in poor-risk patients (b) preparation for surgical resection. 'Subanastomotic cul-de-sac syndrome' (in latero-lateral choledocho-duodenal anastomosis). Caroli disease with common bile duct stones. Acute pancreatitis due to common bile duct stones. Stone removal from the main pancreatic duct.
Hypothetical future indications	Acute relapsing pancreatitis? Obstructive chronic pancreatitis induced by papillary stenosis. Rolling fenestra diverticula responsible for biliary or pancreatic disorder?

From Delmont,[24] with kind permission of the author and Karger Verlag.

age it is possible to wait for a further attempt at extraction of the stone or removal surgically under improved conditions.

Present Limited Indications for Endoscopic Papillotomy

Experience gained so far shows that endoscopic papillotomy is an effective low-risk alternative to surgical treatment of papillary stenosis and for removal of stones from the common bile duct.

With regard to common duct stone removal, the main disadvantage of this non-surgical technique is that it unavoidably damages the sphincter of Oddi. However, this disadvantage is considerably diminished by the fact that, in patients with common bile duct stones, a secondary papillary stenosis is frequently present, which is itself an indication for papillotomy.

Late complications after endoscopic papillotomy are not yet known; possible complications might be ascending infection of the pancreatic and bile duct systems or secretory disturbances of the pancreas and the liver. At the present time, however, there are not enough long-term follow-ups to permit accurate assessment. Preliminary data in 30 patients studied two years after endoscopic papillotomy (Burmeister et al, unpublished data) indicate that the 'bile transport' function of the papilla, as demonstrated by the emptying contractions of the papilla, is preserved in 84 per cent of cases. Its 'valve function' is rarely disturbed; duodenal reflux has been observed in only 21 per cent of these patients. Despite this duodenal reflux, however, neither ascending cholangitis nor pancreatitis has been observed in these patients. In view of the fact that sufficient long-term results are not yet available it would seem desirable, at present, to limit endoscopic papillotomy to patients for whom surgery represents a significant risk. A list of indications for endoscopic papillotomy was produced conjointly by German endoscopists and surgeons during a conference held in Frankfurt in October 1975:

1. Isolated papillary stenosis, verified by clinical and laboratory signs of obstructive jaundice with distension of the extra- and intrahepatic biliary ducts, and, if possible, manometric evidence of an increased duodenobiliary pressure gradient.
2. Common bile duct stones that were either overlooked at one or more surgical operations on the biliary tract or which had formed since operation. In younger patients (under 50 years of age) with an intact papilla of Vater, the surgeons believed that a surgical choledochotomy is preferable to preserve the function of the papilla.
3. Common bile duct stones with symptoms of obstruction in patients with a high surgical

risk; in these cases endoscopic papillotomy may be carried out even though the patient has not been previously subjected to cholecystectomy.

There is, however, a tendency not to be limited to these restricted indications for endoscopic papillotomy; and this procedure has been performed successfully in a variety of other conditions (Table 23.3).

REFERENCES

1. Abbruzzese, A.A. (1974) Retrograde cholangiography and sclerosing cholangitis. *American Journal of Digestive Diseases,* **19,** 571–574.
2. Andrew, D.J. & Johnson, S.E. (1970) Acute suppurative cholangitis. A medical and surgical emergency. *American Journal of Gastroenterology,* **54,** 141–154.
3. Ayoola, E.A., Vennes, J.A., Silvis, J.E., Rohrmann, C.A. & Ansel, M.J. (1976) Endoscopic retrograde intrahepatic cholangiography in liver diseases. *Gastrointestinal Endoscopy,* **22,** 156–159.
4. Belsito, A.A., Marta, J.B., Dickinson, P.B. & Pizinger, R.J. (1975) Endoscopic cholangiogram and intravenous cholangiogram. An analysis of size comparison (Abs.). *Gastroenterology,* **68,** 1018.
5. Bilbao, M.K., Dotter, C.T., Lee, T.G. & Katon, R.M. (1976) Complications of endoscopic retrograde cholangiopancreatography (ERCP). A study of 1000 cases. *Gastroenterology,* **70,** 314–320.
6. Blumgart, L.H. (1975) Duodenoscopy and endoscopy retrograde choledochopancreatography: present position in relation to periampullary and pancreatic cancer. *Journal of Surgery and Oncology,* **7,** 107–119.
7. Blumgart, L.H., Salmon, P.R. & Cotton, P.B. (1974) Endoscopy and retrograde choledochopancreatography in the diagnosis of the patient with jaundice. *Surgery, Gynecology and Obstetrics,* **138,** 565–570.
8. Blumgart, L.H., Salmon, P.R., Cotton, P.B., Davies, G.T., Burwood, R., Beales, J.S.M., Lawrie, B., Skirving, A. & Read, A.E. (1972) Endoscopy and retrograde choledochopancreatography in the diagnosis of the jaundiced patient. *Lancet,* **ii,** 1269–1273.
9. Chavy, A. & Liguory, C. (1975) Duodénoscopie, cholangiographie et wirsungographie rétrograde dans le cancer de l'ampoule de Vater. *Annales de Gastroentérologie et Hépatologie,* **11,** 395–401.
10. Classen, M. & Demling, L. (1974) Endoskopische Sphinkterotomie der Papilla Vateri and Steinextraction aus dem Ductus Choledochus. *Deutsche Medizinische Wochenschrift,* **99,** 496–497.
11. Classen, M. & Demling, L. (1975) Hazards of endoscopic retrograde cholangio-pancreatography (ERCP). *Acta Hepato-Gastroenterologica,* **22,** 1–3.
12. Classen, M. & Safrany, L. (1975) Endoscopic papillotomy and removal of gallstones. *British Medical Journal,* **iv,** 371–374.
13. Classen, M. & Ossenberg, F.W. (1977) Indications for endoscopic papillotomy. In *The Sphincter of Oddi* (Ed.) Delmont, J. pp. 228–231. Basel: Karger.
14. Classen, M. & Ossenberg, F.W. (1977) The nonsurgical removal of common bile duct stones. *Gut,* **18,** 760–769.
15. Classen, M., Frühmorgen, P., Kozu, T. & Demling, L. (1971) Endoscopic–radiologic demonstrations of biliodigestive fistulas. *Endoscopy,* **3,** 138–142.
16. Classen, M., Anacker, H., Stadelmann, O., Seifert, E. & Fritsch, E. (1975) The diagnosis of tumours of the papilla of Vater and of the pancreas by ERCP. In *Efficiency and Limits of Radiologic Examination of the Pancreas.* (Ed.) Anacker, **11,** pp. 203–209. Stuttgart: Thieme.
17. Cotton, P.B. (1972) Cannulations of the papilla of Vater by endoscopy and retrograde cholangiopancreatography (ERCP). *Gut,* **13,** 1014–1025.
18. Cotton, P.B. (1977) Progress report: ERCP. *Gut,* **18,** 316–341.
19. Cotton, P.B., Beales, J.S.M. & Cole, J. (1973) Hazards of endoscopic retrograde cholangio-pancreatography. In *Endoscopy of the Small Intestine with Retrograde Cholangio-Pancreatography* (Ed.) Demling, L. & Classen, M. pp. 74–80. Stuttgart: Thieme.
20. Cotton, P.B., Chapman, M., Whiteside, C.G. & Lequesne, L.P. (1976) Duodenoscopic papillotomy and gallstone removal. *British Journal of Surgery,* **63,** 709–714.
21. Cremer, M., Toussaint, J., Deltenre, M., De Toeuf, J. & Hermanus, A. (1976) Les séquelles de la chirurgie biliaire. *Bordeaux Médical,* **18,** 1463–1469.
22. Cremer, M., Gulbis, A., Toussaint, J., De Toeuf, J., Vanlaethem, A. & Hermanus, A. (1977) Technique of endoscopic papillotomy. In *The Sphincter of Oddi* (Ed.) Delmont, J. pp. 219–227. Basel: Karger.
23. Davis, J.L., Milligan, F.D. & Cameron, J.L. (1975) Septic complications following endoscopic retrograde cholangio-pancreatography. *Surgery, Gynecology and Obstetrics,* **140,** 365–367.
24. Delmont, J. (1977) An attempt to collate. In *The Sphincter of Oddi* (Ed.) Delmont, J. pp. 240–255. Basel: Karger.
25. Demling, L. & Classen, M. (1970) Duodenojejunoskopie. *Deutsche Medizinische Wochenschrift,* **95,** 1427–1428.
26. Demling, L., Classen, M. & Frühmorgen, P. (1974) *Atlas der Enteroskopie.* Berlin: Springer.
27. Elias, E. (1976) Progress report: cholangiography in the jaundiced patient. *Gut,* **17,** 801–811.
28. Elias, E., Summerfield, J.A., Dick, K. & Sherlock, S. (1974) Endoscopic retrograde cholangio-pancreatography in the diagnosis of jaundice associated with ulcerative colitis. *Gastroenterology,* **67,** 907–911.
29. Elias, E., Hamlyn, A.N., Jain, S., Long, R.G., Summerfield, J.A., Dick, R. & Sherlock, S. (1976) A randomized trial of percutaneous transhepatic cholangiography with the Chiba needle versus endoscopic retrograde cholangiography for bile duct visualization in jaundice. *Gastroenterology,* **71,** 439–443.
30. Endo, Y., Morii, T., Tamura, A. & Okuda, S. (1974) Cyto-diagnosis of pancreatic malignant tumors by aspiration, under direct vision, using a duodenal fiberscope. *Gastroenterology,* **67,** 944–951.
31. Falkenstein, D.B., Riccoboni, C., Sidhu, G., Abrams, R.M., Seliger, G. & Zimmon, D.S. (1975) The endoscopic intrahepatic cholangiogram. Clinicopathologic correlation with post mortem cholangiograms. *Investigative Radiology,* **10,** 358–365.

32. Farkas, I., Déak, J., Pálfi, I. & Preisich, P. (1976) Endoscopic retrograde cholangiography in biliodigestive anastomosis. *Endoscopy*, **8**, 127–132.
33. Fischer, M.G., Wolff, W.J., Geffen, A., Shinya, H. & Ozoktay, S. (1974) Antegrade and retrograde visualization of the biliary tree. *American Journal of Gastroenterology*, **61**, 129–132.
34. Fischer, M.G., Wolff, W.J., Geffen, A. & Ozoktay, S. (1975) Combined use of percutaneous transhepatic cholangiography (PTC) and endoscopic ampullary cholangiography in diagnosis of difficult jaundice cases. *American Journal of Gastroenterology*, **63**, 369–380.
35. Fukomoto, K., Nakajima, M., Murakami, K. & Kawai, K. (1974) Diagnosis of pancreatic cancer by endoscopic pancreato-cholangiography. *American Journal of Gastroenterology*, **62**, 210–223.
36. Geenen, J. (1978) Endoscopic papillotomy in the United States. In *International Workshop on Endoscopic Papillotomy, Munich 1976* (Ed.) Demling, L. & Classen, M. Stuttgart: Thieme.
37. Gundel, H., von Fritsch, E. & Koch, H. (1975) Die Bedeutung der endoskopisch-radiologischen Cholangiographie bei Cholestase und Post-cholecystektomie-Syndrom. *Deutsche Medizinische Wochenschrift*, **100**, 1877–1881.
38. Hagenmüller, F., Ossenberg, F.W. & Classen, M. (1977) Duodenoscopic manometry. In *The Sphincter of Oddi* (Ed.) Delmont, J. pp. 72–76. Basel: Karger.
39. Hanafee, W. & Weiner, M. (1967) Transjugular percutaneous cholangiography. *Radiology*, **88**, 35–39.
40. Hatfield, A.R.W., Whittaker, R. & Gibbs, D.D. (1974) The collection of pancreatic fluid for cytodiagnosis using a duodenoscope. *Gut*, **15**, 305–307.
41. Hatfield, A.R.W., Smithies, A., Wilkins, R. & Levi, A.J. (1976) Assessment of endoscopic retrograde cholangio-pancreatography (ERCP) and pure pancreatic juice cytology in patients with pancreatic disease. *Gut*, **17**, 14–21.
42. Haupert, A.P., Carey, L.C., Evans, W.E. & Ellison, E.G. (1967) Acute suppurative cholangitis; experience with 15 consecutive cases. *Archives of Surgery*, **94**, 460–467.
43. Hoffmann, L. & Weiss, W. (1977) Clinical importance of juxta-papillary duodenal diverticula. *Acta Endoscopica*. In press.
44. Huang. T., Bassk, J.A. & Williams, R.D. (1969) The significance of biliary pressure in cholangitis. *Archives of Surgery*, **98**, 629–632.
45. Huchzermeyer, H., Luska, G., Otto, P. & Seifert, I. (1975) The value of the combination of antegrade and retrograde cholangiography in the diagnosis of bile duct obstructions. *Endoscopy*, **7**, 126–133.
46. Hultborn, A., Jacobsson, B. & Rosengren, B. (1962) Cholangio-venous reflux during cholangiography. *Acta Chirurgica Scandinavica*, **123**, 111.
47. Ikeda, S. & Okada, Y. (1975) Classification of choledocho-duodenal fiberscopy and its etiological significance. *Gastroenterology*, **69**, 130–137.
48. Ingelfinger, F.J. (1972) Endoscopic pancreato-cholangiography: progress and problems (Editorial). *New England Journal of Medicine*, **287**, 879–880.
49. Kasugai, T., Kuno, N., Kobayashi, S. & Hattori, K. (1972) Endoscopic pancreatocholangiography. I. The normal pancreato-cholangiogram. *Gastroenterology*, **63**, 217–226.
50. Kasugai, T., Kuno, N., Kizu, M., Kobayashi, S. & Hattori, K. (1972) Endoscopic pancreatocholangiography. II. The pathological pancreatocholangiogram. *Gastroenterology*, **63**, 227–234.
51. Katon, R.M., Bilbao, M.K., Parent, J.A. & Smith, F.W. (1975) Endoscopic retrograde cholangiopancreatography in patients with gastrectomy and gastrojejunostomy (Billroth II), a case for the forward look. *Gastrointestinal Endoscopy*, **21**, 164–165.
52. Kawai, K., Akasaka, Y., Hashimoto, Y. & Nakajima, A. (1973) Preliminary report on endoscopical papillotomy. *Journal of Kyoto Prefectural Medical University*, **82**, 353–355.
53. Kawai, K., Akasaka, Y., Murakami, K., Tada, M., Kohil, Y. & Nakajima, M. (1974) Endoscopic sphincterotomy of the ampulla of Vater. *Gastrointestinal Endoscopy*, **20**, 138–151.
54. Kawai, K., Nakajima, M., Tada, M. & Murakami, K. (1976) Endoscopie opératoire: polypectomie et sphincterotomie endoscopiques. *Endoscopie Digestive*, **1**, 17–22.
55. Kawai, K., Nakajima, M., Akasaka, J., Shimamotu, K. & Murakami, K. (1976) Eine neue endoskopische Technik: die perorale Choledocho-Pancreaticoskopie. *Leber Magen Darm*, **6**, 121–124.
56. Kawanishi, H., Sell, J.E. & Pollard, H.M. (1975) Combined endoscopic pancreatic fluid collection and retrograde pancreatography in the diagnosis of pancreatic cancer and chronic pancreatitis. *Gastrointestinal Endoscopy*, **22**, 82–85.
57. Koch, H. (1975) Endoscopic papillotomy. *Endoscopy*, **7**, 89–93.
58. Koch, H. & Classen, M. (1973) The diagnosis of obstructive jaundice by endoscopic retrograde cholangiopancreatography (ERCP) in malignant tumours. *Acta Gastroenterologica Belgica*, **36**, 676–681.
59. Koch, H., Classen, M. & Demling, L. (1973) Alterations of the biliary duct system in disease of the pancreas. In *Endoscopy of the Small Intestine with Retrograde Pancreatocholangiography*. (Ed.) Demling, L. & Classen, M. pp. 90–94. Stuttgart: Thieme.
60. Koch, H., Belohlavek, D., Schaffner, O. & Demling, L. (1976) Endoskopisch-retrograde Cholangio-Pancreaticographie (ERCP). *Internist*, **17**, 197–203.
61. Kozu, T. (1973) Duodenoscopic collection of intraductal pure pancreatic juice and its application to the cytodiagnosis. In *Endoscopy of the Small Intestine with Retrograde Pancreatocholangiography* (Ed.) Demling, L. & Classen, M. pp. 70–73. Stuttgart: Thieme.
62. Liguory, C., Girault, F. & Coffin, J.C. (1977) Complications of endoscopic sphincterotomy. In *The Sphincter of Oddi* (Ed.) Delmont, J. pp. 232–239. Basel: Karger.
63. Liguory, C., Gouero, H., Chavy, A., Coffin, J.C. & Huguier, M. (1974) Endoscopic retrograde cholangiopancreatography. *British Journal of Surgery*, **61**, 359–362.
64. Liguory, C., Coffin, J.C., Holler, A. & Chavy, A. (1975) Traitement de la lithiase de la voie biliaire principale par voie endoscopique. *Presse Médicale*, **4**, 20.
65. McClelland, D.B.L., Burrell, C.J., Tonkin, R.W. & Heading, R.C. (1978) Hepatitis B absence of transmission by gastrointestinal endoscopy. *British Medical Journal*, **i**, 23–24.

66. McCune, W.S., Shorb, P.E. & Moscovitz, H. (1968) Endoscopic cannulation of the ampulla of Vater: a preliminary report. *Annals of Surgery*, **167**, 752–756.
67. Morissey, J.F. (1972) To cannulate or not to cannulate (Editorial). *Gastroenterology*, **63**, 351–352.
68. Morris, J.M., Cattle, D.S. & Smits, B.J. (1975) Endoscopy and transmission of hepatitis B. *Lancet*, **ii**, 1152.
69. Nebel, O.T. (1975) Manometric evaluation of the papilla of Vater. *Gastrointestinal Endoscopy*, **21**, 126–128.
70. Nebel, O.T., Silvis, S.E., Rogers, G., Sugawa, C. & Mandelstam, P. (1975) Complications associated with endoscopic retrograde cholangio-pancreatography. Results of the 1974 A.S.G.E. survey. *Gastrointestinal Endoscopy*, **22**, 34–36.
71. Nüesch, H.J., Hahnloser, P., Fumagalli, J., Jenny, S. & Deyhle, P. (1973) Endoskopische retrograde Cholangiographie: Methode der Wahl zur Diagnose der Choledochuszyste. *Deutsche Medizinische Wochenschrift*, **98**, 2069–2070.
72. Oi, J., Takemoto, T. & Kondo, T. (1969) Fiberduodenoscope. Direct observations of the papilla of Vater. *Endoscopy*, **1**, 101–103.
73. Okuda, K., Tanikawa, K., Emura, T., Kuratomi, S., Jinnuochi, S., Urabe, K., Sumikoshi, T., Kanda, Y., Fukuyama, Y., Musha, H., Mari, H., Shimukawa, Y., Yakushiji, F. & Matsuura, Y. (1974) Non-surgical percutaneous trans-hepatic cholangiography–diagnostic significance in medical problems of the liver. *American Journal of Digestive Diseases*, **19**, 21–36.
74. Osnes, M., Serck-Hanssen, A. & Myren, J. (1975) Endoscopic retrograde brush cytology (ERBC) of the biliary and pancreatic ducts. *Scandinavian Journal of Gastroenterology*, **10**, 829–831.
75. Ossenberg, F.W. (1977) *Die Pharmakokinetik von Pentobarbital bei Leberschäden.* Baden-Baden: Witzstrock.
76. Ossenberg, F.W., Wurbs, D. & Classen, M. (1977) Risk of complications of endoscopic therapy in biliary tract disease. In press.
77. Ossenberg, F.W., Wurbs, D. & Classen, M. (1977) Endoscopic sphincterotomy in gallstone cholangitis. In *International Symposium on Intensive Care in Hepatology and Gastroenterology*, Marseille 1977.
78. Robbins, A.H., Messian, R.A., Widrich, W.C., Paul, R.E. Jr, Norton, R.A., Schimmel, E.M. & Ogoshi, K. (1974) Endoscopic pancreatography. An analysis of the radiologic findings in pancreatitis. *Radiology*, **113**, 293–296.
79. Rösch, W., Koch, H. & Demling, L. (1976) Manometric studies during ERCP and endoscopic papillotomy. *Endoscopy*, **8**, 30–33.
80. Rösch, W., Koch, H. & Demling, L. (1976) Peroral cholangioscopy. *Endoscopy*, **8**, 172–175.
81. Safrany, L. (1977) Duodenoscopic sphincterotomy and gallstone removal. *Gastroenterology*, **72**, 338–343.
82. Safrany, L., Tari, J., Barna, L. & Torok, J. (1973) Endoscopic retrograde cholangiography: experience of 168 examinations. *Gastrointestinal Endoscopy*, **19**, 163–168.
83. Saik, R.P., Greenburg, A.G., Farris, I.M. & Peskin, G.W. (1975) Spectrum of cholangitis. *American Journal of Surgery*, **130**, 143–150.
84. Salmon, P.R. (1975) Endoscopic retrograde choledocho-pancreatography in the diagnosis of pancreatic disease. *Gut*, **16**, 658–663.
85. Salmon, P.R., Rey, J.F., Baddeley, H., Schiller, K.F.R., Davies, J., Mackenzie, E. & Read, A.E. (1977) ERCP in the diagnosis and management of periampullary carcinoma. In *The Sphincter of Oddi* (Ed.) Delmont, J. pp. 111–114. Basel: Karger.
86. Seifert, E., Urakami, Y. & Elster, K. (1977) Duodenoscopic guided biopsy of the biliary and pancreatic duct. *Endoscopy*, **9**, 154–161.
87. Seifert, E., Stender, H., Safrany, L., Lesch, P., Luska, G. & Misaki, F. (1974) X-ray findings of pancreatic cysts diagnosed by endoscopic pancreato-cholangiography. *Endoscopy*, **6**, 77–83.
88. Seifert, E., Safrany, L., Stender, H.St, Luska, G. & Misaki, F. (1974) Identification of bile duct tumors by means of endoscopic retrograde pancreato-cholangiography (ERCP). *Endoscopy*, **6**, 156–162.
89. Shapiro, H.A. & Cotton, P.B. (1975) Leaving a balloon tip catheter in the bile duct at duodenoscopy. *Lancet*, **ii**, 13–14.
90. Silvis, S.E., Rohrmann, C.A. & Vennes, J.A. (1976) Diagnostic accuracy of endoscopic retrograde cholangiopancreatography in hepatic, biliary and pancreatic malignancy. *Annals of Internal Medicine*, **84**, 438–440.
91. Skude, W., Wehlin, L., Maruyama, T. & Ariyama, J. (1976) Hyperamylasaemia after duodenoscopy and retrograde cholangio-pancreatography. *Gut*, **17**, 127–132.
92. Spängler, H.P. (1968) Die Blutversorgung der Papilla Vateri und des papillennahen Choledochusabschnitts. *Anatomischer Anzeiger*, **122**, 371–376.
93. Stadelmann, O., Safrany, L., Loffler, A., Barna, L., Miederer, S.E., Bopp, D., Kaufer, C. & Sobbe, A. (1974) Endoscopic retrograde cholangio-pancreatography in the diagnosis of pancreatic cancer. Experience with 54 cases. *Endoscopy*, **6**, 84–93.
94. Summerfield, J.A., Elias, E., Hungerford, G.D., Nikapota, V.L.B., Dick, R. & Sherlock, S. (1976) The biliary system in primary biliary cirrhosis: a study by endoscopic retrograde cholangio-pancreatography. *Gastroenterology*, **70**, 240–243.
95. Vennes, J.A., Jacobson, J.R. & Silvis, S.E. (1974) Endoscopic cholangiography for biliary system diagnosis. *Annals of Internal Medicine*, **80**, 61–64.
96. Vondrasek, P., Eberhardt, G. & Classen, M. (1974) Endoskopische Halbleiter-Manometrie. *Innere Medizin*, **3**, 188–192.
97. Weidenhiller, S., Flugel, H. & Rösch, W. (1975) Abrasive cytology of the pancreatic and biliary duct in man. *Endoscopy*, **7**, 72–74.
98. Whorwell, P.J., Smith, C.L. & Foster, K.J. (1976) Arterial blood gas tensions during upper gastro-intestinal endoscopy. *Gut*, **17**, 797–800.
99. Witte, S. & Riegg, H. (1973) Cytological findings in the bile after endoscopic cannulation of the papilla of Vater. In *Endoscopy of the Small Intestine with Retrograde Pancreatocholangiography.* (Ed.) Demling, L. & Classen, M. pp. 94–97. Stuttgart: Thieme.
100. Yamakawa, T., Mieno, K. & Shikata, J. (1975) Improved choledocho-fiberscopes and nonsurgical removal of retained biliary calculi under direct visual control (Abs.). *Gastroenterology*, **68**, 1051.
101. Zimmon, D.S., Falkenstein, D.B. & Kessler, R.E. (1975) Endoscopic papillotomy for choledocholithiasis. *New England Journal of Medicine*, **293**, 1181–1182.
102. Zimmon, D.S., Falkenstein, D.B., Abraham, R.M., Seliger, G. & Kessler, R.E. (1974) Endoscopic retrograde cholangio-pancreatography (ERCP) in the diagnosis of pancreatic inflammatory disease. *Radiology*, **113**, 287–297.

Chapter 24

Choledochoscopy

J. MANNY SHORE
GEORGE BERCI

The problem of retained biliary calculi following choledochotomy has frustrated surgeons since the first common bile duct was opened. This complication is invited by the very nature of the operation, which is essentially one of blind instrumental manipulation. The introduction of cholangiography[11] contributed greatly to the solution of this difficulty but still left an incidence, averaging 10 per cent, of overlooked stones following choledocholithotomy.[6] This limitation becomes significant when one considers the number of patients at risk in the United States alone, where 500 000 cholecystectomies are reported annually.

Despite the introduction of non-operative methods of managing retained biliary calculi,[4, 9, 16, 25] many patients will still require re-exploration with its attendant increased morbidity and mortality. It is apparent that any method with the capability of significantly reducing the incidence of retained stones during the primary operation deserves careful consideration. Direct visualization of any hollow viscus by an endoscope is the most logical way to examine the area in question. While such an approach to the biliary tract was conceived early, successful clinical application had to await technological evolution.

History

The first attempted choledochoscopy was reported by Bakes[1] who constructed a speculum with a mirror and a small proximal light bulb which he inserted into the distal duct. McIver[10] introduced a telescopic system similar to a cystoscope built in a right-angled shape. Unfortunately, this instrument did not gain popularity due to poor visualization from standard lens and lighting systems. Wildegans[26] designed a 60° angled instrument with an improved but standard lens system. Both authors used this instrument[2, 19] but found that the proximity of the rib cage created difficulties during introduction and visualization of the distal duct. This problem was increased during secondary biliary explorations.

With the availability of flexible fibre endoscopes, one of us (JMS) developed the first flexible choledochoscope to overcome these limitations.[19] The main obstacles encountered were lack of control of the floating tip and absence of fixed focus. The invention of rod-lens optics by Hopkins and its introduction to clinical practice[3] (Figure 24.1) paved the way for the return to a rigid but miniaturized instrument.[18]

Instrumentation

The choledochoscope shown in Figure 24.2 incorporates irrigation, lighting and image transmission systems all within a 5 × 3 mm diameter. The horizontal limb measures 40 mm, while the vertical arm measures 300 mm. The standard scope provides complete visualization of the biliary tract in the majority of cases. An identical scope with a 60 mm horizontal limb for longer ducts is also available (Figure 24.2).

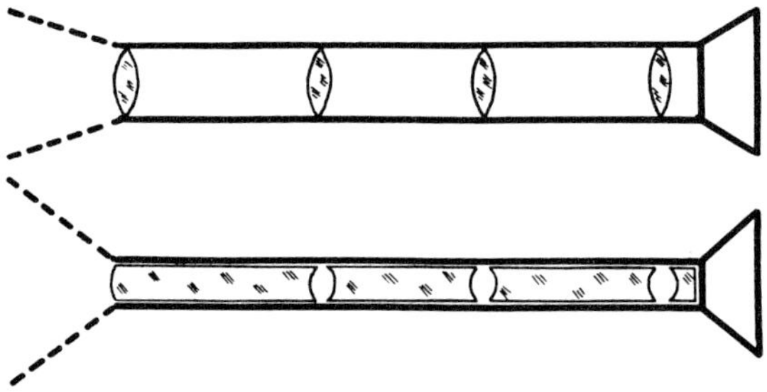

Figure 24.1. Schematic diagram. Top: conventional telescopic system consisting of a series of glass lenses, separated by air spaces. Bottom: Hopkins rod-lens optical system; air and glass are interchanged with rod-lenses, separated by small air interspace. Net result: significant increase in light transmission, larger viewing angle, smaller size, excellent resolution and natural colour display.

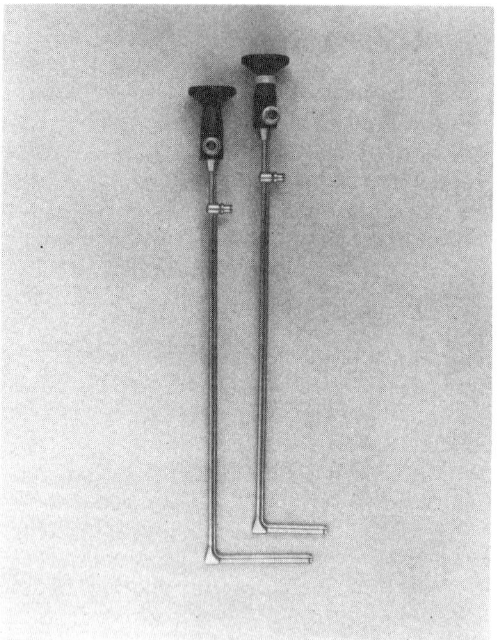

Figure 24.2. The choledochoscope can be obtained in two lengths, with a 40 mm and a 60 mm horizontal limb. The vertical limbs are identical. (K. Storz Endoscope Co.)

The new rod-lens image transmitting system vastly improves visualization because of increased light transmission, extreme depth of field, wide viewing angle, crisp definition and natural colour display. The net result is an exquisite image quality which enhances endoscopic orientation. In addition, the reduced dimensions of the scope facilitate safer introduction and easier manipulation.

Illumination

Any type of light source used for endoscopy in the hospital can be employed. In general, 150 W halogen globes are used. Those which have a reflecting mirror incorporated provide a higher intensity and are therefore preferred. The light is transmitted via a fibreoptic cable which is coupled to the endoscope.

Irrigation

This examination, similar to cystoscopy, is carried out in a viscus filled with fluid. The ductal system has to be dilated to give optimal visualization. Irrigation also helps to clear bile and debris from the lumen. The choledochoscope has a very small irrigation channel because of the compact size of the instrument. A high-pressure irrigation source is therefore required to overcome the resistance while still providing an adequate stream. The Fenwal system (Fenwal Laboratories) used for emergency transfusions or intra-arterial chemotherapy is employed. In principle it is similar to a blood-pressure cuff with a manometer. Normal saline prepacked in litre sterile plastic containers (Fenwal Laboratories) is preferred. The container is placed within the pressure cuff and suspended from an I.V. stand (Figure 24.3). Standard I.V. tubing, coupled to the saline container, delivers the irrigant to the scope through two or three sterile extension tubes. The pressure cuff is inflated to 40 kPa (300 mmHg) and *maintained* at this level. In general, one litre is sufficient for examination. It is worth while to assemble two irrigation systems (a spare one) from the same I.V. pole to avoid running out of fluid in cases requiring repeated scoping for multiple stones. The circulating nurse can then immediately transfer from the empty to the full container.

Accessory instruments

Occasionally, stones discovered by endoscopy cannot be retrieved with conventional instrumental manipulation. In such instances an instrument guide channel can be attached to the scope. This permits extraction of stones under visual control because the manipulating instrument is kept in the visual field. The guide channel increases the instrument diameter to 9 × 5 mm, which is usually readily accommodated by the dilated duct system being explored

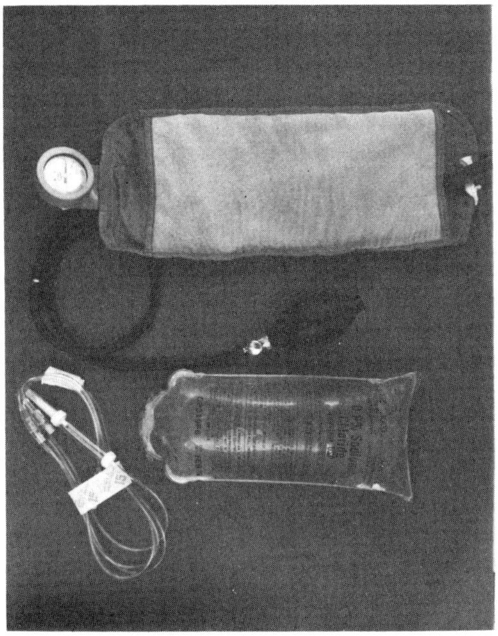

Figure 24.3. The Fenwal pressure cuff with the sterile plastic saline container. The plastic bag is placed in the pressure cuff and suspended from an I.V. stand. Pressure should be kept at 40 kPa (300 mmHg) and maintained at this level.

(Figure 24.4). Various stone-retrieving devices are available.

Flexible stone forceps with alligator jaws (Fr. 7). For small or medium-sized stones, the alligator teeth facilitate a firm grasp on the edge of the stone (Figure 24.4). They can also be used to crush and remove larger calculi piecemeal. If the stone is too large or difficult to grasp, one must resort to other devices.

The Fogarty biliary catheters (Fr. 5 or 6). These can also be introduced through the instrument guide channel and should be advanced beyond the stone, inflated and withdrawn towards the scope, delivering the stone by traction. In the hepatic ducts, they should always be monitored by endoscopic guidance.

Dormia stone basket (Fr. 5). This is a useful tool for larger stones. After positioning the tip beyond the stone, the basket is opened beside the stone; gentle manipulation or rotation brings it into the basket. Pulling the wires then traps the stone and the entire assembly is withdrawn with the scope.

Electrohydraulic lithotomy. This method consists of a small probe through which high-intensity electrical sparks are discharged from a generator. The high-energy shock waves disintegrate stones in a fluid medium. While successfully applied in urology for lithotripsy in the bladder,[15] it is still in an experimental stage for biliary calculi.

Sterilization and Maintenance

Gas sterilization is far preferable to steam autoclaving or chemical disinfection. Gas prolongs the lifetime of the instruments and is more efficient than soaking.[23] Proper maintenance of these delicate optical instruments is of great importance. The endoscope has to be properly rinsed, cleared of debris and blood clots, dried and carefully packed in a metal container to avoid damage in a loaded gas sterilizer.[12]

Preparation of Instrumentation

It is advisable to prepare a separate small sterile table for the choledochoscope and its accessories (Figure 24.5). This will avoid con-

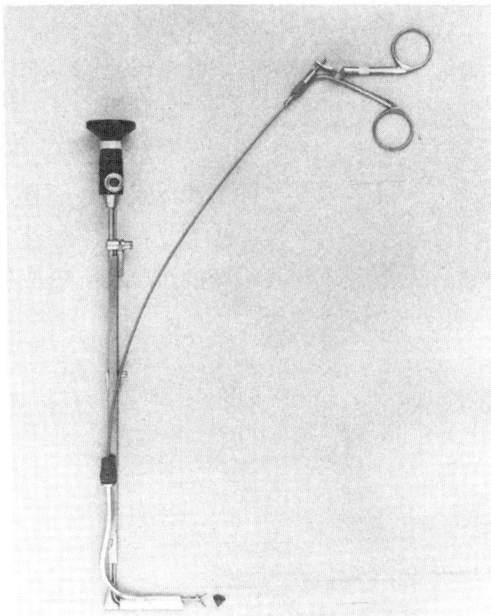

Figure 24.4. The choledochoscope with the attached instrument guide channel. Flexible alligator forceps is advanced and the movements of the jaws can be seen through the eyepiece of the endoscope. The guide channel keeps the manipulating instruments in the visual field. The forceps can be exchanged for the stone basket or Fogarty catheter.

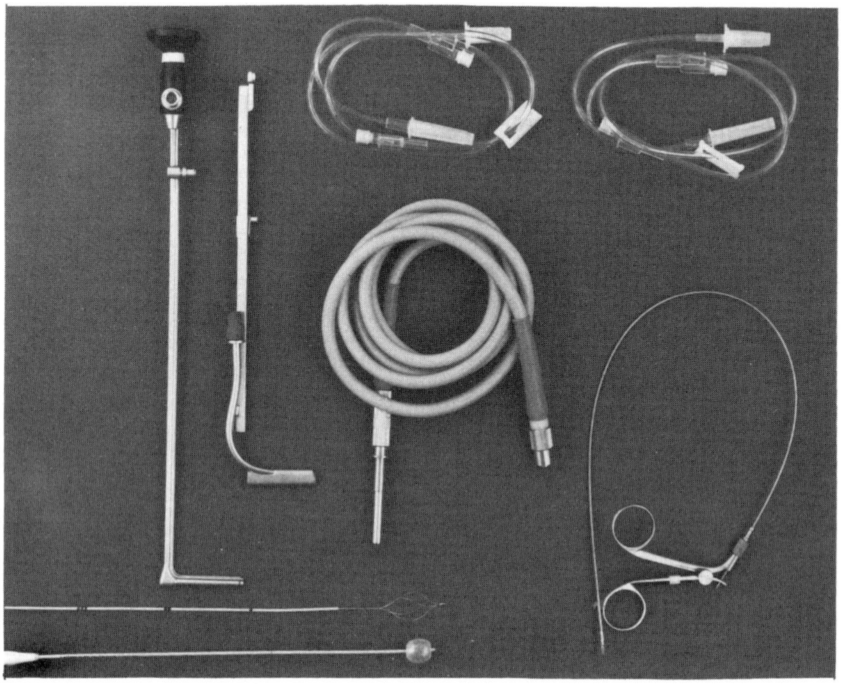

Figure 24.5. Set-up of choledochoscope with accessories: the choledochoscope (40 mm) beside the attachable instrument channel, fibreoptic light cable, two sterile irrigation extension tubes, flexible alligator forceps, Dormia stone basket and Fogarty biliary catheter (Fr. 5).

fusion with the general instrument tables and also coincidental damage caused by mixing delicate optical instruments with heavy steel tools.

TECHNIQUE

Choledochoscopy is a technique which enables the surgeon to see directly into the lumen of the intra- and extrahepatic biliary system. The area of the examination extends from the ampullary orifice to the secondary or tertiary hepatic radicles. The overwhelming majority of stones missed by conventional manipulations can be discovered and removed.

A standard choledochotomy incision is suitable for the introduction of the scope. Ideally, the incision should not exceed 10 mm to avoid excess leakage of irrigating fluid. Endoscopy is best performed from the patient's left side after the duct is felt to be cleared of calculi. A suction tube is placed beside the common bile duct to evacuate the overflow of irrigation fluid. The choledochoscope is assembled by connecting the irrigation tubing as well as the fibreoptic light cable. Introduction of the scope is aided by traction on the stay sutures which open the lumen (Figure 24.6). The tip of the scope is then advanced gently towards the ampulla. Crossing the stay sutures will approximate the common bile duct walls around the scope, decreasing fluid escape and maintaining intraluminal pressure. The image displayed can be clearly seen from a safe distance without contaminating the eyepiece. Observation is easier if the overhead operating lights are switched off, but the room lights may be left on.

The appearance of a yellow or red circle signifies contact of the scope with the wall and is corrected by simply withdrawing or tilting the tip slightly until the lumen is identified (Figure 24.7a). The instrument is then advanced under visual control until the sphincter orifice is seen (Figure 24.7b). This is best achieved by holding the scope with the right hand while applying traction on the distal duct with the left hand on the duodenum. With this manoeuvre the common bile duct will assume a straight line, which is the key to successful distal endoscopy. Attempts to pass the tip into the duodenum are not recommended. The best views are generally obtained during the slow withdrawal of the scope, scanning the area in front of the objective.

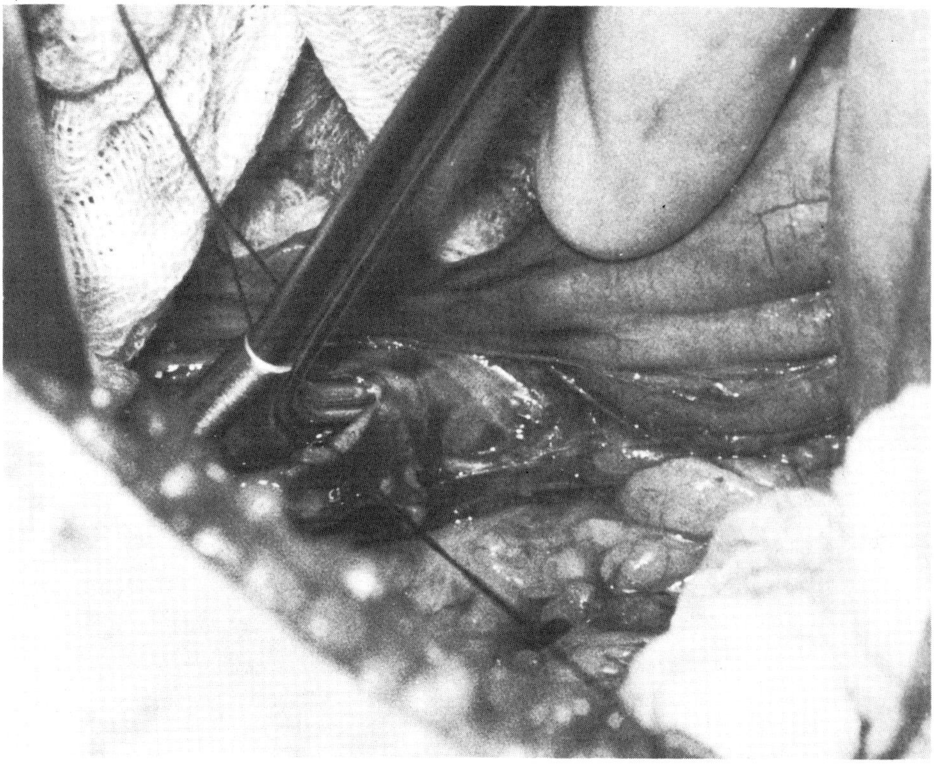

Figure 24.6. The common bile duct is opened and the introduction of the scope is aided by traction on the stay sutures.

In most instances distal endoscopy can be completed without resorting to duodenal mobilization by the Kocher manoeuvre. This may occasionally be necessary if the duct is elongated and the longer (60 mm) scope is not available; after mobilization, the distal duct and the duodenum can be telescoped over the horizontal limb to shorten the duct and bring the ampulla into view. After satisfactory endoscopy of the distal duct, the scope is withdrawn, rotated 180°, and re-introduced towards the hepatic ducts. After identifying the bifurcation (Figure 24.7c and d) the scope is rotated to the left to bring the right main orifice into view. There is a large variation of normal anatomy but after a few cases one accumulates enough experience to examine each orifice systematically. After slow withdrawal of the scope, the bifurcation returns to view. Slight rotation to the right reveals the orifice of the left main duct, which is then followed peripherally. Upon completion of hepatic endoscopy, the instrument is withdrawn and placed on the small sterile table, in case re-examination is required.

ENDOSCOPIC FINDINGS

Normal Anatomy

The mucous membrane of the distal common bile duct has a slightly pitted pale-pinkish appearance (Figure 24.7a). The longitudinal folds are opened by the pressure of the irrigating fluid. As the ampulla is approached the duct becomes funnel-shaped and the mucosa finely papillary. The sphincter must be identified to ensure complete distal examination (Figure 24.7b). The ampullary orifice can be seen in various appearances: stellate, fishmouthed, triangular, pinpoint or patulous. The mucosa is often covered by exudate (debris). Failure to visualize the opening excludes any diagnostic conclusions. The pancreatic duct is rarely seen.

The bifurcation of the common hepatic duct is recognized with ease (Figure 24.7c and d). It is similar in appearance to the bifurcation of the bronchial tree. The right hepatic duct divides into two segmental divisions whereas the left duct usually has no major visible tributaries.

(*Text continued on p. 537*)

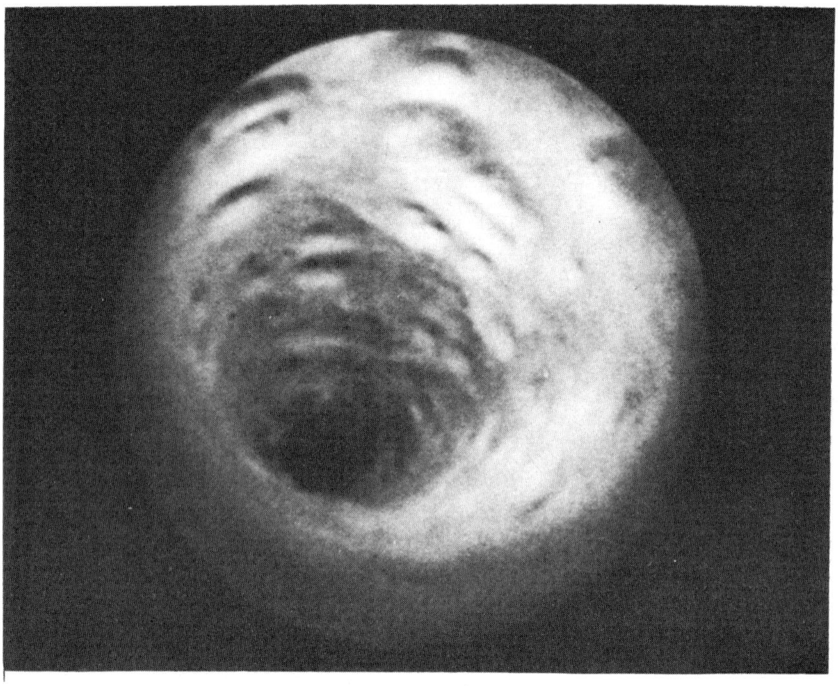

Figure 24.7. Endoscopic views of biliary tract. Figures (a) to (f) are enlargements from single 16 mm colour movie frames. (a) A distal view. Clear tunnel-shaped appearance with the sphincter on the far end. × 14

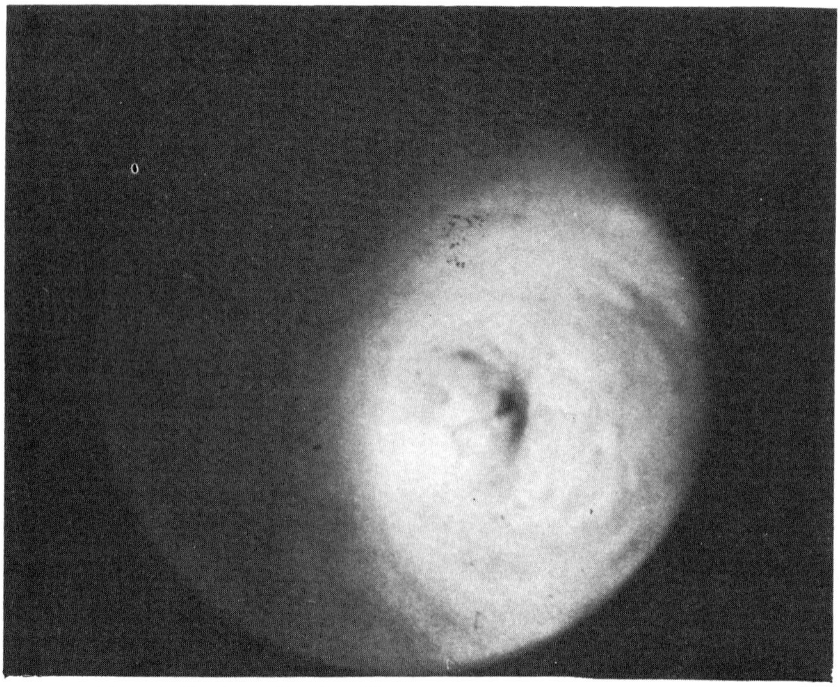

Figure 24.7b. A small stellate-like appearance of sphincter opening. ×14.

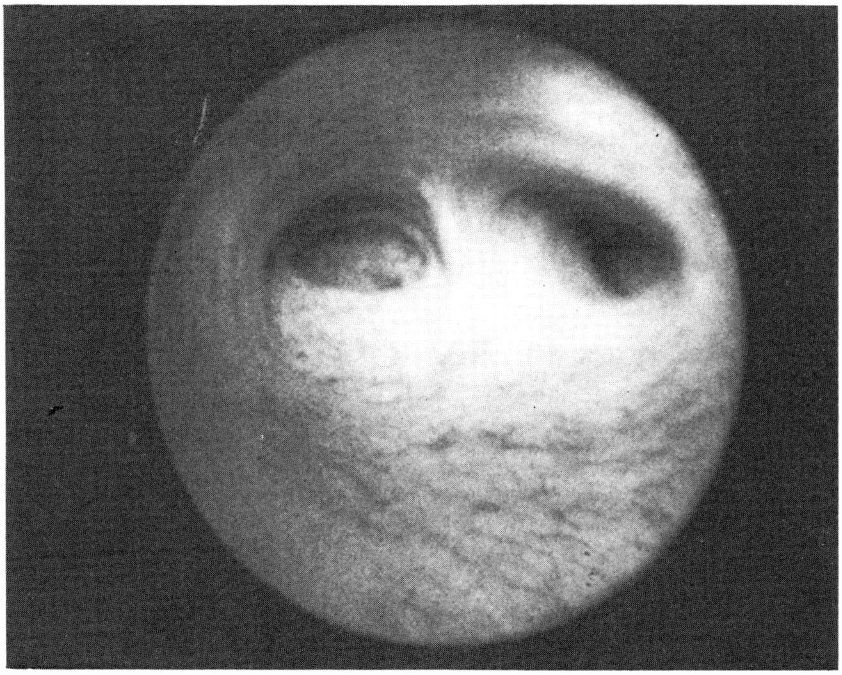

Figure 24.7c. Bifurcation of the main hepatic ducts. × 14.

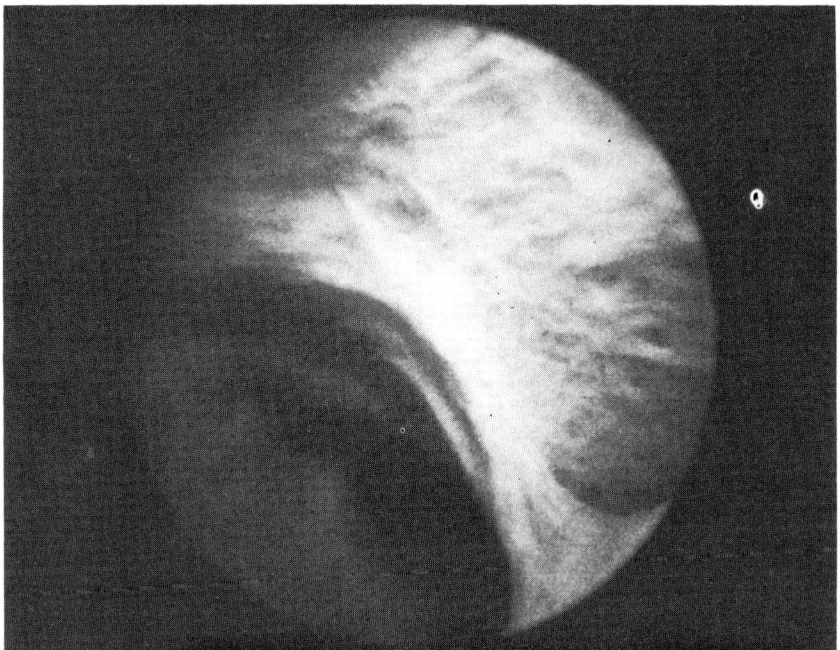

Figure 24.7d. Close-up view of bifurcation. × 14.

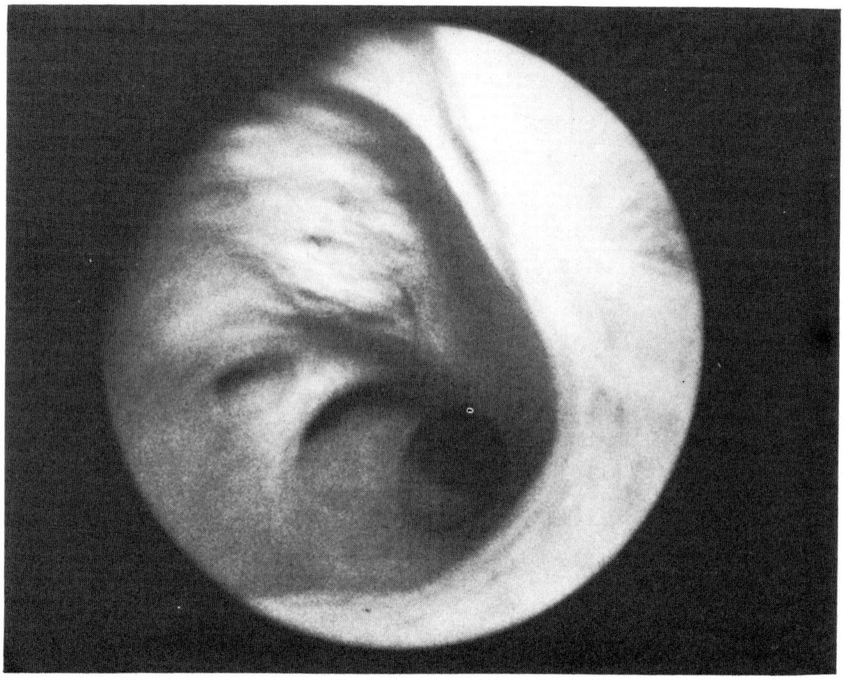

Figure 24.7e. If the duct is clear and distended with the irrigation fluid even tertiary bifurcations can be seen. × 14.

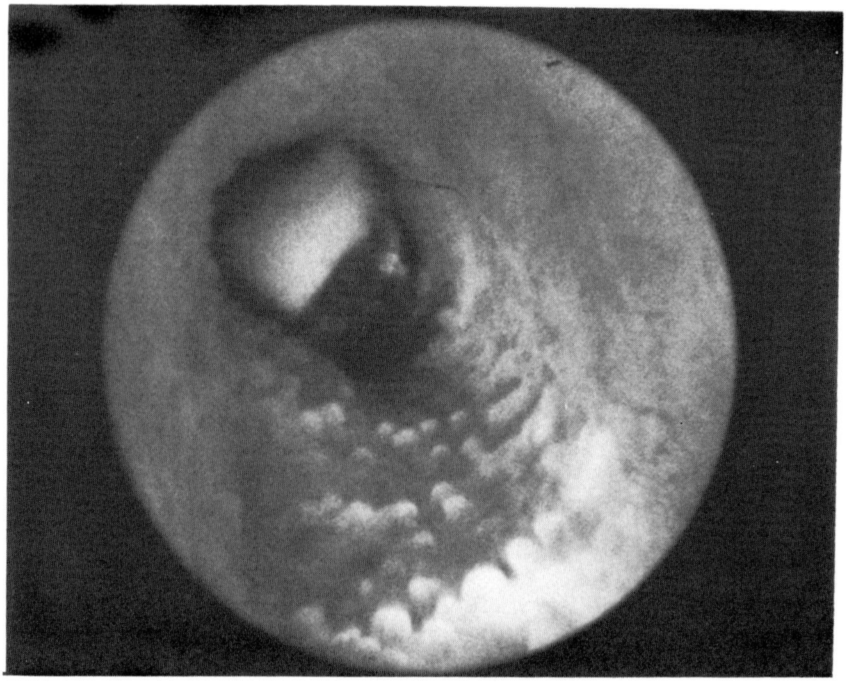

Figure 24.7f. Impacted stone in the distal common duct. × 14.

Variations in the anatomy are common. The junction of the right and left ducts may occur at a wide angle, limiting visualization of the left duct to a few cm, while a narrow union results in a 'trifurcation' endoscopically. When the ducts are dilated one can even see the tertiary hepatic radicles (Figure 24.7e). The major carina is the landmark one must identify to ensure complete hepatic duct visualization.

PATHOLOGY

Cholangitis

Inflammatory reaction is often seen in ducts with stones and varies from congestion and oedema to ulcerative cholangitis with fibrinopurulent exudate. These changes are more prominent in the region of the ampulla, which may be obscured by debris. Removal of these inflammatory products with a stone forceps after withdrawal of the scope is rewarded by improved visualization. These findings are usually less extensive in the hepatic ducts.

Calculi

Calculi may be free-floating, rolling around under the pressure of the irrigating fluid, or fixed, but are always easily identified. If a stone comes into direct contact with the scope, a coloured blur or dark circle will result. At times a stone can be found impacted in the orifice of a hepatic duct or at the ampullary region (Figure 24.7f), partially embedded in the wall or even in a diverticulum or preformed pouch. Multiple calculi or biliary mud are not infrequently encountered behind obstructing calculi. Repeated endoscopic examination will ensure their complete removal.

Ampullary Stenosis

Normally the ampulla is soft and pliable, yielding to the pressure of the irrigating stream. Observation of the characteristic dynamic 'systolic' closing and 'diastolic' opening action identifies the normal sphincter. A stenotic sphincter appears as a fixed circular or pinpoint opening at the end of an easily distended common duct, resembling an oesophageal stricture. This picture, however, is not diagnostic, since it can be mimicked by spasm. Definitive diagnosis must be confirmed by radiological and/or manometric display and histological criteria.

Neoplasms

Tumours protruding into the lumen are very seldom seen. When encountered, they can be biopsied using a flexible forceps advanced through the instrument guide channel. Extrinsic compression of the duct by carcinoma of the pancreas, periductal lymphadenopathy, or carcinoma of the gallbladder is more common. The endoscopic appearance is one of sudden complete occlusion of the lumen. The mucosal lining is smooth and it is difficult to find a site for biopsy. If extrinsic compression results from a process in the pancreas, it is usually impossible to differentiate from the collapsed lumen, whether it is due to a carcinoma of the head of the pancreas or to an inflammatory process.

Other Lesions

Benign tumours or diverticula of the distal duct, congenital webs, foreign bodies (for instance food particles, particularly following biliary–intestinal anastomosis) and parasites are uncommonly seen.

CLINICAL EXPERIENCE

During the past 18 years, the authors have employed choledochoscopy in 359 patients at the Cedars-Sinai Medical Center (Table 24.1). Once the Hopkins-Storz scope became available, the previously used instruments became

Table 24.1. *Experience with Biliary Endoscopy*

	Wildegans Rigid 1960–64	Shore–Lippman Fibreoptic 1965–69	Berci–Shore Rigid 1970–77	Total
Primary choledochotomy	54	160	99	313
Secondary choledochotomy	5	20	21	46
Total	59	180	120	359

obsolete. Because of its superior performance, this new scope is considered to be the definitive diagnostic tool for biliary endoscopy. Evaluation of the results is therefore limited to our experience with this instrument in 120 choledochotomies during the past eight years.

In each patient, the ducts were explored by conventional methods until the surgeon was satisfied that he had cleared them of calculi. Operative biliary endoscopy was then carried out. Overlooked calculi detected by endoscopy were usually readily retrieved with standard common duct instruments; occasionally, removal under direct endoscopic control was required. Completion cholangiograms were obtained on all patients. The final status of the biliary tract was assessed by routine postoperative T-tube cholangiography.

RESULTS

The results are documented in Table 24.2. Ninety-nine patients underwent primary choledochotomy, choledochoscopy and completion operative cholangiography. Calculi were found in 65 patients, while in 20 the results of exploration were negative. In nine patients ampullary stenosis was confirmed, while five harboured a malignant neoplasm. Routine postoperative T-tube cholangiography in this primary group revealed an overlooked stone in one patient (1 per cent). Calculi were also retained in two of 21 patients who underwent secondary choledocholithotomy (10 per cent).

Routine biliary endoscopy during choledochotomy proved to be a valuable adjunct to exploration in several ways:

1. Detection of overlooked stones
2. Endoscopic removal of stones
3. Management of non-removable stones
4. Avoidance of duodenotomy
5. Expediting choledochotomy
6. Diagnosis and 'staging' of biliary tumours.

Detection of Overlooked Stones

It is surprising how often stones are left behind after careful exploration by well-trained surgeons. In our experience additional stones were found by endoscopy in approximately one out of every four cases after conventional instrumentation. It is estimated that 50 per cent of these would have been detected if completion T-tube cholangiography had preceded endoscopy. The supremacy of endoscopy, however, is demonstrated by the extremely low incidence of retained stones (Table 24.2) shown by postoperative T-tube cholangiography. The higher incidence of error in secondary exploration emphasizes the importance of complete ductal evaluation, including endoscopy, during the *initial* operation.

Endoscopic Removal of Stones

In the majority of cases overlooked stones detected by endoscopy can be readily removed by conventional manipulations. In approximately 10 per cent this is not possible for stones lodged in the ampulla or located in the intrahepatic ducts, where retrieval under endoscopic control is the method of choice. The most useful adjuncts for this purpose are the flexible alligator forceps, the Fogarty biliary catheter and the Dormia stone basket. These devices should be used in the hepatic ducts *only* under endoscopic control to avoid injury to these delicate structures.

Management of Non-removable Stones

Rarely, all efforts to extract the 'last' stone from the ductal system fail. Good surgical judgement dictates abandoning further time-consuming fruitless manoeuvres in favour of primary biliary bypass, or leaving a large-diameter T-tube behind for subsequent non-operative stone retrieval[4, 28] if choledocho-enterostomy is not feasible. Although such calculi are retained, their discovery by endoscopy has led to prompt definitive management, thus decreasing the probability of future difficulties.

Table 24.2. *Results of Exploration, Cholangiography and Endoscopy*

Primary choledochotomy		
Calculi found		65
Ducts cleared	64	
Retained calculus	1	
No calculi found		34
Normal duct	20	
Stenosis sphincter	9	
Neoplasm	5	
Secondary choledochotomy		
Calculi found		21
Ducts cleared	19	
Retained calculi	2	
Total		120

Avoidance of Duodenotomy

A variety of conditions may be encountered during choledochotomy which in the past would have required trans-duodenal exploration. The impacted ampullary stone, a questionable mass or filling defect in the distal duct, inability to pass a catheter through the sphincter or non-emptying of contrast material on the completion cholangiogram are examples familiar to every surgeon. Biliary endoscopy permits direct visual diagnosis of the problem in the distal duct, usually leading to appropriate management without duodenotomy.

Expediting Choledochotomy

After direct visualization of the ducts, there is less tendency to prolong the operation; the choledochotomy can be closed early with the expectation that the completion cholangiogram will be negative. Endoscopy thus actually expedites routine common bile duct exploration.

Diagnosis and 'Staging' of Biliary Tumours

Endoscopy and biopsy under visual control is the method of choice for the diagnosis of tumours in the biliary tract. This examination is also valuable for assessing resectability for cure. Tompkins et al[24] have recently reported a significant incidence of multicentricity in biliary carcinomas; the precise information provided by this examination is thus essential for accurate staging prior to radical surgery.

COMPLICATIONS

The incidence of wound infection in this series was within the range usually reported for common duct exploration without endoscopy (2 per cent). There were no endoscopic injuries to the biliary duct system, duodenum, pancreas or liver, although mucosal injury from prior blind instrumentation was occasionally visualized. Three cases of mild postoperative pancreatitis, responding to conservative management, were encountered. No postoperative mortality attributable to biliary endoscopy has been reported.

DISCUSSION

Operative biliary endoscopy has proved to be of immense value in discovering overlooked stones and removing them under visual control. In selected cases it can be of great help in determining whether a biliary bypass should be added to the primary exploration. The degree and extent of cholangitis can be assessed only by looking into the lumen. Since debris and blood clots on the cholangiogram can mimic stones, the endoscopic evaluation will avoid misinterpretation and shorten operating time.

General surgeons are not inclined to extend a tedious operation but biliary endoscopy does not take more than five to ten minutes and the results justify the procedure. Recent reports indicate a significant reduction in the incidence of retained stones to less than 2 per cent in primary choledocholithotomies.[7,13,14,22]

The technique of choledochoscopy can be readily mastered after a minimum of experience. The endoscopic anatomy of the biliary tract is simple, and the major abnormalities encountered are easily recognized. Difficult stone manipulations are rarely necessary.

Rigid or Flexible Instruments?

Every modern rigid rod-lens telescope is superior in image quality to today's flexible fibre endoscopes. These differences are even more obvious (Figure 24.8) when the image-transmitting system is miniaturized. A flexible fibrescope requires greater skill to co-ordinate the various movements because of the more complex design.[28] In addition, the capital outlay and maintenance costs for the latter are excessive: for the price of one flexible choledochoscope, approximately four or five rigid ones can be purchased. The flexible scopes have a limited life-span and the repair costs are significant. In our busy general surgical service, with good instrument care, the original rigid choledochoscope has been used over an eight-year period without repair or exchange. The smaller diameter also permits more universal application.

In Southampton the flexible choledochoscope has been utilized since 1973[5] (Figure 24.9). No cases of retained calculi undetected by the endoscope occurred. Postoperative T-tube cholangiography confirmed the findings of operative biliary endoscopy in all 81 cases where it was employed. The technique was found to be an accurate and safe operative procedure

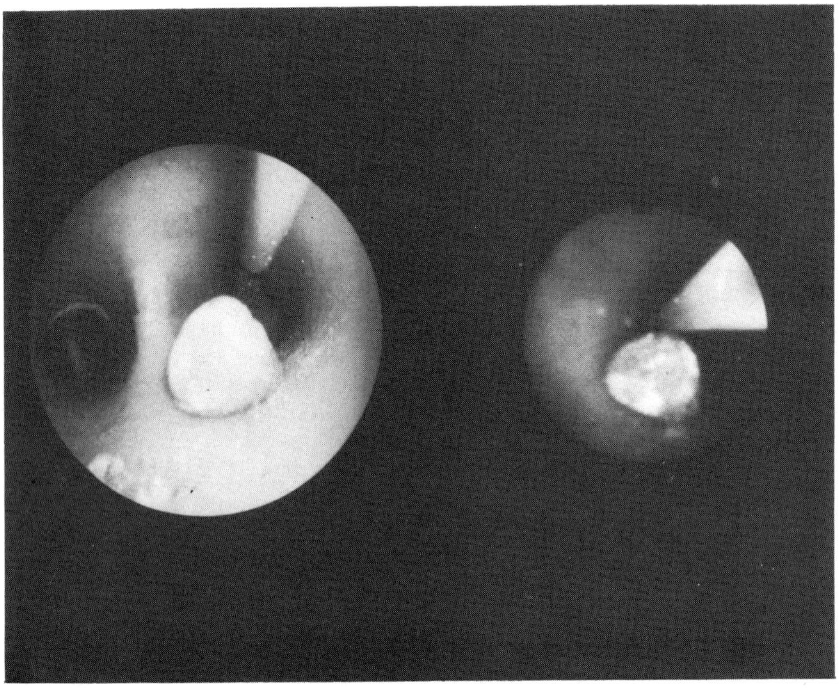

Figure 24.8. Comparative views through rigid and flexible choledochoscopes under identical object distances. Left: rigid choledochoscope. Right: flexible fibre choledochoscope.

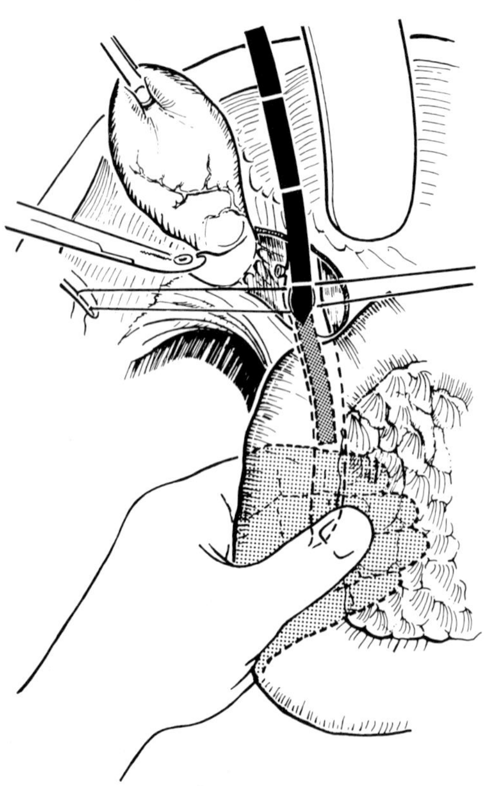

Figure 24.9. Technique of insertion of flexible choledochoscope. Extraluminal control of the tip of the instrument and common duct aids visualization.

capable of eliminating the problem of undetected residual calculi (Table 24.3).

Results obtained by various authors using both the rigid and flexible choledochoscopes are shown in Table 24.4.

Operative Choledochoscopy or Operative Cholangiography?

Many surgeons ask whether completion cholangiography should be eliminated after satisfactory endoscopy. In our experience both procedures are complementary and should be used in every common bile duct exploration. The well-recognized problems of non-emptying and filling defects on cholangiograms can usually be correctly interpreted when interpretation is based on the endoscopic findings. In our series completion cholangiography discovered calculi missed by endoscopy in 2 per cent of the cases, while non-significant filling defects (debris, blood clots) were found in an additional 6 per cent.

Postoperative Choledochoscopy

While the incidence of retained biliary calculi can be minimized by operative chole-

Table 24.3. *Results of Operative Biliary Endoscopy*

Operative findings	No.	Postoperative T-tube cholangiogram	Postoperative x-rays confirmed operative endoscopy
No calculi on exploration or endoscopy	18 (20.5%)	17	17
Endoscopically clear after lithotomy	44 (50%)	40	40
Further calculi on endoscopy →lithotomy →clear	24 (27.3%)	22	22
Endoscopically detected inaccessible calculi	2 (2.2%)	2	2
Total	88	81	81

Table 24.4. *Collected Series: Incidence of Retained Calculi After Choledochoscopy*

	Type of endoscope	No.	Choledochoscopy and postoperative T-tube cholangiogram findings	
			Endo-scopically detected residual calculi	Residual calculi missed endo-scopically
Schein[17]	Rigid	117	0	0
Shore & Shore[21]	Flexible	156	0	4
Longland[8]	Flexible	37	3	2
Leslie[7]	Both	91	0	0
Shore, Berci & Morgenstern[22]	Rigid	120	0	3
Finnis & Rowntree[5]	Flexible	81	2	0
Total		582	5 (0.9%)	9 (1.5%)

dochoscopy, the procedure is not universally employed, leaving a sizeable population of patients with the problem. In recent years a variety of techniques has been developed for the non-operative management of these overlooked stones.[4,25,28] One of the most successful methods for percutaneous extraction of biliary calculi via the T-tube tract was recently reported by Yamakawa and Shikata,[27] using the flexible fibre choledochoscope. Although multiple sessions were often required, complete ductal clearance was achieved in 46 of 48 patients by this method.

CONCLUSION

Biliary endoscopy with newer instrumentation has been found to be of great value in reducing the incidence of retained stones and in diagnosing biliary tumours. The examination is simple, accurate and free of complications. It should be an essential adjunct to every biliary exploration.

REFERENCES

1. Bakes, J. (1923) Die Choledochopapilloskopie nebst Bemerkungen uber Hepaticusdrainage und Dilatation der Papille. *Archiv für Klinische Chirurgie,* **126,** 473 483.
2. Berci, G. (1961) Choledochoscopy. *Medical Journal of Australia,* **2,** 860–863.
3. Berci, G. & Kont, L. (1969) A new optical system in endoscopy with special reference to cystoscopy. *British Journal of Urology,* **41,** 564–571.
4. Burhenne, J.H., Richards, V., Mathewson, C. & Westdale, P.R. (1974) Non-operative extraction of retained biliary tract stones requiring multiple sessions. *American Journal of Surgery,* **128,** 288–292.
5. Finnis, D. & Rowntree, T. (1977) Choledochoscopy in exploration of common bile duct. *British Journal of Surgery,* **64,** 661–664.
6. Glenn, F. (1975) *Common Duct Stones.* p. 68. Springfield, Illinois: Charles Thomas.
7. Leslie, D. (1974) Endoscopy of the bile duct: an evaluation. *Australian and New Zealand Journal of Surgery,* **44,** 340–342.
8. Longland, C.J. (1973) Choledochoscopy in choledocholithiasis. *British Journal of Surgery,* **60,** 626–628.
9. Mazarello, A. (1973) Review of 220 cases of residual biliary tract calculi treated without operation: an eight year study. *Surgery,* **73,** 299–301.
10. McIver, M.A. (1941) An instrument for visualizing the interior of the common duct at operation. *Surgery,* **9,** 112–114.
11. Mirizzi, P.L. (1932) La colangiografie durante las operaciones de las vias bilares. *Boletines y trabajos de la Sociedad de chirugia de Buenos Aires,* **16,** 1133–1161.
12. Nemethy, G. (1976) Instrumentation. III: cleaning, storage, and maintenance and supervision. In *Endoscopy* (Ed.) Berci, G. pp. 133–154. New York: Appleton-Century-Crofts.
13. Nora, P.F., Berci, G., Dorazzio, R.A., Kirshenbaum, G., Shore, J.M., Tompkins, R.K. & Wilson, S.P. (1977) Operative choledochoscopy. *American Journal of Surgery,* **133,** 105–108.

14. Ottinger, L.W., Warshaw, A.L. & Bartlett, M.K. (1974) Intraoperative endoscopic evaluation of the bile ducts. *American Journal of Surgery,* **127,** 465–468.
15. Raney, A.M. (1976) Electrohydraulic cystolithotripsy. *Urology,* **7,** 379–381.
16. Safrany, L. (1977) Duodenoscopic sphincterotomy and gallstone removal. *Gastroenterology,* **72,** 338–343.
17. Schein, C.J.S. (1969) Biliary endoscopy; an appraisal of its value in biliary lithiasis. *Surgery,* **65,** 1004–1006.
18. Shore, J.M. & Berci, G. (1970) The clinical importance of cholangiography. *Endoscopy,* **2,** 117–120.
19. Shore, J.M. & Lippman, H.N. (1962) Operative endoscopy of the biliary tract. *Annals of Surgery,* **156,** 951–955.
20. Shore, J.M. & Lippman, H.N. (1965) A flexible choledochoscope. *Lancet,* **i,** 1200–1201.
21. Shore, J.M. & Shore, S.E. (1970) Operative biliary endoscopy; experience with flexible choledochoscope in 100 consecutive choledocholithotomies. *Annals of Surgery,* **171,** 269–278.
22. Shore, J.M., Berci, G. & Morgenstern, L. (1975) The value of biliary endoscopy. *Surgery, Gynecology and Obstetrics,* **140,** 601–604.
23. Slotnick, I. (1976) Microbiology and sterilization of endoscopes. In *Endoscopy* (Ed.) Berci, G. pp. 155–173. New York: Appleton-Century-Crofts.
24. Tompkins, R.K., Johnson, J., Storm., F.K. & Longmire, W.P. (1976) Operative endoscopy in the management of biliary tract neoplasms. *American Journal of Surgery,* **132,** 174–182.
25. Way, L.W., Admirand, L.G. & Dunphy, J.E. (1972) Management of choledocholithiasis. *Annals of Surgery,* **176,** 347–359.
26. Wildegans, H. (1953) Grenzen der Cholangiography und Aussichten der Cholangioskopie der tiefen Gallenwege. *Medical Klinische,* **48,** 1270–1273.
27. Yamakawa, T. & Shikata, J. (1977) Postoperative choledochoscopy – an appraisal of its clinical value for management of retained biliary stones and intrahepatic stones. *Presented at the American Society for Gastrointestinal Endoscopy Meeting (Digestive Disease Week) Toronto, Canada 1977.*
28. Yamakawa, T., Mieno, K., Shikata, J. (1975) Operative and postoperative choledochoscopy. *Gastroenterology,* **38,** 1052 (abstract).

Chapter 25

Peritoneoscopy

TELFER B. REYNOLDS
RUSSELL E. COWAN

Peritoneoscopy and laparoscopy are synonymous terms though the latter tends to be used more often when the indication is gynaecological. They are defined similarly in medical dictionaries;[5] however, the Cumulative Index Medicus still lists both procedures separately.

HISTORY

The advanced state of development of peritoneoscopy today owes much to the imagination and ingenuity of the originators of this technique. Ott, a gynaecologist, first examined the abdominal cavity in 1901 using a head mirror and speculum and Kelling, in the same year, first used optical instruments to perform what he called 'coelioscopy' in the dog by inflating the abdominal cavity with air and examining the contents with a cystoscope. The technique was published in 1902[16] but its use in humans was not described until 1910 when Jacobaeus[11] published his experience with inspection of the human pleural and peritoneal cavities, again with a cystoscope. One month later Kelling[17] reported his experience with peritoneoscopy in two patients. Two years later Jacobaeus[12] reported on 45 peritoneoscopic examinations of humans but this was followed by a 10-year interval without further progress until Korbsch[18] rediscovered the technique and developed the instruments and methods. Interest in the procedure then flourished, with reports from many peritoneoscopists throughout the world. None contributed more to the technique than Kalk[15] who designed the instrument that has formed the basis of today's peritoneoscopes.

Ruddock[24,25] designed a peritoneoscope with a built-in biopsy facility. He also published his large experience with the procedure. Advances in recent years have stemmed from the introduction of fibreoptics to medical technology whereby glass fibre bundles are used to transmit light from the light source down the shaft of the instrument thus providing 'cold light' illumination of the abdominal cavity.[9]

Peritoneoscopy is used today by gastroenterologists, surgeons and gynaecologists in most countries. There are many excellent reviews of peritoneoscopic experience in the literature, including those by Kalk,[15] Caroli and Ricordeau[4] and Boyce.[2] A colour atlas of peritoneoscopic photographs has been published by Wittman.[30] Developments in the technique and equipment will continue while the desire to perform more functions with the procedure continues to grow.

INDICATIONS

When considering the indications for peritoneoscopy, it is important to know which organs and how much of them can be seen through the peritoneoscope. In general, one can see the anterior surface of the abdominal viscera as when the abdominal wall is removed at autopsy. This includes the entire anterior surface of the left lobe of the liver, the medial two-thirds of the anterior surface of the right lobe, the leading edges and the inferior portion of the posterior surfaces of both lobes, the anterior surface of the gallbladder, the anterior surface of the stomach, parts of the small bowel, colon, mesentery and omentum, and the peritoneum covering the diaphragm, the anterior abdominal wall and the falciform ligament. Not seen are the posterior and lateral surfaces of the right lobe of the liver, the duodenum, the cystic and common bile ducts and the retroperitoneal organs such as kidneys and pancreas. By lifting the left lobe of the liver, Meyer-Burg[19] has been able to visualize and biopsy the pancreas in a number of patients who were not obese. The spleen is visible only if enlarged. The dome of the right lobe of the liver is seen with difficulty. The pelvic organs (bladder, uterus, fallopian tubes and ovaries) are visible, particularly if the patient is placed in the Trendelenberg position and a hand in the vagina or a uterine sound is used to manipulate the uterus. Visualization at peritoneoscopy can be increased by using an examining table that tilts in all directions and by inserting a blunt probe into the peritoneal cavity through a separate abdominal puncture.

Assessment of Liver Disease

A major indication for peritoneoscopy is inspection of the liver surface and evaluation of size and shape of the organ. When combined with liver biopsy this allows the best assessment of the type and severity of chronic liver disease. Cirrhosis is diagnosed if the surface is nodular (Plates 25.1 and 25.2). Small nodules, less than 3 mm in diameter, are most consistent with an alcoholic aetiology while larger, well-developed nodules suggest non-alcoholic cirrhosis. A liver that is paler than normal with an irregular, granular or coarse-sandpaper surface and a thickened leading edge suggests either alcoholic fibrosis or chronic active hepatitis (Plate 25.3). An enlarged liver with a rounded leading edge and a smooth surface is consistent with either a fatty liver or acute alcoholic hepatitis. There is nothing distinctive about the appearance of the liver in acute hepatitis unless the disease is unusually severe with submassive necrosis in which there are often islands of normal-appearing liver surrounded by paler, retracted areas of collapsed parenchyma.

For recording the progression of liver disease, an accurate, objective description of the liver surface is essential. Nodule size can be estimated relatively accurately if the operator knows the magnification produced by his instrument at a specified distance. A photograph is invaluable for recording the appearance of the liver.

In our Liver Unit we use peritoneoscopic visualization for staging chronic liver disease particularly when coagulation defects do not permit liver biopsy. Since bleeding at the peritoneoscopic puncture site is controllable by clamping and tying of blood vessels, we do not regard a low prothrombin time per se as a contraindication to peritoneoscopy.

Liver biopsy under direct vision can be performed either through the peritoneoscope or through a separate puncture site. Direct-vision biopsy is probably no safer than 'blind' biopsy with respect to bleeding except that the peritoneoscopist may have earlier knowledge that bleeding is occurring. Some advise injection of topical thrombin solution into the wound or electrocautery via the biopsy needle.[30] We have had no personal experience with either of these methods. Ruddock[24, 25] obtained forceps biopsies of the leading edge of the liver; these are reputed to contain artefacts more often because of compression of the specimen.

Evaluation of Filling Defects Seen on Hepatic Scan

Filling defects found on radionuclide liver scan and located within the field of vision of the peritoneoscope can be examined, photographed and biopsied. In patients with metastatic cancer there are often small lesions visible on the liver surface but not detectable on scan so that peritoneoscopy may be diagnostic even when the scan is negative (Plate 25.4) or shows a filling defect in an inaccessible area. Tumour masses that are entirely intrahepatic may cause a bulge on the liver surface that helps to guide the biopsy needle. In one study of patients suspected of having hepatic neoplasm, biopsy at peritoneoscopy disclosed malignant tissue in 69 per cent while 'blind' transthoracic liver biopsy performed at the same time was diagnostic in only 39 per cent.[13] An additional advantage to peritoneoscopy in this situation is that liver biopsy can be avoided when a mass lesion looks cystic or extremely vascular.

Hepatocellular carcinoma can usually be differentiated from surrounding cirrhotic nodules by its colour and by its friability and irregularity (Plate 25.5). In some patients, however, the hepatocellular tumour nodules so closely resemble the regenerative nodules of cirrhosis that biopsy is necessary for diagnosis.

Congenital cysts of the liver are easily

diagnosed by their smooth translucent appearance. Other lesions, such as haemangiomas, hydatid cysts, benign tumours and cystadenomas all require experience for ready recognition.

Differential Diagnosis of Ascites

Chronic liver disease causing ascites is usually easily diagnosed at peritoneoscopy. Since much of the peritoneal surface is available for inspection, some of the other causes of ascites can also be identified. In carcinomatous ascites there may be many small neoplastic nodules scattered on the parietal and visceral peritoneum or fewer, larger lesions on the bowel, mesentery or peritoneum (Plate 25.6). In tuberculous or coccidioidal peritonitis there are numerous 0.5 to 2.0 mm yellow or white tubercles on both the visceral and parietal peritoneum (Plate 25.7). Usually the entire peritoneum is involved; occasionally the disease is limited to the upper or lower abdomen. Biopsy of lesions on the intestinal surface is potentially hazardous but a forceps biopsy of a nodule on the peritoneum or mesentery is easy and safe.

Recognition of Portal Hypertension

Portal hypertension is recognized at peritoneoscopy by the presence of portal collateral veins. Occasionally a large vein is seen in the falciform ligament (Plate 25.8); more often numerous tiny vessels are present and appear red in colour though they are venules. Tortuous veins are often seen on the undersurface of the diaphragm or on the lateral or anterior walls of the abdominal cavity. The abdominal wall veins are often visible by transillumination in the darkened precedure room. If there are adhesions in the abdomen in patients with portal hypertension, they frequently contain large collateral veins carrying blood from the mesentery or bowel to the abdominal wall.

Evaluation of Abdominal Masses

Upper abdominal masses that originate in the liver or spleen are readily assessed at peritoneoscopy unless they are obscured by adhesions. Biopsy of hepatic masses under direct vision is relatively easy and, in the epigastric area, may be safer than blind biopsy because of proximity to stomach, intestines and aorta. Mid and lower abdominal masses of non-hepatic origin are often covered by bowel or omentum and evaluation by peritoneoscopy may be unrewarding. Laparotomy is usually preferable for this purpose. Pelvic masses can be examined and biopsied at peritoneoscopy, but whether laparotomy or peritoneoscopy is the best approach to a suspected pelvic mass is a gynaecological decision.

POSSIBLE INDICATIONS

Differential Diagnosis of Jaundice

At times, inspection of the liver surface can be of diagnostic value in a jaundiced patient, particularly when unexpected cirrhosis is encountered. Some authorities believe that the finding of a green liver surface is helpful in indicating chronic bile duct obstruction. Usually, however, examination of the biliary apparatus is necessary to make a diagnosis in a jaundiced patient. A distended 'Courvoisier' gallbladder strongly suggests malignant distal bile duct obstruction (Plate 25.4). However, such enlarged gallbladders are often palpable or can be demonstrated convincingly by ultrasound. Chronic cholecystitis due to gallstone disease is strongly suggested by a small gallbladder that looks white and opaque rather than the usual robin's-egg blue colour. Rarely, carcinoma of the gallbladder is suspected because of a localized abnormality of the gallbladder wall (Plate 25.9). Cholangiography by direct puncture of the gallbladder at peritoneoscopy was introduced years ago by Royer[23] but has not become popular, probably because of the risk of bile leakage. Gaisford[6] modified this procedure by performing the gallbladder puncture transhepatically, with good results in seven patients.

We have not often employed peritoneoscopy for differential diagnosis of jaundice because we consider it of limited value.

Staging of Lymphoma

Some oncology groups have used peritoneoscopy to look at the liver surface for lymphomatous involvement, to obtain multiple liver biopsies and even to biopsy the spleen.[27] However, abdominal lymph nodes cannot be seen or biopsied at peritoneoscopy because of their posterior location in the abdomen and there is insufficient published experience to judge the safety of splenic biopsy.

Portography

It is possible to obtain good-quality portograms by injecting contrast media into a small omental vein that is cannulated after withdrawing a piece of omentum through the peritoneoscopy incision with forceps.[31] We rarely use this method now since arterial portography usually gives excellent results.

CONTRAINDICATIONS

Most contraindications are relative rather than absolute.

Obesity

A thick abdominal wall makes it more difficult to obtain satisfactory anaesthesia of the parietal peritoneum and to penetrate the abdominal wall safely with the peritoneoscopic trocar. Mobility of the peritoneoscope within the abdominal cavity is reduced because the thick abdominal wall tends to hold the instrument in a vertical position. A fatty greater omentum often makes it difficult to view the liver satisfactorily.

Surgical Scars

Adhesions frequently form under surgical scars. After cholecystectomy adhesions often form a curtain in the right upper quadrant preventing visualization of the right lobe of the liver. Similarly, visualization of the left lobe of the liver may be prevented by adhesions under gastric surgery scars. When portal hypertension is present adhesions often contain large collateral veins which, if traumatized by the peritoneoscopic trocar or air needle, can bleed seriously. The peritoneoscope should not be inserted, therefore, into the abdomen close to a scar. Generalized peritonitis or acute pancreatitis can result, throughout the abdominal cavity, in multiple adhesions which impair visualization, limit distensibility of the abdomen with air and constitute a hazard to insertion of the peritoneoscope since loops of bowel can be adherent to the abdominal wall.

Gross Coagulation Defect

Unless a liver biopsy is performed or an adhesion torn the abdominal puncture is the only potential site of bleeding at peritoneoscopy. Since small blood vessels at the puncture site can be clamped and ligated, there is less reason to fear excess bleeding in patients with coagulation defects than there is during percutaneous liver biopsy. However, patients with grossly abnormal prothrombin times tend to be fragile in many respects, so peritoneoscopy should be performed in such patients only when there is a very strong indication. Trauma to a vein on the peritoneal surface of the abdomen at the puncture site can be overlooked at peritoneoscopy since bleeding will be into the abdominal cavity rather than into the wound and may be temporarily prevented by the tamponade effect of the trocar during the procedure, only to start after removal of the instrument.

Uncooperative Patient

Since peritoneoscopy is usually performed without general anaesthesia, some degree of patient cooperation is required. With adequate premedication most apprehensive patients are able to cooperate satisfactorily.

Tense Ascites

Visualization at peritoneoscopy is unsatisfactory through ascitic fluid. When marked ascites is present, therefore, it is necessary to remove much of the fluid and replace it with air. Although, in our experience, the danger from removal of large amounts of ascitic fluid in patients with liver disease is greatly overemphasized, there are occasional instances when signs of hypovolaemia (hypotension, thirst, hyponatraemia, decreased renal function, rise in haematocrit) develop 24 to 48 hours after paracentesis. A second problem in patients with ascites is drainage of fluid from the incision that may persist for several days after the procedure unless the operator is able to suture the hole in the peritoneum. Ascitic fluid extravasation into the tissues of the abdominal wall or into the loose tissues around the male genitalia may also occur if the peritoneal rent is left open while the skin incision is tightly closed.

INSTRUMENTS

Peritoneoscope

Instruments have improved steadily since the introduction of fibreoptic light transmission for endoscopy in 1961.[9] Several excellent instruments are now available, including those made by Storz, Wolff, American Cystoscope Makers, Olympus and Machida. There are both forward oblique and direct-vision telescopes and many contain an operating channel for insertion of a long biopsy needle or a probe. Most instruments are insulated to allow safe conduction of an electric current for coagulation. There are 'paediatric, peritoneoscopes, with an outer diameter of 4.5 mm, that are easier to insert through the abdominal wall; however, they provide less illumination in the abdomen. All makes of peritoneoscopes have photographic capabilities which operate either by using a flash bulb at the distal end of the instrument or by using an electronic flash that is conducted from outside the body down the fibreoptic light bundle. Flexible peritoneoscopic telescopes are in the process of development. Modern instruments are constructed in such a way that they tolerate gas sterilization without loss of optical quality.

Air Insufflation Needle

For air insufflation most operators, including ourselves, prefer the Veress needle which has a blunt retractable cannula inside a sharp-pointed needle. The inner cannula springs forward with a clicking sound and projects beyond the point of the needle when the abdominal cavity is entered.

Acccssorics

Numerous accessories are available, including sterilizable ovens for prewarming telescopes to body temperature. This prevents fogging of the lens after insertion of the telescope into the peritoneal cavity. A suitable alternative is an inexpensive electrical heating pad placed under the tray containing the sterile peritoneoscope. A drop of sterile anti-fog liquid (Ultra-Stop, Sigma Chemic, Vienna) placed on the lens immediately prior to insertion of the telescope into the abdomen is also helpful in preventing fogging. There are automatic gas insufflators that give regulated flow of air or carbon dioxide and provide continuous monitoring of intra-abdominal gas pressure. We prefer hand insufflation with a sterile sphygmomanometer bulb. A variety of biopsy needles is available for insertion through the operating channel of the peritoneoscope or through a separate puncture site. In addition, there are punch-biopsy forceps suitable for biopsying peritoneal nodules.

PREPARATION OF INSTRUMENTS

Care and cleaning of the instruments is best accomplished by a nurse or technician who is familiar with the procedure of peritoneoscopy. Thorough cleaning of the various parts of the instrument after each use is essential. Ethylene oxide gas sterilization clearly provides the greatest possible safety relative to transmission of hepatitis viruses. In this regard, 'wet' sterilization by soaking in activated glutaraldehyde solution poses uncertain risks, although we know of no reported case of transmission of hepatitis with wet-sterilized endoscopes.

TECHNIQUE OF PERITONEOSCOPY

Technique for performance of peritoneoscopy varies considerably and this suggests that the procedure has a large margin of safety and that there are several different ways to achieve the same result. We describe below the method that we have used, with minor modifications, during the past 25 years.

Premedication

We prefer a moderately sedated patient who is not anxious but who is awake enough to respond to commands. Since many patients have severe liver disease and some are habitual drug users the effect of a given dose of premedication varies markedly. Usually we give meperidine, 50 to 100 mg, and promethazine, 25

Plate 23.1. Papilla of Vater. A teflon catheter is inserted in the papillary orifice. Above the papilla is seen a duodenal diverticulum.

Plate 23.2. A large pylorus-like papillary stoma three weeks after endoscopic papillotomy for common bile duct stone removal. A plastic catheter is introduced into the common bile duct.

Plate 25.1. Left lobe of liver in a patient with non-alcoholic cirrhosis. The nodules range from 3 to 6 mm in diameter.

Plate 25.2. Close up view of falciform ligament and medial portions of both left and right liver lobes in a patient with advanced alcoholic cirrhosis. The surface is irregular and lobulated with small regenerative nodules 1 to 2 mm in diameter. Two larger nodules on the left are about 4 mm in diameter.

Plate 25.3. Left lobe of the liver in a patient with alcoholic liver disease and extensive fibrosis on microscopic examination. The liver surface is paler than normal and irregular but without well-defined nodules.

Plate 25.4. Gallbladder and right lobe of liver in a patient with metastatic carcinoma from the pancreas. Numerous small white tumour deposits are evident on the liver surface. These were not seen on $^{99}Tc^{m}$ sulphur colloid liver scan. The gallbladder is markedly distended and projects 6 to 7 cm below the right lobe margin.

Plate 25.5. Right lobe of liver in a patient with cirrhosis due to hepatitis B. On the lower border of the right lobe just above the gallbladder there are two large, pale, irregular, friable masses of hepatocellular carcinoma. There is blood on the omentum at the bottom of the picture resulting from an aspiration biopsy of the tumour.

Plate 25.6. Nodules of metastatic carcinoma 1 to 2 mm in diameter on the parietal peritoneum of a patient with ascites caused by metastatic carcinoma.

Plate 25.7. Parietal peritoneum and surface of the right lobe of the liver in a patient with tuberculous peritonitis. There are numerous small white tubercles on the peritoneum and a few on the liver surface.

Plate 25.8. In the background is the right lobe of the cirrhotic liver. In the foreground is a tortuous blue collateral vein, 4 to 5 mm in diameter, leading towards the base of the falciform ligament (out of view, to the right).

Plate 25.9. Gallbladder, held up by a probe, showing white tumour tissue in its base. The posterior surface of the right lobe of the liver appears at the top of the picture; ascites fluid is seen below the gallbladder.

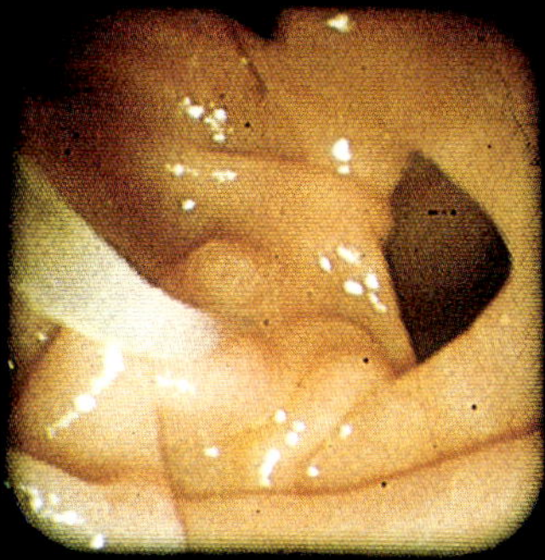
Plate 23.1

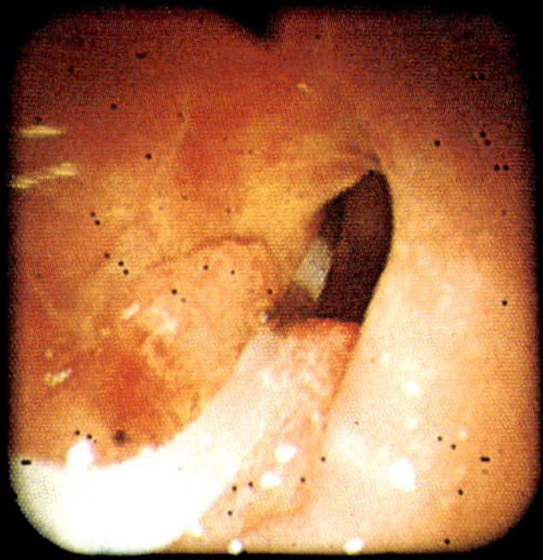
Plate 23.2

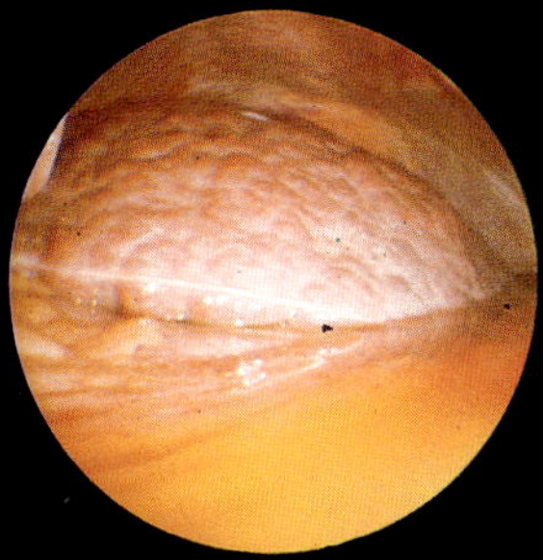
Plate 25.1

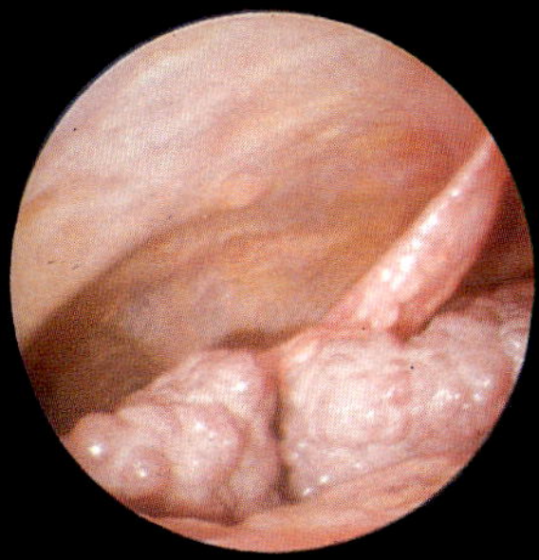
Plate 25.2

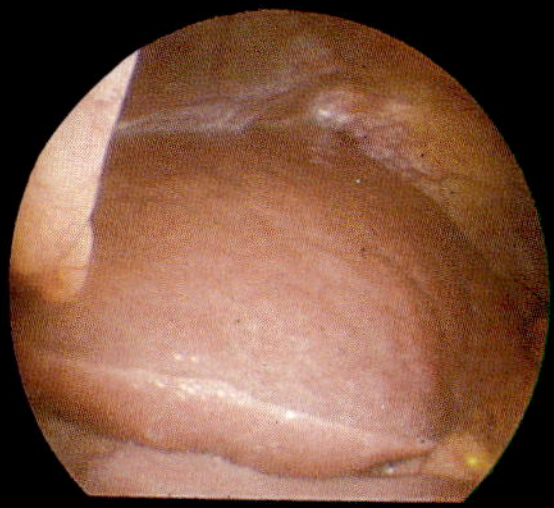
Plate 25.3

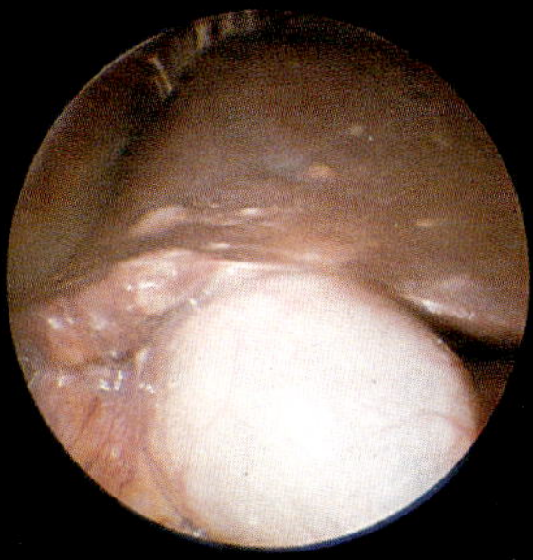
Plate 25.4

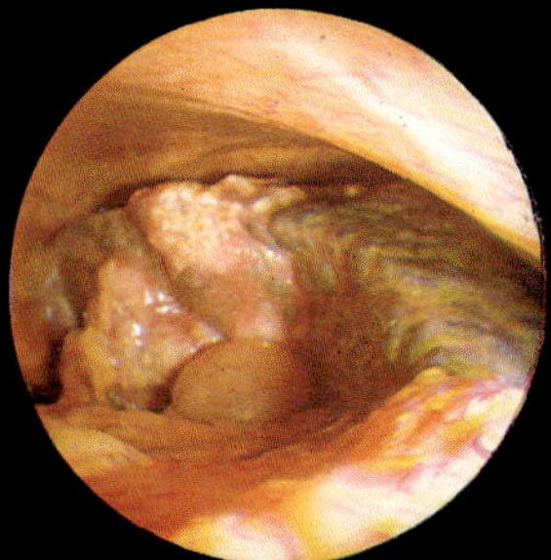
Plate 25.5

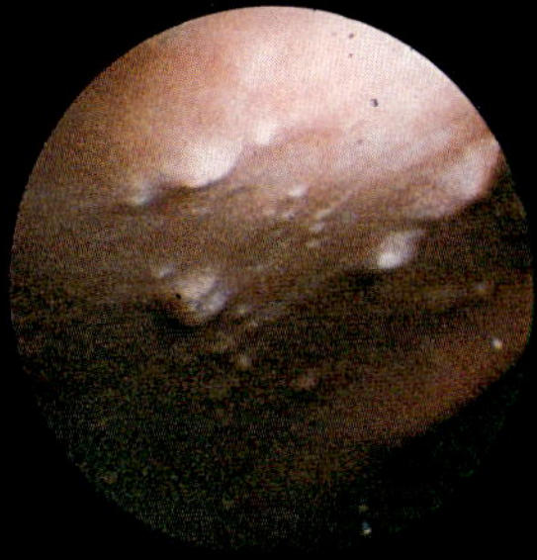
Plate 25.6

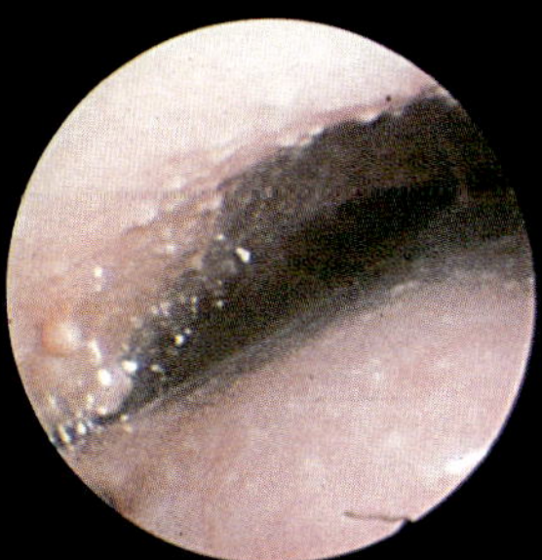
Plate 25.7

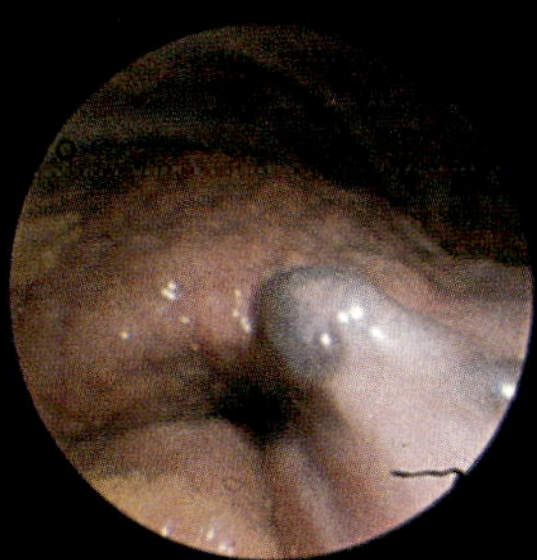
Plate 25.8

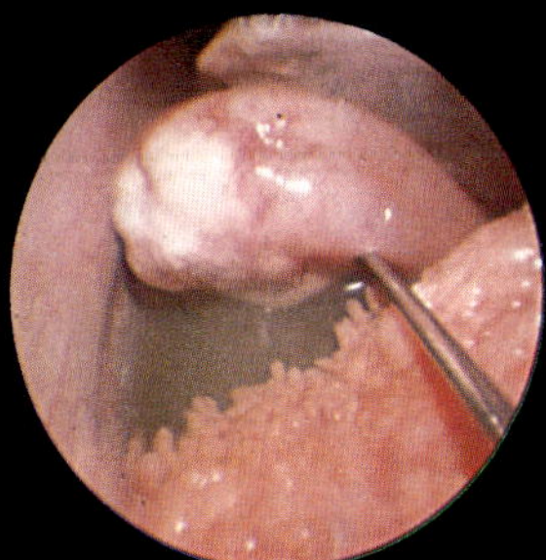
Plate 25.9

to 50 mg, about 45 minutes before peritoneoscopy. If there is anxiety or pain during the procedure, intravenous diazepam (5 to 20 mg) can be added. Some workers give atropine routinely as premedication to prevent vagal reactions which occasionally occur in anxious patients. Most peritoneoscopists do not use general anaesthesia for medical peritoneoscopy since it adds risk and expense and the degree of pain and discomfort seldom warrant it. However, Michel and Raynaud[20] have recently written of the advantages of general anaesthesia of short duration with propanidid. For gynaecological peritoneoscopy general anaesthesia is usually employed because of pain from tubal manipulation and fulguration.

Location

Ideal for peritoneoscopy is a procedure room that can also be used for other endoscopy and minor surgery. There should be an anteroom for changing clothes and a sink for hand scrubbing. The room should contain resuscitation equipment and storage space for the peritoneoscopes and attachments. It should be easily darkened and there should be an automatically adjustable table. The use of a surgical suite is unnecessary and, in most hospitals, impractical.

Performance of Peritoneoscopy

The operator prepares for the procedure with hand and forearm scrubbing and wears a sterile gown and gloves. The patient's abdomen is prepared and draped in a manner that prevents his visualization of the procedure (Figure 25.1). Selection of entry site for the insufflation needle and the peritoneoscopic trocar is important since insertion of these instruments carries the greatest potential risks for serious injury during the procedure. Many experienced peritoneoscopists use separate entry sites for the air needle and the peritoneoscope but it is probably safer and equally satisfactory to use a single entry site. In choosing a location it is important to avoid (a) the epigastric vessels which run in the lateral borders of the rectus muscles, (b) the falciform ligament which may contain large collateral veins, (c) any collateral veins that are visible on the abdominal wall and (d) abdominal scars since these may overlie vascularized adhesions. Obviously, to choose an entry site overlying an abdominal mass or an enlarged liver or spleen will be unwise. We choose most often a point 2 to 4 cm below the umbilicus near the midline (Figure 25.2). Should the patient's size or shape indicate that this location will be too far from the liver for optimum visualization we enter above the umbilicus to the left of the midline to avoid the falciform ligament.

Anaesthesia of the skin and subcutaneous tissue is produced with a local anaesthetic solution. An attempt should be made to anaesthetize the parietal peritoneum. A vertical incision long enough to accommodate the peritoneoscopic trocar is made through the skin and subcutaneous fascia. The Veress needle is then pushed through the abdominal wall, using one hand to exert pressure and the other to keep the needle from abruptly lurching forward when it pierces the parietal peritoneum. When the

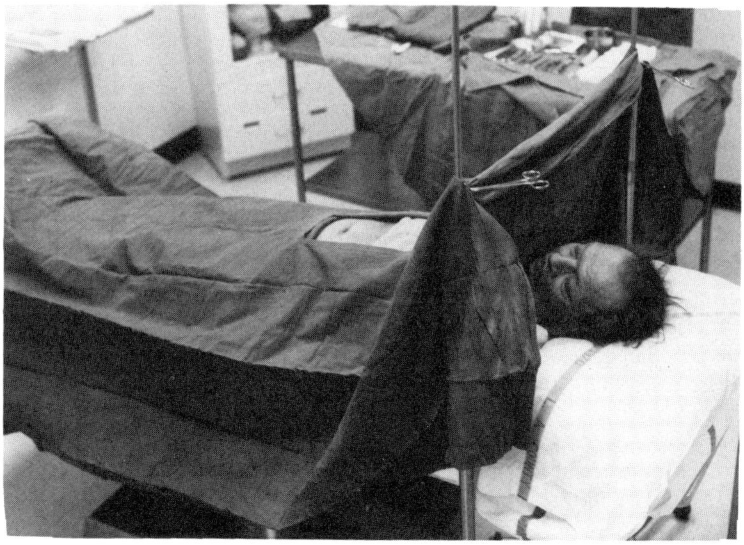

Figure 25.1. Method of draping of the patient for peritoneoscopy.

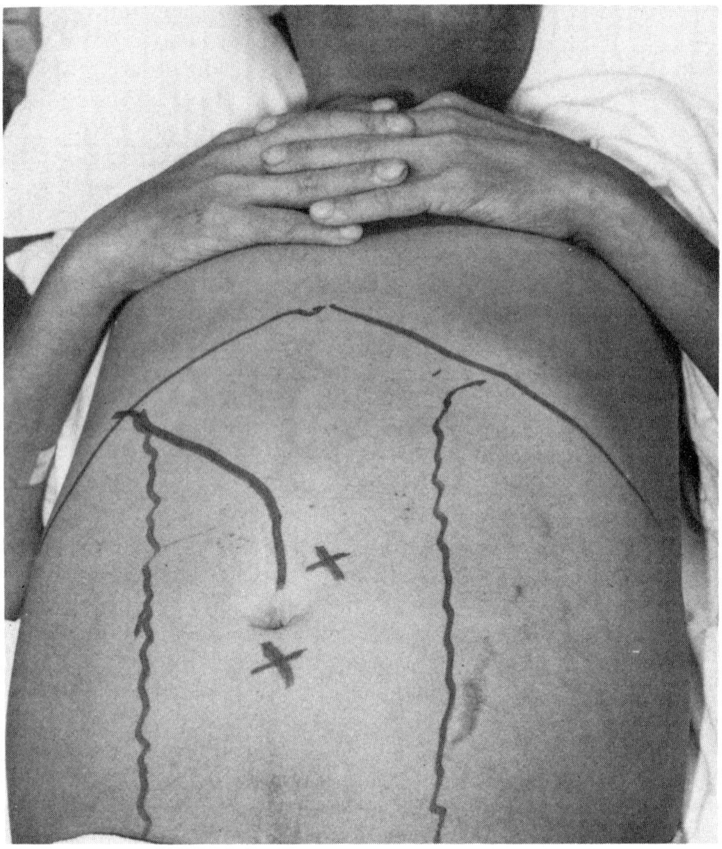

Figure 25.2. Potential entry sites (×) on the abdomen for the air needle and the peritoneoscope. The costal margins and the falciform ligament, represented by the curved line, are outlined in ink. The wavy lines indicate the outer borders of the rectus muscles where the epigastric vessels are located.

abdomen is scaphoid it helps to ask the patient to push the umbilicus forward toward the ceiling during insertion of the needle. When the needle tip is in the peritoneal cavity it should move freely and, unless the abdominal wall is thick, it should lie flat (Figure 25.3). Air or carbon dioxide gas is then introduced with a sphygmomanometer bulb or with an automatic insufflation device. If the air or gas does not enter the abdomen with ease, then the needle point may still be located in the tissues of the abdominal wall. If there is any doubt about this one should listen for escaping gas when the needle hub is open. If there is no return of gas after 100 to 200 ml have been insufflated, then the needle should be removed and another attempt made to enter the peritoneal cavity. In theory, carbon dioxide gas is safer than air since deaths have occurred during peritoneoscopy from air embolism due to pumping air into the liver or into a dilated collateral vein.[8,30] However, carbon dioxide is somewhat irritating to the peritoneum, is more expensive and may cause hypercarbia and arrhythmia under certain circumstances.[1,10,21,26]

After insufflation of enough air or carbon dioxide to distend the abdomen moderately, the needle is removed (or left in place if a different site is used for peritoneoscope insertion). With air in the abdomen it is easier to ensure anaesthesia of the parietal peritoneum if there is doubt that this was satisfactorily achieved initially. Next, the peritoneoscopy trocar is pushed through the abdominal wall. This requires considerable pressure and it is essential to control the instrument with one hand while pushing with the other in order to avoid moving suddenly several centimetres into the abdominal cavity when the resistance from the abdominal wall is overcome. Better control is achieved when the arms are near full extension and the table is low (Figure 25.4). After penetrating the abdominal wall the trocar is removed immediately. The trocar sheath should then move easily into the peritoneal cavity with little resistance. If resistance is more than minimal, it is possible that the end of the sheath is still in the abdominal wall with only the tip of the trocar having pierced the peritoneum. If the sheath is freely movable the peritoneoscopic telescope is

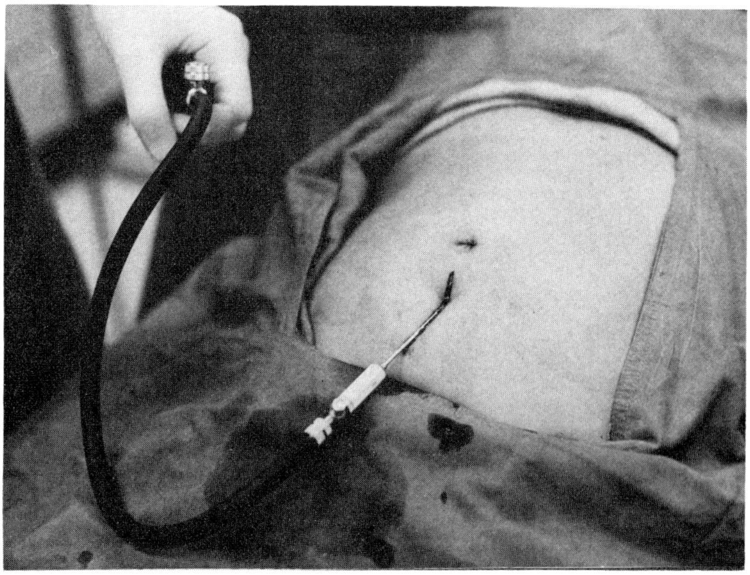

Figure 25.3. When the air needle has penetrated the peritoneum it should lie flat, as pictured, unless the abdominal wall is unusually thick.

next introduced under direct vision with the room darkened. Air or gas is pumped in through the instrument as needed to maintain a satisfactory pneumoperitoneum. The easiest landmark to look for initially is the falciform ligament. Touching the parietal peritoneum, including that over the falciform ligament, causes pain whereas touching the bowel, omentum or liver does not. After initial inspection of the peritoneal cavity visualization can be increased by tilting the table in different directions. Occasionally it is helpful to insert a blunt probe through a second entry site to lift the lower edge of the liver or to move omentum away from a suspected mass. We routinely look at as much of the liver surface as possible, the fundus of the gallbladder, the falciform ligament, the parietal peritoneum and the anterior surface of the stomach and bowel. We attempt to see the spleen when the table is tilted to the right and we scan the pelvis in females. We describe the liver surface as objectively as possible and ordinarily take a colour photograph for a permanent record. If a liver biopsy is indicated it can be performed through the operating channel of the peritoneoscope or through a separate puncture site near the area to be biopsied.

If there is much ascites, it must be aspirated to allow visualization since the fluid prevents adequate light transmission. Most peritoneoscopes have blunt-ended aspiration trocars for removal of ascitic fluid by gentle suction or by siphon drainage. When there is only a small amount of ascites, it is usually possible to see the liver satisfactorily without removing the fluid providing the head of the table is elevated.

At the end of the procedure the peritoneoscope is withdrawn and the air is allowed to escape through the trocar sheath before the latter is finally removed. The wound is closed superficially with interrupted silk sutures. In patients with ascites an attempt should be made to suture the rent in the peritoneum, being careful not to injure the intestine.

Vital signs are recorded immediately before and after the procedure and for two or three hours postoperatively. Though we have not done this, it would be ideal to monitor the patient's vital signs during the peritoneoscopy or, at least, to observe cardiac rhythm on a monitor.

COMPLICATIONS

Peritoneoscopy has a relatively low risk for an invasive procedure. Vilardell, Seres and Marti-Vicente[28] reported a complication rate of 1.2 per cent in 1455 examinations. Bruehl[3] reviewed 63 845 peritoneoscopies performed by 67 physicians and found the complication rate to be 2.5 per cent with a mortality rate of 0.029 per cent. About three-quarters of the procedures included liver biopsy. Similar low rates of serious complications on review of smaller series were reported by Walker, Cooke and Playfair[29] and Handley and Nurick.[7] O'Kieffe and Boyce[22]

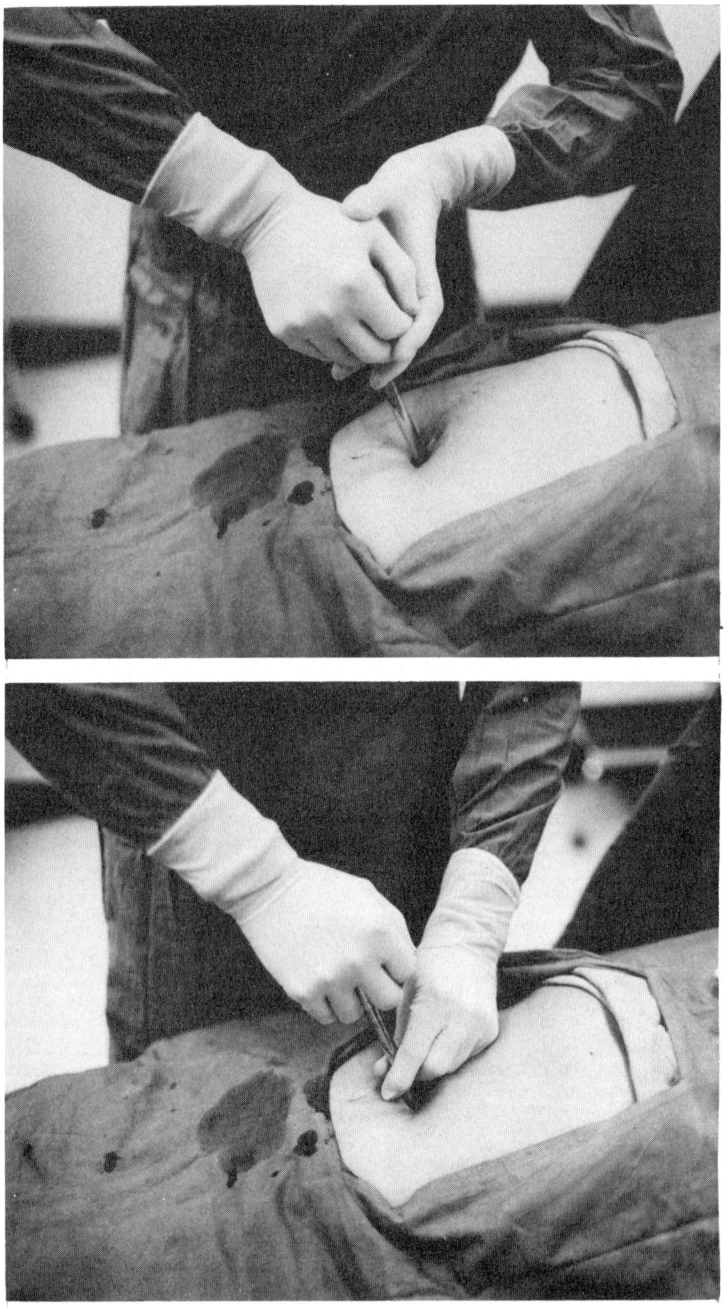

(a)
(b)

Figure 25.4. (a) Insertion of the trocar, with force, in this manner, provides potential for injury of abdominal viscera because of poor control over the depth of insertion. (b) By holding the trocar with one hand while pushing with the other, with the table low and the arms extended, the operator has better control over the depth of insertion.

had an overall incidence of complications of 6 per cent, most of them minor.

Potential major complications are (a) injection of air into the liver or an abdominal vein causing air embolism, (b) bleeding into the abdominal cavity from the puncture site in the abdominal wall, (c) bowel perforation (when the bowel is adherent to the anterior abdominal wall), (d) puncture of an ovarian cyst mistaken for ascites, (e) serious bleeding from a liver biopsy, (f) tearing an adhesion containing a large blood vessel and (g) injury to abdominal viscera (other than bowel adherent to the abdomen) from the insufflation needle or peritoneoscopic trocar. Many different minor complications have been reported, including subcutaneous emphysema, omental emphysema, leakage of ascites from the wound, leakage of ascites into the anterior abdominal wall and genitalia, and vagal reaction with hypotension and bradycardia.

PERSONAL EXPERIENCE

In 25 years we have had eight major complications in approximately 2000 procedures (0.4 per cent), including all of the possibilities mentioned above except the last two. There were four fatalities: one patient died suddenly, presumably from air embolism; one died four hours after the procedure from initially unrecognized abdominal wall bleeding; two patients with hepatocellular carcinoma and advanced liver disease bled persistently from the liver biopsy site and expired two and three days post-peritoneoscopy. Non-fatal major complications were bowel perforation in two patients with tuberculous peritonitis and ovarian cyst perforation in two patients. We have not seen wound infection, peritonitis or hernia formation following peritoneoscopy.

We have reviewed the last 300 consecutive peritoneoscopic examinations performed in our unit during the last three and a half years to examine the indications, completeness, accuracy and safety of this procedure in our hands. Most of the peritoneoscopies were done by resident staff or hepatology fellows under the supervision of one of the authors.

Indications for the procedure in these 300 cases are listed in Table 25.1. This shows that the most common indication was assessment of the type and severity of liver disease, achieved mainly by observation of the surface, leading edge and colour of the liver. Experience with this procedure has enabled us to recognize reliably the appearance of the liver surface with different types of liver disease. This is especially so with alcoholic liver disease which forms a major part of our practice. In some patients the indications were multiple; for example, the assessment of alcoholic liver disease and the search for hepatocellular carcinoma suggested by a filling defect on liver scan or the presence of alpha-fetoprotein in the serum. Seventy-seven examinations were performed for suspected primary or secondary hepatic malignancy, including 34 in whom malignancy was suggested by filling defects on liver scan. In 30 (39 per cent) of these examinations hepatic malignancy was seen with certainty at peritoneoscopy and these included five of the 34 in whom malignancy had been suggested only by liver scan. In another 10 patients hepatic malignancy was detected only by histological examination of liver biopsy tissue taken at peritoneoscopy.

Table 25.1. *Indications for Peritoneoscopy in 300 Consecutive Examinations.*[a]

Indications		No. of cases
Assessment of type and severity of liver disease		145
Suspected hepatic malignancy		77
Hepatocellular carcinoma	49	
Hepatic metastases	28	
Investigation of ascites		43
High protein ascites	20	
Suspected tuberculous peritonitis		15
Suspected peritoneal malignancy		5
TB peritonitis vs peritoneal malignancy		2
Miscellaneous		29

[a] The total number of cases exceeds 300 since in some patients there were multiple indications.

In 43 patients the indication was ascites of uncertain aetiology; 20 had ascites with a high protein content (>30 g/l). In 27 (63 per cent) of these 43 examinations liver disease was the only abnormality found while non-hepatic disease was discovered or confirmed in another eight (19 per cent). In two of the remaining eight cases adenocarcinoma cells were seen in the ascitic fluid, although no evidence of malignancy was seen at peritoneoscopy, and in another patient the clinical diagnosis of ascites was not confirmed at peritoneoscopy.

Miscellaneous indications for peritoneoscopy included undiagnosed jaundice, hepatomegaly of uncertain cause, the evaluation of abdominal masses and, in three patients with liver disease, the examination of pelvic masses.

In 267 patients (89 per cent) complete examination of the abdominal cavity was possible. The examination was incomplete in 25 (8 per cent) because adhesions obscured a part of the abdominal cavity, usually the whole or part of the liver. In eight patients (3 per cent) the procedure was a total failure in that the abdominal cavity was not entered. The gallbladder was seen in 196 examinations (67 per cent) of the remaining 292 patients examined but was not seen in 73 (25 per cent), despite full examination of the right upper quadrant, because of ascites or a large right hepatic lobe. In another 10 patients (3.5 per cent) visualization of the gallbladder was obscured by adhesions in the right upper quadrant. One patient had undergone a cholecystectomy while

Table 25.2. *Assessment of Accuracy of Peritoneoscopic Diagnosis by Histological Confirmation in 165 Patients.*

Peritoneoscopic diagnosis	No. of cases confirmed	No. of cases not confirmed
Alcoholic liver disease	66	6
Non-alcoholic chronic liver disease ± cirrhosis (CAH, cryptogenic cirrhosis)	23	6
Hepatocellular neoplasia (carcinoma, adenoma)	11	5
Hepatic metastases	20	2
Submassive hepatic necrosis with collapse	4	1
Tuberculous peritonitis	2	2
Peritoneal malignancy	4	1
Others	8	4
Total	138 (84%)	27 (16%)

in 12 the gallbladder was not mentioned in the peritoneoscopic report. The spleen was seen in only 50 examinations (17 per cent) whereas it was not visible in 205 cases (70 per cent) despite suitable positioning of the patient. Two patients had undergone splenectomy.

Portal hypertension, diagnosed by the presence of portal collateral circulation, was noted in 134 patients (46 per cent), 120 of whom had ascites before or at the time of the procedure. In 20 cases (7 per cent) there was no comment on the presence of increased vascularity but in the remainder (138) portal hypertension was not diagnosed at peritoneoscopy.

Liver biopsy was performed during only two of the first 65 examinations reviewed and both were by the percutaneous route. This low biopsy rate was due to the lack at that time of a peritoneoscope with an operating channel and it was felt that percutaneous biopsies were best performed as a separate procedure. Since then an instrument with a biopsy channel has been available and also percutaneous biopsies under direct vision have been performed with greater frequency. Thus the liver was biopsied during 108 (46 per cent) of the remaining 235 examinations and the amount of tissue obtained was sufficient to permit a histological diagnosis in 98 (91 per cent). In six patients nodules on the peritoneum were biopsied for suspected tuberculous peritonitis or malignant seeding.

The accuracy of peritoneoscopy as a diagnostic procedure has been assessed by comparing the examination findings with the histological diagnosis. This was possible in 164 (55 per cent) of the 300 examinations reviewed and Table 25.2 shows that a high level of accuracy was achieved in recognizing the various macroscopic appearances of alcoholic liver disease, non-alcoholic chronic liver disease and hepatic metastases. The two cases of incorrectly diagnosed tuberculous peritonitis turned out to have malignant nodules on the peritoneum, whereas the one incorrectly diagnosed peritoneal malignancy had tuberculous peritonitis.

The value of the procedure has been assessed by comparing the clinical diagnosis (based on historical information, laboratory data and physical findings) with the peritoneoscopy findings, together with histological information when available (Table 25.3). The total number of confirmed and unconfirmed clinical diagnoses exceeds 300 since some cases had two possible diagnoses before peritoneoscopy and usually only one was correct. In addition to the clinical diagnoses listed in this table, 20 patients with transudative ascites of unknown cause and nine with undiagnosed jaundice and hepatomegaly were examined.

A major concern with any diagnostic procedure is its safety. Table 25.4 lists the complications encountered and their frequency in the 235 patients in whom records could be readily obtained for review for postoperative problems. There were no serious complications though in two patients with cirrhosis the amount of bleeding from the biopsy site appeared alarming initially. Bleeding stopped spontaneously in both cases under direct vision and no blood replacement was required.

Table 25.3. *Assessment of the Value of Peritoneoscopy by Comparing Clinical Diagnosis with Peritoneoscopic Diagnosis (and Histological Findings when Available) in 300 Patients.*

Clinical diagnosis before peritoneoscopy	Total no.	No. confirmed	No. not confirmed
Alcoholic liver disease	148	131	17
Chronic active hepatitis ± cirrhosis	32	21	11
Chronic non-alcoholic liver disease (type unspecified)	23	16	7
Chronic liver disease + suspected hepatocellular carcinoma	49	13	36
Suspected hepatic metastases	28	17	11
Peritoneal malignancy	7	3	4
Tuberculous peritonitis	17	2	15
Miscellaneous	29	23	6
Total	333	226 (68%)	107 (32%)

Table 25.4. *Complications Occurring with 235 Peritoneoscopy Examinations.*

Complications	No. of patients
Incomplete entry into abdominal cavity	8
Bleeding from entry site	1
Subcutaneous emphysema	5
Vagal attack during procedure	2
Emesis during procedure	2
Ascites leak	11
Pain after procedure	15
Hypotension after procedure	2
Fever	3

Incomplete entry into the peritoneal cavity has been considered a complication since it caused the procedure to be abandoned but in none of these eight cases did any problem follow from the attempt. Leakage of ascites from the wound occurred in 11 patients but ceased quickly with treatment of the ascites and did not interfere with wound healing. Subcutaneous emphysema, usually of the abdominal wall but of the mediastinum as well in one case, spontaneously cleared in a few days and caused no more than aesthetic distress. Pain, usually diffusely abdominal and frequently accompanied by bilateral shoulder tip pain, occurred in 15 patients within the first 24 hours of the procedure but never constituted a worrying problem. The shoulder pain is thought to be due to diaphragmatic irritation from retained air. In three patients there was a transient fever, which did not require treatment, within 24 hours of the procedure. The overall incidence of minor complications was 21 per cent (49 in 235 examinations). This is reduced to 10 per cent (24 in 235) if the eight cases of incomplete entry are excluded, as well as those complications that can occur with any surgical procedure, that is postoperative pain and hypotension in the early postoperative period.

REFERENCES

1. Baratz, R.A. & Karis, J.H. (1969) Blood gas studies during laparoscopy under general anesthesia. *Anesthesiology*, **30**, 463–464.
2. Boyce, H.W. Jr (1975) Laparoscopy. In *Diseases of the Liver* (Ed.) Schiff, L. pp. 272–286. Philadelphia: J.B. Lippincott.
3. Bruehl, W. (1966) Zwischenfälle und Komplikationen bei der Laparoskopie und gezielten Leberpunktion. *Deutsche Medizinische Wochenschrift*, **91**, 2297–2299.
4. Caroli, J. & Ricordeau, P. (1962) Value of peritoneoscopy and peritoneoscopic photography in color and of scintillography in the diagnosis of liver diseases. *Progress in Liver Disease*, **1**, 296–389.
5. *Dorland's Illustrated Medical Dictionary* (1974) Philadelphia: W.B. Saunders.
6. Gaisford, W.D. (1975) Peritoneoscopy: a valuable technic for surgeons. *American Journal of Surgery*, **130**, 671–678.
7. Handley, R.S. & Nurick, A.W. (1956) Peritoneoscopy: evaluation and report of 136 cases. *British Medical Journal*, **ii**, 1211–1214.
8. Hartlieb, J. (1955) Luftembolie bei der Laparoskopie. *Deutsche Medizinische Wochenschrift*, **80**, 1532–1533.
9. Hirschowitz, B.I. (1961) Endoscopic examination of the stomach and duodenal cap with the fiberscope. *Lancet*, **i**, 1074–1078.
10. Hodgson, C., McClelland, R.M.A. & Newton, J.R. (1970) Some effects of the peritoneal insufflation of carbon dioxide at laparoscopy. *Anaesthesia*, **25**, 382–390.
11. Jacobaeus, H.C. (1910) Über die Möglichkeit, die Zystoskopie bei Untersuchungen seröser Höhlungen anzuwenden. *Münchener Medizinische Wochenschrift*, **57**, 2090–2092.
12. Jacobaeus, H.C. (1912) Über Laparo- und Thorakoskopie. *Beiträge zur Klinik der Tuberkulose und spezifischen Tuberkuloseforschung*, **25**, 183–254.
13. Jori, G.P. & Peschle, C. (1972) Combined peritoneoscopy and liver biopsy in the diagnosis of hepatic neoplasm. *Gastroenterology*, **63**, 1016–1019.
14. Kalk, H. (1929) Erfahrungen mit der Laparoskopie (zugleich mit Beischreibung eines neuen Instrumentes). *Zeitschrift für Klinische Medizin*, **111**, 303–348.
15. Kalk, H. (1955) Indikationsstellung und Gefahrenmoment bei der Laparoskopie. *Deutsche Medizinische Wochenschrift*, **61**, 1831–1833.
16. Kelling, G. (1902) Über Oesophagoscopie, Gastroskopie, und Cölioskopie. *Münchener Medizinische Wochenschrift*, **49**, 21–24.
17. Kelling, G. (1910) Über die Möglichkeit, die Zystoskopie bei Untersuchungen seröser Höhlungen anzuwenden. Bemerkung zu dem Artikel von Jacobaeus. *Münchener Medizinische Wochenschrift*, **57**, 2358.
18. Korbsch, R. (1921) Die Laparoskopie nach Jacobaeus. *Berliner Klinische Wochenschrift*, **58**, 696.
19. Meyer-Burg, J. (1972) The inspection, palpation and biopsy of the pancreas by peritoneoscopy. *Endoscopy*, **4**, 99–101.
20. Michel, H. & Raynaud, A. (1977) Intérêt de la laparoscopie sous anesthésie générale. *Endoscopie Digestive*, **2**, 135–136.
21. Motew, M., Ivanovich, A.D., Bieniarz, J., Albrecht, R.F., Zahed, B., Scommegna, A. & Silverman, B. (1973) Cardiovascular effects and acid-base and blood gas changes during laparoscopy. *American Journal of Obstetrics and Gynecology*, **115**, 1002–1012.
22. O'Kieffe, D.A. & Boyce, H.W. Jr (1972) Peritoneoscopy: has this procedure come of age? *Medical Annals of the District of Columbia*, **41**, 437–440.
23. Royer, M. & Solari, A.V. (1947) Cholangiography performed with the help of peritoneoscopy. *Gastroenterology*, **8**, 586–591.
24. Ruddock, J.C. (1934) Peritoneoscopy. *Western Journal of Surgery*, **42**, 392–405.

25. Ruddock, J.C. (1937) Peritoneoscopy. *Surgery, Gynecology and Obstetrics*, **65,** 623–639.
26. Scott, D.B. & Julian, D.G. (1972) Observations on cardiac arrhythmias during laparoscopy. *British Medical Journal*, **i,** 411–413.
27. Veronisi, U., Spinelli, P., Bonadonna, G., Gennari, L., Bajetta, E., Beretta, G. & Tancini, G. (1976) Laparoscopy and laparotomy in staging Hodgkin's and non-Hodgkin's lymphoma. *American Journal of Roentgenology*, **127,** 501–503.
28. Vilardell, F., Seres, I. & Marti-Vicente, A. (1968) Complications of peritoneoscopy. A survey of 1455 examinations. *Gastrointestinal Endoscopy*, **14,** 178–180.
29. Walker, R.M., Cooke, A.M. & Playfair, P.L. (1943) Peritoneoscopy. *Proceedings of the Royal Society of Medicine*, **36,** 445–450.
30. Wittman, I. (1966) *Peritoneoscopy*. Vols. I and II. Budapest: Akdemiai Kiado.
31. Yamamoto, S. & Reynolds, T. B. (1964) Portal venography and pressure measurement at peritoneoscopy. *Gastroenterology*, **47,** 602–603.

Chapter 26

Investigation of the Jaundiced Patient

STEPHEN KARRAN
K.C. DEWBURY
A.E.A. JOSEPH
RALPH WRIGHT

The main problems of diagnosis in the jaundiced patient are:

1. To distinguish between intra- and extrahepatic cholestasis.
2. To identify the site of extrahepatic obstruction.
3. To recognize unusual causes of hepatocellular or haemolytic jaundice which require special management or treatment.
4. To distinguish between acute and chronic hepatocellular disease.

A careful and thorough history and physical examination remain of overriding importance in establishing the diagnosis.

Nevertheless, there have been important technical advances over the past few years which have had a profound effect on the rapidity and accuracy of diagnosis in the jaundiced patient. These include serological tests for hepatitis A and B and autoimmune liver disease, together with radiological and scanning techniques which not only help to distinguish intrahepatic from extrahepatic cholestasis but which also localize accurately the site of extrahepatic obstruction. There have, in addition, been useful advances in techniques for histological staining of liver biopsy material to identify viral markers and to diagnose certain forms of chronic liver disease such as Wilson's disease, primary biliary cirrhosis and alpha-1-antitrypsin deficiency.

By contrast, while biochemical tests of liver function may indicate the severity of hepatic damage they remain disappointing in distinguishing between intra- and extrahepatic cholestasis. Furthermore, certain investigations, such as the standard barium meal, which until relatively recently have been regarded as first-line investigations in the jaundiced patient, are now seldom performed.

The identification of haemolysis as the cause of jaundice is usually not difficult on clinical examination and when simple laboratory investigations are used. The precise cause of the haemolysis may be more difficult to elucidate.

In addition, the extent to which haemolysis contributes to the jaundice may be problematical when it coexists with hepatocellular disease or extrahepatic obstruction. The extent to which breakdown of old red cells from transfused blood contributes to jaundice, particularly in the postoperative period, may also be difficult to determine. When jaundice is mild, and not associated with other symptoms, low grade haemolysis must be distinguished from Gilbert's syndrome, the commonest form of persistent unconjugated hyperbilirubinaemia. In the neonatal period haemolytic disease of the newborn has to be distinguished from physiological jaundice, biliary atresia and neonatal hepatitis.

In the absence of features of cholestasis, the diagnosis of hepatocellular jaundice is seldom a problem, although it may be more difficult to identify its cause. The availability of serological markers for viral hepatitis A and B, EB virus, cytomegalovirus and leptospiral infection have greatly facilitated precise diagnosis (see Chapter 28). The diagnosis of drug-induced jaundice is based largely on the clinical history with limited help from liver biopsy. The identification of chronic liver disease as a cause of jaundice is usually straightforward once the appropriate clinical, biochemical and other investigations have been undertaken (see Chapters 29 and 30). More difficulty may be encountered if the hepatocellular jaundice is part of an unusual systemic disease (see Chapter 37) or due to a tumour (see Chapters 38 and 39), an infection (see Chapter 51) or a parasite (see Chapter 56). Such cases are less likely to be diagnosed if the disorder is unusual in the particular patient's environment.

The identification of extrahepatic obstruction due to gallstones, tumour or stricture is usually straightforward, but diagnostic difficulty may occur when the extrahepatic obstruction results from conditions such as sclerosing cholangitis, intrahepatic bile duct carcinoma (see Chapters 14, 37, 38, 54 and 55) or parasites (see Chapter 56), or when more than one pathology coexist.

Precise diagnosis is particularly difficult when the situation is complex, for example in the postoperative period (see Chapter 47), in the neonate (see Chapters 40 and 41) and when there has been previous biliary tract surgery (see Chapter 54).

It should be emphasized, however, that, in any jaundiced patient in whom the diagnosis is difficult, an unusual presentation of a common cause of jaundice such as hepatitis, drugs, gallstones or tumour is still more likely to be found than a rare condition.

In the majority of patients with jaundice, a careful history and clinical examination, together with simple laboratory tests, will either provide the definitive diagnosis or a guide to the underlying pathology. If more elaborate investigations are required, these should be pursued rapidly so that any necessary operative intervention may be undertaken without delay. A hard core of difficult problems remains requiring extensive investigation. With careful organization in most cases, it should be possible to achieve a definitive diagnosis within three to four days. It is therefore essential to have a well-established plan of investigation. One such simplified scheme is illustrated in Figure 26.1 (see also Chapters 14 and 50). Diagnostic laparotomy should no longer be necessary in specialist centres.

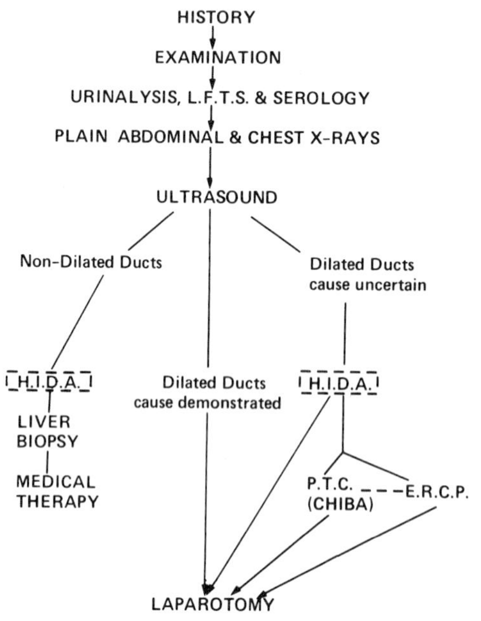

Figure 26.1. Proposed schema for the investigation of the jaundiced patient.

HISTORY

The important points to establish about the jaundice from the history are:

1. Is it cholestatic?
2. Is it painful and, if so, what is the character of the pain?
3. Is it drug-induced or infective?

A patient with cholestatic jaundice will typically have dark urine, pale stools and pruritus. In some patients none of these features may be present, yet either intrahepatic cholestasis may be demonstrated histologically, or an obvious cause of extrahepatic obstruction such as a tumour or a stone may be identified with or without biochemical changes of cholestasis. If the history suggests cholestasis, it is particularly important to determine whether the patient has been taking drugs. Analgesics, tranquillizers, psychotropic drugs and the contraceptive pill are so commonly used that the patient may not regard these as significant. In the very young and in the elderly it is important to obtain a history from the relatives and the general practitioner about the drug intake.

A history of contact with hepatitis, of travel abroad, of eating raw shell fish or of having used parenteral drugs may suggest viral hepatitis. Such patients often have anorexia, distaste for cigarettes, lassitude, joint pains and urticaria but many of these symptoms, particularly distaste for cigarettes, occur with other forms of jaundice, including drug-induced and obstructive jaundice. Fluctuation of the depth of discolouration is suggestive of intermittent obstruction as a result of temporary retention of a calculus at the ampulla of Vater or, rarely, a carcinoma at this site, but it can also occur with intrahepatic cholestasis and, when mild, with Gilbert's syndrome.

Pruritus is an important symptom and, although usually steadily progressive, may fluctuate in both intrahepatic and extrahepatic cholestasis.

A history of biliary 'colic', shoulder tip pain or attacks of acute cholecystitis is strong evidence that the obstructive jaundice is due to calculous disease, although calculi may coexist with neoplastic obstructive lesions or with cirrhosis. Pain of a different nature may indicate more sinister pathology. Pain in the back, for example, is suspicious of pancreatic neoplasm, although penetrating duodenal ulceration may also be responsible. Acute pain referred to the back is suggestive of pancreatitis or gallstones but can also occur with the crises due to rapid haemolysis.

Painless jaundice associated with weight loss is strongly suggestive of neoplasm, particularly of the head of the pancreas.

Bruising may be prominent with decompensated hepatocellular jaundice due to hypoprothrombinaemia or to the low platelet count associated with hypersplenism, but it can also occur in obstructive jaundice as a result of malabsorption of vitamin K.

It is important to obtain a history of foreign travel, not only because such patients are liable to develop viral hepatitis, but they may also be exposed to unusual diseases such as malaria and other parasitic infections which can cause hepatocellular or obstructive jaundice. Even in patients who have not been abroad the diagnosis may be missed because a parasitic infection such as *Fasciola hepatica*, a rare cause of jaundice in the United Kingdom,[3] has not been considered.

An occupational history is also important because this may indicate exposure to a particular infection or to hepatotoxins while a social and occupational history may suggest alcohol or drug abuse. Some forms of jaundice, such as Wilson's disease and Gilbert's syndrome, are familial. In cholelithiasis there is also sometimes a strong family history. A history of putative autoimmune disease in the patient or family suggests chronic active hepatitis or primary biliary cirrhosis.

PHYSICAL EXAMINATION

A careful examination may provide evidence of the severity of the underlying pathology and its aetiology. Hepatocellular dysfunction may be clearly shown by the presence of cutaneous stigmata such as spider naevi, palmar erythema, Dupuytren's contracture. leuconychia and finger clubbing. Dilated cutaneous collateral veins and a palpable spleen may indicate portal hypertension. Ascites can occur in decompensated cirrhosis but also with disseminated neoplasms. The aetiology may be indicated by its systemic manifestations or by a specific feature. Thus, in alcoholic liver disease there may be other signs of alcoholism such as peripheral neuropathy and in drug hypersensitivity reactions there may be other evidence of hypersensitivity such as a skin rash. Kayser–Fleischer rings suggest Wilson's disease and xanthomas and xanthelasmas are associated with primary biliary cirrhosis. Tattoo marks or scarred antecubital veins may provide the clue to hepatitis B infection.

In the assessment of hepatic size, careful palpation and percussion should start in the iliac fossa. If this procedure is not scrupulously followed, the lower edge of a grossly enlarged organ may be missed, particularly in the obese. The upper border of the liver is defined by percussion, and dullness over the liver normally extends upwards as far as the fifth intercostal space. Careful assessment of the consistency of the liver is likewise important. Hard irregular areas, for example, strongly suggest neoplastic involvement. A bruit favours portal hypertension or a neoplasm. Splenomegaly can be detected by palpation commencing in the right iliac fossa and progressing upwards and to the left. In difficult cases, rotation of the patient 45° to the right allows the spleen to fall on the clinician's right hand. The left hand should support the rib cage and relax the skin and abdominal musculature by drawing these down and to the right. Percussion may be useful and, in the presence of ascites, the spleen may be ballottable.

The finding of a palpable gallbladder in the presence of obstructive jaundice suggests malignant obstruction to the biliary tree (Courvoisier's law). This obstruction must obviously be below the junction of the cystic and common hepatic ducts, and carcinoma of the head of the pancreas and ampullary lesions are common causes. It is essential, however, to appreciate that the presence of a palpable gallbladder under these circumstances does *not* exclude calculous disease as the cause of the jaundice. Similarly, failure to palpate the gallbladder does not exclude malignancy either because the biliary tree is involved above the entrance of the cystic duct or the gallbladder itself may be infiltrated, preventing dilatation. A palpable gallbladder simply implies raised intravesical pressure which in most cases is due to neoplastic obstruction of the lower ductal system (see Chapter 53).

LABORATORY INVESTIGATIONS

The haematological, biochemical and serological investigations which may be necessary in the diagnosis of the jaundiced patient are listed in Table 26.1 and have been dealt with in detail in Chapters 8, 13, 14 and 17. Unconjugated hyperbilirubinaemia suggests haemolysis or Gilbert's syndrome or one of the rarer causes such as the Crigler–Najjar syndrome. Haemolysis may be associated with anaemia, spherocytosis, reticulocytosis, reduced red cell survival and a positive Coomb's test. In Gilbert's syndrome, the bilirubin is less than 103 μmol/l (6 mg/dl) and usually of the order of 50 μmol/l (3 mg/dl) and the plasma unconjugated bilirubin concentration shows a two- to threefold increase after fasting or the intravenous administration of 50 mg of nicotinic acid (see Chapter 13).

Standard liver function tests serve only as a general guide in helping to distinguish hepatocellular from obstructive jaundice and are discussed in Chapters 14 and 17. Marked elevation of the aspartate aminotransferase (AST) suggests hepatocellular necrosis, and alkaline phosphatase levels above 30 King Armstrong units extrahepatic obstruction, but the latter can also occur with intrahepatic

Table 26.1. *Laboratory Investigations in the Jaundiced Patient.*

Haematological tests:
 Full blood count; erythrocyte sedimentation rate; reticulocyte count; haptoglobin levels; Coombs' test

Liver function tests:
 Conjugated and unconjugated bilirubin levels; aspartate aminotransferase (AST); alanine aminotransferase (ALT); γ-glutamyl transferase; alkaline phosphatase; bromsulphthalein excretion

Proteins:
 Albumin; globulin; prothrombin time

Immunological and serological tests:
 Mitochondrial antibodies
 Smooth muscle and antinuclear antibody
 Immunoglobulins: IgG, IgM, IgA
 Hepatitis B surface antigen (HB_sAg)
 Cytomegalovirus antibody
 EB virus antibody (monospot)
 Leptospiral agglutinins
 Fasciola complement fixation test
 Amoebic complement fixation test
 Hydatid complement fixation test
 Wassermann reaction and other serological tests for syphilis

Alpha-1-antitrypsin levels

Alpha-fetoprotein levels

Serum amylase

Plasma caeruloplasmin levels

Iron and iron binding capacity

Spot blood alcohol

Urine: urobilin, bilirubin, haemosiderin

Stools: ova and parasites

cholestasis and primary biliary cirrhosis. Low albumin and high globulin levels suggest chronic hepatocellular damage, particularly in association with a prolonged prothrombin time which fails to convert with parenteral vitamin K. Hepatitis B markers suggest acute or chronic hepatitis B infection but markers for hepatitis A are not yet generally available. Strongly positive antinuclear or smooth muscle antibodies suggest chronic active hepatitis (see Chapter 29) and a positive mitochondrial antibody primary biliary cirrhosis (see Chapter 31). Low alpha-1-antitrypsin levels favour the chronic liver disease associated with this deficiency (see Chapter 35) and low caeruloplasmin levels favour Wilson's disease (see Chapter 33).

Clearly, the number and order in which these tests are performed depend on clinical pointers. Laboratory investigations in the jaundiced infant pose special problems and are discussed in Chapter 40 and 41.

RADIOLOGICAL INVESTIGATIONS

Plain abdominal and chest x-rays

Plain x-rays of the abdomen and chest are simple and quick to perform and may give valuable information. Calcification may be seen in 10 to 20 per cent of biliary calculi, occasionally in the gallbladder itself, in hepatic metastases (Figure 26.2) and also in chronic pancreatitis (Figure 26.3). Gas may be seen in the biliary tree, portal venous system or in a subphrenic abcess. On the chest film, a primary neoplasm, secondary deposits or pleural effusions may all be relevant.

Intravenous cholangiography

In this investigation an iodine containing contrast medium, iodipamide (Biligrafin) or ioglycamate (Biligram) is infused over a period

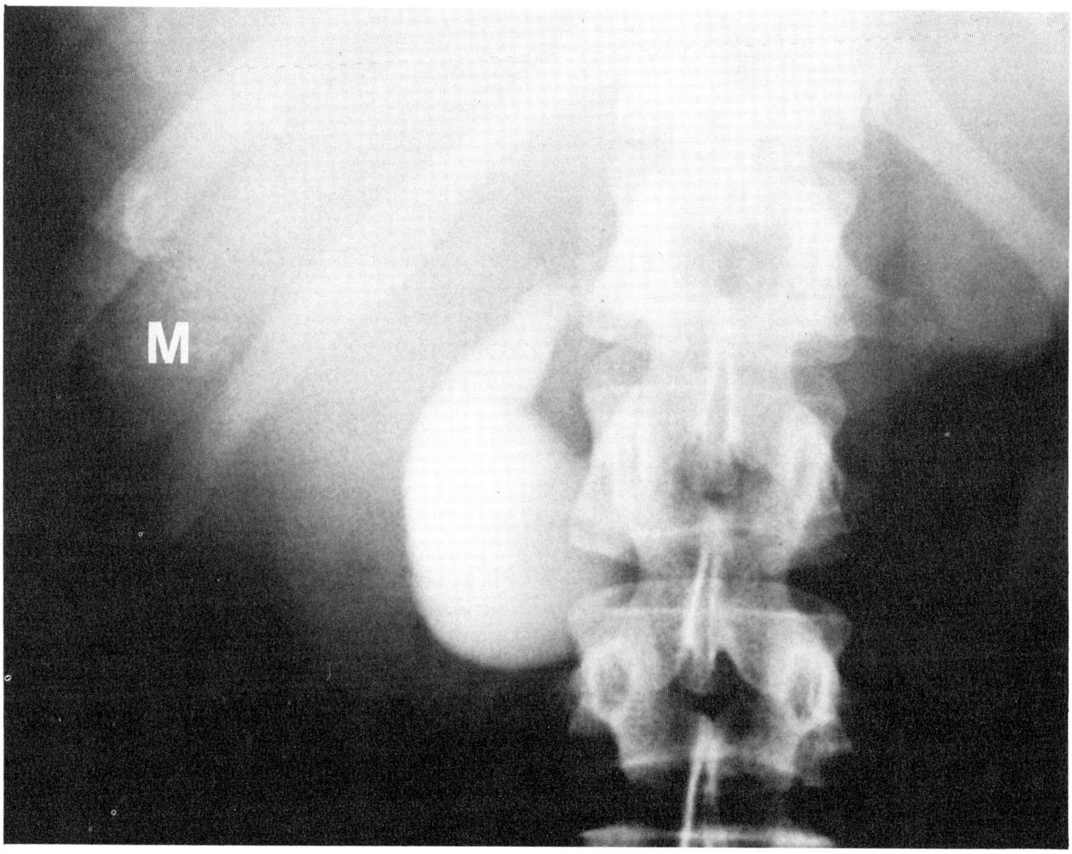

Figure 26.2. Cholecystogram showing calcification in metastases (M) arising from a 'silent' adenocarcinoma of the sigmoid colon in a 35-year-old woman presenting with vague pain in the right hypochondrium.

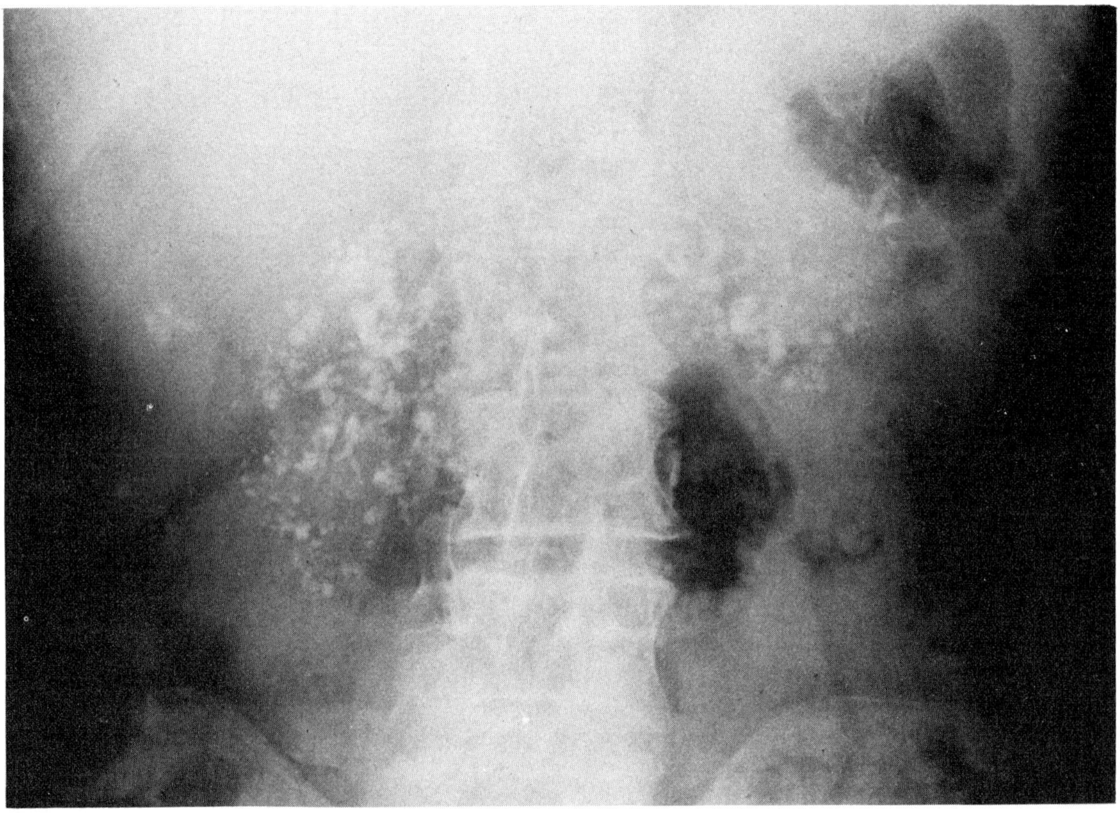

Figure 26.3. Diffuse calcification seen in a case of chronic pancreatitis.

of 30 minutes for optimal results. The contrast medium is bound to protein in the plasma and excreted by the liver cells. Bile ducts are outlined and these are optimally demonstrated by tomography. Gallbladder opacification will be demonstrated if the cystic duct is patent. The probability of duct opacification using intravenous cholangiography diminishes rapidly with bilirubin levels about 50 μmol/l (3 mg/dl).

Intravenous cholangiography plays a small part nowadays in the investigation of the jaundiced patient. Not only is it unsuccessful in the majority of jaundiced patients, but when successful the diagnostic yield is low.[1] Comparative studies have shown it to be less accurate than endoscopic retrograde choledochopancreatography (ERCP) in the diagnosis of patients undergoing surgery for biliary calculi[7] (see Chapter 23).

Ultrasound

This technique is becoming increasingly available and is rapidly establishing itself as an investigation of major importance in the diagnosis of the jaundiced patient (see Chapter 21). It is non-invasive, quick to perform and accurately separates extrahepatic obstruction from other causes of jaundice by the demonstration of dilated biliary radicles.[2,8] In experienced hands the accuracy in detecting ductal dilation is more than 95 per cent. Rarely, diagnostic errors may occur in early acute obstruction because the ducts have not yet become dilated. Ultrasonography is therefore particularly valuable as a screening procedure.

Patients may be separated into three main groups: those without dilated ducts, those with dilated ducts but in whom a definitive cause for the dilation is not shown, and those with dilated ducts in whom the cause of the obstruction is demonstrated (Figure 26.4). For patients in this latter group further investigation should be undertaken as suggested in Figure 26.1. In extrahepatic obstruction ultrasound imaging will establish the *level* of the block in approximately 80 per cent of cases.[2,6] In over 40 per cent of patients, not only the level but the cause of the obstruction will be demonstrated by ultrasound imaging.[2] Difficulties in achieving a definitive diagnosis arise principally with small lesions at the lower end of the common bile duct which is often obscured by gas in the duodenum

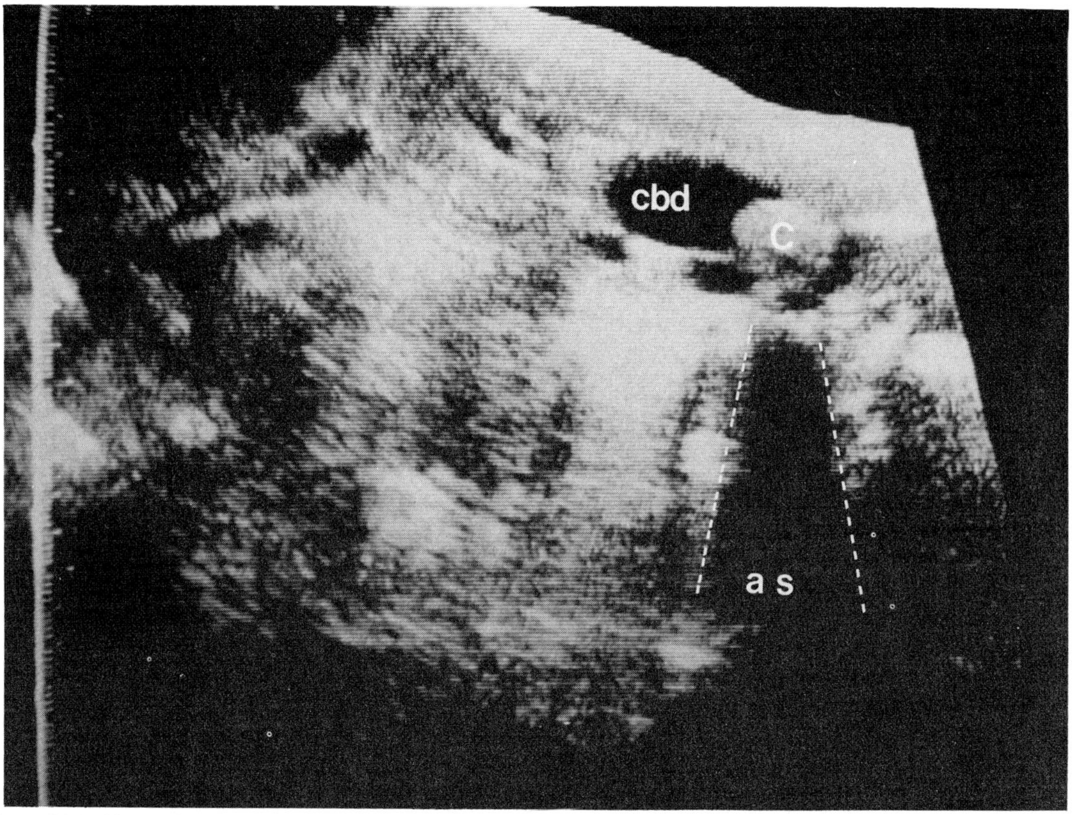

Figure 26.4. Obstructive jaundice produced by a calculus (C) obstructing the dilated common bile duct (cbd). Note the 'acoustic shadow' (as) cast by the stone.

and the colon or when more than one lesion coexists such as gallstones and a carcinoma of the gallbladder (Figure 26.5).

When no dilatation of the biliary radicles is demonstrated the liver may have a normal echo pattern and liver biopsy may be required, but in a significant proportion of patients a specific echo pattern is shown. This is most commonly either the bright, tightly packed echo pattern seen in many cases of cirrhosis or chronic active hepatitis, or, alternatively, the pattern characteristic of diffuse hepatic metastases (Figure 26.6). Further details of this technique are given in Chapter 21.

Radio-isotope imaging (see Chapter 20)

Technetium-99m sulphur colloid imaging is of limited value in the investigation of the jaundiced patient but may confirm the presence of hepatic metastases or suggest an obstructive aetiology with low activity seen in the porta hepatis. ^{131}I rose bengal imaging has also been shown to have prognostic value.

Recently introduced hepatobiliary agents, such as pyridoxylydine glutamate (PGA) and 2:6 dimethylphenylcarbamylmethyl iminodiacetic acid (HIDA) outline the biliary ducts and common bile duct even in the presence of moderately raised bilirubin levels (103 to 120 mmol/l [6 to 7 mg/dl]). With patency of the common bile duct activity is seen in the duct by 60 minutes. In the presence of total obstruction no activity is seen in the duct. In the presence of partial obstruction or jaundice of hepatocellular origin the appearance of activity in the gut is delayed. Ultrasound examination may prove helpful in distinguishing these two situations. The precise significance of delayed appearance of activity in the gut is uncertain. Poor hepatocellular function is associated with impaired excretion and a marked reduction in activity in the gut. This may be confused with partial obstruction. Although in biliary atresia no gut activity is present, there is no good evidence that HIDA studies yield unequivocally diagnostic results.

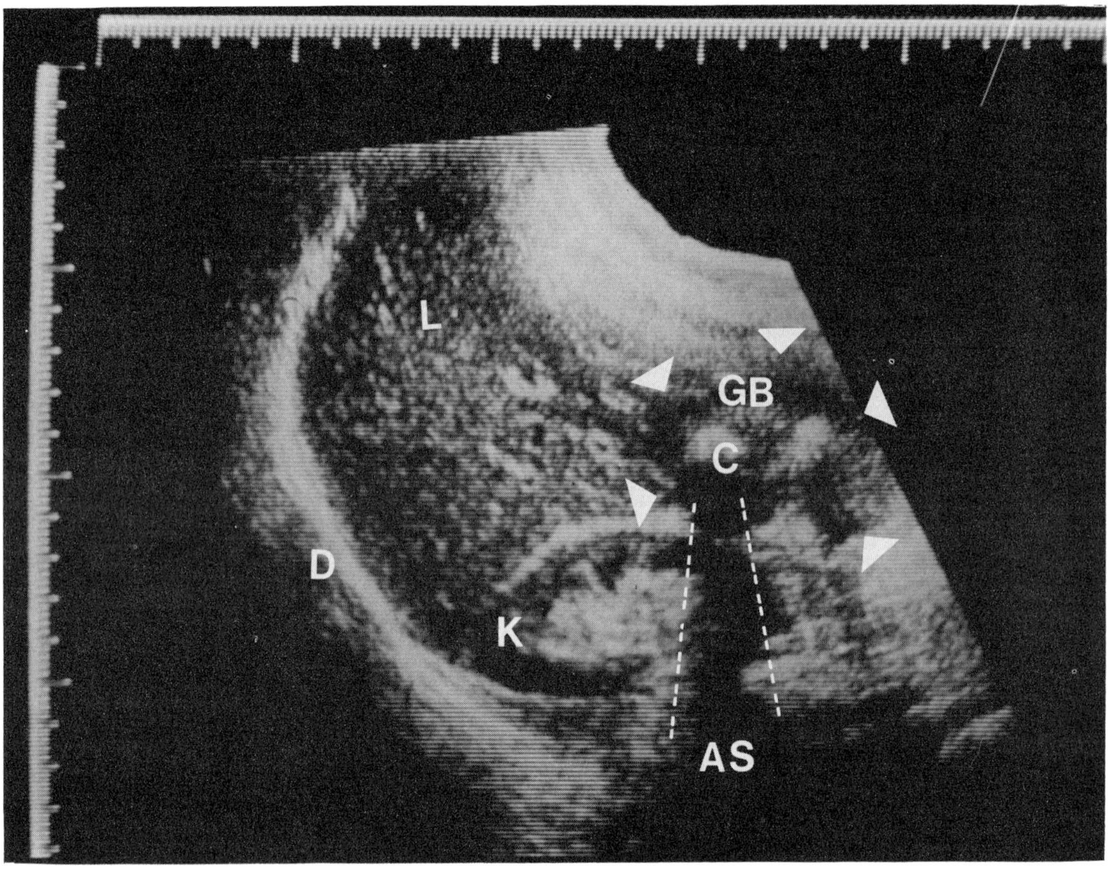

Figure 26.5. Longitudinal scan through right lobe of liver showing a thickened irregular gallbladder containing gallstones and with distal acoustic shadowing. The gallbladder was found to be a carcinoma – diaphragm (D), right kidney (K), liver (L), gallbladder (GB) – outline indicated by arrowheads – calculus (C) and acoustic shadow (AS).

Computerized axial tomographic imaging (CAT) (see Chapter 21)

This non-invasive investigation yields information similar to that obtained with ultrasound. It does not suffer technical failures due to gas in the bowel. At present, however, it remains an expensive investigation and is available only in larger hospitals. When available, it is probably best reserved for problems that cannot be resolved by more simple techniques such as ultrasound and isotope imaging.

Endoscopic retrograde choledochopancreatography (ERCP)

This investigation is described in Chapter 23. In the hands of experienced endoscopists, it is a valuable investigation, particularly in complex postoperative problems (see Chapter 54). Since the development of more accurate non-invasive techniques, particularly ultrasonography, its role is more often secondary and is reserved for those cases where inadequate information has been obtained from simpler investigations.

Percutaneous transhepatic cholangiography (PTC)

Percutaneous transhepatic cholangiography (PTC) with the fine calibre (23 gauge o.d. 0.7 mm) thin-walled Chiba needle is the preferred technique for direct opacification of the biliary duct in the jaundiced patient (Figure 26.7a and b). It is safer and more successful than conventional transhepatic cholangiography.

A lateral approach is used with injection of contrast during withdrawal of the needle. The procedure is carried out under fluoroscopic control to identify entry into a bile duct. Aspiration of bile, though desirable, may not be

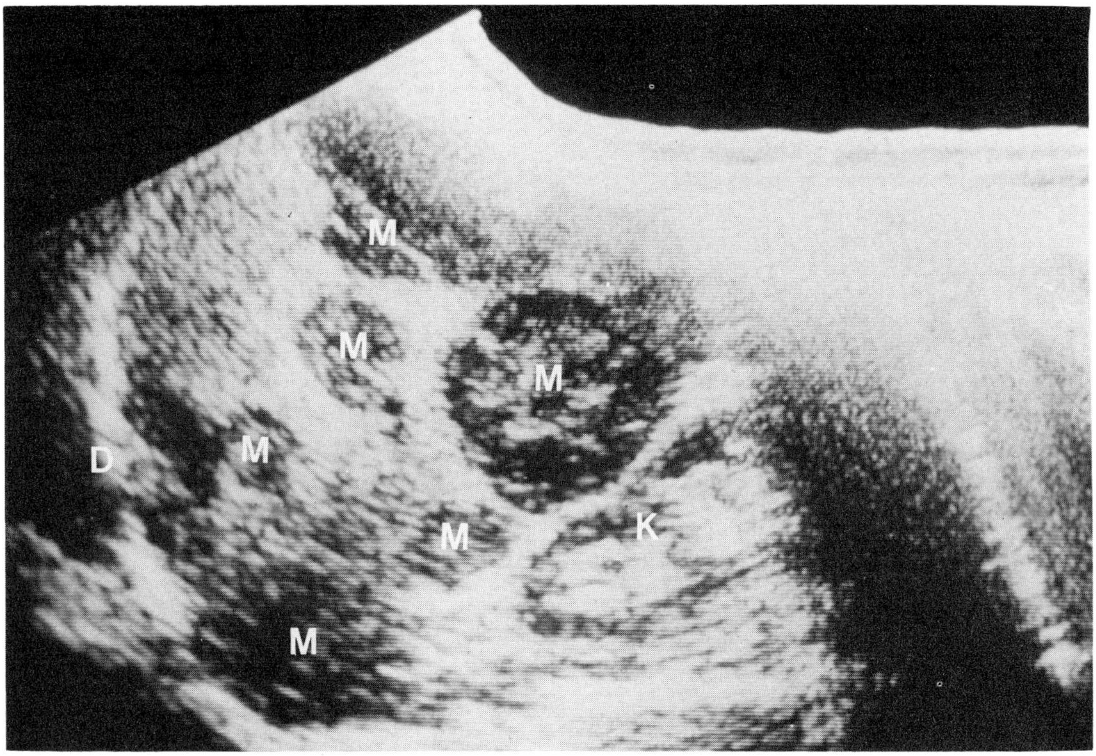

Figure 26.6. Diffuse hepatic metastases (M). Diaphragm (D) and right kidney (K) are also demonstrated.

successful and is not essential. Over-filling of the ducts should be avoided. If a surgical lesion of the biliary ducts is demonstrated immediate laparotomy is not essential but prophylactic antibiotics should be administered while awaiting surgery (see Chapter 53).

Ferrucci and Wittenburg[5] report successful opacification of the bile ducts in 99 per cent of patients with dilated bile ducts and 82 per cent of normal calibre or sclerosed ducts.

In obstruction of the common bile duct the increased viscosity of stagnant bile may cause poor distal flow of contrast medium and prevent adequate mixing of the injected contrast and bile. This may result in false proximal localization of the site of obstruction: delayed and erect films will reduce this error.

When duct dilation is present, fine-needle puncture more consistently produces successful cholangiograms than does ERCP,[4] and it is generally quicker, easier and less expensive to perform. In many centres it is replacing ERCP as the procedure of choice but, occasionally, the combined use of PTC and ERCP may be the only way to produce a definitive answer (Figure 26.8).

When the non-invasive techniques of ultrasound and isotope imaging provide a complete diagnosis, it is not necessary to proceed to either ERCP or PTC.

OTHER DIAGNOSTIC TECHNIQUES

Gastroscopy, sigmoidoscopy, barium studies and angiography may all provide important information in particular patients. These, however, play a secondary role in the specific investigation of jaundice.

Finally, it may be necessary to obtain a diagnosis more directly, either by percutaneous liver biopsy or at laparoscopy or laparotomy.

Liver biopsy

In the absence of dilated ducts, a liver biopsy is often required and should be performed with the usual precautions. The liver biopsy histology will determine the presence, severity and often the aetiology of acute or chronic liver disease

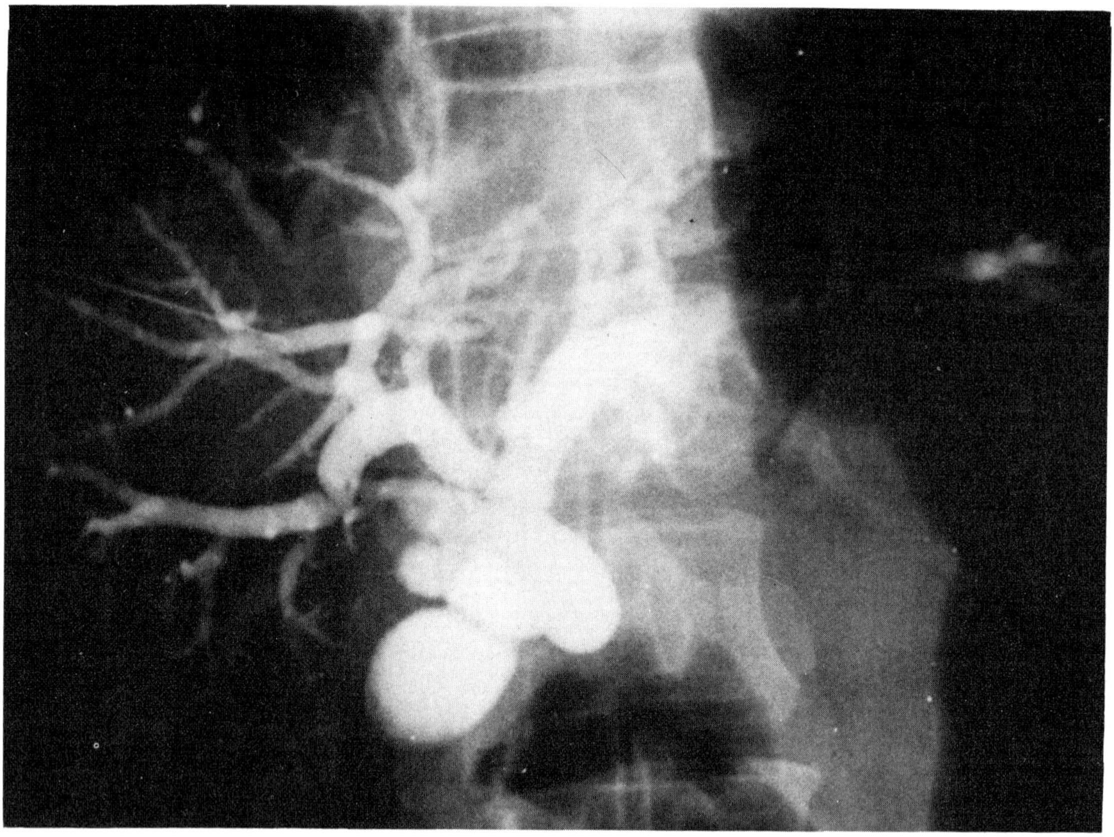

Figure 26.7. (a) Dilated ductal system produced by a carcinoma of the pancreas. (b) Localized stenosis of the common hepatic duct produced by a cholangiocarcinoma causing obstructive jaundice.

and will help to differentiate the various causes of cholestasis (see Chapter 18).

Laparoscopy

For selected patients this investigation may provide valuable information. When used in combination with ERCP, laparoscopy is particularly accurate; it can be combined with liver biopsy under direct vision. The technique is described in detail in Chapter 25.

Laparotomy

Diagnostic laparotomy should be avoidable in nearly all cases now that these other techniques are available. Where such facilities are not readily available, direct visualization and inspection at operation may still be needed. Because it carries a significant morbidity and a definite mortality, particularly in those patients with underlying hepatocellular damage, every effort should be made to reach an accurate diagnosis without recourse to laparotomy.

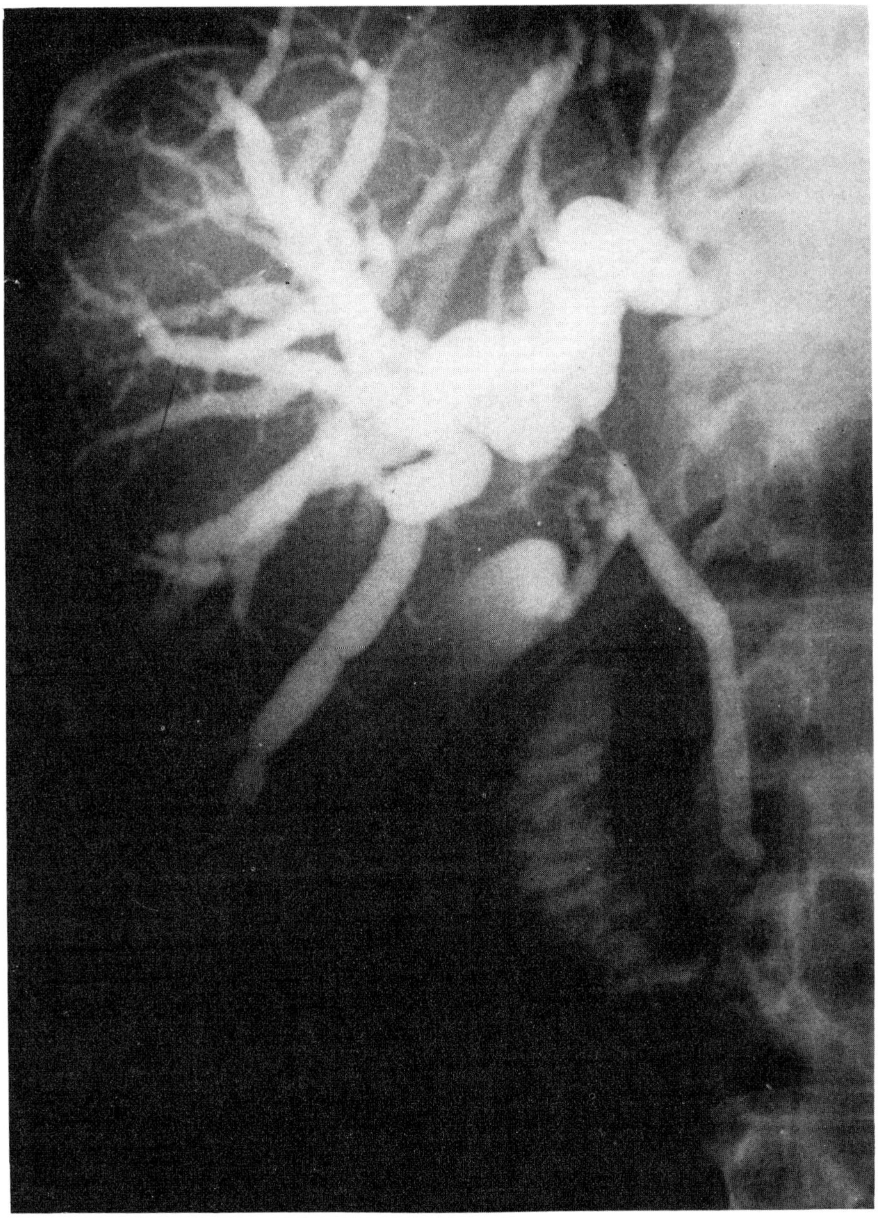

26.7 (b)

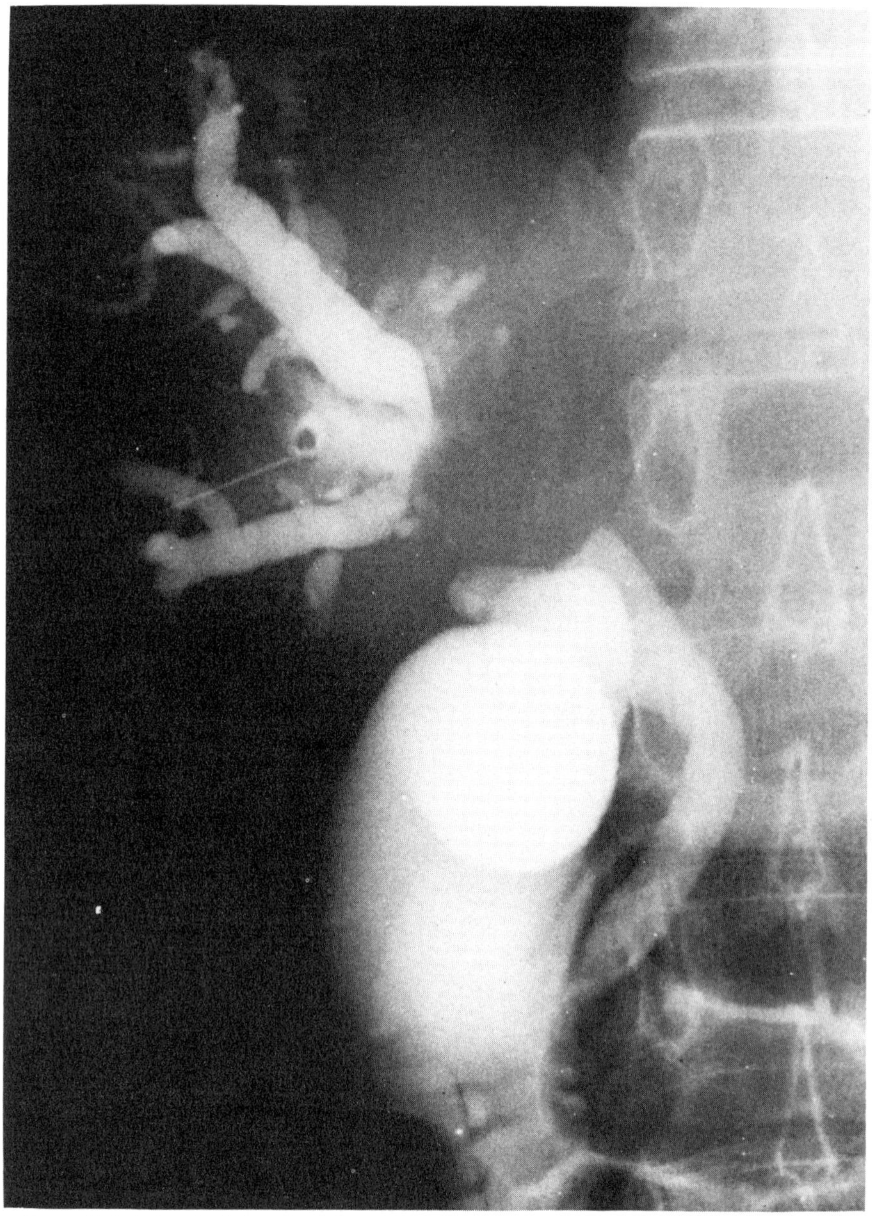

Figure 26.8. A localized ductal carcinoma demonstrated by combination of ERCP and PTC.

REFERENCES

1. Blumgart, L.H., Salmon, P.R. & Cotton, P.B. (1974) Endoscopy and retrograde choledochopancreatography in the diagnosis of the patient with jaundice. *Surgery, Gynecology and Obstetrics*, **138,** 565–570.
2. Dewbury, K.C., Joseph, A.E.A., Hayes, S. & Murray, C. (1979) Ultrasound in the evaluation and diagnosis of jaundice. *British Journal of Radiology*. In press.
3. Editorial (1978) Liver fluke in Britain. *British Medical Journal*, **i,** 1091.
4. Elias, E., Hamlyn, A.N., Jain, S., Long, R.G., Summerfield, J.A., Dick, R. & Sherlock, S. (1976) A randomized trial of percutaneous transhepatic cholangiography with the Chiba needle versus endoscopic retrograde cholangiography for bile duct visualization in jaundice. *Gastroenterology*, **71,** 439–443.
5. Ferrucci, J.T. & Wittenburg, J. (1977) Refinements in Chiba needle transhepatic cholangiography. *American Journal of Roentgenology*, **129,** 11–16.
6. Malini, S. & Sabel, J. (1977) Ultrasonography in obstructive jaundice. *Radiology*, **123,** 429–433.
7. Osnes, M., Larsen, S., Lowe, P., Gronseth, K., Løtveit, T. & Nordhus, T. (1978) Comparison of endoscopic retrograde and intravenous cholangiography in diagnosis of biliary calculi. *Lancet*, **ii,** 230.
8. Taylor, K.J. & Rosenfield, A.T. (1977) Greyscale ultrasonography in the differential diagnosis of jaundice. *Archives of Surgery*, **112,** 820–825.

Chapter 27

Acute Liver Failure

S.J. SAUNDERS
JANET SEGGIE
R.E. KIRSCH
J. TERBLANCHE

Various aspects of acute liver failure have been the subjects of a number of recent reviews.[72,84,95,96,100,125] Our intention in this chapter is to emphasize the most important points in diagnosis and management and to relate them to newer observations and hypotheses.

AETIOLOGY OF ACUTE LIVER FAILURE

The most common cause of acute liver failure is viral hepatitis.[72,96,125] The relative importance of virus A, virus B and the non-A, non-B viruses has still to be elucidated. Williams described 59 cases of acute liver failure due to viral hepatitis; 24 were due to virus A, 17 to virus B and 18 were unclassified.[125] Apart from viral hepatitis, which occurs throughout the world, acute liver failure due to other causes may vary according to the geographic location of the patient. Thus paracetamol overdose constitutes an important aetiological agent in the United Kingdom, while *Amanita phalloides* toxicity is an important cause in France. Toxicity due to other drugs, including halothane-associated hepatotoxicity, is found throughout the world and fatty liver of pregnancy is responsible for a small but significant number of patients.

CLINICAL DIAGNOSIS

Acute liver failure is a rare but overwhelming event in the course of acute hepatitis, whether it be viral in origin or drug or toxin induced. It may develop at any time during the course of hepatitis but usually occurs close to the onset of the illness and, indeed, may occasionally precede the development of jaundice. The characteristics of the syndrome are presented in the following sections.

Encephalopathy

As Plum and Hindfelt[79] have pointed out, the syndrome of hepatic encephalopathy consists of:

(a) personality changes and impaired mental functions;
(b) prominent motor abnormalities (asterixis, tremor, paratonia, hyperactive stretch reflexes, and even decerebrate posturing);
(c) alteration of consciousness;
(d) characteristic neuro-ophthalmological changes, including intact pupils and brisk ocular responses;
(e) a constellation of laboratory abnormalities.

Most clinicians regard the grading of severity of the depressed level of consciousness as being the most important indication of severity and, consequently, of prognosis. Table 27.1 shows one such classification commonly used.

Table 27.1. *Stages in the Onset and Development of Hepatic Coma.*

Grade or stage	Mental stage	Tremor	Electroencephalographic changes
Prodrome or Stage 1 (often diagnosed in retrospect)	Euphoria; occasionally depression; fluctuant, mild confusion; slowness of mentation and affect; untidy, slurred speech; disorder in sleep rhythm.	Slight	Usually absent
Impending coma or Stage 2	Accentuation of Stage 1; drowsiness; inappropriate behaviour; inability to maintain sphincter control.	Present (easily elicited)	Abnormal; generalized slowing
Stupor or Stage 3	Patient sleeps most of the time but is rousable; speech is incoherent; confusion is marked.	Usually present (if patient can co-operate)	Always abnormal
Deep coma or Stage 4	Patient may or may not respond to painful stimuli.	Usually absent	Always abnormal

From Trey, Burns and Saunders,[115] adapted from Adams and Foley,[3] with kind permission of the authors and the editor of *New England Journal of Medicine.*

In the fulminant hepatic failure surveillance study, Trey, Lipworth and Davidson reported that 17.6 per cent of 284 patients in Stage 4 coma survived, as did 48 per cent of 13 patients in Stage 3 and 66 per cent of 21 patients in Stage 2.[116] Most series have shown a mortality of 80 to 90 per cent in patients who have been in Stage 4 for more than a few hours.[11,101,114,117] Plum and Hindfelt have emphasized that the broad categories of drowsiness, stupor or coma are too inclusive for the observer to be able to quantify accurately the day-to-day clinical changes in the severity of the encephalopathy.[79] They have pointed out that the electroencephalogram and biochemical tests may not closely parallel the clinical course and have recommended overall comprehensive evaluation, following the scheme developed by Caronna et al.[20] The outline of the assessment is shown in Table 27.2. The use of this more precise clinical assessment of severity should result in even closer correlation between the extent of neurological involvement and the ultimate prognosis. Such precision is vital in the assessment of new forms of treatment. Even patients with decorticate or decerebrate posturing may recover completely with conventional therapy.[78,94] Conomy and Swash reported the same experience in patients with chronic liver disease.[24]

Fetor hepaticus

This is a very valuable physical sign and is almost invariably present.

Liver size

Clinically, the liver rapidly shrinks in size and soon becomes impalpable. Early in the syndrome no liver dullness is elicitable on percussion. In our experience, those patients dying early in deep coma usually have a liver greatly reduced in weight and showing massive necrosis of the hepatocytes. Nearly all patients are jaundiced and, in some, acute liver failure is heralded by the development of repeated and profuse vomiting.

Haemorrhage

Bleeding is a common complication of acute hepatic necrosis.[52,82,88,116] In our experience, more than half the adults and 70 per cent of the children have a major defect in coagulation, with life-threatening haemorrhage. All these patients have an increase in the one-stage prothrombin time and in one-third of the patients the prothrombin index is less than 20 per cent. The extent of the depression of the prothrombin index is a good indication of the severity of the disease. In states in which there is decompensation of hepatocyte function, impaired hepatic synthesis of some coagulation factors by the liver commonly occurs.[26] Disseminated intravascular coagulation may aggravate the situation.[82] In up to 50 per cent of the patients, the platelet levels may fall below $80 \times 10^9/l$.[96]

Table 27.2. *A Clinical Coma-profile for Bedside Use.*

I.	Verbal response
	none
	incomprehensible sounds
	confused
	normal
II.	Pupils
	non-reactive
	sluggish
	brisk
III.	Eye opening
	none
	to noxious stimuli only
	to verbal stimuli
	spontaneous
IV.	Oculocephalic–oculovestibular responses
	no reaction
	partial or dysconjugate
	full
	normal
V.	Best motor response
	none
	abnormal extensor
	abnormal flexor
	withdrawal or localizes
	obeys commands
VI.	Respiration
	nil on ventilator
	irregular
	regular > 22/min
	regular < 22/min

From Plum and Hindfelt,[79] with kind permission of the authors and the editor of Elsevier/North-Holland Biomedical Press.

Respiratory complications

There is evidence that in humans with hepatic encephalopathy,[68,86] and in goats with carbon tetrachloride (CCl_4)-induced hepatic injury,[105,106,107] hepatic failure is associated with failure of normal cerebral autoregulatory reflexes. In health, a rising $Pa\text{CO}_2$, or a falling $Pa\text{O}_2$, produces cerebral vasodilatation which results in an increase in cerebral metabolic rate for oxygen ($CMRO_2$). Thus $CMRO_2$ is maintained constant over a wide range of arterial gas tensions.

Hypocapnia is often encountered in hepatic failure and parallels the depth of coma. There is a concomitant fall in cerebral blood flow (CBF) and $CMRO_2$. Since the normal autoregulatory response to an increase in $Pa\text{CO}_2$ is an increase in CBF via cerebral vasodilatation, Posner and Plum subjected their patients to inhalation of 5 per cent CO_2 for 30 minutes.[80] The resulting rise in $Pa\text{CO}_2$ produced a fall in CBF and in $CMRO_2$ and a significant clinical deterioration. When CCl_4-treated goats were made hypercapnic by exposure to CO_2-enriched gas mixtures, similar results were obtained. These findings suggest that the usual hypocapnia in hepatic failure is probably beneficial.

Hypoxia is a frequent accompaniment of liver failure. In the healthy individual, transient hypoxia stimulates respiration via the carotid chemoreceptors. Steady state hypoxia exerts its effect upon the brain stem respiratory centres and is the main determinant of respiratory drive. If severe enough, the respiratory stimulant effect of steady state hypoxia is overcome by secondary hypoxic depression of the brain stem centres. In hepatic failure the ventilatory response to transient hypoxia is increased, suggesting heightened sensitivity of peripheral chemoreceptors. This increased ventilatory response is not maintained in the face of prolonged hypoxia consistent with hypoxic depression of the respiratory centres. By implication, any respiratory complication of hepatic failure, such as pneumonia or pulmonary oedema, could lead to a vicious cycle situation in which hypoxic depression of respiratory drive could lead to a further decrease in $Pa\text{O}_2$ and further brain stem depression.

Hypoglycaemia

We have previously emphasized the frequency and importance of hypoglycaemia in these patients.[72,93,96] This hypoglycaemia, it has been suggested, is due to inefficient degradation of insulin by the damaged liver.[40] However, Felig et al have reported a 50 per cent incidence of fasting hypoglycaemia in acute viral hepatitis and have demonstrated an associated 30 per cent decrease in plasma insulin in such patients.[32] The patients also showed a lesser response to glucagon infusion with no improvement of the blood sugar levels by a carbohydrate diet. Biopsy revealed low hepatic glycogen levels and, hence, defects in hepatic glycogen synthesis and in gluconeogenesis were postulated. These metabolic deficiencies are probably greater in patients with massive liver necrosis. In our series, 40 per cent of adults and 44 per cent of children in coma were hypoglycaemic at some time. Several of these patients required very large amounts of oral and intravenous glucose and, even then, hypoglycaemia was controlled with difficulty.

Renal failure (see Chapter 46)

Impairment of renal function frequently accompanies acute hepatic failure. Wilkinson, Blendis and Williams studied 38 of 48 patients who had evidence of renal dysfunction.[122] Thirty-two of these patients could be placed into one of three categories:

1. Prerenal uraemia. The uraemia could be explained on the basis of dehydration or absorption of nitrogenous compounds from the gut following gastrointestinal haemorrhage.
2. Acute tubular necrosis. This diagnosis was based upon the finding of numerous granular and cellular casts in the urine and upon necropsy findings. Urine sodium concentration of over 20 mmol/l (460 mg/l), together with a urine–plasma urea ratio of less than 10, was considered to be additional evidence of this lesion.
3. Functional renal failure. This term was used to describe an otherwise unexplained renal impairment in the presence of low urine sodium concentration (less than 20 mmol/l [460 mg/l]) and a normal urinary sediment. Some of these cases proceeded to acute tubular necrosis as a preterminal event, but in those that did not the kidney was found to be normal at necropsy.

In a follow-up study, Wilkinson et al found a significant correlation between the development of renal failure, intravascular coagulation and endotoxaemia as detected by Limulus lysate assay.[123] Fourteen of 22 patients in fulminant hepatic failure who developed renal failure and disseminated intravascular coagulation had a positive assay, whilst the test in a control group of patients with acute renal failure not associated with liver disease was negative. Furthermore, in two patients in whom serial measurements were carried out, the first signs of renal impairment were noted as the Limulus test became positive. The renal failure was either functional or due to acute tubular necrosis.

Endotoxins, which are powerful triggers of sympathetic nervous vasoconstriction via the kallikrein–bradykinin pathway, of catecholamine release and of renin–angiotensin activation, probably exert their effect by inducing intense renal vasoconstriction.[120] In addition, there is the contribution of disseminated intravascular coagulation which produces severe capillary damage and which itself leads to propagation of vasoconstrictor products. This complication arose in nine out of 14 of Wilkinson's patients, and in two patients coagulation abnormalities became manifest as the Limulus test, which was initially negative, became positive.[123] Liehr studied endotoxaemia intensively and suggested that the development of systemic endotoxaemia following an hepatic insult such as viral hepatitis may convert modest hepatic injury into massive necrosis, leading to fulminant hepatic failure.[64] He has reported on the role of endotoxaemia in acute liver failure, using galactosamine-induced hepatitis as an experimental model. In this model, colectomy, which removes the source of endotoxins, will protect the animals against the development of fulminant hepatic failure. Conversely, the administration of galactosamine with sublethal doses of endotoxins leads promptly to massive hepatic necrosis and death.

The complement system is likely to have a role in the mediation of this endotoxin-induced hepatocellular damage and this would seem to be borne out by the fact that mice which have a congenital complement deficiency are able to resist galactosamine-induced hepatic necrosis even in the presence of endotoxaemia.

Infection

Patients with fulminant hepatic failure have an increased liability to infection. Bailey et al[8] demonstrated a factor in the serum of these patients which was able to inhibit the metabolic activity of the leucocyte–hexose monophosphate shunt as measured by the conversion of ^{14}C-glucose to $^{14}CO_2$. This correlated with neither the low serum complement nor the associated renal failure. They noted that the inhibitory factor was dialysable and could be removed by treatment of the serum with activated charcoal. They were unable to demonstrate any intrinsic leucocyte abnormality in these patients and postulated that various forms of artificial support might improve polymorphonuclear function. Recent work in our laboratory has shown that the serum from eight of 17 patients with acute viral hepatitis was deficient in its ability to support neutrophil bactericidal function in vitro.[97] This defect appeared to be related to the viral infection itself and was not found in patients with drug hepatitis or mechanical obstructive jaundice, nor was it related to the severity of the disease. Our results suggest that the serum factor might not be specific for acute hepatic failure although, of course, more than one factor might be involved. These changes in polymorphonuclear function might play a role in the increased frequency of infection. Lowered complement and other immunological mechanisms are probably also important.

Hypotension

Trewby et al have reported that 82 of 94 consecutive patients with fulminant hepatic failure were significantly hypotensive during their illness.[112] In 60 per cent of these patients the cause of the fall in blood pressure was not due to infection, haemorrhage or other obvious factors. These workers found that most patients had inappropriate systemic vasodilatation. Haemodynamic and radiological studies of the pulmonary circulation suggested that similar changes occurred there, too. They point out that arterial hypotension may cause a reduction in cerebral blood flow and cerebral metabolic rate for oxygen. To try to reduce the incidence of hypotension, adequate volumes of fluid must always be given.

Cerebral oedema

Cerebral oedema as a complication of fulminant hepatic failure was first described in 1944 by Lucké. It has been highlighted in two recent publications.[121,125] Both groups of workers found a high incidence: Ware[121] reported that oedema was present in 16 out of 32 patients dying of massive liver necrosis and Williams[125] recorded its presence in 36 out of 92 patients. Herniation was present in four out of the 32 and eight out of the 92 cases, respectively. Both series found that cerebral oedema occurred with increased frequency in younger patients, while Ware, but not Williams, found a relationship between the duration of Stage 4 coma and the absence of terminal azotaemia. Twenty-five out of the 36 patients reported by Williams had been artificially ventilated, and this may have contributed to the development of cerebral oedema.

The finding that cerebral oedema occurs with a high frequency in fatal cases of Reye's syndrome has led to renewed interest in the pathogenesis and management of such cases (see Chapter 40). In Reye's syndrome there is cytotoxic brain oedema characterized by cellular swelling (neuronal, glial and endothelial) with a decrease of extracellular fluid space. This oedema is associated with a normal cerebrospinal fluid (CSF) protein content and by electron microscopic findings of astrocytic swelling and the appearance of intralamellal blebs in the myelin. These findings, however, have not been described in other forms of hepatic failure.

More recently, two animal models have been developed. A rat model, produced by two-stage hepatectomy, caused cerebral oedema in every case and has been used to demonstrate a defect in the blood–brain barrier.[43] Similarly, a pig model revealed elevation of intracranial pressure when a subdural pressure transducer was used in experimental but not in control animals.[44] In the latter, administration of methylprednisolone 100 mg/kg initially, followed by 25 mg/kg two-hourly at the start of surgery, abolished the rise in intracranial pressure, but the same therapy had no effect when the drug was given four hours after surgery.

While intensive treatment of cerebral oedema permitted a 50 per cent survival rate in patients with Reye's syndrome, patients with fulminant hepatic failure treated with either dexamethasone 16 mg/24 hours, hydrocortisone 600 mg/24 hours or glycerol 1.5 g/kg for 24 hours showed no response to such therapy.

Biochemical changes

The serum transaminases are always elevated early in the syndrome, frequently to high levels. However, the level of the transaminase is not useful in predicting the onset of fulminant hepatic failure. Serum bilirubin usually rises soon after the onset and is mainly conjugated in type. Patients who recover often pass through a phase of marked cholestatic jaundice with very high levels of conjugated bilirubin. Those who die at this stage show large regeneration nodules, the hepatocytes showing intense cholestasis, the aetiology of which is not understood. There is a striking elevation of plasma ligandin levels and the measurement of this cytosol protein in the plasma may prove to be a good index of liver cell necrosis.[10]

Alpha-fetoprotein levels in the plasma may give an indication of the development of regeneration.[7,14,15] Alpha-fetoprotein is synthesized by fetal liver cells[41] and is well established as a serum marker of hepatocarcinoma.[1,81] If a sensitive radio-immunoassay is employed in its detection, alpha-fetoprotein can be found in minute amounts in normal adults.[92] It has been detected in the serum of mice after partial hepatectomy[57] and in patients recovering from acute hepatitis,[5,7] suggesting that it accompanies hepatic regeneration.

Karvountzis and Redeker found raised alpha-fetoprotein levels in 57 per cent of patients with coma complicating fulminant viral hepatitis and in 80 per cent of those who survived.[54] Furthermore, where serial titres were measured, the levels were found to be increasing at the end of the period of coma. In contrast, alpha-fetoprotein was detected in only 37 per cent of those patients who died, despite the fact that some survived up to 10 days. In those patients in whom alpha-fetoprotein was detected before death there was quantitatively more evidence of regeneration at necropsy than in those in whom alpha-fetoprotein was not detected. The presence of alpha-fetoprotein was thought to be a favourable prognostic sign and its absence in fulminant hepatitis to be of ominous significance.

This was not the view of Bloomer et al who studied serial alpha-fetoprotein levels in 12 patients with massive hepatic necrosis due to viral hepatitis, ischaemic necrosis and halothane hepatitis.[15] They noted that alpha-fetoprotein levels were significantly elevated after the eighth day of illness in nine patients, all of whom were shown subsequently at biopsy or necropsy to have histological evidence of hepatic regeneration. Since eight of these patients subsequently died, and only one survived, Bloomer et al have stated that a rising serum alpha-fetoprotein level does not necessarily imply ultimate recovery and that it therefore cannot be used to assess prognosis.[15]

Electrolyte and acid–base disturbances

These patients are particularly prone to hypokalaemia.[72,96] Plum and Hindfelt have suggested that this may be partly nutritional in origin, as a result of poor appetite, nausea and vomiting; partly due to endocrine factors as a consequence of secondary hyperaldosteronism and, in some patients, as a consequence of the use of diuretics.[79] Body stores of potassium have been described as being depleted by as much as 500 mmol (500 mEq).[21] Hypokalaemia enhances the alkalosis which is present due to the primary respiratory drive and it should be noted that the amount of free diffusible ammonia is pH dependent. This theoretical possibility has been confirmed in the experimental animal, in which metabolic alkalosis increased the CSF ammonium content.[104]

We have observed significant hypocalcaemia in these patients and this has also been the experience of others.[74] In a recent study, the sodium, potassium and water content of circulating leucocytes was measured in 30 patients who had fulminant hepatic failure.[6] While potassium levels were depressed, the most striking changes were found in sodium and water content. Serial studies showed that the leucocyte sodium content initially fell with recovery of liver function and returned to the normal range some weeks later. This intracellular shift might contribute to the hyponatraemia seen in some of these patients. Hyponatraemia is also likely to be due in part to haemodilution because of impaired renal excretion of free water.[124]

The CSF glutamine was higher than 0.2 g/l (20 mg/100 ml) in 41 of 43 of our comatose patients. Two patients had levels lower than 0.2 g/l and none had a level lower than 0.16 g/l (16 mg/100 ml).[96] A reasonable correlation between the severity of encephalopathy and CSF glutamine levels was observed by Houvani, Hamlin and Reynolds.[48] In 72 per cent of our patients, the blood urea was below 3.30 mmol/l (20 mg/100 ml).[96]

The neurological signs often appear before the blood ammonia rises, and Plum and Hindfelt point out that this is probably the strongest single argument against ammonia intoxication's being the common denominator of all forms of hepatic encephalopathy.[79] Elevations of blood ammonia are not usually marked at the outset;[111] a more marked elevation tends to occur later in the disease.[23]

Electroencephalogram

The electroencephalogram (EEG) correlates fairly well with the clinical state. Occasionally, the EEG changes are more marked in the early stages of the syndrome than would be suggested by the clinical picture, whereas at a later stage in the illness the EEG may remain abnormal for weeks while the patient's level of consciousness has become normal.[100]

Prognosis in survivors

Karvountzis, Redeker and Peters reported a 3- to 46-month follow-up study in 22 patients who had survived fulminant hepatic failure.[55] Complete clinical and biochemical remission occurred within 45 to 75 days of the onset of the illness. Liver biopsy in 13 patients (2 to 37 months after coma) demonstrated no liver disease except for mild unresolved hepatitis in one patient who was an HB_sAg carrier. The implication is that one severe self-limiting infection does not lead to cirrhosis whereas repeated relatively minor episodes of necrosis frequently do, as in chronic active hepatitis.

MANAGEMENT

It is important to have a good appreciation of the natural history of fulminant hepatic failure in order that the effectiveness of any form of treatment may be assessed. A lack of adequate control data bedevils our knowledge of the effectiveness of most forms of treatment offered in the past and currently in vogue. The most accurate measure of prognosis seems to be based on neurological grading, and a better correlation may be achieved with the more widespread use of the method of assessment recommended by Plum and Hindfelt,[79] coupled with frequent careful clinical observations. As pointed out previously, patients in Stage 4 coma have a mortality of 80 to 90 per cent while in patients in Stage 3 this drops to 50 per cent. Although the very low prothrombin index indicates the severity of the disease initially, this and other laboratory measurements have not been useful in assessing the ultimate prognosis.[95] This was also the experience of Reynolds[87] but is not in keeping with the reports of Rueff and Benhamou,[91] Caroli et al[19] and Robert et al.[89] The duration of deep coma, persistence of overt bleeding and renal failure are usually correlated with a higher mortality but there are no reliable prognostic indices which we may use during the first few days of the syndrome.[95] The aetiology of massive liver cell necrosis is of little help in this regard, with the possible exception of halothane-induced acute liver failure where the survival rate is recorded as 4 per cent.[116] Age seems to have an important bearing on prognosis. In the surveillance study, the survival rate was 34 per cent in patients under the age of 15 years, 22 per cent in patients between 15 and 44 years and only 5 per cent in patients over the age of 45. All patients who were over the age of 60 died.[116] This was also the experience of Rueff and Benhamou[91] and Peters and Edmondson.[77] In contrast, age seemed to have little influence on survival in our own series.[96]

Intensive Care

Intensive care with careful monitoring of vital functions is imperative and may be responsible for any improvement in prognosis in recent years. Cardiac arrhythmias may occur in up to one-third of patients and major gastrointestinal haemorrhage frequently occurs. The early recognition and prompt treatment of these and other complications may influence the prognosis. All attending personnel wear protective gowns, gloves and masks. While we do not follow the rigid precautions suggested by Percy-Robb, Proffitt and Whitby,[76] everyone in contact with the patient is made to understand the nature of the disease and the importance of good personal hygiene.

Fluids and Electrolytes

Initially, all fluids and electrolytes are given intravenously. Particular care must be taken to ensure that adequate potassium is given and some patients require as much as 600 mmol (600 mEq) of potassium daily intravenously to maintain a normal plasma potassium level. Additional calcium and magnesium may also be needed. The fluid always contains 10 per cent dextrose as a continuous infusion and blood sugar levels are monitored hourly by use of dextrostix with frequent chemical confirmation. Additional intravenous glucose is given as required.

Correction of Bleeding Diathesis

Vitamin K_1, administered either intravenously or intramuscularly, has little effect on the low prothrombin index. Three units of fresh frozen plasma are given daily and fresh whole blood as the need arises. The finding of disseminated intravascular coagulation in some patients prompted the use of heparin in the management of bleeding in these patients.[82] A subsequent controlled trial did not confirm the promising early results and heparin has no place in treatment.[39] The upper gastrointestinal tract is the most frequent site of major bleeding which may prove to be fatal either as a direct result of massive blood loss or by exacerbating the encephalopathy. A prospective controlled trial of the H_2-receptor antagonist, cimetidine, showed that this agent was effective in considerably reducing the incidence of this complication.[66] We now use cimetidine routinely.

Avoidance of Excessive Sedation

In our experience, promethazine hydrochloride is the drug of choice. Paraldehyde and diazepam should be avoided, the former because of its liability to cause lactic acidosis in these patients and the latter because its use has been associated with acute respiratory failure in some of our patients with fulminant hepatic failure. This does not seem to be the case in patients with chronic encephalopathy.

Corticosteroids

In 1952, Ducci and Katz[29] reported a 66 per cent survival rate which consisted of two survivors out of three patients. Analysis of their extended series 10 years later showed a 39 per cent survival rate (nine out of 23 patients). All those who recovered were seen during the first half of the study, and this trend for the best results to be obtained during the early part of the series, which was not subsequently borne out in the larger number of patients, has been seen after the introduction of all additional new forms of therapy up to the present time. Benhamou, Rueff and Sicot reviewed 334 patients, including 60 of their own, of whom 190 were treated with steroids, and found no increased survival in the treated group.[11] We do not use corticosteroids in the treatment of our patients (see Chapter 28).

Alleviation of Encephalopathy
(see also Chapter 42)

Mechanisms aimed at reducing the total nitrogenous load

To this end, patients are given no protein by mouth. While certain amino acids given intravenously may prove of benefit in hepatic failure complicating cirrhosis, their administration by mouth may well exacerbate the syndrome. The protein-free diet used in the treatment of hepatic encephalopathy is also very undesirable because it interferes with adequate protein synthesis.

For this reason, the possible use of keto analogues of essential amino acids is of great interest. We have shown that keto isoleucine, keto leucine and keto valine are able to stimulate albumin synthesis both in vitro and in vivo.[58] Walser et al have shown them to be effective in promoting a positive nitrogen balance in severe chronic uraemia in man.[119] Recently, Maddrey et al have studied the effects of keto analogues of essential amino acids in portasystemic encephalopathy.[67] Keto analogues of valine, leucine, isoleucine, methionine and phenylalanine were given either orally or parenterally to 11 patients with portasystemic encephalopathy and high blood ammonia levels. Plasma concentrations of the amino acids corresponding to the infused analogues rose after infusions, while plasma tyrosine and glycine, which were abnormally elevated in the control samples, fell. After one to five daily infusions, the ratio of essential to non-essential amino acids in the fasting plasma increased towards normal and a notable fall in the glutamine also occurred. Arterial blood ammonia and glutamate did not show any change immediately after the infusions. Five patients had eight nitrogen balance studies performed during three to 12 days of oral or intravenous keto-acid therapy and failed to show any consistent improvement in balance. After five courses of oral therapy there was significant improvement in the ratio of essential: non-essential amino acids. Clinical improvement, as assessed by the level of consciousness and psychological testing, occurred in eight of 11 patients. No toxicity was observed. These investigators suggest that the use of keto analogues of essential amino acids may be of benefit to patients in hepatic encephalopathy and have shown that they are converted to the corresponding amino acids in these patients. Alpha-keto analogues of essential amino acids could influence the elevated blood ammonia by combining with amino groups to yield essential amino acids, but it may well be that a more important effect will be the stimulation of protein synthesis by these agents.

One gram of neomycin sulphate is given four-hourly and lactulose 15 to 60 ml every six hours. The latter increases stool frequency, lowers stool pH and may alter gut flora. Its mechanism of action is not fully understood although it is thought to reduce intestinal absorption of ammonia. The dose should be adjusted to achieve two to three stools a day without causing diarrhoea, which is not needed for the therapeutic effect.[16] Enemas are given initially to empty the colon and subsequently in the event of any gastrointestinal haemorrhage, which should be detected by regular aspiration of gastric contents via an indwelling nasogastric tube.

Exchange transfusion

Our first report showed a recovery rate of 71 per cent, i.e. in five out of seven patients so treated.[115] Six years later, the survival rate was 19 per cent, i.e. nine out of 47 patients.[96] Our experience with this form of treatment underlines the difficulty in assessing the results of treatment in the absence of a prospective controlled trial. A large number of reports, including that of the fulminant hepatic failure surveillance study,[113] claimed that this is an effective form of treatment. Redeker and Yamahiro carried out a controlled trial in 29 patients and concluded that exchange transfusion was of no benefit.[85] This was also the conclusion of Benhamou, Rueff and Sicot[11] in their personal series and in their analysis of the published cases from 26 different reports. While exchange transfusion may temporarily improve the neurological status of some of these patients, it has no part to play in therapy.

Plasmaphoresis

Lepore and Martel,[62] Lepore et al[63] and Demeulenare, Barbier and Vermeire[27] have treated patients with plasmaphoresis. Of 23 patients so treated, 12 responded and 10 of these survived. It is doubtful whether more widespread use of this procedure will show better results than those obtained with exchange transfusion.

Total body washout

It is probable that the same conclusions can be drawn concerning treatment with total body washout. This form of therapy has been used by Klebanof[60] and Tobias and Isom.[110] Sixteen patients were treated, 10 of whom had acute liver failure; 11 of the 16 patients survived. Total body washout is a single-pass perfusion performed via closed chest cardiopulmonary bypass and hypothermia. Gocke[42] and Lepore et al[63] used serum containing anti-HB_sAg in an attempt to minimize the ongoing damage produced by the virus, but experience is too limited to be able to assess the value of this procedure.

Cross circulation

The use of human donors is complicated by the risk to the donor, especially when the patient has viral hepatitis. Summers et al used an irreversibly comatose donor because of this danger, but loss of vasomotor tone regulation in the donor proved to be a real disadvantage.[108] Burnell et al noted orthostatic hypotensive episodes in three out of four neurologically normal donors.[18] Although these complications were temporary they were alarming. Immunological and allergic problems do not usually become clinically significant until the fourth day of the procedure.[18,109] Leucopenia, thrombocytopenia, haemolytic anaemia, fever, bronchospasm and pulmonary oedema may all occur.[108] We reported the treatment of one patient by means of cross-circulation with a baboon donor after the latter had been prepared by total replacement with compatible human blood. The result was encouraging.[98] A subsequent review of five papers, in which 13 patients were treated using both humans and baboons as partners, showed a 61.5 per cent recovery rate.[11] The numbers were too small to draw any firm conclusions as to the usefulness of this form of treatment. While the use of human donors is bedevilled by ethical considerations, the use of the baboon partner presents the possible hazard of transmission of simian viruses.[96] There is some experimental support for this form of treatment. Systemic–systemic cross-circulation between control and liverless rats improved the EEG in the latter when flow rates were adequate, while portal–systemic cross-circulation was effective at lower rates of flow.[90]

Extracorporeal liver perfusion

Eiseman, Liem and Raffucci introduced isolated pig liver perfusion in the treatment of this syndrome.[30] Their report was followed by a large number of such procedures carried out in a number of centres, including our own, without striking significant change in the mortality of the treated groups. In Cape Town, five procedures were performed in four patients, none of whom survived but all of whom showed clear neurological improvement after the procedure.[45] The use of the pig liver has given less encouraging results than have livers from other species. Pig liver perfusion resulted in significant thrombocytopenia in all our patients. In subsequent experiments in our laboratory we demonstrated that the experimental perfusion of the isolated pig liver with human blood resulted in approximately 80 per cent of the total circulating platelets being removed from the circulation into the liver within the first half-hour of perfusion.[46] This was not the case when baboon livers were used.[47] Abouna et al used the baboon liver in three patients, two of whom survived.[2] It would appear that homologous liver from a cadaver donor has the fewest immunological complications.[2,99] In the light of current experience there appears to be no indication for the use of this form of treatment.

Liver transplantation

The likelihood of infection of the transplanted organ with the same virus has discouraged the use of orthotopic transplantation as a form of treatment. Auxiliary heterotopic liver transplantation has been suggested by Slapak et al.[103] The possible interference with regeneration which this procedure may cause is a potential problem. Transplantation does not have a part to play in therapy at the present time (see Chapter 52).

Exchange resins and activated charcoal

The use of exchange resins has been suggested in the belief that these will remove toxic substances.[53,127] The King's College Hospital group introduced the use of haemoperfusion through coated, activated charcoal.[128] It is an effective means of removing paracetamol in pigs without loss of leucocytes, platelets or particle embolism, and these workers have used this form of treatment extensively in patients who have fulminant hepatic failure. Their initial favourable results were subsequently not maintained, mainly because of complications of thrombocytopenia, the latter possibly due to a change in the preparation of the charcoal.[125] They are not currently using this form of therapy.[126]

The possible role of neurotransmitters in hepatic encephalopathy: implications for therapy

Many abnormalities in neurotransmitter metabolism occur in the brain in hepatic encephalopathy. These include decreased noradrenaline,[28] increased serotonin,[9] increased octopamine[28,34] and other amines, as well as marked changes in the concentrations of many amino acids.[9,33,35] Intravenously administered amino acids can improve hepatic encephalopathy in the dog[36] and in man.[37] The aromatic amine precursors phenylalanine, tyrosine, tryptophan and methionine are increased in the plasma,[4,51,69,83] and this suggested that the concentration of their metabolites in body fluids would also be increased. Indeed, raised concentrations of 5-hydroxyindole acetic acid, the degradation product of 5-hydroxytryptamine (derived from tryptophan), and of homovanillic acid, the degradation product of dopamine (derived from tyrosine), have been found in the cerebrospinal fluid of patients with acute hepatic encephalopathy. As previously mentioned, octopamine (derived from tyrosine via tyramine) has also been identified as a false neurotransmitter which is present in increased amounts, and all these compounds may be important in the pathogenesis of the encephalopathy.[61] In keeping with these observations, L-dopa caused striking neurological improvement in three patients with fulminant hepatic failure.[75]

The concentration of the branched-chain amino acids valine, leucine and isoleucine is depressed in patients with encephalopathy in the presence of chronic liver disease,[49,50] and in animals with experimental 'encephalopathy'.[4,51] Because of their shared competitive transport mechanisms across the blood–brain barrier, the low concentrations of branched-chain amino acids have been implicated as one of the causes of the increased brain tryptophan in these patients.[34] However, a clear distinction must be drawn between acute and chronic encephalopathy in this respect because in fulminant hepatic failure in man the branched-chain amino acids are normal[37,83] while in the rat they may be elevated.[13] In the study of Record et al, amino acid concentrations were measured in plasma, whole blood, cerebrospinal fluid and brain tissue in 45 patients with Stage 3 or 4 coma due to fulminant hepatic failure.[83] The concentrations of 15 of the 19 amino acids measured were significantly increased in blood, and the increases were greater for the amino acids concerned with neurotransmitter metabolism. There was no correlation between the plasma concentrations of these amino acids and changes in the grade of hepatic coma. Plasma concentrations of the branched-chain amino acids were normal, except in those patients, who subsequently recovered, in whom the levels were slightly decreased. Phenylalanine, tyrosine and methionine were among the 15 out of the 18 amino acids which were significantly increased in cerebrospinal fluid, and among the 15 of the 21 amino acids which were significantly increased in the brain. The increase in tryptophan was associated with significant elevation in the brain 5-hydroxyindole–acetic acid concentration, suggesting an increase in the 5-hydroxytryptamine turnover in hepatic coma. Brain : plasma ratios of most amino acids in hepatic coma patients were similar to those in control subjects, suggesting that plasma concentration is a major factor controlling the cerebral concentration. For the branched-chain amino acids, cerebrospinal fluid and brain concentrations were increased when plasma concentrations were normal, suggesting an increase in brain uptake.[83]

Needle biopsies were taken from the frontal cortex of the brain within an hour of death from 13 of the patients who later had full autopsy examination, and from seven patients dying without evidence of liver disease. Record et al point out that some amino acids are found at a significantly higher concentration in brain obtained at autopsy than in tissue frozen immediately after removal during brain surgery. However, good correlation between their patients and the controls led them to believe that this did not introduce a major error into their study. They suggest that the relatively normal concentration of branched-chain amino acids in their patients may be due to the oxidation of these amino acids by extrahepatic tissues, mainly striated muscle, in those patients who survive.[71] The elevated amino acids in the plasma may arise from the necrotic liver cells or from muscle. The poor nutrition of these patients could result in an increased catabolism of proteins with release of amino acids from voluntary muscle for gluconeogenesis. Under these circumstances, the predominant amino acids are alanine and glutamine, and the raised methionine, phenylalanine and tyrosine suggest that they are of hepatic origin. However, one gets elevated concentrations of plasma and tissue amino acids in dogs after hepatectomy.[38,70,118] In the liverless dog plasma the methionine levels fall very low.[70] It seems likely that the origin of the amino acids in fulminant hepatic failure is from the liver and from increased catabolism in voluntary muscle.

Our own studies in rats which had had a portacaval shunt immediately followed by hepatic artery ligation demonstrated that plasma free tryptophan and brain tryptophan were markedly elevated in hepatic coma, despite *raised* levels of valine, leucine and isoleucine. Concentrations of methionine, tyrosine and phenylalanine were also increased in the plasma, as was glucagon. The concentrations of insulin fell. Brain levels of glutamate increased while cyclic adenosine-3′,5′-monophosphate and γ-aminobutyric acid were unchanged.[13]

There were several possible mechanisms for the rise in brain tryptophan in the presence of increased concentrations of branched-chain amino acids. It may be due to a rise in free tryptophan in the plasma because of its displacement from albumin-binding sites by free fatty acids.[25] The rise in brain tryptophan in rats three weeks after end-to-side portacaval shunt cannot be explained by this as the brain tryptophan : plasma free tryptophan ratio was considerably increased in these animals.

In the patients described in the paper by Record et al the brain tryptophan : plasma total tryptophan ratio was also slightly increased.[83] This suggests that there may be an increased uptake of tryptophan in the brain in hepatic coma. Infusions of amino acid mixtures containing high concentrations of branched-chain amino acids have improved encephalopathy in dogs with portacaval shunts and in man with encephalopathy due to cirrhosis.[36] It has been suggested that the molar ratio of valine, leucine and isoleucine to phenylalanine and tyrosine is important in relating plasma amino acid concentrations to the presence or absence of encephalopathy.[35] The data of Record et al[83] do not suggest that this holds true in man, and our work suggests that this form of therapy is unlikely to be effective in *acute* liver failure. If the mechanisms of amino acid uptake by the brain are disturbed, normalization of plasma amino acid concentrations may not be sufficient. Intravenous amino acids were given to three patients with fulminant hepatic failure. All three initially showed neurological improvement, but no firm conclusions can be derived from this small number.[37]

It is probable that the disturbance in the metabolism of the branched-chain amino acids is not the same in acute hepatic failure as it is in the chronic variety and, in view of the different plasma amino acid pattern in fulminant hepatic failure as compared with chronic portasystemic encephalopathy, it is unlikely that infusions of amino acids will have a direct effect on the neurological signs or ultimate prognosis. Indeed, preliminary results in our laboratory suggest that amino acids, while stimulating albumin synthesis, may at the same time interfere with DNA synthesis after partial hepatectomy in the rat.[59] Whether they would have any deleterious effect on the recovery of human liver is unknown.

Hepatotrophic factors

Bucher and Swaffield showed that hepatic regeneration can be enhanced in laboratory animals by the synergistic action of two pancreatic hormones, insulin and glucagon.[17] Farivar et al showed that intraperitoneal infusion of 16 complement fixation units of A-59 murine hepatitis virus into young mice resulted in the death of more than 80 per cent of the animals within two days, the remainder within four days.[31] Continuous infusion of glucagon and insulin combined, starting immediately after infection with the virus, more than doubled the mean survival time and led to the complete recovery of 40 per cent of the mice. In contrast, insulin alone had a modest effect, and glucagon none. When treatment was delayed for 24 hours, mean survival in the mice treated with both hormones, though less than in the former group, was still significantly enhanced and 15 per cent of the animals recovered. The mechanisms involved are unclear. The hepatic necrosis at 24 hours was much less severe in the treated animals than in the untreated controls, suggesting that the hormones exerted an early protective action. In addition, they probably promoted recovery from hepatitis through the stimulation of hepatic regeneration. Whether any combination of insulin and glucagon, or any other 'hepatotrophic' factors, has a role to play in the treatment of patients with massive liver cell necrosis remains to be seen. Certainly a great deal more experimental animal work needs to be done before any study in man can be undertaken.

Haemodialysis

Results of the treatment of fulminant hepatic failure by routine haemodialysis have been disappointing,[11] although a recent review suggests that the available data are too scanty to justify this conclusion.[12] A recent report by the King's College Hospital group, using polyacrylonitrile-membrane haemodialysis, has been encouraging. Twenty-four patients with fulminant hepatic failure and Stage 4 coma were treated by repeated periods of haemodialysis. Nine fully recovered consciousness, eight of them (33 per cent) surviving. These workers compared their results from using this form of haemodialysis with the results obtained, with conservative treatment alone, in their previous experience (15 per cent survival in 53 patients), and with those obtained initially with charcoal haemoperfusion (38 per cent). Encouraging results have also been obtained by Opolon.[73] Further studies will be needed before a final assessment of this form of treatment can be made.[102] The use and potential of various artificial liver support systems have been reviewed recently.[12]

CONCLUSION

The clinical syndrome of fulminant hepatic failure is easily recognized but its treatment still poses many problems. The final assessment of any new form of therapy for which increased survival rates are claimed must include a prospective controlled trial, as has been emphasized by Chalmers.[22] Such trials can be carried out only in centres where sufficient numbers of patients are seen to make them possible. Thus far, all forms of 'special' treatment assessed in this way have been found wanting.

REFERENCES

1. Abelev, G.I. (1968) Production of embryonal serum α-globulin by hepatomas: review of experimental and clinical data. *Cancer Research,* **28,** 1344–1350.
2. Abouna, G.M., Serrou, B., Boehmigh, H.G., Amemiya, H. & Martineau, G. (1970) Long-term hepatic support by intermittent multi-species liver perfusions. *Lancet,* **ii,** 391–396.
3. Adams, R.D. & Foley, J.M. (1949) Neurological changes in more common types of severe liver disease. *Transactions of the American Neurological Association,* **74,** 217–219.

4. Aguirre, A., Yoshimura, N., Westman, T. & Fischer, J.E. (1974) Plasma amino acids in dogs with two experimental forms of liver damage. *Journal of Surgical Research,* **16,** 339–345.
5. Akeyama, T., Koyama, T. & Kameda, T. (1972) Alpha-fetoprotein in acute hepatitis. *New England Journal of Medicine,* **287,** 989.
6. Alam, A.N., Wilkinson, S.P., Poston, L., Moodie, H. & Williams, R. (1977) Intracellular electrolyte abnormalities in fulminant hepatic failure. *Gastroenterology,* **72,** 914–917.
7. Alexander, M., Kirsch, R.E., Purves, L. & Saunders, S.J. (1977) Alpha foetoprotein in liver disease: Groote Schuur Hospital Experience 1975–1976. *South African Medical Journal* (in press).
8. Bailey, R.J., Wolff, I.L., Cullens, H. & Williams, R. (1976) Metabolic inhibition of polymorphonuclear leucocytes in fulminant hepatic failure. *Lancet,* **i,** 1162–1163.
9. Baldessarini, R.J. & Fischer, J.E. (1973) Serotonin metabolism in rat brain after surgical diversion of portal venous circulation. *Nature New Biology,* **245,** 25–27.
10. Bass, N.M., Kirsch, R.E., Tuff, S.A. & Saunders, S.J. (1976) Plasma ligandin: a sensitive index of experimental hepatic necrosis. *Abstracts of the Twenty-Seventh Annual Meeting of the American Association for the Study of Liver Diseases, Chicago, 1976. Gastroenterology,* **71,** A-2/895.
11. Benhamou, J.-P., Rueff, R.L. & Sicot, C. (1969) Severe hepatic failure: a critical study of current therapy. In *Liver and Drugs* (Ed.) Orlandi, F. & Jezequel, A.M., pp. 213–228. London and New York: Academic Press.
12. Berk, P.D., Martin, J.F., Scharschmidt, B.F. & Plotz, P.D. (1976) Current status of artificial hepatic support systems. In *Progress in Liver Disease* (Ed.) Popper H. & Schaffner, F., pp. 398–417. New York: Grune & Stratton.
13. Biebuyck, J., Mans, A. & Saunders, S.J. (1977) Unpublished observations.
14. Bloomer, J.R., Waldmann, T.A., McIntire, K.R. & Klatskin, G. (1975) Relationship of serum alpha-fetoprotein to the severity and duration of illness in patients with viral hepatitis. *Gastroenterology,* **68,** 342–350.
15. Bloomer, J.R., Waldmann, T.A., McIntire, K.R. & Klatskin, G. (1977) Serum alpha-fetoprotein in patients with massive hepatic necrosis. *Gastroenterology,* **72,** 479–482.
16. Breen, K.J. & Schenker, S. (1972) Hepatic coma: present concepts of pathogenesis and therapy. In *Progress in Liver Disease, 4* (Ed.) Popper, H. & Schaffner, F., pp. 301–332. New York: Grune & Stratton.
17. Bucher, N.L.R. & Swaffield, M.N. (1975) Regulation of hepatic regeneration in rats by synergistic action of insulin and glucagon. *Proceedings of the National Academy of Science of the United States of America,* **72,** 1157–1160.
18. Burnell, J.M., Dawborn, I.K., Epstein, R.B., Gutman, R.A., Leinbeck, G.E., Thomas, E.D. & Volwiler, W. (1967) Acute hepatic coma treated by cross-circulation or exchange transfusion. *New England Journal of Medicine,* **276,** 935–943.
19. Caroli, J., Opolon, P., Scotto, J., Hatchouel, P.E., Thomas, M. & Langeron, A. (1971) Éléments de prognostic au cours des cohas par atrophie hépatique aiguë. *Presse Médicale,* **79,** 463–466.
20. Caronna, J., Shaw, D., Cartlidge, N., Knill-Jones, R. & Plum, F. (1975) The outcome of medical coma: prediction by bedside assessment of physical signs. *Transactions of the American Neurological Association,* **100,** 25–29.
21. Casey, T.H., Summerskill, W.H.J. & Orvis, A.L. (1965) Body and serum potassium in liver disease. I, Relationship to hepatic function of associated factors. *Gastroenterology,* **48,** 198–207.
22. Chalmers, T.C. (1976) A shortage of reliable data. *New England Journal of Medicine,* **294,** 721–722.
23. Colombi, A. (1970) Early diagnosis of fatal hepatitis. *Digestion,* **3,** 129–145.
24. Conomy, J.P. & Swash, M. (1968). Reversible decerebrate and decorticate postures in hepatic coma. *New England Journal of Medicine,* **278,** 876–879.
25. Curzon, G., Kantamaneni, B.D., Winch, J., Rojas-Bueno, A., Murray-Lyon, M. & Williams, R. (1973) Plasma and brain tryptophan changes in experimental acute hepatic failure. *Journal of Neurochemistry,* **21,** 137–145.
26. Davison, G.N.K., Davies, S.H., Darg, A. & Richmond, J. (1969) Coagulation factors in chronic liver disease. *Journal of Clinical Pathology,* **22,** 199–204.
27. Demeulenaere, L., Barbier, F. & Vermeire, P. (1969) Plasmapheresis in hepatic coma. (Letter) *Lancet,* **i,** 152–153.
28. Doddsworth, J.M., James, J.H., Cummings, M.C. & Fischer, J.E. (1974) Depletion of brain norepinephrine in acute hepatic coma. *Surgery,* **75,** 811–820.
29. Ducci, H. & Katz, R. (1952) Cortisone, ACTH and antibiotics in fulminant hepatitis. *Gastroenterology,* **21,** 357–374.
30. Eiseman, B., Liem, D.S. & Raffucci, F. (1965) Heterozogous liver perfusion in treatment of hepatic failure. *Annals of Surgery,* **162,** 329–345.
31. Farivar, N., Wands, J.R., Isselbacher, K.J. & Bucher, N.L.R. (1976) Effect of insulin and glucagon on fulminant murine hepatitis. *New England Journal of Medicine,* **295,** 1517–1519.
32. Felig, P., Brown, V., Levine, R.A. & Klatskin, G. (1970) Glucose homeostasis in viral hepatitis. *New England Journal of Medicine,* **283,** 1436–1440.
33. Fischer, J.E. (1974) Occurrence of false neurotransmitters. *Proceedings of an International Symposium on Artificial Support Systems for Acute Hepatic Failure. Artificial Liver Support* (Ed.) Williams, R. & Murray-Lyon, I.M., pp. 31–50. Tunbridge Wells: Pitman Medical.
34. Fischer, J.E. & Baldessarini, R.J. (1971) False neurotransmitters and hepatic failure. *Lancet,* **ii,** 75–80.
35. Fischer, J.E. & Baldessarini, R.J. (1976) Pathogenesis and therapy in hepatic coma. In *Progress in Liver Disease, V* (Ed.) Popper, H. & Schaffner, F., pp. 363–397. New York and London: Grune & Stratton.
36. Fischer, J.E., Funovic, J.M., Aquirra, J.H., Keane, J.M., Westdorp, R.I.C., Yoshimura, N. & Westman, T. (1975) The role of plasma amino acids in hepatic encephalopathy. *Surgery,* **78,** 276–290.
37. Fischer, J.E., Rosen, H.M., Ebeid, A.M., James, J.H., Keane, J.M. & Soeters, P.B. (1976) The effect of normalization of plasma amino acids on hepatic encephalopathy in man. *Surgery,* **80,** 77–91.
38. Flock, E.V., Lock, M.A., Grundley, J.H., Mann, F.C. & Bollman, J.L. (1953) Changes in free amino

acids in brain after total hepatectomy. *Journal of Biological Chemistry*, **200**, 529–536.

39. Gazzard, B.L., Clark, R., Borirakchanyavat, V. & Williams, R. (1974) A controlled trial of heparin therapy in the coagulation defect of paracetamol-induced hepatic necrosis. *Gut*, **15**, 89–93.
40. Gitler, R.E. (1962) Spontaneous hypoglycaemia. *New York Journal of Medicine*, **62**, 236–250.
41. Gitlin, D. & Boesman, M. (1967) Sites of serum alpha-fetoprotein synthesis in the human and in the rat. *Journal of Clinical Investigation*, **46**, 1010–1016.
42. Gocke, D.J. (1971) Fulminant hepatitis treated with serum containing antibody to Australia antigen. (Letter) *New England Journal of Medicine*, **284**, 919.
43. Goresky, C.A., Livingstone, A.S., Potvin, M., Finlayson, M.H. & Hinchey, E.J. (1977) Changes in the blood brain barrier in hepatic coma following hepatectomy. Reported at *Conference on Fulminant Hepatic Failure, Bethesda*.
44. Hannid, A., MacKenzie, R.L., Mellon, P.J., Davis, M., Silk, D.B.A. & Williams, R. (1977) Cerebral oedema in an experimental model in fulminant hepatic failure: effect of corticosteroids. Reported at *Conference on Fulminant Hepatic Failure, Bethesda*.
45. Hickman, R., Saunders, S.J., King, J.B., Harrison, G.G. & Terblanche, J. (1971) Pig liver perfusion in the treatment of fulminant hepatic necrosis. *Scandinavian Journal of Gastroenterology*, **6**, 563–568.
46. Hickman, R., Parker, J.R., Saunders, S.J. & Terblanche, J. (1972a) Platelet adherence in the pig liver perfused with human blood. *Transplantation*, **13**, 195–196.
47. Hickman, R., Parker, J.R., Saunders, S.J., Goodwin, N.E. & Terblanche, J. (1972b) Heterologous liver perfusion: a comparison of the use of livers from four different species. *British Journal of Surgery*, **59**, 881–884.
48. Houvani, B.T., Hamlin, E.M. & Reynolds, T.B. (1971) Cerebrospinal fluid glutamine as a measure of hepatic encephalopathy. *Archives of Internal Medicine* (Chicago), **127**, 1033–1036.
49. Iber, F.L., Rosen, H., Levenson, S.M. & Chalmers, T.C. (1957) The plasma amino acids in patients with liver failure. *Journal of Laboratory and Clinical Medicine*, **50**, 417–425.
50. Iob, V., Coon, W.W. & Sloan, M. (1966) Altered concentrations of free amino acids from the plasma of patients with cirrhosis of the liver. *Journal of Surgical Research*, **6**, 233–239.
51. Iob, V., Mattson, W.J. Jr, Sloan, M., Coon, W.W., Turcotte, J.G. & Child, G.C. III. (1970) Alterations in plasma-free amino acids in dogs with hepatic insufficiency. *Surgery, Gynecology and Obstetrics*, **130**, 794–801.
52. Jones, E.A., Clain, D., Klink, H.M., MacGillivray, M. & Sherlock, S. (1967) Hepatic coma due to acute hepatic necrosis treated by exchange transfusion. *Lancet*, **ii**, 169–172.
53. Juggi, J.S. (1971) Haemoperfusion through cation exchange columns in the treatment of ammonia intoxication in dogs. *Proceedings of the Society for Experimental Biology and Medicine*, **137**, 39–42.
54. Karvountzis, G. & Redeker, A.G. (1974) Relation of alpha-fetoprotein in acute hepatitis to severity and prognosis. *Annals of Internal Medicine*, **80**, 156–160.
55. Karvountzis, A.A., Redeker, A.G. & Peters, R.L. (1974) Long term follow-up studies of patients surviving fulminant viral hepatitis. *Gastroenterology*, **67**, 870–877.
56. Katz, R., Velasco, M., Klinger, J. & Allesandri, H. (1962) Corticosteroids in the treatment of acute hepatitis in coma. *Gastroenterology*, **42**, 258–265.
57. Kew, M.C., Purves, L.P., Branch, W.R. & Behrson, I. (1973) Alpha-fetoprotein during hepatocellular regeneration. In *Liver* (Ed.) Saunders, S.J. & Terblanche, J., pp. 320–321. London: Pitman Medical.
58. Kirsch, R.E., O'C Frith, L. & Saunders, S.J. (1976) Stimulation of albumin synthesis by keto analogues of amino acids. *Biochimica et Biophysica Acta*, **442**, 437–441.
59. Kirsch, R.E., O'C Frith, L. & Saunders, S.J. (1977) Unpublished observations.
60. Klebanof, G. (1973) Early experience with total body washout for hepatic coma. (Abstract) *Gastroenterology*, **64**, 156.
61. Knell, A.J., Davison, A.R., Williams, R., Kantameni, B.B. & Curzon, S. (1974) Dopamine and serotonin metabolism in hepatic encephalopathy. *British Medical Journal*, **i**, 549–551.
62. Lepore, M.J. & Martel, A.J. (1970) Plasmapheresis with plasma exchange in hepatic coma. Methods and results in five patients with acute fulminant hepatic necrosis. *Annals of Internal Medicine*, **72**, 165–174.
63. Lepore, M.J., McKenna, P.J., Martinez, D.B., Stuttman, L.J., Bonanno, C.A., Conklin, E.F. & Robilotti, J.G. Jr (1972) Fulminant hepatitis with coma successfully treated by plasmapheresis and hyperimmune Australia-antibody-rich plasma. *American Journal of Gastroenterology*, **58**, 381–389.
64. Liehr, J. (1977) As reported at *Conference on Fulminant Hepatic Failure, Bethesda*.
65. Lucké, B. (1944) The pathology of fatal hepatitis. *American Journal of Pathology*, **22**, 471–593.
66. MacDougall, B.R.D., Bailey, R.J. & Williams, R. (1977) H_2-receptor antagonists and antacids in the prevention of acute gastrointestinal haemorrhage in fulminant hepatic failure. *Lancet*, **i**, 617–619.
67. Maddrey, W.C., Weber, F.L., Coulter, A.W., Chura, C.M., Chapanis, N.P. & Walser, M. (1976) The effects of keto analogues of essential amino acids on portal systemic encephalopathy. *Gastroenterology*, **71**, 190–195.
68. Mashford, M.L., Mahon, W.A. & Chalmers, T.C. (1962) Studies of the cardiovascular system in the hypotension of liver failure. *New England Journal of Medicine*, **267**, 1071–1074.
69. Mattson, W.J. Jr, Iob, V., Sloan, M., Coon, W.W., Turcotte, J.G. & Child, G.C. III. (1970) Alteration of individual free amino acids in brain during acute hepatic coma. *Surgery, Gynecology and Obstetrics*, **130**, 263–266.
70. McMenamy, R.H., Vang, J. & Trapanas, T. (1965) Amino acid and alphaketoacid concentration in plasma and blood of the liverless dog. *American Journal of Physiology*, **29**, 1046–1052.
71. Miller, L.L. (1962) The role of the liver and non-hepatic tissue in the regulation of free amino acid levels in the blood. In *Amino Acid Pools* (Ed.) Holden, J.T., pp. 716–717. Amsterdam: Elsevier.
72. Miller, D.J., Saunders, S.J., Hickman, R. & Terblanche, J. (1975) Acute hepatic necrosis: a review of causes and management of fulminant hepatic failure. In *Gastroenterology, V* (Ed.) Reid, A., pp. 64–90. London: Butterworth.
73. Opolon, P. (1977) Personal communication.

74. Parbhoo, S.P., James, I.M., Ajdukiewicz, A., Xanalatos, C., Kennedy, J., Chalstrey, L.J., Brock, P.J., Sayer, P. & Sherlock, S. (1971) Extra corporeal pig liver perfusion in the treatment of hepatic coma due to fulminant hepatitis. *Lancet*, **i**, 659–665.
75. Parkes, J.D., Sharpestone, P. & Williams, R. (1970) Levodopa in hepatic coma. *Lancet*, **ii**, 1341–1343.
76. Percy-Robb, I.W., Proffitt, J. & Whitby, L.J. (1970) Precautions adopted in the clinical chemistry laboratory as a result of an outbreak of serum hepatitis affecting hospital staff. *Journal of Clinical Pathology*, **23**, 751–756.
77. Peters, R.C. & Edmondson, H.A. (1970) Fulminant hepatitis, relationship of patient age to liver morphology. (Abstract) *Gastroenterology*, **58**, 289.
78. Plum, F. (1977) Personal communication.
79. Plum, F. & Hindfelt, B. (1976) The neurological complications of liver disease. In *Handbook of Clinical Neurology, 27, Metabolic and Deficiency Diseases in the Nervous System* (Ed.) Vinken, B.J. & Bruyn, G.W. in collaboration with Klawans, H.L., pp. 349–377. New York: American Elsevier Publishing.
80. Posner, J.B. & Plum, F. (1960) The toxic effects of carbon dioxide and acetazolamide in hepatic encephalopathy. *Journal of Clinical Investigation*, **39**, 1246–1258.
81. Purves, L.R. & Geddes, E.W. (1972) A more sensitive test for alpha-fetoprotein. *Lancet*, **i**, 47–48.
82. Rake, N., Pannell, G., Flute, P.T. & Williams, R. (1970) Intravascular coagulation in acute hepatic necrosis. *Lancet*, **i**, 533–537.
83. Record, C.O., Buxton, C.E., Chase, R.A., Curzon, G.E., Murray-Lyon, I.M. & Williams, R. (1976) Plasma and brain amino acids in fulminant hepatic failure and their relationship to hepatic encephalopathy. *Finnish Journal of Clinical Investigation*, **6**, 387–394.
84. Redeker, A.G. (1974) Fulminant hepatitis. In *The Liver and Its Diseases* (Ed.) Schaffner, F., Sherlock, S. & Carroll, L., pp. 149–155. New York: International Medical Book Corporation.
85. Redeker, A.G. & Yamahiro, H.S. (1973) Controlled trial of exchange-transfusion therapy in fulminant hepatitis. *Lancet*, **i**, 3–6.
86. Reinicke, V., Friis, T. & Mullertz, S. (1963) Respiratory alkalosis and decreased oxygen saturation of arterial blood in patients with acute and chronic hepatitis. *Scandinavian Journal of Clinical and Laboratory Investigation*, **15**, 29–36.
87. Reynolds, T.B. (1969) Exchange transfusion in fulminant hepatic failure. Editorial in *Gastroenterology*, **56**, 170–171.
88. Ritt, D.J., Whelan, G., Werner, D.H., Eigenbrodt, E.H., Schenker, S. & Combes, B. (1969) Acute hepatic necrosis with stupor or coma: an analysis of 31 patients. *Medicine* (Baltimore), **48**, 151–172.
89. Robert, D., Caillat, B., Paliard, P., Motin, J. & Bolot, J.F. (1974) Les facteurs du prognostic de l'insuffisance hépatique aiguë grave. *La Nouvelle Presse Médicale*, **3**, 1207–1210.
90. Roche-Sicot, J., Sicot, C., Peignoux, M., Bourdian, D., Degos, G., Degos, J.-D., Prandi, D., Rueff, B. & Benhamou, J.-P. (1974) Acute encephalopathy in the rat: the effect of cross circulation. *Clinical Science and Molecular Medicine*, **47**, 609–615.
91. Rueff, B. & Benhamou, J.-P. (1973) Acute hepatic necrosis and fulminant hepatic failure. *Gut*, **14**, 805–815.
92. Ruoshlahti, E. & Seppälä, M. (1972) Alpha-fetoprotein in normal human serum. *Nature* (London), **235**, 161–162.
93. Samson, R.I., Trey, C., Timme, A.H. & Saunders, S.J. (1967) Fulminant hepatitis with recurrent hypoglycaemia and haemorrhage. *Gastroenterology*, **54**, 291–300.
94. Saunders, S.J. (1977) Unpublished observations.
95. Saunders, S.J. & Terblanche, J. (1975) Prognosis in acute hepatic failure. In *Artificial Liver Support* (Ed.) Williams, R. & Murray-Lyon, I.M., pp. 217–222. London: Pitman Medical.
96. Saunders, S.J., Hickman, R., MacDonald, R. & Terblanche, J. (1972) The treatment of acute liver failure. In *Progress in Liver Diseases* (Ed.) Popper, H. & Schaffner, F., pp. 333–344. New York and London: Grune & Stratton.
97. Saunders, S.J., Dowdle, E.B.D., Fiskerstrand, C., Bassendine, M. & Walls, R. (1977) Unpublished observations.
98. Saunders, S.J., Terblanche, J., Bosman, S.C.W., Harrison, A.A., Walls, R., Hickman, R., Biebuyck, J., Dent, J., Pearce, S. & Barnard, C.N. (1968) Acute hepatic coma treated by cross-circulation with a baboon and by repeated exchange transfusions. *Lancet*, **ii**, 585–588.
99. Sen, P.K., Bhalerao, R.A., Parulkar, G.P., Samsir, A.B., Shah, B.K. & Kinare, S.G. (1966) Use of isolated perfused cadaveric liver in the management of hepatic failure. *Surgery*, **59**, 774–781.
100. Sherlock, S. (1975) Acute (fulminant) hepatic failure. In *Diseases of the Liver and Biliary System*, 5th ed., pp. 107–121. Oxford: Blackwell Scientific Publications.
101. Sherlock, S. & Parbhoo, S.P. (1971) The management of acute hepatic failure. *Postgraduate Medical Journal*, **47**, 493–498.
102. Silk, D.B.A., Hanid, M.A., Trewby, P.N., Davies, M., Chase, R.A., Langley, P.T., Mellon, P.J., Wheeler, P.G. & Williams, R. (1977) Treatment of fulminant hepatic failure by polyacrylonitrile-membrane haemodialysis. *Lancet*, **ii**, 1–3.
103. Slapak, M., Beaudoin, J.G., Lee, H.M. & Hume, D.M. (1970) Auxiliary liver homotransplantation. A new technique and evaluation of current techniques. *Archives of Surgery*, **100**, 31–41.
104. Stabenau, J.R., Warren, K.S. & Rall, D.P. (1959) The role of pH gradient in the distribution of ammonia between blood and cerebro-spinal fluid, brain and muscle. *Journal of Clinical Investigation*, **38**, 373–383.
105. Stanley, N.N. & Cherniak, N.S. (1976) Effect of liver failure on the cerebral circulatory and metabolic responses to hypoxia in the goat. *Clinical Science and Molecular Medicine*, **50**, 15–24.
106. Stanley, N.N., Kelsen, S.G. & Cherniak, N.S. (1976) Effect of liver failure on the ventilatory response to hypoxia in man and the goat. *Clinical Science and Molecular Medicine*, **50**, 25–35.
107. Stanley, N.N., Salisbury, B.G., McHenry, L.C. & Cherniak, N.S. (1975) Effect of liver failure on the response of ventilation and cerebral circulation to carbon dioxide in man and in the goat. *Clinical Science and Molecular Medicine*, **49**, 157–169.
108. Summers, R.W., Curtis, S.J., Hartford, C.E. & Rubush, J.L. (1970) Acute hepatic coma treated by cross-circulation with irreversibly comatose donor. *Journal of the American Medical Association*, **214**, 2297–2301.

109. Swift, J.E., Ghent, W.R. & Beck, I.T. (1967) Direct transhepatic cross-circulation in hepatic coma in man. *Canadian Medical Association Journal,* **97,** 1435–1445.
110. Tobias, H. & Isom, W. (1973) Total body perfusion in the treatment of hepatic coma secondary to fulminant hepatitis (Abstract). *Gastroenterology,* **64,** 157.
111. Traeger, H.S., Gabuzdas, J., Ballow, A.N. & Davidson, C.S. (1954) Blood ammonia concentration in liver disease and liver coma. *Metabolism,* **3,** 99–109.
112. Trewby, P.M., Chase, R., Davis, M. & Williams, R. (1977) The role of the false neurotransmitter octopamine in the hypotension of fulminant hepatic failure. *Clinical Science and Molecular Medicine,* **52,** 305–310.
113. Trey, C. (1973) The fulminant hepatic failure surveillance study. In *Liver* (Ed.) Saunders, S.J. & Terblanche, J., pp. 120–121. London: Pitman Medical.
114. Trey, C. & Davidson, C.S. (1970) The management of fulminant hepatic failure. In *Progress in Liver Disease,* Vol. III (Ed.) Popper, H. & Schaffner, F., pp. 282–298. New York: Grune & Stratton.
115. Trey, C., Burns, D.G. & Saunders, S.J. (1966) Treatment of hepatic coma by exchange blood transfusions. *New England Journal of Medicine,* **274,** 473–481.
116. Trey, C., Lipworth, L. & Davidson, C.S. (1970) Parameters influencing survival in the first 318 patients reported to the Fulminant Hepatic Failure Surveillance Study (abstract). *Gastroenterology,* **58,** 306.
117. Trey, C., Lipworth, L., Chalmers, T.C., Davidson, C.S., Gottlieb, L.S., Popper, H. & Saunders, S.J. (1968) Fulminant hepatic failure. Presumable contribution of halothane. *New England Journal of Medicine,* **279,** 798–801.
118. Tyce, G.H., Flock, E.V., Owen, C.A., Stobie, E.H. & David, C. (1967) Five hydroxyindole metabolism in the brain after hepatectomy. *Biochemical Pharmacology,* **16,** 979–992.
119. Walser, M., Coulter, A.W., Dighe, S. & Crantz, F.R. (1973) The effect of keto analogues of essential amino acids in severe chronic uraemia. *Journal of Clinical Investigation,* **52,** 678–690.
120. Wardle, E.N. (1975) Endotoxin and acute renal failure. *Nephron,* **14,** 321–332.
121. Ware, A.J., D'Agostino, A.N. & Combes, B. (1971) Cerebral oedema: a major complication of massive hepatic necrosis. *Gastroenterology,* **61,** 877–884.
122. Wilkinson, S.P., Blendis, L.M. & Williams, R. (1974) Frequency and type of renal and electrolyte disorders in fulminant hepatic failure. *British Medical Journal,* **i,** 186–189.
123. Wilkinson, S.P., Gazzard, B.G., Arroyo, V., Moodie, H. & Williams, R. (1974) Relation of renal impairment and haemorrhagic diathesis to endotoxaemia in fulminant hepatic failure. *Lancet,* **i,** 521–524.
124. Wilkinson, S.P., Arroyo, V.A., Moodie, H., Blendis, L.M. & Williams, R. (1976) Abnormalities of sodium excretion and other disorders of renal function in fulminant hepatic failure. *Gut,* **17,** 501–505.
125. Williams, R. (1976) Hepatic failure and development of artificial liver support system. In *Progress in Liver Disease,* Vol. V (Ed.) Popper, H. & Schaffner, F., pp. 418–435. New York: Grune & Stratton.
126. Williams, R. (1977) Personal communication.
127. Willson, R.A., Webster, K.H., Hofmann, A.F. & Summerskill, W.H.J. (1972) Toward an artificial liver: in vitro removal of unbound and protein-bound plasma compounds related to hepatic failure. *Gastroenterology,* **62,** 1191–1199.
128. Willson, R.A., Winch, J., Thompson, R.P.H. & Williams, R. (1973) Rapid removal of paracetamol by haemoperfusion through coated charcoal. *Lancet,* **i,** 77–79.

Chapter 28

Acute Viral Hepatitis

RALPH WRIGHT
G.H. MILLWARD-SADLER

Jaundice is mentioned in the Babylonian Talmud and the writings of Hippocrates, but the first suggestion that it might be infectious in nature came from Pope Zacharias in the 8th century A.D.; he advised that patients with the jaundice should be separated to prevent spread of the contagion.[81] Although Herlitz in Göttingen and Sydenham in London had described epidemics of jaundice, and numerous outbreaks had occurred in the armed forces during the 17th, 18th and 19th centuries, the view was held by Eppinger as late as 1908 that all jaundice was obstructive in origin and due to catarrh in the large bile ducts.[123] McDonald[252] should be credited with first predicting that infective jaundice was produced by an agent smaller than a bacterium, and he postulated that it was due to a virus.

Lürman[234] reported the first recognizable outbreak of serum hepatitis following vaccination of dockers in Bremen with a batch of contaminated vaccine, and during the Second World War a series of outbreaks after the use of measles and yellow fever vaccine established beyond doubt that hepatitis could be spread by the parenteral route.

As a result of transmission experiments in human volunteers in the 1940s, two types of hepatitis were recognized:[235, 236, 237, 288, 389] virus hepatitis type A, which occurred sporadically or in small epidemics and could be transmitted both parenterally and by the faecal–oral route; and hepatitis type B, which was thought to be transmitted by inoculation only, and could progress to the carrier state. These studies were extended by Krugman and associates at the Willowbrook State School in the late 1950s and 1960s.[219] However, despite early claims, neither of the viruses was visualized or grown in tissue culture.

In 1965, Blumberg, Alter and Visnich,[50] when studying the Ag system of serum protein allotypes using a simple immunodiffusion technique, discovered a new precipitin line in the serum of an Australian aborigine. This antigen was unrelated to the Ag system, and was given the eponym 'the Australia antigen'. They subsequently showed that the antigen was present at high frequency in patients with leukaemia, as well as in children with Down's syndrome who were living in large institutions, but not in those who had not been institutionalized, suggesting an environmental factor. They noted that the presence of the antigen correlated with elevation of the serum transaminase levels and anicteric hepatitis on biopsy. This, and the chance development of hepatitis in a laboratory worker who became Australia antigen positive, led to the conclusion that the Australia antigen was associated with hepatitis.[51] Similar and apparently independent conclusions were reached by Prince[304] in New York and Okochi and Murakami[283] in Japan.

Since then, advances have been rapid. The Australia antigen has been characterized and its specific association with hepatitis B established. The development of techniques such as immune electron microscopy has led to the detection of hepatitis A virus in stool specimens. Sensitive serological techniques have been developed for the detection of antibody to hepatitis A, and it has been recognized that some cases of hepatitis are due to non-A non-B infections.

The whole subject of viral hepatitis has been recently reviewed in the Proceedings of the Second Symposium on Viral Hepatitis.[422]

TERMINOLOGY OF HUMAN HEPATITIS VIRUSES (after WHO Technical Report Series[401])

Hepatitis A Virus

HAV. A small virus in the range 25 to 28 nm, possessing cubic symmetry. Identified by immune electron microscopy and other serological tests.

Anti-HAV. Antibody to hepatitis A virus.

Hepatitis B Virus

HBV. The 42 nm double-shelled Dane particle, probably the complete virus.

HB_sAg. Hepatitis B surface antigen. Found on the surface of the Dane particle and on the accompanying unattached spherical 22 nm particles and tubular forms.

HB_cAg. Hepatitis B core antigen; the internal component of the Dane particle.

HB_eAg. The e antigen. Only present in HB_sAg positive sera and closely associated with infectivity.

Anti-HB_s. Antibody to hepatitis B surface antigen.

Anti-HB_c. Antibody to hepatitis B core antigen.

Anti-HB_e. Antibody to the e antigen.

Sub-determinants of hepatitis B surface antigen

The HB_sAg carries a common determinant and a number of sub-types coded by the virus genome and not by the host. These include *ayw*, *ayr*, *adw*, *adr*, *adyw* and *adyr*.

Sub-determinants of hepatitis B_e antigen

Three antigens have been identified. They are designated $HB_eAg/1$, $HB_eAg/2$ and $HB_eAg/3$.[421]

Other Hepatitis Viruses

Other forms of viral hepatitis, clinically indistinguishable from hepatitis type A or type B infection and antigenically unrelated to either, are being recognized (non-A non-B). In addition, several well recognized viral agents affect the liver to a lesser extent and will be dealt with separately. These include cytomegalovirus, Epstein–Barr (EB) virus, herpes virus, yellow fever virus, adenoviruses and enteroviruses, Lassa fever and the Arena viruses.

PROPERTIES OF HEPATITIS A VIRUS (see Table 28.1)

The development of serological techniques for the detection of hepatitis B led to similar attempts to find marker antigens or stool particles associated with hepatitis A. Del Prete, Constantino and Doglia[94] detected an antigen called the 'Milan' antigen by immunodiffusion, which they considered to be specific for hepatitis A, but subsequent studies showed it to be an abnormal lipoprotein unrelated to the virus. At about the same time, Ferris and associates[132] in Australia detected viral particles in acute-phase stool specimens from patients presumed to have hepatitis A, but the results were not reproducible.

In 1973, Feinstone, Kapikian and Purcell,[130] using immune electron microscopy, visualized 27 nm particles in acute-phase stool specimens of two of four subjects inoculated with the MS-1 strain of hepatitis A virus. Faecal shedding of these particles could be demonstrated only in the acute phase, were not present in pre-inoculation specimens, and could be clumped only by hepatitis A convalescent sera. The particles were demonstrated at highest concentration in stools during the prodromal phase and

Table 28.1. *Properties of Hepatitis A Virus.*

25–28 nm particles with cubic symmetry.
'Full' and 'empty' particles.
Isolated from faeces, serum, bile and liver.
Buoyant density 1.48–1.23 g/ml. (Major density 1.34 g/ml.)
Three major polypeptides: 34 000; 25 500 and 23 000 daltons.
RNA or single-stranded DNA but sensitive to RNAse.
Resistant to inactivation by ether, heating at 60°C, acid pH and storage in the cold.
Inactivated by formaldehyde heated at 37°C for 72 hours and ultraviolet irradiation.
Behaves like an enterovirus resembling poliovirus.

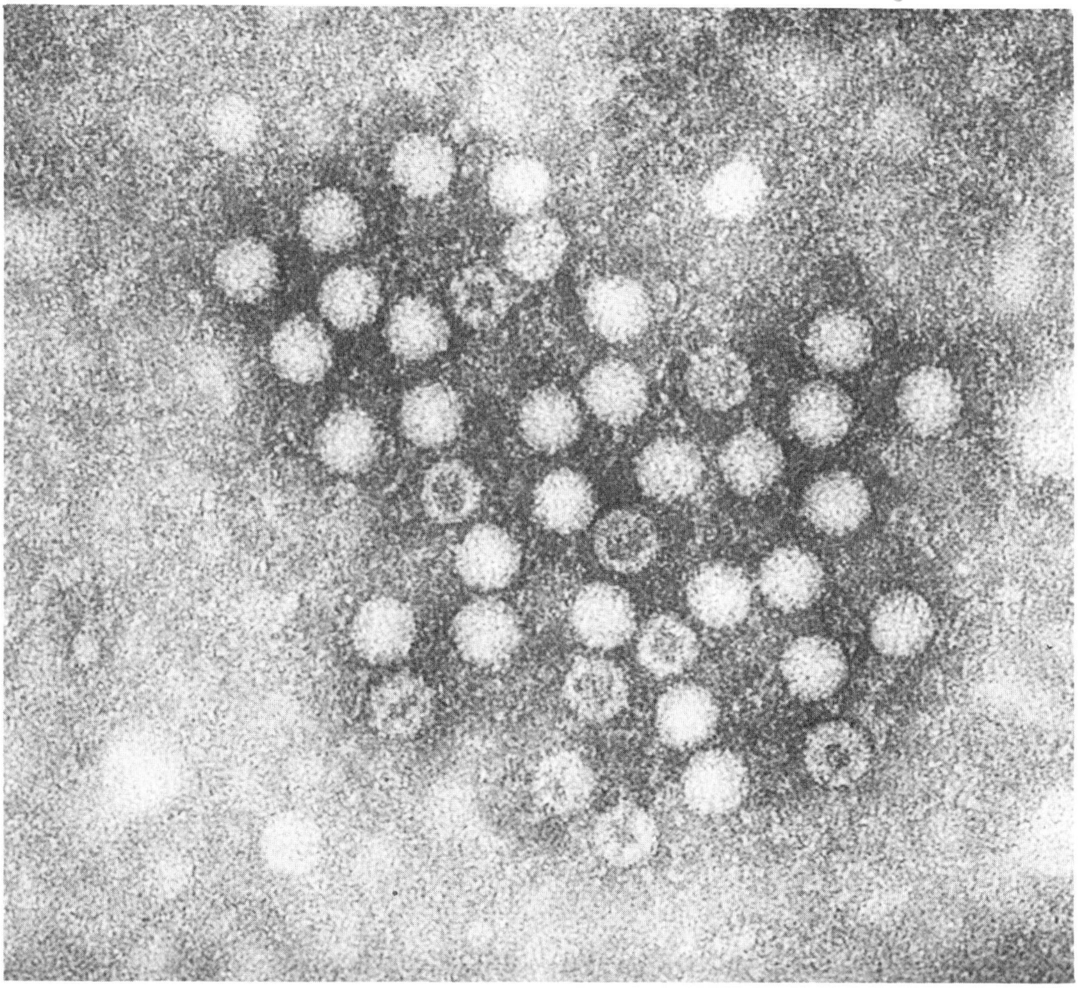

Figure 28.1. Hepatitis A virus showing both full and empty particles. The particles measure 26 to 28 nm in diameter. × 300 000. Electron micrograph from a series by Anthea Thornton and A.J. Zuckerman, London School of Hygiene and Tropical Medicine.

for five days before the onset of jaundice at peak aminotransferase levels, and disappeared during the late acute or early convalescent phase.[101] Antibody, as detected by clumping of these particles, could be demonstrated in sera obtained during well-documented hepatitis A epidemics, experimentally acquired MS-1, and Joliot Prison infections, but not with pre-inoculation specimens or individuals with acute non-bacterial gastroenteritis.[317]

Despite reservations about the specificity of this approach, it is now clear that hepatitis A virus has been isolated and partially characterized from both faeces and serum in man, chimpanzees and marmosets, as well as from the liver of these animals.[58, 105, 262, 311, 333] The virus is approximately 27 nm in diameter (Figure 28.1), has cubic symmetry, structurally resembling RNA-containing picornaviruses and the DNA-containing parvoviruses. 'Full' particles unpenetrated by stain and 'empty' particles can be identified and are antigenically indistinguishable. There are three major particle sizes of 'light' and 'heavy' buoyant density, ranging from 1.48 to 1.23 g/ml (major density 1.34), which has led to the suggestion that they are parvoviruses. Further characterization has revealed three main polypeptides of molecular weight 34 000, 25 500 and 23 000 daltons, thus resembling enteroviruses. Preliminary studies suggest that the nucleic acid of HAV may be either RNA or single-stranded DNA, but it is sensitive to RNAse.

Together with the finding of virus-like particles in the cytoplasm of hepatocytes from marmosets and chimpanzees infected with

HAV, this favours a picornavirus. Until the nucleic acid and polypeptide composition is fully characterized biochemically, it remains uncertain to which viral class HAV belongs, but it has many of the characteristics of an enterovirus resembling poliovirus.

There have been limited studies of the effect of physical changes on its infectivity. It appears to be relatively resistant to inactivation by ether, heating at 60°C for one hour and acid at pH 3. It is not destroyed by storage in the cold and non-ionic detergents do not alter its morphology, but it can be inactivated by formaldehyde solution (0.25 ml/l) heated for 72 hours at 37°C.[311]

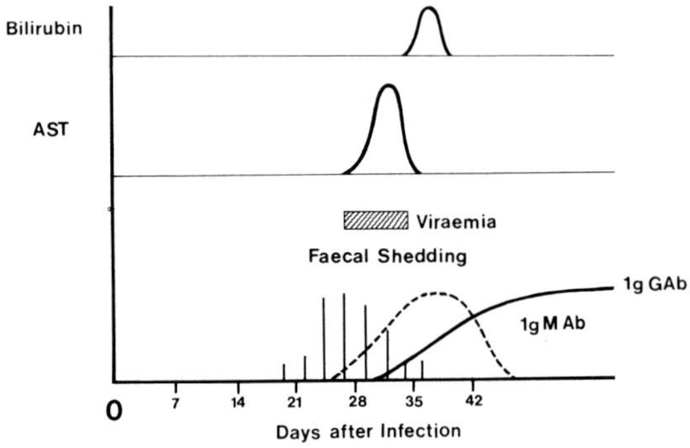

Figure 28.2. Sequence of events after hepatitis A infection.

Laboratory Techniques for the Detection of Hepatitis A Infection

Hepatitis A antigen and antibody can be detected in stools or serum by several techniques. Their widespread application has been limited by the shortage of specific antigen, since this can only be obtained from stools during the acute phase of the illness in man or from the livers or stools of infected animals.

Immune electron microscopy

Although this was the initial technique used for the detection of HAV in stools and remains the only specific method for demonstrating the viral particles, it is too time-consuming for routine screening for antibody.

Complement fixation, immune adherence haemagglutination and radio-immunoassay

Using liver extract from marmosets infected with HAV as a source of antigen, complement fixation[310] and immune adherence haemagglutination techniques (IAHA)[257] have been developed for the detection of anti-HAV in serum. The specificity of the reaction was checked by immune electron microscopy. IAHA depends on the agglutination of human or other primate erythrocytes by specific antigen or antibody in the presence of complement. It is simple to perform, more sensitive than complement fixation, and has been useful in sero-epidemiological studies. However, it requires purified antigen and the caesium chloride used may cause methodological problems. IAHA detects anti-HAV only in the late convalescent stage, whereas the other techniques detect the increases in IgM antibody which occur earlier.

Solid-phase radio-immunoassay (RIA) is potentially the most useful technique for detecting both HAV antigen and antibody. With microtitre plates and ^{125}I-IgG labelled anti-HAV, sensitive and specific techniques have been developed, using chimpanzee or marmoset liver and acute-phase human stools as a source of HAV. For detecting anti-HAV, either blocking techniques[318] or direct coating of the wells with the test serum[180] can be used.

A range of techniques is therefore available for the detection of HAV antigen and antibody in the liver, stools and body fluids of patients and experimental animals with hepatitis A. They are proving useful for studying the epidemiology of hepatitis A and assessing the purity of preparations of HAV. There is now direct evidence that hepatitis A virus appears early in the prodromal phase of the infection, is associated with a transient viraemia, but is usually undetectable in stools or serum once jaundice has appeared. The sequence of events after infection with HAV is summarized in Figure 28.2.

Hepatitis A in Experimental Animals

Despite numerous attempts to culture hepatitis A and claims of success, no consistent results have been achieved. Much effort has therefore been directed at finding an animal model, and it is now clear that certain species of marmosets and chimpanzees are susceptible.

Deinhardt and colleagues[93] transmitted hepatitis to marmosets with the acute-phase human serum GB, and this was confirmed by several other laboratories. However, it differed in certain physical characteristics from the agent in human sera transmitting hepatitis A. Subsequently, this group and others have been able to transmit hepatitis to marmosets using acute-phase sera from children, Joliot Prison volunteers infected with MS-1 virus, or serum from patients in Costa Rica (CR 326) during a natural outbreak of what appeared to be hepatitis A by epidemiological criteria. Serologically, neutralization experiments and the development of specific anti-HAV indicate that the hepatitis produced in marmosets by these three sources is hepatitis A. Furthermore, antisera raised in guinea pigs to human stool-derived HA Ag and marmoset liver-derived HA Ag indicate that they are serologically identical, and that there is apparent homogeneity of HA Ag derived from different sources[105] so that there seems to be only one serotype. By contrast, the hepatitis produced by the GB agent in marmosets is serologically distinct from hepatitis A, and its relationship to human hepatitis is controversial.

Although there was some suggestion from early transmission experiments that chimpanzees were susceptible to hepatitis A and there was indirect evidence of spread from animals to man, conclusive evidence had to await the development of techniques for detecting anti-HAV. It then became apparent that almost all captured chimpanzees have anti-HAV, but transmission has been achieved with animals born and reared in captivity. Such chimpanzees have been inoculated with human stools containing HAV and have subsequently developed hepatitis. The hepatitis is mild, appears 19 to 21 days after inoculation and HAV can be demonstrated in bile, stools and the liver cell cytoplasm by electron microscopy and by radioimmunoassay.[338] Virus particles can be found in faeces nine to 14 days after infection and persist up to the 28th day; antibody appears at the time of transaminase elevation while virus is still being excreted, and thereafter persists.[379] Both groups have found the major density for HAV particles to be 1.34 g/cm^3, which is similar to that in man. There is a close, if not identical, morphological and serological relationship between human and chimpanzee hepatitis A.

PROPERTIES OF HEPATITIS B VIRUS

Electron microscopy of serum containing hepatitis B shows three specific particles: small spherical 22 nm particles first detected in HBV positive sera by Bayer, Blumberg and Werner,[31] tubular or filamentous forms of varying length, and large spherical (Dane) particles 43 nm in diameter.[91] The large Dane particle is thought to be the HB virus itself. It is double-shelled and usually contains a central hexagonal core (HB$_c$Ag) which is immunologically distinct from the outer coat (HB$_s$Ag) (Figure 28.3). The small spherical particles and tubules are probably excess viral protein coat material, which share antigenic determinants with the coat of the Dane particle.

Biophysical and Biochemical Properties of Hepatitis B (see Table 28.2)

The HB$_s$Ag is remarkably resistant to heating, freezing and thawing, treatment with Tween 80 and changes in pH. There is no loss of antigenic activity after heating at 56°C, but antigenicity is lost by heating at 85°C for 60 minutes, by reduction of disulphide bonds and by treatment with butanol. Antigenicity is also impaired by digestion with faeces, intestinal homogenates[293] and certain bacteria.[251]

Anti-HB$_s$ provides passive immunity, so that there has been much interest in the structure of HB$_s$Ag and the antigenicity of its components, with the object of developing a vaccine. There is general agreement that, despite structural diversity, the small particles, the tubular forms and the surface coat of the Dane particle have similar biochemical and biophysical properties. Most attempts at purification have used the more readily available small (22 nm) particles isolated by rate zonal centrifugation on caesium chloride (CsCl) and sucrose density gradients. The HB$_s$Ag has lipoprotein and carbohydrate components, but purified preparations reveal particles varying in size from 17 to 25 nm, with considerable heterogeneity in surface charge, morphology and molecular weight.[110, 143] Since the HB$_s$Ag may contain host components, it is important to try to determine which of the antigenic components are specified by the viral genome and which are host-derived. Normal serum protein constituents have often been found to be associated in variable amounts with the particles purified from serum.[339] Various procedures, including low pH treatment prior to the first CsCl gradient and antibody-coated, immunoabsorbent columns, have been used to dissociate serum components from such particles, as well as to remove anti-HB$_s$. A number of the polypeptides isolated from HB$_s$Ag are immunogenic in experimental animals, but even

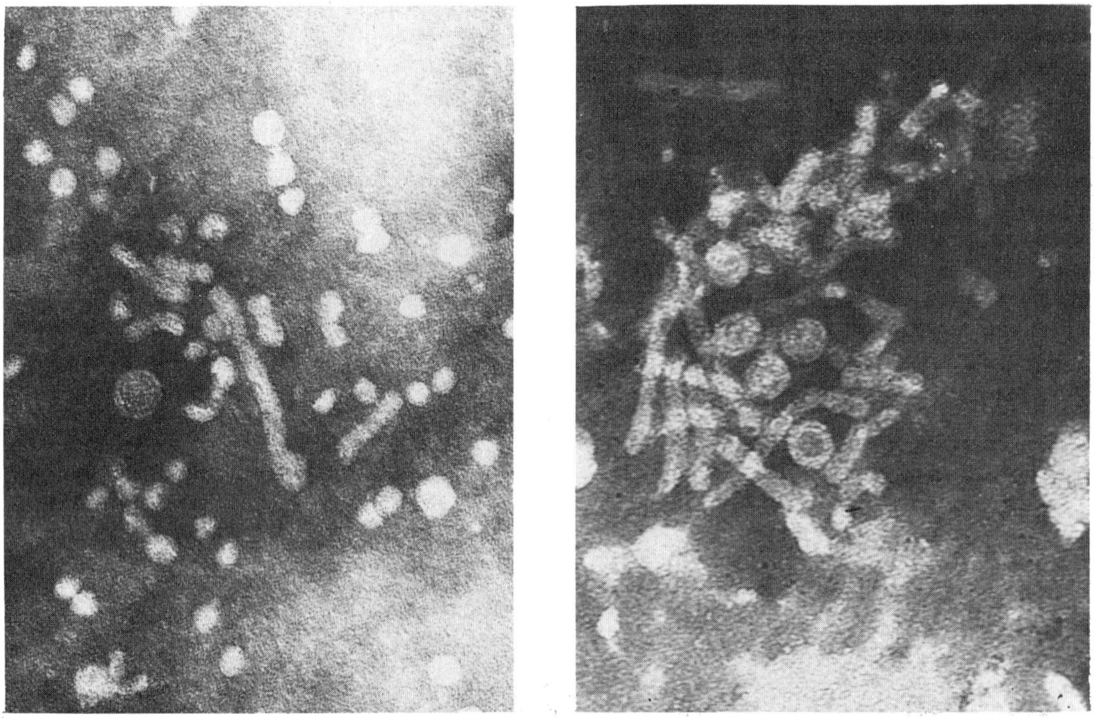

Figure 28.3. Hepatitis B surface antigen in serum. On the left, numerous small spherical particles (19 to 20 nm) predominate and on the right long filamentous particles (40 to 45 nm) are seen. Dane particles are present in both but are most frequent on the right where an 'empty' Dane particle can also be identified.

low molecular weight polypeptides may contain antigenic determinants related to human serum protein.[65]

Seven to nine polypeptides have been shown to be associated with 22 nm particles and they range in molecular weight from 19 000 to 120 000 daltons. Three of these polypeptides are glycoproteins. In addition, HB_sAg contains cholesterol, polar lipids and glycolipids; 3.6 to 6.5 per cent of the antigen is carbohydrate. According to one study buoyant density and molecular weight differ between the two main sub-types of HB_sAg (see below). The *adw* sub-type has a buoyant density of 1.21 g/ml and the *ayw* sub-type a buoyant density of 1.17 g/ml.[110] This has not been confirmed by subsequent studies.[326]

The amino acid composition of HB_sAg particles has been compared with that of known animal viruses and an uninfected mammalian cell lysate. This has shown that the amino acid composition of HB_sAg can differ markedly from known animal viruses and mammalian cells, particularly in terms of the high levels of cystine, proline, leucine and phenylalanine.[110] This supports the view that HB_sAg is a viral product resulting from HBV infection.

Recently, Petersen and associates[292] have isolated two major polypeptides from purified small particles of the *adw* sub-type by acrylamide gel electrophoresis in the presence of sodium dodecyl sulphate. The two polypeptides have molecular weights of 22 000 and 28 000 daltons respectively, and their amino acid content is similar to that of the intact surface antigen. Their difference in molecular weight is apparently due to the addition of a carbohydrate moiety to the second polypeptide. The 22 000-dalton major component is immunogenic when injected into guinea pigs, whereas if carbohydrate is present, as in the 28 000 molecular weight glycopeptide, an antibody response is not induced, thus abrogating the immunogenicity of the major polypeptide. This conflicts with earlier studies which suggest that the carbohydrate moiety is associated with specific antigenic determinants.

It seems likely that the low molecular weight polypeptides are transcribed by the viral genome and that the higher molecular weight components are derived from the host. The wide variation in polypeptide sizes in different studies of HB_sAg particles, all of which contain the same antigenic determinants, has not been described with other viruses, and has led to the suggestion that this might result from

Table 28.2. *Properties of Hepatitis B Virus.*

HB_sAg

Isolated from blood, other body fluids and liver-cell cytoplasm.
Small, spherical, 22 nm particles.
Tubular forms (filaments) 22 nm diameter, variable length.
Envelope of Dane particle.

Buoyant density 1.17–1.21 g/ml.
7–9 polypeptides molecular weight 19 000–120 000 daltons.
2 major polypeptides 22 000–28 000 daltons.
Total size 350 000–494 000 daltons.

Glycoprotein, lipid and carbohydrate with host protein components.
No nucleic acid.
Resistant to heating at 56°C, freezing, thawing, pH changes and ether extraction.
Sensitive to heating at 85°C, butanol, digestion with faeces.

Dane particle

Isolated from serum.
43 nm with central hexagonal core.

Buoyant density:
'full' particles 1.25 g/ml.
'empty' particles 1.20 g/ml.

Molecular weight 1.6×10^6 daltons.
Envelope stripped by detergents.

HB_cAg

Isolated from serum and liver.
27–28 nm hexagonal.

Buoyant density 1.30–1.32 g/ml.

DNA: Dane cores
homogeneous
double-stranded
molecular weight 1.6×10^6 daltons
DNA polymerase present.

Liver cores
heterogeneous
double-stranded
molecular weight 1×10^6 daltons
DNA polymerase absent.

proteolytic degradation of HB_sAg by proteases in serum.[238, 327] Further study of the way in which these polypeptides arise and their exact amino acid sequence is required.

Hepatitis B Sub-types

During the early studies of the Australia antigen, Levene and Blumberg[226] described an additional specificity which they could detect using an antiserum produced in rabbits by the injection of serum from a particular patient with leukaemic reticuloendotheliosis, and which they referred to as Au2. The antigenic heterogeneity of the HB_sAg was confirmed by Le Bouvier,[222, 223] who identified a shared antigenic specificity, *a*, and two mutually exclusive determinants, *d* and *y*, all specimens being either *ad* or *ay*. Subsequently, two additional specificities, *w* and *r*, were described.[25]

Thus there are four major sub-types of HB_sAg (*adw, ayw, adr* and *ayr*) which are specified by distinct genotypes of the virus. However, several additional sub-types have been described, although it is not certain whether these are all determined by the viral genome or whether they reflect the host's reaction.

The HB_sAg sub-types are proving useful in epidemiological studies, and show a striking geographical distribution (Figure 28.4), but they are not directly related to infectivity or severity.

Hepatitis B Core Antigen

Almeida and associates[12] treated pellets from serum rich in Dane particles with 0.5 per cent Tween 80 and released the internal component or core, which could then be specifically clumped by a particular convalescent serum. The core particle, whether obtained from Dane particles in serum or from liver homogenate, reacts with specific antibody. The antibody can be shown by immunofluorescence or immunoperoxidase to react specifically with components in the liver cell nucleus. It therefore forms an antigen/antibody system distinct from that associated with the HB_sAg and its sub-types.

The core particles can be purified at a density of 1.30 to 1.40 g/ml by banding on a CsCl gradient or by rate zonal centrifugation on sucrose.[188, 327] This variation in density may depend upon the source of the particles and whether they are contaminated with HB_sAg. Three major and several minor polypeptide components up to 80 000 daltons in size have been isolated.[327] The core particles are 27 to 28 nm in diameter, have a hexagonal shape with capsomeres and spikes projecting from the surface.

DNA Particle Structure and DNA Polymerase

Hirschman, Vernace and Schaffner[176] first demonstrated DNA polymerase activity in preparations of HB_sAg, and it was subsequently shown to be specific for the core particles. More recently, a double-stranded DNA has been isolated from core particles from human liver and serum.[175]

Irrespective of the method of purification

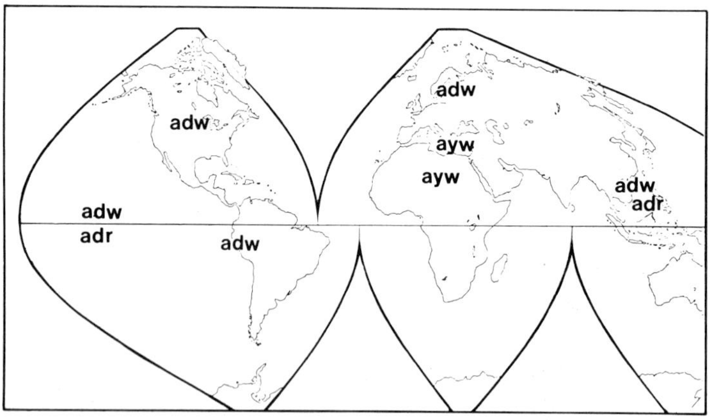

Figure 28.4. Geographical distribution of HB_sAg sub-types.

used, DNA polymerase activity is associated only with the core particles purified from serum but not from human or chimpanzee livers, despite the fact that core particles from liver contain double-stranded DNA.[175] The configuration of the double-stranded DNA, as demonstrated by electron microscopy, depends on the source of the core particles. It is circular in particles purified from human serum and linear in those from the nuclei of human hepatocytes. This raises the possibility that the DNA polymerase found in the Dane particle from serum may be added to the core particle during cytoplasmic maturation and that at the same time the DNA, which is linear in the nucleus of the hepatocyte, adopts a circular configuration.[326]

Another unusual feature of the core particles is that DNA polymerase activity cannot be stimulated by exogenous DNA. This suggests that the DNA polymerase of hepatitis B is specific for its own DNA. In this context it is also of interest that DNA polymerase activity has not been detected in the serum of patients with hepatitis A infection, and this supports the likelihood that it is an RNA virus.

Although it is likely that the Dane particle is the complete hepatitis B virion, its infectivity has not been tested directly and it is still possible that it is a defective virus. If the Dane particle is a complete virus, its uniquely small circular double-stranded DNA and DNA polymerase activity makes it unlike any known virus, and it could represent a new virus class. The double-stranded DNA in the core of the Dane particle from serum has a molecular weight of 1.6×10^6 daltons (2300 nucleotide pairs) and serves as a primer template for the DNA polymerase. This DNA polymerase is a specific marker for the Dane particles.

Recently, Robinson[327] has proposed that the Dane particle DNA molecules consist of a closed circular strand of constant inner length (strand a) and an inner open strand of variable length (strand b) (Figure 28.5). The endogenous DNA polymerase apparently uses the open strand as a primer and the single-stranded gap is closed during the reaction, resulting in a double-stranded DNA of 3200 nucleotide pairs.

HBV is unusual and even unique in several respects:

1. The vast excess of viral protein coat material produced.
2. It has a double-stranded DNA, the inner circle of which is incomplete for a third of its length and is closed by a virion enzyme during DNA synthesis.
3. Robinson[327] has suggested that Dane particles are genetically heterogeneous hepatitis B virions and in support of this concept cites evidence that hepatocytes may vary in their expression of HB_cAg and HB_sAg. Some hepatocytes may produce non-infectious HB_sAg only, others may produce HB_cAg only with or without HB_eAg, and others may produce all three components of the virion.

Hepatitis B_e Antigen and Antibody

A different antigen/antibody system was described by Magnius and Espmark[240] and given the designation e. It was visualized as a precipitin line between two HB_sAg positive sera, was immunologically distinct from the HB_sAg and HB_cAg systems, with different physicochemical properties from HB_sAg.[239] Three determinants have been described.[397, 421] To

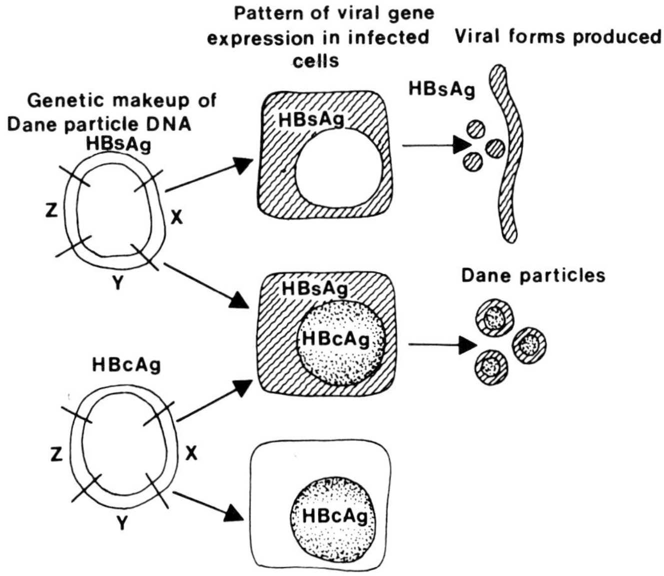

Figure 28.5. Model for replication of defective genetically heterogeneous hepatitis B virions. Dane particles may code for some but not all of the viral components. In the figure, two hepatitis B virions which code for either HB_sAg or HB_cAg as well as for XYZ are represented on the left. Production of Dane particles by a hepatocyte then requires infection by both virion sub-types. From Robinson,[327] with kind permission of the author and the editor of *Annual Review of Microbiology*.

date, e Ag has only been detected in HB_sAg positive sera. As will be discussed later, it appears to correlate with infectivity and with continuing liver damage, and may be a useful guide to prognosis. It is not related to HB_sAg or any of its sub-types, but correlates with the concentration of Dane particles, DNA polymerase activity and HB_cAg in both serum and liver-cell nuclei.[174,278,376] When the e antigen/e antibody system is correlated with subpopulations of Dane particles, namely 'full' particles which contain nucleic acid and DNA polymerase activity, and 'empty' particles without DNA polymerase activity, the majority of e antigen positive sera contain 'full' Dane particles with high DNA polymerase activity, whereas e antibody positive sera contain 'empty' Dane particles or lack Dane particles and have low or absent DNA polymerase activity.[6]

The nature of the e antigen and the mechanism of its formation are still obscure. It has been described as the DNA polymerase of HBV,[254] as an antigenic marker on the surface of the Dane particle or filamentous forms of HB_sAg[272] and as an abnormal isoenzyme of lactic dehydrogenase.[390] Neurath and Strick[271] have claimed that partially purified e antigen has the properties of an immunoglobulin predominantly of the IgG4 sub-class, but this has not been confirmed by others. Clearly some of these explanations are mutually exclusive, and it is still uncertain whether HB_eAg is carried by the viral genome or whether it is an abnormal host protein specifically related to hepatitis B infection.

Magnius[239,414] reported that HB_eAg had a density of 1.29 g/ml with a sedimentation coefficient of 11.6*s* and a molecular weight of 340 000 daltons. If this were so, it would be too large for HB_eAg to be transcribed by the virus. Alternatively, it is possible that HB_eAg represents a hapten or ligand[414] of relatively low molecular weight capable of a degree of self-association or association with serum components. Recent data from Tedder and Bull[378] indicate that this might be the case. These authors partially purified HB_eAg and showed that it behaved as a thermolabile sulphydryl-sensitive protein capable of associating non-specifically with other proteins and lipids, which might account for its heterogeneous physicochemical properties. They estimated that it had a minimal molecular weight of 68 000 daltons in serum and 10 000 daltons under dissociating conditions.

Serological Tests for Hepatitis B-associated Antigens

Hepatitis B surface antigen and antibody

HB_sAg and anti-HB_s were initially detected by a simple immunodiffusion technique. This method was also used for testing the specificity of anti-sera as well as for the detection of HB_sAg sub-types. More sensitive techniques were subsequently developed, including complement fixation, counter-immunoelectrophoresis and rheophoresis. They are cheap, relatively simple to perform, but are insensitive.

These techniques have now largely been replaced by various forms of radio-immuno-assay (RIA), haemagglutination or enzyme immunoassay. RIA is a sensitive and rapid method for the detection of both HB_sAg and anti-HB_s. Either solid-phase RIA or radio-immunoprecipitation is used, and after initial problems with specificity this is now a commonly used technique for screening, but it is expensive and requires the availability of a gamma counter, and the specificity needs to be checked by neutralization with unlabelled anti-HB_s or HB_sAg.[228]

Another widely used simple and sensitive technique is that of reversed passive haemagglutination, using erythrocytes coated with anti-HB_s. A variety of erythrocytes can be used, including human, turkey and sheep, but purity of reagents is important.[72] They are simply and rapidly performed but have limitations when testing for anti-HB_s and occasional false positives occur with HB_sAg because of heterophile agglutinins.

Recently, enzyme-linked immuno-absorbent assays (ELISA) have been developed whereby conjugates of enzyme and antibody degrade a suitable substrate with change in colour, which can be read spectrofluorometrically. These techniques require only relatively simple equipment, are of equal sensitivity to RIA and may have wider application in the future.[399]

Electron microscopy of serum with negative staining, with or without added antibody, is the most specific technique and shows a high degree of sensitivity in expert hands. However, it is too time-consuming for use other than as a research tool.

The clinical relevance of third-generation sensitive techniques such as RIA and haemagglutination depends on the circumstances in which they are employed. If tested early in the course of acute hepatitis, insensitive techniques such as immunodiffusion or complement fixation will have a similar detection rate to third-generation tests. However, the latter will detect a higher proportion of acute cases during convalescence and chronic carriers with low-titre HB_sAg. As will be discussed later, even these techniques are not infallible and it has been suggested that there is an additional need to detect anti-HB_c and DNA polymerase activity which may be positive in occasional sera infectious for HBV but which are HB_sAg negative.

The sensitivity of these techniques is compared in Table 28.3 and has been extensively reviewed.[27, 187, 313]

Sub-typing of hepatitis B surface antigen and antibody

The original micro-Ochterlony immuno-diffusion technique is still the simplest method for sub-typing, using specific anti-sera. The commonest technique used is a counter-immuno-electrophoretic method employing cross-absorbed monovalent reagents. Other techniques include passive haemagglutination and reverse passive haemagglutination. With all these methods, high-titre specific anti-sera are required.

Sub-typing can also be carried out by a double-label radio-immunoassay.[66]

Table 28.3. *Serological Techniques for Detecting Hepatitis B Antigens and Antibodies.*[a]

Technique	Relative sensitivity for detecting:					
	HB_sAg	Anti-HB_s	HB_cAg	Anti-HB_c	HB_eAg	Anti-HB_e
Agar gel immunodiffusion	+	+			+	+
Counter-immuno-electrophoresis	+	++	+	+		
Complement fixation	++	++	+	+		
Rheophoresis	++	++	+	+	+	+
Reversed passive latex agglutination	++					
Passive haemagglutination	++	+++				++
Immune adherence haemagglutination	+++	++	++	+++		
Immune electron microscopy	+++	+++	++	++		
Immunofluorescence microscopy	++	++	++	++		
Reversed passive haemagglutination	+++				+++	
Solid-phase radio-immunoassay	++++	++++	+++	++++	+++	+++
Radio-immunoprecipitation	++++	++++		++++		
Enzyme immunoassay	++++					

[a] After WHO Technical Reports.[400, 401]

Hepatitis B core antigen and antibody

Anti-HB_c is a useful marker of HBV replication. It develops early during the disease and persists with the carrier state. Some individuals have anti-HB_c but are HB_sAg negative, and anti-HB_c may therefore be a useful indication of recent infection.[191]

Techniques which have been developed for the demonstration of anti-HB_c include complement fixation, counter-immuno-electrophoresis and immunofluorescence using infected liver containing core particles as substrate. The most sensitive techniques for the detection of anti-HB_c are radio-immunoassays. One procedure uses core particles containing the tritiated DNA product of the DNA polymerase reaction of the radiolabelled antigen, another a solid-phase radio-immunoassay. These techniques are several hundred times more sensitive than complement fixation, and their use is being considered in screening.[152, 156, 261]

Hepatitis e antigen and antibody

Detection of this antigen is of particular importance because of its correlation with infectivity and the development of chronicity. It is confined to HB_sAg positive sera. At present only insensitive methods such as immunodiffusion and rheophoresis are generally available for its detection and high-titre antibody or antigen is required. Recently, radio-immunoassay[44, 412] and passive haemagglutination techniques have been developed for e and anti-e[377] which increase sensitivity. An association between the HB_eAg/anti-HB_e system and HB_sAg associated albumin binding sites has been reported[415] and it has been claimed that radio-immunoassay for the latter is a more sensitive indicator of infectivity than the HB_eAg.[420]

Hepatitis B in Experimental Animals

Attempts to produce hepatitis B in non-human primates were largely unsuccessful until serological markers of HBV infection became available. This can be explained by the mildness of the infection in susceptible animals and the fact that most animals used for transmission experiments in captivity had already acquired anicteric infection. For practical purposes, the only animals which can be used experimentally are chimpanzees. Some monkeys, including rhesus monkeys, are much less susceptible and do not develop liver damage.[29, 93]

It is necessary to select animals who have no serological markers of HBV. Up to 25 per cent of captive chimpanzees have serological evidence of previous infection and anti-HB_s rises sharply with age. The infection is usually acquired soon after capture and it is not known how frequently these animals develop hepatitis B in the wild.

The chimpanzee model closely resembles HBV infection in man with identical immunological markers, although the hepatic damage seems less severe. Each of the four major sub-types has been transmitted, the sub-type being the same in the infected animal as in the inoculum. Chimpanzee models are providing invaluable information about immunopathological mechanisms, infectivity and the efficacy of active and passive immunization and interferon treatment (see below; see also Chapter 29).

Immunological Response to Hepatitis B Infection

The availability of markers of HBV has provided the opportunity to study the sequence of events during the course of the infection.

The presence of HB_sAg, HB_cAg and HB_eAg, their humoral immune responses and, in the case of HB_sAg, cell-mediated immune responses have been investigated. Systematic observations of the sequence of the early events in man have been limited because patients present clinically only relatively late in the disease. Studies have therefore largely been limited to sera available from experimental transmission as in the Willowbrook Study or following inadvertent transfusion of infected blood or other inoculated material. Giles, McCollum et al[144] showed that the HB_sAg could be detected in serum within one month of exposure, and that it preceded elevation of the serum transaminase, which was first noted at two months. This was followed by studies of anti-HB_s and anti-HB_c using complement fixation or radio-immunoassay,[179, 182, 183, 316] DNA polymerase activity in serum as an index of viral replication,[204, 220] the HB_eAg[4, 241] and anti-HB_e.[4] The chimpanzee model has provided valuable confirmatory information.

Humoral responses

The following sequence of events occurs in a typical infection which is to proceed to a

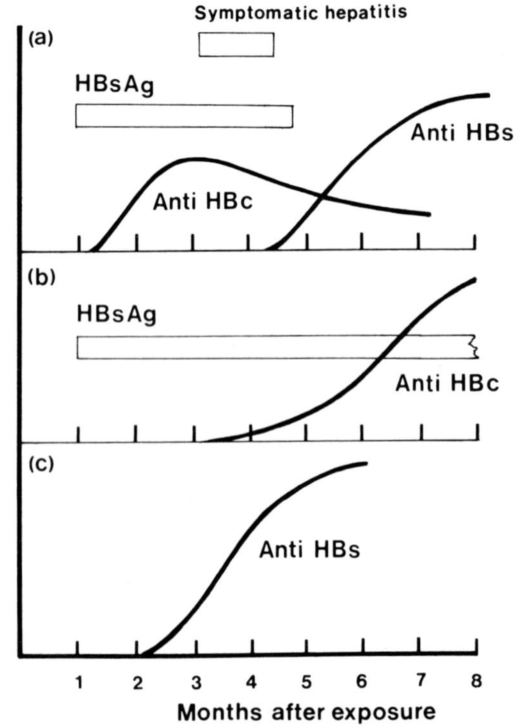

Figure 28.6. Sequence of events after HBV infections: (a) classic acute hepatitis B infection; (b) persistent infection with hepatitis B (carrier state); (c) primary antibody response to HB_sAg. From Wright,[404] with kind permission of Edward Arnold.

clinically overt attack (Figure 28.6; Table 28.4). HB_sAg is detected in the serum three to six weeks after a primary infection and several weeks before biochemical evidence of liver damage or clinical symptoms. HB_sAg persists during the prodromal phase and early acute illness, and is usually cleared from the blood stream during convalescence. Shortly afterwards, at four to eight weeks, DNA polymerase activity, anti-HB_c and the HB_eAg appear in the circulation. DNA polymerase activity and the HB_eAg persist through the prodromal phase and may or may not be present at the time of clinical presentation. Thus, there is evidence of viral replication with production of the HB_eAg and anti-HB_c before there is biochemical or clinical evidence of hepatitis. Anti-HB_c persists during the acute illness, the titre falling gradually during convalescence, long after disappearance of the HB_sAg. Anti-HB_c correlates with the extent and duration of viral replication. Anti-HB_s is the last to appear in the serum and is only detectable as antibody excess once HB_sAg has disappeared from the serum, although complexing with antigen may occur much earlier and the anti-HB_s response may be an important factor in eliminating HB_sAg from the serum. There may therefore be a period when neither HB_sAg nor anti-HB_s is detectable in the serum, and the presence of anti-HB_c may be the only indication of recent infection. Following a minor infection with transient, or possibly absent HB_sAg in serum, anti-HB_c may also be detectable only transiently or not at all. In some instances a primary antibody response to HB_sAg can occur without detectable anti-HB_c. Using a sensitive passive haemagglutination technique Aikawa et al[4] detected HB_eAg in all of seven patients with acute hepatitis early in the illness and some showed seroconversion to anti-HB_e before anti-HB_s became detectable (Figure 28.7; Table 28.4). DNA polymerase activity, the HB_eAg and anti-HB_c all point to continuing infection, although anti-HB_c usually persists for longer than DNA polymerase activity, the HB_eAg or HB_sAg itself. Anti-HB_c may therefore be a more useful marker of recent infection.[191] The highest titre of anti-HB_c is detected in chronic carriers with evidence of continuing replication of the virus.

A secondary response to re-exposure to HBV produces an anamnestic elevation of anti-HB_s titres. It has no effect on the anti-HB_c titres or on the development of DNA polymerase activity or HB_eAg. Similarly, after anti-HB_s is acquired by passive immunity, there is no DNA polymerase activity and anti-HB_c or HB_eAg are not detected (Figure 28.6).

Table 28.4. *Sequence of Events after Infection with Hepatitis B.*

Months after exposure	1	2	3	4	5	6	7	8
SGOT			+	+				
DNA polymerase	+	+	+					
HB_sAg	+	+	+	+				
e Ag	+	+	+					
Anti-HB_c		+	+	+	+	+		
Anti-HB_s					+	+	+	+
Anti-HB_e				+	+	+	+	+

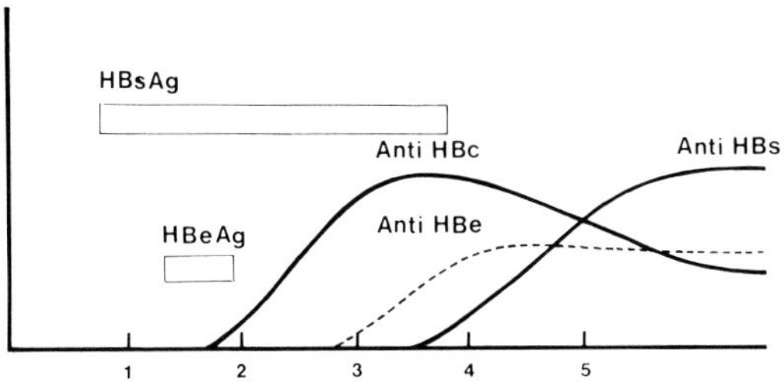

Figure 28.7. Sequence of events, in months, of HB_eAg and anti-e in relation to other HBV markers.

Cell-mediated responses

Cell-mediated responses to HB_sAg can be demonstrated by lymphocyte transformation and leucocyte migration inhibition. It is first detected in the late incubation period and prodromal phase, persists during the acute attack, becomes less pronounced during convalescence and disappears with recovery. It is also present in a proportion of patients with HB_sAg positive chronic active hepatitis, but invariably becomes negative in asymptomatic carriers. It has been suggested that these in vitro techniques reflect cell-mediated immunity to HB_sAg and are important in terminating infection with HBV. They may therefore play a role in the pathogenesis of the hepatic injury but the whole issue is controversial (see Chapter 29).

EPIDEMIOLOGY

As indicated in the previous section, the development of serological markers for hepatitis A and B infections has had a profound effect on our knowledge of the epidemiology of these diseases.

Hitherto, information was largely derived from transmission experiments or clinical studies or from the notification of clinically overt disease. Some of the earlier observations made over many years by such painstaking methods have been confirmed by new laboratory techniques, but it has become apparent that hepatitis B is much more common than was previously thought and its method of spread much more diverse. Furthermore, it is now clear that viruses distinct from hepatitis A and B can produce similar clinical syndromes and the whole subject is in the process of reassessment and review.

Epidemiology of Hepatitis A

This has been fully reviewed by Dienstag et al.[108] Hepatitis A has a worldwide distribution, but the true geographical incidence cannot be determined with accuracy. Studies of the prevalence of anti-HAV in blood donors show that it varies from 29 per cent (in Switzerland) to 90 per cent (in Israel and Yugoslavia), and indicate considerable geographical variation[374] (Figure 28.8). Furthermore, only 5 to 10 per cent of 18- to 19-year-olds in the United States and Switzerland have antibody, compared with over 90 per cent in Israel and Yugoslavia. This confirms reports based on case notification, which suggests an increasing age for acquiring hepatitis A in areas such as the United States. Nevertheless, in most communities the majority of cases occur in childhood. A seasonal incidence, with a peak in late autumn, is usually observed, but is disappearing in the United States.[63]

In most temperate countries, especially in relatively closed communities such as Greenland, hepatitis A occurs in epidemics every five to 25 years, but it is not clear whether the change in incidence being observed in the

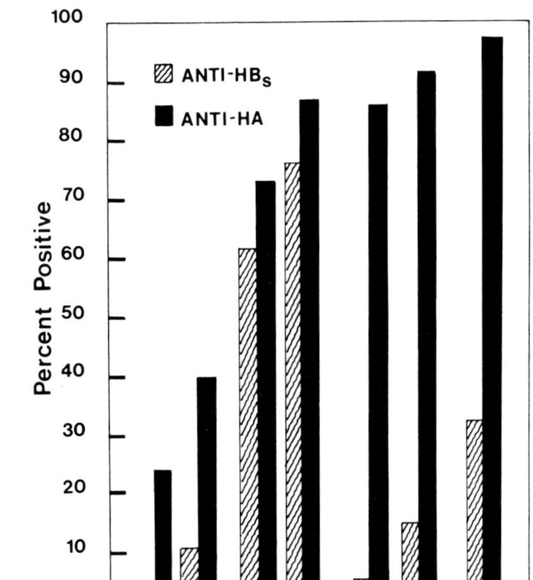

Figure 28.8. Relationships between prevalences of anti-HA and anti-HB_s in young adults by country. From Szmuness et al,[374] with kind permission of the authors and the editor of *American Journal of Epidemiology*.

United States is part of this pattern.[351, 355] It seems likely that it is hyperendemic in tropical countries, particularly in the developing countries where infection occurs at an early age due to poor hygiene. Similarly, in the United States the prevalence of anti-HBV is higher in the lower socio-economic groups, who are affected at an earlier age.[108, 401] In epidemics affecting soldiers, such as in North Africa during the Second World War, the attack rate was higher in the officers than in the enlisted men, suggesting that the latter have a higher degree of immunity, due to previous infection.

Methods of spread of hepatitis A

Documentation of the methods of spread of hepatitis A have been based on transmission experiments and studies of both sporadic and epidemic outbreaks in susceptible communities.[108]

Voegt showed that hepatitis with a short incubation period could be transmitted by duodenal juice.[389] The importance of the faecal–oral route as a mode of transmission was firmly substantiated by the transmission experiments of MacCallum and Bradley,[237] Krugman and associates[219] and others.[235, 236] The periods of infectivity ranged from 14 to 21 days before the onset of jaundice to the seventh or eighth day after jaundice, but were consistently negative thereafter, despite persistence of abnormal liver function tests. Based on these studies, the incubation period, that is the interval to the onset of first symptoms, ranged from 15 to 49 days. Clinical observations produce comparable figures; studies in general practice estimated an incubation period of 26 to 35 days[294] and point-source outbreaks similarly indicated an incubation period of four to six weeks for hepatitis A.[77, 103, 391]

These observations have been confirmed and extended by the direct examination of the shedding of hepatitis A in stools, using immune electron microscopy, and by measuring specific antibody to hepatitis A in serum in transmission experiments or in sporadic outbreaks of hepatitis A in man, as well as in experimental infection of chimpanzees with hepatitis A (Figure 28.2). Dienstag et al studied the pattern of faecal shedding of HA Ag detected by immune electron microscopy in Joliot Prison volunteers inoculated with the MS-1 strain of HAV.[101] Stool shedding of particles was observed 28 to 41 days after inoculation at the time of onset of prodromal symptoms, and peak elevation of the serum transaminase. In one study in chimpanzees faecal shedding of HA Ag was noted 15 to 51 days after intravenous or oral inoculation of infected stools, and correlated with the peak transaminase elevation and histological necrosis in the liver.[102] Anti-HA in serum developed 22 to 47 days after inoculation. Similar results were reported in four other chimpanzees.[379] Spread of infection most commonly occurs sporadically by the faecal–oral route as a result of direct contact. A chronic intestinal carrier state, if it occurs, is rare.[108]

On occasions, in a susceptible community, explosive epidemics can occur. For example, in Greenland in a recent epidemic 93 per cent of those affected were aged between one and 25 years, suggesting widespread immunity in the adult population, probably resulting from a similar epidemic documented in 1947–1948.[355] Similar epidemics have been traced to point-source contamination of food[77] or water supplies[391] and there has recently been serological confirmation of an outbreak of hepatitis A due to ingestion of incompletely cooked mussels contaminated by sewage.[104]

Other modes of spread of hepatitis A

Transient viraemia during the late incubation period and early icteric phase of hepatitis A has been documented repeatedly by transmission experiments or by the inadvertent transfusion of infected blood. Chronic viraemia or progression to chronic liver disease has not been established.

Although circumstantial evidence suggests that transmission by urine can occur, this mode of spread is infrequent and has not been documented directly. Similarly, there have been occasional reports of spread attributable to infected nasopharyngeal secretions, including a recent large food-borne outbreak.[227] This must be regarded as unproven. There is no evidence for an increased incidence in homosexuals, dialysis or multiply-transfused patients.[108]

Epidemiology of Hepatitis B

The facility to detect HBV-associated antigens, including HB_sAg and its sub-types, HB_cAg, HB_eAg and their respective antibodies, has had a profound effect on our understanding of the epidemiology of hepatitis B. This may be summarized as follows:

1. Inapparent inoculation is common.

2. Many infections which would previously have been attributed to hepatitis A are due to hepatitis B.
3. Anicteric infection and chronicity are common, and often established by vertical transmission.
4. There is a striking geographical variation in the carrier state, as well as in cirrhosis and hepatoma related to HBV.

More accurate information is available on the geographical distribution of hepatitis B and its methods of spread than of hepatitis A because of the frequency of the carrier state and the facility for serological testing for HB_sAg and its sub-types.

The prevalence of hepatitis B in the community will depend on a wide range of factors, including social customs such as tribal scarification, parenteral drug abuse and homosexuality, exposure to insect-borne vectors, and population density.

Additional factors to be discussed later facilitate the development of chronicity and the carrier state, including male sex, vertical transmission and immunodeficiency. Thus, in different populations there will be striking differences in the age of acquiring the infection and in whether it is predominantly rural or urban. In western communities it is predominantly urban, whereas in the developing countries it is common in the more primitive rural communities.

Although long-incubation-period acute hepatitis B has been recognized only relatively recently, studies of the carrier state in geographically isolated populations, such as in New Guinea, indicate that it has been well adapted to the human host for thousands of years, transmitted vertically, by scarification or possibly by insect vectors. Such factors play an important role in the widely differing incidence of the carrier state in the community (Table 28.5; see also Chapter 29). Not surprisingly, hepatitis B therefore does not show the seasonal variation and cyclical epidemics that are observed with hepatitis A. For example, in Greenland, hepatitis A occurs in large epidemics 15 to 25 years apart, whereas hepatitis B is endemic.[355]

Table 28.5. *Distribution of HB_sAg in Non-hospitalized (Normal) Population.*[a]

Population	No. tested	HB_sAg positive (%)
North Americans	2412	0.1
Finns	924	0.1
Japanese	1034	0.5
Greeks	857	1.8
Aborigines (Aus.)	1807	2.1
Indians	127	2.4
Bantu (S.A.)	72	2.8
Cebu (P.I.)	764	4.8
Vietnamese	128	6.3
Micronesians	474	7.2

[a] After Blumberg, Sutnick and London.[51]

Sub-typing has provided information not only about spread within a community but also about spread from one community to another. Figure 28.4 illustrates the geographical distribution of HB_sAg sub-types predominant in particular communities. In a Canadian study of 63 symptom-free blood donors, some of whom had emigrated from abroad in childhood, the sub-type correlated with that predominating in their country of birth rather than in their country of domicile.[129] Similarly, retrospective typing of an epidemic in Sweden in 1953 showed it to be predominantly *ad*, which is the usual sub-type in Sweden, whereas another epidemic in 1972 was *ay*, suggesting that it had been introduced from abroad.[196]

Methods of Spread of Hepatitis B

Although spread by blood or blood products accounts for most cases of hepatitis B infection, other methods of spread remain a possibility. Estimates of the incubation period, that is the interval from contact to the first onset of symptoms, have been based on transmission experiments and observations of post-transfusion hepatitis. The period is considered to range from 60 to 180 days with a mean of 90 days.[410] Until methods for detection of the viruses of hepatitis A and B became available, the differences in the incubation period provided the main points of distinction. Some cases of transfusion-associated hepatitis, however, were found to have an incubation period of less than 60 days,[9, 213, 263] but although there are several possible explanations[410] it is most likely that these cases are due to non-A, non-B hepatitis (see below).

The explanation for the wide range of the incubation period is unclear. The size of the inoculum may be a factor but is not a crucial one as there is considerable variation in the incubation period whether HBV is spread by the transfusion of large volumes of blood or by the inoculation of small quantities, for example by needlestick or personal contact. More relevant may be the concentration of Dane particles and anti-HB_s in a particular inoculum. Nevertheless, repeat study of the icterogenic plasma pools and sequential samples of blood from transmission experiments with hepatitis B conducted in 1951–1954 indicate that dilution of the icterogenic pool before inoculation prolongs the time to the first detection of HB_sAg.[28]

It is possible that spread by a route other than inoculation may be associated with a longer incubation period and, in this context, it is of interest that the administration of the MS-2 (HBV) serum pool by mouth is associated with a longer period before elevation of the serum transaminase than when it is given parenterally.[144]

As discussed earlier, infectivity with HBV is maximal at the time of DNA polymerase activity and HB_eAg positivity early in the incubation period of the disease, during the prodromal phase and early clinical course, but may rarely persist as a chronic state.

Spread by blood or blood products

This method of spread was well established following outbreaks of hepatitis in clinics where inadequately sterilized syringes were used, in epidemics following inoculation with contaminated batches of serum or after transfusion with infected blood or blood products: hence the eponyms 'syringe jaundice', 'homologous serum jaundice' and 'transfusional hepatitis'. The use of disposable needles and syringes can eliminate this source of hepatitis unless these are re-used or, as in the case of hardline drug addicts, shared.

The high rate of drug abuse in western society in the late 1960s had an important impact on the epidemiology of viral hepatitis. In the United States this was accompanied by change in the age and sex incidence of hepatitis.[139] Sharing of needles is an important cause of spread of hepatitis B amongst addicts, but other features of their life-style are additional factors. Unusual sub-types of HBV are sometimes encountered because the hepatitis has been introduced from abroad.[395] It is not clear how frequently non-A, non-B hepatitis is responsible for the HB_sAg negative cases.

Scarification is presumed to be an important cause of spread in primitive communities, but the extent to which it contributes to the high frequency of HBV carriers in these communities is not certain. The association between tattooing and hepatitis B has been suspected since the 1950s and recently this has been documented by testing for HB_sAg, both icteric and anicteric cases having been observed, with spread resulting from shared needles or contaminated dye.[268] Infection may also occur following acupuncture. Hepatitis B may result from the accidental inoculation of minute quantities of blood when toothbrushes, razors and hair scissors are used communally. The sporadic hepatitis seen in Swedish track runners, well-documented epidemiologically, is now known to be usually due to hepatitis B, probably resulting from contaminated scrubbing brushes used for cleaning the legs after running.[37]

More controversial is the role of insect vectors which might be an important factor accounting for the high prevalence of hepatitis B in tropical communities. HB_sAg has been detected in mosquitoes[306] and bedbugs,[274] but there is no evidence that the virus replicates in these insects, although HB_sAg has been shown to persist for several weeks in the latter after they have been fed HBV artificially.

Post-transfusion hepatitis

During the Second World War it was recognized that hepatitis could be transmitted by the transfusion of blood or blood products.[35] The attack rate varied from less than 1 per cent to over 10 per cent, depending on the number of donors contributing to the pool with dried human plasma,[248] and in the case of the transfusion of whole blood bore a linear relationship to the number of units transfused, up to six units per patient.[263] Reported attack rates following blood transfusion varied in different countries, and was dependent on factors such as the source of donor blood and the duration of follow-up. In the United States, an incidence as high as 18 per cent has been reported[165] whereas in the United Kingdom it is less than 1 per cent.[253] In the United States, a cooperative study defined a risk which ranged from 0 to 8.6 per 100 patients and confirmed a high risk with transfused blood obtained from commercial donors and a correlation with the volume of blood transfused.[153]

The mortality rate following post-transfusion hepatitis has also varied, from less than 1 per cent to over 20 per cent in elderly patients.[9] It has been estimated that there were 30 000 cases of post-transfusion hepatitis in the United States in 1963 with nearly 3600 deaths.

Hepatitis has also occurred after the administration of other blood derivatives such as commercially prepared plasma fractions and such preparations have also been shown to be contaminated with HB_sAg.[38, 181, 184, 337, 411] These include clotting factor concentrates, cryoprecipitates and fibrinogen including radio-iodinated fibrinogen used in the diagnosis of deep vein thrombosis.[221] The clotting factor concentrates which are most likely to transmit hepatitis are factors II, VII, VIII, IX and X.[194, 282, 360] This may have serious consequences, particularly in haemophiliacs who may develop chronic liver disease after repeated treatment with factor VIII or IX concentrates.[360] Hepatitis is particularly likely to occur with factor VII preparations and its use is therefore restricted. Although albumin fractions were initially thought to be safe, it seems likely that they too may be contaminated with HB_sAg.[181]

From retrospective analyses of the incidence of post-transfusion hepatitis following the use of frozen red blood cells, and one prospective study, these cells were thought to be free of hepatitis risk.[385] This has been questioned following the demonstration of HBV infections in chimpanzees transfused with frozen deglycerolized red blood cells previously inoculated with HBV.[19] Clearly, further prospective studies of the safety of this preparation are needed.[76]

As will be indicated later, screening of donor blood for HB_sAg has only partly decreased the frequency of post-transfusion hepatitis. It is unlikely that hepatitis A, EB virus or cytomegalovirus contributes significantly to post-transfusion hepatitis and the majority of cases, particularly in the United States, are now thought to be due to non-A, non-B viruses (see below).

Haemodialysis and transplantation-associated hepatitis

The dangers of viral hepatitis in association with haemodialysis were not appreciated in the early 1960s when this technique was first introduced until several outbreaks were reported, including some deaths among members of staff.[242]

Once routine testing for HB_sAg became established, it was clear that infection was widespread within many dialysis units, that staff were more severely affected than patients who usually had a mild illness or were asymptomatic, and that there was a high secondary attack rate in the relatives of patients undergoing haemodialysis.[73, 231, 297, 386] For example, in a survey of 583 patients and 451 medical personnel, in 15 haemodialysis centres in the United States, HB_sAg was detected in 16.8 per cent of patients and 2.4 per cent of staff and anti-HB_s in 34 per cent of patients and 31.3 per cent of staff respectively. Sixty-one per cent of family contacts of dialysis patients with a history of hepatitis B infection had one or other of these markers.[371] These studies suggest that although haemodialysis patients may not have overt liver disease, they are likely to transmit more severe infection to contacts, including family members, than do other carriers of the HB_sAg such as blood donors.

The higher infectivity of haemodialysis patients compared to other HB_sAg carriers has been confirmed serologically. In one study almost all the HB_sAg positive haemodialysis patients had HB_eAg and DNA polymerase activity in their serum whereas none of the other carriers had them.[68] A high incidence of HB_eAg in dialysis patients has been confirmed by Miller and co-workers.[255]

The high frequency of dialysis-associated hepatitis B occurs in many European countries as well as in the United States but is now relatively uncommon in the United Kingdom since the introduction of regular screening for HB_sAg (see below).[242]

Although hepatitis B is often introduced into dialysis units by patients who have had previous blood transfusions, cross-infection within units is the chief means of perpetuating hepatitis B.[296] Spread to staff occurs in a variety of ways as a result of contact with patients' blood, usually by inapparent inoculation. There is some evidence that airborne spread may also occur.[14] It is possible that transplantation of an infected kidney may spread hepatitis B although this is not an important cause. The methods of spread of hepatitis in dialysis units and to the household contacts have been thoroughly reviewed.[242, 400]

Although some cases of dialysis-associated hepatitis do not have HBV markers, there is little evidence to implicate hepatitis A.[373] They could, however, be due to non-A, non-B hepatitis.

The outcome of the liver disease in patients who have HB_sAg in their circulation before or after renal transplantation has been variable. In one recent report, there was a fivefold increase in deaths from hepatic failure in HB_sAg positive patients compared with those who were negative[295] although this had not been found in previous studies.[365]

Spread by inapparent inoculation of blood or other body fluids.

The occurrence of sporadic cases of hepatitis in the contacts of patients with serum hepatitis led to the suggestion that spread of hepatitis B might occur other than by inoculation.[59, 260] This was reinforced by the early Willowbrook transmission experiments, in which it was shown that the administration of the MS-2 serum pool by mouth could produce long incubation period hepatitis.[219]

The use of HB_sAg and its sub-types as markers of HBV infection has provided evidence that close personal contact is a common method of spread. Furthermore, testing of body fluids other than blood for HB_sAg has provided indirect evidence to suggest other vehicles of transmission.

Detection of HB_sAg in body fluids other than blood

The possibility that hepatitis B might be transmitted by routes other than those involving overt or inapparent inoculation of serum has led to a search for its presence in other body fluids. Although there is good evidence that hepatitis B can be acquired by the ingestion of the virus by mouth, faecal spread has not been established and could not be achieved in the early transmission experiments. It was therefore of special interest to examine stools and intestinal secretions for HB_sAg. Using immunodiffusion, counter-electrophoresis or radio-immunoassay, HB_sAg and anti-HB_s have been detected in stools of patients with acute viral hepatitis by several groups.[160, 280, 384] HB_sAg was detected both in acute and in chronic hepatitis B, but not in controls or patients with other forms of liver disease. It sometimes persisted in the stools for longer than in the serum.

It is also of interest that faeces and intestinal homogenates,[293] as well as certain bacteria,[251] reduce the antigenicity of HB_sAg by the reduction of disulphide bonds. The antigen has also been detected in bile, where the titre in gallbladder bile is equal to that in the serum, but reports of its presence in duodenal juice have been conflicting, possibly due to the intestinal inhibitor mentioned above.

HB_sAg has been detected in the urine by a number of techniques including immune electron microscopy.[46] The significance of the detection by Heathcote, Tsianides and Sherlock[171] of a urinary substance in patients with acute hepatitis B and their household contacts is uncertain since it has not been clearly shown to be associated with HB_sAg. HB_sAg has also been demonstrated in saliva,[393] in semen[170, 229] and in breast milk.[96]

Clearly, the detection of HB_sAg in body fluids other than blood may be relevant to the possibility of spread by ingestion, venereal spread, vertical transmission and airborne spread, but it must be emphasized that it is difficult to exclude contamination by small quantities of blood in these body fluids and that detection of the HB_sAg does not necessarily imply infectivity. More relevant would be a study of Dane particles, DNA polymerase activity and the HB_eAg.

Contact-associated hepatitis B

Early epidemiological studies indicated that, unlike hepatitis A, spread of hepatitis B by close personal contact was unusual and secondary attack rates were rare in outbreaks of hepatitis following the use of contaminated vaccine.[260] Nevertheless, in the 1940s it was suspected that such spread could occur, for example between spouses and in institutions for the mentally retarded. This has been amply documented by the testing for HB_sAg of contacts of patients with hepatitis B. The e antigen/antibody status is probably highly relevant to transmission. In one series, none of the husbands of women with anti-e developed HBV infections.[354]

Spread by close personal contact is most likely to occur (a) between spouses or other sexual contacts, including prostitutes and homosexuals, and (b) between children, particularly those in institutions for the mentally retarded and family members with prolonged contact.

Spread to a spouse is most common when the primary case has acute viral hepatitis. For example, Koff et al[214] tested prospectively 98 household contacts of 42 patients with acute hepatitis B, and found that three of 13 spouses or sexual partners developed evidence of HBV infection, whereas none of 68 parents, siblings or other household contacts did so. This accords with observations of other workers who have recorded a high incidence in the spouses of patients undergoing haemodialysis[287] or with acute hepatitis B.[264]

The situation regarding the families of carriers is conflicting. In some studies, a higher incidence has been found among siblings of patients than among their spouses, possibly indicating vertical transmission from the mother,[368] whereas in other studies sexual partners have shown the higher incidence.[170]

The importance of sexual spread has been emphasized by studies of the presence of HBV markers in prostitutes and homosexuals.[138, 171, 198, 372] Furthermore, a high incidence of HB_eAg, implying infectivity, has been recorded in male homosexuals.[350] The precise mechanism of spread is uncertain, although true venereal spread during sexual intercourse is a possibility. Salivary spread may be more significant.[388] Although non-parenteral spread of hepatitis B may occur, when epidemics of hepatitis B have been reported, for example in military institutions, it has been difficult to know how many cases were due to unconfessed drug abuse.[8]

Hepatitis B in institutions

It has been recognized for many years that there is a high prevalence of viral hepatitis in institutions for the mentally retarded and this has led to the study of such patients with a view to the development of a hepatitis vaccine.[219]

Several important facts about the epidemiology of hepatitis B have emerged from the examination of patients and staff in such institutions. Although there is variation in the prevalence of HBV markers between institutions, it is usually much higher than in the general population. The frequency of HBV markers increases with the duration of stay in the institution and is greater in patients than in staff although the latter also have an increased incidence (Figure 28.9). The HB_sAg carrier rate in mongols is considerably greater than that for other mentally retarded patients.[52, 210, 367, 369] This is probably due to a defective antibody response and to impaired cell-mediated immunity resulting in a more prolonged carrier state since all patients are equally exposed.[367, 369] The patients in mental institutions often develop anicteric infections; for example none of 26 children who developed HBV markers after admission to one institution were clinically jaundiced.[369]

Mentally retarded carriers, particularly mongols, are more likely to have HB_eAg and less likely to have anti-e than other carriers. Of 26 mentally retarded HB_sAg carriers, 12 had HB_eAg (Figure 28.9) and none had anti-e whereas only one of 50 blood donors or antenatal carriers who were HB_sAg positive had HB_eAg as tested by immunodiffusion.[209] The high frequency of HBV markers is probably due to recurrent exposure by the non-parenteral route, the HB_eAg positive carriers acting as a potent reservoir of infection.

Outbreaks of hepatitis B have also been described in other institutions such as a tuberculosis unit.[133] In this outbreak, 11 of 37 HB_sAg positive patients were jaundiced, a high proportion became carriers and spread occurred to domestic and medical staff as well as to household contacts, particularly spouses.

Hepatitis in medical personnel

The extent to which medical and health care personnel, other than those working in dialysis units or the institutions mentioned above, have

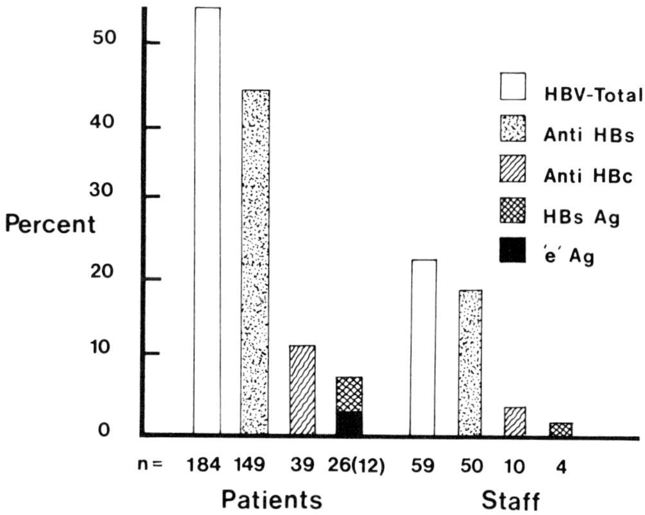

Figure 28.9. HBV markers in patients and staff in an institute for the mentally retarded. From Kingham et al,[210] with kind permission of the editor of *British Medical Journal.*

an excess risk of becoming infected with HBV is difficult to determine. It would depend in part on the closeness of their contact with patients and their blood or other contaminated secretions. In one American survey, dentists and physicians had a three- to fivefold greater rate of HBV markers than volunteer blood donors.[358] Similarly, although laboratory personnel, particularly those handling patients' blood, have an increased risk of developing hepatitis B or markers of infection[159, 286] in areas with a low carrier rate of HB_sAg, the risk is relatively small, and in the United Kingdom is probably no greater than that of acquiring other infectious diseases such as tuberculosis.[166] On the other hand, the carrier rate in Hamburg amongst health care personnel is 2.2 per cent.[197]

Apart from laboratory personnel, those most likely to acquire infection are dentists, anaesthetists and post-mortem attendants, who are in close physical contact with patients. Screening to identify medical personnel who are HB_sAg carriers has been advocated, but this has important implications regarding their continuing occupation if they are found to be HB_sAg positive.[151] Transmission from staff to patients is rare, but has attracted particular attention in dentists. In the United States the HB_sAg carrier rate in dentists is greater than that in volunteer blood donors (0.9 per cent compared with 0.1 to 0.2 per cent[265]). They are considered to be at special risk of acquiring HBV infection from patients because of contact with contaminated blood or saliva directly through small cuts or abrasions on their hands, or possibly by aerosol spread. Even though the HB_sAg carrier rate may be little higher than that of other health care workers[265, 358] the nature of their contact with patients is such as to facilitate spread and examples amongst patients of outbreaks of hepatitis B attributable to HB_sAg positive dentists have been reported in the United States.[323] Clearly, this has important medicolegal implications. The carrier rate in dentists in Denmark, however, is no higher than in the general population.[7]

In addition to staff in haemodialysis units and institutions for the mentally retarded, those involved in the care of other immuno-suppressed patients, for example in oncology units, are specially at risk of developing hepatitis B which may be severe.[392]

Perinatal transmission of hepatitis B

The early literature on transmission of viral hepatitis from mother to infant has been reviewed by Aterman.[24] Although perinatal transmission was then believed to be rare, subsequent studies of HBV markers in the infants of mothers who were either carriers of HB_sAg or who had acute hepatitis B indicate that it is common and may be a major factor in the development of the carrier state. Transmission from carrier mothers to infants is rare in western communities[96, 341] but is much more common in some tropical countries and in Asia.[250, 363] In a study from Birmingham of the infants of HB_sAg positive mothers, nine of 14 Chinese infants, but none of 39 Europeans, became positive for HB_sAg. If the mother has acute hepatitis B during the second and particularly the third trimester, the infant frequently becomes HB_sAg positive with elevated transaminases.[340, 341, 406]

The outcome in the infant bears a striking relationship to the HB_eAg status of the mother.[96, 281, 354] In the study by Okada et al[281] all the babies of 10 mothers who were HB_eAg positive developed HB_sAg, whereas none of seven with anti-e did so. Furthermore, some of the HB_eAg positive mothers had older children who were HB_sAg carriers.

The route of transmission from mother to infant is not clear. Although HB_sAg can be detected by sensitive techniques in cord blood, Dane particles are rare and accidental inapparent inoculation of the infant with maternal blood or liquor seems more likely.[96] Infection is probably not transmitted by breast milk, although it, too, may contain HB_sAg.[96]

It is unusual for infants to develop serious liver disease during the first few years of life, although acute viral hepatitis progressing to cirrhosis can occur.[406] Many infants will become chronic carriers. As will be discussed in Chapter 29, the severity of hepatic abnormality is variable.

Reports of hepatitis in pregnancy have varied in so far as some have suggested that it is no different from hepatitis in non-pregnant women whereas in other series, particularly from India, South-east Asia and Africa, it has been associated with a high mortality.[54, 80, 162] In the latter studies, from Libya, there was a high case-fatality rate of 12.7 per cent in 293 pregnant women compared with 1.6 per cent in 252 non-pregnant women. Several theories, including malnutrition, have been advanced for the greater severity of hepatitis in pregnancy in certain parts of the world but all are speculative. In the Libyan series none of the dead patients was HB_sAg positive and non-A, non-B hepatitis is a possible cause.

NON-A, NON-B HEPATITIS

The availability of markers for both hepatitis A and hepatitis B infection has provided the opportunity to recognize cases of hepatitis which cannot be attributed to either of these infections or to other recognized viruses affecting the liver, such as EB virus and cytomegalovirus. The possibility that such viruses now designated as non-A, non-B existed was suspected from early clinical and epidemiological studies but has become firmly established only in the past few years.[131,307,315] Following widespread introduction of screening of donor blood for HB_sAg, post-transfusion hepatitis was reduced but not eradicated, and it became clear that some cases were due to an unidentified virus or viruses.[60,107] Furthermore, in some patients having multiple bouts of acute viral hepatitis, one or more attacks have occurred which lack serological markers of known viruses.[267]

Recently, non-A, non-B hepatitis has been transmitted to chimpanzees by donors with both acute and chronic hepatitis whose blood had been shown to produce post-transfusional non-A, non-B hepatitis.[18, 375] From these clinical and animal transmission studies, a number of features of non-A, non-B hepatitis have been established, although it is not clear whether it is due to one or more different viruses.

The incubation period of non-A, non-B hepatitis is intermediate between that of hepatitis A and B. Clinically and histologically it bears a closer resemblance to type B than type A hepatitis, and of particular importance is the fact that it appears to be associated with a chronic carrier state and may be a cause of chronic liver disease. Indeed, there is some evidence that abnormal transaminase levels may persist for longer after non-A, non-B hepatitis than after type B.[315] Since hepatitis A is rarely the cause of a transfusional hepatitis and hepatitis B can be greatly reduced by serological testing of donor blood, non-A, non-B is now the commonest cause of post-transfusional hepatitis in areas where screening programmes are undertaken. Although most cases of non-A, non-B hepatitis have been reported from the United States, it has also been observed in a number of other countries, including Great Britain, Australia, Japan and Costa Rica.[102, 315] There have been preliminary reports of localization of an antigen in liver cell nuclei and its detection in serum.[423] Although a virus-specific antigen and antibody have been identified and designated C it is likely that there are at least two non-A, non-B agents.[418]

PATHOLOGY OF ACUTE HEPATITIS

The standard histological changes of acute hepatitis are similar for hepatitis A, B and non-A, non-B both grossly and microscopically, and individual cases cannot be separated other than by techniques for demonstrating the virus.[375]

Macroscopic Changes

The clinically enlarged and tender liver is seen at laparoscopy to be a swollen and reddened organ.[69] These features are sometimes confirmed at inadvertent laparotomy. With more severe degrees of jaundice the liver may also be slightly green but for a given bilirubin level this is always less marked in hepatitis than in large bile duct obstruction.[97]

Microscopic Changes

These have been extensively described.[39, 99, 192, 259, 291, 299] The basic features of inflammation can be identified but the quantitative variation in the changes between cases is considerable. There is cell death and degeneration with a mesenchymal reaction, hepatocyte regeneration and sometimes repair. The overall appearance in a typical biopsy is neatly expressed in the term 'lobular disarray' (Figure 28.10). This reflects the hepatocellular pleomorphism produced by degeneration and loss of hepatocytes, and the disrupted anastomotic cell plate pattern of the lobule and the superimposed features of regeneration. The sinusoids are dilated where loss of hepatocytes has occurred but elsewhere are narrowed by enlarged hepatocytes showing ballooning degeneration and by twinning of cell plates from regeneration. The inflammatory reaction further complicates the histological features by obscuring and filling the sinusoids.

Comparative studies of biopsies have suggested that, quantitatively, parenchymal damage and Kupffer cell reaction are greater in hepatitis B than in non-B hepatitis in which intrahepatic cholestasis is more frequent.[195] Experimental studies in chimpanzees have also suggested that the inflammatory changes in the

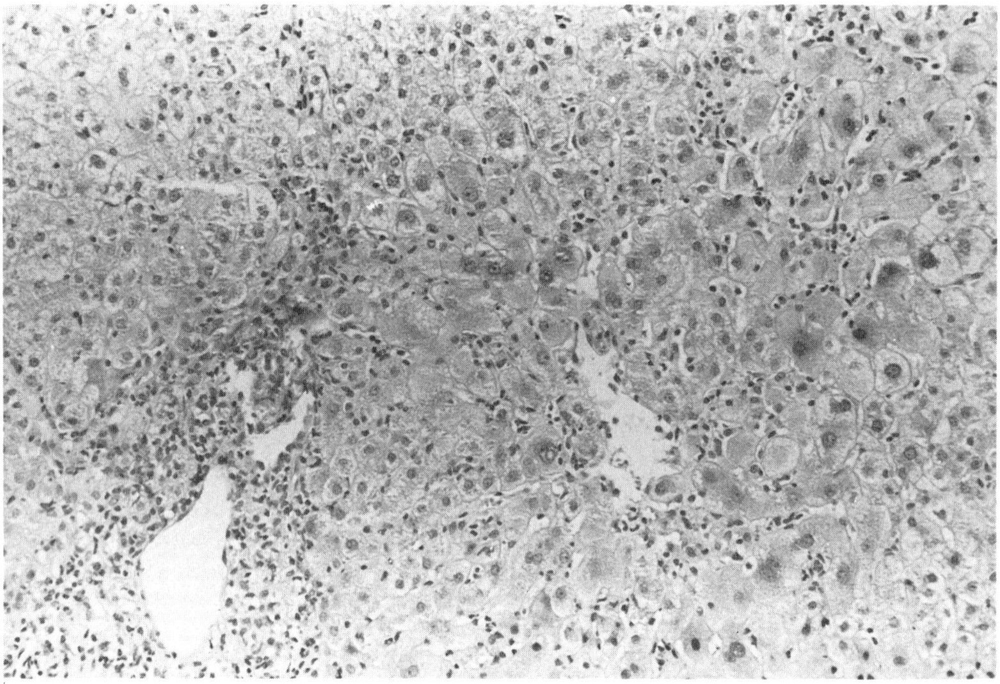

Figure 28.10. Lobule in acute hepatitis with portal tract on bottom left and central vein on centre right. The sinusoids contain mononuclear cells and hyperplastic Kupffer cells and the cell plates are disorganized by loss of hepatocytes and ballooning degeneration. Regeneration is also present and identified by the increased anisonucleosis and numbers of binucleate cells. Haematoxylin and eosin × 120.

centrilobular zone are most prominent in hepatitis B infections while periportal inflammatory changes are most pronounced in hepatitis A.[100]

Cell damage

This is present throughout the lobule and shows considerable variation between cases. It is most striking in the centrilobular area (zone 3 of Rappaport). In mild and anicteric forms of viral hepatitis the damage may be minimal and virtually confined to this zone. Bile stasis is one result of this damage but rarely reflects morphologically the degree of bilirubinaemia. It can be visualized as granules within hepatocytes, mostly centrilobular, and also as thrombi within, and often distending, the bile canaliculi. Some bile is also present in Kupffer cells. While the bile in the canaliculi is conjugated that present in Kupffer cells is unconjugated; a discrepancy attributed to subsequent deconjugation in the Kupffer cell by lysosomal β-glucuronidase.[98] Kupffer cells are also involved in the catabolism of effete red cells and therefore any unconjugated bilirubin present could represent failure of release into the serum.[43]

Damage to hepatocytes can be identified as ballooning degeneration and acidophil degeneration. In ballooning degeneration, hepatocytes are swollen to twice normal or more (Figure 28.11). The nucleus may be normal in appearance but degenerative changes ranging from pyknosis to nuclear inclusions have also been described.[331] It is central in position and surrounded by a cuff of granular cytoplasm. Fine strands of cytoplasm radiate from this cuff to the plasma membrane. There is no staining between the strands and this gives an appearance of peripheral pallor to the cell. The larger the cell the more pronounced is this peripheral zone. The plasma membrane is often sharply defined but focal defects may be seen along its length. Fine granules of bile and lipofuscin may be identified within the cytoplasm. These changes have been attributed to bile retention but where bile is absent cholate stasis has been postulated (see Chapter 14).[301] In the electron microscope there is a striking dilatation of the endoplasmic reticulum, swelling of mitochondria and a loss of ribosomes and glycogen.

A few enlarged cells have abundant granular cytoplasm: it is difficult to decide whether these are degenerative or regenerative in nature.

Ballooning degeneration affects a large

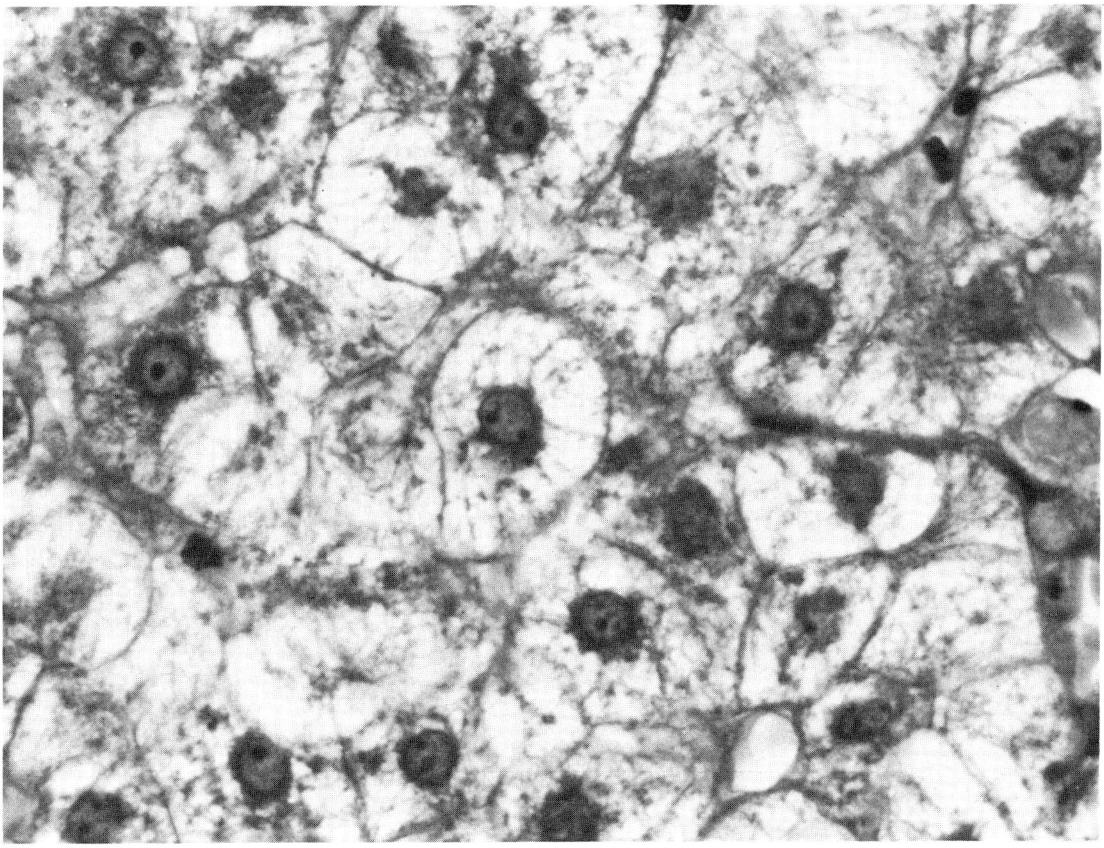

Figure 28.11. Ballooning degeneration. Note the swollen hepatocytes tightly packed together. Strands of cytoplasm pass from the perinuclear condensation to the plasma membrane. Haematoxylin and eosin × 1200.

proportion of the hepatocytes in the lobule and although it is a reversible cell degeneration, lysis may occur. Conversely, acidophil degeneration is irreversible and represents cell death (Figure 28.12). Affected hepatocytes are scattered singly throughout the lobule, are small and have uniformly acidophilic, deeply staining cytoplasm. The cell outline may be angulated at points of residual contact with other hepatocytes but often is rounded and then completely separated by a clear space from its neighbours. Within this condensed cell body the nucleus, if still present, shows either pyknosis or karyorrhexis. In the electron microscope the cells are relatively electron dense with residual organelles compacted together. The membranes of the endoplasmic reticulum are without a lumen, glycogen and ribosomes are absent and surface microvilli are sparse.

Fatty change in hepatocytes (steatosis) is sufficiently rare to question the diagnosis of viral hepatitis if present. When minor degrees occur they are often related to corticosteroid therapy or the later stages of convalescence.

Apart from the active hepatocyte degeneration there is also usually evidence of preceding loss of hepatocytes. This loss results in approximation of the reticulin fibres normally layered along each side of the cell plates and can be visualized on reticulin preparations (Figure 28.13). It may be focal and minor or may represent confluent loss of hepatocytes. In the early stages the reticulin fibres remain slightly apart and regeneration can then reconstitute the cell plate, but otherwise abnormal connective tissue septa may be formed from this passive collapse of the fibre scaffold. The complications which are related to the severity and site of the cell loss are discussed later.

Cell damage may not be confined to hepatocytes. Bile duct damage may be found in a small proportion of cases. Their epithelial cells are enlarged with vacuolated cytoplasm and degenerative changes are present in the nuclei. The damage is usually segmental along a bile duct, may not extend around the whole circumference and when present in a biopsy does not affect all bile ducts.[303] A variable

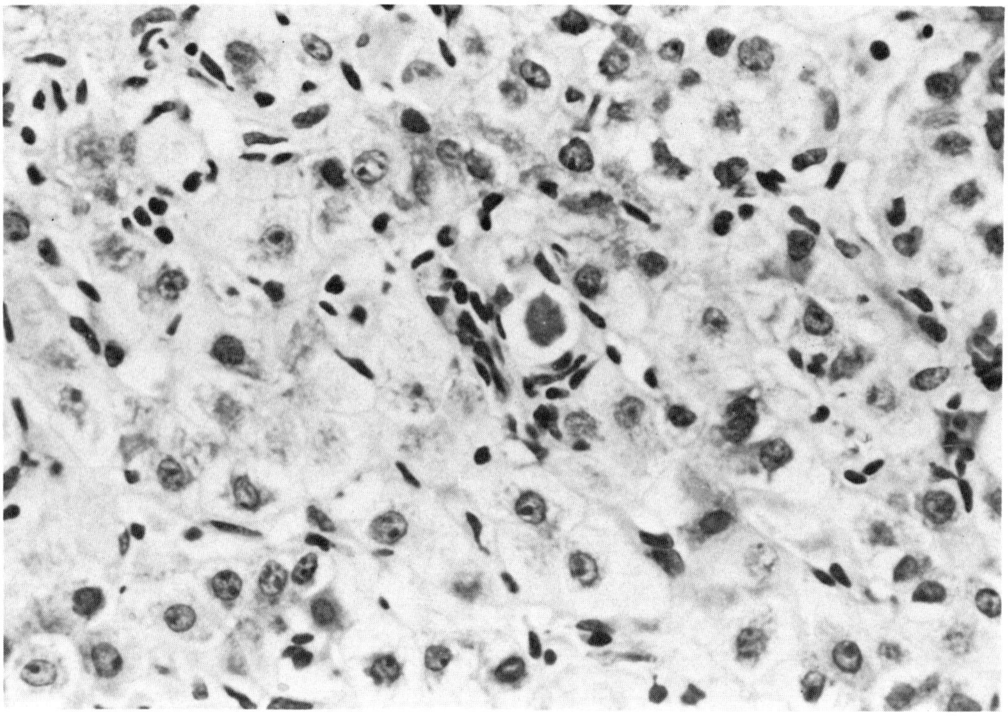

Figure 28.12. Acidophil degeneration. An hepatocyte has rounded off, lost its nucleus and its contact with other hepatocytes and is surrounded by a clear space as though it were in a sinusoid. Note the hyperplasia of mononuclear, probably Kupffer cells around the space. Haematoxylin and eosin × 750.

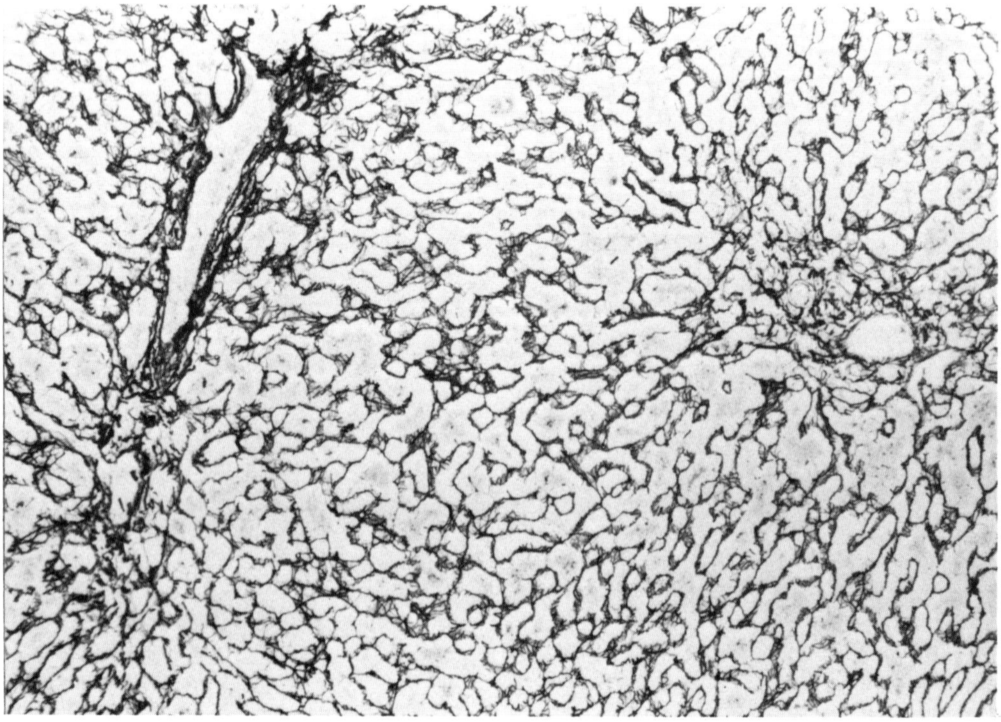

Figure 28.13. Reticulin preparation with portal tract to the right and central vein to the left. Condensed reticulin can be particularly seen around the central vein and results from loss of hepatocytes. Reticulin × 120.

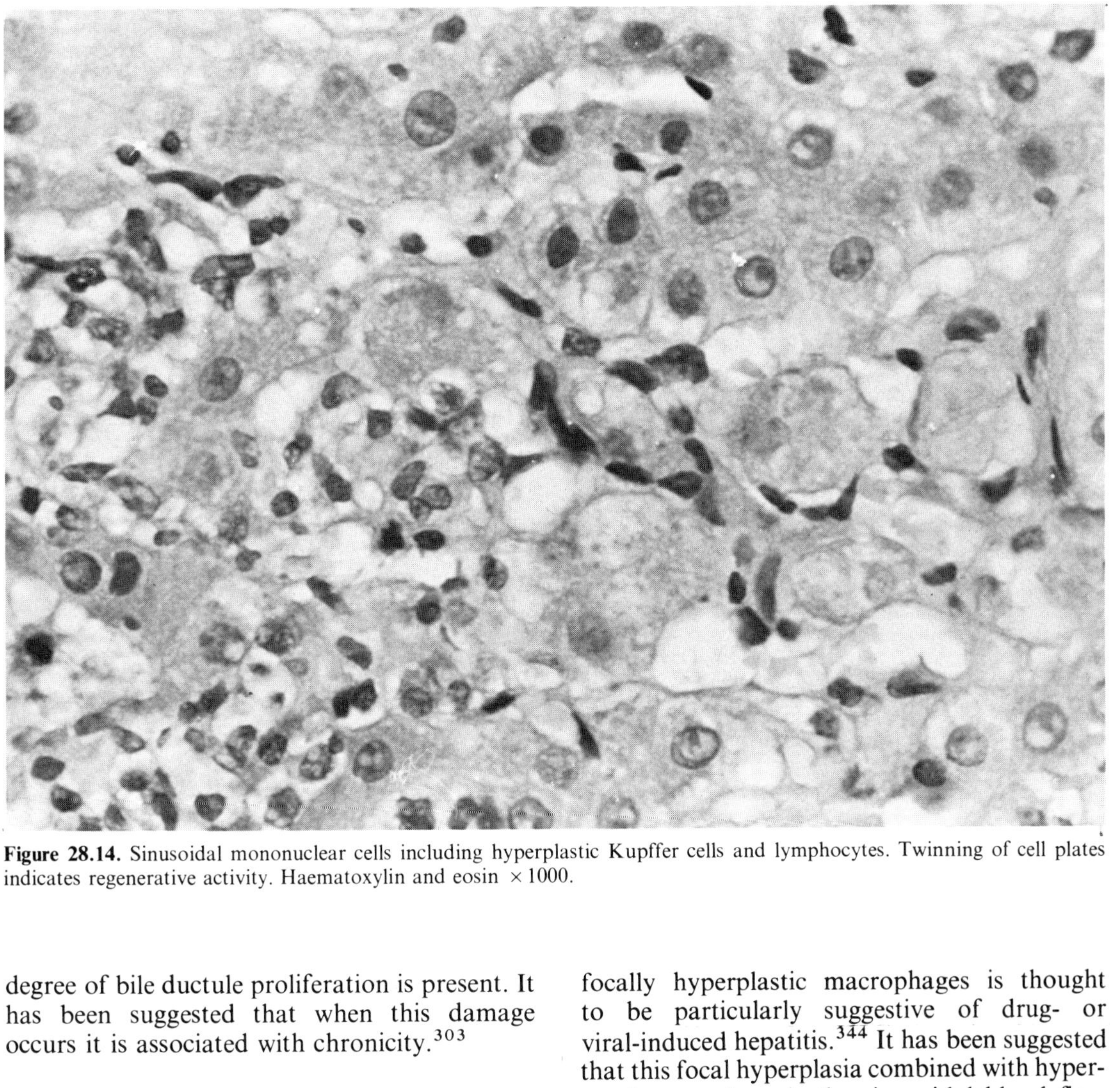

Figure 28.14. Sinusoidal mononuclear cells including hyperplastic Kupffer cells and lymphocytes. Twinning of cell plates indicates regenerative activity. Haematoxylin and eosin ×1000.

degree of bile ductule proliferation is present. It has been suggested that when this damage occurs it is associated with chronicity.[303]

Mesenchymal reaction

There is usually a pronounced inflammatory reaction within the lobule (Figure 28.14). Sinusoids are infiltrated by lymphocytes with occasional plasma cells. The significance of the plasma cells is disputed (see below).[39, 192]

Kupffer cells also show focal proliferation particularly in areas where cell death has been prominent. On occasions they can be found surrounding an acidophil body (Figure 28.12) and aid in the dissolution of this structure.[192] These macrophages are also hypertrophied with bulky cytoplasm laden with phagocytosed debris (Figure 28.15); bile, lipofuscin, ceroid pigments and sometimes haemosiderin pigment have all been identified. The concurrence of both ceroid and haemosiderin pigments within focally hyperplastic macrophages is thought to be particularly suggestive of drug- or viral-induced hepatitis.[344] It has been suggested that this focal hyperplasia combined with hypertrophy may impede the sinusoidal blood flow and that the consequent hypoxia of the adjacent hepatocytes further contributes to the cell damage.[330]

The tracts contain an inflammatory infiltrate, predominantly mononuclear and mostly lymphocytic but with an admixture of plasma cells, macrophages and some neutrophil and eosinophil leucocytes (Figure 28.16). The macrophages, particularly in later stages, contain ceroid pigment and sometimes haemosiderin. There is an overflow of inflammatory cells into periportal sinusoids. The lytic necrosis of hepatocytes may involve the limiting plate and consequently there is dilatation of some periportal sinusoids. Clusters of mononuclear cells fill this area, and blurring of the margins of the portal tract may occur and then be wrongly interpreted as piecemeal necrosis (Figure 28.17).

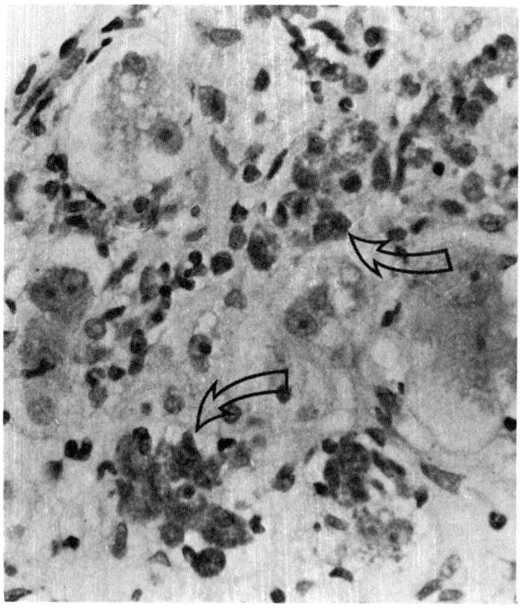

Figure 28.15. Ceroid in Kupffer cells. This is seen as clusters of cells filled with granular pigment (arrows) and obstructing the sinusoids between swollen hepatocytes. Central vein top left. Diastase PAS × 750.

Regeneration

This phenomenon starts within 48 hours of hepatocellular damage (see Chapter 10). Mitotic activity is not often observed in liver biopsies but the results of regenerative activity can be observed. These are: (a) small foci of twinning of cell plates (Figure 28.18) where mitotic activity has occurred, (b) increased numbers of hepatocytes with two or more nuclei and (c) increased variation in size and staining of these hepatocyte nuclei (Figure 28.19). All these features – the thickening of cell plates, the anisonucleosis and the increased numbers of binucleate hepatocytes, with the degenerative changes in hepatocytes of nuclear pyknosis or fragmentation, and cytoplasmic ballooning or acidophil condensation when combined with the inflammatory reaction – are major components of the pleomorphic pattern termed 'lobular disarray'.

Evolution of Changes

The morphological patterns vary between individuals and progress at different rates. Strict chronological or clinical correlations are not possible, but early, middle and late stages can be identified. An overall concept of the morphological evolution has been presented by Bianchi et al.[39]

The features of early viral hepatitis are not well documented but focal liver cell necrosis, many mitoses in hepatocytes, a mononuclear infiltrate in portal tracts and hyperplasia of sinusoidal cells have been described.[97] Biopsies from chimpanzees experimentally infected with hepatitis B virus have demonstrated that a lymphocytic infiltration of sinusoids and portal tracts with hyperplasia of Kupffer cells precedes the parenchymal degenerative changes.[29]

The parenchymal degenerative changes then occur and persist for varying periods, up to several months in some instances (see below), but eventually the active parenchymal degeneration and the cholestasis subside. In these later stages of resolution the emphasis is on previous cell death with prominent regeneration. Focal twinning of cell plates, increased numbers of binucleate hepatocytes and greater nuclear

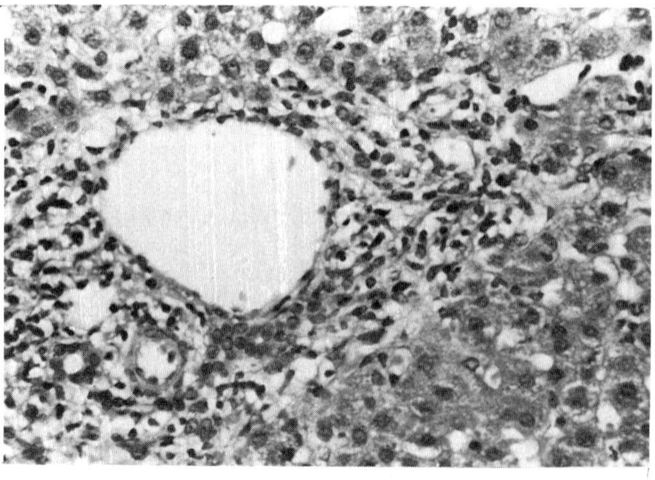

Figure 28.16. Portal tract with vein, bile duct and artery together with a mononuclear cell infiltrate. Haematoxylin and eosin × 390.

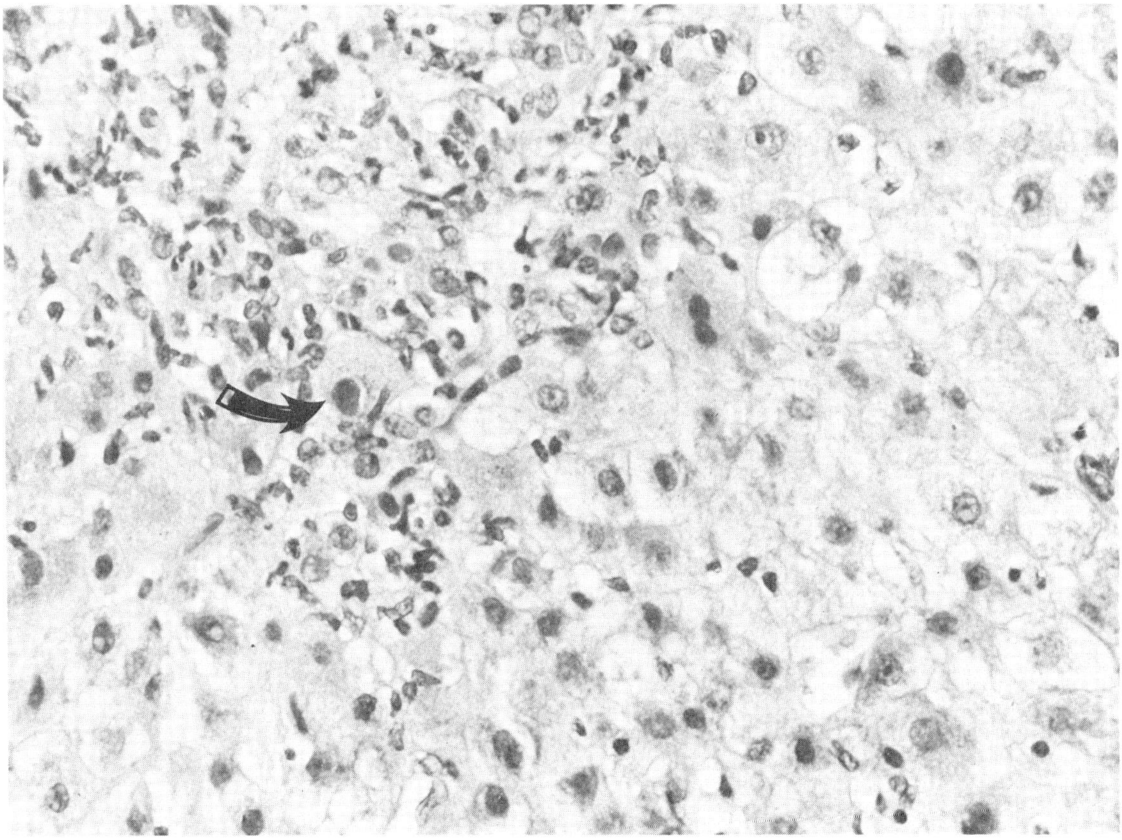

Figure 28.17. Piecemeal necrosis. Edge of portal tract top left with expansion by the inflammatory infiltrate isolating hepatocytes (arrow). Acute hepatocellular damage is still occurring in the lobule. Haematoxylin and eosin × 750.

pleomorphism of hepatocytes are increasingly prominent. There may be a residual lymphocyte infiltrate in portal tracts but more characteristic are the clusters of ceroid-laden macrophages within sinusoids. These persist and may still be present four to six months after the onset of jaundice.

Differential Diagnosis

It has already been indicated that these morphological features will not distinguish between A, B and non-A, non-B hepatitis in the individual cases. An identical histology has also been reported for cytomegalovirus (see later). A drug-induced hepatitis can also be difficult and sometimes impossible to separate by these criteria. Guidelines have been published[41] and drug-induced liver disease is discussed in Chapter 36. A similar morphological pattern of hepatocellular injury has been described with heatstroke.[40] Awareness and a clinical history should identify such cases.

Morphological Variants

Cholestatic hepatitis

Criteria separating cholestatic viral hepatitis from the classical variety are quantitative not qualitative and represent differences in emphasis.[357] Within the lobules there is pronounced cholestasis. The parenchymal changes of viral hepatitis are present but less pronounced. Sometimes only the Kupffer cell reaction and mild hepatocyte anisonucleosis may be identified. The portal tracts show proliferation of bile ductules around the edges and these may be distended and filled with bile. Within the tracts is a mixed inflammatory infiltrate showing an increased proportion of neutrophils. These may surround the proliferating bile ductules and so help to mimic large bile duct obstruction. Interlobular bile ducts have been described as damaged,[97] but this is not a constant feature and in our experience is uncommon.

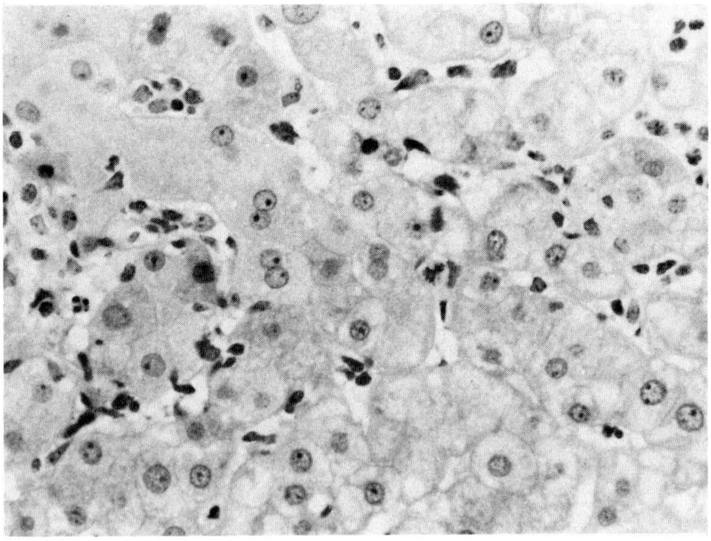

Figure 28.18. Recovery from acute viral hepatitis. There is still persistence of inflammatory cells in the sinusoids and the cell plate pattern is disturbed by the twinning as well as the loss of hepatocytes. Haematoxylin and eosin × 325.

The cholestasis may persist for many months but there is no indication that this variety of hepatitis predisposes to chronic liver disease.

Drug addiction hepatitis

Intravenous injection when employed by drug addicts is frequently associated with a viral hepatitis. Particulate matter such as talc may be mixed with the drug. Classically this produces granulomatous lung disease and right heart endocarditis but sufficient may enter the systemic circulation to reach the liver. A granulomatous reaction around the foreign material may then be found in the portal tracts.[408] Polarized light will facilitate recognition of doubly refractile material such as talc.

Other changes are less characteristic but more frequent and usually involve portal tracts. An intense lymphocytic infiltrate occurs within these tracts and may even form lymphoid follicles, sometimes with a reactive centre. No foreign material is present, no piecemeal necrosis occurs and the reaction appears to relate to the frequency of injection.[117] Both this and the granulomatous reaction may be found after complete resolution of the hepatitis.

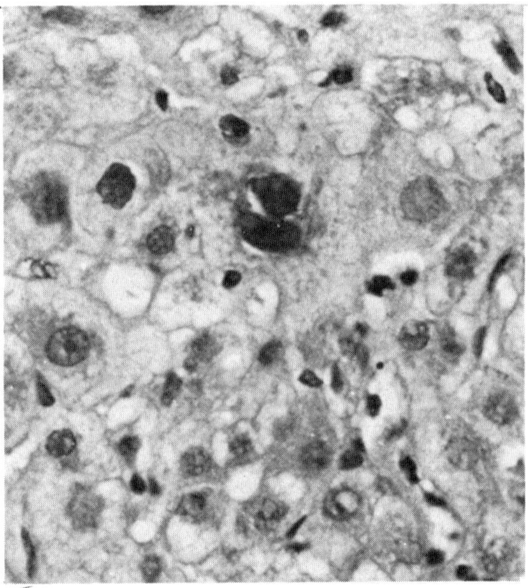

Figure 28.19. Regeneration. There is increased variation in nuclear size and staining in hepatocytes. Haematoxylin and eosin × 1200.

Relapsing hepatitis (chronic lobular hepatitis)

The features described under chronic lobular hepatitis[300] were not recognized as a distinct entity in the Standardization of Nomenclature, Diagnostic Criteria and Diagnostic Methodology.[225] These features are those of a typical acute viral hepatitis on liver biopsy but continuing for more than six months. The condition may be regarded as prolonged or unresolved acute hepatitis. When related to hepatitis B virus infection, scanty orcein-positive hepatocytes may be present.[301] In some cases there may be periods of documented remission but it is difficult to exclude another viral infection in the individual case.

Massive hepatic necrosis

The degree of hepatocellular damage and death varies considerably. In anicteric, asymptomatic viral hepatitis cell death may be minimal whereas fulminating disease results from massive cell death. In these latter instances hepatic failure is profound and survival is rare. Biopsies are rarely performed in the acute stages so that information is derived mostly from autopsy studies such as the classical observations of Lucké.[232, 233] Different gross patterns have been described but these represent the rate of massive necrosis along a time scale rather than variations on a disease process.

In the earliest stages, up to one week, the liver will be approximately normal or only slightly smaller in size and weight because the majority of dead hepatocytes have not disintegrated and the stroma is still separated by this residual effete parenchyma. Loss of hepatocytes will have occurred predominantly around the central veins, and sinusoids will be dilated and passively filled with blood. The overall result is of a soft liver with a wrinkled capsule and congested cut surface.

Submassive hepatic necrosis. Longer survival of between one and four weeks will allow more complete disintegration of hepatocytes with corresponding collapse of the architecture. Macrophages and Kupffer cells are hypertrophied and contain much brown granular pigment as a result of their phagocytic activities. Bile retention is prominent in hepatocytes, canaliculi and Kupffer cells and there is a pronounced lymphoid infiltrate in portal tracts. The cell death in the liver is not uniform; some lobules appear to be totally effaced while others show lesser degrees of damage. Large areas of collapsed stroma contain proliferating bile ductules and show approximation of portal tracts. The consequence of this more complete cell loss is a small and limp liver that is heavily bile stained and has a very wrinkled capsule.

The pattern thus differs from massive hepatic necrosis in which cell death and loss are more uniform and not as advanced. The differences are later further accentuated by hepatocellular regeneration that becomes increasingly obvious with time. Consequently if severe cell damage and death occur for periods of two or three months the liver macroscopically may show large areas of collapse of the reticulin with bulging regenerative masses of parenchyma. Interpretation of the pattern varies. Some workers regard its presence as indicating cirrhosis while others prefer to use the term 'submassive hepatic necrosis'.[118] As the pattern is one of progressive hepatocellular death exceeding regeneration, of relentless clinical deterioration and of increasing liver failure within a relatively well defined and short time scale the latter terminology seems most appropriate. It should be emphasized that these entities, ranging from fulminating hepatic necrosis to submassive hepatic necrosis, are based on clinical and macroscopic pathological appearances in relation to a time scale. The various factors which may help determine the speed of onset and severity of the liver disease or influence its chronicity are discussed below. It must also be emphasized that currently there is no general agreement about the relative merits of each and their interrelationship is even less well understood.

Prognostic Morphological Features

The vast majority of patients with viral hepatitis improve without sequelae and only a small proportion progress to chronic liver disease.[34] Numerous attempts have been made to identify clinical serological and morphological features which might affect prognosis and predict those patients at risk. Clinically the patients who develop cirrhosis are older and include more females than the average.[45] The presence of the hepatitis B virus increases the risk of chronic liver disease. Morphological features that have been associated with an adverse prognosis include confluent necrosis, piecemeal necrosis, an impaired regenerative response, bile duct damage and an excessive proportion of plasma cells. In hepatitis B demonstration of components of the virus or the immunological reaction to it may be of prognostic significance (see below).

Bridging hepatic necrosis

This term, suggested by Conn,[82] has replaced 'sub-acute hepatic necrosis' and should be confined to the appearance of confluent necrosis linking portal tracts with central veins (Figure 28.20). It should not be extended to include the confluent necrosis that either links central veins or links portal tracts together. There is dispute about the relative merits of these three patterns of necrosis and the original term, 'sub-acute hepatic necrosis',[56] did not distinguish between them. Despite this, in their series Boyer and

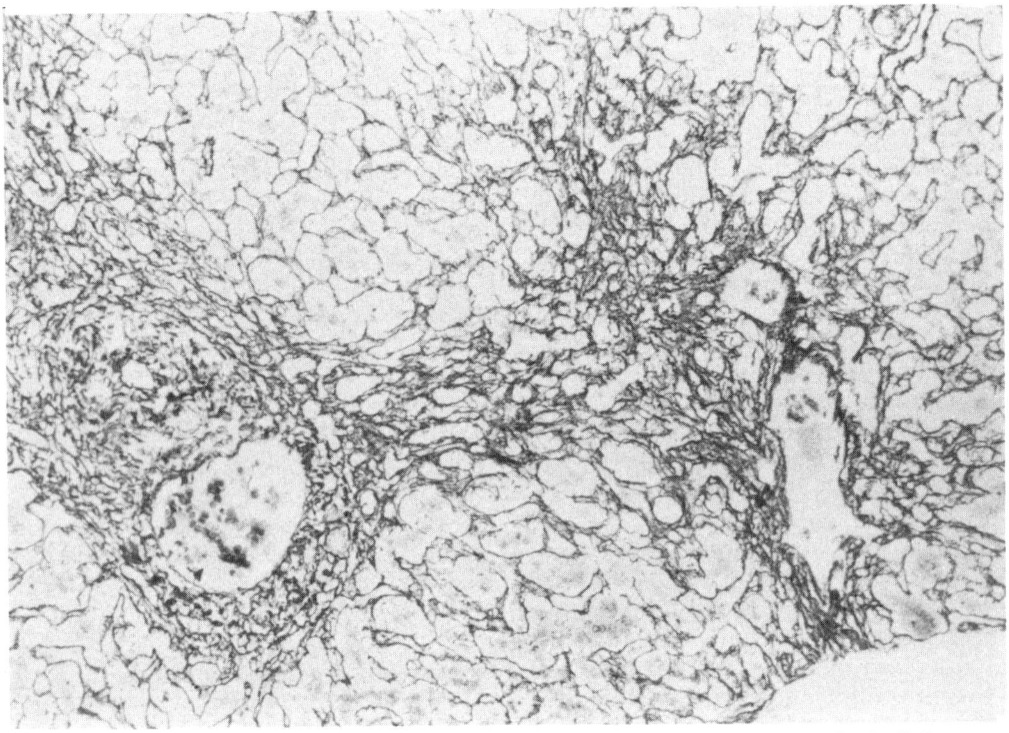

Figure 28.20. Bridging hepatic necrosis. Reticulin preparation showing collapse and condensation of reticulin between central vein (right) and portal tract (left). Numerous plasma cells were also present in this patient's biopsy. × 100.

Klatskin described complications in half of the patients with liver biopsies defined by them as showing this category of confluent necrosis. Many of these patients developed cirrhosis. Similar results but with a lower incidence of complications have been reported by others.[394]

It is perhaps surprising that a single feature representing an acute episode of cell death should be incriminated in the pathogenesis of chronic liver disease and cirrhosis. The known causes of cirrhosis are often present and active for many years before an established cirrhosis ensues. Experimentally it is very difficult, if not impossible, to produce cirrhosis by a single dose of any hepatotoxic agent. Multiple small doses over a long period of time are required. Thus Cameron and Karunaratne[66] demonstrated that a single dose of carbon tetrachloride may produce acute hepatic necrosis and even death, but never cirrhosis, whereas multiple small doses, insufficient to cause necrosis, given over a sufficient period of time could consistently produce a micronodular cirrhosis.[67] Clinically, severe acute hepatic necrosis, whether complicating acute viral hepatitis[205] or drugs such as paracetamol,[302] is not a precursor of cirrhosis.

Bridging hepatic necrosis could predispose to chronic liver disease in several ways. It could provide a septum formed by the passive collapse of reticulin fibres in the space of Disse along which active fibrogenesis produces a bridge of mature collagen between tract and central vein. Blood vessels would form within this collagen bridge, bypass the parenchyma and thus form a vascular shunt. It has been suggested also that the presence of such a pattern of necrosis simply facilitates the progression of a chronic hepatitis so that the architecture is more quickly disrupted.[42] Alternatively, it may be a morphological representation of cell death in excess of regeneration.[118, 291] These three pathogenetic mechanisms are not mutually exclusive and the identification of bridging hepatic necrosis in a liver biopsy should be regarded as a serious adverse prognostic sign requiring, at a minimum, careful follow-up and repeat biopsy in six months.

Impaired regeneration

It is notable that viral hepatitis is frequently much more severe in patients over 40 years of age[56, 118, 205, 243] and that survivors of acute hepatic failure due to viral hepatitis are almost invariably under the age of 30 years.[205] The influence of age upon the relative incidence of fulminating hepatitis and upon survival rates amongst affected patients has been attributed to increasing impairment of hepatocellular regeneration with age.[118,291,416] This is reflected morphologically in zones of confluent necrosis because cell loss is not equally matched by regeneration. The rate at which cell death exceeds regeneration will then determine the clinical and pathological consequences. Extensive simultaneous death of hepatocytes can produce fulminating acute hepatitis before regeneration has had time to develop fully. Such patients, both young and old, will have a high mortality. For lesser degrees of cell death the rate of regeneration may be crucial and in this context it is interesting to note that the average age of patients dying with submassive hepatic necrosis two to four months from the known onset of their illness is 68 years.[118] The argument can be extended further; thus in patients where cell death/regeneration is approximately balanced architectural distortion will be significant, and the bridging necrosis described above will effectively contribute to a subsequent cirrhosis.

A major problem in confirming these ideas is the accurate identification of regenerative capacity in the individual patient particularly histologically. Apart from assessment of the number of mitoses and the twinning of cell plates the *lack* of lobular disarray in the presence of confluent hepatocellular damage may be ominous.[291] This reflects the contribution that regeneration makes to the typical histological pattern of acute viral hepatitis.

Piecemeal necrosis (see Chapter 29)

This is a chronic inflammatory process present at interfaces between parenchyma and connective tissue. It comprises a lymphocytic and plasma cell infiltrate with active fibrogenesis and extends into the parenchyma from the adjacent fibrous tissue. In so doing it isolates small groups of hepatocytes (Figure 28.17). Considerable difficulty arises in separating this lesion from the overspill of inflammatory cells into periportal areas seen in non-complicated acute viral hepatitis. Features of active fibrogenesis, rosette formation of hepatocytes, an intimate relationship between lymphocytes and hepatocytes, and a periportal and portal reaction that is out of proportion to the centrilobular changes suggest piecemeal necrosis. Also, it is rare for hepatocytes to be isolated by simple spillover from portal tracts.

Despite the emphasis on chronicity, piecemeal necrosis may occasionally occur in acute viral hepatitis and then it is postulated that chronicity is likely.[42,109] The rate at which this process then produces significant architectural distortion by fibrosis is influenced by the presence of passive connective tissue septa. These are produced by the collapse of the reticulin architecture that occurs secondary to bridging hepatic necrosis.[42] The process of piecemeal necrosis with its active fibrogenesis then converts these passively collapsed reticulin fibres (type III collagen) into type I collagen (see Chapter 30).

It is unlikely that piecemeal necrosis is present in all cases of chronic liver disease. Only half of the chronic cases reported by Dietrichson and colleagues[109] showed piecemeal necrosis in the biopsy. Nor does the presence of piecemeal necrosis indicate inevitable chronic liver disease.[42,109,128] In a survey of 17 biopsies showing acute hepatocellular damage with chronic aggressive hepatitis taken from patients with acute viral hepatitis only three progressed to chronic liver disease.[128]

Plasma cells

Although these cells are a component of the infiltrate in piecemeal necrosis they are also thought to be an adverse feature when otherwise present.[39,109,193] While present in small numbers in uncomplicated hepatitis they are frequently prominent in biopsies with piecemeal necrosis or bridging hepatic necrosis. Their presence should result in at least a careful search for these features.

Bile duct lesion

Damage to the bile ducts was described in acute hepatitis by Poulsen and Christoffersen[303] who also commented that all these cases progressed to chronic liver disease, and three to cirrhosis. Piecemeal necrosis was a prominent feature (9/14) in many of these 14 cases. The presence of bile duct damage in cholestatic viral hepatitis is not associated with chronicity[97] and the significance of the bile duct lesion per se still requires elucidation.

Specific Demonstration of Hepatitis B Virus in the Liver

Various techniques have been employed to demonstrate hepatitis B or its component parts in the liver, and for some of these an attempt has been made to correlate the appearances with prognosis.

Hepatitis B surface antigen

It is now established that in chronic hepatitis B virus infection of hepatocytes, HB_sAg is only present in the cytoplasm (see Chapter 29). In acute hepatitis both in man and in the chimpanzee HB_sAg has been demonstrated by immunofluorescence in the hepatocyte cytoplasm, particularly around the hepatocyte membrane.[5, 116, 328] No nuclear fluorescence can be demonstrated with purified anti-HB_s,[29, 116, 161, 328] which contradicts earlier reports of nuclear localization.[89, 258, 275, 279] It must be assumed that a variety of other antigen–antibody reactions were being demonstrated in the nucleus. Some workers have been able to demonstrate cytoplasmic fluorescence only when the biopsy shows other features suggesting transition to chronic liver disease,[161, 320, 324] but sequential biopsies in self-limited acute hepatitis in chimpanzees have demonstrated transient cytoplasmic fluorescence with accentuation of staining along the hepatocyte membrane[29, 185] and this supports the observations in man indicating positive cytoplasmic fluorescence only in the early stages of acute hepatitis.[5]

Various histochemical techniques are now known to identify HB_sAg in hepatocyte cytoplasm (see Chapter 29).[348] The two most successful are modifications of stains for elastic tissue – orcein and aldehyde fuchsin. Neither of these techniques is positive in acute hepatitis B[95] and a positive result should either suggest an acute exacerbation of chronic liver disease or a non-B hepatitis occurring in a chronic hepatitis B carrier.[259]

Electron microscopy has consistently failed to demonstrate HB_sAg in hepatocytes in acute hepatitis.

Hepatitis B core antigen

There is now general agreement that the core antigen is predominantly in the nucleus of the hepatocyte in both acute and chronic hepatitis B infection. Immunofluorescent and ultrastructural techniques show that in acute hepatitis many biopsies are negative[161, 284] and even in positive cases electron microscopy demonstrates only scanty intranuclear particles in occasional cells.[279] In experimental studies of acute hepatitis in chimpanzees the core antigen can be demonstrated by immunofluorescence in the nucleus of hepatocytes during the incubation period up to the time of maximal elevation of the serum transaminases – a stage when liver biopsies are unlikely to be obtained in man.[185]

The morphology of intranuclear core particles is identical in acute and chronic hepatitis. They have been extensively studied in chronic hepatitis B where they are much more numerous. They are small (21 to 25 nm diameter) and round with a slightly angular periphery and may have an electron dense core, but this is not always seen (see Chapter 29).

Hepatitis B_e antigen

No satisfactory demonstration of e antigen in the liver in acute hepatitis B has yet been recorded and in chronic hepatitis B the findings are conflicting (see Chapter 29).

Serum components

Both immunoglobulin, particularly IgG, and complement have been demonstrated in the liver by immunofluorescence.[22, 324]

Immunoglobulin, when present, is almost invariably reported in the nucleus and is thought to represent HB_c–anti-HB_c immune complex which may fix complement.[142] Morphological demonstration of complement in acute viral hepatitis may indicate an adverse prognosis. Of 47 patients with acute virus B hepatitis, complement was demonstrated in 10 patients. All progressed to chronic liver disease although it was of varying severity. Of the 37 remaining patients only three developed chronic liver disease.[324]

Specific Demonstration of Hepatitis A Virus in the Liver

After the identification of the virus particle of hepatitis A by immuno-electron microscopy in stools,[103, 107, 130] a similar and antigenically identical 27 nm particle has been demonstrated in the hepatocyte cytoplasm.[338]

Immunofluorescent studies of experimentally infected chimpanzees also showed cytoplasmic localization and failed to demonstrate any nuclear antigen.[246] Positive reactions were obtained before any clinical, biochemical or morphological evidence of hepatitis, and occasionally could be obtained after biochemical resolution of the hepatitis. Initially, many hepatocytes showed faint fluorescence and this progressed to intense fluorescence in a few hepatocytes.

CLINICAL FEATURES

Most cases of infection with either hepatitis A or B are not associated with significant clinical symptoms and often pass unrecognized. There may be no symptoms at all with minimal liver damage, or anicteric infection with non-specific symptoms but with hepatocellular necrosis and biochemical abnormalities. The non-specific symptoms are those seen in the prodromal phase but stop short of frank icterus. Icteric attacks can range in severity from mild to fulminant and fatal. Anicteric infection with hepatitis B may progress to chronic liver disease, but this does not occur with hepatitis A. There are no clear clinical distinctions between hepatitis A and B but hepatitis A usually starts acutely whereas hepatitis B is insidious, more severe and more prolonged (Table 28.6).

Acute Icteric Hepatitis

The prodromal symptoms of hepatitis vary in severity and duration and some patients present only with overt jaundice. The duration of the pre-icteric symptoms range from a few days to two weeks and are mainly respiratory and gastrointestinal. Anorexia, nausea, malaise, weight loss, distaste for cigarettes, dark urine and pale stools, with or without pruritus, are prominent early symptoms. A decreased olfactory acuity appears to be a factor in the anorexia and improves as the illness subsides.[172]

The appearance of jaundice is usually associated with improvement in symptoms; although anorexia, nausea and lassitude may persist, the temperature settles, the pulse becomes slow and hepatic pain prominent.

A serum sickness-like syndrome with arthralgia and arthritis, urticaria and angioneurotic oedema is seen in some patients[147] and is of interest because it is produced by immune complex injury. In one epidemic of hepatitis B 25 per cent of patients had rashes or arthropathy compared with none in an epidemic of hepatitis A.[361] Immune complexes are often associated with cryoglobulinaemia and have been best documented with hepatitis B.[230] Vasculitic and renal lesions are usually seen with chronic hepatitis B but can occasionally be seen in acute hepatitis, including what is presumed to be hepatitis A.[164] The immunopathological mechanisms involved in the extrahepatic manifestations of acute and chronic hepatitis are discussed together in Chapter 29.

The generalized nature of the infection accounts for some exceptional features.[83] These include meningism with a raised protein and lymphocyte count in the cerebrospinal fluid and, rarely, the Guillain–Barré syndrome.[277] Myocarditis, electrocardiographic changes,[36] pancreatitis,[1] pleural effusion[285] and haematological changes also occur (see below and Chapter 8). Renal failure is a rare complication of acute viral hepatitis possibly due to endotoxaemia rather than a direct action of the virus.[396]

In most icteric cases, the liver is enlarged and tender but the spleen is palpable in only about 20 per cent of patients. Lymphadenopathy may be present but is usually insignificant and occasionally there is bruising and purpura; the Schönlein–Henoch syndrome has been reported in three cases during the prodromal phase of acute hepatitis.[145]

Lightening of the urine with a return of the stools to normal colour are early signs of recovery. Appetite improves with a gain in weight but fatigue and lassitude may persist.

Atypical Clinical Forms of Hepatitis

Cholestatic viral hepatitis

Although cholestatic symptoms are a feature in most cases of icteric hepatitis, in some they dominate the clinical picture. Such cases often present acutely with deep jaundice, pronounced pruritus, dark urine and pale stools. In particular, when prodromal symptoms are insignificant they may be difficult to distinguish from extrahepatic cholestasis and drug-induced cholestasis. It is not clear whether the development of this unusual form of viral hepatitis is due to host factors or determined by the strain of virus since in particular outbreaks of both

Table 28.6. *Comparison between Hepatitis A, B and Non-A, Non-B.*

	A	B	Non-A, non-B
Synonyms	Infectious hepatitis MS-1	Serum hepatitis MS-2	—
Incubation period	15–45 days	60–160 days	10–100 days
Spread	Epidemic–sporadic	Sporadic, rarely epidemic	Sporadic
Faecal–oral	V. common	Doubtful	?
Ingestion	V. common	? Common	Unknown
Transfusion	Rare	Common but decreasing	? Common
Sexual	Occasional	Quite common	?
Age of onset			
Western communities	Childhood but increasing	Older age groups	?
Developing countries	Childhood	Any age, often infants	?
Clinical course			
Onset	Usually acute	Insidious	?
Fulminant	Rare	Infrequent	?
Carrier rate and chronicity	None	Common	Yes, but ? frequency
Abnormal LFTs	Short-lived	Prolonged	Prolonged
ESR	High	Normal	?
IgM	High	Normal	?
Animal transmissibility	Chimpanzees, Marmosets	Chimpanzees	Chimpanzees
Viraemia	Transient, early	Early transient or chronic	? Early and chronic
Viral structure	27 nm sphere	43 nm Dane particle + excess viral coat	?
Viral class	Probable enterovirus	? unique	?
Tissue culture	Yes. Preliminary	No	No
Passive immunity	Effective	Variable. Most effective early	?

hepatitis A and B, cholestatic features have been prominent (see Chapter 14). In some cases, the symptoms of cholestasis persist for long periods, but this impression may be due to case selection.[111] Recovery is complete and progression to chronic liver disease is unusual.

The liver is usually not much enlarged and seldom tender, and the biochemical features may be indistinguishable from extrahepatic obstruction.

Fulminant hepatitis

In a small proportion of patients, the onset is acute and the illness rapidly fatal within a period of one to four weeks. Usually the patient becomes deeply jaundiced within a few days, with restlessness, hallucinations, drowsiness, vomiting and convulsions. Rarely the onset may be so abrupt that coma and death may supervene in the absence of marked jaundice. The clinical signs are those of acute fulminant hepatic failure (see Chapter 27), with asterixis, constructional apraxia, progressive deterioration in the level of consciousness, fetor hepaticus, gastrointestinal haemorrhage from acute gastric erosions, bruising and purpura and often renal failure. The liver may shrink in size, which is an ominous sign, as is the development of ascites and oedema.

The serum transaminase, after being very high in the early stages, may fall rapidly to low levels with prolongation of the prothrombin time and a decrease in the serum albumin levels. In contrast to the normal or low count in typical acute viral hepatitis, there is a leucocytosis and occasionally thrombocytopenia associated with intravascular coagulation (see Chapter 8).

Although in most parts of the world the severe cases are due to hepatitis B, in the United Kingdom only about a quarter of cases of fulminant viral hepatitis are HB_sAg positive.[382] Hepatitis A is rarely the cause.[108, 419]

Sub-acute hepatitis

Occasional patients have a severe acute attack and this pursues a more prolonged downhill course with progressive ascites and liver failure, terminating in death over a period of a few months.[419] Even more exceptionally, there may be an apparent period of clinical recovery but with persisting abnormality of liver function before progressive clinical deterioration. Such cases are clearly difficult to distinguish from chronic active hepatitis of unknown aetiology starting acutely, particularly if immunological markers are absent. These patients are often women. Pathologically, such cases often show bridging hepatic necrosis which is sometimes submassive.

Relapsing hepatitis

Following an apparently complete clinical recovery from typical acute viral hepatitis, one or more relapses may occur, with darkening of the urine, a return of symptoms, particularly nausea and anorexia, and with the development of jaundice. This clinicopathological syndrome has been referred to as chronic lobular hepatitis.[301] Occasionally, the liver function tests return to normal in between the acute attack and the relapse, but it is difficult to exclude the possibility that a different virus is the cause of the second attack. It is more usual, despite clinical recovery, for liver function tests to remain abnormal before the next clinical relapse, but here, too, there is a grey area merging with chronic persistent hepatitis (see Chapter 29).

Two attacks of hepatitis due to A, B or non-A, non-B are most likely to occur in drug addicts, haemophiliacs and children in institutions for the mentally retarded. A true relapse of hepatitis is sometimes temporally related to increased physical activity or alcohol abuse.

In some series, an increased relapse rate has been reported in patients following treatment with corticosteroids (see below).

Chronic Sequelae of Acute Viral Hepatitis

Although the overwhelming majority of patients with viral hepatitis recover completely, a proportion progress to chronic liver disease, particularly after hepatitis B infection (see Chapter 29). However, in some patients, there is persistence of symptoms of lethargy, malaise, anorexia and dislike of alcohol and fatty foods, which may last for months. Emotional instability and depression may be a striking feature. The liver may be palpable and tender and liver function tests may or may not be abnormal. There may be post-hepatitic hyperbilirubinaemia. Liver biopsy may be normal or show features of a resolving hepatitis. These symptoms are often referred to as the post-hepatitis syndrome.[244]

BIOCHEMICAL AND IMMUNOLOGICAL DISTURBANCES IN ACUTE VIRAL HEPATITIS

Virtually all the functions of the liver described in Chapter 17 are deranged in acute viral hepatitis. The magnitude of derangement will depend on the severity of hepatocellular necrosis and the degree of cholestasis. Biochemical tests of liver function therefore provide a guide to the diagnosis of acute viral hepatitis and to the assessment of its severity, but have strict limitations and must be interpreted in the light of clinical findings and other investigative procedures in the jaundiced patient (see Chapter 23).

In the typical acute attack of viral hepatitis, serum aspartate aminotransferase (AST) levels become elevated early in the pre-symptomatic period of the disease and may be high in patients who never become icteric. Alanine aminotransferase (ALT) levels are also elevated. When studied serially, the rise in AST is more rapid and less prolonged in hepatitis A infection than in hepatitis B, where the rise is gradual and the fall to normal may take several months.[219] By the time clinically overt jaundice develops, the peak levels of aminotransferase have been achieved and they are usually falling. They are of some value in the differential diagnosis of jaundice, as figures in excess of 500 iu/l are seen only in acute hepatitis from any cause and shock or severe heart failure, but are rare in extrahepatic obstructive jaundice and in chronic liver disease unless severely decompensated.

Serum bilirubin levels are very variable and are dependent not only on hepatocellular damage but on the degree of cholestasis and the presence of associated haemolysis. Although in general the severity of hepatitis is related to the level of the bilirubin, there are striking exceptions, and fulminant hepatitis can occur with relatively little elevation of the bilirubin. In some studies of hepatitis B, a prolonged clinical course has been associated with lower bilirubin levels during the acute attack.[276, 347]

Bilirubinuria appears before the serum bilirubin level is elevated and the urine may clear while jaundice persists. Urobilinogen disappears due to cholestasis at the height of the jaundice in the late pre-icteric phase, and its reappearance may indicate commencing recovery but is of little practical diagnostic value. Similarly, depending on the degree of cholestasis, stools become pale and the reappearance of stercobilin indicates clinical recovery.

Serum alkaline phosphatase levels are increased in acute viral hepatitis. A level of 30 K.A. units has been taken as that distinguishing obstructive from hepatocellular jaundice. This level can be misleading as, although the elevation of alkaline phosphatase is usually only slight in viral hepatitis, some patients, particularly those with the cholestatic variety who clinically are most difficult to distinguish from those with extrahepatic obstruction, may show levels greater than this.

Changes in the plasma lipids and lipoproteins occur in acute viral hepatitis (see Chapter 4), but are not of practical value as tests of liver function.

The serum proteins may provide an important guide to the severity of the hepatitis. Serum albumin levels reflect the ability of the liver to synthesize this protein and are usually normal in the average acute attack of hepatitis. Low levels either indicate fulminating severe hepatic damage, or chronic liver disease. Serum globulin levels are altered in acute viral hepatitis, and formed the basis of some of the early tests of liver function, namely the flocculation tests. In acute viral hepatitis, there is elevation of the IgM levels in HB_sAg negative hepatitis, and of the IgG levels in both hepatitis A and B.[289] Serum complement levels may be low initially, but later rise to normal. The significance of these changes in terms of immune-complex formation is doubtful because of the possibility of decreased synthesis by the damaged liver, with subsequent over-production in response to low levels.[216] Cryoglobulinaemia may be a striking feature.[230]

Apart from the specific immune responses to antigens associated with hepatitis A and B, non-specific immune responses occur in viral hepatitis. There is elevation of antibody titres to gut-associated bacteria such as *E. coli*[383] and to a variety of unidentified viruses and bacteriophage particles present in stools,[11] suggesting a non-specific response to gut-associated antigens, possibly resulting from failure of Kupffer cells in the diseased liver to sequester absorbed antigens (see Chapter 8).

Antibodies to a component of smooth muscle have been demonstrated in a high proportion of patients with both hepatitis A and B.[127, 273, 403] This antibody, which is also detected in other viral infections such as infectious mononucleosis, may react with a component of the liver cell membrane resembling smooth muscle actomyosin.[178] Antibodies to a liver-specific lipoprotein occur transiently in the serum in a high proportion of patients with hepatitis A or B.[199]

HAEMATOLOGICAL CHANGES IN ACUTE VIRAL HEPATITIS

These are described in detail in Chapter 8. Many proteins, important in the coagulation process, are synthesized in the liver, and may provide a sensitive index of hepatocellular dysfunction. As a result of malabsorption of vitamin K, the prothrombin time can be prolonged in cholestasis, whether of extrahepatic or intrahepatic origin, but is readily corrected by its parenteral administration. A prolonged prothrombin time which vitamin K fails to correct is an indication of severe hepatocellular dysfunction.

As with many viral infections, there may be a leucopenia and, in particular, a lymphopenia with atypical lymphocytes, resembling those seen in infectious mononucleosis. Later, there is a relative lymphocytosis, a macrocytosis with a reduced red cell survival[212] and low serum haptoglobulin levels,[356] but marked haemolysis which may be associated with a positive Coombs' test is rare. Thrombocytopenia, agranulocytosis, pancytopenia[163] and transient red cell aplasia have also been reported.[342]

The erythrocyte sedimentation rate is usually high in the pre-icteric phase in HB_sAg negative hepatitis[387] but falls to normal with the appearance of jaundice and thereafter fluctuates until recovery. Serum vitamin B_{12} levels are raised in acute viral hepatitis, presumably due to release from damaged hepatocytes,[319] and serum iron levels may also be elevated.[329] Serum alpha-fetoprotein levels are high and correlate with the severity of the acute hepatitis.[47, 208] The levels rise during the course of the illness as the serum transaminase levels return towards normal, thus favouring the possibility that alpha-fetoprotein is synthesized during hepatocellular regeneration.

DIFFERENTIAL DIAGNOSIS

The main differences between hepatitis A and B are summarized in Table 28.6. They are usually not sufficient to enable a clear clinical distinction to be made, and many sporadic cases previously attributed to hepatitis A can now be shown to be due to hepatitis B. A firm diagnosis is based on the demonstration of the viruses or their serological markers.

Icteric viral hepatitis may be difficult to distinguish from other causes of jaundice, whether discovered incidentally such as one of the constitutional hyperbilirubinaemias, particularly Gilbert's syndrome or the Dubin–Johnson syndrome (see Chapters 13 and 14), or presenting clinically with symptoms of hepatocellular failure or cholestasis.

The approach to the diagnosis of the jaundiced patient is discussed in Chapter 26. Diagnosis may be particularly difficult in infancy, in the elderly, in pregnancy (Chapter 14) and during the postoperative period (Chapter 47). In these situations the patient may be unable to give a good history, may have received many drugs or blood transfusions, and on clinical grounds investigations may have to be limited. In hepatocellular jaundice, the main distinction has usually to be made from drug-induced jaundice (see Chapter 36), infectious mononucleosis (see Chapter 39), leptospirosis and other bacterial infections of the liver (see Chapter 51), and other viral infections where hepatic involvement is a prominent feature (see below). In addition to the clinical features and serological tests, liver biopsy histology provides the most useful information.

The more recent specialized techniques for the investigation of patients presenting with cholestasis, such as ultrasound and total body scanning (see Chapter 21), percutaneous cholangiography with the 'skinny' needle (see Chapter 26) and endoscopic cannulation of the biliary tree (see Chapter 23) have greatly increased the accuracy and speed of diagnosis in such patients.

Anicteric infections or a typical acute attack presenting in the pre-icteric phase are difficult to diagnose clinically. The chief cause of concern is the liability of such cases to spread the infection to health care personnel and patients, and the danger to the patient himself of inadvertent surgery when presenting with gastrointestinal symptoms.

Distinction between acute viral hepatitis and a relapse or decompensation of chronic liver disease is based on clinical, biochemical and histological features.

COURSE AND PROGNOSIS

As indicated earlier, serological markers confirm that anicteric and subclinical infections with hepatitis A and B occur commonly, and this may also apply to non-A non-B hepatitis in some parts of the world.

It is difficult to estimate the proportion of patients infected with HAV who become jaundiced, but it is likely that it is less than 5 per cent.[108] Clinically, overt hepatitis A is more acute than hepatitis B, but resolution is usually rapid; fulminant hepatic failure is rare. Liver function tests are usually back to normal within two months, and chronicity does not occur, although the post-hepatitis syndrome with malaise, lassitude and depression may persist.

Hepatitis B runs a more prolonged course, is responsible for a significant proportion of cases of acute fulminant hepatitis, and may progress to chronicity. The mortality rate of fulminant hepatitis is high. Only 20 to 25 per cent survive, and virtually all are under the age of 40 years, but such patients seldom progress to chronicity. Chronic hepatitis develops in 5 to 10 per cent of patients with acute hepatitis B[276, 321] and is inversely related to the height of the bilirubin.[276] Chronicity is most likely to occur in males, in the very young and in the elderly, in patients on renal dialysis or receiving immunosuppressive therapy or in those with Down's syndrome (Table 28.7).

The presence of the HB_eAg in the serum[276] or bridging necrosis on liver biopsy[56] at the time of the acute attack is associated with the

Table 28.7. *Adverse Prognostic Features in Acute Hepatitis B Infection.*

Clinical	Biochemical and serological	Biopsy
Age Infancy[281, 406] Elderly[45]	Low serum bilirubin and e antigen persistence[276]	Bridging hepatic necrosis[56, 394]
Sex Males[112]	Persistently raised IgG[33]	Piecemeal necrosis[42, 109, 128]
Mild, insidious onset[276]		Impaired regeneration[291, 416]
Immunosuppression[112, 392]		Plasma cells[39, 193]
Renal dialysis[68]		Bile-duct lesions[303]
Mental deficiency[52, 210]		Cytoplasmic HB_sAg[29, 161, 185, 186, 320]
Haemophilia[360]		Complement[324]

development of chronicity. The carrier state of HB_sAg may persist for months or years after an acute attack[405] and is associated with a widely varying appearance on liver biopsy (see Chapter 29).

Non-A non-B hepatitis may also pursue a chronic course, and in one study elevated transaminase levels persisted for longer than after hepatitis B.[315]

TREATMENT OF THE ACUTE ATTACK

In the absence of specific anti-viral agents effective against the viruses responsible for acute hepatitis, treatment has consisted mainly of bed-rest, diet and corticosteroid therapy, although each is controversial.

During the acute attack, patients often have marked malaise, lassitude, anorexia and nausea, and therefore require bed-rest and dietary restriction, particularly of fatty foods. They should be adequately hydrated with a high calorie intake and correction of electrolyte disturbances, if necessary parenterally. In the severe or fulminant case, a treatment regimen for fulminant hepatic failure should be instituted (see Chapter 27).

Whether early ambulation predisposes to relapse and chronicity is open to question. Studies during the Second World War suggesting that early ambulation increased the frequency of relapse were not confirmed, provided the patients had some bed-rest during the day,[75, 270] although there is some suggestion that strenuous physical activity early in the illness might have an untoward effect.[217] While they are acutely ill, we confine patients to bed and permit gradual convalescence with bathroom facilities if symptoms improve, but return to bed-rest if symptoms recur or liver function tests deteriorate sharply. Similarly, we advise patients to reduce their intake of fatty food if it produces nausea, and to abstain from alcohol for six months, although the evidence that either influences the outcome of the illness or progression to chronicity is marginal.

After their introduction into clinical usage, corticosteroids were soon tried in the treatment of viral hepatitis, with improvement in the patients' feeling of well-being and in liver function tests. However, early studies showed that the duration of the illness was unaffected, and unless treatment was continued into convalescence relapse was likely to occur.[126] Because of their side-effects, corticosteroids were therefore seldom recommended in the uncomplicated cases of acute viral hepatitis, although still advocated for prolonged cholestasis and the fulminant form of the disease.[346] Their use has also been advocated in the more severe form of the disease with bridging necrosis which is associated with a relatively poor prognosis.[56]

Recently, in a controlled clinical trial comparing methylprednisolone with placebo in patients with severe acute viral hepatitis and marked abnormalities of liver function, seven of 14 treated patients died, compared with only two of the 15 on placebo. The authors concluded that, far from having a favourable effect, the corticosteroid group had an excess mortality, although the difference did not achieve statistical significance.[158]

In addition to the apparent adverse effect in the controlled clinical trial quoted above, other workers have reported that corticosteroid treatment may be harmful and associated with prominent side-effects.[48, 266]

Nevertheless, there are some patients with chronic active hepatitis who start acutely, and have the histological pattern of piecemeal necrosis, in whom corticosteroids may be effective. If this histology or immunological features such as hyperglobulinaemia with autoantibodies exist and thereby suggest this diagnosis or an established active cirrhosis, then the use of corticosteroids is indicated.

Additional methods that have been tried in a few cases of acute viral hepatitis are treatment with interferon and levamisole, but they have been used more frequently in chronic hepatitis and will be discussed in Chapter 29.

Recently, there has been a report of a controlled trial of (+)-cyanidanol-3 in 100 patients with acute viral hepatitis. The trial was double-blind and it was claimed that the drug, which is a powerful free radical scavenger, accelerated the disappearance of HB_sAg from blood, lowered serum bilirubin levels and relieved symptoms such as anorexia, nausea and pruritus.[49] Although the authors are cautious in their interpretation of the results, they believe that the drug has important advantages over corticosteroids and warrants further study.

In fulminant hepatitis B, specific immunotherapy with anti-HB_s is not beneficial.[2] When pruritus is severe in the cholestatic form of viral hepatitis, it may be relieved by cholestyramine, antihistamines or a short course of corticosteroids.

PREVENTION OF VIRAL HEPATITIS

The measures which should be taken to prevent the spread of viral hepatitis will vary greatly depending on the clinical circumstances. Much attention has been focused on the problem in recent years because of the facility to test for markers of HBV infection and the occurrence of serious outbreaks of hepatitis, particularly in dialysis units. It is important to see the problem in perspective and to recognize that simple, well-established methods are most likely to prevent the spread of infection. Since hepatitis A is spread by the faecal–oral route, measures aimed at good sanitation in the community and scrupulous hygiene amongst those involved in handling water, milk, shellfish and other foods will help to prevent both sporadic cases and common-source epidemics. Special precautions need to be taken to prevent the spread of hepatitis B by the inoculation of blood or blood products and these will be discussed later.

General Measures

There is considerable variation in attitudes regarding the policy for isolation of sporadic cases of acute hepatitis. In western society, mild cases are usually managed at home, but if severe are either admitted to isolation units in infectious disease hospitals or to a side room in a general hospital.

There is little evidence that isolation in the home will reduce the spread of infection to other family members, since it is likely that they will already have been exposed during the incubation period. Simple measures in the home regarding disposal of urine and stools, hand-washing and the use of separate eating utensils are usually advised. The value of passive immunization of contacts is discussed later.

If admitted to hospital, the patient with acute hepatitis should be isolated. Patients are usually admitted to hospital only if the jaundice persists for more than two to three weeks or if they are acutely ill, but if repeated sporadic cases occur in a closed community such as a school, isolation of mild cases may be attempted to contain the spread.

In hospital, the patient with acute hepatitis should be isolated in a single cubicle or at the end of the ward. Adequate facilities should be available for the disposal of urine, faeces, soiled linen, syringes and needles, not only to prevent spread in the hospital ward but to prevent infection of ancillary and laboratory staff. Medical attendants should wear special gowns and gloves when handling patients, particularly if undertaking procedures which involve spillage of blood.

There has also been considerable concern about the management of HB_sAg carriers admitted to hospital. Often the approach is similar to that outlined above. The approach to the management of carriers requiring dental treatment, surgery or obstetric care in hospital also varies. This ranges from the provision of entirely separate facilities to virtually no precautions in geographical areas where the carrier rate is high.

Similarly, the extent to which blood, faeces, urine and other biological fluids from patients with hepatitis or HB_sAg carriers should be identified and specially handled by laboratory staff is controversial. In the United Kingdom, such material is identified and labelled as being a 'hepatitis risk', sent to the laboratory in sealed containers and dealt with separately.

The whole question of the management of patients with acute hepatitis or the chronic HB_sAg carrier in a general hospital and the methods which should be taken to prevent spread should be viewed in relation to the following facts:

1. Many cases of acute hepatitis are no longer infectious at the time of admission to hospital with deep jaundice.
2. Spread from acute cases is most likely to occur if they are admitted to hospital during the incubation period or pre-icteric phase and therefore will not be identified as a hepatitis risk. Furthermore, a high proportion of HB_sAg carriers seen as patients in a general hospital will not be identified. For example, in one survey of consecutive admissions to a general hospital, 84 per cent of the patients found to be HB_sAg positive had not been identified and the test had not been specifically requested.[286] Such patients will therefore be nursed and their blood or other body fluids handled in the laboratory without special precautions.
3. The majority of HB_sAg carriers in a general hospital will be HB_eAg negative and may have anti-e and therefore be unlikely to spread hepatitis B. This does not apply to carriers in dialysis units, mongols or immunosuppressed patients.
4. As discussed earlier, although some surveys have reported a high incidence of HBV markers in hospital personnel, including dentists, the frequency with which they develop clinically overt hepatitis compared with the general population may not be of the same magnitude.

In the authors' view, in a community with a low HB_sAg carrier rate, simple precautions such as those outlined above should be taken when nursing patients with acute hepatitis and if possible they should be accommodated in a side room. HB_sAg carriers requiring dental extraction, endoscopy or surgery should be left to the end of the operating session and the theatre and instruments sterilized after use. Dentists and endoscopists should be encouraged to wear gloves under these circumstances. Laboratory personnel and post-mortem attendants should take simple practical precautions when handling *all* specimens. These include avoidance of mouth-pipetting, eating, smoking and drinking in the laboratory, or the use of equipment or containers that allow spillage of blood. There should be special facilities for handwashing, and clean protective clothing should be worn, including gloves if practicable, particularly if abrasions are present on the hands. Should spillage of potentially contaminated material occur, the work area should be cleaned with hypochlorite, formaldehyde or glutaraldehyde solution as appropriate.

The whole subject is fully reviewed by Cossart,[87] and methods advocated for the control of hepatitis in laboratories have been proposed by the WHO Expert Committee on Viral Hepatitis.[400] We would, however, agree with the view of the WHO Expert Committee on Viral Hepatitis that 'there is no evidence that the identification of patients who are HB_sAg-positive so that their specimens can be specially labelled or handled would lead to any greater reduction of the occupational risk of hepatitis B than would result from the meticulous attention to procedures for the safe handling of all clinical specimens.'[401]

The precautions required to prevent spread of hepatitis by blood or blood products require special consideration.

Prevention of Transfusion-associated Hepatitis

As indicated earlier, the risk of developing transfusion-associated hepatitis is very variable and will depend on the carrier rate of HB_sAg and probably also of non-A non-B viruses in the community, as well as on the presence of naturally acquired immunity to these infections.

There have been reports from several countries indicating that the introduction of routine testing of all blood donations for HB_sAg has resulted in a significant reduction in the frequency of transfusion-associated hepatitis.[16, 146, 152] The techniques which are generally used are radio-immunoassay, particularly in the United States, and passive haemagglutination in the United Kingdom. However, it has become clear that, despite the use of sensitive screening techniques and confining donations to the use of volunteer donors, occasional cases of hepatitis B occur,[149] and a high proportion of cases of post-transfusion hepatitis are due to non-A non-B viruses.[60, 107, 152]

The explanation for the development of hepatitis B despite sensitive screening techniques probably lies in the fact that some specimens may retain infectivity without detectable HB_sAg. It has been proposed that augmenting HB_sAg screening with tests for anti-

HB_c or DNA polymerase activity might reduce the incidence of such cases,[186, 206] but it is unlikely that such screening would be economically viable.[152] Elimination of donations from donors who have a non-specific biochemical abnormality such as raised enzyme levels is also unacceptable because of the high wastage associated with a non-infective cause of such abnormalities. There is optimism that serological tests for non-A non-B viruses will become available, but this too might involve a multiplicity of techniques.

As discussed earlier, it had been hoped that cryopreserved red blood cells would be free of hepatitis risk, but this is open to question[19] and requires further controlled observations.[76]

The screening of plasma fractions, particularly clotting factor concentrates, poses special problems. Factor VIII and IX concentrates used in the treatment of haemophilia are prepared from large pools of several thousand donations and have been associated with the development of hepatitis or asymptomatic chronic liver disease.[90, 360] Although the use of radio-immunoassay to screen the original donations might reduce the frequency of HBV infection, it is unlikely to eliminate it, and non-A non-B hepatitis will still occur.

The use of passive immunity with immune globulin to prevent transfusion-associated hepatitis has aroused controversy and will be discussed below.

Prevention of Dialysis-associated Hepatitis

The introduction of regular screening for HB_sAg and the exclusion of patients and staff with positive tests from 'clean' units has resulted in a considerable reduction in dialysis-associated hepatitis in the United Kingdom.[296] In this survey conducted by the Public Health Laboratory Service there was a sustained decline in the incidence of hepatitis B in dialysis units to 0.3 per cent among patients and 0.1 per cent among staff, a greater than tenfold decrease over a four-year period. This compared very favourably with the 10 per cent HB_sAg carrier rate in European units in 1973, with a further 10 per cent being detected during that year.

Apart from screening, meticulous attention to personal hygiene and sterility during the dialysis procedure is essential, whether carried out at home or in the dialysis unit, so as to reduce HBV and non-A non-B infections. Recommendations for controlling infection in dialysis units have been produced by the WHO Special Committee on Viral Hepatitis.[400]

Control of hepatitis in units in the United States and Europe has been less successful and may not be achieved until active immunization becomes available. During an outbreak, repeated passive immunization of staff with hepatitis B immune globulin (HBIG) may be necessary (see below).

Passive Immunization for Acute Viral Hepatitis

Immunoprophylaxis of hepatitis A

In 1945 several field trials clearly established that normal immune serum globulin (ISG) could prevent hepatitis A infection if given before or within one to two weeks of exposure.[141, 169]

Since then, preparations from widely differing sources in different parts of the world have been shown to be effective either in preventing or attenuating infection.[57, 84, 298] This is presumed to be due to the presence of high-titre anti-HAV in normal serum pools as a result of the frequency of infection in childhood. ISG prepared, for example, from plasma pools in the United States and United Kingdom appears to be effective in preventing hepatitis A acquired abroad. The frequency with which unprotected individuals who travel abroad acquire hepatitis A presumably results from undue exposure rather than variation in strains of hepatitis A in different countries.

By attenuating the infection, rather than preventing it completely, passive–active immunity may result in natural lifelong immunity. Under such circumstances, the immunized individual excretes the virus at some stage, and it has been feared that such undetected ambulant cases might be a hazard to contacts, but this does not appear to be clinically significant. Direct studies of the effect of immunization on excretion of virus in stools should soon be forthcoming.

Since ISG is readily available and is effective in protecting 80 to 90 per cent of contacts if administered before or within one to two weeks of exposure, its widespread use has been advocated. At present, recommendations for the use of ISG are based on epidemiological data identifying groups at risk. If serological techniques for detecting anti-HAV become readily available, advice may be possible on a more rational basis, and similarly the use of batches of high-titre anti-HAV may modify current views about the suggested dosage and need for repeat injections.

The following recommendations are based on those of the Advisory Committee on Immunization Practices[3] and the WHO Expert Committee on Viral Hepatitis.[401]

Close household contacts should all be given ISG unless there is a clear history of hepatitis A infection in the past. Secondary attack rates are highest for children, but although low in adults the disease is often severe and therefore ISG is recommended for them as well.

School and work contacts should not be given ISG routinely unless repeated cases are occurring, suggesting a common-source outbreak.

In prisons or in institutions for the mentally retarded, periodic outbreaks of hepatitis may occur and these may be contained by the administration of ISG to patients and staff.

Hospital and laboratory personnel should not be given routine prophylactic ISG, but reliance on prevention of spread should be based on stringent precautions in dealing with infected material.

Pre-exposure prophylaxis. There is good evidence that travel abroad in tropical areas or developing countries where hepatitis A is common is associated with an increased risk of the infection. It is therefore recommended that ISG should be given in a dose of 0.02 to 0.12 ml/kg body weight intramuscularly and repeated at six months if there is continuing risk of exposure by residence abroad in such countries. There is no evidence that travel on ordinary tourist routes is associated with an increased risk.

Individuals who handle non-human primates, particularly chimpanzees, are liable to develop hepatitis A, and ISG in doses of 0.5 ml/kg body weight administered four-monthly is advisable.

Immunoprophylaxis of hepatitis B

In contrast to the rapid establishment of the efficacy of immune serum globulin in the prevention of type A viral hepatitis, studies in the 1940s and 50s provided little evidence of similar benefit in the prevention of hepatitis B. These studies were chiefly directed at the prevention of post-transfusion hepatitis, and included the administration of large volumes of ISG before and at frequent intervals after blood transfusion. Some provided evidence suggesting that ISG prolonged the incubation period,[113] and there were occasional reports of a reduction in the incidence of post-transfusion hepatitis.[344]

The early reports were undertaken before facilities were available for testing for hepatitis B markers, either in the transfused blood or in the recipients. The availability of such markers has facilitated controlled studies of the use of prophylactic immune globulins in several groups of patients at high risk of developing hepatitis B. These have included needle stick exposure,[345] post-transfusion hepatitis,[344] dialysis-associated hepatitis,[309] non-parenteral transmitted hepatitis B in institutions,[218, 370] after vertical transmission[215] and in spouses.[322]

Despite the fact that hepatitis B markers, including the antigen titre, of infused material and anti-HB_s titre of ISG were sometimes available, these studies have limitations for the following reasons:

1. The volume of infectious virus in the inoculum or the e antigen status was usually not known, and in some instances, such as after needle stick exposure, there was doubt as to whether inoculation of virus had occurred.
2. A placebo group was seldom included and in most studies ISG was compared with hepatitis B immune globulin (HBIG).
3. The duration of follow-up after exposure was sometimes inadequate, and if prolonged the possibility of re-exposure in these high risk categories could not be excluded, i.e. that passive–active immunity had occurred.
4. Finally, the possible effect of non-A non-B infections spread parenterally could not be evaluated.

Despite these deficiencies, it is clear from the controlled experimental study of Krugman and Giles[218] that both HBIG and ISG have a protective effect if administered within *four hours* of the experimental inoculation of a standard dose of the MS-2 serum pool. They showed that all 25 children who received the MS-2 pool, but without prophylactic globulin, developed HB_sAg in their serum, and 24 had elevated transaminase levels. Thirteen of 15 children who received ISG developed circulating HB_sAg, and 12 of these had hepatitis. By comparison, only four of 10 children who received HBIG developed HB_sAg and hepatitis.

Their conclusion, that HBIG had a protective effect, was supported by a large Veterans Administration cooperative study of the prevention of hepatitis following needle stick exposure by the administration of HBIG in two doses.[345]

On the other hand, there is some evidence that both ISG and high-titre HBIG only prolong the incubation period of HBV infection. In earlier studies, the incidence of infection with hepatitis B and circulating HB_sAg was significantly lower in both the patients and staff who received the high-titre material, eight months after admission to the trial, but by 12 months the two groups were similar.[154, 343] In the light of current knowledge, the proposed guidelines for passive immunization for hepatitis B can be summarized as in the following section.[15, 61, 401]

Post-exposure prophylaxis. Following exposure to blood known to be positive for HB_sAg, such as following a needle stick, HBIG should be administered in a dose of 0.05 to 0.07 ml/kg body weight as soon as possible after exposure, and repeated 25 to 30 days later. To be effective it is best given within 24 hours of exposure. Infants born to mothers with acute hepatitis in the third trimester of pregnancy and mothers who are e antigen positive should receive HBIG as a single dose of 0.13 ml/kg body weight immediately after delivery or as soon as possible thereafter.

In both these situations, testing of the recipient for HBV markers might obviate the need for such prophylaxis, and similarly the detection of anti-e in the blood source of exposure would also make prophylaxis unnecessary.

Although it has been shown that there is an increased incidence of hepatitis B in the spouses of individuals with acute HBV infection, and one study has shown a reduction in the attack rate of hepatitis B in spouses following HBIG administration,[322] it is likely that in most cases contact during the incubation period would preclude its effectiveness in these situations.

Similarly, the value of passive immunization with HBIG or ISG in patients or staff on haemodialysis units and in institutions for the mentally retarded is less clear cut, and the recommendations of necessity must be equivocal. If there is clear evidence of an outbreak in a particular institution and especially if patients who are chronically e antigen positive can be identified, it would seem reasonable to administer ISG or HBIG at four-monthly intervals to their non-immune contacts. In such situations, it is suggested that both patients and staff should be monitored for HBV markers at frequent intervals, as a changing status would clearly alter the recommendations made.

Finally, it should be emphasized that routine public health measures involving the handling of infected material and personal hygiene are more important than prophylactic immunization in the control of infection. As regards post-transfusional hepatitis, screening and elimination of donors with HBV markers is more effective in its elimination than the administration of prophylactic globulins.

Active Immunization for Acute Viral Hepatitis

Active immunization for hepatitis A

Although hepatitis A is usually a relatively mild infection acquired in childhood, there is evidence that the age of infection in western communities is increasing. Since attacks may be more severe in the older age group, it can be argued that active immunization in childhood may be indicated if this becomes available.

Active immunization for hepatitis B

The need for developing a vaccine against hepatitis B is much more cogent. As indicated earlier in this chapter, it can be a more serious infection and is liable to chronicity with the possible complications of cirrhosis and hepatoma.

In preliminary studies, Krugman and Giles[218] heated known infective human serum from the MS-2 serum pool at 98°C for one minute to inactivate the virus. When so treated, the serum, if subsequently administered to susceptible individuals on one to three occasions, prevented the development of hepatitis B in two-thirds of individuals after challenge with the original infective serum four to eight months later. Heating at 60°C for 10 hours did not completely inactivate the virus. These studies demonstrated that immunization against hepatitis B was feasible, but inactivated whole human serum containing HBV was unacceptable for general use because of contaminating normal serum or plasma components.

Subsequent attempts at the development of a vaccine have concentrated on purification of the 22 nm spherical particles for use as immunogens. Purified subunit vaccines have been prepared in a number of ways, including repeated isopycnic banding in CsCl and rate zonal centrifugation in sucrose. Purified preparations have then been inactivated with formaldehyde and have been used for studies in chimpanzees. Such vaccines have been shown to be non-infective to susceptible chimpanzees, all animals developing anti-HB_s but no anti-core antibodies. When challenged six months after immunization, these animals have been shown to be wholly immune, irrespective of the subtype of the surface antigen used in the preparation of the vaccine. Some animals were rendered immune by the administration of the vaccine shortly after infection with hepatitis B, so that post-infection vaccination, possibly combined with HBIG, might be feasible.[64, 314]

Although most studies have used purified 22 nm particles, Prince[305] has used a mixed preparation, including Dane particles and e antigen positive serum, which can be completely inactivated by formalin. An alternative approach has been to prepare vaccines from the eight major polypeptides of HB_sAg.

It has been shown that alum-absorbed polypeptide vaccine, if injected into susceptible chimpanzees, will produce circulating anti-HB_s and will render them immune to subsequent challenge with infective virus. Such preparations, however, are difficult to make, and there have been problems with stability, but results are sufficiently encouraging to continue this approach by further characterizing HB_sAg and synthesizing its immunogenic polypeptide components.[417]

Preparations of purified inactivated hepatitis B vaccine have had limited trials in man. Maupas and associates[247] prepared purified HB_sAg by affinity chromatography on antibody-coated gels and inactivated it with formalin. After preliminary testing for safety and efficacy in chimpanzees, they administered it to volunteer patients and staff from a haemodialysis unit with two subcutaneous injections of 1 ml of vaccine at an interval of one month. Thirty-two of 39 subjects free of past infection who were vaccinated developed a specific immunological response. None of the subjects developed any complications following vaccination. Although this report is encouraging, it was uncontrolled, but further studies are imminent.[413]

OTHER VIRUSES

Many other viruses affect the liver and it is impossible to be comprehensive. They range from yellow fever where acidophil degeneration of hepatocytes was first described[88] to the recently identified viruses causing Lassa fever and Ebola haemorrhagic fever. In between this is a range of viruses, some of which produce hepatitis as part of a systemic illness, while others usually produce hepatitis only as an opportunistic infection in immunosuppressed individuals. Many viruses have been isolated from patients presenting clinically with hepatitis but a cause and effect relationship has rarely been established.

Viruses largely confined to neonatal hepatitis are discussed in Chapter 40.

Yellow Fever

This results from infection with an RNA virus transmitted biologically by mosquitoes. Replication of the virus occurs in both vector and host. The virus is endemic in jungle primates of both Africa and the Central and South Americas, and the cycle is between primate and mosquito. Man is involved when incidentally exposed to jungle (or sylvan) yellow fever. An urban variety of yellow fever exists in which the cycle is between man and mosquito and other primates are incidentally involved. The virus is identical for these varieties but the mosquito vectors differ. In the Americas the mosquito *Aedes aegypti* transmits urban yellow fever and *Haemogogus* species complete the jungle cycle. In Africa several species of aedine mosquitoes can transmit both urban and jungle yellow fever.[409]

Most infections are clinically inapparent although usually more severe in older age groups and outbreaks appear to vary in virulence and incidence of complications.[202, 325] Fever, headaches, nausea and vomiting are the most common presenting complaints with jaundice in more severe cases. Abdominal, chest and/or joint pains may be present. Leucopenia is initially found followed by a leucocytosis. Central nervous system involvement, renal failure and evidence of a bleeding diathesis appear to be adverse prognostic features.[202]

The changes in the liver have been documented by biopsy in man[137, 207] and experimentally in monkeys.[380] These confirm the prominent acidophil degeneration of hepatocytes in the midzone (Figure 28.21) as described in the autopsy studies performed by Councilman.[88] Even in severe cases there is sparing of a rim of centrilobular and periportal hepatocytes.[207] In addition there is fatty change and ballooning

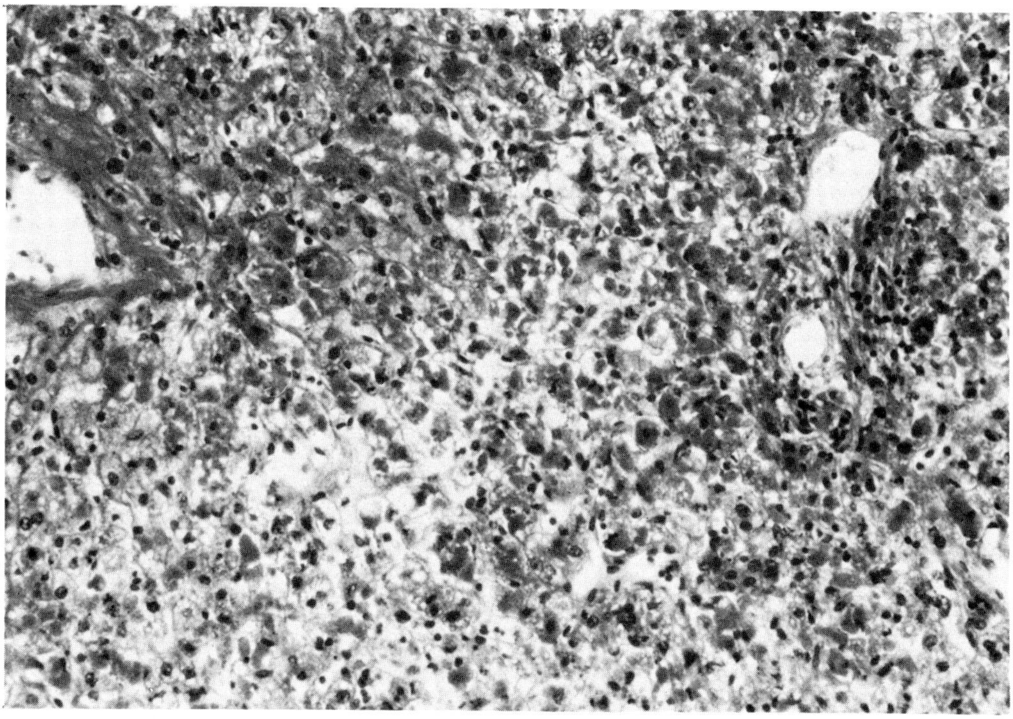

Figure 28.21. Yellow fever. Portal tract to the right and central vein to the left. The pallor of the intervening midzone is due to acidophilic degeneration and disintegration of hepatocytes. (Experimentally infected monkey.) × 200. Courtesy of Dr F.O. MacCallum.

degeneration of other hepatocytes which occurs early in the course of the disease.[137] Experimentally, the earliest feature seen was acidophil necrosis of Kupffer cells 24 hours after inoculation. These were positive in a fluorescent antibody technique using antibody to yellow fever virus. Hepatocyte degeneration did not occur until the third day and then rapidly increased.[380]

There is no well-documented evidence of chronic liver disease resulting from yellow fever. Any such reports must now exclude concomitant infection with hepatitis B virus which is also endemic in these areas.

Treatment is non-specific; supportive measures such as correction of electrolyte imbalance and control of renal failure when necessary are required. Recently, monkeys experimentally infected with a lethal dose of yellow fever have been successfully treated with a nuclease-resistant derivative of a polyriboinosinic polyribocytidytic acid complex.[362] This requires more detailed evaluation. Prophylaxis is obviously more desirable and complete immunity can be achieved by the standard vaccination with an attenuated virus.

Adenoviruses

Many viruses have been isolated from patients with hepatitis in the search for the infective agents of hepatitis A and B. These are often adenoviruses which is not surprising as they are both ubiquitous and relatively easily isolated by current laboratory techniques. Since they are also known to be excreted in the faeces intermittently over many years[134] reactivation of such viruses during an episode of hepatitis is theoretically possible and the isolation of an adenovirus from the faeces during the illness is of dubious significance. It has also been shown that titres of antibody to adenovirus will rise during the course of other primary infections such as viral and mycoplasmal pneumonias.[135] As adenovirus infections of the liver are associated with the presence of hepatocyte intranuclear inclusions which are not described in human viral hepatitis, their aetiological importance seems limited.

The role of adenoviruses and the San Carlos viruses in infectious hepatitis has been reviewed.[409] Now that the probable hepatitis A virus has been identified it is evident that at least one further viral agent (non-A, non-B) is involved. The role of adenoviruses such as adenovirus 5[167] and the San Carlos viruses[92] subsequently identified as adenoviruses types 1 to 3[168] may thus need to be reconsidered.

Herpes Viruses

Infectious mononucleosis

Now well established as an infection with the Epstein–Barr virus (EBV) there is an extensive literature with several reviews.[70,125,177] Typically, infection occurs in adolescence or young adult life and is characterized by fever, malaise, sore throat and adenopathy. Clinically, hepatitis with hepatomegaly occurs in up to 15 per cent of cases but abnormal elevation of serum transaminases is almost universal.[114,140] The clinical presentation may closely mimic infectious hepatitis and then be wrongly diagnosed but the serological reactions are usually characteristic and diagnostic.[177]

The features on liver biopsy have to be distinguished from a malignant lymphomatous infiltrate (see Chapter 39) which they may closely mimic. The portal tracts and sinusoids are heavily infiltrated by mononuclear cells which show morphological variations ranging from mature small lymphocytes to large lymphoblastoid cells. Plasma cells may also be present.[150] Hepatocellular damage is not usually pronounced but regenerative, particularly mitotic, activity may be disproportionately increased. Extensive hepatocellular necrosis can occur[10] but death from hepatic failure is extremely rare as is progression to chronicity.[26]

Cytomegalovirus

This DNA virus is identical on electron microscopy to the herpes viruses with which it is usually grouped. Several antigenic sub-types are thought to exist.[148]

Infection with this virus is very common. It can be transmitted in or around the neonatal period and although overwhelming infection may result most cases are asymptomatic. The peak incidence of infection is in young adult life. Infection may present as a febrile systemic illness, a hepatitis, an atypical mononucleosis syndrome usually with a hepatitis or as the Guillain-Barré syndrome.[336] It is commonly followed by prolonged excretion of the virus which is often intermittent and occurs in the presence of high serum antibody titres.[148] Patients on immunosuppressive therapy are particularly prone to infection, as are those undergoing cardiac surgery. It is not clear whether immunosuppression permits primary infection, infection with a second antigenically distinct sub-type or simply reactivation of the virus.

In the liver the pathological features are identical to those of viral hepatitis with hepatocytes showing acidophil degeneration and a mixed inflammatory cell infiltrate in portal tracts and lobule.[381] A granulomatous hepatitis has also been described.[53] Cytomegalovirus inclusions can be demonstrated in hepatocytes and vascular endothelium but only in approximately 20 per cent of cases.[173] Infected hepatocytes are characteristically strikingly enlarged and contain a prominent large eosinophilic inclusion within the nucleus but not attached to the nuclear membrane. Occasional inclusion bodies within the cytoplasm may also be identified. Visibly infected hepatocytes become surrounded by Kupffer cells and then isolated before morphological changes of acidophil degeneration are visible.

A diagnosis of cytomegalovirus hepatitis as distinct from other forms of viral hepatitis is difficult. It requires either the demonstration of the inclusion bodies in the liver, or isolation of the virus from the patient, or identification of IgM antibody in high titre in the serum.[336]

Herpes simplex

This DNA virus causes disseminated infection with hepatitis in neonatal life.[256] Both strains of herpes simplex virus (HSV-1 and HSV-2) have been isolated from cases of generalized disease.[269] In adults, hepatitis is usually part of a disseminated infection. This usually occurs in individuals immunosuppressed either by therapy[21] or as a result of concurrent illness such as Hodgkin's disease but primary infection in previously healthy individuals and in pregnant women has been recorded.[124,407] The clinical features are fever, a severe disseminated intravascular coagulation syndrome with leucopenia, thrombocytopenia and prolonged prothrombin and partial thromboplastin times as well as evidence of involvement of multiple organs such as encephalitis, myocarditis or hepatitis. The primary focal lesion is most commonly oral, frequently with severe buccal and pharyngeal ulceration,[21] but oeso-

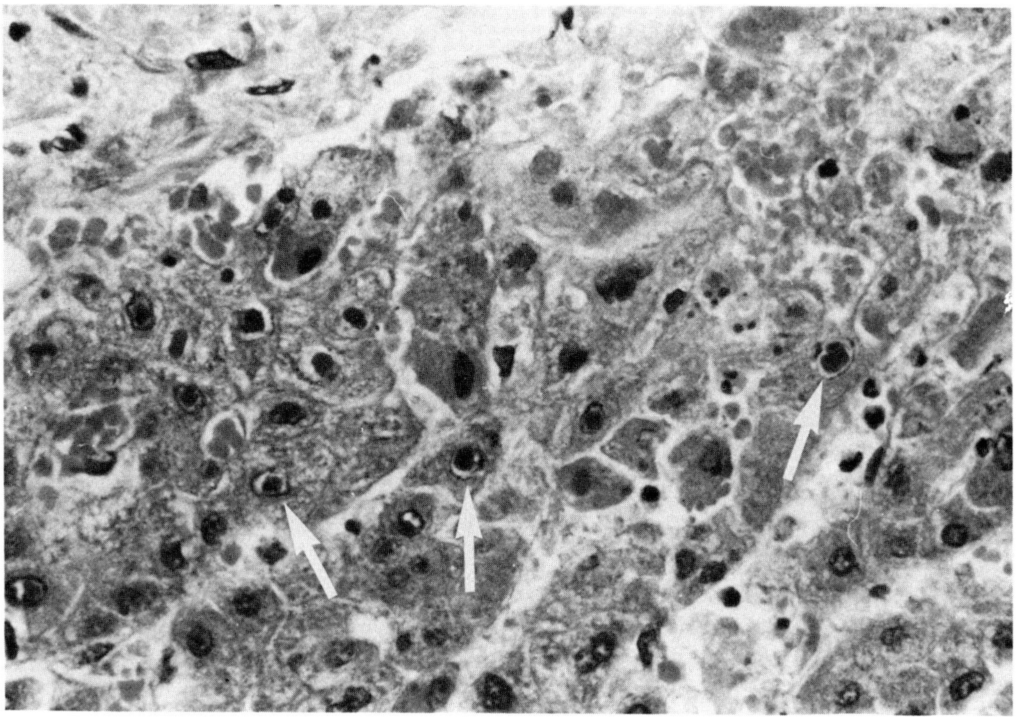

Figure 28.22. Herpes simplex infection. The edge of a portal tract is present, top left, and a zone of coagulative necrosis, top right. Around this zone numerous hepatocytes have large eosinophilic inclusions in their nuclei (arrows). There is usually a halo separating the inclusion from a rim of chromatin and nuclear membrane. Haematoxylin and eosin × 750.

phageal[124] and primary genital infection[407] have been recorded. When associated with pregnancy there is the additional risk of disseminated herpes infection in the fetus. Transplacental infection may occur but most infections are probably acquired during transit through the genital canal.[20] It is of interest that in the case reported by Anuras and Summers[21] there was no evidence of infection of the placenta, amniotic fluid or fetus after caesarian section despite disseminated active maternal infection.

In the liver there are small punctate haemorrhagic foci of necrosis with a variable, usually mononuclear reaction. Hepatocytes around the necrotic focus usually contain the typical intranuclear inclusion bodies (Figure 28.22).[224]

Treatment with cytosine arabinoside is indicated. This is a pyrimidine nucleoside that inhibits DNA synthesis and has antiherpetic activity.[203]

Herpes zoster varicella

This is unusual in adults but may be severe in immunosuppressed individuals. The characteristics of the skin rash with isolation of the virus from the vesicles should establish the diagnosis in doubtful cases. Pneumonitis is the most severe complication. In the liver small foci of necrosis 1 to 3 mm in diameter are found.[78] Nuclear inclusions are readily demonstrable in the epidermal cells of the skin vesicles but their presence in hepatocytes is not so consistent.

Enteroviruses

This group of viruses is one genus of the family of picornaviruses and includes polio virus, coxsackie virus A and B and echoviruses.

The 27 nm hepatitis A virus is morphologically similar to the enteroviruses but its classification is still undecided.

Coxsackie group A viruses

These usually cause herpangina, upper respiratory tract infection or aseptic meningitis but they have also been isolated from patients in epidemics of infectious hepatitis.[121, 200] As for adenoviruses their exact role in the aetiology of infectious hepatitis is debatable, especially as coxsackie viruses are commonly found in the alimentary tract.

Coxsackie B

These viruses classically cause epidemic myalgia but may cause fulminating disease in neonates. They have been associated with a wide variety of syndromes in adults and more recently have been implicated in the pathogenesis of some cardiomyopathies.

Hepatic involvement is documented only rarely despite the widespread organ involvement found in most adult infections. A clinically significant hepatitis has been recorded in two previously healthy young adults and was associated with a myocarditis.[157, 366] Liver biopsy showed a non-specific portal tract inflammation with microabscesses containing neutrophils in the lobule. Electron microscopy demonstrated virus-like particles in hepatocyte cytoplasm.[157]

Echoviruses

Although documented as a cause of hepatic necrosis in neonates,[189] involvement in adults is rarely recorded. Schleissner and Portnoy[335] recorded abnormal liver function tests in one of two adult siblings presenting with pneumonitis and aseptic meningitis.

Arenaviruses

These are a group of morphologically indistinguishable but markedly pleomorphic viruses that have both common and specific antigenic characteristics. They are reviewed by Casals.[71]

Lassa fever

First identified in 1969 this disease attained publicity because of its infectivity and high mortality rate of between one- and two-thirds of cases.[136] Outbreaks have occurred in various parts of West Africa but serological studies

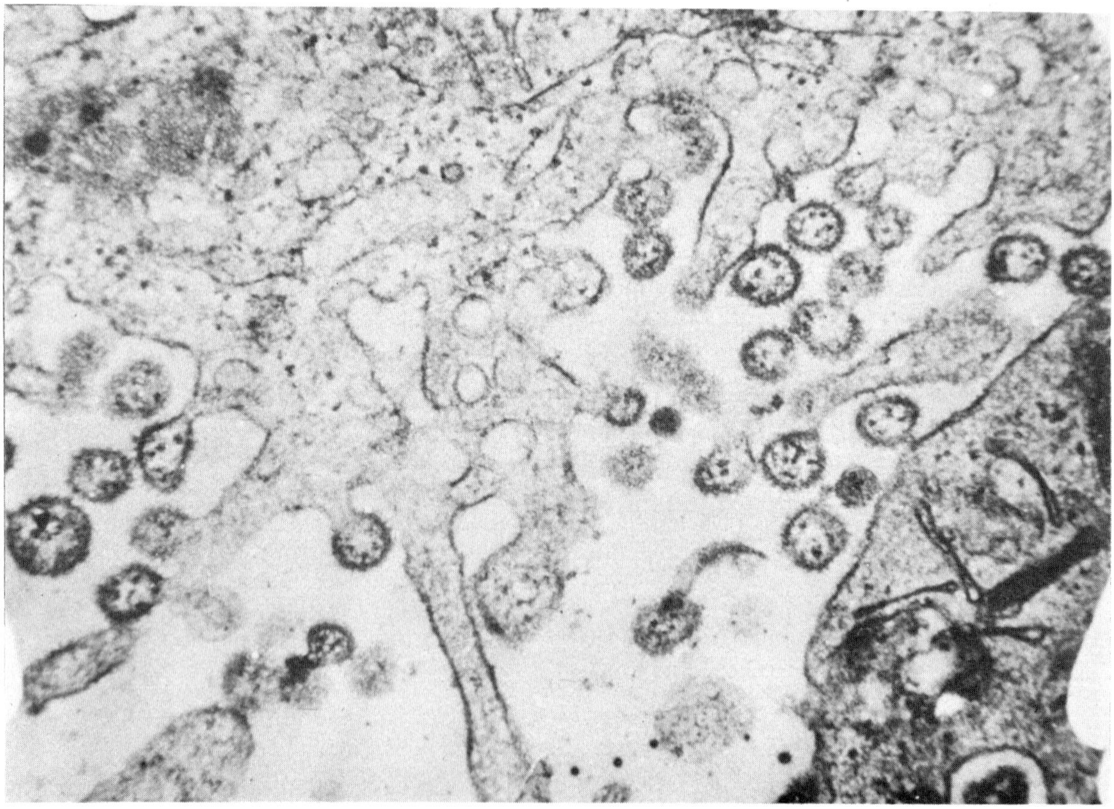

Figure 28.23. Lassa fever. Lassa virus budding out from cell surface. The virus particles contain granules characteristic of the family Arenaviridae and these have been shown to be host ribosomes. Vero cell culture × 98 000. Courtesy of Dr Frederick A. Murphy, C.D.C. Atlanta, and Colonel E.E. Vella, Microbiological Research Establishment, Porton Down, U.K.

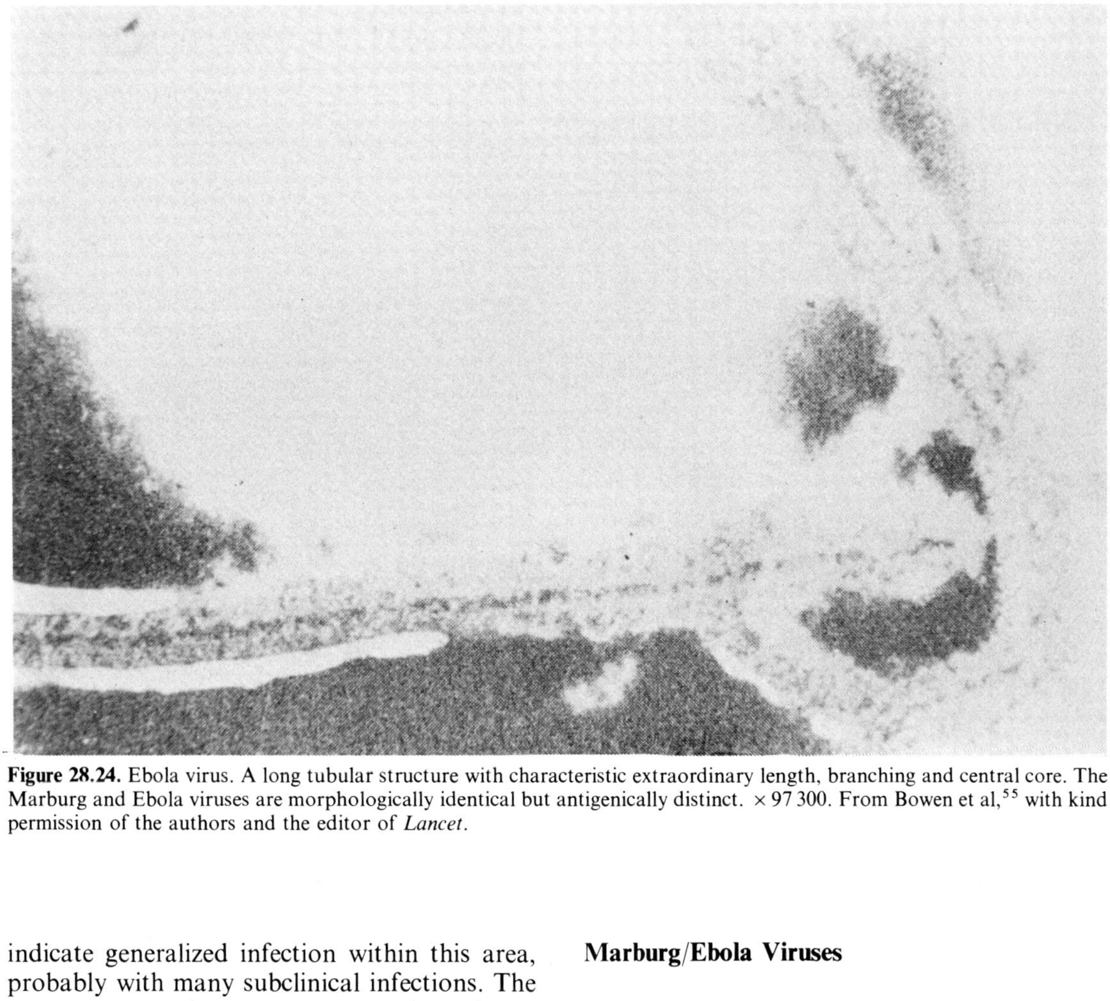

Figure 28.24. Ebola virus. A long tubular structure with characteristic extraordinary length, branching and central core. The Marburg and Ebola viruses are morphologically identical but antigenically distinct. × 97 300. From Bowen et al,[55] with kind permission of the authors and the editor of *Lancet*.

indicate generalized infection within this area, probably with many subclinical infections. The agent, an arenavirus, can be isolated from throat washings for several days (Figure 28.23). Transmission is airborne or by contact. There is fever with generalized organ involvement; pneumonia, myocarditis, encephalopathy, nephropathy and myositis and a haemorrhagic diathesis can all occur. Death is usually from sudden cardiovascular collapse.[71]

In the liver, focal necroses and diffuse hepatocellular damage can be seen with centrilobular accentuation. Acidophil bodies have been described as a prominent feature[115] and virus particles have been demonstrated in the space of Disse and in the bile canaliculus by electron microscopy.[398]

Argentinian and Bolivian haemorrhagic fever

Both these fevers are due to arenaviruses and both are associated with a hepatitis similar to that described for Lassa fever.[79, 120]

Marburg/Ebola Viruses

Marburg virus

In 1967 personnel working with African Green monkeys in Marburg, Frankfurt and Belgrade became seriously ill.[245, 364] Five of the 27 patients died. The early symptoms were high fever, conjunctivitis and an enanthema and were followed by an exanthem with hepatitis, diarrhoea, renal abnormalities and a bleeding tendency. Encephalitis or myocarditis was sometimes clinically present. Leucopenia was characteristically present from the first day of illness and could change to a leucocytosis. There was an atypical lymphocytosis and a profound thrombocytopenia.

The virus has an elongated tubular form 70 to 80 nm diameter in which there is a core of 35 to 40 nm diameter with a hollow centre. The tubules may be branched and spikes may be present on the surface. An enlarged head or torus can be identified on some tubules. Many tubules appear to be incomplete outer coat.[13, 211, 290]

The main changes in the liver are necroses starting off as acidophil degeneration of hepatocytes and occasional acidophil cytoplasmic inclusion bodies may be seen. Mild fatty change is present around these foci. A scanty lymphocytic and histiocytic inflammatory cell infiltrate is present and hyperplastic Kupffer cells around the necrotic foci are laden with ceroid pigment.[32] Long-term complications of the hepatitis have not been described.

Ebola virus

Two simultaneous outbreaks of a severe viral haemorrhagic fever occurred in the Sudan and in Zaire in 1976.[190, 402] The mortality was approximately 70 per cent in over 500 cases. Viruses isolated from these outbreaks were identical to the Marburg virus (Figure 28.24) but antigenically distinct.[201] Clinically, patients presented with high fever, excessive fatigue and gastrointestinal disturbances, and in severe cases developed a tendency to bleed from multiple sites. An extensive morbilliform rash appeared over the back, trunk and limbs.[62] Symptoms and signs may possibly be ameliorated by the use of interferon and convalescent immune serum.[122] Transmission of infection required very close contact with the patient and there is no evidence of droplet transmission. An outbreak can be contained by strict isolation, use of protective clothing and careful handling and disposal of body fluids and excretions. An ultrastructural study of the virus in autopsy tissues has recently been reported.[119] It was abundantly demonstrated in and adjacent to foci of necrosis in the liver in hepatocyte cytoplasm and numerous viral particles were also present in bile canaliculi. The pathology of the viral infection in experimentally infected monkeys has now been studied.[30] Treatment is supportive: the role of immune serum is as yet conjectural.

Miscellaneous

Measles

Elevated transaminase levels with hepatomegaly have been recorded during the course of measles in two adults.[349]

Psittacosis

Hepatomegaly is a relatively common finding in patients with psittacosis.[332] Liver biopsy may show non-specific focal necrosis in the parenchyma or non-caseating epithelioid granulomas.[85]

GB agent

Derived from a patient with acute hepatitis, this agent has been serially passaged in marmosets and is serologically unrelated to any known human virus including the hepatitis A virus.[106] Its identity and significance remain to be established.

REFERENCES

1. Achord, J.L. (1968) Acute pancreatitis with infectious hepatitis. *Journal of the American Medical Association,* **205,** 837–840.
2. Acute Hepatic Failure Study Group (1977) Failure of specific immunotherapy in fulminant type B hepatitis. *Annals of Internal Medicine,* **86,** 272–277.
3. Advisory Committee on Immunization Practices (1978) *Immune Globulins for Protection against Viral Hepatitis.* Atlanta: Center for Disease Control. In Press.
4. Aikawa, T., Sairenji, H., Furuta, S., Kiyosawa, K., Shikata, T., Imai, M., Miyakawa, Y., Yanase, Y. & Mayumi, M. (1978) Seroconversion from hepatitis B e antigen to anti-HB_e in acute hepatitis B virus infection. *Lancet,* **i,** 439–441.
5. Alberti, A., Realdi, G., Tremolada, F. & Spina, G.P. (1976) Liver cell surface localization of hepatitis B antigen and of immunoglobulins in acute and chronic hepatitis and in liver cirrhosis. *Clinical and Experimental Immunology,* **25,** 396–402.
6. Alberti, A., Diana, S., Scullard, G.H., Eddleston, A.L.W.F. & Williams, R. (1977) Full and empty Dane particles in relation to the eAg/eAb system in HB_sAg-positive patients. *Archives Hellenic Medical Societies* (Suppl.), **3,** 6.
7. Aldershvile, J., Brock, A., Dietrichson, O., Hardt, F., Juhl, E., Madsbad, S., Mathiesen, L., Matzen, P., Nielsen, J.O., Schlichting, P., Sorensen, S. & Tage-Jensen, U. (1978) Hepatitis B virus infections among Danish dentists. *Journal of Infectious Diseases,* **137,** 63–66.
8. Allen, A.M., Irwin, G.R., Karwacki, J.J., Warren, D.C. & Levine, R.S. (1975) Epidemic hepatitis B: a sustained outbreak in a large military population. *American Journal of Epidemiology,* **102,** 545–552.
9. Allen, J.G. & Sayman, W.A. (1962) Serum hepatitis from transfusions of blood: epidemiologic study. *Journal of the American Medical Association,* **180,** 1079–1085.
10. Allen, U.R. & Bass, B.H. (1963) Fatal hepatic necrosis in glandular fever. *Journal of Clinical Pathology,* **16,** 339–341.

11. Almeida, J.D., Gay, F.W. & Wreghitt, T.G. (1974) Pitfalls in the study of hepatitis A. *Lancet*, **ii**, 748–751.
12. Almeida, J.D., Rubenstein, D. & Stott, E.J. (1971) New antigen–antibody system in Australia-antigen-positive hepatitis. *Lancet*, **ii**, 1225–1227.
13. Almeida, J.D., Waterson, A.P. & Simpson, D.I.H. (1971) Morphology and morphogenesis of the Marburg agent. In *Marburg Virus Disease. Proceedings of a Symposium* (Ed.) Martini, G.A. & Siegert, R. pp. 84–97. Berlin and New York: Springer.
14. Almeida, J.D., Chisholm, G.D., Kulatilake, A.K., MacGregor, A.B., Mackay, D.H., O'Donaghue, E.P.N., Shackman, R. & Waterson, A.P. (1971) Possible airborne spread of serum hepatitis virus within a haemodialysis unit. *Lancet*, **ii**, 849–850.
15. Alter, H.J., Barker, L.F. & Holland, P.V. (1975) Hepatitis B immune globulin: evaluation of clinical trials and rationale for usage. *New England Journal of Medicine*, **293**, 1093–1094.
16. Alter, H.J., Holland, P.V., Purcell, R.H., Lander, J.J., Feinstone, S.M., Morrow, A.G. & Schmidt, P.J. (1972) Post transfusion hepatitis after exclusion of commercial and hepatitis-B antigen positive donors. *Annals of Internal Medicine*, **77**, 691–699.
17. Alter, H.J., Chalmers, T.C., Freeman, B.M., Lunceford, J.L., Lewis, T.L., Holland, P.V., Pizzo, P.A., Plotz, P.H. & Meyer, W.J. (1975) Health-care workers positive for hepatitis B surface antigen. *New England Journal of Medicine*, **292**, 454–457.
18. Alter, H.J., Purcell, R.H., Holland, P.V. & Popper, H. (1978) Transmissible agent in non-A, non-B hepatitis. *Lancet*, **i**, 459–463.
19. Alter, H.J., Tabor, E., Meryman, H.T., Hoofnagle, J.H., Kahn, R.A., Holland, P.V., Gerety, R.J. & Barker, L.F. (1978) Transmission of hepatitis B by frozen red blood cells. *New England Journal of Medicine*, **298**, 637–642.
20. Amstey, M.S. (1971) Management of pregnancy complicated by genital herpes virus infection. *Obstetrics and Gynecology*, **37**, 515–520.
21. Anuras, S. & Summers, R. (1976) Fulminant herpes simplex hepatitis in an adult: report of a case in renal transplant recipient. *Gastroenterology*, **70**, 425–428.
22. Arnold, W., Meyer zum Büschenfelde, K.H., Hess, G. & Knolle, J. (1975) Intranuclear IgG in hepatocytes of patients with hepatitis-B-core-antigen (HB_cAg) in liver tissue. *Digestion*, **12**, 277.
23. Arnold, W., Nielson, J.O., Hardt, F., Meyer zum Büschenfelde, K.H. (1977) The localisation of e antigen in nuclei of hepatocytes. *Gut*, **18**, 994–996.
24. Aterman, K. (1963) Neonatal hepatitis and its relation to viral hepatitis of mother. *American Journal of Diseases of Children*, **105**, 395–416.
25. Bancroft, W.H., Mundon, F.K. & Russell, P.K. (1972) Detection of additional antigenic determinants of hepatitis B antigen. *Journal of Immunology*, **109**, 842–848.
26. Bar, R.S., Adlard, J. & Thomas, F.B. (1975) Lymphopenic infectious mononucleosis. *Archives of Internal Medicine*, **135**, 334–337.
27. Barbara, J.A.J., Howell, D.R., Cleghorn, T.E., Cameron, C.H., Briggs, M. & Dane, D.S. (1977) A comparison of different methods of screening blood donations for HB_sAg. *Vox Sanguinis*, **32**, 4–9.
28. Barker, L.F. & Murray, R. (1972) Relationship of virus dose to incubation time of clinical hepatitis and time of appearance of hepatitis-associated antigen. *American Journal of the Medical Sciences*, **263**, 27–33.
29. Barker, L.F., Chisari, F.V., McGrath, P.P., Dalgard, D.W., Kirschstein, R.L., Almeida, J.D., Edgington, T.S., Sharp, D.G. & Peterson, M.R. (1973) Transmission of type B viral hepatitis to chimpanzees. *Journal of Infectious Diseases*, **127**, 648–662.
30. Baskerville, A., Bowen, E.T.W., Platt, G.S., McArdell, L.B. & Simpson, D.I.H. (1978) The pathology of experimental Ebola virus infection in monkeys. *Journal of Pathology*, **125**, 131–138.
31. Bayer, M.E., Blumberg, B.S. & Werner, B. (1968) Particles associated with Australia antigen in the sera of patients with leukaemia, Down's syndrome and hepatitis. *Nature*, **218**, 1057–1059.
32. Bechtelsheimer, H., Korb, G. & Gedigk, P. (1972) The morphology and pathogenesis of 'Marburg' virus hepatitis. *Human Pathology*, **3**, 255–264.
33. Becker, M.D., Scheuer, P.J., Baptista, A. & Sherlock, S. (1970) Prognosis of chronic persistent hepatitis. *Lancet*, **i**, 53–57.
34. Beebe, G.W. & Simon, A.H. (1970) Cirrhosis of the liver following viral hepatitis; a 20-year mortality follow-up. *American Journal of Epidemiology*, **62**, 279–286.
35. Beeson, P.B. (1943) Jaundice occurring one to four months after transfusion of blood or plasma. *Journal of the American Medical Association*, **121**, 1332–1334.
36. Bell, H. (1971) Cardiac manifestations of viral hepatitis. *Journal of the American Medical Association*, **218**, 387–391.
37. Berg, R., Ringertz, O. & Espmark, A. (1971) Australia antigen in hepatitis amongst Swedish trail finders. *Acta Pathologica et Microbiologica Scandinavica*, **79B**, 423–427.
38. Berg, J.V.R., Berntsen, K.O., Björling, H., Holmström, B. & Vyas, G.N. (1974) Recovery of hepatitis B antibody from human plasma products separated by a modified Cohn fractionation. *Vox Sanguinis*, **27**, 302–309.
39. Bianchi, L., De Groote, J., Desmet, V.J., Gedigk, P., Korb, G., Popper, H., Poulsen, H., Scheuer, P.J., Schmid, M., Thaler, H. & Wepler, W. (1971) Morphological criteria in viral hepatitis. Review by an International Group. *Lancet*, **i**, 333–337.
40. Bianchi, L., Ohnacker, H., Beck, K. & Zimmerli-Ning, M. (1972) Liver damage in heatstroke and its regression. *Human Pathology*, **3**, 237–248.
41. Bianchi, L., De Groote, J., Desmet, V.J., Gedigk, P., Korb, G., Popper, H., Poulsen, H., Scheuer, P.J., Schmid, M., Thaler, H. & Wepler, W. (1974) Guidelines for diagnosis of therapeutic drug induced liver injury in liver biopsies. Review by an international group. *Lancet*, **i**, 854–857.
42. Bianchi, L., De Groote, J., Desmet, V.J., Gedigk, P., Korb, G., Popper, H., Poulsen, H., Scheuer, P.J., Schmid, M., Thaler, H. & Wepler, W. (1977) Acute and chronic hepatitis revisited. *Lancet*, **ii**, 914–919.
43. Bissell, D.M., Hammaker, L. & Schmid, R. (1972) Hemoglobin and erythrocyte catabolism in rat liver: the separate roles of parenchymal and sinusoidal cells. *Blood*, **40**, 812–822.
44. Biswas, R. & Gerlich, H. (1977) Radioimmunological detection of e-antigen and anti-e in different types of HBV infections. *Archives Hellenic Medical Societies* (Suppl.), **3**, 32.
45. Bjorneboe, M. (1974) Viral hepatitis and cirrhosis. *Clinics in Gastroenterology*, **3**, 409–418.

46. Blainey, J.D., Earle, A., Flewett, T.H. & Williams, L.K.L. (1971) Is the urine infective in serum hepatitis? *Lancet,* **i,** 797.

47. Bloomer, J.R., Waldmann, T.A., McIntyre, K.R. & Klatskin, G. (1975) Relationship of serum alphafetoprotein to the severity and duration of illness in patients with viral hepatitis. *Gastroenterology,* **68,** 342–350.

48. Blum, A.L., Stutz, R. & Haemmerli, U.P. (1969) A fortuitously controlled study of steroid therapy in acute viral hepatitis. *American Journal of Medicine,* **47,** 82–92.

49. Blum, A.L., Berthet, P., Doelle, W., Goebell, H., Kortüm, K., Pelloni, S., Peter, P., Poulsen, H., Strohmeyer, G. & Tygstrup, N. (1977) Treatment of acute viral hepatitis with (+)-Cyanidanol-3. *Lancet,* **ii,** 1153–1155.

50. Blumberg, B.S., Alter, H.J. & Visnich, S. (1965) A 'new' antigen in leukemia sera. *Journal of the American Medical Association,* **191,** 541–546.

51. Blumberg, B.S., Sutnick, A.I. & London, W.T. (1968) Hepatitis and leukemia: their relation to Australia antigen. *Bulletin of the New York Academy of Medicine,* **44,** 1566–1586.

52. Blumberg, B.S., Gerstley, B.J.S., Hungerford, D.A., London, W.T. & Sutnick, A.I. (1967) A serum antigen (Australia antigen) in Down's syndrome, leukaemia and hepatitis. *Annals of Internal Medicine,* **66,** 924–931.

53. Bonkowsky, H.L., Lee, R.V. & Klatskin, G. (1975) Acute granulomatous hepatitis. Occurrence in cytomegalovirus mononucleosis. *Journal of the American Medical Association,* **233,** 1284–1288.

54. Borhanmanesh, F., Haghighi, P., Hekmat, K., Rezaizadeh, K. & Ghavami, A.G. (1973) Viral hepatitis during pregnancy: severity and effect on gestation. *Gastroenterology,* **64,** 304–312.

55. Bowen, E.T.W., Platt, G.S., Lloyd, G., Baskerville, A., Harris, W.J. & Vella, E.E. (1977) Viral haemorrhagic fever in Southern Sudan and Northern Zaire. *Lancet,* **i,** 571–573.

56. Boyer, J.L. & Klatskin, G. (1970) Pattern of necrosis in acute viral hepatitis. *New England Journal of Medicine,* **283,** 1063–1071.

57. Brachott, D., Lifschitz, I., Mosley, J.W., Kendrick, M.A. & Sgouris, J.T. (1975) Potency of fragmented IgG: two studies of postexposure prophylaxis in type A hepatitis. *Journal of Laboratory and Clinical Medicine,* **85,** 281–286.

58. Bradley, D.W., McCaustland, K.A., Schreeder, M.T., Cook, E.H., Gravelle, C.R. & Maynard, J.E. (1977) Multiple buoyant densities of hepatitis A virus in cesium chloride gradients. *Journal of Medical Virology,* **1,** 219–226.

59. Bradley, W.H. (1946) Homologous serum jaundice. *Proceedings of the Royal Society of Medicine,* **39,** 649–654.

60. *British Medical Journal* (1975) The several viruses of post transfusion hepatitis. *British Medical Journal,* **iii,** 663.

61. *British Medical Journal* (1976) High-titre hepatitis B-immune globulin (Editorial). *British Medical Journal,* **i,** 241–242.

62. *British Medical Journal* (1977) Ebola virus infection (Editorial). *British Medical Journal,* **ii,** 539–540.

63. Bryan, J.A. & Gregg, M.B. (1975) Viral hepatitis in the U.S., 1970–73: an analysis of morbidity trends and the impact of HB_sAg testing on surveillance and epidemiology. *American Journal of the Medical Sciences,* **270,** 271–282.

64. Buynak, E.B., Roehm, R.R., Tytell, A.A., Bertland, A.V., Lampson, G.P. & Hilleman, M.R. (1976) Development and chimpanzee testing of a vaccine against human hepatitis B. *Proceedings of the Society for Experimental and Biological Medicine,* **151,** 694–700.

65. Cabral, G.A., Chairez, R., Marciano-Cabral, F., Suarez, M., Dreesman, G.R., Melnick, J.L. & Hollinger, F.B. (1975) Cell-mediated immunity in guinea pigs to subunits derived from hepatitis B surface antigens. *Infections and Immunity,* **12,** 564–570.

66. Cameron, C.H. & Dane, D.S. (1974) Radioimmunoassay and saturation analysis. *British Medical Bulletin,* **30,** 90–92.

67. Cameron, G.R. & Karunaratne, W.A.E. (1936) Carbon tetrachloride cirrhosis in relation to liver regeneration. *Journal of Pathology and Bacteriology,* **42,** 1–21.

68. Cappel, R., De Cuyper, F. & van Beers, D. (1977) e Antigen and antibody, DNA polymerase and inhibitors of DNA polymerase in acute and chronic hepatitis. *Journal of Infectious Diseases,* **136,** 617–622.

69. Caroli, J. & Ricordeau, P. (1961) Value of peritoneoscopy and peritoneoscopic photography in color and of scintillography in the diagnosis of liver diseases. In *Progress in Liver Diseases* (Ed.) Popper, H. & Schaffner, F. Vol. 1, pp. 296–314. New York: Grune & Stratton.

70. Carter, R.L. & Penman, H.G. (Ed.) (1969) *Infectious Mononucleosis.* Oxford: Blackwell.

71. Casals, J. (1976) Arenaviruses. In *Viral Infections in Humans* (Ed.) Evans, A.S. pp. 103–125. New York: Plenum Press.

72. Cayzer, I., Dane, D.S., Cameron, C.H. & Denning, J.V. (1974) A rapid haemagglutination test for hepatitis B antigen. *Lancet,* **i,** 947–949.

73. Chalmers, T.C. (1973) Hemodialysis-associated hepatitis. *Journal of the American Medical Association,* **225,** 412–414.

74. Chalmers, T.C., Koff, R.S. & Grady, G.F. (1965) A note on fatality in serum hepatitis. *Gastroenterology,* **49,** 22–26.

75. Chalmers, T.C., Eckhardt, R.D., Reynolds, W.E., Cigarroa, J.G., Deane, N., Reifenstein, R.W., Smith, C.W. & Davidson, C.S., with the technical assistance of Maloney, M.A., Bonnel, M., Niiya, M., Stang, A. & O'Brien, A.M. (1955) The treatment of acute infectious hepatitis. Controlled studies of the effects of diet, rest and physical reconditioning on the acute course of the disease and on the incidence of relapses and residual abnormalities. *Journal of Clinical Investigation,* **34,** 1163–1235.

76. Chaplin, H. (1978) Frozen blood. *New England Journal of Medicine,* **298,** 679–681.

77. Chaudhuri, A.K.R., Cassie, G. & Silver, M. (1975) Outbreak of food-borne type A hepatitis in Greater Glasgow. *Lancet,* **ii,** 223–225.

78. Cheatham, W.J., Weller, T.H., Dolan, T.F. & Dower, J.C. (1956) Varicella: report of two fatal cases with necropsy, virus isolation and serologic studies. *American Journal of Pathology,* **32,** 1015–1035.

79. Child, P.L., MacKenzie, R.B., Valverde, L.R. & Johnson, K.M. (1967) Bolivian haemorrhagic fever: a pathologic description. *Archives of Pathology,* **83,** 434–445.

80. Christie, A.B., Allam, A.A., Aref, M.K., Muntasser, I.H.El & Nageh, M.El (1976) Pregnancy hepatitis in Libya. *Lancet,* **ii,** 827–829.

81. Cockayne, E.A. (1912) Catarrhal jaundice, sporadic and epidemic and its relation to acute yellow atrophy of the liver. *Quarterly Journal of Medicine,* **6,** 1.

82. Conn, H.O. (1976) Chronic hepatitis: reducing an iatrogenic enigma to a workable puzzle. *Gastroenterology,* **70,** 1182–1184.

83. Conrad, M.E., Schwartz, F.D. & Yound, A.A. (1964) Viral hepatitis: a generalised disease. *American Journal of Gastroenterology,* **42,** 47–51.

84. Co-operative Study (1971) Prophylactic gamma globulin for prevention of endemic hepatitis. Effects of US gamma globulin upon the incidence of viral hepatitis and other infectious diseases in US soldiers abroad. *Archives of Internal Medicine,* **128,** 723–738.

85. Cornog, J.L. & Hanson, C.W. (1968) Psittacosis as a cause of miliary infiltrates of the lung and hepatic granulomas. *American Review of Respiratory Diseases,* **98,** 1033–1036.

86. Cossart, Y.E. (1974) Acquisition of hepatitis B antigen in the newborn period. *Postgraduate Medical Journal,* **50,** 334–337.

87. Cossart, Y.E. (1977) *Virus Hepatitis and its Control.* London: Baillière Tindall.

88. Councilman, W.T. (1890) Pathologic histology of yellow fever. In *Report on Etiology and Prevention of Yellow Fever* (Ed.) Sternberg, G.M. U.S. Marine Hospital Service. Public Health Report Bulletin 2, pp. 151–159.

89. Coyne, V.E. (Zavatone), Millman, I., Cerda, J., Gerstley, B.J.S., London, T., Sutnick, A. & Blumberg, B.S. (1970) The localization of Australia antigen by immunofluorescence. *Journal of Experimental Medicine,* **131,** 307–319.

90. Craske, J., Dilling, N. & Stern, D. (1975) An outbreak of hepatitis associated with intravenous injection of factor VIII concentrate. *Lancet,* **ii,** 221–223.

91. Dane, D.S., Cameron, C.H. & Briggs, M. (1970) Virus-like particles in serum of patients with Australia-antigen-associated hepatitis. *Lancet,* **i,** 695–698.

92. Davis, E.V. (1961) Isolation of viruses from children with infectious hepatitis. *Science,* **133,** 2059–2061.

93. Deinhardt, F. (1976) Hepatitis in primates. *Advances in Virus Research,* **20,** 113–157.

94. Del Prete, S., Constantino, D. & Doglia, M. (1970) Different Australia-antigen determinants in acute viral hepatitis. *Lancet,* **ii,** 292–294.

95. Deodhar, K.P., Tapp, E. & Scheuer, P.J. (1975) Orcein staining of hepatitis B antigen in paraffin sections of liver biopsies. *Journal of Clinical Pathology,* **28,** 66–70.

96. Derso, A., Boxall, E.H., Tarlow, M.J. & Flewett, T.H. (1978) Transmission of HBsAg from mother to infant in four ethnic groups. *British Medical Journal,* **i,** 949–952.

97. Desmet, V.J. & De Groote, J. (1974) Histological diagnosis of viral hepatitis. *Clinics in Gastroenterology,* **3,** 337–354.

98. Desmet, V.J., Bullens, A.M. & De Groote, J. (1970) A clinical and histochemical study of cholestasis. *Gut,* **ii,** 516–523.

99. Dible, J.H., McMichael, J. & Sherlock, S.P.V. (1943) Pathology of acute hepatitis. Aspiration biopsy studies of epidemic, arsenotherapy and serum jaundice. *Lancet,* **ii,** 402–422.

100. Dienstag, J.L., Popper, H. & Purcell, R.H. (1976) The pathology of viral hepatitis types A and B in chimpanzees. A comparison. *American Journal of Pathology,* **85,** 131–148.

101. Dienstag, J.L., Feinstone, S.M., Kapikian, A.Z., Purcell, R.H., Boggs, J.D. & Conrad, M.E. (1975) Faecal shedding of hepatitis-A antigen. *Lancet,* **i,** 765–767.

102. Dienstag, J.L., Feinstone, S.M., Purcell, R.H., Hoofnagle, J.H., Barker, L.F., London, W.T., Popper, H., Peterson, J.M. & Kapikian, A.Z. (1975) Experimental infection of chimpanzees with hepatitis A virus. *Journal of Infectious Diseases,* **132,** 532–545.

103. Dienstag, J.L., Routenberg, J.A., Purcell, R.H., Hooper, R.R. & Harrison, W.O. (1975) Foodhandler-associated outbreak of hepatitis type A. An immune electron microscopic study. *Annals of Internal Medicine,* **83,** 647–650.

104. Dienstag, J.L., Gust, I.D., Lucas, C.R., Wong, D.C. & Purcell, R.H. (1976) Mussel-associated viral hepatitis type A: serological confirmation. *Lancet,* **i,** 561–563.

105. Dienstag, J.L., Schulman, A.N., Gerety, R.J., Hoofnagle, J.H., Lorenz, D.E., Purcell, R.H. & Barker, L.F. (1976) Hepatitis A antigen isolated from liver and stool: immunological comparison of antisera prepared in guinea pigs. *Journal of Immunology,* **117** (3), 876–881.

106. Dienstag, J.L., Wagner, J.A., Purcell, R.H., London, W.T. & Lorenz, D.E. (1976) Virus-like particles and GB agent hepatitis. *Nature,* **264,** 260–261.

107. Dienstag, J.L., Feinstone, S.M., Purcell, R.H., Wong, D.C., Alter, H.J. & Holland, P.V. (1977) Non-A, non-B post-transfusion hepatitis. *Lancet,* **i,** 560–562.

108. Dienstag, J.L., Szmuness, W., Stevens, C.E. & Purcell, R.H. (1978) Hepatitis A virus infection: new insights from seroepidemiologic studies. *Journal of Infectious Diseases,* **137,** 328–340.

109. Dietrichson, O., Juhl, E., Christoffersen, P., Elling, P., Faber, V., Iversen, K., Nielsen, J.O., Petersen, P. & Poulsen, H. (1975) Acute viral hepatitis; factors possibly predicting chronic liver disease. *Acta Pathologica et Microbiologica Scandinavica. Section A: Pathology,* **83,** 183–188.

110. Dreesman, G.R., Hollinger, F.B. & Melnick, J.L. (1975) Biophysical and biochemical properties of purified preparations of hepatitis B surface antigen (HB_sAg). *American Journal of the Medical Sciences,* **270,** 123–129.

111. Dublin, I.N., Sullivan, B.H., LeGolvan, P.C. & Murphy, L.C. (1960) The cholestatic form of viral hepatitis. Experiences with viral hepatitis at Brooke Army Hospital during the years 1951–1953. *American Journal of Medicine,* **29,** 55–72.

112. Dudley, F.J., Scheuer, P.J. & Sherlock, S. (1972) Natural history of hepatitis-associated antigen-positive chronic liver disease. *Lancet,* **ii,** 1388–1393.

113. Duncan, G.C., Christian, H.A., Stokes, J., Rexer, W.F., Nicholson, J.T. & Edgar, A. (1947) Evaluation of immune serum globulin as prophylaxis against homologous serum jaundice. *American Journal of the Medical Sciences,* **213,** 53–57.

114. Dunnet, W.N. (1963) Infectious mononucleosis. *British Medical Journal,* **i,** 1187–1191.

115. Edington, G.M. & White, H.A. (1972) The pathology of Lassa fever. *Transactions of the Royal Society of Tropical Medicine and Hygiene,* **66,** 381–389.

116. Edgington, T.S. & Ritt, D.J. (1971) Intrahepatic expression of serum hepatitis virus-associated antigens. *Journal of Experimental Medicine,* **134,** 871–885.
117. Edland, J.F. (1972) Liver disease in heroin addicts. *Human Pathology,* **3,** 75–84.
118. Edmondson, H. & Peters, R.L. (1977) Liver. In *Pathology* (Ed.) Anderson, W.A.D. & Kissane, J.M. pp. 1321–1438. St Louis: C.V. Mosby.
119. Ellis, D.S., Simpson, D.I.H., Francis, D.P., Knobloch, J., Bowen, E.T.W., Lolik, P. & Deng, I.M. (1978) Ultrastructure of Ebola virus particles in human liver. *Journal of Clinical Pathology,* **31,** 201–208.
120. Elsner, B., Schwarz, E., Mando, O.G., Maiztegui, J. & Vilches, A. (1973) Pathology of 12 fatal cases of Argentine haemorrhagic fever. *American Journal of Tropical Medicine and Hygiene,* **22,** 229–236.
121. Embil, J.A., van Rooyen, C.E. & Nagler, F.P. (1965) Coxsackie A10 virus infection among infectious hepatitis contacts. *Canadian Medical Association Journal,* **93,** 740–742.
122. Emond, R.T.D., Evans, B., Bowen, E.T.W. & Lloyd, G. (1977) A case of Ebola virus infection. *British Medical Journal,* **ii,** 541–544.
123. Eppinger, H. (1908) Die pathogene des Ikterus. *Ergebn. Inn Med. Kinderheilk,* **1,** 107.
124. Epon, L., Kosinski, K. & Hirsch, M.S. (1976) Hepatitis in an adult caused by herpes simplex virus type I. *Gastroenterology,* **71,** 500–504.
125. Evans, A.S. (1974) New discoveries in infectious mononucleosis. *Modern Medicine,* **1,** 18–24.
126. Evans, A.S., Sprinz, H. & Nelson, R.S. (1953) Adrenal hormone therapy in viral hepatitis. I. The effect of ACTH and cortisone in severe and fulminant cases. *Annals of Internal Medicine,* **38,** 1115, 1134, and 1148.
127. Farrow, L.J., Holborow, E.J., Johnson, G.D., Lamb, S.G., Stewart, J.S., Taylor, P.E. & Zuckerman, A.J. (1970) Autoantibodies and the hepatitis-associated antigen in acute infective hepatitis. *British Medical Journal,* **ii,** 693–695.
128. Fauerholdt, L., Asnaes, S., Ranek, L., Schiødt, T. & Tygstrup, N. (1977) Significance of suspected chronic aggressive hepatitis in acute hepatitis. *Gastroenterology,* **73,** 543–548.
129. Feinman, S.V., Berris, B.K., Sinclair, J.C., Wrobel, D.M., Alter, H.J. & Holland, P.V. (1973) Relation of hepatitis B antigen subtypes in symptom-free carriers to geographical origin and liver abnormalities. *Lancet,* **ii,** 867.
130. Feinstone, S.M., Kapikian, A.Z. & Purcell, R.H. (1973) Hepatitis A: detection by immune electron microscopy of virus-like antigen associated with acute illness. *Science,* **182,** 1026–1028.
131. Feinstone, S.M., Kapikian, A.Z., Purcell, R.H., Alter, H.J. & Holland, P.V. (1975) Transfusion associated hepatitis not due to viral hepatitis type A or B. *New England Journal of Medicine,* **292,** 767–770.
132. Ferris, A.A., Kaldor, J., Gust, I.D. & Cross, G. (1970) Faecal antigen in viral hepatitis. *Lancet,* **ii,** 243–244.
133. Fitzgerald, G.R., Grimes, H., Reynolds, M., Hitchcock, H. & McCarthy, C.F. (1975) Hepatitis-associated-antigen-positive hepatitis in a tuberculosis unit. *Gut,* **16,** 421–428.
134. Fox, J.P., Brandt, C.D., Wassermann, F.E., Hall, C.E., Spigland, I., Kogon, A. & Elveback, L.R. (1969) The virus watch program: a continuing surveillance of viral infections in metropolitan New York families. VI. Observations of adenovirus infections: virus excretion patterns, antibody response, efficiency of surveillance patterns of infection and relation to illness. *American Journal of Epidemiology,* **89,** 25–50.
135. Foy, H.M., Cooney, M.K., McMahan, R. & Grayston, J.T. (1973) Viral and mycoplasmal pneumonia in a prepaid medical care group during an 8 year period. *American Journal of Epidemiology,* **97,** 93–102.
136. Frame, J.D., Baldwin, J.M. Jr, Gocke, D.J. & Troup, J.M. (1970) Lassa fever, a new virus disease of man from West Africa. I. Clinical description and pathological findings. *American Journal of Tropical Medicine and Hygiene,* **19,** 670–676.
137. Francis, T.I., Moore, D.L., Edington, G.M. & Smith, J.A. (1972) A clinicopathological study of human yellow fever. *Bulletin of the World Health Organization,* **46,** 659–667.
138. Frösner, G.G., Buchholz, H.M. & Gerth, H.-J. (1975) Prevalence of hepatitis B antibody in prostitutes. *American Journal of Epidemiology,* **102** (3), 241–250.
139. Garibaldi, R.A., Hanson, B. & Gregg, M.B. (1972) Impact of illicit drug-associated hepatitis on viral hepatitis morbidity reports in the U.S. *Journal of Infectious Diseases,* **126,** 288–293.
140. Gelb, D., West, M. & Zimmerman, H.J. (1962) Serum enzymes in disease: IX. Analysis of factors responsible for elevated values in infectious mononucleosis. *American Journal of Medicine,* **33,** 249–261.
141. Gellis, S.S., Stokes, J., Brother, G.M., Hall, W.M., Gilmore, H.R., Beyer, E. & Morrissey, R.A. (1945). The use of human immune serum globulin (γ globulin) in infectious (epidemic) hepatitis in the Mediterranean theater of operations. *Journal of the American Medical Association,* **128,** 1062–1063.
142. Gerber, M.A., Sarno, E. & Vernace, S.J. (1976) Immune complexes in hepatocytic nuclei of HB Ag-positive chronic hepatitis. *New England Journal of Medicine,* **294,** 922–925.
143. Gerin, J.L., Shih, J.W.K. & Kaplan, P.M. (1975) Biophysical and biochemical characterization of hepatitis B antigen. *American Journal of the Medical Sciences,* **270,** 115–121.
144. Giles, J.P., McCollum, R.W., Berndtson, L.W. & Krugman, S. (1969) Viral hepatitis – relation of Australia/SH antigen to the Willowbrook MS-2 strain. *New England Journal of Medicine,* **281,** 119–122.
145. Gitlin, N. (1973) Extrahepatic manifestations of long incubation hepatitis (MS-2 hepatitis): an association with Henoch-Schönlein syndrome. *Liver. Proceedings of the International Liver Conference, Cape Town,* pp. 47–48. London: Pitman Medical.
146. Gocke, D.J. (1972) A prospective study of post-transfusion hepatitis. The role of Australia antigen. *Journal of the American Medical Association,* **219,** 1165–1170.
147. Gocke, D.J. (1975) Extrahepatic manifestations of viral hepatitis. *American Journal of the Medical Sciences,* **270,** 49–52.
148. Gold, E. & Nankervis, G.A. (1976) Cytomegalovirus. In *Viral Infections of Humans* (Ed.) Evans, A.S. pp. 143–161. New York: Plenum Press.
149. Goldfield, M., Black, H.C., Srihongse, S. & Pizzuti, W. (1975) The consequences of administering blood pre-tested for HB_sAg by third generation technique. A progress report. *American Journal of the Medical Sciences,* **270,** 335–342.

150. Gowing, N.F.C. (1975) Infectious mononucleosis: histopathological aspects. In *Haematologic and Lymphoid Pathology Decennial 1966–75* (Ed.) Sommers, S.C. pp. 261–280. New York: Appleton-Century-Crofts.
151. Grady, G.F. (1977) Hepatitis B from medical professionals: how rare? How preventable? *New England Journal of Medicine*, **296** (17), 995–996.
152. Grady, G.F. (1978) Transfusions and hepatitis: update in 1978. *New England Journal of Medicine*, **298**, 1413–1415.
153. Grady, G.F. & Bennett, A.J.E. (1972) National transfusion hepatitis study. Risk of post-transfusion hepatitis in the United States. *Journal of the American Medical Association*, **220**, 692–701.
154. Grady, G.F. & Lee, V.A. (1975) Hepatitis B immune globulin – prevention of hepatitis from accidental exposure among medical workers. *New England Journal of Medicine*, **293**, 1067–1070.
155. Grady, G.F., Bennett, A.J.E., Culhane, P.D., Forrest, J.N. & Iber, F.L. (1972) Eight years of surveillance of patients hospitalised with hepatitis: interpretation of data in light of epidemic parenteral drug abuse and availability of testing for hepatitis-associated antigen. *Journal of Infectious Diseases*, **126**, 87–91.
156. Greeman, R.L., Robinson, W.S. & Vyas, G.N. (1975) A sensitive test for antibody against the hepatitis B core antigen (anti-HB-e). *Vox Sanguinis*, **29**, 77–80.
157. Gregor, G.R., Geller, S.A., Walker, G.F. & Campomanes, B.A. (1975) Coxsackie hepatitis in an adult with ultrastructural demonstration of the virus. *Mount Sinai Journal of Medicine*, **12**, 575–580.
158. Gregory, P.B., Knauer, C.M., Kempson, R.L. & Miller, R. (1976) Steroid therapy in severe viral hepatitis. A double blind, randomized trial of methyl-prednisolone versus placebo. *New England Journal of Medicine*, **294** (13), 681–687.
159. Grist, N.R. (1976) Hepatitis in clinical laboratories, 1973–74. *Journal of Clinical Pathology*, **29**, 480–483.
160. Grob, P.J. & Jemelka, H.I. (1972) Faecal SH-antigen in acute hepatitis. *American Journal of Diseases of Children*, **123**, 400–401.
161. Gudat, F., Bianchi, L., Sonnabend, W., Thiel, G., Aenishaenshin, W. & Stalder, G.A. (1975) Pattern of core and surface expression in liver tissue reflects state of specific immune response in hepatitis B. *Laboratory Investigation*, **32**, 1–9.
162. Haemmerli, U.P. (1966) Jaundice during pregnancy (with special emphasis on recurrent jaundice during pregnancy and its differential diagnosis). *Acta Medica Scandinavica* (Suppl. 444), **179**, 1–111.
163. Hagler, L., Pastore, R.A. & Bergin, J.J. (1975) Aplastic anemia following viral hepatitis: report of two fatal cases and literature review. *Medicine (Baltimore)*, **54** (2), 139–164.
164. Hague, R.V. (1975) Acute glomerulonephritis complicating Australia antigen-negative viral hepatitis. *Scandinavian Journal of Infectious Diseases*, **7**, 277–279.
165. Hampers, C.L., Prager, D. & Senior, J.R. (1964) Post-transfusion anicteric hepatitis. *New England Journal of Medicine*, **271**, 747–754.
166. Harrington, J.M. & Shannon, H.S. (1976) Incidence of tuberculosis, hepatitis, brucellosis, and shigellosis in British medical laboratory workers. *British Medical Journal*, **i**, 759–762.
167. Hartwell, W.V., Love, G.J. & Eidenbock, M.P. (1966) Adenovirus in blood clots from cases of infectious hepatitis. *Science*, **152**, 1390.
168. Hatch, M.H. & Siem, R.A. (1966) Viruses isolated from children with infectious hepatitis. *American Journal of Epidemiology*, **84**, 495–509.
169. Havens, W.P. & Paul, J.R. (1945) Prevention of infectious hepatitis with γ globulin. *Journal of the American Medical Association*, **129**, 270–272.
170. Heathcote, J., Cameron, C.H. & Dane, D.S. (1974) Hepatitis B antigen in saliva and semen. *Lancet*, **i**, 71–73.
171. Heathcote, J., Tsianides, A. & Sherlock, S. (1973) A urinary substance in patients with acute type-B hepatitis and their household contacts. *Lancet*, **ii**, 593–595.
172. Henkin, R.I. & Smith, F.R. (1971) Hyposmia in acute viral hepatitis. *Lancet*, **i**, 823–826.
173. Henson, D.E., Grimley, P.M. & Strano, A.J. (1974) Post natal cytomegalovirus hepatitis. *Human Pathology*, **5**, 93–103.
174. Hess, G., Arnold, W., Shih, J.W.K., Kaplan, P.M., Purcell, R.H., Gerin, J.L. & Meyer zum Büschenfelde, K.H. (1977) Expression of hepatitis B virus-specific markers in asymptomatic hepatitis B surface antigen carriers. *Infection and Immunity*, **17**, 550–554.
175. Hirschman, S.Z., Gerber, M. & Garfinkel, E. (1975) Observations on the core particle of hepatitis B virus and the DNA polymerase associated with hepatitis B antigen. *American Journal of the Medical Sciences*, **270**, 141–149.
176. Hirschman, S.Z., Vernace, S.J. & Schaffner, F. (1971) D.N.A. polymerase in preparations containing Australia antigen. *Lancet*, **i**, 1099–1103.
177. Hoagland, R.J. (1967) *Infectious Mononucleosis*. New York and London: Grune & Stratton.
178. Holborow, E.J. (1972) Immunological aspects of viral hepatitis. *British Medical Bulletin*, **28**, 142–144.
179. Hollinger, F.B., Dreesman,G.R., Fields, H. & Melnick, J.L. (1975) HB_cAg anti-HB_c and DNA polymerase activity in transfused recipients followed prospectively. *Medical Science*, **270**, 343–348.
180. Hollinger, F.B., Bradley, D.W., Dreesman, G.R. & Melnick, J.L. (1976) Detection of viral hepatitis type A. *American Journal of Clinical Pathology*, **65**, 854–865.
181. Hoofnagle, J.H. & Barker, L.F. (1976) Hepatitis B virus and albumin products. *Proceedings of Workshop on Albumin*. WH400 W927, pp. 305–314. Maryland: Bethesda NIH.
182. Hoofnagle, J.H., Gerety, R.J. & Barker, L.F. (1973) Antibody to hepatitis B virus core in man. *Lancet*, **ii**, 869–873.
183. Hoofnagle, J.H., Gerety, R.J. & Barker, L.F. (1975) Hepatitis B core antigen, and antibody. *American Journal of the Medical Sciences*, **270**, 179–187.
184. Hoofnagle, J.H., Gerety, R.J., Thiel, J. & Barker, L.F. (1976) The prevalence of hepatitis B surface antigen in commercially prepared plasma products. *Journal of Laboratory and Clinical Medicine*, **88** (1), 102–113.
185. Hoofnagle, J.H., Michalak, T., Nowoslawski, A., Gerety, R.J. & Barker, L.F. (1978) Immunofluorescence microscopy in experimentally induced type B hepatitis in the chimpanzee. *Gastroenterology*, **74**, 182–187.
186. Hoofnagle, J.H., Seeff, L.B., Bales, Z.B., Zimmerman, H.J. & Veterans Administration Hepatitis Cooperative Study Group (1978) Type B hepatitis after transfusion with blood containing antibody to hepatitis B core antigen. *New England Journal of Medicine*, **298**, 1379–1383.

187. Howard, C.R. & Burrell, C.J. (1976) Structure and nature of hepatitis B antigen. *Progress in Medical Virology,* **22,** 36–103.

188. Howard, C.R. & Zuckerman, A.J. (1977) Core antigen and circulating anti-core antibody in hepatitis B infection. *Journal of Immunological Methods,* **14,** 291–301.

189. Hughes, J.R., Wilfert, C.M., Moore, M., Benirschke, K. & deHoyos-Guevera, E. (1972) Echovirus 14 infection associated with fatal neonatal hepatic necrosis. *American Journal of Diseases of Children,* **123,** 61–67.

190. International Commission (1978) Ebola haemorrhagic fever in Zaire, 1976. Dysentery, malaria, filariasis, measles, amoebiasis, pneumonia, tuberculosis and goitre. *Bulletin of the World Health Organization,* **56,** 271–293.

191. Irwin, G.R., Allen, R.G., Segal, H.G., Allen, A.M., Putnak, J.R., Cannon, H.G. & Top, F.H. (1977) Serodiagnosis of hepatitis B virus infection by antibody to core antigen. *Journal of Infectious Diseases,* **136,** 31–36.

192. Ishak, K.G. (1973) Viral hepatitis: the morphologic spectrum. In *The Liver* (International Academy of Pathology Monograph) (Ed.) Gall, E.A. & Mostofi, F.K. pp. 218–268. Baltimore: Williams & Wilkins.

193. Ishak, K.G. (1976) Light microscopic morphology of viral hepatitis. *American Journal of Clinical Pathology,* **65,** 787–827.

194. Iwarson, S., Kjellman, H. & Teger Nilsson, A.C. (1976) Incidence of viral hepatitis after administration of factor IX concentrates. *Vox Sanguinis,* **31,** 136–140.

195. Iwarson, S., Lundin, P. & Hermodsson, S. (1972) Liver morphology in acute viral hepatitis related to the hepatitis B antigen. *Journal of Clinical Pathology,* **25,** 850–855.

196. Iwarson, S., Magnius, L., Lindholm, A. & Lundin, P. (1973) Subtypes of hepatitis B antigen in blood donors and post-transfusion hepatitis: clinical and epidemiological aspects. *British Medical Journal,* **i,** 84–87.

197. Janzen, J., Tripatzis, I., Wagner, U., Schlieter, M., Müller-Dethard, E. & Wolters, E. (1978) Epidemiology of hepatitis B surface antigen (HB_sAg) and antibody to HB_sAg in hospital personnel. *Journal of Infectious Diseases,* **137,** 261–265.

198. Jeffries, M.D.J., James, W.H., Jeffries, F.J.G., Macleod, K.G. & Wilcox, R.R. (1973) Australia antigen (hepatitis-associated) in patients attending a venereal disease clinic. *British Medical Journal,* **ii,** 455–456.

199. Jensen, D.M., McFarlane, I.G., Portmann, B.S., Eddleston, A.L.W.F. & Williams, R. (1978) Detection of antibodies directed against a liver-specific membrane lipoprotein in patients with acute and chronic active hepatitis. *New England Journal of Medicine,* **299,** 1–7.

200. Jezequel, A.-M. & Steiner, J.W. (1966) Some ultrastructural and histochemical aspects of coxsackie virus–cell interactions. *Laboratory Investigation,* **15,** 1055–1083.

201. Johnson, K.M., Webb, P.A., Lange, J.V. & Murphy, F.A. (1977) Isolation and partial characterisation of a new virus causing acute haemorrhagic fever in Zaire. *Lancet,* **i,** 569–571.

202. Jones, E.M.M. & Wilson, D.C. (1972) Clinical features of yellow fever cases at Vom Christian Hospital during the 1969 epidemic on the Jos Plateau, Nigeria. *Bulletin of the World Health Organization,* **46,** 653–657.

203. Juel-Jensen, B.E. & MacCallum, F.O. (1972) *Herpes Simplex, Varicella and Zoster: Clinical Manifestations and Treatment.* Philadelphia: Lippincott.

204. Kaplan, P.M., Greenman, R.L., Gerin, J.L., Purcell, R.H. & Robinson, W.S. (1973) DNA polymerase associated with human hepatitis B antigen. *Journal of Virology,* **12,** 995–1005.

205. Karvountzis, G.G., Redeker, A.G. & Peters, R.L. (1975) Long term follow-up studies of patients surviving fulminant viral hepatitis. *Gastroenterology,* **67,** 870–877.

206. Katchaki, J.N., Brouwer, R. & Siem, T.H. (1978) Anti-HB_c and blood infectivity. *New England Journal of Medicine,* **298,** 1421–1422.

207. Kerr, J.A. (1973) Liver pathology in yellow fever. *Transactions of the Royal Society of Tropical Medicine and Hygiene,* **67,** 882.

208. Kew, M.C., Purves, L.R. & Bershon, I. (1973) Serum alpha-fetoprotein levels in acute viral hepatitis. *Gut,* **14,** 939–942.

209. Kingham, J.G.C. & Wright, R. (1978) Unpublished observations.

210. Kingham, J.G.C., McGuire, M.J., Paine, D.H.D. & Wright, R. (1978) Hepatitis B in a hospital for the mentally subnormal in Southern England. *British Medical Journal,* **2,** 594–596.

211. Kissling, R.E., Robinson, R.Q., Murphy, F.A. & Whitfield, S. (1968) Green monkey agent of disease. *Science,* **161,** 1364.

212. Kivel, R.M. (1961) Hematologic aspects of acute viral hepatitis. *American Journal of Digestive Diseases,* **6,** 1017–1031.

213. Koff, R.S., Grady, G.F., Chalmers, T.C., Mosley, J.W., Swartz, B.L. & the Boston Inter-Hospital Liver Group (1967) Viral hepatitis in a group of Boston hospitals. *New England Journal of Medicine,* **276,** 703–710.

214. Koff, R.S., Slavin, M.M., Connelly, L.J.D. & Rosen, D.R. (1977) Contagiousness of acute hepatitis B. Secondary attack rates in household contacts. *Gastroenterology,* **72,** 297–300.

215. Kohler, P.F., Dubois, R.S., Merrill, D.A. & Bowes, W.A. (1974) Prevention of chronic neonatal hepatitis B virus infection with antibody to the hepatitis B surface antigen. *New England Journal of Medicine,* **291,** 1378–1380.

216. Kosmidis, J.C. & Leader-Williams, L.K. (1972) Complement levels in acute infectious hepatitis and serum hepatitis. *Clinical and Experimental Immunology,* **11,** 31–35.

217. Krikler, D.M. & Zilberg, B. (1966) Activity and hepatitis. *Lancet,* **ii,** 1046–1047.

218. Krugman, S. & Giles, J.P. (1973) Viral hepatitis, type B (MS-2 strain); further observations on natural history and prevention. *New England Journal of Medicine,* **288,** 755–760.

219. Krugman, S., Giles, J.P. & Hammond, J. (1967) Infectious hepatitis: evidence for two distinctive clinical, epidemiological and immunological types of infection. *Journal of the American Medical Association,* **200,** 365–373.

220. Krugman, S., Hoofnagle, J.H., Gerety, R.J., Purcell, R.G. & Robinson, W.S. (1974) Viral hepatitis B: DNA polymerase activity and antibody to hepatitis B core antigen. *New England Journal of Medicine,* **290,** 1331–1335.

221. Laiwah, A.C.Y., Goudie, R.B., Goldberg, D.M., Davidson, J.F. & Murray, T.S. (1970) Australia antigen in West of Scotland and North of England. *Lancet*, **ii**, 121–123.

222. Le Bouvier, G.L. (1971) The heterogeneity of Australia antigen. *Journal of Infectious Diseases*, **123**, 671–675.

223. Le Bouvier, G.L. (1972) Subspecificities of the Australia antigen complex. *American Journal of Diseases of Children*, **123**, 420–424.

224. Lee, J.C. & Fortuny, I.E. (1972) Adult herpes simplex hepatitis. *Human Pathology*, **3**, 277–281.

225. Leevy, C.M. & Tygstrup, N. (Ed.) (1976) *Standardisation of Nomenclature, Diagnostic Criteria and Diagnostic Methodology*. Basel: S. Karger.

226. Levene, C. & Blumberg, B.S. (1969) Additional specificities of Australia antigen and the possible identification of hepatitis carriers. *Nature*, **221**, 195–196.

227. Levy, B.S., Fontaine, R.E., Smith, C.A., Brinda, J., Hirman, G., Nelson, D.B., Johnson, P.M. & Larson, O. (1975) A large food-borne outbreak of hepatitis A. Possible transmission via oropharyngeal secretions. *Journal of the American Medical Association*, **234**, 289–294.

228. Ling, C.M., Decker, R.H., Foemmel, R.S. & Overby, L.R. (1975) Comparison of confirmation methods for hepatitis B antigen and the nature of false positives detected by ^{125}I immunoglobulins. *Journal of Laboratory and Clinical Medicine*, **86**, 690–699.

229. Linnemann, C.C. & Goldberg, S. (1974) Hepatitis-B antigen in saliva and semen. *Lancet*, **i**, 320.

230. London, T.W. (1977) Hepatitis B virus and antigen–antibody complex diseases. *New England Journal of Medicine*, **296**(26), 1528–1529.

231. London, W.T., Difiglia, M., Sutnick, A.I. & Blumberg, B.S. (1969) An epidemic of hepatitis in a chronic haemodialysis unit. Australia antigen and differences in host response. *New England Journal of Medicine*, **281**, 571–578.

232. Lucké, B. (1944) The pathology of fatal epidemic hepatitis. *American Journal of Pathology*, **20**, 471–593.

233. Lucké, B. & Mallory, T. (1946) The fulminant form of epidemic hepatitis. *American Journal of Pathology*, **22**, 867–945.

234. Lürman (1885) Eine Icterusepidemie. *Berliner Klinische Wochenschrift*, **22**, 20.

235. MacCallum, F.O. (1972) Historical perspectives. *Canadian Medical Association Journal*, **106**, 423–426.

236. MacCallum, F.O. (1972) Early studies of viral hepatitis. *British Medical Bulletin*, **28**, 105–108.

237. MacCallum, F.O. & Bradley, W.H. (1944) Transmission of infective hepatitis to human volunteers. *Lancet*, **ii**, 228.

238. Mackay, P. & Burrell, C.J. (1976) Examination of the polypeptides of hepatitis B surface antigen. *Journal of General Virology*, **33**, 181–191.

239. Magnius, L.O. (1975) Characterization of a new antigen–antibody system associated with hepatitis B. *Clinical and Experimental Immunology*, **20**, 209–216.

240. Magnius, L.O. & Espmark, J.A. (1972) New specificities of Australia antigen positive sera distinct from Le Bouvier determinants. *Journal of Immunology*, **107**, 1017–1021.

241. Magnius, L.O., Lindholm, A., Lundin, P. & Iwarson, S. (1975) A new antigen–antibody system. Clinical significance in long-term carriers of hepatitis B surface antigen. *Journal of the American Medical Association*, **231** (4), 356–359.

242. Marmion, B.P. & Tonkin, R.W. (1972) Control of hepatitis in dialysis units. *British Medical Bulletin*, **28**, 169–179.

243. Martini, G.A. & Baltzer, G. (1972) Complications of viral hepatitis. *Canadian Medical Association Journal*, **106**, 508–512.

244. Martini, G.A. & Strohmeyer, G. (1974) Post hepatitis syndromes. *Clinics in Gastroenterology*, **3**, 377–390.

245. Martini, G.A., Knauff, H.G., Schmidt, H.A., Mayer, G. & Baltzer, G. (1968) A hitherto unknown infectious disease contracted from monkeys. 'Marburg-virus' disease. *German Medical Monthly*, **13**, 457–470.

246. Mathieson, L.R., Feinstone, S.M., Purcell, R.H. & Wagner, J.A. (1977) Detection of hepatitis A antigen by immunofluorescence. *Infection and Immunity*, **18**, 524–530.

247. Maupas, P., Coursaget, P., Goudeau, A., Drucker, J. & Bagros, P. (1976) Immunisation against hepatitis B in man. *Lancet*, **i**, 1367–1370.

248. Maycock, W. d'A. (1965) Control of serum hepatitis. *Report on a European Symposium Convened by the WHO, Prague, 1964*. p. 82. Copenhagen: World Health Organization.

249. Mazzur, S. (1973) Menstrual blood as a vehicle of Australia-antigen transmission. *Lancet*, **i**, 749–751.

250. Mazzur, S. & Watson, T.M. (1974) Excess males among siblings of Australia antigen carriers. *Nature*, **250**, 60–61.

251. Mazzur, S., Corbett, J. & Blumberg, B.S. (1973) Loss of immunologic reactivities of Australia antigen after incubation of bacteria. *Proceedings of the Society for Experimental Biology and Medicine*, **142**, 327–332.

252. McDonald, S. (1908) Acute yellow atrophy. *Edinburgh Medical Journal*. **15**, 208.

253. Medical Research Council Working Party (1974) Post-transfusion hepatitis in a London hospital: results of a two-year prospective study. *Journal of Hygiene (Cambridge)*, **73**, 173–188.

254. Melnick, J.L., Dreesman, G.R. & Hollinger, F.B. (1976) Approaching the control of viral hepatitis type B. *Journal of Infectious Diseases*, **133**, 210–229.

255. Miller, D.J., Williams, A.E., Le Bouvier, G.L., Dwyer, J.M., Grant, J. & Klatskin, G. (1978) Hepatitis B in hemodialysis patients: significance of HB_eAg. *Gastroenterology*, **74**, 1208–1213.

256. Miller, D.R., Hanshaw, J.B., O'Leary, D.S. & Hnilicka, J.V. (1970) Fatal disseminated herpes simplex virus infection and haemorrhage in the neonate. *Journal of Pediatrics*, **76**, 409–415.

257. Miller, W.J., Provost, P.J. & McAleer, W.J. (1975) Specific immune adherence assay for human hepatitis A antibody: application to diagnostic and epidemiologic investigations. *Proceedings of the Society for Experimental Biology and Medicine*, **149**, 254–261.

258. Millman, I., Zavatone, V.E., Gerstley, B.J.S. & Blumberg, B.S. (1969) Australia antigen detected in the nuclei of liver cells of patients with viral hepatitis by the fluorescent antibody technique. *Nature (London)*, **222**, 181–184.

259. Millward-Sadler, G.H. (1976) Pathological aspects of virus hepatitis. In *Topics in Gastroenterology* (Ed.) Truelove, S.C. & Ritchie, J. pp. 29–54. Oxford: Blackwell Scientific Publications.

260. Mirick, G.S. & Shank, R.E. (1959) An epidemic of serum hepatitis studied under controlled conditions. *Transactions of the American Clinical and Climatology Association,* **71,** 176–190.

261. Moritsugu, Y., Gold, J.M.W., Wagner, J., Dodd, R.Y. & Purcell, R.M. (1975) Hepatitis B core antigen. Detection of antibody by radioimmunoprecipitation. *Immunology,* **114,** 1792–1798.

262. Moritsugu, Y., Dienstag, J.L., Valdesuso, J., Wong, D.C., Wagner, J., Routenberg, J.A. & Purcell, R.H. (1976) Purification of hepatitis A antigen from feces and detection of antigen and antibody by immune adherence hemagglutination. *Infection and Immunity,* **13**(3), 898–908.

263. Mosley, J.W. (1965) The surveillance of transfusion-associated viral hepatitis. *Journal of the American Medical Association,* **193,** 1007–1010.

264. Mosley, J.W. (1975) The HBV carrier – a new kind of leper? *New England Journal of Medicine,* **292,** 477–478.

265. Mosley, J.W., Edwards, V.M., Casey, G., Redeker, A.G. & White, E. (1975) Hepatitis B virus infection in dentists. *New England Journal of Medicine,* **293,** 729–734.

266. Mosley, J.W., Combes, B., Volwiler, W. & Zimmerman, H.J. (1976) Corticosteroids in fulminant hepatitis. *New England Journal of Medicine,* **295**(16), 898–899.

267. Mosley, J.W., Redeker, A.G., Feinstone, S.M. & Purcell, R.H. (1977) Multiple hepatitis viruses in multiple attacks of acute viral hepatitis. *New England Journal of Medicine,* **296** (23), 75–78.

268. Mowat, N.A.G., Albert-Recht, F., Brunt, P.W. & Walker, W. (1973) Outbreak of serum hepatitis associated with tattooing. *Lancet,* **i,** 33–34.

269. Nahmias, A.J. & Josey, W.E. (1976) Epidemiology of herpes simplex viruses 1 and 2. In *Viral Infections in Humans* (Ed.) Evans, A.S. pp. 253–271. New York: Plenum Press.

270. Nefzger, M.D. & Chalmers, T.C. (1963) The treatment of acute infectious hepatitis. Ten year follow-up study of the effects of diet. *American Journal of Medicine,* **35,** 299–309.

271. Neurath, A.R. & Strick, N. (1977) Host specificity of a serum marker for hepatitis B: evidence that 'e antigen' has the properties of an immunoglobulin. *Proceedings of the National Academy of Sciences of the United States of America,* **74,** 1702–1706.

272. Neurath, A.R., Trepo, C., Chen, M. & Prince, A.M. (1976) Identification of additional antigenic sites on Dane particles and the tubular forms of hepatitis B surface antigen. *Journal of General Virology,* **30,** 277–285.

273. Newble, D.I., Holmes, K.T., Wangel, A.G. & Forbes, I.J. (1975) Immune reactions in acute viral hepatitis. *Clinical and Experimental Immunology,* **20,** 17–28.

274. Newkirk, M.M., Downe, A.E.R. & Simon, J.B. (1975) Fate of ingested hepatitis B antigen in blood sucking insects. *Gastroenterology,* **69,** 982–987.

275. Nielson, J.O. & Elling, P. (1971) Investigations of liver biopsies for Australia antigen by immunofluorescent technique. *Clinical and Experimental Immunology,* **9,** 699–705.

276. Nielsen, J.O., Dietrichson, O. & Juhl, E. (1974) Incidence and meaning of the 'e' determinant among hepatitis-B-antigen positive patients with acute and chronic liver diseases. *Lancet,* **ii,** 913–915.

277. Niermeijer, P. & Gips, C.H. (1975) Guillain-Barré syndrome in acute HB_sAg positive hepatitis. *British Medical Journal,* **ii,** 732–733.

278. Nordenfelt, E. & Kjellan, L. (1975) Dane particles DNA polymerase and e antigen in two different categories of hepatitis B antigen carriers. *Intervirology,* **5,** 225–232.

279. Nowoslawski, A., Brzosko, W.J., Madalinski, K. & Krawczynski, K. (1970) Cellular localisation of Australia antigen in the liver of patients with lymphoproliferative disorders. *Lancet,* **i,** 494–498.

280. Ogra, P.L. (1973) Immunologic aspects of hepatitis-associated antigen and antibody in human body fluids. *Journal of Immunology,* **110,** 1197–1205.

281. Okada, K., Kamiyama, I., Inomata, M., Imal, M., Miyakawa, Y. & Mayumi, M. (1976) e Antigen and anti-e in the serum of asymptomatic carrier mothers as indicators of positive and negative transmission of hepatitis B virus to their infants. *New England Journal of Medicine,* **294,** 746–749.

282. Oken, M.M., Hootkin, L. & DeJager, R.L. (1972) Hepatitis after Koyne administration. *American Journal of Digestive Diseases,* **17,** 271–274.

283. Okochi, K. & Murakami, S. (1968) Observations on Australia antigen in Japanese. *Vox Sanguinis,* **15,** 374–385.

284. Orr, W. (1974) The detection of hepatitis B antigen in hepatic parenchyma by the fluorescent antibody technique. *American Journal of Clinical Pathology,* **64,** 257–262.

285. Owen, R.L. & Shapiro, H. (1974) Pleural effusion, rash, and anergy in icteric hepatitis. *New England Journal of Medicine,* **291,** 963–965.

286. Pattison, C.P., Maynard, J.E. & Berquist, K.R. (1975) Epidemiology of hepatitis B in hospital personnel. *American Journal of Epidemiology,* **101,** 59–64.

287. Pattison, C.P., Maynard, J.E., Berquist, K.R. & Webster, H.M. (1973) Serological and epidemiological studies of hepatitis B in haemodialysis units. *Lancet,* **ii,** 172–174.

288. Paul, J.R., Havens, W.P., Sabin, A.B. & Philip, C.B. (1945) Transmission experiments in serum jaundice and infectious hepatitis. *Journal of the American Medical Association,* **128,** 911–915.

289. Peters, C.J. & Johnson, K.M. (1972) Serum immunoglobulin levels in Australia antigen positive and Australia antigen negative hepatitis. *Clinical and Experimental Immunology,* **11,** 381–391.

290. Peters, D., Muller, G. & Slenczka, W. (1971) Morphology, development, and classification of the Marburg virus. In *Marburg Virus Disease. Proceedings of a Symposium* (Ed.) Martini, G.A. & Siegert, R. pp. 68–83. New York: Springer-Verlag.

291. Peters, R.L. (1975) Viral hepatitis: a pathologic spectrum. *American Journal of the Medical Sciences,* **270,** 17–31.

292. Petersen, D.L., Roberts, I.M. & Vyas, G.N. (1977) Partial amino acid sequence of two major component polypeptides of hepatitis B surface antigen. *Proceedings of the National Academy of Sciences of the United States of America,* **74,** 1530–1534.

293. Piazza, M., Di Stasio, G., Maio, G. & Marzano, L.A. (1973) Hepatitis B antigen inhibitor in human faeces and intestinal mucosa. *British Medical Journal,* **ii,** 334–337.

294. Pickles, W.N. (1930) Epidemic catarrhal jaundice: outbreak in Yorkshire. *British Medical Journal,* **i,** 1944.

295. Pirson, Y., Alexandre, G.P. & Ypersele, C. (1977) Long-term effect of HBs antigenemia on patient survival after renal transplantation. *New England Journal of Medicine,* **296** (4), 194–196.

296. Polakoff, S. (1976) Hepatitis B in retreat from dialysis units in the United Kingdom in 1973. *British Medical Journal*, **i**, 1579.
297. Polakoff, S., Cossart, Y.E. & Tillett, H.E. (1972) Hepatitis in dialysis units in the U.K. *British Medical Journal*, **ii**, 94.
298. Pollock, T.M. & Reid, D. (1969) Immunoglobulin for the prevention of infective hepatitis in persons working overseas. *Lancet*, **i**, 281.
299. Popper, H. (1972) The pathology of viral hepatitis. *Canadian Medical Association Journal*, **106**, 447–452.
300. Popper, H. & Schaffner, F. (1971) The vocabulary of chronic hepatitis. *New England Journal of Medicine*, **284**, 1154–1156.
301. Popper, H. & Schaffner, F. (1976) Chronic hepatitis: taxonomic, etiologic and therapeutic problems. In *Progress in Liver Diseases*, Vol. 5, pp. 531–558. New York: Grune & Stratton.
302. Portmann, B., Talbot, I.C. & Day, D.W. (1975) Histopathological changes in the liver following a paracetamol overdose: correlation with clinical and biochemical parameters. *Journal of Pathology*, **117**, 169–181.
303. Poulsen, H. & Christoffersen, P. (1969) Abnormal bile duct epithelium in liver biopsies with histological signs of viral hepatitis. *Acta Pathologica et Microbiologica Scandinavica*, **76**, 383–390.
304. Prince, A.M. (1968) An antigen detected in the blood during the incubation period of serum hepatitis. *Proceedings of the National Academy of Sciences (Washington)*, **60**, 814–821.
305. Prince, A.M., Vnek, J., Brotman, B., Hashimoto, N. & van den Ende, M.C. (1978) Comparative evaluations of hepatitis B vaccines in chimpanzees and in man. In *Viral Hepatitis* (Ed.) Vyas, G.N., Cohen, S.N. & Schmid, R. pp. 507–523. Philadelphia: Franklin Institute Press.
306. Prince, A.M., Metselaar, D., Kafuko, G.W., Mukwaya, L.G., Ling, C.M. & Overby, L.R. (1972) Hepatitis B antigen in wild-caught mosquitoes in Africa. *Lancet*, **ii**, 247–250.
307. Prince, A.M., Brotman, B., Grady, G.F., Kuhns, W.J., Hazzi, C., Levine, R.W. & Millian, S.J. (1974) Long-incubation post-transfusion hepatitis without serological evidence of exposure to hepatitis B virus. *Lancet*, **ii**, 241–246.
308. Prince, A.M., Szmuness, W., Mann, M.K., Vyas, G.N., Grady, G.F., Shapiro, F.L., Suki, W.N., Friedman, E.A. & Stenzel, K.H. (1975) Hepatitis B 'immune' globulin: effectiveness in prevention of dialysis-associated hepatitis. *New England Journal of Medicine*, **293** (21), 1063–1067.
309. Prince, A.M., Szmuness, W., Mann, M.K., Vyas, G.N. Grady, G.F., Shapiro, F.L., Suki, W.N., Freidman, E.A., Avram, M.N. & Stenzel, K.H. (1978) Hepatitis B immune globulin: final report of a controlled, multicenter trial of efficacy in prevention of dialysis-associated hepatitis. *Journal of Infectious Diseases*, **137**(2), 131–144.
310. Provost, P.J., Ittensohn, O.L., Villarejos, V.M. & Hilleman, M.R. (1975) A specific complement-fixation test for human hepatitis A employing CR326 virus antigen: diagnosis and epidemiology. *Proceedings of the Society for Experimental Biology and Medicine*, **148**, 962–969.
311. Provost, P.J., Wolanski, B.S., Miller, W.J., Ittensohn, O.L., McAleer, W.J. & Hilleman, M.R. (1975) Physical, chemical and morphologic dimensions of human hepatitis A virus strain CR326. *Proceedings of the Society for Experimental Biology and Medicine*, **148**, 532–539.
312. Purcell, R.H. (1974) Viral hepatitis. *Preventive Medicine*, **3**, 529–534.
313. Purcell, R.H. (1975) Current status of diagnostic tests for viral hepatitis. In *Immunologic Aspects of Anaesthetic and Surgical Practices* (Ed.) Mathieu, A. & Kahan, B.D. pp. 205–226. New York: Grune & Stratton.
314. Purcell, R.H. & Gerin, J.L. (1975) Hepatitis B subunit vaccine: a preliminary report of safety and efficacy tests of chimpanzees. *American Journal of the Medical Sciences*, **270**, 395.
315. Purcell, R.H., Alter, H.J. & Dienstag, J.L. (1976) Non-A, non-B hepatitis. *Yale Journal of Biology and Medicine*, **49**, 243–250.
316. Purcell, R.H., Gerin, J.L., Almeida, J.D. & Holland, P.V. (1974) Radioimmunoassay for detection of the core of the Dane particle and antibody to it. *Intervirology*, **2**, 231–243.
317. Purcell, R.H., Dienstag, J.L., Feinstone, S.M. & Kapikian, A.Z. (1975) Relationship of hepatitis A antigen to viral hepatitis. *American Journal of the Medical Sciences*, **270**, 61–71.
318. Purcell, R.H., Wong, D.C., Mortisugu, Y., Dienstag, J.L., Routenberg, J.A. & Boggs, J.D. (1976) A microtiter solid-phase radioimmunoassay for hepatitis A antigen and antibody. *Journal of Immunology*, **116**, 349–356.
319. Rachmilewitz, M., Moshkowitz, B., Rachmilewitz, B., Grosswicz, N. & Gross, J. (1972) Serum vitamin B12 binding proteins in viral hepatitis. *European Journal of Clinical Investigation*, **2**, 239–242.
320. Ray, M.B., Desmet, V.J., Fevery, J., de Groote, J., Bradburne, A.F. & Desmyter, J. (1976) Distribution patterns of hepatitis B surface antigen (HB_sAg) in the liver of hepatitis patients. *Journal of Clinical Pathology*, **29**, 94–100.
321. Redeker, A.G. (1975) Viral hepatitis: clinical aspects. *American Journal of the Medical Sciences*, **270**, 9–16.
322. Redeker, A.G., Mosley, J.W., Gocke, D.J., McKee, A.P. & Pollack, W. (1975) Hepatitis B immune globulin as a prophylactic measure for spouses exposed to acute type B hepatitis. *New England Journal of Medicine*, **293**, 1055–1059.
323. Rimland, D., Parkin, W.E., Miller, P.H.G.B. & Schrack, W.D. (1977) Hepatitis B outbreak traced to an oral surgeon. *New England Journal of Medicine*, **296**(17), 953–958.
324. Rizzetto, M., Bonino, F., Diana, S. & Verme, G. (1976) Prognostic significance of in-vitro complement fixation in liver biopsy specimens from patients with acute viral hepatitis type B. *Lancet*, **ii**, 436–438.
325. Robbins, F.C., Mahmoud, A.A.F. & Warren, K.S. (1977) Algorithms in the diagnosis and management of exotic diseases. XIX. Major tropical viral infections: smallpox, yellow fever and Lassa fever. *Journal of Infectious Diseases*, **135**, 341–346.
326. Robinson, W.S. (1975) DNA and DNA polymerase in the core of the Dane particle of hepatitis B. *American Journal of the Medical Sciences*, **270**, 151–159.
327. Robinson, W.S. (1977) The genome of hepatitis B virus. *Annual Review of Microbiology*, **31**, 357–377.
328. Roos, C.M., Feltkampf-Vroom, T.M. & Helder, A.W. (1976) The localisation of hepatitis B antigen and immunoglobulin G in liver tissue: an immunofluorescence, light and electron microscopic study. *Journal of Pathology*, **118**, 1–8.

329. Rumball, J.M., Stone, C.M. & Hasset, C. (1959) The behaviour of serum iron in acute hepatitis. *Gastroenterology,* **36,** 219–223.

330. Schaffner, F. (1966) Intralobular changes in hepatocytes and the electron microscopic mesenchymal response in acute viral hepatitis. *Medicine,* **45,** 547–552.

331. Schaffner, F. (1970) The structural basis of altered hepatic function in viral hepatitis. *American Journal of Medicine,* **49,** 658–668.

332. Schaffner, W., Drutz, D.J., Duncan, G.W. & Koenig, M.G. (1967) The clinical spectrum of endemic psittacosis. *Archives of Internal Medicine,* **119,** 433–443.

333. Schaffner, F., Dienstag, J.L., Purcell, R.H. & Popper, H. (1977) Chimpanzee livers after infection with human hepatitis viruses A and B. Ultrastructural studies. *Archives of Pathology and Laboratory Medicine,* **101,** 113–117.

334. Scheuer, P.J. (1973) *Liver Biopsy Interpretation.* pp. 56–65. London: Baillière Tindall.

335. Schleissner, L.A. & Portnoy, L. (1968) Hepatitis and pneumonia associated with echovirus type 9 infection in two adult siblings. *Annals of Internal Medicine,* **68,** 1315–1319.

336. Schmitz, H. & Enders, G. (1977) Cytomegalovirus as a frequent cause of Guillain–Barré syndrome. *Journal of Medical Virology,* **1,** 21–27.

337. Schroeder, D.D. & Mozen, N.M. (1970) Australia antigen: distribution during Cohn ethanol fractionation of human plasma. *Science (New York),* **168,** 1462–1464.

338. Schulman, A.N., Dienstag, J.L., Jackson, D.R., Hoofnagle, J.H., Gerety, R.J., Purcell, R.H. & Barker, L.F. (1976) Hepatitis A antigen particles in liver, bile, and stool of chimpanzees. *Journal of Infectious Diseases,* **134**(1), 80–84.

339. Schuurs, A.H.W.M. & Wolters, G. (1975) Hepatitis B surface antigen and human serum proteins. *American Journal of the Medical Sciences,* **270,** 173–177.

340. Schweitzer, I.L. & Spears, R.L. (1970) Hepatitis associated antigen (Australia antigen) in mother and infant. *New England Journal of Medicine,* **283,** 570–572.

341. Schweitzer, I.L., Mosley, J.W., Edwards, M.A.V.M. & Overby, L.B. (1973) Factors influencing neonatal infection by hepatitis B virus. *Gastroenterology,* **65,** 277–283.

342. Sears, D.A., George, J.N. & Gold, M.S. (1975) Transient red blood cell aplasia in association with viral hepatitis. Occurrence four years apart in siblings. *Archives of Internal Medicine,* **135,** 1585–1589.

343. Seeff, L.B., Zimmerman, H.J., Wright, E.C., Felsher, B.F., Finkelstein, J.D., Garcia-Pont, P., Greenlee, H.B., Dietz, A.A., Hamilton, J., Koff, R.S., Leevy, C.M., Kiernan, T., Tamburro, C.H., Schiff, E.R., Vlahcevic, Z., Zemel, R., Zimmon, D.S. & Nath, N. (1975) Efficacy of hepatitis B immune serum globulin after accidental exposure. Preliminary report of the Veterans Administration Co-operative Study. *Lancet,* **ii,** 939–941.

344. Seeff, L.B., Zimmerman, H.J., Wright, E.C., Finkelstein, J.D., Garcia-Pont, P., Greenlee, H.B., Dietz, A.A., Leevy, C.M., Tamburro, C.H., Schiff, E.R., Schimmel, E.M., Zemel, R., Zimmon, D.S. & McCollum, R.W. (1977) A randomized, double blind controlled trial of the efficacy of immune serum globulin for the prevention of post-transfusion hepatitis. *Gastroenterology,* **72,** 111–121.

345. Seeff, L.B., Wright, E.C., Zimmerman, H.J., Alter, H.J., Dietz, A.A., Felsher, B.F., Finkelstein, J.D., Garcia-Pont, P., Gerin, J.L., Greenlee, H.B., Hamilton, J., Holland, P.V., Kaplan, P.M., Kiernan, T., Koff, R.S., Leevy, C.M., McAuliffe, V.J., Nath, N., Purcell, R.H., Schiff, E.R., Schwartz, C.C., Tamburro, C.H., Vlahcevic, Z., Zemel, R. & Zimmon, D.S. (1978) Type B hepatitis after needle-stick exposure: prevention with hepatitis B immune globulin. Final report of the Veterans Administration Co-operative Study. *Annals of Internal Medicine,* **88**(3), 285–293.

346. Shaldon, S. & Sherlock, S. (1957) Virus hepatitis with features of prolonged bile retention. *British Medical Journal,* **ii,** 734–738.

347. Sherlock, S. (1976) Predicting progression of acute type-B hepatitis to chronicity. *Lancet,* **ii,** 354–356.

348. Shikata, T., Uzawa, T., Yoshiwara, N., Akatsuka, T. & Yamazaki, S. (1974) Staining methods of Australia antigen in paraffin section: detection of cytoplasmic inclusion bodies. *Japanese Journal of Experimental Medicine,* **44,** 25–36.

349. Siegel, D. & Hirschman, S.Z. (1977) Hepatic dysfunction in acute meales infection of adults. *Archives of Internal Medicine,* **137,** 1178–1179.

350. Simmons, P.D., Islam, M.N., Knott, S., Banatvala, J.E. & Supran, M. (1977) e Antigen among male homosexual patients. *British Medical Journal,* **ii,** 1458.

351. Skinhøj, P. (1975) Natural history of viral hepatitis in Greenland. *American Journal of the Medical Sciences,* **270,** 305–307.

352. Skinhøj, P. & Steiness, I. (1972) Hepatitis associated antigen (HAA) in urine from serum HAA positive renal transplant recipients. *Acta Pathologica et Microbiologica Scandinavica, Section B,* **80,** 801–805.

353. Skinhøj, P. & Steiness, I. (1975) Radioimmunoassay of hepatitis B antigen and antibody in dialysis and transplant patients. *Acta Pathologica et Microbiologica Scandinavica,* **83**(2), 125–128.

354. Skinhøj, P., Cohn, J. & Bradburne, A.F. (1976) Transmission of hepatitis type B from healthy HB_sAg-positive mothers. *British Medical Journal,* **i,** 10–11.

355. Skinhøj, P., Mikkelsen, F. & Hollinger, F.B. (1977) Hepatitis A in Greenland: importance of specific antibody testing in epidemiologic surveillance. *American Journal of Epidemiology,* **105**(2), 140–147.

356. Skrede, S., Blomhoff, J.P., Elgjo, K. & Gjone, E. (1973) Biochemical tests in evaluation of liver function. *Scandinavian Journal of Gastroenterology,* **8,** 37–45.

357. Smetana, H.F. (1975) In *Hepatitis Frontiers* (Ed.) Hartmann, F., Lo Grippo, G.A., Mateer, J.G. & Little, B.J. Boston: Brown & Co.

358. Smith, J.L., Maynard, J.E., Berquist, K.R., Doto, I.L., Webster, H.M. & Sheller, M.J. (1976) From the Center for Disease Control: comparative risk of hepatitis B among physicians and dentists. *Journal of Infectious Diseases,* **133**(6), 705–706.

359. Smith, J.L., Murphy, B.L., Auslander, M.O., Maynard, J.E., Schalm, S.S., Summerskill, W.H.J. & Gitnick, G.L. (1976) Studies of the 'e' antigen in acute and chronic hepatitis. *Gastroenterology,* **71,** 208–209.

360. Spero, J.A., Lewis, J.H., van Thiel, D.H., Hasiba, U. & Rabin, B.S. (1978) Asymptomatic structural liver disease in hemophilia. *New England Journal of Medicine,* **298,** 1373–1378.
361. Steigman, A. (1973) Rashes and arthropathy in viral hepatitis. *Mount Sinai Journal of Medicine,* **40,** 752–757.
362. Stephen, E.L., Sammons, M.L., Pannier, W.L., Baron, S., Spertzel, R.O. & Levy, H.B. (1977) Effect of a nuclease-resistant derivative of polyriboinosinic polyribocytidylic acid complex on yellow fever in rhesus monkeys (*Macaca mulatta*). *Journal of Infectious Diseases,* **136,** 122–126.
363. Stevens, C.E., Beasley, R.P., Tsui, J. & Lee, W.-C. (1975) Vertical transmission of hepatitis B antigen in Taiwan. *New England Journal of Medicine,* **292,** 771–774.
364. Stille, W., Böhle, E., Helm, E., van Rey, W. & Siede, W. (1968) An infectious disease transmitted by *Cercopithecus aethiops* (green monkey disease). *German Medical Monthly,* **13,** 470–478.
365. Strom, T.B. & Merrill, J.P. (1977) Hepatitis B, transfusions and renal transplantation (Editorial). *New England Journal of Medicine,* **296**(4), 225–226.
366. Sun, N.C. & Smith, V.M. (1966) Hepatitis associated with myocarditis. Unusual manifestation of infection with coxsackie virus group B type 3. *New England Journal of Medicine,* **274,** 190–193.
367. Sutnick, A.I., Bugbee, S.J., London, T.A., Loeb, L.A., Peyretti, F., Litwin, S. & Blumberg, B.S. (1973) Lymphocyte function in normal people with persistent Australia antigen. *Journal of Laboratory and Clinical Medicine,* **82,** 79–85.
368. Szmuness, W., Harley, E.J. & Prince, A.M. (1975) Intrafamilial spread of asymptomatic hepatitis B. *American Journal of the Medical Sciences,* **270,** 293–304.
369. Szmuness, W., Prince, A.M., Etling, G.F. & Pick, R. (1972) Development and distribution of hemagglutinating antibody against the hepatitis B antigen in institutionalized populations. *Journal of Infectious Diseases,* **126,** 498–506.
370. Szmuness, W., Prince, A.M., Goodman, M., Ehrich, C., Pick, R. & Ansari, M. (1974) Hepatitis B immune serum globulin in prevention of nonparenterally transmitted hepatitis B. *New England Journal of Medicine,* **290,** 701–706.
371. Szmuness, W., Prince, A.M., Grady, G.F., Mann, M.K., Levine, R.W., Friedman, E.A., Jacobs, M.J., Josephson, A., Ribot, S., Shapiro, F.L., Stenzel, K.H., Suki, W.M. & Vyas, G. (1974) Hepatitis B infection. A point-prevalence study in 15 U.S. hemodialysis centers. *Journal of the American Medical Association,* **227,** 901–906.
372. Szmuness, W., Much, I., Prince, A.M., Hoofnagle, J.H., Cherubin, C.E., Harley, E.J. & Block, G.H. (1975) On the role of sexual behaviour in the spread of hepatitis B infection. *Annals of Internal Medicine,* **83**(4), 489–495.
373. Szmuness, W., Dienstag, J.L., Purcell, R.H., Prince, A.M., Stevens, C.E. & Levine, R.W. (1977) Hepatitis type A and hemodialysis: a seroepidemiologic study in 15 U.S. centers. *Annals of Internal Medicine,* **87**(1), 8–12.
374. Szmuness, W., Dienstag, J.L., Purcell, R.H., Stevens, C.E., Wong, D.C., Ikram, H., Bar-Shany, S., Beasley, R.P., Desmyter, J. & Gaon, J.A. (1977) The prevalence of antibody to hepatitis A antigen in various parts of the world. A pilot study. *American Journal of Epidemiology,* **5,** 392–398.
375. Tabor, E., Gerety, R.J., Drucker, J.A., Seeff, L.B., Hoofnagle, J.H., Jackson, D.R., April, M., Barker, L.F. & Pineda-Tamondong, G. (1978) Transmission of non-A, non-B hepatitis from man to chimpanzee. *Lancet,* **i,** 463–466.
376. Takahashi, K., Imai, M., Tsuda, F., Takahashi, T., Miyawaka, Y. & Mayumi, M. (1976) Association of Dane particles with e antigen in the serum of asymptomatic carriers of hepatitis B surface antigen. *Journal of Immunology,* **117,** 102–105.
377. Takahashi, K., Fakuda, M., Baba, K., Imai, M., Mikayawa, Y. & Mayumi, M. (1977) Determination of e antigen and antibody to e by means of passive haemagglutination method. *Journal of Immunology,* **119,** 1556–1561.
378. Tedder, R.S. & Bull, F.G. (1978) Characterisation of 'e' antigen associated with hepatitis B. *Clinical and Experimental Immunology.* In press.
379. Thornton, A., Tsiquaye, K.N. & Zuckerman, A.J. (1977) Studies on human hepatitis A virus in chimpanzees. *British Journal of Experimental Pathology,* **58,** 352–358.
380. Tiggert, W.D., Berge, T.O., Gochenour, W.S., Gleiser, C.A., Eveland, W.C., Vorder Bruegge, C. & Smetana, H.F. (1960) Experimental yellow fever. *Transactions of the New York Academy of Sciences,* **22,** 323–333.
381. Toghill, P.J., Bailey, M.E., Williams, R., Zeegen, R. & Bown, R. (1967) Cytomegalovirus hepatitis in the adult. *Lancet,* **i,** 1351–1354.
382. Trewby, P.N. & Williams, R. (1977) Pathophysiology of hypotension in patients with fulminant hepatic failure. *Gut,* **18,** 1021–1026.
383. Triger, D.R., Alp, M.H. & Wright, R. (1972) Bacterial and dietary antibodies in liver disease. *Lancet,* **i,** 60–63.
384. Tripatzis, I. (1972) Australia antigen in urine and feces. *American Journal of Diseases of Children,* **123,** 401–404.
385. Tullis, J.L., Hinman, J., Sproul, M.T. & Nickerson, R.J. (1970) Incidence of post-transfusion hepatitis in previously frozen blood. *Journal of the American Medical Association,* **214,** 719–723.
386. Turner, G.C. & Bruce White, G.B. (1969) SH antigen in haemodialysis associated hepatitis. *Lancet,* **ii,** 121–124.
387. Vahrman, J. (1971) Viral hepatitis and the E.S.R. *British Medical Journal,* **ii,** 466–467.
388. Villarejos, V.M., Kirsten, P.H., Visona, K.A., Gutierrez, D. & Rodriguez, A. (1974) Role of saliva, urine and feces in the transmission of type B hepatitis. *New England Journal of Medicine,* **291,** 1375–1378.
389. Voegt, H. (1942) Zur aetiologie der hepatitis epidemica. *Munchener Medizinische Wochenscrift,* **89,** 76–79.
390. Vyas, G.N., Peterson, D.L., Townsend, R.M., Damle, S.R. & Magnius, L.O. (1977) Hepatitis B 'e' antigen, apparent association with lactate dehydrogenase isozyme. *Science,* **198,** 1068–1070.
391. Wacker, W.E.C., Riordan, J.F., Snodgrass, P.J., Chang, L.W., Morse, L.J., O'Brien, T.F. & Reddy, W.J. (1972) The Holy Cross hepatitis outbreak: clinical and chemical abnormalities. *Archives of Internal Medicine,* **130,** 357–360.
392. Wands, J.R., Walker, J.A., Davis, T.T., Waterbury, L.A., Owens, A.H. & Carpenter, C.C.J. (1974) Hepatitis B in an oncology unit. *New England Journal of Medicine,* **291**(26), 1371–1374.

393. Ward, R., Borchert, P., Wright, A. & Cline, E. (1972) Hepatitis B antigen in saliva and mouth washings. *Lancet*, **ii**, 726–727.

394. Ware, A.J., Eigenbrodt, E.H. & Combes, B. (1975) Prognostic significance of subacute hepatic necrosis in acute hepatitis. *Gastroenterology*, **68**, 519–524.

395. Wenzel, R.P., Le Bouvier, G.L. & Beam, W.E. (1972) Drug abuse and viral hepatitis in marines. *Journal of the American Medical Association*, **220**, 707–709.

396. Wilkinson, S.P., Davies, M.H., Portmann, B. & Williams, R. (1978) Renal failure in otherwise uncomplicated acute viral hepatitis. *British Medical Journal*, **ii**, 338–341.

397. Williams, A. & Le Bouvier, G. (1976) Heterogeneity and thermolability of 'e'. *Bibliography of Haematology*, **42**, 71–75.

398. Winn, W.C., Monath, T.P., Murphy, F.A. & Whitfield, S.G. (1975) Lassa virus hepatitis. Observations on a fatal case from the 1972 Sierra Leone epidemic. *Archives of Pathology*, **99**, 599–604.

399. Wolters, G., Kuijpers, L.P.C., Kacaki, J. & Schuurs, H.W.M. (1977) Enzyme-linked immunosorbent assay for hepatitis B surface antigen. *Journal of Infectious Diseases*, **136**, 311–317.

400. World Health Organization Technical Report Series, No. 512 (1973) Viral hepatitis: report of a WHO Scientific Group. Geneva.

401. World Health Organization Technical Report Series, No. 602 (1977) Advances in viral hepatitis: report of the WHO Expert Committee on Viral Hepatitis. Geneva.

402. World Health Organization International Study Team (1978) Ebola haemorrhagic fever in Sudan, 1976. *Bulletin of the World Health Organization*, **56**, 247–270.

403. Wright, R. (1970) Australia antigen and smooth-muscle antibody in acute and chronic hepatitis. *Lancet*, **i**, 521–522.

404. Wright, R. (1977) Immunology of gastrointestinal liver disease. In *Current Topics in Immunology* (Ed.) Turk, J. London: Edward Arnold.

405. Wright, R., McCollum, R.W. & Klatskin, G. (1969) Australia antigen in acute and chronic liver disease. *Lancet*, **ii**, 117–121.

406. Wright, R., Perkins, J.R., Bower, B.D. & Jerome, D.W. (1970) Cirrhosis associated with the Australia antigen in an infant who acquired hepatitis from her mother. *British Medical Journal*, **iv**, 719–721.

407. Young, E.J., Killam, A.P. & Greene, J.F. Jr (1976) Disseminated herpes virus infection. Association with primary genital herpes in pregnancy. *Journal of the American Medical Association*, **235**, 2731–2733.

408. Zientara, M. & Moore, S. (1970) Fatal talc embolism in a drug addict. *Human Pathology*, **1**, 324–327.

409. Zuckerman, A.J. (1970) *Virus Diseases of the Liver*. London: Butterworth.

410. Zuckerman, A.J. (1975) In *Human Viral Hepatitis*. Amsterdam and Oxford: North-Holland Publishing Company.

411. Zuckerman, A.J., Taylor, P.E., Bird, G. & Russell, S.M. (1971) The Australia (hepatitis-associated) antigen in fibrinogen and other fractions of human plasma. *Journal of Clinical Pathology*, **24**, 2–7.

412. Fields, H.A., Bradley, D.W., Davis, C.L., Murphy, B.L., Schable, C.A. & Maynard, J.E. (1978) Micro-solid phase immunoradiometric assay (micro-SPIRA) of the detection of HB_eAg and anti-HB_e. In *Viral Hepatitis* (Ed.) Vyas, G.N., Cohen, S.N. & Schmid, R. pp. 173–175. Philadelphia: Franklin Institute Press.

413. Hilleman, M.R., Bertland, A.U., Buynak, E.B., Lampson, G.P., McAleer, W.J., McLean, A.A., Roehn, R.R. & Tytell, A.A. (1978) Clinical and laboratory studies of HB_sAg vaccine. In *Viral Hepatitis* (Ed.) Vyas, G.N., Cohen, S.N. & Schmid, R. pp. 525–537. Philadelphia: Franklin Institute Press.

414. Magnius, L.O. (1978) Structure of HB_eAg. In *Viral Hepatitis* (Ed.) Vyas, G.N., Cohen, S.N. & Schmid, R. pp. 177–182. Philadelphia: Franklin Institute Press.

415. Neurath, A.R. (1978) Discussion: Structure of HB_eAg. In *Viral Hepatitis* (Ed.) Vyas, G.N., Cohen, S.N. & Schmid, R. pp. 183–187. Philadelphia: Franklin Institute Press.

416. Peters, R.L., Omata, M., Aschavai, O. & Liew, C.T. (1978) Protracted viral hepatitis with impaired regeneration. In *Viral Hepatitis* (Ed.) Vyas, G.N., Cohen, S.N. & Schmid, R. pp. 79–84. Philadelphia: Franklin Institute Press.

417. Peterson, D.L., Chien, D.Y., Vyas, G.N., Nitecki, D. & Bond, H.E. (1978) Characterization of polypeptides of HB_sAg for the proposed 'UC vaccine' for hepatitis B. In *Viral Hepatitis* (Ed.) Vyas, G.N., Cohen, S.N. & Schmid, R. pp. 569–573. Philadelphia: Franklin Institute Press.

418. Prince, A.M., Brotman, B., van den Ende, M.C., Richardson, L. & Kellner, A. (1978) Non-A/non-B hepatitis: identification of a virus-specific antigen and antibody. A preliminary report. In *Viral Hepatitis* (Ed.) Vyas, G.N., Cohen, S.N. & Schmid, R. pp. 633–640. Philadelphia: Franklin Institute Press.

419. Redeker, A.G. (1978) Advances in clinical aspects of acute and chronic liver disease of viral origin. In *Viral Hepatitis* (Ed.) Vyas, G.N., Cohen, S.N. & Schmid, R. pp. 425–429. Philadelphia: Franklin Institute Press.

420. Stevens, C.E., Neurath, A.R., Szmuness, W., Beasley, R.P. & Ikram, H. (1978) Correlations between HB_eAg/anti-HB_e, HB_sAg titer, HB_sAg-associated albumin binding sites and infectivity. In *Viral Hepatitis* (Ed.) Vyas, G.N., Cohen, S.N. & Schmid, R. pp. 211–215. Philadelphia: Franklin Institute Press.

421. Trepo, C., Hantz, O., Vitvitski, P., Chevallier, P., Williams, A., Lemaire, J.M. & Sepetjian, M. (1978) Heterogeneity and significance of HB_eAg: characterization of a third specificity (e_3). In *Viral Hepatitis* (Ed.) Vyas, G.N., Cohen, S.N. & Schmid, R. pp. 203–209. Philadelphia: Franklin Institute Press.

422. Vyas, G.N., Cohen, S.N. & Schmid, R. (Ed.) (1978) *Viral Hepatitis*. Philadelphia: Franklin Institute Press.

423. Vitvitsky, L., Prince, A.M., Trepo, C. & Brotman, B. (1979) Detection of virus-associated antigen in serum and liver of patients with non-A, non-B hepatitis. *Lancet*, **ii**, 1263–1267.

Chapter 29

Chronic Hepatitis

RALPH WRIGHT
G.H. MILLWARD-SADLER

The term 'chronic hepatitis' is used to describe an illness associated with continuing inflammation of the liver following viral hepatitis or arising spontaneously, of unknown aetiology, and not due to drugs or toxins. The duration of the biochemical or histological abnormalities before the term 'chronic hepatitis' had been used by different authors has varied from 10 weeks[236] to six months,[166, 222] or even one year.[221] Since the disease may be subclinical, an active cirrhosis at the time of initial presentation also implies chronicity.

It is customary to exclude alcoholic liver disease, Wilson's disease, primary biliary cirrhosis, alpha-1-antitrypsin deficiency and drug-induced chronic active liver disease, although they may show clinical, biochemical and histological features indistinguishable from chronic active (aggressive) hepatitis of unknown aetiology or that due to hepatitis B (HBV).

We therefore use the term 'chronic hepatitis' to include prolonged inflammation of the liver following an attack of acute viral hepatitis, either icteric or anicteric, or chronic active hepatitis of unknown aetiology. We accept the Fogarty proceedings[147] definition of chronic hepatitis as inflammation of the liver for six months or more. The diagnosis is based on the clinical, biochemical, histological and immunological findings. Careful assessment, often with serial liver biopsy, is necessary to determine the clinical course and prognosis and therefore the need for treatment of a particular patient. In prolonged or unresolved viral hepatitis, the outlook is good, providing the adverse prognostic features discussed in Chapter 28 (Table 28.7) are not present. In chronic active hepatitis of unknown aetiology, the prognosis is poor, and in some cases established and irreversible liver damage is present at clinical presentation.

It must be emphasized that the distinction between these different types of chronic hepatitis, clinically or histologically, is not always clear cut, and frequent review and reassessment of the patient are necessary for correct diagnosis and treatment.

CHRONIC HEPATITIS AND POST-HEPATITIC CIRRHOSIS

Although there was circumstantial evidence that patients with acute viral hepatitis, either icteric or anicteric, could progress to chronic active hepatitis and a post-hepatitic cirrhosis, proof of such progression was not forthcoming until it became feasible to test for hepatitis B-associated antigens.

The earlier evidence was based on rare instances where progression of acute viral hepatitis to chronic liver disease could be demonstrated clinically and sometimes histologically on serial liver biopsy.[131, 138, 210, 219] Klatskin[134] emphasized the importance of anicteric infections in the progression of acute viral hepatitis to cirrhosis. More direct evidence arose from the occasional transmission of acute hepatitis to recipients by the transfused blood from donors with cirrhosis.[47] On the other hand, epidemiological studies provided little support for a significant role for viruses in the aetiology of cirrhosis, but most large follow-up studies were probably of outbreaks of hepatitis A and chronicity was therefore not to be expected.[48, 169, 291]

Pathology and Terminology

As the term implies, this is a chronic inflammatory reaction involving the liver. It is usually non-granulomatous and the hallmark of the reaction is the lymphocyte. As in any chronic inflammation, there is cellular damage with regeneration and, particularly in more severe cases, repair. The chronic inflammation and each of its individual components of cell damage, regeneration, inflammation and repair will vary in severity through a continuous spectrum. This variation will be seen not only between patients but also, in an individual patient, between areas of liver and temporally at different times. Arbitrary dividing lines have been drawn separating this spectrum of chronic inflammation into grades which have prognostic significance, but the margins between the groups are frequently blurred and controversy usually arises over those cases which straddle the dividing line.

In chronic hepatitis two types have been described by histopathological criteria[52] termed chronic persistent hepatitis and chronic aggressive hepatitis. The separation of chronic persistent hepatitis and chronic aggressive hepatitis is generally but not universally accepted. Differentiation of these two entities has prognostic implications: chronic aggressive hepatitis destroys the architecture and is a likely cause of cirrhosis, whereas chronic persistent hepatitis does not produce significant architectural distortion.

This division of chronic hepatitis into grades of severity does not have any aetiological significance. Chronic hepatitis B infection in the liver is associated with a spectrum of inflammatory change ranging from normal through chronic persistent hepatitis to chronic aggressive hepatitis with or without cirrhosis. Although follow-up of hepatitis A epidemics has rarely shown more severe lesions than chronic persistent hepatitis (see Chapter 28), the role of non-A, non-B hepatitis in these two groups is not yet determined. It is interesting that both a chronic carrier state and cirrhosis have been related to the latter.[242]

Aetiological classification of chronic hepatitis has also been superimposed on this morphological grading to produce semantic confusion. The term 'chronic active hepatitis', originally used for chronic hepatitis in young females and associated with various serum autoantibodies, has also been used synonymously for chronic aggressive hepatitis. 'Chronic active hepatitis' is now recommended as the official term for the inflammatory process in the liver as well as for a clinical syndrome, with chronic aggressive hepatitis as an acceptable morphological alternative.[147] As the various aetiologies of chronic active hepatitis become more clearly identified, this source of confusion becomes less important. We shall use the term 'chronic active hepatitis' instead of 'chronic aggressive hepatitis'.

CHRONIC PERSISTENT HEPATITIS

Following a typical attack of acute viral hepatitis, a proportion of patients develop persistent symptoms and biochemical abnormalities, which may continue for months or years. The distinction between chronic persistent hepatitis and chronic active hepatitis following viral hepatitis is essentially a histological diagnosis, although there are certain clinical, biochemical and immunological features which may provide a clue to the nature of the underlying liver disease.

Clinical, Biochemical and Immunological Features

Patients may present following a typical acute icteric attack of viral hepatitis, or the initial attack may have been anicteric. Symptoms of fatigue, malaise, lassitude and anorexia with intolerance of fat and alcohol may fluctuate in severity for months or years after the acute attack. There may be failure to regain weight lost during the acute attack. Pain over the liver may be present, particularly after exercise. The liver may be enlarged, tender and slightly firmer than normal, but splenomegaly is unusual. Slight jaundice and dark urine are occasionally present, but this usually indicates a frank relapse of the hepatitis. Palmar erythema, spider naevi, oedema or ascites are not present. The serum transaminase levels are elevated but seldom more than four or five times the upper limit of normal. The prothrombin time is not prolonged, the albumin level is well maintained and hyperglobulinaemia is slight. Autoantibodies, including the smooth muscle antibody, are usually negative.

Because of biochemical screening and screening for hepatitis antigens, the number of patients found to have chronic persistent hepatitis without significant symptoms is increasing. The majority of cases follow hepatitis B infection, usually with persistence of the HB_sAg in the serum, although occasionally the antigen is cleared, but liver cell necrosis and elevated transaminases persist. In a proportion of patients there is no evidence of previous infection with hepatitis B, and it is presumably due to persistence of non-A, non-B hepatitis, since there is little evidence that hepatitis A can progress to chronicity (see Chapter 28).

In one series of 20 patients with chronic inflammation of the liver lasting for more than one year, 13 had a history strongly suggestive of acute viral hepatitis but none was HB_sAg positive.[17] In another study, chronic persistent hepatitis predominated in men, over half were HB_sAg positive, but only one had the e antigen.[37] Some developed a mild chronic aggressive hepatitis, but none progressed to cirrhosis. On the other hand, in another series of 26 cases, three patients showed progression to cirrhosis, but the possibility of sampling error in their initial biopsies could not be excluded.[57]

Pathology

Chronic persistent hepatitis is a histological diagnosis based on the appearances of a normal architecture with a mononuclear, predominantly lymphocytic infiltrate in portal tracts (Figure 29.1). Occasional plasma cells and macrophages may be present. The tracts may be slightly expanded by fibrous spurs, but there is no destruction of the limiting plate by piecemeal necrosis, and this negative feature separates the condition from chronic active hepatitis.

The importance of chronic persistent hepatitis is that it represents a chronic viral infection that is not producing any significant architectural distortion.

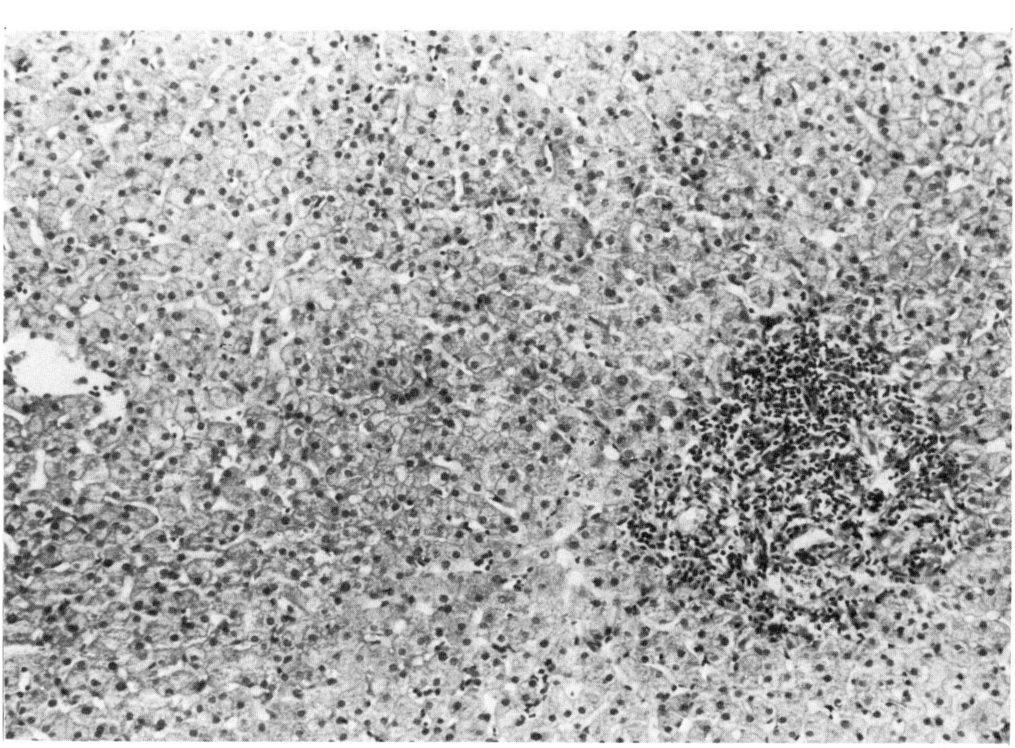

Figure 29.1. Chronic persistent hepatitis with central vein on the left and portal tract on the right. Many lymphocytes fill the slightly enlarged portal tract but there is no piecemeal necrosis. The parenchyma shows focal twinning of cell plates but there is no degeneration and no Kupffer cell activation. Haematoxylin & eosin × 40.

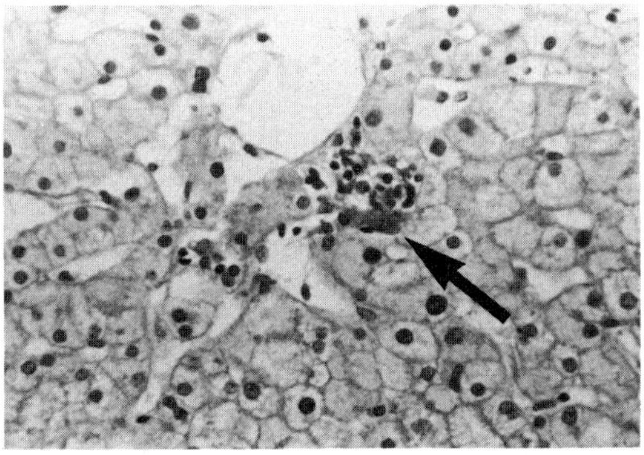

Figure 29.2. Focal necrosis against a central vein. There are lymphocytes with a Kupffer cell containing phagocytosed debris in its abundant cytoplasm (arrow). Diastase-PAS × 250.

Hepatitis B markers can now be demonstrated in paraffin sections of liver biopsies by immunological and histochemical techniques. These are discussed in greater detail below. The histochemical techniques, orcein and aldehyde fuchsin, both of which demonstrate HB_sAg in the hepatocyte cytoplasm,[223] are especially valuable in this category as they are negative in acute but positive in chronic hepatitis B infections of the liver.[54] Therefore, when positively stained hepatocytes are demonstrated there is a chronic hepatitis B infection of the liver which is categorized by the associated morphological changes. 'Ground-glass' hepatocytes, in which there is abundant, finely stippled eosinophilic cytoplasm, are frequently associated with chronic hepatitis B infection,[105] but not all ground-glass hepatocytes are orcein positive and vice versa.[248, 273] Using the basic concept of chronic persistent hepatitis, there are subdivisions of this category, irrespective of the presence or absence of HBV. These are portal triaditis, resolving acute viral hepatitis, persistent or relapsing viral hepatitis and chronic active hepatitis in remission. Some of these have been proposed as separate diagnostic categories distinct from chronic persistent hepatitis.

Portal triaditis

This is an infiltrate predominantly of lymphocytes with some plasma cells and occasional macrophages within portal tracts (Figure 29.1). In smaller portal tracts the infiltrate is uniformly distributed, but in larger ones it is focal and peripheral. Occasional cells may spill over into periportal sinusoids but there is no piecemeal necrosis. There may be a minimal portal tract fibrosis with an occasional slender fibrous spur extending into the lobule. The cell plates are orderly and only interrupted by a very occasional focal cluster of mononuclear cells. These are sometimes seen around a degenerate hepatocyte.

This is the basic minimal change for chronic persistent hepatitis and is present in the other categories. The morphological criteria outlined are not specific and will be found in other conditions that are not due to a persistent viral infection. These include the non-specific reactive changes associated with systemic infections and illnesses, the portal tract lymphoid infiltrates that are related to the frequency of intravenous injections,[72] pericholangitis and congestive cardiac failure. Therefore, if these changes alone are present in the biopsy without demonstrable HBV markers, a morphological diagnosis of chronic persistent hepatitis cannot be made. The changes should be recorded as portal triaditis compatible with chronic persistent hepatitis, and careful correlation made with the clinical, biochemical and serological findings before a diagnosis is established. Even then this must be subject to critical review.

Resolving acute viral hepatitis

Portal triaditis is present with features in the lobule consistent with a preceding episode of acute hepatitis, now resolving or resolved. This acute hepatitis may or may not have been clinically apparent. The features in the biopsy may include active parenchymal degeneration such as acidophil or ballooning degeneration,

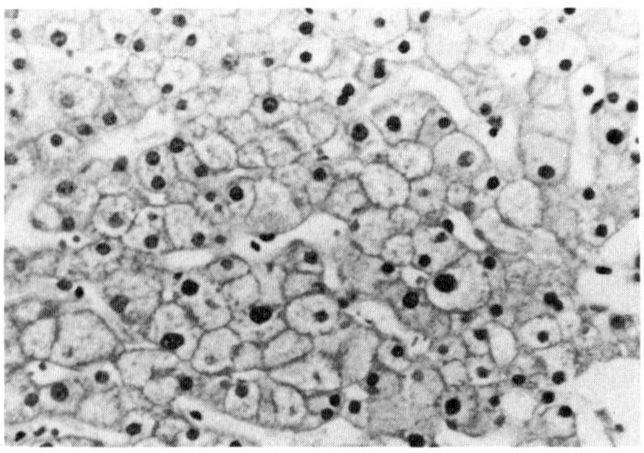

Figure 29.3. The central vein is present in the bottom right corner. Hepatocytes show knots of cells formed from anastomosing twinned cell plates. There is also increased variation in nuclear size and staining for the age of the patient. Haematoxylin & eosin × 250.

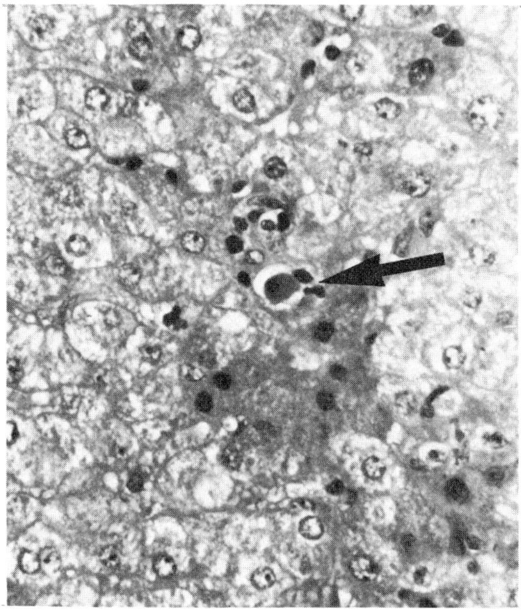

Figure 29.4. Chronic persistent hepatitis: acidophil body (arrow) with pyknotic nucleus that has become rounded off and separated from neighbouring hepatocytes. Haematoxylin & eosin × 1000.

but this is unusual and, even when present, minor or insignificant. Focal collapse of the reticulin architecture around the centrilobular vein, distorting the cell plates, indicates previous loss of hepatocytes. Small focal hyperplastic clusters of hypertrophied and ceroid-laden Kupffer cells can be found within the sinusoids (Figure 29.2) with some similar pigment-laden macrophages in the portal tract. These portal tract macrophages are the last to disappear as the process resolves. Focal 'knots' of hepatocytes three or four cells across are present and reflect the regeneration following cell loss (Figure 29.3). The overall pattern is of residual changes following an acute hepatitis, such as are found commonly at three to four months.

Persistent and relapsing hepatitis

In this group there is direct morphological evidence of chronic hepatitis B infection or presumptive evidence of non-B chronic infection.[121, 182] Most commonly there is an inflammatory infiltrate of lymphocytes and plasma cells in portal tracts in association with mild parenchymal damage. An occasional acidophil body may be seen (Figure 29.4) and the radial cell plate pattern is effaced. This effacement, sometimes termed 'cobblestone'[182] (Figure 29.5), results from a combination of focal loss of hepatocytes with disruption of the cell plate pattern and regenerative hepatocyte activity. The latter is seen as twinning of cell plates with small 'knots' of hepatocytes three to four cells across. Individual hepatocytes throughout the lobule are often slightly larger with more abundant, finely granular eosinophilic cytoplasm. A variable number of orcein positive hepatocytes will be present in cases of chronic hepatitis B infection and some of these cells may also show ground-glass cytoplasmic changes.[105]

Scattered focal necroses with a few lymphocytes and Kupffer cells surrounding a degenerate hepatocyte are present, but the diffuse hyperplasia and hypertrophy of Kupffer cells seen throughout the lobule in acute viral hepatitis are not seen in this case. Pigment phagocytosis is infrequent.

Rarely, liver biopsy may still show the changes of acute viral hepatitis with a history of six months or more of illness. Apart from the length of history, the morphological changes are indistinguishable from the typical acute hepatitis, and this was originally described as chronic lobular hepatitis.[183, 184] These features may reflect a prolonged unresolved course of acute hepatitis[184] or relapsing hepatitis, and probably included are examples of patients who have consecutive but different virus infections of the liver.[167] Until serological or morphological markers of the non-B hepatitis are defined, this must remain an area of speculation.

This more florid chronic lobular hepatitis has been claimed to be distinct from chronic persistent hepatitis.[184] It has also been used to describe the presence of active acidophil and ballooning degenerative changes in the hepatic parenchyma in both chronic active hepatitis[103] and chronic persistent hepatitis.[21,214] The term was not accepted by the Committee for Standardization of Nomenclature, Diagnostic Criteria and Diagnostic Methodology.[147]

Chronic persistent hepatitis in chronic active hepatitis

On occasions, liver biopsy may demonstrate features of chronic persistent hepatitis when the diagnosis has been previously established or is subsequently shown to be chronic active hepatitis. This may result from sampling error, spontaneous remission or successful treatment of chronic active hepatitis,[13] but true progression to chronic active hepatitis from chronic persistent hepatitis has been described.[57,216]

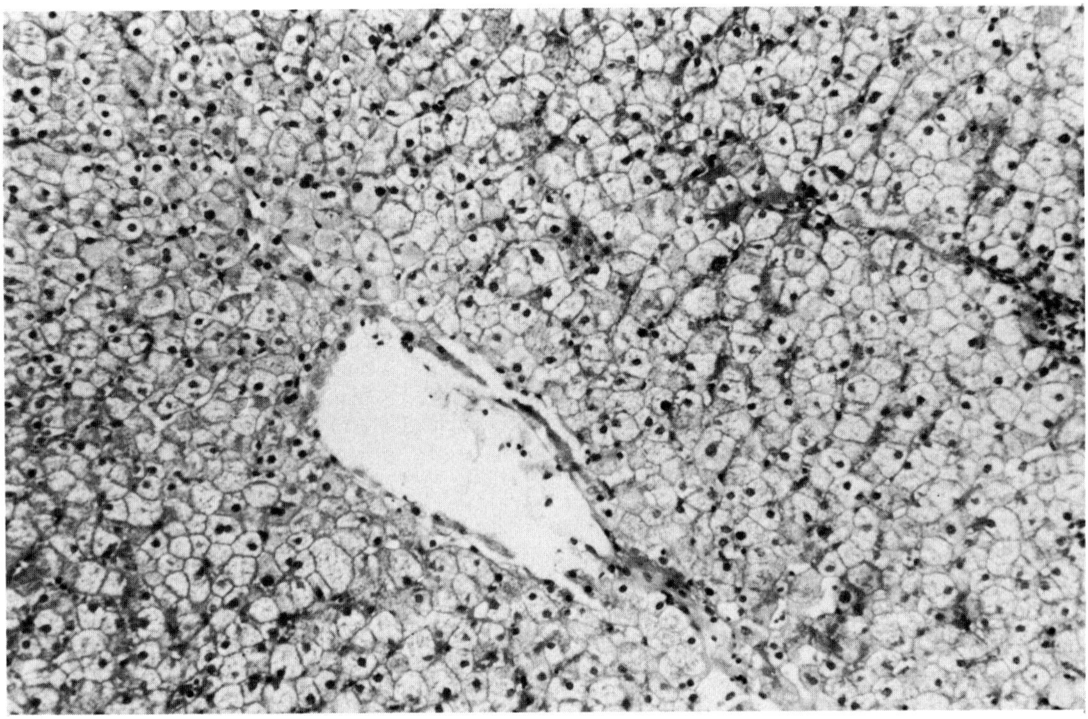

Figure 29.5. HB_sAg positive chronic persistent hepatitis; hepatocytes around the central vein are swollen and sinusoids are more difficult to identify. Consequently there is a masking of the cell plate pattern. Only occasional hepatocytes are orcein positive. Haematoxylin & eosin × 600.

Following spontaneous remission or successful treatment of chronic active hepatitis, residual fibrosis from the preceding piecemeal necrosis may be identified. This will have expanded the portal tracts and may have isolated solitary or small groups of hepatocytes around the periphery.

HB_sAg POSITIVE CHRONIC ACTIVE HEPATITIS

In the initial study of the Australia antigen (HB_sAg) in chronic liver disease from Yale, six of 24 patients with chronic active hepatitis of unknown aetiology were shown to have the hepatitis B antigen in their serum when an insensitive immunodiffusion technique was used.[281] A similar proportion of chronic active hepatitis elsewhere in the United States could be attributed to hepatitis B,[93, 186] but it was rarely observed in patients with chronic active hepatitis in the United Kingdom[69, 82, 277] and in Australia.[158] On the other hand, a high incidence of HB_sAg positive chronic active hepatitis and/or cirrhosis ranging from 25 to 60 per cent has been reported from Greece,[104, 246] Italy,[20] Austria,[139] West Germany,[106, 127] Africa[1,0,159] and Iraq.[31] This striking geographical variation in its frequency (Table 29.1) relates to the prevalence of the carrier state in the community.[279]

Clinical and Biochemical Features

The clinical features of HB_sAg positive chronic active hepatitis, with or without cirrhosis, are very variable. In most series, males have predominated and the disorder often presents over the age of 30 years, but it can occur at any age and one of our own cases was a young female infant who had acquired hepatitis from the mother[282] (Figure 29.6).

The frequency with which a previous history of acute viral hepatitis is found also varies in different series. Clearly, methods of case selection will be an important factor in the clinical presentation and progression of the liver disease. Some series contain patients who are asymptomatic and have been found to have chronic active hepatitis or cirrhosis on routine liver biopsy following the detection of a positive HB_sAg in the serum, hepatomegaly, splenomegaly or abnormal liver function tests. Others

Table 29.1. *HB_sAg in Patients with Chronic Liver Disease.*[a]

Country	Donors	HB_sAg carriage rate: Chronic persistent hepatitis	Chronic active hepatitis	Cirrhosis	Reference
USA	0.1	50	27	–	Wright, McCollum & Klatskin[281]
Germany	0.5	78	61	45	Kaboth et al[127]
Australia	0.1	–	4	–	Mathews & Mackay[158]
Uganda	2.0	–	–	30	Maynard et al[159]
Italy	–	25	51	–	Bianchi et al[20]
Japan	2.0	34	34	24	Hirayama et al[109]
Denmark	0.1	50	30	–	Dietrichson et al[58]
Greece	1.0	–	–	35	Theodoropoulos et al[246]

[a] After Cossart.[46]

will have been followed through from an attack of acute hepatitis B to chronic active hepatitis, with or without cirrhosis.

Finally, some patients with or without a previous history of acute hepatitis will present with the complications of chronic active hepatitis and cirrhosis, such as oedema or ascites, bleeding varices, liver failure, septicaemia or a hepatoma. (The relationship of hepatitis B infection to hepatoma is discussed in Chapter 38.) Another mode of presentation may be with the extrahepatic associations of chronic HBV infection, such as glomerulonephritis or polyarteritis (see below).

The prognosis is very variable (Figure 29.7) and will depend greatly on the mode of presentation. Those cases presenting with the complications of chronic active hepatitis or cirrhosis, such as ascites, bleeding varices and liver failure, will clearly have a poor prognosis. In those who have been discovered incidentally or have been followed through from acute viral hepatitis the prognosis is uncertain but could well be good, since the latent period to the development of clinically overt cirrhosis may be long.

On clinical examination, spider naevi, palmar erythema, acne and endocrinopathies are

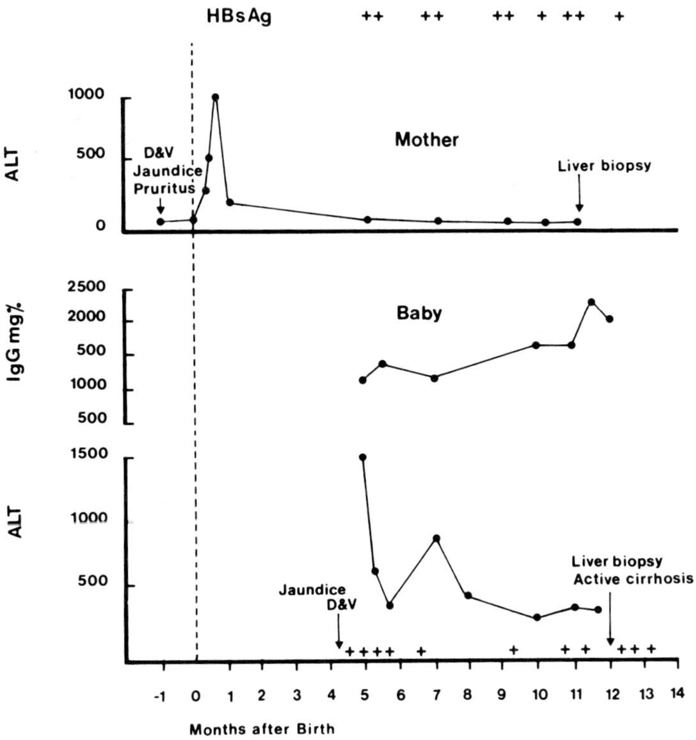

Figure 29.6. Sequence of events in an infant who acquired hepatitis B from her mother who was jaundiced at term. From Wright,[280] with kind permission of Edward Arnold.

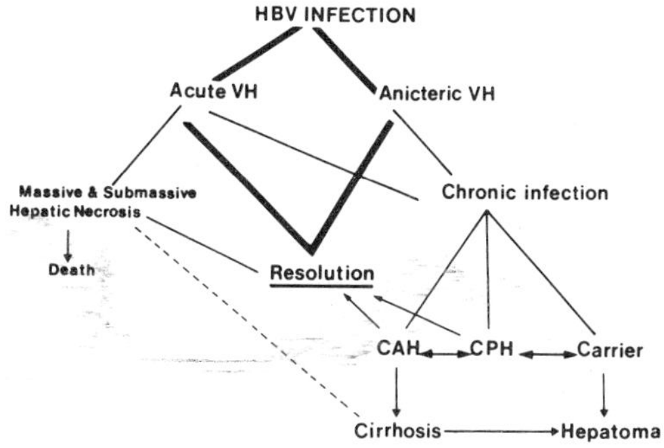

Figure 29.7. Hepatic consequences of HBV infection. Bold lines indicate frequently occurring events.

uncommon, as is the association with putative autoimmune diseases.[65, 103, 135, 277] Tattooing, scarification of the skin, a history of drug abuse or blood transfusion, and medical or paramedical employment may lead to suspicion of the disease.

About a third to half of the patients give a history of jaundice or an episode strongly suggestive of anicteric hepatitis, but usually the jaundice fades and the main biochemical abnormality is persistent elevation of the transaminases, other liver function tests being relatively little deranged until decompensation occurs. Occasionally there are intermittent attacks of acute on chronic hepatitis, but this is relatively infrequent. Hyperglobulinaemia is often not pronounced, and autoantibodies, such as smooth muscle antibody and antinuclear factor, are absent or only present at low titre. DNA-binding antibodies may be present but do not necessarily reflect an autoimmune response.[133]

HBV Markers in Serum

The markers of hepatitis B virus infection include features suggestive of chronicity, but are not sufficiently characteristic to preclude the use of liver biopsy in diagnosis. The titre of HB_sAg is significantly lower in patients with chronic active hepatitis than in chronic persistent hepatitis or in carriers,[20, 38, 62] and in occasional cases these low-titre reactions were detected by radio-immunoassay or haemagglutination techniques when they had been negative by the less sensitive methods.[38,69]

As indicated in Chapter 28, the e antigen and DNA polymerase activity are associated with infectivity, the presence of Dane particles and continuing replication of the virus. The e antigen has often disappeared by the time the patients present clinically with acute hepatitis if insensitive techniques such as immunodiffusion are used for its detection.

Nielsen, Dietrichson and Juhl[172] found that 58 per cent of their patients with chronic hepatitis and 31 per cent with cirrhosis who were HB_sAg positive had the e antigen, compared with only 10 per cent of those with acute hepatitis B. They proposed that the detection of e antigen during the acute symptomatic phase of hepatitis B is associated with a poor prognosis and increases the liability to chronicity. Similarly, Eleftheriou et al[73] detected e antigen in 44 per cent of patients with chronic active hepatitis, whereas only two of 79 such patients had e antibody. They did not detect e antigen in any of 99 cases of acute type B hepatitis who recovered normally. A similar correlation between chronicity, the e antigen and DNA polymerase activity was described by Nordenfelt and Andrén-Sandberg.[173] Feinman et al[76] and Smith et al[229] similarly confirmed the correlation between the presence of e antigen and chronic active liver disease, and showed that many carriers with normal livers have e antibody, but the latter caution against the inference that all e antigen positive individuals develop chronic hepatitis, or, conversely, that the presence of e antibody protects against its development. This is, of course, a different situation from the infectivity of e antigen positive serum as opposed to the relative lack of infectivity of that containing e antibody, which has repeatedly been demonstrated in transmission studies from mother to infant (see Chapter 28) and in the chimpanzee model.[224]

These findings have been confirmed in studies of acute and chronic hepatitis B infection in chimpanzees,[241] but the use of more sensitive techniques, such as haemagglutination, for the detection of e antigen and antibody, as well as the timing of their testing, will be crucial in determining whether these associations are upheld.[3]

The Mayo Clinic group[263] consider that the e antigen is associated with an impaired host response to hepatitis B virus infection and a poor prognosis, and that its disappearance in patients with chronic active liver disease, even with the development of anti-e, can occur with continuing progression of the disease.

Another marker of HBV infection is the antibody to the core antigen (anti-HB_c). This is regarded as a more sensitive indicator of

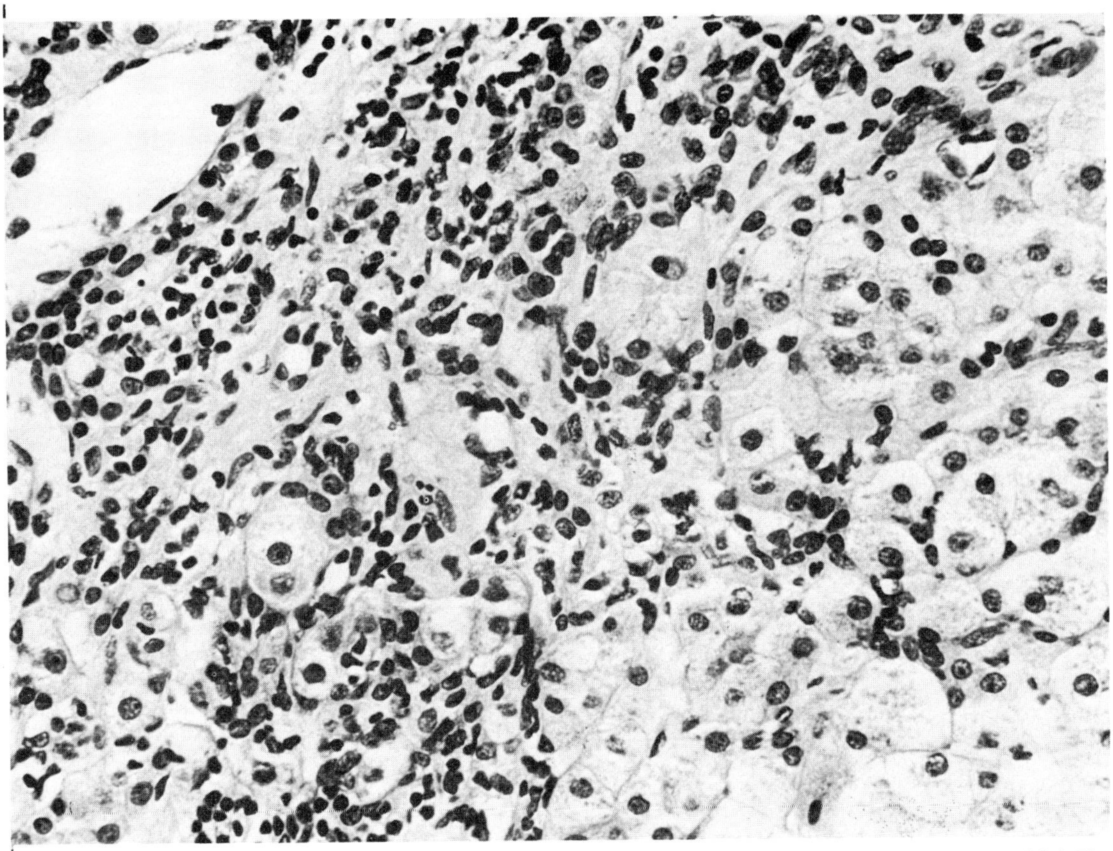

Figure 29.8. Florid piecemeal necrosis in chronic active hepatitis, with portal vein (top left) and parenchyma (bottom right). The interface between the two is blurred by a mononuclear cell infiltrate that is isolating hepatocytes. Haematoxylin & eosin × 1000.

hepatitis virus B replication than hepatitis B surface antigen, and may persist in the serum after HB_sAg has disappeared. It is present in virtually all patients with chronic hepatitis B infection, and because of its continued presence in some HB_sAg negative cases, it has been used as a more sensitive indicator of such infection (see below).

Pathology

The pathology of chronic active hepatitis is basic to several clinical entities and syndromes. Apart from chronic viral infections and idiopathic aetiology, these include Wilson's disease, primary biliary cirrhosis, alpha-1-antitrypsin deficiency and chronic administration of drugs, particularly oxyphenisatin, methyldopa and isoniazid, as well as alcohol. The inflammatory infiltrate and Kupffer cell reaction usually dominate the process, although there is also a variety of degenerative changes in the parenchyma as well as regeneration. Architectural distortion may vary considerably, showing established cirrhosis at presentation or mild enlargement of portal tracts only.

The general features of chronic active hepatitis will be considered here, and variations in emphasis attributed to aetiology noted, but the specific and diagnostic demonstration of HBV markers is considered later.

Mesenchymal reaction

There are three components to the mesenchymal reaction: an inflammatory infiltrate composed of lymphocytes with a variable number of plasma cells and some macrophages, Kupffer cell hyperplasia and increased fibroblastic activity (Figure 29.8). The inflammatory cell infiltrate is variable in intensity in various areas of the biopsy and is mainly centred on portal tracts and established fibrous bands but from these it extends into the parenchyma. Extensive sinusoidal infiltrates of lymphocytes and plasma cells are a feature of the most active disease (Figure 29.9). At the edges of portal tracts and fibrous septa with parenchyma, the lymphocytes

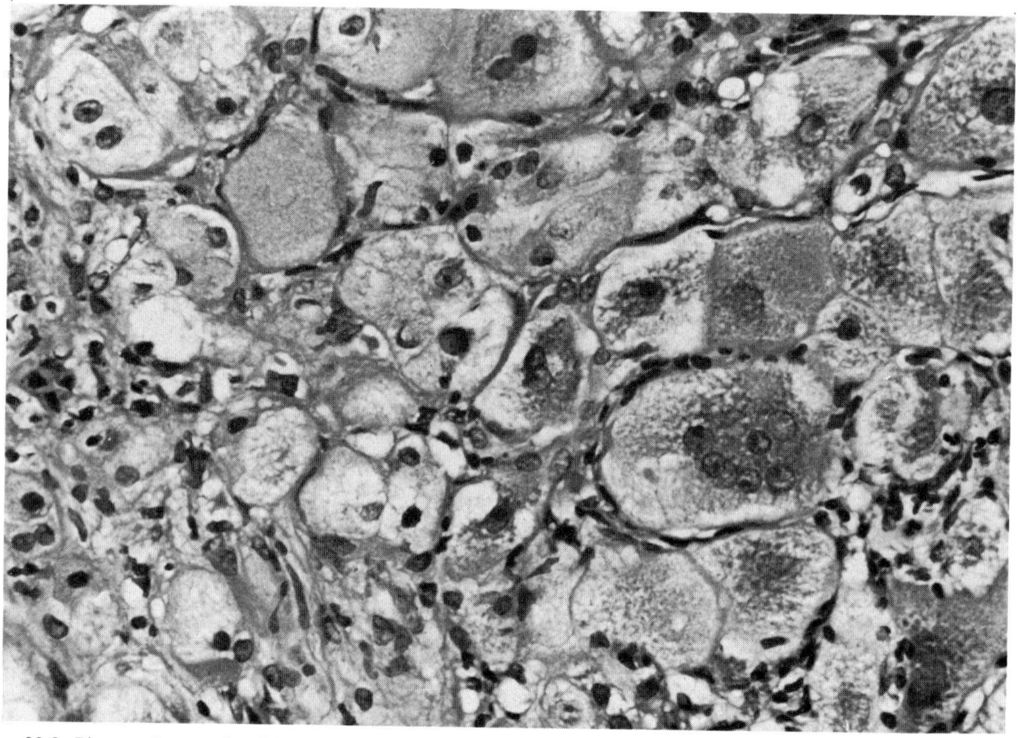

Figure 29.9. Piecemeal necrosis with extensive activity in the parenchyma, which also shows ballooning degeneration and regenerating multinucleate hepatocytes. Haematoxylin & eosin × 1200.

surround and isolate single or small groups of hepatocytes.

Careful study of this intimate association of hepatocyte with lymphocyte suggests that lymphocytes come into direct surface contact with hepatocyte plasma membranes and also invaginate into the hepatocyte. This contact is usually associated with degenerative changes in hepatocyte cytoplasm.[129] Direct extension by lymphocytes into the cytoplasm of degenerating hepatocytes is also observed. Small foci where hepatocytes have been lost or destroyed are marked for a short period by a small collection of lymphocytes with Kupffer cells and occasional plasma cells. Kupffer cells as indicated are hyperplastic in focal areas of cell death but also may be diffusely prominent throughout the sinusoids. There is rarely the hypertrophy with focal proliferation within and obstructing the sinusoids that is a feature of acute viral hepatitis. Similarly, phagocytosis of pigments is not a prominent feature, although small amounts of bile, lipofuscin or ceroid can be demonstrated by specific staining techniques.

The active fibrogenesis which is part of this reaction is responsible for the permanent isolation of single or small groups of hepatocytes. On electron microscopy, new collagen is laid down in the space of Disse, together with a basement membrane-like substance[211] (see Chapter 30).

Piecemeal necrosis. The combination of inflammatory cells and fibroblastic activity destroying parenchyma and surrounding and isolating small groups of hepatocytes at the interfaces between parenchyma and collagen has been termed piecemeal necrosis[181] and is regarded as the hallmark of chronic active hepatitis (Figures 29.8 and 29.9). Piecemeal necrosis occurs irregularly throughout the liver and with varying intensity, so that on biopsy some portal tracts may contain a discrete inflammatory infiltrate mimicking chronic persistent hepatitis with adjacent tracts showing florid piecemeal necrosis. The intensity of the inflammatory cell infiltrate and the extent to which hepatocytes are isolated is the index of activity of the process.

The lesion also varies in intensity with time, so that biopsies showing very little activity may be found at times during the natural course of the disease.[13]

The significance of piecemeal necrosis in the pathogenesis and evolution of chronic active hepatitis has been questioned. Although its significance in the transition of acute into chronic hepatitis has been reaffirmed,[21,60,214] other studies have found that acute hepatitis with piecemeal necrosis usually fails to progress. Only three of 17 such cases progressed to chronic liver disease, and of these one showed chronic persistent hepatitis.[75] Even in established chronic active hepatitis it seems that piecemeal necrosis alone produces only mild or slowly progressive liver disease. This was inferred in the original definition of chronic active hepatitis, which divided the group into moderate and severe:[52] moderate cases showed only mild piecemeal necrosis and severe cases were depicted showing lobular activity. Studies from the Mayo Clinic on chronic active liver disease have emphasized the relatively slow progression and increased remission of disease in patients with biopsies showing only piecemeal necrosis.[13, 213] Unfortunately, they define chronic liver disease as present after 10 weeks of illness, so their series is not strictly comparable.

It is probable that identification of piecemeal necrosis in acute viral hepatitis will mean overdiagnosis of the incidence of chronicity and that when piecemeal necrosis alone is present in chronic disease the clinical course is more indolent. Within such a group of patients, the presence of HB_sAg appears to be an adverse prognostic feature for cirrhosis, although this may also reflect the better response of the non-B group to treatment.[51]

Parenchymal degeneration

All descriptions of chronic active hepatitis have included continuing acidophil and ballooning degeneration of hepatocytes among the features that may be present on biopsy.[13, 21, 52, 103, 120, 121, 165, 183, 184, 214] These are commonly present but not as prominent or as frequent as in acute hepatitis (Figure 29.10). Loss of hepatocytes from lysis with focal clustering of lymphocytes and sinusoidal cells is more variable, but in biopsies showing more 'activity' it can be pronounced.

This cell lysis may become confluent and features resembling bridging hepatic necrosis described in acute viral hepatitis are then found.[13, 21, 213, 217] A zone of collapsed reticulin extends from a portal tract or abnormal fibrous spur into the parenchyma towards an efferent vein. Initially, these reticulin fibres may be slightly apart but in the presence of piecemeal

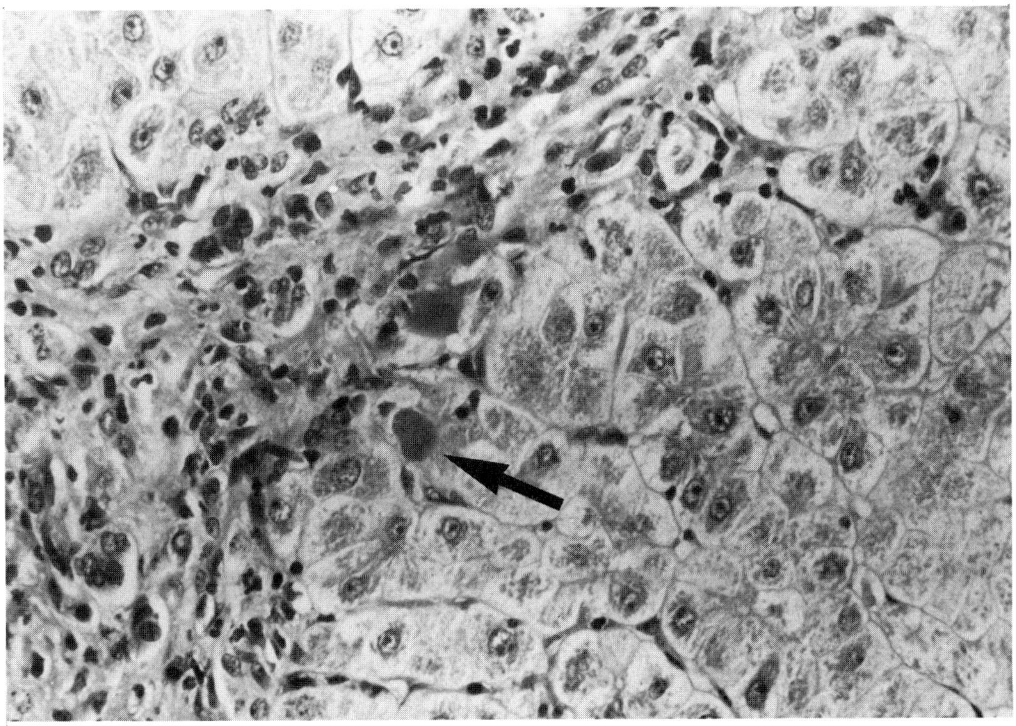

Figure 29.10. Chronic active hepatitis; hepatocytes are swollen with abundant granular cytoplasm, often with peripheral pallor. Acidophil degeneration (arrow) occurs but is relatively infrequent. Prominent twinning of cell plates indicates regenerative activity in the parenchyma. Haematoxylin & eosin × 1200.

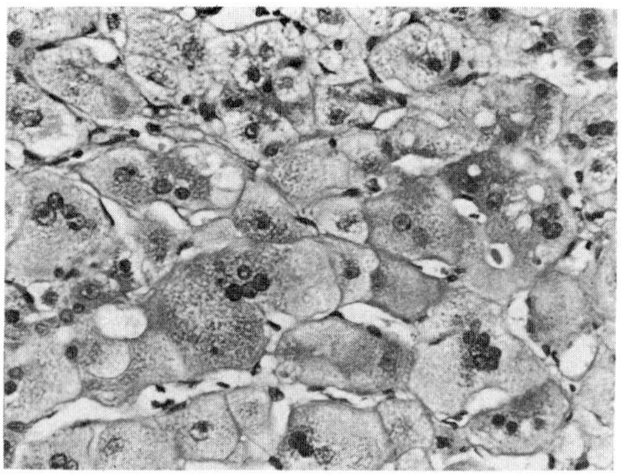

Figure 29.11. Chronic active hepatitis: several hepatocytes contain between four and seven nuclei. Haematoxylin & eosin × 250.

necrosis with its active fibrosis they are rapidly converted to collagen. It has been proposed that these bridges of necrosis permit more rapid spread of piecemeal necrosis throughout the liver so that the architectural distortion is thus rapidly consolidated.[21] The presence of such features in a group of chronic hepatitis patients was associated with a worse prognosis.[213]

Parenchymal regeneration

One of the prominent features in chronic active hepatitis is the regenerative activity identified by twinning of cell plates, formation of knots of hepatocytes and increased variation in hepatocyte nuclear size and staining. More florid regeneration includes the formation of multinucleate hepatocytes (Figure 29.11). These are usually only giant hepatocytes with three or four nuclei but occasionally syncytial hepatocytes with many nuclei may be found.[195] Regenerating hepatocytes may also form rosettes (Figure 29.12). These are usually adjacent to portal tracts and are small groups of four to eight hepatocytes around a central bile canaliculus which is visible as a lumen. A thin fibrous band surrounds this rosette and isolates it from adjacent parenchyma.

Regenerative activity may be irregular in distribution throughout the biopsy, so that active areas with twinning of plates form intraparenchymal nodules compressing adjacent parenchyma[182] and cirrhosis may be simulated.

Bile ducts

Bile-duct lesions have been described in chronic active hepatitis[40] and differ from those found in acute viral hepatitis[185] and the bile-duct damage of primary biliary cirrhosis.[39] The lesion in chronic active hepatitis is segmental, affects both large and small interlobular ducts and consists of focal hyperplasia of the bile-duct epithelium so that the lumen may be narrowed or occluded (Figure 29.13). These hyperplastic epithelial cells have an abundant clear empty cytoplasm and occasional mitoses may be identified.

Differential diagnosis

Excluding the specific demonstration of HBV markers, the morphological differences in chronic active hepatitis between the various aetiologies are minimal. The early descriptions noted an increased plasma cell infiltrate in biopsies associated with autoantibodies in the serum, but the HBV status of these is not known. One direct comparative study of serum HB_sAg positive and negative cases of chronic active hepatitis showed a significantly higher incidence of parenchymal and portal inflammation in non-B chronic hepatitis and a more prominent plasma cell component in the infiltrates in this group,[41] but Schalm and associates[212] failed to demonstrate any significant differences between HBV positive and negative groups.

Separation from primary biliary cirrhosis can be difficult. The destructive bile-duct lesions of primary biliary cirrhosis have been distinguished from those of chronic active hepatitis[39] but are not always present. Active acidophil and ballooning degenerative changes are seldom prominent in primary biliary cirrhosis and cell

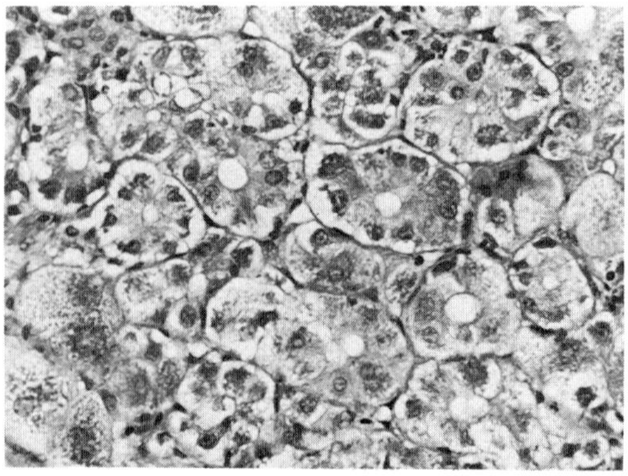

Figure 29.12. Rosettes: hepatocytes are arranged around a central dilated bile canaliculus and surrounded by a thin rim of fibrous tissue. Haematoxylin & eosin × 250.

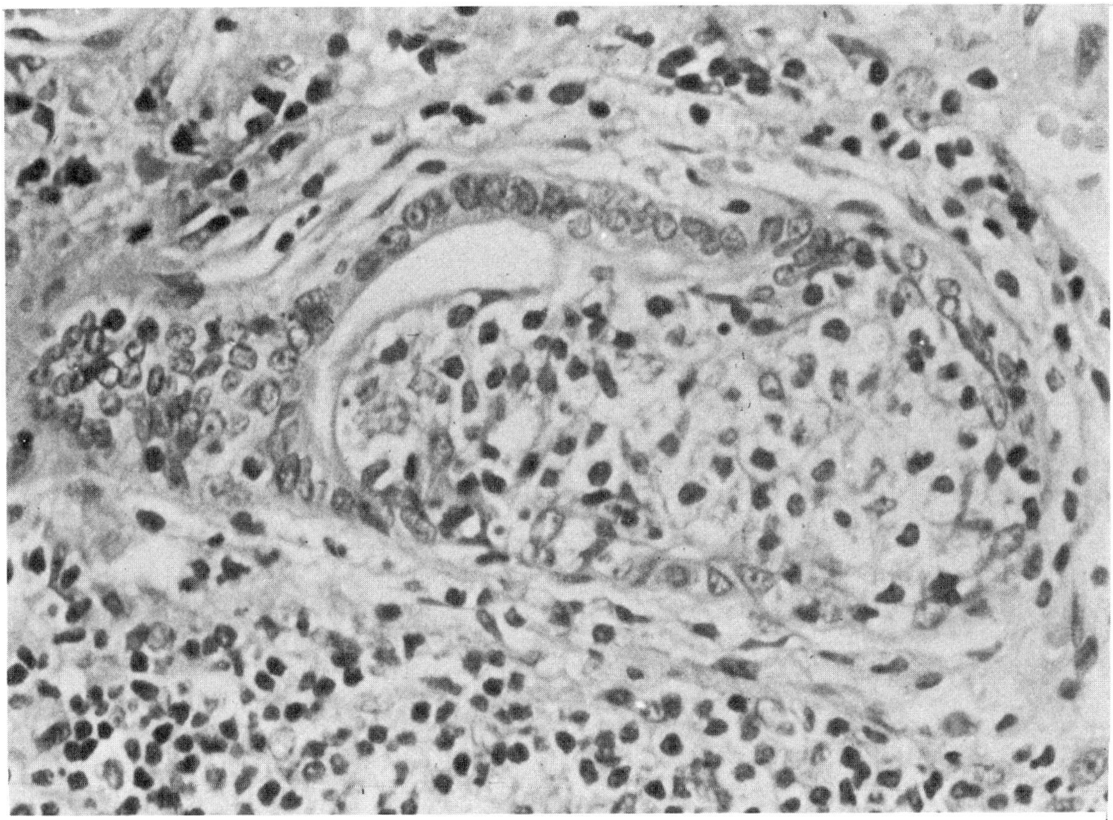

Figure 29.13. Hyperplastic bile-duct epithelium with almost complete obliteration of the lumen. Epithelial cells have abundant vacuolated cytoplasm. Haematoxylin & eosin. From Millward-Sadler,[165] with kind permission of Blackwell Scientific Publications.

plates rarely show the disorganization from cell loss and regeneration that is so prominent in many examples of chronic active hepatitis. Nonetheless, overlap, particularly with milder forms of chronic active hepatitis, occurs. Features favouring primary biliary cirrhosis, particularly in the absence of cirrhosis, include the presence of neutrophils around peripheral proliferating bile ductules in fibrous spurs and periportal or peripheral hepatocytes, showing either cholestasis, an excess of copper or copper-binding protein or Mallory's alcoholic hyalin.

Wilson's disease should be considered in the differential diagnosis, particularly in children and adolescents but also in young adults. Demonstration of excess copper, or its absence, helps considerably, but in rare instances may be misleading (see Chapter 33). Drug-induced liver disease cannot be identified by morphological criteria, but withdrawal of the drug should result in a decrease in activity and a degree of resolution of the chronic hepatitis varying inversely with the preceding architectural damage.

HB_sAg POSITIVE CARRIERS

Once it was recognized that the presence of the HB_sAg in serum is associated with hepatitis B infection, it became apparent that the hepatitis B virus could produce a wide spectrum of hepatic abnormalities, and that carriage of the HB_sAg is very common in some parts of the world. Data already accumulated by Blumberg and associates[23, 24, 25, 238] provided much of the basic information about the racial and geographical distribution, the male sex predominance, possible genetic factors in its inheritance, host factors in its acqusition and the wide range of hepatic abnormalities with which it can be associated.

Although Blumberg and associates used insensitive tests for HB_sAg, such as immunodiffusion, the fact that chronic carriers usually have high-titre HB_sAg enabled them to make these observations, which have subsequently been confirmed and extended by the use of more sensitive techniques as well as by the study of

HB_sAg sub-types, the HB_cAg and eAg systems, and the intrahepatic expression of these HBV markers.

Information about the carrier state has become available as a result of population and family studies and screening programmes, for example of blood donors and pregnant mothers and of patients suspected of having a high carrier rate. These include haemodialysis patients, haemophiliacs and drug addicts, patients with venereal disease, the mentally retarded and immunosuppressed patients.

Genetic Factors

Following the early studies of the Australia antigen in communities in South-east Asia with a high carrier rate, Blumberg et al[27] postulated that susceptibility to the carrier state was inherited as an autosomal recessive trait. There is no doubt that familial clustering can occur; the extent to which environmental and genetic factors contribute is uncertain but has been extensively reviewed.[160, 240, 286] Reports of an excess of blood group A in HB_sAg carriers have been conflicting,[239] and although there appears to be an association between HB_sAg positivity and HLA locus B specificities, further studies are required.[108]

Age and Sex

The age at which infection occurs appears to be important in the development of the carrier state. In tropical communities, where vertical transmission due to perinatal infection is common, the carrier state often develops at an early age. In western communities it is unusual to detect carriers in childhood and the carrier rate increases with age, although it is rare in the elderly, presumably because of spontaneous clearing of HB_sAg.[239, 240]

The proportion of male carriers is substantially greater than female, but it is uncertain whether this is due to a greater liability of males to become infected with HBV because of their life-style, or whether it is a sex-linked genetic phenomenon. This predominance has been explained by postulating cross-reactivity between the HB_sAg and a male determined tissue antigen[288,289] so that the male is tolerant of HBV antigens and therefore has an impaired tissue defence against them.

The Nature of the Carrier State

In addition to the effects of age and sex and possibly an inherited trait, the carrier state is more likely to develop in individuals who are at greatest risk of exposure and those who have defective host responses, probably immunologically mediated, which facilitate persistence of the antigen. The individuals or groups of patients who are at increased risk of exposure to hepatitis B have been outlined in Chapter 28, and include multiply transfused patients, haemophiliacs, haemodialysis patients, drug addicts and those in institutions for the mentally retarded. Patients who have a disease associated with immunodeficiency are liable to become carriers, and an increased carrier rate has been reported in patients with lepromatous leprosy,[26] Down's syndrome,[238] those receiving immunosuppressive therapy[268] and patients with immunodeficiency disorders. The medical and paramedical staff and household contacts involved with such patients will also be at increased risk.

A crucial factor in the spread of infection is the e antigen status of the carrier. There is increasing evidence that carriers who are e antigen positive are more likely to spread the infection than those who have anti-e (see Chapter 28). There are certain groups of patients who are asymptomatic carriers but have a high incidence of e antigen positivity (Table 29.2). When such patients are fully investigated, it is likely that most will have evidence of a chronic active hepatitis on biopsy, as the e antigen is rarely detected in patients with normal histology or only minor abnormalities (see below). The factors responsible for the persistence of e antigen and histological evidence of liver disease are complex and may not be related to the immune response to the HB_sAg. As discussed in Chapter 28, Robinson[200] has proposed that expression of the various HBV markers may occur independently in different hepatocytes and also in different individuals.

Table 29.2. *HB_eAg in HB_sAg Carriers.*

Patients	Total HB_sAg positive	HB_eAg positive
Renal dialysis	17	15
Mongols	26	13
Blood donors	86	1

Clinical Features

When a 'carrier' of the HB_sAg is detected incidentally, there may be a wide variation in clinical and histological appearances. Most will be asymptomatic, but signs of liver disease may or may not be present, and range from complete normality to cirrhosis. The proportion of HB_sAg carriers detected in routine surveys who have histological evidence of liver disease varies considerably in different geographical locations and racial groups, and some or all of the features discussed above may be responsible for this variation.

It can be argued that a carrier of HB_sAg should be defined as someone who is asymptomatic and who has no histological evidence of liver disease. In such individuals, histological evidence of hepatitis may not be present, and indeed it is conceivable that excess viral protein coat is being produced without infectivity.

Pathology

The pathological changes described in the literature vary with the definition of a carrier. In most studies, the carrier is an asymptomatic individual identified in the course of a screening programme usually, but not invariably, for blood donations.[9, 28, 77, 136, 192, 194, 202, 207, 225, 227, 228, 261, 262, 274] Further definition then varies. Some studies exclude individuals with abnormal liver function tests[225] and this affects the spectrum of histological changes that are found (Table 29.3). Asymptomatic individuals who have cirrhosis or chronic active hepatitis on biopsy have almost invariably had abnormal liver function tests. Unfortunately, these biochemical abnormalities are not constantly present, nor does the presence of biochemical abnormalities necessarily indicate significant liver disease. Chronic active hepatitis or cirrhosis are rarely found in individuals with normal liver function tests.

The histopathological changes found commonly in both groups are normal liver, 'ground-glass' hepatocytes, focal necroses and chronic persistent hepatitis. Ground-glass hepatocytes are cells with an increased volume of cytoplasm in which there is a finely granular or stippled, pale-staining eosinophilic zone[105] (Figure 29.14). This zone may form the bulk of the cytoplasm, and then there is usually a halo separating it from the plasma membrane, or it may form a discrete inclusion, sometimes crescentic and occasionally perinuclear in location. These cells may be widely dispersed throughout the biopsy or may form confluent clusters in any part of the lobule. They are most frequent and readily recognized in asymptomatic carriers, but have also been found in chronic active hepatitis and cirrhosis due to HBV. Similar cells had been described in asymptomatic blood donors earlier[136] but Hadziyannis et al[105] were the first to demonstrate that they contained HB_sAg within the cytoplasm. These cells are also orcein positive (Figure 29.15), which separates them from the identical appearances that can be produced by drug-induced hyperplasia of the smooth endoplasmic reticulum.[248, 273] Some biopsies

Table 29.3. *Histology in Asymptomatic HB_sAg Carriers.*

Normal liver function tests				Abnormal liver function tests				
Normal	CPH	CAH & cirrhosis	Other	Normal	CPH	CAH & cirrhosis	Other	Reference
8	15	0	3	0	0	0	0	Shrago, Auslander & Gitnick[225]
12	10	1	1	0	0	0	0	Reinicke et al[192]
14	4	0	3	0	0	0	0	Klinge, Kaboth & Arnold[136]
6	12	0	1	4	9	3	3	Velasco et al[261]
0	0	0	0	0	0	4	0	Sampliner[207]
3	10	0	3	0	14	4	0	Woolf et al[274]
7	11	0	0	0	9	1	1	Feinman et al[77]
3	4	3	0	0	5	2	1	Bolin, Davis & Liddelow[28]
46		0	0	15	4	6	1	Hess et al[107]
1	1	1	1	0	2	2	1	Singleton et al[228]
13	18	0	0	0	11	2	0	Anderson et al[9]
3	3	0	0	1	3	0	1	Russell et al[202]
0	0	0	0	2	28	0	0	Vittal, Dourdourekas & Shobassay[262]
0	2	0	0	0	4	2	1	Simon & Patel[227]

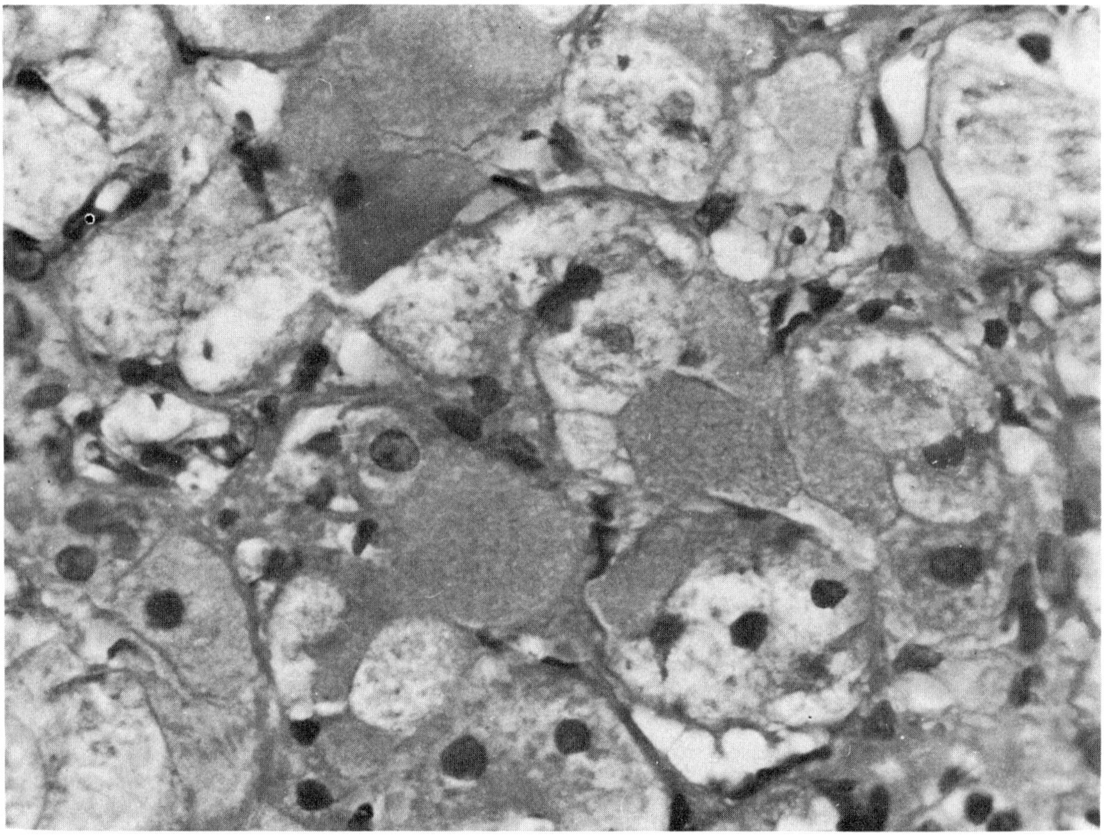

Figure 29.14. Ground-glass hepatocytes: the cell is larger than average because of an increased amount of uniform finely stippled, palely eosinophilic cytoplasm. Haematoxylin & eosin. × 1500.

show only occasional focal necroses without significant portal tract inflammation or generalized parenchymal degeneration. These focal necroses consist of a small cluster of mononuclear cells around a degenerate hepatocyte. Rarely, occasional acidophil bodies may be seen.

In the chronic carrier state, HBV or its markers can be consistently demonstrated histologically by histochemical or immunological techniques, and these show infection not only within 'ground-glass' but also other hepatocytes. Only rarely does failure to demonstrate virus markers result from sampling error in the biopsy.

More recently, chronic hepatitis B infection has been demonstrated in the liver in the absence of HB_sAg and the presence of anti-HB_s in the serum.[232] Of the 13 haemophilic patients described, all had abnormal liver function tests and, on biopsy, eight had chronic persistent hepatitis and four had chronic active hepatitis.

EXTRAHEPATIC MANIFESTATIONS OF HBV INFECTION

Although arthralgia, arthritis and urticaria are well-recognized clinical features of viral hepatitis during the early acute phase, studies of the HB_sAg have re-emphasized their importance and highlighted a variety of other extrahepatic manifestations, chiefly seen in association with chronic liver disease. These include a more chronic polyarthralgia or arthritis, vasculitis, cryoglobulinaemia, glomerulonephritis[151] and acrodermatitis.[94,151]

Arthritis and Arthralgia

Alpert, Isselbacher and Schur[7] measured complement components in 18 patients with acute viral hepatitis B who had initial symptoms of arthralgia, arthritis or urticaria. They found severe depression of total serum haemolytic

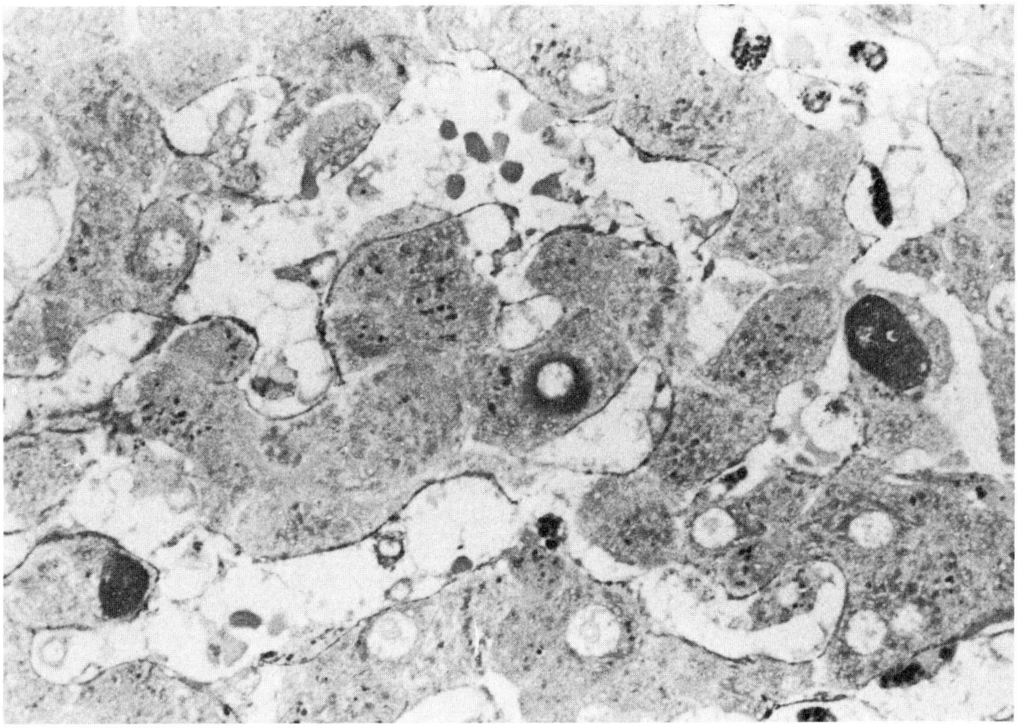

Figure 29.15. Randomly scattered orcein-positive hepatocytes (centre, centre right and lower left). The central hepatocyte shows a perinuclear collar of positive staining, and those to right and left have a microhoneycomb pattern. Orcein × 1500.

complement and C4 in nine patients studied during the acute phase at a time when HB_sAg titres were high, and postulated that immune complexes of HB_sAg and complement played a role in the pathogenesis of the arthritis. In addition, low complement levels have been reported in the synovial fluid of three patients with hepatitis B and arthritis.[175] Subsequently, it was shown that the circulating immune complexes consisted of complement components, immunoglobulins, HB_sAg and anti-HB_s, which activated both the classic and alternate complement pathways in vivo.[269] Similar observations were made in patients with arthritis associated with chronic active hepatitis.[267]

Vasculitis and Cryoglobulinaemia

In 1970, Gocke et al[95] and Trepo and Thivolet[254] described an association between polyarteritis nodosa and circulating HB_sAg, and many additional cases have been reported subsequently.[67, 94, 218] The liver disease is usually chronic but relatively insignificant, the presentation being with fever, polyarthralgia and rashes; peripheral neuropathy, hypertension and azotaemia often develop as the illness progresses. Total haemolytic complement levels in the serum are decreased, there are circulating immune complexes of HB_sAg and anti-HB_s, and complement, immunoglobulin and HB_sAg can be demonstrated in the vessels early in the illness.

Some patients show features resembling a hypersensitivity angiitis rather than polyarteritis nodosa,[218] and in others there is ischaemia on the basis of deposition of cryoproteins.[161] In one such patient with chronic active hepatitis, cryoprotein composed of immunoglobulin and HB_sAg was demonstrated in the small blood vessels in the absence of vasculitis, and it was postulated that it was the cause of the associated peripheral neuropathy.[74] In a study of 30 patients with essential mixed cryoglobulinaemia, a high proportion was found to have anti-HB_s or HB_sAg in the cryoprecipitate, and in four, characteristic HBV particles were observed by electron microscopy.[148] These patients often had purpura, joint symptoms and renal disease, and 26 had hepatomegaly or abnormal liver function tests.

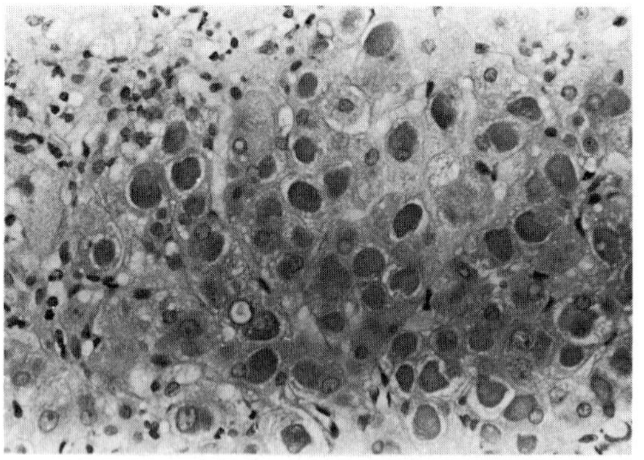

Figure 29.16. Clusters of orcein-positive hepatocytes. Many of these have a thin rim of unstained cytoplasm underneath the plasma membranes. Orcein × 250.

Glomerulonephritis

The association between glomerulonephritis and hepatitis B was described by Combes et al,[43] who demonstrated HB_sAg, IgG and complement in the glomerular basement membrane by immunofluorescence. The deposits are nodular, showing a membrano-proliferative or membranous pattern associated with immune complex deposition.[94] This may be a common cause of glomerulonephritis in certain parts of the world, particularly in children.[33]

HB_sAg or anti-HB_s can be demonstrated directly in blood vessels or the renal glomeruli in these syndromes of vasculitis or cryoprotein precipitation, strongly suggesting immune complex deposition, but the evidence that it produces the lesion is still not conclusive. However, the recognition of these extrahepatic manifestations of HBV infection and the demonstration of immune complexes have important implications in relation to arteritis, glomerulonephritis and arthritis of unknown aetiology.

MORPHOLOGICAL DEMONSTRATION OF HBV MARKERS IN THE LIVER

Most morphological studies of HBV markers have been performed on chronic, as opposed to acute, hepatitis B infections of the liver. These have included histochemical staining, immunological demonstration using either immunofluorescence or immunoperoxidase and direct visualization by electron microscopy. Each of the three known major antigenic components of the virus, HB_sAg, HB_cAg and HB_eAg, will be considered in turn.

HB_sAg

The hepatocytes only contain HB_sAg in the cytoplasm and, as discussed in the preceding section, may have a 'ground-glass' appearance when this antigen is present in excess (Figure 29.14).[105] The number of 'ground-glass' hepatocytes is infrequent when compared with the number of hepatocytes containing HB_sAg demonstrated by these more specific techniques.

Orcein and aldehyde fuchsin stains have been discussed briefly in Chapter 18 and in the section on chronic persistent hepatitis in this chapter. These stains demonstrate HB_sAg in hepatocyte cytoplasm,[54, 165, 223] but also stain elastic fibres and lipofuscin granules. In addition, orcein will demonstrate copper-binding protein as blue-black granules.[205] It has been suggested that these stains demonstrate sulphonic acid groupings formed by oxidation of disulphide bonds.[223] HB_sAg is particularly rich in these bonds.[264] Positive cells are brown or red-brown and often the staining is circumscribed so that a rim of unstained

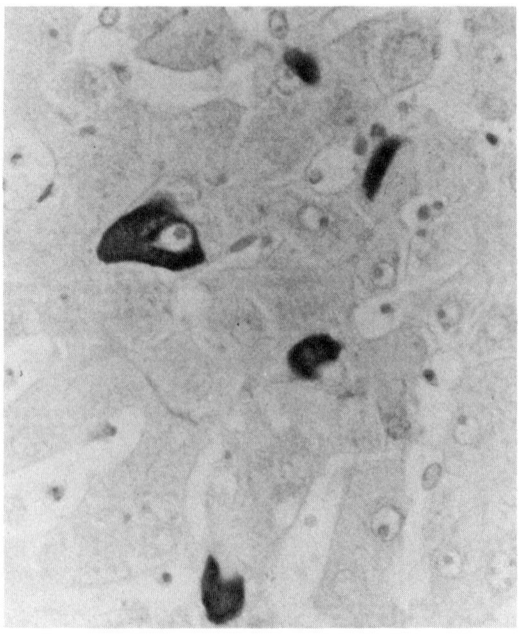

Figure 29.17. Immunoperoxidase (PAP) visualization of HB_sAg in hepatocyte cytoplasm. Note the negative staining of nucleus and nucleolus and also that the positive reaction may be a discrete and localized area within the cell cytoplasm. Rabbit anti-HB_sAg 1/80, Swine antirabbit IgG 1/20, PAP 1/200. Magnification × 1000.

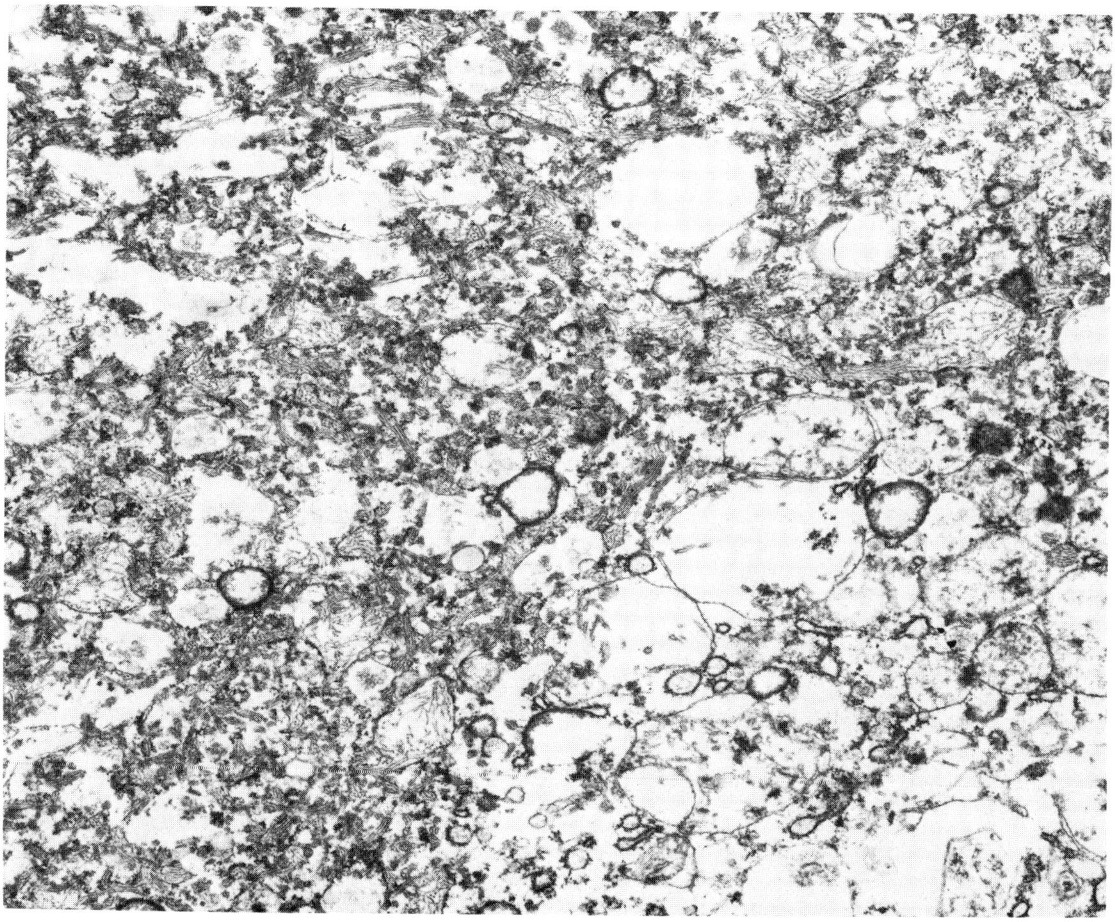

Figure 29.18. Profiles of endoplasmic reticulum containing long filaments sometimes in parallel bundles and 'owl-eye' bodies. Post-mortem liver: uranyl acetate and lead citrate. × 5600.

cytoplasm is present under the plasma membrane. Alternatively, the whole cytoplasm may be stained, or there may be a small positive crescent around the nucleus (Figure 29.15). The staining has an even, non-granular appearance and in some cells is punctuated by many tiny holes, producing a microhoneycomb pattern.

More commonly, orcein positive hepatocytes are scattered throughout the biopsy as isolated positive cells (Figure 29.15) and are randomly distributed in the lobule or nodule, but they may be also found in clusters (Figure 29.16). Karasawa and Shikata[128] have described degenerative changes with an inflammatory reaction occurring in orcein positive hepatocytes in one case but in our experience there is no correlation between orcein positive hepatocytes and either the parenchymal degenerative changes or the distribution of the inflammation.

Although Shikata et al[223] claimed that HB_sAg was demonstrated in both acute and chronic hepatitis B, it is now generally accepted that the antigen is not demonstrable by this technique in acute hepatitis.[54] The positive staining can still be demonstrated if acute hepatocellular damage is superimposed. One of our HBV carriers took an overdose of paracetamol and developed acute hepatic necrosis, confirmed on biopsy. Orcein positive hepatocytes were still demonstrable.

Immunological techniques have been used to demonstrate the HB_sAg. Immunofluorescence has been most frequently employed and demonstrates the antigen in the cytoplasm in both acute and chronic hepatitis.[4, 71, 102, 105, 176, 189, 201, 223] A membrane-staining pattern has been described in acute hepatitis B,[4, 189, 201] but is disputed in chronic hepatitis.[4, 189] Immunoperoxidase techniques also identify the surface antigen in hepatocyte cytoplasm on paraffin sections[1, 35, 165, 244] (Figure 29.17). Membrane localization is rarely noted, but otherwise it compares favourably with fluores-

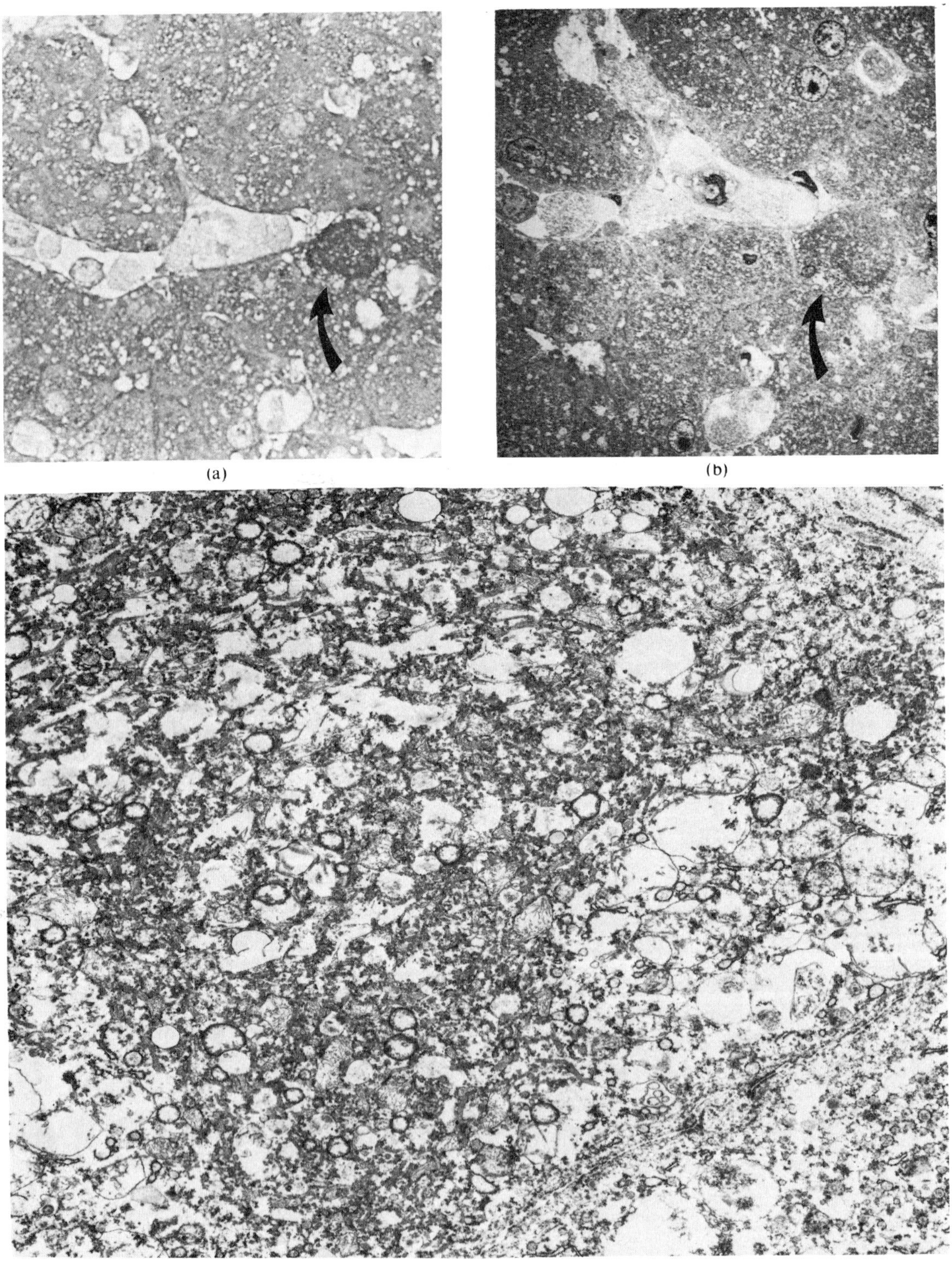

Figure 29.19. Sequence to show (a) orcein staining of 'thick' section, (b) corresponding cell (arrow) on electron microscopy and (c) the filaments in profiles of endoplasmic reticulum within this cell. (a) Orcein staining; (b and c) Uranyl acetate and lead citrate.

cence. A direct comparison suggests that the immunoperoxidase technique is more sensitive than orcein; some orcein negative hepatocytes can be positively stained by the immunoperoxidase method.[165]

Electron microscopy of HB_sAg positive carriers shows parallel arrays of tubular forms, spherical particles and 'owl-eye bodies'[89, 119, 233] within the profiles of the smooth endoplasmic reticulum (Figure 29.18). These 'owl-eye bodies' probably represent the rods cut in cross-section within the cysternae of the SER. The diameters of the tubules and spherical particles correspond to measurements of HB_sAg from the serum. These cytoplasmic inclusions are most readily found in asymptomatic carriers and have not always been found in cases of chronic active hepatitis.[6, 176] This is probably a result of the more scattered distribution of HB_sAg positive hepatocytes in chronic active hepatitis compared with carriers. Confirmation that these cytoplasmic structures are HB_sAg has been provided by immune electron microscopy, and positive staining of associated membranes of the endoplasmic reticulum and cell sinusoidal surface has also been found.[283] Orcein staining of electron microscopic thick sections allows the positive hepatocyte to be identified in the corresponding thin section. Such cells contain these filamentous and spherical forms within profiles of the endoplasmic reticulum (Figure 29.19). Adjacent orcein negative hepatocytes do not contain these structures, although core particles may be visible in the nucleus.

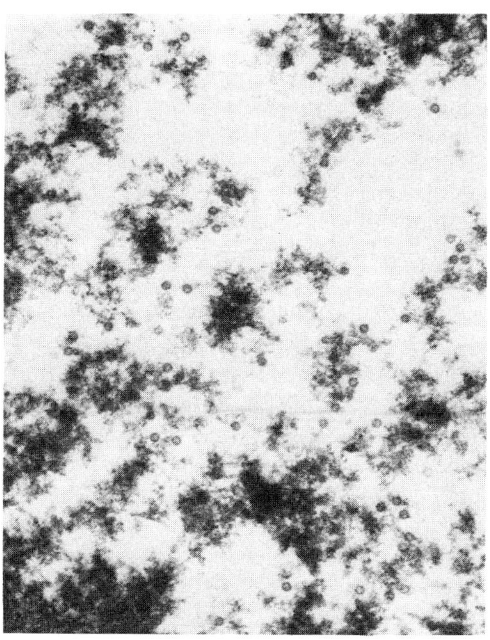

Figure 29.20. Core particles within the nuclear sap.

HB_cAg

The core antigen and particles have been demonstrated by immunofluorescent[11, 102, 107, 118, 189, 197, 198] and immunoperoxidase techniques,[244, 283] and by electron microscopy.[2, 6, 89, 117, 119, 165, 170, 174, 244] Demonstration of HB_cAg usually correlates accurately with the presence of virus-like particles within the nucleus (Figure 29.20). Nuclei with large numbers of core particles can be identified on light microscopy as they have a lightly staining 'sanded' appearance.[18] These core particles are most readily found in patients receiving immunosuppressive therapy (Figure 29.21), and least frequently in acute hepatitis and in the carrier state, but they have been described in all forms of hepatitis B infection.[165] Occasional particles are found in the cytoplasm. They are 21 to 25 nm in size with a slightly angular periphery, suggesting a hexagonal profile, and may appear hollow or have an electron-dense core. The outer margin appears to be formed from subunits approximately 250 nm (25Å) in diameter.[117] They correspond morphologically to the inner component of the Dane particle, and after isolation of these particles from liver nuclei they can be complexed with anti-HB_c.[118] Immune electron microscopy on sections has also shown that these nuclear particles contain core antigen.[88, 283]

Other Antigens

HB_eAg. There is no described morphological counterpart to the HB_eAg. Attempts to localize it within the liver are conflicting: both positive cytoplasmic[171, 255] and nuclear immunofluorescent staining patterns[11] have been described.

HB_δ. A new antigen located to the nucleus but mutually exclusive with HB_c and distinct from the eAg system has been detected by immunofluorescence.[199] Its significance remains to be established.

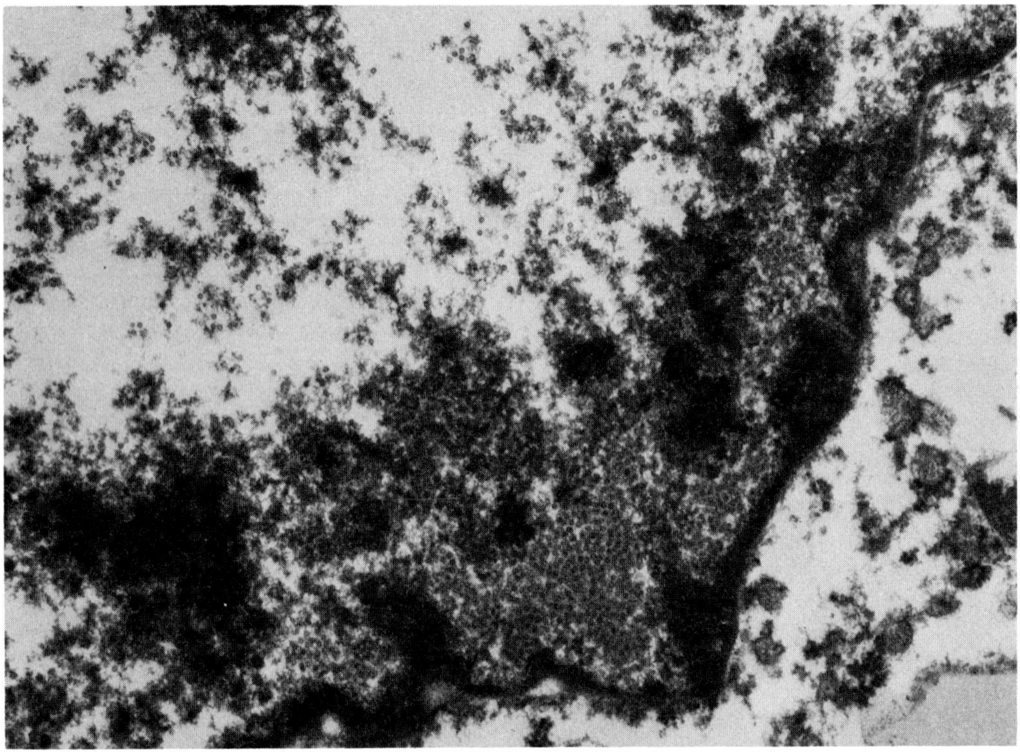

Figure 29.21. Nucleus showing numerous core particles tightly packed along the nuclear membrane. Patient had been treated with corticosteroids for HB_sAg positive chronic active hepatitis. Uranyl acetate & lead citrate × 15 000.

Correlation with Liver Disease
(see Table 29.4)

The demonstration of HB_sAg has been noted to vary with the type of liver disease, but considerable overlap occurs. A peripheral membrane staining described in acute hepatitis is probably transient,[4,114] but has also been related to chronicity.[189,201] This possibly reflects persistence of what is usually a transient phenomenon and is not necessarily a prognostic feature. Diffuse cytoplasmic staining of a hepatocyte is the most common pattern demonstrated in chronic hepatitis, and this may be found in widely scattered hepatocytes or in clusters. The clustering of positive hepatocytes occurs in the carrier state, and relatively quiescent cirrhosis, whereas a scattered distribution is more usual with chronic active hepatitis and chronic persistent hepatitis. The inverse relationship between the number of positive hepatocytes and active liver damage has been repeatedly observed.[102, 105, 189, 244]

Core antigen and particles are relatively scarce in the carrier state,[89, 102, 107, 197, 244] and in acute hepatitis,[102, 197] and an abundance in immunosuppressed individuals has already been noted, but these are not sufficiently dependable to be of diagnostic or prognostic value. There appears to be little difference between chronic persistent and chronic active hepatitis in the frequency or distribution of core antigen alone.

Immunoglobulin, in particular IgG, and complement (or complement binding activity) can be demonstrated in those hepatocyte nuclei containing HB_c in chronic but not acute hepatitis.[87,197,198,201] Most attempts to demonstrate immunoglobulins on the surface membranes or in the cell cytoplasm of HB_sAg positive hepatocytes have failed, but recently success has been claimed using isolated hepatocyte preparations from patients with either acute or chronic hepatitis B infection.[4,116]

The relative distribution of HBV antigens to each other in the types of liver disease has also been studied.[102, 189, 197] Four main groups were identified:

1. Acute self-limited viral hepatitis has minimal expression of HB_c only.
2. Mild chronic, persistent hepatitis and immunosuppression with a gross excess of HB_c and moderate HB_sAg.

Table 29.4. *Demonstration of HB_c and HB_s in Liver Disease.*[a]

	Total	HB_c only	HB_s only	Both HB_c & HB_s
Carrier	16	0	15	1
Acute viral hepatitis	25	8	10	7
Chronic persistent hepatitis	27	5	14	8
Chronic active hepatitis	76	14	6	56
Totals	144	27	45	72

[a] Based on references:
Gudat et al[102]
Rizzetto et al[197]
Rizzetto et al[198]
Arnold et al[11]
Ray et al[189]

3. Chronic persistent hepatitis and carriers have marked excess of HB_sAg and minimal HB_c.
4. Chronic active hepatitis and acute–possibly chronic hepatitis in which both HB_c and HB_sAg can be equally, though randomly, demonstrated.

These studies show that distribution of HBV markers in liver is of limited value (Table 29.5). This may change if the morphological demonstration of HB_e can be definitively established and correlated with other HBV markers in the different categories of liver disease. Correlation of HB_e in the serum with antigens in the liver has demonstrated a close association with nuclear HB_c but no indication of type of liver disease was given.[107]

Obviously, further studies are needed, particularly to localize the e antigen and correlations performed. Two possible areas of value would be the identification of (a) transition to chronicity in an acute infection and (b) chronic active hepatitis masquerading as chronic persistent hepatitis.

IMMUNOPATHOLOGICAL MECHANISMS IN HEPATITIS B INFECTION

As indicated in Chapter 28, there is increasing evidence that HBV is a unique virus in several respects.[200] Much information is available about immunological responses to hepatitis B, but the pathogenesis of the hepatic damage and the explanation for its striking variation in severity remain uncertain. There are two main possibilities. One is that the hepatitis B virus exerts its effect by a direct pathogenic action on hepatocytes, producing cell lysis. The second possibility is that the virus itself is not pathogenic and that the hepatic damage results from a variable immune response of the host to one or more antigenic components of HBV. This abnormal immune response could be mediated in several different ways (Figure 29.22).

Almeida and Waterson[5] suggested that the hepatic damage might be mediated by immune complex injury, a suggestion based on their observations of varying sizes of immune complexes in a small number of patients with HB_sAg positive liver disease. There is no doubt that circulating immune complexes of HB_sAg can be observed in the serum, particularly in acute viral hepatitis, but there is little direct evidence of immune complex damage in the liver as measured by immunofluorescent techniques,[71] as is observed in extrahepatic sites (see above). On the other hand, an enhanced anti-HB_s response has been observed in patients with fulminant hepatitis B,[275] and it has been suggested that this results in an intense ischaemic necrosis of hepatocytes due to an Arthus reaction.

There is more convincing evidence that cell-mediated immune reactions to the HB_sAg may be important in determining the outcome of infection and possibly the pathogenesis of the hepatic injury. It has been suggested that defective T cell function with impaired cell-mediated immunity to HB_sAg may determine whether the infection is self-limited or persists with varying degrees of liver damage.[63] This possibility has been studied extensively in both acute and chronic liver disease, but the results have been conflicting, partly because of the inadequacy of in vitro techniques for assessing T cell function and cell-mediated immunity, and because impure antigens have been used.

A cell-mediated immune reaction to HB_sAg has been reported early in the acute phase of viral hepatitis as measured by lymphocyte transformation[50, 284] and leucocyte migration inhibition.[64, 90, 146] By contrast, chronic carriers of HB_sAg fail to show evidence of cell-mediated immunity. These results suggest that a specific cell-mediated immune reaction to HB_sAg is necessary to eliminate the infection and prevent the carrier state. They do not, however, provide convincing evidence of an abnormal, cell-mediated immune reaction to HB_sAg in the pathogenesis of the hepatocellular necrosis.

The whole question of lymphocyte function and cell-mediated immunity to components of HBV in chronic hepatitis is controversial. The techniques and their interpretation are open to question because of the effect of serum factors on the techniques alleged to demonstrate cell-mediated immunity.[270] Furthermore, it should be noted that there is no information available in man about cell-mediated immune reactions to the core of the Dane particle, which is likely to be the infective agent, although independent cell-mediated immune responses to HB_sAg and HB_cAg have been demonstrated in guinea pigs and rabbits.[91]

As indicated earlier, HB_sAg can be present in liver cells in vast excess without producing hepatocellular necrosis, suggesting that an immune response to the virus causes the tissue damage. In addition, HB_sAg but no HB_cAg can be demonstrated at the hepatocyte surface,[4, 14] but it is not known whether it is present as free particles or as unassembled polypeptides incorporated into the liver-cell membrane. In addition, liver-specific lipoprotein antigens have been localized to the surface membrane of isolated hepatocytes,[115] but there is no evidence to indicate a close association between viral and tissue antigens. Nevertheless, an immune reaction involving both viral and host antigens may mediate the hepatocellular injury.[70,287] It is possible that the virus enters into more than one type of interaction with host cells. The clinical course might then depend on whether there is simple lysis of the hepatocyte or whether there is partial integration of the viral genome into the host cell.[6]

Eddleston and Williams[68] have proposed a unified hypothesis implicating defects in both B and T cell function in the pathogenesis of the liver injury in viral hepatitis. They suggest that tissue injury results from an immune response to both viral and liver-specific antigens. This hypothesis has also been used to advocate the role of HBV in the initiation of chronic active hepatitis of unknown aetiology, but, as will be discussed later, this runs contrary to much other clinical and epidemiological evidence.

Chisari and associates[287] have recently reviewed the possible mechanisms involved. They and others have detected immunoregulatory molecules in the plasma of patients with liver disease and have stressed the interplay between such molecules and suppressor cell activity in the pathogenesis of the liver injury.

An area which has received little attention is the possible role of liver macrophages in terminating infection in acute viral hepatitis. Kupffer cell function appears to be important in acute viral hepatitis in animals, and persistent viral replication may occur in Kupffer cells with spill-over and infection of the hepatocytes or, after transient infection of the Kupffer cells, replication may occur in the hepatocyte itself.[203, 204] It is possible that there may be impaired Kupffer cell function in man, either as a result of an intrinsic abnormality or because of blockade by competitive phagocytosis of auto-antigens or exogenous antigens such as entero-bacteria. Such impairment might result in acute or chronic liver injury, but this hypothesis cannot be tested in man until adequate in vitro tests of macrophage function have been developed.

Another possibility is that there might be a defect in interferon production which results in inability to prevent replication of the virus.

CHRONIC ACTIVE HEPATITIS OF UNKNOWN AETIOLOGY

Clinical and Biochemical Features

Chronic active hepatitis of unknown aetiology occurs predominantly in women, often with florid signs of hepatocellular failure, associated putative autoimmune diseases, hyperglobulinaemia and marked derangement of liver function. It was described initially mainly from Scandinavia, Australia, the United Kingdom and North America. As will be indicated later, this is not surprising, since in these parts of the world chronic active hepatitis due to HBV is relatively uncommon.

Waldenstrom[265] drew attention to chronic liver disease in young women with jaundice, acne, amenorrhoea, hepatosplenomegaly and hyperglobulinaemia. Within the next few years,

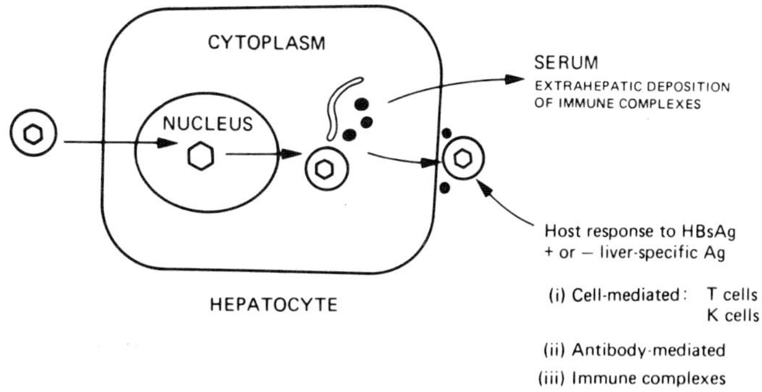

Figure 29.22. Diagram to illustrate immunopathological mechanisms in hepatitis infection. After Wright.[280]

there were several similar reports of chronic active liver disease in young women,[16, 141] and women at the menopause,[36] with features suggesting an immune disturbance. These included a positive LE cell phenomenon,[126] which led to the term 'lupoid hepatitis',[154] and a prominent plasma cell infiltrate in the liver, hence the term 'plasma cell hepatitis'.[99] It is likely that such patients were previously described under the term 'sub-acute or chronic hepatitis of insidious onset' used by Kelsall, Stewart and Witts,[131] and 'sub-chronic atrophy of the liver' by Bjørneboe and Raaschou.[22]

Although the majority of patients in these reports show similarities suggesting a common aetiology, many series included patients in whom a specific aetiology would now be recognized, such as HB_sAg positive chronic active hepatitis,[281] drug-induced chronic active hepatitis,[157] alpha-1-antitrypsin deficiency,[259] Wilson's disease[235] and alcoholic liver disease.[96] Nonetheless, in several large early series such recognized causes are probably in a minority,[166,190,220] and the clinical features which are described match closely with the HB_sAg negative group in whom known viruses and toxins have been excluded.

In the series reported by Read, Sherlock and Harrison[190] and referred to as juvenile cirrhosis, 81 patients were described, of whom 49 were female and 49 were under 21 years of age. In 23 of the 81 patients, the onset was acute, resembling viral hepatitis, but in the remainder it was insidious, with the slow development of jaundice, signs of liver failure, hepatic pain or dyspepsia. In 13 patients, extrahepatic manifestations such as thyroid disease, arthralgia, ulcerative colitis or renal disease were the presenting feature.

On physical examination, the patients often looked well but could have mild jaundice, prominent spider naevi and palmar erythema. Cutaneous striae and gynaecomastia occurred in young males. The spleen was palpable in the majority of patients and the liver usually enlarged, but occasionally it was reduced in size. Amenorrhoea was a common feature in young women, as were acne and skin rashes, including those resembling lupus erythematosus, purpura and splinter haemorrhages. Additional features were arthralgia, pulmonary infiltration and associated diseases such as thyroiditis, ulcerative colitis and diabetes. Renal abnormalities included albuminuria, the nephrotic syndrome and renal tubular acidosis.

The series reported by Mistilis, Skyring and Blackburn[166] was strikingly similar, including the age and sex incidence, mode of presentation, a progressive downhill course, the presence of multisystem involvement and an association with putative autoimmune disease.

Even in those patients who presented insidiously, jaundice and episodes of deteriorating liver function soon developed during the course of the disease. This was often associated with anorexia, marked fatigue, abdominal pain, the development of new spider naevi, fever, haemorrhagic phenomena and ascites. Death usually occurred from liver failure with or without bleeding varices, but in a few patients the course was so unpredictable that remissions occurred even after hepatic failure. In the Australian series, half the deaths occurred in the first few years when the disease was most active, and only six patients survived 10 years.

Biochemically, the height of the bilirubin was variable, but often ran at 50 to 170 μmol/l (3 to 10 mg/dl) for long periods. Serum transaminase levels were moderately elevated to a peak of 500 to 800 iu, but hyperglobulinaemia was almost invariably pronounced, with low serum albumin levels and prolongation of the prothrombin time as the disease progressed.

Haematological changes included an anaemia which was often normochromic, and leucopenia was occasionally observed. A positive LE cell phenomenon was found in 10 of the 81 British patients and nine of 60 cases examined in the

Table 29.5. *Comparison of Two Large Series of Chronic Active Hepatitis.*

	Read, Sherlock & Harrison, 1963	Mistilis, Skyring & Blackburn, 1968
Total number of patients	81	82
Males	32	17
Females	49	65
Age	40 < 20 yrs	32 < 20 yrs
Onset		
acute jaundice	28%	32%
insidious jaundice	37%	48%
anicteric	22%	20%
Splenomegaly	77%	49% (at onset)
Hepatomegaly	72%	75% (at onset)
Spider naevi	nearly 100%	45% (at onset)
Amenorrhoea	all young women	38% (premenopausal)
Ulcerative colitis	6%	11%
Arthralgia	11%	18%
Varices	21%	42%
Ascites	15%	41%
Bilirubin 50–170 μmol/l (3–10 mg)	Most patients	Most patients
Globulin	>5 g 53%	>3.5 g
Albumin	<3 g 33%	mean 3.1 g
LE cells	16%	15%

Australian series. The clinical and biochemical features in these two series are summarized in Table 29.5.

In both of these large series, a limited number of patients were treated with corticosteroids or azathioprine and subsequent series have often established strict criteria for the admission of patients to controlled clinical trials of various therapeutic agents, and so are not strictly comparable. Nevertheless, these clinical and biochemical features have been similar in subsequent series of HB_sAg negative chronic active hepatitis.[135, 212]

Associated conditions

Apart from the high frequency of multisystem disease in idiopathic chronic active hepatitis in the series cited above, there have been systematic studies of their prevalence,[97] and a number of reports of individual cases or of small series. Golding and associates[97] found a high frequency of Sjögren's syndrome, renal tubular acidosis and pulmonary diffusion defects, as well as a small number of patients with peripheral neuropathy, ulcerative colitis, thyroid disorders and arthropathy. Fibrosing alveolitis,[260] ulcerative colitis,[113, 153] arthropathy and arthralgia,[15, 271] myasthenia gravis,[83] Coombs' positive haemolytic anaemia[179] and autoimmune neutropenia[32] are other putative autoimmune diseases with which it has been associated. Chronic active hepatitis associated with urticaria, an allergic capillaritis of the skin[209] and cryoglobulinaemia with immune complex deposition in the kidney,[79] and a monoclonal gammopathy are possible examples in which unknown antigens may be involved.

Immunological Changes

Humoral

Hyperglobulinaemia is one of the most striking immunological abnormalities in chronic active hepatitis, all three major immunoglobulin classes being involved, although the rise is most pronounced in the IgG levels.[78] The mechanism of the hyperglobulinaemia is probably complex. Serum complement levels may be low, but they can be correlated with low serum albumin levels and a prolonged prothrombin time, which suggests that they are due to defective synthesis by the diseased liver, rather than complement utilization in immune complex formation.[80, 177] There is, however, some evidence for in vivo inactivation of C3 in chronic active hepatitis, which favours the latter possibility.[245]

Another striking immunological abnormality is the range of autoantibodies observed.[61] Initial reports were of non-organ-specific autoantibodies, but more recently a liver-specific autoantibody has been described. Antinuclear antibody, often of the IgG class, occurs in over half the patients and is present at high titre; about 10 per cent of patients have a positive LE cell phenomenon. DNA-binding antibodies, which were originally thought to be specific for systemic lupus erythematosus, may also be noted in patients with chronic active hepatitis,[49] including those who are HB_sAg positive.[132] Smooth muscle antibodies were initially described by Johnson, Holborow and Glynn.[125] These antibodies occur in 40 to 60 per cent of HB_sAg negative chronic active hepatitis at high titre,[135, 212, 278] sometimes with concomitant staining of rat renal glomeruli.[272] Although the highest titres and strongest reactions are usually found in chronic active hepatitis, smooth muscle antibodies are also present in other forms of liver disease and in viral infections.[8, 111] The broad reacting high-titre smooth muscle antibody found in chronic active hepatitis has been shown to be directed against actin.[149]

Rizzetto, Swana and Doniach[196] described an antibody reacting with microsomal membranes seen particularly in the sera of young patients with clinically active disease in the absence of other autoantibodies.[230] This antibody is distinct from the mitochondrial (M) antibody (see Chapter 31), which is commonly present in primary biliary cirrhosis but in only a small proportion of patients with chronic active hepatitis.

Of special interest is a serum autoantibody directed against the hepatocyte membrane as demonstrated by indirect immunofluorescence of isolated rabbit hepatocytes. This antibody may be liver-specific and was found in 27 of 72 patients with HB_sAg negative chronic active hepatitis and only very rarely in other forms of hepatic disease.[243] It is directed against the high molecular weight, low-density lipoprotein antigen, LP1, and not the soluble cytoplasmic antigen, LP2.[162]

Jensen et al[124] have developed a specific and sensitive radio-immunoassay for liver-specific membrane lipoprotein antibodies, and have detected it in virtually all patients with chronic active hepatitis, including HB_sAg positive cases. The whole question of the significance of liver-specific antibodies in the pathogenesis of chronic active hepatitis has been critically reviewed by Dienstag and Isselbacher.[56]

High-titre antibodies to a variety of bacterial and viral antigens, particularly enterobacteria, measles, rubella and cytomegalovirus,[256, 258] are also observed in chronic active hepatitis, and there is an overall correlation between the presence of antinuclear antibody, smooth muscle antibody and these viral antibody titres, but no cross-reactivity[257] (see Chapter 9).

Cellular

Patients with chronic active hepatitis often have evidence of impaired cell-mediated immunity, as demonstrated by skin-testing and impaired lymphocyte transformation in response to phytohaemagglutinin, and there is a decrease in the number of circulating T cells.[53, 251] The mechanism and significance of this impairment is uncertain, although it is possible that the diminished peripheral blood concentration of T cells is dependent on the presence of serum inhibitors, which prevent rosette formation, rather than due to the homing of activated T cells to the liver.[208]

Studies of cell-mediated immunity to autologous or heterologous liver tissue have provided some evidence for specific sensitization, but as with circulating autoantibodies it is uncertain whether this is causally related to the liver disease or is a consequence of cell damage. A variety of techniques and preparations of liver antigen has been used. The techniques include lymphocyte transformation[249] and variants of leucocyte migration inhibition. Most recent studies have used the liver-specific lipoprotein antigens of Meyer zum Büschenfelde and Miescher.[162] Miller et al[164] found abnormal leucocyte migration inhibition to LP1 in approximately three-quarters of their patients with chronic active hepatitis but in none of the healthy controls or patients with alcoholic liver disease. On the other hand, Meyer zum Büschenfelde, Knolle and Berger[163] found migration inhibition to a similar antigen in 85 per cent of patients with untreated chronic active hepatitis, but also in 42 per cent of those with cryptogenic cirrhosis.

More recently, this liver-specific antigen has been used in the lymphocyte transformation technique by Thestrup-Pedersen, Ladefoged and Andersen[247] who found specific transformation in 80 per cent of patients with chronic active hepatitis, 40 per cent with cryptogenic cirrhosis and a similar proportion with acute hepatitis, and an occasional control. The sensitization was abolished by treatment with immunosuppressive agents. In chronic active hepatitis, there is a positive correlation between such sensitization and the presence of autoantibodies and HLA-B8.

Studies of lymphocyte cytotoxicity in chronic active hepatitis have also produced a wealth of immunological data which is difficult to interpret. Various target cells have been used, including Chang liver cells,[122, 270] human hepatocytes[92, 180, 266] and rabbit hepatocytes.[42, 130]

In some studies there has been a correlation with leucocyte migration inhibition to liver antigens and the reaction has been shown to be inhibited by blocking factors, presumably antibodies. This will be discussed further when reviewing the possible nature of the immune hepatic damage in chronic active hepatitis.

Patients with chronic active hepatitis have an increased incidence of the histocompatibility antigen HLA-B8.[155] This occurs only in HB_sAg negative chronic active hepatitis,[84] and there is a correlation between the antigen and titres of autoantibodies, as well as antibodies to measles and rubella viruses.[86] These workers suggested that the increased antibody response is a genetically determined increase in immunological responsiveness for which the HLA antigens act as markers. They did not find a correlation between HLA status and *Escherichia coli* antibody titres, which were related to the degree of portasystemic shunting.

Further evidence that genetic factors are associated with chronic active hepatitis stems from the demonstration of a high frequency of autoantibodies in the relatives of such patients.[85] In addition to autoantibodies, Salaspuro et al[206] found very high titre antibodies to measles and rubella in the relatives of patients with chronic active hepatitis.

Pathology

The pathology of idiopathic chronic active hepatitis is indistinguishable from the general features described earlier (page 655). There are no specific morphological features for this disease but obviously the absence of demonstrable HBV, bile duct damage, copper or PAS positive globules are important negative features. More active parenchymal inflammation and an increased proportion of plasma cells are points favouring idiopathic as opposed to HB_sAg positive chronic active hepatitis.

Differential Diagnosis of Chronic Active Hepatitis of Unknown Aetiology

The diagnosis of chronic active hepatitis of unknown aetiology is based on clinical, histological, biochemical and immunological findings, and the failure to identify known causes of this syndrome. Clearly, the proportion of cases falling into this category is being reduced as such factors are identified.

In patients presenting with jaundice or hepatomegaly with abnormal liver function tests of prolonged duration, a distinction from chronic persistent hepatitis or relapsing hepatitis without HBV markers may be difficult. It depends on the histological finding of chronic aggressive hepatitis with piecemeal necrosis but, as indicated earlier, repeat biopsy may be necessary. Spider naevi, palmar erythema, raised globulins and autoantibodies strongly favour chronic active hepatitis.

DISTINCTIONS BETWEEN HB_sAg POSITIVE AND NEGATIVE CHRONIC ACTIVE HEPATITIS (see Table 29.6)

This distinction is important, both on clinical and on epidemiological grounds and in relation

Table 29.6. *Clinical and Immunological Distinctions between HB_sAg Positive and HB_sAg Negative Chronic Active Hepatitis.*[a]

	HB_sAg positive	HB_sAg negative
Age	Often elderly	Often young
Sex	Mostly males	Usually females
Multisystem disease	Rare	Common
Antinuclear factor	Rare	Common
Smooth muscle antibody	Rare	Common
Anti-HB_c	Common	Rare
Liver-specific antibodies	Rare	Common
Hyperglobulinaemia	Moderate	Marked
HLA-B8 distribution	Normal	Increased
Geographical distribution	Variable	Probably universal
Response to corticosteroids	Unknown	Favourable
Prognosis	Unknown	Usually poor

[a] After Wright.[280]

Table 29.7. *Comparison of Chronic Active Hepatitis in Southampton and Baghdad.*[a]

	United Kingdom	Iraq
	31	83
Males	25%	90%
Females	75%	10%
Age (mean)	59 yrs	40 yrs
Jaundice at onset	32%	2%
Fluid retention	12%	25%
Bleeding	9%	9%
Abdominal pain	17%	32%
General malaise	30%	12%
Cutaneous stigmata of chronic liver disease	50%	70%
Varices	20%	42%
Cirrhosis on biopsy	70%	97%
Mean AST	117 iu	57 iu
Mean globulin	41	31
Albumin <3 g	20%	45%
ESR mm/hr	57	37
HB_sAg	6%	81%
HB_sAg neg., anti-HB_c pos.	1 patient	1 patient
Smooth muscle antibody	85%	67%
Antinuclear antibody	58%	5%
Other autoantibodies	58%	5%
Liver membrane antibody	25%	2%
DNA antibody	22	19
Putative autoimmune disease	30%	2%
Diabetes 4, myxoedema 2, rheumatoid 2, pernicious anaemia 1		Diabetes 1

[a] After Holdstock et al.[112]

to treatment. It has been suggested by some that chronic active hepatitis of unknown aetiology might be due to an abnormal immune response initiated by the hepatitis B virus which is no longer detectable. There are, however, important clinical, epidemiological and immunological data which make this unlikely, although histologically the two conditions are indistinguishable, unless HBV markers are specifically demonstrated. Patients with HB_sAg positive chronic active hepatitis are usually males of an older age-group, compared with the idiopathic variety, which occurs particularly in young women and women at the menopause. Furthermore, in HB_sAg positive chronic active hepatitis, multisystem disease of the putative autoimmune type is rare, whereas it occurs commonly in patients who are HB_sAg negative.[65,135,212,279] Although genetic factors may be important in both types, the prevalence of HLA-B8 is increased only in HB_sAg negative chronic active hepatitis.[84,150]

Most studies have shown higher globulin levels and a greater prevalence of circulating autoantibodies, such as antinuclear antibody and anti-smooth muscle antibody, in idiopathic chronic active hepatitis, compared to that with HB_sAg.[34,65,80,135,150,212,278] Others have not found such differences,[20] or they have been related to the fact that the higher prevalence of autoantibodies can be attributed to the larger number of females in the idiopathic variety and that in males this distinction falls away.[69]

The possibility that idiopathic chronic active hepatitis might be induced by HBV has been examined by studying late markers of HBV infection with conflicting findings. Grady, Kaplan and Vyas[100] did not find an increased incidence of anti-HB_c in patients with chronic active hepatitis who did not have the surface antigen in their serum, and therefore concluded that few if any such cases were induced by HBV. Bories et al,[30] Kubo et al,[140] and Zappi et al[285] detected anti-HB_c in about a third of their patients with HB_sAg negative chronic active hepatitis implicating past HBV infections.

Another clinical distinction is the geographical distribution of HB_sAg positive chronic active hepatitis which reflects the prevalence of the carrier state in the community. When we have compared the prevalence of HBV markers in patients with chronic active hepatitis in the United Kingdom with those from Iraq, a striking sex ànd geographical difference has been found, and in both groups only one patient who was HB_sAg negative had anti-HB_c (Table 29.7).

It also seems likely that patients with HB_sAg positive chronic active hepatitis respond less well to treatment with corticosteroid drugs than the idiopathic variety, although their overall prognosis may be better[212] (see below). It is possible that viruses other than HBV might be responsible for some cases of idiopathic chronic active hepatitis, particularly those without immunological markers. As indicated previously, there is no evidence that hepatitis A can proceed to chronicity, though it is likely that non-A, non-B viruses, which behave in a manner similar to HBV, might do so.[291]

OTHER AETIOLOGIES FOR CHRONIC ACTIVE HEPATITIS

Drug-induced Chronic Active Hepatitis

Several drugs have been shown to induce a clinical and histological picture indistinguishable from idiopathic chronic active hepatitis. These include laxatives containing oxyphenisatin,[45, 59, 193] methyldopa,[98, 250] nitrofurantoin,[292] isoniazid[156] and paracetamol.[29] Hyperglobulinaemia and autoantibodies may be present, but the liver lesion usually regresses when the drug is stopped, and is only rarely progressive.[215] The subject has been reviewed by Maddrey and Boitnott[157] (see Chapter 36).

Wilson's Disease

Occasional patients with Wilson's disease, particularly children, may present with the hepatic lesion predominating and clinical and histological features of a chronic active hepatitis. The distinction from the idiopathic variety is clearly important, as treatment is different and diagnosis is based on estimation of the serum copper and caeruloplasmin and liver copper concentration (see Chapter 33).

Alpha-1-antitrypsin Deficiency

This condition, recognized only relatively recently, in both adults and children can pursue a prolonged course with intermittent jaundice and histological features indistinguishable from chronic active hepatitis.[259] The distinction is made on the basis of the detection of PAS positive globules in the liver, which can be shown immunologically to be retained alpha-1-antitrypsin, and the demonstration of low levels in the serum (see Chapter 35).

Alcoholic Liver Disease

Alcoholic liver disease, particularly in women with alcoholic hepatitis, may show clinical features resembling chronic active hepatitis, including intermittent jaundice, prominent spider naevi and palmar erythema, haemorrhagic phenomena, raised globulins and smooth muscle antibodies. Despite the fact that a history of alcoholism may be concealed, other features may be present, such as malnutrition, a peripheral neuropathy or folate deficiency. Histology of the liver usually clinches the diagnosis of alcoholic hepatitis, but recently there have been reports of chronic aggressive or chronic persistent hepatitis on liver biopsy attributable to alcohol.[96]

Primary Biliary and Other Forms of Cirrhosis

Although chronic active hepatitis of unknown aetiology and primary biliary cirrhosis in their classic forms differ clinically and histologically, it is being increasingly recognized that a number of patients show features of both conditions and may be difficult to classify (see Chapter 31). Sampling error on liver biopsy, immunological overlap and the fact that some patients with chronic active hepatitis may show clinical and biochemical features of cholestasis may make the diagnosis difficult. Finally, there is the possibility that patients with cryptogenic or post-necrotic cirrhosis may represent the inactive 'burnt-out' stage of idiopathic chronic active hepatitis, as similar immunological markers and a histological appearance of cellular infiltrate indicating activity may be seen.

TREATMENT OF CHRONIC HEPATITIS

Treatment of Chronic Persistent Hepatitis

Once the diagnosis of chronic persistent hepatitis has been made, if necessary by repeat liver biopsy over a period of six months or a year, patients should be reassured that the prognosis is good. Corticosteroid drugs or azathioprine should not be used, and there need be no restriction on physical activity or diet. Although alcohol is best avoided, there is little evidence that it prolongs the hepatitis.

Treatment of Chronic Active Hepatitis

The mortality from chronic active hepatitis is high, and in most untreated series more than 50 per cent of patients die within five years. Because of the florid histological and immunological features of the disease, immunosuppressive drugs were used in its treatment soon after they were introduced. A beneficial effect of corticosteroids[145, 178] and of azathioprine[152] was reported. These and other early studies were inadequately controlled and in one group of 43 patients treated with corticosteroids it was concluded that using these did not prolong life.[190] Prospective randomized controlled trials of prednisolone and a placebo group therefore seemed justified, as advocated by the Copenhagen Study Group for liver disease.[142]

In one such trial, Cook, Mulligan and Sherlock[44] treated 22 patients with prednisolone and 27 controls, the treated group receiving 15 mg prednisolone initially. The two groups did not differ clinically or in respect of liver function at inclusion in the trial. The most striking finding was a significant reduction in mortality in the treated group compared with the controls. Three patients of the 22 in the treated group died of liver failure, compared with 13 of 27 patients in the control group. Two additional patients in the latter group died of unrelated disorders but with severe liver disease. Of the survivors, the general health of the treated patients at the end of the study was better than that of the controls. The most striking biochemical difference between the two groups was a significantly higher serum albumin in the treated patients than in the controls. The serum bilirubin and total globulins also showed a greater trend towards normality. It was concluded that prednisolone in low dosage is indicated in the early active phase of the disease.

In a large prospective trial of 63 patients from the Mayo Clinic, prednisone 20 mg daily or a combination of 10 mg prednisone and 50 mg azathioprine was shown to be superior to 100 mg azathioprine or placebo. Prednisone alone or in combination with azathioprine significantly improved life expectancy, histological resolution from chronic active hepatitis to non-specific hepatitis and resolution to normal of clinical and biochemical changes.[231] Although most patients receiving azathioprine or placebo deteriorated, 20 per cent resolved spontaneously. The superiority of prednisone over azathioprine was confirmed in another trial of 47 patients.[168] In all these trials, prednisone at a dose of 15 to 20 mg daily was associated with significant and sometimes serious side-effects.

In a further trial, Summerskill et al[237] titrated the dose of prednisone to procure biochemical resolution and administered it on alternate days. They were able to reduce the incidence of side-effects, by comparison with those associated with prednisone in full dosage, but the regimen was not as effective as prednisone 10 mg daily and azathioprine 50 mg daily in producing histological resolution. Furthermore, in the latter group the low incidence of side-effects was maintained.

D-penicillamine has been used in chronic active hepatitis because of its immunosuppressive effect and the possibility that it might improve established cirrhosis, but in a controlled trial it was associated with a higher frequency of side-effects than was prednisolone.[234]

It should be emphasized that these trials are not strictly comparable, in terms both of the treatment regimens used and the criteria for patient selection.

The difficulties associated with conducting controlled clinical trials in liver disease where one is dealing with conditions of multiple aetiology and varying severity have been emphasized by the Copenhagen Study Group for liver disease[142] and in two recent critical reviews.[144, 276] The most effective maintenance regimen would seem to be a combination of prednisone or prednisolone 10 mg daily and azathioprine 50 mg daily, but it is not known whether the use of prednisolone on alternate days will reduce still further the incidence of side-effects. It is also not clear whether a higher dosage of prednisolone should be given initially to achieve biochemical control, although it is our own practice to start with 20 to 40 mg of prednisolone daily, reducing to a maintenance of 10 mg daily over four to six weeks. Using this combined regimen of low-dosage prednisolone and azathioprine, it is likely that the five-year mortality rate can be reduced to 25 per cent or less, but the long-term prognosis is unknown. When assessing the frequency with which 'cures' are achieved, it must be recalled that 20 per cent of patients in the Mayo Clinic trial resolved without treatment, and it is our practice to monitor therapy by liver biopsy done at six months after the start of treatment and thereafter at one to two-yearly intervals.

Haemoglobin, white cell and platelet counts and liver function tests should be checked every two months, but bone marrow depression or hepatotoxicity on the 50-mg maintenance dose of azathioprine is unusual. The usual precautions should be taken to monitor patients on long-term corticosteroids, and complications of the liver disease, such as fluid retention, bleeding varices or hepatic encephalopathy, should be treated appropriately.

Treatment of HB_sAg positive Chronic Active Hepatitis

Most of the trials discussed above contained few if any cases of HB_sAg positive chronic active hepatitis, and adequate controlled clinical trials of the effect of corticosteroids in the treatment of such patients are not available. In one report it was considered that prednisolone might have a favourable effect,[66] but in another it was suggested that prednisone and/or azathioprine had an adverse effect.[12]

Patients admitted to the Mayo Clinic controlled clinical trials of corticosteroids and azathioprine in chronic active hepatitis have recently been analysed by Schalm et al.[212] The numbers of HB_sAg positive cases in the study were small, but the 13 patients who received prednisone failed to respond adequately to treatment with conventional doses and although they often improved with higher doses still did not reach full remission of the disease. In general, this supports clinical impressions, but clearly further controlled studies are required.

Several other approaches have been adopted on a limited number of patients. Reed et al[191] infused high-titre specific immune anti-HB_s globulin into six patients with HB_sAg positive chronic active hepatitis, but did not alter the course of the disease. Attempts have also been made to eliminate the chronic viral infection with hepatitis B by immunostimulation. Transfer factor has been used in a small number of patients with HB_sAg positive chronic liver disease.[123, 137, 226, 253] In the study by Jain, Thomas and Sherlock,[123] four of six patients with HB_sAg positive chronic liver disease developed transient elevation of the serum transaminases in response to the administration of specific transfer factor, suggesting that the transfer factor which they used produced antigen-specific, immunological stimulation. There was, however, no evidence of a therapeutic benefit in these patients or in the other studies cited above, and it is unlikely that it has any place in treatment.

In the absence of specific anti-viral agents, interferon has been used on a small number of patients and experimentally infected chimpanzees. Interferon, which has had limited application as an anti-viral agent in man and has not fulfilled its early promise, inhibits intracellular viral replication and is effective experimentally if cells are exposed to the interferon before being infected with virus. On theoretical grounds, if persistence of HBV in the liver is due to the infection of uninfected hepatocytes, interferon might terminate replication.[110] It is also of interest that the lymphocytes from children with chronic hepatitis have been shown to have a decreased interferon response.[252]

There have been limited studies using both leucocyte and fibroblast interferon in patients with chronic HBV infection. Human leucocyte interferon was used to treat four patients with HB_sAg positive chronic active hepatitis who had high titres of DNA polymerase and high Dane particle counts. The interferon was administered parenterally at a dosage between 6×10^3 and 7×10^4 units per kg per day, and was associated with a rapid and reproducible fall in the titre of HB_cAg and in DNA polymerase activity. However, it required prolonged treatment with interferon to modify the HB_sAg titre and the e antigen.[101] In another study, one patient with HB_sAg positive chronic active hepatitis and two chimpanzee carriers of HB_sAg were given 10^7 iu of human fibroblast interferon over two weeks. The interferon was shown to reduce the expression of HB_cAg in the hepatocytes observed by immunofluorescence on liver biopsy.[55]

In our own study of two patients with HB_sAg positive chronic active hepatitis, we administered human fibroblast interferon 10^7 units daily for two weeks and showed rapid and striking depression of the anti-HB_c titre and in one patient a progressive and sustained fall in the aspartate aminotransferase (AST).[132] In a further experimental study in chimpanzees, an interferon inducer was administered to four animals.[188] This produced a fall in the serum Dane particle-associated DNA polymerase, e antigen and HB_sAg as well as diminution of intrahepatic HB_sAg and HB_cAg during treatment.

These studies must be viewed with caution [110, 143] as all that is being observed is a modification of HBV markers and no clear effect has yet been demonstrated on the disease process. Furthermore, the supplies of interferon are at present extremely limited and the prospects for its synthesis or bulk production are not good. The possibility that interferon might be more effective if combined with a chemical anti-viral agent such as adenine arabinoside is being investigated with encouraging results, but similar reservations apply.

REFERENCES

1. Afrodikas, A.P., Liew, B.S.C.-T. & Peters, R.L. (1976) An immunoperoxidase technic for the demonstration of the hepatitis B surface antigen in human livers. *American Journal of Clinical Pathology*, **65**, 533–539.
2. Ahmed, M.N., Huang, S.N. & Spence, L. (1971) Australia antigen and hepatitis. *Archives of Pathology and Laboratory Medicine*, **92**, 66–72.
3. Aikawa, T., Sairenji, H., Furuta, S., Kiyosawa, K., Shikata, T., Imai, M., Miyakawa, Y., Yanase, Y. & Mayumi, M. (1978) Seroconversion from hepatitis B e antigen to anti-HBe in acute hepatitis B virus infection. *New England Journal of Medicine*, **298**, 439–441.
4. Alberti, A., Realdi, G., Tremolada, F. & Spina, G.P. (1976) Liver cell surface localization of hepatitis B antigen and of immunoglobulins in acute and chronic hepatitis and in liver cirrhosis. *Clinical and Experimental Immunology*, **25**, 396–402.
5. Almeida, J.D. & Waterson, A.P. (1969) Immune complexes in hepatitis. *Lancet*, **ii**, 983–986.
6. Almeida, J.D., Gioannini, P., Scalise, G. & Harrison, C.V. (1973) Electron microscope study of a case of Australia antigen positive chronic hepatitis. *Journal of Clinical Pathology*, **26**, 113–119.
7. Alpert, E., Isselbacher, K.J. & Schur, P.H. (1971) The pathogenesis of arthritis associated with viral hepatitis: complement-component studies. *New England Journal of Medicine*, **285**, 185–189.
8. Andersen, P. (1974) Indirect immunofluorescence studies of smooth muscle antibodies. *Acta Pathologica et Microbiologica Scandinavica*, **82**, 577–584.
9. Anderson, K.E., Sun, S.C., Berg, H.S. & Chang, N.-K. (1974) Liver function and histology in asymptomatic Chinese military personnel with hepatitis B antigenemia. *American Journal of Digestive Diseases*, **19**, 693–703.
10. Anthony, P.P., Vogel, C.L., Sadikali, F., Barber, L.F. & Peterson, M.R. (1972) Hepatitis-associated antigen and antibody in Uganda: correlation of serological testing with histopathology. *British Medical Journal*, **i**, 403–406.
11. Arnold, W., Nielsen, J.O., Hardt, F. & Meyer zum Büschenfelde, K.H. (1977) The localisation of e antigen in nuclei of hepatocytes. *Gut*, **18**, 994–996.
12. Aronoff, A., Gault, M.H., Huang, S.N., Lal, S.W., Moinuddin, K.T., Spence, M.D. & MacLean, L.D. (1973) Hepatitis with Australia antigenemia following renal transplantation. *Canadian Medical Association Journal*, **108**, 43–50.
13. Baggenstoss, A.H., Soloway, R.D., Summerskill, W.H.J., Elveback, L.R. & Schoenfield, L.J. (1972) Chronic active liver disease. The range of histologic lesions, their response to treatment and evolution. *Human Pathology*, **3**, 183–184.
14. Barker, L.F., Maynard, J.E., Purcell, R.H., Hoofnagle, J.H.R., Berquist, K.R. & London, W.T. (1975) Viral hepatitis, type B, in experimental animals. *American Journal of the Medical Sciences*, **270**, 189–195.
15. Barnardo, D.E., Vernon-Roberts, B. & Currey, H.L.F. (1973) A case of active chronic hepatitis with painless erosive arthritis. *Gut*, **14**, 800–804.
16. Bearn, A.G., Kunkel, H.G. & Slater, R.J. (1956) The problem of chronic liver disease in young women. *American Journal of Medicine*, **21**, 3–15.
17. Becker, M.D., Scheuer, P.J., Baptista, A. & Sherlock, S. (1970) Prognosis of chronic persistent hepatitis. *Lancet*, **i**, 53–57.
18. Bianchi, L. & Gudat, F. (1976) Sanded nuclei in hepatitis B. Eosinophilic inclusions in liver cell nuclei due to excess in hepatitis B core antigen formation. *Laboratory Investigation*, **35**, 1–5.
19. Bianchi, L., De Groote, J., Desmet, J.V., Gedigk, P., Korb, G., Popper, H., Poulsen, H., Scheuer, P.J., Schmid, M., Thaler, H. & Wepler, W. (1971) Morphological criteria in viral hepatitis. Review by an International Group. *Lancet*, **i**, 333–337.
20. Bianchi, L., Bianchi Porro, C., Coltorti, M., Dardanoni, L., Del Vecchio Blanco, C., Fagiolo, U., Farini, R., Manozzi, I., Naccarato, R., Pagliaro, L., Spano, G. & Verme, G. (1972) Occurrence of Australia antigen in chronic hepatitis in Italy. *Gastroenterology*, **63**, 482–485.
21. Bianchi, L., De Groote, J., Desmet, V.J., Gedigk, P., Korb, G., Popper, H., Poulsen, H., Scheuer, P.J., Schmid, M. & Thaler, H. (1977) Acute and chronic hepatitis revisited. *Lancet*, **ii**, 914–919.
22. Bjørneboe, M. & Raaschou, F. (1949) The pathology of subchronic atrophy of the liver. A comparison with cirrhosis hepatitis Laennec. *Acta Medica Scandinavica* (Suppl.), **234**, 41–62.
23. Blumberg, B.J., Alter, H.J. & Visnich, S. (1965) A new antigen in leukemia sera. *Journal of the American Medical Association*, **191**, 541–546.
24. Blumberg, B.S., Gerstley, B.J.S., Hungerford, D.A., London, W.T. & Sutnick, A.I. (1967) A serum antigen (Australia antigen) in Down's syndrome, leukaemia and hepatitis. *Annals of Internal Medicine*, **66**, 924–931.
25. Blumberg, B.S., Sutnick, A.I. & London, W.T. (1968) Hepatitis and leukaemia: their relation to Australia antigen. *Bulletin of the New York Academy of Medicine*, **44**, 1566–1586.
26. Blumberg, B.S., Melartin, L., Lechat, M. & Guinto, R.S. (1967) Association between lepromatous leprosy and Australia antigen. *Lancet*, **ii**, 173–176.
27. Blumberg, B.S., Friedlaender, J.S., Woodside, A., Sutnick, A.I. & London, W.T. (1969) Hepatitis and Australia antigen: autosomal recessive inheritance of susceptibility to infection in humans. *Proceedings of the National Academy of Sciences of the United States of America*, **62**, 1108–1115.
28. Bolin, T.D., Davis, A.E. & Liddelow, A.G. (1973) Liver disease and cell mediated immunity in hepatitis-associated antigen (HAA) carriers. *Gut*, **14**, 365–368.

29. Bonkowsky, H.L., Mudge, G.H. & McMurty, R.J. (1978) Chronic hepatic inflammation and fibrosis due to low doses of paracetamol. *Lancet,* **i,** 1016–1018.
30. Bories, P., Coursaget, P., Goudeau, A., Degott, C., Maupas, P. & Benhamou, J.P. (1978) Antibody to hepatitis B core antigen in chronic active hepatitis. *British Medical Journal,* **i,** 396–397.
31. Boxall, E.H., Flewett, T.H., Paton, A. & Rassam, S.W. (1976) Hepatitis B surface antigen and cirrhosis in Iraq. *Gut,* **17,** 119–121.
32. Boxer, L.A., Yokoyama, M. & Wiebe, R.A. (1972) Autoimmune neutropenia associated with chronic active hepatitis. *American Journal of Medicine,* **52,** 279–282.
33. Brzosko, W.J., Krawcyński, K., Nazarewicz, T., Morzycka, M. & Nowosławski, A. (1974) Glomerulonephritis associated with hepatitis-B surface antigen immune complexes in children. *Lancet,* **ii,** 477–482.
34. Bulkley, B.H., Heizer, W.D., Goldfinger, S.E., Isselbacher, K.F. & Shulman, N.P. (1970) Distinctions in chronic active hepatitis based on circulating hepatitis-associated antigen. *Lancet,* **ii,** 1323–1326.
35. Burns, J. (1975) Immunoperoxidase localisation of hepatitis B antigen (HB) in formalin–paraffin processed liver tissue. *Histochemistry,* **44,** 133–135.
36. Cattan, R., Vesin, P. & Bodin, H. (1957) Cirrhoses dysprotéinémiques d'origine inconnue chez la femme. *Bulletin de la Société Médicale des Hôpitaux de Paris,* **73,** 608–616.
37. Chadwick, R.G., Galizzi, J., Heathcote, J., Cohen, P.J., Scheuer, S. & Sherlock, S. (1977) The natural history of chronic persistent hepatitis. *12th Meeting of the E.A.S.L., Archives of the Hellenic Medical Society,* **3,** 3.
38. Chiaramonte, M., Heathcote, J., Crees, M. & Sherlock, S. (1977) Detection by three techniques of hepatitis B surface antigen (HB_sAg) and determination of HB_sAg and anti-HBs titres in patients with chronic liver disease. *Gut,* **18,** 1–6.
39. Christoffersen, P., Poulsen, H. & Scheuer, P.J. (1972) Abnormal bile duct epithelium in chronic aggressive hepatitis and primary biliary cirrhosis. *Human Pathology,* **3,** 227–235.
40. Christoffersen, P., Dietrichson, O., Faber, V. & Poulsen, H. (1972) The occurrence and significance of abnormal bile duct epithelium in chronic aggressive hepatitis. *Acta Pathologica et Microbiologica Scandinavica,* Section A, **80,** 294–303.
41. Christoffersen, P., Dietrichson, O., Nielsen, J.O. & Elling, P. (1973) Histological changes in two serologically defined groups of chronic hepatitis. *Acta Pathologica et Microbiologica Scandinavica,* **81** (Sect. A), 698–702.
42. Cochrane, A.M.G., Moussouros, A., Smith, A., Thomson, A.D., Eddleston, A.L.W.F. & Williams, R. (1976) Autoimmune reaction to a liver specific membrane antigen during acute viral hepatitis. *Gut,* **17** (9), 714–718.
43. Combes, B., Stastny, P., Shorey, J., Eigenbrodt, E.H., Barrera, A., Hull, A.R. & Carter, N.W. (1971) Glomerulonephritis with deposition of Australia antigen–antibody complexes in glomerular basement membrane. *Lancet,* **ii,** 234–237.
44. Cook, C.G., Mulligan, R. & Sherlock, S. (1971) Controlled prospective trial of corticosteroid therapy in active chronic hepatitis. *Quarterly Journal of Medicine,* **40,** 159–185.
45. Cooksley, W.G.E., Cowen, A.E. & Powell, L.W. (1973) The incidence of oxyphenisatin ingestion in active chronic hepatitis: a prospective controlled study of 29 patients. *Australian and New Zealand Journal of Medicine,* **3,** 124–128.
46. Cossart, Y.E. (1977) *Virus Hepatitis and its Control.* London:Baillière-Tindall.
47. Creutzfeldt, W., Schmitt, W., Rickert, J., Kaiser, K. & Matthes, M. (1962) Hepatitis transmissions over a period of ten years by a blood donor with posthepatitis liver cirrhosis. *Deutsche Medizinische Wochenschrift,* **87,** 1801–1804.
48. Cullinan, E.R., King, R.C. & Rivers, J.S. (1958) The prognosis of infective hepatitis. A preliminary account of a long-term follow-up. *British Medical Journal,* **i,** 1315–1317.
49. Davis, P. & Read, A.E. (1975) Antibodies to double stranded (native) DNA in active chronic hepatitis. *Gut,* **16,** 413–415.
50. De Gast, G.C., Houwen, B. & Nieweg, H.O. (1973) Specific lymphocyte stimulation by purified, heat-inactivated hepatitis-B antigen. *British Medical Journal,* **iv,** 707–709.
51. De Groote, J., Fevery, J. & Lepoutre, L. (1978) Long term follow-up of chronic active hepatitis of moderate severity. *Gut,* **19,** 510–513.
52. De Groote, J., Desmet, V.J., Gedigk, P., Korb, G., Popper, H., Poulsen, H., Scheuer, P.J., Schmid, M., Thaler, H. & Uehlinger, E. (1968) A classification of chronic hepatitis. *Lancet,* **ii,** 626–628.
53. DeHoratius, R.J., Strickland, R.G. & Williams, R.C. (1974) T and B lymphocytes in acute and chronic hepatitis. *Clinical Immunology and Immunopathology,* **2,** 353–360.
54. Deodhar, K.P., Tapp, E. & Scheuer, P.J. (1975) Orcein staining of hepatitis B antigen in paraffin sections of liver biopsies. *Journal of Clinical Pathology,* **28,** 66–70.
55. Desmyter, J., Ray, M.B., De Groote, J., Bradburne, A.F., Desmet, V.J., Edy, V.G., Billiau, A., De Somer, P. & Mortelmans, J. (1976) Administration of human fibroblast interferon in chronic hepatitis-B infection. *Lancet,* **ii,** 645–647.
56. Dienstag, J.L. & Isselbacher, K.J. (1978) Liver specific protein: more questions than answers. *New England Journal of Medicine,* **299,** 40–42.
57. Dietrichson, O. (1975) Chronic persistent hepatitis. A clinical, serological and prognostic study. *Scandinavian Journal of Gastroenterology,* **10,** 249–255.
58. Dietrichson, O., Nielsen, J.O., Elling, P. & Christoffersen, P. (1973) The relevance of a serological classification of chronic hepatitis. *Acta Pathologica et Microbiologica Scandinavica,* **81,** 519–524.
59. Dietrichson, O., Juhl, E., Nielsen, J.O., Oxlund, J.J. & Christoffersen, P. (1974) The incidence of oxyphenisatin-induced liver damage in chronic non-alcoholic liver disease. A controlled investigation. *Scandinavian Journal of Gastroenterology,* **9,** 473–478.
60. Dietrichson, O., Juhl, E., Christoffersen, P., Elling, P., Faber, V., Iversen, K., Nielsen, J.O., Petersen, P. & Poulsen, H. (1975) Acute viral hepatitis: factors possibly predicting liver disease. *Acta Pathologica et Microbiologica Scandinavica,* **83** (Sect. A), 183–188.

61. Doniach, D., Roitt, I.M., Walker, J.G. & Sherlock, S. (1966) Tissue antibodies in primary biliary cirrhosis, active chronic lupoid hepatitis, cryptogenic cirrhosis and other liver diseases and their clinical implications. *Clinical and Experimental Immunology*, **1**, 237–262.
62. Dudley, F.J., Fox, R.A. & Sherlock, S. (1971) Relationship of hepatitis-associated antigen (H.A.A.) to acute and chronic liver injury. *Lancet*, **ii**, 1–3.
63. Dudley, F.J., Fox, R.A. & Sherlock, S. (1972) Cellular immunity and hepatitis-associated, Australia antigen liver disease. *Lancet*, **i**, 723–726.
64. Dudley, F.J., Giustino, V. & Sherlock, S. (1972) Cell-mediated immunity in patients positive for hepatitis-associated antigen. *British Medical Journal*, **iv**, 754–756.
65. Dudley, F.J., Scheuer, P.J. & Sherlock, S. (1972) Natural history of hepatitis-associated antigen-positive chronic liver disease. *Lancet*, **ii**, 1388–1393.
66. Dudley, F.J., O'Shea, M.J., Ajdukiewicz, A. & Sherlock, S. (1973) Serum autoantibodies and immunoglobulins in hepatitis-associated antigen (HAA)-positive and -negative liver disease. *Gut*, **14**, 360–364.
67. Duffy, J., Lidsky, M.D., Sharp, J.T., Davis, J.S., Person, D.A., Hollinger, F.B. & Min, K.-W. (1976) Polyarthritis, polyarteritis and hepatitis B. *Medicine (Baltimore)*, **55**, 19–37.
68. Eddleston, A.L.W.F. & Williams, R. (1974) Inadequate antibody response to HBAg or suppressor T-cell defect in development of active chronic hepatitis. *Lancet*, **ii**, 1543–1545.
69. Eddleston, A.L.W.F., Stern, R.B., Reed, W.D., Williams, R., Zuckerman, A.J., Bowes, A. & Earl, P. (1973) Detection of hepatitis-B antigen by radioimmunoassay in chronic liver disease and hepatocellular carcinoma in Great Britain. *Lancet*, **ii**, 690–694.
70. Edgington, T.S. & Chisari, F.V. (1975) Immunological aspects of hepatitis-B virus infection. *American Journal of the Medical Sciences*, **270**, 213–227.
71. Edgington, T.S. & Ritt, D.J. (1971) Intrahepatic expression of serum hepatitis virus-associated antigens. *Journal of Experimental Medicine*, **134**, 871–885.
72. Edland, J.F. (1972) Liver disease in heroin addicts. *Human Pathology*, **3**, 75–84.
73. Eleftheriou, H., Thomas, H.C., Heathcote, J. & Sherlock, S. (1975) Incidence and clinical significance of e antigen and antibody in acute and chronic liver disease. *Lancet*, **ii**, 1171–1173.
74. Farivar, M., Wands, J.R., Benson, G.D., Dienstag, J.L. & Isselbacher, K.J. (1976) Cryoprotein complexes and peripheral neuropathy in a patient with chronic active hepatitis. *Gastroenterology*, **71**, 490–493.
75. Fauerholdt, L., Asnaes, S., Ranek, L., Schiødt, T. & Tygstrup, N. (1977) Significance of suspected 'chronic aggressive hepatitis' in acute hepatitis. *Gastroenterology*, **73**, 543–548.
76. Feinman, S.V., Berris, B., Sinclair, J.C., Wrobel, D.M., Murphy, B.L. & Maynard, J.E. (1975) e Antigen and anti-e in HB_sAg carriers. *Lancet*, **ii**, 1173–1174.
77. Feinman, S.V., Cooter, N., Sinclair, J.C., Wrobel, D.M. & Berris, B. (1975) Clinical and epidemiological significance of the HB_sAg (Australia antigen): carrier state. *Gastroenterology*, **68**, 113–120.
78. Feizi, T. (1968) Immunoglobulins in chronic liver disease. *Gut*, **9**, 193–198.
79. Feizi, T. & Gitlin, N. (1969) Immune-complex disease of the kidney associated with chronic hepatitis and cryoglobulinaemia. *Lancet*, **ii**, 873–876.
80. Finlayson, N.D.C., Krohn, K., Fauconnet, M.H. & Anderson, K.E. (1972) Significance of serum complement levels in chronic liver disease. *Gastroenterology*, **63**, 653–659.
81. Frei, P.C., Desaules, M. & Krafft, T. (1978) Cell-mediated immune response to purified HB_sAg in HBV infections. In *Viral Hepatitis* (Ed.) Vyas, G.N., Cohen, S.N. & Schmid, R. pp. 267–273. Philadelphia: Franklin Institute Press.
82. Fox, R.A., Niazi, S.P. & Sherlock, S. (1969) Hepatitis-associated antigen in chronic liver disease. *Lancet*, **ii**, 609–612.
83. Galbraith, R.F., Summerskill, W.H.J. & Murray, J. (1964) Systemic lupus erythematosus, cirrhosis and ulcerative colitis after thymectomy for myasthenia gravis. *New England Journal of Medicine*, **270**, 229–232.
84. Galbraith, R.M., Eddleston, A.L.W.F., Smith, M.G.M., Williams, R., MacSween, R.N.M., Watkinson, G., Dick, H., Kennedy, L.A. & Batchelor, J.R. (1974) Histocompatibility antigens in active chronic hepatitis and primary biliary cirrhosis. *British Medical Journal*, **iii**, 604–605.
85. Galbraith, R.M., Smith, M., Mackenzie, R.M., Tee, D.E., Doniach, D. & Williams, R. (1974) High prevalence of seroimmunologic abnormalities in relatives of patients with active chronic hepatitis or primary biliary cirrhosis. *New England Journal of Medicine*, **290**, 63–69.
86. Galbraith, R.M., Eddleston, A.L.W.F., Williams, R., Webster, A.D.B., Pattison, J., Doniach, D., Kennedy, L.A. & Batchelor, J.R. (1976) Enhanced antibody responses in active chronic hepatitis: relation to HLA-B8 and HLA-B12 and porto-systemic shunting. *Lancet*, **i**, 930–934.
87. Gerber, M.A., Sarno, E. & Vernace, S.J. (1976) Immune complexes in hepatocytic nuclei of HB_sAg positive chronic hepatitis. *New England Journal of Medicine*, **294**, 922–925.
88. Gerber, M.A., Schaffner, F. & Paronetto, F. (1972) Immuno-electron microscopy of hepatitis B antigen in liver. *Proceedings of the Society for Experimental Biology and Medicine*, **140**, 1334–1339.
89. Gerber, M.A., Hadziyannis, S., Vissoulis, C., Schaffner, F., Paronetto, F. & Popper, H. (1974) Hepatitis B antigen: nature and distribution of cytoplasmic antigen in hepatocytes of carriers. *Proceedings of the Society for Experimental Biology and Medicine*, **145**, 863–867.
90. Gerber, M.J., Phuangsab, A., Vittal, S.B.V., Dourdourekas, D., Steigmann, F. & Clowdus, B.F. (1974) Cell-mediated immune response to hepatitis B antigen in patients with liver disease. *Digestive Diseases*, **19**, 637–643.
91. Gerety, R.J., Hoofnagle, J.H. & Barker, L.F. (1974) Humoral and cell-mediated immune responses to two hepatitis B virus antigens in guinea pigs. *Journal of Immunology*, **113**, 1223–1229.
92. Geubel, A.P., Keller, R.H., Summerskill, W.H.J., Dickson, E.R., Tomasi, T.B. & Shorter, R.G. (1976) Lymphocyte cytotoxicity and inhibition studied with autologous liver cells: observations in chronic active liver disease and the primary biliary cirrhosis syndrome. *Gastroenterology*, **71** (3), 450–456.

93. Gitnick, G.L., Gleich, G.J., Schoenfield, L.J., Baggenstoss, A.H., Sutnick, A.I., Blumberg, B.S., London, W.T. & Summerskill, W.H.J. (1969) Australia antigen in chronic active liver disease with cirrhosis. *Lancet*, **ii,** 285–288.

94. Gocke, D.J. (1978) Immune complex phenomena associated with hepatitis. In *Viral Hepatitis* (Ed.) Vyas, G.N., Cohen, S.N. & Schmid, R. pp. 277–284. Philadelphia: Franklin Institute Press.

95. Gocke, D.J., Hsu, K., Morgan, C., Bombardieri, S., Lockshin, M. & Christian, C.L. (1970) Association between polyarteritis and Australia antigen. *Lancet*, **ii,** 1149–1153.

96. Goldberg, S.J., Mendenhall, C.L., Connell, A.M. & Chedid, A. (1977) 'Nonalcoholic' chronic hepatitis in the alcoholic. *Gastroenterology*, **72** (4), 598–604.

97. Golding, P.L., Smith, M. & Williams, R. (1973) Multisystem involvement in chronic liver disease. Studies on the incidence and pathogenesis. *American Journal of Medicine*, **55,** 772–782.

98. Goldstein, G.B., Lam, K.C. & Mistilis, S.P. (1973) Drug-induced active chronic hepatitis. *Digestive Diseases*, **18,** 177–184.

99. Good, R.A. (1956) Plasma-cell hepatitis and extreme hypergammaglobulinemia in adolescent females. *American Journal of Diseases of Children*, **92,** 508–509.

100. Grady, G.F., Kaplan, M.M. & Vyas, G.N. (1977) Antibody to hepatitis B core antigen in chronic hepatitis and primary biliary cirrhosis: evaluation by a new autologous solid phase radioimmunoassay. *Gastroenterology*, **72,** 590–593.

101. Greenberg, H.B., Pollard, R.B., Lutwick, L.I., Gregory, P.B., Robinson, W.S. & Merigan, T.C. (1976) Effect of human leukocyte interferon on hepatitis B virus infection in patients with chronic active hepatitis. *New England Journal of Medicine*, **295,** 517–522.

102. Gudat, F., Bianchi, L., Sonnabend, W., Thiel, G., Aenishaenslin, W. & Stalder, G.A. (1975) Pattern of core and surface expression in liver tissue reflects state of specific immune response in hepatitis B. *Laboratory Investigation*, **32,** 1–9.

103. Hadziyannis, S. (1974) Chronic viral hepatitis. *Clinics in Gastroenterology*, **3,** 391–408.

104. Hadziyannis, S.J., Merikas, G.E. & Afroudakis, A.P. (1970) Hepatitis-associated antigen in chronic liver disease. *Lancet*, **ii,** 100.

105. Hadziyannis, S., Gerber, M.A., Vissoulis, C. & Popper, H. (1973) Cytoplasmic hepatitis B antigen in 'ground-glass' hepatocytes of carriers. *Archives of Pathology*, **96,** 327–330.

106. Henning, H., Tripatzis, I., Braun, H.H.V. & Luders, C.J. (1973) Hepatitis-B-antigen bei chronischen Leberkrankheiten. *Medizinische Klinik*, **68,** 1503–1510.

107. Hess, G., Nielsen, J.O., Arnold, W. & Meyer zum Büschenfelde, K.H. (1977) e-System and intrahepatocellular HB_cAg and HB_sAg in HB_sAg positive patients with liver diseases and healthy carriers. *Scandinavian Journal of Gastroenterology*, **12,** 325–330.

108. Hillis, W.D., Hillis, A., Bias, W.B. & Walker, W.G. (1977) Associations of hepatitis B surface antigenemia with HLA Locus B specificities. *New England Journal of Medicine*, **296** (23), 1310–1314.

109. Hirayama, C., Tominaga, K., Irisa, T. & Nakamura, M. (1972) Serum gamma globulin and hepatitis-associated antigen in blood donors, chronic liver disease and primary hepatoma. *Digestion*, **7,** 257–265.

110. Ho, M. (1976) Interferon and hepatitis B virus. *New England Journal of Medicine*, **295** (10), 562–563.

111. Holborow, E.J., Hemsted, E.H. & Mead, S.V. (1973) Smooth muscle autoantibodies in infectious mononucleosis. *British Medical Journal*, **iii,** 323–325.

112. Holdstock, G., Rassam, S., Kingham, J.G.C., Sadler, H.M. & Wright, R. (1978) Chronic active hepatitis in the United Kingdom and Iraq. *Gut*. In press.

113. Holdsworth, M.J., Hall, E. & Sherlock, S. (1965) Ulcerative colitis in chronic liver disease. *Quarterly Journal of Medicine*, **34,** 211–227.

114. Hoofnagle, J.H., Michalak, T., Nowaslawski, A., Gerety, R. & Barker, L.F. (1978) Immunofluorescence microscopy in experimentally induced, type B hepatitis in the chimpanzee. *Gastroenterology*, **74,** 182–187.

115. Hopf, U., Meyer zum Büschenfelde, K.H. & Freudenberg, J. (1974) Surface localisation of human liver-specific antigen. *Clinical and Experimental Immunology*, **16,** 117–123.

116. Hopf, U., Arnold, W., Meyer zum Büschenfelde, K.H., Forster, E. & Bolte, J.P. (1975) Studies on the pathogenesis of chronic inflammatory liver diseases. I. Membrane-fixed IgG on isolated hepatocytes from patients. *Clinical and Experimental Immunology*, **22,** 1–8.

117. Huang, S.N. (1971) Hepatitis-associated antigen hepatitis. *American Journal of Pathology*, **64,** 483–491.

118. Huang, S.N. (1975) Structural and immunoreactive characteristics of hepatitis B core antigen. *American Journal of the Medical Sciences*, **270,** 131–139.

119. Huang, S.N., Groh, V., Beaudoin, J.G., Dauphinee, W.D., Guttman, R.D., Morehouse, D.D., Aronoff, A. & Gault, H. (1974) A study of the relationship of virus-like particles and Australia antigen in liver. *Human Pathology*, **5,** 209–222.

120. Ishak, K.G. (1973) Viral hepatitis: the morphologic spectrum. In *The Liver*, I.A.P. Monograph (Ed.) Gall, E.A. & Mostofi, F.K. pp. 218–268. Baltimore: Williams & Wilkins.

121. Ishak, K.G. (1976) Light microscopic morphology of viral hepatitis. *American Journal of Clinical Pathology*, **65,** 787–827.

122. Jacques, E., De Villiers, D., Thomas, H.C. & Sherlock, S. (1976) Lymphocyte mediated cytotoxicity for Chang liver cells in acute and chronic liver disease. *Gut*, **17,** 389.

123. Jain, S., Thomas, H.C. & Sherlock, S. (1977) Transfer factor responses in the attempted treatment of patients with HBsAg positive chronic liver disease. *Clinical and Experimental Immunology*, **30,** 10–15.

124. Jensen, D.M., McFarlane, I.G., Portmann, B.S., Eddleston, A.L.W.F. & Williams, R. (1978) Detection of antibodies directed against a liver-specific membrane lipoprotein in patients with acute and chronic active hepatitis. *New England Journal of Medicine*, **299,** 1–7.

125. Johnson, G.D., Holborow, E.J. & Glynn, L.E. (1965) Antibody to smooth muscle in patients with liver disease. *Lancet*, **ii,** 878–879.

126. Joske, R.A. & King, W.E. (1955) The L.E. cell phenomenon in active chronic viral hepatitis. *Lancet*, **ii,** 477–479.

127. Kaboth, U., Schober, A., Arndt, H.J., Vido, I., Selmair, H., Gallasch, E., Varma, P., Thomsson, R. & Creutzfeldt, W. (1970) Australia (SH) antigen befunder bein Leberkranken und Blutspendern. *Deutsche Medizinische Wochenschrift,* **95,** 2157–2165.
128. Karasawa, T. & Shikata, T. (1977) Necrosis of hepatocytes with hepatitis B surface antigen. *Archives of Pathology and Laboratory Medicine,* **101,** 280–285.
129. Kawanishi, H. (1977) Morphologic association of lymphocytes with hepatocytes in chronic liver disease. *Archives of Pathology and Laboratory Medicine,* **101,** 286–290.
130. Kawanishi, H. & MacDermott, R.P. (1977) Induction of antibody dependent hepatocyte cytotoxicity by chronic active liver disease serum, mediated by normal null cells. *Gastroenterology,* **72,** 1078.
131. Kelsall, A.R., Stewart, A. & Witts, L.J. (1947) Subacute and chronic hepatitis. *Lancet,* **ii,** 195–198.
132. Kingham, J.G.C., Ganguly, N.K., Shaari, Z.D., Mendelson, R., McGuire, M.J., Holgate, S.J., Cartwright, T., Scott, G.M., Richards, B.M. & Wright, R. (1978) Treatment of HBsAg-positive chronic active hepatitis with human fibroblast interferon. *Gut,* **19,** 91–94.
133. Kingham, J.G.C., Rassam, S., Ganguly, N.K., McGuire, M.J., Nasrat, B., Holgate, S.T. & Wright, R. (1978) DNA-binding antibodies and hepatitis B markers in acute and chronic liver disease. *Clinical and Experimental Immunology,* **33,** 204–210.
134. Klatskin, G. (1958) Subacute hepatic necrosis and postnecrotic cirrhosis due to anicteric infections with the hepatitis virus. *American Journal of Medicine,* **25,** 333–358.
135. Klatskin, G. (1975) Persistent HB antigenemia; associated clinical manifestations and hepatic lesions. *American Journal of the Medical Sciences,* **270,** 33–40.
136. Klinge, O., Kaboth, U. & Arnold, R. (1971) Liver histology in healthy carriers of Australia-SH antigen or antibodies. *German Medicine,* **1,** 4–5.
137. Kohler, P.F., Trembath, J., Merrill, D.A., Singleton, J.W. & Dubois, R.S. (1974) Immunotherapy with antibody, lymphocytes and transfer factor in chronic hepatitis B. *Clinical Immunology and Immunopathology,* **2,** 465–471.
138. Krarup, N.B. & Roholm, K. (1941) The development of cirrhosis of the liver after acute hepatitis, elucidated by aspiration biopsy. *Acta Medica Scandinavica,* **108,** 306–331.
139. Krassnitsky, O., Pesendorfer, F. & Wewalka, F. (1970) Australia/SH-antigen und Lebererkrankungen. *Deutsche Medizinische Wochenschrift,* **95,** 249–253.
140. Kubo, Y., Okuda, K., Hashimoto, M., Nagasaki, Y., Ebata, H., Nakajima, Y., Musha, H., Sakuma, K. & Ohtake, H. (1977) Antibody to hepatitis B core antigen in patients with hepatocellular carcinoma. *Gastroenterology,* **72,** 1217–1220.
141. Kunkel, H.G., Ahrens, E.H.Jr, Eisenmenger, W.J., Bongiovanni, A.M. & Slater, R.J. (1951) Extreme hypergammaglobulinemia in young women with liver disease of unknown aetiology. *Journal of Clinical Investigation,* **30,** 654.
142. *Lancet* (1969) Effect of prednisone on the survival of patients with cirrhosis of the liver; a report from the Copenhagen study group for liver disease. *Lancet,* **i,** 119–121.
143. *Lancet* (1976) Interferon therapy in chronic hepatitis B (Editorial). *Lancet,* **ii,** 1122–1124.
144. *Lancet* (1978) Immunosuppressive therapy for chronic active hepatitis. (Editorial). *Lancet,* **ii,** 507–508.
145. Last, P.M. (1957) The treatment of active chronic infectious hepatitis with ACTH (corticotrophin) and cortisone. *Medical Journal of Australia,* **1,** 672–676.
146. Lee, W.M., Reed, W.D., Mitchell, C.G., Galbraith, R.M., Eddleston, A.L.W.F., Zuckerman, A.J. & Williams, R. (1975) Cellular and humoral immunity to hepatitis-B surface antigen in active chronic hepatitis. *British Medical Journal,* **i,** 705–708.
147. Leevy, C.M. & Tygstrup, N. (Ed.) (1976) *Standardisation of Nomenclature, Diagnostic Criteria and Diagnostic Methodology for Diseases of the Liver and Biliary Tree.* Basel: S. Karger.
148. Levo, Y., Gorevic, P.D., Kassab, H.J., Zucker-Franklin, D. & Franklin, E.C. (1977) Association between hepatitis B virus and essential mixed cryoglobulinemia. *New England Journal of Medicine,* **296** (26), 1501–1504.
149. Lidman, K., Biberfeld, G., Fagraeus, A., Norberg, R., Torstensson, R., Utter, G., Carlsson, L., Luca, J. & Lindberg, U. (1976) Anti-actin specificity of human smooth muscle antibodies in chronic active hepatitis. *Clinical and Experimental Immunology,* **24,** 266–272.
150. Lindberg, J., Lindholm., A. & Iwarson, S. (1977) Genetic factors in the development of chronic active hepatitis. *Lancet,* **i,** 67–68.
151. London, T.W. (1977) Hepatitis B virus and antigen-antibody complex diseases. *New England Journal of Medicine,* **296** (26), 1528–1529.
152. Mackay, I.R. (1968) Chronic hepatitis: effect of prolonged suppressive treatment and comparison of azathioprine with prednisolone. *Quarterly Journal of Medicine,* **37,** 379–392.
153. Mackay, I.R. & Wood, I.J. (1962) Lupoid hepatitis: a comparison of 22 cases with other types of chronic liver disease. *Quarterly Journal of Medicine,* **31,** 485–507.
154. Mackay, I.R., Taft, L.I. & Cowling, D.C. (1956) Lupoid hepatitis. *Lancet,* **ii,** 1323–1326.
155. MacKay, J.R. & Morris, P.J. (1972) Association of autoimmune active chronic hepatitis with HL-Al, 8 *Lancet,* **ii,** 793–795.
156. Maddrey, W.C. & Boitnott, J.K. (1973) Isoniazid hepatitis. *Annals of Internal Medicine,* **79,** 1–12.
157. Maddrey, W.C. & Boitnott, J.K. (1977) Progress in hepatology: drug-induced chronic liver disease. *Gastroenterology,* **72** (6), 1348–1353.
158. Mathews, J.D. & Mackay, I.R. (1970) Australia antigen in chronic hepatitis in Australia. *British Medical Journal,* **i,** 259–261.
159. Maynard, E.P., Sadikali, F., Anthony, P.P. & Barker, L.F. (1970) Hepatitis associated antigen and cirrhosis in Uganda. *Lancet,* **ii,** 1326.
160. Mazzur, S. (1976) Genetic mimicry by hepatitis B virus. *Nature,* **261,** 316–317.
161. McIntosh, R.M., Koss, M.N. & Gocke, D.J. (1976) The nature and incidence of cryoproteins in hepatitis B antigen (HBsAg) positive patients. *Quarterly Journal of Medicine,* **177,** 23–38.
162. Meyer zum Büschenfelde, K.H. & Miescher, P.A. (1972) Liver specific antigens: purification and characterization. *Clinical and Experimental Immunology,* **10,** 89–102.

163. Meyer zum Büschenfelde, K.H., Knolle, J. & Berger, J. (1974) Cellulare gegenuber homologen leberspezifischen Antigenen (HLP) bei chronischen Leberentzundungen. *Klinische Wochenschrift,* **52,** 246–248.
164. Miller, J., Smith, M.G.M., Mitchell, C.G., Reed, W.D., Eddleston, A.L.W.F. & Williams, R. (1972) Cell-mediated immunity to a human liver-specific antigen in patients with active chronic hepatitis and primary biliary cirrhosis. *Lancet,* **ii,** 296–297.
165. Millward-Sadler, G.H. (1976) Pathological aspects of virus hepatitis. In *Topics in Gastroenterology* (Ed.) Truelove, S.C. & Ritchie, J.A. Vol. 4, pp. 29–54. Oxford: Blackwell Scientific Publications.
166. Mistilis, S.P., Skyring, A.P. & Blackburn, C.R.B. (1968) Natural history of active chronic hepatitis I. Clinical features, course, diagnostic criteria, morbidity, mortality and survival. *Australasian Annals of Medicine,* **17,** 214–223.
167. Mosley, J.W., Redeker, A.G., Feinstone, S.M. & Purcell, R.H. (1977) Multiple hepatitis viruses in multiple attacks of acute viral hepatitis. *New England Journal of Medicine,* **296,** 75–78.
168. Murray-Lyon, I.A., Stern, R.B. & Williams, R. (1973) Controlled trial of prednisone and azathioprine in active chronic hepatitis. *Lancet,* **i,** 735–737.
169. Nefzger, M.D. & Chalmers, T.C. (1963) Treatment of acute infectious hepatitis: ten-year follow-up study of effects of diet and rest. *American Journal of Medicine,* **35,** 299–309.
170. Nelson, J.M., Barker, L.F. & Danovitch, S.H. (1970) Intranuclear aggregate in the liver of a patient with serum hepatitis, *Lancet,* **ii,** 773–774.
171. Neurath, A.R. (1975) Discussion on viral hepatitis; the agents (hepatitis B virus). *American Journal of the Medical Sciences,* **270,** 205–206.
172. Nielsen, J.O., Dietrichson, O. & Juhl, E. (1974) Incidence and meaning of the 'e' determinant among hepatitis-B-antigen positive patients with acute and chronic liver diseases. Report from the Copenhagen Hepatitis Acuta Programme. *Lancet,* **ii,** (7886), 913–915.
173. Nordenfelt, E. & Andrén-Sandberg, M. (1976) Dane particle-associated DNA polymerase and e antigen: relation to chronic hepatitis among carriers of hepatitis B surface antigen. *Journal of Infectious Diseases,* **134** (1), 85–89.
174. Nowosławski, A., Brzosko, W.J., Madalinski, K. & Krawczynski, K. (1970) Cellular localisation of Australia antigen in the liver of patients with lymphoproliferative disorders. *Lancet,* **i,** 494–498.
175. Onion, D.K., Crumpacker, C.S. & Gilliland, B.C. (1971) Arthritis of hepatitis associated with Australia antigen. *Annals of Internal Medicine,* **75,** 29–33.
176. Orr, W. (1974) The requirement for platelets in the active Arthus reaction. *American Journal of Pathology,* **64,** 257–270.
177. Pagaltsos, A.P., Smith, M.G.M., Eddleston, A.L.W.F. & Williams, R. (1971) Serum total haemolytic complement in liver disease. In *Immunology of the Liver* (Ed.) Smith, M. & Williams, R. pp. 93–100. London: Heinemann.
178. Page, A.R. & Good, R.A. (1960) Plasma-cell hepatitis, with special attention to steroid therapy. *American Journal of Diseases of Children,* **99,** 288–314.
179. Panush, R.S., Wilkinson, L.S. & Fagin, R.R. (1973) Chronic active hepatitis associated with eosinophilia and Coombs' positive hemolytic anemia. *Gastroenterology,* **64,** 1015–1019.
180. Paronetto, F. & Vernace, S. (1975) Immunological studies in patients with chronic active hepatitis. Cytotoxic activity of lymphocytes to autochthonous liver cells grown in tissue culture. *Clinical and Experimental Immunology,* **19,** 99–104.
181. Paronetto, F., Rubin, E. & Popper, H. (1962) Local formation of γ-globulin in the diseased liver and its relation to hepatic necrosis. *Laboratory Investigation,* **11,** 150–158.
182. Peters, R.L. (1975) Viral hepatitis: a pathologic spectrum. *American Journal of the Medical Sciences,* **270,** 17–31.
183. Popper, H. & Schaffner, F. (1971) The vocabulary of chronic hepatitis. *New England Journal of Medicine,* **284,** 1154–1156.
184. Popper, H. & Schaffner, F. (1976) Chronic hepatitis: taxonomic, etiologic and therapeutic problems. In *Progress in Liver Diseases,* Vol. 5, pp. 531–538. New York: Grune & Stratton.
185. Poulsen, H. & Christoffersen, P. (1969) Abnormal bile duct epithelium in liver biopsies with histological signs of viral hepatitis. *Acta Pathologica et Microbiologica Scandinavica,* **76,** 383–390.
186. Prince, A.M. (1971) Role of serum hepatitis virus in chronic liver disease. *Gastroenterology,* **60,** 913–921.
187. Prince, A.M. & Burke, K. (1970) Serum hepatitis antigen (SH): rapid detection by high voltage immunoelectroosmophoresis. *Science,* **169,** 593–595.
188. Purcell, R.H., Gerin, J.L., London, W.T., Wagner, J., McAuliffe, V.J., Popper, H., Palmer, A.E., Lvovsky, E., Kaplan, P.M., Wong, D. & Levy, H.B. (1976) Modification of chronic hepatitis-B virus infection in chimpanzees by administration of an interferon inducer. *Lancet,* **ii,** 757–761.
189. Ray, M.B., Desmet, V.J., De Groote, J., Bradburne, A.F. & Desmyter, J. (1976) Distribution patterns of hepatitis B surface antigen (HBsAg) in the liver of hepatitis patients. *Journal of Clinical Pathology,* **29,** 94–100.
190. Read, A.E., Sherlock, S. & Harrison, C.V. (1963) Active 'juvenile' cirrhosis considered as part of a systemic disease and the effect of corticosteroid therapy. *Gut,* **4,** 378–393.
191. Reed, W.D., Eddleston, A.L.W.F., Cullens, H. & Williams, R. (1973) Infusion of hepatitis B antibody in antigen positive active chronic hepatitis. *Lancet,* **ii,** 1347–1351.
192. Reinicke, V., Dybkjaer, E., Poulsen, H., Banke, O., Lyloff, K. & Nordenfelt, E. (1972) A study of Australia antigen positive blood donors and their recipients with special reference to liver histology. *New England Journal of Medicine,* **286,** 867–870.
193. Reynolds, T.B., Peters, R.L. & Yamada, S. (1971) Chronic active and lupoid hepatitis caused by a laxative oxyphenisatin. *New England Journal of Medicine,* **285,** 813–820.
194. Ricci, G., De Bac, C. & Caramia, F. (1973) Carriers of hepatitis B antigen: an epidemiologic and histologic study. *Journal of Infectious Diseases,* **128,** 125–128.
195. Richey, J., Rogers, S. & Van Thiel, D.H. (1977) Giant multinucleated hepatocytes in an adult with chronic active hepatitis. *Gastroenterology,* **73,** 570–574.
196. Rizzetto, M., Swana, G. & Doniach, D. (1973) Microsomal antibodies in active chronic hepatitis and other disorders. *Clinical and Experimental Immunology,* **15,** 331–344.

197. Rizzetto, M., Bonino, F., Crivelli, O., Canese, M.G. & Verme, G. (1976) Complement fixing hepatitis B core antigen immune complexes in the liver of patients with HBs antigen positive chronic disease. *Gut,* **17,** 837–843.

198. Rizzetto, M., Bonino, F., Diana, S. & Verme, G. (1976) Prognostic significance of in-vitro complement fixation in liver biopsy specimens from patients with acute viral hepatitis type B. *Lancet,* **ii,** 436–438.

199. Rizzetto, M., Canese, M.G., Arnico, S., Crivelli, O., Trepo, C., Bonino, F. & Verme, G. (1977) Immunofluorescence detection of new antigen-antibody system (δ/anti-δ) associated to hepatitis B virus in liver and in serum of HBsAg carriers. *Gut,* **18,** 997–1003.

200. Robinson, W.S. (1977) The genome of hepatitis B virus. *Annual Review of Microbiology,* **31,** 357–377.

201. Roos, C.M., Feltkamp-Vroom, T.M. & Helder, A.W. (1976) The localisation of hepatitis B antigen and immunoglobulin G in liver tissue: an immunofluorescence, light and electron microscopic study. *Journal of Pathology,* **118,** 1–8.

202. Russell, R.I., Goldberg, D.M., Allan, J.G., MacSween, R.N.M. & Wallace, J. (1974) A study of hepatic disease in Australia antigen and antibody-positive blood donors. *American Journal of Digestive Diseases,* **19,** 113–121.

203. Sabesin, S.M. & Koff, R.S. (1974) Pathogenesis of experimental viral hepatitis. I. *New England Journal of Medicine,* **290,** 944–950.

204. Sabesin, S.M. & Koff, R.S. (1974) Pathogenesis of experimental viral hepatitis. II. *New England Journal of Medicine,* **290,** 996–1002.

205. Salaspuro, M. & Sipponen, P. (1976) Demonstration of an intracellular copper-binding protein by orcein staining in long-standing cholestatic liver diseases. *Gut,* **17,** 787–790.

206. Salaspuro, M.P., Laitinen, O.I., Lehtola, J., Makkonen, H., Rasanen, J.A. & Sipponen, P. (1976) Immunological parameters, viral antibodies and biochemical and histological findings in relatives of patients with chronic active hepatitis and primary biliary cirrhosis. *Scandinavian Journal of Gastroenterology,* **11,** 313–320.

207. Sampliner, R. (1977) Chronic active hepatitis in hepatitis B surface antigen (HBsAg) carriers. *Journal of the American Medical Association,* **237,** 50–51.

208. Sanchez-Tapias, J., Thomas, H.C. & Sherlock, S. (1977) Lymphocyte populations in liver biopsy specimens from patients with chronic liver disease. *Gut,* **18,** 474–475.

209. Sarkany, I. (1966) Juvenile cirrhosis and allergic capillaritis of the skin. A hepatocutaneous syndrome. *Lancet,* **ii,** 666–668.

210. Schaefer, J.W., Schiff, L., Gall, E.A. & Oikawa, Y. (1967) Progression of acute hepatitis to postnecrotic cirrhosis. *American Journal of Medicine,* **42,** 348–358.

211. Schaffner, F. & Popper, H. (1963) Capillarization of hepatic sinusoids in man. *Gastroenterology,* **44,** 239–242.

212. Schalm, S.W., Summerskill, W.H.J., Gitnick, G.I. & Elveback, L.R. (1976) Contrasting features and responses to treatment of severe chronic active liver disease with and without hepatitis B_s antigen. *Gut,* **17,** 781–786.

213. Schalm, S.W., Korman, M.G., Summerskill, W.H.J., Czaja, A.J. & Baggenstoss, A.H. (1977) Severe chronic active liver disease. Prognostic significance of initial morphological patterns. *American Journal of Digestive Diseases,* **22,** 973–980.

214. Scheuer, P.J. (1977) Chronic hepatitis: a problem for the pathologist. *Histopathology,* **1,** 5–19.

215. Schweitzer, I.L. & Peters, R.L. (1974) Acute submassive hepatic necrosis due to methyldopa. *Gastroenterology,* **66,** 1203–1211.

216. Seeff, L.B., Zimmerman, H.J., Wright, E.C., Schiff, E.R., Kiernan, T., Leevy, C.M., Tamburro, C.H. & Ishak, K.G. (1975) Hepatic disease in asymptomatic parenteral narcotic drug abusers: a Veterans Administration collaborative study. *American Journal of the Medical Sciences,* **270,** 41–47.

217. Selmair, H., Vido, I., Wildhirt, E. & Ortmans, H. (1970) Die chronisch-nekrotisierende Hepatitis. *Deutsche Medizinische Wochenschrift,* **26,** 1397–1401.

218. Sergent, J.S., Lockshin, M.D., Christian, C.L. & Gocke, D.J. (1976) Vasculitis with hepatitis B antigenemia: long-term observation in nine patients. *Medicine (Baltimore),* **55,** 1–18.

219. Sherlock, S. (1948) Post-hepatitis cirrhosis. *Lancet,* **i,** 817–822.

220. Sherlock, S. (1966) Waldenstrom's chronic active hepatitis. *Acta Medica Scandinavica* (Suppl.), **445,** 426–433.

221. Sherlock, S. (1973) Active chronic hepatitis. In *The Liver,* I.A.P. Monograph (Ed.) Gall, E.A. & Mostofi, F.K. pp. 342–360. Baltimore: Williams & Wilkins Co.

222. Sherlock, S. (1974) Progress report, chronic hepatitis. *Gut,* **15,** 581–597.

223. Shikata, T., Uzawa, T., Yoshiwara, N., Akatsuka, T. & Yamasaki, S. (1974) Staining methods of Australia antigen in paraffin section: detection of cytoplasmic inclusion bodies. *Japanese Journal of Experimental Medicine,* **44,** 25–36.

224. Shikata, T., Karasawa, T., Abe, K., Uzawa, T., Suzuki, H., Oda, T., Imai, M., Mayumi, M. & Moritsugu, Y. (1977) Hepatitis B e antigen and infectivity of hepatitis B virus. *Journal of Infectious Diseases,* **136,** 571–576.

225. Shrago, S.S., Auslander, M.O. & Gitnick, G.L. (1977) Hepatic pathologic condition in asymptomatic Australia antigen carriers. A light microscopical study of 26 cases and a review of the literature. *Archives of Pathology and Laboratory Medicine,* **101,** 648–651.

226. Shulman, S., Schulkind, M. & Ayoub, E. (1974) Transfer-factor therapy of chronic active hepatitis. *Lancet,* **ii,** 650.

227. Simon, J.B. & Patel, S.K. (1974) Liver disease in asymptomatic carriers of hepatitis B antigen. *Gastroenterology,* **66,** 1020–1028.

228. Singleton, J.W., Merrill, D.A., Fitch, R.A., Merrill, D.A., Kohler, P.F. & Rettberg, W.A.H. (1971) Liver disease in Australia-antigen blood donors. *Lancet,* **ii,** 785–787.

229. Smith, J.L., Murphy, B.L., Auslander, M.O., Maynard, J.E., Schalm, S.S., Summerskill, W.H.J. & Gitnick, G.L. (1976) Studies of the 'e' antigen in acute and chronic hepatitis. *Gastroenterology,* **71,** 208–209.

230. Smith, M.G.M., Williams, R., Walker, G., Rizzetto, M. & Doniach, D. (1974) Hepatic disorders, associated with liver/kidney microsomal antibodies. *British Medical Journal,* **ii,** 80–84.

231. Soloway, R.D., Summerskill, W.H.J., Baggenstoss, A.H., Geall, M.G., Gitnick, G.L., Elveback, L.R. & Schoenfield, L.J. (1972) Clinical, biochemical and histological remission of severe chronic active liver disease: a controlled study of treatments and early prognosis. *Gastroenterology,* **63,** 820–833.

232. Spero, J.A., Lewis, J.H., Van Thiel, D.H., Hasiba, U. & Rabin, B.S. (1978) Asymptomatic structural liver disease in haemophilia. *New England Journal of Medicine,* **298,** 1373–1378.

233. Stein, O., Fainaru, M. & Stein, Y. (1972) Visualization of virus-like particles in endoplasmic reticulum of hepatocytes of Australia antigen carriers. *Laboratory Investigation,* **26,** 262–269.

234. Stern, R.B., Wilkinson, S.P., Howorth, P.J.N. & Williams, R. (1977) Controlled trial of synthetic D-penicillamine and prednisone in maintenance therapy for active chronic hepatitis. *Gut,* **18,** 19–22.

235. Sternlieb, I. & Scheinberg, I.H. (1972) Chronic hepatitis as a first manifestation of Wilson's disease. *Annals of Internal Medicine,* **76,** 59–64.

236. Summerskill, W.H.J. (1974) Chronic active liver disease re-examined: prognosis hopeful. *Gastroenterology,* **66,** 450–464.

237. Summerskill, W.H.J., Korman, M.G., Ammon, H.V. & Baggenstoss, A. (1975) Prednisone for chronic active liver disease: dose titration, standard dose and combination with azathioprine compared. *Gut,* **16,** 876–883.

238. Sutnick, A.I., London, W.T., Gerstley, B.J.S., Cronlund, M.M. & Blumberg, B.S. (1968) Anicteric hepatitis associated with Australia antigen. Occurrence in patients with Down's syndrome. *Journal of the American Medical Association,* **205,** 670–674.

239. Szmuness, W. (1975) Recent advances in the study of the epidemiology of hepatitis B. *American Journal of Pathology,* **81,** 629–650.

240. Szmuness, W., Harley, E.J. & Prince, A.M. (1975) Intrafamilial spread of asymptomatic hepatitis. *American Journal of the Medical Sciences,* **270,** 293–304.

241. Tabor, E., Gerety, R.J. & Barker, L.F. (1977) Detection of e antigen during acute and chronic hepatitis B virus infections in chimpanzees. *Journal of Infectious Diseases,* **136,** 541–547.

242. Tabor, E., Gerety, R.J., Drucker, J.A., Seeff, L.B., Hoofnagle, J.H., Jackson, D.R., April, M., Barker, L.F. & Pineda-Tamondong, G. (1978) Transmission of non-A non-B hepatitis from man to chimpanzee. *Lancet,* **i,** 463–466.

243. Tage-Jensen, U., Arnold, W., Dietrichson, O., Hardt, F., Hopf, U., Meyer zum Büschenfelde, K.H. & Nielsen, J.O. (1977) Liver-cell membrane autoantibody specific for inflammatory liver diseases. *British Medical Journal,* **i,** 206–208.

244. Tapp, E. & Jones, D.M. (1977) HBsAg and HBcAg in the livers of asymptomatic HB antigen carriers. *Journal of Clinical Pathology,* **30,** 671–677.

245. Teisberg, P. & Gjone, E. (1973) Circulating conversion products of C3 in liver disease: evidence for in vivo activation of the complement system. *Clinical and Experimental Immunology,* **14,** 509–514.

246. Theodoropoulos, G., Econompoulos, P., Mitakos, S. & Angelopoulos, B. (1974) The relationship between hepatitis-associated antigen and the development of hepatocellular cancer. *Acta Hepato-gastroenterologica,* **21,** 430–432.

247. Thestrup-Pedersen, K., Ladefoged, K. & Andersen, P. (1976) Lymphocyte transformation test with liver-specific protein and phytohaemagglutinin in patients with liver disease. *Clinical and Experimental Immunology,* **24,** 1–8.

248. Thomsen, P., Poulsen, H. & Petersen, P. (1977) Different types of ground glass hepatocytes in human liver biopsies. Morphology, recurrence and diagnostic significance. *Scandinavian Journal of Gastroenterology,* **11,** 113–119.

249. Tobias, H., Safran, A.P. & Schaffner, F. (1967) Lymphocyte stimulation and chronic liver disease. *Lancet,* **i,** 193–195.

250. Toghill, P.J., Smith, P.G., Benton, P., Brown, R.C. & Matthews, H.L. (1974) Methyldopa liver damage. *British Medical Journal,* **iii,** 545–548.

251. Toh, B.H., Roberts-Thomson, I.C., Matthews, J.D., Whittingham, S. & Mackay, I.R. (1975) Depression of cell-mediated immunity in old age and the immunopathic diseases, lupus erythematosus, chronic hepatitis and rheumatoid arthritis. *Clinical and Experimental Immunology,* **14,** 193–202.

252. Tolentino, P., Dianzani, F., Zucca, M. & Giacchino, R. (1975) Decreased interferon response by lymphocyte from children with chronic hepatitis. *Journal of Infectious Diseases,* **132** (4), 459–461.

253. Tong, M.J., Nystrom, J.S., Redeker, A.G. & Marshall, G.J. (1976) Failure of transfer-factor therapy in chronic active type B hepatitis. *New England Journal of Medicine,* **295** (4), 209–211.

254. Trepo, C.H. & Thivolet, J. (1970) Hepatitis associated antigen and periarteritis nodosa. *Vox Sanguinis,* **19,** 410–411.

255. Trepo, C., Vitvitsky, L., Neurath, R., Hashimoto, N., Schaefer, R., Nemoz, G. & Prince, A.M. (1976) Detection of e antigen by immunofluorescence in cytoplasm of hepatocytes of HBsAg carriers. *Lancet,* **i,** 486.

256. Triger, D.R., Alp, M.H. & Wright, R. (1972) Bacterial and dietary antibodies in liver disease. *Lancet,* **i,** 60–63.

257. Triger, D.R., Kurtz, J.B. & Wright, R. (1974) Viral antibodies in chronic liver disease. *Gut,* **15,** 94–98.

258. Triger, D.R., Kurtz, J.B., MacCallum, F.O. & Wright, R. (1972) Raised antibody titres to measles and rubella viruses in chronic active hepatitis. *Lancet,* **i,** 665–667.

259. Triger, D.R., Millward-Sadler, G.H., Czaykowski, A.A., Trowell, J. & Wright, R. (1976) Alpha-1-antitrypsin deficiency and liver disease in adults. *Quarterly Journal of Medicine,* **45,** 351–372.

260. Turner-Warwick, M. (1968) Fibrosing alveolitis and chronic liver disease. *Quarterly Journal of Medicine,* **37,** 133–149.

261. Velasco, M., Gonzalez-Ceron, M., de la Fuente, C., Ruiz, A., Donoso, S. & Katz, R. (1978) Clinical and pathological study of asymptomatic HBsAg carriers in Chile. *Gut,* **19,** 569–571.

262. Vittal, S.B.V., Dourdourekas, D. & Shobassay, N. (1974) Asymptomatic hepatic disease in blood donors with hepatitis B antigenemia. *American Journal of Clinical Pathology,* **62,** 649–654.

263. Vogten, A.J.M., Schalm, S.W., Summerskill, W.H.J., Smith, J.L., Gitnick, G.L., Murphy, B.L. & Maynard, J.E. (1976) Behaviour of e antigen and antibody during chronic active liver disease. Relation to HB antigen-antibody system and prognosis. *Lancet,* **ii,** 126–128.

264. Vyas, G.N., Williams, E.W., Klaus, G.G.B. & Bond, H.E. (1972) Hepatitis-associated Australia antigen, protein, peptides and amino acid composition of

purified antigen with its use in determining sensitivity of the hemagglutination test. *Journal of Immunology*, **108,** 1114.

265. Waldenstrom, J. (1950) Leber, blutproteine und nahrungseweiis stoffwechs. *Sonderband XV Tagung Bad Kissingen*, p. 8.
266. Wands, J.R. & Isselbacher, K.J. (1975) Lymphocyte cytotoxicity to autologous liver cells in chronic active hepatitis. *Proceedings of the National Academy of Science*, **72** (4), 1301–1303.
267. Wands, J.R., Alpert, E. & Isselbacher, K.J. (1975) Arthritis associated with chronic active hepatitis: complement activation and characterization of circulating immune complexes. *Gastroenterology*, **69,** 1286–1291.
268. Wands, J.R., Davis, T.E., Humphrey, R.L., Santos, J.W., Owens, A.H., Alpert, E. & Isselbacher, K.J. (1975) Serial studies on hepatitis B surface antigen and antibody following bone marrow transplantation for acute leukaemia. *Gastroenterology*, **69,** 879.
269. Wands, J.R., Mann, E., Alpert, E. & Isselbacher, K.J. (1975) The pathogenesis of arthritis associated with acute HBsAg positive hepatitis: complement-activation and characterization of circulating immune complexes. *Journal of Clinical Investigation*, **55,** 930–936.
270. Wands, J.R., Perrotto, J.L., Alpert, E. & Isselbacher, K.J. (1975) Cell-mediated immunity in acute and chronic hepatitis. *Journal of Clinical Investigation*, **55,** 921–929.
271. Whelton, M.J. (1970) Arthropathy and liver disease. *British Journal of Hospital Medicine*, **3,** 243–247.
272. Whittingham, S., Mackay, I.R. & Irwin, J. (1966) Autoimmune hepatitis. *Lancet*, **i,** 1333–1335.
273. Winkler, K., Junge, U. & Creutzfeldt, W. (1977) Ground glass hepatocytes in unselected liver biopsies. Ultrastructure and relationship to hepatitis B antigen. *Scandinavian Journal of Gastroenterology*, **ii,** 167–170.
274. Woolf, I.L., Boyes, B.E., Jones, D.M., Whittacker, J.S., Tapp, E., MacSween, R.N.M., Renton, P.H., Stratton, F. & Dymock, I.W. (1974) Asymptomatic liver disease in hepatitis B antigen carriers. *Journal of Clinical Pathology*, **27,** 348–352.
275. Woolf, I.L., El Sheikh, N., Cullens, H., Lee, W.M., Eddleston, A.L.W.F., Williams, R. & Zuckerman, A.V. (1976) Enhanced HB_sAg production in pathogenesis of fulminant viral hepatitis type B. *British Medical Journal*, **ii,** 669–671.
276. Wright, E.C., Seeff, L.B., Berk, P.D., Jones, A. & Plotz, P.H. (1977) Treatment of chronic active hepatitis: an analysis of three controlled trials. *Gastroenterology*, **73,** 1422–1430.
277. Wright, R. (1970) The Australia antigen in chronic active hepatitis. *Vox Sanguinis*, **19,** 320–326.
278. Wright, R. (1970) Australia antigen and smooth-muscle antibody in acute and chronic hepatitis. *Lancet*, **i,** 521–522.
279. Wright, R. (1972) Chronic hepatitis. *British Medical Bulletin*, **28,** 120–124.
280. Wright, R. (1977) Immunology of gastrointestinal and liver disease. In *Current Topics in Immunology* (Ed.) Turk, J. London: Edward Arnold.
281. Wright, R., McCollum, R.W. & Klatskin, G. (1969) Australia antigen in acute and chronic active hepatitis. *Lancet*, **ii,** 117–121.
282. Wright, R., Perkins, J.R., Bower, B.D. & Jerrome, D.W. (1970) Cirrhosis associated with the Australia antigen in an infant who acquired hepatitis from her mother. *British Medical Journal*, **iv,** 719–721.
283. Yamada, G. & Nakane, P.K. (1977) Hepatitis B core and surface antigens in liver tissue. Light and electron microscope localization by the peroxidase-labeled antibody method. *Laboratory Investigation*, **36,** 649–659.
284. Yeung Laiwah, A.A.C. (1971) Lymphocyte transformation by Australia antigen. *Lancet*, **ii,** 470–471.
285. Zappi, T., Vernace, S.J., Gerber, M.A. & Paronetto, F. (1976) Serum antibodies to hepatitis B antigen (anti-HBc) in HBsAg positive and negative chronic hepatitis. *Gastroenterology*, **70,** A–139.
286. Zuckerman, A.J. (1974) Genetic factors in hepatitis. *Nature*, **248,** 377.
287. Chisari, F.V., Edgington, T.S., Routenberg, J.A. & Anderson, D.S. (1978) Cellular immune reactivity in HBV-induced liver disease. In *Viral Hepatitis* (Ed.) Vyas, G.N., Cohen, S.N. & Schmid, R. pp. 245–266. Philadelphia: Franklin Institute Press.
288. Drew, J.S., London, W.T., Lustbader, E.D., Hesser, J.E. & Blumberg, B.S. (1978) Hepatitis B virus and sex ratio of offspring. *Science*, **201,** 687–692.
289. *Lancet* (1978). Son of Australia antigen? *Lancet*, **ii,** 1241–1242.
290. Merigan, T.C. & Robinson, W.S. (1978) Antiviral therapy in HBV infection. In *Viral Hepatitis* (Ed.) Vyas, G.N., Cohen, S.N. & Schmid, R. pp. 575–579. Philadelphia: Franklin Institute Press.
291. Rakela, J. & Redeker, A.G. (1979) Chronic liver disease after acute non-A, non-B viral hepatitis. *Gastroenterology*, **77,** 1200–1202.
292. Black, M., Rabin, L. & Schatz, N. (1980) Nitrofurantoin-induced chronic active hepatitis. *Annals of Internal Medicine*, **92,** 62–64.

Chapter 30

Cirrhosis: an Appraisal

G. H. MILLWARD-SADLER
RALPH WRIGHT

In the evolution of many chronic liver diseases cirrhosis is a stage that is considered to be irreversible. Removal or control of the primary disease process may stabilize the cirrhosis or may slow down its rate of progression, but its presence implies consequences that are unrelated to the primary aetiology of the cirrhosis. These consequences include vascular disturbances such as intrahepatic shunting of blood and obstruction to portal venous blood flow. There is resulting portal venous hypertension (Chapter 43) and impaired parenchymal function, including protein synthesis, hormone metabolism and excretion of bile and bile salts.

The exact point at which a disease process has produced cirrhosis is difficult to define and this problem is magnified by the increasing use of liver biopsy for diagnosis and management. The biopsy itself is small, so that sampling error occurs and diseases are detected by this investigation at a far earlier stage in their evolution. There is an indeterminate zone between severe fibrosis of the liver and cirrhosis that is clearly manifested in biliary obstruction and in schistosomiasis. In these conditions, extensive fibrosis is common and cirrhosis an uncommon or a late sequel, but the fibrosis is often categorized as cirrhosis. Likewise, congenital hepatic fibrosis produces portal hypertension and may be wrongly diagnosed as cirrhosis. This and the allied condition of polycystic disease of the liver are therefore also considered in this chapter.

DEFINITION

Various definitions of cirrhosis have been given.[1,2,37,56,65] The most recent and, because of its conciseness, in our opinion the best available definition states that cirrhosis is *a diffuse process characterized by fibrosis and a conversion of normal architecture into structurally abnormal nodules.*[1,2]

The involvement of the major part of the liver in a diffuse manner and the presence of fibrosis and nodules are all essential for the diagnosis of cirrhosis. Liver biopsy can infer but never determine the first criterion, and so all needle biopsy diagnoses of cirrhosis must be evaluated with this qualification. Usually the clinical manifestations or imaging techniques will indicate the diffuse nature of the process. Fibrosis is an integral part of the definition and essential to the diagnosis because it differentiates cirrhosis from diffuse nodular hyperplasia[32] (see Chapter 38). It is also important in pathogenesis, as will be discussed later.

Structurally abnormal nodules may be obvious on biopsy specimens, but in some cirrhosis is inferred from the more subtle architectural changes present (see Chapter 18). It is in this latter group that there is most difficulty in biopsy interpretation and in achieving diagnostic accuracy. Regeneration is notable by its absence from the definition. The occurrence of regeneration is important in the pathogenesis, but the morphological recognition of regeneration is not essential for the diagnosis. Nodules identified morphologically do not necessarily show features of regeneration and can be formed passively from cell death and collapse of reticulin in combination with fibrosis.

CLASSIFICATION

Any classification of cirrhosis should be purposeful rather than a taxonomic exercise. It

Table 30.1. *Aetiology of Cirrhosis.*

Drugs and toxins	Alcohol		Chapter 32
	Methotrexate		
	Methyldopa		Chapter 36
	Isoniazid		
Infections	Hepatitis B		
	Hepatitis non-A non-B		Chapter 29
	Schistosoma japonicum		Chapter 56
Autoimmune	Chronic active hepatitis		Chapter 29
	Primary biliary cirrhosis		Chapter 31
Metabolic	Wilson's disease		Chapter 33
	Haemochromatosis		Chapter 34
	Alpha-1-antitrypsin deficiency		Chapter 35
	Carbohydrates:	Galactosaemia	
		Type IV glycogen storage	
	Amino acids	Tyrosinosis	Chapter 40
	Urea cycle	ornithine transcarbamylase	Levin et al[38]
	Lipids	abetalipoproteinaemia	Partin et al[52]
	Porphyria		Chapter 15
Biliary obstruction	Atresia		
	Mucoviscidosis		Chapter 40
	Gallstones		Chapter 53 & 54
	Strictures		
Vascular	Chronic right heart failure		
	Budd-Chiari syndrome		Chapter 43
	Veno-occlusive disease		
Miscellaneous	Neonatal hepatitis syndrome		Chapter 40
	Indian childhood cirrhosis		
	Intestinal bypass		Peters, Gay & Reynolds[53]
	Sarcoidosis		Chapter 37
Cryptogenic			

should provide or help to provide information about the aetiology, the pathogenesis, the state of the disease and the probability of complications. Classification also provides the basic information for epidemiological studies.

Cirrhosis is most satisfactorily classified by its aetiology (see Table 30.1), but even then some causes are grouped under a common pathogenesis, for instance biliary obstruction. In this system, cirrhosis is then a stage in liver damage reached in the evolution of a particular disease.

The other system of classification is based upon morphological appearances and is less satisfactory, but these two classifications are not mutually exclusive. Many of the terms that have been used have indicated conjectural pathogenetic mechanisms, and these are now largely superseded by the classification into micronodular, macronodular and mixed nodularity.[1,2,37,71]

Micronodular cirrhosis has uniform nodules of less than 3 mm in diameter, usually separated by definite but indistinct fine bands of fibrosis.

Macronodular cirrhosis has a majority of nodules which are larger than 3 mm in diameter. A small proportion of small nodules are permissible; even large macronodules may appear less than 3 mm in diameter if tangentially sectioned.

This morphological classification is of greatest value in autopsy studies of the whole liver. Microscopic studies of cirrhosis can frequently suggest the aetiological diagnosis but the division into micronodular and macronodular on the basis of nodule size is clumsy and unsatisfactory. This is partly because of sampling error in biopsies and partly because fixation and processing of tissues for histology can produce a considerable shrinkage artefact.

AETIOLOGY

The aetiology of cirrhosis is varied and in individual cases may be unknown. The major causes are listed in Table 30.1. Their importance varies geographically and socially. Alcohol is the most common cause of cirrhosis in the United States and the United Kingdom (see Chapter 32), but is less frequent in most parts of Africa and Asia. Conversely, cirrhosis due to hepatitis B is common in Africa and many parts of Asia (see Chapter 29), and Indian childhood cirrhosis is rare outside the Indian subcontinent, even in immigrant Indian populations to the United Kingdom. Many of these diseases are separately discussed in individual chapters (see Chapters 29, 31, 32, 33, 34, 35, 36 and 40).

MORPHOLOGY

Macroscopic Features

Micronodular cirrhosis

This is an enlarged, very firm or even hard liver. The overall shape and capsular surface of the liver may not be greatly altered and the nodules on the cut surface are usually indistinct, minute in size but uniform in appearance, and fibrosis is diffuse throughout the liver (Figures 30.1 and 30.2). There may be a tan or yellow colour to the liver because of the fatty change in the hepatocytes, but with significant haemosiderosis the liver is dark brown. Alcohol is frequently associated with this pattern, and other causes include haemochromatosis, biliary obstruction and rare examples of chronic active hepatitis.

Macronodular cirrhosis

This varies much more in size. The liver may be enlarged but, particularly when associated clinically with liver failure, is small and may weigh less than 1000 g. The liver shows large bulging nodules of varying and often widely disparate size and these are separated by fibrous bands which may vary considerably in width (Figures 30.3 and 30.4). Included in this group are cirrhosis due to hepatitis B, HB_sAg negative chronic active hepatitis, cryptogenic cirrhosis and the end-stage cirrhosis of almost any aetiology. The cirrhosis of incomplete septal pattern may be less obvious and histology may be required for its identification.

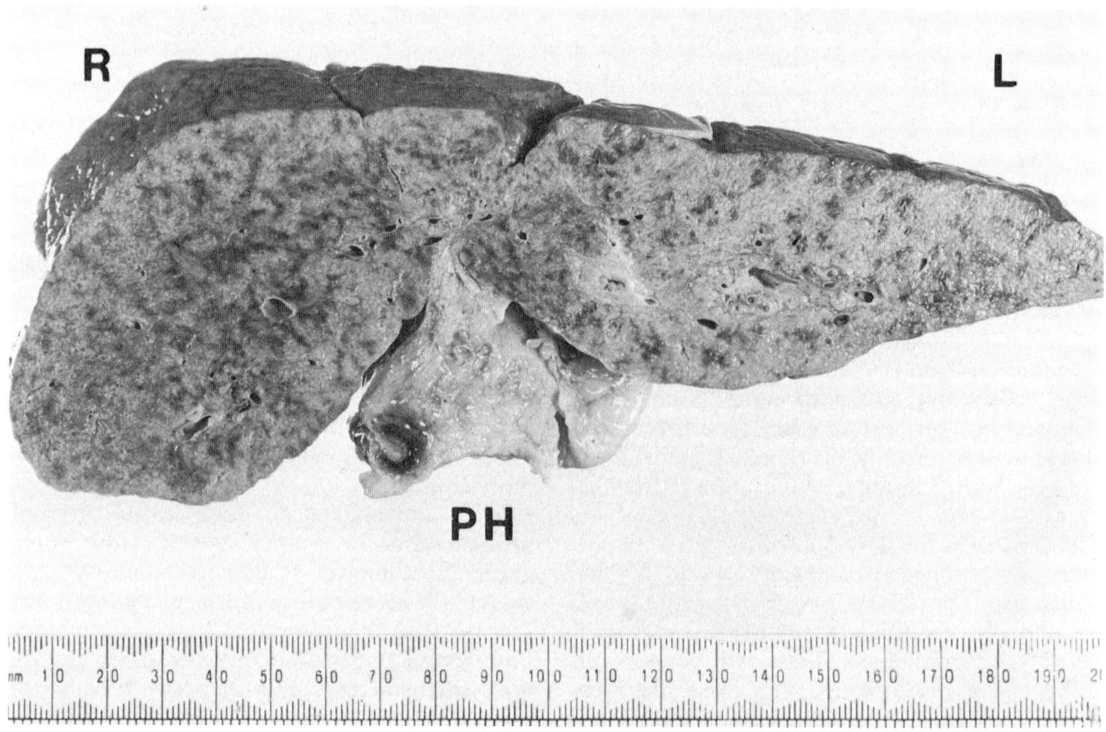

Figure 30.1. Coronal section of liver showing the micronodular cirrhosis of alcoholic liver disease. Note the finely granular capsular surface of the liver. R = right lobe; L = left lobe; PH = porta hepatis.

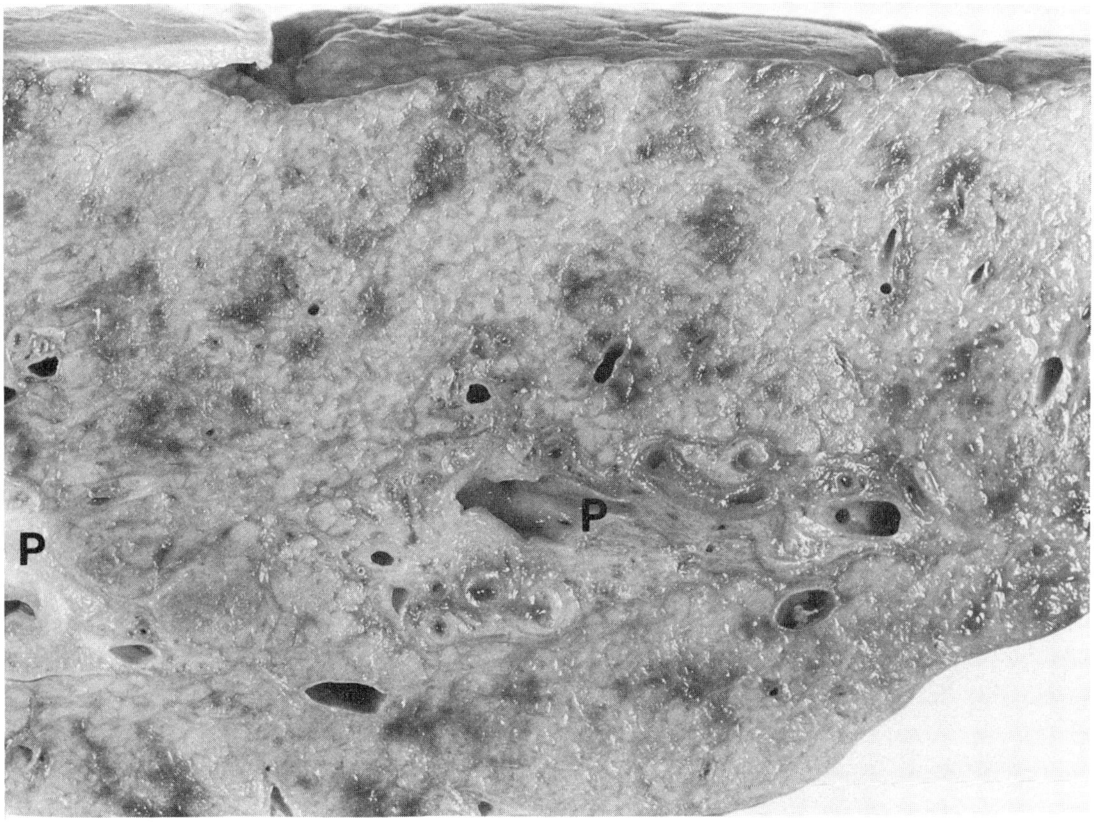

Figure 30.2. Higher power of left lobe of liver illustrated in Figure 30.1. Nodules are most easily seen between the two labelled portal tracts (P) but are present throughout, as can be identified from the slightly irregular capsular surface.

The aetiology or pathogenesis is rarely evident from the macroscopic appearances, although abnormalities of the biliary tree may be demonstrated by dissection and excess iron can be demonstrated grossly by Perls' Prussian blue reaction in appropriate cases.

Necrosis of nodules can be found, particularly in association with clinically significant gastrointestinal bleeding. This necrosis is most easily recognized when they are irregularly distributed throughout the liver so that they contrast with neighbouring nodules. Affected nodules are bright yellow, sometimes with a peripheral red haemorrhagic zone.

Histology

As has already been stated, the simple micronodular/macronodular classification is difficult to apply from routine light microscopy. It is more helpful to relate the architectural distortion to the previous architecture and to identify intralobular and multilobular patterns of disease. This may identify patterns of aetiological significance even in the absence of more specific histological markers or may indicate the stage of a disease process of known aetiology. For instance, alcoholic cirrhosis is usually a micro-micronodular (or intralobular) cirrhosis, but there is evidence that with abstinence this will develop into a macronodular cirrhosis and the complications and prognosis will consequently alter.[36]

Micronodular cirrhosis

Anatomically, lobules are approximately 0.1 cm in diameter. Consequently, micronodular cirrhosis, when defined as nodules less than 0.3 cm in diameter, may contain complete lobules within the nodule. In other cases, nodules may not show any substructure but by their expansive growth appear rounded and surrounded by fibrous tissue that has been orientated into concentric lamellae of collagen. The third and commonest pattern is a micro-micronodular pattern of cirrhosis in which

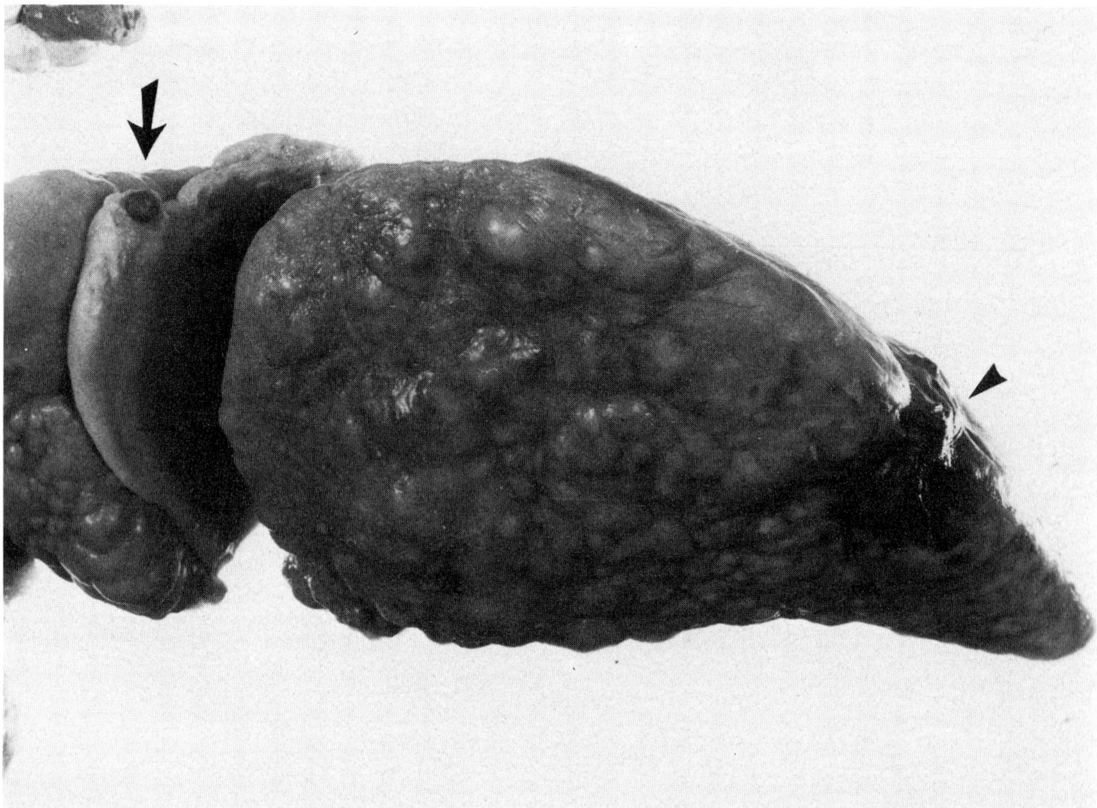

Figure 30.3. Macronodular cirrhosis: the liver is sliced in a coronal plane and shows the inferior margin of the left lobe. Note the thrombosed umbilical vein in the ligamentum teres (arrow) and the biopsy site (arrow head). Numerous large nodules of varying size can be identified on the capsular surface. Adult male aged 62 years with alpha-l-antitrypsin deficiency.

lobules are subdivided into nodules. Virtually every lobule is affected, and this micro-micronodular pattern is associated with alcohol (see Chapter 32), drugs and toxins such as methotrexate[47] and carbon tetrachloride, or metabolic disturbances such as haemochromatosis (see Chapter 34), and many of the inherited childhood causes of cirrhosis, as well as Indian childhood cirrhosis[50] (see Chapter 40).

In this group typically there is fibrosis around the central vein, in the sinusoids and expanding portal tracts so that sub-lobular areas of parenchyma are isolated by irregular centro-portal bridges (Figure 30.5). All major hepatic afferent and efferent channels are then peripheral to these nodules. Features more specific to the aetiology of the cirrhosis can be superimposed upon this basic architectural distortion.

A feature of the majority of these micro-nodular cirrhoses is the relative lack of a significant chronic inflammatory cell infiltrate and frequently the paucity of cells in the areas of fibrosis.

Alcoholic cirrhosis. In active alcoholic cirrhosis, there is fatty change and ballooning degeneration of hepatocytes and Mallory's alcoholic hyalin (Mallory body) is found in many ballooned hepatocytes, but is not exclusive to these cells. In alcoholic hepatitis and in early stages of cirrhosis this hyalin is in hepatocytes in the central area of the lobule (Figure 30.6). Infiltrates of neutrophils are present in the sinusoids and cluster around hepatocytes containing alcoholic hyalin and more especially around apparently extracellular hyalin. Plasma cells, although scanty, are also characteristically present around the central vein in the early stages. More recently, identical histological features associated with a micronodular cirrhosis have been described in intestinal bypass operations for obesity,[53] and in abetalipoproteinaemia.[52]

Cirrhosis due to drugs and toxins other than alcohol must usually be identified by the medical history of occupational, therapeutic or incidental exposure. In methotrexate-induced

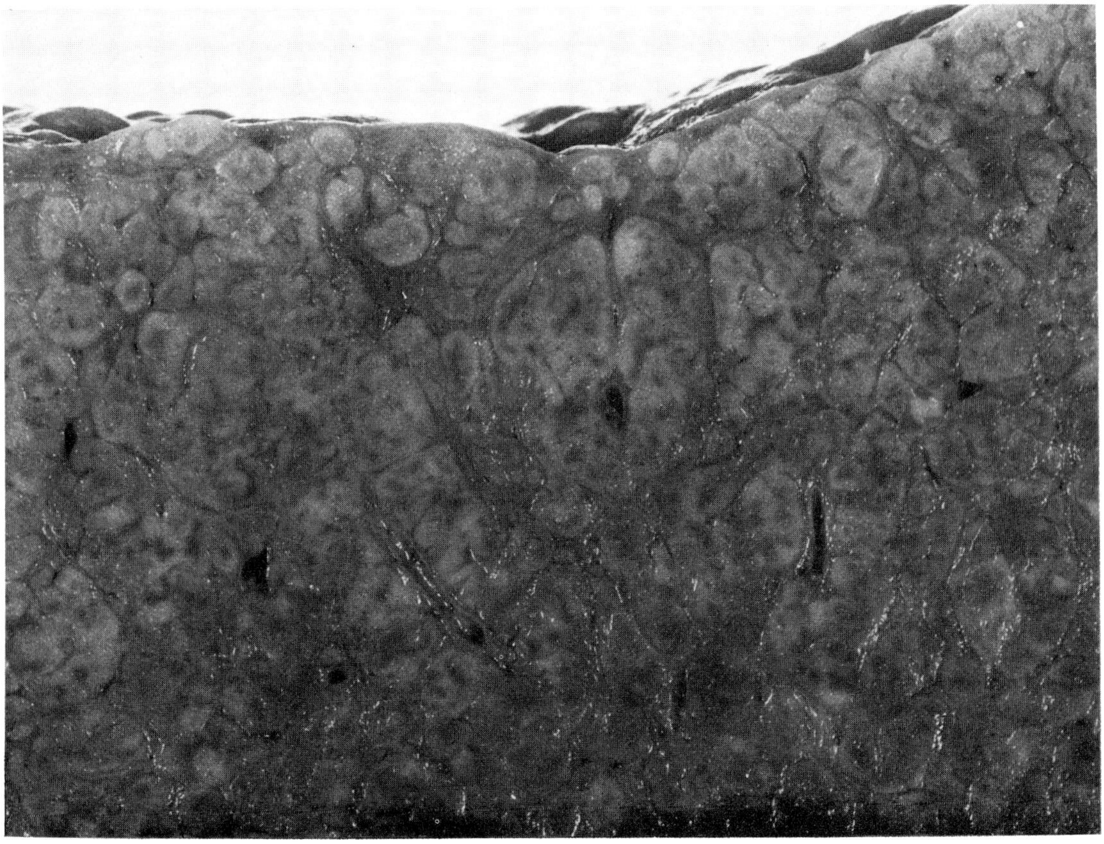

Figure 30.4. Cut surface of liver from Figure 30.3. Note the bosselated capsular surface and the readily identifiable fibrous bands dividing the liver into large nodules.

cirrhosis there is frequently a dramatic nuclear variation in size and shape, partly produced by the gigantism of a few individual nuclei, which possibly results from the anti-folate action of the drug.

Metabolic disorders such as haemochromatosis (Figure 30.7) can be readily identified by specific staining for iron, and deposits of protoporphyrin can be identified by histological examination under polarized light[31] or by electron microscopy.[31,81] Histological features in the childhood carbohydrate, urea cycle and other metabolic disorders are rarely so helpful. Alpha-1-antitrypsin deficiency (see Chapter 35) is a notable exception; the PAS-positive diastase-resistant globules in hepatocytes must be regarded as diagnostic until proved otherwise.

Indian childhood cirrhosis[50] has such a distinctive age range and known racial and geographical features that diagnosis is rarely a problem. Histological features, apart from the fibrosis and architectural distortion, include an abundance of hepatocytes containing Mallory's alcoholic hyalin, vacuolar but not fatty degeneration of hepatocytes, and frequent cholestasis. An extremely high copper-binding protein content can be demonstrated in hepatocytes by the orcein technique[60] (see Chapter 18). The inflammatory infiltrate is mixed and composed of neutrophils in the sinusoids with hepatocytes and histiocytes.

Two other forms of micronodular cirrhosis, chronic biliary obstruction and hepatic venous outflow obstruction, can be identified and result from obstruction to the biliary tree and to the hepatic venous outflow tract. The histological features of these should indicate the pathogenesis if not the exact aetiology.

Chronic biliary obstruction rarely results in cirrhosis. Most commonly the obstruction is due to carcinoma, often inoperable or lethal within a relatively short space of time and before cirrhosis can develop, or due to gallstones when the obstruction is amenable to surgical relief. In addition, chronic biliary obstruction produces portal fibrosis with even-

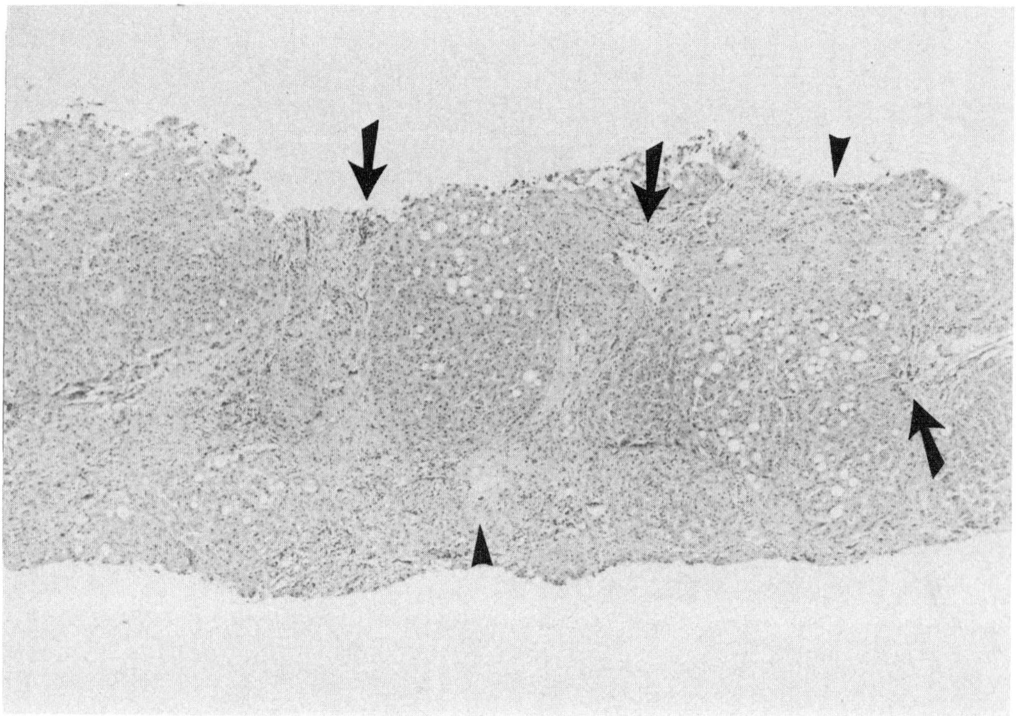

Figure 30.5. Cirrhosis of micronodular pattern. Nodules are formed within the pre-existing lobule by fibrous bridges between central vein (arrowheads) and portal tract (arrows). Haematoxylin and eosin × 100.

tual linking of portal tracts outlining and emphasizing the lobule, as in the pig's liver (Figure 30.8). Cirrhosis is dependent on the interpretation as to when these lobules become abnormal nodules. Such lobules have been interpreted as being indicative of cirrhosis, but it is more commonly accepted that cirrhosis is a later sequel of chronic biliary obstruction.[15]

The histological features are those of acute bile duct obstruction (see Chapter 18) with additional fibrosis, and bile ductule proliferation expanding portal tracts. Bile ducts at this later stage may not be dilated but may show secondary stenosis and periductal fibrosis so that a sclerosing cholangitis may be mimicked. Bile infarcts and old infarcts from which the bile has leaked out may be present. Eventually, a typical 'jigsaw' pattern of secondary biliary cirrhosis (Figure 30.9) is produced.[15]

Extrahepatic obstruction produces a micronodular pattern because the changes are distributed evenly throughout the liver. A different pattern may emerge from focal intrahepatic obstruction, where there will be non-affected areas of liver adjacent to areas showing chronic obstruction. This has been classically described in mucoviscoidosis as 'focal biliary cirrhosis',[14,66] but can also occur in primary biliary cirrhosis. In primary biliary cirrhosis, large bile ducts are affected. When these are destroyed, obstructive changes are produced in the drainage area so that the advanced disease with many ducts affected becomes micronodular in pattern.

Hepatic venous outflow obstruction produces severe congestive changes in centrilobular areas. These changes are associated with pressure atrophy and ischaemic necrosis of centrilobular hepatocytes so that portal tracts with periportal hepatocytes become isolated from each other. Chronic venous obstruction of lesser severity replaces centrilobular areas by bland fibrosis (Figure 30.10) and a pattern of reversed lobulation is seen. This fibrosis is a common complication of chronic obstruction and eventually extends towards portal tracts which also show mild scarring. Cirrhosis is a rare event, primarily because the most common causes of hepatic venous obstruction – right heart and congestive heart failure – are nowadays rarely of sufficient duration unless of non-ischaemic aetiology. Apart from a raised central venous pressure, these changes may be produced by hepatic venous diseases which range from the microscopic veno-occlusive disease affecting

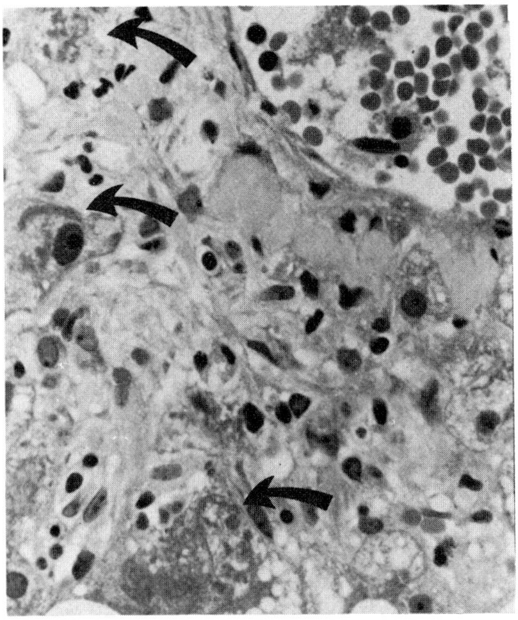

Figure 30.6. Mallory bodies (arrows) in hepatocytes adjacent to the central vein in alcoholic liver disease. Haematoxylin and eosin × 1250.

small centrilobular venous radicles to obstruction of the major hepatic veins as they approach or enter the inferior vena cava (Budd–Chiari syndrome). Causes of veno-occlusive disease include irradiation, Jamaican 'bush-tea' intoxication and the contraceptive pill, while causes of the Budd–Chiari syndrome include strategically situated tumours within the liver and of the inferior vena cava, venous thrombosis associated with myeloproliferative diseases, and a congenital web across the lumen of the hepatic vein (see Chapter 43).

Macronodular cirrhosis

Two basic patterns of macronodular cirrhosis can be demonstrated, and each of these has had a multitude of names.

The post-necrotic, advanced or regenerative pattern. In this, the nodules are separated by dense collagen arranged in bands of varying but often broad width (Figure 30.11). Within these areas of fibrosis there is bile ductule proliferation and a lymphocytic inflammatory cell infiltrate. Thin-walled vascular channels and lymphatics are dilated and often prominent. Juxtaposition of several portal tracts within this fibrosis without intervening parenchyma is frequent and has been interpreted as collapse of the lobular architecture from confluent necrosis. The nodules are usually surrounded by a narrow zone of collagen fibres arranged as concentric lamellae, producing an impression of encapsulation (Figure 30.12). This pseudo-encapsulation may result from the rapid growth of the nodules, and this interpretation is also suggested by their frequently rounded appearance and by

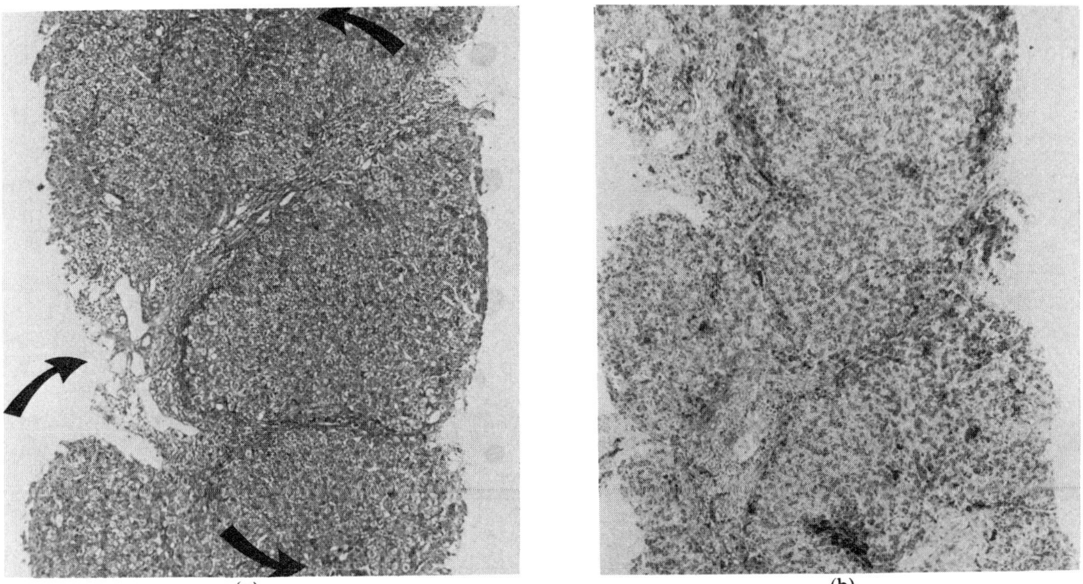

(a) (b)

Figure 30.7. (a) Haemochromatosis. There is increased fibrosis which radiates out from portal tracts (arrows). The gross excess of iron in hepatocytes here can only be identified as a dark rim along the edges of the portal tracts. It is more clearly identified when specific stains are used, as in Figure 30.7b. Haematoxylin and eosin × 100. (b) Perls' Prussian blue reaction. All hepatocytes contain increased amounts of iron. The greatest excess is seen here in periportal hepatocytes and collections of macrophages as a black pigment. Perls' Prussian blue × 100.

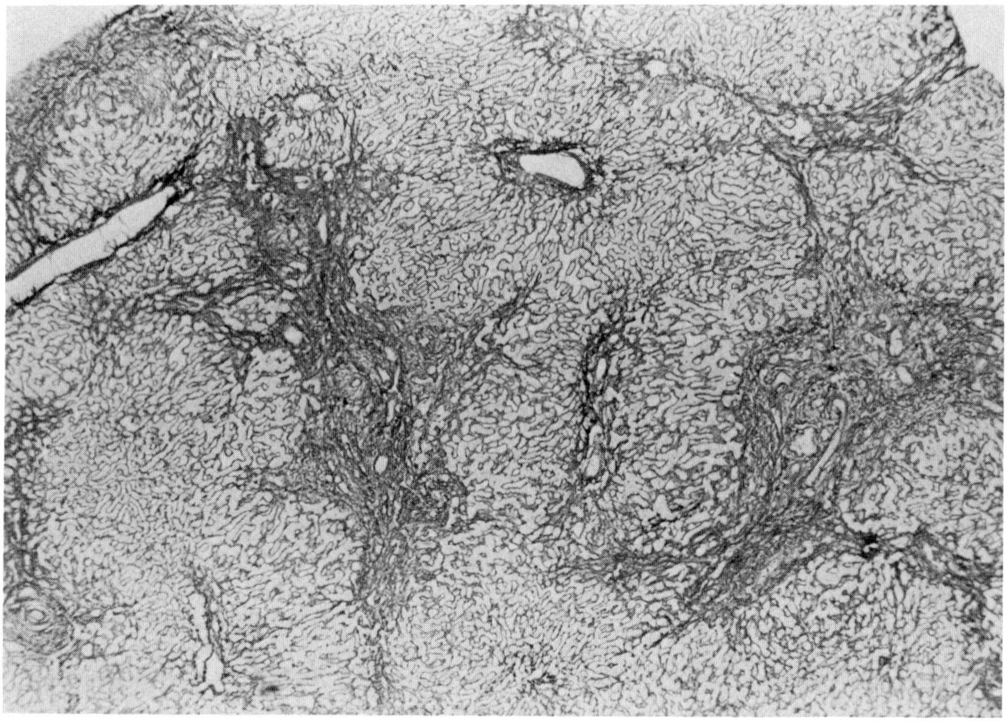

Figure 30.8. Chronic biliary obstruction. Portal tracts are linked together by the formation of new fibrous tissue. The cell plates are still single and radially orientated although there is now collapse of centrilobular reticulin from loss of bile-damaged hepatocytes. Reticulin × 100.

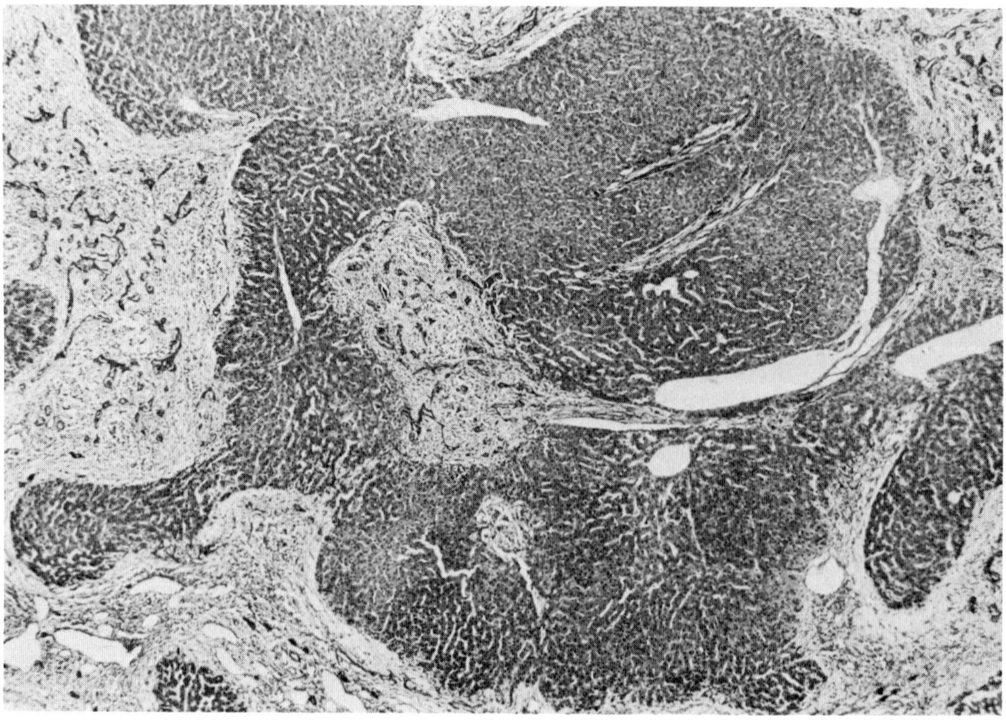

Figure 30.9. Advanced pattern of biliary cirrhosis showing the typical 'jig-saw puzzle' pattern of parenchyma separated by broad bands of fibrous tissue. Haematoxylin and eosin × 100.

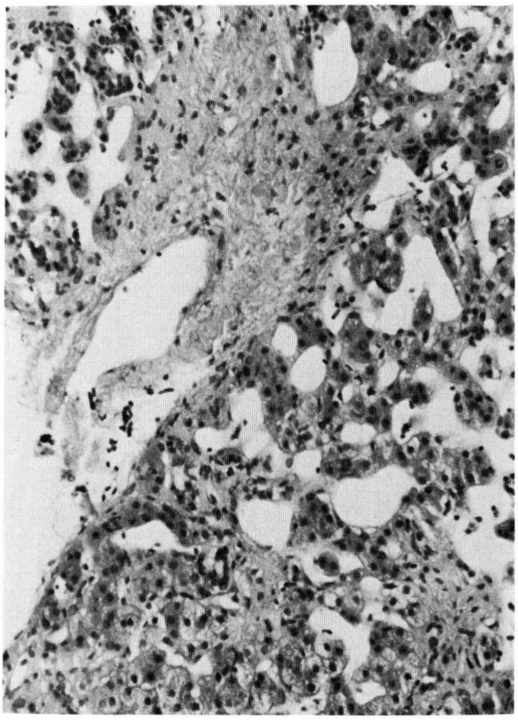

Figure 30.10. Bland centrilobular fibrosis associated with dilation of sinusoids in centrilobular zones. Patient with constrictive pericarditis of long duration. Haematoxylin and eosin × 400.

the twinning of cell plates within the nodule. Larger nodules may develop a few incomplete fibrous septa in which an arteriole and miniscule bile ductule can be found (Figure 30.13). These are not true portal tracts and can usually be identified by the miniature nature of the structures.

Bile retention is sometimes seen within hepatocytes and canaliculi. In such instances, oedema of the pseudo-capsule and neutrophils around adjacent proliferating bile ductules may suggest biliary obstruction, but extrahepatic obstruction in these circumstances is rare and the features are presumably intrahepatic and focal in origin.

Within the nodules all forms of hepatocellular degeneration may be found, and sometimes Mallory's alcoholic hyalin can be identified within hepatocytes. These forms are usually found in peripheral hepatocytes and do not imply an alcoholic aetiology.

These nodules are especially susceptible to infarction following gastrointestinal haemorrhage. The appearances do not differ from infarction in other organs; there is uniform coagulative necrosis of hepatocytes throughout the nodule, with a vascular and neutrophil exudative response to the cell death, varying according to the time elapsed between infarction and examination.

The aetiology of this pattern of macronodular cirrhosis is hard to determine unless some specific or strongly indicative histological feature is present, such as a gross excess of copper or iron, globules of alpha-1-antitrypsin deficiency or the hepatitis B surface antigen. This regenerative or postnecrotic pattern occurs most frequently in autopsy studies of patients who have died in terminal hepatic failure and is probably a final common end-stage cirrhosis that can evolve from any other preceding pattern of cirrhosis. It corresponds with macronodular cirrhosis that may develop in alcoholics with cirrhosis who stop drinking.[36]

The other multilobular macronodular pattern shows large nodules of parenchyma within which some semblance of lobular architecture can be identified. The presence of several portal tracts, either normal or only slightly expanded by fibrosis, together with efferent veins in the nodule, indicates a multilobular macronodular cirrhosis. These nodules show a deranged cell plate pattern and contain an excess of efferent veins which also show an abnormally close approximation to portal tracts and fibrous bands (Figure 30.14).

Fibrous bands may vary considerably in width and distribution. When they are very fine and slender, have short blind spurs extending into nodules and are clearly demarcated from the parenchyma with minimal, if any, piecemeal necrosis, the term 'incomplete septal' cirrhosis is used (Figure 30.15). More commonly found, especially in the United Kingdom, are broader bands of fibrous tissue and these can be associated with piecemeal necrosis at the junction with parenchyma.

The presence of piecemeal necrosis (chronic active hepatitis) indicates a pathological process, not a disease entity, and is found in several diseases or syndromes, including chronic hepatitis B infection, idiopathic chronic active (autoimmune) hepatitis, primary biliary cirrhosis, Wilson's disease, and some examples of drugs, alcohol and alpha-1-antitrypsin deficiency. Of these, specific histological features are usually present in chronic hepatitis B infection (see Chapter 29), primary biliary cirrhosis (see Chapter 31), Wilson's disease (see Chapter 33) and alpha-1-antitrypsin deficiency (see Chapter 35).

Cryptogenic cirrhosis is usually macronodular

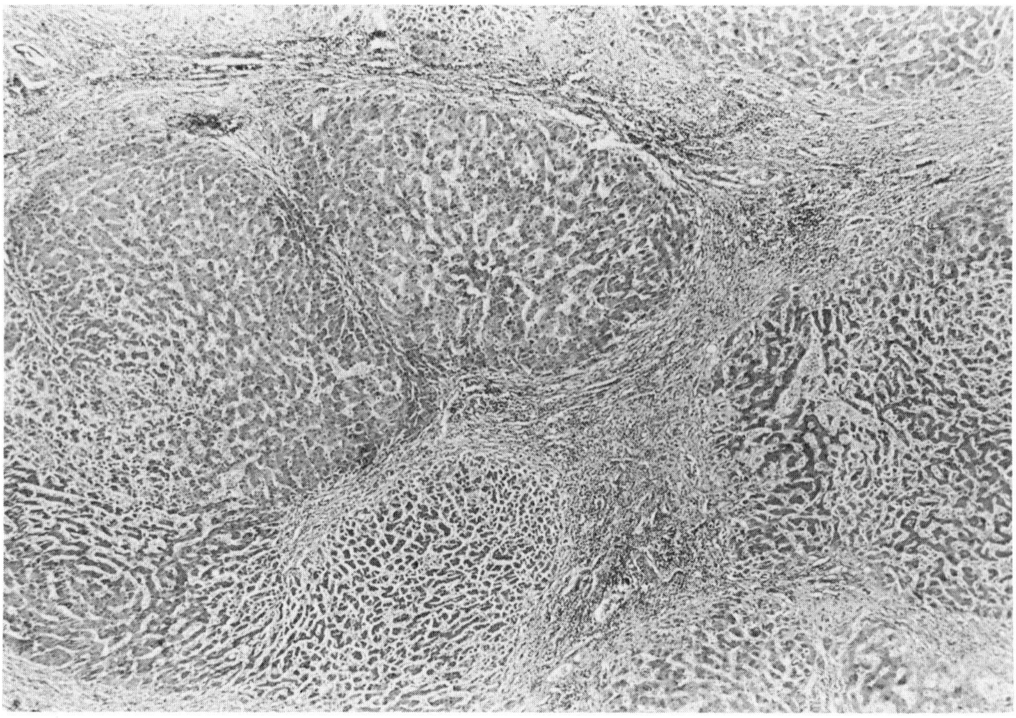

Figure 30.11. Cirrhosis of postnecrotic (advanced) pattern with nodules separated by broad bands of dense fibrous tissue. Haematoxylin and eosin × 100.

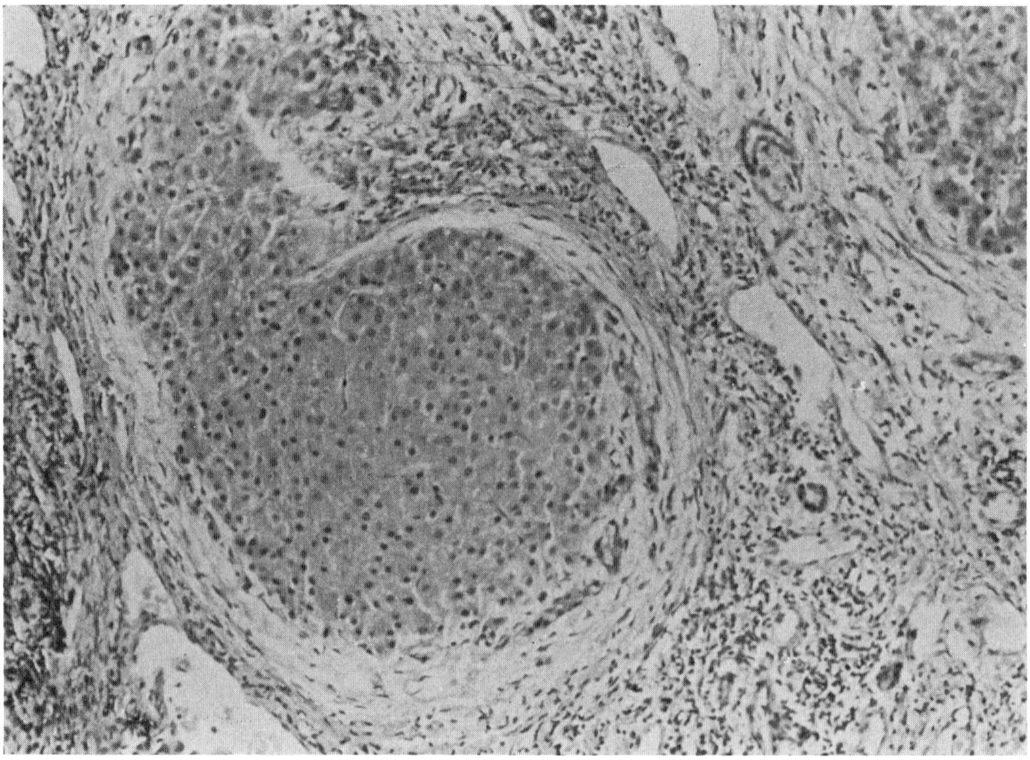

Figure 30.12. Cirrhotic nodule surrounded by a zone of concentric oedematous connective tissue. Haematoxylin and eosin × 400.

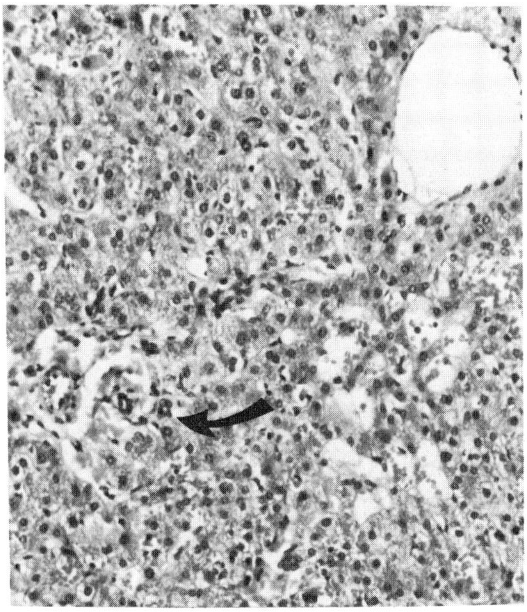

Figure 30.13. Hypoplastic 'portal tract' (arrow) in a macronodular cirrhosis. The arteriole is far larger than the bile duct and the portal vein tributary is collapsed. The efferent vein (top right) is too close to this tract and in the parenchyma there is twinning of cell plates with sinusoidal ectasia. Haematoxylin and eosin × 400.

but may be either of an incomplete septal pattern or postnecrotic following hepatic damage which at this end stage is no longer identifiable.

With a multilobular macronodular cirrhosis of incomplete septal type, no specific pathological features can usually be identified and the disorder in these patients seems to follow a quiescent, indolent course for many years. Portal hypertension and gastrointestinal bleeding, rather than impaired liver function, are the major causes of symptoms and complications. The aetiology is obscure, but claims for an association with hepatitis in Africa and Asia[1] and with alcohol in western societies[55] have been made. In our experience, there is rarely any evidence for either of these conditions, although we have followed one patient whose first biopsy showed cirrhosis with florid piecemeal necrosis and whose second needle biopsy six years later showed a quiescent multilobular cirrhosis suggestive of an incomplete septal pattern (Figures 30.16 and 30.17).

PATHOGENESIS

Cirrhosis evolves slowly over a period of time that can rarely be quantified but usually spans years, and its development depends upon constant stimulation by the aetiological factor. This stimulus is usually the regularly induced damage and death of hepatocytes, which in turn evoke the classic mechanisms of regeneration and repair.

Architectural Changes

Although by definition the whole liver must be involved, there are two ways in which this may be achieved. In the first of these, the liver lobules are uniformly affected throughout and the changes in any one unit of liver at any one moment are representative of the changes in the liver as a whole. In the second, the process is focal within the liver and produces local distortion of the architecture with fibrosis, while other areas of liver are unaffected. Cirrhosis in such instances develops as and when the majority of the liver becomes involved.

Examples of the first mechanism are alcohol and cytotoxic drugs such as methotrexate. Both these toxins are evenly distributed throughout the liver by the portal venous blood flow, and the effects will be simultaneous throughout the liver. Many of the known causes of micro-

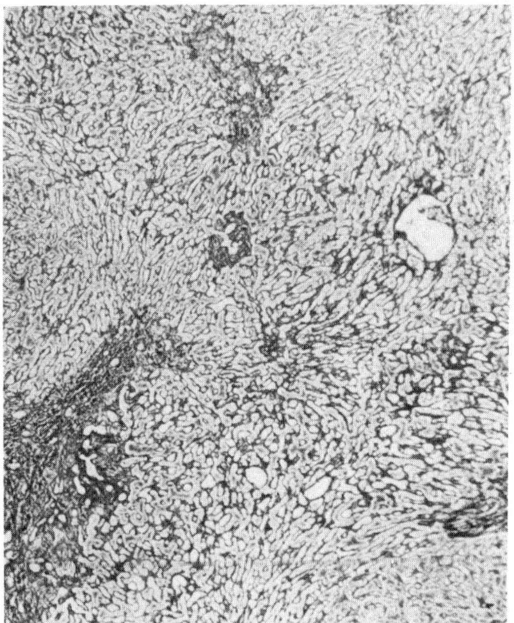

Figure 30.14. Macronodular cirrhosis showing abnormal fibrosis and an excess of efferent veins, some of which are too close to the band of fibrosis (bottom left). The cell plate pattern is also haphazardly orientated although twinning of cell plates in this area is not a prominent feature. Reticulin × 100.

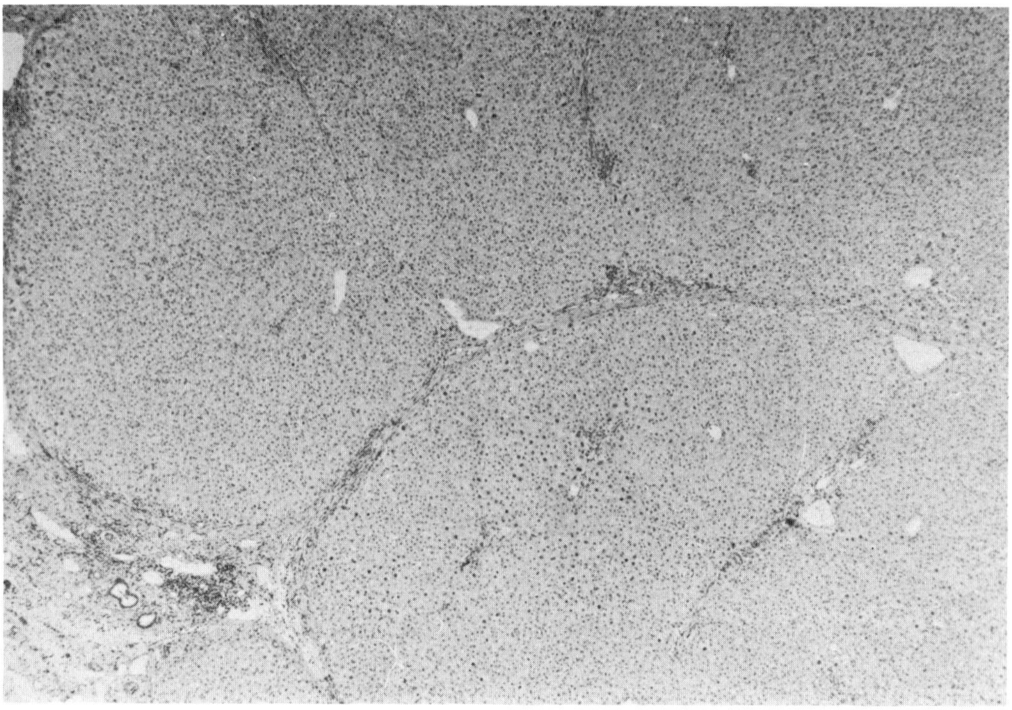

Figure 30.15. Cirrhosis of incomplete septal pattern. A portal tract can be clearly identified on the left. The parenchyma is intersected by several slender bands of fibrous tissue which often 'peter' and are thus 'incomplete'. There is also an excess of dilated efferent veins. Haematoxylin and eosin × 100.

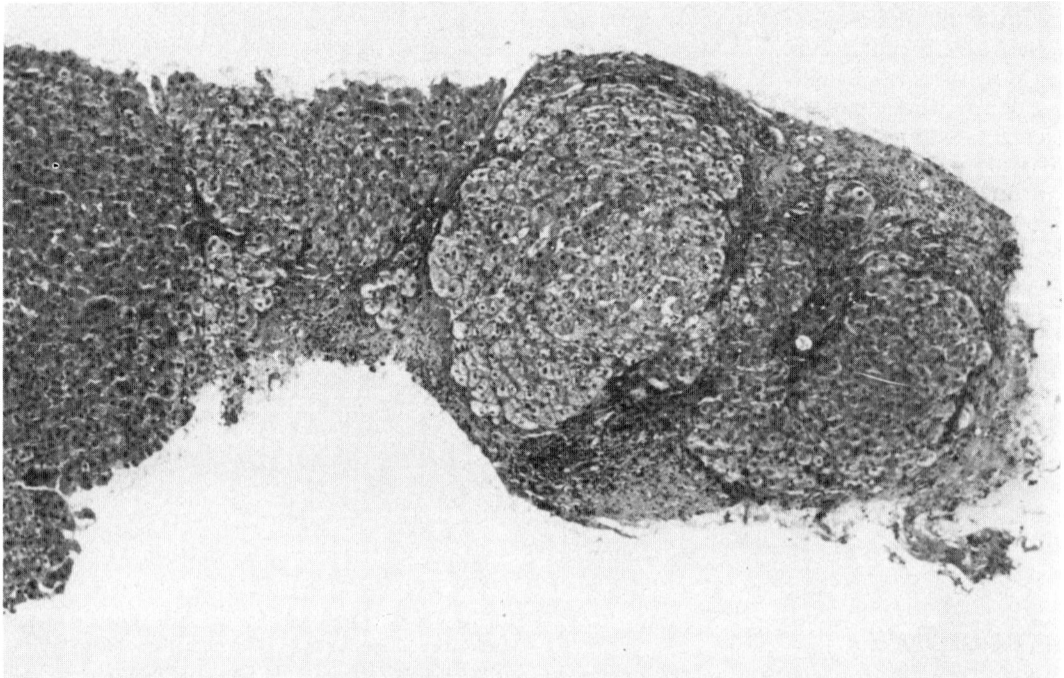

Figure 30.16. A biopsy showing cirrhosis and piecemeal necrosis from a patient with HB_sAg negative chronic active hepatitis. Haematoxylin and eosin × 125.

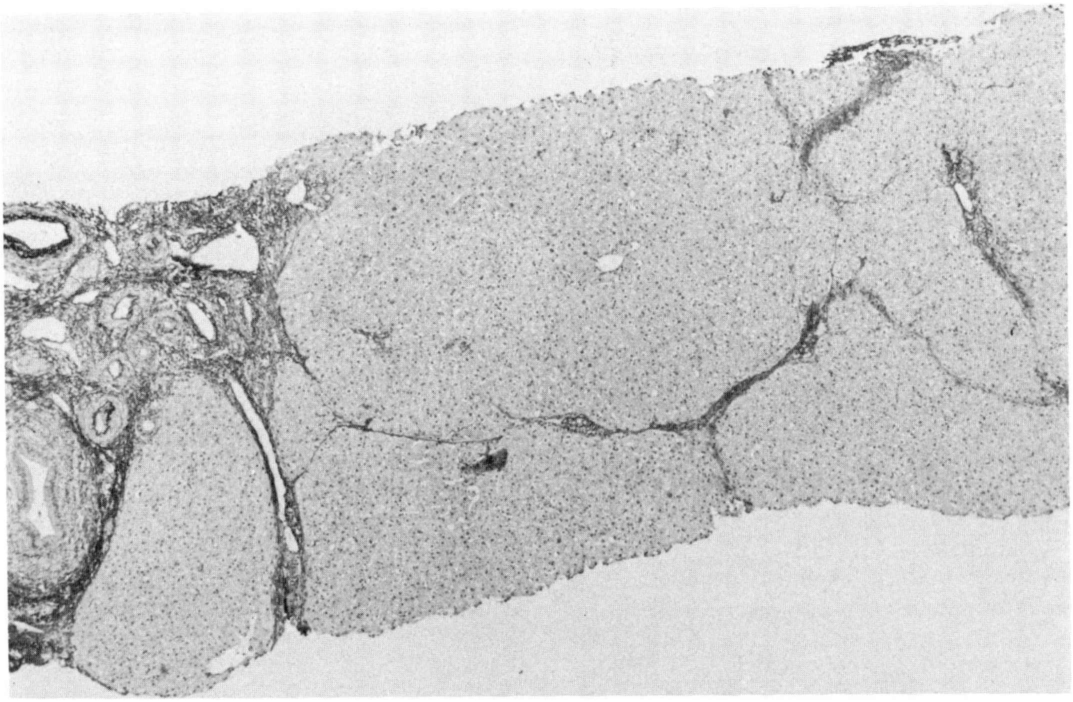

Figure 30.17. A second liver biopsy six years after the biopsy illustrated in Figure 30.16 shows a cirrhosis apparently of incomplete septal pattern. There is no piecemeal necrosis or other evidence of activity in the biopsy. Orcein × 125.

micronodular cirrhosis are conditions that fulfil these criteria. This alone suggests that the unknown mechanisms of Indian childhood cirrhosis are of toxic or metabolic origin although, despite a careful search for known hepatotoxins, none has so far been identified.[50]

This pattern of cirrhosis, once established, will have a rapid clinical course unless the aetiological agent is treated or removed. Once cirrhosis is present, only 40 per cent of alcoholics who continue drinking survive five years, whereas of those who stop, 63 per cent survive five years.[62] Removal of the aetiological agent will also decrease the rate of cell damage and death and allow regeneration to proceed relatively unopposed towards a macronodular cirrhosis.[36] The micronodules will thus enlarge and in so doing will compress bands of fibrous tissue, close vascular channels and obstruct bile ducts. The net result will be to produce large nodules separated by dense fibrous bands. The vascular obstruction will induce ischaemic changes in other nodules of parenchyma and so produce a self-perpetuating cycle. The obstructed bile ducts may also induce zones of oedema with bile ductule proliferation around affected nodules and this can heal by scarring.

The second mechanism might be expected to produce a multilobular macronodular cirrhosis. Some of the larger nodules surrounded by fibrous tissue will be areas of liver with the original architecture showing only minor changes while other areas will show nodular regeneration. As these undamaged areas of liver are involved in the disease process, so the multilobular nodule is subdivided, but at the same time the earlier nodules are growing and enlarging. The cirrhosis can thus evolve into the other, postnecrotic pattern of macronodular cirrhosis. Alternatively, if the disease process is accelerated or regeneration impaired, the multilobular macronodules may be subdivided before significant enlargement of the earliest nodules occurs and the overall pattern then becomes micronodular.

Chronic active hepatitis commonly produces a macronodular cirrhosis and occasionally a micronodular cirrhosis. In chronic active hepatitis, the activity, as judged by the severity of piecemeal necrosis, varies widely throughout the liver. Areas in which activity is minimal are commonly found and are adjacent to areas of intense piecemeal necrosis with architectural distortion. The rationale for the seemingly random activity of this process throughout the liver is not understood. Certainly in HB_sAg positive chronic active hepatitis the distribution of the inflammatory reaction is not related to the distribution of any of the hepatitis B markers that can be morphologically demonstrated.

The cirrhosis associated with mucoviscidosis, aptly termed 'focal biliary cirrhosis', also illustrates this mechanism.[14,51] In this condition, the mucus secreted by the bile duct epithelium is abnormally viscid and gives rise to random plugging of intrahepatic bile ducts. That area of liver distal to the obstruction then shows the changes of chronic biliary obstruction and eventually secondary biliary cirrhosis. Slowly, other areas of liver are also affected and eventually the whole liver is involved.

Vascular Changes

It has been postulated that the major factor in the determination of cirrhosis is the alteration of the vascular pattern. Cirrhosis develops when nodules of parenchyma are formed with all the pre-existing vascular afferents and efferents on the periphery.[56] The confluent loss of hepatocytes, combined with fibrosis, can bridge the portal tracts with central veins. Blood flowing in these bridges may thus bypass the sinusoidal system completely and pass directly from hepatic artery and portal vein to the central vein or may enter the sinusoidal system close to the central vein.

These new intrahepatic vascular channels shunt blood from the hepatic artery to the central vein, from the portal vein to the central vein and also from the hepatic artery to the portal vein.[48] Functional studies of blood flow have confirmed the existence of these shunts,[19,20,22,23,73] and demonstrated that, on average, 20 per cent of hepatic arterial blood flow is shunted through the liver, although over 50 per cent may be shunted in individual examples;[20] a similar proportion of portal venous blood is shunted.[19]

Apart from these intrahepatic shunts, anastomoses between the portal and systemic venous circulations are also formed as a result of the portal venous hypertension. When these collaterals are established, up to 80 per cent of blood from the portal venous bed may never enter the liver. As a consequence, there is both a real and an apparent increase in that proportion of the total hepatic blood flow supplied by the hepatic artery.

These intra- and extrahepatic shunts have various consequences. Metabolites and toxins may escape into the systemic circulation[9,10] (see Chapter 42), and particulate matter is not adequately filtered by the Kupffer cells. The escape of antigens into the systemic circulation is one explanation of the hypergammaglobulinaemia that occurs (see Chapter 9), and similarly the unimpeded passage of bacteria through the liver accounts for the increased incidence of spontaneous bacteraemia and peritonitis (see below).[10,79]

Cell Death

In all these situations, the basic features of cell death, regeneration and fibrosis are involved and these may vary in their relative proportions. The factors governing the variation are poorly understood.

Death of hepatocytes is not always evident morphologically but is the predisposing factor for cirrhosis. The damage must be continually inflicted and there is no good evidence that an acute isolated episode of hepatic necrosis will produce cirrhosis even if the extent of the damage clinically precipitates hepatic failure. Thus, hepatic necrosis due to paracetamol overdosage may cause death in acute hepatic failure but does not result in chronic sequelae.[59] Likewise, acute viral hepatitis proceeding to hepatic failure is often fatal, but survivors regain normal liver function and structure.[28] Hepatitis A virus infection is self-limiting and terminates with a rising anti-HAV titre; it is not associated with chronic liver disease or cirrhosis, nor with a chronic carrier state (see Chapter 28). Conversely, hepatitis B virus infection may be chronic and then can be associated with a cirrhosis or a chronic HBV carrier state, but there is no evidence that cirrhosis is a sequel to acute self-limiting hepatitis B infection (see Chapters 28 and 29).

Evidence from studies of methotrexate-induced cirrhosis also suggests that the hepatocellular insult needs to be continuous rather than repetitive and gives some idea of the minimal time interval required to produce cirrhosis.[12,47] Methotrexate administered as a large dose parenterally every fourteenth day produces hepatocellular damage and cell death in relation to this bolus of therapy,[70] but rarely produces cirrhosis.[12,47] The administration of the same total dosage as a series of small aliquots spread over seven to ten days of the fortnight is associated with cirrhosis. Although this could reflect increased exposure of the liver to the drug in the portal vein an alternative explanation is related to the poor hepatic uptake of methotrexate.[25] Following a single dose of the drug, there is a sharp rise in serum levels followed by an equally sharp fall with much of the drug excreted in the urine. Within 24 hours, the serum level has returned to zero. Hepatocyte uptake of methotrexate is very slow and it has been estimated that 72 hours are required for maximum cellular concentration. Even with such continuing exposure to an efficient cytotoxic drug, the average period of exposure documented to cirrhosis is 48 months.

Cell death leading to cirrhosis has been achieved by ischaemia in cardiac cirrhosis, drugs and toxins, metabolic abnormalities, immunological reactions, metals, bile and bile salts. The mechanisms by which these various agents damage the cell are varied.

Alcohol can alter the whole redox potential within the cell by overwhelming the hydrogen ion receptor, nicotine adenine dinucleotide (NAD), and so minimizing the availability of NAD for other processes that require this compound. At the same time, it promotes those processes that oxidize the reduced form, $NADH_2$, into NAD (see Chapter 32). Carbon tetrachloride produces cell damage by the action of its intermediary metabolites and so its hepatotoxic action is potentiated by barbiturates and other inducers of microsomal activity. Paradoxically, the administration of a small dose of carbon tetrachloride within 12 hours prior to an established LD_{50} dose will decrease the toxicity of this larger dose. This effect is produced because the microsomal activity is blocked by the small priming dose and therefore there is a less rapid accumulation of metabolites. The nature of these metabolites and their site of action are still unknown.

Many congenital metabolic abnormalities are associated with cirrhosis (see Chapter 40), but as a group they are not a common cause of cirrhosis. The precise defect may have been defined in any one particular condition, but the reason for cell death and cirrhosis may still be unclear. For instance, in alpha-1-antitrypsin (A1AT) deficiency there is probably a single amino acid substitution in the M-allotype protein that changes it into a Z-allotype protein.[24, 83] This substitution results in an accumulation of the A1AT in the hepatocytes and this is detectable morphologically. Such accumulation can also be identified in heterozygotes. It is argued that because there is no known association between the heterozygous condition and cirrhosis this accumulation of A1AT is not the critical factor. We believe that cirrhosis is associated with the heterozygous condition and that the above argument is not valid for this reason. Nonetheless, a simple accumulation of A1AT within the hepatocytes cannot satisfactorily explain all the features of the cirrhosis in this disease (see Chapter 35).

Immune and autoimmune mechanisms that may occur in liver disease are discussed in Chapters 9 and 29. It is noticeable that liver damage in viral hepatitis corresponds to the onset of the immune response to the virus and that in the absence of an effective immune response a carrier state of persistent viral infection occurs. These immune mechanisms may be humoral or cellular. So far, there is no evidence that immune complexes are important in the pathogenesis of chronic liver disease, but the role of antibody in lymphocyte cytotoxicity mechanisms is still undetermined. A cellular immune response appears to be important in controlling infection, but the exact mechanisms by which the lymphocytes act are still speculative. Recently it has been suggested that in the various forms of viral and non-viral hepatitis the hepatocellular damage and death may be produced by activation of macrophages recruited into the liver by helper T-lymphocytes. Activation may be achieved by various means, ranging from endotoxin to immune complexes. These activated macrophages then release one or more cytotoxins which produce the critical damage.[17] The existence of such cytotoxins has not yet been demonstrated.

The mechanism of the cell damage is more clearly defined in Wilson's disease (and in haemochromatosis). Copper is an essential factor in many enzyme systems, but equally in high concentrations it is toxic to such systems (see Chapter 33). Interference with such enzymes as membrane-bound ATPase alters the potential of the plasma membrane and its ability to control the flux of ions and water.

Cell damage occurs in association with retention of bile and bile salts, but it is not clear whether this damage is attributable to the bile or associated with it. Cell death is not a conspicuous feature of acute bile-duct obstruction, although cell damage has been recorded in biochemical surveys in this condition and morphological evidence of such damage is eventually seen. It has also been postulated that bile salts without bile may accumulate and be equally toxic and that such bile salt retention could account for the ballooning degeneration of hepatocytes seen in some chronic liver diseases.

Death of hepatocytes is usually the trigger for the mechanisms of inflammation, regeneration and repair, but the factors stimulating the process are not known. Recently, collagen synthesis has been experimentally stimulated by factors of low molecular weight (< 5000 daltons) extracted from the livers of alcoholic cirrhosis and experimental carbon tetrachloride damage,[41,43] but the nature, significance and mode of action of these factors is as yet unknown.

Inflammation

The 'activity' of a cirrhosis is usually judged by a combination of features of cell death and, more especially, the cellular inflammatory infiltrate. Thus there are many neutrophils around bile ductules in 'active' biliary cirrhosis or within the sinusoids and around Mallory bodies in 'active' alcoholic cirrhosis. The degree of activity in the various diseases in which piecemeal necrosis is found is assessed by the intensity of the mononuclear cell infiltrate at the interface of stroma and parenchyma and by the degree and extent of the sinusoidal involvement in the nodule. It is this activity that is suppressed by corticosteroid therapy although other manifestations of the disease process may not be involved.

Cell Regeneration

Regeneration is fully discussed in Chapter 10; although many factors are known which influence regeneration, the critical events which initiate this phenomenon after cell death are still uncertain.

It must be emphasized that not all abnormal nodules are regenerative in origin and that some are formed passively by the isolation of an area of parenchyma by fibrosis, initially with minimal cell death or regeneration. Conversely, actively regenerating nodules of non-neoplastic hepatocytes may form in the absence of fibrosis or cell death. This is a feature noted clinically as nodular transformation (see Chapter 38).[69]

In cirrhosis, regeneration is identified morphologically by the formation of cell plates two or more cells thick and by abnormal irregular cell plate patterns. Instead of showing an orderly anastomosing radial pattern, the plates are more haphazardly arranged. There may be different growth rates in the parenchymal nodules, so that some cell plates may become compressed by the more rapid growth elsewhere.

Cytologically, there are increased numbers of binucleate hepatocytes, as well as an increased variation in the size of the nuclei. This variation in size corresponds to the degree of ploidy in the hepatocyte. Octoploid nuclei are not uncommon. In the electron microscope, the consistent feature of hepatocytes from cirrhotic nodules is the deeper extension of the perisinusoidal recess between hepatocytes so that the bile canaliculus is approached. Microvillous processes identical to those on the sinusoidal surface of the hepatocytes are formed on these lateral cell membranes.[54] This is probably an adaptation of the cell to its altered anatomical and functional environment rather than a feature of regeneration.

Regenerative activity within a nodule may be exceeded or balanced by the cell death or, alternatively, regeneration may exceed cell death within the nodule. If cell death is in excess of regeneration and is representative, then rapid clinical deterioration may be expected. This is frequently seen in alcoholics with cirrhosis who drink heavily, and the excessive cell death is one of the factors contributing to the shorter survival recorded in alcoholics who continue drinking.[62] A balance between cell death and regeneration in the individual regenerative nodules is not usually recognized. When regenerative activity more than compensates for the loss of hepatocytes, growth of the nodule and compression of the surrounding fibrous tissue occur. This expansile growth will help to condense the fibrous stroma and approximate portal tract structures. It will also stretch and compress the vascular channels and shunts that have been formed, as well as the bile ducts. This impedance of blood flow by compression and by stretching the channel over the nodule will affect the low pressure system most severely and so accentuate the portal venous hypertension and accelerate the formation of collaterals. In addition, the distal distribution of blood through that channel will be impaired and nodules will become increasingly dependent upon hepatic arterial blood flow. When this arterial flow is impaired, for instance by further growth and compression of the nodules or by hypovolaemic shock from bleeding varices, then further cell death due to ischaemia will occur and a vicious cycle is created.

Fibrosis

Collagen

Structure. Knowledge about the structure and biosynthesis of collagen has rapidly expanded in the last few years.[5,18,33,57,64] Collagen is a triple helix of polypeptide chains secreted by the cell in a precursor form, procollagen. Each chain contains approximately 1000 amino acids and is rich in glycine, hydroxyproline and hydroxylysine. Glycine is present in every third position along the chain, although the full amino acid sequences have not been completed. Each polypeptide chain of the procollagen has non-helical terminals: at the amino-terminal this contains approximately 200 residues and at the carboxy-terminal 350 residues. Conversion to collagen involves the removal of these non-helical terminals by collagen peptidases. The tensile strength and the stability of collagen are then produced by cross-linkages both within and between these triple helices.

Four types of collagen are now described,[18] although there could be more.[7,46] These four are labelled types I to IV. Types I and III are the predominant collagens in liver; type II collagen is found only in cartilage and type IV collagen constitutes basement membranes. Type I collagen corresponds to the mature, doubly refractile collagen of portal tracts and is widespread throughout the body from dermis to bone. The triple helix is composed of two identical polypeptide chains, each termed α_1(I) with an α_2 chain. Types II to IV collagen are each composed of three identical polypeptides which are termed respectively α_1(II), α_1(III) and α_1(IV). Type III collagen in the liver corresponds to the reticulin framework in the sinusoids but is also present in portal tracts; small amounts of type IV collagen can be readily identified as the basement membrane material around bile ducts.

Collagen in human liver. In normal human liver, type I and type III collagen are present in at least approximately equal proportions,[72] although the proportion of type I is claimed to be as much as 80 per cent.[67] In cirrhosis, the total amount of collagen increases, but the proportions of type I to type III collagen are debated.[67,72] Both a relative increase of type I[72] and a relative increase of type III collagen[67] are claimed in alcoholic cirrhosis. It is not known if there are any diagnostic or prognostic differences in the types of collagen induced in cirrhosis or indeed if there are different patterns of biosynthesis related to aetiology.

Synthesis of collagen is usually attributed to the fibroblast, but there is increasing evidence that many other cells can be involved.[35] These include macrophages and histiocytes, smooth muscle cells[68] and epithelial cells[35] from various sites of the body, as well as the perisinusoidal cells of the liver (see Chapters 2 and 17).[42]

Regulation of collagen synthesis. Several factors capable of stimulating collagen synthesis have been identified, but these and the subsequent regulation of synthesis are not well understood. Of these, cell death is most important, but the stimulus could be possibly related as much to the cause of the cell necrosis as to the death of the cell. Alcohol has been incriminated as one factor. Not only is the degree of fibrosis in human alcoholic liver disease extreme and frequently out of proportion to the cellular damage, but the administration of alcohol to rats quickly results in a rapid rise in fibrosis and hepatic prolyl-hydroxylase activity.[45] Several low molecular weight factors (all less than 5000 daltons) have been found in both human cirrhosis and experimentally induced cirrhosis and all these can stimulate fibrosis.[41,43]

Macrophages and lymphocytes have also been incriminated in the induction of fibrosis.[61] If lymphocytes cultured from patients with chronic active liver disease are exposed to autologous liver, they will release lymphokines capable of stimulating fibroblastic activity.[8] Similar lymphokine-induced collagen formation can be produced by normal human lymphocytes stimulated by phytohaemagglutinin.[27] In *Schistosoma mansoni* infection of mice, extracts and culture supernatants of isolated egg granulomas have been shown to stimulate proliferation of fibroblasts.[82]

Architectural patterns of fibrosis

Fibrosis is the usual method of repair of any form of chronic inflammation and so may be found in the liver in the absence of cirrhosis. It is nonetheless a prerequisite of cirrhosis that the amount of fibrous tissue be abnormally increased, and the patterns of fibrosis within a cirrhotic liver – fine incomplete septal, broad postnecrotic scars and diffuse sinusoidal fibrosis – have already been indicated.

Two ways of producing fibrosis are described: passive and active.[58] In the passive variety, death of confluent areas of parenchyma results in the collapse of the reticulin architecture with apposition of the fibres. In the active form, new collagen fibres are formed directly by mesenchymal biosynthetic activity. It is generally accepted that the passive collapse of reticulin fibres can revert if adequate parenchymal regeneration occurs within a short space of time, but that active fibrogenesis will otherwise produce an irreversible scar. It seems therefore that passive collapse will promote cirrhosis by producing scarring more deeply within the lobule and this will accelerate the subdivision of the architecture. Bridging hepatic necrosis therefore results in fibrosis in all parts of the lobule, while piecemeal necrosis alone is at first confined to the edges of the portal tracts and should be more slowly progressive. This could account for the relatively benign course of piecemeal necrosis in acute viral hepatitis unless other adverse prognostic features are present (see Chapter 28). Likewise, fibrosis expands portal tracts in biliary obstruction but the lobular structure is preserved until a late stage and often the central vein can be identified surrounded by hepatocytes and then encircled by the fibrosis of the linked portal tracts. Cirrhosis in diseases of the biliary tract is therefore a late event and occurs only after considerable fibrosis has been produced.

Fibrosis may occur in the liver without cirrhosis and usually this is clearly separable from cirrhosis. Even excluding diseases where severe fibrosis occurs prior to the cirrhosis, there are instances when distinction from cirrhosis is difficult. The two classic instances are hepar lobatum (see Chapter 56), which is increasingly rare in western societies, and congenital hepatic fibrosis (see Chapter 40).

Congenital hepatic fibrosis

This condition has to be considered in the differential diagnosis of cirrhosis and because it frequently produces symptoms, signs and complications of portal venous hypertension. Originally described in children,[29,30] it is now apparent that it may occur in asymptomatic adults.[3] We have also identified this condition in three adults, all of whom had good liver function but who presented with severe portal hypertension (Figure 30.18).

The condition probably represents one end of a pathological spectrum, with polycystic liver at the other end. Linking these two extremes is the biliary microhamartoma, the von Meyenburg complex. These are relatively common incidental findings at autopsy and in biopsy specimens, but they can be mistaken at operation for minute metastases (approximately 2 to 3 mm in diameter), and infection and

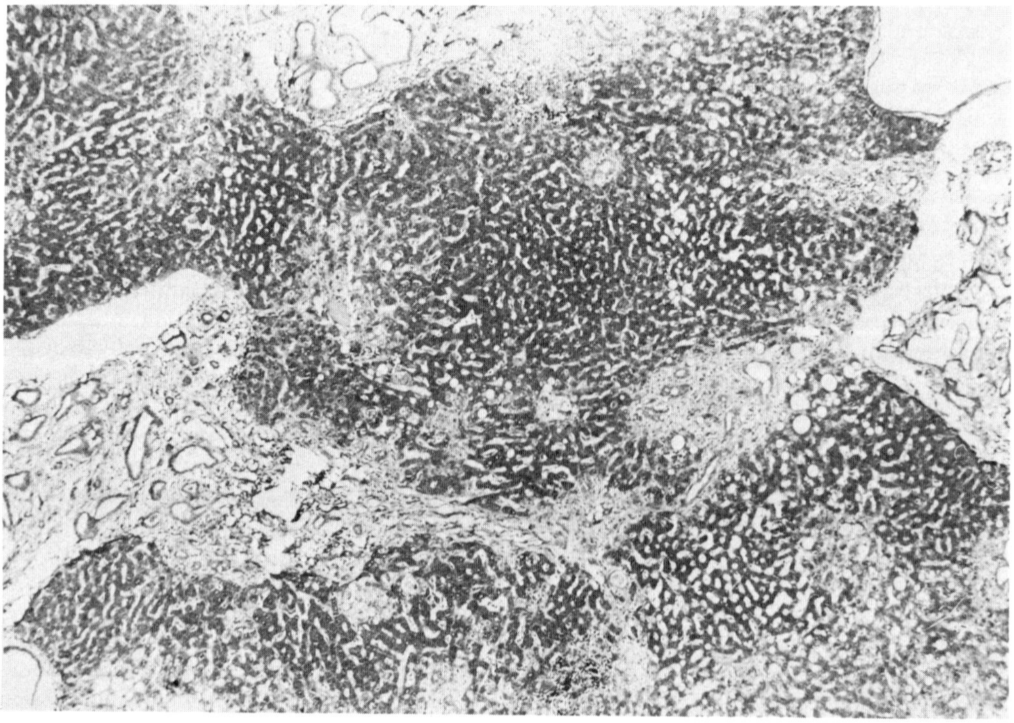

Figure 30.18. Congenital hepatic fibrosis. Excessive fibrosis is present. Focal aggregates of irregular, angular, dilated bile ducts are present in these bands of fibrous tissue. Haematoxylin and eosin × 150.

carcinomatous transformation[11] are rare complications. They have fibrous and epithelial components; the dense fibrous stroma contains irregular angular spaces lined by bile duct epithelium. These spaces sometimes contain bile. The complex expands, or is adjacent to, a portal tract.

Congenital hepatic fibrosis is that end of the spectrum in which there is considerable increase in the amount of fibrous stroma, and this can extensively distort the architecture. For the diagnosis it is essential to identify the more focal epithelial components. A relative increase in the epithelial component probably accounts for polycystic disease of the liver. In this condition there are many cysts, usually filled with clear fluid and lined by an atrophic epithelium. In many places the epithelium is sufficiently preserved to show identity with biliary epithelium, and von Meyenburg complexes can often be found in non-cystic portions of liver.

The relationship of these conditions to polycystic disease of the kidneys is discussed in Chapter 40, but it is interesting to note that in the experimental production of polycystic kidneys in rats, cystic lesions were also produced in the liver.[44]

CLINICAL FEATURES

The clinical features of cirrhosis will depend on the underlying cause and whether or not the two major complications, hepatocellular failure and portal hypertension, have developed. As indicated above, cirrhosis results from hepatocellular damage followed by regeneration and fibrosis. This process usually takes place over a period of many years. In most instances, it is due to persistence of the damaging agent, for example continued alcohol consumption, chronic hepatitis B infection, or the continued deposition of iron or copper. Rarely, there is an acute, relatively short-lived episode of hepatocellular damage followed by the late presentation of cirrhosis. A single episode of hepatocellular damage, such as occurs with toxins, even though severe, rarely if ever leads to cirrhosis.

The progression of the disease may be intermittent, for example due to varying alcohol consumption or to modification by treatment such as with corticosteroids in chronic active hepatitis.

Clinical presentation may occur at any time during this period of progression to cirrhosis as a result of a temporary exacerbation of hepatocellular damage or as an incidental clinical or laboratory finding, but usually presentation is with hepatocellular failure or portal hypertension when the disease is well established. A proportion of cirrhotics are detected incidentally at post-mortem without any antecedent history of liver disease. Clinically, the disease may therefore be latent and well compensated or active and decompensated.

It is particularly important to recognize patients in the latent phase of the disease, or even before cirrhosis has developed. Clinical situations in which this might occur are as follows:

1. In alcoholics presenting with other features of alcohol abuse such as depression, obesity, malnutrition, folate or other vitamin deficiencies, pancreatitis, peripheral neuropathy, peptic ulceration, anorexia, loss of libido, or with incidental physical or laboratory findings (see Chapter 32);
2. In patients with associated diseases such as autoimmune or collagen diseases (see Chapters 29 and 31), inflammatory bowel disease and sarcoidosis (see Chapter 37), systemic infections, for example tuberculosis, septicaemia or spontaneous bacterial peritonitis (see below and Chapter 51), the neurological features of Wilson's disease (see Chapter 33) and the diabetes or endocrinopathies of haemochromatosis (see Chapter 34);
3. The incidental physical finding of spider naevi, Dupuytren's contracture, gynaecomastia, pigmentation, hepatomegaly or splenomegaly;
4. The incidental laboratory finding of abnormal liver function tests, raised globulins, a positive mitochondrial antibody or hepatitis B surface antigen; and
5. In the course of screening the relatives of patients with familial disorders such as Wilson's disease (see Chapter 33), haemochromatosis (see Chapter 34), alpha-1-antitrypsin deficiency (see Chapter 35), cystic fibrosis and polycystic disease of the liver and kidney (see below).

Most patients present clinically with the consequences of hepatocellular failure or portal hypertension. The two are often interrelated.

Cirrhosis usually presents in the fourth, fifth or sixth decades, but chronic active hepatitis and Wilson's disease often present in the teens

Table 30.2. *Comparison of EARLY Clinical Features in Common Forms of Cirrhosis.*[a]

	Alcoholic	Chronic active hepatitis		Primary biliary cirrhosis	Cryptogenic cirrhosis	Haemo-chromatosis
		HB_sAg Neg.	HB_sAg Pos.			
Sex ratio: male to female	2 to 10:1	1:3	9:1	1:9	1:1 or 2	5 to 10:1
Malaise, lethargy and dyspepsia	80%	60%	30%	40%	50%	60%
Abdominal pain	25%	10–20%	30%	rare	20%	30%
Loss of libido	60%	rare	?common	rare	uncommon	80%
Jaundice	20%	30%	10%	50% (mild)	10%	rare
Pruritus	rare	rare	rare	80%	occasional	rare
Fever	5–10%	rare	rare	rare	rare	rare
Fluid retention	50%	20–30%	20–30%	5%	30%	10%
Gastrointestinal haemorrhage	25%	10–20%	10–20%	5%	20%	5%
Pigmentation	25%	uncommon	uncommon	75%	25%	90%
Spider naevi	50%	70%	50%	20%	30%	10%
Dupuytren's contracture	10–30%	uncommon	uncommon	uncommon	10%	10%
Gynaecomastia and testicular atrophy	20–30%	rare	10–20%	rare	5%	80%
Hepatomegaly	90%	70%	50%	80%	40%	90%
Splenomegaly	20%	60%	50%	40%	25%	20%
Incidental findings	5–10%	<5%	5–10%	10%	5%	5–10%

[a]Based on references in the text and personal series.

or twenties, and the various forms of cirrhosis of childhood present even earlier.

The male to female sex ratio in alcoholic liver disease ranges widely, from 2 to 10 : 1,[6,21,62,63] although its frequency in women appears to be increasing.[49] It is universally accepted that haemochromatosis is considerably more common in males than in females, figures ranging from 5 to 10 : 1 (see Chapter 34). Similarly, there is a striking male preponderance in HB_sAg positive chronic active hepatitis (see Chapter 29). This predominance has been explained by postulating cross-reactivity between the HB_sAg and a male determined tissue antigen[16,34] so that the male is tolerant of HB_sAg and therefore has an impaired immune defence against it. HB_sAg negative chronic active hepatitis has a female to male ratio of 2 to 3 : 1 (see Chapter 29) and primary biliary cirrhosis is predominantly a disease of women, fewer than 10 per cent of cases occurring in men (see Chapter 31). In most series of postnecrotic or cryptogenic cirrhosis, the sex ratio is either equal[63] or there is a slight female preponderance.[21,74]

Presenting symptoms are very variable, depending on the aetiology and whether hepatocellular failure or portal hypertension predominates. As indicated earlier, some patients present incidentally while their cirrhosis is latent and well compensated. Late clinical features at the stage of liver failure, bleeding varices, ascites and infection may be similar, irrespective of the aetiology. Comparison between series is difficult because of variation in the stage at which clinical and laboratory information has been collected. The common symptoms and signs early in the course of the disease are compared in alcoholic cirrhosis, chronic active hepatitis, primary biliary cirrhosis, cryptogenic cirrhosis and haemochromatosis (Table 30.2).

Non-specific symptoms such as malaise and lethargy are common at the onset in all types of cirrhosis, but are most pronounced in alcoholic cirrhosis and HB_sAg negative chronic active hepatitis. Vague gastrointestinal symptoms including dyspepsia, bloating and nausea are also common, and, in the alcoholic, anorexia, vomiting and weight loss may be prominent. Abdominal pain and pain over the liver are occasional early symptoms, particularly in the alcoholic, in whom associated peptic ulceration may be the cause. Loss of libido is common in the male alcoholic and in haemochromatosis, but is rare in other forms of cirrhosis except possibly HB_sAg positive chronic active hepatitis. Jaundice is an early symptom and sign in primary biliary cirrhosis but is mild. It occurs in about 30 per cent of patients with chronic active hepatitis and will vary in frequency in the alcoholic, depending on the severity of associated hepatitis. It is uncommon in cryptogenic cirrhosis and rare early in the disease in haemochromatosis. Pruritus is infrequent, except in primary biliary cirrhosis, where it is present in the vast majority of patients at the onset. Some cases of cryptogenic cirrhosis also have cholestatic features.[13] Fever in the absence of infection is rare early in the course of the disease, except in the alcoholic. Fluid retention manifested as peripheral oedema or ascites occurs in a quarter to half the patients, but is uncommon early in primary biliary cirrhosis and haemochromatosis.

The frequency with which patients present with gastrointestinal haemorrhage varies widely in different series, ranging from 5 to 20 per cent. It is common in alcoholics, who may bleed from acute gastric erosions, peptic ulceration or varices. Variceal bleeding may also be a presenting feature in cryptogenic cirrhosis; it is unusual in primary biliary cirrhosis, although reports have been conflicting.[75,84]

Pigmentation is very common in primary biliary cirrhosis and haemochromatosis, and also occurs in a high proportion of alcoholics and patients with cryptogenic cirrhosis. Spider naevi are common in patients with chronic active hepatitis and alcoholic cirrhosis, but are less frequent and less florid in the other forms of cirrhosis. They are confined to the upper part of the body above the nipple-line in the distribution drained by the superior vena cava; it is important to demonstrate their arteriolar nature so as to distinguish them from other forms of vascular malformation. Palmar erythema is frequently associated. Dupuytren's contracture is most common in alcoholic cirrhosis, but the frequency has varied widely, from 4.6 per cent[62] to 66 per cent,[80] and is related to alcohol consumption, social class and occupations involving manual labour. It is generally considered to be uncommon in other forms of cirrhosis, but in our own experience, if carefully looked for, thickening of the palmar fascia is not infrequent.

Gynaecomastia, testicular atrophy and loss of body hair are commonly observed in haemochromatosis and in the alcoholic. Hepatomegaly is almost invariable in patients with haemochromatosis and alcoholic cirrhosis, where the liver may be grossly enlarged. Moderate hepatomegaly is frequent in primary biliary cirrhosis and chronic active hepatitis, but patients with cryptogenic cirrhosis may have normal-sized or small livers at presentation. Splenomegaly is present significantly more often in chronic active hepatitis than in alcoholic cirrhosis,[63] and with variable frequency in other forms of cirrhosis. Other physical signs that may be noted in any form of cirrhosis are finger-clubbing, leuconychia and abdominal herniae. Superficial venous collaterals are frequent in patients with portal hypertension and there may be a venous hum over the liver.

Associated clinical features not necessarily directly related to the cirrhosis may be present early in the course of the disease, particularly with alcoholic cirrhosis, haemochromatosis and primary biliary cirrhosis. Alcoholics may show other features of malnutrition and vitamin deficiency, including Wernicke's encephalopathy, peripheral neuritis, parotid enlargement and folate deficiency. Alcoholic pancreatitis and myopathy are other associations. Patients with haemochromatosis often have overt or biochemical diabetes at the onset (see Chapter 34) and may have an arthropathy and cardiomyopathy. In primary biliary cirrhosis, xanthelasma are frequently present early in the disease and xanthomas with or without a neuropathy develop later (see Chapter 31). Other putative autoimmune diseases may be associated with HB_SAg negative chronic active hepatitis, primary biliary cirrhosis and, less frequently, with cryptogenic cirrhosis. Patients with HB_SAg positive chronic active hepatitis may have a chronic arthritis, vasculitis or glomerulonephritis due to extrahepatic deposition of immune complexes (see Chapter 29).

As cirrhosis progresses, the clinical features merge irrespective of the aetiology and are dominated by liver failure, ascites, oedema, variceal bleeding, haemorrhagic phenomena and secondary infections. In some advanced cases, the original aetiology is undetermined and such cases are labelled as cryptogenic or postnecrotic cirrhosis. They are undoubtedly a heterogeneous group, representing the end stage of many pathological processes of differing aetiology. As new causes or associations of cirrhosis are recognized, the number of unknown aetiology will diminish. For example, some such cases are now recognized as being due to hepatitis B; some may be due to non-A, non-B viruses. Others are associated with alpha-1-antitrypsin deficiency and the high incidence of autoantibodies observed (one-third in some series) raises the probability that some cases may represent burnt-out autoimmune hepatitis. Not surprisingly, such patients often present with the complications of cirrhosis.

DIAGNOSIS

The diagnosis is based on the clinical features, laboratory investigations, liver biopsy histology and radiological and scanning techniques.

There are no definitive laboratory tests which indicate cirrhosis, but it should be suspected if there is reversal of the albumin/globulin ratio, if there are haematological features of hypersplenism or unexplained macrocytosis and target cells on the peripheral film (see Chapter 8) and if there are serological abnormalities such as low alpha-1-antitrypsin levels or a positive mitochondrial antibody or HB_SAg in the serum. Cirrhosis may be suspected on a colloid liver scan if there is patchy liver uptake and redistribution into the bone marrow and spleen (see Chapter 20) and on ultrasound scan if there is a bright echo pattern or a dilated portal vein (see Chapter 21). Occasionally varices are detected incidentally during an upper gastrointestinal barium study.

Often the definitive diagnosis will be made on liver biopsy (see Chapter 18) at laparoscopy, at surgery or at post-mortem.

COMPLICATIONS

The main complications of cirrhosis are gastrointestinal haemorrhage (see Chapter 43), hepatic failure (see Chapters 27 and 42), hepatocellular carcinoma (see Chapter 38), bacterial infection and renal failure (see Chapter 46). The relative frequency of these complications in the different forms of cirrhosis is difficult to determine. It will depend in part on the stage of the disease at which comparisons are made. Gastrointestinal haemorrhage is commoner in the alcoholic cirrhotic than in other forms of cirrhosis, and is not infrequently due to lesions other than bleeding varices, such as a peptic ulcer.

Hepatic failure is often precipitated by gastrointestinal haemorrhage, bacterial infection or episodes of heavy alcohol abuse, and the injudicious treatment of ascites with diuretics. The picture is dominated by increasing jaundice, acute or chronic encephalopathy, haemorrhagic phenomena, ascites and renal failure. Hepatocellular carcinoma is an important complication to recognize as a cause of decompensation, as the cirrhosis may be relatively mild and the carcinoma potentially treatable by transplantation or resection (see Chapters 49 and 52), although the results have not been encouraging.

According to one recent study, hepatocellular carcinoma occurs most commonly in HB_SAg positive chronic active hepatitis and haemochromatosis (42 and 36 per cent respectively), in about one-quarter of the patients with alcoholic or cryptogenic cirrhosis, but is infrequent in primary biliary cirrhosis (3 per cent) and HB_SAg negative chronic active hepatitis.[26] Johnson et al's overall figure of 24 per cent[26] is similar to that in other British series,[36,40,77] but is much higher than in series from the United States.

Bacterial infection is a reversible complication of cirrhosis, and its early diagnosis and vigorous treatment offers the best hope of improving hepatic and renal failure. The Kupffer cells normally remove bacteria passing through the liver in the blood stream,[4] particularly those absorbed from the gut. There is a high incidence of septicaemia due to enterobacteria in cirrhotics and endotoxaemia from gut-derived bacteria may be a factor in the renal failure associated with cirrhosis (see Chapter 46). An increased incidence of bacterial endocarditis in cirrhosis has been reported,[76] presumably because of the high frequency of bacteraemia. There is also an increased incidence of spontaneous peritonitis due to anaerobic bacteria in cirrhosis[79] (see Chapter 46). Tuberculosis is still occasionally encountered in association with cirrhosis, particularly of the alcoholic, as is inhalational pneumonia and lung abscess.

COURSE AND PROGNOSIS

There have been few unselected comparative studies of the prognosis of different forms of cirrhosis. In a follow-up study of liver cirrhosis in Malmo, Sweden, less than half the patients survived one year and only one-tenth survived six years.[21] Similar figures were reported by Stone, Islam and Paton,[77] in a series of unselected patients seen in a general hospital in Birmingham, England, between 1959 and 1964; only 14.3 per cent survived five years. In one series the prognosis in patients with cryptogenic cirrhosis was better than that with alcoholic cirrhosis,[78] but in others the reverse has been the case.[63,77] For example, Powell, Mortimer and Harris[63] found the cumulative five-year survival to be 25.4 per cent in cryptogenic cirrhosis, compared with 47 per cent in alcoholic cirrhosis; survival of patients with chronic active hepatitis was similar to the alcoholics and in those with haemochromatosis was still better, at 67.8 per cent.

There is also good evidence that the prognosis in the alcoholic is greatly improved in those who stop drinking[62] (see Chapter 32). Similarly, treatment of chronic active hepatitis (see Chapter 29), haemochromatosis (see Chapter 34) and Wilson's disease (see Chapter 33) significantly improves the prognosis.

TREATMENT

This is both specific and general. Specific treatment is aimed at removal of the aetiological agent, such as alcohol, iron, copper or drugs. Increasingly, alcoholic liver disease is being recognized in social classes I and II, rather than in the 'Skid Row' down-and-out alcoholic. Recognition of such cases and aggressive rehabilitation offer greater hope of successful treatment than previously (see Chapter 32). Removal of iron from patients with haemochromatosis (see Chapter 34) and copper in Wilson's disease (see Chapter 33) is also advantageous therapeutically. HB_SAg negative chronic active hepatitis may respond to corticosteroid drugs, though the effect on established cirrhosis is less certain (see Chapter 29), and penicillamine improves the prognosis in primary biliary cirrhosis (see Chapter 31). At present, no specific therapy exists for HB_SAg positive chronic liver disease, though interferon and antiviral agents are potentially useful (see Chapter 29), and there is no way of modifying the liver disease associated with alpha-1-antitrypsin deficiency (see Chapter 35).

Treatment of the complications of cirrhosis are dealt with under appropriate chapters, including liver failure (see Chapters 27 and 42), gastrointestinal haemorrhage (see Chapters 43 and 44), ascites, fluid retention and renal failure (see Chapter 46). As indicated above, treatment of complicating bacterial infections may be of great benefit.

REFERENCES

1. Anthony, P.P., Ishak, K.G., Nayak, N.C., Poulsen, H.E., Scheuer, P.J. & Sobin, L.H. (1977) The morphology of cirrhosis: definition, nomenclature and classification. *Bulletin of the World Health Organization*, **55**, 521–540.

2. Anthony, P.P., Ishak, K.G., Nayak, N.C., Poulsen, H.E., Scheuer, P.J. & Sobin, L.H. (1978) The morphology of cirrhosis. *Journal of Clinical Pathology,* **31,** 395–414.
3. Averback, P. (1977) Congenital hepatic fibrosis. Asymptomatic adults without renal anomaly. *Archives of Pathology and Laboratory Medicine,* **101,** 260–261.
4. Beeson, P.B., Brannon, E.S. & Warren, J.V. (1945) Observations on the sites of removal of bacteria from the blood in patients with bacterial endocarditis. *Journal of Experimental Medicine,* **81,** 9–23.
5. Bornstein, P. (1974) The biosynthesis of collagen. *Annual Review of Biochemistry,* **43,** 567–603.
6. Brunt, P.W., Kew, M.C., Scheuer, P.J. & Sherlock, S. (1974) Studies in alcoholic liver disease in Britain. 1. Clinical and pathological patterns related to natural history. *Gut,* **15,** 52–58.
7. Burgeson, R.E., El Adli, F., Kartila, I. & Hollister, D.W. (1976) Fetal membrane collagens: identification of two new collagen alpha-chains. *Proceedings of the National Academy of Sciences of the United States of America,* **73,** 2579–2583.
8. Chen, T., Zetterman, R. & Leevy, C.M. (1973) Sensitized lymphocyte and hepatic fibrogenesis. *Gastroenterology,* **65,** 532–533.
9. Conn, H.O. (1961) Ammonia tolerance as an index of portal-systemic collateral circulation in cirrhosis. *Gastroenterology,* **41,** 97–106.
10. Conn, H.O. & Fessel, J.M. (1971) Spontaneous bacterial peritonitis in cirrhosis: variations on a theme. *Medicine,* **50,** 161–197.
11. Cruikshank, A.H. & Sparshott, S.M. (1971) Malignancy in natural and experimental hepatic cysts: experiments with aflotoxin in rats and the malignant transformation of cysts in human livers. *Journal of Pathology,* **104,** 185–190.
12. Dahl, M.G.C., Gregory, M.M. & Scheuer, P.J. (1972) Methotrexate hepatotoxicity in psoriasis comparison of different dose regimens. *British Medical Journal,* **i,** 654–656.
13. Datta, D.V., Scheuer, P.J. & Sherlock, S. (1963) Postnecrotic cirrhosis with chronic cholestasis. *Gut,* **4,** 223–230.
14. di Sant'Agnese, P.A. & Blanc, W.A. (1956) A distinctive type of biliary cirrhosis of the liver associated with cystic fibrosis of the pancreas. *Pediatrics,* **18,** 387–409.
15. Doehlert, C.A. Jr, Baggenstoss, A.H. & Cain, J.C. (1955) Obstructive biliary cirrhosis and alcoholic cirrhosis: comparison of clinical and pathological features. *American Journal of Clinical Pathology,* **25,** 902–914.
16. Drew, J.S., London, W.T., Lustbader, E.D., Hesser, J.E. & Blumberg, B.S. (1978) Hepatitis B virus and sex ratio of offspring. *Science,* **201,** 687–692.
17. Ferluga, J. & Allison, A.C. (1978) Role of mononuclear infiltrating cells in pathogenesis of hepatitis. *Lancet,* **ii,** 610–611.
18. Gallop, P.M., Blumenfeld, O.O. & Seifter, S. (1972) Structure and metabolism of connective tissue proteins. *Annual Review of Biochemistry,* **41,** 617–672.
19. Gross, G. & Perrier, C.V. (1975) Intrahepatic portasystemic shunting in cirrhotic patients. *New England Journal of Medicine,* **293,** 1046–1047.
20. Groszmann, R.J., Kravetz, D. & Parysow, O. (1977) Intrahepatic arteriovenous shunting in cirrhosis of the liver. *Gastroenterology,* **73,** 201–204.
21. Hällén, J. & Krook, H. (1963) Follow-up studies on an unselected ten-year material of 360 patients with cirrhosis in one community. *Acta Medica Scandinavica,* **173,** 479–493.
22. Horisawa, M., Goldstein, G., Waxman, A. & Reynolds, T. (1976) The abnormal hepatic scan of chronic liver disease: its relationship to hepatic hemodynamics and colloid extraction. *Gastroenterology,* **71,** 210–213.
23. Huet, P.M., Marleau, D., Lavoie, P. & Viallet, A. (1976) Extraction of ^{125}I-albumin microaggregates from portal blood: an index of functional portal blood supply in cirrhotics. *Gastroenterology,* **70,** 74–81.
24. Jeppsson, J.O. (1976) Aminoacid substitution glu-lys in A1AT PiZ. *Federation of European Biochemical Societies' Letters,* **65,** 195–197.
25. Johns, D.G., Hollingsworth, J.W., Cashmore, A.R., Plenderleith, I.H. & Bertino, J.R. (1964) Methotrexate displacement in man. *Journal of Clinical Investigation,* **43,** 621–629.
26. Johnson, P.L. Krasner, N., Portmann, B., Eddleston, A.L.W.F. & Williams, R. (1978) Hepatocellular carcinoma in Great Britain: influence of age, sex, HB_sAg status, and aetiology of underlying cirrhosis. *Gut,* **19,** 1022–1026.
27. Johnson, R.L. & Ziff, M. (1976) Lymphokine stimulation of collagen accumulation. *Journal of Clinical Investigation,* **58,** 240–252.
28. Karvountzis, G.G., Redeker, A.G., & Peters, R.L. (1974) Long term follow-up studies of patients surviving fulminant viral hepatitis. *Gastroenterology,* **67,** 870–877.
29. Kerr, D.N.S., Okoukwo, S. & Choa, R.G. (1978) Congenital hepatic fibrosis: the long term prognosis. *Gut,* **19,** 514–520.
30. Kerr, D.N.S., Harrison, C.V., Sherlock, S. & Milnes-Walker, R. (1961) Congenital hepatic fibrosis. *Quarterly Journal of Medicine,* **30,** 91–117.
31. Klatskin, G. & Bloomer, J.R. (1974) Birefringence of hepatic pigment deposits in erythropoietic protoporphyria. Specificity of polarization microscopy in the identification of hepatic protoporphyrin deposits. *Gastroenterology,* **67,** 294–302.
32. Knowles, D.M., Kaye, G.I. & Godman, G.C. (1975) Nodular regenerative hyperplasia of the liver. *Gastroenterology,* **69,** 746–751.
33. *Lancet* (1978) Collagen in health and disease (Editorial). *Lancet,* **i,** 1077–1078.
34. *Lancet* (1978) Son of Australia antigen (Editorial). *Lancet,* **ii,** 1241–1242.
35. Langness, U. & Undenfriend, S. (1974) Collagen biosynthesis of non-fibroblastic cell lines (propyl hydroxylase). *Proceedings of the National Academy of Sciences of the United States of America,* **71,** 50–51.
36. Lee, F.I. (1966) Cirrhosis and hepatoma in alcoholics. *Gut,* **7,** 77–85.
37. Leevy, C.M. & Tygstrup, N. (1976) Standardization of nomenclature, diagnostic criteria and diagnostic methodology for diseases of the liver and biliary tract. S. Karger, Basel. *Fogarty International Centre Proceedings,* No. 22, DHEW Publication No. (NIH) 76–725, Washington, D.C.: U.S. Government Printing Office.
38. Levin, B., Dobbs, R.H., Burgess, A. & Palmer, T. (1969) Hyperammonaemia. A variant type of deficiency of liver ornithine transcarbamylase. *Archives of Disease in Childhood,* **44,** 162–169.
39. Liebovich, S.J. & Ross, R. (1976) A macrophage-dependent factor that stimulates the proliferation of fibroblasts in vitro. *American Journal of Pathology,* **84,** 501–513.

40. MacSween, R.N.M. (1974) A clinico-pathological review of 100 cases of primary malignant tumours of the liver. *Journal of Clinical Pathology,* **27,** 669–682.
41. McGee, J.O'D. (1977) Collagen deposition in liver disease. *Annals of the Rheumatic Diseases,* **36** (Suppl.), 29–36.
42. McGee, J.O'D. & Patrick, R.S. (1972) The role of perisinusoidal cells in hepatic fibrogenesis: an electron microscopic study of acute carbon tetrachloride liver injury. *Laboratory Investigation,* **26,** 429–440.
43. McGee, J.O'D., O'Hare, R.P. & Patrick, R.S. (1973) Stimulation of the collagen biosynthetic pathway by factors isolated from experimentally-injured liver. *Nature,* **243,** 121–123.
44. McGeoch, J.E.M. & Darmady, E.M. (1976) Polycystic disease of kidney, liver and pancreas: a possible pathogenesis. *Journal of Pathology,* **119,** 221–228.
45. Mezey, E., Potter, J.J. & Maddrey, W.C. (1976) Hepatic collagen proline hydroxylase activity in alcoholic liver disease. *Clinica Chimica Acta,* **68,** 313–320.
46. Miller, E.J. (1976) Biochemical characteristics and biological significance of the genetically-distinct collagens. *Molecular and Cellular Biochemistry,* **13,** 165–192.
47. Millward-Sadler, G.H. & Ryan, T.J. (1974) Methotrexate-induced liver disease in psoriasis. *British Journal of Dermatology,* **90,** 661–667.
48. Mitra, S.K. (1966) Hepatic vascular changes in human and experimental cirrhosis. *Journal of Pathology and Bacteriology,* **92,** 405–414.
49. Morgan, M.Y. & Sherlock, S. (1971) Sex-related differences among 100 patients with alcoholic liver disease. *British Medical Journal,* **i,** 939–941.
50. Nayak, N.C. & Ramalingaswami, V. (1975) Indian childhood cirrhosis. *Clinics in Gastroenterology,* **4**(2), 333–349.
51. Oppenheimer, E.H. & Esterly, J.R. (1975) Hepatic changes in young infants with cystic fibrosis: possible relation to focal biliary cirrhosis. *Journal of Pediatrics,* **86,** 683–689.
52. Partin, J.S., Partin, J.C., Schubert, W.K. & McAdams, A.J. (1974) Liver ultrastructure in abetalipoproteinaemia: evolution of micronodular cirrhosis. *Gastroenterology,* **67,** 107–118.
53. Peters, R.L., Gay, T. & Reynolds, T.B. (1975) Post-jejuno-ileal bypass hepatic disease: its similarity to alcoholic hepatic disease.. *American Journal of Clinical Pathology,* **63,** 318–331.
54. Phillips, M.J. & Steiner, J.W. (1965) Electron microscopy of liver cells in cirrhotic nodules. I. The lateral cell membranes. *American Journal of Pathology,* **46,** 985–1005.
55. Popper, H. & Kent, G. (1975) Fibrosis in chronic liver disease. *Clinics in Gastroenterology,* **4**(2), 315–332.
56. Popper, H. & Orr, W. (1970) Current concepts in cirrhosis. *Scandinavian Journal of Gastroenterology,* **6,** 203–222.
57. Popper, H. & Piez, K.A. (Eds.) (1978) Collagen metabolism in the liver. An annotated and supplemented report of a workshop at the National Institutes of Health on 28th February and 1st March, 1977. *American Journal of Digestive Diseases,* **23,** 641–659.
58. Popper, H. & Undenfriend, S. (1970) Hepatic fibrosis: correlation of biochemical and morphological investigations. *American Journal of Medicine,* **49,** 707–721.
59. Portmann, B., Talbot, I.C., Day, D.W., Davidson, A.R., Murray-Lyon, I.M. & Williams, R. (1975) Histopathological changes in the liver following a paracetamol overdose: correlation with clinical and biochemical parameters. *Journal of Pathology,* **117,** 169–181.
60. Portmann, B., Tanner, M.S. Mowat, A.P. & Williams, R. (1978) Orcein positive liver deposits in Indian childhood cirrhosis *Lancet,* **i,** 1338–1340.
61. Postlethwaite, A.E., Snyderman, R. & Kang, A.H. (1976) The chemotactic attraction of human fibroblasts to a lymphocyte derived factor. *Journal of Experimental Medicine,* **144,** 1188–1203.
62. Powell, W.J. Jr. & Klatskin, G. (1968) Duration of survival in patients with Laennec's cirrhosis: influence of alcohol withdrawal, and possible effects of recent changes in general management of the disease. *American Journal of Medicine,* **44,** 406–420.
63. Powell, L.W., Mortimer, R. & Harris, O.D. (1971) Cirrhosis of the liver. A comparative study of the four major aetiological groups. *Medical Journal of Australia,* **1,** 941–950.
64. Ramachandran, G.N. & Reddi, A.H. (Eds.) (1976) *Biochemisty of Collagen,* New York: Plenum Press.
65. Report of the Board of Classification and Nomenclature of Cirrhosis of the Liver. 5th Pan-American Congress of Gastroenterology, La Habana, Cuba, 1956. *Gastroenterology,* **31,** 213–216.
66. Roberts, W.C. (1962) The hepatic cirrhosis of cystic fibrosis of the pancreas. *American Journal of Medicine,* **32,** 324–328.
67. Rojkind, M. & Martinez-Palomo, A. (1976) Increase in type I and type III collagens in human alcoholic liver cirrhosis. *Proceedings of the National Academy of Sciences of the United States of America,* **73,** 539–543.
68. Ross, R. & Glomset, J. (1976) The pathogenesis of atherosclerosis. *New England Journal of Medicine,* **295,** 369–377; 420–425.
69. Rougier, P., Degott, C., Rueff, B. & Benhamou, J.-P. (1978) Nodular regenerative hyperplasia of the liver. Report of six cases and review of the literature. *Gastroenterology,* **75,** 169–172.
70. Ryan, T.J., Vickers, H.R., Salem, S.N., Callender, S.T. & Badenoch, J. (1964) The treatment of psoriasis with folic acid antagonists. *British Journal of Dermatology,* **76,** 555–564.
71. Scheuer, P.J. (1970) Liver biopsy in the diagnosis of cirrhosis. *Gut,* **11,** 275–278.
72. Seyer, J.M., Hutcheson, E.T. & Kang, A.H. (1977) Collagen polymorphism in normal and cirrhotic human liver. *Journal of Clinical Investigation,* **59,** 241–248.
73. Shaldon, S., Chiandussi, L., Guevara, L., Caesar, J. & Sherlock, S. (1961) The estimation of hepatic blood flow and intrahepatic shunted blood flow by colloidal heat-denatured human serum albumin labelled with I^{131}. *Journal of Clinical Investigation,* **40,** 1346–1354.
74. Sherlock, S (1975) *Diseases of the Liver and Biliary System,* 5th ed. Oxford and Edinburgh: Blackwell.
75. Sherlock, S. & Scheuer, P.J. (1973) The presentation and diagnosis of 100 patients with primary biliary cirrhosis. *New England Journal of Medicine,* **289,** 674–678.
76. Snyder, N., Atterbury, C.E., Correia, J.P. & Conn, H.O. (1977) Increased concurrence of cirrhosis and bacterial endocarditis. *Gastroenterology,* **73,** 1107–1113.

77. Stone, W.D., Islam, N.R.K. & Paton, A. (1968) The natural history of cirrhosis. Experience with an unselected group of patients. *Quarterly Journal of Medicine,* **145,** 119–132.
78. Summerskill, W.H., Davidson, C.S., Dible, J.H., Mallory, G.K., Sherlock, S., Turner, M.D. & Wolfe, S.J. (1960) Cirrhosis of the liver: a study of alcoholic and non-alcoholic patients in Boston and London. *New England Journal of Medicine,* **262,** 1–9.
79. Targan, S.R., Chow, A.W. & Guze, L.B. (1977) Anaerobic bacteria in spontaneous peritonitis of cirrhosis. *American Journal of Medicine,* **62,** 397–403.
80. Wolfe, S.J., Summerskill, W.H.J. & Davidson, C.S. (1956) Thickening and contraction of the palmar fascia (Dupuytren's contracture) associated with alcoholism and hepatic cirrhosis. *New England Journal of Medicine,* **255,** 559.
81. Wolff, K., Wolff-Schreiner, E. & Gschnaitt, F. (1975) Liver inclusions in erythropoietic protoporphyria. *European Journal of Clinical Investigation,* **5,** 21–26.
82. Wyler, D.J., Wahl, S.M. & Wahl, L.M. (1978) Hepatic fibrosis in schistosomiasis: egg granulomas secrete fibroblast-stimulating factor in vitro. *Science,* **202,** 438–440.
83. Yoshida, A., Lieberman, J., Gaidulis, L. & Ewing, C. (1976) Molecular abnormality of human AIAT variant PiZZ associated with plasma activity deficiency. *Proceedings of the National Academy of Sciences of the United States of America,* **73,** 1324–1328.
84. Zeegen, R., Stansfeld, A.G., Dawson, A.M. & Hunt, A.H. (1969) Bleeding oesophageal varices as the presenting feature in primary biliary cirrhosis. *Lancet,* **ii,** 9–13.

Chapter 31

Primary Biliary Cirrhosis

SHEILA SHERLOCK

This condition was first described in 1851 by Addison and Gull and later by Hanot.[41] The association with high serum cholesterol levels and skin xanthomas led to the term 'xanthomatous biliary cirrhosis'.[61] Ahrens et al[2] termed the condition 'primary biliary cirrhosis'. However, in the early stages, nodular regeneration in the liver is inconspicuous and the anatomical criteria needed for the diagnosis of cirrhosis are not fulfilled.[80] Recent pathological studies make the term 'chronic non-suppurative destructive cholangitis'[74] a better one, although it is unlikely that it will replace the shorter, more popular one of 'primary biliary cirrhosis'.

The aetiology is unsolved. Any answer must take into account the predilection of the disease for middle-aged women. In one series of 100 patients, 90 were women and, in 73, the diagnosis was made between the ages of 40 and 59.[81] Earlier diagnosis at an asymptomatic stage is lowering the age of presentation. Any answer must also explain the association of the disease with other conditions with disturbed immunity, such as chronic active hepatitis and cryptogenic cirrhosis.[20] The regular, consistent demonstration, in high titre, of serum antibodies, such as antinuclear antibody (ANA), smooth muscle and mitochondrial antibodies, are virtually confined to three liver diseases, primary biliary cirrhosis, chronic active hepatitis and cryptogenic cirrhosis – particularly in women.

A possible immunological basis for the injury to small bile ducts and its perpetuation has not been proved. Cell-based immunity is considerably disturbed in primary biliary cirrhosis. This suggests that sensitized T-lymphocytes might be the basis of the bile duct injury. The histological reaction round injured bile ducts is predominantly monocytic with lymphocytic accumulations prominent. Well-formed granulomas are included and, indeed, extrahepatic granulomas are found in lymph nodes, lung and even bone marrow.[29] Granulomas are the hallmark of disturbed cell-based immunity. Skin tests using tuberculin or dinitrochlorobenzene (DNCB) show that many patients with primary biliary cirrhosis are anergic.[29] Phytohaemagglutinin (PHA)-stimulated lymphocytes show impaired transformation in patients with primary biliary cirrhosis.[29] Using a single dose of PHA and with culture in autologous plasma, 23 of 30 patients showed impaired lymphocyte transformation. There is no correlation between the histological stage of the disease and the degree of impairment. Indeed, two presymptomatic patients had normal mechanisms of delayed hypersensitivity.[28] This raised the possibility that the anergy was the result rather than the cause of the disease. The subnormal in vitro lymphocyte reactivity to PHA has been confirmed.[63] Similarly, abnormal cell-mediated responses in the leucocyte migration test have been found in 64 per cent of patients with primary biliary cirrhosis.[85]

In a further study, the humoral and cellular immune response to haemocyanin was measured in normal subjects and in patients with primary biliary cirrhosis.[27] The incidence of positive skin tests was reduced and a poor antibody response was also noted. Both impaired T cell function and a poor humoral response were therefore found, and lack of T and B cell cooperation was postulated.

There is no relationship between the various serological autoantibody markers, and particularly between the positive mitochondrial antibody test, which is so valuable in diagnosis, and the aetiology of the disease. Similarly, disturbances in cell-based immunity seem to bear little relationship to severity. Studies of a daughter who was symptomatic and a mother with primary biliary cirrhosis, who was not, showed strikingly similar immunological changes.[93] The immunological aspects of primary biliary cirrhosis have been discussed in more detail in Chapter 9.

GENETIC AND EPIDEMIOLOGICAL ASPECTS

Familial instances of primary biliary cirrhosis are rare. Two sisters have been reported, one of whom had fairly typical disease and the other a picture very suggestive of primary biliary cirrhosis.[98] Both had high titres of serological mitochondrial antibodies. Other instances, in brothers, have been noted, and in twin sisters.[13] Primary biliary cirrhosis and chronic active hepatitis have been reported in elderly sisters.[100] The possible familial nature of the disease is better emphasized by surveys for the presence of serum autoimmune tests in family members of sufferers. Feizi et al noted a significant increase in mitochondrial antibodies among the relatives of 26 patients with primary biliary cirrhosis.[25] In a larger study, 260 family members of sufferers from chronic active hepatitis or primary biliary cirrhosis were studied and mitochondrial and smooth muscle antibodies were much more frequent than in controls matched for age and sex.[32] Surprisingly, the prevalence of positive mitochondrial antibody tests was not greater in the primary biliary cirrhosis relatives than in those with chronic active hepatitis. Seven to eight per cent of symptomless relatives of patients with primary biliary cirrhosis showed a positive mitochondrial antibody test, which is 10 times more than that found in the general population. The reason for this familial incidence is uncertain. Equally unsure is the trigger that leads to clinically overt primary biliary cirrhosis in some but not all of these susceptible family members. Some factor or factors presumably sensitizes the biliary epithelium to injury.

The frequency of the histocompatibility antigens HLA-A1 and HLA-B8 in Australia,[60] South-east England and Glasgow was greater in patients with chronic active hepatitis than in controls.[34] But this did not apply to patients with primary biliary cirrhosis. There is no excess of any particular ABO blood group or of rhesus negativity.[40]

There are very few epidemiological studies of incidence. Certainly, the disease has been reported from all parts of the world. Chinese, Europeans, Indians, Japanese, Jews and Negroes are among those affected. The death-rates from primary biliary cirrhosis in various countries are difficult to assess but are probably of the order of 0.6 to 2.00 per cent of those dying with cirrhosis.[39] In an epidemiological study conducted in England, it was concluded that primary biliary cirrhosis predominantly affects middle-aged women of social classes 1 and 2, living in an urban situation.[39] There is an undoubted sampling error in such studies. Further detailed epidemiological surveys are essential in different parts of the world.

Relationship between Primary Biliary Cirrhosis, Chronic Active Hepatitis and Cryptogenic Cirrhosis

The regular and consistent demonstration in high titre of antibody tests such as ANA, smooth muscle and mitochondrial antibodies is virtually confined to sera from patients with three liver diseases – primary biliary cirrhosis, chronic active hepatitis and cryptogenic cirrhosis – particularly in women.[20] Results are negative in such conditions as alcoholic liver disease, Wilson's disease, sclerosing cholangitis and biliary atresia, even though the extent of hepatocellular or biliary damage may be as great. This suggests that the increases do not simply represent antibodies developing as a response to constituents of damaged liver cells or bile ducts.

PATHOLOGY

The liver is large and green. At operation or laparoscopy the surface appears smooth but, as time passes, it becomes nodular. The gallbladder and bile ducts are normal. Enlarged fleshy lymph glands in the porta hepatis and along the common bile duct often lead to a mistaken diagnosis of reticulosis. Such lymph nodes show only a reticulum cell hyperplasia with phagocytes loaded with bile pigment. The spleen shows pulp hyperplasia and the changes associated with portal hypertension.

Hepatic Histology[74, 78]

The disease is essentially one of progressive granulomatous injury and, finally, disappear-

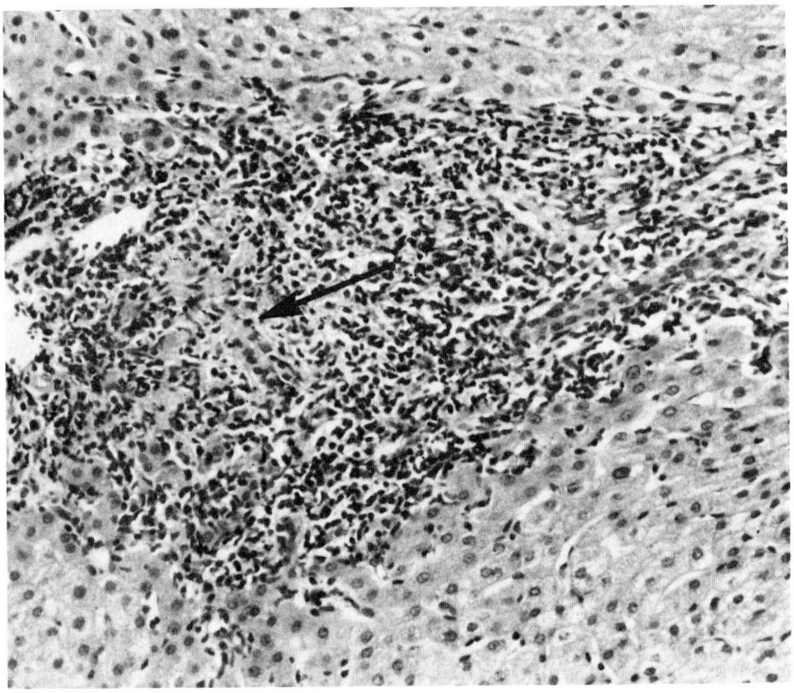

Figure 31.1. Primary biliary cirrhosis. Diagnostic stage 1 lesion with damaged bile ducts (arrow), surrounded by a mononuclear cell infiltrate. Haematoxylin and eosin × 120.

ance of septal and interlobular bile ducts within the liver. Four stages can be recognized.

Stage 1: the florid duct lesion. This is pathognomonic. Septal and larger interlobular bile ducts are damaged and surrounded by a dense infiltrate of lymphocytes, large histiocytes or epithelioid cells, plasma cells and a few eosinophils (Figure 31.1). Lymphoid aggregates, with or without germinal centres, may be found. Granulomas are often seen as poorly defined collections of histiocytes or as well-organized tuberculoid lesions with giant cells but without central necrosis. They are usually near a damaged duct in the portal tract. This damage is seen as swelling, proliferation and crowding of epithelial cells and as rupture. The bile ducts are swollen with finely granular eosinophilic cytoplasm with little or no vacuolation. They are in a single layer. The bile duct lesions must be distinguished from those found in chronic aggressive hepatitis.[14] This disease involves medium-sized ducts which may show ballooning, vacuolation and stratification of the epithelial cells. Germinal centres may be seen, but never granulomas. Duct rupture is absent. Nuclear pleomorphism is more common than in primary biliary cirrhosis and fibrosis surrounding the duct is unusual.

The portal tract is otherwise normal and the limiting liver cell plates are intact. Within the lobules there may be slight mononuclear cell infiltration and regenerative hyperplasia seen as double liver cell plates. Centrizonal cholestasis may be seen but is often absent and is rarely severe.

Stage 2: ductular proliferation. The lesions are now more widespread throughout the expanded portal tracts but are less specific. There is fibrosis, acute and chronic inflammatory infiltration and ductular proliferation. Ducts are reduced and their place is taken by ill-defined lymphoid aggregates which, together with the fibrosis and inflammation, give a rather characteristic appearance. The appearances are often compatible with, or suggestive of, primary biliary cirrhosis rather than being diagnostic. Granulomas are less common. Periportal areas show a slight to moderate degree of liver cell necrosis, swelling and cholestasis. Lipid-laden histiocytes are sometimes seen.

Stage 3: scarring. The inflammation subsides and relatively acellular septa extend from the portal tracts into and around the lobules. Lymphoid aggregates are still seen and periportal cholestasis may be severe. Here, again, the appearances are not pathognomonic of primary biliary cirrhosis but can be interpreted as highly suggestive and compatible.

Stage 4: cirrhosis. Regeneration nodules are seen and the picture is of end-stage liver disease. The diagnosis may still be suggested by paucity of bile ducts or by accumulations of lymphocytes. There is much overlap between the stages to the extent that stage 1 lesions are occasionally seen in stage 4 livers with well-established cirrhosis.[38]

Hepatocellular hyaline deposits.[33,62] Hyaline inclusions similar to those of alcoholic disease are found in the hepatocytes in about 25 per cent of cases. They are usually adjacent to portal tracts and connective tissue septa. Their presence does not correlate with any other clinical or biochemical parameter of the disease.

Ultrastructural Changes

Primary biliary cirrhosis shows distinctive features on electron microscopy compared with extrahepatic biliary obstruction.[11] These include changes in the small and medium-sized bile ducts. The bile duct epithelium shows intracytoplasmic filamentous structures grouped into bundles. The mitochondria are swollen and exhibit fewer circular cristae. The rough endoplasmic reticulum is vesicular and ribosomes are scanty. The luminal microvilli are at first blunted and scanty and finally disappear. In the final stage, the basement membranes of the bile ducts are disrupted and invaded by polymorphonuclear leucocytes. Some of the changes observed in the bile ducts are also seen to a minor degree in other pathological entities, but their prominence and progression are distinctive in primary biliary cirrhosis and possibly make them features of diagnostic significance.

Diagnosis on Liver Biopsy Specimens

The only hepatic lesion pathognomonic of primary biliary cirrhosis is the injured septal or interlobular bile duct. Such ducts are not often seen in sections of liver obtained by needle biopsy but are usually well represented in the larger wedge biopsy obtained surgically. Histopathological diagnosis of primary biliary cirrhosis is therefore more confident with operative biopsies than with needle ones. Yet the number of such specimens is decreasing with the greater emphasis on cholangiography for demonstration of main bile ducts and the decreasing number of laparotomies. Great importance is being placed in the reading of the needle biopsy section and the experience of the histopathologist.[79] Local, portal-zone lymphocyte accumulations with a 'biliary type' of fibrosis and peripheral cholestasis are very suggestive of primary biliary cirrhosis. The distinction between diagnostic changes, i.e. destructive lesions of larger bile ducts, and compatible ones is very helpful. The report of a compatible histology can be slotted into place with the clinical, biochemical and immunological findings to provide a diagnostic whole.

The florid duct lesion of stage 1 must be distinguished from the peribiliary infiltration of long-standing large duct obstruction in which duct damage is generally absent and granulomas are rare. In the pericholangitis associated with ulcerative colitis, the ducts are not destroyed, granulomas are absent and the infiltrate is predominantly lymphocytic with few or no plasma cells. A somewhat similar bile duct lesion, but generally without granulomas, is found in a few patients with acute or chronic viral hepatitis.[14] Piecemeal necrosis in the later stages, may make it difficult to distinguish between primary biliary cirrhosis and chronic active hepatitis, and there are mixed forms.[68] Features favouring primary biliary cirrhosis include intact lobules, slight piecemeal necrosis, periseptal cholestasis and lymphoid aggregates. When cirrhosis has developed and clinical features are atypical, cryptogenic cirrhosis may be wrongly diagnosed.

CLINICAL FEATURES AND INVESTIGATION

Criteria for diagnosis

Clinically, primary biliary cirrhosis is a disease of middle-aged women who present with a slow onset of cholestasis. The serum mitochondrial antibody test is positive. Needle liver biopsy histology shows small bile duct destruction, which is diagnostic, or features which are compatible with the diagnosis. The main bile ducts have been shown to be patent by some form of cholangiography. Additional presence of diseases known to be associated with primary biliary cirrhosis may add diagnostic weight. This description is of the 'ideal' case. In practice, of course, all these criteria may not be met. After weighing the evidence, the physician uses clinical judgement and decides whether or not the patient is suffering from primary biliary cirrhosis.

Presentation

In the past, the patient presented at a late, icteric stage. One or more laparotomies had usually been performed to exclude surgical jaundice. Now, the disease can usually be recognized earlier and without surgery. In a series published in 1959,[80] 20 per cent of the patients diagnosed were anicteric and this proportion had risen to 41 per cent by 1973.[81] By 1977, 20 patients could be diagnosed at a stage when they had no symptoms of hepatobiliary disease.[59]

The patient is usually female, but about 10 per cent are male.[81] Male sex should not exclude the diagnosis. Nevertheless, more detailed investigations are necessary, and the main bile ducts, in particular, must be shown to be patent before a diagnosis of primary biliary cirrhosis in males, compared with females, is made. The reason for the sex preference is unknown. Other hepatic diseases with circulating autoantibodies, such as chronic active (lupoid) hepatitis and cryptogenic cirrhosis, are also more common in females, but the predilection for the female sex in these conditions is not so great as in primary biliary cirrhosis.

The disease usually presents between the ages of 40 and 60, but has been diagnosed at the age of 23 in an asymptomatic patient,[59] and even up to the age of 72.[81]

The usual onset is as insidious pruritus. This is commonly diffuse, but may commence in the perianal or genital regions. It is enhanced by warm weather, or at night, or by wearing coarse, woollen underwear. This symptom usually brings the patient to her physician and often to the dermatologist. Unless the medical attendant is alert to the possibility of primary biliary cirrhosis, many months of local skin treatment can ensue before the underlying cholestasis is recognized.

The pruritus may appear during pregnancy, especially during the last trimester. Pregnancy is always a condition which is potentially, although subclinically, cholestatic and this is progressive. The cholestasis is shown by the reduction of the transport maximum (Tm) for bromsulphthalein by 27 per cent during the last half of pregnancy while the bromsulphthalein storage (S) increases.[15] Primary biliary cirrhosis adds its own component of cholestasis to that of normal pregnancy, and pruritus develops. Primary biliary cirrhosis may then be confused with cholestatic jaundice of the last trimester. In contrast to that condition, however, the pruritus usually persists when the patient is delivered. Occasionally, the itching of primary biliary cirrhosis disappears after delivery only to return months or years later.

Similarly, the pruritus of primary biliary cirrhosis may become manifest when the asymptomatic patient is given birth-control pills containing cholestatic hormones.

Jaundice may appear at the same time as the pruritus, but very rarely antedates it. The jaundice usually appears six months to two years after the itching, but delays of 10 to 20 years can occur. The jaundice is rarely deep at presentation. It is cholestatic in type with darkening of the urine and pallor of the stools. Jaundice without itching is very rare.

Although bleeding from oesophageal varices has been reported as a frequent initial complaint,[101] in our experience it is rare.[52] Portal hypertension, of course, is common as the disease advances and this will be discussed later.

Primary biliary cirrhosis may be diagnosed when the patient is under investigation for another condition known to be associated with it. Early diagnosis has been made in some patients with no cholestasis or other hepatic symptoms who were being investigated for such conditions as rheumatoid arthritis, arthropathy, dermatomyositis, keratoconjunctivitis sicca, or familial hyperparathyroidism, pernicious anaemia or telangiectasia.[56] Such patients tended to be younger than those diagnosed when symptomatic. The increasing use of biochemical screening procedures which include serum alkaline phosphatase values allows more patients to be diagnosed at an early stage. Any elevation of such values in a middle-aged woman should always raise the suspicion of primary biliary cirrhosis. It must be followed by confirmation that the raised alkaline phosphatase is of hepatic origin. This is done either by isoenzyme techniques or by showing a raised serum 5′-nucleotidase or γ-glutamyl transpeptidase value. Routine screening for serum autoantibodies when a positive mitochondrial antibody test is found may be another mode of presentation.

The patient is usually pigmented from the outset. The liver is variably enlarged, non-tender and the edge has a firm consistency. The spleen is usually enlarged.

Xanthomas are never marked at presentation and, if present, are usually seen only as xanthelasma.

Biochemical Changes

Serum bilirubin values are rarely very high at the outset, and in about one-half of patients are less than 34 μmol/l (2 mg/100 ml) (Figure 31.2). Serum alkaline phosphatase is always markedly raised, exceeding 6 μmol/s/l (50 KA units) in about 71 per cent of patients (Figure 31.3). Raised serum 5′-nucleotidase confirms that the phosphatase is of biliary origin. The serum bilirubin levels may fluctuate and may be within normal limits for some months. The serum alkaline phosphatase, however, continues elevated. Asymptomatic patients may have normal or only minimally raised alkaline phosphatase, cholesterol and aspartate transaminase levels while the serum bilirubin level may be normal.[59]

Serum bile acid levels may be a more sensitive index of cholestasis than the serum alkaline phosphatases. One patient with asymptomatic primary biliary cirrhosis had a normal serum alkaline phosphatase and other biochemical tests, yet the post-prandial serum bile acid value was increased.[90]

The total serum cholesterol concentration increases, but not constantly, and is an unreliable diagnostic test. The total serum lipids are greatly increased and this particularly involves the phospholipid and total cholesterol fractions. Neutral fat is very slightly increased. In spite of the high lipid content, the serum is characteristically clear and not milky. This may be due to the surface-tension-lowering effect of phospholipid which keeps the other lipids in solution.

The serum albumin level is usually normal at presentation. The total serum globulin may be moderately increased.

Serum lipoproteins are increased due to a rise in the low density (α_2, β) fraction. The high-density lipoproteins are decreased. The increase consists largely of an abnormal lipoprotein which contains a high proportion of unesterified cholesterol and phospholipid and has been called lipoprotein X. The origin is unknown but it may be an intestinal lipoprotein, normally catabolized in the liver and accumulating as a result of hepatic dysfunction. It appears by electron microscopy as a disc-shaped particle. Serum lipoprotein X is usually found in patients with primary biliary cirrhosis, and certainly in the icteric stage.

Serum immunoglobulin M (IgM) is usually raised, often to very high values.[24,67] The estimation has even been suggested for diagnosis.[8] However, in about 25 per cent of patients, values do not exceed the upper limit of 1.95 g/l (195 mg/100 ml).[81] Serum IgM levels can in no sense be regarded as reliable for diagnosis of primary biliary cirrhosis. However, increased values are found in 84 per cent of asymptomatic cases so that high values in the presence of slightly raised serum bilirubin levels are supporting evidence for the diagnosis of primary biliary cirrhosis.

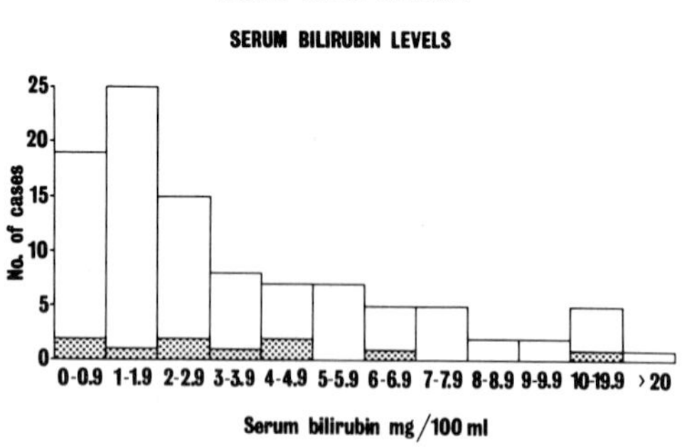

Figure 31.2. Serum bilirubin levels at presentation in 100 patients with primary biliary cirrhosis. Note that the serum bilirubin level was less than 34 μmol/l (2 mg/100 ml) in 41 per cent. Males are in hatched columns. From Sherlock and Scheuer,[81] with kind permission of the editor of *New England Journal of Medicine*.

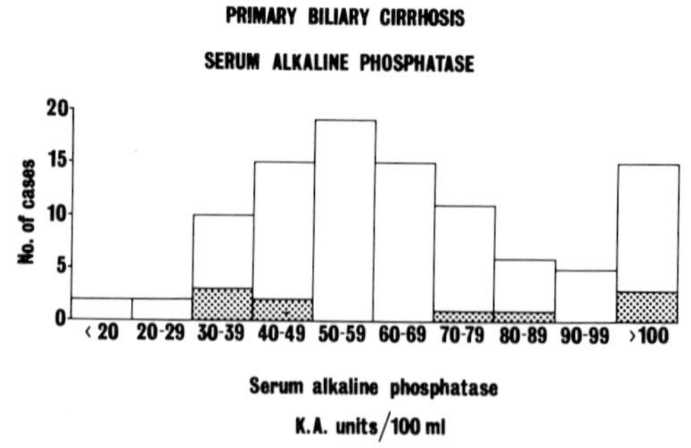

Figure 31.3. Serum alkaline phosphatase levels (normal 0.36 to 1.68 μmol/s/l [3 to 14 KA units]) at presentation in 100 patients with primary biliary cirrhosis. The level exceeded 6 μmol/s/l (50 KA units) in 71 per cent. Males are in hatched columns. From Sherlock and Scheuer,[81] with kind permission of the editor of *New England Journal of Medicine*.

Haematological Changes

These are in general non-contributory. The erythrocyte sedimentation rate is usually markedly increased. The erythrocytes show reduced osmotic fragility. Target cells have been related to an accumulation of cholesterol in the red cell membrane, thus increasing red cell surface area and leading to target formation.[17]

Mitochondrial Antibodies

In 1965, it was recognized that patients with primary biliary cirrhosis had in their serum an antibody against mitochondria.[97] This was shown by granular fluorescence in an immunofluorescent technique on tissue sections. The staining reactions were neither organ- nor species-specific. The test section currently employed is human kidney where the reaction is seen to be strongest in the ascending loop of Henle and in the distal tubules. The sera are usually tested at 1 : 10 since undiluted specimens may give non-specific fluorescence and, occasionally, strongly positive sera show prozone effects and appear negative until diluted. The use of non-specific anti-IgG conjugate probably increases the diagnostic accuracy but also reduces the number of positives in cases of primary biliary cirrhosis.

The antigen is a component of the mitochondrial inner membrane.[7] It is a lipoprotein which may be a membrane transport protein. It has recently been purified.[6] The molecular weight is 180 000 to 200 000. This purification may be of use if an automated radioimmunoassay were to prove sensitive and specific for the detection of mitochondrial antibody. The aetiological importance of the antibody is unknown but is probably slight, for it is not related either to the stage of the disease or to other immunological phenomena, particularly those concerning cell-based immunity.[29] It is possibly related to a cross-reaction with an unknown microorganism whose primitive enzyme systems resemble those of mitochondria. The test is positive in 84 to 96 per cent of patients with primary biliary cirrhosis.[22,37,53] It is negative in mechanical obstruction to bile ducts, however prolonged.[73] Reports suggesting positive results in long-standing biliary obstruction are probably due to technical differences, particularly in the tissue used and its species-source.[64] In one series of patients with surgical cholestatic jaundice, the test was positive preoperatively but remained so after relief of the obstruction, suggesting an underlying positivity irrespective of the block. The extrahepatic biliary obstruction was probably a complication of mitochondrial antibody positive liver disease.[50]

The mitochondrial antibody test is also positive in about 20 per cent of patients with hepatitis B antigen negative chronic active hepatitis. It may also be found in some patients with cryptogenic cirrhosis. These are usually middle-aged women who have some points in common with primary biliary cirrhosis in terms of hepatic histology and cholestatic biochemistry.[21,53] It has also been described in some women with collagenoses and diseases of 'autoimmune' type such as thyroiditis and gastritis.[97] In these patients, liver histology shows a non-specific hepatitis. The significance remains uncertain but primary biliary cirrhosis is known to be associated with collagen diseases such as rheumatoid arthritis, Sjögren's disease and scleroderma.

The practical diagnostic importance of the mitochondrial antibody test is twofold. In a patient with cholestasis, a negative result always arouses suspicion that primary biliary cirrhosis is not the correct diagnosis (Figure 31.4). Secondly, a positive result in an icteric patient throws considerable doubt that the jaundice is due to a mechanical block to main bile passages.

Cholangiography

If possible, the main bile ducts should be demonstrated to be patent. In the anicteric or mildly jaundiced patient, the intravenous cholangiographic perfusion technique with

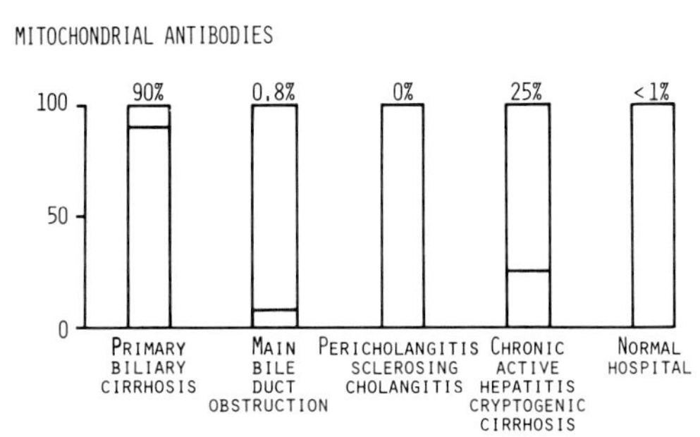

Figure 31.4. The percentage positivity of the serum mitochondrial antibody tests in primary biliary cirrhosis, main bile duct obstruction, pericholangitis and sclerosing cholangitis, chronic active hepatitis and cryptogenic cirrhosis and in a normal hospital population.

Table 31.1. *The Calibre of the Bile Ducts in Normals and Primary Biliary Cirrhosis.*

	No.	Diameter of ducts (mm)		
		Common bile	Right hepatic	Left hepatic
Normal	10	9.1 ± 2.4	5.6 ± 2.2	5.9 ± 1.7
Primary biliary cirrhosis	23	9.5 ± 2.5	5.0 ± 2.1	5.2 ± 1.9

Differences not significant.
From Summerfield et al,[89] with kind permission of the authors and the editor of *Gastroenterology*.

tomography of the bile ducts is often successful. In the more deeply jaundiced patient, endoscopic retrograde cholangiography or percutaneous cholangiography must be considered.

Endoscopic retrograde cholangiography

This technique is particularly useful in patients with primary biliary cirrhosis.[89] It has the advantage over the percutaneous technique in that oesophagus, stomach, duodenum and pancreatic ducts may also be visualized. If the endoscope head (10 mm) is used as a standard of reference, the approximate maximum and minimum size of the main bile ducts can be assessed. The calibre of the common bile duct, right hepatic duct and left hepatic duct do not differ from those observed in control subjects (Table 31.1).[89] However, differences from control subjects are seen in the main intrahepatic bile ducts (Table 31.2). In some instances, the ducts are irregular in calibre and run a tortuous course.[76,89] Similar irregularities have been observed in operative cholangiograms from patients with primary biliary cirrhosis. These duct irregularities correlated well with histologically-proven biliary cirrhosis.[89] Narrowing and tortuosity indicate that cirrhosis has developed. Duct changes probably result from distortion of hepatic parenchymal architecture with nodule formation (Figure 31.5).

Endoscopic retrograde cholangiography is also useful in diagnosing gallstones in patients with primary biliary cirrhosis and in defining their location, whether in gallbladder or common bile duct. The high incidence of gallstones in patients with primary biliary cirrhosis will be discussed later.

Percutaneous cholangiography

This technique, performed with the Okuda 'skinny needle', often allows normal-sized bile ducts to be visualized.[23,66] Refinements in technique and increased operative facility with practice now allow the technique frequently to succeed in the patient with primary biliary cirrhosis who has non-dilated ducts in the liver.[47] This is a less costly procedure and is technically easier than endoscopic retrograde cholangiography. It is playing an increasing role in establishing patent bile ducts in patients with intrahepatic cholestasis and particularly in those with primary biliary cirrhosis.

The Place of Laparotomy

This has the advantage of visualizing the bile ducts, gallbladder and noting any other pathological condition in the abdominal cavity. It also allows a wedge biopsy of the liver to be obtained and this is likely to give more diagnostic histological appearances than a needle one. However, with the advent of endoscopic and percutaneous cholangiography and more widespread availability of the mitochondrial antibody test, laparotomy is rarely needed for the diagnosis of primary biliary cirrhosis. Certain circumstances, and particularly combinations of circumstances, may make the procedure useful. Indications include the early development of deep jaundice, particularly in a man. Persistent pain and fever are both unusual features of primary biliary cirrhosis and may indicate the need for laparotomy. Ingestion of cholestatic drugs in close relation to the development of pruritus may cause a confusing picture. Primary biliary cirrhosis in the presence of a negative mitochondrial antibody test always demands

Table 31.2. *Intrahepatic Ducts and Gallstones in Primary Biliary Cirrhosis.*

Fibrosis	No.	Duct abnormality		
		Calibre	Course	Gallstones
Slight	3	1	0	1
Extensive	4	0	1	0
Cirrhosis	14	7	7	8

From Summerfield et al,[89] with kind permission of the authors and the editor of *Gastroenterology*.

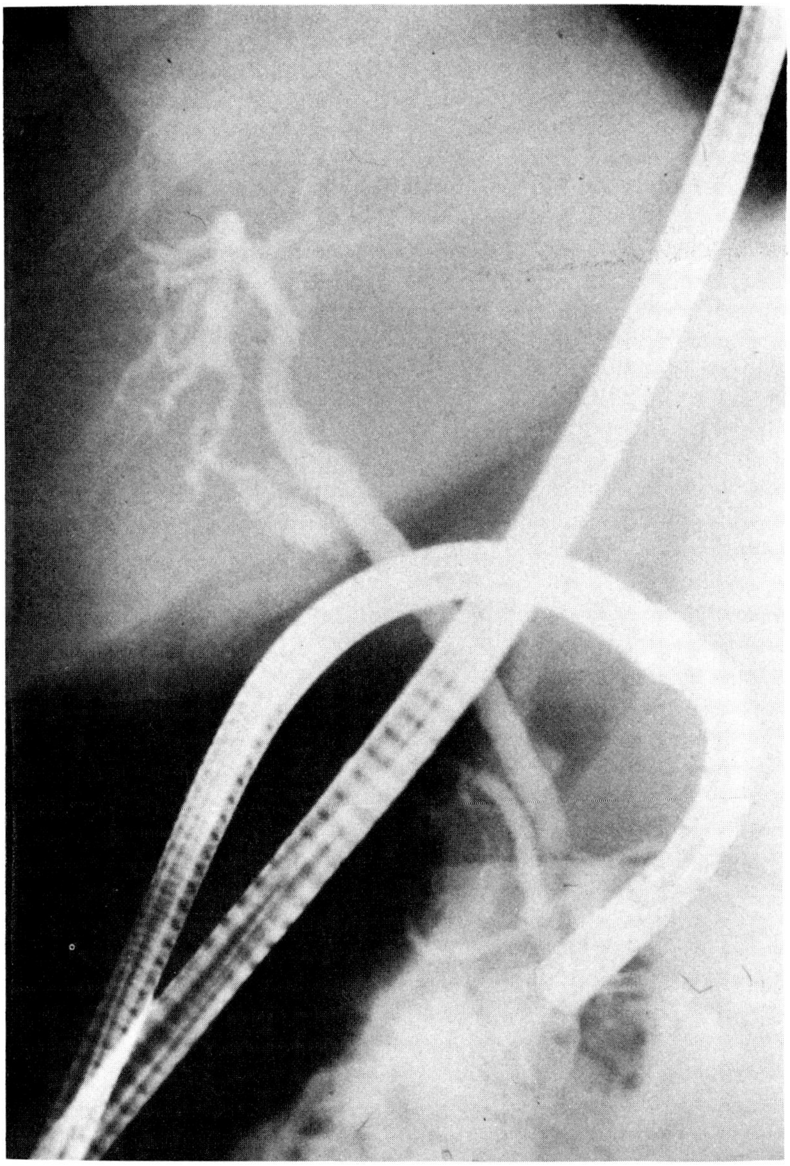

Figure 31.5. Endoscopic retrograde cholangiopancreatography in a patient with late-stage primary biliary cirrhosis. Note the patent common bile duct. The intrahepatic bile ducts are distorted and stretched round nodules, indicating that cirrhosis has already developed. From Summerfield et al,[89] with kind permission of the authors and the editor of *Gastroenterology*.

visualization of the bile ducts, and if this is impossible by non-invasive techniques, laparotomy may be needed.

Scanning Procedures

The grey wedge ultrasonic scanning or the more sophisticated scanning by computerized axial tomography may be used to demonstrate dilated intrahepatic ducts and so diagnose obstruction to main bile ducts and exclude the diagnosis of primary biliary cirrhosis.

Gallstones

In one series of 23 patients with primary biliary cirrhosis studied by endoscopic cholangiography, 39 per cent had gallstones in the gallbladder but not in the common bile duct.[89] Cirrhotic patients are known to have an increased frequency of gallstone formation. In one autopsy study, 29.4 per cent of all cirrhotics and 30.8 per cent (4 of 13) of the patients with primary biliary cirrhosis had gallstones, compared with 12.8 per cent of the non-cirrhotic population.[9] In contrast to the findings in non-cirrhotic patients, most of the gallstones were of pigment type. This type would be unexpected if decreased bile acid concentration in bile was playing a part. Analysis of the last 21 autopsies on patients with primary biliary cirrhosis at the Royal Free Hospital showed that eight of 21 (38 per cent) had gallstones; this figure agrees closely with the figure obtained by endoscopic retrograde cholangiography.[89]

The decision whether or not to recommend surgical exploration in patients with primary biliary cirrhosis who also have gallstones is extremely difficult. If the gallstones are asymptomatic, and in the gallbladder, they are probably best left alone. If they are in the common bile duct, surgical intervention is probably indicated. If the gallstones in the gallbladder are producing symptoms, the decision is particularly difficult. Patients with underlying chronic liver disease, even if it is only primary biliary cirrhosis, tolerate surgery poorly. In the presence of primary biliary cirrhosis, liver histology obtained by needle biopsy is not particularly helpful in making the distinction between gallstone obstruction and primary biliary cirrhosis. Indeed, liver biopsy may confuse the decision as to whether gallstones are, or are not, causing biliary obstruction. Each case has to be decided on its merits, and great clinical experience is needed for the decision-making.

Portal Hypertension

Bleeding from oesophageal varices is generally believed to be a late feature of primary biliary cirrhosis.[82] This is not always so, and presentation as bleeding varices was noted in 15 of 23 patients in one series.[101] These patients, however, were in a highly selected group referred to a surgeon for possible relief of portal hypertension. Nevertheless, if portal hypertension is sought, it is frequently demonstrated even quite early in the course. In one series of 109 patients, 50 showed oesophageal varices radiologically.[52] Intrasplenic pressures cannot be measured with safety because of the danger of bleeding from the splenic puncture site. In only four was bleeding the initial manifestation of disease. In another 17, however, it was recognized within two years of the first symptom. The presence of bleeding varices considerably worsens the prognosis, particularly when ascites is an associated factor. In general, portal hypertension is related to nodular regeneration in the liver and to cirrhosis. Nodules are generally believed to be late features of primary biliary cirrhosis and, in fact, the portal hypertension frequently antedates nodule formation.[52,82,101] The mechanism of the early portal hypertension in these patients is therefore difficult to understand. It could be related to obstruction to portal venous flow by portal tract lesions, and hence be at a presinusoidal level.[101] However, marked or moderate portal fibrosis is not more common in patients with varices and there is no difference in other factors, such as cellular infiltration or lymphoid aggregates in portal tracts or septa, which might cause obstruction at a presinusoidal level.[52] Nor is there a difference in the number of thin-walled vessels or arterioles in the portal tracts of patients with and without varices. Obstruction to efferent veins or at a sinusoidal level by mononuclear cell infiltration, hypertrophy of Kupffer cells or narrowing of sinusoids by consistent twin hepatocyte plates cannot be demonstrated. The mechanism of the portal hypertension therefore remains most obscure.

COURSE

The course of the disease is marked by all the complications of cholestasis. These include pruritus, xanthomas and various other skin lesions. The effects of diminished bile salt concentration in the intestinal lumen include diarrhoea, steatorrhoea and fat-soluble vitamin and calcium deficiency. Ultimately, hepatocellular failure becomes overt. The course is afebrile and abdominal pain is, in general, unusual, although occasionally pain over the liver, in the absence of gallstones, may be a problem. In spite of the jaundice, patients feel surprisingly well and have a good appetite. Weight loss is slow.

Jaundice is variable. It tends to fluctuate for the first five years or so and then deepens progressively during the last year of illness. Skin pigmentation is progressive. It is particularly marked in those with a racial or other predisposition to pigmentation. The increase in pigment is particularly obvious in the face, in flexures and in the scars of trauma or previous surgery.

Pruritus results in scratch marks on the skin and these may become secondarily infected. A butterfly area over the back may be devoid of scratch marks as it is usually inaccessible to the fingers.[71] The skin becomes thickened over fingers, ankles and legs.

Xanthomas develop frequently and sometimes acutely, but many patients remain in the pre-xanthomatous state throughout their illness. The planous variety occurs characteristically as xanthelasma. These lesions are flat or slightly raised, bright yellow and soft, around the eyes and on the upper lid. They may also be seen in the palmar creases, below the breasts and on the neck, chest or back. The tuberous lesions appear later and are characteristically found on extensor surfaces, especially the wrists, elbows, knees, ankles and buttocks, on pressure points and in scars. The xanthomas associated with cholestatic jaundice rarely affect tendon sheaths. The development of skin xanthomas is in proportion to the level of the total serum lipids. If the level is greater than 18 g/l (1800 mg/100 ml) for longer than three months, then skin xanthomas become generalized. Local xanthelasma may develop at levels of 13 to 18 g/l (1300 to 1800 mg/100 ml). Lowering of the serum lipid and cholesterol values results in disappearance of the xanthomas. In the later stages, when hepatocellular failure results in a fall of serum lipid and cholesterol levels, the xanthomas disappear.

Pain in the fingers, especially on opening doors, and in the toes may be due to xanthomatous involvement of peripheral nerves causing a xanthomatous neuropathy.[91]

Easy bruising with minimal trauma is related to hypoprothombinaemia following vitamin K deficiency.

Diarrhoea is related to steatorrhoea. The fingers show clubbing in the later stages.

In dogs, ligation of the common bile duct is associated with an increased incidence of peptic ulcers, and such animals often die from perforation or haemorrhage. Diversion of alkaline bile from the duodenum is probably important. Duodenal ulcer is frequent in patients with primary biliary cirrhosis. The defect in blood coagulation adds to the severity of bleeding.

Bone Changes and Calcium Metabolism

Bone changes are common in long-standing primary biliary cirrhosis.[4,55] At the early stages, these present simply as pain, particularly backache. Later, the vertebral bodies become crushed and wedge-shaped and kyphosis is gross. The thoracic cage is decalcified and pseudo-fractures are frequent. Ribbon-like areas of decalcification (Looser zones), often symmetrical, are found, particularly in the axillary border of the scapula, in the pelvis, femoral neck and ribs. Pain over the ribs may indicate a pathological fracture. The hands also show rarefaction. The lamina dura around the teeth disappears and the teeth loosen and fall out. Proximal myopathy may be an associated feature.

The bony lesion is usually osteomalacia but can be osteoporosis. Osteomalacia is characterized by reduced mineralization and excessive production of osteoid. Osteoporosis is characterized by diminished bone volume. Using a computerized technique, the osteoid and total bone volume proportion with osteoblastic and osteoclastic surface extent may be quantified. Using this method, 18 of 25 patients with chronic cholestatic disease had osteomalacia and 10 of 25 had osteoporosis.[59]

The diagnosis of the type of bone change is very difficult without biopsy of bone. There is no correlation of the biopsy findings with clinical data, plasma calcium, phosphorus, magnesium or bone alkaline phosphatase isoenzyme.[59] Clinical evidence of bone disease is slow to develop and unlikely unless the cholestasis is deep and has lasted longer than two years. Ill-advised prednisolone therapy may hasten the progress of bone changes. Painful osteoarthropathy may develop in wrists and ankles.[99]

When the serum cholesterol levels are very high for a long time, erosions are seen in the heads of the digits on x-ray. These represent bone xanthomas.

Mechanisms of the bone changes. Where intestinal fat is excessive, dietary calcium forms insoluble soaps and is not absorbed. Bile acids are essential for the absorption of vitamin D in man, and hence this vitamin will not be absorbed properly in cholestasis. A poor diet and lack of sunshine adds to the vitamin D deficiency. The understanding of the metabolism of vitamin D compounds has advanced considerably. After synthesis in the skin or absorption from the gut, ergocalciferol (vitamin D_2) and cholecalciferol (vitamin D_3) are transported to the liver (Figure 31.6). Hydroxylation in the C25 position takes place predominantly in the liver by a 25-hydroxylase enzyme

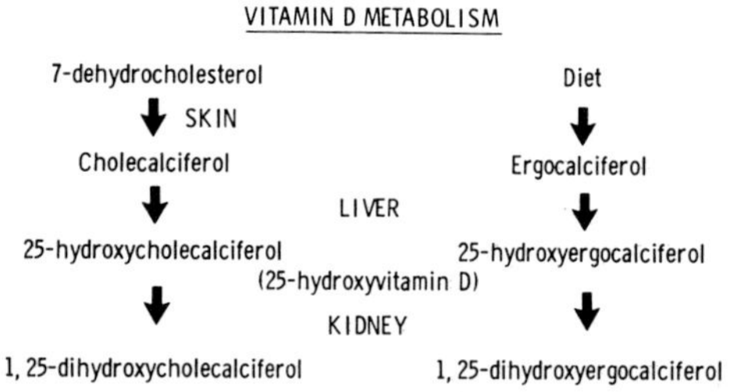

Figure 31.6. The metabolism of vitamin D.

with the formation of 25-hydroxy derivatives. With chronic hepatocellular disease, this metabolism could be disturbed and might account for the osteomalacia seen in some patients. Low levels of 25-hydroxy-vitamin D (including both 25-hydroxy D_2 and 25-hydroxy D_3) are found in cholestatic liver disease (Figure 31.7).[58] These low levels are returned to normal by regular monthly injections of vitamin D, indicating that the liver in primary biliary cirrhosis is usually able to hydroxylate vitamin D adequately if sufficient amounts of substrate are provided.[83] In the later stages of liver failure, this hydroxylation may become inadequate, as is reported in advanced alcoholic liver disease.[44] The 25-hydroxy-vitamin D undergoes enterohepatic circulation, and deficiency of this metabolite may be increased by failure of intestinal reabsorption. This could be further interrupted by the administration of cholestyramine.[16]

Parathyroid hormone, measured by radioimmunoassay, is normal in cholestatic patients with liver disease.[57]

The osteoporosis is not adequately explained. It is presumably related to the general failure of protein synthesis as the liver cell fails.

The proximal myopathy is due to vitamin D deficiency.

Kayser–Fleischer Rings

The Kayser–Fleischer ring associated with Wilson's disease is a light brown ring at the periphery of the cornea. During the early stages it may be seen only by slit-lamp examination, when it is easily recognizable by its colour, granular appearance and situation in a layer deep in the cornea (Descemet's membrane). The granules contain copper and may consist of copper chelates.[42] In view of the increased copper concentration in the liver in chronic cholestasis generally, it is perhaps not surprising that Kayser–Fleischer rings have been reported in primary biliary cirrhosis,[26] and in a patient whose disease resembled primary biliary cirrhosis in some respects but in others was nearer to chronic active hepatitis.[30]

Associated Diseases

Primary biliary cirrhosis is associated with many other conditions. In one series, 69 per cent of 47 patients had a non-hepatic association.[35] The most commonly associated conditions are the collagen diseases. Articular symptoms were found in 4 per cent of one series[35] and rheumatoid arthritis in 5 per cent of 100 patients in another.[81] In general, the severity of the arthritic symptoms is the inverse of that of the primary biliary cirrhosis.[12] Serological tests for rheumatoid factor are positive.[12] The possibility that cholesterol crystals play a part in the arthritis has been considered but the relationship of these to symptoms is unclear. Dermatomyositis has also been an associated condition.[81]

In 1964, primary biliary cirrhosis was first described with scleroderma.[5] This observation has been confirmed.[65] Later, the association of the whole CRST syndrome of calcinosis cutis, Raynaud's phenomenon, sclerodactyly and telangiectasia was noted.[72] The telangiectasia resembles that seen in the Rendu–Osler–Weber syndrome, being on finger pads and lips and occasionally on the mucosa of the upper gastrointestinal tract. Concomitant polymyositis has also been noted.[95] The association

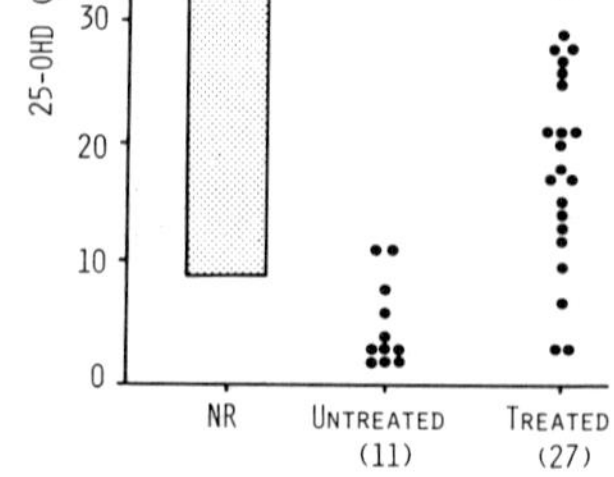

Figure 31.7. Serum 25-hydroxy-vitamin D values in primary biliary cirrhosis. Values in 27 treated patients are contrasted with values in 11 patients untreated with parenteral vitamin D_2. N.R. is the normal range. From Skinner et al,[83] with kind permission of the authors and the editor of *Lancet*.

of CRST with primary biliary cirrhosis was noted in three of 100 patients[81] and, conversely, primary biliary cirrhosis was found in 11 of 29 patients with CRST.[53] The underlying hepatic disease is more likely to determine the prognosis than is the scleroderma.

The 'sicca complex' of dry eyes and mouth, with or without the arthritis completing the Sjögren syndrome, was found in about 75 per cent of patients with primary biliary cirrhosis.[36] Schirmer's test for lacrymal function should be performed in all patients with primary biliary cirrhosis. Investigations of this sicca component of the Sjögren syndrome with a battery of tests showed abnormalities which do not correlate with duration or degree of liver disease, presence of autoantibodies or serum immunoglobulin levels.

Autoimmune thyroiditis is another association.

Renal tubular acidosis may be found, but is more frequent with chronic active hepatitis.[34] Circulating antibodies to the loop of Henle have been seen in one patient.[10]

One patient showed a papular and vesicular lesion of the skin, biopsy of which revealed capillaritis associated with IgM and C3. The biochemical features of renal tubular acidosis and the nephrotic syndrome were present and biopsy of the kidney showed IgM-associated membranous glomerulonephritis.[69] Possibly, deposition of circulating immune complexes, including IgG and IgM, might account for both the renal glomerular lesion and the cutaneous capillaritis.

DIAGNOSIS

This is usually easy if all ancillary diagnostic tests are available. These must include the serum mitochondrial antibody test, needle liver biopsy, cholangiography, whether endoscopic or percutaneous, and hepatic scanning.

In the presymptomatic stage the diagnosis must be made from other causes of a raised serum alkaline phosphatase, such as Paget's disease. The raised serum 5′-nucleotidase in primary biliary cirrhosis usually makes the distinction. Before jaundice appears, distinction from other causes of chronic pruritus must be made.

In the later stages, the diagnosis from chronic active hepatitis and cryptogenic cirrhosis may be exceedingly difficult. Indeed, there is some overlap between the three conditions. Occasionally, patients with cryptogenic cirrhosis show predominantly cholestatic features.[18] The pattern of biochemical tests of liver function and the liver biopsy appearances are usually diagnostic. However, liver biopsy can show the classical features of chronic active hepatitis in one area and those of primary biliary cirrhosis in another.

Ulcerative colitis with pericholangitis and/or sclerosing cholangitis may cause diagnostic difficulty. In sclerosing cholangitis, the mitochondrial antibody test is always negative and cholangiography demonstrates the typical bile duct irregularities. Investigation of the large bowel by sigmoidoscopy, biopsy and radiology establishes the presence of chronic inflammatory bowel disease.

Chronic drug jaundice, particularly that related to chlorpromazine, may simulate primary biliary cirrhosis.[70] The onset, however, is much more acute, with rapidly deepening jaundice occurring four to six weeks after the drug is first used.

Widespread tissue granulomas may suggest sarcoidosis.[87] Chronic intrahepatic cholestasis has been described in sarcoidosis.[75] In sarcoidosis, however, the Kveim skin test is positive (75 per cent) and the mitochondrial antibody test is negative. Bile duct destruction is not seen on liver biopsy.

PROGNOSIS

This is extremely variable and the outlook when the patient is first seen may be unpredictable, except that the disease is not curable at present. There seems to be no correlation between the extent and severity of the histological liver lesion and the duration of symptoms. In 1959, the mean duration of 35 fatal cases was $5\frac{1}{2}$ years (range three to 11 years) from diagnosis.[80] This applied to patients symptomatic at presentation and jaundiced before diagnosis was made. They were already far along the course of the disease. Over the years, diagnosis has become possible at an asymptomatic stage, and it has become apparent that primary biliary cirrhosis runs a much longer course.

Twenty patients were diagnosed at an asymptomatic stage (Figure 31.8).[59] A mean of 4.5 years after diagnosis, ten of the patients had not developed hepatobiliary symptoms; four of these ten have survived six to ten years. Ten patients developed symptoms after a mean of

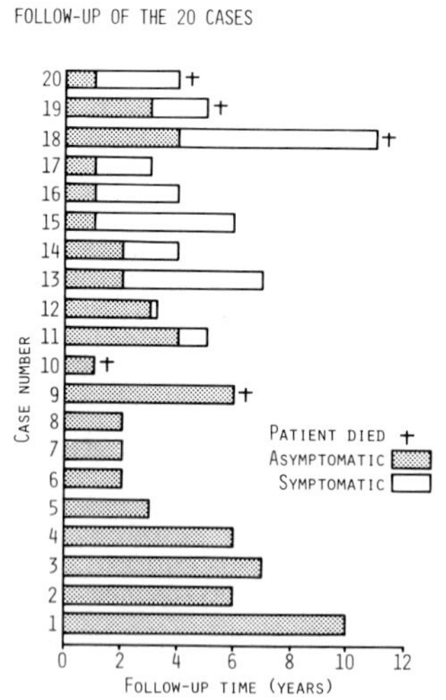

Figure 31.8. The course of 20 patients presenting with asymptomatic primary biliary cirrhosis. The duration of follow-up and asymptomatic and symptomatic disease is indicated. From Long et al,[56] with kind permission of the authors and the editor of *Gastroenterology*.

2.2 years from initial diagnosis; seven are still alive, but three have died from liver failure. The development of symptoms could not be predicted by either serum biochemical tests or hepatic histology. The diagnosis of asymptomatic primary biliary cirrhosis is compatible with ten or more asymptomatic years.

The final year or so of the disease is marked by progressive liver failure. Jaundice deepens rapidly. Total serum cholesterol levels fall and xanthomas disappear. Pruritus is no longer experienced. Serum albumin values decrease and oedema and ascites appear. The fluid retention becomes less and less responsive to diuretic therapy and dietary sodium restriction. The hepatorenal syndrome may ensue. The intellect deteriorates and episodes of frank encephalopathy are seen. Death results from liver failure marked by the ominous triad of bleeding, ascites and coma, usually with renal failure. Septicaemias, particularly those which are gram-negative, may be terminal.

TREATMENT

General measures and nutrition

The problem is essentially that of intestinal bile salt deficiency. Calorie intake should be maintained and protein must be adequate. Neutral fat is poorly tolerated and badly absorbed, and steatorrhoea reduces calcium absorption. Dietary fat should be restricted to 40 g daily in the jaundiced patient. Additional fat is supplied by medium-chain triglycerides (MCT) which are digested and absorbed quite well, in the absence of bile salts, presumably into the portal vein as free fatty acids. They can be given as Portagen (Mead Johnson) or as MCT (coconut oil).

If there is evidence of bruising or haemorrhage associated with a prolonged prothrombin time, vitamin K, 10 mg intramuscularly, may be administered daily until the deficiency is corrected. It is then given in a dose of ten mg intramuscularly every four weeks. Vitamin A, 100 000 units, should be given every four weeks intramuscularly. The problem of bone thinning will be discussed later.

Patients must be encouraged to lead as normal a life as possible, since the disease is compatible with a full domestic and professional life, often for many years. Skilful make-up may be necessary to conceal facial icterus. Plasmaphoresis has been used to relieve xanthomatosis with intractable neuropathy.[94]

Control of pruritus

Cholestyramine is used to control pruritus. This drug will have its maximum benefit when bile salt concentration in the small bowel is greatest. This is at breakfast time, when the gallbladder discharges its overnight reservoir of bile into the duodenum.[49] Cholestyramine should therefore be given as one satchet immediately before and another after the first meal of the day and one satchet before the midday and one before the evening meal. Cholestyramine may also be beneficial as a choleretic in increasing bile salt flow and perhaps in reducing the injurious effects of retained (toxic) bile salts on the liver cell. A case should be made for giving cholestyramine even in those who are not itching. Phenobarbital also increases bile flow but is not as effective as cholestyramine.

On no account must clofibrate be given as a cholesterol-reducing agent. In primary biliary cirrhosis, there is a paradoxical increase in serum cholesterol, the mechanism being uncertain.[77] Xanthomas become more severe. Gallstones may form even in the bile ducts.[88]

Treatment of bone changes

Patients with primary biliary cirrhosis should be encouraged to be in sunlight as much as possible. The diet should be generally nutritious. The patient should take extra (preferably low-fat or skimmed) milk, at least 500 ml daily.

Jaundiced patients should take extra calcium in the form of calcium gluconate or, preferably, effervescent calcium (Sandoz), eight tablets daily, equivalent to 30 g calcium gluconate. Calcium should, if possible, be given in milk between meals when it is better absorbed, and not at the same time as cholestyramine. Vitamin D is given intramuscularly, 100 000 units every four weeks. This is adequate to maintain normal serum 25-hydroxycholecalciferol levels (Figure 31.7).[83] It will restore the intestinal absorption of calcium to normal.[51]

In spite of these measures, bone thinning with pain and fractures can develop. A course of intravenous calcium injections may afford relief for two to three months.[3] Fifteen mg calcium per kg body weight is given as calcium gluconate in 500 ml 5 per cent dextrose over four hours. The infusion is given daily for about seven days and repeated as necessary.

25-hydroxycholecalciferol is several times more potent than its parent vitamin.[86] It may be of value in patients with bony complications of primary biliary cirrhosis when given in a daily dose of 50 to 100 μg by mouth. 1,25-dihydroxycholecalciferol is biologically the most active vitamin D derivative. It is formed in the kidney from the hepatic metabolite, 25-hydroxy-vitamin D. This derivative has been given to patients with primary biliary cirrhosis who had received regular intramuscular vitamin D_2, but who still suffered bone pain and myopathy and whose bone biopsy gave evidence of osteomalacia.[59] Serum 25-hydroxycholecalciferol levels were normal. Fifteen to 30 μg were given intramuscularly in arachis oil every four weeks. After one to five months bone pain was relieved and the myopathy sometimes resolved. Bone biopsy showed reduction in osteoid tissue indicating healing of osteomalacia. It appears, therefore, that 1,25-dihydroxycholecalciferol may have a beneficial effect on bone and muscle in hepatic osteomalacia. This response suggests either a failure of vitamin D_1 hydroxylation, or that hepatic osteomalacia is vitamin D_2 resistant.

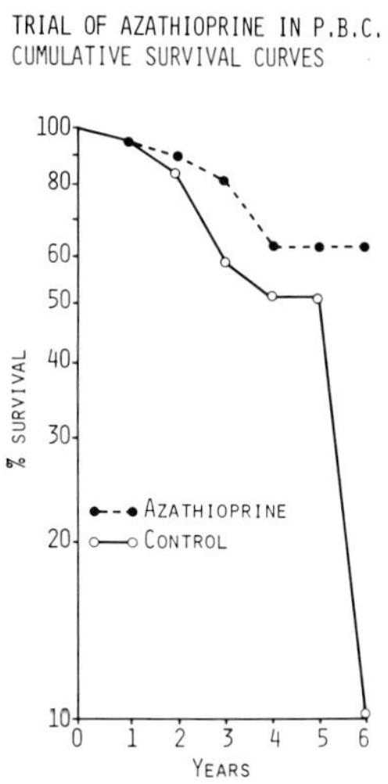

Figure 31.9. Results of a controlled prospective trial of azathioprine in primary biliary cirrhosis. Cumulative survival curves show no significant differences between treated and control groups except at the sixth year, when the number of patients in both groups is very small. From Heathcote et al,[43] with kind permission of the authors and the editor of *Gastroenterology*.

Azathioprine

Primary biliary cirrhosis is one of three hepatic conditions where serum autoantibodies can be demonstrated with some regularity. The others are chronic active hepatitis and cryptogenic cirrhosis. This disturbance in humoral immunity is accompanied by granulomas in the liver and the evidence for depression of cell-based immunity has already been discussed. Prednisolone, with or without azathioprine, is of proven benefit in chronic active hepatitis and the use of both in primary biliary cirrhosis should therefore be considered. Corticosteroid therapy increases bone thinning and, indeed, devastating spinal collapse and pathological fractures may follow its use in primary biliary cirrhosis where a tendency to such complications already exists. Moreover, various uncontrolled reports suggest that prednisolone does not seem to have beneficial effects in primary biliary cirrhosis and does not even reduce the depth of jaundice. Azathioprine has also been used. This does not produce the increase in skeletal thinning associated with corticosteroids. A controlled trial was conducted at the Royal Free Hospital over a four-year period (1969–1973) in patients with symptomatic but not end-stage primary biliary cirrhosis.[43] There were 22 patients given azathioprine (2 mg/kg body weight) and 23 controls. Clinical evaluation of the two groups demonstrated no difference in the degree of pruritus; there was some improvement in the degree of physical activity in the treated group. The serum alkaline phosphatase and transaminase levels fell significantly in the treated group after six months in the trial; however, this trend was no longer seen at 1½ and 2½ years after entry to the trial. Serum bilirubin levels were similar in both groups and tended to remain constant. An initial fall in serum IgM levels was seen in the treated group but these later rose to pre-treatment values. Review of serial liver biopsies showed the expected decrease in inflammatory cells in treated subjects but cirrhosis developed in both groups. Finally, the length of survival in the treated group, using the life table method, was no greater than in the control group (Figure 31.9). This emphasizes the importance of conducting controlled trials of any proposed therapy, and of allowing sufficient time for assessing the results. The azathioprine trial has now been abandoned. Azathioprine may be of benefit in the exceptional case where pruritus cannot be controlled by other agents such as cholestyramine.

PRE-TRIAL LIVER COPPER CONCENTRATIONS

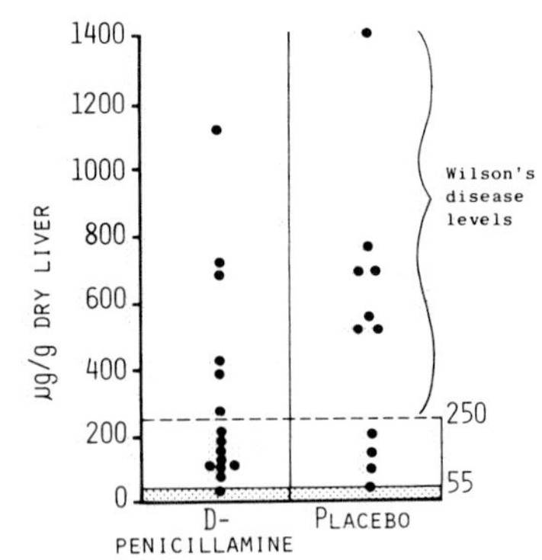

Figure 31.10. A controlled prospective trial of D-penicillamine in patients with primary biliary cirrhosis. Results for liver copper concentration at the commencement of the trial. Patients in both groups had levels above the upper limits of normal of 0.90 mmol/g (approx. 55 mg/g) dry liver. In many instances, the values exceeded the range found in Wilson's disease, which is above 4 µmol/g (250 µg/g). From Jain et al,[47] with kind permission of the authors and the editor of *Lancet*.

Copper metabolism and D-penicillamine therapy

Copper, an essential trace element, behaves as a hepatotoxin in experimental animals and in patients with Wilson's disease. It exerts its toxic effect by an inhibitory action on intracellular enzyme systems. Approximately 80 per cent of absorbed copper is normally excreted in the bile. In chronic cholestasis, hepatobiliary excretion of copper is decreased and it is not surprising that hepatic copper concentrations increase.[45,84] In primary biliary cirrhosis, the levels of hepatic copper are increased to levels found in Wilson's disease, i.e. above 4 mmol/g (approx. 250 mg/g) dried liver (Figure 31.10).[47] The normal range is 0.25 to 0.90 mmol/g (approx. 15 to 55 mg/g) dried liver. Urinary copper is raised, the level correlating with the hepatic copper concentration.[19] Serum caeruloplasmin levels are also increased, but these do not correlate with urinary copper or hepatic copper concentrations.[19]

D-penicillamine therapy has been shown to be of considerable benefit in the treatment of Wilson's disease. The hepatic concentration of copper in primary biliary cirrhosis can be as high or even higher than that found in Wilson's disease. Moreover, in this condition, copper extravasation from disrupted ducts and ductules has been postulated as an important aetiological factor leading to the development of cirrhosis.[19,54] Copper chelation therapy must therefore be carefully considered for the treatment of primary biliary cirrhosis. Early workers had reported marked increases in urinary copper in patients with primary biliary cirrhosis given penicillamine.[45,54] Two controlled randomized prospective trials of the use of penicillamine in primary biliary cirrhosis have been reported.[19,47] Jain and co-workers reported that D-penicillamine 900 mg/24 hr reduced liver copper concentration (Figure 31.11). Serum transaminases were lower than in the placebo-treated group. Liver biopsies showed less cholestasis, but inflammation and necrosis were unchanged. Deering and colleagues, 1977, reported that D-penicillamine 250 to 1000 mg/24 hr increased urinary copper and reduced liver copper concentrations. Both groups reported side-effects, some of them serious. They included nausea and vomiting, proteinuria, lymphadenopathy, thrombocytopenia, rashes and transient taste loss. Urticaria could be suppressed by corticosteroid treatment. D-penicillamine also prevents formation of some types of cross-linkage between collagen molecules during the extracellular phase of collagen maturation. The drug reduces the amount of connective tissue formed in experimentally-induced rat cirrhosis. Whether or not D-penicillamine might prevent collagen deposition in primary biliary cirrhosis cannot be predicted since the predominant type of cross-

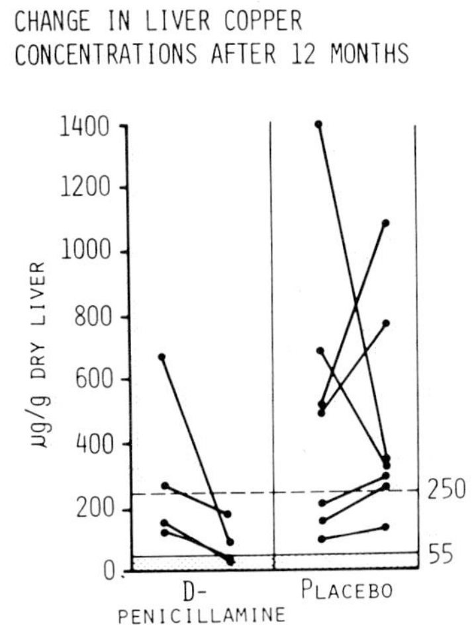

Figure 31.11. A controlled trial of D-penicillamine treatment in primary biliary cirrhosis. The changes in liver copper concentration in both treated and placebo groups after 12 months are indicated. From Jain et al,[47] with kind permission of the authors and the editor of *Lancet*.

linking of the collagen has not been characterized. Some of the benefits reported after its use, however, might be related to the anti-inflammatory action.

Before penicillamine is commenced liver copper should, if possible, be estimated. The best method of determining this is on liver biopsy samples by neutron activation[92] or by atomic absorption spectrophotometry. The needle used for biopsy must be prepared by washing in 1 per cent ethylenediaminetetra-acetic acid to remove surface copper. If such methods are not available, copper can be assessed in liver biopsies by histochemical means.[47] Copper staining of liver biopsies by rubeanic acid or rhodanine can be graded.[47] The rhodanine method may be slightly less sensitive than the rubeanic acid, but has the advantage that a positive result is an orange-red colour which is easy to distinguish from bile. The dark greenish-black of rubeanic acid tends to mimic other intracellular pigments. The rubeanic acid or rhodanine staining does not give a reliable indication of the actual liver copper concentration, but a strongly positive staining reaction has been associated only with liver copper levels exceeding 3.23 μmol/g (approx. 205 μg/g). In Wilson's disease, rubeanic acid and rhodanine stains are unreliable in detecting excess copper.[47] Strongly positive rhodanine staining reaction should be present before penicillamine is started. If liver biopsy is not possible, a fair estimation of liver copper excess can be obtained by 24-hour urinary copper concentrations.[19] The D-penicillamine is started in a dose of 200 mg/24 hr and increased slowly to a maintenance dose of 600 mg/24 hr. If cholestyramine is needed, it should be given at least one hour after taking the D-penicillamine. During the first four weeks of treatment, urine must be checked repeatedly for protein, and white cell and platelet counts performed. Treatment must continue for at least one year. At that time, a further liver biopsy analysis for copper should be made and urinary copper determined.

Because of the variable and often long natural history of primary biliary cirrhosis, and the longer-observed survival resulting from earlier diagnosis, many years must elapse before it is known whether or not cirrhosis, portal hypertension and liver failure are prevented by D-penicillamine and whether survival is prolonged. In the meantime, for an illness for which no other form of therapy seems to offer the prospect of halting or delaying progressive liver damage, treatment with D-penicillamine is recommended in spite of the high incidence of toxicity.

REFERENCES

1. Addison, T. & Gull, W. (1851) On a certain affection of the skin – vitiligoidea α plana, β tuberosa. *Guys Hospital Reports*, **7**, 265–276.
2. Ahrens, E.H. Jr, Payne, M.A., Hunkel, H.G., Eisenmenger, W.J. & Blondheim, S.H. (1950) Primary biliary cirrhosis. *Medicine (Baltimore)*, **29**, 299–336.
3. Ajdukiewicz, A.B., Agnew, J.E., Byers, P.D., Wills, M.R. & Sherlock, S. (1974) The relief of bone pain in primary biliary cirrhosis with calcium infusions. *Gut*, **15**, 788–793.
4. Atkinson, M., Nordin, B.E.C. & Sherlock, S. (1956) Malabsorption and bone disease in prolonged obstructive jaundice. *Quarterly Journal of Medicine*, **25**, 299–312.
5. Bartholomew, L.G., Cain, J.C., Winkelmann, R.K. & Baggenstoss, A.H. (1964) Chronic disease of the liver associated with systemic scleroderma. *American Journal of Digestive Diseases*, **9**, 43–55.
6. Ben-Yoseph, Y., Shapira, E. & Doniach, D. (1974) Further purification of the mitochondrial inner membrane autoantigen reacting with primary biliary cirrhosis sera. *Immunology*, **26**, 311–321.
7. Berg, P.A., Roitt, I.M., Doniach, D. & Horne, R.W. (1969) Mitochondrial antibodies in primary biliary cirrhosis. III. Characterisation of the inner membrane complement fixing antigen. *Clinical and Experimental Immunology*, **4**, 511–525.
8. Bevan, G., Baldus, W.P. & Gleich, G.J. (1969) Serum immunoglobulin levels in cholestasis. *Gastroenterology*, **56**, 1040–1046.

9. Bouchier, I.A.D. (1969) Postmortem study of the frequency of gallstones in patients with cirrhosis of the liver. *Gut*, **10**, 705–710.
10. Chanarin, I., Loewi, G., Tavill, A.S., Swain, C.P. & Tidmarsh, E. (1973) Defect of renal tubular acidification with antibody to loop of Henle. *Lancet*, **ii**, 317–318..
11. Chedid, A., Spellberg, M.A. & DeBeer, R.A. (1974) Ultrastructural aspects of primary biliary cirrhosis and other types of cholestatic liver disease. *Gastroenterology*, **67**, 858–869.
12. Child, D.L., Matthews, J.A. & Thompson, R.P.H. (1977) Arthritis and primary biliary cirrhosis. *British Medical Journal*, **ii**, 557.
13. Chohan, M.R. (1973) Primary biliary cirrhosis in twin sisters. *Gut*, **14**, 213–214.
14. Christoffersen, P., Poulsen, H. & Scheuer, P.J. (1972) Abnormal bile duct epithelium in chronic aggressive hepatitis and primary biliary cirrhosis. *Human Pathology*, **3**, 227–235.
15. Combes, B., Shibata, H., Adams, R., Mitchell, B.D. & Trammell, V. (1963) Alterations in sulfobromophthalein sodium-removal mechanisms from blood during normal pregnancy. *Journal of Clinical Investigation*, **42**, 1431–1442.
16. Compston, J.E. & Thompson, R.P.H. (1977) Intestinal absorption of 25-hydroxyvitamin D and osteomalacia in primary biliary cirrhosis. *Lancet*, **i**, 721–723.
17. Cooper, R.A. & Jandl, J.H. (1968) Bile salts and cholesterol in the pathogenesis of target cells in obstructive jaundice. *Journal of Clinical Investigation*, **47**, 809.
18. Datta, D.V., Scheuer, P.J. & Sherlock, S. (1963) Postnecrotic cirrhosis with chronic cholestasis. *Gut*, **4**, 223–230.
19. Deering, T.B., Dickson, E.R., Fleming, C.R., Geall, M.G., McCall, J.T. & Baggenstoss, A.H. (1977) Effect of D-penicillamine on copper retention in patients with primary biliary cirrhosis. *Gastroenterology*, **72**, 1208–1212.
20. Doniach, D. & Walker, J.G. (1969) A unified concept of autoimmune hepatitis. *Lancet*, **i**, 813–815.
21. Doniach, D. & Walker, J.G. (1974) Progress report. Mitochondrial antibodies (AMA). *Gut*, **15**, 664–668.
22. Doniach, D., Roitt, I.M., Walker, J.G. & Sherlock, S. (1966) Tissue antibodies in primary biliary cirrhosis, active chronic (lupoid) hepatitis, cryptogenic cirrhosis and other liver diseases and their clinical implications. *Clinical and Experimental Immunology*, **1**, 237–262.
23. Elias, E., Hamlyn, A.N., Jain, S., Dick, R. & Sherlock, S. (1976) A randomized trial of percutaneous transhepatic cholangiography with the chiba needle versus endoscopic retrograde cholangiography for bile duct visualization in jaundice. *Gastroenterology*, **71**, 439–443.
24. Feizi, T. (1968) Immunoglobulins in chronic liver disease. *Gut*, **9**, 193–198.
25. Feizi, T., Naccarato, R., Sherlock, S. & Doniach, D. (1972) Mitochondrial and other tissue antibodies in relatives of patients with primary biliary cirrhosis. *Clinical and Experimental Immunology*, **10**, 609–622.
26. Fleming, C.R., Dickson, E.R., Hollenhorst, R.W., Goldstein, N.P., McCall, J.T. & Baggenstoss, A.H. (1975) Pigmented corneal rings in a patient with primary biliary cirrhosis. *Gastroenterology*, **69**, 220–225.
27. Fox, R.A., Dudley, F.J. & Sherlock, S. (1973) The primary immune response to haemocyanin in patients with primary biliary cirrhosis. *Clinical and Experimental Immunology*, **14**, 437–480.
28. Fox, R.A., Scheuer, P.J. & Sherlock, S. (1973) Asymptomatic primary biliary cirrhosis. *Gut*, **14**, 444–447.
29. Fox, R.A., James, D.G., Scheuer, P.J., Sharma, O. & Sherlock, S. (1969) Impaired delayed hypersensitivity in primary biliary cirrhosis. *Lancet*, **i**, 959–962.
30. Frommer, D., Morris, J., Sherlock, S., Abrams, J. & Newman, S. (1977) Kayser–Fleischer-like rings in patients without Wilson's disease. *Gastroenterology*, **73**, 1331–1335.
31. Galbraith, R.M., Eddleston, A.L.W.F., Smith, M.G.M., Williams, R., MacSween, R.N.M., Watkinson, G., Dick, H., Kennedy, L.A. & Batchelor, J.R. (1974) Histocompatibility antigens in active chronic hepatitis and primary biliary cirrhosis. *British Medical Journal*, **ii**, 604–605.
32. Galbraith, R.M., Smith, M., Mackenzie, R.M., Tee, D.E., Doniach, D. & Williams, R. (1974) High prevalence of seroimmunologic abnormalities in relatives of patients with active chronic hepatitis or primary biliary cirrhosis. *New England Journal of Medicine*, **290**, 63–69.
33. Gerber, M.A., Orr, W., Denk, H., Schaffner, F. & Popper, H. (1973) Hepatocellular hyalin in cholestasis and cirrhosis; its diagnostic significance. *Gastroenterology*, **64**, 89–98.
34. Golding, P.L. & Mason, A.M.S. (1971) Renal tubular acidosis and autoimmune liver disease. *Gut*, **12**, 153–157.
35. Golding, P.L., Smith, M. & Williams, R. (1973) Multisystem involvement in chronic liver disease. *American Journal of Medicine*, **55**, 772–782.
36. Golding, P.L., Bown, R., Mason, A.M.S. & Taylor, E. (1970) 'Sicca complex' in liver disease. *British Medical Journal*, **ii**, 340–343.
37. Goudie, R.B., MacSween, R.N.M. & Goldberg, D.M. (1966) Serological and histological diagnosis of primary biliary cirrhosis. *Journal of Clinical Pathology*, **19**, 527–538.
38. Hadziyannis, S., Scheuer, P.J., Feizi, T., Naccarato, R., Doniach, D. & Sherlock, S. (1970) Immunological and histological studies in primary biliary cirrhosis. *Journal of Clinical Pathology*, **23**, 95–98.
39. Hamlyn, A.N. & Sherlock, S. (1974) The epidemiology of primary biliary cirrhosis: a survey of mortality in England and Wales. *Gut*, **15**, 473–479.
40. Hamlyn, A.N., Morris, J.S. & Sherlock, S. (1974) ABO blood groups. Rhesus negativity and primary biliary cirrhosis. *Gut*, **15**, 480–481.
41. Hanot, V. (1876) *Étude sur une Forme de Cirrhose Hypertrophique du Foie (Cirrhose Hypertrophique avec Ictère Chronique)*. Paris: J.B. Ballière.
42. Harry, J. & Tripathi, R. (1970) The Kayser–Fleischer ring. A pathological study. *British Journal of Ophthalmology*, **54**, 794–800.
43. Heathcote, J., Ross, A. & Sherlock, S. (1976) A prospective controlled trial of azathioprine in primary biliary cirrhosis. *Gastroenterology*, **70**, 656–660.
44. Hepner, G.W., Roginsky, M. & Moo, H.F. (1976) Abnormal vitamin D metabolism in patients with cirrhosis. *Digestive Diseases*, **21**, 527–532.

45. Hunt, A.H., Parr, R.M., Taylor, D.M. & Trott, N.G. (1963) Relation between cirrhosis and trace metal content of liver with special reference to primary biliary cirrhosis and copper. *British Medical Journal*, **iii**, 344–346.

46. Jain, S., Long, R.G., Scott, J., Dick, R. & Sherlock, S. (1977) Percutaneous transhepatic cholangiography using the 'Chiba' needle – 80 cases. *British Journal of Radiology*, **50**, 175–180.

47. Jain, S., Scheuer, P.J., Samourian, S., McGee, J.O'D. & Sherlock, S. (1977) A controlled trial of D-penicillamine therapy in primary biliary cirrhosis. *Lancet*, **i**, 831–834.

48. Jain, S., Scheuer, P.J., Archer, B., Newman, S.P. & Sherlock, S. (1978) Histological demonstration of copper and copper-binding protein in chronic liver diseases. In preparation.

49. Javitt, N.B. (1974) Timing of cholestyramine doses in cholestatic liver disease. *New England Journal of Medicine*, **23**, 1328–1329.

50. Kaplowitz, N., Finlayson, N.D.C., Walmsley, P., Thurnherr, N. & Javitt, N.B. (1973) Hepato-biliary diseases associated with serum antimitochondrial antibody (AMA). *American Journal of Medicine*, **54**, 725–730.

51. Kehayoglou, A.K., Agnew, J.E., Holdsworth, C.D., Whelton, M.J. & Sherlock, S. (1968) Bone disease and calcium absorption in primary biliary cirrhosis. *Lancet*, **i**, 715–718.

52. Kew, M.C., Varma, R.R., Dos Santos, H.A., Scheuer, P.J. & Sherlock, S. (1971) Portal hypertension in primary biliary cirrhosis. *Gut*, **22**, 830–834.

53. Klatskin, G. & Kantor, F.S. (1972) Mitochondrial antibodies in primary biliary cirrhosis and other diseases. *Annals of Internal Medicine*, **II**, 533–541.

54. Leeson, P.M. & Fourman, P. (1967) A disorder of copper metabolism treated with penicillamine in a patient with primary biliary cirrhosis and renal tubular acidosis. *American Journal of Medicine*, **43**, 620–635.

55. Lichtwitz, A., Cachin, M., Hioco, D., Tutin, M. & de Sèze, S. (1959) Le syndrome phosphocalcique des cirrhoses. *Semaines des Hôpitaux de Paris*, **35**, 2399–2409.

56. Long, R.G., Scheuer, P.J. & Sherlock, S. (1977) Presentation and course of asymptomatic primary biliary cirrhosis. *Gastroenterology*, **72**, 1204–1207.

57. Long, R.G., Meinhard, E., Varghese, Z., Skinner, R.K., Wills, M.R. & Sherlock, S. (1978) Osteomalacia, osteoporosis and parathyroid function in chronic liver disease. In Press.

58. Long, R.G., Skinner, R.K., Wills, M.R. & Sherlock, S. (1976) Serum 1-25-hydroxy-vitamin-D in untreated parenchymal and cholestatic liver disease. *Lancet*, **ii**, 650–652.

59. Long, R.G., Varghese, Z., Meinhard, E., Skinner, R.K., Wills, M.R. & Sherlock, S. (1978) Parenteral 1-25-dihydroxy cholecalciferol in hepatic osteomalacia. *British Medical Journal*, **i**, 75–77.

60. Mackay, I.R. & Morris, P.J. (1972) Association of autoimmune active chronic hepatitis with HL-Al, 8. *Lancet*, **ii**, 793–795.

61. MacMahon, H.E. & Thannhauser, S.J. (1949) Xanthomatous biliary cirrhosis (a clinical syndrome). *Annals of Internal Medicine*, **30**, 121–179.

62. MacSween, R.N.M. (1973) Mallory's ('alcoholic') hyaline in primary biliary cirrhosis. *Journal of Clinical Pathology*, **23**, 95–98.

63. MacSween, R.N.M., Galbraith, I., Thomas, M.A., Watkinson, G. & Ludlam, G.B. (1973) Phytohaemagglutinin (PHA) induced lymphocyte transformation and *Toxoplasma gondii* antibody studies in primary biliary cirrhosis. Evidence of impaired cell-mediated immunity. *Clinical and Experimental Immunology*, **15**, 35–42.

64. Mistilis, S.P. (1973) Positive tissue antibody tests in patients with prolonged extrahepatic biliary obstruction. *Gastroenterology*, **64**, 664–665.

65. Murray-Lyon, J.M., Thompson, R.P., Ansell, I.D. & Williams, R. (1970) Scleroderma and primary biliary cirrhosis. *British Medical Journal*, **iii**, 258–259.

66. Okuda, K., Tanikawa, K., Emura, T. & Kuratomi, S. (1974) Non-surgical percutaneous transhepatic cholangiography – diagnostic significance in medical problems of the liver. *American Journal of Digestive Diseases*, **19**, 21–36.

67. Paronetto, F., Schaffner, F. & Popper, H. (1964) Immunocytochemical and serologic observations in primary biliary cirrhosis. *New England Journal of Medicine*, **27**, 1123–1128.

68. Popper, H. & Schaffner, F. (1970) Non-suppurative destructive chronic cholangitis and chronic hepatitis. In *Progress in Liver Diseases*, Vol. 3 (Ed.) Popper, H. & Schaffner, F., pp. 336–354. New York: Grune & Stratton.

69. Rai, G.S., Hamlyn, A.N., Dahl, M.G.C., Morley, A.R. & Wilkinson, R. (1977) Primary biliary cirrhosis, cutaneous capillaritis and IgM-associated membranous glomerulonephritis. *British Medical Journal*, **i**, 817.

70. Read, A.E., Harrison, C.V. & Sherlock, S. (1961) Chronic chlorpromazine jaundice with particular reference to its relationship to primary biliary cirrhosis. *American Journal of Medicine*, **31**, 249–258.

71. Reynolds, T.B. (1973) The 'butterfly' sign in patients with chronic jaundice and pruritus. *Annals of Internal Medicine*, **78**, 545–546.

72. Reynolds, T.B., Denison, E.K., Frankl, H.D., Lieberman, F.L. & Peters, R.L. (1971) Primary biliary cirrhosis with scleroderma, Raynaud's phenomenon and telangiectasia. *American Journal of Medicine*, **50**, 302–312.

73. Richer, G. & Viallet, A. (1974) Mitochondrial antibodies in extrahepatic biliary obstruction. *American Journal of Digestive Diseases*, **19**, 740–744.

74. Rubin, E., Schaffner, F. & Popper, H. (1965) Primary biliary cirrhosis. Chronic non-suppurative destructive cholangitis. *American Journal of Pathology*, **46**, 387–407.

75. Rudzki, C., Ishak, K.G. & Zimmerman, H.J. (1975) Chronic intrahepatic cholestasis of sarcoidosis. *American Journal of Medicine*, **59**, 373–387.

76. Safrany, L., Ambrus, C. & Barna, L. (1974) Veranderungen im retrograden Cholangiogramm bei primar biliarer Leberzirrhose. *Fortschrift Rontgen*, **120**, 258.

77. Schaffner, F. (1969) Paradoxical elevation of serum cholesterol by clofibrate in patients with primary biliary cirrhosis. *Gastroenterology*, **57**, 253–255.

78. Scheuer, P.J. (1967) Primary biliary cirrhosis. *Proceedings of the Royal Society of Medicine*, **60**, 1257–1260.

79. Scheuer, P.J. (1973) *Liver Biopsy Interpretation*. 2nd Ed. London: Baillière, Tindall & Cassell.

80. Sherlock, S. (1959) Primary biliary cirrhosis (chronic intrahepatic obstructive jaundice). *Gastroenterology*, **31**, 574–586.
81. Sherlock, S. & Scheuer, P.J. (1973) The presentation and diagnosis of 100 patients with primary biliary cirrhosis. *New England Journal of Medicine*, **289**, 674–678.
82. Sicot, C. & Benhamou, J.P. (1970) Portal hypertension and primary biliary cirrhosis. *Proceedings 5th Meeting European Association for the Study of the Liver*, pp. 25–26.
83. Skinner, R.K., Long, R.G., Sherlock, S. & Wills, M.R. (1977) 25-hydroxylation of vitamin D in primary biliary cirrhosis. *Lancet*, **i**, 720–721.
84. Smallwood, R.A., Williams, H.A., Rosenoer, V.M. & Sherlock, S. (1968) Liver-copper levels in liver disease: studies using neutron activation analysis. *Lancet*, **ii**, 1310–1313.
85. Smith, M.G.M., Golding, P.L., Eddleston, A.L.W.F., Mitchell, C.G., Kemp, A. & Williams, R.L. (1972) Cell-mediated immune responses in chronic liver diseases. *British Medical Journal*, **i**, 527–530.
86. Stamp, T.C.B., Haddad, J.G. & Twigg, C.A. (1977) Comparison of oral 25-hydroxycholecalciferol, vitamin D_2 and ultraviolet light as determinants of circulating 25-hydroxy vitamin D. *Lancet*, **i**, 1341–1343.
87. Stanley, N.N., Fox, R.A., Whimster, W.F., Sherlock, S. & James, D.G. (1972) Primary biliary cirrhosis or sarcoidosis or both. *New England Journal of Medicine*, **287**, 1282–1284.
88. Summerfield, J.A., Elias, E. & Sherlock, S. (1975) Effects of clofibrate in primary biliary cirrhosis, hypercholesterolemia and gallstones. *Gastroenterology*, **69**, 998–1000.
89. Summerfield, J.A., Elias, E., Hungerford, G.D., Nikapota, V.L.B., Dick, R. & Sherlock, S. (1976) The biliary system in primary biliary cirrhosis. *Gastroenterology*, **70**, 240–243.
90. Thjodleifsson, B., Barnes, S., Chitranukroh, A., Billing, B.H. & Sherlock, S. (1977) Assessment of the plasma disappearance of cholyl-114 C-glycine as a text of hepatocellular disease. *Gut*, **18**, 697–702.
91. Thomas, P.K. & Walker, J.G. (1965) Xanthomatous neuropathy in primary biliary cirrhosis. *Brain*, **88**, 1079–1088.
92. Todd, A.P., Thorpe, M.E.C. & Rosenoer, V.M. (1967) Tissue copper determinations by neutron activation analysis. *Journal of Clinical Pathology*, **20**, 276–279.
93. Tong, M.J., Nies, K.M., Reynolds, T.B. & Quismorio, F.P. (1976) Immunological studies in familial primary biliary cirrhosis. *Gastroenterology*, **71**, 305–307.
94. Turnberg, L.A., Mahoney, M.P., Gleeson, M.H., Freeman, C.B. & Gowenlock, A.H. (1972) Plasmaphoresis and plasma exchange in the treatment of hyperlipaemia and xanthomatous neuropathy in patients with primary biliary cirrhosis. *Gut*, **13**, 976–981.
95. Uhl, G.S., Baldwin, J.L. & Arnett, F.C. (1974) Primary biliary cirrhosis in systemic sclerosis (scleroderma) and polymyositis. *The Johns Hopkins Medical Journal*, **135**, 191–198.
96. Walker, J.G., Doniach, D. & Doniach, I. (1970) Mitochondrial antibodies and subclinical liver disease. *Quarterly Journal of Medicine*, **39**, 31–48.
97. Walker, J.G., Doniach, D., Roitt, I.M. & Sherlock, S. (1965) Serological tests in the diagnosis of primary biliary cirrhosis. *Lancet*, **i**, 827–831.
98. Walker, J.G., Bates, D., Doniach, D., Ball, P.A.J. & Sherlock, S. (1972) Chronic liver disease and mitochondrial antibodies: a family study. *British Medical Journal*, **i**, 146–148.
99. Whelton, M.J. (1970) Arthropathy and liver disease. *British Journal of Hospital Medicine*, **3**, 243–247.
100. Williams, M., Smith, P.M. & Doniach, D. (1976) Primary biliary cirrhosis and chronic active hepatitis in two sisters. *British Medical Journal*, **ii**, 566.
101. Zeegen, R., Stansfeld, A.G., Dawson, A.M. & Hunt, A.H. (1969) Bleeding oesophageal varices as the presenting feature in primary biliary cirrhosis. *Lancet*, **ii**, 9–13.

Chapter 32

Alcoholic Liver Disease

MIKKO P. SALASPURO
CHARLES S. LIEBER

The association of alcohol abuse and liver damage was known by the ancient Greeks and was also recognized in Indian manuscripts dealing with the Ayerveda system of medicine.[313] The relation of alcoholism to fatty liver was described by Addison[1] and Rokitansky.[318] Early literature on alcoholic cirrhosis covering clinical, pathological and experimental factors was reviewed extensively by Jollife and Jellinek.[157] They concluded that the association between chronic alcoholism and cirrhosis of the liver was well established, that a direct causation through alcohol toxicity had been ruled out, and that none of the rival theories of indirect causation had been sufficiently documented to warrant acceptance.

Numerous subsequent reviews and books cover epidemiological[195, 349] and aetiopathological[206, 212] as well as statistical, geographical and clinical aspects of alcoholic liver disease,[94,404,405,406] and most of them will be cited subsequently in this chapter.

EPIDEMIOLOGY OF ALCOHOLIC LIVER DISEASE

Mortality and Prevalence

In the early sixties it was estimated that the worldwide annual mortality from cirrhosis was at least 310 000.[370] Morbidity from all types of alcoholic liver disease is of course much higher, but no valid data or even rough estimations in a given population are available. From studies of clinical and autopsy series it can be stated that a majority of cases of cirrhosis is due to alcohol.[194, 247] In North and South America the aetiological role of alcoholism in liver cirrhosis is somewhat higher than in Europe (66 and 42 per cent respectively), whereas in Asia its contribution is only 11 per cent.[194]

The mortality rates for cirrhosis vary greatly from country to country; for example, according to 1972 WHO statistics they were 7.5/100 000 in Finland and 57.2/100 000 in France. Corresponding per capita alcohol consumptions were 5.1 and 16.8 l of absolute alcohol respectively.[142] The most menacing trend, however, is that while deaths from other causes such as cardiovascular diseases decreased from 1950 to 1974 by 2 per cent in the United States, deaths from cirrhosis climbed 71.7 per cent. In Canada, cirrhosis has been the most rapidly increasing cause of death in the population over 25 years of age, followed by lung and bronchial cancer and suicide[349] and it is now the fifth major cause of death for men in the productive years from 25 to 64.[310] The concentration of mortality of alcoholic cirrhosis to a rather young population group occurs also in the United States of America. In Baltimore, it was the fifth leading cause of death for persons 25 to 44 years of age[182] and the third leading cause of death for those 25 to 64 years of age in New York City.[267]

The male to female preponderance of mortality is more than 2 : 1 for all cases of cirrhosis and it is even greater when restricted to alcoholic cirrhosis.[127,156] However, there is recent evidence that the progression to more severe liver injury is accelerated in women.[310] For both males and females mortality from cirrhosis in the non-white population is at least double that of the white population in urban areas of the United States of America.[182]

The incidence of liver cirrhosis has recently been calculated in 16 areas of the United States of America.[110] In the Baltimore area during 1973 the age-adjusted incidence rates (first hospitalizations) for all alcoholic liver diseases per 100 000 population over 20 years were: 36.3 for white males, 19.8 for white females, 60.0 for non-white males and 25.4 for non-white females. The increasing incidence of alcoholic liver diseases, especially among women, has also been demonstrated in Great Britain,[265] where it is now the major cause of liver damage. The morbidity of liver cirrhosis has been reported to be 28 times higher among the problem drinkers than among the non-drinkers in a survey of factory workers.[283]

Relation to Alcohol Consumption

Despite the high incidence of alcoholism in cirrhosis throughout the world the prevalence of cirrhosis in alcoholics is relatively low. According to autopsy the prevalence of cirrhosis is about 18 per cent and in series based on liver biopsy it ranges from 17 to 30.8 per cent.[189,192,193,403] This discrepancy can at least partly be explained on the basis that the development of alcoholic liver disease correlates both with the magnitude and duration of alcohol consumption, as illustrated in Figure 32.1. Pequignot[284] and Pequignot et al[285] estimated that the average 'cirrhogenic dose' is 180 g ethanol/day consumed regularly for approximately 25 years. The risk is increased five times with a consumption between 80 and 160 g/day and 25 times if daily ethanol consumption exceeds 160 g. As mentioned before, the average cirrhogenic dose as well as the threshold doses are lower in females than males (see Chapter 6).

As already mentioned, the prevalence and mortality from liver cirrhosis varies from country to country. A close correlation exists between the per capita alcohol consumption and cirrhosis mortality.[156,195,348,349] Both in Finland and Canada liver cirrhosis mortality has been used as a means to measure the prevalence of alcoholism.[44,298]

The availability of alcoholic beverages has

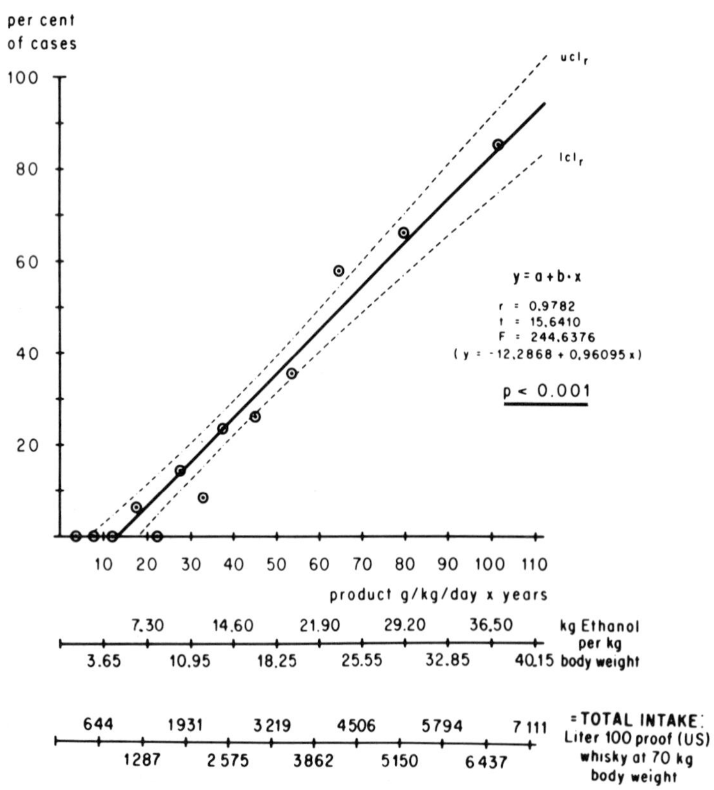

Figure 32.1. Correlation between total amounts of ethanol consumed per kilogram of body weight during drinking life and incidence of cirrhosis of the liver (n=39) in 265 alcoholics (ucl, lcl = upper and lower confidence limits of regression). From Lelbach,[194] with kind permission of the author and the editor of *Annals of the New York Academy of Sciences*.

been shown to correlate with liver disease prevalence in various countries. During the First and Second World Wars in Europe and in the time of prohibition in the United States there was a clear decrease in mortality from cirrhosis.[247] Licensing laws, economic factors and environmental conditions have also been shown to influence both per capita alcohol consumption and mortality from cirrhosis. High alcohol taxes were associated with decreased death-rates from cirrhosis in England and Wales from 12/100 000 in 1914 to 2/100 000 in 1945.[372] Similarly, the termination of alcohol rationing in Sweden in 1955 was followed by an increase in deaths attributable to cirrhosis.[127] Wine as an inexpensive source of ethanol plays a dominant role in alcoholic liver diseases in some economically disadvantaged countries such as Chile and Portugal, where mortality from cirrhosis is particularly high. On the other hand economic growth in such countries as West Germany resulted in an increase of problem drinkers and cirrhosis mortality.[247] The incidence of liver damage in Austrian brewery workers with free daily allowance of beer (144 g ethanol) was 26 per cent as opposed to only 9.3 per cent of a group of metal workers.[100]

It is now generally accepted that both the consumption and rates of alcohol problems can be regulated by means of various restrictions and tax policies. Both in Canada and Finland the potential usefulness of the many diverse restrictions through which control can be exercised has recently been examined in great detail.[45, 299]

There is no valid epidemiological or clinical evidence to suggest that drinking habits – continuous versus periodic – or the type of alcoholic beverage influence mortality from cirrhosis.[348]

PATTERNS AND PATHOLOGY OF ALCOHOLIC LIVER INJURY

The spectrum of alcoholic liver injury involves hepatic steatosis (fatty liver), central venous sclerosis, alcoholic hepatitis and cirrhosis.

Fatty Liver

Fat accumulation in the liver cells is the earliest and most common response to alcohol and alcohol is its most common aetiological

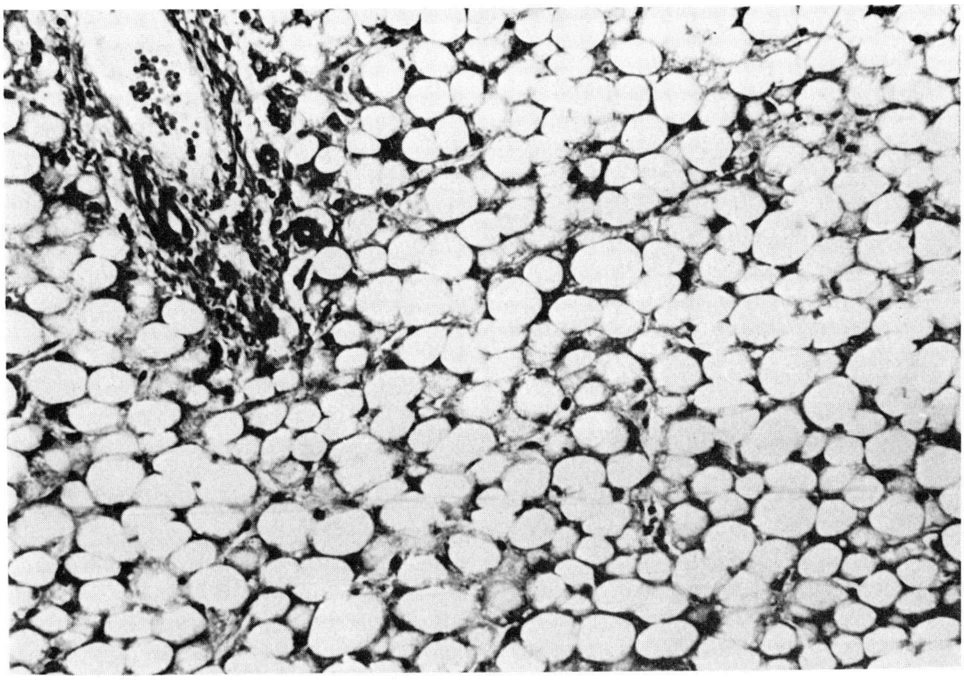

Figure 32.2. Severe fatty liver of an alcoholic. The hepatocytes are uniformly filled by large fat droplets and nuclei are eccentrically placed. Numerous fatty cysts are present.

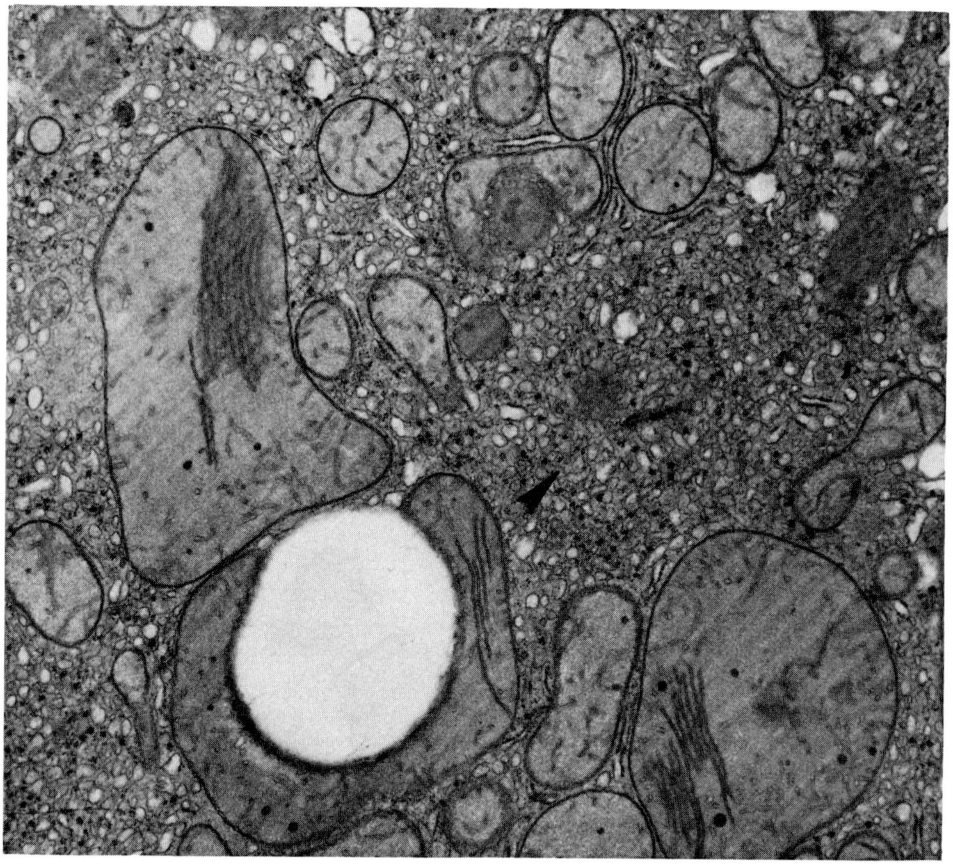

Figure 32.3. Ultrastructural changes after prolonged ethanol ingestion in a baboon. Note the prominence of endoplasmic reticulum (arrow). Mitochondrial changes include swelling, pallor of the matrix, shortening of the cristae, and diminution or absence of matrix granules. Some normal sized mitochondria are still present. Disruptions of mitochondrial membranes are common. × 17 600. Courtesy of Dr Y. Matsuda.

factor.[188] The normal liver weighs about 1.5 kg, whereas the alcoholic fatty liver weighs 2.0 to 2.5 kg. In rare cases massive accumulation of fat may occur, resulting in livers weighing from 4.0 to 6.0 kg. On hematoxylin and eosin stained sections parenchymal accumulation of lipid is seen as clear intracytoplasmic vacuoles, or as black globules with various Sudan stains. In massive steatosis the hepatocytes are uniformly filled by large fat droplets, the cell nucleus may be eccentrically placed and when the cell membranes between adjacent hepatocytes rupture numerous fatty cysts are formed (Figure 32.2). Increased hepatic lipid content may be demonstrated by biochemical measurements before it becomes histologically apparent. Evidence of necrosis is usually sparse but sometimes hepatocytes are surrounded by mononuclear cells indicating a mild inflammatory response. These formations are called 'lipogranulomas'.

Characteristic ultrastructural changes reveal enlarged and distorted mitochondria with shortened cristae containing crystalline inclusions.[373] The endoplasmic reticulum shows vacuolar dilatation and proliferation. Despite adequate nutrition, alcohol can induce these alterations in baboons and in both alcoholic and non-alcoholic human volunteers[184,323] (Figures 32.3 and 32.4).

Pericentral Venous Sclerosis

Sclerosis around central veins can be isolated or associated with a necrotizing process called 'sclerosing hyaline necrosis'.[77] When intensive, it may obliterate central veins and lead to post-sinusoidal portal hypertension with ascites prior to the development of cirrhosis. In a recent series pericentral sclerosis was observed in 40 per cent of alcoholics with simple fatty liver without evidence of diffuse alcoholic hepatitis (Figure 32.5). Sequential biopsies in the baboon

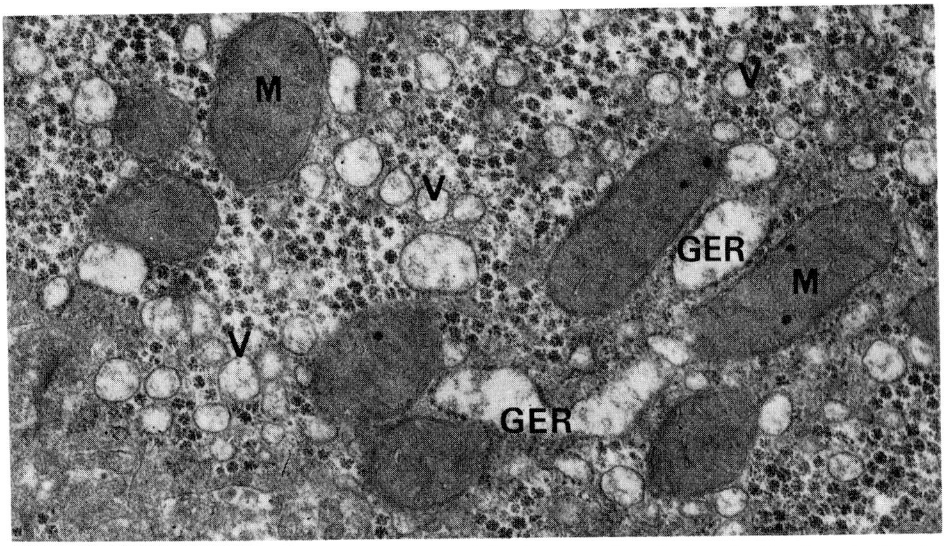

Figure 32.4. Ultrastructural alterations in human hepatocytes following ingestion of ethanol with adequate diets for 18 days. Numerous smooth membrane-bound vesicles (V) several times the diameter of the fine tubules of agranular endoplasmic reticulum in control biopsies are distributed among the glycogen rosettes. Mitochondrial changes include the variety in size and forms. Granular endoplasmic reticulum (GER); mitochondria (M). ×17 000. From Lane and Lieber,[184] with kind permission of the authors and *American Journal of Pathology*.

model of alcoholic liver injury have confirmed these findings. This may be of practical importance, since pericentral venous sclerosis may indicate progression towards cirrhosis.[397]

Alcoholic Hepatitis

From either clinical or pathological signs this inflammatory response of the liver to alcohol has been called 'florid cirrhosis', 'acute hepatic insufficiency', 'progressive alcoholic cirrhosis', or 'steatonecrosis – Mallory body type'. The term 'alcoholic hepatitis' used by Beckett, Livingston and Hill[22] is nowadays widely accepted by most pathologists and clinicians. While the incidence of fatty liver in alcoholics is very common, alcoholic hepatitis develops in only a proportion of heavy drinkers, even after decades of abuse.[183,194]

Histological characteristics of alcoholic hepatitis are ballooning and great disarray of hepatocytes, predominantly in centrilobular areas, parenchymal and portal infiltration with polymorphonuclear leucocytes, varying degrees of steatosis, necrosis, fibrosis, and cholestasis (Figure 32.6). Mallory's alcoholic hyaline – irregular cytoplasmic bodies – can be considered as a diagnostic hallmark[77,126,130,229,291,303] but it is not always present. Ultrastructural changes in alcoholic hepatitis are similar but more severe than the ones seen in fatty liver.[373] Collagenous material may be found in the space of Disse and may be associated with loss of microvilli that normally project from the hepatocyte.[78,177]

Mallory's alcoholic hyaline

This was first defined by Mallory[242] as an irregular, coarse, hyaline meshwork which stains deeply with eosin. Cells containing these bodies may be surrounded by numerous polymorphonuclear leucocytes (Figure 32.7). Electron microscopically alcoholic hyaline is fibrillar, is not surrounded by a limiting membrane and is readily distinguished from giant mitochondria[29,95,102,144,290,412] (Figure 32.8). They have been related to actin,[271] but this has not been confirmed by recent biochemical and immunological studies.[276,356] The nearest morphological cytosolic counterpart of Mallory bodies might be the intermediate filament, as suggested by Sim et al.[356] Although the real origin of Mallory bodies has not yet been resolved, it is interesting that the antitubulin agents colchicine and griseofulvin also induce Mallory body formation in mice.[69,70,103]

Although alcoholic hyaline is a characteristic of alcoholic hepatitis, it has also been demonstrated in primary biliary cirrhosis,[264] in cholestasis and cirrhosis,[111] in hepatocellular carcinoma,[167] in Wilson's disease,[301] in abetalipoproteinaemia[282] and in Indian child-

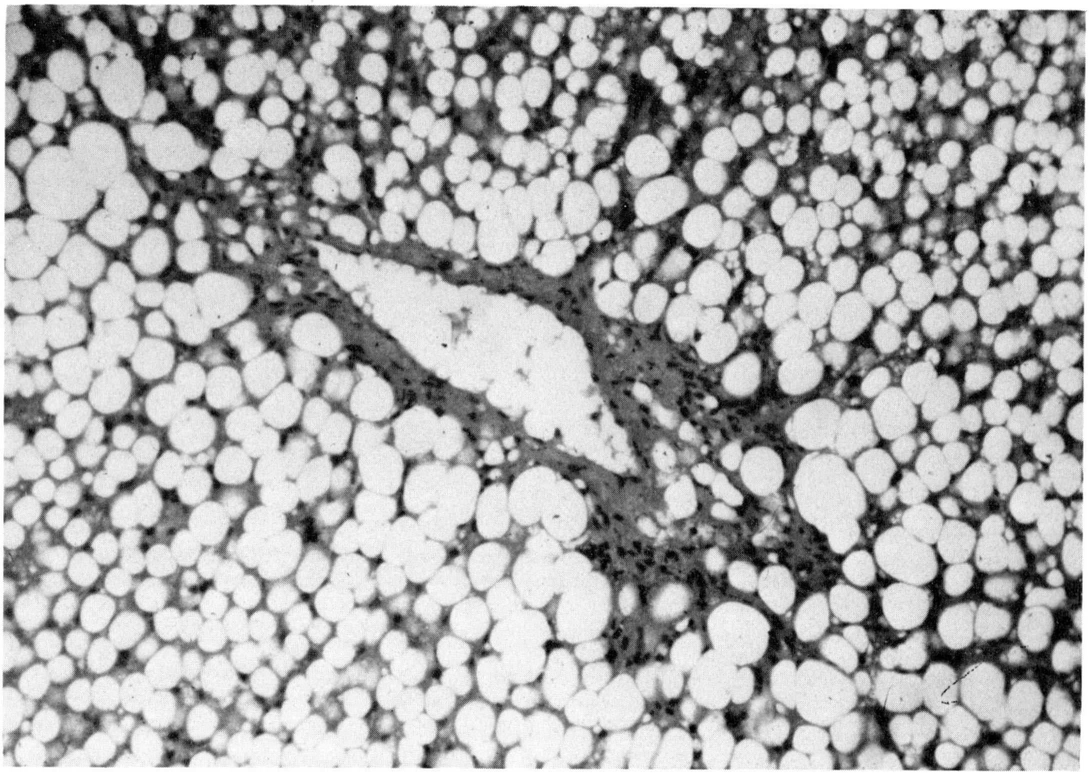

Figure 32.5. Pericentral venous sclerosis of a baboon fed alcohol. Note the broad fibrotic zone around the central vein. Fat accumulation can also be seen.

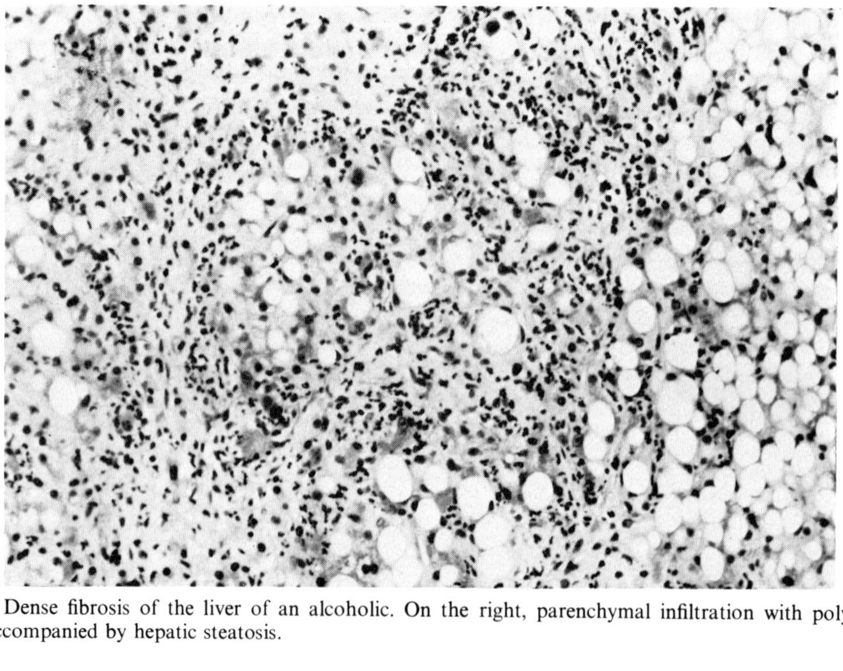

Figure 32.6. Dense fibrosis of the liver of an alcoholic. On the right, parenchymal infiltration with polymorphonuclear leucocytes accompanied by hepatic steatosis.

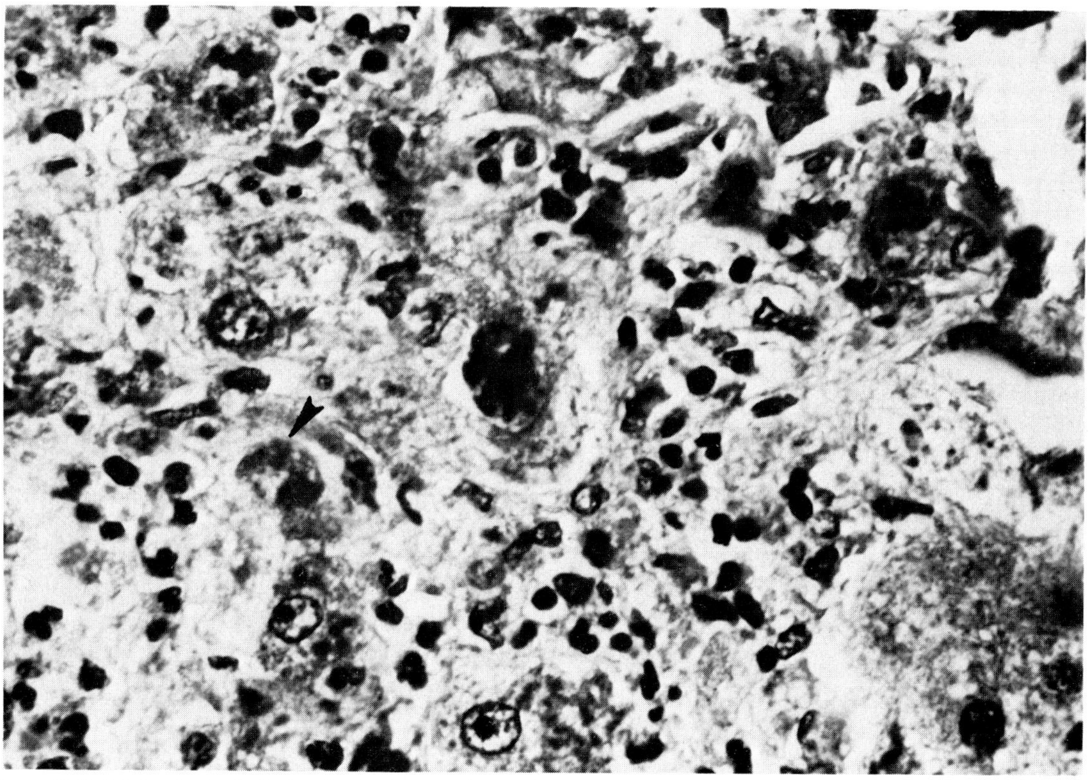

Figure 32.7. Mallory's alcoholic hyaline in human liver cell. Several cells contain dark-staining hyaline masses (arrow). Some of them are partly surrounded by polymorphonuclear leucocytes. Note the ballooning and disarray of hepatocytes. Courtesy of Dr F. Paronetto.

hood cirrhosis.[322] On the other hand, hyaline is not required for the diagnosis of alcoholic hepatitis.[52,53] The diagnosis of alcoholic hepatitis is often based on clinical findings (see below) associated with histological changes of parenchymal inflammation with polymorphonuclear leucocytes. In these cases alcoholic hyaline is found in approximately 30 per cent of patients.[229] The appearance of Mallory bodies does not correlate with mortality rates either retrospectively[130] or prospectively,[30] but they are accompanied by more severe degrees of necrosis, cholestasis and steatosis. The possible pathogenetic role of alcoholic hyaline will be discussed in the section 'Pathogenesis of alcoholic liver disease'.

Cirrhosis

Macroscopically the early cirrhotic liver is golden yellow with fine uniform nodules (from 1 to 5 mm) on the surface. Traditionally this type of cirrhosis is called 'micronodular' or 'Laennec's cirrhosis'. The size of the liver varies, depending on the degree of fibrosis, inflammation and steatosis, from a small, shrunken and hard liver to a large organ weighing up to 4 kg. In later stages the size of the nodules increases ranging from 5 to 50 mm and deep scars appear. This macronodular cirrhosis resembles the postnecrotic cirrhosis.

Microscopically, scar tissue distorts the normal architecture of the liver by forming bands of connective tissue joining portal and central zones. At first, nodules are regular in size and shape (Figure 32.9).[324] In more advanced cirrhosis nodules become larger and frequently irregular in size and shape. The nodules eventually become 'relobulized' through formation of small portal tracts and efferent venous channels.

One of the most characteristic pathological features of cirrhosis are the changes in the hepatic blood circulation. The regenerative nodules may compress the hepatic veins, preventing the flow of blood out of the liver resulting in post-sinusoidal portal hypertension. With the progression of the fibrosis the outflow is further depressed.[311] In addition, the total as well as the effective blood flow in the liver decreases in cirrhosis.[40,60] The total blood flow

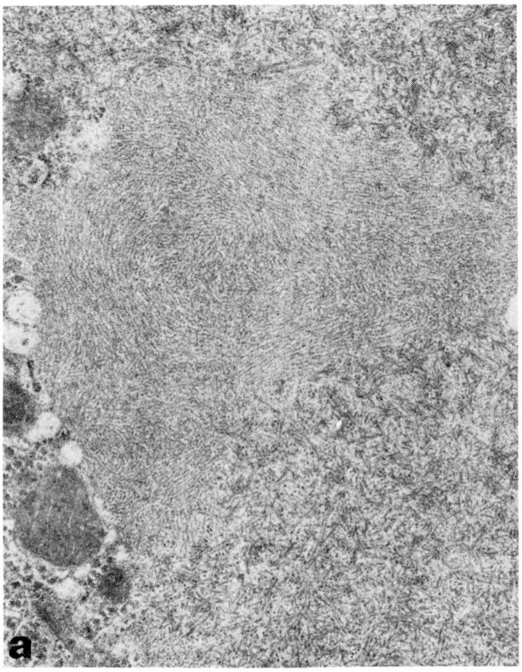

(a)

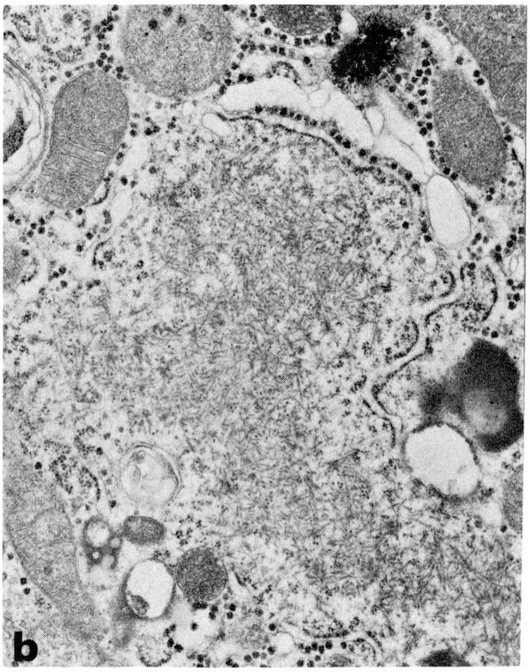

(b)

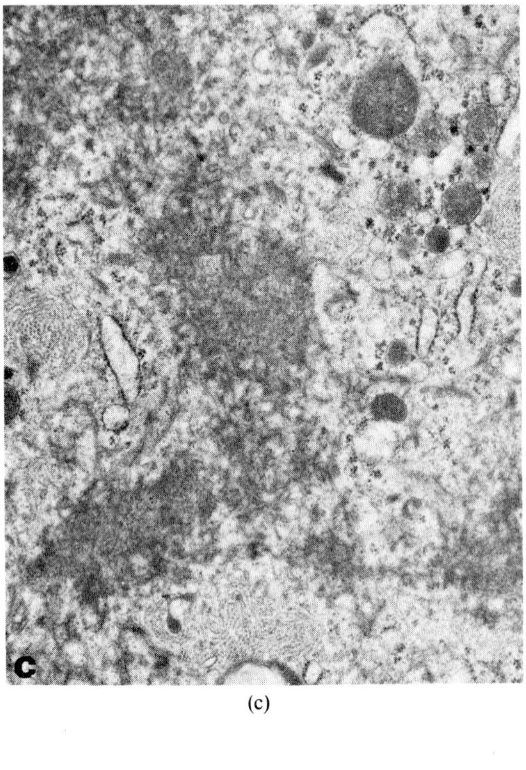

(c)

Figure 32.8. Electron micrographs (× 19 000) of alcoholic hyaline demonstrating the three types of filaments as classified by Yokoo et al.[412] (a) In a parallel manner arranged light, sharp filaments (young), type I. (b) Randomly oriented darker filaments (older), type II. (c) Homogeneous amorphous osmiophilic material (oldest), type III. Courtesy of Dr Oscar A. Iseri.

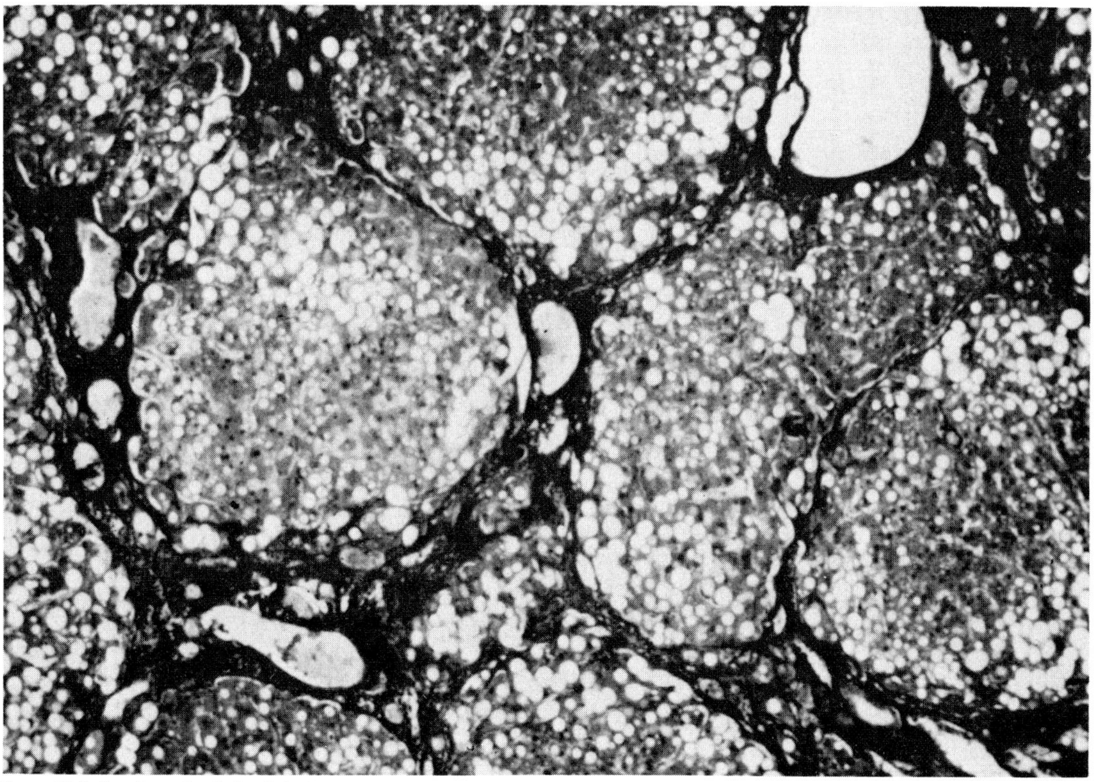

Figure 32.9. Section of a cirrhotic baboon liver. Note the typical regenerative nodules of regular size and shape. Portal tracts or central veins cannot be demonstrated. Cirrhosis is accompanied by moderate steatosis.

is reduced by extrahepatic portasystemic shunts and the effective circulation is limited by neovascularization of connective tissue septae which form anastomoses between the afferent branches of the portal vein and hepatic artery and the efferent tributaries of the hepatic veins.[300] Collagen deposits in the space of Disse may further isolate the hepatocyte from its blood supply.[78,177] As a result of these changes marked deterioration in residual hepatic function may occur, especially if either the cardiac output or circulating blood volume changes.

In addition to fibrosis, various admixtures of fat, inflammatory reactions, and cholestasis may be seen. Histologically stainable iron deposits are common in cirrhotic livers, especially in alcoholic subjects[24,307] and in patients who have undergone portacaval shunts.[384] The exact mechanism leading to iron accumulation is, however, unclear.[119] Quantitative measurements of hepatic iron content in these disorders have demonstrated that iron stores are very seldom increased and never exceed 179 mmol (10 g). In some cases the finding can possibly be related to the high iron content of alcoholic beverages, especially red wines[288] and Kaffir beer used by the Bantu in South Africa.[143] The differentiation from primary haemochromatosis is possible by measuring the total hepatic iron content from liver biopsies. Venesections are not indicated. Copper accumulations can sometimes be demonstrated with orcein or copper staining methods,[334] particularly in those cases of alcoholic cirrhosis which are characterized by long-standing cholestasis.[338]

Primary hepatic carcinoma is a frequent finding in liver cirrhosis, presumably because of improved management and prolonged survival.[108,187] Pathogenetically, it probably relates to cirrhosis rather than to the effect of alcohol itself, although possible carcinogen properties of alcohol have not been ruled out.

PATHWAYS OF ALCOHOL METABOLISM

Alcohol Dehydrogenase

Most ingested alcohol is metabolized in the liver[237] by the cytosolic enzyme *alcohol*

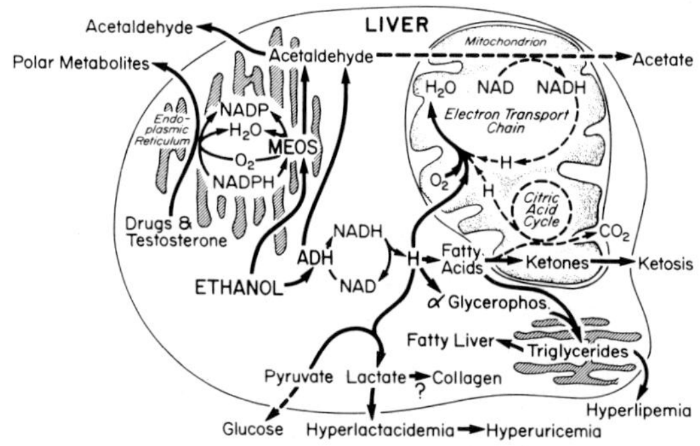

Figure 32.10. Schematic representation of the metabolism and metabolic effects of ethanol in the hepatocyte. ADH = alcohol dehydrogenase; MEOS = microsomal ethanol oxidizing system; NAD = nicotinamide-adenine dinucleotide; NADH = nicotinamide-adenine dinucleotide, reduced form; NADP = nicotinamide-adenine dinucleotide phosphate; NADPH = nicotinamide-adenine dinucleotide phosphate, reduced form. Pathways decreased by acute or chronic administration of ethanol are represented by dotted lines. From Lieber,[207] with kind permission of the editor of *New England Journal of Medicine*.

dehydrogenase (*ADH*) (Figure 32.10). The contribution of other tissues, as well as the renal and pulmonary excretion, to ethanol elimination is under 10 per cent.[404,405,406] The activity of hepatic ADH is low during fetal life; adult levels are reached during the first years after birth.[294,295] In addition to alcohol, ADH also catalyses other reactions and, furthermore, several isoenzymes have been described in human liver.[203,293,345,361,362]

ADH catalyses the conversion of ethanol to acetaldehyde in a reaction which requires NAD as a cofactor[379,380] (Figure 32.10). As a net result, ethanol oxidation generates an excess of reducing equivalents as free NADH in hepatic cytosol, primarily because the metabolic systems involved in NADH removal are not normally able to prevent fully the accumulation of NADH. The acetaldehyde produced in the reaction is further converted to acetate by acetaldehyde dehydrogenase, which is mainly located in mitochondria.[245,387] In addition, in this reaction step NAD functions as a coenzyme and NADH is formed. The increased NADH/NAD ratio is a sign of major change in liver metabolism during ethanol oxidation, as discussed below. As a net result ethanol is converted in the liver to acetate which is released into the blood stream to be further oxidized to CO_2 and water in the peripheral tissues. For detailed characteristics of the ADH pathway see Lundquist[235,236] and Lieber.[206]

Microsomal Ethanol Oxidizing System and Catalase

Alternate pathways for ethanol oxidation are the *microsomal ethanol oxidizing system* (*MEOS*)[206,208,377] and catalase.[381,382] The quantitative role of these alternate pathways for ethanol oxidation is probably low in normal conditions. However, there is growing evidence of an adaptive increase of MEOS during chronic alcohol consumption. MEOS is localized in the endoplasmic reticulum and utilizes NADPH and oxygen (Figure 32.10). Its increase in activity after chronic ethanol consumption is associated with a proliferation of the smooth endoplasmic reticulum (see above).[146] Compared to ADH, MEOS requires higher ethanol levels for full saturation and maximal velocity and therefore at higher blood ethanol concentrations the contribution of this non-ADH pathway is strikingly increased, at least in vitro.[125]

Catalase is also capable of oxidizing ethanol in vitro in the presence of an H_2O_2-generating system.[168,169] It is generally accepted that the H_2O_2-mediated ethanol peroxidation by catalase is limited by the rate of H_2O_2 generated and, since the physiological rate of H_2O_2 production is rather low, the contribution of catalase to in vivo ethanol elimination is not quantitatively significant.[206]

Accelerated Ethanol Metabolism after Chronic Alcohol Consumption

Regular drinkers tolerate larger amounts of alcoholic beverages, mainly because of central nervous system adaptation.[405] In addition, alcoholics develop increased rates of blood ethanol clearance, the so-called metabolic tolerance.[165,394] Experimental ethanol administration also results in an increased rate of ethanol metabolism.[262,386] The contribution, however, of different pathways of ethanol metabolism in the adaptive increase of alcohol elimination is controversial.

It is commonly accepted that hepatic ADH activity is not a rate limiting step in ethanol metabolism. Examples of the lack of correlation between the rates of ethanol oxidation and hepatic ADH activity are numerous.[93,121,208,210,393,399] Even in human subjects who have the atypical ADH, which shows a much higher activity than normal ADH,[407] the rate of alcohol metabolism is not higher than normal.[79] From the kinetic results of Theorell and Chance[380] it can be calculated that when the NADH produced in ADH reaction can no longer be removed, its concentration increases with subsequent inhibition of ADH reaction. On this basis ethanol oxidation rate is normally regulated by the speed of the re-oxidation of the ADH-NADH complex.

On the other hand, if hepatic ADH activity is decreased by protein deficiency or by 4-methylpyrazole (ADH inhibitor) it may become a rate-limiting step in the ADH pathway. Consequently, NADH does not accumulate in hepatic cytosol, and redox related metabolic changes during ethanol oxidation are attenuated.[332, 333, 335, 336] In experiments with isolated hepatocytes the rate of ethanol oxidation may also be limited by the V_{max} of liver ADH in situations which are not associated with substrate deficiencies.[66]

It has been claimed that the adaptive increase in ethanol elimination is due to a 'hypermetabolic state' of the liver, the primary cause being an increased activity of NA^+–K^+-activated ATPase leading to an increased ATP consumption, a decreased phosphorylation potential and an increased oxygen consumption.[147, 148] This in turn should increase mitochondrial NADH re-oxidation. Others, however, have not been able to confirm the increase of ATPase activity associated with increased oxygen consumption.[116]

The recent interesting demonstration by Bosron et al[38] of an anodic form of human liver alcohol dehydrogenase awaits further studies. This has a higher activity and much higher Km for ethanol than the other forms and, on this basis, could theoretically contribute significantly to alcohol elimination in man, particularly at high ethanol concentrations.

The role of increased microsomal function in the acceleration of ethanol metabolism after chronic ethanol consumption has been discussed recently in detail by Matsuzaki et al.[250] This concept is further supported by the finding that 4-methylpyrazole (a specific inhibitor of alcohol dehydrogenase) does not decrease ethanol elimination rate to the same extent in all alcoholics, indicating that the proportional contribution of ADH pathway to total elimination is smaller in alcoholics with poor nutrition.[335, 336] Moreover, recent experiments with rats,[88] baboons and human volunteers[330] indicate that the ethanol elimination increases with rising concentration beyond those required for full ADH saturation. This non-uniformity is augmented after chronic ethanol consumption. If it is assumed that ethanol is oxidized only by the classic low Km alcohol dehydrogenase, the ethanol elimination curve should be virtually uniform at all ethanol concentrations above 5 mmol/l. The non-uniformity of ethanol elimination curve favours the existence of a non-ADH pathway with a higher Km value for ethanol oxidation.

Whatever the mechanism of the acceleration of ethanol metabolism after chronic consumption, its role in the pathogenesis of alcoholic liver disease remains to be resolved. The adaptive increase in ethanol elimination rate (far beyond the generally accepted 7 g/hr) as well as the apparent non-linearity of ethanol elimination curve may, however, have some clinical implications. At present a constant rate of ethanol elimination curve is widely assumed for various medico-legal purposes in order to determine retrospectively the blood ethanol concentration at a given time. In view of the recent findings calculations based on linearity and constant ethanol elimination rate should be interpreted with caution. It should also be emphasized that ethanol elimination rate may remain elevated even in relatively severe alcoholic liver damage if the measurement has been made within 30 days from abstinence.[394]

ACUTE AND CHRONIC METABOLIC EFFECTS OF ALCOHOL

Most of the acute effects of ethanol on liver metabolism can be explained by the effect it exerts on the redox levels (an increased NADH/NAD ratio; Figure 32.10) of the cytosol and mitochondria. This redox change was first demonstrated in baker's yeast by Holzer, Schultz and Lynen[140] and in rat liver by Forsander, Räihä and Suomalainen.[97] Several other changes in liver metabolism caused by acute ethanol administration are secondary to this basic phenomenon.

There is, however, recent information which indicates that chronic ethanol consumption itself results in an acceleration of the removal of cytosolic free NADH. This 'adaptation' may further be associated with a decrease in hepatic ADH concentration with the consequence that instead of the rate of NADH removal it is hepatic ADH activity which finally becomes rate limiting in the ADH pathway.[331] In this situation there is no more accumulation of NADH in hepatic cytosol after the acute administration of alcohol, and this results in an attenuation of the redox mediated metabolic changes. At present, it is not known which of the acute metabolic effects of alcohol still occur in the chronic situation; this should be borne in mind whenever the results of metabolic experiments performed in alcoholics or in alcohol fed animals are interpreted.

Hyperlactacidaemia; Hyperuricaemia

The enhanced NADH/NAD ratio reflects itself in an increased lactate/pyruvate ratio[352] with *hyperlactacidaemia*.[138,220] As a rule the blood lactate levels are only moderately elevated and the acidosis, accordingly, is not severe. Some cases of moderately severe lactic acidosis have, however, been described.[277] Theoretically, other agents known to induce lactic acidosis (for instance, fructose infusion or phenformin) might exaggerate lactic acidosis caused by alcohol; on this basis they should be avoided in the treatment of alcohol intoxication.

The hyperlactacidaemia may lead to secondary *hyperuricaemia* caused by decreased urinary excretion of uric acid.[220] This can be related to the common association of alcohol abuse and gouty attacks.[272] Simultaneous ketosis may further promote alcoholic hyperuricaemia.[238] Alcoholic hyperuricaemia can be readily differentiated from the primary variety because of its reversibility upon discontinuation of alcohol abuse.

Inhibition of Citric Acid Cycle

When ethanol is oxidised in the liver the carbon dioxide production is almost totally inhibited.[99,214,222,237,392] This indicates a depression of the citric acid cycle caused by slowing of the reactions of the cycle that requires NAD.[96,226] This interpretation accords with the finding that in protein deficiency, when ethanol oxidation does not result in an increased cytosolic free NADH, the citric acid cycle is not inhibited any more by ethanol.[333] A major site of inhibition by this mechanism is 2-oxoglutarate dehydrogenase.[279] The end result is a decreased fatty acid oxidation,[214,222] a key mechanism in the genesis of fatty liver (see the section on the pathogenesis of fatty liver, below).

Hyper- and Hypoglycaemia (see also Chapter 3)

In fed animals and man, acute alcohol administration results in hyperglycaemia.[98,251] This is caused by the release of glucose from the glycogen reserves of the liver into the blood and is mediated mostly by the adrenal medulla and the sympathetic nervous system,[5,251] although decreased peripheral utilization of glucose may also contribute to it.[232]

A particularly dramatic complication of acute alcohol abuse is hypoglycaemia which may be responsible for some of the unexplained sudden deaths in acute alcoholic intoxication. A prompt diagnosis and initiation of therapy is mandatory in view of the reported mortality rate of 11 per cent in adults and 25 per cent in children.[239] Extensive clinical and in vivo studies have established that hypoglycaemia following alcohol administration during a state of fasting is a normal reaction in man and experimental animals.[92,101] Hypoglycaemia is due to decreased reserves of hepatic glycogen and the inhibition of hepatic gluconeogenesis from various precursors as a consequence of the increased NADH/NAD ratio.[181] In clinical practice, however, severe alcoholic hypoglycaemia is uncommon. In several conditions, refractiveness to alcohol hypoglycaemia can be demonstrated: in non-diabetic obese subjects,[8] in some alcoholics with a diabetic glucose pattern[136] and during steroid therapy.[7] Refractiveness has also been demonstrated in chronic malnourished alcoholics.[328,329] This presumably can be related to the attenuation of alcohol-induced hepatic redox changes after chronic alcohol consumption, as stated in the beginning of this chapter. Similarly, alcohol-induced hypoglycaemia can also be suppressed by 4-methylpyrazole (alcohol dehydrogenase inhibitor).[337] The treatment of choice of alcohol-induced hypoglycaemia is the intravenous infusion of glucose.

Alcoholic Ketosis and Ketoacidosis

Alcoholic ketosis was formerly attributed to poor nutrition.[74] Now it is clear that ketonaemia may be induced by the chronic administration of ethanol in association with calorically adequate diets.[190] The biochemical mechanism of ketoacidosis is obscure, but there is evidence that it reflects a persistent effect of alcohol, perhaps an alteration in mitochondrial function.[50,205]

Most individuals with alcoholic ketoacidosis

have been drinking recently.[63] Clinically, the patients have a history of nausea, vomiting and diminished food consumption. Physical signs typical of ketoacidosis include dehydration, tachycardia, Kussmaul respiration, diffuse abdominal tenderness and confusion. Initial laboratory values are consistent with metabolic acidosis. 3-Hydroxybutyrate/aceto-acetate ratio is increased and on this basis the nitroprusside test (Acetest) may be negative or only slightly positive because of its insensitivity to 3-hydroxybutyrate.[202] Alcoholic hypoglycaemia, acute pancreatitis, lactic acidosis and hepatic coma should be considered in the differential diagnosis. Blood glucose and insulin levels are generally depressed.[63] Insulin therapy is not required. Treatment is supportive and consists of correction of dehydration. Small amounts of bicarbonate can be used to correct the acidosis.

Alcoholic Hyperlipaemia (see also Chapter 4)

The oral or intravenous administration of ethanol produces a consistent and rapid increase in fasting serum lipoproteins, primarily very low-density lipoproteins (VLDL) containing mainly triglycerides.[160] This effect is enhanced if alcohol is administered together with a fat-containing meal.[409] Chronic alcohol abuse results in a lipaemic response which varies according to the duration and dose of alcohol intake.[221,343] There is also evidence that the hyperlipaemic effect of alcohol is more intensive in hypertriglyceridaemic persons.[112,253] Recently it was demonstrated that alcohol consumption is positively associated with high-density lipoprotein cholesterol level in all populations.[49]

According to animal experiments the primary mechanism of alcoholic hyperlipaemia appears to be the increased hepatic production of VLDL.[15,16,17,19] On the other hand, an acute large dose of alcohol may produce a decrease in serum triglycerides and VLDL.[6,240] This phenomenon could be related to decreased lipoprotein secretion or synthesis as discussed later (see the section on pathogenesis of fatty liver, below). Individual lipaemic response to alcohol varies greatly in relation to the dietary habits, obesity, diabetes or prediabetes, pancreatitis or essential hyperlipaemia.[212]

The changes in plasma free fatty acids (FFA) produced by ethanol are dose dependent. The decrease in plasma FFA with moderate amounts of ethanol is due to inhibition of FFA release from adipose tissue[86,159,221] and is mediated by acetate.[65] The increase in plasma FFA concentration after administration of a high dose of alcohol may result from mobilization of depot fat due to adrenergic stimulation since the stimulatory response is inhibited by β-adrenergic blocking agents.[39]

Ethanol consumption may also interfere with plasma cholesterol. Increased cholesterol synthesis after ethanol ingestion[191] may have a microsomal basis akin to that after barbiturate[350] and may explain, in part, the accumulation of cholesterol ester observed in the liver after feeding of alcohol. In hyperlipaemic patients the cholesterol content of the LDL-fraction has been reported to decrease and that of the VLDL-fraction to increase with an unchanged total cholesterol.[112] In the same study a statistically significant increase of plasma cholesterol caused by alcohol in normal subjects was demonstrated. Chronic alcohol consumption results in increased HDL blood levels,[49] which may be of importance in the protection against athero sclerosis.[260]

Transient haemolytic anaemia can accompany episodes of hyperlipaemia in alcoholics – the so-called Zieve's syndrome.[415] In rats chronically fed with alcohol, reticulocytosis and increased osmotic fragility of the erythrocytes, which correlate with the degree of hyperlipaemia, have also been reported.[14] Recent critical reviews, however, have questioned the syndrome.[80,224]

Progression of alcoholic liver disease results in changes of both lipoproteins and lipids. Characteristically, the absence of alpha- and pre-beta-lipoprotein bands with the presence of a single band with abnormal motility can be demonstrated.[327] The changes are associated with a decrease in plasma lecithin : cholesterol acyltransferase (LCAT) activity, resulting in greatly reduced levels of plasma cholesterol esters and increased levels of unesterified cholesterol. The decrease or absence of pre-beta-lipoproteins and increased chylomicrons has recently been confirmed in patients with alcoholic cirrhosis and also in baboons in which the progressive liver damage was produced by feeding liquid diets containing ethanol.[36] The results suggest impaired release of triglyceride-carrying lipoproteins from the liver with advancing alcoholic liver injury.

In cholestatic stages of alcoholic hepatitis, serum cholesterol levels may increase due to decreased biliary secretion but, if the injury of parenchymal cells prevails, the synthesis of cholesterol decreases and the end result may be either a normal or a decreased serum cholesterol level.[257,258]

The incidence of alcoholic hyperlipaemia has been reported to be as high as 34 per cent in one series of consecutive patients, hospitalized because of alcoholism, within 24 to 48 hours of alcohol withdrawal.[268] The incidence is also influenced by the type of associated alcoholic liver damage, the frequency being greatest in the patients with fatty liver.[248]

Usually, alcoholic hyperlipaemia is first suspected because of the incidental observation of serum lactescence or of hypercholesterolaemia. It is commonly associated with hepatic, gastrointestinal or pancreatic complications of alcoholism, and on this basis a varying combination of symptoms is seen. Most frequent ones are anorexia, nausea, vomiting, abdominal pain, fever, jaundice and transient haemolysis. Paroxysms of crampy or dull pain in the upper abdomen may lead to explorative laparotomy.[171] The differentiation from acute pancreatitis may be difficult because serum lactescence interferes with the enzyme determinations.[82,122] The diagnosis of alcoholic hyperlipaemia is based on the visible turbidity or lactescence of the fasting serum and on the chemical determination of serum lipids and lipoproteins. Normally triglycerides and VLDLs predominate, but lipid patterns can vary.[17,234] Management of the patient is symptomatic and supportive and withdrawal of alcohol rapidly normalizes serum lipids.

Epidemiological studies concerning the aetiological role of alcoholic hyperlipaemia in atherosclerosis are controversial, showing positive correlations,[383] no correlations[269] or negative correlations.[411] A rise in HDL associated with both experimental alcohol administration[15] and with increased human alcohol consumption[49] has been demonstrated. This association may be significant in view of the correlation between HDL blood levels and possible protection against ischaemic heart disease.[260]

Alcohol as a Source of Calories

At the beginning of this century Atwater and Benedict[9] showed that the caloric value of alcohol can be utilized by the human body. Le Breton and Tremolières[186] calculated that the average alcohol consumption for a man in France covers between 10 and 15 per cent of the daily caloric need. An average oxidation of 7 g of alcohol per hour produces about 210 kJ (50C), and if alcohol is used in quantities allowing a day-long metabolism 5040 kJ (1200 C) can be derived from ethanol. Depending on the basal energy requirements alcohol may furnish from 40 to 80 per cent of the average caloric requirement. In the liver the oxidation of ethanol to acetate may cover up to 80 per cent of the energy requirements of this organ and on this basis the proportional consumption of other energy sources (mainly fatty acids) decreases. In this situation about 75 per cent of the normal oxygen uptake of the liver is utilized for the oxidation of alcohol.[196,237] The most evident clinical implication of the high caloric value of alcohol is its contribution in the genesis of obesity.

In alcoholics, however, the situation is different. As stated in the section 'Accelerated ethanol metabolism after chronic alcohol consumption', the contribution of a NADPH and O_2-consuming non-ADH pathway to ethanol oxidation may be increased during chronic consumption. Since this microsomal ethanol oxidation is not coupled with oxidative phosphorylation, it generates only heat without conservation of chemical energy. This is one reason why ethanol produces a greater increase in oxygen consumption in alcoholics than in normal individuals.[388] Enhanced oxygen consumption has also been produced by experimental chronic ethanol or barbiturate feeding to rats.[296,297] The existence and induction of a microsomal energy-wasting pathway explain the lesser growth of ethanol-fed animals as compared to isocalorically-fed controls.[217,340] In human volunteers the isocaloric substitution of food by ethanol resulted in a relative failure to gain weight as compared to the effect of other calories.[296]

Interference of Alcohol with Drug Metabolism

The well-known combination of drug abuse and alcoholism emphasizes the clinical importance of ethanol and drug interactions. It is obvious that many of the central nervous effects of various drugs may be potentiated by simultaneous alcohol use. On the other hand it is now known that the elimination rates of various drugs are influenced both by chronic ethanol consumption and by the possible liver injury. Detailed information of individual drug interactions with ethanol can be obtained from Wallgren and Berry.[406]

As already mentioned, chronic ethanol administration results in adaptive hypertrophy of the hepatic smooth endoplasmic reticulum. This hypertrophy is accompanied by an increased content of microsomal cytochrome P-450[325] and of NADPH-cytochrome P-450 reductase.[158] These components play a key role in the microsomal hydroxylation of various drugs and explain the well-documented enhanced clearance of such drugs as meprobamate, pentobarbital and tolbutamide.[48, 166, 262, 398] This metabolic adaptation evidently contributes to the tolerance of alcoholics for drugs, including sedatives.[363] Alcoholic liver injury may, however, interfere with their elimination.[200] Furthermore, the adaptive response is seen only when the alcoholic is sober. Simultaneous ethanol and drug administration (for instance, ethanol and tranquillizers) results in additive or even in synergistic effects by additive action of central nervous system effects and by the inhibition of drug metabolism.[326]

Interference of Alcohol with Hormone Metabolism (see also Chapter 7)

Hypogonadism and gynaecomastia are commonly associated with alcoholic cirrhosis in the male.[230, 246] Both primary gonadal and hypothalamic–pituitary suppression are demonstrable in men with alcoholic liver injury.[395] Recent observations indicate that alcohol itself also markedly affects testosterone metabolism independently of cirrhosis or nutritional factors through decreased production and enhanced catabolism.[117] On this basis the direct metabolic effects of alcohol may at least partly contribute to the pattern of endocrine abnormalities in alcoholic liver disease. Furthermore, profound disturbances in hepatic metabolism of oestrogens are associated with hepatic injury.[2]

PATHOGENESIS OF ALCOHOLIC LIVER DISEASE

Aetiological Role of Ethanol

On the basis of some animal experiments it was generally believed until 20 years ago that liver disease of the alcoholic was due exclusively to malnutrition and not to direct toxic effects of alcohol itself.[28, 61, 67] Characteristically, alcoholic cirrhosis was called 'fatty nutritional cirrhosis'.Alcoholics undoubtedly suffer from malnutrition for a variety of reasons. Alcohol has a high caloric value, but alcoholic calories are so-called 'empty calories' since alcoholic beverages are usually devoid of minerals, vitamins and proteins. Because alcohol fulfils much of the caloric requirements by providing a large fraction of the daily caloric intake,[252] it may decrease the intake of other nutrients and, in addition, associated poor appetite, nausea, secondary maldigestion and malabsorption may contribute to secondary malnutrition.[18] During the last 20 years, however, many experimental studies have shown that ethanol can also affect the liver independently of malnutrition.[212] The culmination of these studies was the reproduction of the entire spectrum of alcoholic liver disease, including cirrhosis, in the baboon chronically fed an alcohol-containing diet without protein or other deficiencies.[211,216]

The basis of the feeding technique is to incorporate ethanol in a totally liquid diet. In order to quench either thirst or hunger the experimental animals have to ingest the alcohol. In rats the amount of ethanol consumed was increased to 36 per cent and in baboons to 50 per cent of total calories, a proportion comparable to moderate or extensive alcohol intake in man. Isocaloric replacement of sucrose or other carbohydrate by ethanol produced a progressive increase in hepatic lipid content during the first month of alcohol administration in rats.[217] Fatty liver, however, did not develop if the ethanol intake was decreased from 36 to 20 per cent of the total calories. It has not been possible to produce more advanced alcoholic liver injury in rats. This is probably due to the shorter life span and lower alcohol intake of the rat as compared to the baboon. On the basis of these animal experiments and the epidemiological studies discussed before it is apparent that ethanol itself must play a major role in the pathogenesis of alcoholic liver disease.

The deleterious effect of alcohol on the liver has also been confirmed in controlled studies with human volunteers under metabolic ward conditions. Morphological and biochemical increase in hepatic lipid was demonstrated when ethanol was given either as a supplement or as an isocaloric substitution for carbohydrate together with an otherwise nutritionally adequate diet. Hepatic steatosis was produced even with a high-protein, vitamin-supplemented diet and was accompanied by striking ultrastructural liver changes and by elevations of hepatic transaminases in blood.[184, 213, 217, 221]

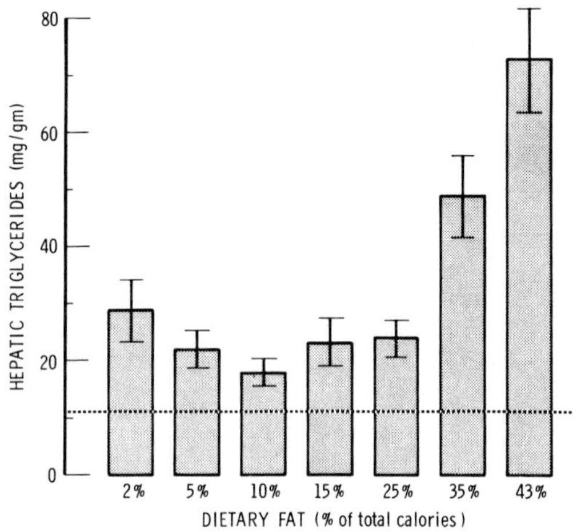

Figure 32.11. Effects of varying amounts of dietary fat with standard dose of ethanol on hepatic triglyceride accumulation. Hepatic triglycerides in seven groups of rats given ethanol (36 per cent of calories) with a diet of normal protein (18 per cent of calories). Average hepatic triglyceride concentration in the control animals is indicated by a dotted line. From Lieber and DeCarli,[209] with kind permission of the authors and the editor of *American Journal of Clinical Nutrition.*

Role of Fat, Protein and Lipotropic Factors

If the fat content of liquid diet is decreased from 35 to 25 per cent hepatic triglyceride accumulation significantly decreases[209] (Figure 32.11). In addition, the chain length of the dietary fatty acids is important. Replacement of dietary triglycerides containing long chain fatty acids (LCT) by fat containing medium chain fatty acids (MCT) markedly reduced the capacity of alcohol to produce a fatty liver in rats.[222]

As already mentioned, until 20 years ago malnutrition was considered the main pathogenetic factor of alcoholic liver disease. This concept was based on animal experiments, but there was no evidence that malnutrition or, especially, protein deficiency could lead to liver cirrhosis in man. On the contrary, both epidemiological and histological findings failed to establish a connection between kwashiorkor and liver cirrhosis.[62, 309] In adolescent baboons protein restriction to 7 per cent of total calories did not result in conspicuous liver injury when assessed either by biochemical analysis or by light and electron microscopic examination after 19 months.[223] Significant steatosis was observed only when the protein intake was reduced to 4 per cent of total calories. Furthermore, an excess of protein (25 per cent of total calories, or twice the recommended amount) did not prevent ethanol from producing fat accumulation in human volunteers[204] (Figure 32.12).

Both in rat and man protein deficiency may result in decreased hepatic alcohol dehydrogenase activity,[35] which in turn prevents some acute metabolic effects of alcohol such as the inhibition of citric acid cycle, the increase in lactate/pyruvate ratio,[333] ethanol-induced fasting hypoglycaemia[328,329] and ethanol-induced inhibition in galactose elimination.[332] However, in a chronic situation a combination of ethanol and a diet deficient in both protein and lipotropic factors leads to more pronounced hepatic steatosis than either deficiency alone.[176,219] In some other studies, the combination of alcohol and protein deficiency significantly increased the mortality of the experimental animals without demonstrating differences in hepatic fat accumulation.[28, 178, 304]

Deficiencies in *lipotropic factors* (choline and methionine) can produce fatty liver and cirrhosis in growing rats[28] but primates are far less susceptible to protein and lipotropic deficiency than rodents.[139] Furthermore, both clinical data from patients with alcoholic liver disease as well as experiments in human volunteers have shown the ineffectiveness of lipotropic factors in the prevention of alcoholic liver injury.[278, 323] This is not surprising, since there is no evidence that a diet which is deficient in choline is deleterious to adult man. On the other hand there are several biochemical and ultrastructural differences between liver diseases produced either by choline deficiency or ethanol feeding.[212] Thus, hepatic injury induced by choline deficiency appears to be primarily an experimental disease of rats with little, if any, relevance to alcoholic liver injury, particularly in humans.

Fatty Liver: Biochemical Mechanisms of Fat Accumulation

Fatty liver can be induced by either acute or chronic administration of alcohol both in laboratory animals and man. Lipids accumulating in the liver may originate from (a) dietary lipids as chylomicrons, (b) adipose tissue as free fatty acids (FFA) or (c) they may be synthesized in the liver itself (Figure 32.13). Depending on experimental conditions alcohol may (a) increase peripheral fat mobilization, (b) enhance hepatic triglyceride synthesis, (c) decrease lipid oxidation in the liver and (d) decrease hepatic lipoprotein release.

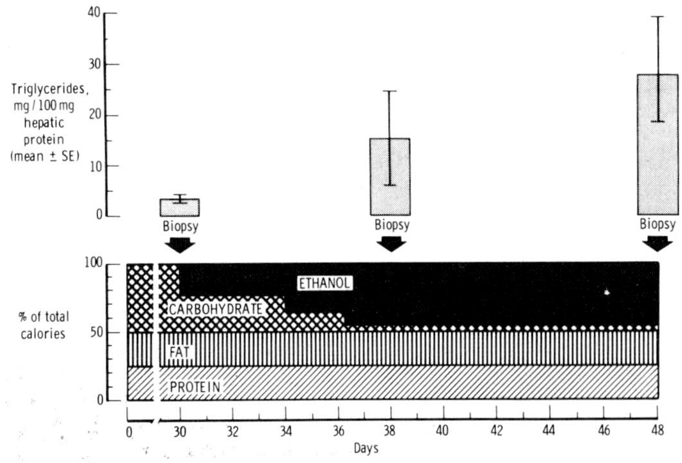

Figure 32.12. Effect of ethanol on hepatic triglycerides in five volunteers given a high-protein, low-fat diet. From Lieber,[204] with kind permission of the editor of *Federation Proceedings*.

Increased peripheral fat mobilization

One large sublethal dose of ethanol induces a temporary increase of hepatic triglycerides.[244] Fatty acid mobilization in this condition, however, represents a non-specific stress reaction, and it can be produced only in the presence of adrenocortical and pituitary hormones.[42, 243, 314] On the other hand, peripheral fat mobilization is of little clinical relevance after chronic ethanol consumption in which the fatty acids deposited in the liver do not derive primarily from adipose tissue but tend to reflect the lipids in the diet.[215, 218]

Enhanced hepatic lipogenesis

The oxidation of ethanol results in an increase of hepatic NADH/NAD ratio (see above, 'Pathways of alcohol metabolism'; Figure 32.10). Consequently, in addition, the concentration of hepatic alpha-glycerophosphate increases[273] and this favours triglyceride accumulation in the liver by trapping fatty acids.[155] Furthermore, excess NADH promotes fatty acid synthesis,[115, 214] possibly by the elongation pathway or transhydrogenation to nicotinamide-adenine dinucleotide phosphate (NADP). Both NADH and NADPH may serve as hydrogen donors in the elongation of fatty acid chains. On this basis enhanced lipogenesis can be considered a means for disposing of the excess hydrogen. The role of increased hepatic fatty acid synthesis in ethanol-induced triacylglycerol accumulation has, however, recently been questioned.[341]

Decreased lipid oxidation

Decreased fatty acid oxidation by ethanol has been demonstrated in liver slices,[214] perfused liver,[222] isolated hepatocytes,[279] human liver

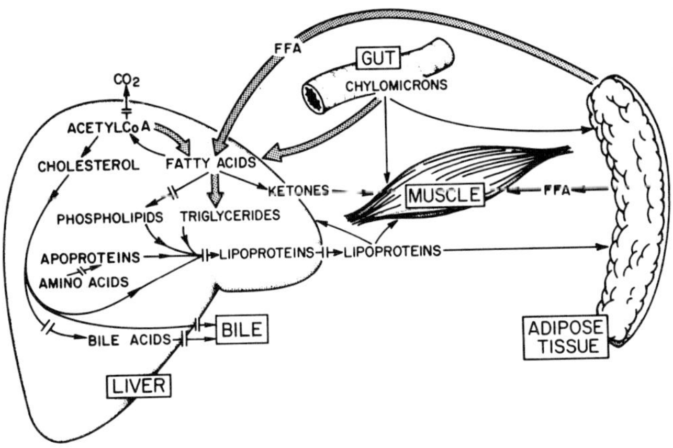

Figure 32.13. Possible mechanisms of fatty liver production through either increase (⇨) or decrease (⊣⊢→) of lipid transport and metabolism.

biopsy tissue[275] and in man in vivo.[33] During ethanol oxidation, fatty acids that normally serve as the main energy source for the liver are supplanted by ethanol.[105] The mitochondria use the hydrogen equivalents originating from ethanol, since the normal source of NADH, the citric acid cycle, is depressed (see 'Inhibition of citric acid cycle', above). The end result is the deposition in the liver of dietary fat, when available, or fatty acids derived from endogenous synthesis in the absence of dietary fat.[212, 255] This mechanism can be considered as a major cause for the development of alcoholic fatty liver.

Hepatic protein (including lipoprotein) production and release

Fat accumulates inside the liver cells as triglycerides, first as small liposomes and later as larger lipid collections seen sometimes even in the space of Disse.[11, 274, 367] In addition to the greatly depressed fatty acid oxidation caused by hepatic ethanol metabolism the only possibility for the liver cells to reduce fat accumulation is by increased transport of fat from the liver to peripheral tissues. The normal mechanism is to combine triglycerides with protein and phospholipids to form VLDLs. These synthetic and transport processes occur in endoplasmic reticulum; in ribosomes,[46] microsomal membranes[366] and the Golgi apparatus.[231] As stated before, these cell organelles have been shown to be 'induced', both morphologically and biochemically, during chronic ethanol feeding.[145,146,184] The last step in the transport system, secretion, is mediated by the microtubular–microfilament system, which has been shown to be of importance for the intracellular movement and the possible release of VLDL particles.[197] This conclusion was drawn from studies carried out with colchicine which is a well-known inhibitor of the microtubular system. The concept is further supported by the finding that colchicine treatment leads to the accumulation of Golgi-derived secretory vesicles containing VLDL particles[368] and, moreover, colchicine has been shown to interfere also with the intracellular transport and secretion of other proteins.[90,198,358,369]

It is well known that the main mechanism of fatty liver induced by choline deficiency,[233] protein deficiency[351] or various toxic agents, such as ethionine and carbon tetrachloride,[83, 84] is a decreased production of lipoproteins. There is also evidence that an acute large dose of ethanol may produce a decrease either in lipoprotein synthesis or secretion.[6, 240, 342] However, in man and animals fed chronically with alcohol both increases[15,19,160] and decreases[68] have been reported. Evidently the role of lipoproteins in ethanol-induced fatty liver is complex, but speculations to clarify some of the findings are in order.

The pathogenetic mechanism of alcoholic fatty liver is an over-supply of fatty acids. In the acute situation they are mainly derived from adipose tissue. In the chronic situation both the decreased fatty acid oxidation and increased synthesis of fatty acids lead to over-supply. This may be further enhanced by fat load from dietary sources. The expected response is an enhanced lipoprotein synthesis and secretion.

In animals an acute dose of alcohol decreases protein (albumin) synthesis in perfused liver,[320,321] in isolated cells[154,266] and in liver slices.[287] Similarly, lipoprotein synthesis may be inhibited. The mechanism of inhibition can presumably be related to the ethanol-induced increase in NADH/NAD ratio.[286] However, in the chronic situation lipoprotein synthesis may not be decreased because (a) hepatic redox changes caused by ethanol oxidation are less prominent both in human alcoholics[332, 335, 336] and in chronically alcohol-fed rats[75] or baboons,[330] and (b) the inhibition is also offset by the proliferation of hepatic endoplasmic reticulum.[145, 184]

The effect of ethanol on lipoprotein secretion mediated by the microtubular–microfilament system may also be significant. Baraona et al[20, 21] found that chronically ethanol-fed rats retain export protein (i.e. albumin and transferrin) in the soluble fraction of the liver cells and at the same time colchicine-binding protein (microtubules) was decreased. The loss of microtubular function could explain the retention of export proteins including lipoproteins by the liver cells.

Transitional Lesions from Alcoholic Fatty Liver to More Advanced Injury

The relationship between alcoholic fatty liver, alcoholic hepatitis and cirrhosis has not yet been elucidated. Although hepatic fat accumulation itself is not necessarily harmful, it reflects a metabolic disturbance of the liver. It is possible that this disturbance, when exaggerated, may eventually lead to irreversible damage of the hepatocyte. Necrosis in turn could lead to inflammation, resulting in alcoholic hepatitis. A number of biochemical, morphological and immunological data concerning the hepatic effects of alcohol have accumulated in vivo and in vitro in human and animal experiments. The most prominent findings in various cell organelles will be summarized here.

Alcohol-induced changes in the cytosol

Hepatomegaly is one of the earliest manifestations of chronic alcohol abuse. This phenomenon was attributed to fat accumulation which, however, accounted for only half of the increase.[217] Baraona et al[20] demonstrated that part of the enlargement of the liver was due to protein accumulation with a concomitant retention of water in the cytosol of the liver cell leading to an overall increase in the size of the hepatocyte. Typical export proteins, such as albumin and transferrin, were increased, whereas constituent proteins, such as ferritin, did not increase. Subsequent studies indicated that the incorporation of labelled amino acids into plasma proteins was delayed in animals fed alcohol chronically, whereas the simultaneous accumulation of labelled proteins, including prealbumin, was increased in the liver.[21] The accumulation of protein was associated with a decreased amount of polymerized tubulin in hepatic cytosol, which may explain the defect in protein secretion (see above, 'Hepatic protein production and release'). The accumulation of protein, together with the concomitant retention of water and an overall increase in the size of the hepatocyte, leads to the so-called 'ballooning' of the hepatocyte. The end result may be the necrosis of the cell.

Alcohol-induced changes in mitochondria

Striking morphological alterations, including swelling and abnormal cristae, have been demonstrated in electron microscopical studies of human alcoholic livers.[175,373] Controlled studies in man,[184] rats[145] and baboons[216,223] have shown that these changes are due to alcohol itself rather than to other factors (such as malnutrition). The structural abnormalities are associated with functional impairment.[135,173,174]

As mentioned above, the first metabolite of ethanol oxidation, *acetaldehyde*, is further metabolized by a mitochondrial enzyme, acetaldehyde dehydrogenase. On this basis several alterations due to acetaldehyde oxidation occur, including a change in the mitochondrial redox state.[227,228] Numerous toxic effects have also been attributed to acetaldehyde.[390] In this respect the finding that blood acetaldehyde levels during ethanol oxidation are elevated in alcoholics may be of importance,[180] especially since acetaldehyde has been shown to depress a variety of important mitochondrial functions such as respiration[172] and fatty acid oxidation.[50] Furthermore, the depressing effect of acetaldehyde on mitochondrial respiration with NAD-dependent substrates – even with the low acetaldehyde concentration likely to occur in vivo – has recently been demonstrated.[249] The elevation of blood acetaldehyde in alcoholics may perhaps be related to mitochondrial damage and decreased acetaldehyde oxidation caused by chronic alcohol consumption.[135] Whether ethanol-induced mitochondrial injury can be related to cell death or not is still unresolved, but a vicious circle of progressive mitochondrial damage mediated by acetaldehyde could be one mechanism, as suggested by Hasumura, Teschke and Lieber.[134]

Israel et al[149] have suggested that alcohol-induced liver damage may be caused by a hypermetabolic state of the liver with increased oxygen consumption, which leads to hypoxaemia and death of the liver cells. The theory involves an increased utilization of ATP by the Na^+–K^+-activated ATPase after chronic ethanol feeding. Contradictory findings from other laboratories,[51,116] however, indicate that the hypermetabolic state does not fully explain all changes in ethanol metabolism during chronic alcohol feeding.

Alterations of the endoplasmic reticulum and Golgi apparatus

The well-documented proliferation of the membranes of the smooth endoplasmic reticulum has been interpreted as an adaptive process, but theoretically it may have also some injurious consequences. Some compounds acquire hepatotoxicity only after metabolism or activation by the microsomal enzymes. For instance, the hepatotoxicity of carbon tetrachloride is known to be much more pronounced in alcoholics, presumably due to enhanced activation by the microsomes.[133] Through a similar mechanism, alcoholics may be more susceptible to the hepatotoxic actions of a variety of compounds present in our environment, including a number of commonly used drugs.

The morphological prominence[263] and increased biochemical activity[109] of the Golgi apparatus caused by chronic ethanol administration can be considered as adaptive phenomena promoting hepatic lipoprotein secretion.

Plasma membrane and cAMP

The effect of acute or chronic ethanol administration either on the plasmalemma of the hepatocyte or on mitochondrial or other membranes is not well understood. However, possible interference with membrane function, especially as to hormone actions, could play an essential role in various cell functions.

High alcohol concentrations achieved in vitro have been shown to increase cAMP levels both by the stimulation of its synthesis via membrane-bound adenylate cyclase and also by inhibiting its degradation by phosphodiesterase.[118,123,374] In vivo findings are controversial; an acute dose of ethanol has been reported to decrease cAMP level in the liver[402] and there is evidence that the effect is time or dose-dependent.[371] Other workers have found an elevation in hepatic cAMP concentration after an acute dose of ethanol.[153] Chronic alcohol treatment with liquid diet has been shown to result in a decrease of hepatic cAMP level[402] but this may be due to the high fat content of the diet.[341] There is also evidence from experiments with isolated cells which indicates that the decrease might be mediated by the most typical metabolic effect of ethanol, i.e. the increase of the hepatic NADH/NAD ratio.[413]

Lipid peroxidation

The microsomal pathway requiring O_2 is also capable of generating lipid peroxides. Enhanced lipid peroxidation has been proposed as a mechanism for ethanol-induced fatty liver[72] and also as a cause of peroxidative injury of hepatic mitochondria (membrane lipids) mediated through acetaldehyde.[73] Theoretically, increased activity of microsomal NADPH oxidase following chronic ethanol consumption[210] could result in enhanced H_2O_2 production, thereby also favouring lipid peroxidation. However, contradictory results have been reported.[34,132,344] Furthermore, ethanol was found actually to exert a sparing action on vitamin E deficiency (a common cause of lipid peroxidation).[199]

Alterations in immune mechanisms in alcoholic liver disease (see also Chapter 9)

Over the last few years, increasing evidence suggests that immunological mechanisms play an important role in the pathogenesis and potentiation of alcoholic liver injury. Serum immunoglobulins, especially IgA, are usually elevated in patients with alcoholic liver disease.[150,359] This is associated with an increased incidence of auto-antibodies, both bacterial[389] and tissue antibodies.[12] Cell-mediated mechanisms have also been implicated. Loss of delayed hypersensitivity was reported by Berenyi, Straus and Cruz.[26] Other studies include the inhibition of PHA-stimulated lymphocyte transformation,[141] decreased active T-rosette formation,[25] and a pronounced decrease in peripheral blood T-lymphocytes in patients with alcoholic hepatitis.[27] More recently, an altered cell-mediated immunity to liver antigens has been described in patients with alcoholic liver disease, in studies using either autologous liver,[365] normal human liver[259] or alcoholic hyaline.[414] Furthermore, the existence of alcoholic hyaline antigen and its antibody has been reported by Kanagasundram et al[164] and, finally, it has been shown that lymphocytes from baboons with alcoholic liver injury are cytotoxic against autologous liver cells in tissue culture.[281] The latter finding is consistent with human studies.[56,163] These observations suggest that immunological mechanisms may be involved in the perpetuation of hepatic damage produced by alcohol. While the findings do not differentiate primary events from changes secondary to pre-existing liver injury, they justify further investigation directed at determining the role of immunological factors in the development and progression of alcoholic liver disease.

Scarring; relationship between fatty liver, alcoholic hepatitis and cirrhosis

Sequential histological studies have shown that alcoholic hepatitis is a potentially precirrhotic lesion.[106] Necrosis and inflammation function as a trigger of collagen fibre formation or scarring. An unresolved question, however, is whether fatty infiltration of the liver (usually a reversible lesion) can progress to cirrhosis without an intermediate alcoholic hepatitis. In the baboon model of alcoholic liver disease it was observed that although some animals displayed mild hepatitis, as indicated by necrosis and polymorphonuclear infiltration, 'florid' alcoholic hepatitis was not seen, yet cirrhosis developed in one out of three animals.[216] This experimental observation supports the morphological concept that alcoholic hepatitis may not be a necessary precursor of Laennec's cirrhosis in the alcoholic.[206] It also raises the possibility that the extensive necrosis and inflammation is not the only trigger for the development of fibrosis and cirrhosis. It is possible that the low grade of necrosis and inflammation seen in many alcoholics and also in the baboons fed with alcohol may suffice to promote the scarring. In this respect the demonstration of pericentral or perivenular sclerosis (see above, 'Pericentral venous sclerosis'), even in the absence of widespread inflammation and necrosis both in baboons and humans,[397] may be of importance.

The progression of pericentral sclerosis to cirrhosis without diffuse inflammation[397] indicates that one should also consider other mechanisms whereby alcohol may trigger the development of cirrhosis. In this respect the effect of ethanol on the metabolism of *collagen*, the predominant and key protein of fibrous tissue, is important. Such a possibility is supported by the observation that, after experimental alcohol administration to either rats or baboons, an increase in liver collagen is already detectable chemically at the fatty liver stage, prior to any inflammation, necrosis or visible fibrosis or even pericentral sclerosis.[87] The mechanism responsible for this collagen accumulation has not yet been elucidated. Evidence was found in favour of increased production of collagen, associated with enhanced activity of peptidylproline hydroxylase.[87] Theoretically, the activation of this could be mediated by lactate, which is a known activator of the enzyme and, as stated before, alcohol consumption is associated with elevation of blood lactate. The enhanced production of collagen may be associated with accelerated degradation, since urinary excretion of hydroxyproline and glycosaminoglycans is increased by chronic alcohol feeding to rats.[256] The pathogenetic implication of collagen accumulation is further supported by findings which indicate that the fibrotic process of alcoholic liver disease in humans is accompanied by alterations in collagen polymorphism. Seyer, Hutcheson and Kang[353] demonstrated that the relative amount of collagen type I is increased in cirrhotic livers.

Many epidemiological, clinical and experimental data emphasize the role of individual susceptibility to the hepatotoxic effect of alcohol. It was stated in the epidemiological part of this chapter that severe alcoholic liver disease manifests itself in only one-third of the alcoholics. The incidence of fatty liver is presumably higher but is mostly reversible. Furthermore, in serial biopsies of human alcoholics, it has been shown that only 38 per cent of cases with alcoholic hepatitis develop liver cirrhosis. In 52 per cent alcoholic hepatitis may persist for several years and 10 per cent of patients may even heal although some alcohol consumption continues.[106] In the baboon model of alcoholic liver disease also, only one-third developed liver cirrhosis.[216] Evidence supports a sex difference in the hepatotoxic effect of alcohol. Several studies indicate that females are particularly susceptible to alcohol-induced liver injury.[229, 408] However, further studies to elucidate the role and mechanism of different susceptibilities for alcoholic liver injury are still needed.

CLINICAL MANIFESTATIONS OF ALCOHOLIC LIVER DISEASE

The commonest histological finding in an alcoholic patient in whom liver injury is suspected is the fatty infiltration of hepatic parenchymal cells. In some cases this may be the only manifestation of hepatic involvement, but often fatty liver is accompanied by moderate or severe alcoholic hepatitis, cirrhosis without hepatitis or scarring and hepatitis without evidence of cirrhosis.[43]

Alcoholic Fatty Liver

The clinical spectrum of alcoholic fatty liver may extend from silent non-symptomatic hepatomegaly to severe hepatocellular failure with cholestasis and portal hypertension. Most of the patients with pure fatty liver are virtually asymptomatic. Hepatomegaly is the commonest clinical sign, present on physical examination in 75 per cent of patients.[188] In more advanced cases hepatic tenderness, anorexia, nausea, emesis, jaundice, fluid accumulation and even spider angiomas are present. In many of these cases an associated alcoholic hepatitis may contribute to the clinical picture and laboratory findings.

The typical patient with more severe alcoholic fatty liver is young or middle aged with a history of drinking alcohol heavily for weeks or months. The liver edge may be a few cm below the costal margin or may extend to the iliac crest. The liver is usually solid and its surface is smooth. Mild tenderness is common, associated sometimes with severe epigastric or right upper quadrant pain.[113] Severe forms of fatty liver may present a clinical picture mimicking extrahepatic obstructive jaundice, especially if associated with dark urine and acholic stools.[13,292] Typical abnormalities in laboratory tests are slightly or moderately elevated serum transaminases SGOT and SGPT and slight retention of bromsulphthalein (BSP).[71,188] However, the correlation between the pathological and laboratory findings and the degree of hepatic steatosis is rather poor.[41] Serum prothrombin concentrations are frequently low, even in mild cases of alcoholic fatty liver. In cases of associated malnutrition or malabsorption the prothrombin time can be corrected by administration of vitamin K. Both decreased and normal serum albumin values have been reported in alcoholic fatty liver.[71,188] Serum protein values should be interpreted cautiously, however, since they may be influenced by direct metabolic effects of alcohol as well as by nutritional factors. In contrast to more advanced alcoholic liver injury all the abnormalities in laboratory tests tend to return to normal rapidly within the first days of hospitalization. Transient anaemia and albuminuria can be detected in about 25 per cent of patients with fatty liver at the time of initial hospitalization. Albuminuria disappears within 24 to 72 hours and its mechanism has not been resolved.[188] Anaemia is usually due to associated nutritional deficiencies or gastrointestinal haemorrhage (see Chapter 6).

Rarely, alcoholic fatty liver may be complicated by hyperlipaemia, haemolytic anaemia and jaundice (Zieve's syndrome).[415] As stated in 'Alcoholic hyperlipaemia', above, the syndrome consists of a combination of symptoms with a common aetiological factor, ethanol. The possible simultaneous manifestation of various metabolic abnormalities (such as hypoglycaemia, alcoholic ketoacidosis and lactic acidosis) was discussed.

Alcoholic Hepatitis

The fulminant and fatal nature of alcoholic hepatitis was stressed by early studies based on autopsy materials. In those cases patients were acutely ill, with fever, anorexia, nausea, abdominal pain, jaundice, tender hepatomegaly, ascites, oedema of lower extremities or even liver coma.[77,129] In subsequent studies when the diagnosis was based on histological criteria the clinical picture was characterized by milder symptomatology and a less dismal prognosis.[4,22,23,55,120,131] The spectrum of alcoholic hepatitis may thus range from mild anicteric hepatomegaly to fatal disease with jaundice, ascites, liver coma, gastrointestinal haemorrhage and with all the complications of severe hepatic insufficiency. The only clinical difference between the mild and severe form of alcoholic hepatitis is in the intensity and frequency of various symptoms.[124,131,137,229] The most frequent symptoms of the milder cases include anorexia, fatigue, intermittent fever, right epigastric pain and hepatomegaly. In general, patients with alcoholic hepatitis are more ill than those with a simple fatty liver, and there is a correlation between the severity of the histological features of alcoholic hepatitis (hepatocellular necrosis, leucocytic infiltration, frequency of alcoholic hyaline) and the degree of hepatomegaly, leukocytosis and elevations of serum transaminases and in the intensity of symptoms.[55,130] Occasional clinical findings are Dupuytren's contractures[270] and parotid swelling.[37] Patients with central hyaline sclerosis may have portal hypertension, splenomegaly, ascites and oesophageal and gastric varices, even in the absence of cirrhosis.[316]

Characteristic *laboratory findings* (see also Chapter 17) include the elevations of serum *enzymes*. γ-Glutamyl transpeptidase (γ-GTP), ornithine carbamyl transferase (OCT), aspartate aminotransferase (AST) and alanine aminotransferase (ALT) are elevated in all cases and alkaline phosphatases (ALP) in 80 per cent.[359] In contrast to non-alcoholic liver diseases AST/ALP or, even more clearly, γ-GTP/ALP ratios are increased,[359] and this may be important in the differential diagnosis. The role of these ratios as quantitative reflectors of liver cell damage can be questioned, however, since the origin of AST is at least in part extrahepatic[179] and the increased serum activity of γ-GTP may be partly due to the well-known induction of microsomal enzymes.[376] A better correlation between the degree of liver necrosis and inflammation was observed when the serum level of a mitochondrial enzyme, glutamic dehydrogenase, was measured.[396]

Serum *protein changes* include a decrease in serum albumin in about half of the patients, while haptoglobin and complement 3 are usually increased, whereas serum transferrin concentration is relatively low.[360] Serum immunoglobulin IgA is usually elevated and seems to correlate with the degree of liver damage as assessed from histological liver specimens.[150] In addition, the depression of serum albumin and prolongation of the prothrombin time has been shown to correlate with the severity of the histological lesion.[137]

Other common laboratory findings include serum *bilirubin* elevations (90 per cent of patients). It should, however, be remembered that serum bilirubin may also be increased in the absence of alcoholic hepatitis (for instance, because of haemolysis or alcoholic pancreatitis). Even more sensitive indicators of alcoholic liver injury are serum *bile acids*. The concentration of chenodeoxycholic acid, especially, is increased, but the correlation to the degree of liver cell necrosis is poor.[261] The clinical value of *postprandial bile acid* measurements,[85] as well as the role of bile acid tolerance tests,[185] in the evaluation of the degree of alcoholic liver injury remains to be clarified (see Chapter 12). The same pertains to a variety of other quantitative liver function tests. Although BSP, galactose, indocyanine green and antipyrine tests have been reported to be abnormal in liver damage, especially in cirrhosis, they lack practical discriminative value in the evaluation of initial alcoholic liver injury, fatty liver, central venous sclerosis or alcoholic hepatitis.

Alcoholic Cirrhosis

Alcoholic cirrhosis is predominantly a disease of males.[127, 312] It becomes symptomatic at an average age of 50 years especially when it is not complicated by acute fatty liver or alcoholic hepatitis. Most patients are detected when they seek treatment for complications. However, according to autopsy studies cirrhosis may remain unrecognized ante-mortem in 40 per cent of cirrhotic patients and in about 20 per cent it is discovered fortuitously on routine examination or during the evaluation of some other, unrelated, disease.

The most common signs of cirrhosis are weight loss (unless masked by ascites), weakness and anorexia.[312] Jaundice can be detected in about two-thirds of patients when first admitted to hospital and is often the main reason for more extensive examination. Low-grade and continuous fever is also common in decompensated cirrhosis.[385]

Jaundice and hepatomegaly are typical primary physical signs of cirrhosis. Secondary phenomena include portal hypertension with splenomegaly and ascites, encephalopathy with asterixis and other neurological signs, gastrointestinal haemorrhage from oesophageal or gastric varices, caput medusae and oedema or bleeding tendencies due to clotting factor abnormalities. Tertiary complications include spontaneous peritonitis caused by anaerobic bacteria[375] and, in males, gynaecomastia and a female pattern of pubic hair distribution resulting from testicular atrophy and hormonal imbalance. Other manifestations include spider angiomas, palmar erythema, parotid enlargement and Dupuytren's contracture. A more detailed review of these common clinical features of cirrhosis can be found in Chapter 30.

Abnormalities found on laboratory examination range from mild BSP retention to profound hyperbilirubinaemia, hypoalbuminaemia, hypoprothrombinaemia and hyperglobulinaemia. Typically, serum electrophoresis reveals a decrease in serum albumin and pre-albumin and a broad elevation of the beta and gamma globulins.[359] Frequently, IgA and also IgG and IgM are elevated.[3, 89, 150, 360] With more advanced liver injury a depression or even absence of alpha- and pre-beta-lipoprotein bands can be demonstrated.[327] This is associated with a decrease of the esterified fraction of plasma cholesterol secondary to depressed lecithin : cholesterol acyltransferase (LCAT) activity.[32,161,357] Serum transaminases and alkaline phosphatases are usually only mildly elevated. An impaired glucose tolerance and an increased incidence of diabetes have been described in patients with Laennec's cirrhosis.[58, 59]

DIAGNOSIS AND DIFFERENTIAL DIAGNOSIS OF ALCOHOLIC LIVER DISEASES

In addition to the features of alcoholic liver disease described above, these patients may have other symptoms and signs as a result of alcohol abuse which are of value in diagnosis. These include a peripheral neuropathy, other neurological symptoms such as cerebellar atrophy, Wernicke's encephalopathy, an alcoholic myopathy, chronic relapsing pancreatitis, alcoholic cardiomyopathy and an anaemia due to folate deficiency or a direct toxic effect of alcohol on the bone marrow (see Chapter 8).

1. At each stage of alcoholic liver disease (fatty liver, alcoholic hepatitis, cirrhosis) the clinician must distinguish between alcoholic and non-alcoholic causes of liver injury. This is important for the subsequent treatment of the patient as exemplified by a case of chronic active hepatitis in an alcoholic.[114]
2. The clinician must differentiate between the acute, reversible forms of alcoholic liver disease such as fatty liver and alcoholic hepatitis, and the chronic, mainly irreversible, cirrhosis.

History, Clinical Signs and Laboratory Findings

In the evaluation of the patient with either an incidental finding of pathological laboratory values pointing to liver damage or with more advanced symptomatology requiring hospitalization *the history of heavy alcohol intake* for weeks or months before hospital admission is strongly suggestive for the alcoholic aetiology of liver injury. For this purpose simplified screening questions such as 'Has your family ever objected to your drinking?', 'Did you ever think you drank too much in general?', 'Have others (i.e. friends, physicians, clergymen) ever said you drink too much for your own good?' can be used. With these questions true alcoholics can be identified in more than 90 per cent of cases.[410] The clinician, however, should realize that estimation of alcohol consumption even in a careful interview reveals only about 40 per cent of total alcohol consumption.[241] Furthermore, the casual estimation of blood ethanol seldom reveals heavy drinkers and does not differentiate between chronic and acute alcohol consumption.[128] Serum enzyme elevations can be used to detect alcoholics, but do not differentiate alcoholic liver injury from other liver diseases.[319] In this respect the recent demonstration that increased plasma α-amino-N-butyric acid relative to leucine is a useful marker of prolonged heavy drinking as defined by history,[354,355] the National Council of Alcoholism criteria on alcoholism,[162] or psychological testing, may in the future provide new possibilities in the evaluation of a patient with liver disease. In advanced liver disease, however, false positive findings may occur because of depressed plasma leucine.

At present, there is no definite biochemical marker, which can differentiate the alcoholic liver diseases from the non-alcoholic ones even when different test combinations are analysed by the discriminant analysis.[359,364]

Laboratory tests are not much better for the differentiation of various stages of alcoholic liver disease. This is due to the great variability in the severity of both alcoholic hepatitis and fatty liver. In extreme cases both of them may simulate the clinical picture of liver cirrhosis or even extrahepatic biliary obstruction.

The most characteristic clinical signs and laboratory test or test combinations in the diagnosis and differential diagnosis of alcoholic liver diseases are summarized in Tables 32.1 and 32.2. The histological confirmation of the diagnosis by liver biopsy obtained either blindly or during laparoscopy is essential. Laparoscopy and endoscopic retrograde cholangiography are indicated in rare cases simulating extrahepatic biliary obstruction. The diagnostic laparotomy

Table 32.1. *Clinical Findings in Alcoholic Liver Diseases.*

	Fatty liver %	Alcoholic hepatitis %	Cirrhosis %
Anorexia, nausea, fatigue	2–10	70	35
Abdominal pain	2–10	50	34
Fever	2–10	50 (intermittent)	24 (low grade, continuous)
Hepatomegaly	75	95	67
Jaundice	2	55	49
Signs of portal hypertension (ascites, splenomegaly)	2	40	50
Spider angiomas	8	30	38

Data are based on references cited in the text.
The percentages represent mean values. A wide range in the incidence of various symptoms is common in alcoholic hepatitis and depends on the selection of patient material.

Table 32.2. *Laboratory Findings in Alcoholic Liver Diseases.*

I. Suggestive for the alcohol aetiology of liver disease:	
ASAT (GOT) and ALAT (GPT):	Both enzymes are elevated in about 50% of patients with alcoholic steatosis and cirrhosis and in about 95% of patients with alcoholic hepatitis. ASAT/ALAT ratio increases in alcoholic hepatitis (in 40% of cases) and in alcoholic cirrhosis (59%).
γ-GTP and alkaline phosphatase (ALP)	γ-GTP is greatly elevated in almost all cases and every stage of alcoholic liver disease. ALP is increased in 80% of patients with alcoholic hepatitis and cirrhosis but in only 28% of patients with alcoholic fatty liver. The γ-GPT/ALP ratio ranges from one to three in non-alcoholic liver diseases but from five to 35 in alcoholic liver diseases, even in alcoholic steatosis.
Tissue antibodies (smooth muscle, antinuclear, mitochondrial):	The incidence of tissue antibodies has been reported to be both increased and normal in alcoholic liver diseases. However, the incidence as well as titres are generally low. On this basis the occurrence of tissue antibodies is highly suggestive to a non-alcoholic aetiology or pathogenetic mechanism of the liver injury.
IgA (immunoglob.):	Frequently increased in alcoholic liver injury. The magnitude of increase and IgA/IgG ratio can be used to differentiate alcoholic from non-alcoholic liver diseases
Plasma alpha-amino-n-butyric acid relative to leucine:	An increase is strongly suggestive of the recent heavy alcohol consumption. Severe non-alcoholic liver injury may give a false positive finding.
II. Differentiation between the various stages of alcoholic liver disease:	
Glutamate dehydrogenase (GLDH)	A mitochondrial enzyme, which correlates better with the degree of liver cell necrosis and inflammation than the other enzymes.
Albumin, pre-albumin, coagulation factors, elimination tests, NH_3:	A negative correlation between the progression and the severity of the liver injury. In fatty liver and alcoholic hepatitis abnormal values normalize after the acute phase of the disease. In cirrhosis abnormal findings are more constant.
IgA (immunoglob.):	The degree of increase correlates positively to the severity of histological damage.
Lipoproteins:	Pre-beta lipoproteins are increased in fatty liver. In severe liver damage (cirrhosis) the pre-beta band disappears almost completely, and often all lipoproteins migrate as a single wide band.
III. Others:	Anaemia, leucocytosis and hyperbilirubinaemia are common non-specific findings in alcoholic hepatitis and cirrhosis.

Data are based on references cited in the text.

should be avoided, since it constitutes a great hazard in acute alcoholic liver disease.[170]

The Role of Histology in the Differential Diagnosis of Alcoholic Liver Diseases

The aims of the histological interpretation of liver biopsy specimens in alcoholic liver disease are threefold: (a) to differentiate between non-alcoholic and alcoholic liver diseases; (b) to determine the stage of alcoholic liver disease (fatty liver, pericentral venous sclerosis, alcoholic cirrhosis); and (c) to evaluate the possible progression of the liver injury in serial biopsies.

The first of these goals is clearly emphasized by two recent studies. Goldberg et al[114] found 10 alcoholic patients whose biopsies demonstrated chronic active or chronic persistent hepatitis. Ethanol may be involved in the pathogenesis as a trigger (see above, 'Pathogenesis of alcoholic liver disease') or there may be a coincidental association of two diseases. In any event, the overlap of laboratory abnormalities was too extensive to allow differentiation. Levin et al[201] reported that in their population one out of five subjects with alcoholism and chronic abnormalities of liver function has a non-alcoholic liver disease. Furthermore, they concluded that liver biopsy is necessary to establish the diagnosis since non-alcoholic liver disease could not be detected by the clinical data.

The determination of the stage of the alcoholic liver disease is important both for prognosis and treatment. As stated earlier, in 'Patterns and Pathology of Alcoholic Liver Injuries',[397] the demonstration of pericentral sclerosis, even in the absence of more severe liver lesions, may predict the development of cirrhosis upon continued drinking, at least in baboons. If these results can be extrapolated to man, the presence of pericentral sclerosis could be regarded as a warning sign which might enable us to detect those individuals prone to develop cirrhosis. For differential diagnostic purposes it should, however, be noted that both fatty liver and pericentral fibrosis, even with subsequent development of liver cirrhosis, have also been described in association with obesity, diabetes and after ileojejunal bypass.[76,81,289,302,378]

Liver biopsy is certainly indicated when the laboratory abnormalities have persisted for three to six months. The frequency of subsequent biopsies can be decided individually, depending on the initial diagnosis. If the diagnosis of liver cirrhosis is certain, further biopsies are not indicated unless a complication such as hepatic carcinoma is suspected. In cases of fatty liver and alcoholic hepatitis liver biopsy should be repeated once a year if the drinking habits cannot be controlled or the history is unreliable. Changes in laboratory patterns are crucial for making a decision.

Peritoneoscopy

There is wide disagreement concerning the technique of liver biopsy and the reliability of the histological interpretation, especially in cirrhosis.[10] In patients with simple fatty liver and/or alcoholic hepatitis a blind biopsy with a Menghini needle is the method of choice. However, in cirrhosis blind biopsy is much more unreliable. Vido and Wildhirt[400] failed to establish with blind biopsy the diagnosis of cirrhosis in about half of 272 patients. Similar failure was reported in several other studies.[104,225,346,401] On this basis the prevailing view in Europe is that laparoscopy with guided biopsy is a better method in the diagnosis of liver cirrhosis. False negative results of needle biopsy result from the tendency of the needle to slide off hard fibrous tissue and selectively to sample the softer parenchyma. False positive diagnoses can result from the biopsy of an area of focal fibrosis. Furthermore, needle biopsies from cirrhotic liver very often tend to be small and broken up. The diagnosis of liver cirrhosis can be made macroscopically at laparoscopy and it enables photographic follow-up of the course of the alcoholic liver disease.

On this basis *the indications for peritoneoscopy* in alcoholic liver disease are as follows: (a) to establish the diagnosis of liver cirrhosis when blind biopsy has failed or when the liver specimen is too small for definitive diagnosis; (b) to establish the diagnosis of fatty liver or alcoholic cirrhosis with guided biopsy when a blind biopsy has failed; (c) to make a macroscopic and also, if needed, microscopic diagnosis in cases in which a blind biopsy is contraindicated, for example in clotting disorders or in jaundice. Peritoneoscopy can be performed even when the prothrombin is 10 to 20 per cent of normal because electrocoagulation can be performed, if required; (d) to exclude malignancy if it is suspected.

TREATMENT AND PROGNOSIS OF ALCOHOLIC LIVER DISEASE

Several studies have demonstrated that the prognosis for acute and chronic alcoholic liver disease is dramatically improved by abstinence from alcohol, while continued consumption is associated with increased morbidity and mortality.

Fatty Liver

Alcoholic steatosis is completely reversible in most cases. In some extremely severe cases alcoholic fatty liver may have a fatal outcome, but as a rule even those cases needing hospitalization improve within a few days or weeks after cessation of alcohol consumption. In contrast to alcoholic hepatitis, laboratory abnormalities rapidly return to normal levels and hepatomegaly decreases.[54,71,188] Fat mobilization may be delayed only if steatosis has been extreme, with fatty cysts, or if it is complicated by obesity or prediabetes.

In addition to alcohol withdrawal and the provision of a diet with sufficient calories, vitamins and protein no other treatment is needed. The addition of lipotropes such as choline to the diet has no beneficial value in treating alcoholic fatty liver.[306] Anabolic steroids have been found to be efficacious in the treatment of alcoholic fatty liver by Jabbari and Leevy[151] and Mendenhall[254] but not by Fenster.[91] On the other hand, anabolic steroids are relatively contraindicated because of their known hepatotoxicity.

Alcoholic Hepatitis

The survival of patients with alcoholic hepatitis is dramatically improved by the discontinuation or reduction of alcohol consumption. Galambos[107] reported that the seven year survival is 50 per cent with continued drinking and 80 per cent with reduced drinking. This finding has been confirmed by others.[43] The reported mortality rates for acute alcoholic hepatitis depend on the material selected. Early reports were drawn from autopsy material. Accordingly, an early mortality of two-thirds to three-quarters was reported by Phillips and Davidson,[291] and about 30 per cent by Hardison and Lee.[129] More recently a mortality of from 1.5 to 8 per cent in individuals with alcoholic hepatitis ill enough to require hospitalization but well enough to permit liver biopsy has been found.[55, 120, 130, 229]

Clinical and pathological signs of alcoholic hepatitis regress within weeks or months in most cases. A poorer short-term prognosis can be expected in patients with a prolonged prothrombin time and ascites.[107] The long-term prognosis is unfavourably influenced by the presence of severe histological inflammation and fibrosis in the initial liver biopsy specimen.[107] Elevations of serum enzymes are less valuable prognostic indicators.

The general treatment of the patient with alcoholic hepatitis is the same as for alcoholic steatosis. The role of adrenocorticosteroid therapy of acute alcoholic hepatitis has been the subject of debate for years. Helman et al,[137] in a controlled prospective study, reported significant improvement in survival of steroid-treated patients with encephalopathy, but not in those with milder illness. Several subsequent controlled studies, however, have not confirmed these findings.[47,305,347] Indeed, in one of the controlled studies an increased risk of fungal infection associated with corticosteroid therapy was reported.[31] Therefore, we do not recommend corticosteroid treatment in most cases of acute alcoholic hepatitis. Further studies are still needed to establish the role of steroids in those cases of alcoholic hepatitis (mostly females) which simulate chronic active hepatitis either histologically or immunologically. Propylthiouracil has recently been suggested for the treatment of alcoholic hepatitis.[280] These preliminary findings await further confirmation.

Alcoholic Cirrhosis

In patients with histologically proven cirrhosis the five-year survival rate for patients without jaundice, ascites or haematemesis is 88.9 per cent for abstainers and 62.8 per cent for drinkers.[308] The five-year survival rates are unfavourably affected by jaundice, ascites and haematemesis in abstainers (57.5, 52.4 and 35 per cent, respectively) and in drinkers 33.3, 32.7 and 21 per cent, respectively. The prognosis is still poor during the first year after the discontinuation of drinking. The survival rate of patients who live beyond the first year and who continue to abstain from alcohol is 86.2 per cent for the subsequent four years, which is close to the expected survival for individuals of a similar age.

Corticosteroids did not prolong survival of patients with alcoholic cirrhosis in a controlled study performed by the Copenhagen Study Group for Liver diseases.[347, 391] Colchicine may provide a new approach for the treatment of alcoholic liver injury[317] but results of controlled trials are still awaited.

Prophylactic portasystemic shunting in unselected cirrhotic patients does not improve the overall survival although the terminal event may alter from haemorrhage to hepatic failure.[57, 60, 152, 315]

Prevention of Alcoholic Liver Disease

The main goal in management of alcoholic liver disease is the withdrawal of alcohol. This is the only effective way both to prevent the progression and to improve the prognosis. On this basis a clinician who treats alcoholic liver injuries should not limit his efforts to the hepatic symptomatology but should refer his patient to those community organizations willing to take care of alcohol problems. Furthermore, it should be borne in mind that changes in the overall consumption of alcoholic beverages bear a close relationship to liver cirrhosis mortality and that alcohol control measures can be used to limit consumption: thus control of alcohol availability is becoming a public health issue.[45]

REFERENCES

1. Addison, T. (1836) Observations on fatty degeneration of the liver. *Guy's Hospital Reports*, **1**, 476–485.
2. Adlercreutz, H. (1974) Hepatic metabolism of estrogens in health and disease. *New England Journal of Medicine*, **290**, 1081–1083.
3. Agostini, A., Vergani, C., Stabilini, R. & Marasini, B. (1969) Determination of seven serum proteins in alcoholic cirrhosis. *Clinica Chimica Acta*, **26**, 351–355.
4. Alexander, J.F., Lischner, M.W. & Galambos, J.T. (1971) Natural history of alcoholic hepatitis. II. The long term prognosis. *American Journal of Gastroenterology*, **56**, 515–525.

5. Ammon, H.P.T. & Estler, C.J. (1968) Inhibition of ethanol-induced glycogenolysis in brain and liver by adrenergic β-blockade. *Journal of Pharmacy and Pharmacology,* **20,** 164–165.
6. Annable, W. & Cooper, C. (1974) Inhibition of release of hepatic triglyceride by ethanol. *Biochemical Pharmacology,* **23,** 2063–2068.
7. Arky, R.A. & Freinkel, N. (1966) Alcohol hypoglycemia. V. Alcohol infusion to test gluconeogenesis in starvation with special reference to obesity. *New England Journal of Medicine,* **274,** 426–433.
8. Arky, R.A., Abramson, E.A. & Freinkel, N. (1968) Alcohol hypoglycemia. VII. Further studies on the refractoriness of obese subjects. *Metabolism: Clinical and Experimental,***17,** 977–987.
9. Atwater, W.O. & Benedict, F.C. (1902) An experimental inquiry regarding the nutritive value of alcohol. *Memorial National Academy of Science,* **8,** 335–397.
10. Baggenstoss, A.H. (1975) Morphological features: their usefulness in the diagnosis, prognosis, and management of cirrhosis. *Clinics in Gastroenterology,* **4,** 227–245.
11. Baglio, C.M. & Farber, E. (1965) Reversal by adenine of the ethionine-induced lipid accumulation in the endoplasmic reticulum of the rat liver. *Journal of Cell Biology,* **27,** 591–601.
12. Bailey, R.J., Krasner, N., Eddleston, A.L.W.F., Williams, R., Tee, D.E.H., Doniach, D., Kennedy, L.A. & Batchelor, J.R. (1976) Histocompatibility antigens, auto-antibodies and immunoglobulins in alcoholic liver disease. *British Medical Journal,* **ii,** 727–731.
13. Ballard, H., Bernstein, M. & Farrar, J.T. (1961) Fatty liver presenting as obstructive jaundice. *American Journal of Medicine,* **30,** 196–201.
14. Baraona, E. & Lieber, C.S. (1969) Fatty liver, hyperlipemia and erythrocyte alterations produced by ethanol feeding in the rat. *American Journal of Clinical Nutrition,* **22,** 356–357.
15. Baraona, E. & Lieber, C.S. (1970) Effects of chronic ethanol feeding on serum lipoprotein metabolism in the rat. *Journal of Clinical Investigation,* **49,** 769–778.
16. Baraona, E. & Lieber, C.S. (1975) Intestinal lymph formation and fat absorption: stimulation by acute ethanol administration and inhibition by chronic ethanol feeding. *Gastroenterology,* **68,** 495–502.
17. Baraona, E. & Lieber, C.S. (1976) Alcoholic hyperlipemia. In *Handbuch der Inneren Medizin Band VHC/4 Fettstoffwechsel* (Ed.) Schettler, G., Greten, H., Schlierf, G. & Seidel, D. pp. 389–407. Berlin and Heidelberg: Springer-Verlag.
18. Baraona, E. & Lindenbaum, J. (1977) Metabolic effects of alcohol on the intestine. In *Metabolic Aspects of Alcoholism* (Ed.) Lieber, C.S. pp. 81–116. Baltimore: University Park Press.
19. Baraona, E., Pirola, R.C. & Lieber, C.S. (1973) The pathogenesis of postprandial hyperlipemia in rats fed ethanol containing diets. *Journal of Clinical Investigation,* **52,** 296–303.
20. Baraona, E., Leo, M.A., Borowsky, S.A. & Lieber, C.S. (1975) Alcoholic hepatomegaly: accumulation of protein in the liver. *Science,* **190,** 794–795.
21. Baraona, E., Leo, M.A., Borowsky, S.A. & Lieber, C.S. (1977) Pathogenesis of alcohol-induced accumulation of protein in the liver. *Journal of Clinical Investigation,* **60,** 546–554.
22. Beckett, A.G., Livingston, A.V. & Hill, K.R. (1961) Acute alcoholic hepatitis. *British Medical Journal,* **ii,** 1113–1119.
23. Beckett, A.G., Livingston, A.V. & Hill, K.R. (1962) Acute alcoholic hepatitis without jaundice. *British Medical Journal,* **ii,** 580–582.
24. Bell, E.T. (1955) Relation of portal cirrhosis to hemochromatosis and to diabetes mellitus. *Diabetes,* **4,** 435–446.
25. Berenyi, M.R., Straus, B. & Avila, L. (1975) T rosettes in alcoholic cirrhosis of the liver. *Journal of the American Medical Association,* **232,** 44–46.
26. Berenyi, M.R., Straus, B. & Cruz, D. (1974) In vitro and vivo studies of cellular immunity in alcoholic cirrhosis. *American Journal of Digestive Diseases,* **19,** 199–205.
27. Bernstein, I.M., Webster, K.H., Williams, R.C. & Strickland, R.G. (1974) Reduction in circulating T lymphocytes in alcoholic liver disease. *Lancet,* **ii,** 488–490.
28.. Best, C.H., Hartroft, W.S., Lucas, S.S. & Ridout, J.H. (1949) Liver damage produced by feeding alcohol or sugar and its prevention by choline. *British Medical Journal,* **ii,** 1001–1006.
29. Biava, C. (1964) Mallory alcoholic hyalin: a heretofore unique lesion of hepatocellular ergastoplasm. *Laboratory Investigation,* **13,** 301–320.
30. Birschbach, H.R., Harinasuta, U. & Zimmerman, H.J. (1974) Alcoholic steatonecrosis. II. Prospective study of prevalence of Mallory bodies in biopsy specimens and comparison of severity of hepatic disease in patients with and without this histological feature. *Gastroenterology,* **66,** 1195–1202.
31. Blitzer, B.L., Mutchnick, M.G., Joshi, P.H., Phillips, M.M., Fessell, M. & Conn, H.O. (1977) Adrenocorticosteroid therapy in alcoholic hepatitis. A prospective double-blind randomized study. *American Journal of Digestive Diseases,* **22,** 477-484.
32. Blomhoff, J.P., Skrede, S. & Ritland, S. (1974) Lecithin: cholesterol acyltransferase and plasma proteins in liver diseases. *Clinica Chimica Acta,* **53,** 197–207.
33. Blomstrand, R. & Kager, L. (1973) The combustion of triolein-l-^{14}C and its inhibition by alcohol in man. *Life Sciences,* **13,** 113–123.
34. Bloom, R.J. & Westerfield, W.W. (1971) The thiobarbituric acid reaction in relation to fatty livers. *Archives of Biochemistry and Biophysics,* **145,** 669–675.
35. Bode, C.H., Buchwald, B. & Goebell, H. (1971) Inhibition of ethanol breakdown due to protein deficiency in man. *German Medical Monthly,* **1,** 149–150.
36. Borowsky, S., Perlow, W., Baraona, E. & Lieber, C.S. (1980) Relationship of alcoholic hypertriglyceridemia to stage of liver disease and dietary lipid. *Dig. Dis. and Sci.,* **25,** 22–27.
37. Borsanyi, S.U. & Blanchard, C.L. (1961) Asymptomatic enlargement of the parotid glands in alcoholic cirrhosis. *Southern Medical Journal (Birmingham),* **54,** 678–682.
38. Bosron, W.F., Li, T.-K., Lange, L.G., Dafeldecker, W.P. & Vallee, B.L. (1977) Isolation and characterization of an anodic form of human liver alcohol dehydrogenase. *Biochemical and Biophysical Research Communications,* **74,** 85–90.
39. Bouchier, I.A. & Dawson, A.M. (1964) The effect of infusions of ethanol on the plasma free fatty acids in man. *Clinical Science,* **26,** 47–54.
40. Bradley, S.E., Ingelfinger, F.J. & Bradley, G.P. (1952) Hepatic circulation in cirrhosis of the liver. *Circulation,* **5,** 419–429.

41. Bradus, S., Korn, R.J., Chomet, B. & West, M. (1963) Hepatic function and serum enzyme levels in association with fatty metamorphosis of the liver. *American Journal of the Medical Sciences,* **246,** 35–41.

42. Brodie, B.B., Butler, W.M., Horning, M.G., Maickel, R.P. & Maling, H.M. (1961) Alcohol-induced triglyceride deposition in liver through derangement of fat transport. *American Journal of Clinical Nutrition,* **9,** 432–435.

43. Brunt, P.W., Kew, M.C., Scheuer, P.J. & Sherlock, S. (1974) Studies in alcoholic liver disease in Britain. 1. Clinical and pathological patterns related to natural history. *Gut,* **15,** 52–58.

44. Bruun, K., Koura, E., Popham, R.E. & Seeley, J.R. (1960) *Liver Cirrhosis Mortality as a Means to Measure the Prevalence of Alcoholism.* Helsinki: The Finnish Foundation for Alcohol Studies.

45. Bruun, K., Edwards, G., Lumio, M., Mäkelä, K., Österberg, E., Pan, L., Popham, R.E., Room, R., Schmidt, W., Skog, O.-J., Sulkunen, P. & Österberg, E. (1975) *Alcohol Control Policies in Public Health Perspective, Report of an International Working Group.* Helsinki: The Finnish Foundation for Alcohol Studies.

46. Bungenberg de Jong, J.J. & Marsh, J.B. (1968) Biosynthesis of plasma lipoproteins by rat liver ribosomes. *Journal of Biological Chemistry,* **243,** 192–199.

47. Campra, J.L., Hamlin, E.M., Kirshbaum, R.J., Olivier, M., Redecker, A.J. & Reynolds, T.B. (1973) Prednisone therapy of acute alcoholic hepatitis. Report of a controlled trial. *Annals of Internal Medicine,* **79,** 625–631.

48. Carulli, N., Manenti, F., Gallo, M. & Salvioli, G.F. (1971) Alcohol–drugs interaction in man: alcohol and tolbutamide. *Journal of Clinical Investigation,* **1,** 421–424.

49. Castelli, W.P., Doyle, J.T., Gordon, T., Hamnes, C., Hjortland, M.C., Hulley, S.B., Kagan, A. & Zukel, W.J. (1977) Alcohol and blood lipids. The cooperative phenotyping study. *Lancet,* **ii,** 153–155.

50. Cederbaum, A.I., Lieber, C.S., Beattie, D.S. & Rubin, E. (1975) Effect of chronic ethanol ingestion on fatty acid oxidation by hepatic mitochondria. *Journal of Biological Chemistry,* **250,** 5122–5129.

51. Cederbaum, A.I., Dicker, E., Lieber, C.S. & Rubin, E. (1977) Factors contributing to the adaptive increase in ethanol metabolism due to chronic consumption of ethanol. *Alcoholism: Clinical and Experimental Research,* **1,** 27–31.

52. Christoffersen, P. & Juhl, E. (1971) Mallory bodies in liver biopsies with fatty changes but no cirrhosis. *Acta Pathologica et Microbiologica Scandinavica,* **79,** 201–207.

53. Christoffersen, P. & Nielsen, K. (1971) The frequency of Mallory bodies in liver biopsies from chronic alcoholics. *Acta Pathologica et Microbiologica Scandinavica,* **79,** 274–278.

54. Christoffersen, P. & Nielsen, K. (1972) Histological changes in human liver biopsies from chronic alcoholics. *Acta Pathologica et Microbiologica Scandinavica,* **80,** 557–565.

55. Christoffersen, P., Iversen, K. & Nielsen, K. (1970) A comparative study of two groups of patients with Mallory bodies with and without liver cell necrosis and neutrophilic infiltration. *Scandinavian Journal of Gastroenterology,* **5,** 633–638.

56. Cochran, A.G., Moussouros, A., Portmann, B., McFarlane, I.G., Thomson, A.D., Eddleston, A.L.W.F. & Williams, R. (1977) Lymphocyte cytotoxicity for isolated hepatocytes in alcoholic liver disease. *Gastroenterology,* **72,** 918–923.

57. Conn, H.O. & Lindenmuth, W.W. (1968) Prophylactic portacaval anastomosis in cirrhotic patients with esophageal varices. *New England Journal of Medicine,* **279,** 725–732.

58. Conn, H.O., Schreiber, W. & Elkington, S.G. (1969) Cirrhosis and diabetes. I. Increased incidence of diabetes in patients with Laennec's cirrhosis. *American Journal of Digestive Diseases,* **14,** 837–852.

59. Conn, H.O., Schreiber, W. & Elkington, S.G. (1971) Cirrhosis and diabetes. II. Association of impaired glucose tolerance with portal–systemic shunting in Laennec's cirrhosis. *American Journal of Digestive Diseases,* **16,** 227–239.

60. Conn, H.O., Lindenmuth, W.W., May, C. & Ramsby, G.R. (1972) Prophylactic portacaval anastomosis: a tale of two studies. *Medicine,* **51,** 27–40.

61. Connor, C.L. & Chaikoff, L. (1938) Production of cirrhosis in fatty livers with alcohol. *Proceedings of the Society for Experimental Biology and Medicine,* **32,** 356–359.

62. Cook, G.C. & Hutt, M.S.R. (1967) The liver after kwashiorkor. *British Medical Journal,* **iii,** 454–457.

63. Cooperman, M.T., Davidoff, E., Spark, R. & Pallota, J. (1974) Clinical studies of alcoholic ketoacidosis. *Diabetes,* **23,** 433–439.

64. Copenhagen Study Group for Liver Diseases (1974) Sex, ascites, and alcoholism in survival of patients with cirrhosis: effect of prednisone. *New England Journal of Medicine,* **291,** 271–273.

65. Crouse, J.R., Gerson, C.D., DeCarli, L.M. & Lieber, C.S. (1968) Role of acetate in the reduction of plasma free fatty acids produced by ethanol in man. *Journal of Lipid Research,* **2,** 509–512.

66. Crow, K.E., Cornell, N.W. & Veech, R.L. (1977) The rate of ethanol metabolism in isolated rat hepatocytes. *Alcoholism: Clinical Experimental Research,* **1,** 43–47.

67. Daft, F.S., Sebrell, W.H. & Lillie, R.D. (1941) Production and apparent prevention of a dietary liver cirrhosis in rats. *Proceedings of the Society for Experimental Biology and Medicine,* **48,** 228–229.

68. Dajani, R.M. & Kouyoumjian, C. (1967) A probable direct role of ethanol in the pathogenesis of fat infiltration in the rat. *Journal of Nutrition,* **91,** 535–539.

69. Denk, H. & Echerstorfer, R. (1977) Colchicine-induced Mallory body formation in the mouse. *Laboratory Investigation,* **36,** 563–565.

70. Denk, H., Gschnait, F. & Wolff, K. (1975) Hepatocellular hyalin (Mallory bodies) in long term griseofulvin-treated mice. A new experimental model for the study of hyalin formation. *Laboratory Investigation,* **32,** 773–776.

71. Devenyi, P., Rutherdale, J., Sereny, G. & Olin, J.S. (1970) Clinical diagnosis of alcoholic fatty liver. *American Journal of Gastroenterology,* **54,** 597–602.

72. Di Luzio, N.R. (1966) A mechanism of acute ethanol-induced fatty liver and the modification of liver injury by antioxidants. *Laboratory Investigation,* **15,** 50–63.

73. Di Luzio, N.R. & Stege, T.E. (1977) The role of ethanol metabolites in hepatic lipid peroxidation. In *Alcohol and the Liver* (Ed.) Fisher, M.M. & Rankin, J.G. pp. 42–62. New York: Plenum Press.

74. Dillon, E.S., Dyer, W.W. & Smelo, L.S. (1940) Ketone acidosis in nondiabetic adults. *Medical Clinics of North America*, **24**, 1813–1822.

75. Domschke, S., Domschke, W. & Lieber, C.S. (1974) Hepatic redox state: attenuation of the acute effects of ethanol induced by chronic ethanol consumption. *Life Sciences*, **15**, 1327–1334.

76. Drenick, E.J., Simmons, M.D. & Murphy, J.F. (1970) Effect on hepatic morphology of treatment of obesity by fasting, reducing diets and small-bowel bypass. *New England Journal of Medicine*, **289**, 829–834.

77. Edmondson, H.A., Peters, R.L., Reynolds, T.B. & Kuzma, O.T. (1963) Sclerosing hyaline necrosis of the liver. A recognizable clinical syndrome. *Annals of Internal Medicine*, **59**, 646–673.

78. Edmondson, H.A., Peters, R.L., Frankel, H.H. & Borowsky, S. (1967) The early stage of liver injury in the alcoholic. *Medicine*, **46**, 119–129.

79. Edwards, J.A. & Price Evans, D.A. (1967) Ethanol metabolism in subjects possessing typical and atypical liver alcohol dehydrogenase. *Clinical Pharmacology and Therapeutics*, **8**, 824–829.

80. Eichner, E.R. (1973) The hematologic disorders of alcoholism. *American Journal of Medicine*, **54**, 621–630.

81. Falchuk, K.R., Fiske, S., Trey, C., Haggitt, R. & Federman, M. (1977) Pericentral hepatic fibrosis in diabetes mellitus. *Gastroenterology*, **72**, 1174 (abstract 151).

82. Fallat, R.W., Vester, J.W. & Glueck, C.J. (1973) Suppression of amylase activity by hypertriglyceridemia. *Journal of the American Medical Association*. **225**, 1331–1334.

83. Farber, E. (1967) Ethionine fatty liver. *Advances in Lipid Research*, **5**, 119–183.

84. Farber, E. (1971) Response of cells to inhibition of synthesis of DNA, RNA and protein. *Biochemical Pharmacology*, **20**, 1023–1026.

85. Fausa, O. & Gjone, E. (1976) Serum bile acid concentrations in patients with liver disease. *Scandinavian Journal of Gastroenterology*, **11**, 537–543.

86. Feinman, L. & Lieber, C.S. (1967) Effect of ethanol on plasma glycerol in man. *American Journal of Clinical Nutrition*, **20**, 400–403.

87. Feinman, L. & Lieber, C.S. (1972) Hepatic collagen metabolism: effect of alcohol consumption in rats and baboons. *Science*, **176**, 795.

88. Feinman, L., Baraona, E., Matsuzaki, S., Korsten, M. & Lieber, C.S. (1978) Concentration dependence of ethanol metabolism in vivo in rats and man. *Alcoholism: Clinical and Experimental Research*, **2**, 381–385.

89. Feizi, T. (1968) Immunoglobulins in chronic liver disease. *Gut*, **9**, 193–198.

90. Feldman, G., Maurice, M., Sapin, C. & Benhamou, J.-P. (1975) Inhibition by colchicine of fibrinogen translocation in hepatocytes. *Journal of Cell Biology*, **67**, 237–243.

91. Fenster, L.F. (1966) The nonefficacy of short-term anabolic steroid therapy in alcoholic liver disease. *Annals of Internal Medicine*, **65**, 738–744.

92. Field, J.B., Williams, H.E. & Mortimore, G.E. (1963) Studies on the mechanism of ethanol induced hypoglycemia. *Journal of Clinical Investigation*, **42**, 497–506.

93. Figueroa, R.B. & Klotz, A.P. (1962) Alterations of alcohol dehydrogenase and other hepatic enzymes in alcoholic cirrhosis. *Metabolism*, **11**, 1169–1180.

94. Fisher, M.M. & Rankin, J.G. (Ed.) (1977) *Alcohol and the Liver*, Vol. 3, New York: Plenum Press.

95. Flax, M.H. & Tisdale, W.A. (1964) An electron microscopic study of alcoholic hyalin. *American Journal of Pathology*, **44**, 441–453.

96. Forsander, O.A. (1970) Influence of ethanol on the redox state of the liver. *Quarterly Journal of Studies on Alcohol*, **31**, 550–570.

97. Forsander, O.A., Räihä, N. & Soumalainen, H. (1958) Alkoholoxydation und Bildung von Acetoacetat in normaler und glycogen-armer intakter Rattenleber. *Hoppe-Seylers Zeitschrift für Physiologische Chemie*, **312**, 243–248.

98. Forsander, O., Vartia, K.O. & Krusius, F.E. (1958) Experimentelle Studien über die biologische Wirkung von Alcohol. 1. Alcohol und Blutzucker. *Annales Medicinae Experimentalis et Biologiae Fenniae*, **36**, 416–434.

99. Forsander, O.A., Räihä, N., Salaspuro, M. & Mäenpää, P. (1965) Influence of ethanol on the liver metabolism of fed and starved rats. *Biochemical Journal*, **94**, 259–265.

100. Frank, H., Heil, W. & Leodolter, I. (1967) Leber und Bierkonsum vergleichende Untersuchungen an 450 Arbeitern. *Müchener Medizinische Wochenschrift*, **109**, 892–897.

101. Frienkel, N., Arky, R.A., Singer, D.L., Cohen, A.K., Bleicher, S.J., Anderson, J.B., Silbert, L.K. & Foster, A.E. (1965) Alcohol hypoglycemia: IV. Current concepts of its pathogenesis. *Diabetes*, **14**, 350–361.

102. French, S.W. & Davies, P.L. (1975) The Mallory body in the pathogenesis of alcoholic liver disease. In *Alcoholic Liver Pathology* (Ed.) Khanna, J.M., Israel, Y. & Kalant, H. pp. 113–144. Toronto: Addiction Research Foundation.

103. French, S.W., Sim, J.S., Franks, K.E., Barbige, E.J., Deuton, T. & Caldwell, M.G. (1977) Alcoholic hepatitis. In *Alcohol and the Liver* (Ed.) Fisher, M.M. & Rankin, J.G. pp. 261–286. New York: Plenum Press.

104. Fritsch, W.-P., Herms, W., Hurth, F., Wetzels, E. & Hausamen, T.-U. (1972) Die Wertigkeit von Laparoskopie und Leberpunktion für die Diagnostik der chronischer Hepatopathien. *Deutsche Medizinische Wochenschrift*, **97**, 1635–1637.

105. Fritz, J.B. (1961) Factors influencing the rates of long-chain fatty acid oxidation and synthesis in mammalian systems. *Physiological Reviews*, **41**, 52–129.

106. Galambos, J.T. (1972) Natural history of alcoholic hepatitis. III. Histological changes. *Gastroenterology*, **63**, 1026–1035.

107. Galambos, J.T. (1974) Alcoholic hepatitis. In *The liver and its diseases* (Ed.) Schaffner, F., Sherlock, S. & Leevy, C.M. pp. 255–267. New York: Intercontinental Medical Book.

108. Gall, E.A. (1960) Primary and metastic carcinoma of liver – relationship to hepatic cirrhosis. *Archives of Pathology*, **70**, 226–232.

109. Gang, H., Lieber, C.S. & Rubin, E. (1973) Ethanol increases glycosyl transferase activity in the hepatic Golgi apparatus. *Nature (New Biology)*, **243**, 123–125.

110. Garagliano, C.F., Mendeloff, A.I. & Lilienfeld, A.M. (1977) Incidence of liver cirrhosis in 16 areas of the U.S. *Gastroenterology*, **72**, 1060 (abstract 37).

111. Gerber, M.A., Orr, W., Denk, H., Schaffner, F. & Popper, H. (1973) Hepatocellular hyalin in cholestasis and cirrhosis: its diagnostic significance. *Gastroenterology*, **64,** 89–98.

112. Ginsberg, H.H., Olefsky, J., Fahrquhar, J.W. & Reaven, G.M. (1974) Moderate ethanol ingestion and plasma triglyceride levels. A study in normal and hypertriglyceridemic persons. *Annals of Internal Medicine*, **80,** 143–149.

113. Goldberg, M. & Thompson, C.M. (1961) Acute fatty metamorphosis of the liver. *Annals of Internal Medicine*, **55,** 416–432.

114. Goldberg, S.I., Mendenhall, C.L., Connell, A.M. & Chedid, A. (1977) 'Nonalcoholic' chronic hepatitis in the alcoholic. *Gastroenterology*, **72,** 598–604.

115. Gordon, E.R. (1972) Effect of an intoxicating dose of ethanol on lipid metabolism in an isolated, perfused rat liver. *Biochemical Pharmacology*, **21,** 2991–3004.

116. Gordon, E.R. (1977) ATP metabolism in an ethanol-induced fatty liver. *Alcoholism: Clinical Experimental Research*, **1,** 21–25.

117. Gordon, G.G., Altman, K., Southern, A.L., Rubin, E. & Lieber, C.S. (1976) Effect of alcohol (ethanol) administration on sex-hormone metabolism in normal man. *New England Journal of Medicine*, **225,** 793–797.

118. Gorman, R.E. & Bitensky, M.W. (1970) Selective activation by short chain alcohols of glucagon responsive adenyl cyclase in liver. *Endocrinology*, **87,** 1075–1081.

119. Grace, N.D. & Powell, L.W. (1974) Iron storage disorders of the liver. *Gastroenterology*, **64,** 1257–1283.

120. Green, J., Mistilis, S. & Schiff, L. (1963) Acute alcoholic hepatitis. *Archives of Internal Medicine*, **112,** 67–78.

121. Greenberger, N.J., Cohen, R.B. & Isselbacher, K.J. (1965) The effect of chronic alcohol administration on liver alcohol dehydrogenase activity in the rat. *Laboratory Investigation*, **14,** 264–271.

122. Greenberger, N.J., Hatch, F.T., Drummey, G.D. & Isselbacher, K.J. (1966) Pancreatitis and hyperlipemia: a study of serum lipid alterations in 25 patients with acute pancreatitis. *Medicine (Baltimore)*, **45,** 161–174.

123. Greene, H.L., Herman, R.H. & Kramer, S. (1971) Stimulation of jejunal cyclase by ethanol. *Journal of Laboratory and Clinical Medicine*, **78,** 336–342.

124. Gregory, D.H. & Levi, D.F. (1972) The clinical–pathologic spectrum of alcoholic hepatitis. *American Journal of Digestive Diseases*, **17,** 479–488.

125. Grunnet, N., Quistorff, B. & Thieden, H.I.D. (1973) Rate-limiting factors in ethanol oxidation by isolated rat-liver parenchymal cells. Effect of ethanol concentration, fructose, pyruvate and pyrazol. *European Journal of Biochemistry*, **40,** 275–282.

126. Hall, E.M. & Ophuls, W. (1925) Progressive alcoholic cirrhosis. Report of four cases. *American Journal of Pathology*, **1,** 477–493.

127. Hällen, J. & Krook, H. (1963) Follow-up studies on an unselected ten-year material of 360 patients with liver cirrhosis in one community. *Acta Medica Scandinavica*, **173,** 479–493.

128. Hamlyn, A.N., Brown, A.J., Sherlock, S. & Baron, D.N. (1975) Casual blood ethanol estimations in patients with chronic liver disease. *Lancet*, **ii,** 345–347.

129. Hardison, W.G. & Lee, F.I. (1966) Prognosis in acute liver disease of the alcoholic patient. *New England Journal of Medicine*, **275,** 61–66.

130. Harinasuta, U. & Zimmerman, H.J. (1971) Alcoholic steatonecrosis. I. Relationship between severity of hepatic disease and presence of Mallory bodies in the liver. *Gastroenterology*, **60,** 1036–1046.

131. Harinasuta, U., Chomet, B., Ishak, K. & Zimmerman, H.J. (1967) Steatonecrosis – Mallory body type. *Medicine*, **46,** 141–162.

132. Hashimoto, S. & Recknagel, R.O. (1968) No chemical evidence of hepatic lipid peroxidation in acute ethanol toxicity. *Experimental and Molecular Pathology*, **8,** 225–242.

133. Hasumura, Y., Teschke, R. & Lieber, C.S. (1974) Increased carbon tetrachloride hepatotoxicity, and its mechanism after chronic ethanol consumption. *Gastroenterology*, **66,** 415–422.

134. Hasumura, Y., Teschke, R. & Lieber, C.S. (1975) Acetaldehyde oxidation by hepatic mitochondria: its decrease after chronic ethanol consumption. *Science*, **189,** 727–729.

135. Hasumura, Y., Teschke, R. & Lieber, C.S. (1976) Characteristics of acetaldehyde oxidation in rat liver mitochondria. *Journal of Biological Chemistry*, **251,** 4908–4913.

136. Hed, R. & Nygren, A. (1968) Alcohol induced hypoglycemia in chronic alcoholics with liver disease. *Acta Medica Scandinavica*, **183,** 507–510.

137. Helman, R.A., Temko, M.H., Nye, S.W. & Fallon, H.J. (1971) Alcoholic hepatitis: natural history and evaluation of prednisolone therapy. *Annals of Internal Medicine*, **74,** 311–321.

138. Himwich, H.E., Nahum, L.H., Rakieten, N., Fazekas, J.F. & Du Bois, H. (1932) Effects of alcohol on metabolism. *American Journal of Physiology*, **101,** 57.

139. Hoffbauer, F.W. & Zaki, G. (1965) Choline deficiency in baboon and rat compared. *Archives of Pathology*, **79,** 364–369.

140. Holzer, H., Schultz, G. & Lynen, F. (1956) Bestimmung des Quatienten DPNH/DPN in lebenden Hefezellen durch Analyse stationäres Alkohol- und Acetaldehyd-Konzentrationen. *Biochemische Zeitschrift*, **328,** 259–263.

141. Hsu, C.C.S. & Leevy, C.M. (1971) Inhibition of PHA stimulated lymphocyte transformation by plasma from patients with advanced alcoholic cirrhosis. *Clinical and Experimental Immunology*, **8,** 749–760.

142. International Statistics on Alcoholic Beverages; Production Trade and Consumption 1950–1979 (1977) *The Finnish Foundation for Alcohol Studies and the World Health Organization Regional Office for Europe*. Forssa, Finland: Aurasen Kirjapaino. Distributed by the Finnish Foundation for Alcohol Studies (Alkoholitutkimussäätiö: Kalevankatu 12, 00100 Helsinki 10, Finland).

143. Isaacson, C., Seftel, H.C., Kelley, K.J. & Well, T.H. (1961) Siderosis in the Bantu: the relationship between iron overload and cirrhosis. *Journal of Laboratory and Clinical Medicine*, **58,** 845–853.

144. Iseri, O.A. & Gottlieb, L.S. (1971) Alcoholic hyaline and megamitochondria as separate and distinct entities in liver disease associated with alcoholism. *Gastroenterology*, **60,** 1027–1035.

145. Iseri, O.A., Lieber, C.S. & Gottlieb, L.S. (1966) The ultrastructure of fatty liver induced by prolonged ethanol ingestion. *American Journal of Pathology*, **48,** 535–555.

146. Ishii, H., Joly, J.G. & Lieber, C.S. (1973) Effect of ethanol on the amount and enzyme activities of hepatic rough and smooth microsomal membranes. *Biochimica et Biophysica Acta,* **291,** 411–420.
147. Israel, Y., Videla, L. & Bernstein, J. (1975) Hypermetabolic state after chronic ethanol consumption. Hormonal interrelations and pathogenic implications. *Federation Proceedings,* **34,** 2052–2059.
148. Israel, Y., Khanna, J.M., Kalant, H., Stewart, D.J., MacDonald, J.A., Rachamim, G., Wahid, S. & Orrego, H. (1977) The spontaneously hypertensive rat as a model for studies on metabolic tolerance to ethanol. *Alcoholism: Clinical and Experimental Research,* **1,** 39–42.
149. Israel, Y., Orrego, H., Khanna, J.M., Stewart, D.J., Phillips, M.J. & Kalant, H. (1977) Alcohol induced susceptibility to hypoxic liver damage: possible role in the pathogenesis of alcoholic liver disease. In *Alcohol and the Liver* (Ed.) Fisher, M.M. & Rankin, J.G. pp. 323–346. New York: Plenum Press,
150. Iturriaga, H., Pereda, T., Estévez, A. & Ugarte, G. (1977) Serum immunoglobulin changes in alcoholic patients. *Annals of Clinical Research,* **9,** 39–43.
151. Jabbari, M. & Leevy, C.M. (1967) Protein anabolism and fatty liver of the alcoholic. *Medicine,* **46,** 131–139.
152. Jackson, F.C., Perrin, E.B., Smith, A.G., Dagradi, A.E. & Wadal, H.M. (1968) A clinical investigation of the portacaval shunt. II. Survival analyses of the prophylactic operation. *American Journal of Surgery,* **115,** 22–42.
153. Jauhonen, V.P., Savolainen, M.J. & Hassinen, I.E. (1975) Cyclic AMP-linked mechanisms in ethanol-induced derangements of metabolism in rat liver and adipose tissue. *Biochemical Pharmacology,* **24,** 1879–1883.
154. Jeejeebhoy, K.N., Ho, J., Sodkte, U., Phillips, M.J., Greenberg, G.R. & Bruce-Robertson, A. (1975) Free liver cells in the study of albumin synthesis and the effect of ethanol. In *Alcoholic Liver Pathology* (Ed.) Khanna, J.M., Israel, Y. & Kalant, H. pp. 351–356. Canada: Addiction Research Foundation of Ontario.
155. Johnson, O. (1974) Influence of the blood ethanol concentration on the acute ethanol-induced liver triglyceride accumulation in rats. *Scandinavian Journal of Gastroenterology,* **2,** 207–213.
156. Jollife, N. & Jellinek, E.M. (1941) Vitamin deficiencies and liver cirrhosis in alcoholism. Part VII: Cirrhosis of the liver. *Quarterly Journal of Studies on Alcohol.* **2,** 544–583.
157. Jolliffe, N. & Jellinek, E.M. (1942) Cirrhosis of the liver. In *Alcohol addiction and Chronic Alcoholism* (Ed.) Jellinek, E.M. pp. 273–309. New Haven: Yale University Press.
158. Joly, J.G., Ishii, H., Teschke, R., Hasumura, Y. & Lieber, C.S. (1973) Effect of chronic ethanol feeding on the activities and submicrosomal distribution of reduced nicotinamide adenine dinucleotide phosphate (NADPH)-cytochrome P-450 reductase and the demethylases for aminopyrine and ethyl morphine. *Biochemical Pharmacology,* **22,** 1532–1535.
159. Jones, D.P., Perman, E.S. & Lieber, C.S. (1965) Free fatty acid turnover and triglyceride metabolism after ethanol ingestion in man. *Journal of Laboratory and Clinical Medicine,* **66,** 804–814.
160. Jones, D.P., Losowsky, M.S., Davidson, C.S. & Lieber, C.S. (1963) Effects of ethanol on plasma lipids in man. *Journal of Laboratory and Clinical Medicine,* **62,** 675–682.
161. Jones, D.P., Sosa, F.R., Shartsis, J., Shah, P.T., Skromak, E. & Beher, W.T. (1971) Serum cholesterol esterifying and cholesterol ester hydrolyzing activities in liver diseases: relationships to cholesterol, bilirubin and bile salt concentrations. *Journal of Clinical Investigation,* **50,** 259–265.
162. Kaim, S.C. (1972) Criteria for the diagnosis of alcoholism. *Annals of Internal Medicine,* **77,** 249–258.
163. Kakumu, S. & Leevy, C.M. (1977) Lymphocyte cytotoxicity in alcoholic hepatitis. *Gastroenterology,* **72,** 594–597.
164. Kanagasundaram, N., Kakumu, S., Chen, T. & Leevy, C.M. (1976) Alcoholic hyalin antigen (AHAg) and its antibody (AHAb) in alcoholic liver disease. *Clinical Research,* **24,** 478A (abstract).
165. Kater, R.M.H., Carulli, N. & Iber, F.L. (1969) Difference in the rate of ethanol metabolism in recently drinking alcoholic and nondrinking subjects. *American Journal of Clinical Nutrition,* **22,** 1608–1617.
166. Kater, R.M.H., Roggin, G., Tobon, F., Zieve, P. & Iber, F.L. (1969) Increased rate of clearance of drugs from the circulation of alcoholics. *American Journal of the Medical Sciences,* **258,** 35–39.
167. Keeley, A.F., Iseri, O.A. & Gottlieb, L.S. (1972) Ultrastructure of hyaline cytoplasmic inclusions in a human hepatoma: relationship to Mallory's alcoholic hyalin. *Gastroenterology,* **62,** 280–293.
168. Keilin, D. & Hartree, E.F. (1936) Couple oxidation of alcohol. *Proceedings of the Royal Society (London),* Series B, **119,** 141–159.
169. Keilin, D. & Hartree, E.F. (1945) Properties of catalase. Catalysis of coupled oxidation of alcohols. *Biochemical Journal,* **39,** 293–301.
170. Kern, W.H., Mikkelsen, W.P. & Turrill, F.L. (1969) The significance of hyaline necrosis in liver biopsies. *Surgery, Gynecology and Obstetrics,* **129,** 749–754.
171. Kessel, L. (1962) Acute transient hyperlipemia due to hepatopancreatic damage in chronic alcoholics (Zieve's syndrome). *American Journal of Medicine,* **32,** 747–757.
172. Kiessling, K.-H. (1963) The effect of acetaldehyde on mitochondrial respiration. *Experimental Cell Research,* **30,** 569–576.
173. Kiessling, K.-H. & Pilström, L. (1966) Effect of ethanol on rat liver. I. Enzymatic and histological studies of liver mitochondria. *Quarterly Journal of Studies on Alcohol,* **27,** 189–200.
174. Kiessling, K.-H. & Tilander, K. (1963) The effect of prolonged alcohol treatment on the respiration of liver and brain mitochondria from male and female rats. *Experimental Cell Research,* **30,** 476–480.
175. Kiessling, K.-H., Lindgren, L., Strandberg, B. & Tobe, U. (1964) Electron microscopic study of liver mitochondria from human alcoholics. *Acta Medica Scandinavica,* **176,** 595–598.
176. Klatskin, G., Krehl, W.A. & Conn, H.O. (1954) The effect of alcohol on the choline requirement. I. Changes in the rat's liver following prolonged ingestion of alcohol. *Journal of Experimental Medicine,* **100,** 605–614.
177. Klion, F.M. & Schaffner, F. (1968) Ultrastructural studies in alcoholic liver disease. *Digestion,* **1,** 2–14.
178. Koch, O.R., Porta, E.A. & Hartroft, W.S. (1968) A new experimental approach in the study of alcoholism. *Laboratory Investigation,* **18,** 379–386.

179. Konttinen, A., Härtel, G. & Louhija, A. (1970) Multiple serum enzyme analyses in chronic alcoholics. *Acta Medica Scandinavica*, **188,** 257–264.
180. Korsten, M.A., Matsuzaki, S., Feinman, L. & Lieber, C.S. (1975) High blood acetaldehyde levels following ethanol administration: differences between alcoholic and non-alcoholic subjects. *New England Journal of Medicine*, **292,** 386–389.
181. Krebs, H.A., Freedland, R.A., Hems, R. & Stubbs, M. (1969) Inhibition of hepatic gluconeogenesis by ethanol. *Biochemical Journal*, **112,** 117–124.
182. Kuller, L., Kramer, K. & Fisher, R. (1969) Changing trends in cirrhosis and fatty liver mortality. *American Journal of Public Health and the Nation's Health*, **59,** 1124–1133.
183. Kyösola, K. & Salorinne, Y. (1975) Liver biopsy and liver function tests in 28 consecutive long-term alcoholics. *Annals of Clinical Research*, **7,** 80–84.
184. Lane, B.P. & Lieber, C.S. (1966) Ultrastructural alterations in human hepatocytes following ingestion of ethanol with adequate diets. *American Journal of Pathology*, **49,** 593–603.
185. laRusso, N.F., Hoffman, N.E., Hofmann, A.F. & Korman, M.G. (1975) Validity and sensitivity of an intravenous bile acid tolerance test in patients with liver disease. *New England Journal of Medicine*, **222,** 1209–1214.
186. Le Breton, E. & Tremolières, J. (1955) Part de l'alcool dans la dépense calorique. *Proceedings of the Nutrition Society*, **14,** 97.
187. Lee, F.I. (1966) Cirrhosis and hepatoma in alcoholics, *Gut*, **7,** 77–85.
188. Leevy, C.M. (1962) Fatty liver: a study of 270 patients with biopsy proven fatty liver and a review of the literature. *Medicine*, **41,** 249–276.
189. Leevy, C.M. (1968) Cirrhosis in alcoholics. *Medical Clinics of North America*, **52,** 1445–1451.
190. Lefevre, A.F., Adler, H.M. & Lieber, C.S. (1970) Effect of ethanol on ketone metabolism. *Journal of Clinical Investigation*, **49,** 1775–1782.
191. Lefevre, A.F., DeCarli, L.M. & Lieber, C.S. (1972) Effect of ethanol on cholesterol and bile acid metabolism. *Journal of Lipid Research*, **13,** 48–55.
192. Lelbach, W.K. (1966) Leberschäden bei chronischem Alkoholismuss, I-III. *Acta Hepatosplenologica*, **13,** 321–349.
193. Lelbach, W.K. (1967) Leberschäden bei chronischem Alkoholismuss. *Acta Hepatosplenologica*, **14,** 9–39.
194. Lelbach, W.K. (1975) Cirrhosis in the alcoholic and its relation to the volume of alcohol abuse. *Annals of the New York Academy of Sciences*, **252,** 85–105.
195. Lelbach, W.K. (1976) Epidemiology of alcoholic liver disease. In *Progress in Liver Diseases* (Ed.) Popper, H. & Schaffner, F. pp. 494–515. New York: Grune & Stratton.
196. Leloir, L.F. & Munoz, J.M. (1938) Ethyl alcohol metabolism in animal tissues. *Biochemical Journal*, **31,** 299–307.
197. LeMarchand, Y., Singh, M., Assimacopoulus-Jeannet, F., Orci, L., Rouiller, C. & Jeanrenaud, B. (1973) A role of microtubular system in the release of very low density lipoproteins by perfused mouse livers. *Journal of Biological Chemistry*, **248,** 6862–6870.
198. LeMarchand, Y., Patzelt, C., Assimacopoulos-Jeannet, F., Loten, E.G. & Jeanrenaud, B. (1974) Evidence for a role of the microtubular system in the secretion of newly synthesized albumin and other proteins by the liver. *Journal of Clinical Investigation*, **53,** 1512–1517.
199. Levander, O.A., Morris, V.C., Higgs, D.Y. & Varma, R.N. (1973) Nutritional·interrelationships among vitamin E, selenium, antioxidants and ethyl alcohol in the rat. *Journal of Nutrition*, **103,** 536–542.
200. Levi, A.J., Sherlock, S. & Walker, D. (1968) Phenylbutazone and isoniazide metabolism in patients with liver disease in relation to previous drug therapy. *Lancet*, **i,** 1275–1279.
201. Levin, D.M., Baker, A.L., Rochman, H. & Boyer, J.L. (1977) Alcoholic patients with chronic abnormalities in liver function harbor unsuspected non-alcoholic liver diseases, detectable only by liver biopsy. *Gastroenterology*, **72,** 1172 (abstract 149).
202. Levy, L.J., Duga, J., Girgis, M. & Gordon, E.E. (1973) Ketoacidosis associated with alcoholism in non-diabetic subjects. *Annals of Internal Medicine*, **78,** 213–219.
203. Li, T.-K. & Magnes, L.J. (1975) Identification of a distinctive molecular form of alcohol dehydrogenase in human livers with high activity. *Biochemical and Biophysical Research Communications*, **63,** 202–208.
204. Lieber, C.S. (1967) Chronic alcoholic hepatic injury in experimental animals and man: biochemical pathways and nutritional factors. *Federation Proceedings*, **26,** 1443–1448.
205. Lieber, C.S. (1974) Effects of ethanol upon lipid metabolism. *Lipids*, **9,** 103–116.
206. Lieber, C.S. (1977) Metabolism of ethanol. In *Metabolic Aspects of Alcoholism* (Ed.) Lieber, C.S. pp. 1–29. Baltimore: University Park Press.
207. Lieber, C.S. (1978) Pathogenesis and early diagnosis of alcoholic liver injury. *New England Journal of Medicine*, **288,** 888–893.
208. Lieber, C.S. & DeCarli, L.M. (1968) Ethanol oxidation by hepatic microsomes: adaptive increase after ethanol feeding. *Science*, **162,** 917–918.
209. Lieber, C.S. & DeCarli, L.M. (1970) Quantitative relationship between the amount of dietary fat and the severity of the alcoholic fatty liver. *American Journal of Clinical Nutrition*, **23,** 474–478.
210. Lieber, C.S. & DeCarli, L.M. (1970) Reduced nicotinamide-adenine dinucleotide phosphate oxidase: activity enhanced by ethanol consumption. *Science*, **170,** 78–79.
211. Lieber, C.S. & DeCarli, L.M. (1974) An experimental model of alcohol feeding and liver injury in the baboon. *Journal of Medical Primatology*, **3,** 153–163.
212. Lieber, C.S. & DeCarli, L.M. (1977) Metabolic effects of alcohol on the liver. In *Metabolic Aspects of Alcoholism* (Ed.) Lieber, C.S. pp. 31–79. Baltimore: University Park Press.
213. Lieber, C.S. & Rubin, E. (1968) Alcoholic fatty liver in man on high protein-low fat diet. *American Journal of Medicine*, **44,** 200–206.
214. Lieber, C.S. & Schmid, R. (1961) The effect of ethanol on fatty acid metabolism: stimulation of hepatic fatty acid synthesis in vitro. *Journal of Clinical Investigation*, **40,** 394–399.
215. Lieber, C.S. & Spritz, N. (1966) Effects of prolonged ethanol intake in man: role of dietary, adipose, and endogenously synthesized fatty acids in the pathogenesis of alcoholic fatty liver. *Journal of Clinical Investigation*, **45,** 1400–1411.
216. Lieber, C.S., DeCarli, L.M. & Rubin, E. (1975) Sequential production of fatty liver, hepatitis, and cirrhosis in sub-human primates fed ethanol with adequate diets. *Proceedings of the National Academy of Sciences of the United States of America*, **72,** 437–441.

217. Lieber, C.S., Jones, D.P. & DeCarli, L.M. (1965) Effects of prolonged ethanol intake: production of fatty liver despite adequate diets. *Journal of Clinical Investigation,* **44,** 1009–1021.

218. Lieber, C.S., Spritz, N. & DeCarli, L.M. (1966) Role of dietary, adipose and endogenously synthesized fatty acids in the pathogenesis of the alcoholic fatty liver. *Journal of Clinical Investigation,* **45,** 51–62.

219. Lieber, C.S., Spritz, N. & DeCarli, L.M. (1969) Fatty liver produced by dietary deficiencies: its pathogenesis and potentiation by ethanol. *Journal of Lipid Research,* **10,** 283–287.

220. Lieber, C.S., Jones, D.P., Losowsky, M.S. & Davidson, C.S. (1962) Interrelation of uric acid and ethanol metabolism in man. *Journal of Clinical Investigation,* **41,** 1863–1870.

221. Lieber, C.S., Jones, D.P., Mendelson, J. & DeCarli, L.M. (1963) Fatty liver, hyperlipemia, and hyperuricemia produced by prolonged alcohol consumption, despite adequate dietary intake. *Transactions of the Association of American Physicians,* **76,** 289–300.

222. Lieber, C.S., Lefevre, A., Spritz, N., Feinman, L. & DeCarli, L.M. (1967) Difference in hepatic metabolism of long- and medium-chain fatty acids: the role of fatty acid chain length in the production of the alcoholic fatty liver. *Journal of Clinical Investigation,* **46,** 1451–1460.

223. Lieber, C.S., DeCarli, L.M., Gang, H., Walker, G. & Rubin, E. (1972) Hepatic effects of long term ethanol consumption in primates. In *Medical Primatology—1972.* Part 3 (Ed.) Goldsmith, E.I. & Moor-Jankowski, J. pp. 270–278. Basel: Karger.

224. Lindenbaum, J. (1977) Metabolic effects of alcohol on the blood and bone marrow. In *Metabolic Aspects of Alcoholism* (Ed.) Lieber, C.S. pp. 215–247. Baltimore: University Park Press.

225. Lindenfelser, R. & Breining, H. (1970) Diagnostische Zuberlässigkeit der Leber punktion bei Zirrhose. *Medizinische Klinik,* **65,** 2021–2025.

226. Lindros, K.O. (1972) Role of the redox state in ethanol-induced suppression of citrate-cycle flux in the perfused liver of normal, hyper-, and hypothyroid rats. *European Journal of Biochemistry,* **26,** 338–346.

227. Lindros, K.O. (1974) Acetaldehyde oxidation and its role in the overall metabolic effects of ethanol in the liver. In *Regulation of Hepatic Metabolism* (Ed.) Lundquist, F. & Tygstrup, N. pp. 417–432. Copenhagen: Munksgaard.

228. Lindros, K.O., Vihma, R. & Forsander, O.A. (1972) Utilization and metabolic effects of acetaldehyde and ethanol in the perfused rat liver. *Biochemical Journal,* **126,** 945–952.

229. Lischner, M.W., Alexander, J.F. & Galambos, J.T. (1971) Natural history of alcoholic hepatitis. I. The acute disease. *American Journal of Digestive Diseases,* **16,** 481–494.

230. Lloyd, C.W. & Williams, R.H. (1948) Endocrine changes associated with Laennec's cirrhosis of the liver. *American Journal of Medicine,* **4,** 315–330.

231. Lo, C.-H. & Marsh, J.B. (1970) Biosynthesis of plasma lipoproteins. Incorporation of ^{14}C-glucosamine by cells and subcellular fractions of rat liver. *Journal of Biological Chemistry,* **245,** 5001–5006.

232. Lochner, A., Wulff, J. & Madison, L.L. (1967) Ethanol-induced hypoglycemia. I. The acute effects of ethanol on hepatic glucose output and peripheral glucose utilization in fasted dogs. *Metabolism: Clinical and Experimental,* **16,** 1–18.

233. Lombardi, B.P., Pani, P. & Schlunk, F.F. (1968) Choline-deficiency fatty liver: impaired release of hepatic triglycerides. *Journal of Lipid Research,* **9,** 437–446.

234. Losowsky, M.S., Jones, D.P., Davidson, C.S. & Lieber, C.S. (1963) Studies of alcoholic hyperlipemia and its mechanism. *American Journal of Medicine,* **35,** 794–803.

235. Lundquist, F. (1971) The metabolism of alcohol. In *Biological Basis of Alcoholism* (Ed.) Israel, Y. & Mardones, J. pp. 1–52. New York: John Wiley.

236. Lundquist, F. (1975) Interference of ethanol in cellular metabolism. *Annals of the New York Academy of Sciences,* **252,** 11–20.

237. Lundsgaard, E. (1938) Alcohol oxidation as a function of the liver. *Comptes Rendus des Travaux du Laboratoire Carlsberg (Kobenhavn),* **22,** 333–337.

238. MacLachlan, M.J. & Rodan, G.P. (1967) Effect of food, fast, and alcohol on serum uric acid and acute attacks of gout. *American Journal of Medicine,* **42,** 38–57.

239. Madison, L.L., Lochner, A. & Wulff, J. (1967) Ethanol induced hypoglycemia. II. Mechanism of suppression of hepatic gluconeogenesis. *Diabetes,* **16,** 252–258.

240. Madsen, N.P. (1969) Reduced serum very low-density lipoprotein levels after acute ethanol administration. *Biochemical Pharmacology,* **18,** 261–262.

241. Mäkelä, K. (1971) Measuring the consumption of alcohol in the 1968–1969 alcohol consumption study. *Social Research Institute of Alcohol Studies,* No. 2. Helsinki: Oy Alko Ab, Box 350.

242. Mallory, F.B. (1911) Cirrhosis of the liver. Five different types of lesions from which it may arise. *Bulletin of the Johns Hopkins Hospital,* **22,** 69–75.

243. Mallow, S. (1957) Effect of adrenalectomy on ethanol and fat metabolism in the rat. *American Journal of Physiology,* **189,** 428–432.

244. Mallow, S. & Block, J.F. (1956) Role of hypophysis and adrenals in fatty infiltration of liver resulting from acute ethanol intoxication. *American Journal of Physiology,* **184,** 29–34.

245. Marjanen, L. (1972) Intracellular localization of aldehyde dehydrogenase in rat liver. *Biochemical Journal,* **127,** 633–639.

246. Martini, G.A. (1975) Extrahepatic manifestations of cirrhosis. *Clinics in Gastroenterology,* **4,** 439–460.

247. Martini, G.A. & Bode, C.H. (1970) The epidemiology of cirrhosis of the liver. In *Alcoholic Cirrhosis and Other Toxic Hepatopathies* (Ed.) Engel, A. & Larsson, T. pp. 315–335. Stockholm: Nordiska Bokhandelns Förlag.

248. Marzo, S., Ghirardi, P., Sardini, D., Prandini, B.D. & Albertini, A. (1970) Serum lipids and total fatty acids in chronic alcoholic liver disease at different states of cell damage. *Klinische Wochenschrift (Berlin),* **48,** 949–950.

249. Matsuzaki, S. & Lieber, C.S. (1977) Increased susceptibility of hepatic mitochondria to the toxicity of acetaldehyde after chronic ethanol consumption. *Biochemical and Biophysical Research Communications,* **75,** 1059–1065.

250. Matsuzaki, S., Teschke, R., Ohnishi, K. & Lieber, C.S. (1976) Acceleration of ethanol metabolism by high ethanol concentrations and chronic alcohol consumption: role of the microsomal ethanol oxidizing system (MEOS). In *Alcohol and the Liver* (Ed.) Fisher, M.M. & Rankin, J.G. pp. 119–143. New York: Plenum Press.

251. Matunaga, H. (1942) Experimentelle Untersuchungen über den Einfluss des Alkohols auf den Kohlenhydratstoffwechsel. I. Über die Wirkung des Alkohols auf den Blutzuckerspiegel und den Glykogenhalt der Leber, mit besonderer Berücksichtigung seines Wirkungsmechanismus. *Tohoku Journal of Experimental Medicine,* **44,** 130–157.
252. Mendelson, J.H. & LaDou, J. (1964) Experimentally induced chronic intoxication and withdrawal in alcoholism. Part 2. Psychophysiological findings. *Quarterly Journal of Studies on Alcohol* (Suppl. No. 2), 14–39.
253. Mendelson, J.H. & Mello, N.K. (1973) Alcohol-induced hyperlipidemia and beta lipoproteins. *Science,* **180,** 1372–1374.
254. Mendenhall, C.L. (1968) Anabolic steroid therapy as an adjunct to diet in alcoholic hepatic steatosis. *American Journal of Digestive Diseases,* **13,** 783–791.
255. Mendenhall, C.L. (1972) Origin of hepatic triglyceride fatty acids; quantitative estimation of the relative contributions of linoleic acid by diet and adipose tissue in normal and ethanol-fed rats. *Journal of Lipid Research,* **13,** 177–183.
256. Mezey, E., Potter, J.J., Slusser, R.J. & Abdi, W. (1977) Changes in hepatic collagen metabolism in rats produced by chronic ethanol feeding. *Laboratory Investigation,* **36,** 206–214.
257. Miettinen, T.A. (1973) Clinical implications of bile acid metabolism in man. In *The Bile Acids,* Vol. 2 (Ed.) Nair, P.P. & Kritchevsky, D. pp. 191–247. New York: Plenum Press.
258. Miettinen, T. (1975) Bile acid metabolism. In *Handbook of Experimental Pharmacology,* New Series, Vol. 41 (Ed.) Born, G.V.R., Eichler, O., Farah, A., Herken, H. & Welch, A.D. pp. 109–150. Berlin: Springer-Verlag.
259. Mihas, A.A., Bull, D.M. & Davidson, C.S. (1975) Cell-mediated immunity to liver in patients with alcoholic hepatitis. *Lancet,* **i,** 951–956.
260. Miller, G.J. & Miller, N.E. (1975) Plasma-high-density-lipoprotein concentration and development of ischaemic heart-disease. *Lancet,* **i,** 16–19.
261. Milstein, H.J., Bloomer, J.R. & Klatskin, G. (1976) Serum bile acids in alcoholic liver disease, comparison with histological features of the disease. *Journal of Digestive Diseases,* **21,** 281–285.
262. Misra, P.S., Lefevre, A., Ishii, H., Rubin, E. & Lieber, C.S. (1971) Increase of ethanol, meprobamate and pentobarbital metabolism after chronic ethanol administration in man and in rats. *American Journal of Medicine,* **51,** 346–351.
263. Mollenhauer, H.H., Morre, D.J. & Kogut, C. (1969) Dietary modification of the stability of rat liver Golgi apparatus. *Exper. Molecular Pathology,* **2,** 113–122.
264. Monroe, S., French, S.W. & Zamboni, L. (1973) Mallory bodies in a case of primary biliary cirrhosis. An ultrastructural and morphogenetic study. *American Journal of Clinical Pathology,* **59,** 254–262.
265. Morgan, M.Y. & Sherlock, S. (1977) Sex-related differences among 100 patients with alcoholic liver disease. *British Medical Journal,* **i,** 939–941.
266. Mörland, J. & Bessesen, A. (1977) Inhibition of protein synthesis by ethanol in isolated rat liver parenchymal cells. *Biochimica et Biophysica Acta,* **474,** 312–320.
267. *Mortality from cirrhosis of the liver–New York City 1949–1968* (1969) City of New York Department of Health Bureau of Records and Statistics, Statistical Division.
268. Myers, G.E., Rosen, A., Fend, L.Y. & Kuo, P.T. (1969) Incidence and type of hyperlipoproteinemia in chronic alcoholism. *Federation Proceedings,* **28,** 696.
269. Myrhed, M. (1974) Alcohol consumption in relation to factors associated with ischemic heart disease. *Acta Medica Scandinavica* (Suppl. 567), 1-93.
270. Nazari, B. (1966) Dupuytren's contractures associated with liver disease. *Journal of the Mount Sinai Hospital,* **33,** 69–72.
271. Nenci, I. (1975) Identification of actin-like protein in alcoholic hyalin by immunofluorescence. *Laboratory Investigation,* **32,** 257–260.
272. Newcombe, D.S. (1972) Ethanol metabolism and uric acid. *Metabolism: Clinical and Experimental,* **21,** 1193–1203.
273. Nikkilä, E.A. & Ojala, K. (1963) Role of hepatic L-alpha-glycerophosphate and triglyceride synthesis in production of fatty liver by ethanol. *Proceedings of the Society for Experimental Biology and Medicine,* **113,** 814–817.
274. Novikoff, A.B., Roheim, P.S. & Quintana, N. (1966) Changes in rat liver cells induced by orotic acid feeding. *Laboratory Investigation,* **15,** 27–49.
275. Oette, K. (1974) Experimentelle Untersuchungen an menschlichen Leberpunktaten und Rattenleberschnitten zur Oxidation von Fettsäuren mit unterschiedlicher Kettenlänge und Zahl von Doppelbindungen. *Research in Experimental Medicine (Berlin),* **162,** 185–203.
276. Okamura, K., Harwood, T.R. & Yokoo, H. (1975) Isolation and electrophoretic study on Mallory bodies from the livers of alcoholic cirrhosis. *Laboratory Investigation,* **33,** 193–199.
277. Oliva, R.B. (1970) Lactic acidosis. *The American Journal of Medicine,* **48,** 209–225.
278. Olson, R.E. (1964) Nutrition and alcoholism. In *Modern Nutrition in Health and Disease* (Ed.) Goodhart, R.S. & Shils, M.E. pp. 1037–1050. Philadelphia: Lea & Febiger.
279. Ontko, J.A. (1973) Effects of ethanol on the metabolism of free fatty acids in isolated liver cells. *Journal of Lipid Research,* **14,** 78–86.
280. Orrego, H., Kalant, H., Israel, Y., Medline, A., Rankin, J., Armstrong, A. & Kapur, B. (1979) Effect of short-term therapy with propylthiouracil in patients with alcoholic liver disease. *Gastroenterology,* **76,** 105–115.
281. Paronetto, F. & Lieber, C.S. (1976) Cytotoxicity of lymphocytes in experimental alcoholic liver injury in the baboon. *Proceedings of the Society for Experimental Biology and Medicine,* **153,** 495–497.
282. Partin, J.S., Partin, J.C., Schubert, W.K. & McAdams, A.J. (1974) Liver ultrastructure in abetalipoproteinemia: evolution of micronodular cirrhosis. *Gastroenterology,* **67,** 107–118.
283. Pell, S. & D'Alonzo, C.A. (1968) The prevalence of chronic disease among problem drinkers. *Archives of Environmental Health,* **16,** 679–684.
284. Péquignot, G. (1958) Enquête par interrogatoire sur les circonstances diététiques de la cirrhose alcoolique en France. *Bulletin of the Institute of National Hygiene,* **13,** 719–939.
285. Péquignot, G., Chabert, C., Eydoux, H. & Corcowl, M.A. (1974) Increased risk of liver cirrhosis with intake of alcohol. *Revue in Alcoholism,* **20,** 191–202.

286. Perin, A. & Sessa, A. (1975) In vitro effects of ethanol and acetaldehyde on tissue protein synthesis. In *The Role of Acetaldehyde in the Actions of Ethanol.* (Ed.) Lindros, K.O. & Eriksson, C.J.P. pp. 105–122. Helsinki: Kauppakirjapaino.
287. Perin, A., Scalabrino, G., Sessa, A. & Arnaboldi, A. (1974) In vitro inhibition of protein synthesis in rat liver as a consequence of ethanol metabolism. *Biochimica et Biophysica Acta,* **366,** 101–108.
288. Perman, G. (1967) Hemochromatosis and red wine. *Acta Medica Scandinavica,* **182,** 281–284.
289. Peters, R.L., Gay, T. & Reynolds, T.B. (1975) Post-jejunoileal bypass hepatic disease. *American Journal of Clinical Pathology,* **63,** 318–331.
290. Petersen, P.U. (1977) Alcoholic hyalin, microfilaments and microtubules in alcoholic hepatitis. *Acta Pathologica et Microbiologica Scandinavica,* **85,** 384–394.
291. Phillips, G.B. & Davidson, C.S. (1954) Acute hepatic insufficiency of the chronic alcoholic. *Archives of Internal Medicine,* **94,** 585–603.
292. Phillips, G.B. & Davidson, C.S. (1957) Liver disease of the chronic alcoholic simulating extrahepatic biliary obstruction. *Gastroenterology,* **33,** 236–244.
293. Pietruszko, R., Theorell, H. & de Zalenski, C. (1972) Heterogeneity of alcohol dehydrogenase from human liver. *Archives of Biochemistry and Biophysics,* **153,** 279–293.
294. Pikkarainen, P. & Räihä, N.C.R. (1967) Development of alcohol dehydrogenase activity in the human liver. *Pediatric Research,* **1,** 165–168.
295. Pikkarainen, P. & Räihä, N.C.R. (1969) Change in alcohol dehydrogenase isoenzyme pattern during development of human liver. *Nature,* **222,** 563–564.
296. Pirola, R.C. & Lieber, C.S. (1972) The energy cost of the metabolism of drugs, including ethanol. *Pharmacology,* **7,** 185–196.
297. Pirola, R.C. & Lieber, C.S. (1976) Energy wastage in rats given drugs that induce microsomal enzymes. *Journal of Nutrition,* **105,** 1544–1548.
298. Popham, R.E. (1970) Indirect methods of alcoholism prevalence estimation: a critical evaluation. In *Alcohol and Alcoholism* (Ed.) Popham, R.E. Toronto: University of Toronto Press.
299. Popham, R.E., Schmidt, W. & DeLint, J.E. (1976) The effect of legal restraint on drinking. In *Biology of Alcoholism, Vol. 4: Social Biology* (Ed.) Kissin, B. & Begleiter, H. pp. 579–625. New York: Plenum Press.
300. Popper, H. (1977) The pathogenesis of alcoholic cirrhosis. In *Alcohol and the Liver* (Ed.) Fisher, M.M. & Rankin, J.G. pp. 289–305. New York: Plenum Press.
301. Popper, H. & Schaffner, F. (1961) The hepatic lesion in Wilson's disease. In *Wilson's Disease, Some Current Concepts* (Ed.) Walshe, J.M. & Cummings, J.N. pp. 192–197. Oxford: Blackwell.
302. Popper, H. & Schaffner, F. (1971) Nutritional cirrhosis in man. *New England Journal of Medicine,* **285,** 577–578.
303. Popper, H., Szanto, P.B. & Parthasarathy, M. (1955) Florid cirrhosis. A review of 35 cases. *American Journal of Clinical Pathology,* **25,** 889–901.
304. Porta, E.A. & Gomez-Dumm, C.L.A. (1968) A new experimental approach in the study of chronic alcoholism. I. Effects of high alcohol intake in rats fed a commercial laboratory diet. *Journal of Laboratory Investigation,* **18,** 352–364.
305. Porter, H.P., Simon, F.R., Pope, C.E., Volwiler, W. & Fenster, F. (1971) Corticosteroid therapy in severe alcoholic hepatitis: a double-blind drug trial. *New England Journal of Medicine,* **284,** 1350–1355.
306. Post, J., Benton, J., Breatstone, R. & Hoffman, J. (1952) The effects of diet and choline on fatty infiltration of the human liver. *Gastroenterology,* **20,** 403–410.
307. Powell, L.W. (1975) The role of alcoholism in hepatic iron storage disease. *Annals of the New York Academy of Sciences,* **252,** 124–134.
308. Powell, W.J. & Klatskin, G. (1968) Duration of survival in patients with Laennec's cirrhosis. Influence of alcohol withdrawal and possible effects of recent changes in general management of the disease. *American Journal of Medicine,* **44,** 406–420.
309. Ramalingaswami, V. (1964) Perspectives in protein malnutrition. *Nature,* **201,** 546–551.
310. Rankin, J.G. (1977) The natural history and management of the patient with alcoholic liver disease. In *Alcohol and the Liver* (Ed.) Fisher, M.M. & Rankin, J.G. pp. 365–381. New York: Plenum Press.
311. Rappaport, A.M. (1975) Liver architecture and microcirculation. In *Alcoholic Liver Pathology* (Ed.) Khanna, J.M., Israel, Y. & Kalant, H. pp. 43–67. Ontario: The Addiction Research Foundation of Ontario.
312. Ratnoff, O.D. & Patek, A.J. Jr (1942) Natural history of Laennec's cirrhosis of the liver. An analysis of 386 cases. *Medicine (Baltimore),* **21,** 207–268.
313. Ravi Varma, L.A. (1950) Alcoholism in Ayerveda. *Quarterly Journal of Studies on Alcohol,* **11,** 484–491.
314. Reboucas, J. & Isselbacher, K.J. (1961) Studies on the pathogenesis of the ethanol induced fatty liver. I. Synthesis and oxidation of fatty acids by the liver. *Journal of Clinical Investigation,* **40,** 1355–1362.
315. Resnick, R.H., Chalmers, T.C., Ishihara, A.M., Garceau, A.J., Callow, A.D., Schimmel, E.M. & O'Hara, E.T. (1969) A controlled study of the prophylactic portacaval shunt: a final report. *Annals of Internal Medicine,* **70,** 675–688.
316. Reynolds, T.B., Hidemura, R., Michel, H. & Peters, R. (1969) Portal hypertension without cirrhosis in alcoholic liver disease. *Annals of Internal Medicine,* **70,** 497–506.
317. Rojkind, M. & Kershenobich, D. (1976) Hepatic fibrosis. In *Progress in Liver Diseases* (Ed.) Popper H. & Schaffner, F. pp. 294–310. New York: Grune & Stratton.
318. Rokitansky, C. (1849) *A Manual of Pathological Anatomy, 2,* p. 145. London: Sydenham Society.
319. Rollason, J.G., Pincherle, G. & Robinson, D. (1972) Serum gamma glutamyl transpeptidase in relation to alcohol consumption. *Clinica Chimica Acta,* **39,** 75–80.
320. Rothschild, M.A., Oratz, M. & Schreiber, S.S. (1974) Alcohol, amino acids, and albumin synthesis. *Gastroenterology,* **67,** 1200–1213.
321. Rothschild, M.A., Oratz, M. & Schreiber, S.S. (1977) The influence of ethanol on albumin metabolism. In *Alcohol and The Liver* (Ed.) Fisher, M.M. & Rankin, J.G. pp. 79–100. New York: Plenum Press.
322. Roy, S., Ramalingaswami, V. & Nayak, N.C. (1971) An ultrastructural study of the liver in Indian childhood cirrhosis with particular reference to the structure of cytoplasmic hyaline. *Gut,* **12,** 693–701.

323. Rubin, E. & Lieber, C.S. (1968) Alcohol-induced hepatic injury in non-alcoholic volunteers. *New England Journal of Medicine*, **278**, 869–876.
324. Rubin, E. & Popper, H. (1967) The evolution of human cirrhosis deduced from observations in experimental animals. *Medicine*, **46**, 163–183.
325. Rubin, E., Bacchin, P., Gang, H. & Lieber, C.S. (1970) Induction and inhibition of hepatic microsomal and mitochondrial enzymes by ethanol. *Laboratory Investigation*, **22**, 569–580.
326. Rubin, E., Gang, H., Misra, P.S. & Lieber, C.S. (1970) Inhibition of drug metabolism by acute ethanol intoxication. A hepatic microsomal mechanism. *American Journal of Medicine*, **49**, 801–806.
327. Sabesin, S.M., Hawkins, H.L., Kuiken, L. & Ragland, J.B. (1977) Abnormal plasma lipoproteins and lecithin–cholesterol acyltransferase deficiency in alcoholic liver disease. *Gastroenterology*, **72**, 510–518.
328. Salaspuro, M. (1970) Influence of the unchanged redox state of the liver during ethanol oxidation, on galactose and glucose metabolism in protein deficiency. In *Alcohol and the Liver* (Ed.) Gerok, W., Sickinger, K. & Hennekeuser, H.H. pp. 58–64. Stuttgart and New York: Schattauer Verlag.
329. Salaspuro, M.P. (1971) Influence of ethanol on the metabolism of the pathological liver. In *Biological Basis of Alcoholism* (Ed.) Israel, Y. & Mardones, J. pp. 163–182. New York and London: John Wiley.
330. Salaspuro, M. & Lieber, C.S. (1978) Non-uniformity of blood ethanol elimination: its exaggeration after chronic consumption. *Annals of Clinical Research*, **10**, 294–297.
331. Salaspuro, M.P. & Lieber, C.S. (1979) Metabolic consequences of chronic alcohol consumption: attenuation of hepatic redox changes despite enhanced capacity to eliminate ethanol. In *Currents in Alcoholism* (Ed.) Galanter, M. pp. 109–118. New York: Grune & Stratton.
332. Salaspuro, M.P. & Kesäniemi, Y.A. (1973) Intravenous galactose elimination tests with and without ethanol loading in various clinical conditions. *Scandinavian Journal of Gastroenterology*, **8**, 681–686.
333. Salaspuro, M.P. & Mäenpää, P. H. (1966) Influence of ethanol on the metabolism of perfused normal, fatty and cirrhotic rat livers. *Biochemical Journal*, **100**, 768–774.
334. Salaspuro, M. & Sipponen, P. (1976) Demonstration of an intracellular copper-binding protein by orcein staining in long-standing cholestatic liver diseases. *Gut*, **17**, 787–790.
335. Salaspuro, M.P., Lindros, K.O. & Pikkarainen, P. (1975) Ethanol and galactose metabolism as influenced by 4-methylpyrazole in alcoholics with and without nutritional deficiencies. *Annals of Clinical Research*, **7**, 269–272.
336. Salaspuro, M.P., Lindros, K.O. & Pikkarainen, P.H. (1978) Effect of 4-methylpyrazole on ethanol elimination rate and hepatic redox changes in alcoholics with adequate or inadequate nutrition and in nonalcoholic controls. *Metabolism: Clinical and Experimental*, **27**, 631–639.
337. Salaspuro, M.P., Pikkarainen, P. & Lindros, K. (1977) Ethanol-induced hypoglycemia in man: its suppression by the alcohol dehydrogenase inhibitor 4-methylpyrazole. *European Journal of Clinical Investigation*, **7**, 487–490.
338. Salaspuro, M.P., Sipponen, P. & Makkonen, H. (1976) The occurrence of orcein-positive hepatocellular material in various liver diseases. *Scandinavian Journal of Gastroenterology*, **11**, 677–681.
339. Samaan, N.A., Stone, D.B. & Eckhardt, R.D. (1969) Serum glucose, insulin and growth hormone in chronic hepatic cirrhosis. *Archives of Internal Medicine*, **124**, 149–152.
340. Saville, P.D. & Lieber, C.S. (1965) Effect of alcohol on growth, bone density and muscle magnesium in the rat. *Journal of Nutrition*, **87**, 477–488.
341. Savolainen, M.J., Hiltunen, K.J. & Hassinen, I.E. (1977) Effect of prolonged ethanol ingestion on hepatic lipogenesis and related enzyme activities. *Biochemical Journal*, **164**, 169–177.
342. Schapiro, R.H., Drummey, G.D., Shimizu, Y. & Isselbacher, K.J. (1964) Studies on the pathogenesis of ethanol-induced fatty liver. II. Effect of ethanol on palmitate-1-C14 metabolism by isolated perfused rat liver. *Journal of Clinical Investigation*, **43**, 1338–1347.
343. Schapiro, R.H., Scheig, R.L., Drummey, G.D., Mendelson, J.H. & Isselbacher, K.J. (1965) Effect of prolonged ethanol ingestion on the transport and metabolism of lipids in man. *New England Journal of Medicine*, **272**, 610–615.
344. Scheig, R. & Klatskin, G. (1969) Some effects of ethanol and carbon tetrachloride on lipoperoxidation in rat liver. *Life Sciences*, **8**, 855–865.
345. Schenker, T.M., Teeple, L.J. & von Wartburg, J.-P. (1971) Heterogeneity and polymorphism of human-liver alcohol dehydrogenase. *European Journal of Biochemistry*, **24**, 271–279.
346. Scheuer, P.J. (1970) Liver biopsy in the diagnosis of cirrhosis. *Gut*, **11**, 275–278.
347. Schlichling, P., Juhl, E., Poulsen, H. & Winkel, P. (1976) Alcoholic hepatitis superimposed on cirrhosis: clinical significance and effect of long-term prednisone treatment. *Scandinavian Journal of Gastroenterology*, **11**, 305–312
348. Schmidt, W. (1975) Agreement, disagreement in experimental, clinical and epidemiological evidence on the etiology of alcoholic liver cirrhosis: a comment. In *Alcoholic Liver Pathology* (Ed.) Khanna, J.M., Israel, Y. & Kalant, H. pp. 19–30. Toronto: Addiction Research Foundation.
349. Schmidt, W. (1977) The epidemiology of cirrhosis of the liver: a statistical analysis of mortality data with special reference to Canada. In *Alcohol and the Liver* (Ed.) Fisher, M.M. & Rankin, J.G. pp. 1–26. New York: Plenum Press.
350. Schoenfield, L.J., Bonorris, G.G. & Ganz, P. (1973) Induced alterations in the rate limiting enzymes of hepatic cholesterol and bile acid synthesis in the hamster. *Journal of Laboratory and Clinical Medicine*, **82**, 858–868.
351. Seakins, A. & Waterlow, J.C. (1972) Effect of a low-protein diet on the incorporation of amino acids into rat serum lipoproteins. *Biochemical Journal*, **129**, 793–795.
352. Seligson, D., Stone, H.H. & Nemir, P. Jr (1957) The metabolism of ethanol in man. *Surgical Forum*, **9**, 85–88.
353. Seyer, J.M., Hutcheson, E.T. & Kang, A.H. (1977) Collagen polymorphism in normal and cirrhotic human liver. *Journal of Clinical Investigation*, **59**, 241–248.

354. Shaw, S., Stimmel, B. & Lieber, C.S. (1976) Plasma alpha amino-n-butyric acid to leucine ratio. An empirical biochemical marker of alcoholism. *Science,* **194,** 1057–1058.

355. Shaw, S., Lue, S.-L. & Lieber, C.S. (1978) Biochemical tests for the detection of alcoholism: comparison of plasma alpha-amino-n-butyric acid with other available tests. *Alcoholism: Clinical and Experimental Research,* **2,** 3–7.

356. Sim, J.S., Franks, K.E., French, S.W. & Caldwell, M.G. (1977) Mallory bodies compared with microfilament hyperplasia. *Archives of Pathology and Laboratory Medicine,* **101,** 401–404.

357. Simon, J.B. & Scheig, R. (1970) Serum cholesterol esterification in liver disease. *New England Journal of Medicine,* **283,** 841–846.

358. Singh, A., LeMarchand, Y., Orci, L. & Jeanrenaud, B. (1975) Colchicine administration to mice: a metabolic and ultrastructural study. *European Journal of Clinical Investigation,* **5,** 495–505.

359. Skrede, S., Blomhoff, J.P. & Gjone, E. (1976) Biochemical features of acute and chronic hepatitis. *Annals of Clinical Research,* **8,** 182–199.

360. Skrede, S., Blomhoff, J.P., Elgjo, K. & Gjone, E. (1975) Serum proteins in diseases of the liver. *Scandinavian Journal of Clinical and Laboratory Investigation,* **35,** 399–406.

361. Smith, M., Hopkinson, D.A. & Harris, H. (1971) Developmental changes and polymorphism in human alcohol dehydrogenase. *Annals of Human Genetics (London),* **34,** 251–271.

362. Smith, M., Hopkinson, D.A. & Harris, H. (1972) Alcohol dehydrogenase in adult human stomach and liver evidence for the activity of the ADH_3 locus. *Annals of Human Genetics (London),* **35,** 243–253.

363. Soehring, K. & Schuppel, R. (1966) Wechselwirkungen zwischen Alkohol und Arzneimitteln. *Deutsche Medizinische Wochenschrift,* **91,** 1892–1898.

364. Solberg, H.E., Skrede, S. & Blomhof, J.P. (1975) Diagnosis of liver diseases by laboratory results and discriminant analysis. *Scandinavian Journal of Clinical and Laboratory Investigation,* **35,** 713–719.

365. Sorrell, M. & Leevy, C.M. (1972) Lymphocyte transformation and alcoholic liver injury. *Gastroenterology,* **63,** 1020–1025.

366. Stein, Y. & Shapiro, B. (1958) Glyceride synthesis by microsome fractions of rat liver. *Biochimica et Biophysica Acta,* **30,** 271–277.

367. Stein, O. & Stein, Y. (1965) Fine structure of the ethanol induced fatty liver in the rat. *Israel Journal of Medical Science,* **1,** 378–388.

368. Stein, O. & Stein, Y. (1973) Colchicine-induced inhibition of very low density lipoprotein release by rat liver in vivo. *Biochimica et Biophysica Acta,* **306,** 142–147.

369. Stein, O., Sanger, L. & Stein, Y. (1974) Colchicine-induced inhibition of lipoprotein and protein secretion into the serum and lack of interference with secretion of biliary phospholipids and cholesterol by rat liver in vivo. *Journal of Cell Biology,* **62,** 90–103.

370. Steiner, P.E. (1964) World problem in the cirrhotic diseases of the liver. Their incidence, frequency, types and aetiology. *Tropical and Geographical Medicine,* **16,** 175–205.

371. Stifel, F.B., Greene, H.L., Lufkein, E.G., Hagler, R. & Herman, R.H. (1974) Acute effects of oral and intravenous ethanol on rat hepatic enzyme activities. *Biochimica et Biophysica Acta,* **428,** 633–638.

372. Stone, W.D., Islam, N.R.K. & Paton, A. (1968) The natural history of cirrhosis. *Quarterly Journal of Medicine,* **37,** 119–132.

373. Svoboda, D.J. & Manning, R.T. (1964) Chronic alcoholism with fatty metamorphosis of the liver. *American Journal of Pathology,* **44,** 645–662.

374. Tague, L.L. & Shanbour, L.L. (1973) Alterations of gastric mucosal cAMP system in presence of ethanol. *Texas Reports on Biology and Medicine,* **31,** 103–104.

375. Targan, S.R., Chow, A.W. & Guze, L.B. (1977) Role of anaerobic bacteria in spontaneous peritonitis of cirrhosis. Report of two cases and review of the literature. *American Journal of Medicine,* **62,** 397–403.

376. Teschke, R., Brand, A. & Strohmeyer, G. (1977) Induction of hepatic microsomal gamma-glutamyl transferase activity following chronic alcohol consumption. *Biochemical and Biophysical Research Communications,* **75,** 718–724.

377. Teschke, R., Matsuzaki, S., Ohnishi, K., DeCarli, L.M. & Lieber, C.S. (1977) Microsomal ethanol oxidizing system (MEOS): current status of its characterization and its role. *Alcoholism: Clinical and Experimental Research,* **1,** 7–15.

378. Thaler, H. (1975) Relation of steatosis to cirrhosis. *Clinics in Gastroenterology,* **4,** 273–280.

379. Theorell, H. & Bonnichsen, R. (1951) Studies on liver alcohol dehydrogenase. I. Equilibria and initial reaction velocities. *Acta Chemica Scandinavica,* **5,** 1105–1126.

380. Theorell, H.S. & Chance, B. (1951) Studies on liver alcohol dehydrogenase. II. The kinetics of the compound of horse liver alcohol dehydrogenase and reduced diphosphopyridine nucleotide. *Acta Chemica Scandinavica,* **5,** 1127–1144.

381. Thurman, R.G. & Brentzel, H.J. (1977) The role of alcohol dehydrogenase in microsomal ethanol oxidation and the adaptive increase in ethanol metabolism due to chronic treatment with ethanol. *Alcoholism: Clinical and Experimental Research,* **1,** 33–38.

382. Thurman, R.G., Ley, H.G. & Scholz, R. (1972) Hepatic microsomal ethanol oxidation. Hydrogen peroxide formation and the role of catalase. *European Journal of Biochemistry,* **25,** 420–430.

383. Tibblin, G., Wilhelmsen, L. & Werkö, L. (1975) Risk factors for myocardial infarction and death due to ischemic heart disease and other causes. *American Journal of Cardiology,* **35,** 514–522.

384. Tisdale, W.A. (1961) Parenchymal siderosis in patients with cirrhosis after portosystemic shunt surgery. *New England Journal of Medicine,* **265,** 928–932.

385. Tisdale, W.A. & Klatskin, G. (1960) The fever of Laennec's cirrhosis. *Yale Journal of Biology and Medicine,* **33,** 94–106.

386. Tobon, F. & Mezey, E. (1971) Effect of ethanol administration on hepatic ethanol and drug metabolizing enzymes and on rates of ethanol degradation. *Journal of Laboratory and Clinical Medicine,* **77,** 110–121.

387. Tottmar, S.O.C., Petterson, H. & Kiessling, K.H. (1973) The subcellular distribution and properties of aldehyde dehydrogenases in rat liver. *Biochemical Journal,* **135,** 577–586.

388. Tremolières, J. & Carré, L. (1961) Études, sur les modalités d'oxydation de l'alcool chez l'homme normal et alcoolique. *Revue de l'Alcoolisme,* **7,** 202–227.

389. Triger, D.R. (1976) Bacterial, viral and auto antibodies in acute and chronic liver disease. *Annals of Clinical Research,* **8,** 174–181.
390. Truitt, E.B. Jr & Walsh, M.J. (1971) The role of acetaldehyde in the actions of ethanol. In *The Biology of Alcoholism* (Ed.) Kissin, B. & Begleiter, H. pp. 161–196. New York: Plenum Press.
391. Tygstrup, N., Juhl, E. & The Copenhagen Study Group for Liver Diseases (1971) The treatment of alcoholic cirrhosis. The effect of continued drinking and prednisone on survival. In *Alcohol and the Liver* (Ed.) Gerok, W., Sickinger, K. & Henneheuser, H.H. pp. 519–526. New York and Stuttgart: Schattauer Verlag.
392. Tygstrup, N., Winkler, K. & Lundquist, F. (1965) The mechanism of the fructose effect on the ethanol metabolism of the human liver. *Journal of Clinical Investigation,* **44,** 817–830.
393. Ugarte, G., Pino, M.E. & Insunza, J. (1967) Hepatic alcohol dehydrogenase in alcoholic addicts with and without hepatic damage. *American Journal of Digestive Diseases,* **12,** 589–599.
394. Ugarte, G., Iturriaga, H. & Pereda, T. (1977) Possible relationship between the rate of ethanol metabolism and the severity of hepatic damage in chronic alcoholics. *Digestive Diseases,* **22,** 406–410.
395. van Thiel, D.H., Lester, R. & Sherins, R.J. (1974) Hypogonadism in alcoholic liver disease: evidence for a double effect. *Gastroenterology,* **67,** 1188–1199.
396. Van Waes, L. & Lieber, C.S. (1977) Glutamate dehydrogenase, a reliable marker of liver cell necrosis in the alcoholic. *British Medical Journal,* **ii,** 1508–1510.
397. Van Waes, L. & Lieber, C.S. (1977) Early perivenular sclerosis in alcoholic fatty liver: an index of progressive liver injury. *Gastroenterology,* **73,** 646–650.
398. Vesell, E.S., Page, J.G. & Passananti, G.T. (1971) Genetic and environmental factors affecting ethanol metabolism in man. *Clinical Pharmacology and Therapeutics,* **12,** 192–201.
399. Videla, L. & Israel, Y. (1970) Factors that modify the metabolism of ethanol in rat liver and adaptive changes produced by its chronic administration. *Biochemical Journal,* **118,** 275–281.
400. Vido, I. & Wildhirt, E. (1969) Korrelation des Laparoskopischen und histologischen Befundes bei chronischer Hepatitis und Leberzirrhose. *Deutsche Medizinische Wochenschrift,* **94,** 1633–1637.
401. Vido, I. & Winckler, K. (1972) Diagnose der Leberzirrhose anhand laparoskopischer und histologischer Befunde. *Medizinische Klinik,* **67,** 400–402.
402. Volicer, L. & Gold, B.J. (1975) Interactions of ethanol with cyclic AMP. In *Advances in Experimental Medicine and Biology* (Ed.) Majchrowicz, E. Vol. 56, pp. 211–237. New York: Plenum Press.
403. Von Oldershausen, H.F. (1970) Alkoholische Leberschäden. *Therapiewoche,* **20,** 58–73.
404. Wallgren, H. & Barry, H. III (1970) Some basic data on the chemistry and pharmacology of ethyl alcohol. In *Actions of Alcohol* (Ed.) Wallgren, H. & Barry, H. III. Vol. I, pp. 17–73. Amsterdam, London and New York: Elsevier Publishing.
405. Wallgren, H. & Barry, H. III (1970) Prolonged exposure to alcohol. In *Actions of Alcohol* (Ed.) Wallgren, H. & Barry, H. III. Vol. II, pp. 480–583. Amsterdam, London and New York: Elsevier Publishing.
406. Wallgren, H. & Barry, H. III (1970) Drug actions in relation to alcohol effects. In *Actions of Alcohol* (Ed.) Wallgren, H. & Barry, H. III. Vol. II, pp. 621–714. Amsterdam, London and New York: Elsevier Publishing.
407. Wartburg, J.-P., Papenberg, J. & Aebi, H. (1965) An atypical human alcohol dehydrogenase. *Canadian Journal of Biochemistry,* **43,** 889–898.
408. Wilkinson, P., Santamaria, J.N. & Rankin, J.G. (1969) Epidemiology of alcoholic cirrhosis. *Australian Annals of Medicine,* **18,** 222–226.
409. Wilson, D.E., Schreibman, P.H., Brewster, A.C. & Arky, R.A. (1970) The enhancement of alimentary lipemia by ethanol in man. *Journal of Laboratory and Clinical Medicine,* **75,** 264–274.
410. Woodruff, R.A., Clayton, P.J., Cloninger, C.R. & Guze, S.B. (1977) A brief method of screening for alcoholism. *Diseases of the Nervous System,* **37,** 434–435.
411. Yano, K., Rhoads, G.G. & Kagan, A. (1977) Coffee, alcohol and risk of coronary heart disease among Japanese men living in Hawaii. *New England Journal of Medicine,* **297,** 405–409.
412. Yokoo, H., Minick, O.T., Batti, F. & Kent, G. (1972) Morphologic variants of alcoholic hyalin. *American Journal of Pathology,* **69,** 25–40.
413. Zederman, R., Löw, H. & Kerstin Hall (1977) Effect of ethanol and lactate on the basal and glucagon-activated cyclic AMP formation in isolated hepatocytes. *Febs Letters,* **75,** 291–294.
414. Zetterman, R.K., Luisada-Opper, A. & Leevy, C.M. (1976) Alcoholic hepatitis. Cell-mediated immunologic response to alcoholic hyalin. *Gastroenterology,* **70,** 382–384.
415. Zieve, L. (1958) Jaundice, hyperlipemia, and hemolytic anemia: a heretofore unrecognized syndrome associated with alcoholic fatty liver and cirrhosis. *Annals of Internal Medicine,* **48,** 471–496.

Chapter 33

Wilson's Disease

IRMIN STERNLIEB
I. HERBERT SCHEINBERG

DEFINITION

Wilson's disease (hepatolenticular or hepatocerebral degeneration) is a fatal defect in copper metabolism, with a world-wide prevalence of about one in 200 000, and is present in individuals who have inherited a specific pair of abnormal recessive genes. Concentrations of tissue copper, increasing with time, eventually become directly toxic to the liver, brain, kidney and eye and produce indirect pathological changes in several other tissues and organs, including the skeletal system. The liver, however, is unique in being the organ that is not only the most frequently and catastrophically affected by the copper toxicity that constitutes the disease clinically, but is also the site of the aetiological biochemical abnormality. This chapter, therefore, will concern itself almost exclusively with the interrelationship of Wilson's disease and the liver, except where it is patently artificial to omit reference to the neurological effects of a disease that was first recognized and defined by a neurologist, or when inclusion of extrahepatic phenomena is helpful. Curiously, although Wilson[92] denied that the hepatic disease was clinically significant in any of his six patients, not only did three manifest liver disease – indeed, one died of exsanguinating haemorrhage – but Frerichs[23] described cirrhosis in a case reported 51 years earlier.

COPPER METABOLISM AND THE PATHOGENESIS OF WILSON'S DISEASE

At least two distinct homeostatic mechanisms must control the balance and metabolism of copper in man, since Wilson's disease and Menkes' disease are each caused by one of two different genetic defects. In one, a mechanism that seems to control excretion has gone awry and the resulting accumulation of copper causes Wilson's disease. In Menkes' disease, the regulation of the transport of this essential metal from the intestine is faulty and results in fatal deficiency of copper in certain vital organs or tissues that cannot function without this metal.[15]

Despite the abundance of copper in almost every diet, chronic copper toxicosis is seen only in those individuals who possess a pair of 'Wilson's disease genes' because of the extraordinary efficiency of the homeostatic mechanism that controls the balance of copper in individuals with a pair, or even one, of the normal alleles of this gene. While such people remain in virtually zero copper balance throughout life, copper accumulates progressively in the liver of the Wilson's disease patient-to-be, although its positive balance is small, amounting to only about 2 to 3 per cent of the average copper intake (2 to 5 mg/day).

In an individual with normal copper metabolism, about 60 to 90 per cent of an oral dose of radiocopper is deposited in the liver four hours after its ingestion,[73] having been transported there loosely bound to albumin[4] and perhaps to amino acids.[53] Two proteins of the hepatic cytosol, hepatocuprein (superoxide dismutase)[8] and L-6-D (copper LP),[45] incorporate about 80 per cent of the absorbed radiocopper,[79] while 20 per cent is either incorporated into specific copper proteins, such as cytochrome *c* oxidase, or is sequestered by lysosomes before being excreted in bile.

In several studies, the concentration of copper in the bile of patients with Wilson's disease was consistently less than in that of control subjects.[47,79] Frommer[24] found that the patients excreted about 9.5 μmol (0.6 mg) of copper in the bile daily while control subjects excreted about 19 μmol (1.2 mg). The excess copper retained by the patient, though two to four times more than is needed to account for the average accumulation of copper in patients with the disease, suggests that a defect in biliary excretion of the metal causes Wilson's disease.

Sternlieb et al[79] administered radiocopper to a patient with Wilson's disease and to a control subject 18 hours before cholecystectomy. From analyses of bile and biopsy samples of liver taken at operation, it appeared that (1) the hepatic lysosomal fraction of the patient contained 43 times the concentration of copper present in that of the control subject; (2) the biliary concentration of copper in the patient was six times less than in the control; and (3) the specific activity of radiocopper in the bile of the Wilson's disease patient was different from that in every subcellular fraction except that containing lysosomes, to which it was virtually identical. The tentative conclusion from the foregoing is that defective excretion of copper from hepatic lysosomes to bile underlies the accumulation of excess copper in Wilson's disease. In an as yet unexplained fashion, this defect is associated with diminished hepatic synthesis of the plasma copper glycoprotein, caeruloplasmin,[54] but with no abnormality in any of the other dozen or so human copper proteins.[1,10]

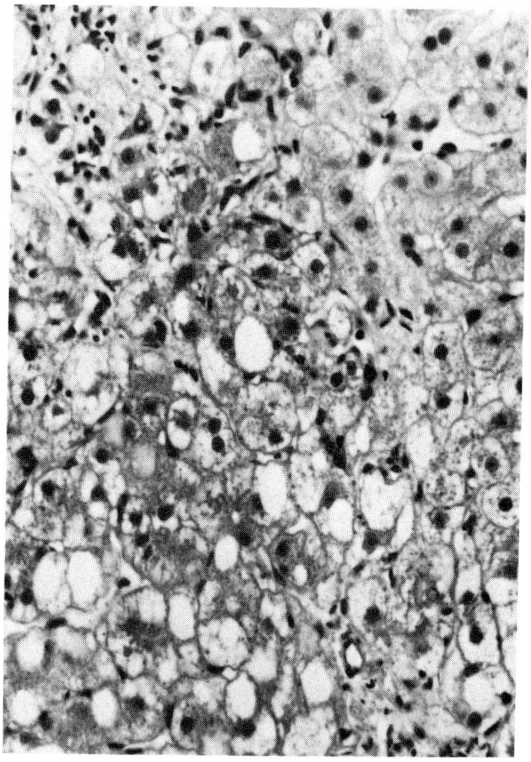

Figure 33.1. Light micrograph of section of liver biopsy specimen obtained from an asymptomatic 13-year-old girl with a six-year history of persistent elevations of aminotransferases. At the time of diagnosis her serum caeruloplasmin concentration was 230 mg/l and the hepatic copper concentration 8.86 μmol/g (563 μg/g) dry tissue. Note fatty changes, prominence of Kupffer cells and scattered mononuclear cell infiltrates. Haematoxylin and eosin. × 250.

NATURAL HISTORY OF WILSON'S DISEASE

The accumulation of toxic amounts of copper begins in infancy, but the deposits are limited for years to the liver.[71] Yet hepatic signs and symptoms never appear before six years of age; neurological effects occur generally later in childhood; and the most usual age of onset of clinical disease is adolescence. Occasionally, a patient may remain in apparent good health until the sixth decade.[20] During these years of latency, as much as 50 times the normal concentration of 30 μg of copper per gram dry liver can be present with no indication of extrahepatic toxicity and only minimal anatomical or functional evidence of damage by copper to the liver itself.[2,56] The full-blown syndrome which Wilson[92] described and named 'progressive lenticular degeneration' is now recognized as including psychiatric manifestations;[31,60] deposits of copper in Descemet's membrane of the cornea, known as Kayser–Fleischer rings;[35] sunflower cataracts; and the renal,[3,26,27] haematological, endocrine, osseous, and articular pathological

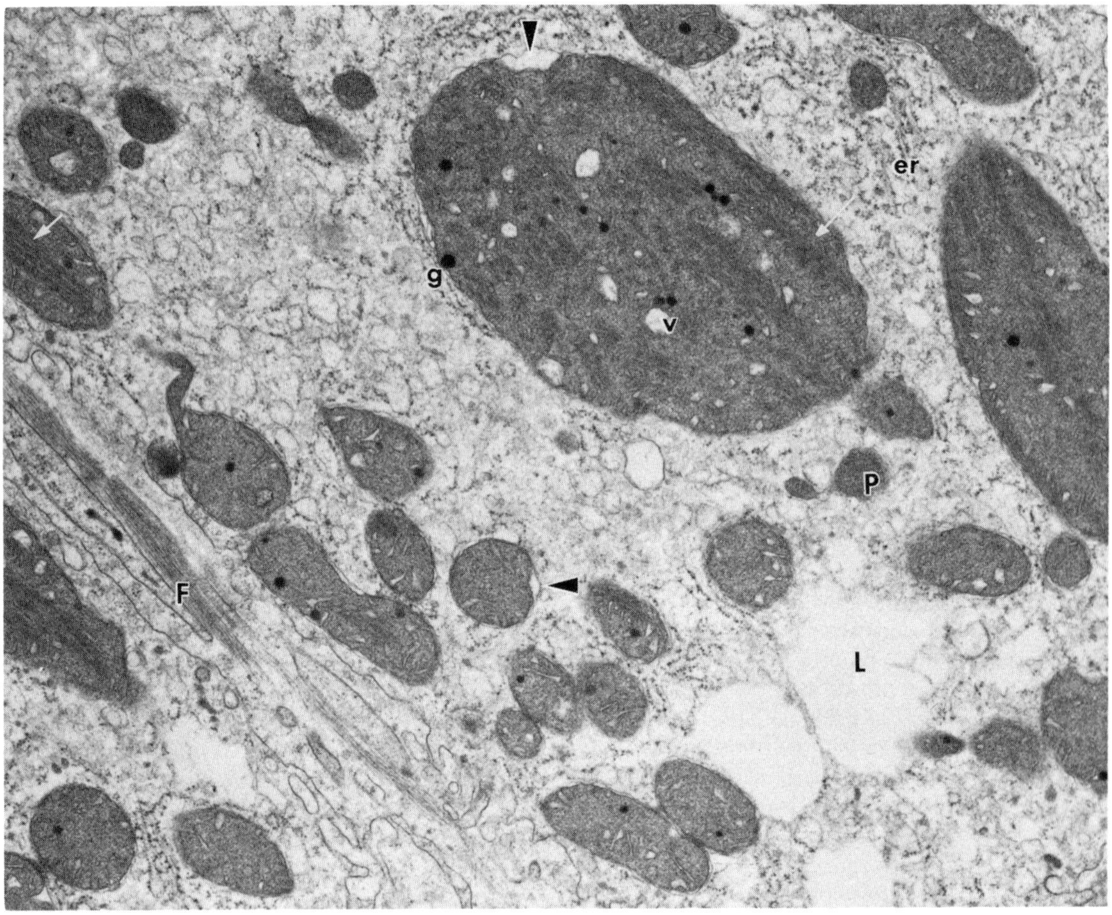

Figure 33.2. Electron micrograph of fine section of liver biopsy specimen, obtained from a 24-year-old woman with symptomatic Wilson's disease, showing portions of two hepatocytes. There is striking pleomorphism of mitochondria that display features noted in the text: v, vacuole in megamitochondrion with distorted and dilated cristae, numerous crystals (white arrows) and enlarged dense granules (g), and separations of outer from inner membranes (arrowheads). F, abnormal bundles of intercellular filaments; L, lipid droplet; er, endoplasmic reticulum. Osmium tetroxide; Epon; uranyl acetate and lead citrate; Siemens Elmiskop Ia. × 28 000.

effects[3, 29, 44] – some direct, some indirect – of copper toxicosis.

ANATOMICAL AND CLINICAL PATHOLOGY

The earliest hepatocellular lesions detectable by light microscopy of liver biopsy samples reveal droplets of triglycerides in the cytoplasm and ballooned nuclei filled with glycogen (Figure 33.1).[2, 56] Occasionally, nuclear ballooning results from cytoplasmic invagination of the nucleus (Chapter 2). At this stage, in spite of its high tissue concentration, copper is only detectable histochemically by sensitive methods, such as Timm's silver sulfide stain, because it is diffusely distributed in the cytoplasm.[28] The effectiveness of the sensitive and more specific rhodanine method[38] has yet to be evaluated. This is also the stage when hepatocellular mitochondria are markedly pleomorphic, and exhibit increased matrix density, separation of the normally apposed inner and outer mitochondrial membranes, widened intercristal spaces, enlarged granules and crystalline, vacuolated or dense inclusions;[64, 65] changes that are probably pathogenetically related to the steatosis (Figure 33.2). In some specimens, the peroxisomes – organelles also involved in cellular lipid metabolism – are enlarged, rounded or misshapen, and contain a granular, flocculent, rather than a homogeneous, matrix (Figure 33.3) of varying electron density.[69]

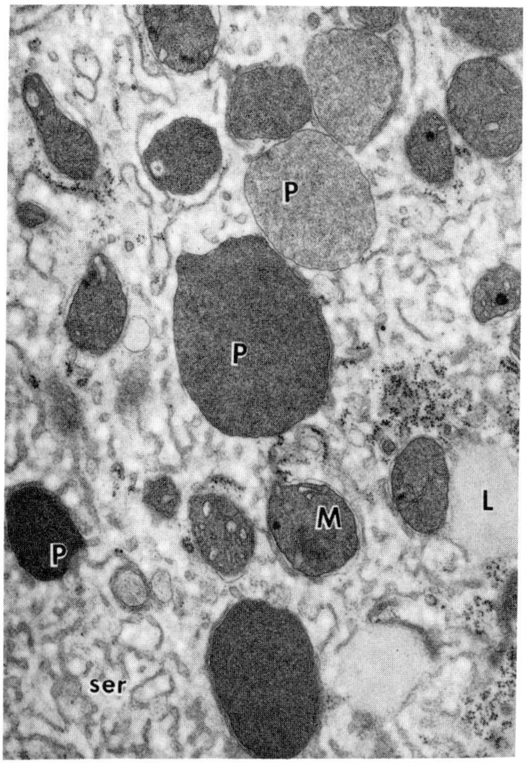

Figure 33.3. Electron micrograph from an eight-year-old asymptomatic boy with Wilson's disease, showing portion of hepatocyte containing a cluster of enlarged, abnormal peroxisomes (P) with matrices of differing electron density. Note that these peroxisomes are considerably larger than the adjacent mitochondria, and contrast with the normal, reverse relationship shown in Figure 33.7. M, mitochondrion; ser, smooth endoplasmic reticulum. Same processing as in Figure 33.2. × 8000.

Often the number of lipolysosomes seems to be increased.[34] Hyperplasia of Kupffer cells is occasionally present. There may be no overt symptoms; nothing more than hepatomegaly; and perhaps a few inconspicuous spider naevi on physical examination and elevations of aminotransferase activities in the blood.

The rate and mode of progression from this initial steatosis to fibrosis and, ultimately, cirrhosis are variable. Modest infiltrates of mononuclear cells are not uncommonly associated with abnormal collagen deposits. In other instances, a clinical and histological picture of chronic active hepatitis with prominent round cell infiltrates, piecemeal necrosis, erosion of marginal plates, Councilman-like bodies and parenchymal collapse develops (Figure 33.4), associated with elevated serum gammaglobulin levels and other evidence of hepatic dysfunction.[72] This florid hepatitis may subside spontaneously, with late evolution towards postnecrotic cirrhosis, or escalate suddenly into fulminant hepatitis, with some hepatocytes displaying Mallory's cytoplasmic hyalin.[2]

Inexplicably, however, many patients, in whom the disease first manifests itself neurologically, give no history whatever of clinical liver disease, though the liver – occasionally slightly enlarged, more often shrunken, with a finely or coarsely nodular surface and bands of fibrous tissue – always shows histological evidence of damage. Round cell infiltrates and abundant proliferated bile ductules may be distributed within the bands of collagen (Figure 33.5). Excess fat and glycogen nuclei may still be found in the hepatocytes of some nodules (Figure 33.6). At this stage, the copper is considerably more easily detectable histochemically because it is now sequestered in hepatocellular lysosomes rather than being diffusely distributed throughout the cytoplasm, and only in certain nodules, others apparently being spared.[28,68]

Now, too, in contrast to the earlier appearance, except for the abundance of lipofuscin granules (Figure 33.7), the ultrastructure of the individual hepatocytes in cirrhotic specimens is almost normal. Collagen fibrils or basement membrane material may be found in sinusoidal spaces and, in some specimens, abnormal separation of hepatocytes and pseudo-glandular formations are seen (Table 33.1).

Hepatocellular carcinoma has been reported in only two,[39,84] or possibly three, patients with Wilson's disease, in striking contrast to its high frequency in haemochromatosis (see Chapter 34).

Extrahepatic pathological changes of major clinical significance are limited to the central nervous system and the kidneys. They are well described by Wilson[92] and other workers.[3,7,40,80,82,89]

CLINICAL MANIFESTATIONS

In 151 symptomatic patients, the initial clinical manifestation was hepatic in 42 per cent; neurological in 34 per cent; psychiatric in 10 per cent; renal in 1 per cent; and haematological or endocrine, secondary to hepatic dysfunction, in 12 per cent. Two or more of these types were seen in about 25 per cent of patients.[58] This

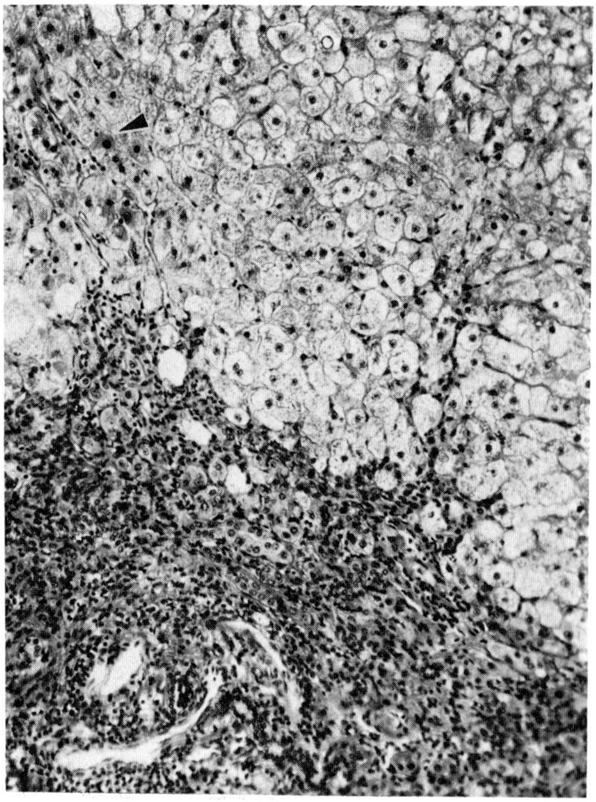

Figure 33.4. Light micrograph of section of surgical liver biopsy specimen obtained from a previously healthy 12-year-old boy three months after the onset of an acute haemolytic episode. Liver dysfunction, Kayser–Fleischer rings and deficiency of serum caeruloplasmin (153.0 mg/l) were found. Liver biopsy revealed a hepatic copper of 15.9 μmol/g (971 μg/g) dry tissue. An abundant round cell infiltrate, erosion of the marginal plate, proliferated bile ductules and an occasional Councilman body (arrowhead) – findings indistinguishable from those of chronic active hepatitis – are evident. There is a vacuolated, glycogen-filled nucleus near the top. Haematoxylin and eosin. ×225.

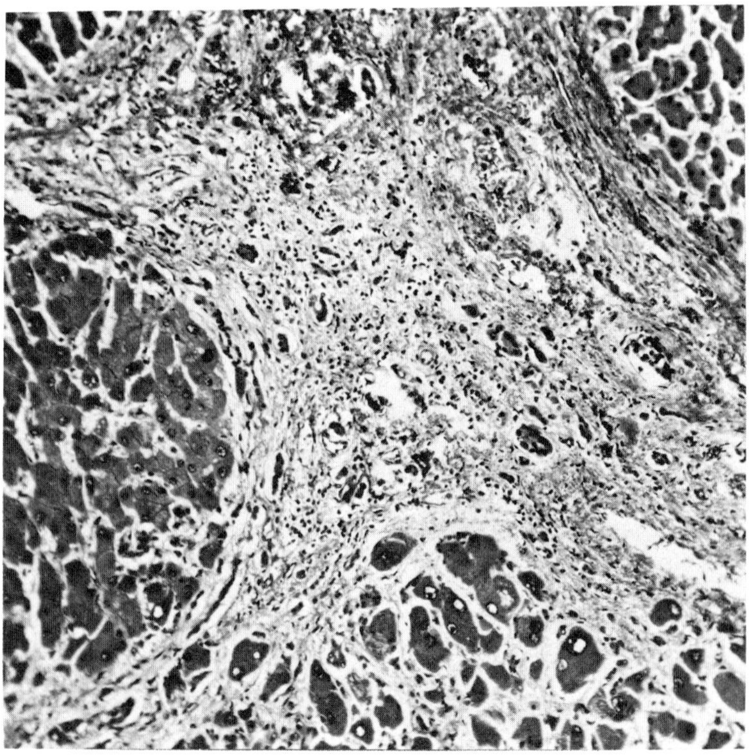

Figure 33.5. Low power light micrograph of histological section of liver obtained at autopsy from a 41-year-old woman with neurological Wilson's disease, who was treated with D-penicillamine for the last three years of her life. In spite of marked neurological improvement hepatic insufficiency developed, causing her death within six months. Broad fibrous septa containing small bile ductules and round cells separate discrete regenerative nodules. Glycogen nuclei and degeneration of hepatocytes are conspicuous in the nodule at the bottom of this illustration. Haematoxylin and eosin. ×150.

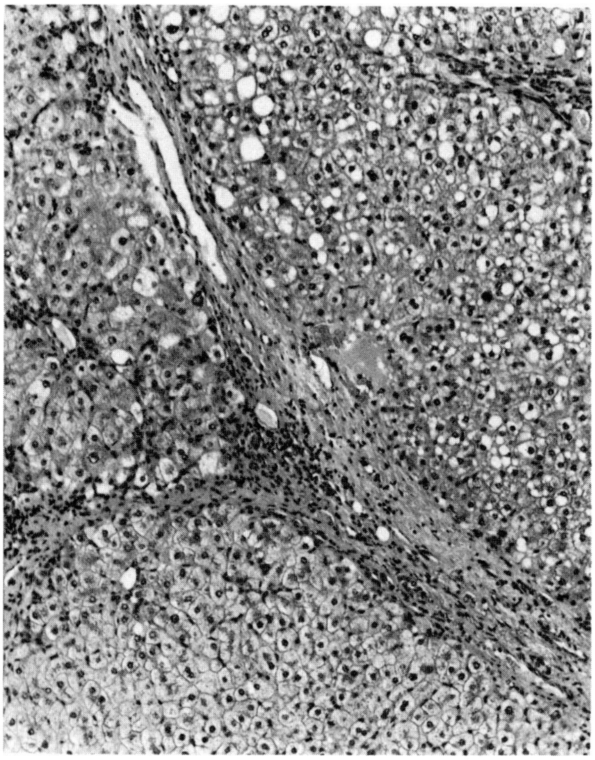

Figure 33.6. Inactive cirrhosis with contrasting appearances of hepatocytes in adjacent nodules, some displaying moderate steatosis, in the liver biopsy specimen obtained from a 15-year-old boy at the time of splenectomy for suspected idiopathic thrombocytopenic purpura. Haematoxylin and eosin. × 125.

distribution of modes of onset is quite similar to that observed by Walshe[89] in a series of European patients.

As expected from the natural history of the disease, the hepatic manifestations – fatigue, lassitude, abdominal pains, spider angiomas, jaundice, oedema, ascites, malnutrition, variceal haemorrhages and splenomegaly – tend to appear at an earlier age than does disease of the CNS. Acute or chronic hepatitis,[72] infectious mononucleosis, juvenile or alcoholic cirrhosis with hepatic encephalopathy, or a rapidly fatal massive hepatic necrosis[43, 52] may be diagnosed instead of Wilson's disease. Abnormalities of liver function may be non-existent or nothing more than elevations of alanine and aspartate aminotransferases (Figure 33.1), or there may be generalized hepatic derangement with hyperbilirubinaemia, hypoalbuminaemia, hypoprothrombinaemia and other laboratory evidence of defective hepatocellular excretion and synthesis. Yet in some patients who have Wilson's disease with advanced neurological manifestations, despite the omnipresent cirrhosis referred to above, almost all liver function tests, including the clearance of bromsulphthalein (BSP), may yield normal results.[61] In these instances, the clearance of infusions of glycine conjugates of cholic acid probably provides the most sensitive indicator of the presence of hepatic pathophysiology.[11]

Bleeding and easy bruising, due to deficiencies of fibrinogen, factors II, V, VII and X and prothrombin, are caused by hepatic insufficiency, portal hypertension and hypersplenism. The last accounts for the leucopenia, anaemia and thrombocytopenia encountered in some patients, although defects in platelet function have also been described.[49] Shortened red cell survival, similar to that seen in other forms of cirrhosis,[14, 81] may be responsible for an apparent increased incidence of bilirubin calculi in patients with Wilson's disease. Hepatic necrosis can release enough copper from the liver to cause a severe, but not invariably fatal, haemolytic anaemia.[16, 51, 52]

Primary or secondary amenorrhoea in women and delayed puberty and gynaecomastia in boys, sometimes the first symptoms for which medical help is sought, are very probably secondary to the hepatic dysfunction since they are usually corrected as the underlying liver disease improves.

Some patients succumb rapidly, after their first clinical manifestation, to a syndrome of massive hepatic necrosis, haemolysis and consequent renal insufficiency, and some exsanguinate from uncontrollable variceal bleeding. Generally, however, physical deterioration and invalidism progress slowly in the untreated patient to hepatic insufficiency, electrolyte imbalance, renal insufficiency, sepsis (often from spontaneous peritonitis or as a complication of surgery) or prolonged coma. In the terminally ill patient it may be impossible to determine the part played by hepatic encephalopathy and that related to cerebral coma.

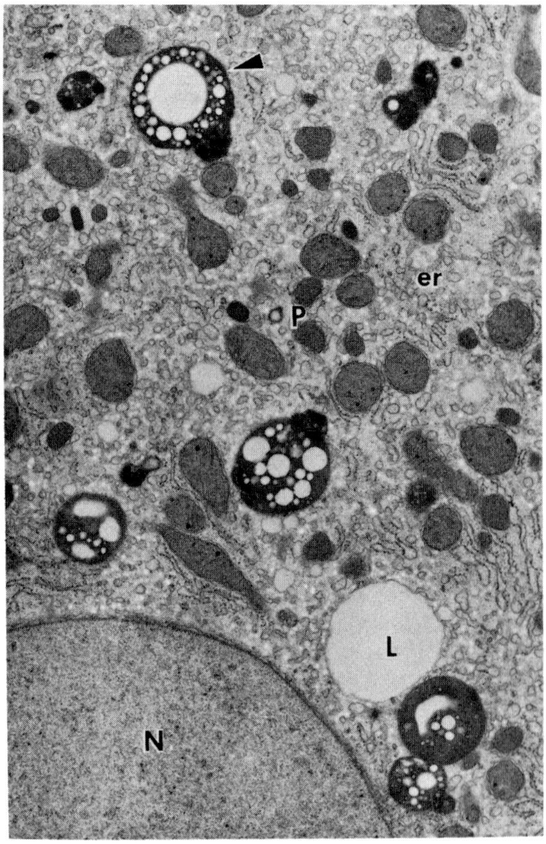

Figure 33.7. Electron micrograph showing portion of hepatocyte from a 14-year-old patient with symptomatic Wilson's disease. The cytoplasmic organelles appear normal, except for the presence of an increased number of peculiar, vacuolated, osmiophilic lysosomal granules (arrowhead). L, lipid; N, nucleus; P, peroxisomes; er, endoplasmic reticulum. Osmium tetroxide; araldite; uranyl acetate and lead citrate; RCA EMU-3H. ×5100.

BIOCHEMICAL ABNORMALITIES

The biochemical abnormalities associated with Wilson's disease can be classified into the primary, and probably direct, effects of the underlying genetic defect, and the secondary abnormalities resulting from copper toxicosis of various organs and tissues.

Primary abnormalities

Deficiency of caeruloplasmin. This blue copper glycoprotein possessing oxidase activity toward a number of substrates is present in the plasma of normal, healthy adults in a concentration of 200 to 400 mg/l. Since in vivo the protein irreversibly binds a constant 0.3 per cent of copper, by weight, 9.5 to 19 μmol/l (60 to 120 μg/dl) of copper will necessarily be present in the plasma of these subjects, with rarely more than an additional 0.8 to 1.6 μmol/l (5 to 10 μg/dl) of non-caeruloplasmin copper.[55] Ninety-five per cent of patients with Wilson's disease exhibit concentrations of caeruloplasmin below 200 mg/l at the time of diagnosis (Table 33.2). The low normal concentrations of caeruloplasmin (usually between 200 and 300 mg/l) found in the others may represent a temporary result of the stimulus to synthesis of caeruloplasmin, which is an acute phase reactant, provided by the inflammatory process in the liver (or elsewhere) or by an excess of circulating oestrogens. Treatment with D-penicillamine is frequently followed by a further reduction of the concentration of caeruloplasmin in plasma.[58]

About 10 per cent of heterozygous carriers of one Wilson's disease gene also exhibit hypocaeruloplasminaemia (Table 33.1). Neither structural differences between caeruloplasmin from normal subjects and patients with Wilson's disease,[46] nor the presence of low concentrations of apocaeruloplasmin in patients,[37] nor quantitative discrepancies between the oxidase activity in plasma[36] and the amount of material precipitable by antibodies to caeruloplasmin[32] have been confirmed to be characteristic of the disorder.

Excess of hepatic copper. Normal human hepatic copper concentrations are between 0.3 and 0.8 μmol/g (20 and 50 μg/g) dry liver. Untreated patients with Wilson's disease almost always exhibit from 4 to 47 μmol/g (250 to 3000 μg) of copper per gram of dry hepatic biopsy sample.[10,13,71] Rare lower values, as low as 1.6 μmol/g (100 μg/g), are probably due to sampling since the copper is not uniformly

Table 33.1. *Pathological Features Observed in Livers of Patients at Three Stages of the Evolution of Wilson's Disease.*

	Early	Intermediate ('acute')	Late
Size	Normal or enlarged	Normal, irregularly enlarged, or shrunken	Normal or shrunken
Gross appearance	±Normal	Finely or coarsely nodular	Hobnailed
Histological characteristics	Fatty changes, inflammation, fibrosis	Collapse of parenchyma, fibrosis, mesenchymal infiltration, proliferation of bile ductules	Cirrhosis
Predominant hepatocellular abnormalities	Fatty changes	Scattered fatty changes, necrosis, Councilman or Mallory bodies	Pigment granules
Abnormalities of organelles	In mitochondria and peroxisomes	Insufficiently studied	Excess lipofuscin
Copper concentration, dry wt, mean±s.d. (n)	15.47±5.79 μmol/g (983±368 μg/g) (36)	Insufficiently studied	7.76±4.09 μmol/g (493±260 μg/g) (21)
Copper distribution	Diffuse in cytoplasm	Diffuse in some lobules, concentrated in lysosomes in others	Concentrated in lysosomes
Rubeanic acid stain (specific)	Negative	May be positive	Positive
Timm's silver sulfide (not specific)	Positive	Positive	Positive

From Sternlieb and Scheinberg,[74] with kind permission of the editor of Intercontinental Book Corporation.

distributed throughout the liver. Concentrations indistinguishable from those of Wilson's disease are seen in patients with biliary cirrhosis and chronic cholestasis.[21]

Heterozygous carriers of one Wilson's disease gene who never show signs of copper toxicosis may nevertheless show slightly elevated concentrations of hepatic copper, and occasionally this reaches 4 μmol/g (250 μg/g) dry liver.[71]

Excess of non-caeruloplasmin serum copper. This copper, often termed 'free' despite its loose binding to albumin or amino acids of serum, can be as high as 8 μmol/l (50 μg/dl). It almost surely represents excess copper that has diffused from liver to blood. Since Wilson's disease is characterized by a reduction in caeruloplasmin copper and an increase in non-caeruloplasmin copper, total serum copper may be only slightly less than normal.[9] Non-caeruloplasmin copper may not be increased in untreated asymptomatic patients because their excess copper is still confined in the liver.

Excess of urinary copper. The normal subject excretes about 0.47 μmol/24 hr (30 μg/24 hr) of copper in the urine. Almost all symptomatic patients with Wilson's disease excrete in excess of 1.6 μmol/24 hr (100 μg/24 hr)[9] which is derived from the non-caeruloplasmin copper in serum. Considerably larger amounts are excreted when massive necrosis suddenly releases much copper from hepatic stores.

Decreased incorporation of radiocopper into caeruloplasmin. Following oral administration of radiocopper to a normal subject, the concentration of non-caeruloplasmin radiocopper in plasma rises rapidly, reaching a maximum in one to two hours; then falls; and rises again, over the next two days, as caeruloplasmin copper, to a concentration exceeding that reached initially by the non-caeruloplasmin nuclide.[5,73,77,78] In patients with Wilson's disease there is little or no incorporation of radiocopper into newly synthesized caeruloplasmin, while in heterozygotes incorporation is intermediate between that seen in control subjects and patients with Wilson's disease.[48,74,78]

Secondary abnormalities

In addition to the effects of copper toxicosis on the liver (considered now as a target organ), renal dysfunction, due to copper-induced

Table 33.2. *Distribution of Serum Caeruloplasmin Concentrations in 273 Symptomatic Homozygotes and 88 Obligatory Heterozygotes[a] for the Wilson's Disease Gene.*

Range of serum caeruloplasmin concentrations mg/l	Homozygotes %	Heterozygotes %
0–9	22	0
10–49	28.9	1.1
50–99	24.6	1.1
100–149	12.8	2.3
150–199	6.6	15.9
>200	5.1	79.6

[a]Parents and offspring of homozygotes.

glomerular or tubular damage, can be manifested as haematuria, aminoaciduria, uricosuria (often with hypo-uricaemia), renal glycosuria, phosphaturia (with hypophosphataemia), hypercalciuria, proteinuria and/or renal tubular acidosis.[3,6,26,42]

DIAGNOSIS

Patients with neurological manifestations. There should be no difficulty in establishing a diagnosis of Wilson's disease in patients with clear-cut neurological manifestations. Kayser–Fleischer rings[35,62] always accompany neurological Wilson's disease, and serum caeruloplasmin concentrations below 200 mg/l are seen in 95 per cent of these patients.[54] If Kayser–Fleischer rings are absent, on slit-lamp examination by an ophthalmologist, in patients with neurological signs, the patient does not have Wilson's disease.

Patients with hepatic manifestations. In patients with liver disease, a family history of Wilson's disease, fatal hepatitis or juvenile cirrhosis; absence of a history of relevant exposure and lack of prodromal symptoms of viral hepatitis; a poor response to customary therapeutic measures; a protracted course; the presence of neurological abnormalities, such as a fixed grin (sometimes mistaken for an ingratiating effort); behavioural changes; or, above all, the presence of an unexplained haemolytic process with anaemia, should alert the physician to the possibility that Wilson's disease is the diagnosis.

Most, but not all, Wilsonian patients presenting with a clinical picture resembling acute or chronic hepatitis, juvenile cirrhosis or other hepatic disorders have Kayser–Fleischer rings, low serum caeruloplasmin concentrations and a urinary copper excretion in excess of 1.57 μmol/24 hr (100 μg/24 hr). But any one, or even two, of these characteristic findings may be absent. Moreover, the combination of Kayser–Fleischer-like rings, elevated hepatic copper concentration and increased urinary copper excretion is seen in some patients suffering from primary biliary cirrhosis or chronic cholestatic syndromes,[21,22,25] though almost always with elevated serum caeruloplasmin concentrations which should suggest that Wilson's disease is not the diagnosis.[41] Furthermore, the correct diagnosis can generally be made on clinical and histopathological grounds. If uncertainty remains, or if biopsy is precluded by clotting abnormalities or other clinical considerations, measurement of the incorporation of radiocopper into caeruloplasmin will almost always settle the question (Figure 33.8).[73,78]

In patients who present with massive hepatic necrosis, but without Kayser–Fleischer rings, a low serum caeruloplasmin concentration is not sufficient to establish a diagnosis of Wilson's disease, since marked depression of synthesis, due to hepatic necrosis of any aetiology, can cause temporary hypocaeruloplasminaemia.[91]

Except in patients in whom rigidity of the abdominal muscles limits palpation, scintiscans with $^{99}Tc^{m}$ sulphur colloid contribute little to the diagnosis beyond the information regarding the configuration and sizes of liver and spleen. Radiocopper scans are also of limited clinical value. Correlated measurements of portal and wedged hepatic vein pressures may suggest the existence of a presinusoidal block in patients with Wilson's disease.

Asymptomatic patients. It is mandatory that all siblings and children of patients with Wilson's disease be screened for the disorder and it is desirable to do this in any blood relative. Slit-lamp examination of the cornea and a measurement of serum caeruloplasmin concentration will be sufficient in most adults, but serum aminotransferase activities should also be determined in children who may have asymptomatic hepatic Wilson's disease. Measurement of urinary copper excretion is unreliable for screening relatives of patients.

If a concentration of caeruloplasmin of less than 200 mg/l of serum is found (a necessary, but not sufficient, criterion for diagnosis, since about 10 per cent of heterozygous carriers exhibit caeruloplasmin deficiency), or if either of

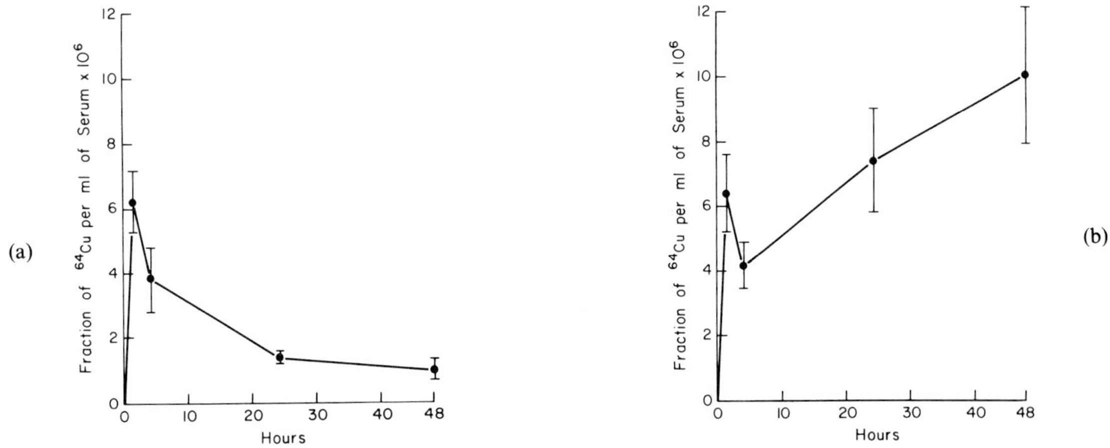

Figure 33.8. Mean $\pm$s.e. of the concentrations of ^{64}Cu in whole serum vs time following the oral administration of 2 mg of ^{64}Cu ion in eight patients with Wilson's disease with serum caeruloplasmin concentrations ranging from 151 to 293 mg/l (Figure 33.8a) and in 10 patients with other types of liver disease who were suspected of suffering from Wilson's disease because of confusing laboratory or clinical findings (Figure 33.8b). Their caeruloplasmin concentrations ranged from 245 to 571 mg/l. Samples of serum were obtained at 1, 2, 4, 24 and 48 hours and measured for radioactivity. The higher value at either 1 or 2 hours was selected for the calculation of the mean $\pm$s.e. of the initial peak. Note the positive slope of ^{64}Cu, indicating incorporation of the isotope into caeruloplasmin in the non-Wilsonian patients, in contrast to the low concentration of ^{64}Cu at 48 hours in the patients with Wilson's disease. The mean $\pm$s.e. of the ratio (R) of the concentrations of ^{64}Cu at 48 hours to the initial peak in the non-Wilsonian patients (2.02 ± 0.58) is strikingly different from that of the patients with Wilson's disease (0.21 ± 0.08). (Sternlieb and Scheinberg, 1977, unpublished observations.)

the two other tests yield abnormal results in a blood relative of a patient, analyses of a hepatic biopsy sample for copper, quantitatively, and for histological changes by light (and, if possible, electron) microscopy are required. A concentration in excess of 250 μg/g dry liver confirms the diagnosis of Wilson's disease in a hypocaeruloplasminaemic subject[66, 71] and histopathological changes in the biopsy sample will be found in the great majority of biopsy samples from such patients.

TREATMENT

With the introduction of BAL (2,3-dimercaptopropanol)[12, 18] and penicillamine[85] the relentless progression of Wilson's disease to illness, disability and death has been drastically changed. These agents increase the output of copper in the urine, thereby reducing the concentration of the metal in the body; they reverse clinical abnormalities in the majority of symptomatic patients, and prevent the appearance of overt disease in the asymptomatic patient.[57, 86] Numerous studies have established D-penicillamine as the drug of choice.[17, 30, 57, 89] Improvement of neurological, hepatic and psychiatric abnormalities may often lead to health and activity that are normal in all observable respects. In asymptomatic patients, effective prevention of clinical disease requires adherence to the therapeutic regimen indefinitely.[66]

The initial daily dose of 1 to 2 g D-penicillamine produces urinary copper excretion of several milligrams, though the cupriuresis diminishes with time as less tissue copper is available for chelation.[57] To maximize the cupriuretic effect, the drug is administered in four divided doses, on an empty stomach, about half an hour before meals and before retiring. In some patients a gratifying response to therapy occurs in a matter of weeks, but in others temporary worsening of neurological symptoms may be observed for several months before improvement takes place.[30, 89] When therapy produces disappointing results, particularly in a severely ill patient, the daily dosage of penicillamine can be increased, for a period of several weeks, to as much as 4 g. Short courses of daily intramuscular injections of BAL (3 ml of 10 per cent suspension) may also be beneficial in very sick patients. For the long term, a daily dose of penicillamine greater than 1 g is not advisable.

A low copper diet, in which a few foods with a particularly high copper content (liver, shellfish, mushrooms, nuts and chocolate) are limited, may be of value.

When oedema, ascites or anasarca is present, non-specific therapy, i.e. restriction of salt intake, spironolactone and diuretics, should be instituted. Vitamin K supplementation is often ineffective in correcting the hypoprothrombinaemia. Salt-poor albumin infusions may be of benefit as a temporary measure in severely hypo-albuminaemic patients.

When symptoms are controlled, usually after years of therapy, and the patient's condition is stable, the dosage of D-penicillamine can be reduced to 0·75 g daily. But administration of penicillamine must be lifelong since withdrawal of the drug can be fatal. Even temporary interruption of therapy should be avoided since sensitivity may occur on its re-institution. Fading or disappearance of Kayser–Fleischer rings provides visible evidence that copper removal is occurring and is commonly seen in younger patients.[83] The rings may not change, however, in spite of marked clinical improvement. Abnormalities of liver function may be slow in subsiding, but generally abate within a year. Improvement, even disappearance, of cytological abnormalities can also be demonstrated in treated patients.[67] Therapy should be continued during pregnancy.[59,90]

Apart from monitoring the cupriuretic response of D-penicillamine at intervals of a few months, the most useful indicator of both the drug's continued effectiveness and the patient's faithfulness to the prescribed regimen is the reduction in the concentration of non-caeruloplasmin plasma copper to virtually zero. This concentration is the difference between that of total serum copper, and that of caeruloplasmin copper, and can be calculated only if both measurements are made.

About 20 per cent of patients experience sensitivity reactions to D-penicillamine and these occur within the first few weeks of treatment, most often between the seventh and twelfth days. Fever, erythematous eruptions, urticaria, lymphadenopathy, malaise, leukopenia or thrombocytopenia, or any combination of these, can occur. All are reversible if the drug is promptly discontinued. The patient can always be desensitized if slowly increasing doses of D-penicillamine are given together with 20 to 30 mg of prednisone, though there may be several bouts of sensitivity, requiring cessation of penicillamine administration, before the drug can be given successfully after prednisone has been tapered to zero. During the first six to eight weeks of treatment, white blood cell and platelet counts should be obtained twice weekly; at monthly intervals for the next four months; and at longer intervals thereafter. Routine urinalysis, in addition to occasional determinations of 24-hour urinary copper output, should be carried out when blood counts are obtained.

Small doses of pyridoxine, 25 mg daily at most, should be given to patients in order to compensate for the weak anti-pyridoxine effect of D-penicillamine. In growing children and menstruating women occasional iron supplements may be required, but the administration of mineral or vitamin supplements is unnecessary in the absence of appropriate clinical indications.

Nausea, temporary loss of taste, friability of the skin,[70] aphthous lesions of the mouth, arthralgias and elastosis perforans serpiginosa[50] are comparatively minor side-effects of D-penicillamine. However, D-penicillamine can produce the nephrotic syndrome,[63] fatal Goodpasture's syndrome[75] or disseminated lupus erythematosus.[89] The appearance, or the exacerbation, of pre-treatment proteinuria (several grams daily) or haematuria (of significant degree) requires discontinuation of D-penicillamine therapy. Lupus, or troublesome arthralgias, however, may generally be kept in check with small doses of prednisone while continuing D-penicillamine at a reduced dose.

If intolerance to D-penicillamine is serious, triethylenetetramine, a chelating agent developed by Walshe,[87] can be substituted. Although its cupriuretic effect is less marked than that of D-penicillamine, it seems to be clinically effective.[89]

The asymptomatic patient must be treated for life, and just as diligently as the overtly ill patient.

Surgery

Untreated patients with Wilson's disease tolerate major surgical procedures poorly. In particular, the creation of a portasystemic shunt or splenectomy should be avoided since either is frequently followed by neurological deterioration and death.[76]

The indications for other elective surgery should be carefully evaluated and when necessary – for example, for cholelithiasis or cancer – the dosage of D-penicillamine should be reduced temporarily in order to minimize the effects of the drug on cross-linking of collagen and wound-healing.

Long-term survival, by now six years, of one boy with Wilson's disease, in whom an orthotopic liver transplant was performed, has been reported.[33]

REFERENCES

1. Alexander, N.M. & Benson, G.D. (1975) Superoxide dismutase activity (erythrocuprein) in Wilson's disease. *Life Sciences,* **16,** 1025–1032.
2. Anderson, P.J. & Popper, H. (1960) Changes in hepatic structure in Wilson's disease. *American Journal of Pathology,* **36,** 483–497.
3. Bearn, A.G. (1972) Wilson's disease. In *The Metabolic Basis of Inherited Disease,* 3rd ed. (Ed.) Stanbury, J.G. & Fredrickson, D.S., pp. 1033–1050. New York: McGraw Hill.
4. Bearn, A.G. & Kunkel, H.G. (1954) Localization of Cu^{64} in serum fractions following oral administration: an alteration in Wilson's disease. *Proceedings of the Society for Experimental Biology and Medicine,* **85,** 44–48.
5. Bearn, A.G. & Kunkel, H.G. (1955) Metabolic studies in Wilson's disease using Cu^{64}. *Journal of Laboratory and Clinical Medicine,* **45,** 623–631.
6. Bearn, A.G., Yü, T.-F. & Gutman, A.B. (1957) Renal function in Wilson's disease. *Journal of Clinical Investigation,* **36,** 1107–1114.
7. Boudin, G. & Pepin, B. (1959) *Dégénérescence Hépatolenticulaire.* Paris: Masson.
8. Carrico, R.J. & Deutsch, H.F. (1969) Isolation of human hepatocuprein and cerebrocuprein. Their identity with erythrocuprein. *Journal of Biological Chemistry,* **244,** 6087–6093.
9. Cartwright, G.E., Hodges, R.E., Gubler, C.J., Mahoney, J.P., Daum, K., Wintrobe, M.M. & Bean, W.B. (1954) Studies on copper metabolism. XIII. Hepatolenticular degeneration. *Journal of Clinical Investigation,* **33,** 1487–1501.
10. Committee on Medical and Biologic Effects of Environmental Pollutants (1977) *Copper.* Washington: National Academy of Sciences.
11. Cowen, A.E., Korman, M.G., Hofmann, A.F. & Goldstein, N.P. (1975) Biliary bile acid composition in Wilson's disease. *Mayo Clinic Proceedings,* **50,** 229–233.
12. Cumings, J.N. (1951) The effects of B.A.L. in hepatolenticular degeneration. *Brain,* **74,** 10–22.
13. Cumings, J.N. (1959) *Heavy Metals and the Brain.* Springfield: C. Thomas.
14. Czlonkowska, A. (1972) A study of haemolysis in Wilson's disease. *Journal of the Neurological Sciences,* **16,** 303–314.
15. Danks, D.M., Cartwright, E., Stevens, B.J. & Townley, R.R.W. (1973) Menkes' kinky-hair disease: further definition of the defect in copper transport. *Science,* **179,** 1140–1142.
16. Deiss, A.G., Lee, G.R. & Cartwright, G.E. (1970) Hemolytic anemia in Wilson's disease. *Annals of Internal Medicine,* **73,** 413–418.
17. Deiss, A., Lynch, R.E., Lee, G.R. & Cartwright, G.E. (1971) Long-term therapy of Wilson's disease. *Annals of Internal Medicine,* **75,** 57–65.
18. Denny-Brown, D. & Porter, H. (1951) The effect of BAL (2,3-dimercaptopropanol) on hepatolenticular degeneration (Wilson's disease). *New England Journal of Medicine,* **245,** 917–925.
19. Finby, N. & Bearn, A.G. (1958) Roentgenographic abnormalities of the skeletal system in Wilson's disease (Hepatolenticular degeneration). *American Journal of Roentgenology,* **79,** 603–611.
20. Fitzgerald, M.A., Gross, J.B., Goldstein, N.P., Wahner, H.W. & McCall, J.T. (1975) Wilson's disease (hepatolenticular degeneration) of late adult onset. *Mayo Clinic Proceedings,* **50,** 438–442.
21. Fleming, C.R., Dickson, E.R., Baggenstoss, A.H. & McCall, J.T. (1974) Copper and primary biliary cirrhosis. *Gastroenterology,* **67,** 1152–1187.
22. Fleming, C.R., Dickson, E.R., Wahner, H.W., Hollenhorst, R.W. & McCall, J.T. (1977) Pigmented corneal rings in non-Wilsonian liver disease. *Annals of Internal Medicine,* **86,** 285–288.
23. Frerichs, F.T. (1861) *A Clinical Treatise on Diseases of the Liver,* Vol. II, pp. 60–62, London: The New Sydenham Society.
24. Frommer, D.J. (1974) Defective biliary excretion of copper in Wilson's disease. *Gut,* **15,** 125–129.
25. Frommer, D.J., Morris, J., Sherlock, S., Abrams, J. & Newman, S. (1977) Kayser–Fleischer-like rings in patients without Wilson's disease. *Gastroenterology,* **72,** 1331–1335.
26. Fulop, M., Sternlieb, I. & Scheinberg, I.H. (1968) Defective urinary acidification in Wilson's disease. *Annals of Internal Medicine,* **68,** 770–777.
27. Gilsanz, V., Barrera, A. & Anaya, A. (1960) The renal biopsy in Wilson's disease. *American Medical Association Archives of Internal Medicine,* **105,** 758–761.
28. Goldfischer, S. & Sternlieb, I. (1968) Changes in the distribution of hepatic copper in relation to the progression of Wilson's disease (hepatolenticular degeneration). *American Journal of Pathology,* **53,** 883–901.
29. Golding, D.N. & Walshe, J.M. (1977) Arthropathy of Wilson's disease. *Annals of the Rheumatic Diseases,* **36,** 99–111.
30. Goldstein, N.P. & Gross, J.B. (1977) Treatment of Wilson's disease. In *Clinical Neuropharmacology,* Vol. 2 (Ed.) Klawans, H.L., pp. 99–112, New York: Raven Press.
31. Goldstein, N.P., Ewert, J.C., Randall, R.V. & Gross, J.B. (1968) Psychiatric aspects of Wilson's disease (hepatolenticular degeneration): results of psychometric tests during long-term therapy. *American Journal of Psychiatry,* **124,** 1555–1561.
32. Gollan, J.L., Stocks, J., Dormandy, T.L. & Sherlock, S. (1977) Reduced oxidase activity in the caeruloplasmin of two families with Wilson's disease. *Journal of Clinical Pathology,* **30,** 81–83.
33. Groth, C.G., Dubois, R.S., Corman, J., Halgrimson, C., Rodgerson, D.O. & Starzl, T.E. (1973) Hepatic transplantation in Wilson disease. In *Enzyme Therapy in Genetic Diseases. Birth Defects Original Article Series,* Vol. IX, No. 2. New York: The National Foundation.
34. Hayashi, H. & Sternlieb, I. (1975) Lipolysosomes in human hepatocytes. Ultrastructural and cytochemical studies of patients with Wilson's disease. *Laboratory Investigation,* **33,** 1–7.
35. Herron, B.E. (1976) Wilson's disease (hepatolenticular degeneration). *Ophthalmic Seminars,* **1,** 63–99.
36. Holmberg, C.G. & Laurell, C.-B. (1951) Oxidase reactions in human plasma caused by caeruloplasmin. *Scandinavian Journal of Clinical and Laboratory Investigation,* **3,** 105–107.

37. Holtzman, N.A. & Gaumnitz, B.M. (1970) Identification of an apoceruloplasmin like substance in the plasma of copper-deficient rats. *Journal of Biological Chemistry*, **245**, 2350–2353.
38. Irons, R.D., Schenk, E.A. & Lee, J.C.K. (1977) Cytochemical methods for copper. *Archives of Pathology and Laboratory Medicine*, **101**, 298–301.
39. Kamakura, K., Kimura, S., Igarashi, S., Fujiwara, K., Oda, T., Yoshitoshi, Y. & Shoti, S. (1975) A case of Wilson's disease with hepatoma. *Journal of the Japanese Society of Internal Medicine*, **64**, 232–238.
40. Konovalov, N.V. (1960) *Hepatolenticular Degeneration.* Moscow: Medgiz (in Russian).
41. LaRusso, N.F., Summerskill, W.H.J. & McCall, J.T. (1976) Abnormalities of chemical tests for copper metabolism in chronic active liver disease: differentiation from Wilson's disease. *Gastroenterology*, **70**, 653–655.
42. Leu, M.L., Strickland, G.T. & Gutman, R.A. (1970) Renal function in Wilson's disease: response to penicillamine therapy. *American Journal of the Medical Sciences*, **260**, 381–398.
43. McIntyre, N., Clink, H.M., Levi, A.J., Cumings, J.N. & Sherlock, S. (1967) Hemolytic anemia in Wilson's disease. *New England Journal of Medicine*, **276**, 439–444.
44. Mindelzun, R., Elkin, M., Scheinberg, I.H. & Sternlieb, I. (1970) Skeletal changes in Wilson's disease. A radiologic study. *Radiology*, **94**, 127–134.
45. Morell, A.G., Shapiro, J.R. & Scheinberg, I.H. (1961) Copper binding protein of human liver. In *Wilson's Disease. Some Current Concepts* (Ed.) Walshe, J.M. & Cumings, J.N., pp. 36–42. Oxford: Blackwell Scientific Publications.
46. Neifakh, S.A., Vasiletz, I.M. & Shavlovsky, M.M. (1972) Molecular pathology of ceruloplasmin. *Biochemical Genetics*, **6**, 231–238.
47. O'Reilly, S., Weber, P.M., Oswald, M. & Shipley, L. (1971) Abnormalities of the physiology of copper in Wilson's disease. III. The excretion of copper. *Archives of Neurology*, **25**, 28–32.
48. Osborn, S.B. & Walshe, J.M. (1967) Studies with radioactive copper (^{64}Cu and ^{67}Cu) in relation to the natural history of Wilson's disease. *Lancet*, **i**, 346–350.
49. Owen, C.A., Goldstein, N.P. & Bowie, E.J.W. (1976) Platelet function and coagulation in patients with Wilson's disease. *Archives of Internal Medicine*, **136**, 148–152.
50. Pass, F., Goldfischer, S., Sternlieb, I. & Scheinberg, I.H. (1973) Elastosis perforans serpiginosa during penicillamine therapy for Wilson's disease. *Archives of Dermatology* (Chicago), **108**, 713–715.
51. Robitaille, G.A., Piscatelli, R.L., Majeski, E.J. & Gelehrter, T.D. (1977) Hemolytic anemia in Wilson's disease. *Journal of the American Medical Association*, **237**, 2402–2403.
52. Roche-Sicot, J. & Benhamou, J.-P. (1977) Acute intravascular hemolysis and acute liver failure associated as a first manifestation of Wilson's disease. *Annals of Internal Medicine*, **83**, 301–303.
53. Sass-Kortsak, A. (1965) Copper metabolism. *Advances in Clinical Chemistry*, **8**, 1–67.
54. Scheinberg, I.H. & Gitlin, D. (1952) Deficiency of ceruloplasmin in patients with hepatolenticular degeneration (Wilson's disease). *Science*, **116**, 484–485.
55. Scheinberg, I.H. & Morell, A.G. (1973) Ceruloplasmin. In *Inorganic Biochemistry* (Ed.) Eichhorn, G.L., pp. 306–319. Amsterdam: Elsevier.
56. Scheinberg, I.H. & Sternlieb, I. (1959) The liver in Wilson's disease. *Gastroenterology*, **37**, 550–564.
57. Scheinberg, I.H. & Sternlieb, I. (1960) The long term management of hepatolenticular degeneration (Wilson's disease). *American Journal of Medicine*, **29**, 316–333.
58. Scheinberg, I.H. & Sternlieb, I. (1975) Unpublished observations.
59. Scheinberg, I.H. & Sternlieb, I. (1975) Pregnancy in penicillamine-treated patients with Wilson's disease. *New England Journal of Medicine*, **293**, 1300–1302.
60. Scheinberg, I.H., Sternlieb, I. & Richman, J. (1968) Psychiatric manifestations in patients with Wilson's disease. In *Wilson's Disease* (Ed.) Bergsma, D., Scheinberg, I.H. & Sternlieb, I., pp. 85–87. New York: The National Foundation–March of Dimes.
61. Schoenfield, L.J., Onstad, G.R. & Goldstein, N.P. (1970) Normal sulfobromophthalein retention in established liver disease. *American Journal of Digestive Diseases*, **15**, 337–342.
62. Sternlieb, I. (1966) The Kayser–Fleischer ring. *Medical Radiography and Photography*, **42**, 14–15.
63. Sternlieb, I. (1966) Penicillamine and the nephrotic syndrome. *Journal of the American Medical Association*, **198**, 1311–1312.
64. Sternlieb, I. (1968) Mitochondrial and fatty changes in hepatocytes of patients with Wilson's disease. *Gastroenterology*, **55**, 354–367.
65. Sternlieb, I. (1972) Evolution of the hepatic lesion in Wilson's disease (hepatolenticular degeneration). In *Progress in Liver Diseases* (Ed.) Popper, H. & Schaffner, F., Vol. 4, pp. 511–525. New York: Grune & Stratton.
66. Sternlieb, I. (1976) Present status of diagnosis and prophylaxis of asymptomatic patients with Wilson's disease. In *Diseases of the Liver and Biliary Tract* (Ed.) Leevy, C.M., pp. 137–142. Basel: Karger.
67. Sternlieb, I. & Feldmann, G. (1976) Effect of anticopper therapy on hepatocellular mitochondria in patients with Wilson's disease. *Gastroenterology*, **71**, 457–461.
68. Sternlieb, I. & Goldfischer, S. (1976) Heavy metals and lysosomes. In *Lysosomes in Biology and Pathology*, Vol. 5. (Ed.) Dingle, J.T. & Dean, R.T., Ch. 7, pp. 185–200. Oxford: North Holland.
69. Sternlieb, I. & Quintana, N. (1977) The peroxisomes of human hepatocytes. *Laboratory Investigation*, **36**, 140–149.
70. Sternlieb, I. & Scheinberg, I.H. (1964) Penicillamine therapy in hepatolenticular degeneration. *Journal of the American Medical Association*, **189**, 748–754.
71. Sternlieb, I. & Scheinberg, I.H. (1968) Prevention of Wilson's disease in asymptomatic patients. *New England Journal of Medicine*, **278**, 352–359.
72. Sternlieb, I. & Scheinberg, I.H. (1972) Chronic hepatitis as a first manifestation of Wilson's disease. *Annals of Internal Medicine*, **76**, 59–64.
73. Sternlieb, I. & Scheinberg, I.H. (1972) Radiocopper in diagnosing liver disease. *Seminars in Nuclear Medicine*, **2**, 176–188.
74. Sternlieb, I. & Scheinberg, I.H. (1974) Wilson's disease. In *The Liver and its Diseases* (Ed.) Schaffner, F., Sherlock, S. & Leevy, C.M., pp. 328–336. New York: Intercontinental Medical Book Corporation.
75. Sternlieb, I., Bennett, B. & Scheinberg, I.H. (1975) D-penicillamine induced Goodpasture's syndrome in Wilson's disease. *Annals of Internal Medicine*, **82**, 673–676.
76. Sternlieb, I., Scheinberg, I.H. & Walshe, J.M. (1970) Bleeding oesophageal varices in patients with Wilson's disease. *Lancet*, **i**, 638–641.

77. Sternlieb, I., Morell, A.G., Tucker, W.D., Greene, M.W. & Scheinberg, I.H. (1961) The incorporation of copper into ceruloplasmin *in vivo*: studies with copper^{64} and copper^{67}. *Journal of Clinical Investigation*, **40**, 1834–1840.
78. Sternlieb, I. & Scheinberg, I.H. (1979) The role of radiocopper in the diagnosis of Wilson's disease, *Gastroenterology*, **77**, 138–142.
79. Sternlieb, I., van den Hamer, C.J.A., Morell, A.G., Alpert, S., Gregoriadis, G. & Scheinberg, I.H. (1973) Lysosomal defect of hepatic copper excretion in Wilson's disease (hepatolenticular degeneration). *Gastroenterology*, **64**, 99–105.
80. Strickland, G.T. & Leu, M.L. (1975) Wilson's disease: clinical and laboratory manifestations in 40 patients. *Medicine* (Baltimore), **54**, 113–137.
81. Strickland, G.T., Chang, N.-K. & Beckner, W.M. (1972) Hypersplenism in Wilson's disease. *Gut*, **13**, 220–224.
82. Strickland, G.T., Frommer, D., Leu, M.L., Pollard, R., Sherlock, S. & Cumings, J.N. (1973) Wilson's disease in the United Kingdom and Taiwan. *Quarterly Journal of Medicine*, **42**, 619–638.
83. Sussman, W. & Scheinberg, I.H. (1969) Disappearance of Kayser–Fleischer rings. Effects of penicillamine. *Archives of Ophthalmology*, **83**, 738–741.
84. Vachon, A., Paliard, P., Barthe, J., Grimaud, J.A., Peyrol, G.L. & Reiss, Th. (1973) Les étapes de l'atteinte hépatique de la dégénérescence hépatolenticulaire: lésions précoces, hypertension portale et dégénérescence cancéreuse. À propos de 4 observations. *Lyon Médical*, **230**, 591–598.
85. Walshe, J.M. (1956) Penicillamine, a new oral therapy for Wilson's disease. *American Journal of Medicine*, **21**, 487–495.
86. Walshe, J.M. (1966) Wilson's disease, a review. In *The Biochemistry of Copper* (Ed.) Peisach, J., Aisen, P. & Blumberg, W.E., pp. 495–498. New York: Academic Press.
87. Walshe, J.M. (1969) Management of penicillamine nephropathy in Wilson's disease: a new chelating agent. *Lancet*, **ii**, 1401–1402.
88. Walshe, J.M. (1973) Copper chelation in patients with Wilson's disease. *Quarterly Journal of Medicine*, **42**, 441–452.
89. Walshe, J.M. (1976) Wilson's disease (hepatolenticular degeneration). In *Handbook of Clinical Neurology* (Ed.) Vinken, P.J. & Bruyn, G.W., pp. 379–414. Oxford: North-Holland.
90. Walshe, J.M. (1977) Pregnancy in Wilson's disease. *Quarterly Journal of Medicine*, **46**, 73–83.
91. Walshe, J.M. & Briggs, J. (1962) Caeruloplasmin in liver disease. A diagnostic pitfall. *Lancet*, **ii**, 263–265.
92. Wilson, S.A.K. (1912) Progressive lenticular degeneration: a familial nervous disease associated with cirrhosis of the liver. *Brain*, **34**, 295–509.

Chapter 34

Haemochromatosis and Related Iron Storage Diseases

L.W. POWELL

The association between cirrhosis, hepatic pigment deposits and diabetes mellitus was recognized just over a century ago. The early descriptions of the syndrome reflected the various beliefs as to whether the disorder was primarily hepatic, pancreatic or haematological in origin. Troisier, who was the first to describe the syndrome, used the title 'la cirrhose pigmentaire dans le diabète sucré'.[92] Hanot suggested the term 'bronze diabetes' for the disorder because he believed that the diabetes was of primary importance, being the likely cause of both the cirrhosis and the skin pigmentation.[41] In contrast, von Recklinghausen, the main advocate of the haemic theory of aetiology, coined the term 'haemochromatosis' for the disease.[95] The French hepatologist, Gilbert, considered that the disorder was merely a form of alcoholic cirrhosis: 'la cirrhose alcoolique hypertrophique pigmentaire'.[36] Sheldon was the first to emphasize that all these terms probably referred to the same condition and further suggested that 'the title haemochromatosis is, in spite of its implicit but unproved assumptions, the best name for the disease'.[87] Largely because of Sheldon's authoritative monograph (1935) this misnomer has been generally retained for the disorder.

Sheldon's classic monograph was the first major review of the disease and surveyed the available literature of some 300 cases to that time. He concluded that the disease resulted from an inborn error of iron metabolism leading, after many years of slowly progressive iron accumulation, to the distinctive clinicopathological features of the disease. This concept was seriously questioned when, largely as a result of the introduction of percutaneous needle biopsy of the liver, pathologists recognized that cirrhosis of the liver could be associated with varying grades of iron deposition up to the gross amounts seen in idiopathic haemochromatosis and that the complete clinicopathological picture of haemochromatosis could follow secondary accumulation of iron in patients with pre-existing cirrhosis,[55,82,106] especially within a few years of portacaval anastomosis.[83,94] Furthermore, the syndrome was shown to result from prolonged exposure to a high dietary intake of iron and alcohol, as in the negroes of Southern Africa, without a demonstrable metabolic defect in iron absorption.[13,96] This and other evidence led to the postulate that so-called 'idiopathic haemochromatosis' was the result of two conditions, hepatic cirrhosis and iron deposition, occurring together but not causally related.[62]

Thus, the concept propounded by Sheldon that haemochromatosis is the result of a specific metabolic abnormality has been expanded to include a number of other forms of iron overload. Indeed, it is now generally accepted that the full syndrome of haemochromatosis may result from secondary iron overload superimposed upon hepatic cirrhosis, without the presence of a primary underlying disturbance of iron metabolism. However, there is also general acceptance that the disorder now known as 'idiopathic haemochromatosis' is a disease sui generis resulting from at least one inborn error of iron metabolism. This view has been considerably strengthened by the recent demonstration of a strong statistical association between certain histocompatibility antigens on chromosome number 5 and the development of the disease.[10,88] This association is not present in patients with alcoholic cirrhosis and secondary iron deposition.

An understanding of the pathophysiology of idiopathic haemochromatosis and the various causes of secondary haemochromatosis requires a knowledge of basic concepts of normal iron metabolism and, in particular, how iron balance is regulated normally.

BASIC CONCEPTS OF IRON METABOLISM

Iron Storage and Balance

The body of a healthy adult male normally contains about 90 mmol (5 g) of iron.[12] Two-thirds of this are present in compounds such as haemoglobin, myoglobin and tissue enzymes, while the remainder represents a store which is located primarily in the reticuloendothelial system and which can be drawn upon as need arises. Storage iron exists in two forms. Firstly, in the large iron-storage protein, ferritin, and secondly as haemosiderin, a poorly defined molecule which consists of aggregates derived from ferritin. When the amounts of storage iron are within the physiological range there is some preponderance of ferritin over haemosiderin, but as the stores enlarge the haemosiderin content increases to a greater extent than ferritin.[66]

Ferritin has both a protective and a reserve function. A protective role is required because free iron is toxic and daily losses are small (see below). Iron stored as ferritin and haemosiderin is accessible for haemoglobin production although iron mobilization is a relatively slow process. Normally only 18 μmol (1 mg) (0.1 per cent) of iron enters and leaves the storage compartment each day.[45]

The liver is a major storage organ for iron, containing about one-third of the total body iron content.[12] Other important storage sites are skeletal muscle and bone marrow. Small amounts of iron may be visible in the liver either within the Kupffer cells (macrophages) or in parenchymal cells. The relative importance of the two sites of storage is still unclear. There is increasing evidence, however, that different structural and metabolic forms of ferritin occur in different tissues and even within the same tissue.[25] Gabuzda and Pearson concluded from double-isotopic tracer studies in bone marrow that one form of ferritin, which they termed 'anabolic', accepted iron from transferrin, whereas the other or 'catabolic' form accepted its iron from phagocytosed red cells.[35] It is known that deposits of iron in macrophages are largely derived from the breakdown of red cells while parenchymal iron stores appear to originate from free haemoglobin, from the haemoglobin bound to haptoglobin and from transferrin.[34,47]

Recently, ferritin has been detected in both human and rat serum and its concentration has been shown to be proportional to body iron stores.[50] The serum ferritin concentration is also elevated in some disease states not related to increased iron loading, including, especially, alcoholic liver disease, malignant hepatoma and leukaemia.[49] However, the origin and function of serum ferritin remains one of the enigmas of iron metabolism.

The rate of iron absorption is regulated via poorly understood mechanisms to maintain body iron stores at optimal levels. The rate of absorption is greater than normal when the stores are depleted and diminished when stores are increased. In the adult, the amounts of iron in stores remain relatively constant. The obligatory daily iron losses are of the order of 18 μmol (1 mg) in adult males. Approximately two-thirds of this are lost via the gut and most of the remainder in the urine and skin. These obligatory losses are reduced by about half in iron deficiency and may rise to figures of up to three times normal in states of iron overload.[39] In the female, of course, additional losses are incurred through menstruation and pregnancy. The mean normal menstrual losses, when expressed in terms of daily iron balance, are approximately 9 μmol (0.5 mg), although there is much variation. During pregnancy the requirement is even greater. It has been calculated that approximately 18 mmol (1 g) of iron is needed for each pregnancy. This is equivalent to an average daily requirement of between 90 and 110 μmol (between 5 and 6 mg) throughout the last two trimesters.

Iron Absorption

The mechanism by which the body regulates iron absorption by the intestine so that iron balance is maintained remains a mystery despite much investigation of the subject. The available data suggest that the control of iron uptake and transport by the intestine lies primarily within the intestinal cell itself and that this is influenced by other factors such as the degree of erythropoiesis.[70] Both the availability of dietary iron for absorption and amount of iron in the diet vary greatly so that approximately only 10 per cent of iron in food is absorbed, especially iron of vegetable origin. About 10 per cent of iron taken up by the intestinal cell is normally retained, and this may rise to 20 per cent or more in iron deficiency. Highly refined foods commonly used in western countries contain approximately 90 μmol (5 mg) iron per 1000 calories.[18] Normal males consuming 3000 calories per day would therefore obtain, at most, 270 μmol (15 mg) iron per day, of which 9 to 27 μmol (0.5 to 1.5 mg) would be absorbed. The maximum which could be absorbed in the iron-deficient subject could thus be little more than 54 μmol (3 mg) per day. It is thus apparent that the possible range of absorption from the normal diet is quite narrow, extending from less than 9 μmol (0.5 mg) daily in the iron-replete subject to approximately 72 μmol (4 mg) in the iron deficient subject.

Iron Excretion

Iron losses are difficult to measure accurately but studies using ^{55}Fe calculated that the mean daily iron loss was 11 μmol (0.6 mg) in men and non-menstruating women and 22 μmol (1.2 mg) in menstruating women.[32] Higher losses have been found in the negroes of Southern Africa due to dietary iron overload. The major route of loss of iron is through the gastrointestinal tract, 6.8 μmol (0.38 mg) per day from blood loss, 4.7 μmol (0.26 mg) in the bile and 1.8 μmol (0.1 mg) in exfoliated epithelial cells.[39] Skin losses have been estimated as a maximum of 3.6 to 5.4 μmol (0.2 to 0.3 mg) per day, with the assumption that all radioactive iron incorporated in the skin after injection is eventually exfoliated. Urinary losses of iron are about 1.8 μmol (0.1 mg) per day.[39] The wide variation in iron losses and requirements among various groups in the community causes considerable difficulty in planning programmes for the fortification with iron in order to eliminate iron deficiency. In clinical practice, the measurement of iron loss by whole-body counting may be of use in confirming and quantifying excess blood loss in those patients where this has proved difficult by other methods.

Pathogenesis of Iron Overload

An absolute increase in total body iron content may arise in several different ways:

1. In idiopathic haemochromatosis, the outstanding example of a regulatory abnormality in iron storage, the absorption of iron is inappropriately high, permitting the accumulation of 270 to 900 mmol (15 to 50 g) of body iron over a period of 25 to 50 years. With increasing body iron stores, absorption decreases towards the level found in the normal individual. However, this amount is still greater than that absorbed by an individual without this disorder who has a similar iron load; a point of some diagnostic significance. When iron is removed by phlebotomy, absorption regains its former high level.[59] The cause of the abnormal iron absorption in idiopathic haemochromatosis has not been identified. Despite much research on possible gastric, pancreatic and other factors, convincing evidence is lacking and the most recent evidence suggests that the primary defect may lie in the reticuloendothelial (RE) system with secondary effects on the intestinal mucosa, resulting in increased iron absorption.[16]
2. Disorders of erythropoiesis are also associated with increased iron absorption. However, gross iron overload is usually restricted to those conditions with ineffective erythropoiesis, as in hereditary sideroblastic anaemia and thalassaemia major (see below).
3. The association of liver disease and various degrees of iron overload has been recognized for over a century and, indeed, has resulted in much confusion as to its distinction from idiopathic haemochromatosis, as discussed earlier. The precise pathogenesis of the increased iron storage is still uncertain. Liver disease associated with excess iron storage is

usually complicated by factors such as ineffective erythropoiesis, folate deficiency or the ingestion of excessive iron from alcoholic beverages. Some evidence that increased iron absorption is directly related to liver disease also exists.[40] This subject has recently been reviewed in some detail.[38]

4. Whether significant iron overload can be produced in the normal individual by prolonged oral iron intake is uncertain. Clearly, if the oral intake is sufficient to overcome mucosal regulation, probably an amount of 1.8 mmol (100 mg) per day or more over a period of many years, iron overload will result. In Ethiopia, the ingestion of up to 3.6 mmol (200 mg) of iron per day of dirt iron causes only a modest increase in RE stores.[48] In contrast, a similar amount in the Kaffir beer of South African negroes produces massive iron overload associated with disease.[15] Several reports have stated that the syndrome of haemochromatosis has occurred in caucasian subjects following medicinal iron intake totalling more than 18 mol (1000 g) over many years, but other evidence suggests that the disease is rare even with such a dose.[52] Until the basic metabolic defect in this disorder is known, it remains uncertain whether such subjects are heterozygous for the inherited trait of idiopathic haemochromatosis with consequent marginal increase in iron absorption. This was suggested by the study of Powell who investigated iron metabolism in relatives of patients with idiopathic haemochromatosis and also relatives of patients with alcoholic liver disease.[69] In both groups of relatives there were two women who had taken iron tablets for more than 10 years. The two in the first group showed evidence of increased body iron stores, whereas both women in the second group had normal iron stores.
5. Parenteral iron administration also results in iron overload. Since iron excretion is limited to about 3 6 μmol (2 mg) per day, iron overload is easily produced by repeated blood transfusions or injections of iron preparations. Parenterally administered iron undergoes RE processing before its iron becomes available to other body tissues and usually results in predominantly RE haemosiderosis. This tends to be relatively innocuous since cellular dysfunction and tissue injury appear to be related more closely to parenchymal iron loading.[64]

The site of iron storage is determined by the plasma iron levels. When the plasma iron level is within normal limits, excessive iron is located predominantly in the RE system. In contrast, if the plasma iron level is elevated and the saturation of transferrin is greater than 60 per cent, iron is deposited in parenchymal cells. Thus, the degree of parenchymal iron overload is more important than the total amount of iron involved.

The conditions which produce iron overload vary greatly in their effect on the iron distribution. In idiopathic haemochromatosis, there appears to be impaired RE ability to store iron and to regulate plasma iron level. Thus, during the early stages of this disease the plasma iron level is high and parenchymal iron overload occurs with little or no demonstrable increase in RE iron.[14] In haemochromatosis secondary to chronic anaemia associated with increased erythropoiesis, the plasma iron level is also high and both RE and parenchymal storage systems are usually iron loaded. In liver disease, RE overload predominates although, in those patients where the plasma iron level is high and transferrin saturation increased, both types of storage iron may be seen. Excessive intake of oral iron usually induces a moderate increase in RE storage.

Iron Toxicity

The medical literature contains much controversy over the question of whether the excess tissue iron in haemochromatosis is responsible for the tissue damage and complications of the disease. The subject has recently been reviewed in depth.[37,38] The hesitancy to accept iron as a cause of tissue damage results from several factors. Firstly, an animal model of the disease is absent. Until recently it has not been possible to produce comparable tissue damage in animals by injection of iron alone. However, two recent reports[58,97] suggest that the duration of iron overload may be the important factor in addition to the total parenchymal iron content achieved, since large quantities of iron given to dogs over many years have produced fibrosis or cirrhosis. Secondly, in humans, there is still controversy over whether the administration of iron over long periods of time results in tissue damage. As indicated above, much confusion has arisen because of failure to distinguish between predominantly parenchymal and predominantly RE iron overload when considering the pathophysiology of iron storage. Haemochromatosis in this context is a disorder of parenchymal iron overload, whereas RE iron overload is comparatively innocuous.[64] In patients with anaemia associated with hyperplastic bone marrow, heavy parenchymal distribution of iron occurs and numerous reports of such patients exhibiting all the classical clinical features of haemochromatosis have been described (see below). This, together with the impressive clinical, biochemical and histological improvement which follows iron removal, represents strong circumstantial evidence for an aetiological role of iron in the pathogenesis of the tissue injury in this disease.

Recent elegant studies by Peters and Seymour have revealed a possible biochemical basis for the clinical observations given above.[68] They demonstrated significantly elevated lysosomal enzymes and more fragile lysosomes in liver biopsies from patients with primary or secondary haemochromatosis. They suggested that iron accumulation damages the lysosomal membrane, releasing acid hydrolases into the cytoplasm and initiating cell damage.

Thus, in summary, there is increasing evidence that the presence of iron in parenchymal cells over many years is an important aetiological factor in determining tissue damage. However, other metals and undefined constitutional factors may also be important in individual cases in determining the extent of hepatic damage and which particular organs are affected, as, for example, in relation to the development of diabetes mellitus.[91]

DEFINITIONS AND CLASSIFICATION

The terms 'haemosiderosis' and 'siderosis' are widely used to indicate the deposition of varying quantities of haemosiderin in tissues without associated tissue damage. The terms do not necessarily imply that the total iron content of the body is increased. There are two situations in particular in which hepatic siderosis is seen with no or little increase in total body iron stores. Firstly, in alcoholic liver disease variable amounts of stainable iron may be present in the liver.[8] The precise reason for the excess stainable iron is uncertain. Secondly, in any anaemia not due to blood loss or to dietary iron deficiency, there is a redistribution of body iron with less in haemoglobin and more in the iron stores (relative haemosiderosis). Under such circumstances, hepatic iron stores may increase to two to three times the normal amount. Haemosiderosis may be localized to other organs; for example, the lungs in idiopathic pulmonary siderosis, and the kidneys in paroxysmal nocturnal haemoglobinuria. An absolute increase in body iron stores is commonly referred to as 'iron overload'. This implies that the regulatory mechanisms for controlling the iron content of the body are deranged or have been bypassed.

The term 'haemochromatosis' has come to be applied to the condition in which the liver and other organs contain grossly excessive amounts of storage iron, usually 1 per cent dry weight or more, and show pathological evidence of damage, usually in the form of diffuse fibrosis. *Thus, haemochromatosis may be defined as a pathological entity characterized by the deposition of excess iron in parenchymal cells of the liver and in the parenchymal cells of various other organs, including pancreas, heart and pituitary gland, with eventual fibrosis and functional inefficiency of the organs involved.* Diabetes mellitus and skin pigmentation are often present but are not necessary for the diagnosis. Practical clinical and pathological criteria are given in Table 34.1 and a classification of causes of the syndrome in Table 34.2.

Table 34.1. *Classification of Haemochromatosis: Definitions.*

1. Haemochromatosis
   Increased total body iron stores with tissue injury.
   Clinical criteria: fibrosis or cirrhosis (biopsy) and increased body iron assessed by response to repeated venesections, injection of a chelating agent, serum ferritin concentration or hepatic iron concentration.
   Pathological criteria: fibrosis or cirrhosis with grossly increased iron concentration in parenchymal and other cells of the liver and other organs, e.g. pancreas and heart (preferably assessed by chemical analyses).
2. Idiopathic haemochromatosis
   Haemochromatosis developing in the absence of known causes of secondary iron overload, usually in association with a family history of iron storage disease.
3. Latent or precirrhotic idiopathic haemochromatosis
   Increased body iron stores associated with increased iron absorption and a family history of iron storage disease.
4. Haemosiderosis
   Increased stainable tissue iron without tissue damage.

Table 34.2. *Classification of Haemochromatosis: Aetiology.*

1. Primary or idiopathic haemochromatosis
   (a) Latent or precirrhotic stage
   (b) Cirrhotic stage
2. Secondary haemochromatosis
   (a) Hepatic cirrhosis with gross secondary iron accumulation
   (b) Hepatic cirrhosis and iron overload associated with chronic anaemias
   (c) Chronic alcohol ingestion associated with excess dietary iron ('Bantu-type' haemochromatosis)

Increasingly, idiopathic haemochromatosis is being diagnosed during its early stages when the iron overload is of lesser degree and organ damage slight or absent.[43] At this stage, the condition is best referred to as 'latent or precirrhotic haemochromatosis'.[30,70,101]

IDIOPATHIC HAEMOCHROMATOSIS

Definition and Prevalence

By definition, the term 'idiopathic haemochromatosis' should be used for those patients in whom there is no apparent cause for the iron accumulation. This diagnosis is considerably strengthened by

1. A strong family history of iron storage disease.
2. Lack of a history of increased alcohol intake.
3. Significant cardiac or endocrine involvement.

Estimates of the prevalence of the disease have ranged from one in 20 000 hospital admissions and one in 7000 hospital deaths[33] to 2.5 per 10 000 necropsies performed in Johannesburg[7] and one in 10 000 of the Australian population.[70]

Aetiology and Mode of Inheritance

The concept proposed by Sheldon,[87] that idiopathic haemochromatosis results from an inborn error of metabolism which leads to a daily iron absorption slightly in excess of excretion, was reinforced by the extensive review of Finch and Finch.[33] From their review of 787 cases previously reported, these authors concluded that haemochromatosis was the result of excessive iron storage over many years, with consequent pathological changes, and that the degree and rapidity of iron overload in any particular individual was influenced not only by an inherited defect leading to increased iron absorption but also by extraneous factors, such as the amount of iron in the diet, the age of the subject and the rate of iron lost by menstruation. Numerous family studies which have subsequently been reported collectively present persuasive evidence for an inherited defect in iron metabolism leading to gradual accumulation of unwanted iron.[21] Systematic examination of families reveals that up to 12 per cent of siblings manifest the full syndrome while about a further 25 per cent of siblings and 10 per cent of children have one or more detectable abnormalities in iron metabolism.[43,65,69,104]

The most recent addition to the mounting evidence for a genetic basis for the disease has been the demonstration of an increased incidence of histocompatibility antigens HLA-A3 and B14 in this disease.[10,88] In a controlled study, Simon and colleagues have shown that this association is not present in subjects with alcoholic cirrhosis and mild to moderate haemosiderosis.[89]

Since the concept that idiopathic haemochromatosis is a disease entity has been challenged in the past[62] it may be of interest to summarize the evidence now available in support of the concept (Table 34.3).

The mode of inheritance of idiopathic haemochromatosis is uncertain and is likely to remain so until the basic defect or defects have been determined. However, two patterns of inheritance seem to be emerging. Firstly, in most families only one or two relatives are affected.

Table 34.3. *Summary of Evidence that Idiopathic Haemochromatosis Exists as an Entity Distinct from Alcoholic Cirrhosis.*

1. Well-documented cases have been reported in teetotallers.
2. Well-documented cases have been reported in children with normal siblings living under the same environmental conditions.
3. Abnormalities of iron metabolism (including increased iron absorption) occur in relatives of patients with idiopathic haemochromatosis but not in relatives of patients with alcoholic cirrhosis.
4. Patients with idiopathic haemochromatosis differ from patients with cirrhosis with respect to carbohydrate tolerance, insulin sensitivity and endocrine status.
5. Differences in prognosis have been reported between the two diseases and reversal of most features of haemochromatosis following intensive venesection therapy.
6. Differences in incidence of histocompatibility antigens.

In other families numerous siblings and children are affected and the pattern of inheritance is clearly dominant. The former group would fit the pattern of inheritance of a recessive trait as suggested by Walsh and his colleagues,[99] Schienberg[84] and Powell.[70] Families in the second group have been reported more often and this has led to conclusions that the disease has a dominant mode of inheritance.[81] There is increasing evidence that the disorder is a heterogeneous one with different abnormalities of iron and ferritin metabolism and possibly different modes of inheritance.[74,75]

The various hypotheses that have been advanced for the underlying metabolic defect in this disease have included: (a) an abnormal avidity of liver and other tissues for iron;[17] (b) abnormal kinetics of the iron transferrin complex;[80] (c) aberrant reticuloendothelial function;[14] (d) abnormal luminal factors, including abnormalities in pancreatic and gastric secretions;[9,23,24] and (e) abnormal mucosal cell function.[76] To summarize, the available evidence suggests that iron absorption increases inappropriately at an early stage in idiopathic haemochromatosis as a result of increased iron transfer across the intestinal mucosal cell. It is not known whether this is due to a primary intestinal cell defect, to a generalized metabolic defect or to an abnormality in reticuloendothelial cell function which secondarily affects mucosal iron absorption. Thus, whatever the fundamental error or errors in iron metabolism in patients with idiopathic haemochromatosis, there seems little doubt that the control of iron absorption is involved and that the disorder causes a slight increase in iron absorption from the diet and a gradual accumulation of iron over many years.

Pathology

In the fully-established disease, the total iron content of the body is usually between 360 and 720 mmol (20 and 40 g).[33,87] Iron deposits are heaviest in the liver and pancreas, in which the iron concentration is 50 to 100 times normal. The iron content of other organs is also elevated from 5 to 25 times normal, particularly in the endocrine glands, cardiac muscle and skin. A notable exception is the testis, the iron content of which is relatively low[87] despite the fact that impaired gonadal function is a characteristic and early feature of the disease.[78]

The detailed pathological findings in the disease have been described elsewhere.[33,54,56,72,87] The most characteristic and diagnostically the most important findings are seen in the liver. This is usually greatly enlarged, weighing over 2000 g. The cut surface has a reddish-brown colour and it is firm in consistency. Histologically, the two outstanding features are extensive pigmentation and fibrosis. The appearances are best appreciated in autopsy or wedge biopsy specimens.[72] They show a characteristic pattern of fibrosis and iron deposition with dense fibrous septa forming a network surrounding groups of lobules, somewhat analogous to that seen in chronic biliary disease. A fully-established cirrhosis with nodularity develops comparatively late in the disease. The haemosiderin deposits characteristically appear first in the periportal parenchyma, being found within lysosomes in the pericanalicular cytoplasm of the hepatocytes. Later, they are distributed widely throughout the lobules as well as in biliary duct epithelium, Kupffer cells and connective tissue.

Microscopic examination of the pancreas usually shows heavy deposits of haemosiderin in the acinar cells and, to a lesser extent, in the islets of Langerhans, with the number of islets diminished. Haemosiderin is also found in the heart muscle fibres in nearly all cases of well-established haemochromatosis. Fibrosis is relatively rare. Haemosiderin is also deposited in the conducting fibres of the arteriovenous node, as opposed to the sinoatrial node, and is presumably responsible for the cardiac arrhythmias which occur in this disease. The pituitary, adrenal, thyroid and parathyroid glands frequently contain extensive haemosiderin deposits, although evidence of functional impairment is usually confined to the pituitary.

Clinical Features and their Pathogenesis

For many years the disease is latent and the course depends on a number of factors, including sex, dietary intake of iron, presence of associated hepatotoxins (especially alcohol) and, probably, on whether the subject is heterozygous or homozygous for the inherited trait.[84] The overt clinical manifestations occur more frequently in men than in women. The current sex ratio is about 5:1 (males to females).[70] This is one-half of that reported in 1955 by Finch and Finch.[33] The reason is unknown. The less common incidence in women is explained in part by physiological blood loss and probably also by the fact that women ingest less iron than men since iron intake is closely linked to caloric intake. The majority of patients present in the fifth decade and women usually present after the menopause. Rarely, the disease may present in the second or third decades and in such patients it is commonly associated with endocrine or cardiac manifestations.

Powell, Mortimer and Harris analysed the symptoms and signs at presentation of an unselected group of patients with haemochromatosis compared with those seen in other forms of cirrhosis.[78] In the majority of patients the classical triad described by Sheldon[87] (pigmentation of the skin, hepatomegaly and diabetes mellitus) was present (see Figures 34.1 and 34.2). The major differences between the clinical features of patients with haemochromatosis and other forms of cirrhosis were the relatively high incidence of gonadal atrophy, skin pigmentation, hepatomegaly, and the relatively prolonged and benign course of the liver disease. Indeed, in the series studied by Powell and colleagues, more than 50 per cent of patients had no symptoms other than lethargy and loss of libido, and no physical signs other than hepatomegaly, skin pigmentation and testicular atrophy. Furthermore, over half the patients have little or no laboratory evidence of functional liver impairment in spite of the presence of cirrhosis.[78] Thus, haemochromatosis should be considered in any patient with skin pigmentation and an enlarged firm liver, especially in males if testicular atrophy is present. The skin pigmentation manifests either as a bronze hue due to melanin or the characteristic slaty, bluish-grey metallic colour. The latter is not necessarily caused by iron and possibly results from melanin in an atrophic skin.

Carbohydrate intolerance occurs in up to 80 per cent of patients with idiopathic haemochromatosis, but overt diabetes mellitus presents in only about 60 per cent. This appears to be multifactorial in origin with variable contributions from hepatic cirrhosis, pancreatic islet cell damage from iron and the inheritance of the gene for idiopathic diabetes mellitus.[2,27,81,91] This contrasts with the other causes of cirrhosis in which carbohydrate intolerance is due to insulin insensitivity. Clinically, the diabetes of haemochromatosis may be mild or severe and is occasionally resistant to insulin. Associated complications such as retinopathy, nephropathy and peripheral neuropathy occur as in idiopathic diabetes mellitus.

Evidence of endocrine involvement in addition to decreased gonadal function is occasionally seen, most commonly as hypopituitarism. Haemosiderin is almost invariably found in the pituitary gland[87] and deficiency of other pituitary hormones has been demonstrated in this disease.[90] Hypoparathyroidism, hypothyroidism and Addison's disease have also been described but are exceedingly rare.

Cardiac manifestations occur in about 15 per cent of patients and characteristically take the

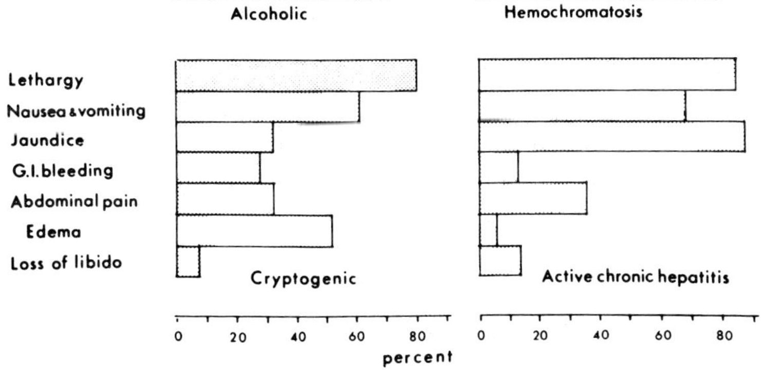

Figure 34.1. Symptoms of patients with haemochromatosis or other causes of cirrhosis during the first month of the illness. From Powell, Mortimer and Harris,[78] with the kind permission of the editor of *Medical Journal of Australia*.

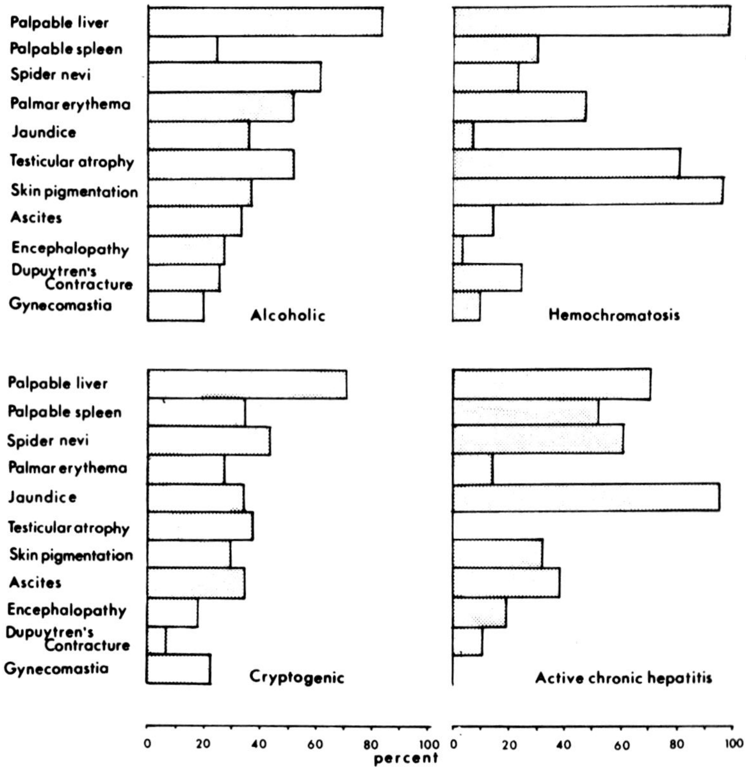

Figure 34.2. Physical signs present at the first examination of patients with haemochromatosis or other forms of cirrhosis. From Powell, Mortimer and Harris,[78] with the kind permission of the editor of *Medical Journal of Australia*.

form of arrhythmias or progressively severe heart failure. However, with the widespread use of phlebotomy therapy, these complications appear to be much less common than 20 years ago.[33]

A recently described and characteristic feature in some 25 to 50 per cent of cases is the presence of an arthropathy characterized by the deposition of calcium pyrophosphate and iron in the synovium – *chondrocalcinosis.* Both small and large joints are involved, with pain, swelling and limitation of movement. There is a correlation between the degree of chondrocalcinosis and the severity of the joint disease, but the exact relationship of the iron deposition to the arthritis is uncertain. For a detailed description of this complication the reader is referred to several recent large studies.[26,44,98] Recently osteoporosis and vertebral collapse have also been described, frequently in association with ascorbic acid depletion, presumably because of the oxidative effects of body iron.[86,102] However, this complication appears to be confined almost exclusively to the negroes of Southern Africa.

Primary liver cell cancer is increasing as a complication of haemochromatosis and this is probably related to the increase in human life span as a result of more effective therapy of diabetes mellitus and cardiac failure. Hepatic cirrhosis appears to be an important prerequisite for the development of malignant hepatoma.[73] This has obvious important implications for the early diagnosis of the disease.

Precirrhotic or Latent Haemochromatosis

There is increasing evidence that iron has an aetiological role in producing tissue damage and that early detection and treatment of the disease prolongs life and may delay or prevent irreversible complications.[70,105] For this reason, and because cirrhosis represents a critical and largely irreversible stage in the development of idiopathic haemochromatosis,[73] the physician who diagnoses the disease has an ethical responsibility to inform all the patient's blood relatives and to see that they are screened for the disease. There is therefore much interest in non-invasive methods for detecting the early precirrhotic stage of the disease (see below) and also in the natural history of the disease. Since there are no reported sequential or longitudinal studies of haemochromatosis, the sequence of

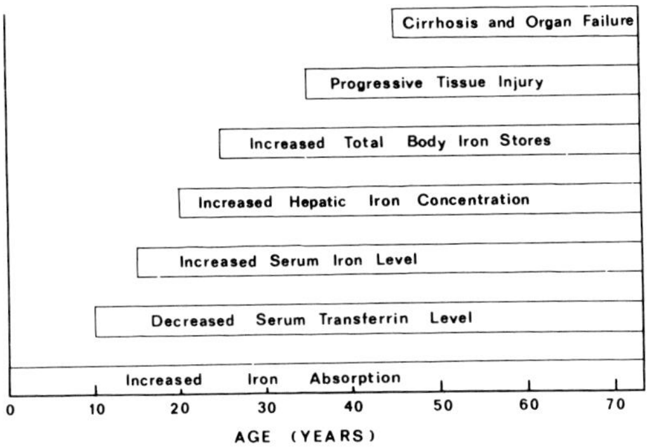

Figure 34.3. Suggested natural history of idiopathic haemochromatosis on the basis of available data (see text).

changes is uncertain. However, from a personal study of 140 families with this disease and from a review of the literature the following schematic representation of events is proposed (Figure 34.3).

Diagnosis and Differential Diagnosis

The diagnosis of haemochromatosis is usually made on the basis of the above clinical features together with laboratory investigations indicative of excessive iron stores and tissue damage. These include an elevated serum iron level > 30 μmol/l (> 170 μg/100 ml) associated with a reduction in the total iron-binding capacity of the serum and complete or almost complete transferrin saturation, excessive parenchymal iron deposits identified by tests using iron-chelating agents, the serum ferritin concentration, and liver biopsy. Hepatic biopsy is important in defining the extent of tissue damage as well as in permitting both histochemical assessment of tissue iron and measurement of hepatic iron concentration. The ultimate diagnosis rests on the pathology and the demonstration of a hepatic iron concentration in excess of 180 μmol/g (1 g/100 g) dry weight.[38,87]

Uncertainty concerning the minimum acceptable criteria necessary for the diagnosis of haemochromatosis has followed the realization that patients with hepatic cirrhosis may develop skin pigmentation, diabetes mellitus, a high serum iron level with saturation of the iron-binding protein, and various degrees of parenchymal iron deposition in the liver and other organs. For this reason the diagnosis of haemochromatosis should not be based merely on the presence of suggestive clinical features in association with some parenchymal iron deposition in the liver and cirrhosis. An attempt should be made to quantify the degree of iron excess. In this respect the serum iron concentration and percentage transferrin saturation are of little help and greater reliance should be placed on the semi-quantitative tests employing iron chelating agents, on the measurement of the serum ferritin concentration, on chemical analysis of tissue obtained by biopsy or at necropsy and, of course, retrospectively on the amount of iron removed by phlebotomy.[38,46,75] A 24-hour urinary excretion of iron in excess of 36 μmol (2 mg) following an intramuscular injection of 0.5 g of desferrioxamine is indicative of excess parenchymal iron deposits. In patients with untreated haemochromatosis the amount usually exceeds 180 μmol (10 mg) in 24 hours. More complex chelation tests have been devised, such as the differential ferrioxamine test,[4,31] in an attempt to define the degree of iron overload more precisely. However, these tests are too cumbersome for routine clinical use.

The recent development of sensitive immunological assays for ferritin[1,42] has resulted in the demonstration that this protein is present in serum in proportion to body iron stores.[50,100] A recent extensive study of 43 families with idiopathic haemochromatosis showed that the serum ferritin concentration was elevated in all 42 probands studied and in 98 per cent of relatives with increased iron stores. Further, increased iron stores were reflected in increased serum ferritin levels in subjects as young as 14 years, in subjects in whom the hepatic iron concentration was only twice normal, and before there was any architectural damage of the liver.[43] The authors concluded that the serum ferritin concentration is a useful non-invasive screening test for precirrhotic idiopathic haemochromatosis and it is predicted that this test will replace the more cumbersome screening tests involving urinary iron excretion. However, two notes of caution should be sounded. Firstly, the serum level may be elevated out of proportion to body iron stores when there is hepatocellular necrosis, especially in alcoholic liver disease. Secondly, at least three families have been reported in which the serum ferritin concentration has been normal in relatives despite unequivocal increase in body iron stores.[30,74,101] The reason for this is uncertain. It would appear to be an exceptional situation, however, since a further recent family study has confirmed that the serum ferritin concentration is usually elevated to levels of 1000 ng/ml or more when body iron stores are increased.[28] The distinction between haemochromatosis and alcoholic cirrhosis with secondary iron accumulation of only mild to moderate degree can usually be made on the basis of the above tests of body iron stores. In contrast to patients with haemochromatosis, those with cirrhosis and secondary haemosiderosis have usually only a slight increase in chelatable body iron, a normal or modestly increased serum ferritin level and normal or slightly increased amounts (18 to 45 mmol [1 to 2.5 g]) of iron mobilizable by repeated venesections.[75,79]

Additional information may be obtained from family studies. Abnormalities of iron metabolism occur in over 25 per cent of first-degree relatives of patients with idiopathic haemochromatosis, whereas such abnormalities are very infrequent in relatives of patients with cirrhosis and haemosiderosis, even in those relatives who consume alcohol to excess.[69] The importance of checking other family members is obvious because early and often asymptomatic cases with reversible disease may be detected in this way.

In summary, the diagnosis of haemochromatosis should be made on the basis of histological proof of tissue damage, that is, well-established fibrosis or cirrhosis, associated with convincing evidence of grossly increased body iron stores. Idiopathic haemochromatosis is diagnosed by excluding the known causes of secondary haemochromatosis, such as chronic refractory or haemolytic anaemia, and by family studies. The causes of secondary haemochromatosis are usually easily recognized. However, diagnostic problems may arise in alcoholic patients for whom family studies reveal no abnormality of iron metabolism and for whom previous histological material is unavailable. In such patients it may be impossible to distinguish with certainty between idiopathic haemochromatosis aggravated by alcoholism and haemochromatosis of the Bantu type. Wedge biopsies of the liver or HLA antigen typing may be of additional help.

Treatment and Prognosis

The prognosis of haemochromatosis, treated or untreated, is significantly better than that of alcoholic cirrhosis. In addition, there is now strong circumstantial evidence that venesection therapy prolongs life and that established tissue damage is at least partially reversible.[70,73,105] Because the evidence (discussed above) that iron accumulation causes hepatic damage, a controlled trial of venesection therapy in asymptomatic relatives with the early manifestations of the disease does not seem justified. Therapy should be pursued energetically and the excess iron removed as rapidly as possible to minimize the risk of complications, especially primary liver cell cancer. Twice-weekly phlebotomies, each of 500 ml, are usually well tolerated. Manifestations of the disease usually improve or disappear except for diabetes, testicular atrophy and articular chondrocalcinosis. Therefore, in addition to removal of iron, replacement therapy with testosterone may be helpful. Insulin requirements in diabetic patients frequently decrease after venesection therapy. Therapy with desferrioxamine is not practical in idiopathic haemochromatosis because the amount of iron excreted, 270 to 360 μmol/day (15 to 20 mg/day) does not compare with that removed by venesections. However, when venesection therapy is not feasible, for example in haemochromatosis secondary to chronic anaemia, therapy with iron-chelating agents should be used.[5] For example, desferrioxamine can be given intravenously in glucose-saline following each transfusion (e.g. 1 g eight-hourly) and up to 18 mmol (1 g) of iron may be excreted over two to three days during such therapy.

Since the average patient with idiopathic haemochromatosis has 360 to 720 mmol (20 to 40 g) of stored iron, the weekly phlebotomy schedule usually has to be continued for two to three years. During this period the plasma iron remains high and falls only when available iron stores are depleted. Bleeding should therefore be continued as required to keep the plasma iron level below 27 μmol/l (150 μg/100 ml) and the serum ferritin level normal.

The ultimate prognosis appears to depend on the amount and rapidity of parenchymal iron loading and the presence of associated liver disease of other aetiology. The mean survival after diagnosis in 1935 was 4.4 years[33] when treatment was limited to the supportive measures for diabetes, liver disease and cardiac failure. At that time 14 per cent of patients developed primary liver cell cancer. In 1969, Williams and co-workers demonstrated that of 28 patients treated by phlebotomy during the preceding 20 years, 89 per cent had a five-year survival rate from the time of diagnosis.[105] In another analysis of 26 non-alcoholic patients with haemochromatosis, Powell found a significant difference in mortality, with only three deaths of 19 in the treated group compared with four deaths of seven in the untreated group.[70] There is suggestive evidence, though no absolute proof, that the disease may be prevented in individuals whose tissues are overloaded with iron but not yet damaged, as long as the excess iron is removed and future accumulation of iron prevented. Malignant hepatoma does not appear to develop if the disease is treated in the precirrhotic phase.[72] Thus, especially in relatives of patients and in those patients with early disease, the complications and natural course of haemochromatosis should be entirely preventable.

SECONDARY HAEMOCHROMATOSIS

Cirrhosis with Subsequent Gross Secondary Iron Overload

As discussed above, it has long been recognized that patients with hepatic cirrhosis may secondarily develop increased hepatic iron stores. Indeed, MacDonald and Mallory[63] at the Boston City Hospital were so impressed with the histological similarities between their cases of portal cirrhosis and the cases of haemochromatosis reported by Sheldon[87] that they concluded that idiopathic haemochromatosis was not an inherited disease of iron metabolism but rather a variant of alcoholic cirrhosis, the iron and the liver disease being unrelated causally. Although this hypothesis oversimplified the case, it did result in more intensive research into iron metabolism in patients with cirrhosis and the recognition that the full syndrome of haemochromatosis as defined above could, albeit rarely, result from iron accumulation secondary to pre-existing cirrhosis.[82] The situation may be summarized as follows:

1. A variable proportion of patients with hepatic cirrhosis accumulate iron secondarily, but rarely do the body iron stores or hepatic iron concentrations reach levels comparable with those seen in patients with haemochromatosis. When they do, the clinical and pathological features are almost indistinguishable from those seen in idiopathic haemochromatosis. The distinction then requires the demonstration of
   (a) a family history of iron storage disease (idiopathic haemochromatosis);
   (b) serial liver biopsies showing cirrhosis preceding the iron accumulation in alcoholic cirrhosis or the reverse in idiopathic haemochromatosis;
   (c) wedge biopsy of the liver showing the characteristic appearances of early non-alcoholic idiopathic haemochromatosis, as described above, with dense fibrous septa and large areas of preserved parenchyma without frank nodularity.[73]
2. A much more common diagnostic problem for the physician or hepatologist is the distinction between idiopathic haemochromatosis and alcoholic cirrhosis with only mild to moderate increase in stainable liver iron or body iron stores. This differentiation can be made by evaluating the degree of iron loading using the various tests discussed above.
3. The factors that have been implicated as contributing to increased iron absorption and iron accumulation in patients with cirrhosis of the liver are
   (a) increased oral iron intake in alcoholic beverages or iron tablets;
   (b) stimulation of absorption of inorganic iron by alcohol;
   (c) pancreatic insufficiency;
   (d) folic acid deficiency;
   (e) portacaval shunt surgery.
   Each of these factors and the relevant literature have been discussed in depth elsewhere.[38]
4. There is an increased incidence of alcoholism in patients with idiopathic haemochromatosis, varying from between 25 and 50 per cent of patients.[70,97] This has contributed to the confusion, which is discussed in detail above, between this disease and alcoholic cirrhosis. However, a systematic comparison of alcoholic and non-alcoholic subjects with haemochromatosis as defined above showed no significant difference between the two groups with respect to the clinical and pathological features or to the degree of iron overload, except for the presence of active hepatocellular disease in some alcoholic patients.[70,71] Furthermore, a detailed study of the pathology of the liver in haemochromatosis[73] revealed that the hepatic findings were the same in alcoholic and non-

alcoholic patients, except that in about 25 per cent of the alcoholic patients there were changes of alcoholic liver disease superimposed on the underlying haemochromatosis. This is, of course, an incidence of alcoholic liver disease very similar to that reported amongst heavy drinkers in the general population.

The inescapable conclusion is that the majority of alcoholic subjects with haemochromatosis possess the basic genetic defect of iron metabolism and that the iron accumulation has been accelerated by alcoholism.[70] Scheinberg suggested that such subjects were heterozygous for the inherited trait whereas non-alcoholic subjects were homozygous.[84] This is consistent with reported family studies.[76]

5. Phlebotomy therapy should be performed in all patients with primary idiopathic haemochromatosis, whether alcoholic or non-alcoholic, unless contraindicated by the presence of ischaemic heart disease, etc. However, depletion of excess iron has no role in the treatment of the alcoholic cirrhotic with excess iron stores.[38]

Haemochromatosis Associated with Chronic Anaemias ('Erythropoietic Haemochromatosis')

Increased erythropoiesis induced experimentally in animals results in increased iron absorption.[20] In man, such increased iron absorption occurs primarily in those forms of haemolytic anaemia associated with ineffective erythropoiesis as in hereditary sideroblastic anaemia and thalassaemia major.[3] However, haemochromatosis has also been described in association with other chronic refractory anaemias such as congenital spherocytosis.[6] Causative factors for the excess storage iron, in addition to increased absorption, include iron released from the breakdown of excess haemoglobin and exogenous iron from blood transfusions or from the inadvertent administration of oral iron compounds.

Various degrees of iron overload are found in these patients. Those with diseases associated with ineffective erythropoiesis and increased iron absorption have predominant parenchymal iron loading whereas in those whose iron load has been acquired primarily parenterally, there is predominantly RE cell involvement.[73] Fibrosis and functional impairment of the affected organs, although uncommon overall, are seen more often in the former group. The full clinicopathological syndrome of haemochromatosis, including cardiac failure, diabetes mellitus and hypopituitarism, has been described in such patients.[3,6]

Treatment is rather unsatisfactory at present. Cautious phlebotomy, pyridoxine and chelating agents may be tried.[103] Intensive regular chelation therapy with desferrioxamine has been shown in a controlled trial to be effective in reducing the iron load and delaying the onset of hepatic fibrosis[5] but the development of more effective chelating agents is eagerly awaited for this group of patients. At present, intravenous or subcutaneous infusions of desferrioxamine are the most effective form of chelation therapy.

Dietary Iron Overload

Gross iron overload resulting from excess absorption of dietary iron is very rare in all populations that have been studied with the single exception of the negroes of Southern Africa among whom it is common (so-called 'Bantu-type haemochromatosis'). The disease in that population has been extensively reviewed recently[11] and will not be discussed further here. In caucasians, the setting in which haemochromatosis may be seen solely as a result of secondary iron accumulation from dietary sources is the patient with alcoholic cirrhosis who is mildly anaemic, usually due to folic acid and *not* iron deficiency, and who is given oral iron supplements by his physician. Jandl, Davidson and Abelmann reported such a patient who developed haemochromatosis otherwise indistinguishable from the idiopathic variety and complicated by polycythaemia and a malignant hepatoma.[51]

PORPHYRIA CUTANEA TARDA

This is a chronic disorder of porphyrin metabolism characterized by blistering, fragility, hyperpigmentation, hirsutism and, occasionally, sclerodermoid changes of the sun-exposed skin. It is most commonly seen in males with a history of excessive alcohol consumption. Biochemically, it is characterized by excessive hepatic synthesis and faecal and urinary excretion of uroporphyrin I.[67,85]

The degree of iron overload amongst these patients is increased to about 90 mmol (5 g) in toto.[61] There is strong circumstantial clinical evidence and experimental support for the concept of a pathogenetic relationship between the increased iron stores and the porphyria.[57,93] The removal of excess iron stores by phlebotomy frequently has a beneficial effect on the disease, including a marked reduction in urinary uroporphyrin excretion.[29] It is of particular interest that this therapy benefits some patients with *normal* iron stores, is independent of alcohol intake, and that replenishing the iron stores has induced a biochemical relapse which improved with a second course of phlebotomy.[60] It has been suggested on the basis of in vitro studies of the effects of iron on porphyrin metabolism that the biochemical explanation for the role of iron in this disease is the inactivation of uroporphyrinogen III cosynthetase activity, resulting in increased amounts of uroporphyrin I.[53] It should be emphasized, nevertheless, that there is no evidence that iron causes liver disease in porphyria cutanea tarda, and that the cirrhosis found in some of these patients is more likely to be related to excess alcohol intake.

REFERENCES

1. Addison, G.M., Beamish, M.R., Hales, C.N., Hodgkins, M., Jacobs, A. & Llewellin, P. (1972) An immunoradiometric assay for ferritin in the serum of normal subjects and patients with iron deficiency and iron overload. *Journal of Clinical Pathology*, **25**, 326–329.
2. Balcerzak, S.P., Mintz, D.H. & Westerman, M.P. (1968) Diabetes mellitus and idiopathic hemochromatosis. *American Journal of the Medical Sciences*, **255**, 53–62.
3. Bannerman, R.B., Keusch, G., Kreimer-Birnbaum, M., Vance, V.K. & Vaughan, S. (1967) Thalassemia intermedia with iron overload, cardiac failure, diabetes mellitus, hypopituitarism and porphyrinuria. *American Journal of Medicine*, **42**, 476–486.
4. Barry, M., Cartei, G. & Sherlock, S. (1969) Differential ferrioxamine test in haemochromatosis and liver disease. *Gut*, **10**, 697–704.
5. Barry, M., Flynn, D. & Risdon, R. (1974) Long-term chelation therapy in thalassaemia major: liver iron concentration, histology and clinical progress. *British Medical Journal*, **ii**, 16.
6. Barry, M., Scheuer, P.J., Sherlock, S., Ross, C.F. & Williams, R. (1968) Hereditary spherocytosis with secondary haemochromatosis. *Lancet*, **ii**, 481–485.
7. Becker, B.J. & Chatgidakis, C.B. (1961) Cirrhosis of the liver in Johannesburg. *Acta Unionis Internationalis contra Cancrum*, **17**, 639.
8. Bell, E.T. (1955) Relation of portal cirrhosis to hemochromatosis and to diabetes mellitus. *Diabetes*, **4**, 435–446.
9. Biggs, J.C. & Davis, A.E. (1963) Relationship of diminished pancreatic secretion to haemochromatosis. *Lancet*, **ii**, 814.
10. Bomford, A., Eddleston, A.L.W.F., Kennedy, L.A., Batchelor, J.R. & Williams, R. (1977) Histocompatibility antigens as markers of abnormal iron metabolism in patients with idiopathic haemochromatosis and their relatives. *Lancet*, **ii**, 327–329.
11. Bothwell, T.H. & Charlton, R.W. (1976) Hemochromatosis. In *Diseases of the Liver* (Ed.) Schiff, L. 5th ed. Philadelphia and Toronto: Lippincott.
12. Bothwell, T.H. & Finch, C.A. (1962) *Iron Metabolism*. Boston: Little, Brown.
13. Bothwell, T.H. & Isaacson, C. (1962) Siderosis in the Bantu. A comparison of the incidence in males and females. *British Medical Journal*, **i**, 522.
14. Bothwell, T.H., Cohen, I., Abrahams, O.H. & Perold, S.M. (1959) A familial study in idiopathic hemochromatosis. *American Journal of Medicine*, **27**, 730–738.
15. Bothwell, T.H., Seftel, H., Jacobs, P., Torrance, J.D. & Baumslag, N. (1964) Iron overload in Bantu subjects. *American Journal of Clinical Nutrition*, **14**, 47.
16. Brink, B., Disler, P., Lynch, S., Jacobs, P., Charlton, R. & Bothwell, T. (1976) Patterns of iron storage in dietary iron overload and idiopathic hemochromatosis. *Journal of Laboratory and Clinical Medicine*, **88**, 725–731.
17. Charlton, R.W. & Bothwell, T.H. (1966) Hemochromatosis: dietary and genetic aspects. In *Progress in Hematology*. pp. 298–323. New York: Grune & Stratton.
18. Charlton, R.W., Hawkins, D.M. & Mavor, W.O. (1970) Hepatic storage iron concentrations in different population groups. *American Journal of Clinical Nutrition*, **23**, 358.
19. Charlton, R.W., Jacobs, P., Seftel, H. & Bothwell, T.H. (1964) Effect of alcohol on iron absorption. *British Medical Journal*, **ii**, 1427–1429.
20. Conrad, M.E., Weintraub, L.R. & Crosby, W.H. (1965) Iron metabolism in rats with phenylhydrazine-induced hemolytic disease. *Blood*, **25**, 990.
21. Crosby, W.H. (1966) Heredity of hemochromatosis. In *Controversy in Internal Medicine*. (Ed.) Ingelfinger, F.J., Relman, A.S. & Finland, M. pp. 261–270. Philadelphia: W.B. Saunders.
22. Crosby, W.H. (1976) Normal serum ferritin in precirrhotic hemochromatosis. *New England Journal of Medicine*, **294**, 1116.
23. Davis, A.E. (1961) Relationship of disturbed pancreatic function to haemosiderosis. *Lancet*, **ii**, 749–750.
24. Davis, P.S., Luke, C.G. & Deller, D.J. (1966) Reduction of gastric iron-binding protein in haemochromatosis – a previously unrecognized metabolic defect. *Lancet*, **ii**, 1431–1433.
25. Drysdale, J.W., Adelman, T.G., Arosio, P., Casareale, D., Fitzpatrick, P., Hazard, J.T. & Yokota, M. (1977) Human isoferritins in normal and disease states. *Seminars in Hematology*, **14**, 71–88.

26. Dymock, I.W., Hamilton, E.B.D., Laws, J.W. & Williams, R. (1970) Arthropathy of haemochromatosis: clinical and radiological analysis of 73 patients with iron overload. *Annals of the Rheumatic Diseases*, **29**, 469–476.

27. Dymock, I.W., Cassar, J., Pyke, D.A., Oakley, W.G. & Williams, R. (1972) Observations on the pathogenesis, complications and treatment of diabetes in 115 cases of hemochromatosis. *American Journal of Medicine*, **52**, 203–210.

28. Edwards, C.Q., Carroll, M., Bray, P. & Cartwright, G.E. (1977) Hereditary hemochromatosis. *New England Journal of Medicine*, **297**, 7–13.

29. Epstein, J.H. & Redeker, A.G. (1968) Porphyria cutanea tarda: a study of the effect of phlebotomy. *New England Journal of Medicine*, **279**, 1301–1304.

30. Feller, E.R., Pont, A., Wands, J.R., Carter, E.A., Foster, G., Kourides, I.A. & Isselbacher, K.J. (1977) Familial hemochromatosis. *New England Journal of Medicine*, **296**, 1422–1426.

31. Fielding, J. (1965) Differential ferrioxamine test for measuring chelatable body iron. *Journal of Clinical Pathology*, **18**, 88–97.

32. Finch, C.A. (1959) Body iron exchange in man. *Journal of Clinical Investigation*, **38**, 392–396.

33. Finch, S.C. & Finch, C.A. (1955) Idiopathic hemochromatosis, an iron storage disease. A. Iron metabolism in hemochromatosis. *Medicine (Baltimore)*, **34**, 381.

34. Finch, C.A., Denbelbeiss, K., Cook, J.D., Eshbach, J.W., Harker, L.A., Funk, D.D., Mansaglia, G., Hillman, R.S., Slichter, S., Adamson, J.W., Ganzoni, A. & Giblett, E.R. (1970) Ferrokinetics in man. *Medicine*, **49**, 17–53.

35. Gabuzda, T.G. & Pearson, J. (1969) Metabolic and molecular heterogeneity of marrow ferritin. *Biochimica et Biophysica Acta*, **194**, 50–54.

36. Gilbert, A. & Grenet, A. (1896) *Semaine Médecine*, **16**, 514 (in French).

37. Grace, N.D. (1978) Evidence for hepatic toxicity of iron. In *Metals and the Liver: Health and Disease* (Ed.) Powell, L.W. New York: Marcel Dekker.

38. Grace, N.D. & Powell, L.W. (1974) Iron storage disorders of the liver. *Gastroenterology*, **64**, 1257–1283.

39. Green, R., Charlton, R., Seftel, H., Bothwell, T., Mayet, F., Adams, B., Finch, C. & Layrisse, M. (1968) Body iron excretion in man: a collaborative study. *American Journal of Medicine*, **45**, 336.

40. Greenberg, M.S., Strohmeyer, G., Hine, G.J., Keene, W.R., Curtis, G. & Chalmers, T.C. (1964) Studies in iron absorption III: body radioactivity measurements in patients with liver disease. *Gastroenterology*, **46**, 651–661.

41. Hanot, V. & Schachmann, M. (1886) *Arch Physiol Norm Path*, **7**, 50.

42. Halliday, J.W., Gera, K.L. & Powell, L.W. (1975) A sensitive radioimmunoassay for serum ferritin. *Clinica Chimica Acta*, **58**, 207.

43. Halliday, J.W., Russo, A., Cowlishaw, J. & Powell, L.W. (1977) Serum ferritin in the diagnosis of early haemochromatosis: a study of 43 families. *Lancet*, **ii**, 621–623.

44. Hamilton, E., Williams, R., Barlow, K.A. & Smith, P.M. (1968) The arthropathy of idiopathic haemochromatosis. *Quarterly Journal of Medicine*, **37**, 171–182.

45. Harrison, P.M. (1977) Ferritin: an iron-storage molecule. *Seminars in Hematology*, **14**, 55–70.

46. Haskins, D., Stevens, A.R. Jr, Finch, S. & Finch, C.A. (1952) Iron metabolism. Iron stores in man as measured by phlebotomy. *Journal of Clinical Investigation*, **31**, 543–547.

47. Hershko, C., Cook, J.D. & Finch, C.A. (1972) Storage iron kinetics. II. The uptake of hemoglobin iron by hepatic parenchymal cells. *Journal of Laboratory and Clinical Medicine*, **80**, 624.

48. Hofvander, Y. (1968) Hematological investigations in Ethiopia with special reference to a high iron intake. *Acta Medica Scandinavica* (Suppl.), **494**, 1.

49. Jacobs, A. & Worwood, M. (1975) Ferritin in serum. *New England Journal of Medicine*, **292**, 951.

50. Jacobs, A., Miller, F., Worwood, M., Beamish, M.R. & Wardrop, C.A. (1972) Ferritin in the serum of normal subjects and patients with iron deficiency and iron overload. *British Medical Journal*, **iv**, 206.

51. Jandl, J.H., Davidson, C.S., Abelmann, W.H. & MacDonald, R.A. (1963) Hemochromatosis terminating in polycythemia and hepatoma, with observations on the natural history of hemochromatosis. *New England Journal of Medicine*, **269**, 1054–1059.

52. Johnson, B.F. (1968) Haemochromatosis resulting from prolonged oral iron therapy. *New England Journal of Medicine*, **278**, 1100.

53. Kalivos, J.T., Pathak, M.A. & Fitzpatrick, T.B. (1969) Phlebotomy and iron overload in porphyria cutanea tarda. *Lancet*, **i**, 1184–1187.

54. Kent, G. & Pepper, H. (1968) Liver biopsy in diagnosis of hemochromatosis. *American Journal of Medicine*, **44**, 837–841.

55. Klion, F.M. & Schaffner, F. (1968) Hemochromatosis following hepatitis in a patient with systemic iron overload. *Archives of Pathology*, **86**, 342–347.

56. Knoblauch, M. & Hedinger, C. (1963) Die Hamochromatoseleber. *Virchows Archiv a Pathologische Anatomie*, **337**, 205–214.

57. Kushner, J.P., Lee, G.R. & Nacht, S. (1972) The role of iron in the pathogenesis of porphyria cutanea tarda: an in vitro model. *Journal of Clinical Investigation*, **51**, 3044–3051.

58. Lisboa, P.E. (1971) Experimental hepatic cirrhosis in dogs caused by chronic massive iron overload. *Gut*, **12**, 363.

59. Losowsky, M.S. & Wilson, A.R. (1967) Whole-body counting of the absorption and distribution of iron in haemochromatosis. *Clinical Science*, **32**, 151.

60. Lundvall, O. (1971) The effect of replenishment of iron stores after phlebotomy therapy in porphyria cutanea tarda. *Acta Medica Scandinavica*, **189**, 51–63.

61. Lundvall, O., Weinfeld, A. & Lundin, P. (1970) Iron storage in porphyria cutanea tarda. *Acta Medica Scandinavica*, **188**, 37–53.

62. MacDonald, R.A. (1964) *Hemochromatosis and Hemosiderosis*. Springfield, Illinois: C. Thomas.

63. MacDonald, R.A. & Mallory, G.K. (1960) Hemochromatosis and hemosiderosis: study of 211 autopsied cases. *Archives of Internal Medicine*, **105**, 686–700.

64. Mendel, G.A. (1964) Iron metabolism and etiology of iron-storage diseases. *Journal of the American Medical Association*, **189**, 45.

65. Morgan, E.H. (1961) Idiopathic haemochromatosis – a family study. *Australasian Annals of Medicine*, **10**, 114–120.

66. Morgan, E.H. & Walters, M.N.I. (1963) Iron storage in human disease. Fractionation of hepatic and splenic iron into ferritin and hemosiderin with histochemical correlations. *Journal of Clinical Pathology*, **16,** 101.
67. Nacht, S., San Martin DeViale, L.C. & Grimstein, J. (1970) Human porphyria cutanea tarda. Isolation and properties of the urinary porphyrins. *Clinica Chimica Acta*, **27,** 445–452.
68. Peters, T.J. & Seymour, C.A. (1976) Acid hydrolase activities and lysosomal integrity in liver biopsies from patients with iron overload. *Clinical Science and Molecular Medicine*, **50,** 75–78.
69. Powell, L.W. (1965) Iron storage in relatives of patients with haemochromatosis and in relatives of patients with alcoholic cirrhosis and haemosiderosis. *Quarterly Journal of Medicine*, **34,** 427–442.
70. Powell, L.W. (1970) Changing concepts in haemochromatosis. *Postgraduate Medical Journal*, **46,** 200–209.
71. Powell, L.W. (1975) The role of alcoholism in hepatic iron storage disease. *Annals of the New York Academy of Sciences*, **252,** 124–134.
72. Powell, L.W. & Kerr, J.F.R. (1970) Reversal of 'cirrhosis' in idiopathic haemochromatosis following long-term intensive venesection therapy. *Australasian Annals of Medicine*, **1,** 54–57.
73. Powell, L.W. & Kerr, J.F.R. (1975) The pathology of the liver in hemochromatosis. *Pathobiology Annual* (Ed.) Joacim, H. New York: Allenbury Century Crofts.
74. Powell, L.W. & Halliday, J.W. (1976) Serum ferritin in haemochromatosis. *New England Journal of Medicine*, **294,** 1185.
75. Powell, L.W., Halliday, J.W. & Cowlishaw, J.L. (1978) The relationship between serum ferritin and total body iron stores in idiopathic haemochromatosis. *Gut*, June.
76. Powell, L.W. & Lloyd, H.M. (1975) Haemochromatosis. *Archives of Internal Medicine*, **135,** 1269.
77. Powell, L.W., Campbell, C.B. & Wilson, E. (1970) Intestinal mucosal uptake of iron and iron retention in idiopathic haemochromatosis as evidence for a mucosal abnormality. *Gut*, **11,** 727–731.
78. Powell, L.W., Mortimer, R. & Harris, O.D. (1971) Cirrhosis of the liver: a comparative study of the four major aetiological groups. *Medical Journal of Australia*, **1,** 941–950.
79. Prieto, J., Barry, M. & Sherlock, S. (1975) Serum ferritin in patients with iron overload and with acute and chronic liver diseases. *Gastroenterology*, **68,** 525–533.
80. Ross, J., Kochwa, S. & Wasserman, L.R. (1964) Kinetics of iron transferrin complex formation (abstract). *Blood*, **24,** 850–851.
81. Rowe, J.W., Wands, J.R., Mezey, E., Waterbury, L.A., Wright, J.R., Tobin, J. & Andres, R. (1977) Familial hemochromatosis: characteristics of the precirrhotic stage in a large kindred. *Medicine*, **56,** 1197–2027.
82. Sabesin, S.M. & Thomas, L.B. (1964) Parenchymal siderosis in patients with pre-existing portal cirrhosis. A pathologic entity simulating idiopathic and transfusional hemochromatosis. *Gastroenterology*, **46,** 477–485.
83. Schaeffer, J.W., Amick, C.J., Oikawa, Y. & Schiff, L. (1962) The development of hemochromatosis following portacaval anastomosis. *Gastroenterology*, **42,** 181–188.
84. Scheinberg, H. (1973) The genetics of hemochromatosis. *Archives of Internal Medicine*, **132,** 126–128.
85. Schmid, R. (1966) The porphyria and hyperbilirubinemia. In *The Metabolic Basis of Inherited Disease* (Ed.) Sternburg, J.B., Wyngaarden, J.B. & Frederickson, D.S. pp. 813–871. New York: McGraw-Hill.
86. Seftel, H.C., Malkin, C., Schmaman, A., Abrahams, C., Lynch, S.R., Charlton, R.W. & Bothwell, T.H. (1966) Osteoporosis, scurvy and siderosis in Johannesburg Bantu. *British Medical Journal*, **i,** 642–646.
87. Sheldon, J.H. (1935) *Haemochromatosis*. London: Oxford University Press.
88. Simon, M., Bourel, M., Fauchet, R. & Genetet, B. (1976) Association of HLA-A3 and HLA-B14 antigens with idiopathic haemochromatosis. *Gut*, **17,** 332–334.
89. Simon, M., Bourel, M., Genetet, B., Fauchet, R., Edan, G. & Brissot, P. (1977) Idiopathic hemochromatosis and iron overload in alcoholic liver disease: differentiation by HLA phenotype. *Gastroenterology*, **73,** 655–658.
90. Stocks, A.E. & Martin, F.I.R. (1968) Pituitary function in hemochromatosis. *American Journal of Medicine*, **45,** 839–845.
91. Stocks, A.E. & Powell, L.W. (1973) Carbohydrate intolerance in idiopathic haemochromatosis and cirrhosis of the liver. *Quarterly Journal of Medicine*, **42,** 733–749.
92. Troisier, M. (1871) Diabète sucré. *Bulletin de la Société d'Anatomie Paris*, **44,** 231–235.
93. Turnbull, A., Baker, H., Vernon-Roberts, B. & Magnus, I.A. (1973) Iron metabolism in porphyria cutanea tarda and in erythropoietic protoporphyria. *Quarterly Journal of Medicine*, **42,** 341–355.
94. Tuttle, S.G., Figueroa, W.G. & Gorssman, M.I. (1959) Development of hemochromatosis in a patient with Laennec's cirrhosis. *American Journal of Medicine*, **26,** 655–658.
95. von Recklinghausen, F.D. (1889) *Tageblatt der (62) Versammlung Deutsch, Naturforscher und Arzte in Heidleberg*, p. 324 (in German).
96. Wainwright, J. (1957) Siderosis in the African. *South African Journal of Laboratory and Clinical Medicine*, **3,** 1–28.
97. Walker, R.J. & Williams, R. (1974) Haemochromatosis and iron overload. In *Iron in Biochemistry and Medicine* (Ed.) Jacobs, A. & Worwood, M. pp. 589–612. London: Academic Press.
98. Walker, R.J., Dymock, I.W., Ansell, I.D., Hamilton, E.B.D. & Williams, R. (1972) Synovial biopsy in haemochromatosis arthropathy. Histological findings and iron deposition in relation to total body iron overload. *Annals of the Rheumatic Diseases*, **31,** 98–102.
99. Walsh, R.J., Perkins, K.W. & Blackburn, C.R.B. (1965). A genetic study of hemochromatosis. In *Tenth International Congress of Hematology, Stockholm 1964*. Basel: Karger.
100. Walters, G.O., Miller, F.M. & Worwood, M. (1973) Serum ferritin concentration and iron stores in normal subjects. *Journal of Clinical Pathology*, **26,** 770–775.
101. Wands, J.R., Rowe, J.A., Mezey, S.E., Waterbury, L.A., Wright, J.R., Halliday, June, Isselbacher, K.J. & Powell, L.W. (1976) Normal serum ferritin concentrations in precirrhotic hemochromatosis. *New England Journal of Medicine*, **294,** 302.

102. Wapnick, A.A., Lynch, S.R., Kravitz, P., Seftel, H.C., Charlton, R.W. & Bothwell, T.H. (1968). Effects of iron overload on ascorbic acid metabolism. *British Medical Journal,* **iii,** 704–707.
103. Weintraub, L.R., Conrad, M.E. & Crosby, W.H. (1966) Iron-loading anemia. Treatment with repeated phlebotomies and pyridoxine. *New England Journal of Medicine,* **275,** 169–176.
104. Williams, R., Scheuer, P.J. & Sherlock, S. (1962) The inheritance of idiopathic haemochromatosis. A clinical and liver biopsy study of 16 families. *Quarterly Journal of Medicine,* **31,** 249–265.
105. Williams, R., Smith, P.M., Spicer, E.J.F., Barry, M. & Sherlock, S. (1969) Venesection therapy in idiopathic haemochromatosis. *Quarterly Journal of Medicine,* **38,** 1–16.
106. Zimmerman, H.J., Chomet, B., Kulesch, M.H. & McWhorter, C.A. (1961) Hepatic hemosiderin deposits. Incidence in 558 biopsies from patients with and without intrinsic hepatic disease. *Archives of Internal Medicine,* **197,** 494–503.

Chapter 35

Alpha-1-antitrypsin Deficiency and Liver Disease

D.R. TRIGER
G.H. MILLWARD-SADLER

Clinical interest in the serum globulin alpha-1-antitrypsin (A1AT) arose following the discovery in Sweden of an association between pulmonary emphysema of early adulthood and deficiency of this protein.[51] Subsequently, studies have shown that this deficiency is associated with some of the variants of A1AT. The original cases of early onset pulmonary emphysema were homozygous deficient, and although subsequently many workers have suggested that heterozygous deficiency also predisposes to pulmonary emphysema this aspect remains controversial.

Although Ganrot and colleagues[32] noted two cases of cirrhosis and one hepatocellular carcinoma in their series of adults with lung disease, the association between the enzyme defect and liver disease was first suggested in children.[75] A further survey showed that childhood or juvenile cirrhosis was commonly preceded by a history of neonatal hepatitis.[74] Reports of cirrhosis in adults soon followed and several cases of hepatic carcinoma in association with A1AT deficiency have been described. More recently, cirrhosis has been found in heterozygous patients. While there is little doubt that deficiency of A1AT may be associated with liver disease both in children and adults, the pathogenesis is uncertain.

GENETICS OF ALPHA-1-ANTITRYPSIN

Variants of A1AT can be recognized by their differing protein mobility on electrophoresis (Figure 35.1). Faster-moving proteins are identified by earlier letters of the alphabet, and the slowest-moving variant is labelled Z. The individual phenotype is described by the letters Pi (protease inhibitor) followed by the letters describing the particular variant. The common phenotýpe, PiMM, is found in 80 to 95 per cent of the population and is accompanied by normal serum levels. At least 24 alleles have been identified, of which the most important clinically are S and Z, and inheritance follows an autosomal co-dominant pattern.

A rare variant termed Pi nul (Pi–) has no detectable A1AT in the serum.[82] Since this is impossible to detect by electrophoresis, it has become the habit of some authors to describe the phenotype of homozygous patients by a single letter (i.e., PiZ or PiM) and to use the full description (PiZZ or PiMM) when the second allele has been determined by family studies.

Extensive population studies conducted in different countries have revealed quite significant variations in the frequency of certain phenotypes.[17, 28] Most notable among these has

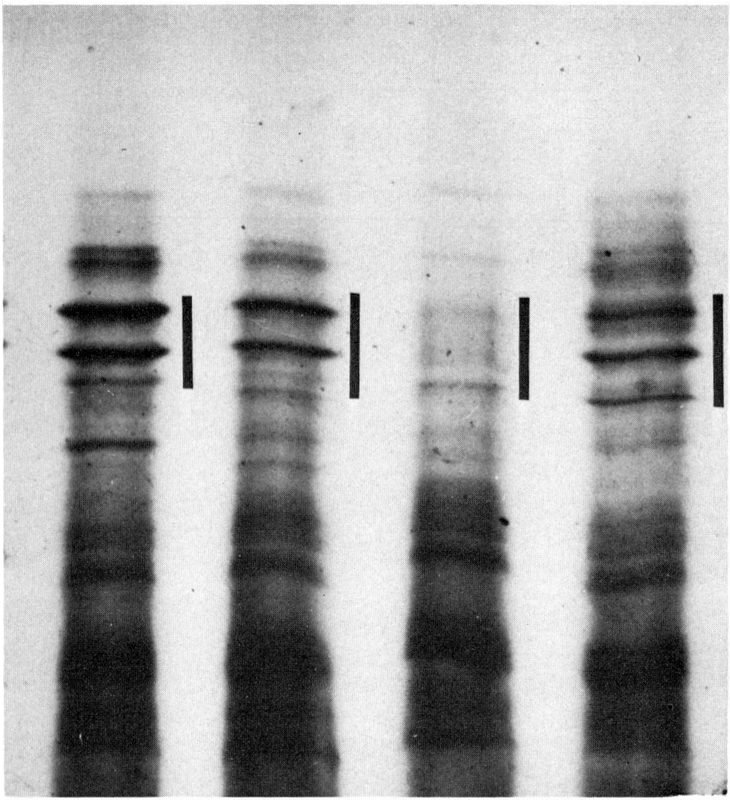

Figure 35.1. Isoelectric focusing plate showing A1AT phenotypes. The vertical bars indicate the region showing the characteristic pattern for each phenotype (from left to right M; MZ; ZZ; MS). Courtesy of Dr A. Milford Ward, Supraregional Protein Reference Laboratory, Sheffield.

been a high frequency of PiS in Spain and a very low incidence of abnormal phenotypes in negroes[68] and American Indians.[86] The largest population studies have found a frequency of 0.06 per cent for the homozygous Z phenotype and a gene frequency of 2.4 per cent for the Z allele.[52, 78]

Liver disease has been reported in association with very few of the phenotypes and the approximate incidence of these is shown in Table 35.1. PiZZ appears to be the most common type, particularly in childhood liver disease and, with few exceptions, liver abnormalities have been found only in association with the Z allele.

BIOCHEMISTRY AND PHYSIOLOGY

Alpha-1-antitrypsin is a glycoprotein (mol.wt 50000) synthesized only in the liver. The carbohydrate moiety which comprises about 12 per cent of the molecule consists of galactose, mannose, *N*-acetyl glucosamine and sialic acid. It is thought that six sialic acid residues are

Table 35.1. *Abnormal alpha-1-antitrypsin Phenotypes. Incidence and Reported Relationship to Clinical Liver Disease.*

Phenotype	Approximate incidence (%)	Serum concentration (% of normal)	Neonatal hepatitis	Childhood cirrhosis	Adult liver disease	Hepatoma
ZZ	0.01–0.06	15	+ + +	+ + +	+ + +	+ + +
MZ	0.5–4.7	60	+	+	+ +	+
SZ	0.1–0.2	40	+	+	+	–
FZ	0.02	60	–	–	+	–
SS	0.1–1.6	60	–	–	+	–

– = not reported; + = isolated case reports; + + = several case reports; + + + = well recognized association.

attached to the molecule in the normal PiM phenotype, but fewer, probably only four residues, are attached to the Z variant.[19] Fingerprinting has demonstrated differences in the amino acid composition of the polypeptide chains of some variants when compared with PiM. In PiZ the amino acid lysine has been substituted for glutamic acid,[43,89] and in PiS valine has been similarly exchanged for glutamic acid.[67]

As the name implies, A1AT is the major trypsin inhibitor in the serum and has a concentration in normal healthy individuals of 200 to 300 mg/dl. Apart from trypsin it also inhibits numerous other enzymes, notably elastase, collagenase, plasmin and chymotrypsin. Increased synthesis and transport of A1AT to the site of injury occur during inflammation when it is thought to neutralize proteolytic enzymes released as a consequence of tissue damage. Levels also rise in response to various drugs and non-specific stimuli and are commonly elevated in acute and chronic liver disease.[40] Rarely, levels may be severely depressed in acute hepatic necrosis and in protein-losing states.[13]

The half-life of normal A1AT is four to six days[57] and is slightly less for the PiZ variant but this difference is insufficient to account for the marked variation in serum levels.[53]

Measurement of Serum Alpha-1-antitrypsin

Since A1AT forms 90 per cent of the normal alpha-1-globulin band a marked deficiency is reflected in the electrophoretic strip. Unfortunately, this simple test is not a reliable technique since (a) it will detect only the most severely deficient subjects and (b) the globulin increase which commonly accompanies liver disease may be so diffuse as to conceal a deficiency in the α_1 moiety.

A more direct method is to measure the trypsin inhibitory effect of the serum:[51] alterations in serum levels of the protein are readily reflected by this functional measurement.

Serum A1AT can be measured immunochemically. The commonly used method is single radial immunodiffusion for which agar gel plates and quantitative standards are widely available commercially.[58] We have found the alternative technique of electro-immunoassay – involving the electrophoresis of serum samples into agarose gel-containing antibody – to be a more sensitive and reproducible test which, in addition, gives a permanent record for future comparison.[85]

Phenotyping

Measurement of the serum level of A1AT alone may indicate, but it cannot identify, the individual's phenotype. Under conditions mentioned earlier the serum levels may be artificially elevated or depressed, particularly in the case of MM and MZ phenotypes.[81] In order to confirm the alleles it is necessary to examine the electrophoretic mobility of the A1AT. Acid starch gel electrophoresis enables separation of A1AT into three major and five minor bands.[29] Antigen–antibody crossed electrophoresis may be used as an additional technique for distinguishing the more difficult cases.[49] It should be emphasized that these electrophoretic techniques are time consuming, have technical problems and should be carried out in specialized centres possessing both considerable experience and adequate control sera. Because of the doubts raised by the present techniques many authorities recommend that any unusual phenotypes should be supported by family studies whenever possible. More recently a technique involving isoelectric focusing on polyacrylamide gel slabs has been described.[3] It appears to be a much simpler procedure and is much quicker to perform. It also appears to be more sensitive, as Kueppers[45] has been able to subdivide the M genotype into M and M_1 by this technique, and it is likely to become the standard method (Figure 35.1).

CLINICAL FEATURES

Neonatal Hepatitis

Neonatal jaundice is a common presentation of liver disease associated with A1AT deficiency, and has also proved to be a significant diagnostic category in this heterogeneous syndrome. The differential diagnosis of neonatal hepatitis is discussed in detail elsewhere in this book, and the diagnosis depends upon establishing deficiency of A1AT in the serum or finding characteristic histological features on liver biopsy. This should enable the physician to distinguish the condition from biliary atresia which otherwise can be impossible to separate on clinical grounds although the two conditions

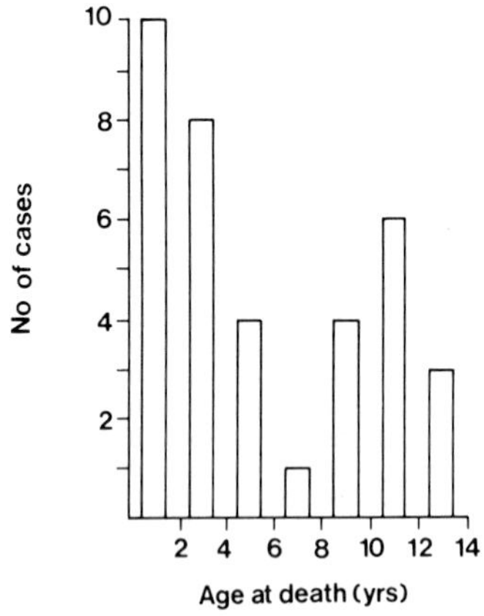

Figure 35.2. Childhood deaths associated with ZZ A1AT deficiency and liver disease. Data include 25 cases reported in the literature and 11 unpublished cases from the South-east England Epidemiological Survey on Neonatal Hepatitis.[18] Courtesy of Dr A.P. Mowat.

may occur simultaneously.[16,66] A1AT deficiency appears to be a significant cause of neonatal hepatitis, accounting for 13 to 40 per cent of cases.[1,18,64] Although most of the children appear to be normal at birth, retrospective analysis in several series has shown that their birth weight tends to be below normal.[69,78] The typical symptoms of jaundice, pale stools and dark urine usually appear between one and six weeks after birth, although it may be present at birth or develop as late as two or three months of age. The increase in serum bilirubin is invariably accompanied by elevations in aspartate transaminase (AST) and in alkaline phosphatase. In the majority of cases the jaundice is transient and the other liver function tests return to normal although hepatosplenomegaly may persist. Long-term follow-up of these cases has shown that many of them present in later childhood with cirrhosis and progressive hepatic failure.

Despite the initial gloomy reports of prognosis[74] the literature contains very few reports of children with A1AT deficiency dying of liver failure. Analysis of these deaths (Figure 35.2) shows that the mortality is slightly higher in the first four years of life and is followed by a fairly even distribution throughout the years of childhood, suggesting that the rate of progress of liver disease is very variable.

Kumar et al[48] report one patient who presented with jaundice at six weeks and, apart from requiring a portacaval anastomosis at the age of 16 for bleeding oesophageal varices, is well and at work at 25 years. We have seen a patient who died at the age of 27 years of liver failure secondary to homozygous A1AT deficiency.[85] She was jaundiced during the first two months of life, and the jaundice resolved only to recur intermittently from the age of 12 onwards. Several teenagers have been reported as alive and well with varying degrees of hepatic abnormality up to 19 years after neonatal hepatitis.[64]

Certain criteria may give some idea of prognosis. Children with an early onset of cirrhosis (i.e., within the first year) develop jaundice earlier in the neonatal period and the jaundice persists for longer than in those with a more benign course.[18] In addition, the maximum abnormalities in standard liver function tests (bilirubin, AST and alkaline phosphatase) are greater in those with a poorer prognosis. Moroz and colleagues[64] claim that persistent elevation in AST during the second year of life is a poor prognostic sign. These conclusions are based on relatively small series of patients and confirmation is required before any definite prognostic guidelines can be established. Similarly prognostic features have been suggested in liver biopsies (see below).[39] Clinical presentation in the neonatal period has been reported mostly in children with the homozygous PiZ defect although individual reports in association with PiSZ[88] and MZ[24] have appeared. However, not all children with PiZZ genotype develop neonatal hepatitis. Cottrall, Cook and Mowat,[18] in an epidemiological survey in South-east England, have calculated that one in seven of these homozygous-deficient infants develop clinical features of neonatal hepatitis. This is comparable with the current results from the larger and more comprehensive prospective study being conducted in Sweden.[78] In this study, over 95 per cent of all infants born between January 1972 and November 1974 have been screened during the first few days of life and all those with serum A1AT levels less than 40 per cent of normal were referred for phenotyping. One-hundred and twenty out of 200000 were found to possess the PiZZ phenotype and, of these, 22 infants developed jaundice and abnormal liver function tests during the first three months of life. This corresponds closely to the figures obtained in the English study, but may underestimate the true incidence of liver disease associated with the enzyme deficiency since elevated SGOT levels were reported in 44 out of 84 of all ZZ infants at three months and 36 out of 60 at six months. Follow-up studies on this group of children over the next few years will undoubtedly assess the risk of a ZZ child developing liver disease in addition to defining the significance of the elevated AST levels in early childhood.

Although the screening technique employed in this study was able to detect all infants with PiZZ, the cut-off level of 40 per cent was too low to pick up reliably any other phenotype except for SZ. Forty-eight infants with this type were detected (representing about half the calculated incidence) and there were no cases of neonatal hepatitis among this group. However, 10 out of 42 at three months and one out of 22 at six months had abnormal liver function tests, although usually of a lower magnitude than that found in ZZ infants. Again, it is hoped that follow-up over a number of years will define the risk of developing liver disease for children of SZ genotype.

Childhood Cirrhosis

Although neonatal hepatitis is known to predispose to the development of childhood cirrhosis, in at least 50 per cent of children presenting with cirrhosis associated with A1AT deficiency there is no antecedent history of jaundice during the first few months of life.[1] The clinical features of the liver disease are similar to those noted in cirrhosis secondary to any other cause. A chance finding of hepatosplenomegaly in an asymptomatic child is a common feature. Other presenting symptoms include pruritus, progressive hepatic failure or haematemesis from bleeding oesophageal varices. Death may occur from bleeding, hepatic coma or intercurrent infection. The cirrhosis can be grossly macronodular or micronodular in type and death from haemoperitoneum following rupture of a non-malignant nodule has been reported.[85] Once again, most cases have been reported in association with the PiZZ phenotype although a few reports of cirrhosis in this age group in association with MZ have appeared.[22,56] The prognosis of this condition, as discussed in the previous section, appears to be very variable but many more data are required. Although pulmonary emphysema is often seen in conjunction with the liver disease, either may be independently found. There seems little doubt from the literature that the presence of liver disease has a much greater effect on survival than does pulmonary involvement.

Adult Cirrhosis

The fact that many of the cases detected in childhood are found by chance in asymptomatic individuals suggests that the rate of progression is very variable and many other cases could be expected to present in adulthood. Review of the literature, together with our own unpublished cases, has yielded 39 adults with documented liver disease and PiZZ A1AT deficiency.

The age of these patients ranges up to 83 years and the slight predominance of males over females (23:16) is consistent with the male preponderance noted by Sveger[78] in neonatal hepatitis. Cirrhosis was documented in 25 cases, portal fibrosis in 12, and a curious cholangiolar hyperplasia in two instances.[35,79] Hepatic carcinoma has been noted in a number of cases and this will be considered later in greater detail.

The clinical presentation of these patients is similar to that encountered with any type of chronic liver disease. Signs of liver disease in a patient with long-standing pulmonary symptoms should alert the clinician to the possibility of the disorder even though the significance may be obscured by a history of heavy cigarette consumption. However, only 26 of the 39 adults reviewed in the literature had evidence of chest disease. In the younger patient it is often possible to elicit a history of jaundice during early childhood; but this has not been reported in the older patients. This may simply reflect the difficulty in obtaining information about self-limiting illness which occurred 40 or more years previously. Alternatively, these patients might belong to the sub-group of PiZZ infants who develop little or no abnormality in liver function during the neonatal period. This question may be answered by the prospective study in Sweden. To date, however, even individual case reports of cirrhosis progressing slowly over a number of years in adults are lacking. Eriksson and Hagerstrand[25] described nine adults who presented with a rapidly progressive downhill course to death from variceal bleeding or hepatic coma. Six out of eight patients who died within two years of presentation had hepatocellular carcinoma which may have accounted for the rapid decompensation. Our personal experience of older patients who present with cirrhosis (as opposed to hepatic fibrosis) suggests that once the patients have developed clinical evidence of hepatic disturbance the prognosis is relatively poor. Further long-term studies should show whether this is due to a sudden deterioration of relatively benign hepatic state, or whether it reflects the quiescent asymptomatic nature of hepatic cirrhosis which manifests itself only when it is very advanced.

As in the childhood liver disease cirrhosis in adults associated with the homozygous ZZ state is better recognized and documented than the association with other phenotypes. Nevertheless, cirrhosis has been reported in adults with MZ,[71,85] SZ[14] and FZ phenotypes.[11] In addition, we have observed a further case of macronodular cirrhosis associated with MZ phenotype as well as cases of hepatic fibrosis associated with SZ and SS phenotypes (each with characteristic A1AT globules in the liver). The paucity of clinical reports to date may reflect the rarity of such occurrences, but more awareness of a possible association between liver disease and other A1AT variants may lead to greater detection.

How much liver disease in adults and neonates can be attributed to either the homozygous or heterozygous condition is still not known. As the gene frequency varies among ethnic groups and the incidence of liver disease is affected by social, cultural and environmental variation this will reflect the proportion of liver disease due to PiZ. Fisher, Taylor and Sherlock[31] in a prospective study of 469 patients with hepatobiliary disease found five patients of PiZZ phenotype and an additional 22 patients (4.7 per cent) with other abnormal phenotypes compared with 6.1 per cent in a control population. However, this is a relatively small sample reflecting the spectrum seen in a specialist centre.

In 5 years in a busy general hospital we have found 12 patients with histopathological evidence of both liver disease and A1AT deficiency in whom serum phenotyping substantiated the diagnosis. Cirrhosis was found in 166 liver biopsies of which seven (4.2 per cent) had A1AT deficiency and fibrosis was recorded in 73 biopsies with A1AT deficiency in five (6.9 per cent) of these. Unfortunately, we do not know the incidence of the gene in our sampling population although Cook[17] has established a gene frequency of 2 per cent for parts of South and South-east England.

Another approach to the problem is by retrospective examination of autopsy material. In a recently published study Blenkinsopp and Haffenden[9] reviewed all the necropsy liver specimens over a 15-year period from patients with cirrhosis, hepatic fibrosis and hepatocellular carcinoma. Out of 4895 necropsies, 64 adults had cirrhosis. Ten of these contained periodic acid Schiff (PAS)-positive globules antigenically identical to A1AT. Four out of nine cases with hepatic fibrosis were similarly

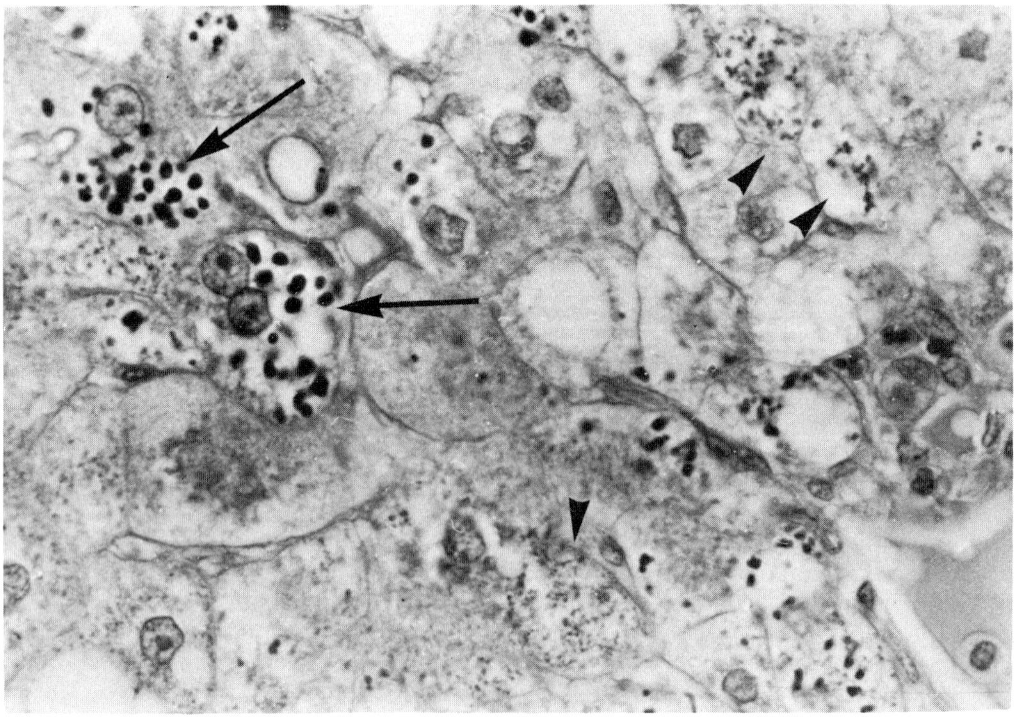

Figure 35.3. Numerous PAS-positive diastase-resistant globules (arrows) within hepatocytes adjacent to a fibrous band. The edge of this is present at bottom right. Apart from these obvious globules there are hepatocytes with a fine PAS-positive diastase-resistant granularity (arrowheads) that react positively in immunocytochemical techniques. DPAS technique × 600.

positive. This would suggest that A1AT deficiency plays a significant part in the aetiology of chronic liver disease, but the study is limited by the inability to measure the serum A1AT level or to establish the phenotype.

Hepatoma

Although Ganrot, Laurell and Eriksson[32] noted that one patient with ZZ phenotype and pulmonary emphysema had a primary hepatic carcinoma, Berg and Eriksson,[8] observing two hepatocellular and one cholangiocellular carcinomas among eight patients with PiZZ deficiency and cirrhosis or fibrosis, were the first to suggest an association. In a retrospective review of 75 liver cell carcinomas, these authors found seven cases in which the characteristic morphology of A1AT was demonstrable in the liver. Other workers have reported the presence of PAS-positive globules in four out of 15 hepatic carcinomas examined at autopsy. No phenotyping was available and there was no difference in frequency from hepatomas arising in cirrhotic livers of different aetiology.[9] A subsequent report from the Swedish group cites six hepatomas among nine patients with cirrhosis and PiZZ phenotype.[25] The rarity with which both primary hepatocellular carcinomas and PiZZ occur in Sweden suggests that there is a significant association between the two conditions. The occurrence has not only been associated with cirrhosis but has also been reported in the presence of hepatic fibrosis[91] and normal hepatic architecture.[72] Hepatocellular carcinoma may also occur in association with the MZ phenotype.[56, 71] Despite the suggestion from the autopsy studies that the enzyme deficiency might be present in 20 to 30 per cent of cases of liver cell cancer, two prospective studies have failed to support this. Theodoropoulos et al[84] have shown no increase in the frequency of PiZ phenotype in 50 patients with hepatic carcinoma and cirrhosis, although they did observe a significant increase in the frequency of PiFM (14 per cent). This finding requires confirmation, especially as Cook[17] noted that an artefact resembling the FM genotype could be found in plasma samples that either contained haemolysed blood or had been at the ambient temperature for several days. Charlionet et al,[15] studying Pi phenotype in 19 European and 38 West African patients with hepatoma, were unable to detect any cases of PiZ. In these patients no comment was made on either the morphology of the livers or the incidence of other predisposing factors to hepatocellular carcinoma. We have found only one case of hepatoma amongst our cases of liver disease associated with the Z allele: autopsies have been performed on nine of the 10 who have died (unpublished observations).

PATHOLOGY

The histopathology of the liver in homozygous PiZ deficiency is characterized by the almost constant presence within hepatocytes of globules which are diastase resistant and strongly PAS positive. These acidophilic globules are not readily identified on routine haematoxylin and eosin (H & E) sections as they merge with the general cytoplasmic staining. They are concentrated within hepatocytes adjacent to portal tracts and abnormal fibrous tissue and may be single large globules that distend the cytoplasm and displace the nucleus to one side or multiple small globules within the cytoplasm (Figure 35.3). In general, the globules increase in size and the number of involved hepatocytes increases with the severity of the associated liver disease. The largest globules and the highest proportion of affected hepatocytes are usually demonstrated in autopsy specimens, probably because A1AT is an acute phase reactant protein so that more pronounced retention may result from any stressful stimulus.

The globules can also be demonstrated in the livers from PiMZ patients but the number of involved hepatocytes is usually much smaller. The globules may be very small both in size and in number and may be found in only a few of the hepatocytes. Although these are periportal in distribution none may be demonstrated against some or even several portal tracts. In H & E sections involved hepatocytes frequently have palely staining cytoplasm and are fractionally larger but it is very easy to overlook their presence even after appropriate histochemical staining.

Occasional cells within the low cuboidal epithelium of a peripherally positioned bile ductule sometimes contain a cluster of globules.

Histochemically, the globules are identified as glycoprotein without a lipid component[23, 37] and are antigenically identical to A1AT by immunofluorescent and immunoperoxidase techniques[85] (Figure 35.4). By both these techniques it is interesting that the rim of the

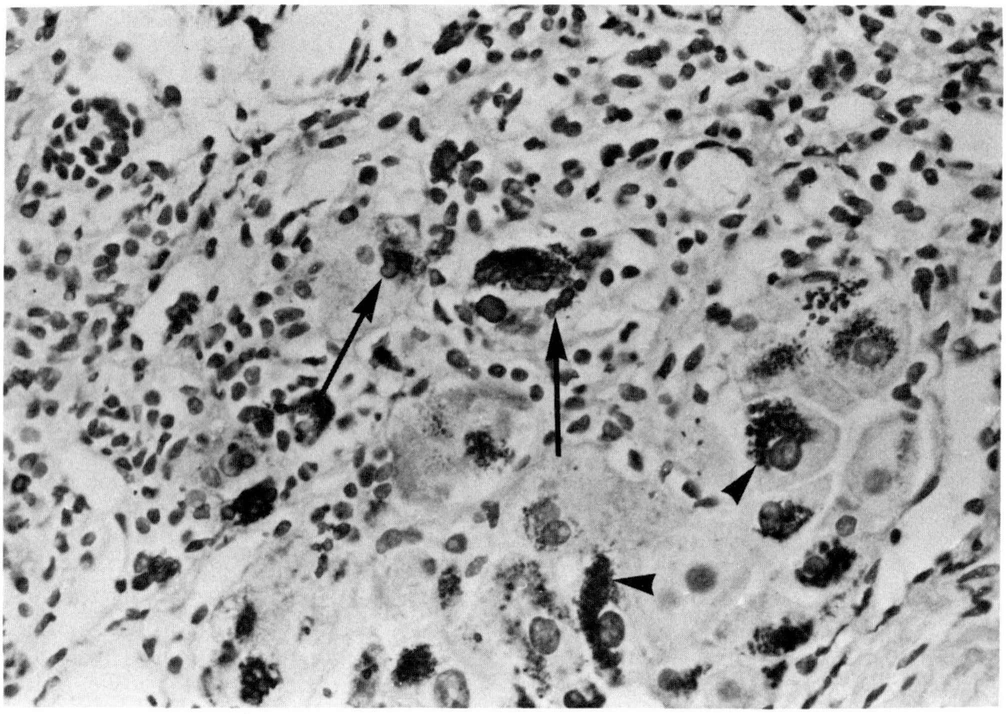

Figure 35.4. Edge of cirrhotic nodule with hepatocytes irregularly separated by fibrosis. Clusters of globules can be seen: the larger ones have an intensely staining rim (arrows). Smaller ones are seen as tightly packed granules (arrowheads). Peroxidase–antiperoxidase technique × 400.

globule is more strongly stained than the contents. Ultrastructurally, the globules are identified as amorphous electron-dense material within dilated saccular endoplasmic reticulum (Figure 35.5). Both rough and smooth components of endoplasmic reticulum are involved and the earliest and greatest accumulation appears to occur in the smooth endoplasmic reticulum.[30,73,90] No dilatation or accumulation of material within the Golgi apparatus has been seen. Confirmation that this amorphous material is A1AT has been provided at the ultrastructural level using an immunoperoxidase technique when positive staining of the contents of the dilated endoplasmic reticulum and also of any attached ribosomes was obtained.[30]

Although PAS-positive globules are a characteristic feature in the livers of these deficient patients they unfortunately are not diagnostic. They have been described in periportal hepatocytes of patients of PiM phenotype with normal serum levels of A1AT. The globules may contain A1AT, demonstrated by the peroxidase–anti-peroxidase technique[10] or, using less sensitive techniques, may not react with antibodies to A1AT.[60] An abnormal A1AT which electrophoretically migrates as PiM is associated with extreme deficiency in the homozygote but low normal serum levels in the heterozygote.[20, 54] In the family study reported by Lieberman, Gaidulis and Klotz[54] PAS-positive globules were present in the homozygote's liver but immunocytochemical studies were not recorded. An interrelationship of these cases is an intriguing possibility.

Globules are said not to occur in hepatocytes of PiS patients except in association with the Z allele, and the case recorded by Lieberman, Mittman and Gordon[55] was subsequently retyped as PiSZ.[37] However, we have seen a patient with PiSS genotype and with no evidence of the Z allele in either him or his family and whose liver contained PAS-positive and immunoperoxidase-positive globules.

Despite these exceptions we always regard the presence of amylase-resistant PAS-positive globules in hepatocytes as evidence of A1AT deficiency until proved otherwise and then we proceed to at least immunoperoxidase identification and serological confirmation with family studies whenever possible.

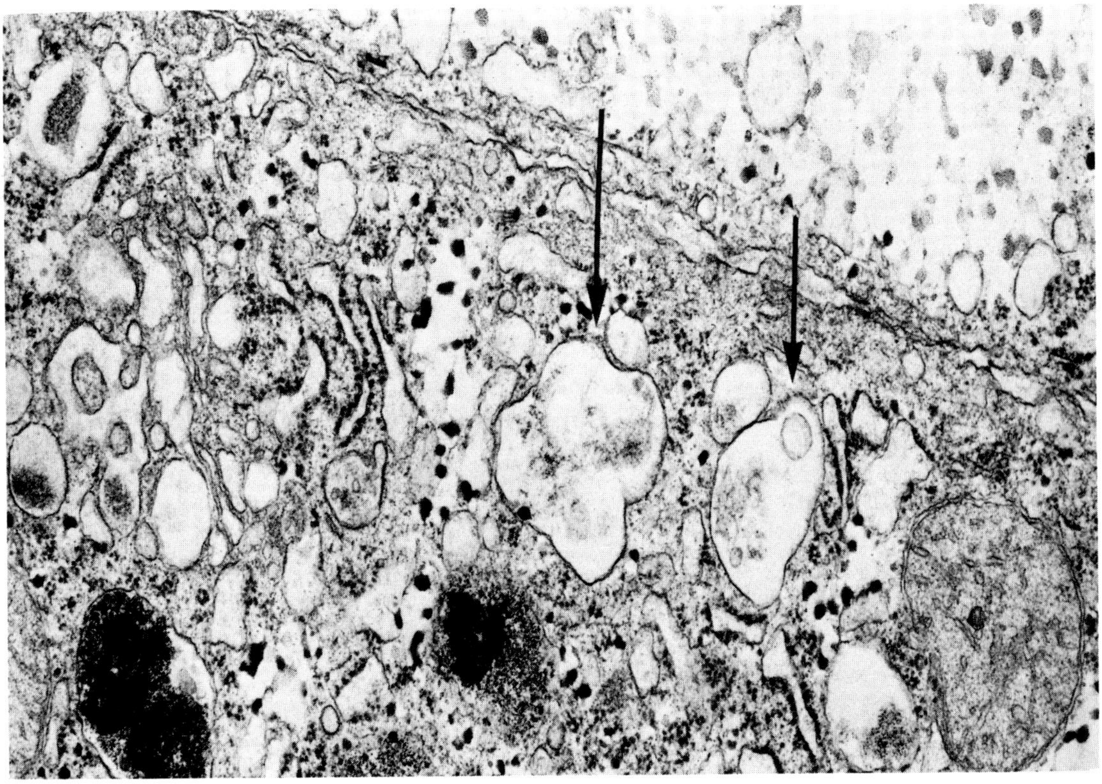

Figure 35.5. Hepatocyte with floccular material contained within dilated endoplasmic reticulum (arrows). Uranyl acetate and lead citrate × 33000.

Neonatal Hepatitis Syndrome

In the homozygous PiZZ with neonatal jaundice the liver is enlarged and green and may be smooth or finely granular. The extrahepatic biliary tree is usually patent although well-documented cases of hypoplasia have been noted.[12, 16, 59, 90]

It is difficult to assess the severity of this reported extrahepatic biliary hypoplasia and whether these lesions on their own would have been sufficient to cause jaundice. Cases such as that described by Christen, Bau and Halsband,[16] where the patency of the bile ducts has increased by the time of the second laparotomy, suggest either that the condition could be under-diagnosed or that the range of normal in the neonatal biliary tree is not appreciated. However, the occasional presence of intrahepatic biliary hypoplasia (see below) indicates that there may be a genuine association.

The histological manifestations of the neonatal liver disease vary, with appearances ranging from secondary biliary cirrhosis to classical giant cell neonatal hepatitis.[83] The unifying feature is the constant presence of the PAS-positive globules in periportal hepatocytes. Although Talbot and Mowat[83] failed to demonstrate these globules in patients less than 12 weeks old, others have frequently identified them in patients as young as one month old.[12, 39, 66]

The most common pattern is a cholestatic jaundice with portal tract expansion and little evidence of parenchymal disturbances (Figure 35.6). In the lobule bile is retained within canaliculi and hepatocytes and, though most severe in centrilobular areas, can be identified in periportal zones and even triads. Periportal hepatocytes may be rearranged to form rosettes or pseudo-acini[83] (Figure 35.7). Centrilobular hepatocytes maintain their normal cell plate pattern with uniformity of nuclear and cell size even though very occasional multinucleate hepatocytes may be seen. Kupffer cells, however, are grossly hypertrophied, contain abundant phagocytosed pigments, including bile, lipofuscins, ceroid and haemosiderin, and form a prominent feature in the lobule. This

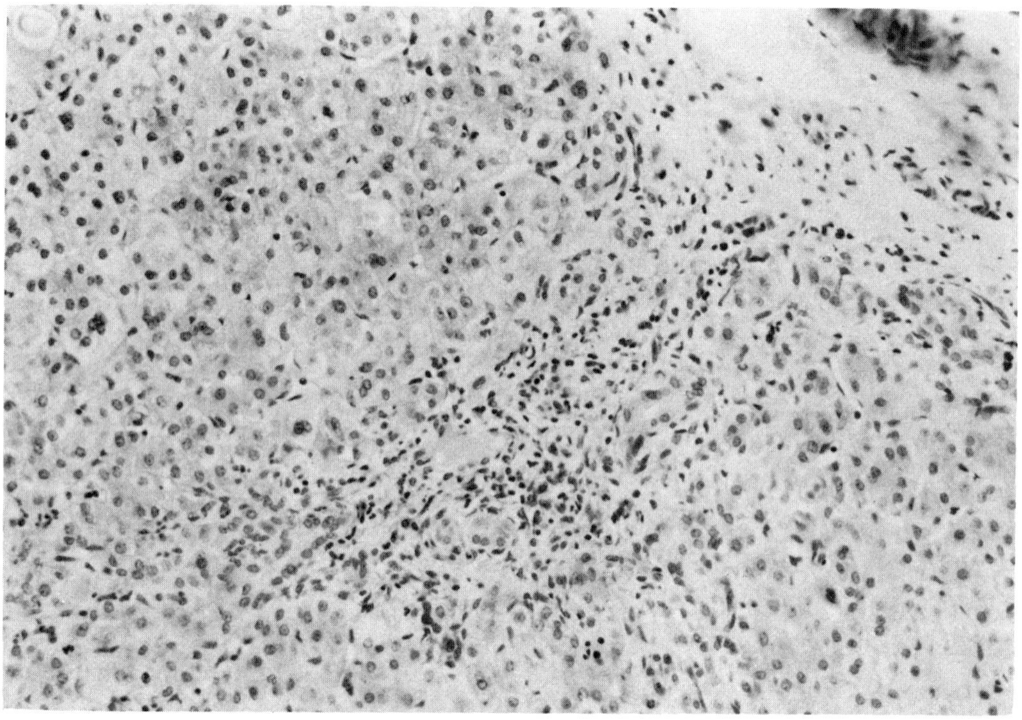

Figure 35.6. Portal tract top right with expansion and bile duct proliferation seen as a spur passing down towards bottom left. Hepatocytes are arranged in the normal neonatal twinned cell plates: giant multinucleate hepatocytes are not a feature. Haematoxylin and eosin × 200.

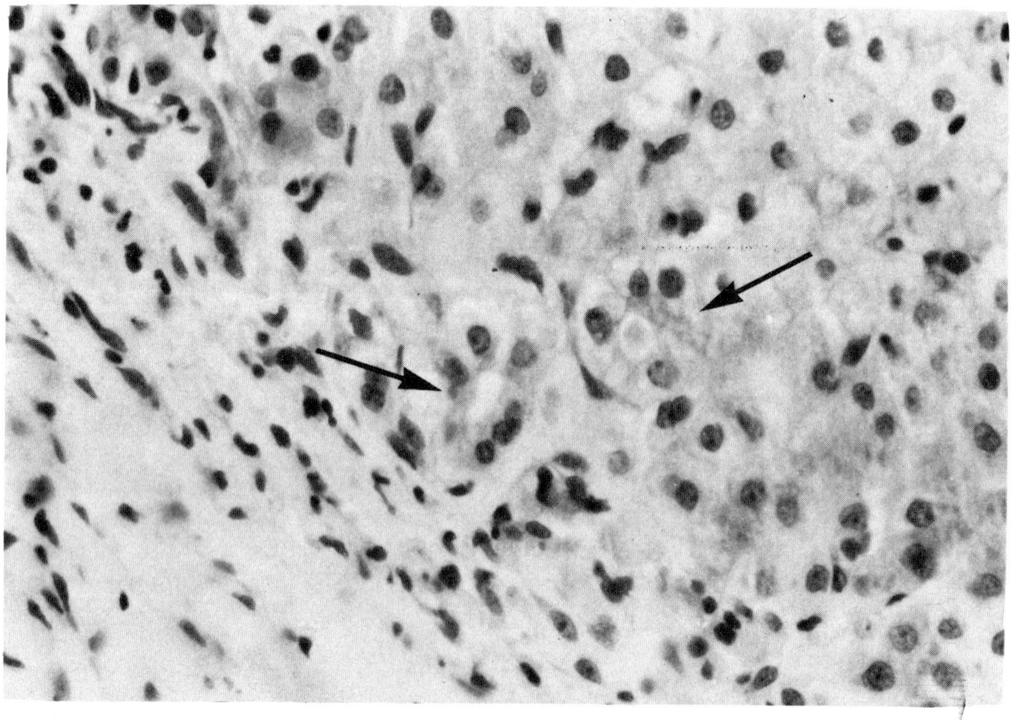

Figure 35.7. Hepatocytes arranged in periportal rosettes: one contains bile within the central lumen (arrows). Haematoxylin and eosin × 400.

prominence is accentuated in amylase digested PAS preparations when much of the phagocytosed pigment is positively stained, as sometimes is the lipofuscin within hepatocytes. This makes it difficult to identify the globules in the hepatocytes in some cases. In such instances the immunoperoxidase technique will clearly demonstrate the globules with their intensely stained rim and confirm the diagnosis.

Portal tracts are expanded by new fibrous tissue and contain a scanty mixture of inflammatory cells including pigment-laden macrophages, neutrophils and lymphocytes. Bile duct proliferation can be identified at the edge of these expanded portal tracts and these bile ductules are composed of two opposed cell plates without a central lumen. Centrally within the tract the branches of the portal vein and hepatic artery can be identified but the concomitant bile ducts may be present, absent or hypoplastic. Cases of intrahepatic hypoplasia of bile ducts in association with A1AT deficiency have been occasionally reported. Hadchouel and Gautier,[39] however, describe intrahepatic biliary hypoplasia as a distinct subgroup. Among their 15 cases of A1AT deficiency were five in whom repeat liver biopsies consistently showed a paucity of bile ducts within portal tracts. This appeared to be associated with relatively asymptomatic survival into the late teens. Strangely, proliferation of bile ductules was not a feature associated with this paucity. Rather, proliferation when present was an adverse sign indicating the presence of portal tract fibrosis sometimes sufficiently severe to be termed 'cirrhosis'. Clearly, careful assessment of biopsy features and correlation with subsequent progress are required in a larger number of cases.

Childhood Cirrhosis

Many cases of childhood cirrhosis directly follow from an episode of neonatal jaundice. The most frequent pattern is a micronodular cirrhosis, but only rarely have sequential changes through to autopsy been documented.[5,12,83] In one such case over a period of five years a micronodular cirrhosis became macronodular with large regeneration nodules separated by broad bands of fibrous tissue.[5]

In the micronodular cirrhosis all lobules are apparently equally affected by fibrous bands of varying width which link portal areas and occasionally extend towards central veins. Bile ductular proliferation can be identified within these fibrous bands and there is also an inflammatory infiltrate, usually composed of lymphocytes and some neutrophils, which may blur the junction of parenchyma with fibrous tissue. Bile ductules, sometimes containing bile, may be particularly prominent and with neutrophils in the surrounding stroma a pattern of biliary cirrhosis secondary to obstruction is produced.[69,83]

A paucity of interlobular bile ducts has been noted[33,36] but it is not known if at this stage this feature identified children of the subgroup described by Hadchouel and Gautier.[39]

Adult Liver Disease

This may be fibrosis or cirrhosis. The fibrosis expands portal tracts irregularly and not every tract is involved. Globules are most prominent against abnormal tracts.

When present, the cirrhosis is most frequently macronodular but descriptions in the literature are brief and usually confirm the cirrhosis and demonstrate the globules on appropriate histological examination. Two patterns of macronodular cirrhosis may be identified. One is multilobular in character with large areas of parenchyma enclosed by fibrous bands and in which portal tracts and central veins alternate. In some there is an excess of central veins. These macronodules are adjacent to areas of liver showing 'true' nodular regeneration but separated by slender bands of fibrosis. Fibrous bands also expand and link portal tracts to a variable degree (Figure 35.8). It is not determined whether any of these multilobular macronodules are as yet uninvolved areas of liver or represent new 'portal tracts' in reorganizing regenerative macronodules. In our series this pattern of cirrhosis at autopsy was found in patients with minimal evidence of preceding hepatocellular dysfunction who had died of the lung disease or complications of portal hypertension.[85] Other cases of cirrhosis have macronodules that are regenerative in nature with prominent twinning of cell plates and compression of the adjacent stroma from the expansile growth of the nodule. These are separated by broad bands of fibrous tissue in which bile ductular proliferation is prominent. This is usually present in the abnormal fibrous tissue and is most prominent with this pattern of cirrhosis. Most of these patients died with parenchymal liver failure or terminal infection.

So far, no paucity of interlobular bile ducts in adult cases has been described. The cholangiolar

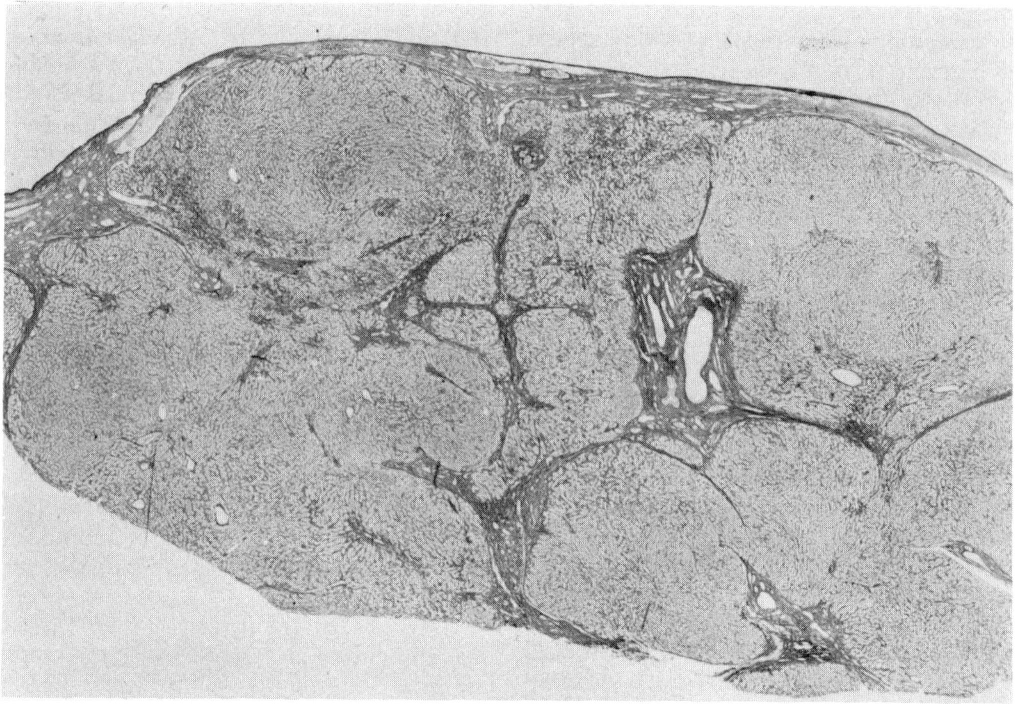

Figure 35.8. Wedge biopsy of liver showing capsule along the top and slender bands of fibrous tissue separating large areas of parenchyma. Nodules are present and there is an excess of efferent veins. Reticulin × 14.

hyperplasia described by Gherardi[35] was seen in two of our patients with cirrhosis: it was focal in the biopsy and both patients were in the terminal stage of their illness.

The lymphocytic infiltrate in the stroma is usually scanty or moderate but may be associated with piecemeal necrosis. A notable feature is the relative absence of neutrophils: when present in numbers they usually indicate the presence of a complicating factor. In the two cases we have recorded one had an associated gram-negative septicaemia and the other was in terminal liver failure.[85] Since then we have found them in two further biopsies. Both are from alcoholics who have the classical features of alcoholic hepatitis with *centrilobular* fibrosis. They happen to be heterozygous MZ on phenotyping and have only scanty tiny globules against occasional portal tracts (unpublished observations). Since mild to moderate fatty change is a common finding in the hepatocytes and Mallory's alcoholic hyalin may be found in hepatocytes, a pattern of alcoholic liver disease can be mimicked. In A1AT deficiency, however, the Mallory bodies occur in the peripheral hepatocytes of cases of cirrhosis which are usually macro- and not micronodular. In alcoholic liver disease the Mallory bodies are characteristically centrilobular in distribution or in a micronodular cirrhosis (see Chapter 32).

Iron could be demonstrated histochemically in small amounts in approximately half of our cases. It was never more severe than grade II. Orcein staining for the hepatitis B surface antigen was consistently negative.

Hepatoma

Apart from the characteristic globules in the cirrhosis there are no specific gross or microscopic features of the hepatomas that distinguish them from hepatomas with other associations (see Chapter 38).

PATHOGENESIS

Because of the variable rate of progression of the liver disease, with some homozygous children presenting with neonatal jaundice and progressing to cirrhosis and death within a few years while others never apparently develop clinical disease, ancillary/synergistic factors have been proposed.[2] These include hepatitis B virus,[69] iron[42] and copper.[41] None of these has been confirmed.[85] It is postulated that the lack of circulating A1AT allows an almost unopposed action of proteases, collagenases and elastases on the fabric of the lung and this results in a panacinar emphysema. The proteolytic enzymes are thought to be derived from neutrophil leucocytes. The lung bears the brunt of this failed physiological inhibition because it is (a) being constantly exposed to exogenous stimuli likely to result in a neutrophil chemotaxis and (b) it is normally a site of leucocyte sequestration, particularly in the lower lobes. It is difficult to use or modify this hypothesis to account for the liver disease because any damage to hepatocytes should immediately result in the local release of the accumulated A1AT with consequent inactivation of the proteolytic enzymes. It has been suggested that, as a function of Kupffer cells is to screen the portal vein blood for bacteria, A1AT may be necessary to limit any damage that occurs to these phagocytes and that without this limitation fibrogenesis may be stimulated and the hepatocyte damage then will follow the fibrosis.[74] Regrettably, this attractive hypothesis lacks experimental proof and does not satisfactorily account for the rapid onset of the neonatal jaundice. In addition, at the other end of the spectrum it is still difficult to see how any homozygote Z could survive into late adult life without developing cirrhosis.

The alteration in amino acid constitution of A1AT which occurs in both PiZ and PiS variants could alter the steric configuration of the protein chain and affect attachment of the carbohydrate side chain. The result is a net deficit of sialic acid attached to the molecule and this is thought to impede release from the endoplasmic reticulum of the hepatocyte where, consequently, the protein accumulates and is demonstrable.[6,19] Such an accumulation of protein within the hepatocytes might be cytotoxic with continuing cell death resulting in regeneration, fibrosis and eventually cirrhosis. This still does not explain the differential rate of progression of the liver disease, nor does it explain the apparent normality of livers in heterozygous MZ patients despite the demonstrable presence of globules of retained A1AT within hepatocytes. Additional biochemical abnormalities such as a defect in sialyltransferase have been implicated,[47] and although this particular defect is not found in most cases[26] it is conceivable that other abnormalities in A1AT metabolism may ultimately explain the discrepancies in this condition.

Despite the clearly established association of cirrhosis and homozygous Z deficiency the risk in the heterozygote MZ is not known. Although cases of cirrhosis in heterozygotes have been reported[85] chance association of the two has not been excluded. There is no evidence of an association with other liver disease such as alcoholic cirrhosis[63] or chronic active liver disease and primary biliary cirrhosis.[46] The numbers studied, however, are small so an association, though unlikely, is not excluded. For instance, MZ occurred in 2 to 3 per cent of the control patients studied by Kueppers et al, so that, by chance, two of their 85 patients in the study group should have been heterozygotes. None was found and this was not statistically significant. If, for example, the heterozygous state doubles the risk of developing chronic active liver disease, only four or five cases would have been present in their study group, but this, too, would not be statistically significant.

EXTRAHEPATIC MANIFESTATIONS

The association between A1AT deficiency and pulmonary emphysema is well recognized and has been widely reviewed elsewhere.[62] Low serum A1AT levels have been reported in children with untreated coeliac disease but no phenotyping was carried out.[87] Since the serum levels were higher in a group of treated coeliacs it is possible that the lower levels were due to the protein-losing enteropathy which may accompany this disorder. Nevertheless, intestinal mucosal atrophy has been reported in association with cirrhosis and pulmonary emphysema in a patient with PiZZ deficiency.[38] Membranous glomerulonephritis has been described both in a clinical[61,64,85] and in a subclinical entity.[74] Moroz and colleagues[64] examined the kidneys by immunofluorescence and observed subendothelial deposits of complement and immunoglobulin on the glomerular basement membrane. There were no such lesions on the glomeruli of children dying with cirrhosis due to other causes. Several other conditions have been reported associated with A1AT deficiency, including gastric or duodenal ulcer,[4] chronic pancreatitis,[65] fibrosing alveolitis[34] and rheumatoid arthritis,[21] although the latter has not been substantiated.[34,77]

TREATMENT

No definitive treatment is currently available for A1AT deficiency. Since the half-life is only four to six days, replacement with purified enzymes would be impractical even if large amounts of such material were available. The possibility of a synthetic enzyme inhibitor has been considered but this has not yet been developed and it is unlikely that such a substance would in any way influence established liver disease.[80]

In the case of neonatal hepatitis and juvenile cirrhosis genetic counselling of the parents is recommended. For established cirrhosis treatment should be directed towards the complications of chronic liver disease as with any other form of cirrhosis. Treatment with phenobarbitone in an effort to induce enzyme turnover has been unsuccessful[69,74] and, similarly, corticosteroids have been tried without benefit by Porter et al.[69]

Bleeding from oesophageal varices has been reported in many of the children and at least 11 cases of portal venous decompression surgery for this condition have been reported in the literature. Reasonable follow-up data are available for seven of these. Deaths from rebleeding varices are reported at $4\frac{1}{2}$ years and six years, while three other cases are alive and well after five, eight and ten years respectively, suggesting that this may be a useful therapeutic manoeuvre. From an empirical point of view, it seems logical to advise patients with liver disease, or those at risk of developing it, to avoid potentially hepatotoxic substances such as alcohol although no scientific evidence supports this advice.

Since it appears that the liver is the site of the defect, liver transplantation offers the possibility of a cure not only of the liver disease but also of the enzyme deficiency (see Chapter 52). To date two such cases have been reported, one surviving for only a few days[74] and the other surviving for two years.[70] In both cases transplantation was followed by immediate and sustained rise in A1AT levels with conversion from ZZ to MM phenotype. Future advances in the techniques of liver transplantation may ultimately establish this as the treatment of choice for the juvenile or young adult with progressive liver disease.

A GUIDE TO THE INVESTIGATION AND DIAGNOSIS OF A1AT DEFICIENCY AND LIVER DISEASE

From all that has been written in this chapter, it is clear that the present status of A1AT deficiency in liver disease is far from accurately defined, and that this will depend upon the careful and systematic diagnosis and investigation of such cases. As a guide to the problem we offer the following approach, which is shown in a diagrammatic form in Figure 35.9. A clinical suspicion of the diagnosis may be aroused by history of neonatal hepatitis or of early onset pulmonary emphysema. A family history of cirrhosis or emphysema may also alert the clinician to the possibility of A1AT deficiency. Many cases, however, will have no such clues but the diagnosis should always be considered in any case of chronic liver disease of unknown aetiology. Having considered the possibility, either serological or histological investigations may be pursued. The serum A1AT level can be easily measured and is a useful screening test, if

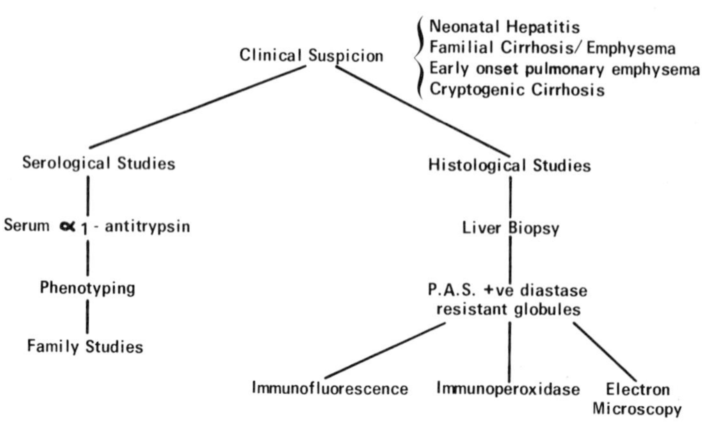

Figure 35.9. Guide to the investigation and diagnosis of liver disease associated with A1AT deficiency.

the situations which may elevate or depress the value are appreciated. Any low or equivocally low values should always be checked by phenotyping. The presence of unusual phenotypes can be strengthened, if not confirmed, by family studies. Histological confirmation of the diagnosis is based on the demonstration of characteristic PAS-positive diastase-resistant globules in relation to portal tracts in the liver. The specific protein content of the globules should be identified by immunocytochemical methods whenever possible. Although sampling error may occur the absence of the globules in a patient with liver disease must raise considerable doubts as to the diagnosis.

REFERENCES

1. Aagenaes, O., Matlary, A., Elgjo, K., Munthe, E. & Fagerhol, M. (1972) Neonatal cholestasis in α1AT deficient children: clinical, genetic, histological and immunohistochemical findings. *Acta Paediatrica Scandinavica*, **61**, 632–642.
2. Aagenaes, O., Fagerhol, M., Elgjo, K., Munthe, E. & Hovig, T. (1974) Pathology and pathogenesis of liver disease in α1AT deficient individuals. *Postgraduate Medical Journal*, **50**, 365–375.
3. Allen, R.C., Harley, R.A. & Talamo, R.C. (1974) A new method for determination of α1AT phenotypes using isoelectric focusing on polyacrylamide gel slabs. *American Journal of Clinical Pathology*, **62**, 732–739.
4. André, F., André, C., Lambert, R. & Descos, F. (1974) Prevalence of α1AT deficiency in patients with gastric or duodenal ulcer. *Biomedicine* (*Express*), **21**, 222–224.
5. Asarian, J., Archibald, R.W. & Lieberman, J. (1975) Childhood cirrhosis is associated with α1AT deficiency. A genetic biochemical and morphologic study. *Journal of Pediatrics*, **86**, 844–850.
6. Bell, O.F. & Carrell, R.W. (1973) Basis of the defect in α1 antitrypsin deficiency. *Nature*, **243**, 410–411.
7. Benn, R.T. & Wood, P.H. (1976) Rheumatoid arthritis and α1AT. *Lancet*, **ii**, 147.
8. Berg, N.O. & Eriksson, S. (1972) Liver disease in adults with α1AT deficiency. *New England Journal of Medicine*, **287**, 1264–1267.
9. Blenkinsopp, W.K. & Haffenden, G.P. (1977) α1AT bodies in the liver. *Journal of Clinical Pathology*, **30**, 132–137.
10. Bradfield, J.W.B. & Blenkinsopp, W.K. (1977) α1AT globules in the liver and PiM phenotype. *Journal of Clinical Pathology*, **30**, 464–466.
11. Brand, B., Bezahler, G.H. & Gould, R. (1974) Cirrhosis and heterozygous FZ α1AT deficiency in an adult. Case report and review of the literature. *Gastroenterology*, **66**, 264–268.
12. Burke, J.A., Kiesel, J.L. & Blair, J.D. (1976) α1AT deficiency and liver disease in children. *American Journal of Diseases of Children*, **130**, 621–629.
13. Campra, J.L., Ashcavai, M., Peters, R.L. & Redeker, A. (1973) Serum α1AT levels in acute hepatic necrosis. *British Medical Journal*, **ii**, 616.
14. Campra, J.L., Craig, J.R., Peters, R.L. & Reynolds, T.B. (1973) Cirrhosis associated with partial deficiency of α1AT in an adult. *Annals of Internal Medicine*, **78**, 233–238.
15. Charlionet, R., Martin, J.P., Sesboué, R. & Ropartz, C. (1976) Is there a relationship between alpha-1-antitrypsin PiMZ phenotype and hepatoma? *Biomedicine* (*Express*), **25** (4), 126.
16. Christen, H., Bau, J. & Halsband, H. (1975) Hereditary α1AT deficiency associated with congenital extrahepatic bile duct hypoplasia. *Klinische Wochenschrift*, **53**, 90–91.
17. Cook, P.J.L. (1975) The genetics of α1AT: a family study in England and Scotland. *Annals of Human Genetics* (*London*), **38**, 275–287.
18. Cottrall, K., Cook, P.J. & Mowat, A.P. (1974) Neonatal hepatitis syndrome and α1AT deficiency: an epidemiological study in South-east England. *Postgraduate Medical Journal*, **50**, 376–380.
19. Cox, D.W. (1973) Defect in α1AT deficiency. *Lancet*, **ii**, 844–845.
20. Cox, D.W. (1975) A new deficiency allele of α1AT: PiM Malton. In *Protides of Biological Fluids* (Ed.) Peeters, H. Vol. 23, pp. 375–378. New York: Pergamon Press.
21. Cox, D.W. & Huber, O. (1976) Rheumatoid arthritis and α1AT. *Lancet*, **i**, 1216–1217.
22. Cruz, M., Molina, J.A., Pedrola, D. & Munoz Lopez, F. (1975) Cirrhosis and heterozygous α1AT deficiency in a 4 year old girl. *Helvetica Paediatrica Acta*, **30**, 501–507.
23. De Lellis, R.A., Balough, K. & Merk, F.B. (1972) Distinctive hepatic cell globules in adult α1AT deficiency: a histochemical, immuno histochemical and ultrastructural study. *Archives of Pathology*, **94**, 308–316.
24. Elema, J.D., Boersma, R. & Reerink-Bronkers, E. (1975) Proceedings: clinical observations and histopathology of the liver in infants and children with α1AT deficiency. *Archives of Diseases in Childhood*, **50**, 663.
25. Eriksson, S. & Hagerstrand, I. (1974) Cirrhosis and malignant hepatoma in α1AT deficiency. *Acta Medica Scandinavica*, **195**, 451–458.
26. Eriksson, S. & Larsson, C. (1975) Role of sialyltransferase in α_1AT deficiency. *New England Journal of Medicine*, **292**, 925–926.
27. Evans, H.E., Bognacki, N.S., Perrott, L.M. & Glass, L. (1977) Prevalence of α1AT Pi types among newborn infants of different ethnic backgrounds. *Journal of Pediatrics*, **90**, 621–624.
28. Fagerhol, M.K. (1976) The genetics of α1AT and its implications. *Postgraduate Medical Journal*, **52** (Suppl. 2), 73–83.
29. Fagerhol, M.K. & Laurell, C.B. (1967) The polymorphism of prealbumins and α_1 antitrypsin in human sera. *Clinica Chimica Acta*, **16**, 199–203.
30. Feldmann, G., Bignon, J., Chahinian, P., Degott, C. & Benhamou, J.P. (1974) Hepatocyte ultrastructural changes in α1AT deficiency. *Gastroenterology*, **67**, 1214–1224.
31. Fisher, R.L., Taylor, L. & Sherlock, S. (1976) α1AT deficiency in liver disease: the extent of the problem. *Gastroenterology*, **71**, 646–651.
32. Ganrot, P.O., Laurell, C.B. & Eriksson, S. (1967) Obstructive lung disease and trypsin inhibitor in α1AT deficiency. *Scandinavian Journal of Clinical Investigation*, **19**, 205–208.

33. Gans, H., Sharp, H.L. & Tan, B.H. (1969) Antiprotease deficiency and familial infantile liver cirrhosis. *Surgery, Gynecology and Obstetrics,* **129,** 289–299.
34. Geddes, D.M., Webley, M., Brewerton, D.A., Turton, C.W., Turner-Warwick, M., Murphy, A.H. & Milford Ward, A. (1977) α-1-antitrypsin phenotypes in fibrosing alveolitis and rheumatoid arthritis. *Lancet,* **ii,** 1049–1050.
35. Gherardi, G.J. (1971) α1AT deficiency and its effect on the liver. *Human Pathology,* **2,** 173–175.
36. Glasgow, J.F.T., Lynch, M.J., Hercz, A., Levison, H. & Sass-Kortsak, A. (1976) α1AT deficiency in association with both cirrhosis and chronic obstructive lung disease in two sibs. *American Journal of Medicine,* **54,** 181–194.
37. Gordon, H.W., Dixon, J., Rogers, J.C., Mittman, C. & Lieberman, J. (1972) α1AT accumulation in livers of emphysematous patients with α1AT deficiency. *Human Pathology,* **3,** 361–370.
38. Greenwald, A.J., Johnson, D.S., Oskvig, R.M., Aschenbrener, C.A. & Randa, D.C. (1975) α1AT deficiency, emphysema, cirrhosis and intestinal mucosal atrophy. *Journal of the American Medical Association,* **231,** 273–276.
39. Hadchouel, M. & Gautier, M. (1976) Histopathologic study of the liver in the early cholestatic phase of α1AT deficiency. *Journal of Pediatrics,* **89,** 211–215.
40. Heidelberger, K.P. (1976) α1AT deficiency: a review 1963–75. *Annals of Clinical and Laboratory Sciences,* **6,** 110–117.
41. Ishak, K.G., Jenis, E.H., Marshall, M.L., Bolton, B.H. & Battistone, G.C. (1972) Cirrhosis of the liver associated with α1AT deficiency. *Archives of Pathology,* **94,** 445–455.
42. Janus, E.D. & Carrell, R.W. (1975) Alpha-1-antitrypsin deficiency in New Zealand. *New Zealand Medical Journal,* **81,** 461–467.
43. Jeppsson, J.O. (1976) Amino acid substitution glu–lys in α1AT PiZ. *FEBS Letters,* **65,** 195–197.
44. Jeppsson, J.O., Larsson, C. & Eriksson, S. (1975) Characterisation of α1AT deficiency. *New England Journal of Medicine,* **293,** 576–579.
45. Kueppers, F. (1976) α1AT M1 – a new common genetically determined variant. *American Journal of Human Genetics,* **28** (4), 370–377.
46. Kueppers, F., Dickson, E.R. & Summerskill, W.H.J. (1976) α1AT phenotypes in chronic active liver disease and primary biliary cirrhosis. *Mayo Clinic Proceedings,* **51**(5), 286–288.
47. Kuhlenschmidt, M.S., Yunis, E.J., Iammarino, R.M., Turco, S.J., Peters, S.P. & Glew, R.H. (1974) Demonstration of sialyltransferase deficiency in the serum of a patient with α1AT deficiency and cirrhosis. *Laboratory Investigation,* **31,** 413–419.
48. Kumar, P., Lancaster-Smith, M., Cook, P., Stansfield, A., Clark, M.L. & Dawson, A.M. (1974) α1AT deficiency in chronic liver disease and a report of cirrhosis and emphysema in adult members of a family. *British Medical Journal,* **i,** 366–367.
49. Laurell, C.B. (1965) Effect of neuraminidase, acetone and chloroform on α1AT. *Scandinavian Journal of Clinical and Laboratory Investigation,* **17,** 297–298.
50. Laurell, C.B. (1972) Variations of the α1AT level of plasma. In *Pulmonary Emphysema and Proteolysis* (Ed.) Mittman, C. pp. 161–166. London: Academic Press.
51. Laurell, C.B. & Eriksson, S. (1963) The electrophoretic α_1 globulin pattern of serum in α1AT deficiency. *Scandinavian Journal of Clinical Laboratory Investigation,* **15,** 132–140.
52. Laurell, C.B. & Sveger, T. (1975) Mass screening of newborn Swedish infants for α1AT deficiency. *American Journal of Human Genetics,* **27,** 213–217.
53. Laurell, C.B., Nosslin, B. & Jeppsson, J.O. (1977) Catabolic rate of α1AT of Pi type M and Z in man. *Clinical Science and Molecular Medicine,* **52,** 457–461.
54. Lieberman, J., Gaidulis, L. & Klotz, S.D. (1976) A new deficient variant of α1AT (M. Duarte). *American Review of Respiratory Diseases,* **113,** 31–36.
55. Lieberman, J., Mittman, C. & Gordon, H.W. (1972) α1AT in the liver of patients with emphysema. *Science,* **175,** 63–65.
56. Lieberman, J., Silton, R.M., Agliozzo, C.M. & McMahon, J. (1975) Hepatocellular carcinoma and intermediate α1AT deficiency (MZ phenotype). *American Journal of Clinical Pathology,* **64,** 304–310.
57. Makino, S. & Reed, C.E. (1970) Distribution and elimination of exogenous α1AT. *Journal of Laboratory and Clinical Medicine,* **75,** 742–746.
58. Mancini, G., Carbonara, A.O. & Heremans, J.F. (1965) Immuno chemical quantitation of antigens by single radial immunodiffusion. *Immunochemistry,* **2,** 235–254.
59. McPhie, J.L., Binnie, S. & Brunt, P.W. (1976) α1AT deficiency and infantile liver disease. *Archives of Diseases in Childhood,* **51,** 584–588.
60. Millward-Sadler, G.H., Czaykowski, A.A. & Wright, R. (1975) Diagnosis of α1AT deficiency. *Lancet,* **ii,** 1050.
61. Miller, F. & Kuschner, M. (1969) α1AT deficiency emphysema, necrotizing angiitis and glomerulonephritis. *American Journal of Medicine,* **46,** 615–623.
62. Mittman, C. (1972) *Pulmonary Emphysema and Proteolysis.* London: Academic Press.
63. Morin, T., Martin, J.P., Feldmann, G., Rueff, B., Benhamou, J.P. & Ropartz, C. (1975) Heterozygous α1AT deficiency and cirrhosis in adults, a fortuitous association. *Lancet,* **i,** 250–251.
64. Moroz, S.P., Cutz, E., Cox, D.W. & Sass-Kortsak, A. (1976) Liver disease associated with α1AT deficiency in childhood. *Journal of Pediatrics,* **88,** 19–25.
65. Novis, B.H., Young, G.O., Bank, S. & Marks, I.N. (1975) Chronic pancreatitis and α1AT. *Lancet,* **ii,** 748–749.
66. Odièvre, M., Martin, J.P., Hadchouel, M. & Alagille, D. (1976) α1AT deficiency and liver disease in children. Phenotypes, manifestations and prognosis. *Pediatrics,* **57,** 226–231.
67. Owen, M.C. & Carrell, R.W. (1976) α1AT: molecular abnormality of S variant. *British Medical Journal,* **i,** 130–131.
68. Pierce, J.A., Eradio, B. & Dew, T.A. (1975) Antitrypsin phenotypes in St Louis. *Journal of the American Medical Association,* **231,** 609–612.
69. Porter, C.A., Mowat, A.P., Cook, P.J., Haynes, D.W., Shilkin, K.B. & Williams, R. (1972) α1 Antitrypsin deficiency and neonatal hepatitis. *British Medical Journal,* **iii,** 435–439.
70. Putman, C.W., Porter, K.A., Peters, R.L., Aschcavai, M., Redeker, A.G. & Starzl, T.E. (1977) Liver replacement of α1 antitrypsin deficiency. *Surgery,* **81,** 258–261.
71. Rawlings, W. Jr, Moss, J., Cooper, S. & Hamilton, S.R. (1974) Hepatocellular carcinoma and partial deficiency of α1AT. *American Journal of Internal Medicine,* **81,** 771–773.
72. Schleissner, L.A. & Cohen, A.L. (1975) α1AT deficiency and hepatic carcinoma. *American Review of Respiratory Diseases,* **3,** 863–868.

73. Scotto, J.M., Stralin, H.G. & Alagille, D. (1975) Deficit en α-1-antitrypsine chez l'enfant. Ultrastructure du foie et spéculations. *Virchows Archiv a Pathologische Anatomie*, **369**, 19.
74. Sharp, H.L. (1976) α1 antitrypsin deficiency. *Hospital Practice*, **6**, 83–96.
75. Sharp, H.L., Bridges, R.A., Krivit, W. & Freier, E.M. (1969) Cirrhosis associated with α1AT deficiency – a previously unrecognised inherited disorder. *Journal of Laboratory and Clinical Medicine*, **73**, 934–939.
76. Sharp, H.L., Mathis, R., Krivit, W. & Freier, E. (1971) The liver in non-cirrhotic α1AT deficiency. *Journal of Laboratory and Clinical Medicine*, **78**, 1012–1013.
77. Sjöblom, K.G. & Wollheim, F.A. (1977) α-1-antitrypsin phenotypes and rheumatic diseases. *Lancet*, **ii**, 41–42.
78. Sveger, T. (1976) Liver disease in α1AT deficiency detected by screening of 20 000 infants. *New England Journal of Medicine*, **294**, 1316–1321.
79. Sweeney, E.C. (1975) Adult α1 antitrypsin deficiency. *Journal of Clinical Pathology*, **28**, 613–619.
80. Talamo, R.C. (1975) Basic and clinical aspects of the α1AT. *Pediatrics*, **56**, 91–99.
81. Talamo, R.C., Langley, C.E., Levine, B.W. & Kazemi, H. (1972) Genetics vs quantitative analysis of serum α1 antitrypsin. *New England Journal of Medicine*, **287**, 1067–69.
82. Talamo, R.C., Langley, C.E., Reed, C.E. & Makino, S. (1973) α1AT deficiency: a variant with no detectable α1 antitrypsin. *Science (New York)*, **181**, 70–71.
83. Talbot, I.C. & Mowat, A.P. (1975) Liver disease in infancy: histological features and relationship to α1AT phenotype. *Journal of Clinical Pathology*, **28**, 559–563.
84. Theodoropoulos, G., Fertakis, A., Archimandritis, A., Karpordelis, C. & Angelopoulos, B. (1976) α1AT phenotypes in cirrhosis and hepatoma. *Acta Hepato-gastroenterologica (Stuttgart)*, **23**(2), 114–117.
85. Triger, D.R., Millward-Sadler, G.H., Czaykowski, A.A., Trowell, J. & Wright, R. (1976) α1AT deficiency and liver disease in adults. *Quarterly Journal of Medicine*, **45**, 351–372.
86. Vandeville, D., Martin, J.P., Lebreton, J.P. & Ropartz, C. (1972) Le système Pi dans les populations normande et amérindienne. *Revue Française de Transfusion*, **15**, 213–218.
87. Walker-Smith, J. & Andrews, J. (1972) α1AT autism and coeliac disease. *Lancet*, **ii**, 883–884.
88. Wilkinson, E.J., Raab, K., Browning, C.A. & Hosty, T.A. (1974) Familial hepatic cirrhosis in infants associated with α1AT SZ phenotype. *Journal of Pediatrics*, **85**, 159–164.
89. Yoshida, A., Lieberman, J., Gaidulis, L. & Ewing, C. (1976) Molecular abnormality of human α1AT variant, PiZZ associated with plasma activity deficiency. *Proceedings of the National Academy of Science of the United States of America*, **73**, 1324–1328.
90. Yunis, E.J., Agostini, R.M. Jr, & Glew, R.H. (1976) Fine structural alterations of the liver in α1AT deficiency. *American Journal of Pathology*, **82**, 265–286.
91. Zwi, S., Hurwitz, S.S., Cohen, C., Prinsloo, I. & Kagan, E. (1975) α1AT deficiency: an association with hepatic malignancy. *South African Medical Journal*, **49**, 1887–1890.

Chapter 36

The Liver and Drugs

ALAN E. READ

The liver occupies a key position in the metabolism of drugs. Its function is to change these largely lipid-soluble agents to water-soluble ones for biliary and urinary excretion. This it does with a highly adaptable series of drug-oxidizing enzymes,[111] principally cytochrome P-450, situated on the smooth endoplasmic reticulum of the hepatocyte. The first change produced by this enzyme system is the insertion of reactive groups into the drug molecule (phase one reaction) which is then detoxified, and the second is a linking of the resultant reactive metabolite to a conjugating agent such as glucuronide or gluthathione. This conjugating (or phase two) reaction renders the drug water-soluble and therefore accessible for excretion because of its loss of lipid (renal tubular epithelial) penetrating powers. This system of enzymes is also employed for the metabolism of steroids, hormones and bilirubin itself (see Chapters 13 and 16).

Damage to the liver by drugs is often referred to as either *predictable* or *non-predictable*. In the former, liver injury is a normal consequence of the administration of a drug or poison. The severity of this damage is often dose-related and, where due to a drug metabolite rather than the parent drug, dependent on rates of metabolism. In non-predictable drug injury a harmful effect on liver structure and function is seen in only a small percentage of patients treated with that agent and the causes for this are largely unknown.

Though an increasingly elaborate system of testing, both in animals and man, ensures that the toxic effects are kept to a minimum, such a scheme is not foolproof. Furthermore, the continuing introduction of large numbers of new drugs means that the chances of drug toxicity are steadily increasing. The problem of drug-induced liver disease should be seen in perspective, however. It is obvious, on the one hand, that some patients with serious underlying diseases may develop abnormalities of liver cell function which are due to drugs administered to them and yet they are not permanently affected by these changes. On the other hand, a few patients suffer severe effects from drug-induced liver disease and may be seriously ill or die as a consequence. It is generally stated that, in hospital practice, in about 10 per cent of patients jaundice is due to drugs, but the picture in the country as a whole is less clear because identification of drug-induced liver disease is largely hospital-based. The Committee for the Safety of Medicines (CSM) publishes a register of drug reactions (Table 36.1). The relevant headings of the CSM data showed that there were 324 deaths between 1964 and 1976 attributable to hepatotoxicity of drugs. Thus approximately 25 adult patients die per annum from drug-induced liver disease in this country. This is worth bearing in mind when one considers, for example, that prescriptions for chlorpromazine from general practice alone are approximately $10^6 \times 6$ per annum.

Within the total number of patients with liver injury due to drugs there is obviously an extremely variable frequency of lesions from drug to drug. For example, only seven of over 100 listed agents account for 10 or more examples of 'abnormal hepatic function', these being halothane, acetylsalicylic acid, indomethacin, suxamethonium, ethinyloestradiol, rifampicin and isoniazid. In the list of those drugs causing 'jaundice' (Table 36.2) over 400

Table 36.1. *The Major Relevant CSM Headings and Drug Hepatotoxicity.*

	Total cases due to drugs 1964–76	Total deaths
Hepatic failure	9	8
Abnormal hepatic function	131	4
Hepatic necrosis	149	125
Drug hepatitis	154	31
Hepatocellular damage	64	10
Jaundice	1390	141
Jaundice cholestatic	101	4
Raised AST	54	0
Raised ALT	60	0
Totals	2112	323

are to be found, but only 16 of these drugs were known to produce 50 or more cases in the period of study, or more than four cases per year. Of these, by far and away the most commonly reported were chlorpromazine (240 cases, 38 deaths) and halothane (254 cases, 83 deaths), the other drugs lagging very much behind these two. The percentage of drug reactions which involve the liver as opposed to other organs is about 10 per cent, but sometimes multiple organ involvement which may include the liver is seen.

The CSM points out that these statistics are not necessarily accurate; they measure what the medical profession cares to report and only the overall results can be used to show rough trends. In the above lists, for example, the relatively high number of cases of jaundice due to atropine and thiopentone, drugs not normally felt to have hepatotoxicity, are perhaps a reflection of part of the profession's failure to accept the hepatic toxicity of halothane and to over-respond by recording jaundice due to other anaesthetic agents. In any case, jaundice in the postoperative period is exceptionally difficult to ascribe to any single agent or event (see Chapter 47) and for this reason inaccuracies may readily occur.

It is important to be able to identify drug jaundice. In examples with cholestasis, the patient may be subjected to complex investigations and surgical interference with all its subsequent hazards. In patients with liver cell damage due to drugs, these procedures are less likely to be performed unless there is diagnostic difficulty. However, on the whole, drug-induced acute hepatocellular damage carries a worse prognosis than its viral counterparts.

One further aspect concerning the diagnosis is also important. Unlike most cases of virus A hepatitis, progression of drug-induced liver injury to chronic liver disease is probably not a rarity. Increasing numbers of drugs, such as oxyphenisatin, methyldopa and isoniazid, are being recognized as a cause of chronic hepatitis and cirrhosis in susceptible people, whilst there is a clear relationship between other drugs and hepatic neoplasia.

PATHOLOGY

Though drugs may interfere with bilirubin metabolism and produce jaundice by many potential mechanisms, two major types of pathological lesions are found on microscopic examination of the liver. These two histological disorders are *cholestasis*, i.e. intralobular bile retention, and *hepatocellular damage*, though in some examples these lesions merge. Drug disorders in the liver produce a complete spectrum ranging from pure cholestasis (without significant cell degeneration or portal tract infiltrate) through drug hepatitis (with or without cholestatic features), which mimics closely the picture seen in acute viral hepatitis, to liver tissue necrosis which is zonal, lobular or massive. Unlike hepatitis of viral origin, however, in drug lesions there is often a variable degree of fatty change in hepatocytes which, with some agents, becomes the dominant lesion. In *pure cholestasis* due to drugs such as the 17α substituted testosterones and nortestosterones the outstanding feature is bile retention. Bile

Table 36.2. *Jaundice Due to Drugs Reported to CSM 1964–76. The 17 Major Drugs.*

Drug	Number of reports	Fatalities
Nitrous oxide	75	22
Halothane	234	83
Thiopentone	74	21
Chlorpromazine	240	38
Diazepam	50	3
Amitryptyline	54	0
Pethidine	50	14
Paracetamol	63	2
Atropine	62	15
Methyldopa	73	2
Ethynyloestradiol	69	1
Ampicillin	72	11
Isoniazid	51	3
Sulphamethoxazole	65	2
Suxamethonium	52	16
Norethisterone	59	1
Trimethoprim	65	2

These data do not include figures under headings such as hepatic necrosis, etc.

pigment is seen in canaliculi, liver cells and Kupffer cells, the lobular architecture remains undisturbed and there is no portal tract or sinusoidal infiltration by inflammatory cells. In patients with a mixed picture such as is found with jaundice due to phenothiazines, differences from pure cholestasis are noted in that there is a variable but definite accompanying hepatitis which shows a distinct portal tract inflammatory reaction, sometimes with a high eosinophilic content. There is also evidence of liver cell destruction, with swollen and multinucleated hepatocytes. Prominent centrilobular cholestasis is also seen and with the later disappearance of the inflammatory reaction in the portal tracts this may then mimic 'pure' cholestasis. Furthermore, corticosteroid drugs given as misguided therapy may suppress the inflammatory infiltrate and render diagnosis more difficult.

In patients with hepatocellular injury there is either prominent fatty change (e.g. tetracycline or carbon tetrachloride) or the lesion resembles viral hepatitis. The presence of eosinophils and the appearance of confluent zones of necrosis are suggestive of a drug cause but differentiation from viral hepatitis can be difficult. In such cases, evidence of focal fatty change or a zonal pattern to the lesions might also be particularly helpful in ascribing the liver disorder to a drug. A guide to the morphological features of drug-induced liver disease has been produced by an international group of pathologists.[13]

MECHANISMS

Cholestasis (see also Chapter 14)

It must be admitted that the major causes for hepatic drug toxicity have not been elucidated. Although some drugs produce a cholestatic and others a hepatitis-like picture, a clear differentiation between these two mechanisms is not possible because a pure cholestatic or hepatitic lesion is not always seen. Drugs tend to produce hepatic disorders with a mixture of pathological features so that this makes both diagnosis and any unifying concept regarding aetiology equally problematical.

In the early days of research on cholestatic liver disease due to drugs it was thought that the lesion resulted from changes in the very fine radicles of the biliary tree, the biliary canaliculus. Postulated causes included stunting and loss of canalicular villi, from the presence of bile plugging which occluded canaliculi or the swelling of hepatocytes which acted similarly. It is now known that many of these changes, particularly those of the microvilli, are the result rather than the cause of obstruction. An interesting hypothesis was first put forward by Schaffner and Popper[119] to explain the biochemical and histological features of cholestasis due to drugs. These workers suggested that the site of the lesion lay in the liver cell (smooth endoplasmic reticulum – SER) rather than in the bile canaliculus itself. Here the fault was a qualitative and quantitative failure of bile salt secretion into bile. This failure of bile salt production produced a failure of biliary flow with secondary bile plugging and resultant changes in the microvilli. Both experimentally and in human subjects with cholestasis, changes in the SER can be seen on electron microscopy. The SER is hypertrophied, although, in respect of drug and bile salt metabolism, this organelle functions subnormally. The concept of a hypertrophied but hypofunctioning SER as a cause of drug cholestasis, with the drug being responsible for the SER lesion and the cholestasis resulting from impaired biliary flow, is an attractive one. Such a hypothesis does not, of course, explain all cases of cholestasis and this is perhaps particularly true of drugs which produce 'pure' cholestasis. A close link obviously exists between the cholestasis of certain steroid drugs and that seen occasionally in pregnancy. It seems possible that direct interference with non-bile-salt-mediated biliary flow could occur. Drugs such as the oestrogens are known to affect this part of biliary excretion and it seems eminently possible that an action at this site may account for some pure cholestatic lesions.

Evidence suggests that drugs may alter bile salt excretion by directly precipitating bile salts – again producing impaired biliary flow and promoting cholestasis. Such an action is known to occur experimentally with chlorpromazine which is, of course, a cause of cholestatic hepatitis. The drug jaundice related to chlorpromazine is a particularly good example of the complexity of the problem. Excess bilirubin production and impaired bilirubin conjugation can also be demonstrated as experimental causes of jaundice when chlorpromazine is administered to rats,[65] over and above any action on the biliary tree.

Hepatocellular Dysfunction

The precise manner in which drugs and toxic compounds cause damage is also unknown. It is generally supposed for drugs where hepatic dysfunction is only an occasional finding that some hypersensitivity either of an immunological or biochemical variety exists. A further link in such a mechanism was perhaps highlighted by the effects of protein depletion in modifying the hepatotoxicity of some drugs. Thus McLean[79] produced hepatotoxicity in rats with carbon tetrachloride and found that protein deficiency gave protection against liver damage and that phenobarbitone and other enzyme-inducing agents accentuated it. It seemed from these and other studies that, in some cases, hepatotoxicity was in fact due to metabolites of a drug which were produced in the liver rather than to the original drug itself. Modification of drug metabolism by protein deficiency and enzyme induction, which respectively decreased and increased drug-metabolizing enzymes, had a considerable effect on the degree of hepatotoxicity produced.

The fact that drug toxicity could equally be due to toxic metabolites of the parent drug led to further investigation of the ways in which damage was produced. Toxic metabolites are implicated as mediators of hepatic damage resulting from a variety of drugs. These metabolites appear to be highly reactive and, if not cleared from the liver by conjugation, fix covalently to cellular organelles and produce hepatic damage and necrosis. The conjugation mechanism can therefore be seriously compromised if large doses of some drugs are given, whilst with smaller doses conjugation ensures rapid elimination. In this respect, glutathione, glucuronide and sulphate occupy key places as materials for drug conjugation and their rapid depletion – as, for example, by a large dose of paracetamol – allows the persistence of other toxic metabolites which fix with components of the liver cell.

Drug metabolism is widely influenced by such factors as nutrition and enzyme induction. Genetic effects are also important. Acetylation and several other hepatic drug-metabolizing processes are known to be affected by genetic influences. An increase in the rate of drug acetylation allows a more rapid production of acetyl derivatives in the liver. If these bind covalently, as seems to be so for isoniazid and the monoamine oxidase inhibitors in general, then hepatotoxicity becomes a particular problem in those who acetylate rapidly or in whom this process is stimulated by concurrent administration of enzyme inducers such as alcohol. This may, in fact, be a partial explanation for the increased numbers of black and oriental subjects who have suffered from hepatitis and hepatic necrosis associated with isonicotinic acid hydroxide (INAH) therapy.[83] The incidence of fast acetylators is increased in these populations, compared with caucasians.

It is possible, too, that immunological factors may be important in the pathogenesis of both cholestatic and hepatic drug-induced liver disease. A drug or its metabolites, by functioning as an antigen, could excite a damaging immunological attack upon itself and part or all of the hepatocyte. The drug or a metabolite derived from it would have to fix with components of the hepatocyte membrane and then form an antigenically active complex against which an immune attack could be mounted. Where drug fixation occurs on bile canalicular membrane the immunological attack might result in a predominantly cholestatic picture, whilst localization to other parts of the hepatocyte membrane might determine a clinical picture showing hepatocellular features. The severity of this attack would presumably determine the amount and character of the damage to the hepatocyte, whilst genetic factors might determine which subjects are susceptible to immune reactions of this type.

Once an immunological reaction has been mounted to a complex of drug and/or metabolite linked to hepatocyte membrane, this mechanism could mushroom if other damaged intracellular components act as antigenic stimulants.

DRUGS AND TOXINS CAUSING HEPATIC DAMAGE

The following groups of drugs will be dealt with in this chapter although, on some occasions, grouping may have little to do with the chemical properties or pharmacological activities of the individual agents. The classification is for ease of presentation only.

1. Antituberculous drugs
2. Steroid drugs
3. Psychotropic drugs
4. Antibiotic and chemotherapeutic agents
5. Analgesic and anti-inflammatory drugs
6. Anaesthetic agents (excluding halothane) and anticonvulsant drugs
7. Antimetabolite and immunosuppressive drugs
8. Drugs used in cardiovascular disorders

9. Drugs used in the treatment of diabetes and endocrine disorders
10. Industrial agents and toxins
11. Other drugs and therapeutic agents

Antituberculous Drugs

Since the introduction of effective chemotherapy for tuberculosis in the late 1940s it has become increasingly recognized that most of these agents can, in susceptible patients, cause hepatic damage. The picture is complicated somewhat by the fact that the drugs are usually administered together in order to prevent the emergence of resistant bacterial strains. Hepatic damage under such circumstances may occasionally be attributed to the wrong drug or there may be drug interaction so that toxicity is potentiated. Further, it is known that patients with tuberculosis are often poorly nourished, sometimes with significant liver disease due to alcohol and other factors, and the relationship of liver damage to any specific drug may be difficult to define. Nevertheless there is a generalized pattern of liver cell damage, often mimicking viral hepatitis, common to many of these drugs. Though features of damage to other organs, such as the skin, lungs and lymph nodes, make a hypersensitivity type of damage likely, this group shows evidence, too, of toxicity due to products formed by hepatic biotransformation.

Para-aminosalicylic acid (PAS)

It is often said that about 1 to 1.3 per cent of patients treated with this drug develop a drug hepatitis, usually within two months of the commencement of therapy.[11,101] Hepatomegaly and fever occur, and skin rashes, arthropathy and pneumonitis are recognized, suggesting, as does an accompanying eosinophilia, a hypersensitivity type of drug damage. This type of disorder is occasionally complicated by fatal hepatic necrosis but, normally, recovery rapidly follows removal of the drug. PAS is the major cause of drug hepatitis within the antituberculous group,[117] but hepatitis is comparatively rare compared with the overall figure for drug sensitivity which ranges up to 15 per cent. The mortality, though non-existent in 16 patients recorded by Rossouw and Saunders, ranges up to 21 per cent,[127] but the reasons for this finding in some series are not known. Fever may precede the onset of jaundice by up to one month and if drug therapy is stopped early, hepatitis may not occur. Early recognition is obviously important.

Histologically, PAS hepatitis shows a predominant picture of liver cell injury, but cholestatic features do occur, and when toxicity cannot be defined as being due to PAS or INAH the histological picture shows less cholestasis and a rise in the mortality rate. There is the possibility, too, that hepatitis in patients on PAS and INAH represents the combined hepatotoxic effect of both drugs. It is difficult, as with other antituberculous drugs, to monitor therapy with a view to preventing hepatitis since asymptomatic self-limited elevations of transaminases are a feature of antituberculous and some other types of drug therapy. Certainly, in regard to PAS, monitoring must be concentrated in the first two to three months and all drugs should be stopped if a drug sensitivity develops. The drugs can be re-introduced one at a time in order to detect the harmful one by giving a single dose and monitoring the aspartate aminotransferase (AST) three and seven days later. Because para-aminosalicylic acid is the most likely drug to cause hepatitis and because of its poor acceptability by the patient, its continuing use as first-time antituberculous therapy is questionable.

Isonicotinic acid hydrazide (INAH)

Reactions causing hepatic damage from this drug have been recognized since its introduction but, generally speaking, these have been confined to the occurrence of raised transaminases in 10 to 20 per cent of those treated.[18] Raised transaminase levels occasionally settle spontaneously, despite continuation of the drug. The elevated transaminase levels are accompanied, in cases where biopsies have been performed, by scattered necrosis of liver cells.[120] Where more severe reactions to INAH have been recorded cases have usually been treated with other antituberculous drugs which are hepatotoxic and, in particular, with PAS. Recently, INAH has been used alone in the treatment of patients with positive tuberculin reactivity and large series of patients treated in this way have been recorded from the United States. Black et al,[14] in a series of 13 838 patients in one American survey treated with INAH 300 mg daily, found 114 cases of hepatocellular jaundice which in 13 patients caused death. Twenty other patients who sustained liver damage were shown to have severe degrees of hepatic necrosis. In over 50 per cent of patients with liver damage the onset of the hepatic disease was between two and 11 months after the commencement of drug therapy. Furthermore, the incidence of eosinophilia was less than 4 per cent. Both of these latter features suggest a non-allergic cause for the hepatic reaction. Late onset and a serum bilirubin greater than 340 μmol/l (20 mg/dl) had a particularly bad prognosis and there was a high mortality in blacks, particularly black females. These observations fit in well with the possibility that the cause of INAH hepatitis lay in a biochemical, not in an immunological, susceptibility to the drug. In particular, it raised the possibility that genetic variability of INAH metabolism determined hepatic damage. This ties in well, too, with the known individual variability of acetylation (acetylator status). In the series of patients recorded by Mitchell et al,[83] the incidence of severe reactions was higher in a non-caucasian group of patients, where rapid acetylation is more common, than in caucasians. Similar evidence linking INAH hepatitis to rapid acetylator status comes from evidence of increased toxicity in orientals (where 90 per cent of subjects are of rapid acetylator status). Presumably, the acetylated derivatives of INAH (chiefly acetylhydrazine) are responsible for the hepatic toxicity. They could act in one of two major ways: firstly, by covalent binding to organelles in the hepatocytes or, possibly, by the development of an immunological reaction to damaged hepatic macromolecules.

The newer evidence concerning an apparently increased incidence of INAH hepatoxicity needs further evaluation in Britain where INAH is hardly ever employed singly. Perhaps this fact and the suggested inhibiting action of PAS on INAH metabolism means that therapy with this agent in combination is safe – as clinical evidence to prove otherwise outside the United States is lacking. Alcohol, phenobarbitone and the antituberculous drug rifampicin may all potentiate the toxicity of INAH by speeding drug metabolism.

Rifampicin

This important antituberculous drug was introduced into this country in the early 1970s. It soon became recognized as the cause of a drug-induced hepatitis in a small percentage, e.g. 1 to 4 per cent, of patients treated solely with this drug.[123] The lesion often starts early during therapy and those who are affected within three weeks of starting treatment are particularly likely to show evidence of severe disease. The usual biochemical features of a drug-induced cell disorder are seen, with elevation of the serum bilirubin and transaminases being most important. The histological features include evidence of a mild hepatitis and a portal infiltration, the latter showing sparing of some portal zones. Cholestasis is mild, whilst acidophilic bodies are prominent. Toxicity due to rifampicin is probably more common than is recognized by the clinical detection of jaundice and the prognosis of this generally mild disorder seems good. There is evidence, too, that continuation of rifampicin therapy is compatible with recovery from hepatitis. The dose of the drug may also be important since hepatitis is an accompaniment of higher dosage, a feature of the hepatotoxicity of a number of antituberculous drugs.

A further hepatic disorder is seen in patients treated with rifampicin.[19] This is an unconjugated and conjugated hyperbilirubinaemia which is thought to result from interference by the drug with the uptake of bilirubin into liver cells, as well as with bilirubin excretion. The initial rise in bilirubin is then followed by a significant fall, this being due to an effect of rifampicin in producing hypertrophy of the drug-oxidizing enzyme system with subsequent enzyme induction. The enzyme induction produced by rifampicin may be important in the production of INAH hepatitis.[73] The drug is excreted in high concentrations in bile.[3]

Other antituberculous drugs

Pyrazinamide is not now used in the treatment of tuberculosis because it is a known hepatotoxin, producing a drug hepatitis in 1 to 3 per cent of patients given the drug alone or in combination. The mechanism is uncertain and the lesion is serious enough for the drug to be stopped if liver function tests become abnormal. Several deaths are recorded and, rather like INAH, the onset of the hepatic disorder may be delayed for five or six months from the start of therapy.[77] Ethionamide similarly may produce a late onset type of hepatitis which may be fatal,[26] whilst cycloserine, neomycin and streptomycin are probably never hepatotoxic in man and such reactions as occur are likely to be due to the accompanying therapy. Ethambutol is similarly non-hepatotoxic.

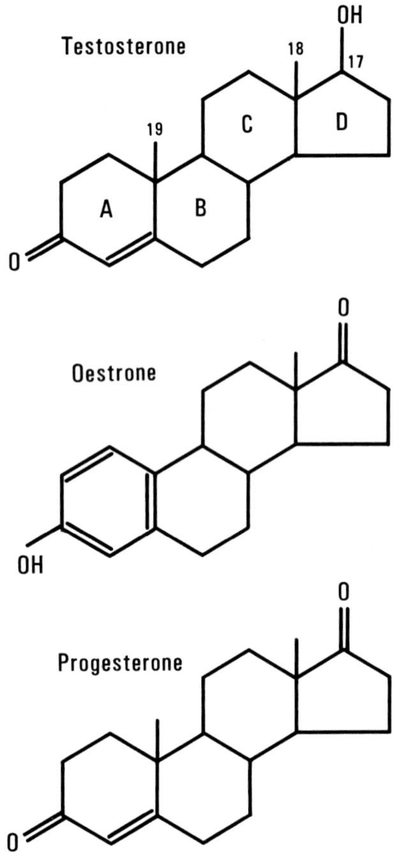

Figure 36.1. The chemical structure of some natural sex steroids.

Steroid Drugs

Certain drugs bearing the steroid (cyclopentanophenanthrene) nucleus are icterogenic. The parent compounds from which these agents have developed are shown (Figure 36.1). It will be seen that the major differences between them are few and that testosterone, oestrone and progesterone differ mainly in the possession of methyl groups at the 19 and 18 positions and the degree of unsaturation of the A ring. Though natural steroids may occasionally be icterogenic it is the compounds which have been developed from them which are most hepatotoxic. In particular, certain changes in the basic structure are known to be associated with hepatotoxicity. These changes include:

1. The conjugation of the steroid with alkyl or ethynyl groupings at the C-17α position (C-17α-alkyl/ethinyl substituted compounds).[95]
2. The possession of one as opposed to two CH_3 groups at the 18 and 19 positions (the 19-nortestosterone compounds).

The possession of both of these characteristics in 19-nortestosterones that are 17α-alkyl substituted reinforces the icterogenic effect. Drugs which are 19-nortestosterones which are not C-17α-alkyl/ethinyl substituted, e.g. chlormadinone (which is a 17α-acetate substituted progestogen), are not icterogenic. The jaundice produced with all these drugs is cholestatic in type.

Testosterone and anabolic steroids

Methyltestosterone liver disease. This agent produces cholestasis when given therapeutically.[17] Other preparations of testosterone which do not possess the 17α-alkyl grouping do not produce this effect, e.g. testosterone propionate. The jaundice is related to the dosage of the agent and the duration of time over which it is used. Where the cumulative dosage is insufficient to produce jaundice, changes in BSP excretion can be detected and the alkaline phosphatase may be raised. The clinical picture is of an obstructive jaundice, whilst liver biopsy shows simple cholestasis with bile plugs, but without evidence of hepatocellular necrosis or of a portal tract inflammation. Cholestasis gradually clears once therapy is stopped and even long-term cholestasis remits in this way. Some examples of more chronic liver disease due to methyltestosterone are peliosis hepatis[10,53] and liver cell carcinoma (hepatoma) (see below). These have usually been reported where methyltestosterone and other anabolic agents have been used in the therapy of hypoplastic anaemia, e.g. Fanconi's anaemia in childhood. More recently, long-term high dosage therapy has been associated with the development of adenomas and the presence of a layer of hepatocytes within the lumen of the central veins.[99] Amongst the other substituted testosterones which produce cholestasis are C-17α-ethynyl substituted norethandrolone (17α-ethyl-19-nortestosterone) and norethisterone (17α-ethinyl-19-nortestosterone), whilst nadrolone, a phenylpropionate ester of 19-nortestosterone, is usually non-icterogenic.

Prior to the introduction of cholestyramine and other bile salt chelating agents for the treatment of the icterus of biliary obstruction, some of the above 17α-substituted testosterones and nortestosterones were used in the treatment of the pruritus accompanying biliary obstruction. They are effective in relieving this, but this desirable relief is obtained at the expense of a further rise in the serum bilirubin level. These combined antipruritic and cholestatic effects suggest that a biochemical mechanism may underlie both of these actions, perhaps directed at bile salt excretion at the canalicular level.

Oestrogens

Natural and synthetic oestrogens have a variety of deleterious effects on the liver. These include (a) cholestasis and/or a defect of BSP excretion,[96,118] (b) the production of hepatic tumours (adenoma, hamartoma and hepatoma)[8] (see Chapter 38), (c) an exacerbation of the cutaneous manifestation of porphyria cutanea tarda[76] and (d) an increased incidence of gallstones.[15] As the need for large doses of oestrogens is limited to males with carcinoma of the prostate and some postmenopausal patients with breast cancer, the only major problem is the occasional patient with cholestasis or porphyria cutanea tarda.[66] Furthermore, long-term oestrogen therapy has been associated with hepatic tumours only in patients using the contraceptive pill where duration of therapy is obviously important.

The cholestasis which accompanies pregnancy, 'recurrent intrahepatic cholestasis of pregnancy',[132] is of uncertain cause but a biochemical disorder is likely and oestrogens or some other steroid hormone produced in pregnancy are the likely causes. Typically, jaundice appears in the third trimester, when it is of variable severity and may cause only skin irritation. Hepatic histology shows pure cholestasis without evidence of a portal infiltrate or liver cell necrosis. Patients who suffer from this disorder often do so with subsequent pregnancies and on exposure to the contraceptive pill (see Chapter 14). Furthermore, there is a not inconsiderable risk of prematurity for the fetus.[110]

The mechanism by which oestrogens and related steroids produce cholestasis is uncertain. Experimentally they interfere with canalicular biliary flow and in particular that part which is independent of bile salt secretion. The close relationship between the effects of large doses of oestrogens in normal subjects – jaundice due to taking the contraceptive pill – and the form found in the last trimester of pregnancy suggests a common mechanism in these three situations.

Jaundice and the contraceptive pill. With the widespread acceptance of this convenient and acceptable method of birth control (there were 3.1×10^6 women 'on the pill' in England and Wales alone in 1975) has come the recognition of a variety of hepatic disorders associated with its use. The commonest of these contraceptive-induced cholestasis, 'pill jaundice',[94,136] usually occurs within two or three months of starting therapy. The jaundice is cholestatic, with itching, pale stools and dark urine, and it is usually mild. However, some cases are reported where the serum bilirubin is high and liver cell damage in the form of scattered areas of liver cell necrosis and high serum transaminases are found. The prognosis of this disorder is excellent, a slow resolution of the jaundice following the removal of this type of therapy. Cholestasis resulting from the pill is rare in Britain. An increased incidence is seen in Scandinavia and in parts of South America, suggesting the presence of a genetic factor. The fact that sufferers from cholestasis of pregnancy, idiopathic cholestasis[34] and those with congenital conjugated hyperbilirubinaemia, e.g. Dubin–Johnson syndrome, may show deepening jaundice on cyclical hormone therapy of this type suggests some action of the pill on bilirubin excretion from the liver cell. Most oral contraceptives contain a mixture of a synthetic oestrogen and a synthetic progestin which are given simultaneously or sequentially. The components may both be 17α-ethynyl substituted and this, no doubt, is one factor in determining their hepatotoxicity. Furthermore, progestins are metabolized to oestrogens, though it seems clear that the toxic effect resides largely, if not entirely, with the oestrogen component of the pill. The cholestatic action is therefore entirely in line with that described for the natural oestrogens, though an additive effect due to the progestin therapy cannot be excluded.

Further actions of the contraceptive pill on the liver must be mentioned.

Hepatic tumour formation (see also Chapter 38). Increased numbers of hepatic adenomas are described in patients taking the contraceptive pill. These tumours, which are usually solitary, sometimes grow to a large size. They present either as an abdominal mass with some localized pain or, more dramatically, with shock due to rupture and subsequent intraperitoneal haemorrhage. Carcinoma of the liver is also recorded in women taking the contraceptive pill,[31] as are localized areas of benign regenerative foci (benign focal hyperplasia, hamartoma).

Gallstones. There is also an increased incidence of gallstones in patients taking the pill, a feature which perhaps ties in with the increased incidence of gallstones with repeated pregnancies.

Peliosis hepatis. This condition, in which the hepatic sinusoids communicate with blood-filled lacunae, is also a feature in some patients on cyclical hormonal therapy.[142] Its precise cause is unknown and it is also recorded in patients taking anabolic steroids[91] as well as in patients with severe malnutrition or cachexia.

The Budd–Chiari syndrome.[131, 144] This may be caused by thrombosis of the major hepatic veins and this thrombotic tendency is presumably due to the recognized increased incidence of venous thrombosis in these subjects.

Progesterone and progestins

Progesterone produces no deleterious effect on hepatic function, though it may be a powerful inducer of drug-metabolizing enzymes. One form of jaundice in the neonate – breast milk jaundice – may bear some relationship to the presence in human milk of 3α-20β-pregnanediol (a progesterone derivative).[6] This steroid is certainly capable of inhibiting glucuronide formation, using artificial substrates as well as bilirubin. It could conceivably be associated with the prolonged unconjugated hyperbilirubinaemia seen in less than 1 per cent of breast-fed infants. Bilirubin levels of up to 342 μmol/l (20 mg/dl) are recorded but jaundice subsides following cessation of breast feeding. Successive infants may be affected. In view of the profound effects that nutrition may have on bilirubin disposition and the fact that glucuronide inhibitors other than 3α-20β-pregnanediol may be produced, the precise cause of this syndrome, which may remit even though breast feeding continues, is uncertain.

Psychotropic Drugs

Over the past two decades, the number of drugs available for the treatment of the minor and major psychiatric disorders has increased considerably. The drugs largely fall into two major groups, that is, those used in the treatment of the depressive disorders, e.g. monoamine oxidase inhibitors and iminobenzyl derivatives (tricyclic antidepressants), and those used as tranquillizers, e.g. the phenothiazines and benzodiazepins. All four groups of agents can produce significant hepatotoxicity, with ensuing features either of cholestasis or liver cell disease or both.

Table 36.3. *Available Monoamine Oxidase Inhibitors.*

Commercial preparation	Approved name
Marplan	Isocarboxazid
Marsilid	Iproniazid
Nardil	Phenelzine
Niamid	Nialamide
Parnate	Tranylcypromine
Parstelin	Tranylcypromine Trifluoperazine (phenothiazine)

Monoamine oxidase inhibitors

With the introduction of iproniazid for the treatment of pulmonary tuberculosis came the recognition that severe and occasionally fatal liver necrosis sometimes resulted from this agent.[104, 116] It was hardly surprising, therefore, that this and structurally similar agents used for the treatment of depressive illness led to the detection of further similar examples[7] and the subsequent banning of a certain number of these agents. Few are now available (see Table 36.3).

The toxic effect is not confined to the hydrazine derivative of this family of drugs as was originally thought, but certainly hepatotoxicity is more commonly seen with this group. Typically, jaundice occurs in 1 to 2 per cent of those treated with these drugs. The onset may follow some months after starting therapy, but is most commonly seen after an interval of about four weeks. In every way the condition mimics viral hepatitis, though comment has been made about the rarity of fever as compared to viral hepatitis and the greater severity of the drug-induced disorder. Serum bilirubin values are often in excess of those seen in 'average' cases of hepatitis, whilst transaminase levels are often less marked. None of these distinguishing features is absolute, however. The severity of the drug-induced disorder is mirrored by the mortality of about 20 per cent. Death, which is often accompanied by coma, deepening jaundice, haemorrhagic phenomena and reduction in liver size, is due to massive hepatic necrosis. Therapy has little or no effect once this stage has been reached and death is then to be expected.

Argument concerning the cause of this serious type of liver cell disease is considerable. The low incidence – at least of clinically apparent cases – suggests some immunological or biochemical sensitivity, but the lack of features such as eosinophilia, skin rashes, etc., makes the former cause less likely. These agents may share with isoniazid the biochemical potential for causing hepatotoxicity and metabolic conversion in the liver may determine this. Certainly, acetylation is the major route of metabolism, and factors which alter this, such as genetic acetylator status or the concurrent administration of drugs which might alter the speed of the acetylation process, could all be important. The relatively few numbers of cases with hepatotoxicity might then be explained on the basis of biochemical sensitivity due either to direct or indirect liver cell damage consequent upon covalent binding to hepatocyte fractions or to an immunological attack directed against a metabolite/liver cell complex.

Phenothiazines

The phenothiazine drugs produce a cholestatic hepatitis in a certain number (1 to 2 per cent) of patients who are treated with them.[24] Usually appearing two to four weeks after administration,[64] the lesion has been most classically associated with chlorpromazine (Largactil), but an identical type of reaction can occur with other drugs of this family, such as mepazine, perphenazine, prochlorperazine and promazine. These drugs have often been used subsequent to chlorpromazine. Typically, the onset is acute, with fever, and in a significant number of patients eosinophilia and eosinophil infiltration in the portal tracts at liver biopsy have been noted. These suggestions of a hypersensitivity type of reaction have been countered by the fact that a remission may occur despite a continuation of therapy and the observation of an elevation of transaminase levels in 20 to 50 per cent of patients treated with these agents.

The lesion is of variable severity. A significant number of patients show biochemical and histological evidence of liver cell damage and necrosis. This may be in accord with the fact that several fatalities are documented as resulting from use of this drug (see Table 36.1) and, in at least some of these, extensive necrosis has been demonstrated. Obviously, many of these patients may have had other serious debilitating disorders which may have completely or partially explained the liver cell damage, but it should not be forgotten that this group of drugs causes liver damage which is potentially both cholestatic and hepatocellular in type. Further peculiarities recorded in patients with phenothiazine jaundice include an onset after only one dose of the drug and a positive skin patch test in a number of patients.

In certain patients, an alarming and prolonged clinical picture is produced. Jaundice with pruritus and hepatosplenomegaly persists, widespread xanthomas are found, the clinical and histological picture resembles that of primary biliary cirrhosis with positive mitochondrial antibodies in the serum. Jaundice has been reported as lasting up to six years[108, 138] and opinions differ as to whether complete remission is or is not possible once this stage has been reached. Certainly, no treatment is known to play any significant part in hastening resolution. Cholestyramine to combat itching and fat-soluble vitamins to prevent bleeding and osteomalacia are recommended symptomatic and prophylactic measures.

It has generally been thought that an immunological hypersensitivity is the basis of this lesion and such an explanation might be in accord with the eosinophilia, neutropenia and skin rashes that are sometimes seen. It seems possible, too, that the considerable portal tract infiltrate which is a feature of some established cases could act as a further obstructive lesion to biliary flow. Nevertheless, other mechanisms, usually based on the results of animal experiments, continue to be discovered. An effect on bile salt excretion, related to precipitation of bile salts by chlorpromazine and other derivatives, might diminish bile flow.[20] Experimental evidence of increased bilirubin loading due to haemolysis and of defective glucuronidation may also play a significant but, at the moment, uncertain part in the production of jaundice.[65]

Tricyclic antidepressants (*dibenzazepines*)

Included in this group are imipramine (Tofranil), amitriptyline (Tryptizol), iprindole (Prondol) and their desmethyl derivatives desipramine, nortriptyline (Aventyl, Motival), protriptyline (Concordin) and doxepin (Sinequan). They are chemically closely related to the phenothiazines (Figure 36.2) and it is therefore not surprising that they occasionally cause jaundice. Thus amitriptyline,[54, 87] iprindole[4] and imipramine[125] cause a cholestatic hepatitis, and in about 20 per cent of patients treated with the latter drug a symptomless rise in transaminases occurs. Similar findings are noted with desipramine but these drugs

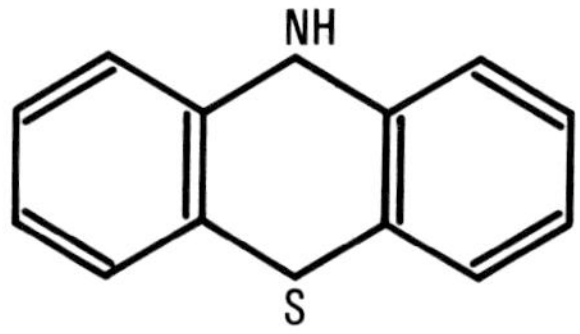

Phenothiazine Nucleus

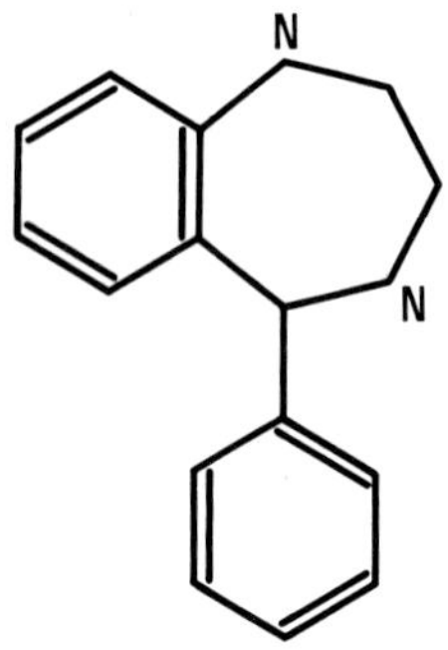

Diazepin Nucleus

Figure 36.2. The chemical structure of the two major groups of tranquillizers.

occasionally cause a severe and fatal hepatic necrosis.[105]

Anxiolytic agents (benzodiazepines)

These agents include diazepam (Valium), chlordiazepoxide (Librium), nitrazepam (Mogadon) and flurazepam (Dalmane). They can cause a cholestatic hepatitis with fever and eosinophilia but, considering their widespread use, this is extremely rare.[74]

Antibiotic and Chemotherapeutic Agents

Tetracycline

This valuable antibiotic can cause a serious form of liver disease, with accompanying azotaemia and pancreatitis.[25] Histologically, the hepatic disorder is characterized by a fine droplet fatty infiltration of the hepatocytes. Characteristically, the nucleus remains central and is not displaced to one side. The majority of cases have been in pregnant women where urinary tract infection has been a common cause for the use of this drug. Toxicity is the result of the appearance of excessive levels of tetracycline in the blood and thus has usually, but not always, been associated with I.V. administration. It should be stressed, however, that males and non-pregnant females can be affected to some degree, even when the tetracycline is given orally. The reason why pregnant women seem to be susceptible is uncertain, but animals given oestrogens are more liable to damage than are untreated ones; it is certainly not due to a difference in drug removal rates in pregnant and non-pregnant women. Great caution is therefore necessary when tetracycline is given, particularly in large doses, and where it is used I.V. a suitable reduction in dose must be made.

Clinically, two to three days after tetracycline I.V., nausea, vomiting, abdominal pain and jaundice occur. In some cases death due to acute liver failure and signs of renal failure and pancreatitis also occur. In pregnancy this condition mimics very closely the acute (idiopathic) fatty liver of pregnancy and a history of tetracycline therapy is then of diagnostic value. Treatment is supportive and, in patients dying of this condition, both the liver and kidneys may show fatty change.

Toxic hepatic injury due to tetracycline can be produced in animals and it can be clearly demonstrated that the fatty infiltration is associated with a reduction of triglyceride output by the liver. It has been suggested that this is, in turn, due to a decreased production of the apoprotein of hepatic very low-density lipoprotein (VLDL) with subsequent retention of unbound lipid in the liver.[121] The disease is certainly preventable by avoiding this antibiotic as an intravenous medication.

Similar effects can be seen with oxytetracycline (Terramycin) and chlortetracycline (Aureomycin), but they are usually of no clinical consequence when the drugs are given orally, though I.V. chlortetracycline can produce a lesion as severe as that produced by I.V. tetracycline.

Chloramphenicol

Apart from its well-recognized effects on the blood and bone marrow and its toxicity in the newborn, chloramphenicol is sometimes also the cause of hepatotoxicity, but in this case there is a well-defined hepatitis rather than fatty infiltration.[49]

Penicillin

A hepatitis may occasionally accompany the skin rashes, lymphadenopathy, arthralgia and purpura seen in patients with penicillin hypersensitivity, [137] and sometimes, too, a prolonged cholestatic illness with a long recovery phase may follow this. Ampicillin, despite the frequency of cutaneous hypersensitivity phenomena, is a rare cause of drug hepatitis.

Sulphonamides

All sulphonamide drugs may cause drug-induced hepatitis,[45] but the overall incidence is less than 5 per cent. Toxicity is seen with the short-acting and long-acting sulpha drugs and with drugs containing sulphonamides in combination, e.g. co-trimoxazole. The onset, which usually occurs two to six weeks after commencing therapy, is sudden and in every way mimics viral hepatitis unless skin rashes and other hypersensitivity phenomena appear. In severe cases death may be caused by hepatic necrosis, whilst milder cases show scattered foci of hepatocellular necrosis and granulomas.[21]

Novobiocin

This antibiotic causes an increase in the serum unconjugated bilirubin level and when this occurs in neonates there may be frank jaundice. The lesion seems to result from an impairment of bilirubin conjugation which can be demonstrated in vitro, but inhibiting effects on hepatocyte uptake and excretion of bilirubin are also possible.[2] Over and above this disorder a true drug-induced hepatitis, which may be fatal, is sometimes seen.

Erythromycin estolate

Unlike erythromycin, this ester may produce a cholestatic hepatitis,[44] presumably due to hypersensitivity. The cholestasis subsides when the drug, which is now rarely used, is withdrawn.

Griseofulvin

This antifungal agent is important because of its ability to produce a porphyria-like syndrome in rodents as well as to exacerbate the clinical state of patients with porphyria cutanea tarda. The mechanism is uncertain and may be due merely to an exacerbation of the liver disease that accompanies this syndrome or there may be an interference with the feedback mechanism controlling ALA synthetase production which, though not the primary disturbance in this condition, is an important factor in determining clinical severity (see also Chapter 15).

Nitrofurantoin

This urinary antiseptic is known to produce important side-effects (particularly skin reactions, peripheral neuropathy when blood levels are high and pulmonary infiltration). It is a rare cause, too, of cholestatic hepatitis which seems to be part of a generalized hypersensitivity picture. Obstructive jaundice usually settles within two months of the cessation of therapy.[12,41]

Arsenic

Several hepatotoxic effects result from the use of this agent. When it was used before the Second World War in the treatment of syphilis, serum hepatitis (virus B hepatitis) was extremely common due to the use of contaminated syringes. A small proportion of those treated developed a sensitivity reaction, with fever, rash, arthralgia and eosinophilia and, on occasions, an accompanying hepatitis. This constitutes Milian's syndrome and is of importance because it was commonly associated with cholestasis which sometimes became chronic. Pruritus and hepatomegaly were then complicated by obstructive liver function tests and hypercholesterolaemia and xanthomatosis. This, as with the similar type of reaction seen after chlorpromazine therapy, becomes indistinguishable in some cases from primary biliary cirrhosis.

Delayed hepatotoxic effects of arsenic have become recognized only in the last few years. Apart from early evidence that arsenic contained in insecticides was a possible cause of cirrhosis (other than alcohol) in German vineyard workers, it is also reported that arsenic – usually given as Fowler's solution – produced portal tract fibrosis with portal venous block and accompanying intrahepatic portal hypertension.[89] A further and more sinister complication was the development in one patient of angiosarcoma following 15 years' daily therapy with Fowler's solution.[71] Death was due to liver cell failure and systemic spread of the tumour. In this patient there was no significant hepatic fibrosis present. This sequence of events is remarkably similar to that accompanying the hepatic lesion of vinyl chloride and Thorotrast (see below).

Niridazole (*Ambilhar*)

This non-antimonial drug used in the treatment of schistosomiasis has been associated with elevated serum transaminases[63] and may cause alarming side-effects in patients with liver involvement (infection with *S. mansoni* or *S. japonicum*). The side-effects include hallucinations, delirium and coma, confusion and, occasionally, loss of consciousness. These effects are presumably due to raised drug levels in the systemic circulation consequent on portal hypertension and portasystemic shunting.

Hycanthone

This drug is used for schistosomiasis and may produce abnormal serum transaminase levels within 24 hours of injection. Liver biopsy appearances after five days showed fatty change, occasional acidophil bodies and an infiltrate of lymphocytes in portal tracts.[42]

Sulphones

These drugs, particularly dapsone, are used in the treatment of leprosy. They have also been used by dermatologists to treat a variety of skin disorders including dematitis herpetiformis and pustular psoriasis. Rarely, a cholestatic hepatitis complicates the therapy.[81]

Analgesic and Anti-inflammatory Drugs

Paracetamol (*Acetaminophen*)

This drug now contributes significantly to the list of agents used by patients attempting suicide. Hospital admissions in England and Wales rose from 150 in 1968 to about 10 times that number in 1971 with over 50 deaths. The effect on the liver is predictable and dose-dependent. The drug causes massive hepatic necrosis and in less severe cases there is a well-defined centrilobular death of hepatocytes. Recovery in non-fatal cases is complete and cirrhosis is not an end-result. The dosage required to produce fatal hepatic necrosis may be as low as 15 g, whilst hepatic injury may be noted on biochemical testing after only 6 g. The toxicity of paracetamol is increased by taking enzyme-inducing agents, particularly alcohol, and reduced by nausea, vomiting and gastric lavage. The effect on the liver is thought to be produced by a reactive metabolite of paracetamol rather than the parent compound itself.

There is a clinically characteristic sequence of time changes. After initial anorexia, nausea and vomiting, symptoms settle and two or three days after ingestion the only evidence of liver damage is biochemical, with raised transaminases, an extended prothrombin time and a mildly raised and largely unconjugated hyperbilirubinaemia. The clinician may well be lulled into a sense of false security by these changes, but they may herald the onset of worsening liver failure. In a study by Clark,[23] 17 of 19 patients with a serum bilirubin > 68 µmol/l (4 mg/dl) and with a prothrombin ratio of 2.2 or greater, developed encephalopathy and 12 died. The severity of the coagulation defect has been interpreted as evidence of a disseminated intravascular coagulation as much as simply a failure to synthesize coagulation factors. Overall mortality will depend on the dosage taken, the state of hepatic enzyme induction, etc., but it varies in different series from 2 to 13 per cent (mean 2 to 3 per cent).

The mechanism of toxicity is important as it dictates the treatment.[30] Normally, paracetamol is conjugated with glucuronide and glutathione and rendered water-soluble for excretion. Sulphation is a further method of disposal, but all of these excretory pathways are readily overpowered by an overdose of the drug. As a result, paracetamol forms active unconjugated metabolites (possibly an *N*-hydroxy derivative) which, by covalent binding, damage hepatocytes. Other conjugates of paracetamol are formed with cysteine and acetylcysteine and these appear in the urine after intoxication in greatly increased amounts. Attempts at therapy are therefore based on increasing the liver's ability to detoxify paracetamol. This can theoretically be done by giving agents such as cysteamine, methionine or more recently *N*-acetyl cysteine. These agents have been shown to be of value in certain patients.

Patients who have taken an overdose of paracetamol need early assessment of probable severity following initial gastric wash-out. Patients with blood levels of 200 µg/ml or more at 4 hours and 50 µg or more at 12 hours after ingestion have a 60 per cent chance of developing severe liver damage. In practice, the drawing of a line between these two points separates a high-risk group in whom treatment is required, providing it is given early (< 8 hrs), from less severe groups with levels below this range. The most useful treatment now is with *N*-acetyl cyteine which is available as a 20 per cent solution for I.V. use (Parvolex). It is given at a dose of 150 mg/kg body weight I.V. over 15 minutes, followed by 50 mg/kg in 500 ml dextrose solution over the next 4 hours, then 100 mg/kg body weight in 1 litre of 5 per cent dextrose (total: 300 mg/kg in 20 hrs). It is most effective when given within 8 hours of poisoning, and is ineffective after 15 hours when it may actually be harmful. It is otherwise non-toxic.

Phenylbutazone

This widely used pyrazole anti-inflammatory analgesic causes a wide variety of toxic effects. Hepatitis is a rare manifestation of toxicity and when it occurs there is often evidence of multi-organ involvement, e.g. drug rashes, fever, lymphadenopathy and thrombocytopenia, making a drug hypersensitivity likely. The picture is that of a hepatitis with liver cell dysfunction, though occasionally there may be significant cholestasis.[39] Liver biopsy may demonstrate epithelioid granulomas with giant cells and a large number of eosinophils. The granulomas may be transient.[57] It is reported that cirrhosis can follow and fatalities certainly occur.

Indomethacin

Despite the fact that side-effects from this drug are common, it is a very rare cause of drug hepatitis.[43] This is also seen with a number of proprionic acid derivatives (Table 36.4) used as anti-inflammatory drugs and with a profound effect on prostaglandin synthetase.

Aspirin

Aspirin and other salicylates in high dosage may also cause focal hepatic damage histologically with accompanying abnormalities of the liver function tests – particularly elevation of the transaminases.[124]

Carbamazepine (Tegretol)

This analgesic and anticonvulsant, used principally in the treatment of painful neuralgias, can also cause a cholestatic drug hepatitis.[107]

Gold

Colloidal gold has been extensively used in the treatment of rheumatoid arthritis. Jaundice and hepatomegaly have been rarely reported. Hepatitis was described in the original records but it is difficult to exclude viral hepatitis in these reports. More recently, jaundice of obstructive pattern with intrahepatic cholestasis and minimal hepatocellular damage has been described.[122]

Anaesthetic Agents and Anticonvulsant Drugs

The historically well-known hepatic necrosis due to chloroform seems to be caused by the parent drug itself, because protein depletion potentiates hepatotoxicity (cf. carbon tetrachloride) and further indicates the important dependence of the drug-metabolizing enzyme system on protein metabolism. This has been followed by hepatic reactions to several other anaesthetic agents. Such reactions include transient alterations of hepatic function due to cyclopropane and much more dramatic and serious effects related to the use of halothane and, to a lesser extent, methoxyflurane (Penthrane)[60] with which there appears to be a cross-sensitivity.[62] The problem of hepatotoxicity induced by halothane is dealt with in Chapter 47.

It is important to realize that changes in liver structure and function after surgical treatment

Table 36.4. *Analgesic and Anti-inflammatory Drugs.*

Drug	Hepatic lesion	Incidence
Paracetamol (acetaminophen)	Zonal (centrilobular) necrosis Massive hepatic necrosis	Dose-related
Phenylbutazone	Granulomatous hepatitis ± cholestasis ? Cirrhosis	Rare
Indomethacin	Hepatitis	Rare
Proprionic acid derivatives		
Ibuprofen	Nil	
Ketoprofen	Hepatitis	Rare
Naproxen	Cholestatic hepatitis	Rare
Carbamazepine	Cholestatic hepatitis	Rare
Salicylates	Hepatitis	Dose-related (blood level 20–45 mg/dl)
Gold	Cholestasis	Rare

have multiple causes (see Chapter 47) and the direct implication of anaesthetic agents is of necessity difficult.

Phenytoin

Amongst the many recorded side-effects of this drug is hepatocellular necrosis. Though much rarer than skin sensitivity, hepatitis seems to be as common as the nephrotic syndrome and blood dyscrasias. Liver biopsy shows a diffuse hepatitis with acidophil bodies, focal necroses and an eosinophil infiltrate.[52] It must be stressed that these are acute hypersensitivity reactions and have nothing to do with long-term side-effects.

Antimetabolite and Immunosuppressive Drugs

In view of their action in preventing cellular division and diminishing the cellular immune response, it is perhaps hardly surprising that these agents sometimes cause hepatocellular damage. In addition, the diseases for which these agents are used means that liver damage can be due to infiltration, infection, anaemia and a variety of other therapeutic agents. This makes the effects of the underlying disease difficult to unravel from the effects of therapy. Knowledge of the effects of some of the anti-cancer and immunosuppressive agents therefore becomes very important.

Azathioprine (*Imuran*)

This drug is metabolized by the liver to produce 6-mercaptopurine and thioinosinic acid which are potent immunosuppressives. This action is utilized in a variety of immunological disorders, including chronic active hepatitis where, in combination with corticosteroids, it has been shown to be effective in reducing both mortality and morbidity in this disease.[27] Experimentally in dogs it produces, after an interval of eight to nine weeks, both histological and biochemical evidence of liver cell and cholestatic hepato-toxicity. Similarly, in patients with chronic liver cell disease such as chronic active hepatitis and in primary biliary cirrhosis – in both of which diseases it has been used therapeutically – evidence of a deterioration of liver function with cholestatic features is sometimes recorded,[130] though it may be difficult to attribute these changes specifically to the drug. A few cases occur, however, where the relationship seems clear cut. When used alone, azathioprine has also occasionally been shown to produce evidence of deterioration of liver function as measured by removal of indocyanine green (ICG).[113] Rarely, too, fatal hepatic necrosis occurs.[145]

Because the immunosuppressive activity of azathioprine is dependent on effective hepatic metabolism, it might be supposed that poor liver function could be associated with a high incidence of toxicity due to unmetabolized azathioprine and poor immunosuppression. Interestingly enough, clinical improvement in patients with chronic liver disease is not necessarily related to immunosuppressive action, at least as measured by the red cell rosette test.[141]

Peliosis hepatis in renal transplant patients has been attributed to azathioprine.[32]

6-Mercaptopurine

This produces a drug hepatitis rather more commonly, particularly if high doses ($>$ 2.5 mg/kg daily) are used.[37] Sometimes this is accompanied by leucopenia and the disease can be fatal. The patient with chronic liver cell disease – perhaps because of impaired meta-bolism of 6-mercaptopurine – is particularly likely to develop this effect and it should be used very cautiously in those with chronic liver disease. It may be the reason for the occasional reaction of patients with chronic liver disease to azathiopurine (see 'Azathioprine').

Methotrexate

There is a serious risk of hepatic damage when methotrexate is given over a long period of time, as has occurred in the treatment of severe psoriasis.[28, 82, 139]

Liver cell damage with fatty change, fibrosis of the portal tracts and the eventual develop-ment of cirrhosis are all recognized com-plications. The relationship between the dura-tion of therapy and the severity of the liver disease is fairly close, such that the risk of fibrosis and cirrhosis is considerable after two years of therapy.[28] In this respect, too, treatment with small doses of continuous rather than intermittent (weekly) high dosage therapy seems the more dangerous.[28,82,102] The severity of the psoriasis may influence the likelihood of methotrexate-induced fibrosis and cirrhosis.[82]

Obviously, patients treated with this drug over a considerable period need careful monitoring and, because of the risks, alternative methods of treatment are usually employed.

Corticosteroids

Patients with Cushing's syndrome may show severe fatty infiltration of the liver and this type of damage may occur in patients treated with corticosteroids. In patients with viral hepatitis, fat is also only seen in the liver biopsies of those patients who are treated with corticosteroid drugs. The manner by which corticosteroids cause fatty infiltration of the liver is uncertain. Two mechanisms, either singly or combined, may be responsible, namely, increased mobilization of fat from peripheral fat depots or decreased esterification and release of fat from the liver.[58]

Chlorambucil

Chlorambucil may, on occasions, produce hepatocellular necrosis and patients being treated with this agent for chronic lymphatic leukaemia may develop jaundice with resultant diagnostic difficulty. In addition, cirrhosis may sometimes follow the acute reaction.[5]

Drugs Used in Cardiovascular Disorders

α-Methyldopa (*Aldomet*)

Hepatitis due to the administration of α-methyldopa is unusual[38] and in 1976 there were

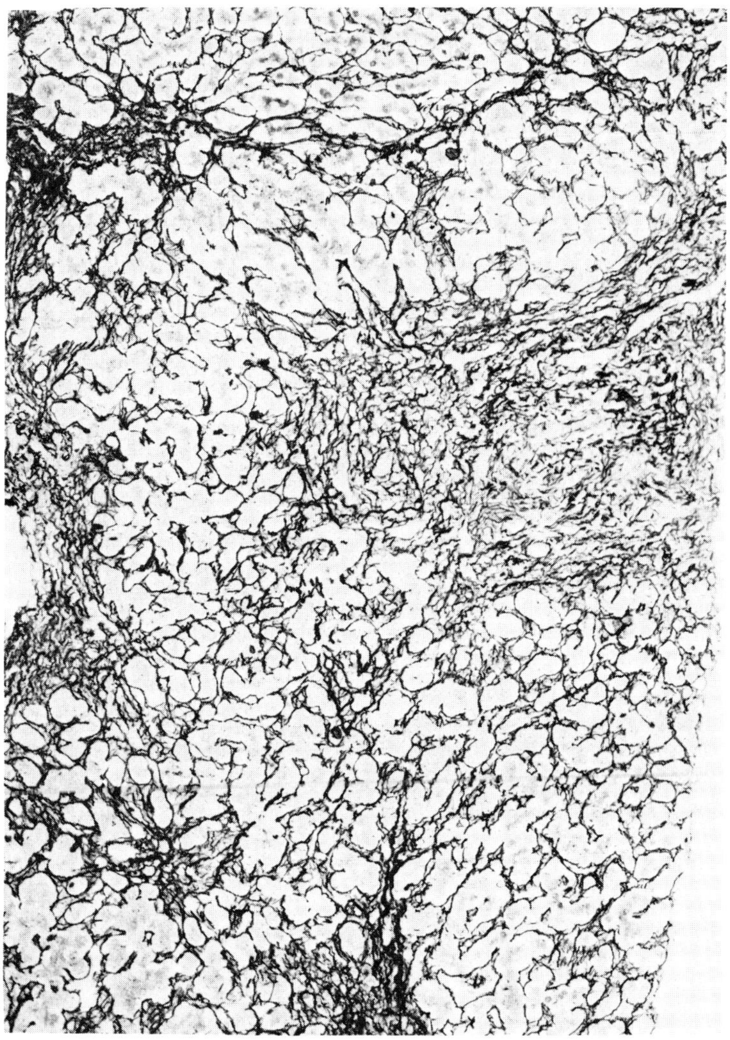

Figure 36.3. Fibrosis with disruption of lobular reticulin by piecemeal necrosis in methyldopa hepatitis. Gordon and Sweet's reticulin × 135.

reports of fewer than 100 cases, despite a vast usage of this drug for the treatment of hypertension.[115] Despite the rarity of hepatitis following administration of this drug, it should be discussed because the reaction may, rarely, be fatal and, perhaps more important, hepatitis may proceed to chronic liver disease (Figure 36.3). Early on, too, the disease is reversible, whilst later, when cirrhosis is present, it is not. In its subacute state it closely mimics chronic active (aggressive) hepatitis and recognition of the cause may result in complete resolution when the drug is withdrawn.

The mechanism of methyldopa-induced liver disease is unknown, but it has generally been thought to be immunological in type and its occasional association with rash and fever supports such a view. However, apart from patients who develop a multi-organ sensitivity, a larger number (5 per cent) show a rise in transaminases and other abnormal LFTs which is of uncertain cause and prognosis. Positive LE cell preparations have been found in some patients. Smooth muscle antibodies may also be found.

Nausea and vomiting one or two weeks after the administration of the drug herald the onset of jaundice, which may follow one to five weeks later. The disease may therefore follow shortly after the drug has been started, unlike, for example, most cases of hepatitis due to isoniazid, but there are exceptions to this rule. Striking evidence of diffuse hepatic inflammation may be seen and bridging necrosis is common, perhaps heralding the onset of cirrhosis in some cases. Rarely, progression can occur after administration of the drug has ceased.

The importance of drugs in the causation of chronic active hepatitis is stressed in the report from Australia by Goldstein, Lam and Mistilis.[50] Of 21 patients with chronic active hepatitis no fewer than 14 were taking drugs which could have caused the lesion (nine oxyphenisatin and five methyldopa). Further, it seems likely that patients with chronic liver disease due to methyldopa may be misdiagnosed as the abnormality of the liver function tests may be attributed to the effects of heart failure secondary to heart disease.

Perhexiline maleate

This vasodilator agent has been shown to be of value in some patients with angina pectoris. An early report that abnormalities of hepatic enzymes can occur from its use was made by Howard and Russell Rees.[55] These workers followed 16 male patients on 200 or 400 mg of perhexiline daily and noted a rise in transaminases in seven of them, this elevation sometimes subsiding with therapy. Recent reports show that hepatomegaly may occur[68] and may be accompanied by liver and Kupffer cell swelling with retention of lipid and mild non-specific hepatitis. The intracellular material was similar to that found in Niemann–Pick disease and was shown to be ganglioside, whilst an increase in cytoplasmic glycogen and decreased glucose-6-phosphatase suggested a minor form of type I glycogen storage disease.[70]

Not all histological studies of the liver have demonstrated this change and some similarity to the changes found in alcoholics has raised the possibility of synergistic liver damage due to these agents. Peripheral neuropathy,[103] weight loss and hypoglycaemia are other accompaniments of this complex toxic reaction due to perhexiline.

Benzothiadiazine diuretics

Cholestatic hepatitis, sometimes running a protracted course, is an occasional result of the administration of chlorothiazide[56] and a similar type of illness, accompanied by fever and skin rash, is seen with the closely related agent chlorthalidone. The more powerful diuretics such as ethacrynic acid may also cause hepatitis, with either cholestatic or hepatocellular features being seen.[29] All diuretic drugs may also produce hepatic encephalopathy in patients with chronic liver cell failure.

Anticoagulants

Hypersensitivity reactions to the oral anticoagulant phenindione are common. The spectrum of abnormalities includes agranulocytosis, nephropathy and thrombocytopenia. Hepatitis with both cholestatic and hepatocellular features is also seen[84,100] and has also been described for phenprocoumon.[33] For these reasons sodium warfarin is now usually preferred.

Drugs Used in the Treatment of Diabetes and Endocrine Disorders

Oral antidiabetic agents

The earlier oral antidiabetic agents, notably carbutamide, produce a drug hepatitis. This group of agents is closely related to the sulphonamides and it is perhaps not surprising that such reactions occur. Unfortunately this type of reaction is also seen with some of the currently popular agents and, at least with chlorpropamide, cholestatic hepatitis is reckoned to be a complication of therapy in about 5 per cent of patients[109] and a granulomatous reaction has also been described.[114] The hepatitis is sometimes accompanied by skin rashes, fever and eosinophilia. When this happens, diagnosis is facilitated, but the differential diagnosis from pancreatic cancer, in which diabetes may be an early symptom and subsequent obstructive jaundice the result of bile duct compression by the tumour, can be difficult. Pancreatic cancer often produces diabetes which is variable and difficult to control,[69] whilst jaundice due to chlorpropamide is usually seen within two to three months of starting therapy. It seems likely that many patients (perhaps up to 25 per cent) when treated with chlorpropamide will show abnormalities of liver function (particularly an elevated alkaline phosphatase), though not necessarily developing the clinical features of jaundice. The development of jaundice due to chlorpropamide in a patient with diabetes is an indication for the use of tolbutamide or glibenclamide, neither of which causes significant hepatotoxicity.

Antithyroid drugs

Hepatitis and other features which suggest a hypersensitivity reaction, e.g. skin rashes, neutropenia, salivary gland enlargement, lymphadenopathy, and even polyarteritis, are rare complications of some of the earlier drugs used for the control of thyrotoxicosis, such as methamizole, thiouracil and propylthiouracil. The hepatitis may be cholestatic or predominantly hepatocellular. It is not a feature of carbimazole therapy.

Industrial Agents and Toxins

Vinyl chloride

The manufacture of polyvinyl chloride (PVC) from its monomer vinyl chloride (VC) has exposed the workers involved in this process to a variety of diseases directly due to VC. These involve disorders of the skin, bone and liver, of which angiosarcoma and fibrosis with resulting portal hypertension are the most important hepatic ones. In an analysis of 161 deceased workers at two plants using vinyl chloride in the United States there was a 50 per cent excess of deaths due to cancer of all types, with the greatest excess in the liver and biliary tract, lungs and brain.[86] Five patients with angiosarcoma of the liver were noted by these authors and it may therefore be that vinyl chloride induces a generalized increase in cancer incidence.

The first case of angiosarcoma of the liver in Britain occurred in a 71-year-old man who had been a process worker in the manufacture of PVC from VC for 20 years.[72] At that time 19 cases of VC-induced angiosarcoma of the liver had been recorded, the tumour being composed of a honeycomb of vascular channels with lining spheroidal cells and intervening areas where sheets of spindle and spheroidal cells had infiltrated and disrupted the liver structure. Most of the angiosarcoma patients had worked in polymer plants for periods from 12 to 27 years.

Early work in rats had shown that liver damage, together with angiosarcoma and parenchymal changes in organs such as the skeletal and connective tissues, can be produced by concentrations of VC in the atmosphere of 250 parts per million when this is administered for a year. It is uncertain what factors other than concentration and duration of exposure lead to the onset of malignant change, but it is conceivable that alcohol or other drugs could be additional factors. Certainly stringent regulations that set a new upper limit for exposure to VC at 50 p.p.m. are now in force, but demands for a much lower level have already been made. Though PVC is harmless, there remains a possibility that some VC is given off from newly manufactured PVC and the latter's very widespread use has alerted the manufacturers to possible large-scale contamination.

Apart from angiosarcoma, attention has been drawn to a syndrome in VC workers where splenomegaly and portal hypertension can be attributed to non-cirrhotic fibrosis of the liver.[128] In this series, seven patients with portal

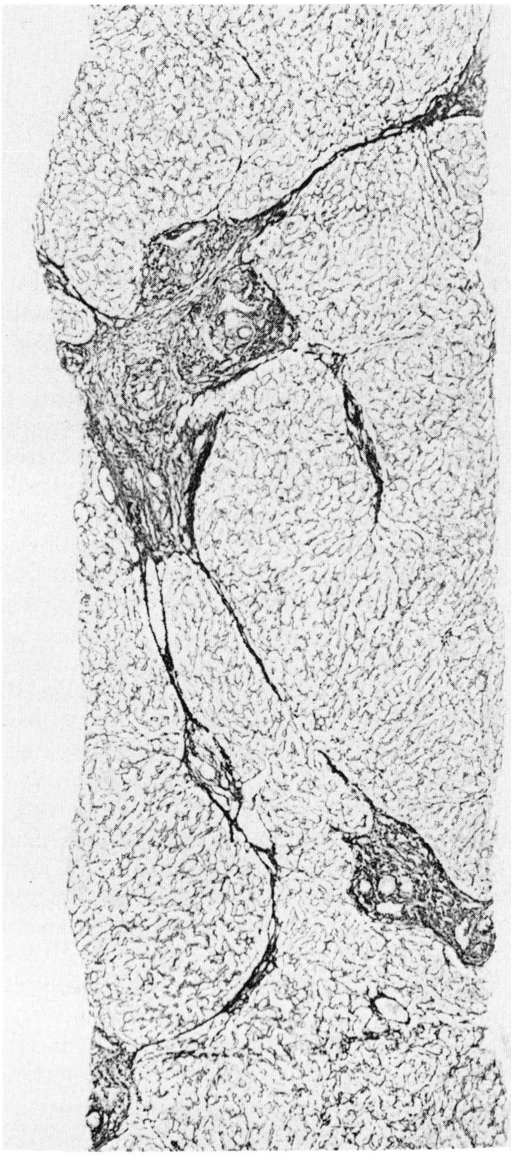

Figure 36.4. Non-cirrhotic extension of fibrous bands from portal tracts in needle biopsy from a vinyl chloride worker. Reticulin stain × 50.

hypertension, of whom four had bled from varices, were found in a survey of one workplace and four patients required shunt surgery. This seemed to be well tolerated with a good survival and no encephalopathy, presumably because of good (non-cirrhotic) liver cell function (Figure 36.4).

The occurrence of malignant angiosarcoma of the liver in Britain has recently been reviewed.[9] It is reported as a complication of vinyl chloride, arsenic and Thorotrast. In each case there is a long latent interval, which can be very accurately determined in the case of Thorotrast since this was used as a contrast medium for angiography.[16]

Thorotrast

This diagnostic x-ray medium was widely used until the end of the Second World War when the long-term sequelae became apparent. It is a colloidal suspension of thorium dioxide which emits predominantly alpha particles and has a half-life of 1.4×10^{10} years. After injection it is retained within the reticuloendothelial system and is therefore concentrated in liver, spleen, lymph nodes and bone marrow. A wide variety of tumours has been described arising either at the site of local deposition or from liver, kidney or spleen. Within the liver these tumours include hepatocellular carcinomas, intrahepatic cholangiocarcinomas, carcinomas of the gallbladder and biliary tree and sarcomas – usually of vascular origin (see Chapter 38).

Fibrosis of the liver is also described and is sometimes associated with cirrhosis. Diagnosis can be established by the presence of large clusters of cells containing the dense black Thorotrast pigment characteristically within an area of fibrosis. Autoradiography will confirm the radioactive nature of the particles.

The subject has been extensively reviewed.[51,134]

Carbon tetrachloride

This substance, which is used as a fat solvent and in dry-cleaning and fire-fighting equipment, is a well recognized cause of hepatic necrosis. Poisoning is by inhalation or ingestion and the risk from inhalation is increased where it is used in a confined space lacking proper ventilation. The variability in suceptibility to this toxin is remarkable and some of the factors responsible for this include those related to the functional activity of the cytochrome P-450 enzyme-inducing system in the liver.

Within a few hours of ingestion or inhalation, dizziness, headache, nausea and vomiting are followed by jaundice and hepatomegaly, which usually first appears after about two days. This may be followed, too, by renal involvement (with azotaemia and oligura) and this may then be complicated by pulmonary oedema and death. Death is usually due to renal rather than hepatic failure. Histologically the liver shows a diffuse fatty infiltration with centrilobular necrosis, haemorrhage and leucocyte infiltration.

Sometimes, particularly as a result of chronic exposure, a chemically induced hepatic cirrhosis results.

Much interest has centred on the mechanism of toxicity of this agent, which has acted as a model to demonstrate that hepatotoxicity can be due to a toxic metabolite rather than to the parent compound. This has certainly been proven for carbon tetrachloride as it can be demonstrated in animals that carbon tetrachloride toxicity is potentiated where the drug-oxidizing enzyme system in the liver is artificially stimulated by agents such as phenobarbitone and alcohol.[61] This is in full accord with clinical experience, where patients taking these agents are particularly likely to develop hepatotoxicity.

Conversely, for any condition where the drug-metabolizing system is hypoactive, as in the protein deficiency of starvation, carbon tetrachloride has a protective effect and spares experimental animals from liver damage. The effect of phenobarbitone has been used experimentally as a means of producing cirrhosis in carbon tetrachloride-treated rats.

Other chlorinated hydrocarbons are nowadays rare causes of hepatic injury; examples include *tetrachlorethane* (used originally in the aircraft industry), which causes subacute or massive hepatic necrosis, and *trichlorethylene* (a dry-cleaning agent), which causes a fatty infiltration of the liver and, in those addicted to sniffing this compound in glues,[93] more serious centrilobular hepatic necrosis.

The Epping jaundice (4,4-diaminodiphenylmethane)

In 1965 an outbreak of jaundice occurred in people purchasing bread from a single baker in Epping (England). He used flour which had been contaminated in transit by 4,4-diaminodiphenylmethane, an aromatic amine used in the plastics industry.[67] Eighty-four subjects were involved, the illness being sudden in onset and, in most, accompanied by abdominal pain, fever rigors, limb pains and hepatomegaly with a mild obstructive jaundice. The onset with pain made for diagnostic difficulties in the early cases and, as some patients had an eosinophilia, a diagnosis of parasitic biliary obstruction was considered in some patients. A portal tract infiltrate of eosinophils was also seen on liver biopsy, suggesting a hypersensitivity reaction. On the other hand, the fairly large number of patients involved (there were 84 clinical cases out of a potential 400, apart from the sub-clinical cases) is rather unlike such a hypersensitivity reaction.

Other histological features included cholestasis, increased numbers of hepatocyte mitotic figures and some evidence of liver cell damage. All 84 patients recovered.

Tannic acid

When tannic acid application was popular for the treatment of burns, it was uncertain whether the occasional cases of severe liver cell necrosis that were seen were due to burns themselves, perhaps acting by diminishing hepatic blood flow following plasma loss, or to the toxicity of tannic acid. In 1963 interest in the hepatotoxicity of tannic acid was rekindled when eight deaths from hepatic failure were reported from Canada.[75] All these subjects had been investigated by barium enema examination, the contrast material containing up to 2 per cent tannic acid. This agent was used because it facilitates adherence of barium to the colonic mucosa and improves the quality of the radiological pictures. It soon became apparent that the tannic acid was to blame and that diseases such as ulcerative colitis probably increased the absorption of this agent. This agent is now either not used for large bowel radiology or its concentration is kept below 0.5 per cent.

Iron

Iron tablets are often taken mistakenly by children who, following an acute phase with vomiting, often complicated by haematemesis, develop jaundice and an associated periportal hepatic necrosis.

Copper

Apart from the chronic effects of an excess of copper (see Chapter 33), hepatomegaly and jaundice with centrilobular necrosis and cholestasis have occurred following acute copper sulphate poisoning.[22]

Phosphorus

Poisoning by yellow phosphorus is by inhalation and ingestion. It produces a marked and usually peripheral fatty degeneration of hepatic lobules. Poisoning carries a high mortality.

Beryllium

Exposure to beryllium results in acute and/or chronic pulmonary disease. The acute syndrome is more common, follows inhalation of fumes or dust containing beryllium and produces a desquamative pneumonitis. The chronic disease follows prolonged exposure and is a generalized granulomatous disease resembling sarcoidosis.[129] Numerous small epithelioid and giant cell granulomas are found throughout the liver and lungs. Although pulmonary fibrosis occurs, significant fibrosis of the liver is rare. The diagnosis can be confirmed by the patient's occupational history or by demonstrating beryllium in the granulomas by microemission spectography.[106]

Pesticides

Despite their widespread use and well-documented toxicity there is little evidence of liver disease. Initial experiments demonstrated centrilobular necrosis in animals given large doses of DDT[92] but the long-term administration of DDT to rats failed to produce necrosis, cirrhosis or tumours.[97] In humans, equivocal differences in liver function tests were found when workers exposed to pesticides were compared to controls, despite their having very high serum levels of DDT and dieldrin.[88]

Mycotoxins

Many mycotoxins have been described although only a few have been isolated. The subject has been extensively reviewed.[46] Although many are toxic very few are *hepatotoxic* to man, and species variation is considerable. For instance, sporidesmins produce an acute cholangitis progressing to fibrous obliteration in sheep, but horses, pigs, rats and mice are resistant.[35] Two groups of mycotoxins deserve particular attention: the aflatoxins for their well-documented carcinogenic potential and the toxins associated with ingestion of the death cap toadstool, *Amanita phalloides*.

Aflatoxins. These toxins are derived from species of *Aspergillus* and are known to contaminate stored foods and groundnuts. Chronic effects are considered in Chapter 38. Acute toxicity, consisting of fatty change and focal hepatocellular necrosis, has been shown in animals.[133] Aflatoxins also experimentally reduce the uptake of RNA precursors and the synthesis of RNA, probably by inhibiting RNA polymerase activity.[143]

Amanita. In Britain three species of the genus *Amanita* (*A. muscaria*, *A. pantherina* and *A. phalloides*) are toxic but only *A. phalloides* is known to be hepatotoxic. Two toxins have been described, amanitotoxin which is heat stable and phalloidin which is heat labile.

Following ingestion of *A. phalloides* there is a lag of several hours before the onset of symptoms. These vary in severity with the quantity ingested but start as nausea, vomiting, abdominal pain and diarrhoea, are variably followed within the first week by dehydration and shock and frequently progress to coma with convulsions and death. Signs of renal damage are also common and may result in oliguria and uraemia.

The pathological features again vary. Experimentally chronic administration of phalloidin in small doses has produced a striking increase in the microfilament network in the hepatocyte, initially around the bile canaliculus,[47] and is associated with canalicular changes and cholestasis.[40] Clinically, liver biopsy in mild cases has shown centrilobular necrosis without steatosis and with striking ceroid pigment accumulation in Kupffer cells around the necrosis. Complete recovery of these cases occurred.[140] Fatal cases show severe steatosis and more extensive or massive hepatic necrosis.

No antitoxin is available and treatment is empirical. Supportive measures include the restoration of fluid and electrolyte balance treatment and prevention of hypoglycaemia. Further measures may be required for renal failure and/or hepatic failure.

Other Drugs and Therapeutic Agents

Laxative (oxyphenisatin) jaundice

In 1949 C.V. Munthe-Fog first suggested that chronic ingestion of laxatives and chronic hepatitis might be related.[90] In 1971 first reports of a syndrome resembling infective hepatitis and related to the prolonged use of a specific laxative, oxyphenisatin, were described. The clinical picture is that of a mild or moderately severe hepatitis with anorexia, fatigue, upper abdominal pain and jaundice. It is commonest in women, who have usually taken laxatives daily for 6 to 12 years or more before symptoms of hepatic disease appear. This liver disorder usually subsides when the drug is withdrawn. Histologically the lesion is identical with that of acute viral hepatitis.[78]

A chronic liver disease which is identical clinically, histologically and immunologically to chronic active (aggressive) hepatitis is seen in patients who continue to take oxyphenisatin for longer periods.[50] Accompanying this disorder are immunological abnormalities such as positive LE cells and antinuclear factor tests. Occasionally, as in the 'immunological' variety of chronic active hepatitis, systemic disorders such as polyarthritis can be seen and in these subjects the impersonation of non-drug-induced chronic active hepatitis is complete.

The acute and chronic examples of oxyphenisatin hepatic damage are important as they may both respond to removal of the toxic agent. In a follow-up of 27 patients recorded by Reynolds and co-workers[112] all save two showed a remarkable improvement on cessation of therapy, and thus an accurate drug history must be taken in all patients with acute and chronic liver disease. Oxyphenisatin is no longer available in Britain, the United States or Australia. Most cases have been recorded from these last two countries.

Other Important Drug Effects on the Liver

Cholestasis and hepatitis are not the only hepatic lesions attributable to drugs. The importance of chronic active hepatitis, cirrhosis, hepatic venous occlusion and tumours, both benign and malignant, resulting from a variety of drugs, has already been stressed in this chapter. There remains a number of unrelated disorders associated with drug administration that need to be described.

Granulomatous hepatitis and drugs

Granulomas in the liver are found both in apparently normal patients and in a wide variety of disease processes. A granuloma consists of a central area of macrophages and epithelioid cells surrounded by a collar of lymphocytes and they contain, on occasions, one or more giant cells from epithelioid cell fusion. The key process in granuloma formation is the transformation of macrophages to epithelioid cells. Granulomas may occur anywhere in the liver lobule, though in general they tend to accumulate in and around the portal tracts.

Granulomas due to the action of drugs may be transient or longer-lasting. The important drugs involved include the sulphonamides,[21] phenylbutazone,[57] penicillin,[137] allopurinol,[126] methyldopa,[80] halothane,[36] chlorpropamide,[114] hydralazine[59] and quinidine,[48] though these make up only a small percentage of the cases of granulomatous hepatitis.

Pigment deposition

A variety of intravenously administered plasma expanders may be taken up and deposited in Kupffer cells. These include polyvinylpyrrolidone (PVP) and dextran. A syndrome of the increased accumulation of lipofuscin (wear and tear) pigment, particularly in the hepatocytes in the centrilobular zone, is a feature of the prolonged administration of analgesics, particularly phenacetin. Looking at a consecutive series of needle biopsies, Tygstrup, Schiødt and Winkler[135] found marked lipofuscin pigment in 15 per cent of those biopsied, but accurate details of drug ingestion were not given, though it was pointed out that hepatomegaly may be a feature of this condition.

Abrahams et al, [1] commenting on the hepatic morphological appearances in four patients who had consumed 3 g of phenacetin, noted lipofuscin accumulation and distension of the rough endoplasmic reticulum and secondary damage to mitochondria. Both ceroid and lipofuscin are highly oxidized products of fatty acids and it was suggested that increased production might involve intermediary methaemoglobin formation.

Alterations in bilirubin metabolism

Drugs may act at several points in the metabolic cycle of bilirubin to produce changes in the serum bilirubin level. Thus drugs like rifampicin, radiographic agents[85] used for cholecystography and flavaspidic acid compete with bilirubin for liver cell uptake and their use results in a mildly raised serum bilirubin. Conjugation of bilirubin can be altered by drug action. It may be slowed by drugs such as novobiocin, with a resultant unconjugated hyperbilirubinaemia, and may be accelerated by phenobarbitone. Serum bilirubin levels are also lower than normal in patients taking anticonvulsant drugs.

REFERENCES

1. Abrahams, C., Wheatley, A., Rubenstein, A.H. & Stables, D. (1964) Hepatocellular lipofuscin after excessive ingestion of analgesics. *Lancet*, **ii**, 621–622.
2. Acocella, G. & Billing, B.H. (1965) Effect of drugs on the hepatic transport of bilirubin. In *Therapeutic Agents and the Liver* (Ed.) McIntyre, N. & Sherlock, S. pp. 1–8. Oxford: Blackwell Scientific Publications.
3. Acocella, G., Mattiussi, R., Nicholis, F.B., Pallanza, R. & Tenconi, L.T. (1968) Biliary excretion of antibiotics in man. *Gut*, **9**, 536–545.
4. Ajdukiewicz, A.B., Grainger, J., Scheuer, P.J. & Sherlock, S. (1971) Jaundice due to iprindol. *Gut*, **12**, 705–708.
5. Amromin, G.D., Deliman, R.M. & Shanbrom, E. (1962) Liver damage after chemotherapy for leukaemia and lymphoma. *Gastroenterology*, **42**, 401–410.
6. Arias, I.M. (1964) Prolonged neonatal unconjugated hyperbilirubinaemia associated with breast feeding and a steroid pregnane-3α,20β-diol in maternal milk that inhibits glucuronide conjugation in vitro. *Journal of Clinical Investigation*, **43**, 2037–2047.
7. Bandt, C. & Hoffbauer, F.W. (1964) Liver injury associated with tranylcypromine therapy. *Journal of the American Medical Association*, **188**, 752–753.
8. Baum, J.K., Holtz, F., Bookstein, J.J. & Klein, E.W. (1973) Possible association between benign hepatomas and oral contraceptives. *Lancet*, **ii**, 926–929.
9. Baxter, P.J., Anthony, P.P., MacSween, R.N.M. & Scheuer, P.J. (1977) Angiosarcoma of the liver in Great Britain 1963–73. *British Medical Journal*, **ii**, 919–921.
10. Bernstein, M.S. (1971) Hepatoma and peliosis hepatis developing in a patient with Fanconi's anaemia. *New England Journal of Medicine*, **284**, 1135–1136.
11. Berte, S.J., Dimase, J.D. & Christiansen, C.S. (1964) Isoniazid para-aminosalicylic acid and streptomycin intolerance in 1744 patients. *American Review of Respiratory Diseases*, **90**, 598–606.
12. Bhagwat, A.G. & Warren, R.E. (1969) Hepatic reaction to nitrofurantoin. *Lancet*, **ii**, 1369.
13. Bianchi, L., De Groote, J., Desmet, V., Gedgick, P., Korb, G., Popper, H., Poulsen, H., Scheuer, P.J., Schmid, M., Thaler, H. & Wepler, W. (1974) Guidelines for diagnosis of therapeutic drug induced liver injury in liver biopsies. Review by an International Group. *Lancet*, **i**, 854–857.
14. Black, M., Mitchell, J.R., Zimmerman, H.J., Ishak, K.G. & Epler, G.R. (1975) Isoniazid associated hepatitis in 114 patients. *Gastroenterology*, **69**, 289–302.
15. Boston Collaborative Drug Surveillance Programme (1973) *Lancet*, **i**, 1399–1404.
16. Boyd, J.T., Langlands, A.O. & Maccabe, J.J. (1968) Long term hazards of Thorotrast. *British Medical Journal*, **ii**, 517–521.
17. Brick, I.B. & Kyle, L.H. (1952) Jaundice of hepatic origin during the course of methyltestosterone therapy. *New England Journal of Medicine*, **246**, 176–179.
18. Brummer, D.L. (1971) Isoniazid and liver disease. *Annals of Internal Medicine*, **75**, 643.
19. Capelle, P., Dhumeaux, D., Mora, M., Feldmann, G. & Berthelot, P. (1972) Effect of rifampicin on liver function in man. *Gut*, **13**, 366–371.
20. Carey, M.C., Hirom, P.C. & Small, D.M. (1974) Precipitation of bile salts by chlorpromazine CPZ. The protective effect of lecithin. *Proceedings of the American Association for the Study of Liver Disease. Gastroenterology*, **66**, 671.
21. Carmelita, R.E., Kim, T.S. & Levene, R.A. (1968) Granulomatous hepatitis associated with sulphadimethoxine hypersensitivity. *Journal of the American Medical Association*, **202**, 985–988.
22. Chuttani, H.K., Gupta, P.S., Gulati, S. & Gupta, D.N. (1965) Acute copper sulphate poisoning. *American Journal of Medicine*, **39**, 849–854.
23. Clark, R., Thompson, R.P.H., Borirakchanyavat, V., Widdop, B., Davidson, A.R., Goulding, R. & Williams, R. (1973) Hepatic damage and death from overdose of paracetamol. *Lancet*, **i**, 66–69.
24. Cohen, I.M. & Archer, J.D. (1955) Liver function and hepatic complications in patients receiving chlorpromazine. *Journal of the American Medical Association*, **159**, 99–101.
25. Combes, B. (1973) Tetracycline in man. In *Proceedings III International Symposium – Drugs and the Liver*. (Ed.) Gerok, W. & Sickinger, K. pp. 263–268. Stuttgart: Schattauer.
26. Conn, H.O., Binder, H.J. & Orr, H.D. (1964) Ethionamide-induced hepatitis: a review with a report of an additional case. *American Review of Respiratory Diseases*, **90**, 542–552.
27. Cook, G.C., Mulligan, R. & Sherlock, S. (1971) Controlled prospective trial of corticosteroid therapy in active chronic hepatitis. *Quarterly Journal of Medicine*, **40**, 159–185.
28. Dahl, M.G.C., Gregory, M.M. & Scheuer, P.J. (1972) Methotrexate toxicity in psoriasis – a comparison of different dose regimes. *British Medical Journal*, **i**, 654–656.
29. Datey, K.K., Deshmukh, S.N., Dalvi, C.P. & Purandarc, N.M. (1967) Hepatocellular damage with ethacrynic acid. *British Medical Journal*, **iii**, 152–153.
30. Davis, M. & Williams, R. (1975) Paracetamol and liver damage. In *Modern Trends in Gastroenterology*. (Ed.) Read, A.E. pp. 318–344. London: Butterworths.
31. Davis, M., Portmann, B., Searle, M., Wright, R. & Williams, R. (1975) Histological evidence of malignancy in a primary hepatic tumour associated with oral contraceptives. *British Medical Journal*, **iv**, 496–498.
32. Degott, C., Potet, F., Feldmann, G. & Rueff, B. (1977) Peliosis hepatitis: a pathological study of 12 cases after renal transplantation. *Digestion*, **15**, 228.
33. den Boer, W. & Loeliger, E.H. (1976) Phenprocoumon induced jaundice. *Lancet*, **i**, 912.
34. de Pagter, A.G.F., van Berg Henegouwen, G.P., ten Bokkel Huinink, J.A. & Brandt, K.-H. (1976) Familial benign recurrent intrahepatic cholestasis. *Gastroenterology*, **71**, 202–207.
35. Done, J., Mortimer, P.H. & Taylor, A. (1961) The production of sporidesmin and sporidesmolides by *Pithomyces chartarum*. *Journal of General Microbiology*, **26**, 207–222.

36. Dordal, E., Glagor, S., Orlando, R.A. & Platz, C. (1970) Fatal halothane hepatitis with transient granulomas. *New England Journal of Medicine,* **283,** 357–359.
37. Einhorn, M. & Davidsohn, J. (1964) Hepatotoxicity of mercaptopurine. *Journal of the American Medical Association,* **188,** 802–806.
38. Elkington, S.G., Schreiber, W.M. & Conn, H.O. (1969) Hepatic injury caused by L-α-methyldopa. *Circulation,* **40,** 589–595.
39. Engleman, E.P. (1954) Hepatitis following the ingestion of phenylbutazone. *Journal of the American Medical Association,* **156,** 98–111.
40. Erlinger, S. (1978) Cholestasis: pump failure, microvilli defect or both. *Lancet,* **i,** 533–534.
41. Ernaelsteen, D. & Williams, R. (1961) Jaundice due to nitrofurantoin. *Gastroenterology,* **41,** 590–593.
42. Farid, Z., Smith, J.H., Bassily, S. & Sparks, H.A. (1972) Hepatoxicity after treatment of schistosomiasis with hycanthone. *British Medical Journal,* **ii,** 88–89.
43. Ferich, F.T., Bannister, W.H. & Grech, J.L. (1967) Hepatitis with biliverdinaemia in association with indomethacin therapy. *British Medical Journal,* **iii,** 155–156.
44. Fischer, H.W. & Hoak, J.C. (1964) Mimicry of acute cholecystitis by erythromycin estolate reaction. *American Journal of the Medical Sciences,* **247,** 283–285.
45. Fries, J. & Sinaganian, R. (1966) Sulphonamide hepatitis: report of a case due to sulphamethoxazole and sulphoxasole. *New England Journal of Medicine,* **274,** 95–97.
46. Fuell, A.J. (1969) Types of mycotoxins in foods and feeds. In *Aflatoxin – Scientific Background, Control and Implications* (Ed.) Goldblatt, L.A. New York: Academic Press.
47. Gabbiani, G., Montesano, R., Tuchweber, B., Salas, M. & Orci, L. (1975) Phalloidin induced hyperplasia of actin filaments in rat hepatocytes. *Laboratory Investigation,* **33,** 562–569.
48. Geltner, D., Chajek, T., Rubinger, D. & Levij, I.S. (1976) Quinidine hypersensitivity and liver involvement. *Gastroenterology,* **70,** 650–652.
49. Gjone, E. & Orning, O.M. (1966) Jaundice due to chloramphenicol. *Acta Hepatosplenologica (Stuttgart),* **13,** 288–292.
50. Goldstein, G.B., Lam, K.C. & Mistilis, S.P. (1973) Drug induced active chronic hepatitis. *American Journal of Digestive Diseases,* **18,** 177–184.
51. Grampa, G. (1971) Radiation injury with particular reference to Thorotrast. In *Pathology Annual* (Ed.) Sheldon, C. pp. 147–169. New York: Sommers. Appleton Century-Crofts.
52. Harinasuta, U. & Zimmerman, H. (1968) Diphenylhydantoin sodium hepatitis. *Journal of the American Medical Association,* **203,** 1015–1018.
53. Henderson, J.T. (1973) Androgenic–anabolic steroid therapy and hepatocellular carcinoma. *Lancet,* **i,** 934.
54. Hoaken, P.C.S. (1964) Jaundice during imipramine treatment. *Canadian Medical Association Journal,* **90,** 1367.
55. Howard, D.J. & Russell Rees, J. (1976) Long term perhexiline maleate and liver function. *British Medical Journal,* **i,** 133.
56. Husebye, K.G. (1964) Jaundice with persisting pericholangiolitic inflammation in a patient treated with chlorothiazide. *American Journal of Digestive Diseases,* **9,** 439–446.
57. Ishak, K.G., Kirchner, J.P. & Dahr, J.K. (1977) Granulomas and cholestatic hepatocellular injury associated with phenylbutazone: report of two cases. *American Journal of Digestive Diseases,* **22,** 611–617.
58. Jeanrenaud, B. (1967) Effect of glucocorticoid hormones on fatty acid mobilization and re-esterifications in rat adipose tissue. *Biochemical Journal,* **103,** 627–633.
59. Jori, G.P. & Peschle, C. (1973) Hydralazine disease associated with transient granulomas in the liver. *Gastroenterology,* **64,** 1163–1167.
60. Joshi, P.H. & Conn, H.O. (1974) The syndrome of methoxyflurane hepatitis. *Annals of Internal Medicine,* **80,** 395–401.
61. Judah, J.D., McLean, A.E.M. & McLean, E.K. (1970) Biochemical mechanisms of liver injury. *American Journal of Medicine,* **49,** 609–616.
62. Judson, J.A., de Jongh, H.J. & Walmsley, J.B.W. (1971) Possible cross sensitivity between halothane and methoxyflurane: report of a case. *Anesthesiology,* **35,** 527–532.
63. Kanani, S.R., Knight, R. & Woodruff, A.W. (1970) The treatment of schistosomiasis with niridazole in Britain. *Journal of Tropical Medicine and Hygiene,* **73,** 162–169.
64. Kelsey, J.R., Moyer, J.H., Brown, W.G. & Bennett, H.D. (1955) Chlorpromazine jaundice. *Gastroenterology,* **29,** 865–875.
65. Knodell, R.G. (1975) Effects of chlorpromazine on bilirubin metabolism and biliary secretion in the rat. *Gastroenterology,* **69,** 965–972.
66. Kontturi, M. & Sotaniemi, E. (1969) Effect of oestrogen on liver function of prostatic cancer patients. *British Medical Journal,* **iv,** 204–205.
67. Kopelman, H., Scheuer, P.J. & Williams, R. (1966) The liver lesion of the Epping jaundice. *British Journal of Medicine,* **35,** 553–564.
68. Kopelman, P. & Morgan, P.G.M. (1977) Liver damage after perhexiline maleate. *Lancet,* **i,** 705.
69. Kyle, J. & Karmody, A. (1968) Association between carcinoma of the pancreas and diabetes mellitus. Proceedings of a meeting of the British Society of Gastroenterology. *Gut,* **9,** 366.
70. Lageron, A., Poupon, R., de Saint Maur, P.P. & Levy, V.G. (1977) Liver ganglioside storage after perhexiline maleate. *Lancet,* **i,** 483.
71. Lander, J.J., Stanley, R.J., Hatton, W.S., Boswell, D.C. & Aach, R.D. (1975) Angiosarcoma of the liver associated with Fowler's solution. *Gastroenterology,* **68,** 1582–1586.
72. Lee, F.I. & Harry, D.S. (1974) Angiosarcoma of the liver in a vinyl chloride worker. *Lancet,* **i,** 1316–1317.
73. Lees, A.W., Asgher, B., Hasheim, M.A. & Sinha, B.N. (1970) Jaundice after rifampicin. *British Journal of Diseases of the Chest,* **64,** 85–89.
74. Lo, K.J., Eastwood, I.R. & Eidelman, S. (1967) Cholestatic jaundice associated with chlordiazepoxide hydrochloride (Librium) therapy. *American Journal of Digestive Diseases,* **12,** 845–849.
75. Lucke, H.H., Hodge, K.E. & Patt, N.L. (1963) Fatal liver damage after barium enemas containing tannic acid. *Canadian Medical Association Journal,* **89,** 1111–1114.
76. Marver, H.S. & Schmid, R. (1972) The porphyrias. In *Metabolic Basis of Inherited Disease.* 3rd ed. (Ed.) Stanbury, J.B., Wyngaarden, J.B. & Fredrickson, D.S. pp. 1087. New York: McGraw-Hill.

77. McDermot, W. (1954) Pyrazinamide–isoniazid in tuberculosis. *American Review of Tuberculosis,* **69,** 319–350.

78. McHardy, G. & Balart, L.A. (1970) Jaundice and oxyphenisatin. *Journal of the American Medical Association,* **211,** 82–85.

79. McLean, A.E.M. & McLean, E.K. (1966) The effect of diet and DDT on microsomal hydroxylation and on sensitivity of rats to CCl_4 poisoning. *Biochemical Journal,* **100,** 564–571.

80. Miller, A.G. & Reid, W.M. (1976) Methyl dopa induced granulomatous hepatitis. *Journal of the American Medical Association,* **235,** 2001–2002.

81. Millikan, L.E. & Harrell, E.R. (1970) Drug reactions to the sulfones. *Archives of Dermatology,* **102,** 220–224.

82. Millward-Sadler, G.H. & Ryan, T.J. (1974) Methotrexate induced liver disease in psoriasis. *British Journal of Dermatology,* **90,** 661–667.

83. Mitchell, J.R., Thorgeirsson, U.P., Black, M., Timbrell, J.A., Potter, W.Z. & Snodgrass, W.R. (1975) Increased incidence of isoniazid hepatitis in rapid acetylators. Possible relation to hydrazine metabolites. *Clinical Pharmacology and Therapeutics,* **180,** 70–79.

84. Mohamed, S.D. (1965) Sensitivity reaction to phenindamine with urticaria, hepatitis and pancytopenia. *British Medical Journal,* **iii,** 1475–1476.

85. Monroe, L.S. & Longmore, W.J. (1966) Inhibition of sulphbromophthalein (BSP) conjugates with glutathione by ipanoic acid (Telepaque). *Gastroenterology,* **50,** 396.

86. Monson, R.R., Peters, J.M. & Johnson, M.M. (1974) Proportional mortality among vinyl chloride workers. *Lancet,* **ii,** 397–398.

87. Morgan, D.H. (1969) Jaundice associated with amitriptyline. *British Journal of Psychiatry,* **115,** 105–106.

88. Morgan, D.P. & Roan, C.C. (1974) Liver function in workers having high tissue stores in chlorinated hydrocarbon pesticides. *Archives of Environmental Health,* **29,** 14–17.

89. Morris, J.S., Schmid, M., Newman, S., Scheuer, P.J. & Sherlock, S. (1974) Arsenic and non-cirrhotic portal hypertension. *Gastroenterology,* **64,** 86–94.

90. Munthe-Fog, C.V. (1949) On protein intake hepatitis and consumption of laxatives. *Acta Medica Scandinavica Supplement,* **234,** 125–129.

91. Nadell, J. & Kosek, J. (1977) Peliosis hepatitis. Twelve cases associated with oral androgen therapy. *Archives of Pathology and Laboratory Medicine,* **101,** 405–410.

92. Nelson, A.A., Draize, J.H., Woodward, G., FitzHugh, O.G., Smith, R.B. Jr & Calvery, H.D. (1944) Histopathological changes following administration of D.D.T. to several species of animals. *Public Health Report,* **59,** 1009.

93. O'Brien, E.T., Yeoman, W.B. & Hobby, J.A.E. (1971) Hepatorenal damage from toluene in a glue sniffer. *British Medical Journal,* **ii,** 29–30.

94. Ockner, R.K. & Davidson, C.S. (1967) Hepatic effects of oral contraceptives. *New England Journal of Medicine,* **276,** 331–334.

95. O'Connor, J.A. (1976) Hepatotoxicity and the oral contraceptives. *Annals of Internal Medicine,* **86,** 118–119.

96. Orellana-Alcade, J.M. & Dominguez, J.P. (1966) Jaundice and oral contraceptive drugs. *Lancet,* **ii,** 1278–1280.

97. Ortega, P. (1966) Light and electron microscopy of dichlorodiphenyltrichloroethane (D.D.T.) poisoning in the rat liver. *Laboratory Investigation,* **15,** 657–679.

98. Paracetamol Symposium Addendum (1976) The recommended management of a case of paracetamol overdose. *Journal of International Medical Research,* Suppl. 4, 157–158.

99. Paradinas, F.J., Bull, T.B., Westaby, D. & Murray-Lyon, I.M. (1977) Hyperplasia and prolapse of hepatocytes into hepatic veins during long term methyl testosterone therapy: possible relationships of these changes to the development of peliosis hepatitis and liver tumours. *Histopathology,* **1,** 225–246.

100. Perkins, J. (1962) Phenindione jaundice. *Lancet,* **i,** 125–127.

101. Pernod, J. (1965) Hepatic tolerance of ethionamide. *American Review of Respiratory Diseases,* **92,** 39–42.

102. Podurgiel, B.J., McGill, D.B., Ludwig, J., Taylor, W.F. & Muller, S.A. (1973) Liver injury associated with methotrexate therapy for psoriasis. *Gastroenterology,* **64,** 190.

103. Pollet, S., Haun, J.J., Escourolle, R. & Baumann, D. (1977) Peripheral nerve lipid abnormalities in patients on perhexiline maleate. *Lancet,* **i,** 1258.

104. Popper, H. (1959) Hepatic injury in patients who have received iproniazid. *Annals of the New York Academy of Sciences,* **80,** 928–938.

105. Powell, W.J. (1968) Lethal hepatic necrosis after therapy with imipramine and desipramine. *Journal of the American Medical Association,* **206,** 642–645.

106. Prine, J.R., Brokeshoulder, S.F., McVean, D.E. & Robinson, F.R. (1966) Demonstration of the presence of beryllium in pulmonary granulomas. *American Journal of Clinical Pathology,* **45,** 448–454.

107. Ramsay, I.D. (1967) Carbamezapine induced jaundice. *British Medical Journal,* **iv,** 155.

108. Read, A.E., Harrison, C.V. & Sherlock, S. (1961) Chronic chlorpromazine jaundice with particular reference to its relationship to primary biliary cirrhosis. *American Journal of Medicine,* **31,** 249–258.

109. Reichel, J., Goldberg, S.B., Ellenberg, M. & Schaffner, F. (1960) Intrahepatic cholestasis following administration of chlorpropamide. *American Journal of Medicine,* **28,** 654–660.

110. Reid, R., Ivey, K.J., Rencore, R.H. & Storey, B. (1976) Fetal complications of obstetric cholestasis. *British Medical Journal,* **i,** 870–872.

111. Remmer, H. (1970) The role of the liver in drug metabolism. *American Journal of Medicine,* **49,** 617–629.

112. Reynolds, T.B., Peters, R.L. & Yamada, S. (1971) Chronic active and lupoid hepatitis caused by a laxative oxyphenisatin. *New England Journal of Medicine,* **285,** 813–820.

113. Rickers, L. & Sherlock, S. (1975) Influence of azathioprine on hepatic reserve in chronic active liver disease. *Gut,* **16,** 214–219.

114. Rigberg, L.A., Robinson, M.J. & Espiritu, C.R. (1976) Chlorpropamide induced granulomas. *Journal of the American Medical Association,* **235,** 409–410.

115. Rodman, J.S., Deutsch, D.J. & Gutman, S.I. (1976) Methyldopa hepatitis. A report of six cases and review of the literature. *American Journal of Medicine,* **60,** 941–948.

116. Rosenblum, L.E., Korn, R.J. & Zimmerman, H.J. (1960) Hepatocellular jaundice as a complication of iproniazid therapy. *Archives of Internal Medicine*, **105,** 583–593.
117. Rossouw, J.E. & Saunders, S.J. (1975) Hepatic complications of antituberculous therapy. *Quarterly Journal of Medicine*, **44,** 8–15.
118. Schaffner, F. (1966) The effect of oral contraceptives on the liver. *Journal of the American Medical Association*, **198,** 1019–1021.
119. Schaffner, F. & Popper, H. (1969) Cholestasis is the result of hypoactive hypertrophic smooth endoplasmic reticulum in the hepatocyte. *Lancet*, **ii,** 355–359.
120. Scharer, L. & Smith, J.P. (1969) Serum transaminase elevations and other hepatic abnormalities in patients receiving isoniazid. *Annals of Internal Medicine*, **71,** 1113–1120.
121. Schenker, S., Breen, J. & Heimberg, M. (1973) Pathogenesis of tetracycline induced fatty liver. In *Proceedings III International Symposium on Drugs and the Liver*. (Ed.) Gerok, W. & Sickinger, K. pp. 269–280. Stuttgart: Schatauer.
122. Schenker, S., Olson, K.N., Dunn, D., Breen, K.J. & Combes, B. (1973) Intrahepatic cholestasis due to therapy of rheumatoid arthritis. *Gastroenterology*, **64,** 622–629.
123. Scheuer, P.J., Lal, S., Sommerfield, J.A. & Sherlock, S. (1974) Rifampicin hepatitis. *Lancet*, **i,** 421–425.
124. Seaman, W.E., Ishak, K.G. & Plotz, P.H. (1974) Aspirin induced hepatotoxicity in patients with systemic lupus erythematosus. *Annals of Internal Medicine*, **80,** 1–8.
125. Short, M.H., Burns, J.M. & Harris, M.E. (1968) Cholestatic jaundice during imipramine therapy. *Journal of the American Medical Association*, **206,** 1791–1792.
126. Simmons, F., Feldman, B. & Gerety, D. (1972) Granulomatous hepatitis in a patient receiving allopurinol. *Gastroenterology*, **62,** 101–104.
127. Simpson, D.G. & Walker, J.H. (1960) Hypersensitivity to para-aminosalicylic acid. *American Journal of Medicine*, **29,** 297–306.
128. Smith, P.M., Williams, D.M.J. & Crossley, I.P. (1975) Portal hypertension induced by vinyl chloride. *Gut*, **16,** 402–403.
129. Sneddon, I.B. (1955) Berylliosis: a case report. *British Medical Journal*, **i,** 1448–1450.
130. Sparberg, M., Simon, N. & Del Greco, F. (1969) Intrahepatic cholestasis due to azathioprine. *Gastroenterology*, **57,** 439–441.
131. Sterup, K. & Mosbech, J. (1967) Budd Chiari syndrome after taking oral contraceptives. *British Medical Journal*, **iv,** 660.
132. Svanborg, A. & Ohlsson, S. (1959) Recurrent jaundice of pregnancy – a clinical study of 22 cases. *American Journal of Medicine*, **27,** 40–49.
133. Svoboda, D., Grady, H.J. & Higginson, J. (1966) Aflatoxin B_1 injury in rat and monkey liver. *American Journal of Pathology*, **49,** 1023–1951.
134. Swarm, R.L. Conference Chairman (1967) Distribution, retention and late effects of thorium dioxide. *Annals of the New York Academy of Sciences*, **145,** 523–858.
135. Tygstrup, N., Schiødt, T. & Winkler, K. (1965) Correlation between pathological and clinical findings in 195 consecutive liver biopsies showing brown pigment. *Gut*, **6,** 194–199.
136. Urban, E., Frank, B.W. & Kern, F. Jr (1968) Liver dysfunction with mestranol but not with norethynodrel in a patient with Enovid-induced jaundice. *Annals of Internal Medicine*, **68,** 598–602.
137. Vardivia-Barriga, V., Feldman, A. & Orellana, J. (1963) Generalised hypersensitivity with hepatitis and jaundice after the use of penicillin and streptomycin. *Gastroenterology*, **45,** 114–117.
138. Walker, C.O. & Coombes, B. (1966) Biliary cirrhosis induced by chlorpromazine. *Gastroenterology*, **51,** 631–640.
139. Weinstein, G.D. & Frost, P. (1971) Methotrexate for psoriasis. A new therapeutic schedule. *Archives of Dermatology*, **103,** 33–38.
140. Wepler, W. & Opitz, K. (1972) Histologic changes in the liver biopsy in *Amanita phalloides* intoxication. *Human Pathology*, **3,** 249–254.
141. Whelan, G. & Sherlock, S. (1972) Immunosuppressive activity in patients with active chronic hepatitis and primary biliary cirrhosis treated with azathioprine. *Gut*, **13,** 907–914.
142. Winkler, K. & Poulsen, H. (1975) Liver disease with periportal sinusoidal dilatation. A possible complication to contraceptive steroids. *Scandinavian Journal of Gastroenterology*, **10,** 699–704.
143. Wogan, G.N. (1973) Mycotoxins and liver injury. In *The Liver* (Ed.) Gall, E.A. & Mostofi, F.K. pp. 161–181. Baltimore: Williams & Wilkins.
144. Wu, S.-M., Spurny, O.M. & Klotz, A.P. (1977) Budd–Chiari syndrome after taking oral contraceptives. *American Journal of Digestive Diseases*, **22,** 622–628.
145. Zaraday, Z., Veith, F.J., Gleidman, M.L. & Soberman, R. (1972) Irreversible liver damage after azathioprine. *Journal of the American Medical Association*, **222,** 690–691.

Chapter 37

Hepatic Changes in Systemic Disease

GREG HOLDSTOCK
G.H. MILLWARD-SADLER
RALPH WRIGHT

The liver is frequently involved in systemic diseases. There are several reasons why this should be so. Firstly, the Kupffer cells of the liver form a major component of the reticulo-endothelial system and are responsible for phagocytosis and degradation of circulating bacteria, viruses and other antigens (see Chapter 9). Secondly, the hepatocytes have a variety of functions in normal metabolic processes and in the detoxication of drugs and other chemicals. They are therefore exposed to many different, potentially toxic agents. Thirdly, the cellular components of the liver are exposed to substances reaching it by the systemic and portal circulation. The pathogenesis of many of the abnormalities cannot be fully explained, but episodes of anoxia, toxin release, haemolysis and a direct effect of infective organisms may all play a significant role.

In some instances, structural and functional changes affect the liver as a part of a non-specific effect on all systems of the body, and these will be considered only briefly. In other situations, the liver is involved as part of a specific systemic disease process. This hepatic involvement may be of clinical significance, either because the consequences impair hepatic function and contribute to the clinical syndrome, or because the changes in the liver may provide a clue to the underlying diagnosis.

In the first part of this chapter, we will deal with non-specific changes, such as fatty change and granulomatous hepatitis. The second part of the chapter deals with clinical, functional and pathological changes occurring in the liver during the course of a variety of conditions. Many are proven associations, but even in these cases the true incidence of the hepatic abnormalities is far from clear, as all reports have dealt with a selected population. Some suggested associations are based on isolated case reports, many of which are likely to be no more than coincidental.

FATTY CHANGE (see also Chapters 4, 6 and 32)

Fatty change, otherwise known as fatty infiltration or steatosis, is one of the commonest abnormalities encountered on liver biopsy. Fatty liver has been described in a multitude of conditions, including pregnancy, drug therapy (for example, tetracycline and corticosteroids), and toxins (for example, carbon tetrachloride, phosphorus and alcohol).[5, 131] It is seen in diabetes, obesity and malnutrition, especially kwashiorkor. It is also seen during hyperalimentation and following hepatic resection and jejunal bypass surgery. In many cases, fatty liver is simply a measure of the degree of debility caused by the underlying illness, rather than a direct effect of the disease process.

Pathogenesis

The exact pathogenesis of fatty liver is not fully understood. The liver receives fat in the form of chylomicrons from the gut via the portal circulation, or as lipoproteins via the systemic circulation resulting from the breakdown of adipose tissue. There is also some synthesis in the liver itself. The fat is then either oxidized in the liver to carbon dioxide, water and ketones, or leaves via the hepatic vein in the form of very low-density lipoprotein. Interference with any of these steps in fat metabolism can result in fatty liver. The pathogenesis has recently been reviewed.[5, 131]

In alcoholic liver disease, there appears to be a direct toxic effect resulting in reduced oxidation of fat in the liver. Other factors, including the effects of malnutrition, increased breakdown of adipose tissue, increased hepatic fatty acid synthesis and decreased triglyceride secretion from the liver, may all be important.[175, 253] Coexistent malnutrition can significantly contribute to the severity of the fatty change,[176] but on its own is thought not to be a cause of cirrhosis.[52]

In carbon tetrachloride poisoning, fatty change is associated with diminished protein synthesis.[238] Many of the other conditions which are commonly associated with fatty change are discussed elsewhere in this book. Table 37.1 summarizes some of the pathological findings and the suggested pathogenesis of fatty liver in various conditions.

Pathology

In the normal liver, fat accounts for only 5 per cent of the total weight and cannot usually be seen unless specific stains are employed. In severe cases of fatty change, fat can account for up to 50 per cent of the total weight of the liver and is mainly in the form of fatty acids and triglycerides, although small amounts of phospholipids, cholesterol and cholesterol esters may also be present. Histology reveals multiple vacuoles that enlarge the hepatocyte and displace the nucleus to one side (Figure 37.1). Often there may be only one single large vacuole. Affected hepatocytes are most frequently centrilobular in position or do not show any zonal distribution but a periportal distribution (Figure 37.2) reflects hypoproteinaemia or phosphorus poisoning. The steatosis of tetracycline poisoning is unusual because the fat is finely dispersed within the cytoplasm so that the hepatocyte has a foamy appearance and the nucleus remains central within the cells. Apart from these minor differences, the aetiology of fatty change cannot be identified from its appearance or distribution and is usually distinguished by other morphological features.

In severe steatosis, small foci of mononuclear cells including lymphocytes and macrophages may be seen in the lobule gathered around fat or fat spaces. These are termed 'lipogranulomas' and are associated with mild collapse of the reticulin architecture. The most florid examples show fat-laden macrophages which

Table 37.1. *Some Common Causes of Fatty Change, with Suggested Pathogenesis and Distinguishing Features.*

Aetiology	Pathogenesis	Distribution of fat	Location of hepatic nucleus	Other helpful features
Alcohol	↓ Oxygenation of fatty acids	Random–diffuse	Peripheral	Neutrophil infiltrate, Mallory bodies, ballooning degeneration, centrilobular fibrosis
Kwashiorkor	↓ Secretion of VLDL	Periportal–diffuse	Peripheral	Non-specific
Obesity	↑ Dietary fat	Centrilobular–diffuse	Peripheral	Non-specific
Jejunoileal bypass	Not known	Diffuse	Peripheral	Inflammatory infiltrate, cell necrosis, bile-duct proliferation, fibrosis
Diabetes mellitus	↓ Lipogenesis in mature onset ↑ Lipolysis in juvenile onset	Random–diffuse	Peripheral	Non-specific
Pregnancy	Not known	Centrilobular–diffuse	Central	Non-specific
Tetracycline	↓ Secretion of VLDL	Diffuse and finely dispersed	Central	Non-specific

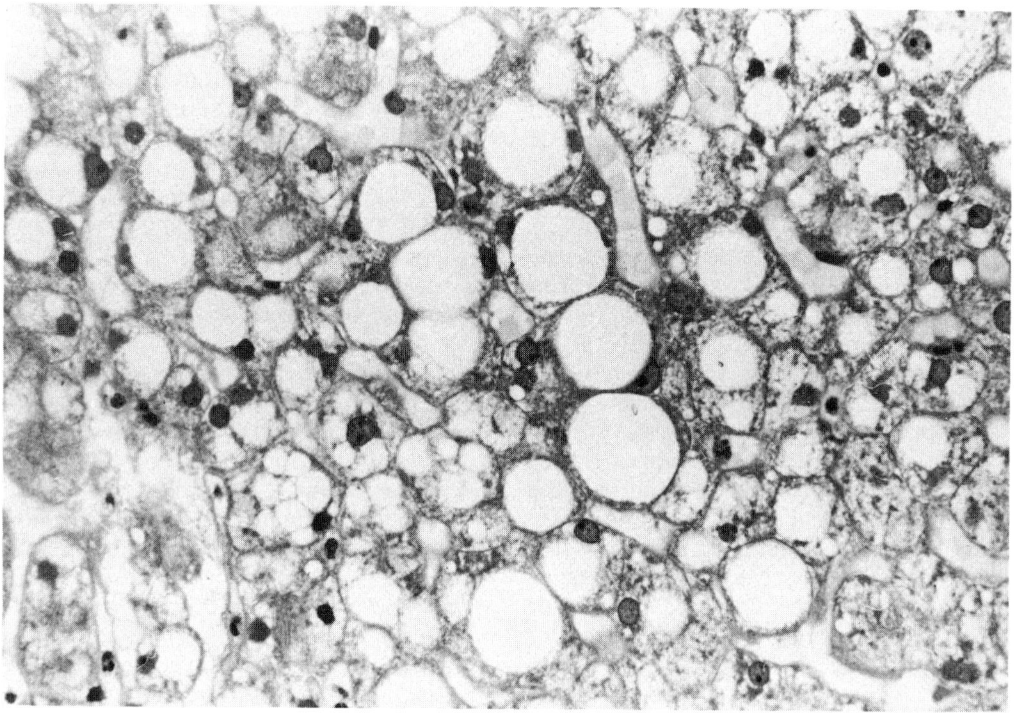

Figure 37.1. Accumulation of fat within the hepatocyte can produce a large vacuole that displaces the nucleus to the periphery but may also be identified as several small vacuoles within the cytoplasm. Haematoxylin and eosin × 1200.

have sometimes fused to form a multinucleate giant cells. When this happens, a small fibrous scar results.[43]

Clinical Aspects

In idiopathic fatty liver of pregnancy and in Reye's syndrome there can be an acute, fulminating and often fatal course, but these conditions are rare and unexplained. In most cases of fatty liver, clinical features are insignificant. Symptoms and signs, when they do occur, are often a feature of the underlying condition, such as alcoholism. In one study of patients with fatty liver,[167] 18 per cent had symptoms, namely abdominal discomfort and tenderness over the liver, attributed to distension of the liver by fat. There may be mild abnormalities of the liver function tests, such as slight elevation of the bilirubin, alkaline phosphatase or the transaminases.[27] Occasionally, obstructive jaundice[13] or jaundice with other features of hepatic cell failure have been described,[167] but again these should be interpreted with caution. In most conditions, fatty change is a reversible benign condition. No specific therapy is required other than that of the underlying condition and measures to improve general health. The fat content in obese patients is reduced by their losing weight.[69] Although the diagnosis is usually based on histological examination, with the advent of ultrasound scanning it may be possible to diagnose fatty liver by non-invasive means.[94]

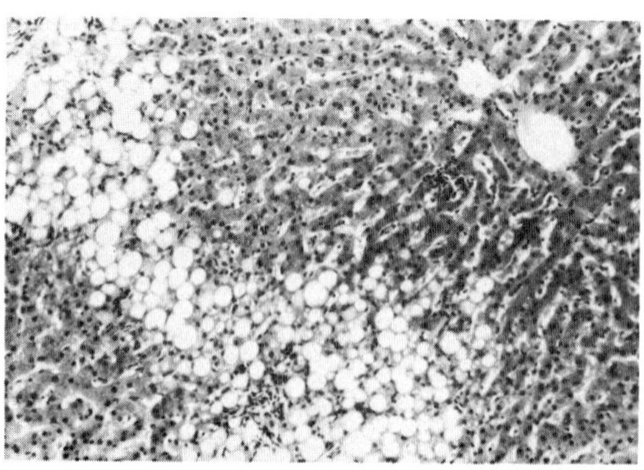

Figure 37.2. The central 'efferent' vein is top right and two portal tracts are present at top left and bottom centre. Fatty change is confined to the periportal zone in a pattern approximating to zone 1 of the liver acinus. Haematoxylin and eosin × 50.

NON-SPECIFIC REACTIVE HEPATITIS

This is also a common finding in liver biopsies, and is encountered in a wide variety of conditions, ranging from infections to collagen disorders (see Table 37.2). It can also be found adjacent to focal lesions of the liver, such as tumours or abscesses. Clinical features vary, but liver biopsy is usually performed in the course of the investigation of unexplained abnormal liver function tests or hepatomegaly.

Table 37.2. *Common Conditions Associated with Non-specific Reactive Hepatitis.*

1. Infection: (a) disseminated, including fungal, bacterial, viral
   (b) localized
2. Collagen disorders
3. Congestive cardiac failure
4. Inflammatory bowel disease
5. Adjacent to focal intrahepatic lesions

Histology shows mononuclear cell inflammatory infiltrate, mainly in the portal tracts and often associated with mild fatty change and focal liver cell necrosis. The Kupffer cell proliferation may, rarely, form an ill-defined granuloma.

Although reactive hepatitis is a common abnormality it is usually clinically insignificant, and in some communities where parasitic infections are endemic it is a frequent incidental finding on liver biopsy.[133]

In secondary carcinoma of the liver there may be a reactive hepatitis adjacent to the focal lesions, or there can be changes in the liver unrelated to the presence of secondary deposits. In the case of hypernephroma, a clear-cut syndrome has been defined[289] where the patient frequently has a non-specific illness consisting of fever, general malaise and weight loss. There may be hepatomegaly with elevation of the alkaline phosphatase or the bilirubin, a prolonged prothrombin time and a non-specific increase in the gammaglobulins. Biopsy in these patients shows a non-specific reactive hepatitis with mild degenerative hepatocellular changes. These abnormalities return to normal if the primary tumour is treated.[204, 310, 321] There has been one case report of unexplained progressive hepatic failure associated with hypernephroma in which liver biopsy merely showed the non-specific changes described above.[297]

GRANULOMATOUS HEPATITIS

Although this is a term often used, 'granulomatous hepatitis' is a misnomer, as the liver parenchymal cells are usually normal, but there may in addition be reactive changes. Granulomas are defined as focal nodular collections of chronic inflammatory cells which are predominantly macrophages but frequently include lymphocytes and plasma cells. These macrophages may or may not fuse to form multinucleate giant cells and may or may not show change into epithelioid cells. Multinucleate giant cell formation is more common in association with epithelioid cell change or with foreign body reactions. Granulomas are found in a wide spectrum of disorders[90] (see Table 37.3) and may be present in between 2 and 7 per cent of all liver biopsies.[226] In several large series of hepatic granulomas, up to 60 per cent of cases have been attributed to tuberculosis or to sarcoidosis,[111, 319] but in 20 per cent of cases no associated disorder may be defined. In the literature, distinction is not always made between non-epithelioid and epithelioid cell granulomas. Although epithelioid cell change is not a specific feature, it does occur in some of these granulomatous conditions, for example sarcoidosis, more frequently than in others. Those conditions more commonly or consistently associated with epithelioid granulomas are listed in Table 37.4. Because of its high frequency, sarcoidosis will be discussed separately.

Clinical Features

In most patients, in addition to the hepatic abnormality, symptoms of the appropriate underlying condition may be present. In those patients where no associated disorder can be identified, there may be hepatomegaly, occasionally with splenomegaly, and mild abnormalities of liver function tests, particularly elevation of the alkaline phosphatase. Such cases may be regarded as granulomatous hepatitis of unknown aetiology.

A syndrome of hepatic granulomas associated with a pyrexia of unknown origin and a polymyalgia-like illness has been described.[85, 98, 278] All five patients described by Eliakim[85] failed to respond to broad-spectrum antibiotics, but all made an uneventful recovery in a matter of weeks. Of the 13 cases intensively investigated by Simmons, Feldman and

Table 37.3. *Diseases Associated with a Granulomatous Hepatitis.*

Systemic disease:

- Sarcoid[280]
- Collagen diseases, e.g. polymyalgia[181]
- Wegener's granuloma[89, 284]
- Granulomatous disease of childhood[39, 107]
- Hypogammaglobulinaemia[248]

Bacterial:

- Mycobacterial (typical and atypical)[159, 319]
- Leprosy[143]
- Tularaemia[234]
- Brucellosis[139]
- Granuloma inguinale[184]
- Meliodosis[25]
- Listerosis[237]
- Staphylococcal septicaemia[128]

Rickettsial:

- Q fever[74]

Spirochaetal:

- Syphilis (early and late)[270]

Fungal:

- Histoplasmosis[199, 227]
- Coccidiodomycosis[56, 262]
- Blastomycosis[333]
- Aspergillus[40]
- Actinomycosis[155]
- Nocardiasis[119]
- Cryptococcus[273]
- Candidiasis[220]

Parasitic:

- Ascaris[148]
- Toxocara[70]
- Schistosomiasis[114, 323]
- Amylostoma[111]
- Amoebiasis[67]
- Tongueworm (*Linguatala serrata*)[70]
- *Stronglyloides stercoralis*[230]

Viral:

- Cytomegalovirus[242]
- Lymphogranuloma venerum[319]
- Influenza B[155]
- Infectious mononucleosis[155]

Drug-induced:

- Phenylbutazone[136]
- Sulphonamide[235]
- Sulphonamide derivation[245]
- Penicillin[327]
- Allopurinol[195, 278]
- Halothane[66]
- Hydralazine[138]
- Quinidine[99]
- Diazepam[154]
- Methyldopa[196]

Neoplasm:

- Hodgkin's[140, 279]

Others:

- Primary biliary cirrhosis[92]
- Crohn's disease[192]
- Berylliosis[155]
- Erythema nodosum[155]
- Drug addicts[79]
- Haemophiliacs[233]
- Ileal bypass operations[343]

Gerety[278] one was later found to have Hodgkin's disease. Nine out of ten responded well to moderate doses of corticosteroids, but the response to antituberculous therapy was disappointing. Those patients who responded to steroids might be at one end of a spectrum of disease related to temporal arteritis, since granulomatous liver disease is a not uncommon finding in these patients.[181]

Pathology

Histology shows sharply defined lesions composed of macrophages or of pale-staining epithelioid cells and giant cells surrounded by lymphocytes (Figure 37.3). In long-standing cases fibrosis may occur. The appearance and distribution of the granulomas are rarely

Table 37.4. *Common Causes of Sarcoid-like Epithelioid Granulomas in the Liver.*

Infections:

- Tuberculosis
- Brucellosis
- Histoplasmosis
- Schistosomiasis

Drugs:

- Phenylbutazone
- Sulphonamides
- Chlorpropamide

Others:

- Sarcoid
- Primary biliary cirrhosis
- Tumour (Hodgkin's disease)
- Crohn's disease
- Collagen diseases

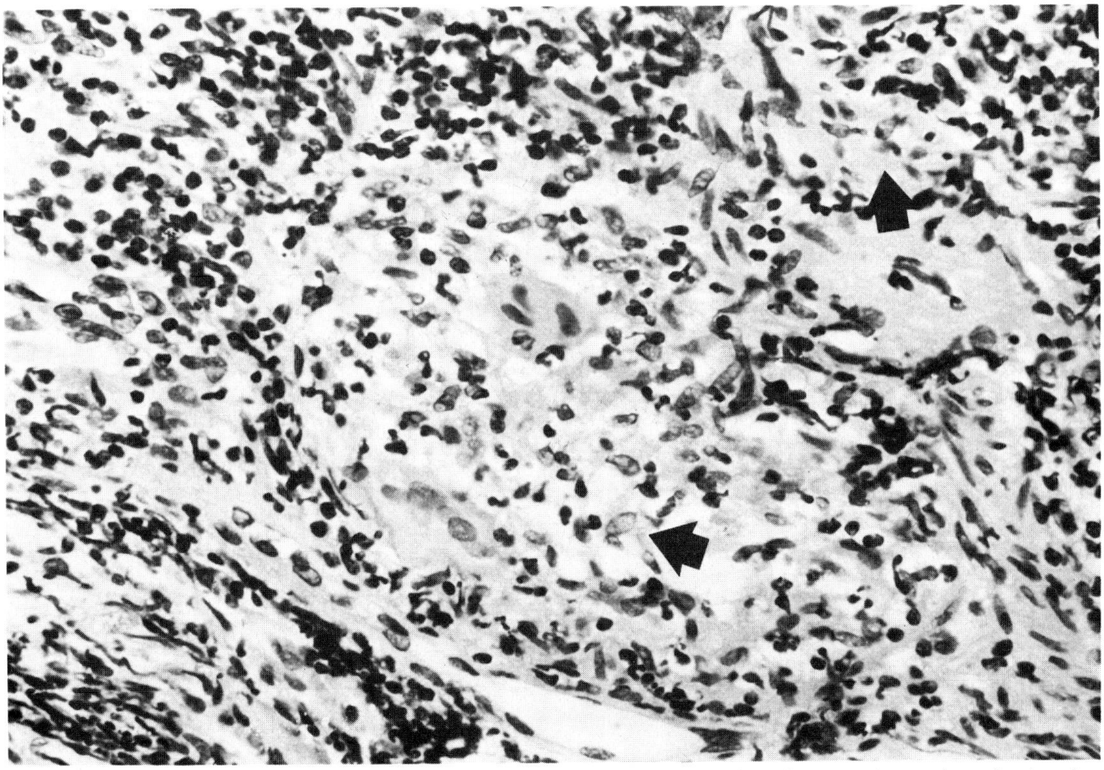

Figure 37.3. Detail of an epithelioid granuloma showing the large pale epithelioid cells (arrows) sometimes fused to form multinucleate giant cells and admixed with lymphocytes. Haematoxylin and eosin × 1500.

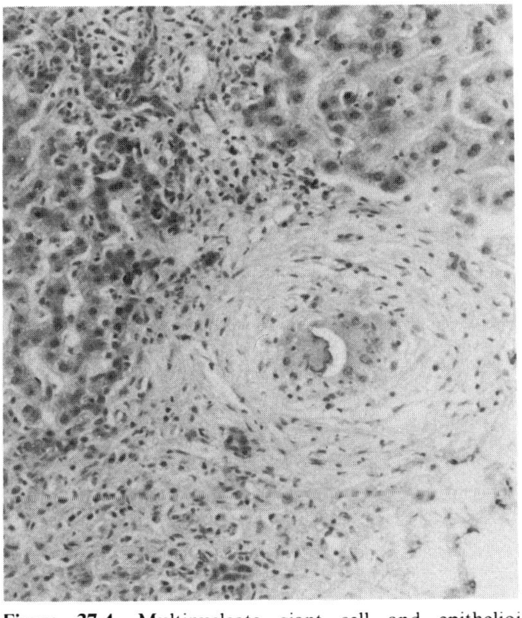

Figure 37.4. Multinucleate giant cell and epithelioid granuloma surrounding the remnant of a schistosomal ovum. Fibrous tissue arranged in concentric lamellae around the granuloma is characteristic in this late stage of a schistosomal granuloma. Haematoxylin and eosin × 500.

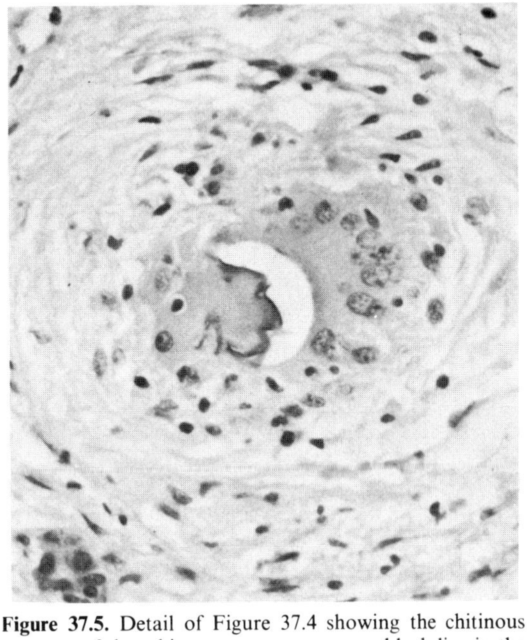

Figure 37.5. Detail of Figure 37.4 showing the chitinous remnant of the schistome ovum as a wavy black line in the centre of the multinucleate giant cell. Haematoxylin and eosin × 1250.

pathognomonic of the underlying disease process unless caseation is present or a specific infective agent is demonstrated.

Caseation is virtually diagnostic of tuberculosis, though infrequent even in florid cases. Acid alcohol-fast bacilli are rarely found even in non-caseating granulomas. The presence of hepatic granulomas in tuberculosis implies miliary spread since they are rare with other forms of tuberculosis. Granulomas in schistosomiasis are characteristic and the ova may be demonstrated (Figures 37.4 and 37.5).

In other bacterial and fungal infections, organisms can sometimes be demonstrated (see Chapter 51).

In granulomatous reactions to drugs such as phenylbutazone,[136] the presence of an eosinophilic infiltrate may suggest the diagnosis. Intravenous drug addiction may be associated with foreign body granulomas in portal tracts.[79] Doubly refractile talc can sometimes be identified within these granulomas. Granulomas have also been noted in the portal tracts of liver biopsies from haemophiliacs treated with cryoglobulins.[233]

Investigation and Treatment

A history of drug-taking or exposure to an infection such as tuberculosis, brucellosis or leprosy is helpful. A chest x-ray may indicate tuberculosis or sarcoidosis. Other appropriate investigations include blood culture, examination of stools and skin and serological tests. Isolation of a specific organism from a liver biopsy is rare.

The investigation of granulomatous hepatitis is often unrewarding, and the extent of investigation will vary depending on the geographical area. Appropriate treatment will depend on identification of the cause. Faced with a deteriorating patient, empirical treatment with antituberculous therapy or corticosteroids may be necessary.

SARCOIDOSIS

Sarcoidosis is a generalized granulomatous disease of unknown origin with a widely varying presentation. Although patients with sarcoidosis seldom present with symptoms of liver disease, the liver is frequently the site of sarcoid granulomas, and only the lungs and lymph nodes are more commonly affected.

Clinical Features

Despite frequent involvement of the liver in sarcoidosis, symptoms and signs rarely result. Hepatomegaly and splenomegaly occur in about 20 per cent of all cases of sarcoidosis.[193, 232] There may be elevation of the alkaline phosphatase or, less commonly, of the transaminases. Jaundice is extremely rare,[29, 189, 212, 215, 254] but when present it may take the form of intrahepatic cholestasis.[130, 254] It can be difficult to differentiate sarcoidosis from primary biliary cirrhosis, a condition also associated with granulomas.

Hepatocellular failure is rare, but has been reported.[211,212,232] Sarcoidosis has been documented as a rare cause of portal hypertension[201,232] which is usually pre-sinusoidal,[201] although obstruction at sinusoidal or hepatic venous levels may occur.[189] The portal hypertension is usually presumed to be the end result of a granulomatous cirrhosis,[155, 211] but sometimes there may be little fibrosis present.[201] In these cases, portal hypertension may be the result of compression of the portal vein branches by granulomas.

In sarcoidosis, ascites is rare and may be the result of liver failure or of peritoneal involvement.[334] Occasionally, the gallbladder can be involved, in which case the clinical presentation is undistinguishable from cholecystitis.[179]

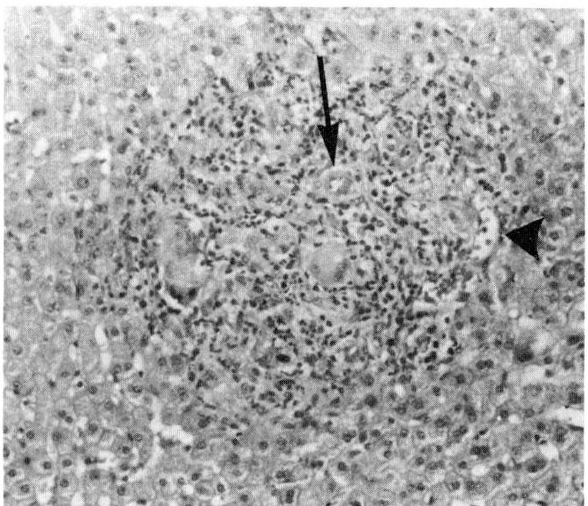

Figure 37.6. A portal tract in which the artery (arrow) is still visible and contains multinucleate giant cells and epithelioid cells. The portal vein (arrowhead) is displaced to the edge of the tract. The tract is a common location for granulomas. Haematoxylin and eosin × 450.

Pathology

Early studies showed that granulomas were present in the liver in about two-thirds of patients with sarcoidosis who came to autopsy. Studies on living patients indicated that it was equally common.[155, 191] Because of the discrete nature of the lesion, examination of multiple sections from the liver biopsy may be required to minimize the number of false negatives.

Granulomas are most commonly found in relation to the portal tract (Figure 37.6) and are rare around the central veins. They are discrete and consist of large epithelioid cells and multinucleate giant cells with surrounding lymphocytes. The rest of the liver is usually normal, although hepatocytes adjacent to the granulomas are occasionally damaged. There may be small areas of apparent necrosis at the centre of these granulomas, but caseation necrosis, as seen in tuberculosis, is not a feature. Kupffer cell proliferation is sometimes seen. The granulomas may disappear without trace, but many lesions heal by fibrosis and leave a cellular hyaline scar.

Diagnosis and Treatment

Often the diagnosis is easy and readily made from the clinical features or radiological findings. The diagnosis should be confirmed by a Kveim test. The granulomas seen in sarcoidosis cannot be readily distinguished from those in other types of granulomatous hepatitis. Sarcoidosis in the liver can be confused with primary biliary cirrhosis but in primary biliary cirrhosis the granulomas are usually adjacent to bile ducts, and a mitochondrial antibody is present in the serum. The results of treatment are difficult to assess as sarcoidosis runs such a variable course, but corticosteroids are often used in severe cases, sometimes with benefit. The abnormalities of liver function tests usually rapidly improve following corticosteroid therapy, and hepatomegaly and splenomegaly regress, although this is not necessarily associated with a decrease in the portal pressure.[100] Portacaval shunts have been performed with some success on patients who develop portal hypertension.[72]

It is difficult to assess the effect of corticosteroid therapy on the number of granulomas present because of sampling errors. Some workers have reported a reduction in size and number of granulomas following corticosteroid treatment,[145, 191] but others have reported an increase in fibrosis under the same circumstances.[42] It would appear that mild hepatic abnormalities do respond, although it is unlikely that these patients would develop complications from the liver involvement. Those patients with severe and progressive disease usually do not respond to corticosteroids.[189] Under some circumstances, when there is doubt about the diagnosis of sarcoidosis, a trial of antituberculous therapy may be justified.

In summary, corticosteroid therapy should be given only for patients with severe liver disease, although there is little hope of arresting the disease process. Sarcoidosis is a generalized disease, and there may be indications other than the liver involvement for corticosteroid therapy.

Prognosis

Despite the frequent involvement of the liver in sarcoidosis, progression to serious chronic liver disease is rare and the prognosis is usually good. In the rare instances of progression to cirrhosis with portal hypertension, the prognosis will be poor.

COLLAGEN DISEASES

These are systemic disorders which may have an autoimmune basis. The systemic manifestations vary and there is frequent overlap between the syndromes. Clinically overt liver disease is unusual, although in many instances hepatomegaly or mild abnormalities of liver function tests occur. Even in the absence of overt liver disease, gamma globulin levels are often increased, which in theory may result from impaired Kupffer cell function.[307] On liver biopsy, non-specific changes, including fatty change and reactive hepatitis, are commonly present, but interpretation of their significance must be guarded as they may be secondary to debility or drug therapy rather than part of the basic disease process. It is of interest that the tissue-type HLA-B8 is common to many of these collagen disorders and also to some forms of chronic liver disease, notably chronic active hepatitis.

Rheumatoid Arthritis

Although in 1969 Hart stated that the liver was not involved in rheumatoid arthritis,[116] soon afterwards several patients were reported with elevation of alkaline phosphatase levels.[146] This elevation appeared to correspond to the activity of the underlying rheumatoid arthritis. In more recent series, hepatomegaly or minor abnormalities of liver function tests occur in up to 20 per cent of cases.[47, 328] On liver biopsy, there may be fatty change, an inflammatory infiltrate or occasional fibrosis.[63, 328] Various forms of chronic liver disease have been reported in patients with rheumatoid arthritis, including primary biliary cirrhosis and chronic active hepatitis, but these are extremely rare.[83, 87, 296]

Felty's Syndrome

This is a syndrome of severe seropositive rheumatoid arthritis, splenomegaly and hypersplenism. Abnormalities of liver function tests are more common than in rheumatoid arthritis alone,[22] but the exact incidence is unknown. Histological changes range from a pronounced sinusoidal lymphocytic infiltration (Figure 37.7) to occasional macronodular cirrhosis. Portal tract fibrosis and Kupffer cell proliferation are also encountered.[22] Nodular regenerative (adenomatous) hyperplasia (Figure 37.8) in Felty's syndrome is unusual,[23] and has been reported in patients with rheumatoid arthritis without Felty's syndrome.[115] It is characterized by a normal architecture within which are nodules of parenchyma compressing the surrounding cell plates. There is no fibrosis. It can also occur as an isolated condition and usually presents with symptoms and signs of portal hypertension.[252] Amyloidosis can occasionally complicate both rheumatoid arthritis and Felty's syndrome.[168]

Still's Disease (Juvenile Rheumatoid Arthritis)

This presents more acutely than adult rheumatoid arthritis, and hepatosplenomegaly and jaundice are common. Available histological reports show lymphocytic and plasma cell infiltration and Kupffer cell proliferation.[160, 258]

Sjögren's Syndrome

Although Sjögren defined his syndrome as 'keratoconjunctivitis sicca, xerostomia and rheumatoid arthritis', it is now clear that the first two changes occur in patients who have no rheumatoid arthritis but have other putative

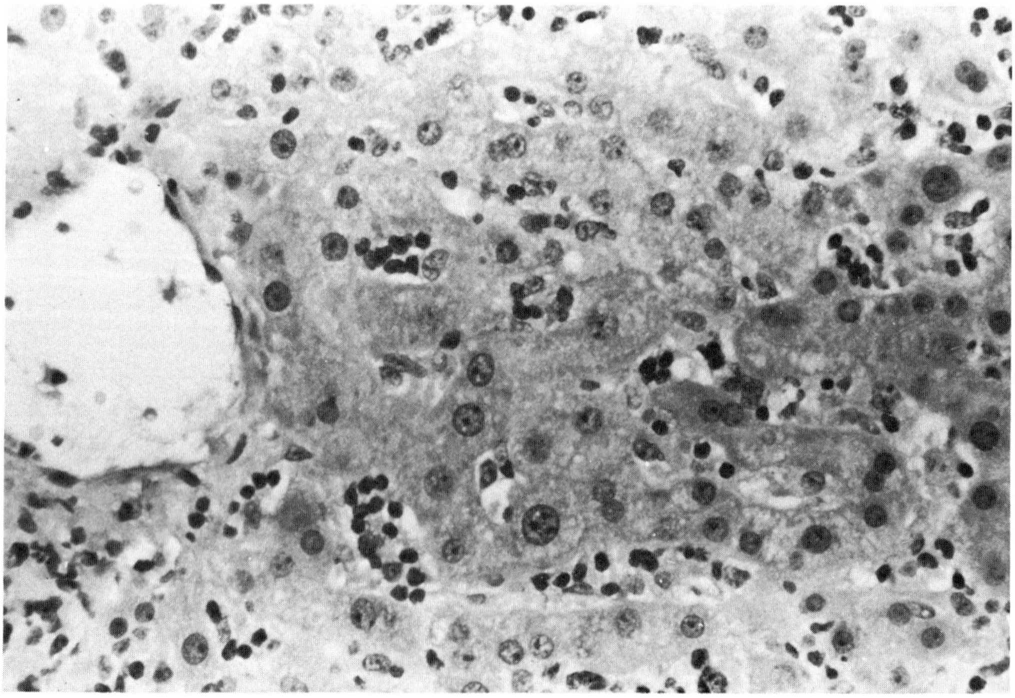

Figure 37.7. Numerous lymphocytes infiltrate the sinusoids in Felty's syndrome. Hepatocytes show increased nuclear variation and mitotic activity may also be increased. A central vein is present on the left. Haematoxylin and eosin × 1250.

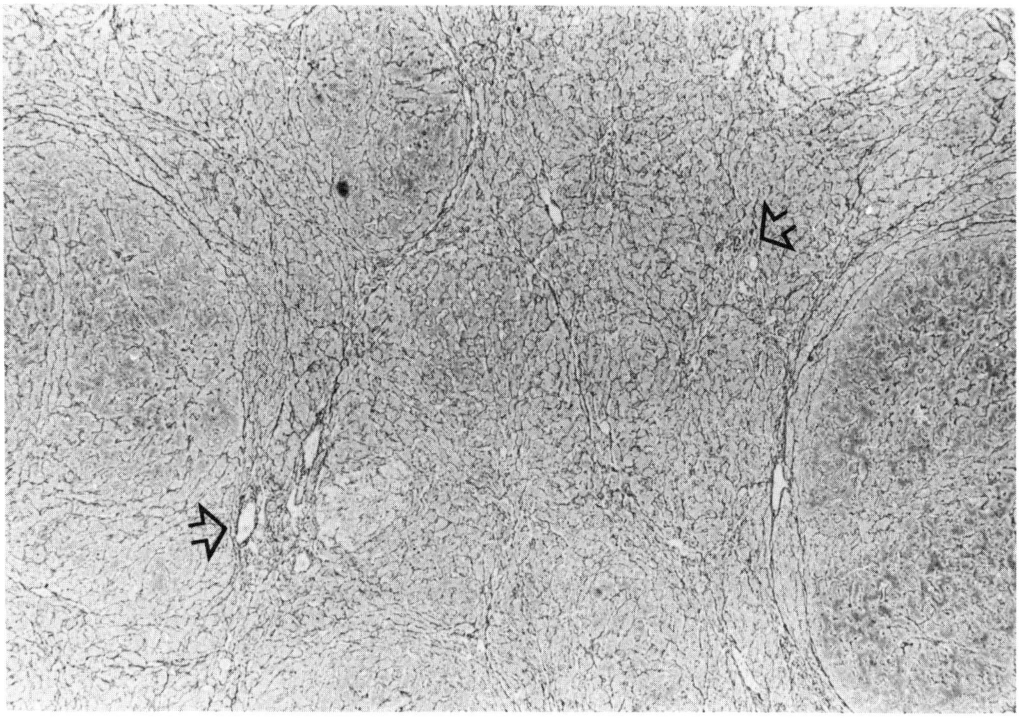

Figure 37.8. Nodular hyperplasia. The lobular architecture is distorted by the presence of numerous hyperplastic nodules of liver parenchyma. These have compressed intervening parenchyma with some condensation of reticulin but there is no fibrosis. Two portal tracts are indicated by arrows. Reticulin × 120.

autoimmune conditions. Keratoconjunctivitis sicca is commonly seen in liver disease; about 42 per cent of patients with chronic active hepatitis, 40 per cent with cryptogenic cirrhosis and up to 75 per cent with primary biliary cirrhosis had some features of this syndrome.[3, 106] Conversely, in a study of patients with keratoconjunctivitis sicca evidence of liver disease was found in 6 per cent.[331] The most common findings are mild hepatomegaly[312, 331] and elevation of the alkaline phosphatase.[339] Histology of the liver showed non-specific changes, including lymphocytic infiltration.[331]

Systemic Sclerosis

The incidence of liver disease is low. In one series of 727 patients, only eight had chronic liver disease.[16] These included cases of chronic active hepatitis. In another report, liver disease was more common in a control group than in patients with systemic sclerosis.[58] More recently, several cases of primary biliary cirrhosis and systemic sclerosis have been described, and this seems more common when scleroderma takes the form of the CRST (calcinosis cutis, Raynaud's phenomenon, sclerodactyly and telangiectasis) syndrome.[205,208,243] The liver may be calcified in these patients[118] and the biliary tract is occasionally the site of fibrosis.[53]

Systemic Lupus Erythematosus (SLE)

The exact relationship between chronic liver disease and systemic lupus erythematosus is obscure, as many symptoms, for example arthralgia and glomerulonephritis, and some laboratory features, including the LE phenomenon, are common to both disorders.

Early studies of patients with SLE reported cellular infiltration of the portal tract and steatosis.[117] Localized lymphoid aggregation, focal necrosis and reactive hepatitis have also been described.[187, 188] Clinically, some minor abnormalities are not unusual, including hepatomegaly in 20 per cent of cases and jaundice in up to 3 per cent.[71] Chronic active hepatitis is rarely seen, although there are several reports of lupoid nephritis occurring in patients with chronic active hepatitis.[95, 277]

Spontaneous rupture of the liver[172] or spleen[161] occasionally occurs. There is at least one report of SLE presenting with a similar clinical and histological appearance to that of acute viral hepatitis,[268] but a similar appearance has been attributed to aspirin by others.[264] Interpretation of these non-specific changes is difficult because there is some evidence that patients with SLE are liable to become chronic carriers of HB_sAg because of their impaired immunological competence.[4]

Polyarteritis Nodosum

In one study only 6 per cent had abnormal liver function tests.[207] The relationship between chronic hepatitis and polyarteritis nodosum is complicated because of the association with hepatitis B infection (see Chapter 29).

Patients with polyarteritis nodosum may present with obscure illnesses, pyrexia of unknown origin and abnormal liver function tests,[55] or more acutely, as occurs in hepatic infarction.[38, 141] Occasionally, spontaneous rupture of the liver can occur. Polyarteritis nodosum can also present with a similar picture to that of acute viral hepatitis.[268]

Even when multiple hepatic artery aneurysms have been demonstrated, needle biopsy can be entirely normal,[32] and surgical wedge biopsies are frequently needed to confirm the diagnosis. The arteritis may affect vessels of varying calibre, ranging from medium-sized vascular arteries down to arterioles. There is extensive inflammatory destruction of the wall of the vessel (Figure 37.9). Neutrophils, lymphocytes, plasma cells and eosinophils are all present and may be associated with the presence of fibrinoid necrosis.[55] All layers of the artery are involved and healing is by fibrosis.

The gallbladder may also be the site of an arteritis and may present as a case of cholecystitis.

Polymyalgia Rheumatica

Liver abnormalities are well recognized in polymyalgia rheumatica,[34, 62, 101, 104] but histological studies are limited. A granulomatous hepatitis,[178,181] a portal lymphocytic infiltration or liver-cell necrosis may be found.[144, 181] All these changes return to normal following treatment with corticosteroids.[62] Rarely, hepatic disease may be the main presenting feature of the illness, and headaches and polymyalgia may be insignificant features. A high incidence of anti-HB_s has been reported in patients with polymyalgia,[10] but has not been confirmed by others.[174]

(a) 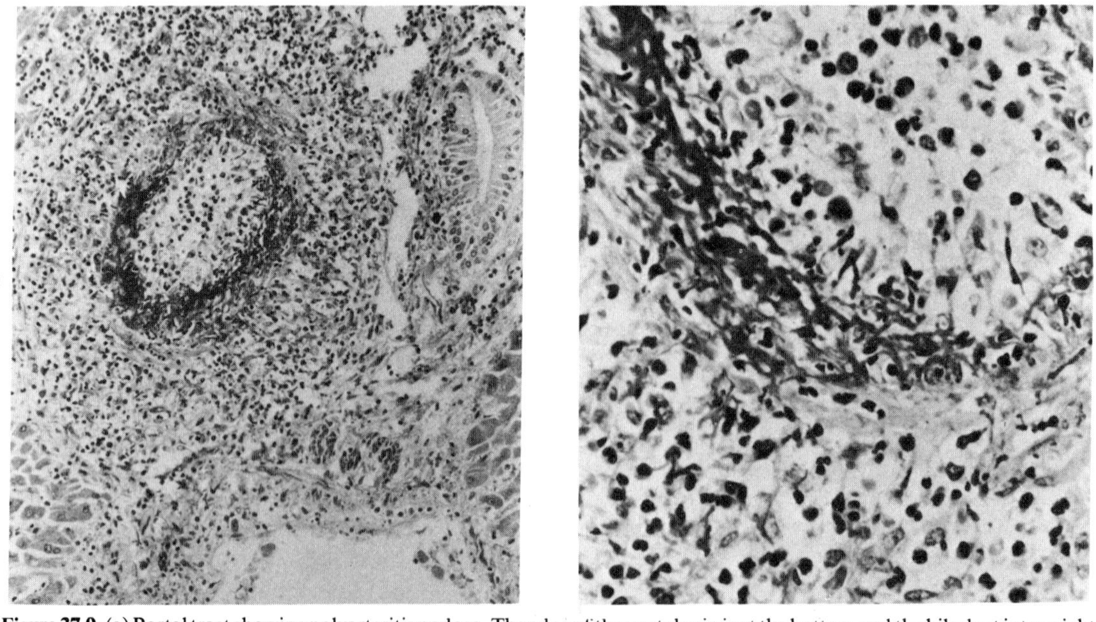 (b)

Figure 37.9. (a) Portal tract showing polyarteritis nodosa. The edge of the portal vein is at the bottom and the bile duct is top right. Fibrinoid necrosis of the arterial wall is seen as the dark band and numerous inflammatory cells surround the artery and infiltrate the wall. Haematoxylin and eosin × 120. (b) High power detail of the arterial wall in Figure 37.9a showing the destruction of the arterial wall with fibrinoid necrosis extending from top left to centre and numerous inflammatory cells in all areas. Haematoxylin and eosin × 1250.

Polymyositis and Dermatomyositis

In secondary dermatomyositis, liver involvement with tumour is common. In the primary form, abnormalities of the liver are rare. Hepatomegaly with or without abnormal liver function tests is well described[20] and non-specific histological changes, including portal tract inflammation, fatty change and focal hepatic necrosis have been recorded.[152] Amyloid is extremely rare.[342]

AMYLOIDOSIS

This is defined as the extracellular deposition of the protein amyloid in one or more sites of the body. Amyloidosis was recognized early in the 19th century and the liver was described as being grossly enlarged, waxy and elastic. Recognition of amyloidosis as a disease is usually credited to Rokitansky, but the term amyloid was coined by Virchow because the tissue became blue-black when treated with dilute sulphuric acid and iodine and so resembled vegetable starch. Early studies dealt purely with post-mortem findings, and it was not until biopsy procedures were used, and the solubility of amyloid in 6 M guanidine hydrochloride[103] and the staining properties of amyloid with Congo red were discovered, that real advances in understanding the disease were made.

Classification

There have been several different classifications of amyloidosis. Originally, clinical features divided patients into groups classified as either primary or secondary amyloidosis, and others made minor changes to this classification,[57, 151] but still used clinical criteria.

In the primary form there is no detected antecedent or coexistent disease and the amyloid is mainly deposited in mesodermal tissue, such as nerve and muscle of the cardiovascular system and the gastrointestinal tract. Macroglossia is a classic feature.

Secondary amyloidosis usually follows a long-standing chronic inflammatory process and amyloid distribution is predominantly in the liver, spleen, kidneys and adrenal glands. Separate entities of amyloidosis associated with multiple myeloma and with other tumours are also described.[241]

A different classification is based on the observation that amyloid tissue is deposited along pre-existing fibrils.[121] Amyloidosis is again divided into two groups, pericollagen and perireticular, approximately corresponding to primary and secondary amyloid of the clinical classification.

Neither system is satisfactory, and a more recent classification is based on the actual structure of the amyloid tissues.[48, 84, 132, 137] Two major structural forms of amyloid tissue designated as pattern 1 and pattern 2, which again correspond to primary and secondary amyloidosis, have been identified.

In pattern 1, the amyloid tissue has amino acid sequences identical to the light-chain component of immunoglobulin and is the result of light-chain abnormalities[102] associated with a plasma cell dyscrasia or overt multiple myeloma. In pattern 2, the amyloid is protein A[124, 170] which is a new protein with an amino acid sequence unlike any other previously described peptide. A simple method depending on the difference in resistance of the Congo red staining to decolourization by potassium permanganate and dilute sulphuric acid separates the two conditions. With this technique, pattern 1 is resistant to the potassium permanganate whilst pattern 2 is not.[335] The various schemes of classification are summarized in Table 37.5.

As well as the two major groups described above, there is a distinct form of amyloidosis associated with tumours, particularly medullary carcinoma of the thyroid.[283] There are also various familial forms, including Mediterranean fever. The more general aspects of the disease are the subject of several reviews.[48,93,163,293]

The Liver in Amyloidosis

The liver was probably the first organ in which amyloidosis was noted. The first description in which liver involvement was the major feature is that of Waldenström,[320] but in other early series the liver was not noted to be a frequent site of deposition of amyloidosis.[250, 305] Improved techniques established that the liver was commonly affected, and up to two-thirds of patients with amyloidosis had liver involvement at autopsy.[287, 341]

The liver is involved almost as frequently in the primary as in the secondary form,[171, 291] and 85 per cent of patients dying with primary amyloidosis and 98 per cent of patients with secondary amyloidosis have hepatic

Table 37.5. *Simplified Classification of Amyloidosis, excluding Tumour-associated and Familial Forms.*

	Other classifications	Associated conditions	Type of amyloid
Pattern 1	Primary Pericollagen Atypical	Plasma cell dyscrasia including multiple myeloma	Immunoglobulin
Pattern 2	Secondary Perireticular Typical	Chronic infections Paraplegia Collagen disorders Inflammatory bowel disease Diabetes	Protein A

involvement.[30] The incidence of liver disease could be higher, as minimal deposition may be detectable only by electron microscopy.[281]

Clinical Features

The clinical presentation is varied and depends on the anatomical distribution of amyloid tissue.[48] Common features include general malaise, fatigue, proteinuria, nephrotic syndrome, renal and cardiovascular failure.[162] Overt liver disease is rare, although on examination hepatomegaly is relatively common. In one series 90 per cent of patients with primary amyloidosis and 60 per cent with secondary amyloidosis had clinical evidence of hepatomegaly.[28] More recently, in a large series 50 per cent of all patients with amyloidosis were found to have hepatomegaly.[163]

Symptoms and signs of chronic liver disease are extremely rare, although there have been occasional reports of hepatic cell failure[265] and the development of portal hypertension.[28, 142] Ascites may occur in up to 30 per cent of cases as a terminal event,[110, 171] but it can usually be attributed to involvement of the kidneys and heart, resulting in the nephrotic syndrome and heart failure respectively.

Despite extensive deposition of the amyloid tissue in the liver, liver function tests are often entirely normal. Abnormalities encountered in severe cases include elevation of the transaminases and alkaline phosphatase. In a recent report, nearly 50 per cent of patients with amyloidosis were found to have some abnormality of liver function tests.[163] Jaundice occurs in less than 5 per cent of cases.[28, 171, 257] Occasionally the jaundice may be severe and due to intrahepatic biliary obstruction by the amyloid tissue.[173]

Diagnosis

The classic diagnostic tests using Evans blue or Congo red dye are now obsolete. Many cases will be suspected clinically and confirmed by rectal biopsy[96] or, in patients in whom renal involvement is the predominant abnormality, by renal biopsy. In those patients in whom the liver abnormalities predominate, diagnosis can usually be made on liver biopsy, although the procedure is alleged to have an increased risk of haemorrhage in patients with amyloidosis.[318] In many patients with known and proven amyloidosis presenting with hepatomegaly or abnormalities of liver function tests, invasive investigations are unnecessary.

Liver and spleen scans can show features varying from a normal appearance to gross enlargement of the liver. Occasionally, the pattern of multiple filling defects can be encountered and mistaken for multiple metastases.[105,286] Grey-scale ultrasound scanning may show hepatomegaly with a generalized increase in echo pattern.

Pathology

Macroscopically, the liver may be grossly enlarged, weigh up to 9000 g, and be smooth, pale and waxy in appearance. Histologically, amyloid is a homogeneous, amorphous, eosinophilic material found in the portal tracts and between endothelial and parenchymal cells in the space of Disse (Figure 37.10). Electron microscopic studies have confirmed this localization within the space of Disse.[281] Although the hepatocytes are not involved, in severe cases they may be atrophic either from ischaemia or compression, particularly in the mid-zonal or portal regions. Amyloid deposition around

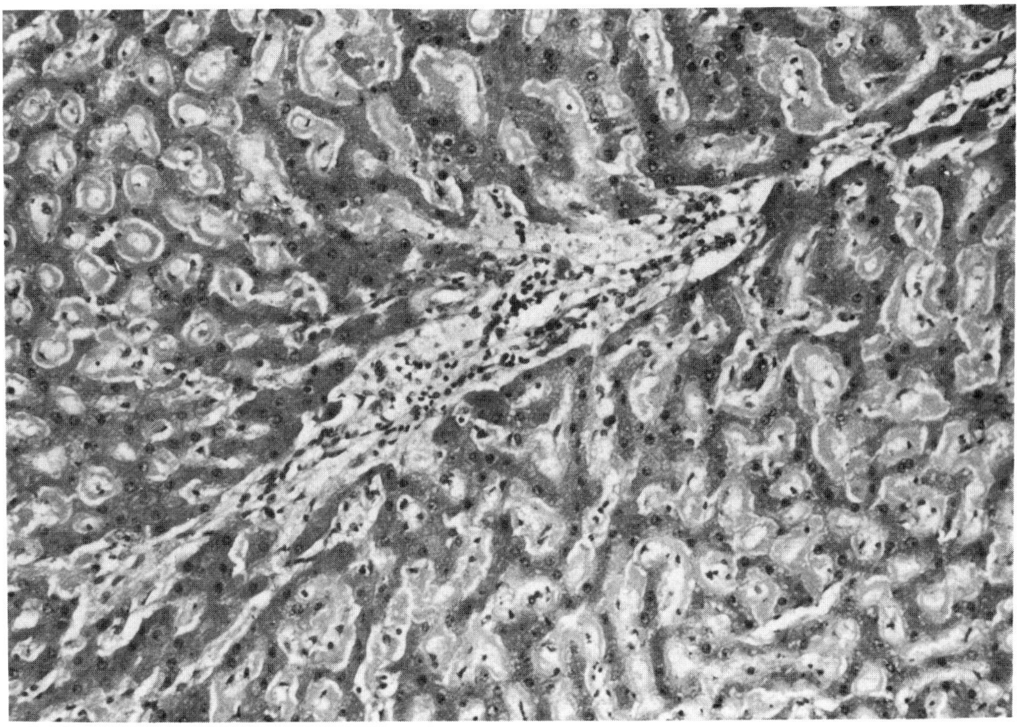

Figure 37.10. Amyloid is diffusely deposited as an acellular amorphous and hyaline eosinophilic material in the space of Disse between the endothelial cells and hepatocytes. The hepatocytes are atrophic. Haematoxylin and eosin × 750.

arteries and portal veins is common, and it has been suggested that this is more a feature of primary than of secondary amyloidosis.[290] Sampling differences between biopsy specimens are not unusual.[259]

Amyloid is salmon-pink when stained with alkaline Congo red and if it is then viewed with polarized light (Figure 37.11) a variable blue/green to yellow birefringence is seen, which is typical of amyloid tissue. As mentioned above, it is possible to separate the immunoglobulin form from protein A, depending on the resistance of the staining to potassium permanganate and dilute sulphuric acid.[335] On electron microscopy the features are diagnostic. Amyloid is a non-branching fibrillar protein 7.5 nm in diameter, with random orientation of the fibrils. Each fibril is composed of five protofibrils which are intertwined and produce a characteristic 10 nm periodicity.[274]

Treatment and Prognosis

There is no specific treatment for amyloidosis. Treatment of the underlying disease has led to resolution of the amyloid reaction,[64, 91, 182, 222] but this is the exception rather than the rule. Corticosteroid therapy is indicated only in those cases complicated by Addison's disease. Prognosis is poor and depends on the stage and extent of the amyloid deposition. If there is evidence of proteinuria or other serious complications, 90 per cent of patients are dead within two years. Death usually results from the underlying disease or from amyloid-induced renal failure. Hepatic failure is extremely rare.

THE LIVER IN HEART FAILURE

There is close anatomical proximity of the hepatic vein to the right atrium, so that the venous drainage of the liver is dependent on the central venous pressure. This can easily be demonstrated in patients with incipient heart failure by the hepatojugular reflex. Conversely, a significant rise in the central venous pressure will produce changes in the liver.

The classic 'nutmeg liver' of severe heart failure was first reported in 1833.[149] Other reports soon followed, demonstrating the frequent abnormalities of liver function tests that can occur. The physiological and anatomical basis for these changes have been thoroughly investigated and documented.[272]

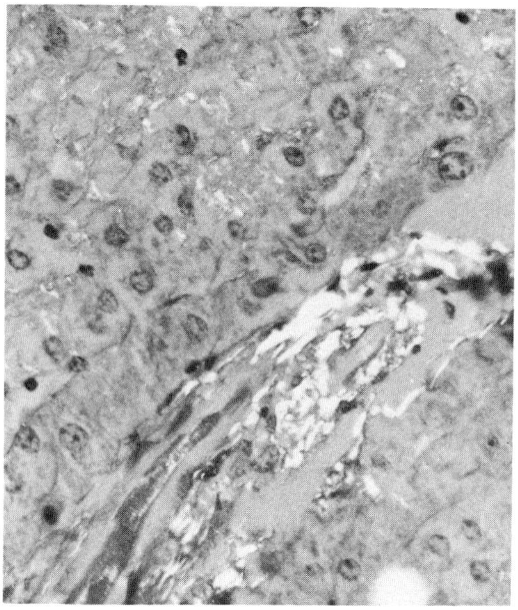

Figure 37.11. In polarized light amyloid stained by Congo red shows anomalous colours ranging from yellow to green to blue. Here it can be identified predominantly in the arterial wall in a portal tract but is also present in small amounts in the space of Disse. Congo red in polarized light × 1250.

Pathogenesis

Hepatocytes are sensitive even to shortlived periods of ischaemia,[267] and three factors have been incriminated in the pathogenesis of the changes occurring in heart failure. These are (a) arterial hypoxia; (b) a fall in the cardiac output; and (c) peripheral venous hypertension with sinusoidal congestion and oedema, resulting in reduced oxygen diffusion.

Arterial hypoxia

This may be only a minor factor.[332] If for any reason the cardiac output is reduced, there is a proportional decrease in hepatic blood flow.[209] The liver can compensate to a degree by increasing oxygen extraction, but eventually there will be excess lactate production and ischaemia will result.[261]

Acute heart failure

In acute heart failure or shock, the predominant factor in the pathogenesis of the liver abnormality is a fall in the cardiac output. Hepatic necrosis is inevitable if hypotension is prolonged.

Peripheral venous hypertension

This is more important in chronic heart failure, but there is also a reduction in cardiac output. The $P\text{O}_2$ may be reduced both in the hepatic and the portal vein,[209] and the liver is therefore perfused with less blood containing less oxygen. The centrilobular liver cells receive blood at a lower tension than peripheral hepatocytes and are more vulnerable to the ischaemia.

Pathology

In acute heart failure or shock, the hepatic vein and the sinusoids are seen to be markedly congested with occasional local haemorrhage, necrosis or atrophy of the parenchyma. The necrosis is usually focal and centrizonal, although it can spread into the mid-zonal region. In particularly severe cases, there may be bridging necrosis.[35] Hepatocytes around these necrotic zones frequently contain palely staining PAS positive diastase-resistant globules. The contents of these globules can be shown to be alpha-1-antitrypsin by immunological techniques[197] (Figure 37.12).

Lipofuscin pigment is present in the hepatic cells and in the Kupffer cells. A polymorphonuclear inflammatory infiltrate is occasionally

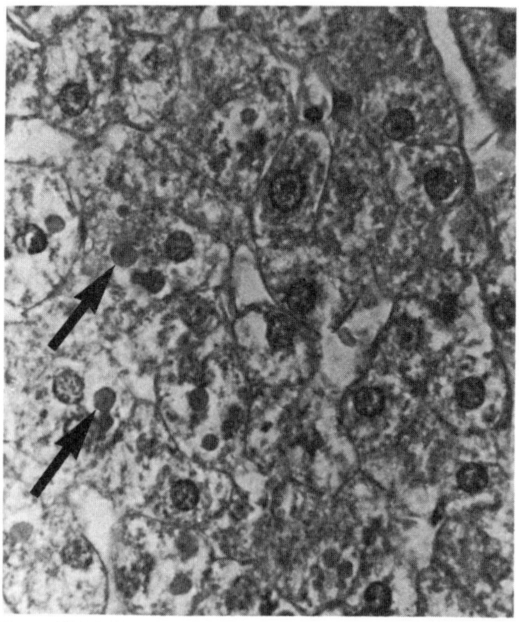

Figure 37.12. Swollen palely staining hepatocytes adjacent to areas of necrosis may contain scanty globules (arrows) which are weakly PAS positive and diastase resistant. Immunohistochemical studies demonstrate that they contain alpha-l-antitrypsin. DPAS × 1500.

present but never severe. The reticulin structure remains intact and fatty change is not a feature. In severe cases of heart failure, changes are similar to those found in the Budd–Chiari syndrome, where most of the lobule is replaced by blood, leaving just a peripheral rim of surrounding liver cells. The presence of red blood cells in the space of Disse has been described as pathognomonic of the Budd–Chiari syndrome and veno-occlusive disease of the liver,[169] but similar changes are seen in particularly severe right heart failure. More recently, well-documented examples of left ventricular failure without right ventricular failure have also been associated with centrilobular parenchymal atrophy, sinusoidal dilatation and red cells in the space of Disse.[49]

In chronic heart failure, the liver is macroscopically grossly enlarged and congested. Many of the changes are similar to those found in acute heart failure. The classic nutmeg appearance of red and yellow is caused by centrilobular congestion with fatty change peripheral to this zone. There is progressive atrophy of the parenchymal cell plates towards the central zone with sinusoidal dilatation and congestion. Cholestasis may be present and Kupffer cells and macrophages are laden with lipofuscin and ceroid pigment. In acute heart failure these macrophages separate the reticulin fibres, but with chronicity this framework collapses and is replaced by bland, fibrous tissue (Figure 37.13). The fibrosis progresses so that in severe and longstanding cases all the central veins are linked. There is usually mild fibrous enlargement and sclerosis of the portal tracts. The centrizonal distribution, the relative lack of inflammatory infiltrate and the lack of nodular regeneration help to distinguish and identify these advanced cases. Rarely, fibrosis does bridge central veins and portal tracts and nodular regeneration may be found so that a true cardiac cirrhosis is produced.

With the advent of potent diuretics, the severe changes mentioned above are encountered only rarely, and then usually in association with inoperable mitral or tricuspid valve disease or constrictive pericarditis.

Electron microscopy studies have shown dilatation of the endoplasmic reticulum and swelling of the mitochondria. Lysosomes are larger and more frequent.[127] There are central vacuoles which do not contain alkaline phosphatase. The centrizonal parenchymal cells are atrophic.[256]

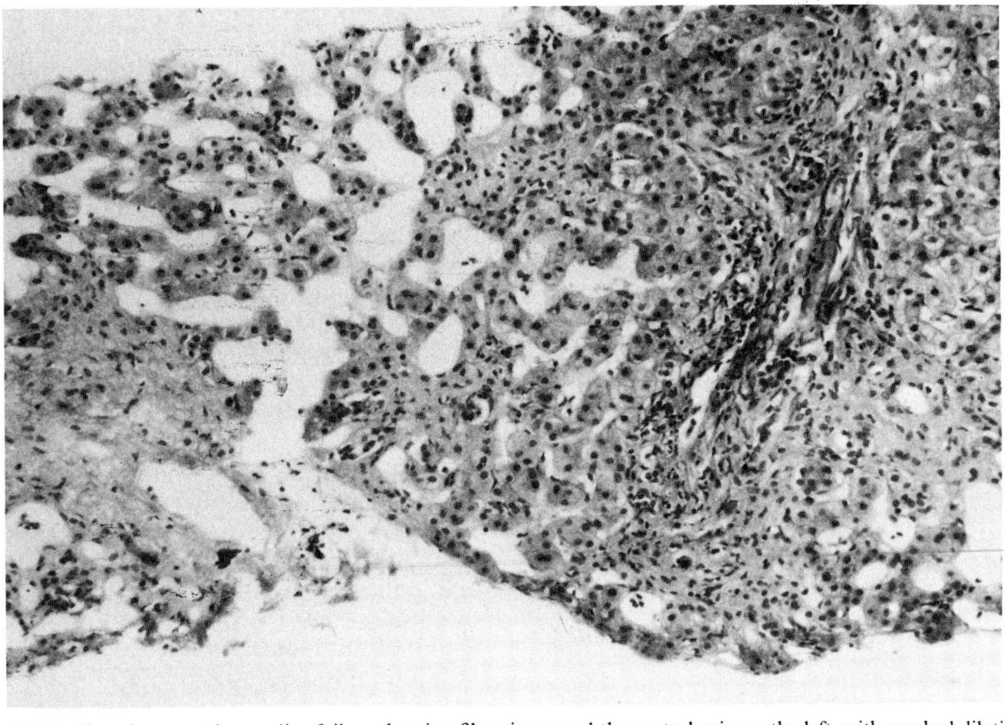

Figure 37.13. Chronic congestive cardiac failure showing fibrosis around the central vein on the left, with marked dilation of centrilobular sinusoids and atrophy of hepatocytes. Mild fibrosis expands the portal tract on the right. Haematoxylin and eosin × 600.

Clinical Features

Common causes of acute heart failure or shock include trauma, blood loss, burns, myocardial ischaemia, pulmonary embolus and septicaemia. Under these circumstances, liver abnormalities are not of great clinical significance, as other organs, especially the brain, are more sensitive to periods of anoxia. Hepatomegaly may be present and unexpectedly abnormal liver function tests may be found. In chronic heart failure, patients may present with pain in the right upper quadrant. Hepatomegaly is a common finding and the liver may be tender. Splenomegaly can also be present.[73] The bilirubin is usually only mildly elevated and rarely exceeds 50 μmol/l (3 mg/dl) and may in part be due to haemolysis. Both the alkaline phosphatase and the transaminase can be increased.[244] Elevation of the transaminase is usually only mild to moderate, but on occasion can be more severe and suggestive of acute hepatitis.[49] The prothrombin time can be disproportionately prolonged and patients may be unduly sensitive to anticoagulants,[157] but plasma protein, immunoglobulins and the autoimmune profile are usually normal. Clinical jaundice and stigmata of chronic liver disease are rare but have been reported.[153]

It has recently been shown that quite severe changes in liver function can be encountered, not only in patients with obvious right ventricular failure but also in those with left ventricular failure in whom there is no evidence of right heart failure.[49]

Prognosis usually depends more on the underlying condition than the state of liver function. It is important for the clinician to be aware of the abnormalities of liver function that can occur, in order to avoid unnecessary investigation. Some of the abnormalities described, including hepatomegaly, can persist some time after the heart failure appears to have been adequately treated. Portal hypertension occasionally occurs, particularly in patients with constrictive pericarditis. In one study, 5 per cent of all cases of congestive cardiac failure had evidence of varices, sometimes even in the absence of cirrhosis.[183]

THE CARDIOVASCULAR SYSTEM IN LIVER FAILURE

In one study, 37 per cent of patients with fulminating hepatic failure, mostly as the result of paracetamol overdose, were found to have clinical or radiological evidence of pulmonary oedema.[300] In many of these cases, the terminal event is a cardiac dysrhythmia,[330] although this may be the result of paracetamol toxicity rather than the direct effect of the liver failure. The cause of the heart failure appears to be central in origin, possibly similar to that seen in severe head injury.

Intrapulmonary vascular shunts occur in both acute and chronic liver cell failure.[17] These are often clinically insignificant, but cyanosis attributable to these shunts has been found in approximately one-third of all patients with cirrhosis.[247]

OTHER VASCULAR ABNORMALITIES OF THE LIVER

Some conditions, including the Budd–Chiari syndrome and veno-occlusive disease, are discussed in Chapter 43.

Hepatic Artery Thrombosis

Hepatic infarcts are the result of thrombosis of branches of the hepatic artery. The relative infrequency of these infarcts in clinical practice can be explained in two ways: firstly, by the dual blood supply to the liver via the hepatic artery and portal vein, and secondly, by the rapid development of collateral blood flow following thrombosis.[194]

Many instances of hepatic artery thrombosis are likely to go unnoticed and undiagnosed, as symptoms and signs may be minimal and even in severe cases there can be a full recovery. There is usually an underlying disease process, most commonly SLE, polyarteritis nodosa or a vasculitis.[63, 141]

Symptoms. When they occur, symptoms usually consist of right upper quadrant abdominal discomfort or pain. Frequently patients are debilitated from the underlying illness. In severe cases there may be collapse and hypertension, and in the days that follow there may be a mild pyrexia, a leucocytosis and elevated transaminases. On examination, there may be tender hepatomegaly and occasionally a hepatic bruit. Although there is no specific treatment, attention should be given to relief of pain and treatment of the underlying disease.

Prognosis. This is good with small infarcts, and even if there has been extensive infarction complete recovery can occur.[214] Recovery can also occur if the hepatic artery is transected during surgery, especially if the artery is occluded distal to the origins of the gastroduodenal and the right gastric artery. Unusual conditions which may be complicated by hepatic infarction include liver transplantation[288] and blunt abdominal trauma.[36]

Hepatic Artery Aneurysm

Aneurysms of the hepatic artery are rare. Seventy-five per cent are extrahepatic and 25 per cent are intrahepatic. They can vary enormously in size, from very small to very large. They are usually the result of biliary surgery or some underlying systemic illness, the most common being infections, atherosclerosis and polyarteritis nodosum.[112] They are usually incidental findings, either at laparotomy or at post-mortem, and only rarely give rise to symptoms in life. As a result, many go undiagnosed.

Symptoms, when they occur, form the classic triad of pain, jaundice and haematemesis. The jaundice is the result of pressure on the bile duct by the aneurysm and the haematemesis results from rupture of the aneurysm into the biliary tract. Hepatic artery aneurysm should be suspected in patients presenting with haematemesis some time after gallbladder surgery.[185] Primary aneurysms of the hepatic artery are almost unknown and again are seldom diagnosed during life. Diagnosis is by arteriography,[32] although recently ultrasound and isotopic scans have been utilized.[294]

When an aneurysm is diagnosed during life, it can be difficult to decide between active treatment and conservative management. The aneurysms can either be excised or wrapped in cellophane.[112] In the absence of pain or life-threatening emergencies such as haemorrhage, an expectant policy is probably best. Occasionally, aneurysms of the hepatic artery can dissect.[125]

Infarcts of Zahn

Portal vein thrombosis is discussed in Chapter 43. Although hepatic artery ligation results in hepatic infarction, portal vein occlusion does not.[221, 223] Occlusions of the smaller branches of the portal vein result in so-called pseudo-infarcts, otherwise known as Zahn's infarcts.[337] These pseudo-infarcts are occasionally seen following splenectomy, but are nearly always asymptomatic.[299] Histology shows that, although the sinusoids are dilated and the lobule and hepatocytes atrophic, there is no necrosis. It is possible that pseudo-infarcts occur only when both the portal and the systemic circulations are embarrassed[299] but in animal studies, it has been shown that the hepatocytes atrophy soon after occlusion of the portal vein.[329]

Congenital Haemorrhagic Telangiectasia (Rendu–Osler–Weber Disease)

Cirrhosis is relatively common in patients with congenital haemorrhagic telangiectasia.[190] About 50 per cent of patients have symptoms, usually of pain or discomfort in the right upper quadrant of the abdomen. On examination, about the same number have hepatosplenomegaly. Liver function is usually well preserved, the most frequent abnormality being elevation of the alkaline phosphatase or of the bilirubin. Portal hypertension and hepatic encephalopathy are occasionally encountered. Histology may show a coarse, nodular cirrhosis. In the fibrous bands there are multiple telangiectases of varying sizes,[340] and prominent subcapsular vascularity may be seen.[26] There may also be an associated inflammatory infiltrate.

Other abnormalities of the liver have been described in association with congenital haemorrhagic telangiectasia, including cavernous haemangiomas, hepatic artery aneurysms and arteriovenous fistulae.[306] The pathogenesis of all of these abnormalities remains obscure.

Peliósis Hepatis and Sinusoidal Ectasia

Peliosis hepatis

This is a pathological entity that is usually an incidental finding at autopsy or laparotomy.[11,338] Until recently, the majority of cases were associated with tuberculosis and terminal cachexia, particularly from carcinomatosis. Peliosis is now also associated with the contraceptive pill and with androgenic steroid therapy, and probably the commonest condition in which peliosis is now seen is an aplastic anaemia treated with long-term androgenic steroids.[11] The relationship between peliosis and the hepatomas and adenomas that occur in

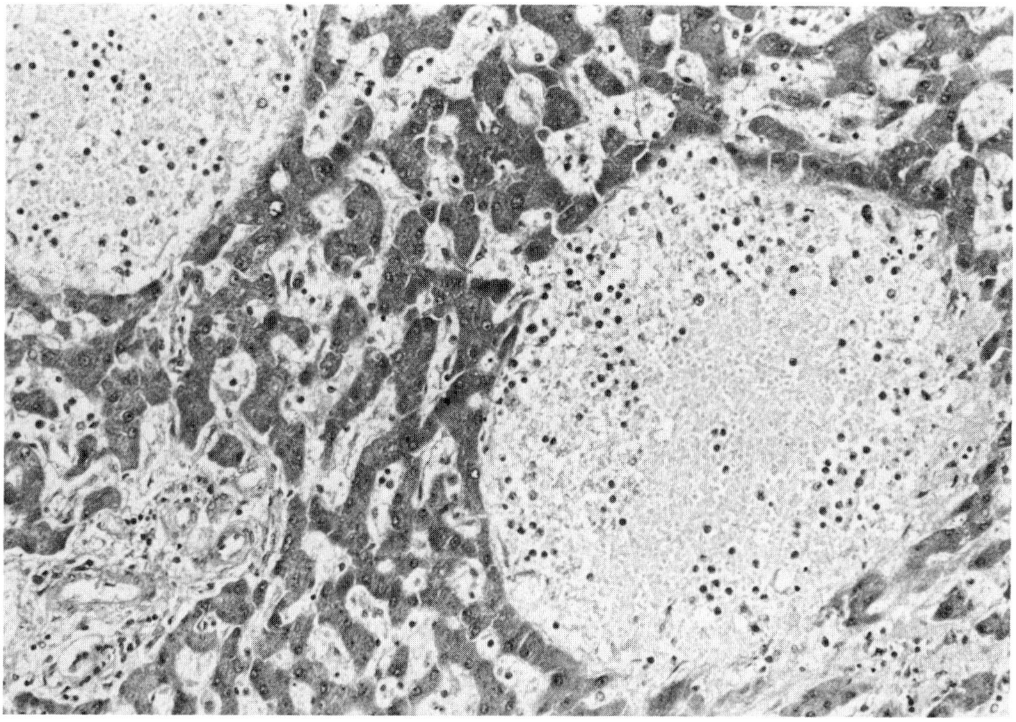

Figure 37.14. Peliosis hepatis: Two large blood-filled cystic spaces are present in the parenchyma. They are in direct continuity with adjacent sinusoids. A portal tract is present bottom left. Haematoxylin and eosin × 600.

patients taking anabolic steroids[11, 88] or oral contraceptives[158, 217] is uncertain. These conditions can sometimes occur in the same patient.[11] Peliosis has also been recorded in renal transplant patients and attributed to their azathioprine therapy.[61]

Clinical features. These vary considerably. In one series, six out of seven patients developed hepatomegaly and three out of seven developed jaundice.[11] There may be mild or moderate elevation of the transaminases and the albumin may be low. The prothrombin time can be prolonged.

Macroscopic examination of the liver. This shows obvious lakes filled with blood, varying in size but sometimes larger than 4 mm.

Light microscopy. This shows blood-filled cavernous cysts (Figure 37.14) which are in continuity with the sinusoids and which may exhibit a centrilobular emphasis. It is unlikely that the division into phlebectatic and parenchymal types[336] really exists.[210] Hepatocytes are basically normal, although they may show minor changes and, immediately adjacent to the peliosis, may show mild atrophy. Electron microscopy studies have shown that the cells lining the sinusoids contain numerous vacuoles and dense bodies which may be lysosomes.

Pathogenesis of peliosis is uncertain, but a direct toxic effect on the lining cells of the sinusoids, rather than on the hepatocytes, has been suggested.[210]

Diagnosis can be confirmed by liver biopsy, although theoretically there is an increased risk of haemorrhage complicating the procedure. Suspicion of peliosis hepatis should be high in any patient on long-term androgenic steroids who develops symptoms or signs of liver disease.

Prognosis is dependent on the underlying condition, although on occasions patients have developed hepatic failure.[210]

Sinusoidal ectasia (see also Chapters 18 and 38)

This is a closely allied phenomenon and probably represents a less extreme version of peliosis hepatis. In sinusoidal ectasia, hepatocytes are atrophied and the sinusoids are widened, sometimes abruptly and dramatically so (Figure 37.15). It can occur in any part of the

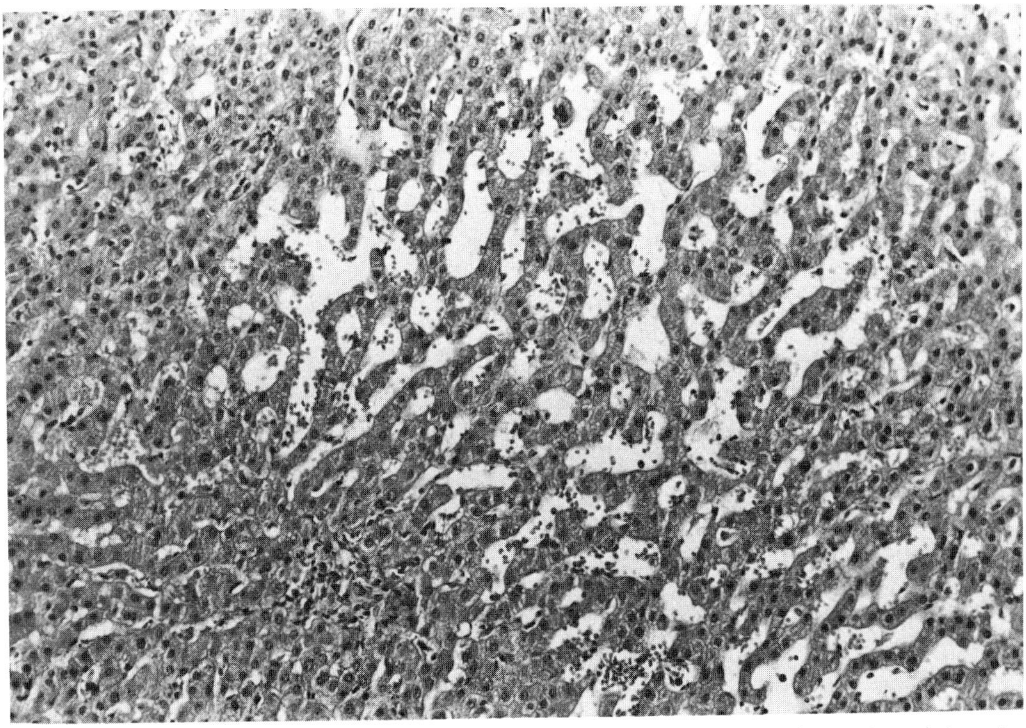

Figure 37.15. Sinusoidal ectasia. Sinusoids are dilated and may have a diameter greater than the intervening cell plates. A non-zoned distribution is particularly common in association with malignancy. Haematoxylin and eosin × 500.

lobule. The aetiological associations are the same as those of peliosis hepatis, but this lesion also occurs in cirrhosis, is particularly common around tumour deposits within the liver, and is the major histological feature in the parenchyma following portal vein occlusion (infarct of Zahn).

The lesion is asymptomatic, usually being a chance histological finding, but it may occasionally be identified as the dark halo around a reflective metastasis on ultrasound examination of the liver.[198] Recognition of this lesion in the biopsy without any obvious or known association should provoke a careful history and a meticulous search for tumour in the specimen. Treatment is dependent upon the aetiology.

HAEMATOLOGICAL DISORDERS

These are discussed in detail in Chapter 8.

Haemolytic Anaemias

Jaundice can occur in any haemolytic anaemia, due to an increase in the level of the unconjugated bilirubin. There is an associated increase in the incidence of gallstones in these conditions. Patients undergoing repeated blood transfusions may also develop haemosiderosis. Initially this is in Kupffer cells, but the parenchyma may eventually become involved (see Chapter 34). Intravascular haemolysis releases iron that is phagocytosed by and demonstrable within Kupffer cells.

Sickle-cell Disease

In sickle-cell disease the liver is often enlarged and tender during crisis. There may be abnormalities of liver function tests, including elevation of the alkaline phosphatase, bilirubin and transaminases.[249] Histology reveals clumps of erythrocytes, platelets and fibrin in the sinusoids with areas of focal necrosis.[12,249,285] Occasionally, an acute crisis can be mistaken for cholecystitis.[7]

Extramedullary Haemopoiesis

The liver is often the site of extramedullary haemopoiesis in conditions such as the myeloproliferative disorders. It is also a common occurrence in neonatal and childhood anaemias.

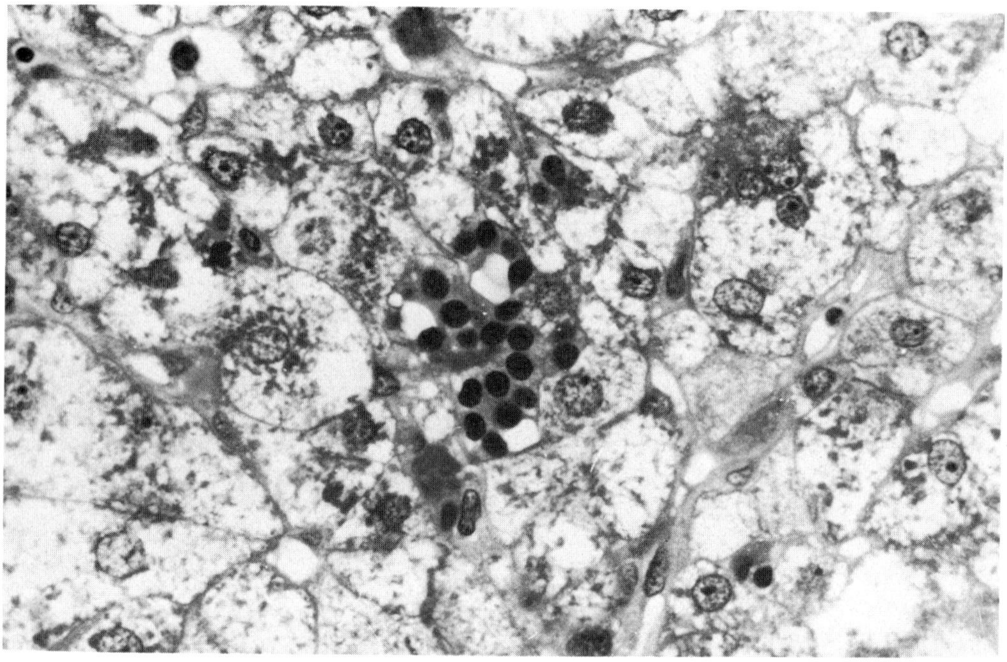

Figure 37.16. Extramedullary haemopoiesis in the sinusoid. Haematoxylin and eosin × 2000.

Thirty per cent of the lobule may be occupied. Erythropoiesis is concentrated mainly in the lobule, and erythroblasts and normoblasts with some megakaryocytes can be seen in the hepatic sinusoids (Figure 37.16). Granulocytic precursors are located primarily in the portal triads.[322] The clinical features are those of the underlying condition together with hepatosplenomegaly which may be massive. The commonest abnormality of liver function is elevation of the alkaline phosphatase, which in one series occurred in nearly 50 per cent of patients.[322] The transaminases and bilirubin are usually normal. Portal hypertension can occur in many of these conditions, notably chronic myeloid leukaemia, polycythaemia and myelosclerosis, and often is the result of portal vein thrombosis due to an increased clotting tendency. In other cases it is either due to infiltration of the portal tracts and sinusoids[269] or to increased portal blood flow, when splenectomy can be curative.[295]

HYPERPYREXIAS

Heat Stroke

This is only rarely encountered in clinical practice, and with the lack of an adequate history diagnosis can be difficult. Prostration with cerebral symptoms are most common, but liver abnormalities may be a prominent feature, with elevation of the transaminases and the alkaline phosphatase. Jaundice is relatively rare, normally occurring on about the third day of the illness and reaching a peak within the first week. In one large series of 244 patients, only 10 had jaundice while 17 had some evidence of hepatic abnormality.[123]

Pathological investigation reveals centrilobular zonal necrosis with marked hydropic degeneration and sometimes extensive cholestasis. Other features occasionally found include bile-duct proliferation and cholangiolitis.[19, 313] Fatty change is not a feature, and occasionally the histological appearance can be mistaken for viral hepatitis with confluent necrosis.

The prognosis for heat stroke is generally not very good, but the liver abnormalities are overshadowed by the systemic effects. The pathogenesis of the liver abnormalities has not been fully explained, although hypoxia and hypovolaemia may be important factors. The subject of heat stroke has recently been well reviewed.[46]

Malignant Hyperpyrexia

This is an anaesthetic complication related to suxamethonium sensitivity, and although similar in some respects to heat stroke, abnormalities of liver function tests are rare.[31] There are a few reports of liver histology which shows non-specific changes.[302]

CHRONIC INFLAMMATORY BOWEL DISEASE

General Considerations

Even before ulcerative colitis was recognized as a clinical entity, fatty change in the liver associated with diffuse ulceration of the colon had been described.[301] Later, Lister[177] reported interstitial hepatitis in a patient with ulcerative colitis. An autopsy study in 1948 established the association between liver abnormalities and ulcerative colitis.[228] In Crohn's disease, several early studies found no evidence of hepatic involvement,[54, 82, 311] but subsequently it became apparent that the distribution of hepatic abnormalities in Crohn's disease was similar to that in ulcerative colitis.[41, 156, 224, 225]

The true incidence is difficult to determine, since it would have to include an unselected survey of both liver function and histology. Most figures concerning the incidence of hepatic abnormalities have been based either on autopsy studies,[41, 59, 156, 219, 228] or on surgical biopsies[60, 65, 75, 77, 78] obtained at laparotomy, but these are both inevitably highly selected series.

The highest incidence is found in surgical specimens, where up to 95 per cent of biopsies may show some form of hepatic abnormality.[75, 200] An incidence of up to 50 per cent has been reported from autopsy specimens,[219] but such patients have severe disease and are often debilitated. The most realistic estimate of the frequency of liver abnormalities is obtained by screening patients for clinical or laboratory evidence of liver disease and submitting those with abnormalities to routine liver biopsy. In such studies, between 15 and 25 per cent of all patients have abnormal liver function tests, and of those undergoing liver biopsy, about 30 per cent have pericholangitis and a further 30 per cent have fatty change.

In one such study, Perrett and coworkers[224, 225] screened 300 unselected patients with ulcerative colitis and 100 unselected patients with Crohn's disease for clinical and laboratory evidence of liver disease. Forty-five ulcerative colitics and 26 patients with Crohn's disease had biochemical evidence of liver abnormalities, and 50 patients with ulcerative colitis and 39 with Crohn's underwent liver biopsy. The distribution of the histological changes is shown in Table 37.6 A poor correlation was found between abnormal liver function tests and histological abnormality, when relatively minor changes were present. A random group of patients without abnormality of liver function were biopsied, and the histological changes found were similar to those in patients with abnormal liver function tests. Overall, there was a striking similarity in the hepatic changes in ulcerative colitis and Crohn's disease.

Clinically overt liver disease is much less common and is present in less than 5 per cent of all patients with inflammatory bowel disease.[109]

There is no consistent temporal relationship between the length of symptoms of the inflammatory bowel disease and the liver abnormalities. On average, ulcerative colitis has been present for about eight years when the liver disease is detected.[65] The liver abnormalities may precede or occur decades after the onset of the bowel disease, including the severe form of liver disease.[81, 304] The exact relationship in time is difficult to define, as both conditions may be asymptomatic for many years prior to their actual diagnosis.

The more severe forms of liver disease tend to occur in patients with long-standing, often quiescent, total colitis,[224] but there is no close relationship to the extent or duration of the colitis. The distribution of minor hepatic abnormalities appears to be independent of the extent or severity of the colitis.[6, 224]

The distribution of abnormalities in Crohn's disease of the colon is similar to that found in ulcerative colitis. It is of interest that if the Crohn's disease is restricted to the small bowel,

Table 37.6. *Liver Abnormalities Reported in a Large Series of Patients with Inflammatory Bowel Disease.*[224, 225]

	Ulcerative colitis	Crohn's disease
Total number screened	300	100
Abnormal LFTs	45	26
Liver biopsy		
total	50	39
Normal	19	20
Focal necrosis	3	6
Fatty change	19	8
Pericholangitis	15	8
Chronic active hepatitis	4	1
Cirrhosis	3	1
Amyloidosis	1	0

Table 37.7. *Liver and Biliary Abnormalities Found in Inflammatory Bowel Disease.*

	Ulcerative colitis	Crohn's disease
Pericholangitis	Common	Common
Fatty liver	Common	Common
Hepatoportal fibrosis	Unusual	Unusual
Chronic active hepatitis	Unusual	Unusual
Sclerosing cholangitis	Unusual	Case reports only
Cryptogenic cirrhosis	Unusual	Unusual
Granulomatous hepatitis	Not reported	Rare
Amyloidosis	Very rare	Rare
Bile-duct carcinoma	Rare	Not reported
Cholelithiasis	Normal incidence 5%	Increased incidence 13–30%

liver involvement is unusual,[75] and this may explain the infrequency of hepatic changes found in the early reports, which included few cases of colonic Crohn's disease. The liver abnormalities in Crohn's disease and ulcerative colitis are summarized in Table 37.7.

Fatty change and pericholangitis occur in a similar proportion in the two diseases. Sclerosing cholangitis is only rarely associated with Crohn's disease,[9] and bile-duct carcinoma has not been reported, whereas chronic active hepatitis and cirrhosis have a similar incidence in the two conditions. Granulomatous hepatitis and amyloidosis are more common in Crohn's disease than in ulcerative colitis.[65, 192] There is also an increased incidence of gallstones in patients with Crohn's disease, but not in ulcerative colitis.[109]

Although salazopyrine is occasionally hepatotoxic and patients with inflammatory bowel disease are at risk of developing hepatitis from repeated blood transfusions, the incidence of hepatic abnormalities is independent of the type of treatment used.

The aetiology of inflammatory bowel disease is unknown, as is that of most of the hepatic abnormalities with which it is associated. The relationship of the extra-intestinal manifestations of the disease, including the hepatic changes, to the bowel involvement is unclear. It is not known whether these manifestations indicate that inflammatory bowel disease is a generalized disorder or whether they are true complications of the colitis, possibly related to the presence of immune complexes.

Fatty Change

Fatty liver is common and may be found in up to 30 per cent of liver biopsies in patients with inflammatory bowel disease. Its presence is probably related more to general ill health and the severity of the underlying colitis than to any more specific factors. The incidence of fatty change in patients with ulcerative colitis at autopsy is similar to that of other debilitated patients.[219]

There are no symptoms, although on examination there may be hepatomegaly. Liver function tests are usually normal. Changes on light microscopy can be distinguished from fatty liver occurring in other conditions only if some diagnostic features of the other disease are present; for example, Mallory bodies and inflammatory infiltrate in alcoholics. No specific treatment is required and measures should be directed at improving general health and treating the underlying bowel disorder. Fatty change is a reversible condition and will return to normal when the patient's general health improves.

Pericholangitis

Otherwise known as portal triaditis, this is probably the commonest liver lesion associated with inflammatory bowel disease, and occurs in up to 30 per cent of cases with abnormal liver function tests.[50, 65] It is not confined to inflammatory bowel disease and is non-specific, occurring in other conditions, such as pancreatitis, abdominal sepsis and typhoid fever.

The histological appearance shows some similarity to non-specific reactive hepatitis, changes of early primary biliary cirrhosis,[231] benign idiopathic recurrent cholestasis[271, 308] and some cases of drug-induced hepatitis.

Pathogenesis

The nature and site of the inflammatory infiltrate has led to the hypothesis that pericholangitis is secondary to portal bacteraemia.[24, 33, 76] In support of this hypothesis, when enterobacteria, particularly *Escherichia coli*, have been cultured from portal blood taken at laparotomy from patients with inflammatory bowel disease, simultaneous cultures of liver biopsy tissue and systemic blood were sterile.[33] Subsequently, it was shown that a portal bacteraemia occurs in patients undergoing other abdominal operations who do not have inflammatory bowel disease or liver disease. Furthermore, there is no relationship between the presence of portal bacteraemia and the hepatic abnormalities.[76]

An alternative approach has been to attempt to produce pericholangitis in experimental models. This has been achieved by injection of *E. coli* and other bacteria. If *E. coli* are perfused into the portal vein of a calf's liver, an appearance resembling pericholangitis can be produced,[316] but these studies must be interpreted with caution.[147] Similar lesions have been produced around rodent bile ducts after injection of 1-phenylenedi-isothiocyanate.[266]

Early reports of broad-spectrum antibiotic therapy were encouraging,[236] but subsequent studies were disappointing.[203] These clinical studies make it doubtful that a portal bacteraemia, as a direct infection, is the cause of the pericholangitis.

Other theories of pathogenesis include the absorption of a potentially toxic substance, such as lithocolic acid,[218] and an autoimmune disturbance, but all are speculative.[147]

Clinical features

Usually pericholangitis is asymptomatic and liver function is normal.[202] When symptoms occur, they are often episodic and consist of jaundice, mild pruritus and fever with hepatomegaly. The commonest abnormality of liver function tests is mild elevation of the alkaline phosphatase.[315] Although it has been claimed that pericholangitis can progress to cirrhosis, with symptoms and signs of portal hypertension and hepatic cell failure,[200] it is usually reversible.[282] It is likely that the apparent progression to cirrhosis is sometimes due to sampling error on the initial liver biopsy. Radiography of the biliary tract may be needed to exclude obstructive jaundice. In a recent study on a selected group of patients, retrograde cholangiography showed abnormalities of the bile duct similar to those of sclerosing cholangitis.[21] This is an important finding and suggests that pericholangitis and sclerosing cholangitis may be the same condition, differing only in severity and distribution. Further studies on unselected patients, comparing histology with retrograde cholangiography, are needed.

Pathology

Acute and chronic pericholangitis have been described.[224, 225] The histological appearance of acute pericholangitis is of an inflammatory process limited to the portal tract and consisting of a mixed infiltrate of large and small lymphocytes, plasma cells, macrophages, neutrophils and occasional eosinophils. The infiltration surrounds the interlobular bile ducts, but it may be evenly distributed throughout the portal tract. The latter distribution cannot be distinguished from nonspecific reactive changes. Damage to bile-duct epithelium is unusual. In severe cases,

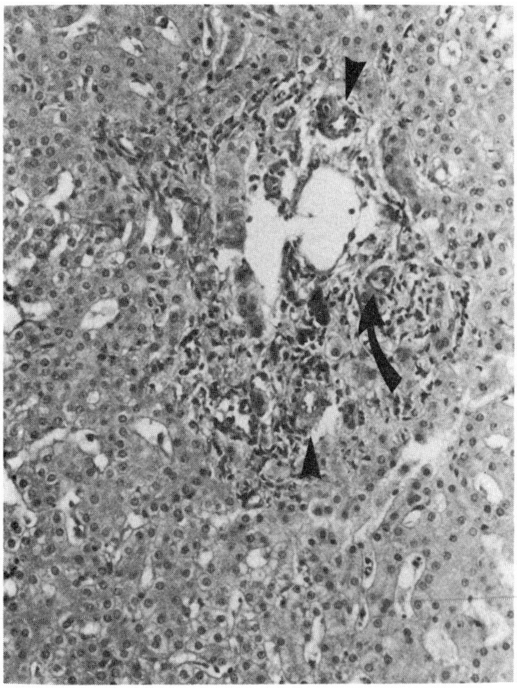

Figure 37.17. Portal tract showing chronic pericholangitis. The tract is expanded by new fibrous tissue with some bile ductule proliferation. There is a scanty mononuclear inflammatory infiltrate and the interlobular bile duct (arrow) is narrowed compared with the size of the arteries (arrowheads). The basement membrane around the bile duct is thickened. PAS × 500.

particularly if the biopsy coincides with a period of jaundice, there may be bile plugging of the canaliculi. Chronic pericholangitis shows sclerosis occurring around the bile duct with an associated chronic inflammatory cell infiltrate surrounding the bile duct (Figure 37.17) but the concentric collar of collagen that usually surrounds bile ducts can easily be mistaken for this feature of sclerosis.

There is also peripheral ductular proliferation expanding the portal tract, and the inflammatory process is less in evidence. Fibrosis may even traverse the hepatic lobules and when particularly severe this can resemble cryptogenic cirrhosis and may be difficult, purely on histological grounds, to distinguish from primary biliary cirrhosis. These changes can suggest chronic biliary obstruction and may result from the intrahepatic sclerosis of the bile ducts.

Treatment

Despite early reports, there is no evidence that antibiotics, corticosteroids or colectomy influence the course of the disease.[77, 225] The course is usually benign and once other causes of obstructive jaundice have been excluded treatment should be aimed at the relief of symptoms of cholestasis (see Chapter 54).

Sclerosing Cholangitis

This is a rare condition, occurring in less than 1 per cent of patients with ulcerative colitis.[324, 325] About one-third of all patients with sclerosing cholangitis have ulcerative colitis, and other associations include retroperitoneal fibrosis, sclerosing mediastinitis,[122, 260] Reidel's thyroiditis[15] and relapsing pancreatitis.[263] It has also been reported in immunodeficient states.[239] There have been only occasional case reports of sclerosing cholangitis occurring in patients with Crohn's disease.[9]

Clinical features

Clinical features are similar, with or without the presence of ulcerative colitis. The usual presentation is with jaundice, right-sided hypochondrial discomfort, pruritus and occasional fever. Weight loss and general malaise are common. Symptoms are frequently intermittent but can be progressive. In later stages, symptoms and

(a)

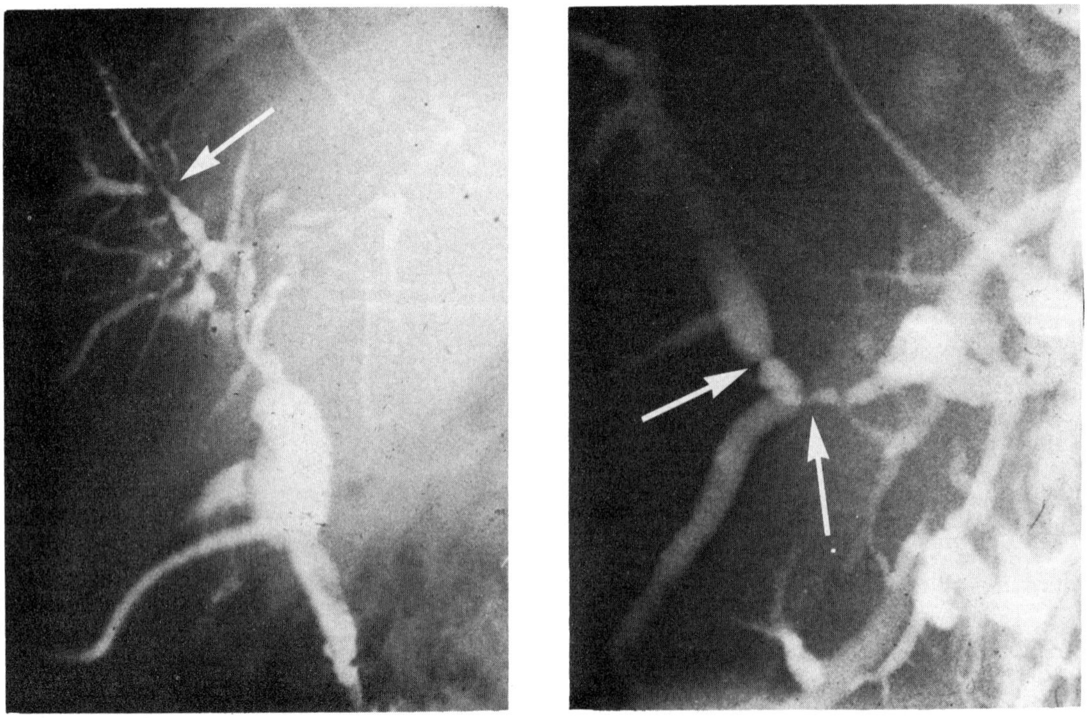

(b)

Figure 37.18. (a) Retrograde cholangiogram showing marked irregularity of the intrahepatic biliary tree with areas of stenosis (arrow) in sclerosing cholangitis. (b) High power detail of the stenotic intrahepatic lesion seen in Figure 37.18a.

signs of portal hypertension and liver-cell failure can occur. On examination, there may be hepatomegaly or jaundice. No specific features distinguish this condition from any other cause of obstructive jaundice, and the history can be suggestive of cholecystitis. The commonest abnormality of liver function tests is elevation of the alkaline phosphatase. There is no specific abnormality of immunoglobulins or autoantibodies.

The sclerosis usually affects both intra- and extrahepatic ducts and even the gallbladder.[304] Rarely, the intrahepatic ducts alone are affected.[18] We have seen one such patient where the intrahepatic ducts failed to fill adequately at endoscopic retrograde cholangiopancreatography (ERCP) and the gallbladder became distended; at autopsy she was found to have typical sclerosing cholangitis of the intrahepatic ducts with fibrous obliteration but without evidence of bile-duct carcinoma.

Until recently, sclerosing cholangitis was often diagnosed only at laparotomy for obstructive jaundice, but now an accurate diagnosis should be made, either by transhepatic percutaneous cholangiography (TPC) or ERCP. ERCP is thought by some to be better at detecting early changes than TPC. There may be irregular narrowing of the common bile duct with dilatation of the intrahepatic branches or, in the earlier cases, the intrahepatic ducts are diffusely and irregularly beaded and narrowed[97, 255] (Figure 37.18). Ultrasound or CAT scanning may show features of cirrhosis and occasionally irregular areas of intrahepatic bile-duct dilatation.[44] An important differential diagnosis is sclerosing carcinoma of the bile duct.

Pathology

Further support for the diagnosis can be obtained on liver biopsy, which may show narrowed ducts surrounded by dense fibrous tissue with features of large duct biliary obstruction (Figure 37.19) and sometimes secondary biliary cirrhosis. Rarely, there is intrahepatic sclerosis of the bile duct (Figure 37.20). Pericholangitis and primary sclerosing cholangitis are sometimes found in the same biopsy.[21, 304] There is considerable overlap histologically between chronic pericholangitis and sclerosing cholangitis. Even with the benefit of these investigations, laparotomy may still be necessary to establish thc diagnosis and finally to exclude gallstones or an intrahepatic bile-duct carcinoma.

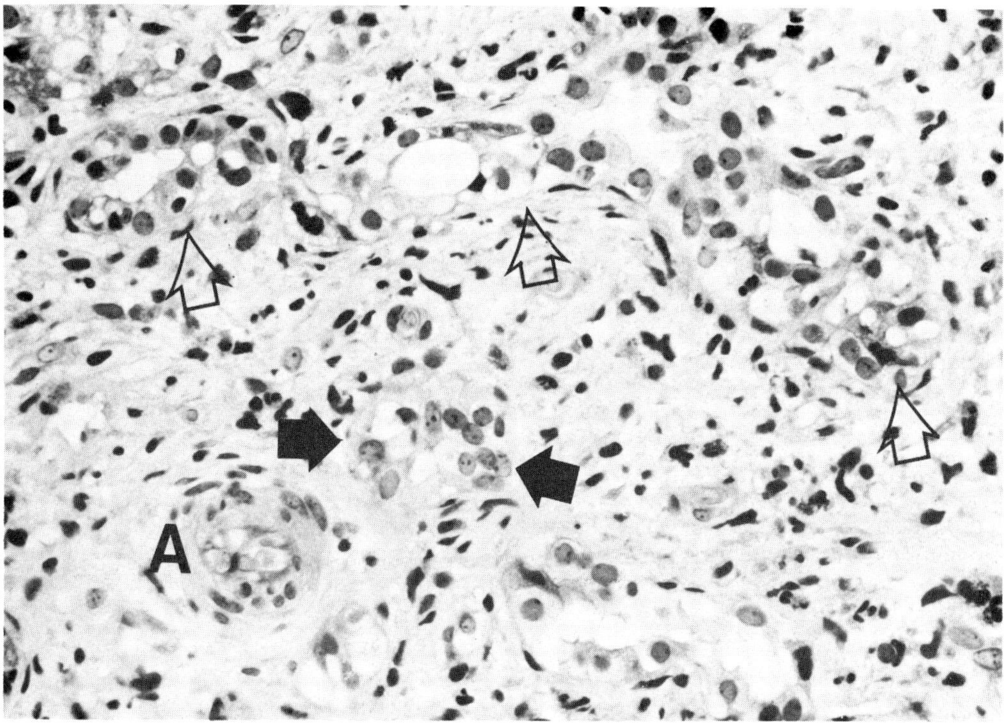

Figure 37.19. The interlobular bile duct (thick arrows) adjacent to the artery (A) is compressed and the lumen is further compromised by the degenerative and regenerative features in the epithelium. By contrast the bile duct (open arrows) along the edge of the portal tract is distended with a prominent lumen despite similar epithelial changes. Haematoxylin and eosin × 1250.

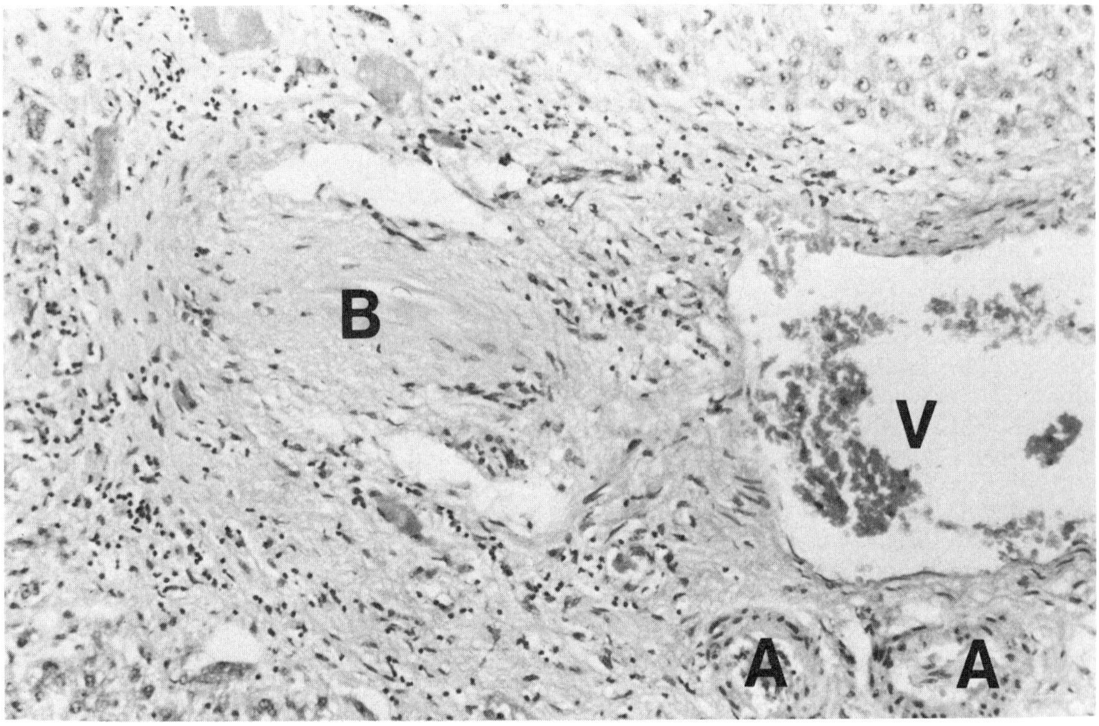

Figure 37.20. Portal tract showing portal vein (V), hepatic arteries (A) and a relatively acellular hyaline scar (B) marking the site of a missing bile duct of large interlobular or septal calibre. Haematoxylin and eosin × 750.

Treatment and prognosis

Medical treatment is unsatisfactory. Both steroids and broad-spectrum antibiotics have been used without benefit. In severe and progressive cases, surgical drainage of one of the large bile ducts should be attempted (see Chapter 54). There are few reports on prognosis, but this is usually poor, and if jaundice is present survival beyond four years is rare. Death is usually from portal hypertension or hepatic cell failure.[303, 324]

Cirrhosis

The complications of cirrhosis accounted for 10 per cent of all deaths in patients with ulcerative colitis over a 20-year period in one study.[80] In one autopsy study, cirrhosis occurred 12 times more commonly than in a control group.[219] In another series of 590 patients with cirrhosis, 20 were found to have inflammatory bowel disease.[129] The overall incidence of cirrhosis in inflammatory bowel disease is estimated to lie between 1 and 2 per cent.

The histological appearance is of a cryptogenic cirrhosis, and sometimes the features of chronic active hepatitis or sclerosing cholangitis may be recognized. As indicated above, the relationship between the pericholangitis and cirrhosis is unclear.

The clinical presentation and diagnosis of cirrhosis complicating inflammatory bowel disease is similar to that of other forms of cryptogenic cirrhosis or chronic active hepatitis. Although there have been reports of patients with inflammatory bowel disease developing primary biliary cirrhosis,[129, 314] it is doubtful whether a true association exists.

Chronic Active Hepatitis

This is an uncommon, although increasingly recognized, association of inflammatory bowel disease, occurring in about 1 per cent of patients.[80,224,225] The clinical features, histology and laboratory investigations of the liver disease are similar to chronic active hepatitis of unknown aetiology without inflammatory bowel disease[186] (see Chapter 29).

Granulomatous Hepatitis

This is occasionally seen in patients with Crohn's disease but is less frequently associated with ulcerative colitis.[65, 192] The clinical presentation is usually with mild pyrexia, hepatomegaly or non-specific abnormalities of liver function tests. Histologically, the epithelioid granulomas are randomly distributed throughout the liver lobule and cannot be distinguished from those occurring in a variety of other conditions.

Amyloidosis

This is a rare complication, occurring in less than 1 per cent of patients with inflammatory bowel disease. It is more commonly associated with Crohn's disease than ulcerative colitis.[275] Inflammatory bowel disease has been present on average for 10 years before amyloidosis develops, but this time interval can vary from one to 21 years. Although long-term survivals have been reported, and there has been one report of amyloidosis regressing following colectomy, this is exceptional and the prognosis is generally poor.[91]

Bile-duct Carcinoma

Although this is a rare complication of ulcerative colitis, carcinoma of the bile duct is estimated to occur about 10 times more frequently than in the general population.[2, 51, 81, 206, 251] There is no relationship to other pre-existing liver diseases, and cholelithiasis is not a feature. An increased incidence has not been reported in Crohn's disease.

Any part of the biliary tract, including the gallbladder, can be the site of the tumour. The ulcerative colitis is of long duration, having been present on average for approximately 15 years. Such patients tend to be about 20 years younger than those with bile-duct carcinoma without inflammatory bowel disease. Colectomy does not appear to protect against the development of the tumour.[246] The prognosis is poor and management is similar to that for other bile-duct carcinomas (see Chapter 54).

Cholelithiasis

The incidence of gallstones is increased in patients with Crohn's disease of the small bowel. The figure often quoted, about 30 per cent,[50, 120] is probably greater than the true incidence because of case selection. A more realistic figure is about 13 per cent.[109] The incidence of gallstones in ulcerative colitis and in Crohn's disease confined to the colon is around 5 per cent and is similar to that in the general population.[109]

The increased incidence of gallstones is due to a disturbance of bile salt metabolism as a result of disease of the terminal ileum.[1, 50, 68, 126, 317] Bile-salt absorption is reduced, due to disease of the terminal ileum or to surgical resection. Diarrhoea results, with excessive faecal loss of deoxycholic acid and other bile salts. The resulting fall in the bile-salt/cholesterol ratio in the gallbladder produces increased cholesterol precipitation and results in the formation of gallstones.

The Investigation of Jaundice in Inflammatory Bowel Disease

In patients with inflammatory bowel disease, liver biopsy is indicated if there is any clinical or laboratory evidence of underlying liver disease. If jaundice develops, it is investigated along the usual lines (see Chapter 26). If the features are those of an obstructive jaundice, a diagnosis of sclerosing cholangitis or bile-duct carcinoma should be considered, although other causes are numerically more common.

In patients with sclerosing cholangitis, TPC may be difficult, even with the 'skinny needle', so that endoscopic retrograde cholangiography is the investigation of choice.[86] It has the added advantage of showing early changes more readily. Histologically, there may be difficulty in identifying the aetiology and pathogenesis of an advanced cirrhosis, and diagnosis may then depend on clinical features. Associated autoantibodies and autoimmune conditions are helpful in diagnosis, as they are unusual in pericholangitis or sclerosing cholangitis.[164]

The Place of Colectomy in the Treatment of the Liver Disease

There has been much discussion about the role of colectomy in the treatment of the liver disease associated with inflammatory bowel disease. Some extra-intestinal manifestations of inflammatory bowel disease, such as arthritis and pyoderma gangrenosum, appear to be true complications of the intestinal lesion and respond dramatically to colectomy. It has been suggested that radical surgery might have a similar beneficial effect on the course of the liver disease,[75] but this is open to question.[166]

Clearly, established cirrhosis will not be affected, and the lost hepatic function will not be regained. The effect of colectomy on fatty infiltration and pericholangitis is clinically unimportant as these are benign conditions. Following colectomy, pericholangitis has been shown to stabilize[77, 202, 292] or progress.[202]

Of the more serious liver abnormalities, there have been occasional case reports of benefit following colectomy. It has been suggested but not proved that early surgery benefits patients with sclerosing cholangitis,[213] and chronic active hepatitis.[216] Unfortunately, the natural history of both conditions is variable and these reports must be taken with some scepticism. Colectomy does not prevent the development of bile-duct carcinoma.[246] There has been one report of regression of amyloidosis following surgery for inflammatory bowel disease.[91]

In our opinion, there is no indication at present to recommend colectomy on the grounds of possible benefit to the associated liver disease.

MALABSORPTION

The jejunal mucosa may show minor abnormalities in cirrhotic patients.[8, 14] Recently, interest has been shown in abnormalities of the liver in patients with coeliac disease. In one study, four out of 124 patients with coeliac disease were found to have abnormalities of liver function tests,[108] and these findings have been confirmed by others.[229] There have been case reports of coeliac disease associated with primary biliary cirrhosis,[180] cryptogenic cirrhosis,[45] chronic hepatitis[113] and hepatoma.[165] It is not clear whether these associations are coincidental or represent a true increase in incidence. Severe cases of coeliac disease show fatty change resulting from their malnutrition.

HLA-B8 is common in both coeliac disease and some forms of chronic liver disease, and an association on an autoimmune basis might be one explanation. Finally, in patients with coeliac disease who develop lymphoma, the liver is a common site of tumour spread.[135]
37.21).

Whipple's Disease

The liver is occasionally involved in Whipple's disease.[276]

RADIOTHERAPY AND THE LIVER

The liver is a relatively radio-resistant organ,[326] but hepatic abnormalities do occur occasionally, usually as the result of high doses of radiation such as are given to patients with lymphoma undergoing total abdominal irradiation. The changes appear to be dose-related[134] but are rare, although they can occur in patients having as little as 3000 rads. In one study, only two out of 117 patients undergoing total abdominal radiation developed any liver problems.[150]

Clinical Features

The clinical features vary, but the onset of symptoms usually occurs two to six weeks after completion of the radiation therapy. The most common features are abdominal discomfort, increasing abdominal girth and weight gain. On examination, there may be ascites, oedema and gross hepatomegaly. Non-specific abnormalities of all liver function tests occur, the most common being elevated alkaline phosphatase levels.[134, 150] Liver scan may show hepatomegaly and may suggest the presence of a space-occupying lesion.[150, 309]

Pathology

The liver shows changes, mainly in the centrilobular region. The general lobular architecture remains intact, but in the centrilobular region sinusoidal congestion and haemorrhage, together with atrophy of hepatocytes, may be found. There may also be intimal fibrous

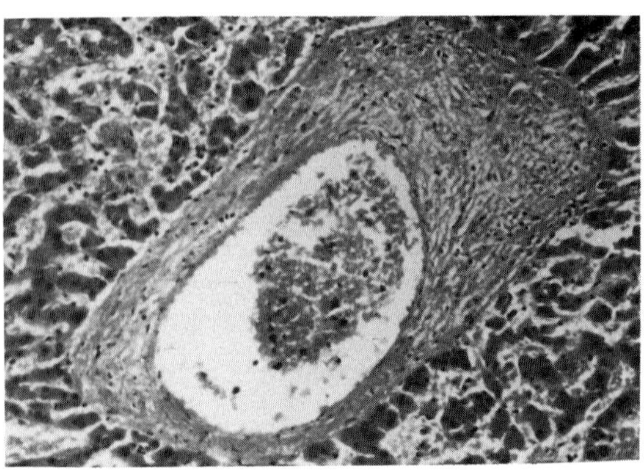

Figure 37.21. Radiation damage to the liver: there is a bland intimal fibrosis which considerably encroaches upon the lumen of the efferent central vein.

obliteration of the smaller branches of the hepatic vein[240] (Figure 37.21). These changes are reversible, and abnormalities of liver function, liver scans and histology usually disappear in a matter of weeks or months.

Pathogenesis

The pathogenesis of the hepatic changes is not clear-cut and could be either a direct effect of radiotherapy on the parenchymal cells or an indirect effect resulting from altered blood supply. Although tissue-specific antigen/antibody complexes may follow radiation, it is doubtful whether they play any significant role in the pathogenesis.

REFERENCES

1. Admirand, W.H. & Small, D. (1968) The physio-chemical basis for cholesterol gallstone formation in man. *Journal of Clinical Investigation,* **47,** 1043–1052.
2. Akwari, O.E., Van Heerden, J.A., Adson, M.A., Foulk, W. & Baggenstoss, A.H. (1976) Bile-duct carcinoma associated with ulcerative colitis. *Review of Surgery,* **33** (4), 289–293.
3. Alarcón-Segovia, D., Diaz-Jouanen, E. & Fishbein, E. (1973) Features of Sjögren's syndrome in primary biliary cirrhosis. *Annals of Internal Medicine,* **79,** 31–36.
4. Alarcón-Segovia, D., Fishbein, E. & Diaz-Jouanen, E. (1972) Presence of hepatitis-associated antigen in systemic lupus erythematosus. *Clinical and Experimental Immunology,* **12,** 9–19.
5. Alpers, D.H. & Isselbacher, K.J. (1975) Lipid metabolism and the liver. In *Diseases of the Liver* (Ed.) Schiff, L. 4th ed., pp. 815–832. Philadelphia: Lippincott.
6. Anthonisen, P., Christoffersen, P., Riis, P., Schourup, K. & Schwartz, M. (1966) Liver histology in ulcerative colitis. *Acta Medica Scandinavica,* **180,** 551–559.
7. Ariyan, S., Shessel, F.S. & Pickett, L.K. (1976) Cholecystitis and cholelithiasis masking as abdominal crisis in sickle cell disease. *Pediatrics,* **58,** 252–258.
8. Astaldi, G. & Strosselli, E. (1960) Peroral biopsy of the intestinal mucosa in hepatic cirrhosis. *American Journal of Digestive Diseases,* **5,** 603–612.
9. Atkinson, A.J. & Carroll, W.W. (1964) Sclerosing cholangitis. Association with regional enteritis. *Journal of the American Medical Association,* **188,** 183–184.
10. Bacon, P.A., Doherty, S.M. & Zuckerman, A.J. (1975) Hepatitis B antibody in polymyalgia rheumatica. *Lancet,* **ii,** 476–478.
11. Bagheri, S.A. & Boyer, J.L. (1974) Peliosis hepatitis associated with androgenic-anabolic steroid therapy. A severe form of hepatic injury. *Annals of Internal Medicine,* **81,** 610–618.
12. Bagoch, A., Casselman, W.G.B., Margolies, M.P. & Bockus, H.L. (1955) Liver disease in sickle cell anaemia. A correlation of clinical, biochemical, histological and histochemical observations. *American Journal of Medicine,* **19,** 583–609.
13. Ballard, H., Bernstein, M. & Farrar, T. (1961) Fatty liver presenting as obstructive jaundice. *American Journal of Medicine,* **30,** 196–201.
14. Baraona, E., Orreggo, H., Fernandez, O., Amenabar, E., Maldonado, E., Tag, F. & Salinas, A. (1967) Absorptive function of the small intestine in liver cirrhosis. *American Journal of Digestive Diseases,* **7,** 318–330.
15. Bartholomew, L., Cain, J., Woolner, L., Utz, O. & Ferris, D. (1963) Sclerosing cholangitis: its possible association with Riedel's strauma and fibrous retroperitonitis. Report of two cases. *New England Journal of Medicine,* **269,** 8–12.
16. Bartholomew, L.G., Cain, J.C., Winkleman, R.K. & Baggenstoss, A.H. (1964) Chronic disease of the liver associated with systemic scleroderma. *American Journal of Digestive Diseases,* **9,** 43–55.
17. Berthelot, P., Walker, J.G., Sherlock, S. & Reid, L. (1966) Arterial changes in the lungs in cirrhosis of the liver – lung spider naevi. *New England Journal of Medicine,* **274,** 291–298.
18. Bhathal, P.S. & Powell, L.W. (1969) Primary intrahepatic obliterating cholangitis. A possible variant of sclerosing cholangitis. *Gut,* **10,** 886–893.
19. Bianchi, L., Ohnacker, H., Beck, K. & Zimmerli-Ning, M. (1972) Liver damage in heatstroke and its regression. A biopsy study. *Human Pathology,* **3,** 237–248.
20. Bitnum, S., Daeschner, C.W., Travis, L.B., Dodge, W.F. & Hopps, H.C. (1964) Dermatomyositis. *Journal of Pediatrics,* **64,** 101–131.
21. Blackstone, M.O. & Nemchausky, B.A. (1978) Cholangiographic abnormalities in ulcerative colitis-associated pericholangitis which resembles sclerosing cholangitis. *American Journal of Digestive Diseases,* **23,** 579–585.
22. Blendis, L.M., Ansell, I.D., Lloyd-Jones, K., Hamilton, E. & Williams, R. (1970) Liver in Felty's syndrome. *British Medical Journal,* **i,** 131–135.
23. Blendis, L.M., Parkinson, M.C., Shilkin, K.B. & Williams, R. (1974) Nodular regenerative hyperplasia of the liver in Felty's syndrome. *Quarterly Journal of Medicine,* **43,** 25–32.
24. Boden, R.W., Rankin, J.G., Goulston, S.J.M. & Morrow, W. (1959) The liver in ulcerative colitis: the significance of raised serum alkaline phosphatase levels. *Lancet,* **ii,** 245–248.
25. Borchadt, K.A., Stansifer, P. & Albano, P.M. (1966) Osteomyelitis due to *Pseudomonas pseudomallei. Journal of the American Medical Association,* **196,** 660–663.
26. Bousser, J., Littoum, R., Patarin, J.M. & Sultan, C. (1964) Angiome et cirrhose hépatique dans la maladie du Rendu Osler. *Semaine des Hôpitaux de Paris,* **40,** 2716–2721.
27. Bradus, S., Korn, R.J., Chomet, B., West, M. & Zimmerman, H.J. (1963) Hepatic function and serum enzyme levels in association with fatty metamorphosis of the liver. *American Journal of the Medical Sciences,* **246,** 35–41.
28. Brandt, K., Cathcart, E. & Cohen, A.S. (1968) Clinical analysis of the course and prognosis of 42 patients with amyloidosis. *American Journal of Medicine,* **44,** 955–969.

29. Branson, J.H. & Park, J.H. (1954) Sarcoidosis – hepatic involvement: presentation of a case with fatal liver involvement, including autopsy findings and review of the evidence for sarcoid involvement of the liver as found in the literature. *Annals of Internal Medicine,* **40,** 111–145.
30. Briggs, W.G. (1961) Amyloidosis. *Annals of Internal Medicine,* **55,** 943–957.
31. Britt, B.A. (1975) Malignant hyperthermia. In *Metabolic Aspects of Anaesthesia* (Ed.) Cohen, P.J. pp. 61–74. Philadelphia: F.A. Davis.
32. Bron, K.M. & Gajaraj, A. (1970) Demonstration of hepatic aneurysm in polyarthritis nodosum by arteriography. *New England Journal of Medicine,* **282,** 1024–1025.
33. Brooke, B.N. & Slaney, G. (1958) Portal bacteraemia in ulcerative colitis. *Lancet,* **i,** 1206–1207.
34. Buerk, K. & Smith, M. (1972) Polymyalgia rheumatica. *Lancet,* **ii,** 715–716.
35. Buhac, I., Agrawal, A.B. & Park, S.K. (1976) Jaundice and bridging centrilobular necrosis of liver in circulating failure. *New York State Journal of Medicine,* **76,** 678–682.
36. Bushkin, F.L., MacGregor, A.M.C., Hawkins, I.F. & Kelley, M.J. (1972) Hepatic artery dissection as a result of abdominal trauma. *Surgery, Gynecology and Obstetrics,* **135,** 721–726.
37. Bruckstein, A.H. (1978) Oxacillin hepatitis: two patients with liver biopsy, and review of the literature. *American Journal of Medicine,* **64,** 519–522.
38. Carroll, R. (1963) Infarction of the human liver. *Journal of Clinical Pathology,* **16,** 133–136.
39. Carson, M.J., Chadwick, D.L., Brubaker, C.A., Cheland, R.S. & Landing, B.H. (1965) Thirteen boys with progressive septic granulomatosis. *Pediatrics,* **35,** 405–412.
40. Cawley, E.P. (1947) Aspergillosis and aspergilli; report of a unique case of the disease. *Archives of Internal Medicine,* **80,** 423–434.
41. Chapin, L.E., Scudamore, H.H., Baggenstoss, A.H. & Bargen, J.A. (1956) Regional enteritis, associated visceral changes. *Gastroenterology,* **30,** 404–415.
42. Cheitlin, M.D., Sullivan, B.H., Myers, J.E. & Hench, R.F. (1960) Portal hypertension in hepatic sarcoidosis. *Gastroenterology,* **38,** 60–69.
43. Christoffersen, P., Braendstrup, O., Juhl, E. & Poulsen, H. (1971) Lipogranulomas in human liver biopsies with fatty change. *Acta Pathologica et Microbiologica Scandinavica,* **79,** 150–158.
44. Clinical-Gastroenterology Conference, Cello, J.P. (1977) Cholestasis in ulcerative colitis. *Gastroenterology,* **73,** 357–374.
45. Clinical-pathological Conference (1970) A case of malabsorption; intestinal mucosal atrophy and ulceration, cirrhosis and emphysema. *British Medical Journal,* **iii,** 207–212.
46. Clowes, G.H. & O'Donnell, T.F. (1974) Heat stroke. *New England Journal of Medicine,* **291,** 564–567.
47. Cockel, R., Kendall, M.J., Becker, J.F. & Hawkins, C.F. (1971) Serum biochemical values in rheumatoid arthritis. *Annals of the Rheumatic Diseases,* **30,** 166–170.
48. Cohen, A.E. (1967) Amyloidosis. *New England Journal of Medicine,* **277,** 522–530; 574–583; 628–638.
49. Cohen, J.A. & Kaplan, M.N. (1978) Left-sided heart failure presenting as hepatitis. *Gastroenterology,* **74,** 583–587.
50. Cohen, S., Kaplan, M., Gottlieb, L. & Patterson, J. (1971) Liver disease and gallstones in regional enteritis. *Gastroenterology,* **60,** 237–245.
51. Converse, C.F., Reagan, J.W. & De Cosse, J.J. (1971) Ulcerative colitis and carcinoma of the bile duct. *American Journal of Surgery,* **121,** 39–45.
52. Cook, G.C. & Hutt, M.S.R. (1967) The liver after kwashiorkor. *British Medical Journal,* **iii,** 454–457.
53. Copeman, P.W.M. & Medd, W.E. (1967) Diffuse systemic sclerosis with abnormal liver and gall bladder. *British Medical Journal,* **iii,** 353–354.
54. Cornes, J.S. & Stecher, M. (1961) Primary Crohn's disease of the colon and rectum. *Gut,* **2,** 189–201.
55. Cowan, R.E., Mallinson, C.N., Thomas, G.E. & Thomson, A.D. (1977) Polyarteritis nodosa of the liver; a report of two cases. *Postgraduate Medical Journal,* **53,** 89–93.
56. Craig, J.R., Hillberg, R.H. & Balchum, O.J. (1975) Disseminated coccidiodomycosis. Diagnosis by needle biopsy. *Western Journal of Medicine,* **122,** 171–174.
57. Dahlin, D.C. (1950) Classification and general aspects of amyloidosis. *Medical Clinics of North America,* **34,** 1107–1111.
58. D'Angelo, W.A., Fries, J.F., Masi, A.T. & Shulman, L.E. (1969) Pathologic observations in systemic sclerosis (scleroderma). *American Journal of Medicine,* **46,** 428–440.
59. Dawson, B., Tidy, H.L. & Spicer, J.E. (1909) Statistics of ulcerative colitis from the London Hospital. *Proceedings of the Royal Society of Medicine,* **2,** 107–109.
60. Dedombal, F.T., Goldie, W., Watts, J.McK. & Golliger, J.C. (1966) Hepatic histological changes in ulcerative colitis. *Scandinavian Journal of Gastroenterology,* **1,** 220–227.
61. Degott, C., Rueff, B., Kreis, H., Du Boust, A., Fotet, F. & Benhamou, J.P. (1978) Peliosis hepatis in recipients of renal transplants. *Gut,* **19,** 748–753.
62. Dickson, E.R., Maldonado, J.E. & Sheps, S.G. (1973) Systemic giant-cell arteritis with polymyalgia rheumatica. Reversible abnormalities of liver function. *Journal of the American Medical Association,* **224,** 1496–1498.
63. Dietrichson, O., From, A., Christoffersen, P. & Juhl, E. (1976) Morphological changes in liver biopsies from patients with rheumatoid arthritis. *Scandinavian Journal of Rheumatology,* **5,** 65–69.
64. Dikman, S.H., Kahn, T., Gribetz, D. & Churg, J. (1977) Resolution of renal amyloidosis. *American Journal of Medicine,* **63,** 430–433.
65. Dordal, E., Glagov, S. & Kirsner, J.B. (1967) Hepatic lesions in chronic inflammatory bowel disease. I. Clinical correlations with liver biopsy diagnoses in 103 patients. *Gastroenterology,* **52,** 239–253.
66. Dordal, E., Glagov, S., Orlando, R.A. & Platz, C. (1970) Fatal halothane hepatitis with transient granulomas. *New England Journal of Medicine,* **283,** 357–359.
67. Doxiades, T., Candreviotis, N., Yiotsas, Z.D. & Smyrniotis, F.E. (1963) Chronic amoebic hepatitis. Clinical and experimental observations. *Archives of Internal Medicine,* **111,** 219–225.
68. Dowling, R.H., Bell, G.D. & White, J. (1972) Lithogenic bile in patients with ileal dysfunction. *Gut,* **13,** 415–420.
69. Drenick, E.J. (1970) Effect on hepatic morphology and treatment of obesity by fasting, reducing diets and small bowel .bypass. *New England Journal of Medicine,* **282,** 829–834.

70. Drury, R.A.B. (1962) Larval granulomata in the liver. *Gut*, **3**, 289–294.
71. Dubois, E.L. & Tuffanelli, D.L. (1964) Clinical manifestations of systemic lupus erythematosus; computer analysis of 520 patients. *Journal of the American Medical Association*, **190**, 104–111.
72. Dunlap, R.W., Hallenbeck, G.A. & Hanlon, D.G. (1952) Portal hypertension associated with sarcoidosis and with hemochromatosis. Report of two cases with splenectomy and splenorenal anastomosis. *Proceedings of Staff Meeting, Mayo Clinic*, **27**, 266–272.
73. Dunn, G.D., Hayes, P., Breen, K.J. & Schenker, S. (1973) The liver in congestive heart failure – a review. *American Journal of Medical Science*, **265**, 174–189.
74. Dupont, H.L., Hornick, R.B., Levin, H.S., Rapaport, M.I. & Woodward, T.E. (1971) Q fever hepatitis. *Annals of Internal Medicine*, **74**, 198–206.
75. Eade, M.N. (1970) Liver disease in ulcerative colitis. I. Analysis of operative liver biopsy in 138 consecutive patients having colectomy. *Annals of Internal Medicine*, **72**, 475–487.
76. Eade, M.N. & Brooke, B.N. (1969) Portal bacteraemia in cases of ulcerative colitis submitted to colectomy. *Lancet*, **i**, 1008–1010.
77. Eade, M.N., Cooke, W.T. & Brooke, B.N. (1970) Liver disease and ulcerative colitis. II. The long-term effect of colectomy. *Annals of Internal Medicine*, **72**, 489–497.
78. Eade, M.N., Cooke, W.T., Brooke, B.N. & Thompson, H. (1971) Liver disease in Crohn's colitis. A study of 21 consecutive patients having colectomy. *Annals of Internal Medicine*, **74**, 518.
79. Edland, J.F. (1972) Liver disease in heroin addicts. *Human Pathology*, **3**, 75–84.
80. Edwards, F.C. & Truelove, S.C. (1963) The course and prognosis of ulcerative colitis. *Gut*, **4**, 299–315.
81. Edwards, F.C. & Truelove, S.C. (1964) The course and prognosis of ulcerative colitis. Part III. Complications. *Gut*, **5**, 1–15.
82. Edwards, H. (1964) Crohn's disease. *Journal of the Royal College of Surgeons, Edinburgh*, **9**, 115–127.
83. Ehrlick, G. (1976) Sjögren's syndrome and liver disease in rheumatoid arthritis. In *Non-articular Forms of Rheumatoid Arthritis* (Ed.) Feltkamp, T.E.W. pp. 242–244. Leyden: Staffen's Scientific Publishing.
84. Ein, D., Kimura, S. & Terry, W.D. (1972) Aminoacid sequence of an amyloid fibril protein of unknown origin. *Journal of Biological Chemistry*, **247**, 5653–5655.
85. Eliakim, M., Eisenberg, S., Levij, I. & Sacks, T. (1968) Granulomatous hepatitis accompanying a self-limited febrile illness. *Lancet*, **i**, 1348–1352.
86. Elias, E., Summerfield, J.A., Dick, R. & Sherlock, S. (1974) Endoscopic retrograde cholangiopancreatography in the diagnosis of jaundice associated with ulcerative colitis. *Gastroenterology*, **67**, 907–911.
87. Ellman, M.H., Weis, M.J. & Spellberg, M.A. (1974) Liver disease in rheumatoid arthritis. *American Journal of Gastroenterology*, **62**, 46–53.
88. Farrell, G.C., Uren, R.F., Perkins, K.W., Joshua, D.G., Baird, P.J. & Kronenberg, H. (1975) Androgen-induced hepatoma. *Lancet*, **i**, 430–432.
89. Fauci, A.S. & Wolff, S.M. (1973) Wegener's granulomatoma: studies in 18 patients and a review of the literature. *Medicine*, **52**, 535–561.
90. Fauci, A.S. & Wolff, S.M. (1976) Granulomatous hepatitis. In *Progress in Liver Diseases* (Ed.) Popper, H. & Schaffner, F. Vol. 5, pp. 609–621. New York: Grune & Stratton.
91. Fitcher, J.H. (1975) Amyloidosis and granulomatous ileocolitis. Regression after surgical removal of the involved bowel. *New England Journal of Medicine*, **292**, 352–353.
92. Fox, R.A., James, D.G., Scheuer, P.J., Sharm, O. & Sherlock, S. (1969) Impaired delayed hypersensitivity in primary biliary cirrhosis. *Lancet*, **i**, 959–962.
93. Franklyn, E.C. (1974) The complexity of amyloid. *New England Journal of Medicine*, **290**, 512–513.
94. Freese, M. & Lyons, E.A. (1977) Ultrasound bankscatter from human liver: its dependence on frequency and protein/lipid components. *Journal of Clinical Ultrasound*, **5**, 307–312.
95. Fung, W.P., Chew, B.K. & Tan, K.K. (1969) Active chronic hepatitis with positive LE cell test and lupus nephritis. *Australasian Annals of Medicine*, **18**, 288–291.
96. Gafni, J. & Sohar, E. (1960) Rectal biopsy for the diagnosis of amyloidosis. *American Journal of the Medical Sciences*, **240**, 332–336.
97. Geisse, G., Nelson, G.C., Tedesco, F.J., Kelly, J.J. & Stanley, R.J. (1975) Sclerosing lesions of the biliary tree: evaluation with endoscopic retrograde cholangiography (ERC) and percutaneous transhepatic cholangiography. *American Journal of Roentgenology, Radiotherapy and Nuclear Medicine*, **123**, 378–385.
98. Gelb, A.M., Brazenas, N., Sussman, H. & Wallach, R. (1970) Acute granulomatous disease of the liver. *American Journal of Digestive Diseases*, **15**, 844–847.
99. Geltner, D., Chajek, T. & Rubinger, D. (1976) Quinidine hypersensitivity and liver involvement. A survey of 32 patients. *Gastroenterology*, **70**, 650–652.
100. Gerard, A.G., Roth, A.L., Becker, S.M. & Shih, C.S. (1968) Regression of sarcoid hepatosplenomegaly on corticosteroid therapy. *Journal of the Medical Society of New Jersey*, **65**, 64–67.
101. Gibbs, P. (1974) Polymyalgia rheumatica and liver disease. *Lancet*, **i**, 351–352.
102. Glenner, G.G., Terry, W.D. & Isersky, C. (1973) Amyloidosis: its nature and pathogenesis. *Seminars in Hematology*, **10**, 65–86.
103. Glenner, G.G., Cuatrecasas, P., Isersky, C., Bladen, H.A. & Eanes, E.D. (1969) Physical and chemical properties of amyloid fibres. II. Isolation of a unique protein constituting the major component from human splenic amyloid fibril concentrates. *Journal of Histochemistry and Cytochemistry*, **17**, 769–780.
104. Glick, E.N. (1972) Raised serum alkaline phosphatase levels in polymyalgia rheumatica. *Lancet*, **ii**, 328.
105. Goergen, T.G., Taylor, A. & Alazraki, N. (1976) Lack of gallium uptake in primary hepatic amyloidosis. *American Journal of Roentgenology*, **126**, 1246–1248.
106. Golding, P.L., Brown, R., Mason, A.M.S. & Taylor, E. (1970) 'Sicca complex' in liver disease. *British Medical Journal*, **iii**, 340–344.
107. Good, R.A., Quie, P.G., Windhorst, D.B., Page, A.R., Rodez, G.E. & White, J. (1968) Fatal (chronic) granulomatous disease of childhood: a hereditary defect of leukocyte function. *Seminars in Hematology*, **5**, 215–254.

108. Green, P.A. & Wollaeger, E.E. (1960). The clinical behaviour of sprue in the United States. *Gastroenterology*, **38,** 399–418.
109. Greenstein, A.J., Jarowitz, H. & Sachar, D. (1976) Extraintestinal complications of Crohn's disease and ulcerative colitis: a study of 700 patients. *Medicine*, **55,** 401–412.
110. Gregg, J.A., Herskovic, T. & Bartholomew, L.G. (1965) Ascites in systemic amyloidosis. *Archives of Internal Medicine*, **116,** 605–610.
111. Guckian, J.C. & Perry, J.E. (1966) Granulomatous hepatitis. An analysis of 63 cases and review of the literature. *Annals of Internal Medicine*, **65,** 1081–1100.
112. Guida, P.M. & Moore, S.W. (1966) Aneurysm of the hepatic artery. Report of five cases with a brief review of the previously reported cases. *Surgery*, **60,** 299–310.
113. Hagander, B., Berg, N.O., Brandt, L., Norden, A., Sjolund, K. & Stenstam, M. (1977) Hepatic injury in adult coeliac disease. *Lancet*, **ii,** 270–272.
114. Hamilton, P.K., Hutchison, H.S., Jamieson, P.W. & Jones, H.L. (1959) The pathology and pathogenesis of the hepatosplenic disease associated with schistosomiasis; Egyptian splenomegaly. *American Journal of Clinical Pathology*, **32** (1), 18–33.
115. Harris, M., Rash, R.M. & Dymock, I.W. (1974) Nodular, non-cirrhotic liver associated with portal hypertension in a patient with rheumatoid arthritis. *Journal of Clinical Pathology*, **27,** 963–966.
116. Hart, F.D. (1969) Rheumatoid arthritis, extra-articular manifestations. *British Medical Journal*, **iii,** 131–136.
117. Harvey, A.M., Schulman, L.E., Tumulty, P.A., Conley, C.L. & Schoenrick, E.H. (1954) Systemic lupus erythematosus. Review of the literature and clinical analysis of 138 patients. *Medicine*, **33,** 291–437.
118. Harvier, P. & Borduelle, M. (1947) Sclérodermie progressive avec calcification hépato-splénique. *Presse Médicale*, **55,** 369–370.
119. Hathaway, B.M. & Mason, K.N. (1962) Nocardiosis: study of fourteen cases. *American Journal of Medicine*, **32,** 903–909.
120. Heaton, K.W. & Read, A.E. (1969) Gall stones in patients with disorders of the terminal ileum and disturbed bile salt metabolism. *British Medical Journal*, **iii,** 494–496.
121. Heller, H., Missmahl, H.P., Sohar, E. & Gafni, J. (1964) Amyloidosis: its differentiation into peri-reticulin and peri collagen types. *Journal of Pathology and Bacteriology*, **88,** 15–34.
122. Hellstrom, H.R. & Perez-Stable, E.C. (1966) Retroperitoneal fibrosis with disseminated vasculitis and intrahepatic sclerosing cholangitis. *American Journal of Medicine*, **40,** 184–187.
123. Herman, R.H. & Sullivan, B.H. (1959) Heatstroke and jaundice. *American Journal of Medicine*, **27,** 154–166.
124. Hermodson, M.A., Kuhn, R.W. & Walsh, K.A. (1972) Aminoacid sequence of monkey amyloid protein. *Biochemistry*, **11,** 2934–2938.
125. Hill, D.E., Lobell, M. & Edwards, J.E. (1974) Primary dissecting aneurysm of the hepatic artery. *Archives of Internal Medicine*, **133,** 471–474.
126. Hill, G.L., Mair, W.S.J. & Goligher, J.C. (1975) Gallstones after ileostomy and ileal resection. *Gut*, **16,** 932–936.
127. Holden, W.D., De Palma, R.G., Drucker, W.R. & McKalen, A. (1968) Ultrastructural changes in haemorrhagic shock: electron microscopic study of liver, kidney and striated muscle cells in rats. *Annals of Surgery*, **162,** 517–536.
128. Holdstock, G. & Wright, R. (1978) Unpublished observation.
129. Holdsworth, C.D., Hall, E.W., Dawson, A.M. & Sherlock, S. (1965) Ulcerative colitis in chronic liver disease. *Quarterly Journal of Medicine*, **34,** 211–227.
130. Holtzman, I.N. (1961) Sarcoidosis followed by biliary cirrhosis and xanthelomatosis. *New York Journal of Medicine*, **61,** 1757–1764.
131. Hoylumpa, A.N., Greene, H.L., Dunn, D. & Schernher, S. (1975) Fatty liver: biochemical and clinical considerations. *American Journal of Digestive Diseases*, **20,** 1142–1170.
132. Husby, G., Sletten, K. & Michaelsen, T.E. (1972) Antigenic and chemical characterisation of non-immunoglobulin amyloid proteins. *Scandinavian Journal of Immunology*, **1,** 393–400.
133. Hutt, M.S. (1971) Some aspects of liver disease in Ugandan Africans. *Transactions of the Royal Society of Tropical Medicine and Hygiene*, **65,** 273–285.
134. Ingold, J.A., Reed, G.B., Kaplan, H.S. & Bagshaw, M.A. (1965) Radiation hepatitis. *American Journal of Roentgenology*, **93,** 200–208.
135. Isaacson, P. & Wright, D.H. (1978) Intestinal lymphoma associated with malabsorption. *Lancet*, **i,** 67–70.
136. Ishak, K.G., Kirchner, J.P. & Dhar, J.K. (1977) Granulomas and cholestatic-hepatocellular injury associated with phenylbutazone. Report of two cases. *American Journal of Digestive Diseases*, **22,** 611–617.
137. Isobe, T. & Osserman, E. (1974) Patterns of amyloidosis and their association with plasma cell dyscrasia, monoclonal immunoglobulins and Bence Jones proteins. *New England Journal of Medicine*, **290,** 473–477.
138. Jori, G.P. & Peschle, C. (1973) Hydralazine disease associated with transient granulomas in the liver. *Gastroenterology*, **64,** 1163–1167.
139. Joske, R.A. & Finckh, E.S. (1955) Hepatic changes in human brucellosis. *Medical Journal of Australasia*, **1,** 266–269.
140. Kadin, M.E., Donaldson, S.S. & Dorfman, R.F. (1970) Isolated granulomas in Hodgkin's disease. *New England Journal of Medicine*, **283,** 859–861.
141. Kanter, D.M. (1965) Hepatic infarction. *Archives of Internal Medicine*, **115,** 479–481.
142. Kapp, J.P. (1965) Hepatic amyloidosis with portal hypertension. *Journal of the American Medical Association*, **191,** 497–499.
143. Karat, A.B.A., Job, C.K. & Rao, P.S.S. (1971) Liver in leprosy; histological and biochemical findings. *British Medical Journal*, **i,** 307–310.
144. Kasolcharoen, P. & Magnia, G.F. (1976) Liver dysfunction in polymyalgia rheumatica: a case report. *Journal of Rheumatology*, **3,** 50–53.
145. Kelley, M.L. & McHardy, R.J. (1955) An unusual case of fatal hepatic sarcoidosis. *American Journal of Medicine*, **18,** 842–850.
146. Kendall, M.J., Bold, A.M., Farr, M. & Hawkins, C.F. (1971) 5-nucleotidase in the serum and synovial fluid of patients with rheumatoid disease. *Lancet*, **ii,** 1012–1013.

147. Kern, F. (1976) Hepatobiliary disorders in inflammatory bowel disease. In *Progress in Liver Diseases* (Ed.) Popper, H. & Schaffner, F. Vol. 5, pp. 575–589. New York: Grune & Stratton.
148. Khaleque, K.A. & Alam, K.S. (1963) Hepatic granuloma caused by Ascaris ova. *Journal of Tropical Medicine and Hygiene,* **66,** 249–251.
149. Kiernan, F. (1833) The anatomy and physiology of the liver. J.H. Green, *Philosophical Transactions,* Royal Society of London.
150. Kim, T.H., Panahon, A.M., Friedman, M. & Webster, J.H. (1976) Acute transient radiation hepatitis following whole abdominal irradiation. *Clinical Radiology,* **27,** 449–454.
151. King, L.S. (1948) Atypical amyloid disease; with observations on a new silver stain for amyloid. *American Journal of Pathology,* **24,** 1095–1115.
152. Kinney, T.D. & Marker, M.M. (1940) Dermatomyositis – a study of five cases. *American Journal of Pathology,* **16,** 561–594.
153. Kisloff, B. & Schaffer, G. (1976) Fulminant hepatic failure secondary to congestive heart failure. *American Journal of Digestive Diseases,* **21,** 895–900.
154. Klatskin, G. (1975) Toxic and drug-induced hepatitis. In *Diseases of the Liver* (Ed.) Schiff, L. 4th ed., pp. 604–710. Philadelphia: Lippincott.
155. Klatskin, G. & Yesner, R. (1950) Hepatic manifestations of sarcoidosis and other granulomatous diseases. A study based on histological examination of tissue obtained by needle biopsy of the liver. *Yale Journal of Biology and Medicine,* **23,** 207–248.
156. Kleckner, M.S., Stauffer, M.H., Bargen, J.A. & Docherty, M.B. (1952) Hepatic lesions in the living patients with chronic ulcerative colitis as demonstrated by needle biopsy. *Gastroenterology,* **22,** 13–33.
157. Kliesch, W.F., Young, P.C. & Davis, W.D. (1969) Dangers of prolonged anticoagulant therapy in hepatic disease. *Journal of the American Medical Association,* **209,** 1186–1190.
158. Knapp, W.A. & Ruebner, B.H. (1974) Hepatomas and oral contraceptives. *Lancet,* **i,** 270–271.
159. Koenig, M.G., Collins, R.D. & Heyszel, R. (1966) Disseminated mycobacteriosis caused by Battey type mycobacteria. *Annals of Internal Medicine,* **64,** 145–154.
160. Kornreich, H., Malouf, N.N. & Hanson, V. (1971) Acute hepatic dysfunction in juvenile rheumatoid arthritis. *Journal of Pediatrics,* **79,** 27–35.
161. Krauser, R.E. (1976) Spontaneous rupture of the spleen in lupus erythematosus. *Journal of the American Medical Association,* **236** (10), 1149.
162. Kuhlbäck, B. & Wegelius, O. (1966) Secondary amyloidosis. A study of clinical and pathological findings. *Acta Medica Scandinavica,* **180,** 737–745.
163. Kyle, R.A. & Bayrd, E. (1975) Amyloidosis. Review of 236 cases. *Medicine,* **54,** 271–299.
164. Lam, K., Mistilis, S.P. & Perrett, N. (1972) Positive tissue antibody tests in patients with prolonged extrahepatic biliary obstruction. *New England Journal of Medicine,* **286,** 1400–1402.
165. Lancaster-Smith, M.J., Perrin, J., Swarbrick, E.T. & Wright, J.T. (1974) Coeliac disease and autoimmunity. *Postgraduate Medical Journal,* **50,** 45–48.
166. *Lancet* (1970) The liver in ulcerative colitis (Editorial). *Lancet,* **ii,** 402–403.
167. Leevy, C.M. (1962) Fatty liver: a study of 270 patients with biopsy-proven fatty liver and a review of the literature. *Medicine,* **41,** 249–276.
168. Lender, M. & Wolf, E. (1972) Incidence of amyloidosis in rheumatoid arthritis. *Scandinavian Journal of Rheumatology,* **1,** 109–112.
169. Leopold, J.G., Parry, T.E. & Storring, F.F. (1971) A change in the sinusoid trabecular structure of the liver with hepatic venous outflow block. *Journal of Pathology,* **100,** 87–98.
170. Levin, M., Franklyn, E.C. & Frangione, B. (1972) The aminoacid sequence of a major non-immunoglobulin component of some amyloid fibrils. *Journal of Clinical Investigation,* **51,** 2773–2776.
171. Levine, R.A. (1962) Amyloid disease of the liver. Correlation of clinical, functional and morphologic features in 47 patients. *American Journal of Medicine,* **33,** 349–357.
172. Levitin, P.M., Sweet, D., Brunner, C.M., Kathou, R.E. & Bolton, W.K. (1977) Spontaneous rupture of the liver: an unusual complication of SLE. *Arthritis and Rheumatism,* **20,** 748–750.
173. Levy, M., Fry, D.C. & Eliakin, M. (1971) Intrahepatic obstructive jaundice. *Gastroenterology,* **61,** 234–238.
174. Liang, M., Greenberg, H., Pincus, T. & Robinson, W.S. (1976) Hepatitis B antibody in polymyalgia rheumatica. *Lancet,* **i,** 43.
175. Lieber, C.S. (1974) Effects of ethanol upon lipid metabolism. *Lipids,* **9,** 103–116.
176. Lieber, C.S., Spritz, N. & De Carli, L.M. (1966) Role of dietary, adipose and endogenously synthesized fatty acids in the pathogenesis of the alcoholic fatty liver. *Journal of Clinical Investigation,* **45,** 51–62.
177. Lister, J.D. (1899) A specimen of diffuse ulcerative colitis with secondary diffuse hepatitis. *Transactions of the Pathology Society of London,* **50,** 130–135.
178. Litwack, K.D., Bohan, A. & Silverman, L. (1977) Granulomatous liver disease and giant cell arteritis. Case report and literature review. *Journal of Rheumatology,* **4,** 307–312.
179. Lloyd-Davies, R.W. & Forbes, G.B. (1965) Sarcoidosis of the gall bladder. *Gastroenterology,* **49,** 287–290.
180. Logan, R., Ferguson, A., Finlayson, N. & Weir, D.G. (1978) Primary biliary cirrhosis and coeliac disease. *Lancet,* **i,** 230–233.
181. Long, R. & James, O. (1974) Polymyalgia rheumatica and liver disease. *Lancet,* **i,** 77–79.
182. Lowenstein, J. & Gallo, G. (1970) Remission of the nephrotic syndrome in renal amyloidosis. *New England Journal of Medicine,* **28,** 128–132.
183. Luna, A., Meister, H.P. & Zanto, P.B. (1968) Oesophageal varices in the absence of cirrhosis. Incidence and characteristics of congestive heart failure and neoplasm of the liver. *American Journal of Clinical Pathology,* **49,** 710–717.
184. Lyford, J., Johnson, R.W., Blackman, S. & Scott, R.B. (1946) Pathologic findings in a fatal case of disseminated granuloma inguinale with miliary bone and joint involvement. *Bulletin of the Johns Hopkins Hospital,* **79,** 349–357.
185. MacKay, A.G. & Page, H.G. (1959) Hematemesis associated with hemobilia. *New England Journal of Medicine,* **260,** 468–471.
186. MacKay, I.R. & Wood, I.J. (1962) Lupoid hepatitis: a comparison of 22 cases with other types of chronic liver disease. *Quarterly Journal of Medicine,* **31,** 485–507.
187. MacKay, I.R., Taft, L. & Cowling, D.C. (1959) Lupoid hepatitis and the hepatic lesions of systemic lupus erythematosus. *Lancet,* **i,** 65–69.

188. MacKay, I.R., Waden, F. & Husker, J. (1965) Autoimmune hepatitis. *Annals of the New York Academy of Sciences,* **124,** 767–768.

189. Maddrey, W., Johns, C., Boitnott, J. & Iber, F. (1970) Sarcoidosis and chronic hepatitic disease: a clinical and pathological study of 20 patients. *Medicine,* **49,** 375–395.

190. Martini, G.A. (1978) The liver in hereditary haemorrhagic telangiectasia: an inborn error of vascular structure with multiple manifestation – a reappraisal. *Gut,* **19,** 531–537.

191. Mather, G., Dawson, J. & Hoyle, C. (1955) Liver biopsy in sarcoidosis. *Quarterly Journal of Medicine,* **24,** 331–350.

192. Maurier, L.H., Hughes, R.W., Folley, J.H. & Mosenthal, W.T. (1967) Granulomatous hepatitis associated with regional enteritis. *Gastroenterology,* **53,** 301–305.

193. Mayock, R.L., Bertrand, P., Morrison, C.E. & Scott, J.H. (1963) Manifestations of sarcoidosis. Analysis of 145 patients, with a review of nine series selected from the literature. *American Journal of Medicine,* **35,** 67–89.

194. Mays, E.T. & Wheeler, C.S. (1974) Demonstration of collateral arterial flow after interruption of hepatic arteries in man. *New England Journal of Medicine,* **290,** 993–996.

195. Medline, A., Cohen, L.B., Tobe, B.A. & Sellars, E.N. (1978) Liver granulomas and allopurinol. *British Medical Journal,* **ii,** 1320–1321.

196. Miller, A.C. & Reid, W.M. (1976) Methyldopa-induced granulomatous hepatitis. *Journal of the American Medical Association,* **235,** 2001–2002.

197. Millward-Sadler, G.H. (1978) Personal observation.

198. Millward-Sadler, G.H., Clarke, C.W. & Joseph, A.E. (1978) Unpublished observation.

199. Mir-Madjlessi, S.H., Farmer, R.G. & Hawk, W.A. (1973) Granulomatous hepatitis. A review of 50 cases. *American Journal of Gastroenterology,* **60,** 122–133.

200. Mistilis, S.P. (1965) Pericholangitis and ulcerative colitis. I. Pathology, etiology and pathogenesis. *Annals of Internal Medicine,* **63,** 1–16.

201. Mistilis, S.P., Green, J.R. & Schriff, L. (1964) Hepatic sarcoidosis with portal hypertension. *American Journal of Medicine,* **36,** 470–475.

202. Mistilis, S.P., Skyring, A.P. & Goulston, S.J.M. (1965) Pericholangitis and ulcerative colitis. II. Clinical aspects. *Annals of Internal Medicine,* **63,** 17–26.

203. Mistilis, S.P., Skyring, A.P. & Goulston, S.J.M. (1965) Effect of long-term tetracycline therapy, steroid therapy and colectomy in pericholangitis associated with ulcerative colitis. *Australasian Annals of Medicine,* **14,** 286–294.

204. Mohammed, S.D. (1965) Reversible non-metastatic liver-cell dysfunction and thrombocytosis from a hypernephroma. *Lancet,* **ii,** 621–623.

205. Morgan, M.Y. (1973) Primary biliary cirrhosis, scleroderma and kerato-conjunctivitis sicca. *Proceedings of the Royal Society of Medicine,* **66,** 1112.

206. Morowitz, D.A., Glagov, S., Dordal, E. & Kirsner, J.B. (1971) Carcinoma of the biliary tract complicating chronic ulcerative colitis. *Cancer,* **27,** 356–361.

207. Mowrey, F.H. & Lundberg, E.A. (1954) The clinical manifestations of essential polyangiitis (periarteritis nodosa) with emphasis on the hepatic manifestations. *Annals of Internal Medicine,* **40,** 1145–1164.

208. Murray-Lyon, I.M., Thompson, R.P.H., Ansell, I.D. & Williams, R. (1970) Scleroderma and primary biliary cirrhosis. *British Medical Journal,* **iii,** 258–261.

209. Myers, J.D. & Hickam, J.B. (1948) An estimation of the hepatic blood flow and splanchnic oxygen consumption in heart failure. *Journal of Clinical Investigation,* **27,** 620–627.

210. Nadell, J. & Kosek, J. (1977) Peliosis hepatitis. *Archives of Pathological and Laboratory Medicine,* **101,** 405–410.

211. Nelson, R.S. & Schwabe, A.D. (1966) Progressive hepatic decompensation with terminal hepatic coma in sarcoidosis. Report of a case. *American Journal of Digestive Diseases,* **11,** 495–501.

212. Nelson, R.S. & Sears, M.E. (1968) Massive sarcoidosis of the liver. Report of two cases. *American Journal of Digestive Diseases,* **13,** 95–106.

213. Nugent, F.W., Shea, J.A., Haggitt, R.C. & Glaser, D. (1976) Sclerosing cholangitis in inflammatory bowel disease. *Gastroenterology,* **70,** 972 (Abstract 114).

214. O'Connor, P.J., Buhac, I. & Balint, J.A. (1976) Spontaneous hepatic artery thrombosis with infarction of the liver. *Gastroenterology,* **70,** 599–601.

215. Oliai, A. & Koff, R.S. (1972) Primary amyloidosis presenting as 'sicca complex' and severe intrahepatic cholestasis. *American Journal of Digestive Diseases,* **17,** 1033–1036.

216. Olson, R. & Hulten, L. (1975) Concurrence of ulcerative colitis and chronic active hepatitis – clinical course and result of colectomy. *Scandinavian Journal of Gastroenterology,* **10,** 331–334.

217. O'Sullivan, J.P. & Wilding, R.P. (1974) Liver hamartomas in patients on oral contraceptives. *British Medical Journal,* **iii,** 7–10.

218. Palmer, R.H. (1972) Bile acids, liver injury and liver disease. *Archives of Internal Medicine,* **130,** 606–617.

219. Palmer, W.L., Kirsner, J.B., Goldgraber, M.B. & Fuentes, S.S. (1964) Disease of the liver in chronic ulcerative colitis. *American Journal of Medicine,* **36,** 856–866.

220. Parker, J.C., McCloskey, J.J. & Knauer, K.A. (1976) Pathobiologic features of human candidiasis. *American Journal of Clinical Pathology,* **65,** 91–100.

221. Parker, R.G.F. (1955) Arterial infarction of liver in man. *Journal of Pathology and Bacteriology,* **70,** 521–528.

222. Parkins, R.A. & Bywaters, E.G.L. (1959) Regression of amyloidosis secondary to rheumatoid arthritis. *British Medical Journal,* **i,** 536–540.

223. Parr, I.J. (1935) Infarction of liver. *American Journal of Pathology,* **11,** 503.

224. Perrett, A.D., Higgins, G., Johnston, H.H., Massarella, G.R., Truelove, S.C. & Wright, R. (1971) The liver in Crohn's disease. *Quarterly Journal of Medicine,* **40,** 187–209.

225. Perrett, A.D., Higgins, G., Johnston, H.H., Massarella, G.R., Truelove, S.C. & Wright, R. (1971) The liver in ulcerative colitis. *Quarterly Journal of Medicine,* **40,** 211–238.

226. Petersdorf, R.G. & Beeson, P.B. (1961) Fever of unexplained origin – report on 100 cases. *Medicine,* **40,** 1–30.

227. Pinkerton, H. & Iverson, L. (1952) Histoplasmosis; three fatal cases with disseminated sarcoid-like lesions. *American Medical Association Archives of Internal Medicine,* **90,** 456–467.

228. Pollard, H.M. & Block, M. (1948) Association of hepatic insufficiency with chronic ulcerative colitis. *Archives of Internal Medicine,* **82,** 159–174.
229. Pollock, D.J. (1977) The liver in coeliac disease. *Histopathology,* **1,** 421–424.
230. Poltera, A.A. & Katsimbura, N. (1974) Granulomatous hepatitis due to *Strongyloides stercoralis. Journal of Pathology,* **113,** 241–246.
231. Popper, H. & Schaffner, F. (1957) *The Liver Structure and Function.* New York: McGraw Hill. 404 pp.
232. Porter, G.H. (1961) Hepatic sarcoidosis. A cause of portal hypertension and liver failure; review. *Archives of Internal Medicine,* **108,** 483–495.
233. Preston, F.E., Triger, D.R., Underwood, J.C.E., Bardhan, G., Mitchell, V.E., Stewart, R.M. & Blackburn, E.K. (1978) Percutaneous liver biopsy and chronic liver disease in haemophiliacs. *Lancet,* **ii,** 592–594.
234. Pullen, R.L. & Stuart, B.N. (1945) Tularemia – analysis of 225 cases. *Journal of the American Medical Association,* **129,** 495–500.
235. Rafoth, R.J. (1974) Systemic granulomatous reaction to salicylazosulfapyridine (AZULFIDINE) in a patient with Crohn's disease. *American Journal of Digestive Diseases,* **19,** 465–469.
236. Rankin, J.G., Boden, R.W., Goulston, S. & Morrow, A.W. (1959) The liver in ulcerative colitis. Treatment of pericholangitis in patients with tetracycline. *Lancet,* **ii,** 1110–1112.
237. Ray, C.J. & Wedgewood, R.J. (1964) Neonatal listeriosis: six case reports and a review of the literature. *Pediatrics,* **34,** 378–392.
238. Recknagel, R.D. (1967) Carbon tetrachloride hepatotoxicity. *Pharmacological Review,* **19,** 145–208.
239. Record, L.O., Eddleston, A.L.W.F., Shilkin, K.B. & Williams, R. (1973) Intrahepatic sclerosing cholangitis associated with a familial immunodeficiency syndrome. *Lancet,* **ii,** 18–20.
240. Reed, G.B. & Cox, A.J. (1966) The human liver after radiation injury. *American Journal of Pathology,* **48,** 597–611.
241. Reimann, H.A., Koncky, R.F. & Eklund, C.M. (1935) Primary amyloidosis limited to tissue of mesodermal origin. *American Journal of Pathology,* **ii,** 977–988.
242. Reller, L.B. (1973) Granulomatous hepatitis associated with acute cytomegalovirus infection. *Lancet,* **i,** 20–22.
243. Reynolds, T.B., Denison, E.K., Frankl, H.D., Lieberman, F.L. & Peters, R.L. (1971) Primary biliary cirrhosis with scleroderma, Raynaud's phenomenon and telangectasia. New syndrome. *American Journal of Medicine,* **50,** 302–312.
244. Richman, S.M., Delman, A.J. & Grob, D. (1961) Alteration in indices of liver function in congestive heart failure with particular reference to serum enzymes. *American Journal of Medicine,* **30,** 211–225.
245. Rigberg, L.A., Robinson, M.J. & Espiritu, C.R. (1976) Chlorpropamide-induced granulomas. A probable hypersensitivity reaction in liver and bone marrow. *Journal of the American Medical Association,* **235,** 409–410.
246. Ritchie, J.K., Allan, R.N., Macartney, J., Thompson, H., Hawley, P.R. & Cooke, W.T. (1974) Biliary tract carcinoma associated with ulcerative colitis. *Quarterly Journal of Medicine,* **43,** 263–279.
247. Rodman, T., Sobel, M. & Close, H.P. (1960) Arterial oxygen unsaturation and the ventilation-perfusion defect of Laennec's cirrhosis. *New England Journal of Medicine,* **263,** 73–77.
248. Rosen, R.S. & Janeway, C.A. (1966) The gamma-globulin. III. The antibody deficiency syndrome. *New England Journal of Medicine,* **275,** 769–775.
249. Rosenblate, H.J., Eisenstein, R. & Holmes, A.W. (1970) The liver in sickle cell anemia. A clinical-pathologic study. *Archives of Pathology,* **90,** 235–245.
250. Rosenblatt, M.B. (1934) The clinical manifestations of amyloidosis. *Annals of Internal Medicine,* **8,** 678–689.
251. Ross, A.P. & Braasch, J.W. (1973) Ulcerative colitis and carcinoma of the proximal bile ducts. *Gut,* **14,** 94–97.
252. Rougier, P., Degott, C., Rueff, B. & Benhamou, J.P. (1978) Nodular regenerative hyperplasia of the liver. *Gastroenterology,* **75,** 169–172.
253. Rubin, E. & Lieber, C.S. (1968) Alcohol-induced hepatic injury in non-alcoholic volunteers. *New England Journal of Medicine,* **278,** 869–876.
254. Rudzki, C., Ishak, K.G. & Zimerman, H.J. (1975) Chronic intrahepatic cholestasis of sarcoidosis. *American Journal of Medicine,* **59,** 373–387.
255. Ruskin, R., Katon, R., Bilboa, M.K. & Smith, F. (1976) Evaluation of sclerosing cholangitis by endoscopic retrograde cholangiopancreatography. *Annals of Internal Medicine,* **136,** 232–235.
256. Safran, A.P. & Shaffner, F. (1967) Chronic passive congestion of the liver in man. Electron microscopic study of cell atrophy and intralobular fibrosis. *American Journal of Pathology,* **50,** 447–463.
257. Sanders, R. & Child, C. (1960) Primary amyloidosis with jaundice. *Journal of the American Medical Association,* **174,** 1202–1204.
258. Schaller, J., Beckwith, B. & Wedgewood, R.J. (1970) Hepatic involvement in juvenile rheumatoid arthritis. *Journal of Pediatrics,* **77,** 203–210.
259. Scheuer, P.J. (1972) Systemic disease, pregnancy and organ transplantation. In *Liver Biopsy Interpretation.* p. 130. London: Baillière Tindall.
260. Schneider, C.F. (1964) Idiopathic retroperitoneal fibrosis producing vena caval, biliary, ureteral and duodenal obstructions. *Annals of Surgery,* **159,** 316–320.
261. Schroder, R., Eltringham, W.K., Gumpert, J.R.W., Plath, J.R. & Zollinger, R.M.J. (1969) The role of the liver in the development of lactic acidosis in low flow states. *Postgraduate Medical Journal,* **45,** 566–570.
262. Schwarz, J. & Muth, J. (1951) Coccidiomycocis: review. *American Journal of Medical Science,* **221,** 89–107.
263. Schwartz, S.I. & Dale, W.A. (1958) Primary sclerosing cholangitis; review and report of six cases. *American Medical Association Archives of Surgery,* **77** (3), 439–451.
264. Seaman, W.E., Ishak, K.G. & Plotz, P.H. (1974) Aspirin-induced hepatotoxicity in patients with systemic lupus erythematosus. *Annals of Internal Medicine,* **8,** 1–8.
265. Seki, H., Takamara, Y. & Kono, T. (1975) An autopsy case of systemic amyloidosis with hepatic failure. *Japanese Journal of Gastroenterology,* **72,** 385–391.
266. Selye, H. & Szabo, S. (1972) Experimental production of cholangitis by 1.4 phenylenedisothiocyanate. *Annals of Pathology,* **94,** 486–488.
267. Seneviratne, R.D. (1949) Physiological and pathological responses in the blood vessels of the liver. *Quarterly Journal of Experimental Physiology,* **35,** 77–110.

268. Sestoft, L., Poulsen, H. & Winkler, K. (1971) Collagen disease debuting as acute hepatitis. *Scandinavian Journal of Gastroenterology,* **6,** 495–500.

269. Shaldon, S. & Sherlock, S. (1962) Portal hypertension in the myeloproliferative syndrome and the reticuloses. *American Journal of Medicine,* **32,** 758–764.

270. Shapiro, E. & Weiner, H. (1951) The diagnosis of tertiary syphilis of liver: 25 years after McCrae. *American Journal of the Medical Sciences,* **222,** 494–499.

271. Shapiro, R. & Isselbacher, K.J. (1963) Benign recurrent intrahepatic colestasis. *New England Journal of Medicine,* **268,** 708–711.

272. Sherlock, S. (1951) The liver in heart failure; relation of anatomical, functional and circulatory changes. *British Heart Journal,* **13,** 273–293.

273. Shields, L.H. (1959) Disseminated cryptococcus producing a sarcoid-type reaction: the report of a case treated with Amphotericin B. *Archives of Internal Medicine,* **104,** 763–770.

274. Shirahama, T. & Cohen, A.S. (1967) High resolution electron microscopic analysis of the amyloid fibril. *Journal of Cellular Biology,* **33,** 679–708.

275. Shorvan, P.J. (1977) Amyloidosis and inflammatory bowel disease. *Digestive Diseases,* **22** (3), 209–213.

276. Sieracki, J.C. & Fine, G. (1959) Whipple's disease – observations on systemic involvement. II. Gross and histologic observations. *American Medical Association Archives of Pathology,* **67,** 81–93.

277. Silver, H., Hall, E., Hill, K., Shaldon, S. & Sherlock, S. (1965) Renal involvement in active juvenile cirrhosis. *Journal of Clinical Pathology,* **18,** 157–163.

278. Simmons, F., Feldman, B. & Gerety, D. (1972) Granulomatous hepatitis in a patient receiving allopurinol. *Gastroenterology,* **62,** 101–104.

279. Simon, H.B. & Wolfe, S. (1973) Granulomatous hepatitis and prolonged fever of unknown origin. A study of 13 patients. *Medicine,* **52,** 1–21.

280. Simon, H.B. & Wolfe, S. (1974) Sarcoidosis and hepatic granulomatosis. *Annals of Internal Medicine,* **80,** 560–561.

281. Skinner, M.S., Kattine, A.A. & Spurlock, B.O. (1966) Electron microscopic observations of early amyloidosis in human liver. *Gastroenterology,* **50,** 243–247.

282. Slavin, S. & Keynan, A. (1972) Acute pericholangitis as the initial manifestation of fulminant ulcerative colitis. *Israel Journal of Medical Science,* **8,** 1716–1720.

283. Sletten, K., Westermark, P. & Natvig, J.B. (1976) Characteristics of amyloid fibril proteins from medullary carcinoma of the thyroid. *Journal of Experimental Medicine,* **143,** 993–998.

284. Sokolov, R.A., Rachmaninoff, N. & Kaine, H.D. (1962) Allergic granulomatosis. *American Journal of Medicine,* **32,** 131–141.

285. Song, Y.S. (1957) Hepatic lesions in sickle cell anemia. *American Journal of Pathology,* **33,** 331–352.

286. Sostre, S., Martin, N.D., Lucas, R.N. & Strauss, H.W. (1975) Scintigraphic findings in primary amyloidosis. An analysis of 7 cases. *Radiology,* **115,** 675–677.

287. Spain, D.M. & Riley, R.L. (1944) Jaundice in amyloidosis of the liver. *American Journal of Clinical Pathology,* **14,** 284–288.

288. Starzl, T.E., Groth, G.C., Brettschneider, L., Moon, J.B., Fulginiti, V.A., Cotton, E.K. & Porter, K.A. (1968) Extended survival in 3 cases of orthopic homotransplantation of the human liver. *Surgery,* **63,** 549–563.

289. Stauffer, M.H. (1961) Nephrogenic hepatosplenomegaly. *Gastroenterology,* **40,** 694.

290. Stauffer, M.H. & Dahlin, D.C. (1969) Amyloidosis of the liver. In *Diseases of the Liver* (Ed.) Schiff, L. 3rd ed., pp. 965–973. Philadelphia: Lippincott.

291. Stauffer, M.H., Gross, J.B., Foulk, W.T. & Dahlin, D.C. (1961) Amyloidosis: diagnosis with needle biopsy of the liver in 18 patients. *Gastroenterology,* **41,** 92–96.

292. Stauffer, M.H., Sauer, W.G., Dearing, W.H. & Baggenstoss, A.H. (1965) The spectrum of cholestatic hepatic disease. *Journal of the American Medical Association,* **191,** 829–837.

293. Stirling, W.A. (1975) Amyloidosis. In *Recent Advances in Pathology* (Ed.) Harrison, C.V. & Weinbeck, K. pp. 249–272. London: Churchill.

294. Sukerkar, A., Dulay, C.G., Anandappa, E. & Asokan, S. (1977) Mycotic aneurysm of the hepatic artery. *Radiology,* **124,** 444.

295. Sullivan, A., Rheinlander, H. & Weintraub, L.R. (1974) Esophageal varices in agnogenic myeloid metaplasia. Disappearance after splenectomy. *Gastroenterology,* **66,** 429–432.

296. Sullivan, S., Hamilton, E.B.D. & Williams, R. (1978) Rheumatoid arthritis and liver involvement. *Journal of the Royal College of Physicians,* **12,** 418–422.

297. Summerskill, W.H.J. & Shorter, R.G. (1967) Progressive hepatic failure. Its association with undifferentiated renal tumour. *Archives of Internal Medicine,* **120,** 81–84.

298. Sweeny, E.C. (1975) Adult (α_1) antitrypsin deficiency. *Journal of Clinical Pathology,* **28,** 613–619.

299. Symmers, W. St C. (1950–51) Portal embolism following thrombosis of splenic vein, and causing infarct-like cyanotic atrophy ('Zahn's infarcts') of the liver. A complication of splenectomy performed in the course of total gastrectomy. *British Journal of Surgery,* **38,** 498–502.

300. Tewby, P.N., Warren, R., Contini, S., Crosby, W., Wilkinson, S.P., Laws, J.N. & Williams, R. (1978) Incidence and pathophysiology of pulmonary oedema in fulminant hepatic failure. *Gastroenterology,* **74,** 859–865.

301. Thomas, G.H. (1874) Ulceration of the colon with enlarged fatty liver. *Transactions of the Pathology Society, Philadelphia,* **4,** 87–93.

302. Thomford, N.R., Hamelberg, W.E. & Wielderholt, W.C. (1969) Sudden hyperpyrexia during general anaesthesia. *Surgery,* **66,** 850–855.

303. Thompson, B.W., Read, R.C. & White, H.J. (1972) Sclerosing cholangitis. *Archives of Surgery,* **104,** 460–463.

304. Thorpe, M.E.C., Scheuer, P.J. & Sherlock, S. (1967) Primary sclerosing cholangitis, the biliary tree, and ulcerative colitis. *Gut,* **8,** 435–448.

305. Tiber, A.M., Pearlman, A.W. & Cohen, S.E. (1941) Hepatic function in patients with amyloidosis. *Archives of Internal Medicine,* **68,** 309–324.

306. Trell, E., Johansson, B.W., Linell, F. & Ripa, J. (1972) Familial pulmonary hypertension and multiple abnormalities of large systemic arteries in Osler's disease. *American Journal of Medicine,* **53,** 50–63.

307. Triger, D.R. & Wright, R. (1973) Hyperglobulinaemia in liver disease. *Lancet,* **i,** 1494–1496.

308. Tygstrup, N. (1960) Intermittent possibly familial intrahepatic cholestatic jaundice. *Lancet,* **i,** 1171–1172.
309. Usselman, J.A. (1966) Liver scanning in the assessment of liver damage from therapeutic external radiation. *Journal of Nuclear Medicine,* **7,** 761–772.
310. Utz, D.C., Warren, M.M., Gregg, J.A., Ludwig, J. & Kelalis, P. (1970) Reversible hepatic dysfunction associated with hypernephroma. *Mayo Clinic, Proceedings,* **45,** 161–169.
311. Van Patter, W.N., Bargen, J.A., Docherty, M.D., Feldman, W.H., Maye, C.W. & Waugh, J.M. (1954) Regional enteritis. *Gastroenterology,* **26,** 347–350.
312. Vanselow, N.A., Dodson, V.N., Angell, D.C. & Duff, I.F. (1963) A clinical study of Sjögren's syndrome. *Annals of Internal Medicine,* **58,** 124–135.
313. Vescia, F.G. & Peck, O.C. (1962) Liver disease from heat stroke. *Gastroenterology,* **43,** 340–343.
314. Vinnik, I.E. & Kern, F. (1963) Biliary cirrhosis in a patient with chronic ulcerative colitis. *Gastroenterology,* **45,** 529–534.
315. Vinnik, I.E., Kern, F. & Gorley, W.D. (1963) Serum 5-nucleotidase and pericholangitis in patients with chronic ulcerative colitis. *Gastroenterology,* **45,** 492–498.
316. Vinnik, I.E., Kern, F., Struthers, J.E., Hills, R.B. & Guzak, S. (1964) Experimental chronic portal vein bacteraemia. *Proceedings of the Society for Experimental and Biological Medicine,* **115,** 311–314.
317. Vlahcevic, Z.R., Bell, C., Buhac, I., Farrar, J.T. & Swell, L. (1970) Diminished bile acid pool size in patients with gallstones. *Gastroenterology,* **59,** 165–173.
318. Volwiler, W. & Jones, C.M. (1947) The diagnostic and therapeutic value of liver biopsies, with particular reference to trocar biopsy. *New England Journal of Medicine,* **237,** 651–656.
319. Wagoner, G., Anton, A., Gall, E. & Shiff, L. (1953) Needle biopsy of the liver; experiences with hepatic granulomata. *Gastroenterology,* **25,** 487–494.
320. Waldenström, H. (1928) Formation and disappearance of amyloid in man. *Acta Chirurgica Scandinavica,* **63,** 479–530.
321. Walsh, P.N. & Kissane, J.M. (1968) Non-metastatic hypernephroma with reversible hepatic dysfunction. *Archives of Internal Medicine,* **122,** 214–222.
322. Ward, H.P. & Block, M.H. (1971) The natural history of agnogenic myeloid metaplasia (AMM) and a critical evaluation of its relationship with the myeloproliferative syndrome. *Medicine,* **50,** 357–420.
323. Warren, K.S., Domingo, E.O. & Cowan, R.B.J. (1967) Granuloma formation around schistosoma eggs as a manifestation of delayed hypersensitivity. *American Journal of Pathology,* **51,** 735–756.
324. Warren, K.W. & Tan, E.C.G. (1975) Disease of the gall bladder and bile-ducts. In *Diseases of the Liver* (Ed.) Schiff, L. 4th ed., pp. 1319–1323. Philadelphia: Lippincott.
325. Warren, K.W., Athanassiades, S. & Monge, J.I. (1966) Primary sclerosing cholangitis. A study of forty-two cases. *American Journal of Surgery,* **111,** 23–38.
326. Warren, S. (1942) Effects of radiation on normal tissues. IV. Effects of radiation on gastrointestinal tract, including salivary glands, liver and pancreas. *Archives of Pathology,* **34,** 749–787.
327. Waugh, D. (1952) Myocarditis, arteritis and focal hepatic, splenic and renal granulomas apparently due to penicillin sensitivity. *American Journal of Pathology,* **28,** 437–447.
328. Webb, J., Whaley, K., MacSween, R.N.M., Nuki, G., Dick, W.C. & Buchanan, W.W. (1975) Liver disease in rheumatoid arthritis and Sjögren's syndrome. Prospective study using biochemical and serological markers of hepatic dysfunction. *Annals of the Rheumatic Diseases,* **34,** 70–81.
329. Weinbren, K. & Tarsh, E. (1964) The mitotic response in the rat liver after different regenerative stimuli. *British Journal of Experimental Pathology,* **45,** 475–480.
330. Weston, M.J., Talbot, I.C., Howorth, P.J.N., Mant, A.K., Capildeo, R. & Williams, R. (1976) Frequency of arrhythmias and other cardiac abnormalities in fulminant hepatic failure. *British Heart Journal,* **38,** 1179–1188.
331. Whaley, K., Goudie, R.B., Williamson, J., Nuki, G., Dick, W.C. & Buchanan, L.W. (1970) Liver disease in Sjögren's syndrome and rheumatoid arthritis. *Lancet,* **i,** 861–863.
332. Whelan, G., Pierce, A.K., Schenker, S. & Combes, B. (1969) Hepatic function in patients with hypoxaemia due to chronic pulmonary disease. *Australasian Annals of Medicine,* **18,** 243–247.
333. Witorsch, P. & Utz, J.P. (1968) North American blastomycosis. A study of 40 patients. *Medicine,* **47,** 169–200.
334. Wong, M. & Rosen, S.W. (1962) Ascites in sarcoidosis due to peritoneal involvement. *Annals of Internal Medicine,* **57,** 277–280.
335. Wright, J.R., Calkins, E. & Humphrey, R.L. (1977) Potassium permanganate reaction in amyloidosis. A histologic method to assist in differentiating forms of this disease. *Laboratory Investigation,* **36,** 274–281.
336. Yanoff, M. & Rawson, A.J. (1967) Peliosis hepatitis: an anatomic study with demonstration of two varieties. *Archives of Pathology,* **77,** 159–165.
337. Zahn, F.W. (1898) *Verhardlungen der Gesellschaft deutscher Naturforscher und Arzte Braunschweig,* **2,** 9–15.
338. Zak, F.G. (1950) Peliosis hepatis. *American Journal of Pathology,* **26,** 1–15.
339. Zawadzki, Z.A. & Edwards, G.A. (1970) Dysimmunoglobulinaemia associated with hepatobiliary disorders. *American Journal of Medicine,* **48,** 196–202.
340. Zelman, S. (1962) Liver fibrosis in hereditary hemorrhagic telangiectasia; fibrosis of diffuse insular character. *Archives of Pathology,* **74,** 66–72.
341. Zetzel, L. (1947) Hepatomegaly with jaundice due to primary amyloidosis. *Gastroenterology,* **8,** 783–787.
342. Zilko, P.J. & Dawkins, R.L. (1975) Amyloidosis associated with dermatomyositis and features of multiple myeloma. *American Journal of Medicine,* **59,** 448–452.
343. Banner, B.F. & Banner, A.S. (1979) Hepatic granulomas following ileal bypass for obesity. *Archives of Pathology and Laboratory Medicine,* **102,** 655–657.

Chapter 38

Hepatic Tumours

M.M. SCHONLAND
G.H. MILLWARD-SADLER
D.H. WRIGHT
RALPH WRIGHT

Consideration of liver tumours provides a study of contrasts. Neoplasms of childhood differ greatly from those of adulthood. Primary tumours dominate the picture in children, whereas in adults a majority of tumours are metastatic. Benign liver tumours are rare, except for the haemangioma. Primary malignant liver tumours are also rare except for hepatocellular carcinomas, which are exceedingly common in some communities.

The ease of production of liver tumours in experimental animals facilitates investigation of aetiological and surgical problems.[21, 48, 100] Improved diagnostic aids and operative techniques[15, 117] (see Chapters 15 to 22) encourage surgical approaches to the liver, and liver transplants are becoming feasible[114] (see Chapters 45 and 48).

Liver tumours are classified in Table 38.1. Those which develop especially in childhood are marked (*a*). An American study showed that carcinomas comprised 90 per cent of primary hepatic neoplasms seen in a 36-year period (after exclusion of haemangiomas).[42] This was also true of a large series of cases seen on the east coast of Southern Africa; 92 per cent of 442 primary liver tumours shown in Natal during 1970–76 were hepatocellular carcinomas.[162] This neoplasm is thus of prime importance in the spectrum of hepatic tumours, and will be discussed first.

HEPATOCELLULAR CARCINOMA

Incidence

Hepatocellular carcinomas (HCC) show a striking variation in frequency in different parts of the world. The standardized liver cancer incidence rates for 13 countries are given in Table 38.2. These rates are generally taken to reflect variations in the frequency of hepatocellular carcinoma (although, strictly speaking, they include all primary hepatic tumours) as HCC is the predominant tumour in all regions. The incidence of HCC in Africa, especially along the south-east coast of Mozambique and Natal, is very high indeed, and fairly high rates are also found in Asian and Pacific areas.

Geographical variations in the frequency of HCC are more closely related to socio-economic and cultural factors than geographical ones. Examination of the rates for South Africa, New Zealand, Hawaii and California reveals very different rates for sub-communities in the same geographical region (Table 38.3).

A pronounced male predominance, of the order of about 3:1, is found throughout the world among HCC cases although female rates in areas of high liver cancer incidence are higher than male rates in areas of low incidence (see Table 38.2). Male predominance is usually

Table 38.1. *Classification of Primary Liver Tumours.*

1. Malignant	2. Benign
A. Epithelial tumours	
Hepatocellular carcinoma	Liver cell adenoma
Cholangiocarcinoma	Focal nodular hyperplasia
Combined carcinoma	(Adenomatous hyperplasia)
Cholangiolocellular carcinoma	(Partial nodular transformation)
Carcinoid tumour	
Squamous carcinoma	Bile duct adenoma
	Biliary cystadenoma
	Microhamartoma
[a]Hepatoblastoma	Heterotopic rest tumours
B. Mesodermal tumours	
Malignant haemangio-endothelioma	Cavernous haemangioma
Malignant mesenchymoma[a]	Infantile haemangio-endothelioma[a]
Other sarcomas	Mesenchymal hamartoma[a]
	Other benign tumours
C. Mixed tumours	
Malignant mixed hepatic tumour[a]	Benign teratoma[a]
Carcinosarcoma	

[a] Found in childhood.

Table 38.2. *The Geographical Variation in Standardized Incidence*[a] *Rates for Liver Cancer.*[b]

	Males	Females
African areas		
Mozambique – Maputo	103.8	30.8
South Africa – Natal (Africans)	28.4	6.9
South Africa – Johannesburg (Africans)	19.2	9.9
Nigeria – Ibadan	11.2	4.8
Uganda – Kyodondo	6.2	2.3
Asian and Pacific areas		
Singapore (Chinese)	8.6	1.2
Japan	6.0	4.7
New Zealand (Maori)	7.8	1.7
American areas		
Canada – five provinces	1.0	0.5
United States – Nevada	1.6	0.3
Jamaica	3.3	0.9
Europe and Middle East		
United Kingdom – south-west region	1.7	0.6
Finland	1.4	0.8
Israel	2.1	1.0

[a] Standardized to World Standard Population; cases per annum per 100 000 population.
[b] From Doll et al.[38, 39]

Table 38.3. *The Incidence[a] of Primary Liver Cancer in Sub-communities of Different Countries.[b]*

	Males	Females
South Africa		
Caucasian	1.2	0.6
Indian	9.5	3.8
African	28.4	6.9
New Zealand		
Caucasian	1.5	0.6
Maori	7.8	1.7
California		
Caucasian	2.4	0.9
African	8.8	1.2
Hawaii		
Hawaiian	15.2	4.0
Chinese	7.3	0.0
Japanese	6.7	1.1
Filipino	6.1	5.3
Caucasian	4.3	1.9

[a]Annual incidence per 100000 people, adjusted to World Standard Population.
[b] From Doll, Muir and Waterhouse.[38]

explained by the fact that alcoholism, chronic liver disease, and in particular chronic hepatitis B virus infections (see Chapter 29) are more prevalent among males. In addition, experiments have shown that female rats tolerate greater doses of aflatoxin than do male rats, suggesting that hepatic endoplasmic reticulum in the female is better adapted to deal with some carcinogens.[148]

In communities with a high rate of HCC, patients with this disease are younger than those in communities with a low HCC rate. Age-specific rates for liver cancer in Mozambique are highest in Africans aged 35 to 44 years, and, in Natal, in Africans aged 45 to 54 years. These figures can be compared with age-specific rates in areas where HCC is uncommon, such as the south-west region of England, where the highest age-specific rates are found in the decade 75 to 84 years.[38, 39]

Among 407 Natal cases of HCC, nine were aged between 11 and 18 years. The frequency of HCC in young subjects in regions where HCC is common suggests that a carcinogenic stimulus is not only acting upon more people, but also acting upon them at a younger age, and that they are less able to resist this stimulus. Higginson[60] considered that the liver in young individuals is more susceptible to carcinogens than the liver of adults, and put forward a two-stage hypothesis that damage to the liver in early life renders it subsequently more susceptible to carcinogens encountered later on.

Aetiology

Cirrhosis and haemosiderosis

In communities with a low liver cancer incidence, only 4 to 10 per cent of cirrhotics develop neoplasia, whereas in communities with a high incidence, malignancy supervenes in up to 50 per cent of cirrhotics.[13, 46, 59] In Cape Town Thomson[156] found cirrhosis to be almost equally common in caucasians and Africans (6.2 per cent and 8.3 per cent of male necropsies in the two respective groups) but noted that 2.6 per cent of caucasians and 54.5 per cent of Africans had liver carcinomas as well. Among Natal Africans in the period 1970–76, HCC was found in 277 liver biopsies (usually with cirrhosis), and cirrhosis alone was found in 564 biopsies, indicating that roughly one-third of Natal African cirrhotics develop HCC. This difference in susceptibility to HCC among cirrhotics in sub-communities of the same region suggests that a factor(s) additional to cirrhosis is cancer-promoting in some sub-communities.

Most observers find that macronodular cirrhosis is most frequently associated with HCC[8, 82, 139] although an early study by Edmondson[42] showed micronodular cirrhosis to be more common. Peters and colleagues[121] report a rising incidence in recent years of hepatitis B in Californian cases of HCC, which could account for the greater frequency of macronodular cirrhosis with HCC in later studies. In Natal, among Africans with HCC (Table 38.4) only 5 per cent had no concomitant liver abnormality, portal fibrosis was present in 18 per cent, and cirrhosis, most often of the micronodular type, was found in 77 per cent of cases.

Warren and Drake[165] and Purtilo and Gottlieb[130] found that the risk of hepatic neoplasia was higher in patients with pigmentary micronodular cirrhosis than in those with non-siderotic cirrhosis. Siderosis of the liver (acquired haemochromatosis) may contribute significantly to the high liver cancer incidence among Africans of Southern Africa, as it is common, especially in male subjects. Much of the high dietary iron is received in local beers.[64] Pigmentary micronodular cirrhosis, which often ensues, may be related as closely to the alcoholic habit as to iron overload. Of Natal African cases with HCC, approximately half were

Table 38.4. *Types of Cirrhosis Seen in 100 Natal African Patients with Primary Carcinomas of the Liver and Percentage who were Siderotic.*

	Males		Females		Both sexes	
	Total	No. with siderosis	Total	No. with siderosis	Total	No. with siderosis
No cirrhosis or scarring	3 (4%)	3 (100%)	1 (7%)	1 (100%)	4 (5%)	4 (100%)
Portal fibrosis	13 (18%)	8 (61%)	3 (21%)	1 (33%)	16 (18%)	9 (56%)
Macronodular cirrhosis	15 (20%)	7 (47%)	3 (21%)	0 (0%)	18 (20%)	7 (39%)
Micronodular cirrhosis	28 (37%)	18 (64%)	4 (29%)	4 (100%)	32 (37%)	22 (69%)
Cirrhosis, but type not known	15 (20%)	6 (40%)	3 (21%)	0 (0%)	18 (20%)	6 (33%)
No information about cirrhosis or fibrosis	10 –	5 (50%)	2 –	1 (50%)	12 –	6 (50%)
Totals	84 (99%)	47 (56%)	16 (99%)	7 (44%)	100 (100%)	(54%)

siderotic (see Table 38.4). Siderosis least often accompanied macronodular cirrhosis, and was seen most often with micronodular cirrhosis or portal fibrosis. All four cases of carcinoma without cirrhosis or scarring were siderotic.

Hepatitis B viral infection

In 1969 Smith and Blumberg[144] suggested that HB_sAg might be associated with HCC but failed to find an increased incidence in the serum of three different population groups. Shortly afterwards, Vogel and colleagues[160] reported a very high incidence of HB_sAg (40 per cent) in Ugandan HCC cases compared with 3 per cent in the general Ugandan population. A number of other studies from different areas followed, and most of these confirmed that a strikingly high percentage of HCC cases had HBV markers in their serum when compared with the general population or with blood donors. Table 38.5 gives comparable results from several of these studies.[18, 27, 85, 90, 126, 128, 142, 152, 161] If such studies of the incidence of HB_sAg in patients with HCC are extended to include anti-HB_c, the incidence in highly endemic areas ranges from 60 to 95 per cent of patients with HCC.[74] The percentage of HB_sAg carriers in the control population is usually high in areas where HCC has a high incidence. It has been calculated that there is a 33 times greater chance of developing HCC for HBV positive carriers when compared with negative controls matched for age, sex and race.[126]

HB_eAg is not a common finding in HB_sAg positive patients with HCC. It is possible that this partly reflects the insensitivity of commonly used techniques for detecting HB_eAg. The risk of developing HCC is considerably increased in HBV carriers compared with controls and is approximately 20 to 30 per cent. This increased risk ratio is the same for patients from the United Kingdom and United States as for patients from Africa.[74]

Techniques for identifying differing components of the hepatitis B virus (HBV) in histological tissue sections have been developed[63, 140] (Chapter 29) and can be used when serum is not available. In Singapore, a five-year retrospective study of autopsy material from Chinese males demonstrated HBV components (orcein positive cells) in 4 per cent of normal livers, 42 per cent of cirrhotic livers, and 74 per cent of livers with HCC. In addition, HCC was noted in a higher proportion of orcein positive (56 per cent) than orcein negative (25 per cent) cirrhotic livers. There were 12 cases of HCC arising in non-cirrhotic livers; in 9 (75 per cent) of these, orcein positive hepatocytes were present.[153] Similarly, Nayak and colleagues[108] have shown in India that 94 per cent of HCC cases, 71 per cent of cirrhotics, and 2 per cent of control cases have evidence of HBV in liver biopsies. Viral components identified by these methods are far more often found in liver cells than in tumour cells, suggesting that either hepatoma cells are not permissive to viral growth[56] or that HBV is occult in hepatoma cells. MacNab and her colleagues[84] have cultured a human hepatoma cell line which consistently produces HB_sAg, but not the Dane particle.

The prevalence of HBV infection in the tropics, especially in the early years of life, may be due to cultural traditions of scarification or circumcision[127] or to exposure to blood-sucking

Table 38.5. *Geographical Variation in Incidence of HB_sAg in Liver Cancer and Controls.*

	Percentage positive for HB_sAg	
	Cases of hepatocellular carcinoma	Blood donors and other controls
Africa		
Senegal[a,b]	42–61	11
Nigeria[c]	40	1.9– 6.3
Ghana[d]	32	5.9– 9.5
Uganda[a]	40	3
Kenya[a]	26	5.6
Mozambique[a,e]	60	9.0–15.0
South Africa[f]	59.5	9
Ethiopia[a]	2.6	4.2
Asia		
Japan[a]	37.3	2.6
Taiwan[b]	80	15
Singapore[a,b]	33.6–35.0	7.8
Vietnam[b]	70	19
Hong Kong[b]	5	4
America and Europe		
Philadelphia, USA[g]	24	4
United Kingdom[a,b]	16–23	1
Greece[b]	31–76	1.8– 4

[a] Williams[168]
[b] Peters, Afroudakis and Tatter.[121]
[c] Prince.[125]
[d] Blumberg, Sutnick and London.[17]
[e] Kew, Marcus and Geddes.[74]
[f] MacNab.[85]
[g] Maupas.[90]

arthropod vectors such as the mosquito or the common bedbug (see Chapter 28). Prince and colleagues[127] found HB_sAg in eight species of East African mosquitoes, and it has also been identified in bedbugs in South Africa.[72]

Larouze and colleagues[80] and Ohbayashi[111] investigated familial cryptogenic cirrhosis and HCC, and found a high incidence of HB_sAg in relatives, especially in mothers and their children. It is suggested that transmission by mothers to their offspring in the perinatal period (see Chapter 28) gives rise to families of HBV carriers, some of whom subsequently develop chronic liver disease and HCC.

Ingested carcinogens

Hepatocellular carcinoma is readily produced by plant alkaloids and fungal metabolites in experimental animals.[78, 137] These substances may also be carcinogenic in man, possibly acting synergistically with other factors. In Africa, herbal medicines are often taken by adults and children, and several are hepatotoxic.[98, 109, 163] Aflatoxins are frequently demonstrable in food consumed in Africa and Asia.[170] In animals, a delay of approximately two years is noted between the administration of a dose of aflatoxin and the development of hepatic neoplasia;[23] this delay makes assessment of the carcinogenic effects of ingested substances in human subjects very difficult. Peers and Linsell[119] showed an association between high aflatoxin ingestion and liver cancer in some districts of Kenya, and a similar association was found in Uganda by Alpert and colleagues.[7] Many plant alkaloids cause hepatic cirrhosis or scarring.[41, 98] In the West Indies and South America where these are also often taken, the incidence of HCC is not high, but the position may differ in Africa.

Other aetiological factors

Other factors have been implicated in the aetiology of HCC. These may be grouped as

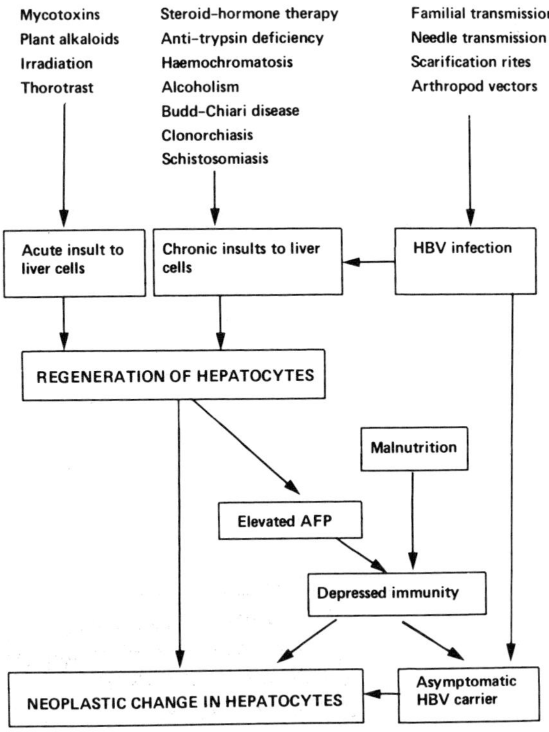

Figure 38.1. Diagram illustrating the interplay of various aetiological factors in the pathogenesis of hepatocellular carcinoma. HBV = hepatitis B virus; AFP = alpha-fetoprotein.

pharmacological, metabolic, physical and infective causes. Pharmacological preparations which have been implicated in the aetiology of hepatomas include contraceptive pills[35, 76, 110] and androgenic–anabolic steroids.[70, 75] Metabolic states which may be aetiologically related to HCC are the alpha-1-antitrypsin deficiency states (see Chapter 35) and that of chronic liver disease with raised alpha-fetoprotein levels.[1, 131] Physical causes include irradiation and Thorotrast administration:[159] infective conditions include clonorchiasis[129] and schistosomiasis.[104] The possibility that protozoal and schistosomal infections depress immunological competence and thus permit neoplastic change or HBV infection to develop is of interest.[79, 164] In Natal, although schistosomiasis is endemic, with a high incidence among schoolchildren, no association with liver cancer has been detected, since in 100 consecutive necropsy cases of liver cancer, schistosomiasis was present in only two cases.

Interplay of aetiological factors

The hypothesis that HBV is the aetiological agent of HCC links cirrhosis and neoplasia, and provides an explanation for the variable geographical distribution, the differences in cultural and socio-economic sub-groups, the occurrence in young patients, and may account for sex differences (see Chapter 29). Other factors may also play their part, and Larouze and colleagues[81] have proposed a possible sequence of events for the pathogenesis of HCC, which has been modified and extended in Figure 38.1.

The acquisition of HBV infection in the perinatal period may induce tolerance to the virus, and an asymptomatic carrier state. A number of factors may depress the immune response and facilitate the development of HCC. These include alpha-fetoprotein produced by regenerating hepatocytes,[27, 45, 107] a liver-derived alpha-2-globulin,[20] protein-calorie deficiency states or protozoal infections.[79, 146] This may explain why cirrhotic patients with elevated alpha-fetoprotein levels have a high risk of developing HCC.[131] MacSween and coworkers[86] were successful in showing disturbances of both cellular and humoral immunity in a model of cirrhosis in the rat, although Primack and colleagues[124] could not demonstrate immunological depression in Ugandan HCC cases.

The evidence points to an interplay of factors in the aetiology and pathogenesis of HCC, with chronic liver disease and HBV infection playing the most important roles, although the asymptomatic HBV carrier state combined with another factor such as haemochromatosis or malnutrition might also lead to the development of HCC.

Clinical Features

The onset of symptoms in cases with HCC may be insidious or sudden. Usually years of ill-health attributable to chronic liver disease precede more acute symptoms such as abdominal pain or jaundice. A majority of HCC patients experience abdominal discomfort or pain, and malaise, anorexia, weight loss, nausea, fever and jaundice may also be noted.[25, 36, 112] Clinical signs are most often those of tender hepatomegaly, often with a palpable hepatic mass, ascites, jaundice, vascular naevi and distended abdominal surface veins. Less constant signs are splenomegaly (15 to 20 per cent of cases), pyrexia, palmar erythema, gynaecomastia and increased skin pigmentation. Many of these features are due to concomitant cirrhosis, but hepatic pain is characteristic of an enlarging hepatic lesion. A bruit is heard over the liver in about 25 per cent of cases.

Occasionally the initial presentation is one of an abdominal catastrophe, such as haematemesis or haemoperitoneum. Okuda[112] notes that extensive carcinoma in a non-cirrhotic liver may produce few symptoms, whereas the patient with early or occult HCC and advanced cirrhosis may show features of decompensated liver disease. He divides patients with HCC into clinical sub-types, such as the frankly evident, the occult, the cirrhotic, the hepatitic and the cholestatic types.

Investigations

Haematological changes are mostly related to the cirrhosis and accompanying splenomegaly but, rarely, other haematological syndromes occur (see below; and see also Chapter 8).

Biochemical investigations can show abnormal levels of bilirubin, alkaline phosphatase, transaminases and serum proteins in both cirrhosis and hepatocellular carcinoma and do not distinguish between these conditions. In a patient known to have cirrhosis an abrupt change in these values suggests a complicating hepatocellular carcinoma, particularly if there is unexplained elevation of the alkaline phosphatase.

Alpha-fetoprotein (AFP) was first reported to be raised in the blood of mice with hepatomas by Abelev and co-workers.[2] The diagnostic usefulness of raised AFP levels was soon established; although raised AFP levels are also found in acute and chronic liver disease and in other malignancies,[3, 5, 134] very high levels are suggestive of HCC. Vogel and colleagues[161] noted an association between high AFP levels and HB_sAg positivity, and high AFP levels are also associated with rapid tumour growth and tumour anaplasia.[1, 5]

Radiological investigations and imaging techniques are important in the diagnosis of suspected primary hepatic tumours and are considered in Chapters 20, 21 and 22. Calcification of hepatocellular carcinoma noted on a plain x-ray of the abdomen has been recorded.[112]

Extrahepatic Manifestations

Margolis and Homcy[88] and Cochrane and Williams[29] have discussed the various and numerous syndromes associated with HCC. These may be grouped as endocrine manifestations, metabolic changes and haematological syndromes.

Endocrine manifestations include erythrocytosis, possibly due to production of erythropoietin or its substrate by tumour cells, or to decreased inactivation of erythropoietin by the diseased liver; hypercalcaemia, due to multiple skeletal metastases or to production of parathormone-like substances by tumour; sexual precocity and gynaecomastia, due to production by the tumour of gonadotrophin and somatotrophin-like hormones.

Metabolic changes include hypoglycaemia, due either to increased glucose utilization by the tumour or to decreased glucose production by the diseased liver; hyperlipidaemia, possibly due to uncontrolled cholesterogenesis by tumour cells; increased alpha-fetoproteinaemia, increased serum alkaline phosphatase, macroglobulinaemia and porphyria.

Haematological syndromes include dysfibrinogenaemia, possibly due to release of an anti-fibrinolytic substance, and dysproteinaemias such as raised levels of cryofibrinogen, haptoglobin or caeruloplasmin.[29]

Erythrocytosis and hypoglycaemia are more often seen in patients in Asia, while hyperlipidaemia is common in African patients.[29] This finding is not yet explicable.

Pathology

Macroscopic appearances

The liver with HCC is usually vastly increased in weight and is nodular, due in part to tumour deposits but also to cirrhosis, which is present in 80 to 90 per cent of cases. The largest focus of tumour tissue is generally taken to be the primary focus of HCC. In spite of tumour necrosis, umbilication of subcapsular tumour nodules is not seen, and this is a helpful point in distinguishing primary from metastatic neoplasms. Macroscopically, the tumour may be described as nodular, massive or diffuse in type.

The nodular pattern (Figure 38.2) is most common, and is characterized by the presence of

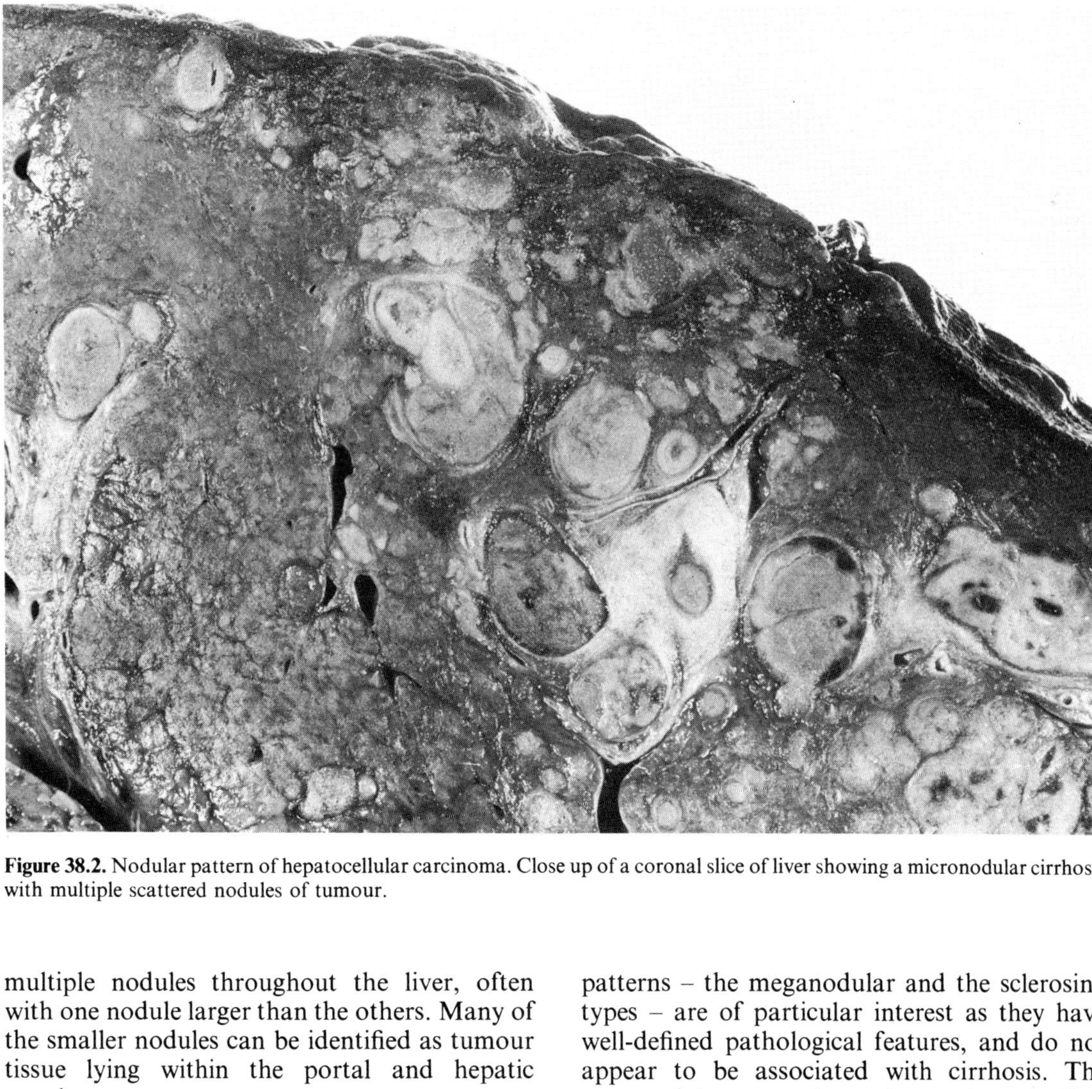

Figure 38.2. Nodular pattern of hepatocellular carcinoma. Close up of a coronal slice of liver showing a micronodular cirrhosis with multiple scattered nodules of tumour.

multiple nodules throughout the liver, often with one nodule larger than the others. Many of the smaller nodules can be identified as tumour tissue lying within the portal and hepatic venules.

The massive pattern (Figure 38.3) is also common, in which a very large tumour is found, often replacing all of one lobe. There may be some immediately peripheral satellite nodules. This type of tumour is most often associated with capsular rupture and intraperitoneal haemorrhage.

The diffuse pattern (Figure 38.4) is rare. In this type, tiny indistinct nodules are scattered throughout the liver, and are difficult to distinguish from regenerative nodules of cirrhosis. Disparity of nodule size, necrotic softening, undue haemorrhage or bile-staining, and freedom from siderosis may suggest the neoplastic nature of a nodule.

Peters[120] has suggested an alternative classification into six groups of which two patterns – the meganodular and the sclerosing types – are of particular interest as they have well-defined pathological features, and do not appear to be associated with cirrhosis. The meganodular type shows large circumscribed nodules which have a very uniform bulging cut surface (Figure 38.5). The sclerosing type is firm due to pronounced desmoplasia, and may be confused with cholangiocarcinoma or with metastatic scirrhous carcinoma. This type is frequently associated with non-metastatic hypercalcaemia.

Hepatocellular carcinomas readily invade the hepatic vasculature (Figure 38.4). Tumour tissue can often be identified inside the main portal vein, often exacerbating ascites and oesophageal varicosities. Tumour tissue within the branches of the hepatic veins may produce lobular or massive centrilobular congestion, and tumour masses may occlude the inferior vena cava and extend into the right atrium.

The pattern of spread seen at necropsy in 96 Natal cases of HCC is shown in Table 38.6. In 20 cases there was no spread beyond the liver; in

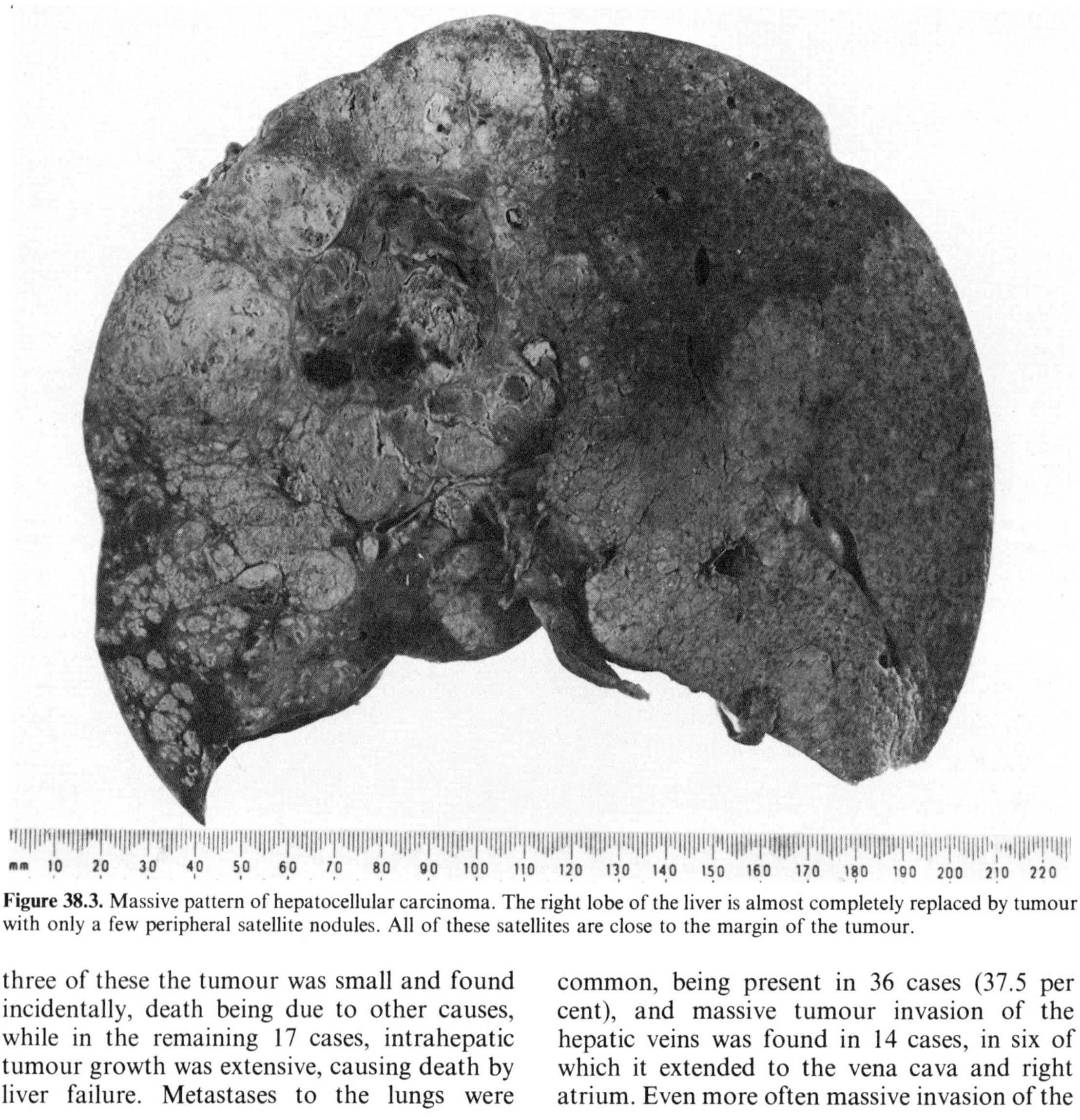

Figure 38.3. Massive pattern of hepatocellular carcinoma. The right lobe of the liver is almost completely replaced by tumour with only a few peripheral satellite nodules. All of these satellites are close to the margin of the tumour.

three of these the tumour was small and found incidentally, death being due to other causes, while in the remaining 17 cases, intrahepatic tumour growth was extensive, causing death by liver failure. Metastases to the lungs were common, being present in 36 cases (37.5 per cent), and massive tumour invasion of the hepatic veins was found in 14 cases, in six of which it extended to the vena cava and right atrium. Even more often massive invasion of the

Table 38.6. *The Spread of Primary Liver Carcinoma in 100 African Patients in Natal.*[a]

	Hepatocellular carcinoma (96 cases)	Cholangiocellular carcinoma (4 cases)
A. No spread outside the liver	20	0
B. Pulmonary metastases	36	3
Portal vein invasion (main trunk)	34	0
Hepatic vein invasion (main trunk)	14	0
Vena caval and right atrial invasion	6	0
Abdominal lymph nodes involved	22	3
Contiguous spread in abdomen	14	1
Thoracic and cervical lymph node involvement	8	1
Renal and/or adrenal involvement	6	0
Vertebral metastases	7	0
Other bone metastases	3	0
Cerebral metastases	2	0
Splenic metastases	1	0

[a] Wainwright and Schonland.[162]

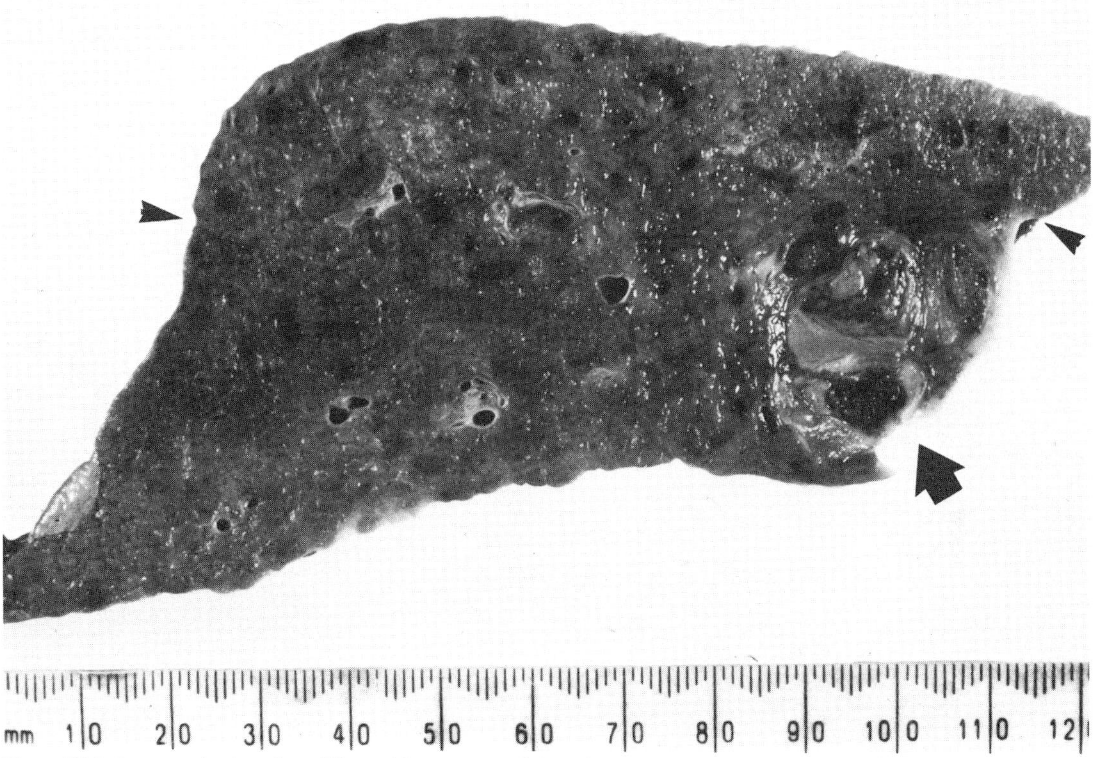

Figure 38.4. A parasagittal section of liver with tumour and thrombus occluding the portal vein in the porta hepatis (arrow). There is a micronodular cirrhosis evident along the lower half of the liver with a diffuse nodular hepatoma along the upper half. The approximate line of division is marked by arrowheads. Areas of this tumour were paler and had a yellow/brown hue compared with the light brown colour of the cirrhotic areas.

portal vein was seen (34 cases). Involvement of intra-abdominal lymph nodes was much more common than involvement of nodes above the diaphragm, while spread to brain, bone, kidney, spleen or other distant sites was rare.

Microscopic features

The commonest arrangement of hepatocellular carcinoma is the characteristic trabecular (or sinusoidal) pattern, in which groups and columns of malignant liver cells lie in a blood-filled sinusoidal stroma, each cluster of tumour cells being covered by a delicate layer of flat endothelial cells (Figure 38.6). The tumour may assume other appearances such as an acinar (tubular) pattern (Figure 38.7), a bizarre giant-cell pattern, a clear-cell pattern (Figure 38.8), a spindle cell pattern, or a sclerosing pattern. About 10 per cent of HCC show bile-producing cells, and sometimes a well-differentiated type produces proteinaceous material or bile in the tubule lumina. Bile production is the hallmark of HCC, whatever the pattern, and a mixed hepatocellular and cholangiocellular pattern is regarded as HCC.[42]

Tumour cells vary in appearance from easily recognized bile-producing cells to highly anaplastic dedifferentiated cells. They are seldom fatty, and usually do not show haemosiderin granules, possibly because they are so newly formed. Nuclear or cytoplasmic vacuolation may be present, and the cytoplasm may contain material resembling Mallory's hyalin.[73] In 15 per cent of tumours hepatocytes may contain PAS positive and diastase-resistant globules, and immunoperoxidase studies have shown that these contain alpha-1-antitrypsin (Figures 38.9 and 38.10).[118] Rarely orcein and immunoperoxidase stains may show components of HBV in both the nucleus and cytoplasm of carcinoma cells, although these are much more often found in adjacent non-malignant hepatocytes.[106,135]

When comparing carcinomatous cells with hepatocytes in adjacent liver nodules, the tumour cells appear denser and more basophilic than the hepatocytes, with less glycogen in the cytoplasm. Occasional tumours are composed of clear cells,[19] and clear cells may form a variable proportion of any histological pattern. Kupffer cells are absent in tumour nodules.[58]

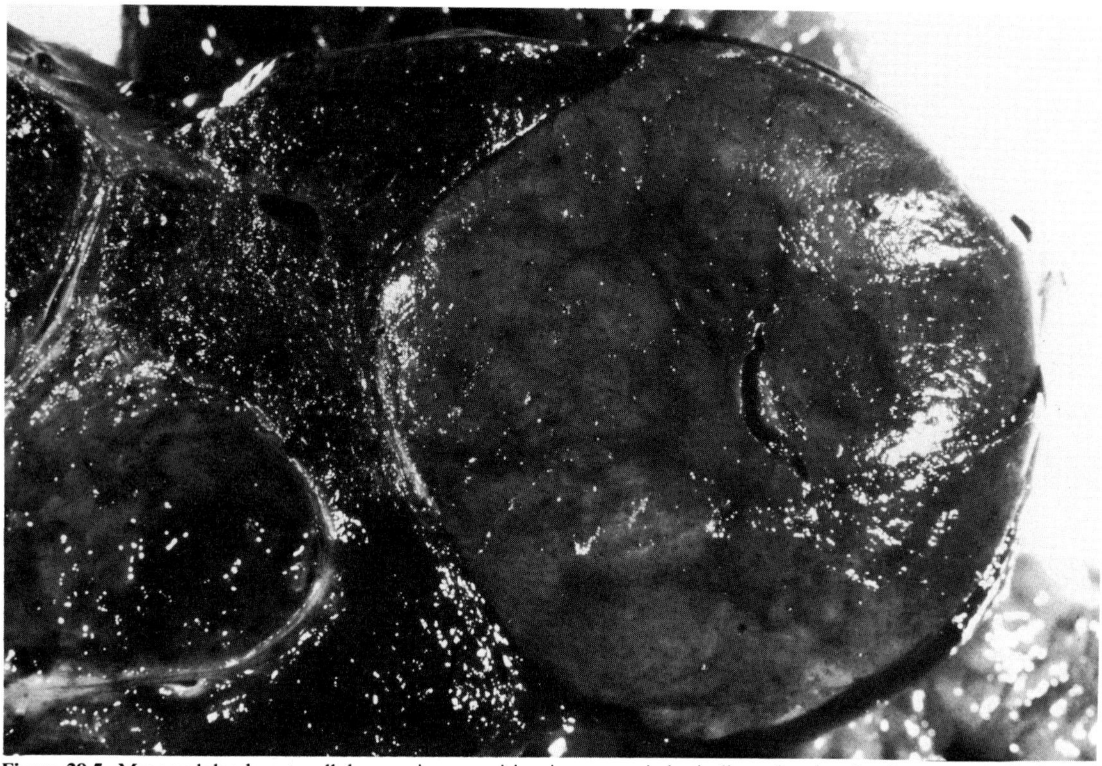

Figure 38.5. Meganodular hepatocellular carcinoma arising in a non-cirrhotic liver showing focal segmental dilation of intrahepatic bile ducts. A large dilated bile duct is seen top right. The tumour is rounded and has a bulging uniform cut surface.

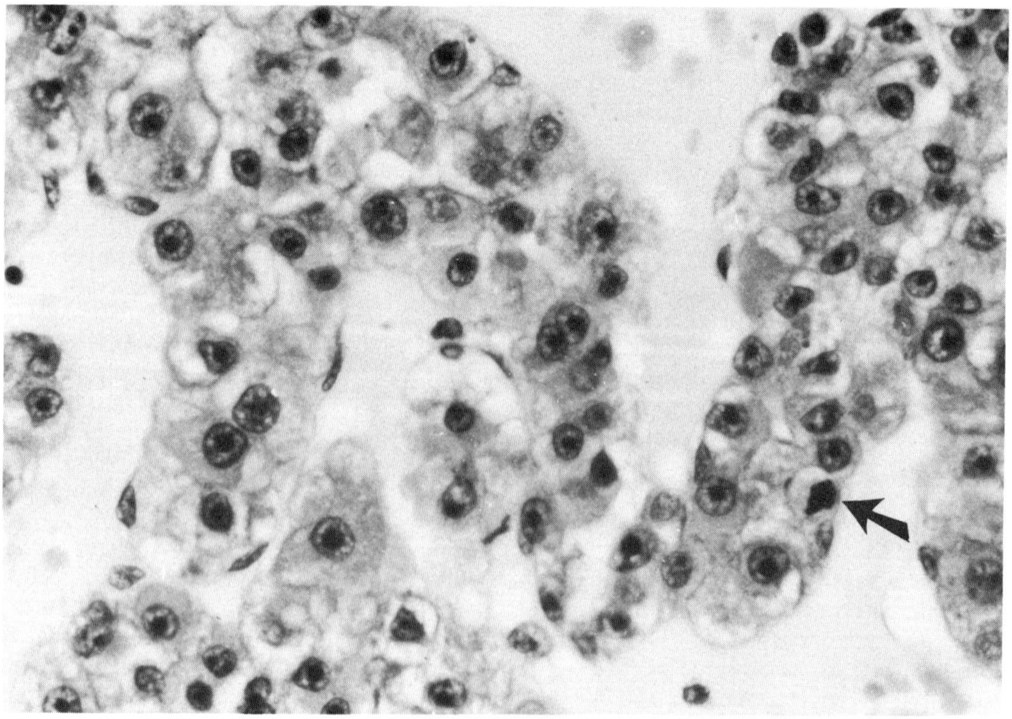

Figure 38.6. Trabecular (sinusoidal) pattern of hepatocellular carcinoma showing tumour cells closely resembling hepatocytes arranged in plates at least two cells thick and covered by endothelial cells. Note the large nucleoli and the mitosis (arrow). Haematoxylin and eosin × 1500.

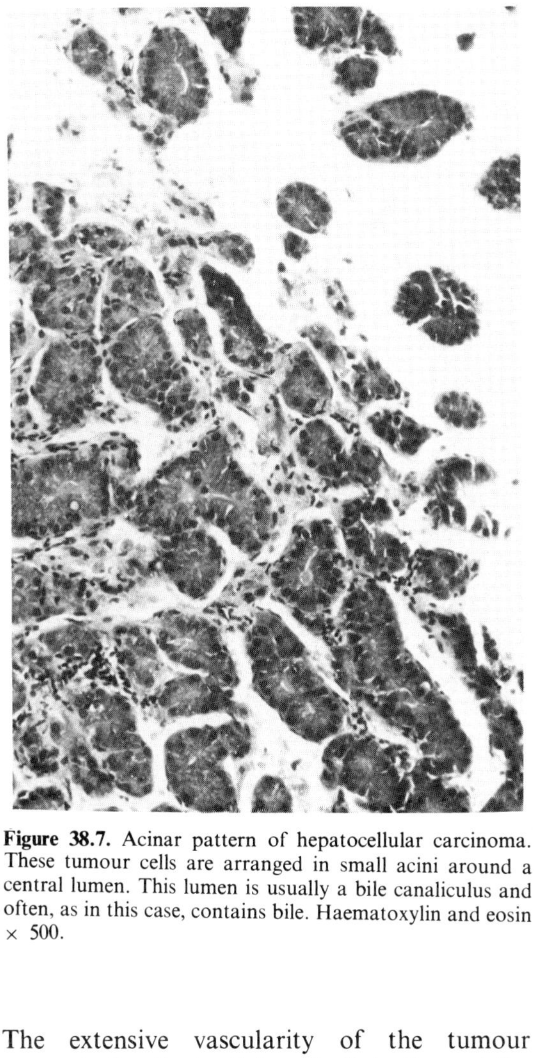

Figure 38.7. Acinar pattern of hepatocellular carcinoma. These tumour cells are arranged in small acini around a central lumen. This lumen is usually a bile canaliculus and often, as in this case, contains bile. Haematoxylin and eosin × 500.

The extensive vascularity of the tumour accounts for the bruit heard clinically, and for the tendency to bleed into the peritoneum after capsular invasion.

Course and Prognosis

The course of the disease in HCC patients varies from case to case, but is usually rapidly fatal, most observers noting a mean survival time of about six months.[25, 36, 112] Surgical extirpation of the tumour is usually impossible as rapid spread within the liver produces a multicentric carcinoma at an early stage of the disease. Rupture of oesophageal varices is often hastened by tumour invasion of the larger branches of the portal vein; intraperitoneal haemorrhage following capsular infiltration by the tumour is not infrequent. In Natal African patients with HCC, liver failure was the immediate cause of death in 36 per cent, pulmonary metastases in 21 per cent, ruptured oesophageal varices in 16 per cent and haemoperitoneum in 9 per cent.

Treatment

Some hepatocellular carcinomas are amenable to resection (see Chapter 49) or transplantation (see Chapter 52) and the principal alternative forms of therapy are indicated below (see 'Prognosis and treatment of hepatic tumours').

CHOLANGIOCARCINOMA

Intrahepatic carcinomas of the cholangiocellular type are much less often seen than hepatocellular carcinomas. An American study reported that 75 per cent of primary liver carcinomas were of the hepatocellular type[43] and a Natal series of 442 hepatic neoplasms contained 30 examples of cholangiocarcinoma (7 per cent).[162] Cholangiocarcinomas are distributed fairly uniformly in the world, unlike HCC,[8] occur most frequently in the sixth decade, and no male predominance is noted.[113]

Aetiology

Cirrhosis is less often present in cholangiocarcinoma than in HCC,[8,42,129,139] a relationship to HBV infection has not been demonstrated, and hepatic siderosis (haemochromatosis) is less frequent. Analysis of four necropsy and 26 biopsy cases in Natal indicated that siderosis was present in only 20 per cent of these cases, as compared with a 54 per cent incidence of siderosis in HCC cases (see Table 38.4). In the Far East an aetiological association is recognized with clonorchiasis. The liver fluke (*Clonorchis sinensis*) resides in bile ducts and releases ova into the hepatic parenchyma, causing suppurative cholangitis and hepatic scarring. Purtilo[129] described 38 cases of clonorchiasis in Hong Kong, of which 10 had HCC, seven had cholangiocarcinoma, one had carcinoma of the common bile duct and one had lymphoma. Gallagher and colleagues[51] reported two cases in which cholangiocarcinoma had developed in subjects with congenital dilatation of the intrahepatic bile ducts. Cruickshank and Sparshott[34] note that the microhamartomas of von Meyenberg have a

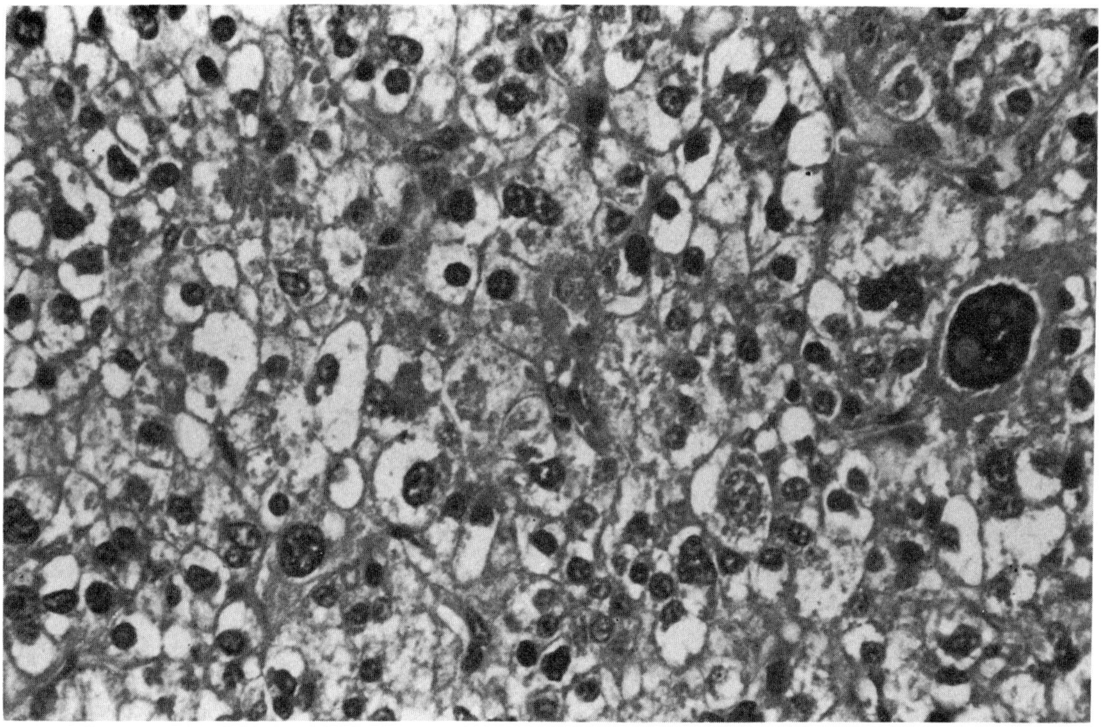

Figure 38.8. Clear cell hepatocellular carcinoma simply describes the non-staining appearances of the cytoplasm of the tumour cells. The cells may form only a small proportion of the tumour or may be the dominant feature when distinction from renal cell carcinoma may be difficult. Tumour giant cells as seen on the right can also be a prominent feature in hepatocellular carcinoma. Haematoxylin and eosin × 1250.

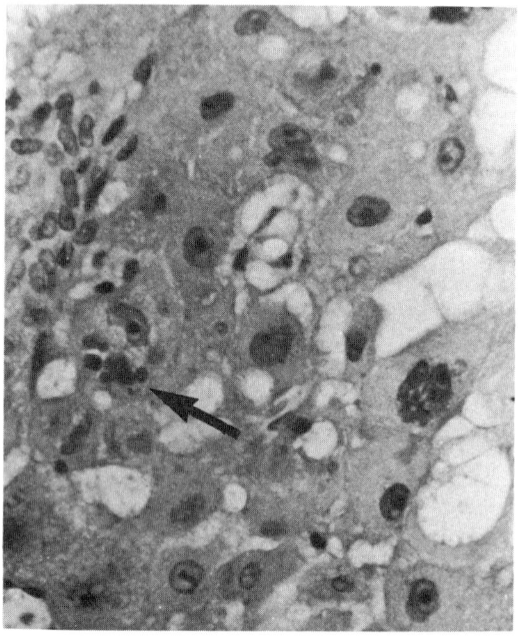

Figure 38.9. Hepatocellular carcinoma with PAS positive diastase resistant globules (arrow) in tumour cells. Diastase PAS × 1500.

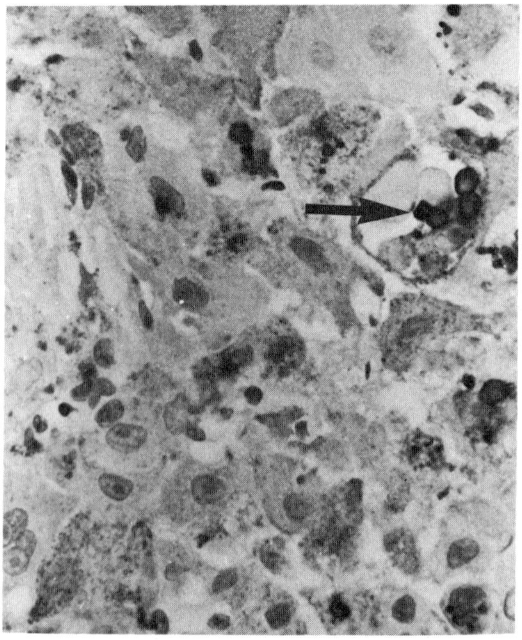

Figure 38.10. Same tumour as in Figure 38.9. The globules are stained by an immunoperoxidase technique using primary antibody against alpha-1-antitrypsin. (Rabbit anti-human A1AT $\frac{1}{400}$, swine anti-rabbit IgG $\frac{1}{20}$, peroxidase antiperoxidase complex $\frac{1}{200}$.) × 1500.

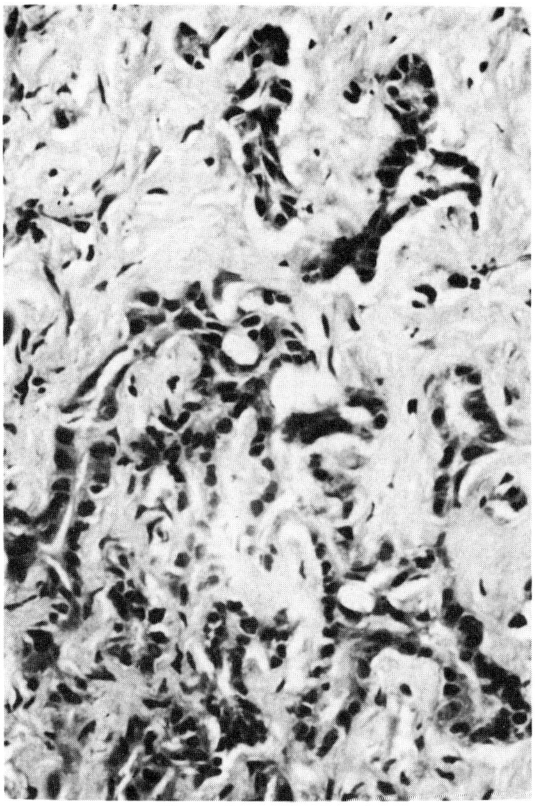

Figure 38.11. Intrahepatic cholangiocarcinoma is composed of small irregular acini lined by low cuboidal tumour cells within an abundant dense fibrous stroma. Tumour cell pleomorphism and atypicality may be only slight and distinction of a small focus of such a tumour from proliferating bile ductules in a needle biopsy specimen can be difficult. Haematoxylin and eosin × 900.

tendency to undergo malignant transformation to cholangiocarcinoma. Cholangiocarcinoma rarely has been associated with the previous administration of thorium dioxide.[11]

It seems apparent that these lesions are aetiologically different from HCC, and may develop in association with distension and infection in the intrahepatic biliary tree.

Clinical Features

Tumours at the hilum usually present as problems in the differential diagnosis of obstructive jaundice, and peripheral cholangiocarcinomas present with abdominal pain, anorexia and jaundice. In both groups jaundice is a much more frequent initial symptom than in HCC[113] but otherwise the clinical presentation is similar to that of HCC. Alpha-fetoprotein is not produced by these tumours[8] and a clinical suspicion of cholangiocarcinoma may be entertained in the absence of both an elevated AFP and a bruit.

Pathology

Macroscopic appearances

On naked-eye examination of the liver, cholangiocarcinoma may be suspected because of the fibrous stroma which usually accompanies the tumour, giving a firm and whitish appearance. These tumours can also be classed as massive, nodular or diffuse in type; the edges of the carcinoma tissue are less well defined than in HCC, and show an infiltrating pattern of growth. Necrosis, bile-staining, haemorrhage, and vascular invasion are not so evident as in HCC. Most cholangiocarcinomas arise peripherally but a hilar type has been described which presents as obstructive jaundice.[166]

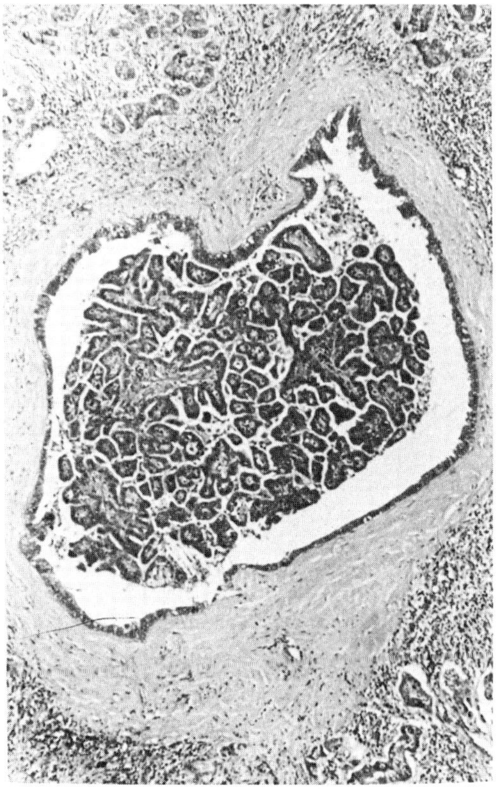

Figure 38.12. Intrahepatic cholangiocarcinoma with a papillary pattern. More conventional tumour acini can be seen on the margins. Elsewhere papillary areas also showed psammoma body formation. Haematoxylin and eosin × 175.

Microscopic appearances

Histologically, cholangiocarcinomas are usually well-differentiated sclerosing adenocarcinomas, with a well-marked acinar pattern and much collagenized stroma (Figure 38.11). They may be mucin-producing but never secrete bile. A few exhibit a papillary pattern (Figure 38.12) and some are anaplastic. In biopsy material it may be difficult to distinguish these tumours from metastatic adenocarcinomas, especially those arising in the extrahepatic biliary system, or from sclerosing acinar forms of HCC. When the tumour invades blood vessels, it utilizes the vascular endothelium as a basement membrane, and creates cyst-like spaces rather than solid intravascular tumour nodules as seen in HCC.[42] Extensive invasion of larger vessels is not seen (see Table 38.6).

Treatment

This is discussed below (see 'Prognosis and treatment of hepatic tumours') and in Chapter 55.

OTHER PRIMARY CARCINOMAS

Combined Carcinomas

Carcinomas of mixed HCC and cholangiocellular (CCC) pattern are sometimes encountered; they are thought to arise from the canals of Hering (the cholangioles). The recognition of malignant hepatocytes in a mixed tumour indicates that the case should be regarded as one of HCC.[42] Very rarely, separate but contiguous carcinomas of HCC and CCC types are seen in the same patient, and these can be regarded as true combined tumours or, if far apart, as double carcinomas.

Cholangiolocellular Carcinoma

A cholangiolocellular carcinoma, probably derived from cholangioles, has been described as a separate entity by Steiner and Higginson.[147] This carcinoma resembles and is difficult to distinguish from cholangiocarcinoma but has uniformly cuboidal-celled acini scattered in a fibrotic stroma, rather than the flattened and pleomorphic malignant acinar cells of the cholangiocarcinoma. There is some uncertainty about this rare entity, as it is also difficult to distinguish from sclerosing HCC. Peters[120] observed that all three types of sclerosing carcinoma have an association with hypercalcaemia.

Biliary Cystadenocarcinoma

A rare biliary cystadenocarcinoma has been described.[68] It is claimed that this arises from the cystadenoma.

Primary Hepatic Carcinoid Tumour

This is very rare and may produce a carcinoid syndrome. Hypoglycaemia has also been a recorded association.[4] It arises from scattered argentaffin cells which are found in bile duct and gallbladder epithelium.[42]

Primary Squamous Carcinoma

This arises in the wall of a solitary developmental cyst and was reported as a very rare entity by Edmondson.[42]

HEPATOBLASTOMA

These tumours (sometimes called embryonal hepatic tumours) occur in the first two years of life but have been recorded in adult life.[9, 66, 94]

Clinical Features

Hepatoblastoma usually presents with abdominal swelling with hepatomegaly, but anorexia, diarrhoea and vomiting may occur. The tumour may rupture and present as an acute abdominal emergency with a haemoperitoneum. There is no association with cirrhosis.[66] Rarely, a thrombocytosis may be present in the peripheral blood.[105] A variety of conditions and congenital abnormalities has been described in patients with hepatoblastoma.[66,105] These include hemihypertrophy, renal abnormalities, osteoporosis and precocious virilization in males.

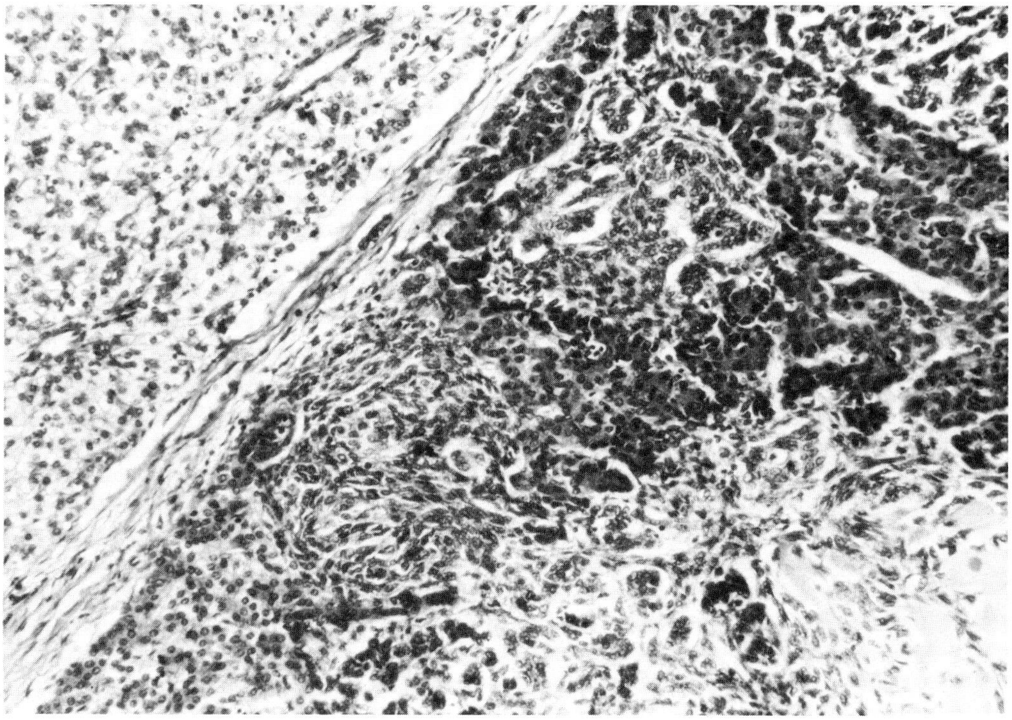

Figure 38.13. Edge of an epithelial hepatoblastoma with non-tumour liver in the top left. The tumour is composed of spindle fetal hepatocytes with more polygonal embryonal hepatocytes. Haematoxylin and eosin × 600.

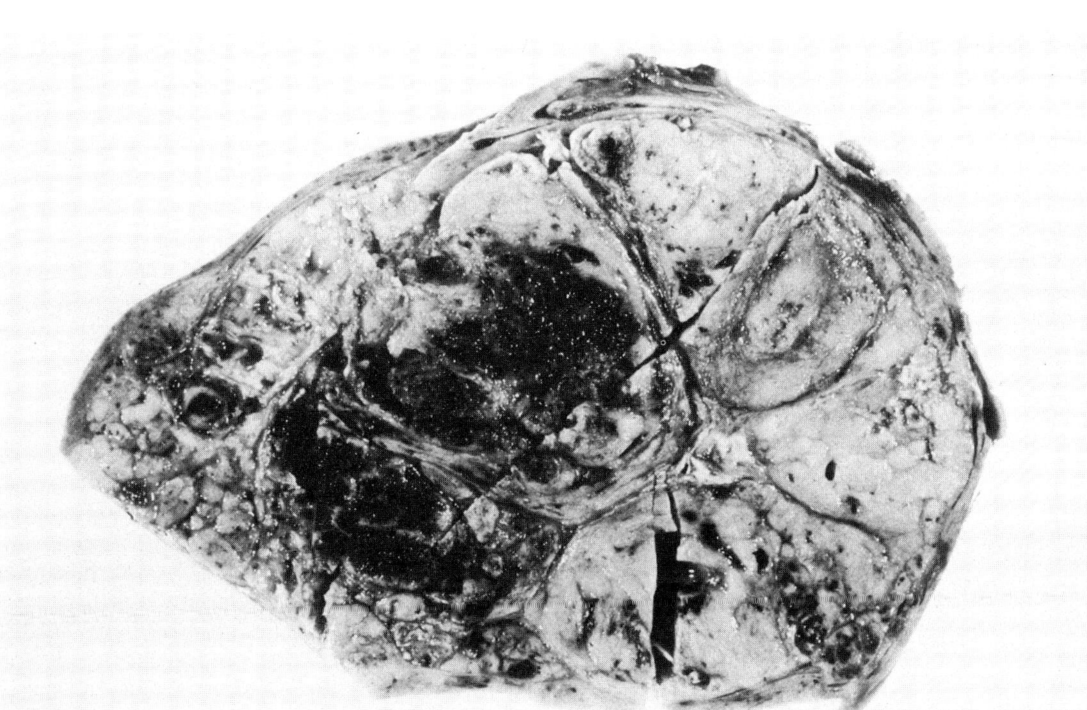

Figure 38.14. A mixed type of hepatoblastoma showing a lobular tumour with a variegated appearance to the cut surface.

Pathology

The tumour mass is usually single, but in a few cases multiple nodules have been seen. The tumour is usually situated in the right lobe, and may vary in size from 6 to 17 cm in diameter, with a soft consistency in two-thirds of cases.[9] Two types of hepatoblastoma have been identified by Ishak and Glunz:[66] the epithelial and the mixed types.

The epithelial type shows a rather uniform cut surface. Histologically it is composed of varied proportions of fetal and embryonal cells (Figure 38.13). Fetal hepatocytes resemble small hepatocytes and are arranged in cords separated by sinusoids. Embryonal liver cells are primitive blast-like cells, small and dark, with a tendency to form rosettes and imperfect acinar structures. They often form and surround small vascular lakes. Fetal hepatocytes, unlike embryonal hepatocytes, may contain fat and glycogen and secrete bile. Foci of haematopoiesis are found in the sinusoids between the fetal liver cells, but are not seen in the uninvolved liver or among the embryonal hepatocytes.

The mixed type of hepatoblastoma is macroscopically a lobulated tumour of variegated colouring (tan, haemorrhagic or greenish-grey) (Figure 38.14) which may contain foci of calcification. Histologically the tumour is composed of the epithelial elements mentioned above together with mesenchymal elements of peculiar type: a primitive mesenchymal stroma (Figure 38.15) contains foci of osteoid, cartilage or striated muscle, and this stroma surrounds tubular elements, often mucus-secreting duct-like structures. This type of hepatoblastoma is more often seen in females. Silverman and colleagues[141] and Ito and Johnson[69] reported on the ultrastructural features of these tumours, noting that the primitive hepatocytes contained numerous intracytoplasmic fibrils which enabled cases to be distinguished from HCC in children. The mixed type of hepatoblastoma is similar to, and sometimes confused with, the malignant hepatic mixed tumour (see below) which contains a well-differentiated hepatocellular carcinomatous element among its components.

At present there is no known difference in prognosis between the epithelial and mixed types of hepatoblastoma. If untreated, they are uniformly fatal, although successful resections are now being reported.[9, 47] About one-third of cases show histological evidence of vascular invasion, and metastases develop in the lungs, the abdominal lymph nodes and the brain.

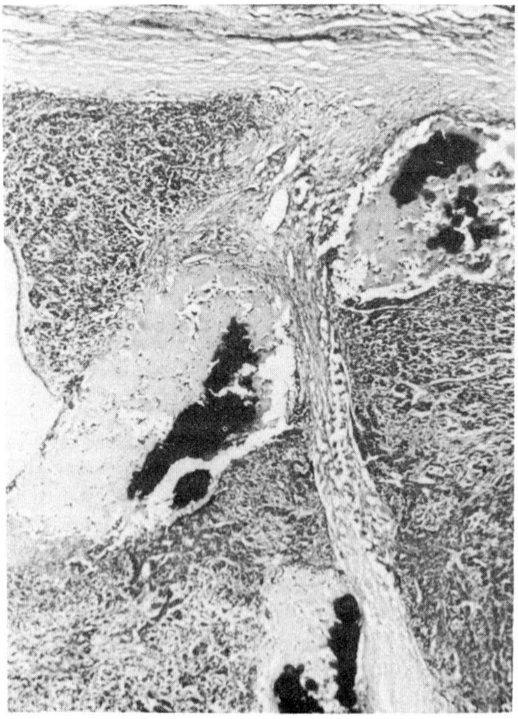

Figure 38.15. Stromal osteoid is a frequent finding in a mixed type of hepatoblastoma. Calcification commonly occurs within such areas. Haematoxylin and eosin × 150.

LIVER CELL ADENOMA

These once rare tumours have shown an increased incidence in the last 15 years. They are usually solitary but may be multiple and are more often seen in young women.

Aetiology

Baum and her co-workers[12] first reported seven cases of this tumour in women who were taking oral contraceptive pills, and subsequent observers[24, 26, 44, 49, 50, 53, 115, 158] confirmed that oral contraceptives are aetiologically very important. The risk of adenomas rises with the duration of use of the contraceptive pill and with the age of the patient.[24] Women over 27 years of age are more likely to develop these tumours. There are also more adenomas reported in women taking mestranol-containing compounds[44, 76] or compounds of high hormonal potency[24] but this might simply reflect

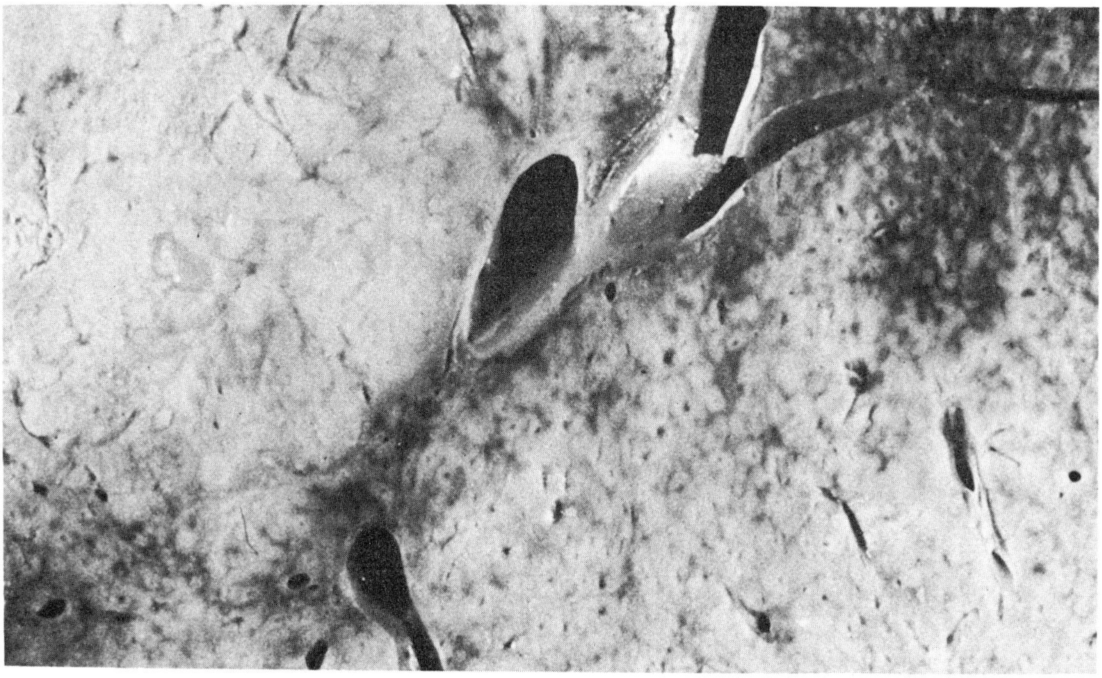

Figure 38.16. High power detail of the non-encapsulated edge of an adenoma with its paler more homogeneous cut surface (top left) and adjacent liver parenchyma. The patient, an American negress on 'the pill' for many years, died in right heart failure due to idiopathic pulmonary hypertension. The dilated central veins are readily seen in the non-tumour liver.

the market distribution of these compounds in the populations studied.[158]

Clinical Features

Clinically these patients may present with abdominal pain, or in a shocked state secondary to intraperitoneal bleeding from a ruptured nodule, or they may be asymptomatic with hepatomegaly discovered as an incidental chance finding. Many adenomas present with haemoperitoneum, and can be successfully resected.[57, 76] On laparoscopy or laparotomy a solitary, subcapsular, large, bile-stained, bleeding tumour in a non-cirrhotic liver can be suspected to be an adenoma, although histological confirmation is essential. Alpha-fetoprotein was produced in only one of five cases.[101]

Pathology

Macroscopically (Figure 38.16) the adenoma may or may not be encapsulated and is frequently subcapsular, bile-stained and of quite large size (6 to 30 cm in diameter) at the time of diagnosis. Histologically, the adenoma is composed of normal-looking well-differentiated hepatocytes arranged in sheets or cords (Figure 38.17), sometimes producing bile and sometimes having a clear 'hypernephroid' appearance. Sinusoids are present but frequently difficult to define. A genuine capsule can be found in some adenomas, while others are clearly demarcated only on gross examination. These latter tumours do not have a genuine capsule, and although some may show compression of normal liver by the growth of the adenoma, in others the normal hepatocytes appear to be in direct continuity with tumour cells. The tumours are vascular and often bleed into their substance or into adjacent normal liver tissue, and this can further obscure the junction between adenoma and surrounding liver parenchyma on microscopy. The adenoma may be subdivided by slender fibrous septa but there are no bile ducts or portal tracts in the tumours, and cholestasis can result.

These tumours have to be distinguished from focal nodular hyperplasia and from well-differentiated hepatocellular carcinomas. The distinction from focal nodular hyperplasia can be made on the larger size, the absence of central scars, and the lack of bile ducts in the adenoma. Differentiation from carcinoma may be suggested by features such as lack of alpha-fetoprotein but requires histological evidence of the tumour's benign nature.

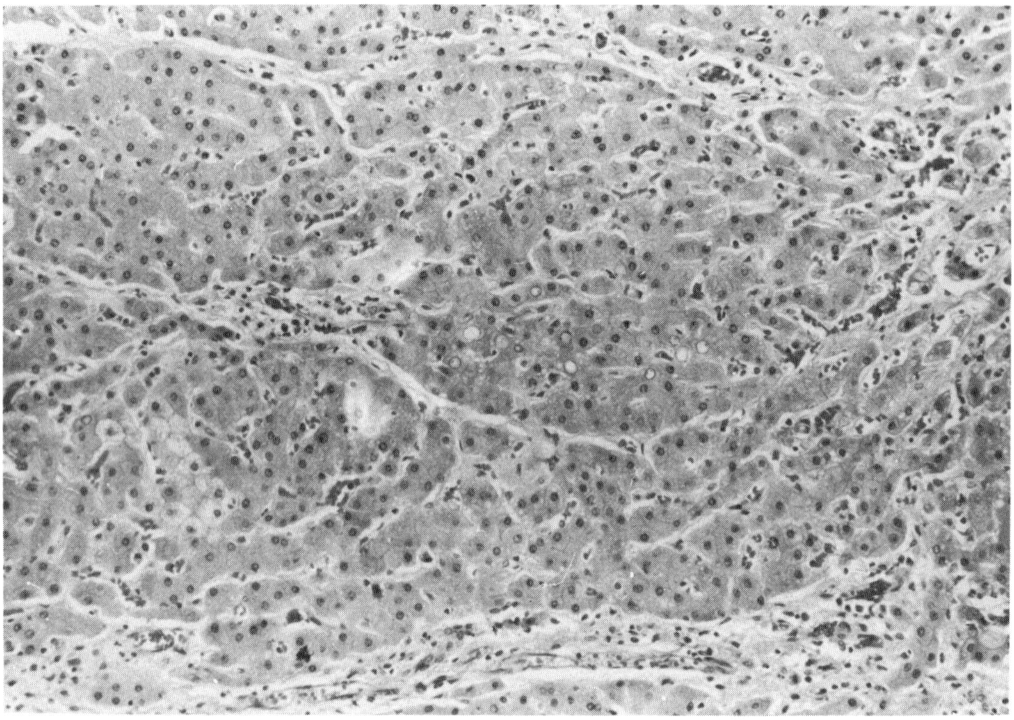

Figure 38.17. Hepatocytes from an adenoma show an irregular cell plate pattern and twinning of cell plates but are cytologically normal. There are no portal tracts. Haematoxylin and eosin × 600.

Prognosis and Treatment

While adenomas are the most frequently encountered hepatic tumours in women taking oral contraceptives, hepatocellular carcinoma may sometimes develop, occasionally in intimate association with an adenoma.[35,76,110]

Although regression of the tumour has been related to stopping the contraceptive pill[44] this is rare. Treatment (see below) should be aimed at removal of the tumour but it is feasible to observe the progress of a small nodule after stopping 'the pill', before a decision is taken.

FOCAL NODULAR HYPERPLASIA

Focal nodular hyperplasia was well defined by Edmondson[42,44] and confirmed by others.[49,50,97] It has been variously regarded as a benign hepatoma,[61] an adenoma[52] and more usually as a hamartoma.[122,154]

Aetiology

The aetiology is obscure and, more recently, controversial, as there are many individual reports associating this lesion with oral contraceptive therapy.[26,92] Fechner[49,50] has cogently argued that the incidence of focal nodular hyperplasia has not altered from the pre-contraceptive pill era. He believes that the current association with oral contraceptives is due to an accentuation of the vascular abnormalities by the pill, with a consequent increase in clinical symptoms and signs; such patients are then selected as case reports, and a self-fulfilling association with oral contraceptives becomes apparent. This viewpoint is supported by a retrospective survey of all cases of focal nodular hyperplasia from the combined files of three hospital pathology departments.[97] Eighteen cases were found with a 5:1 female preponderance, but only four women were using oral contraceptives and one of the men was receiving oestrogens for prostatic carcinoma. Vascular changes were particularly prominent in this 'oestrogen group'. Only five lesions, including four from the 'oestrogen group' were not chance discoveries at autopsy; of these, three were incidentally discovered during cholecystectomy, one during caesarean section, and one lesion produced symptoms. It is clear that further large consecutive studies are required and that careful correlation of detailed and accurate morphological observations with clinical features is necessary.

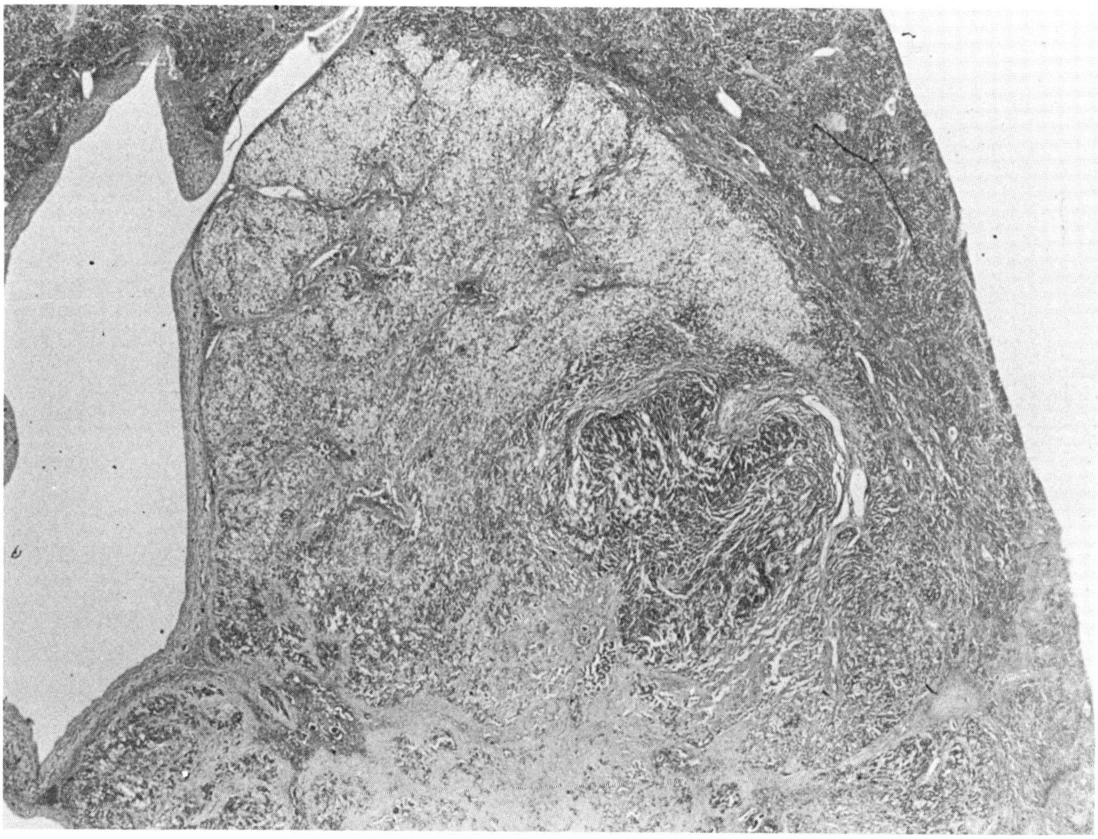

Figure 38.18. Low power view of focal nodular hyperplasia with the capsular surface on the right and a large central vein on the left. The centre of the nodule along the bottom margin shows sclerosis and contains dilated vascular channels and proliferating bile ductules. Peripherally, hepatocytes in the nodule are clearly demarcated from adjacent liver. Haematoxylin and eosin × 150.

Clinical Features

Clinically, a majority of nodules are asymptomatic, and are chance findings at operation or autopsy,[97] although since the advent of oral contraception in 1960 reports of intraperitoneal bleeding following rupture of these lesions have increased.[50]

Pathology

This lesion forms a discrete, usually subcapsular, nodule (Figure 38.18) within an otherwise normal liver. Multiple nodules are found in approximately 15 per cent of cases.[14, 97] Each nodule has a characteristic fibrous stellate centre with slender septa radiating out to the periphery. Within the central and radiating fibrous bands there are numerous bile ductules (Figure 38.19) and in the fibrous centre there are many abnormal dilated vascular channels, which may give an angiomatous appearance. Other vascular changes may also be prominent, including intimal proliferation in arterioles and venules, thrombosis in small vessels, and pronounced arterial medial hypertrophy[92, 116] (Figure 38.20). Hepatocytes in the lesion resemble normal liver cells, or may be slightly larger, and they may show considerable fatty change. There is usually a clear line of demarcation from the surrounding liver parenchyma.

MISCELLANEOUS EPITHELIAL TUMOURS

Adenomatous Hyperplasia

Rarely, the liver may show extensive multiple, ill-defined, non-encapsulated nodules of hepatic parenchyma not associated with fibrosis (Figure 38.21). Although this appearance has been

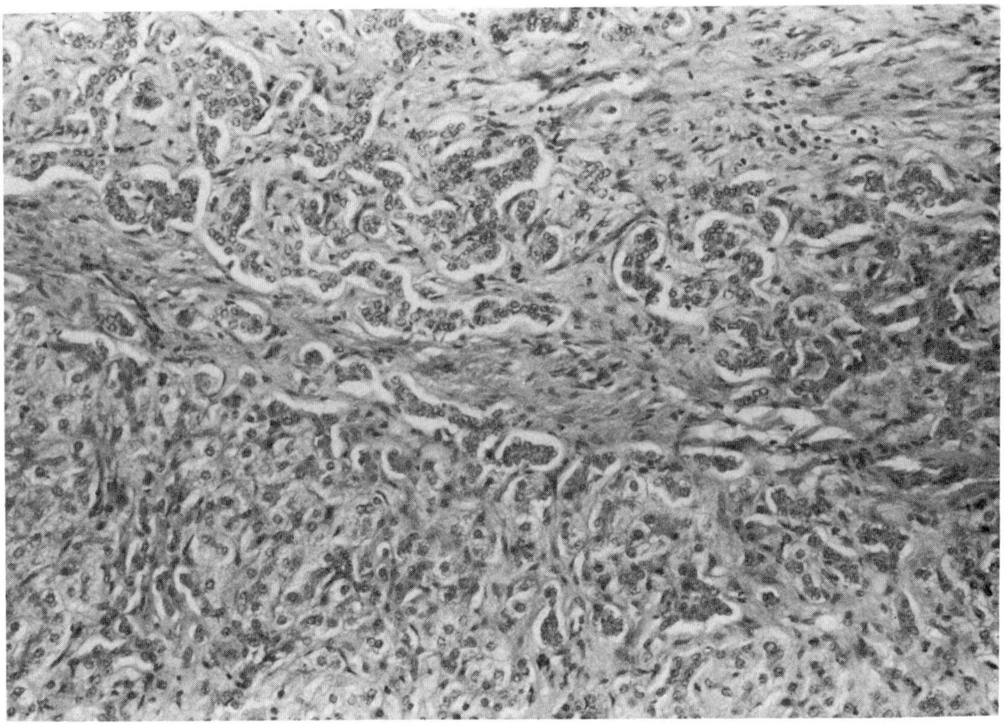

Figure 38.19. Numerous proliferating bile ductules within a fibrous septum in focal nodular hyperplasia. Haematoxylin and eosin × 600.

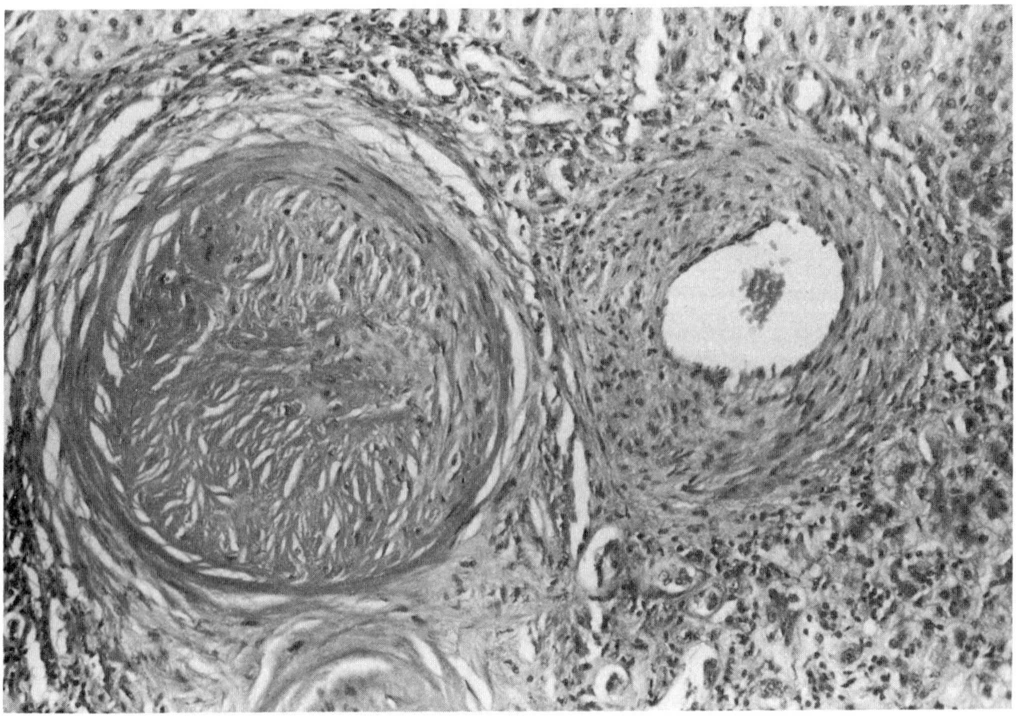

Figure 38.20. Gross smooth muscle hyperplasia in arteries. Such abnormal vessels and dilated vascular channels are more common in 'pill' associated tumours. Haematoxylin and eosin × 600.

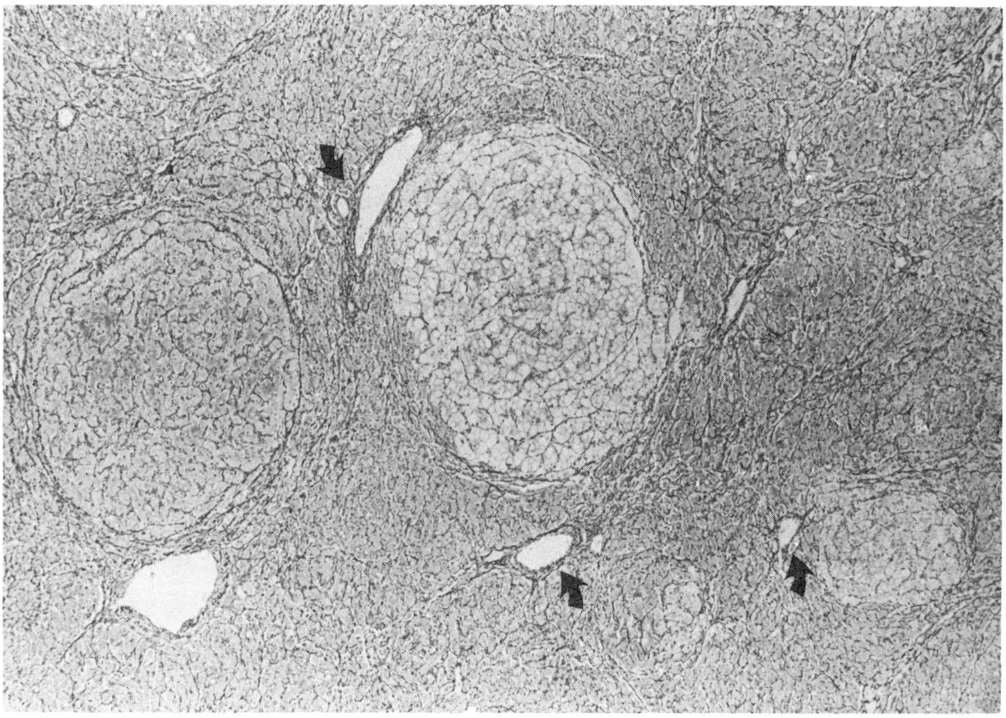

Figure 38.21. Adenomatous hyperplasia. Nodular regenerative activity of the parenchyma with compression of surrounding liver but no fibrosis. Some portal tracts are arrowed. Reticulin × 150.

reported in association with rheumatoid arthritis[16] this association is not present in all cases.[77, 150]

Partial nodular transformation may be an example of idiopathic adenomatous hyperplasia critically situated around the hilum of the liver and thus creating portal hypertension.[138]

Bile Duct Adenomas, Cystadenomas and Microhamartomas

Bile duct adenomas. These rare tumours are encountered by chance in middle-aged patients, most often males, at the time of laparotomy or autopsy. They are usually single and small, pale, firm, circumscribed nodules, being less than one cm in diameter, and 90 per cent of cases are subcapsular and are easy to resect. They are composed of numbers of small duct-like structures separated by a moderate amount of mature connective tissue stroma; the ductular epithelium is non-malignant in character, and in some cases the stroma is abundant; normal portal tract structures may be present within the adenoma. This tumour is regarded by many as a hamartoma.[9, 67] It is important to distinguish this tumour from a cholangiocellular or a cholangiolocellular carcinoma; the size and location of the lesion, the absence of symptoms, and the histological appearance should enable the distinction to be made.

Biliary cystadenomas are also rare; reported cases have been in older females.[67, 68, 99] Cystadenomas are usually large multilocular cystic tumours; the locules are lined by a single layer of columnar, mucin-producing epithelium, which may be flattened in tense cysts. The adjacent stroma is collagenized, and may contain smooth muscle cells and cholesterol clefts. The large size and cystic nature of this tumour enables it to be detected on liver scanning, and it has been successfully resected on several occasions.[67]

Microhamartomas, or von Meyenburg complexes (Figure 38.22) are not uncommonly seen, especially in wedge biopsies. They are tiny lesions and are usually multiple; each complex is composed of cystically dilated bile ducts lying in a stroma of mature collagenized fibrous tissue; the ducts may contain bile, and are lined by normal cuboidal epithelium. These complexes develop in or near portal tracts. They are usually symptomless, but occasionally produce portal hypertension. This lesion is akin to that of congenital hepatic fibrosis.[93,136] Von Meyenburg complexes may undergo malignant transformation into cholangiocellular carcinomas.[34, 62]

Heterotopic Rest Tumours

Heterotopic rests of epithelium from other sites occasionally provide further examples of benign epithelial tumours. Adrenal rest tumours are rare, but well documented.[42, 167] These benign tumours are usually located subcapsularly and may be difficult to distinguish histologically from liver cell adenomas. Evidence of adrenal cortical hyperfunction or identification of hormonal activity in the tumour is an essential criterion for diagnosis.

Pancreatic heterotopia has been reported in the liver, with a retention cyst of one of the aberrant pancreatic ducts.[67]

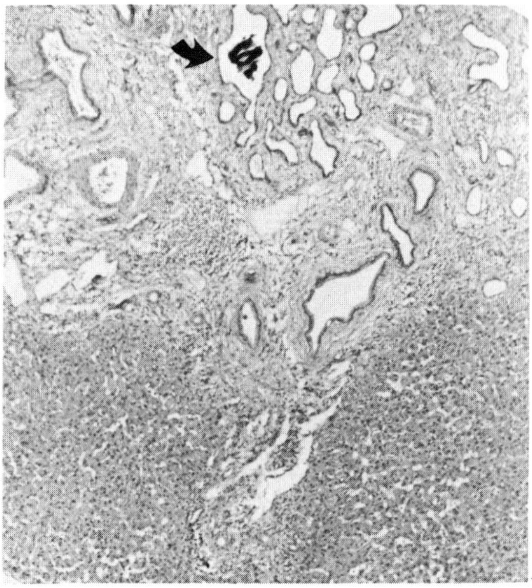

Figure 38.22. A von Meyenburg complex (top right) expands the portal tract (top left). It is composed of numerous irregular spaces lined by biliary epithelium and contained within a fibrous stroma. Bile (arrow) is present in one of the larger spaces indicating a communication with the normal biliary tree. Haematoxylin and eosin × 150.

MALIGNANT HAEMANGIO-ENDOTHELIOMA

Aetiology

Although a rare tumour, the malignant haemangio-endothelioma has recently been reported in males working with the polymerization of vinyl chloride.[33, 40, 87] The period of exposure had been from four to 28 years. Prior to these reports, the tumour had been associated with cirrhosis,[123] arsenic ingestion[132] and thorium dioxide administration.[155, 159] Most early reports of this tumour came from wine-producing countries in Europe, where arsenic was used by vineyard workers in insecticide sprays and dusts.[132]

Clinical Features

Symptoms are usually non-specific with malaise, anorexia, weight loss and right upper quadrant pain. Jaundice and abdominal swelling from ascites are late features. Hepatomegaly and splenomegaly are present on initial examination.

The patients may have anaemia, and microangiopathic haemolysis has been recorded.[6, 123]

Pathology

This tumour is composed of vasoformative angiosarcomatous tissue. Macroscopically, the tumour is composed of greyish-white or haemorrhagic nodules (Figure 38.23). The tumour is occasionally a solitary one. It spreads to the lungs, to the nodes of the porta hepatis, and occasionally to the spleen.[87] Involvement of bone marrow and peritoneal surfaces has also been recorded.[123] Rupture of a superficial nodule in the liver may result in haemoperitoneum. The microscopic appearance can resemble the infantile haemangio-endothelioma, being composed of vasoformative tissue infiltrating the hepatic parenchyma. The endothelial cells which line the vascular channels are plump pleomorphic cells, and have a clearly malignant appearance (Figure 38.24). These cells can be seen at the edges of the tumour invading and extending along the hepatic sinusoids (Figure 38.25). In the deeper parts of the tumour, the dilated vascular channels resemble blood lakes, and islands of residual hepatic parenchyma appear to float in these lakes. Extramedullary haematopoiesis is a regular feature of the tumour sinusoids.[42,87,123] Some observers regard these tumours as Kupffer cell sarcomas, having noted multinucleated pigment-laden cells in the more

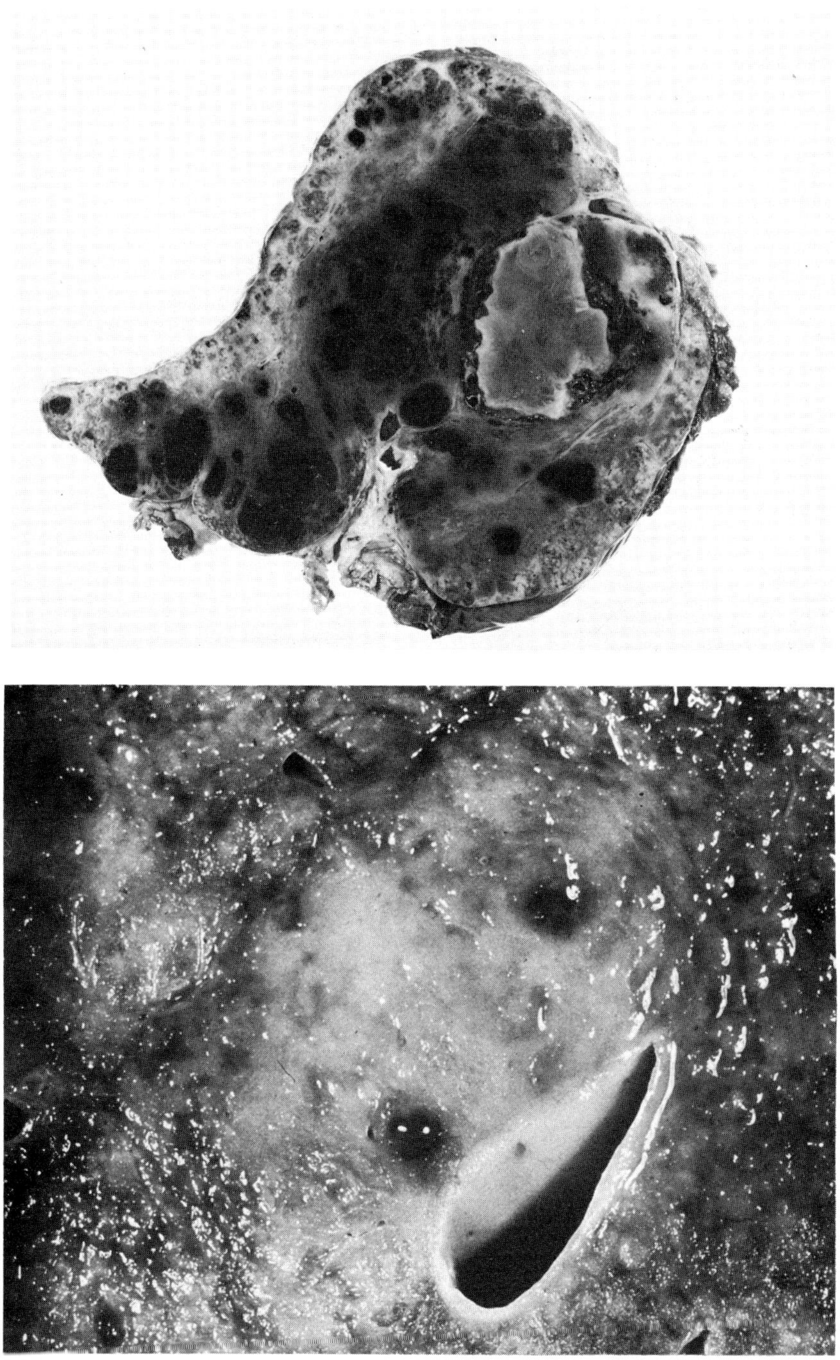

(a)

(b)

Figure 38.23. (a) Malignant haemangio-endothelioma of the liver containing many blood-filled tumour nodules, including one large nodule showing thrombosis. From Pollard and Millward-Sadler[123] with kind permission of the editor of *Journal of Clinical Pathology*. (b) Detailed view of small white nodule of malignant haemangio-endothelioma in which two small dark blood-filled spaces can be seen.

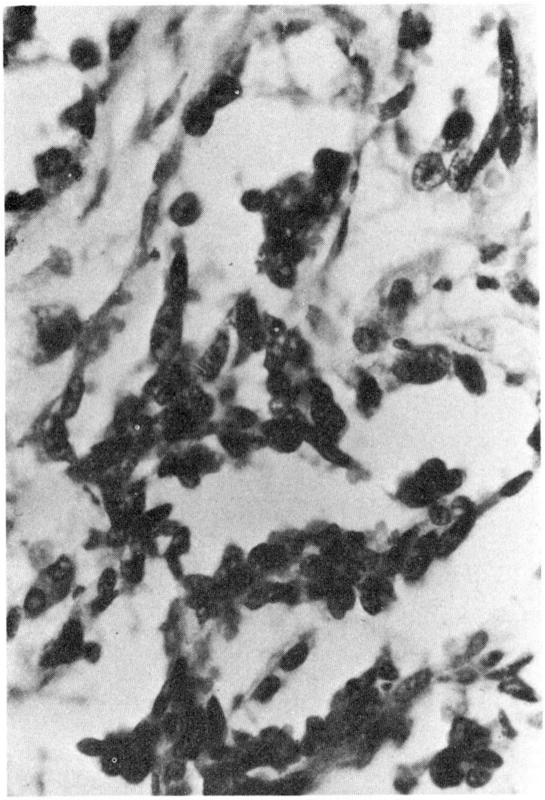

Figure 38.24. Vascular channels lined by and containing proliferating spindle tumour cells of malignant haemangio-endothelioma. Haematoxylin and eosin × 700.

solid areas of tumour tissue,[22, 58] but this feature is not always seen.[87]

Course and prognosis

The tumour is rapidly progressive and patient survival time is short, being usually less than one year after presentation.[10, 123]

OTHER PRIMARY SARCOMAS

The malignant mesenchymoma is rare and is found only in children. It is a rapidly growing sarcoma, and on gross inspection varies in colour from greyish-white to reddish-purple. It does not metastasize. Histologically, the malignant mesenchymoma is composed of undifferentiated mesenchymal tissue (Figure 38.26) often associated with extramedullary haematopoiesis, differentiated smooth or striated muscle fibres (Figure 38.27) and fibroblastic and myxoid connective tissue. Any of the spindle cell elements may be sarcomatous, and muscle cells may appear as giant myoblasts, sometimes with cross-striations. Osteoid tissue and bone are not seen in this tumour.

Monomorphic sarcomas are discussed by Ishak.[65] They are rare but have been occasionally reported in elderly subjects. A predominance of myoblasts in some tumours classes them as hepatic rhabdomyosarcomas or leiomyosarcomas, while in other cases a fibrosarcomatous pattern is evident. Sarcomas arising in the ligamentum teres have been seen in younger patients, and are more accessible to resection. Rhabdomyosarcomas of childhood are rare, and the botryoid type preponderates in girls.

Undifferentiated (embryonal) sarcomas. Stocker and Ishak[149] recently reported 31 cases of undifferentiated (embryonal) sarcoma of the liver, of which 71 per cent occurred in the six to 15 year age group, 13 per cent in the 16 years or

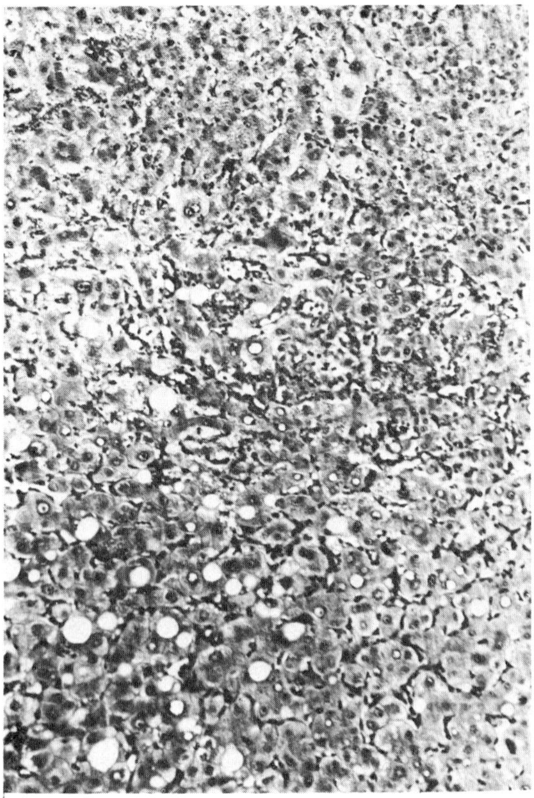

Figure 38.25. Typical pattern of sinusoidal infiltration by tumour cells at the advancing margin of malignant haemangio-endothelioma. Superficially, there can be a resemblance to the florid mesenchymal reaction seen in the later stages of acute viral hepatitis. Haematoxylin and eosin × 280.

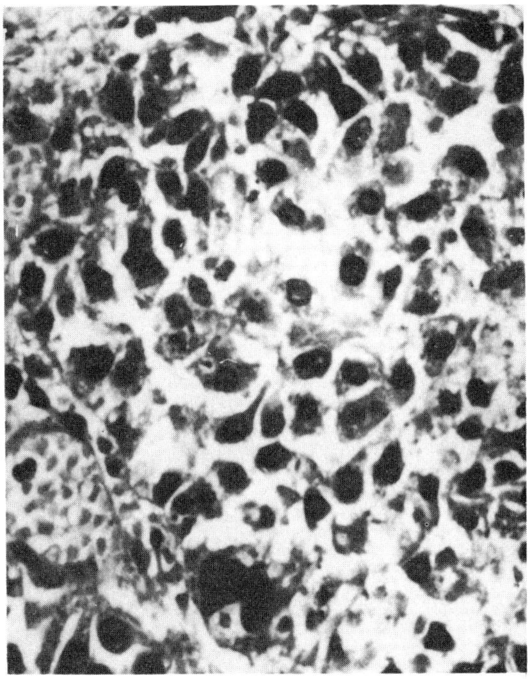

Figure 38.26. Predominantly small undifferentiated mesenchymal cells of a malignant mesenchymoma. Haematoxylin and eosin × 900.

more age group and 16 per cent in the group less than six years old. This rare sarcoma is seen as a large, single globular tumour macroscopically, the cut surface showing areas of necrosis, haemorrhage and gelatinous degeneration (Figure 38.28). A pseudocapsule demarcates the tumour. On microscopy (Figure 38.29), the main component is undifferentiated sarcomatous tissue, with stellate or spindle cells packed in fascicles or lying loosely in a myxoid stroma. Characteristically, within this are single or small groups of large polygonal cells which contain PAS positive and diastase resistant globules in their cytoplasm. At the edges of the mass, degenerating dilated bile duct and islands of hepatocytes are seen, giving a resemblance to the mesenchymal hamartoma, of which this may be the malignant counterpart. Ninety per cent of these cases presented as an abdominal mass and/or abdominal pain, and the average prognosis was less than one year.[149]

Differential Diagnosis of Malignant Mesenchymal Tumours

At times it may be difficult to identify the type of hepatic neoplasm and to distinguish between primary and metastatic tumour. Identification of striated muscle cells in a tumour has the following differential diagnosis:

1. Malignant mesenchymoma: children, pleomorphic mesodermal tissues.
2. Rhabdomyosarcoma: all ages; monomorphic pattern.
3. Hepatoblastoma (mixed type): infants; fetal or embryonal epithelial elements are also present, possibly with osteoid.
4. Malignant hepatic mixed tumour: children; a malignant teratoid tumour, with a mature carcinomatous element.
5. Metastatic rhabdomyosarcoma: botryoid type in first decade, the alveolar type in the first two decades, the adult pleomorphic type in older adults.

The jumbled well-differentiated teratoid pattern of the benign teratoma is not likely to cause confusion; carcino-sarcomas have spindle-cell sarcomatous tissue associated with hepatocellular carcinoma.

CAVERNOUS HAEMANGIOMA

Edmondson[42] found this to be the most common hepatic tumour at autopsy and it is

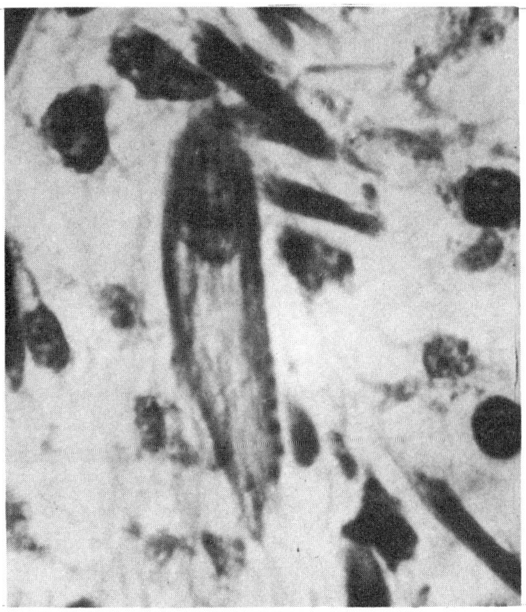

Figure 38.27. Cross-striations in a strap cell in a malignant mesenchymoma. Phosphotungstic acid haematoxylin × 1500.

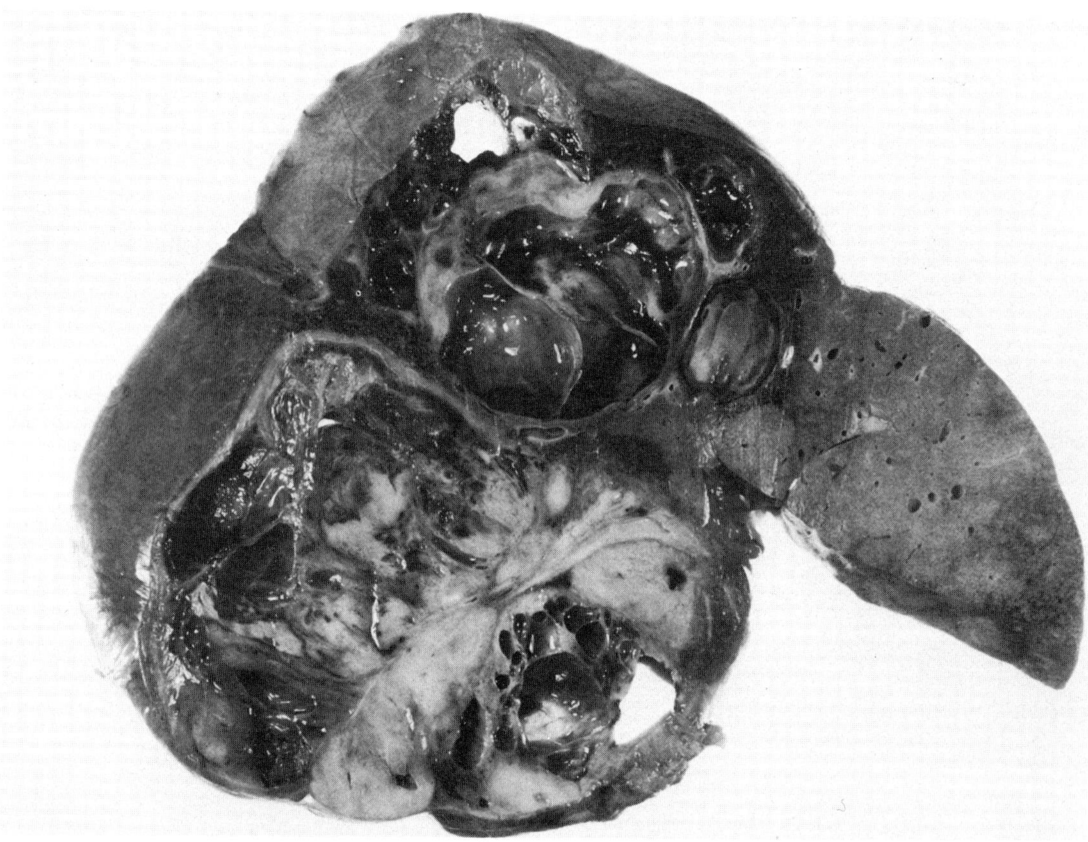

Figure 38.28. A large multicystic tumour with solid areas and areas of mucinous and haemorrhagic degeneration completely replaces the right lobe of the liver. Embryonal sarcoma of liver.

(a) 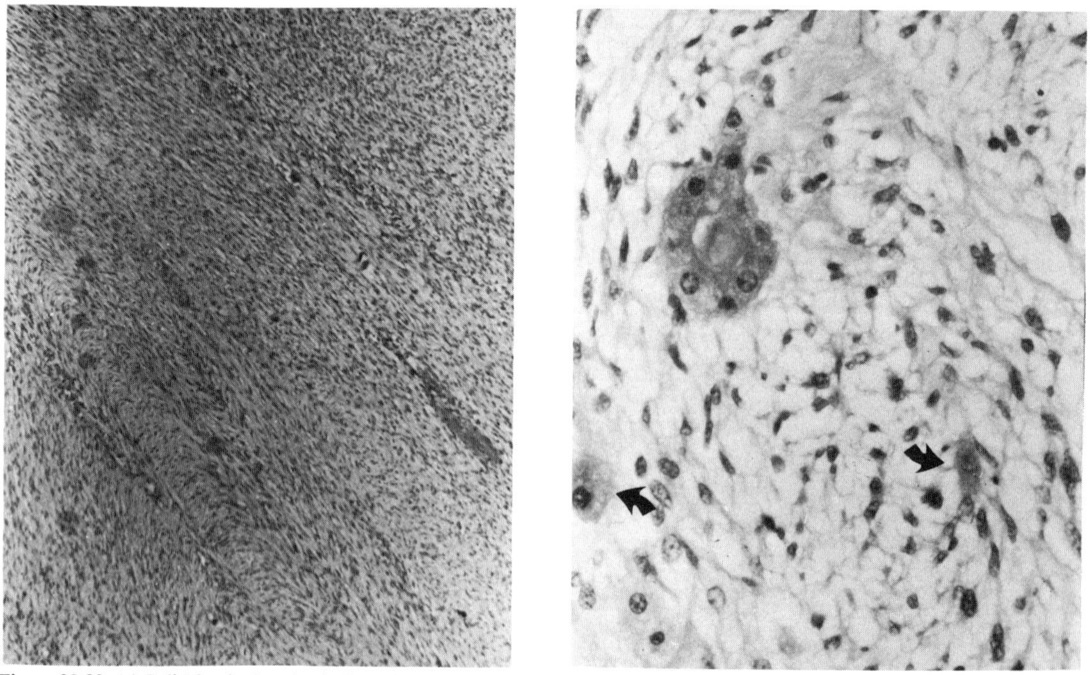 (b)

Figure 38.29. (a) Solid fasciculated spindle cell areas of tumour illustrated in Figure 38.28. Haematoxylin and eosin × 150. (b) Area of tumour composed of stellate cells in a myxoid stroma. Larger polygonal tumour cells are also present (arrows) and contain PAS positive diastase resistant globules. The tumour may trap bile ducts or, as here, small groups of hepatocytes. Those illustrated have bile in a central lumen. Haematoxylin and eosin × 600.

certainly the commonest mesodermal tumour of the liver.

Pathology

Macroscopically, haemangiomas are usually quite small, from 1 to 4 cm in diameter, but occasionally may be enormous.[42] The tumours are single, well-defined, dark, blood-filled lesions, with a soft spongy consistency. Multiple tumours are very rare. On microscopic examination they are composed of fairly large vascular channels, lined by mature, flattened endothelial cells, enclosed in a loose fibroblastic stroma with a variable amount of collagenization. The tumour is separated from the surrounding hepatic parenchyma by a pseudo-capsule of fibrous tissue. The vascular channels may contain thrombi, sometimes showing organization or dystrophic calcification, or sclerosis may be extensive. Most lesions are situated within the liver substance, and there is no tendency to haemorrhage.

Clinical Features

Clinical manifestations are rare, and the tumours are discovered only by chance, usually at autopsy. Patients are usually middle-aged but occasionally these tumours cause hepatomegaly in neonates.[54] The frequency of haemangiomas in multiparous females (four to five times the incidence in males) suggests that the aetiology may be related to hormonal influences during pregnancy.[9]

Differential Diagnosis

Hereditary haemorrhagic telangiectasia is a haemangiomatous lesion composed of multiple foci of dilated vascular channels with irregular portal fibrosis, and can be distinguished from haemangiomas because the latter are usually single lesions[89, 171] (see Chapter 37). The distinction from infantile haemangio-endothelioma is discussed in the following section.

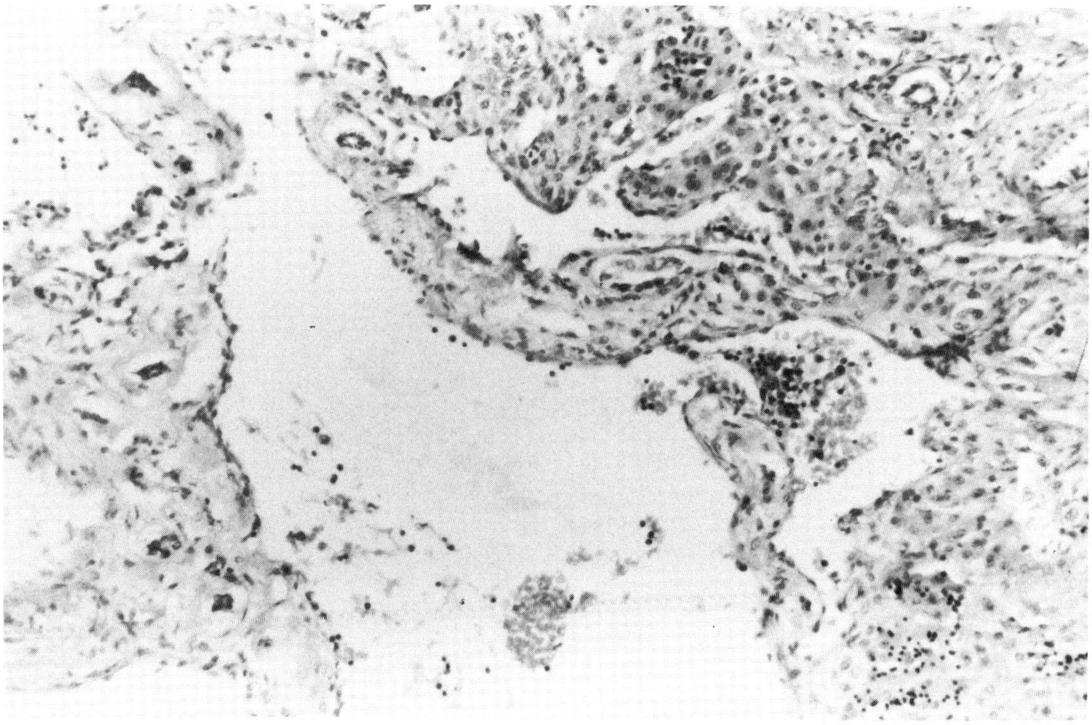

Figure 38.30. Portal tract (top right), a thin rim of hepatocytes and large cavernous vascular spaces lined by a single layer of flattened epithelium. The extension of these vascular channels between the hepatocytes distinguishes this type I infantile haemangio-endothelioma from a cavernous haemangioma. Small bile ductules are also trapped in the fibrous stroma of the tumour and can be seen bottom left. Haematoxylin and eosin × 600.

INFANTILE HAEMANGIO-ENDOTHELIOMA

This benign tumour is most often seen in infants during the first six months of life.

Clinical Features

The vascular structure of the tumour produces a haemodynamic disturbance similar to an arteriovenous shunt in the infant with a bruit. Many children present as cases of congestive cardiac failure with hepatomegaly. Some tumours have produced microangiopathic haemolytic anaemia or profound thrombocytopenia, and jaundice of the haemolytic type is seen in one-third of cases.[67] Angiography is of value in revealing the tumour, and foci of calcification may be seen on abdominal radiographs. In about half of reported cases cutaneous haemangiomas are also present.

Pathology

This can be a solitary nodule, or a multicentric tumour, which is well demarcated but not encapsulated. The cut surface is reddish-brown with a spongy consistency, and may show haemorrhages, scarring or calcified foci in the central areas. Tumour nodules vary in size from a few millimetres to over 15 cm in diameter. On microscopy, the tumour is composed of anastamosing vascular channels lined by one or more layers of plump endothelial cells, single layers being known as the type I pattern, while several endothelial layers represent the type II pattern. Growth is infiltrative between hepatic cell plates (Figure 38.30) and this distinguishes the tumour from a cavernous haemangioma. The tumour cells are benign and uniform in character, and mitotic figures are rare.[67] Type I tumours have to be distinguished histologically from cavernous haemangiomas and type II tumours from malignant haemangio-endotheliomas.

Prognosis and Treatment

Occasional cases have involuted spontaneously; a few have metastasized. Successful results have been variously reported with x-irradiation, corticosteroid therapy, hepatic artery ligation, and resection of solitary tumour nodules.[67]

MISCELLANEOUS MESENCHYMAL AND MIXED TUMOURS

Mesenchymal hamartoma

These rare benign tumours may present macroscopically as firm fibroadenomatous tumours or, more often, as soft 'lymphangiomatoid' lesions. Edmondson[42] regards these lesions as fibrodysplasias of liver tissue, rather than as true tumours. They are encountered most often in the first two years of life, and the oldest case has been five years old. The liver often increases suddenly in size as fluid accumulates in the degenerating mesenchymal tissue of the lesion. Histologically they are composed mainly of oedematous connective tissue and serous-filled cyst-like spaces; variable amounts of mature collagenized connective tissue, loose primitive mesenchymal tissue, and fluid-filled unlined pseudocysts. Branching or dilated bile ducts are present in the stroma, and islands of hepatic parenchyma lie between the oedematous mesenchymal areas (Figure 38.31). Sutton and Eller[151] reported four cases, and

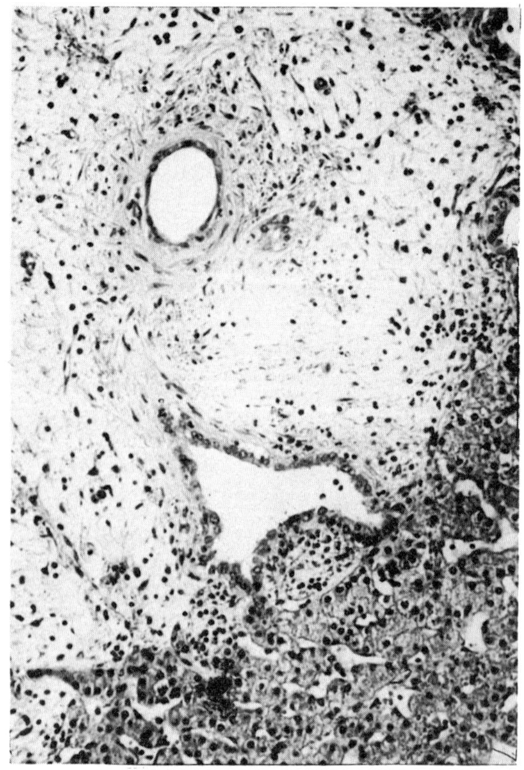

Figure 38.31. Mesenchymal hamartoma showing the myxoid stromal tissue and containing abnormal dilated bile ducts. Haematoxylin and eosin × 250.

suggested that the tendency for these tumours to enlarge rapidly in the process of becoming cystic was a helpful clinical diagnostic point. As these tumours are not malignant, if successful resection is achieved the prognosis is good.

Malignant hepatic mixed tumour

These tumours generally develop during childhood but are exceedingly rare. They characteristically contain a mixture of mesenchymal and epithelial elements. Any of several components may be malignant. The epithelial components are well-differentiated mature tissues and produce hepatocellular, squamous or papillary carcinomatous patterns. The mesenchymal components are usually poorly differentiated, although foci of osteoid or bone may be present. Malignant hepatic mixed tumours with a hepatocellular carcinomatous element and a benign mesenchymal element (such as foci of osteoid or bone) have sometimes been called 'liver cell carcinomas of childhood', but this term is not preferred.[42]

Differentiation from other possible tumours is made on the following points:

1. Hepatoblastoma (mixed type): the epithelial component is of fetal or embryonic type, with ultrastructural points of difference.
2. Malignant mesenchymoma: does not contain an epithelial element, and bone or osteoid have not been reported.
3. Carcinosarcoma: is seen in adults; components are not intimately mixed; the epithelial element is always hepatocellular, while the mesenchymal element is fibrosarcomatous, and osteoid or bone is not present.

Carcinosarcoma

In adults, mixed tumours are occasionally encountered which contain both hepatocellular carcinoma and spindle-cell sarcomatous elements. The two malignancies are not very intimately mixed, and some may in fact be separate malignancies; in others both elements are present in metastases.[42] These rare tumours must be distinguished, where possible, from spindle-cell variants of hepatocellular carcinoma and from malignant hepatic mixed tumours of childhood.

Teratomas

These tumours are rare, and occur at birth or in infancy; they usually prove fatal because of their size, in spite of their benign character.[96] Macroscopically they have a bizarre lobulated structure. Histologically they show benign differentiated mesodermal elements together with benign epithelial components, such as liver cells, ductular structures, brain, skin, respiratory tissue and even teeth. They must be distinguished from hepatoblastomas of the mixed type which may also contain bone or cartilage.

Other benign mesodermal tumours

Rare instances of lipomas, angiomyolipomas and myelolipomas are discussed by Ishak.[65] These are usually small, well-demarcated yellow tumours related to the capsule. Mesotheliomas may occasionally arise from Glisson's capsule.[42]

METASTATIC TUMOURS OF THE LIVER

In western societies, malignancy within the liver is most commonly metastatic in origin and frequently is asymptomatic or incidental to other features of the primary tumour. Occasionally, symptoms and signs due to the involvement of the liver may be the presenting feature of an otherwise occult primary tumour. In such cases, the likely symptoms are malaise, weight loss, hepatic pain and abdominal distension. Physical examination may then confirm the weight loss and usually demonstrates a large liver with an irregular edge. Despite this, liver involvement may not be established even in known cases of disseminated malignancy until autopsy.

Investigations

Biochemical

Liver function tests are too insensitive to detect hepatic metastases. The most consistent abnormality is a raised serum alkaline phosphatase, but extensive metastatic disease may be present in the absence of such biochemical abnormalities.

Radio-isotope imaging

Techniques of liver scintigraphy have improved (see Chapter 20), and Ruiter et al[133] found an 83 per cent accuracy in 59 patients who came to autopsy within a few weeks of their liver scans. They quote accuracy rates for scintigraphy in six series, including their own, as varying from 72 to 95 per cent, though not all these series used post-mortems to evaluate their results. The majority of false negative results, six out of 33 in the series reported by Ruiter et al,[133] were accounted for by lesions under 2.5 cm in diameter. Maxfield et al[91] noted that cysts, abscesses and enlarged lymph nodes in the hilum of the liver may give false positive results on scintigraphy, and they advocate scans as an adjunct to needle biopsy.

Ultrasound and computed tomography (CT)

Ultrasound and CT scanning (see Chapter 21) also accurately identify space-occupying lesions in the liver, and a correct diagnosis has been claimed in 93 per cent of cases.[145] They have advantages because cystic lesions can be differentiated from solid lesions and also because they are safe, non-invasive techniques.

Liver biopsy

Tissue tests are often necessary to confirm the diagnosis. Direct visualization of the liver at laparotomy or laparoscopy with biopsy of suspicious areas is most reliable, but sometimes metastases may be present only on the distant, non-visible surface of the liver or deep within its substance.

Percutaneous needle biopsy of the liver is much more widely practised and yields a sample representing one-500 000th of the total liver mass.[31] The potential sampling error may be reduced by directing the needle biopsy at presenting tumour nodules that are clinically apparent or detected either by ultrasound or by scintigraphy. Several studies have been performed on cadavers to compare the results of needle biopsy with subsequent examination of the liver at autopsy. In a series of 100 patients, Dixon and Burns[37] obtained a positive needle biopsy in 50 per cent of those with hepatic metastases. Not surprisingly, the yield was highest in those with extensive metastases. Seven cases with a single tumour nodule in their series all yielded negative biopsies.

Several authors have advocated taking two biopsies through a single subcostal entry point, each in a different direction.[31, 32, 55] There were more positive results after two biopsies compared with the findings on one alone. Since these were post-mortem studies, they did not show whether the double biopsy technique had an increased morbidity or mortality over the single biopsy.

Cytological preparations of the fluid obtained with the biopsy tissue have been advocated. In a series of 67 patients, 39 of whom had liver metastases, 15 per cent were positive on a cytological preparation but negative on both biopsies. The total yield of positive results was thus increased to 69 per cent.[55] It is surprising that, despite its apparent usefulness without increasing the risk to the patient, this simple technique does not appear to be widely practised.

Conn[31] advocated serial sectioning of the needle biopsies, noting that, although in 90 per cent of his positive biopsies tumour was present in all sections, in 10 per cent it was found in some levels and not others. Thus, from these studies it would appear that even with minimal involvement of the liver by a tumour the needle biopsy is positive in approximately 15 per cent of cases,[31] and that overall the technique has an accuracy rate of approximately 50 per cent, but that this might be significantly improved by combining histology with cytology.

Frequency

Fine slicing of the liver at autopsy with appropriate microscopy is the most accurate method of confirming metastases within the liver. In his classic study of 500 carefully

Table 38.7. *Origin of Hepatic Metastases.*[a]

Primary	Percentage of cases
Stomach	22
Intestines	18
Breast	12
Lung	9
Head and neck	8
Oesophagus	4
Pancreas	4
Biliary tree/liver	4
Kidney	3
Melanomas	1
Sarcomas	4
Other	11

[a] After Willis.[169]

documented autopsies on patients dying with neoplastic disease, Willis[169] found the liver to be the most frequent site for metastatic growths. These were present in 36 per cent of his cases, the corresponding figure for the lungs being 29 per cent. The incidence of hepatic metastases was greatest for primary tumours lying within the portal venous drainage (48 per cent), although after excluding cranial tumours it was considerable for those in extraportal sites (37 per cent) (Table 38.7).

It can be seen from Table 38.7 that, outside the portal venous drainage, lung and breast are the most common primary sites of metastases in the liver at autopsy and that melanoma is rare. These frequencies are not necessarily those found in series based on liver biopsy diagnoses,[55] presumably because of bias in the selection of patients.

Willis[169] noted that the high incidence of blood-borne secondary tumours in the liver from primary neoplasms not within the portal area was in striking contrast to the paucity of the hepatic arterial blood supply, and suggested that this was due to particularly favourable conditions within the liver for the establishment and growth of tumour emboli. Despite the suggested segregation of portal venous blood, so that a disproportionate volume of splenic blood goes to the left lobe and intestinal blood to the right lobe, Willis was unable to find the corresponding segregation of early hepatic metastases from primary tumours in the intestine.

Pathology

Macroscopic appearances

Metastases may be single but are most frequently multiple discrete lesions (Figure 38.32) and often grossly enlarge the liver, up to three or four times. Nearly all metastatic deposits are pearly grey-white in appearance, although exceptions occur, particularly with melanomas. Central necrosis often occurs within the tumour and may result in an accumulation of clear fluid or of blood within the centre of the metastasis. In subcapsular metastases, central necrosis can be seen as an umbilication of the nodule and this feature is

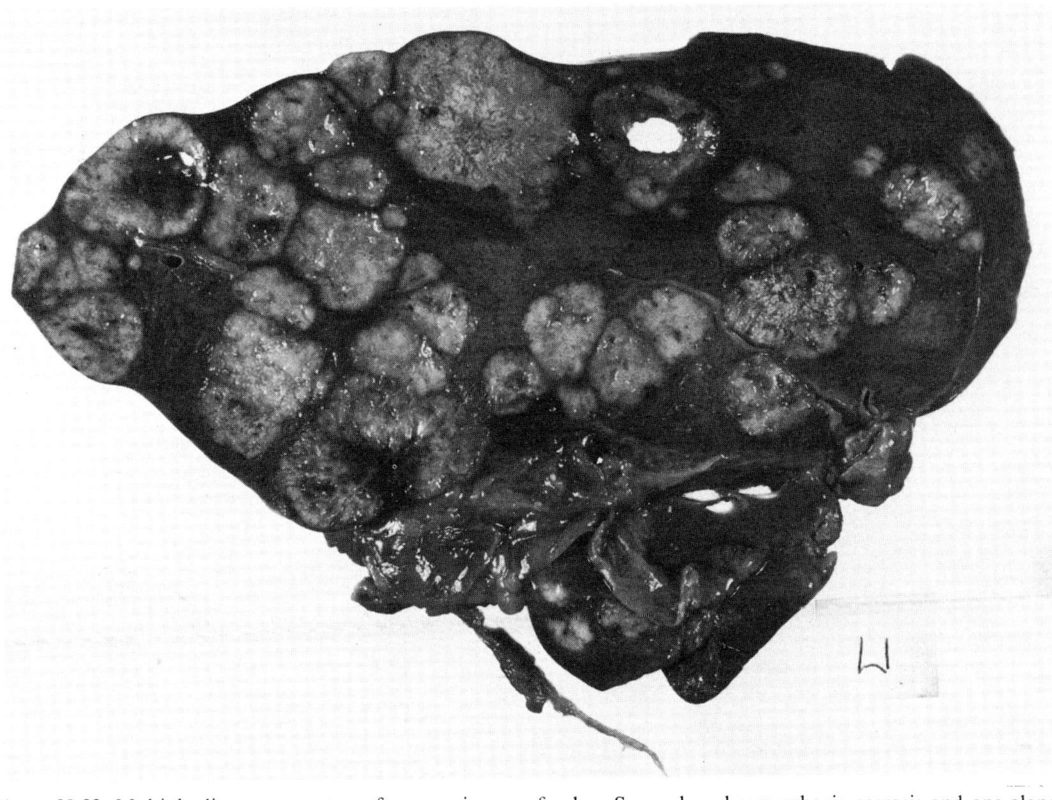

Figure 38.32. Multiple discrete metastases from carcinoma of colon. Some show haemorrhagic necrosis and one along the superior border shows liquefacture necrosis.

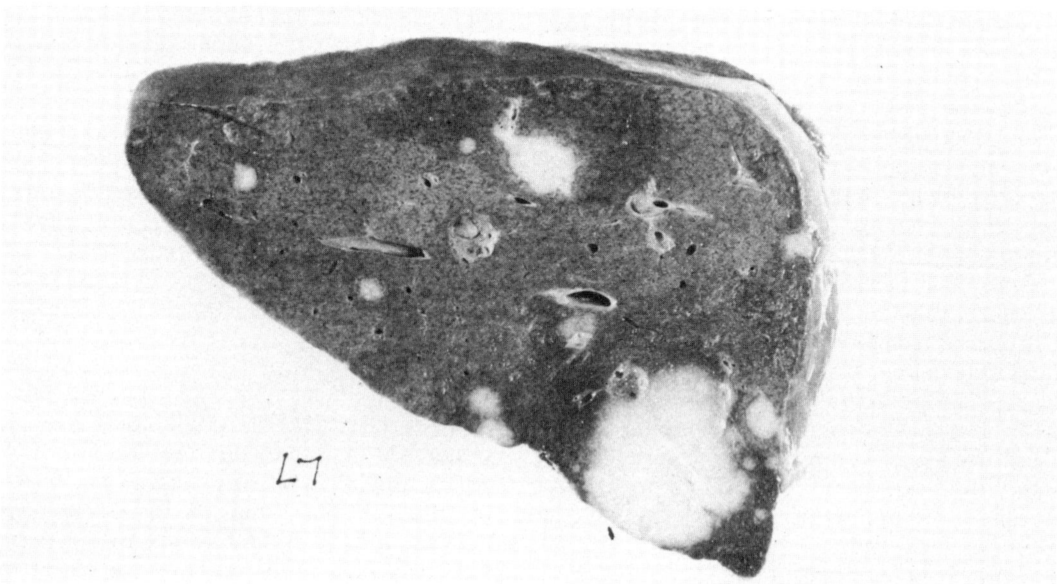

Figure 38.33. White metastatic nodules of carcinoma present in the liver are surrounded by a dark haemorrhagic zone of liver.

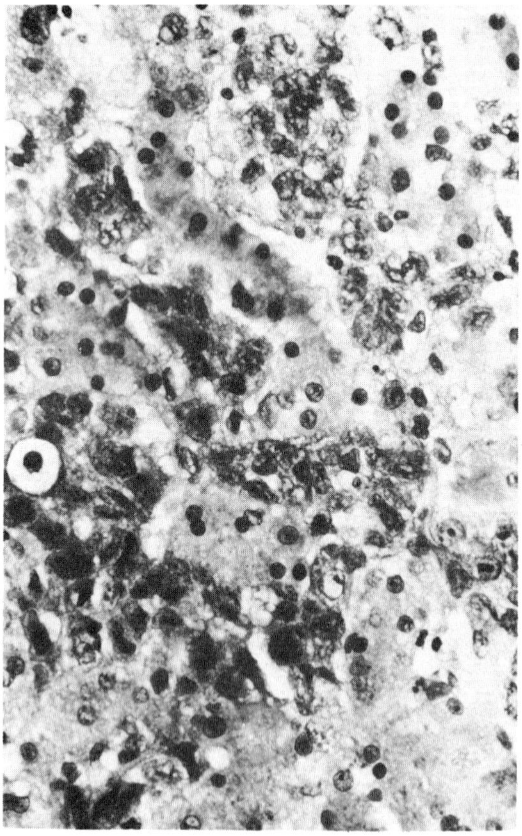

Figure 38.34. Oat cell carcinoma of bronchus. The core of liver shows diffuse permeation of sinusoids by carcinoma cells. Haematoxylin and eosin × 1250.

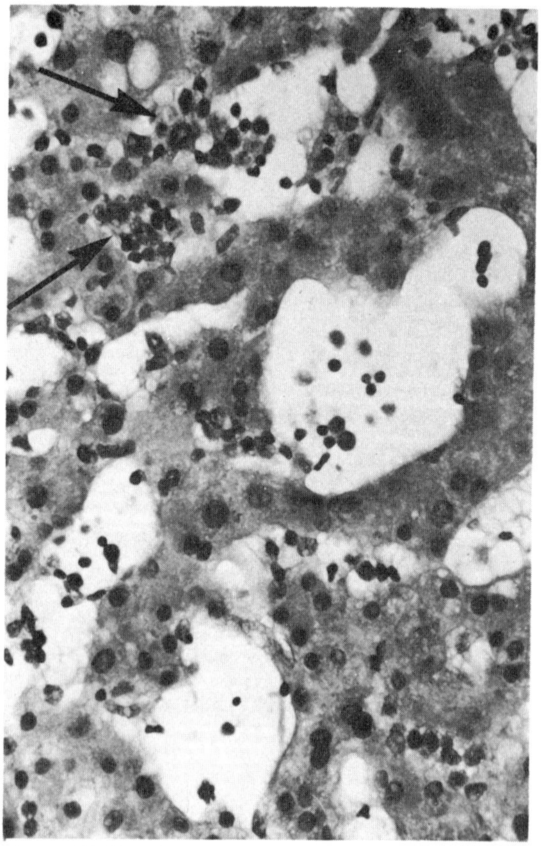

Figure 38.35. Metastatic oat cell carcinoma. Marked sinusoidal dilatation. Sinusoids contain haematopoietic cells, related to bone marrow infiltration by the tumour. Occasional carcinoma cells seen (arrows). Needle biopsy. Haematoxylin and eosin × 1250.

rare in primary tumours. The liver parenchyma around the metastases shows compression and sometimes there is a haemorrhagic zone (Figure 38.33). The latter microscopically corresponds to sinusoidal ectasia.

Microscopic

The histology will obviously vary according to the tumour's primary origin and cannot be detailed here. The majority of tumours are either adenocarcinomas or anaplastic carcinomas. Occasional neoplasms, in addition to generating metastatic tumour nodules, may disseminate throughout the sinusoids in a diffuse fashion. The most common of these are neuroblastomas in childhood and oat cell carcinoma of the bronchus in adults (Figure 38.34). If the initial sections of the liver biopsy are negative, serial section through the specimen is indicated, particularly in the presence of known space-occupying lesions of the liver, and the presence histologically of focal sinusoidal ectasia (Figure 38.35) or focal biliary obstruction.

DIFFERENTIAL DIAGNOSIS OF HEPATIC TUMOURS

The primary duty of the clinician in the management of patients with suspected hepatic tumours is to exclude other treatable disorders with which they may be confused and to identify the benign or malignant tumours which are amenable to hepatic resection. The conditions which are most likely to be misdiagnosed as hepatic neoplasms are cysts, abscesses, tuberculomas and gummas and the infiltrative or storage disorders.

In geographical areas where hepatoma is common, patients usually present with abdominal pain, ascites, malaise, weight loss and a rapidly enlarging liver, often with jaundice. Fever is frequent and there may be a raised right diaphragm, so that a distinction from amoebic liver abscess is important. Hydatid disease is another important benign condition which must be excluded.

Ultrasonography or CT scanning is a crucial investigation in such cases, since they readily distinguish cysts and solid tumours (see Chapter 21), and should be supplemented by serological tests for amoebic abscess and hydatid disease. Polycystic disease of the liver will also be identified by these techniques, and, if suspected, the pancreas and kidney should also be examined.

In childhood, hepatoma must be distinguished from other causes of marked hepatomegaly, such as the infiltrative and storage diseases, and in particular benign conditions, including liver abscess, tuberculomas and congenital syphilis (hepar lobatum).

In the cirrhotic patient, a complicating hepatoma should be suspected if there is decompensation of otherwise well-stabilized liver disease. This may be manifested as rapidly developing varices with or without bleeding, ascites, unexplained fever and undue elevation of the alkaline phosphatase.

Although the distinction between primary and secondary malignant hepatic tumours may be of little relevance in terms of patient care at present, an increasingly aggressive approach to treatment, whether by resection, transplantation or chemotherapy, is being adopted. Investigation should therefore be aimed not only at excluding benign causes of an hepatic mass which might otherwise be attributed to malignant disease, but at identifying patients who have a lesion, either primary or secondary, which is localized and potentially treatable surgically. As indicated in Chapter 49, the results to date have been disappointing, but early detection and a combined approach of resection and more effective chemotherapy or transplantation should be explored.

Benign hepatic tumours, particularly those associated with the contraceptive pill, are being recognized with increasing frequency. As indicated earlier, they present in a variety of ways, ranging from an incidental finding on physical examination and surgery or on hepatic scanning to an abdominal emergency as a result of intraperitoneal haemorrhage.

Investigations which should be undertaken in patients presenting with a suspected hepatic neoplasm are as follows:

1. Full blood count, erythrocyte sedimentation rate, liver function tests and coagulation screen;
2. Alpha-fetoprotein;
3. Serological and other tests appropriate to exclude infections such as hepatitis, tuberculosis, syphilis, amoebic liver abscess and hydatid disease;
4. Autoimmune profile;
5. Plain abdominal film and chest x-ray;
6. Colloid liver scan, ultrasonography, CT scanning and, if necessary, angiography;
7. Liver biopsy with or without laparoscopy;

8. Appropriate investigation to identify a primary site, particularly of the gastrointestinal tract, lung and breast.

PROGNOSIS AND TREATMENT OF HEPATIC TUMOURS

Large benign hepatic tumours should be resected to exclude malignant change and because of the danger of intraperitoneal haemorrhage. If they are associated with taking contraceptive pills, the drug should be stopped. As regression may occur in the 'pill-associated' adenomas after stopping the drug, it may be feasible in individual patients to observe smaller lesions by repeated scans before a decision is reached. There is no evidence that subsequent pregnancy is contraindicated. Large haemangiomas and infantile haemangio-endotheliomas may not be resectable and treatment by radiotherapy or corticosteroids may be necessary (see Chapter 41).

The prognosis of primary hepatocellular carcinoma is poor, and the longest survivals occur after partial hepatectomy or transplantation (see Chapters 49 and 52). The majority of patients have an associated cirrhosis, and in such circumstances partial hepatectomy is impracticable. Similarly, the number of patients who are suitable for transplantation is small, and although long-term survival has occurred in a few patients (see Chapter 52), an alternative approach is necessary for the majority. Cochrane and associates[28] showed by means of controlled trials that a combination of quadruple chemotherapy using 5-fluorouracil, cyclophosphamide, methotrexate and vincristine gave a significantly longer survival time than that of patients given radiotherapy followed by the same regimen of chemotherapy. In a subsequent study, Johnson and associates[71] were able to induce clinical remission in 14 of 44 patients with hepatocellular carcinoma, using doxorubicin (60 mg/m^2 at three-weekly intervals). They also noted that patients whose serum alpha-fetoprotein level fell after the initial injection of doxorubicin had a favourable clinical response, whereas in those patients who did not respond the level continued to rise.

Hepatic artery ligation has been used for the treatment of both primary and secondary neoplasms which are not amenable to resection.[102] This can be combined with postoperative chemotherapy[103] with apparent tumour regression as monitored by liver scanning and serial measurements of alpha-fetoprotein levels. Success has also been claimed with the intra-arterial infusion of cytotoxic agents.

Although regimens employing cytotoxic agents appear to be associated with a regression in tumour size, intensive chemotherapy for primary or secondary liver neoplasms has not met with the same success achieved by the aggressive treatment of Hodgkin's disease. It is therefore important to assess any proposed regimens of treatment by carefully controlled clinical trials.

REFERENCES

1. Abelev, G.I. (1971) Alphafetoprotein in ontogenesis and its association with malignant tumours. *Cancer Research,* **14,** 295–357.
2. Abelev, G.I., Perova, S.P., Khramkova, N.I., Postnikova, Z.A. & Irlin, I.S. (1963) Production of embryonal alpha-globulin by transplantable mouse hepatomas. *Transplantation,* **1,** 174–180.
3. Alexander, M.G., Purves, L.R., Kirsch, R.R., Bass, N.M., Gitlin, N., Terblanche, J. & Saunders, S.J. (1978) Alpha-fetoprotein in liver disease. *South African Medical Journal,* **53,** 433–436.
4. Ali, M., Fayeuci, A.O. & Braun, E.V. (1978) Malignant apudoma of the liver with symptomatic intractable hypoglycaemia, *Cancer,* **42,** 686–692.
5. Alpert, E. (1976) Human alpha-1-fetoprotein. In *Hepatocellular Carcinoma* (Ed.) Okuda, K. & Peters, R.L. pp. 353–367. London: John Wiley and Sons.
6. Alpert, L.I. & Benisch, B. (1970) Hemangioendothelioma of the liver associated with microangiopathic hemolytic anemia. *American Journal of Medicine,* **48,** 624–628.
7. Alpert, M.E., Hutt, M.S.R., Wogan, G.N. & Davidson, C.S. (1971) Association between aflatoxin content of food and hepatoma frequency in Uganda. *Cancer,* **28,** 253–260.
8. Anthony, P.P. (1976) Primary carcinoma of the liver. *Annals of the Royal College of Surgery of England,* **58,** 285–292.
9. Baggenstoss, A.H. (1970) The pathology of tumours of the liver in infancy and childhood. In *Tumours of the Liver* (Ed.) Pack, G.T. & Islami, A.H. pp. 240–258. London: William Heinemann.
10. Baker, H. de C., Paget, G.E. & Dawson, J. (1956) Haemangioendothelioma (Kupffer cell sarcoma) of the liver. *Journal of Pathology and Bacteriology,* **72,** 173–182.
11. Battifora, H.A. (1976) Thorotrast and tumours of the liver. In *Hepatocellular Carcinoma* (Ed.) Okuda, K. & Peters, R.L. pp. 83–94. New York: John Wiley & Sons.
12. Baum, J.K., Holtz, F., Brookstein, J.J. & Klein, E.W. (1973) Possible association between benign hepatomas and oral contraceptives. *Lancet,* **ii,** 926–929.
13. Becker, B.T.P. & Chatgidakis, C.B. (1961) Primary carcinoma of the liver in Johannesburg. *Acta Unionis Internationalis contra Cancrum,* **17,** 650–653.

14. Benz, E.J. & Baggenstoss, A.H. (1953) Focal cirrhosis of the liver: its relation to the so-called hamartoma (adenoma, benign hepatoma). *Cancer,* **6,** 743–755.
15. Black, M. (1975) Diagnostic methods in liver disease. *Medical Clinics of North America,* **59,** 1015–1024.
16. Blendis, L.M., Ansell, I.D., Lloyd-Jones, K., Hamilton, E. & Williams, R. (1970) Liver in Felty's syndrome. *British Medical Journal,* **i,** 131–135.
17. Blumberg, B.S., Sutnick, A.I. & London, W.T. (1970) Australia antigen as a hepatitis virus. *American Journal of Medicine,* **48,** 1–8.
18. Blumberg, B.S., Larouze, B., London, W.T., Werner, B., Hesser, J., Millman, I., Saimot, G. & Payet, M. (1975) The relation of infection with hepatitis B agent to primary hepatic carcinoma. *American Journal of Pathology,* **81,** 669–682.
19. Buchanan, T.F. & Huvos, A.G. (1974) Clear cell carcinoma of the liver. *American Journal of Clinical Pathology,* **61,** 529–539.
20. Buffe, D. & Rimbaud, C. (1975) Immunosuppressive effect of a human hepatic glycoferroprotein, alpha-2H-globulin. *Immunology,* **29,** 175–184.
21. Burdette, W.J. (1970) Hepatic carcinogenesis. In *Tumours of the Liver* (Ed.) Pack, G.T. & Islami, A.H. pp. 53–71. London: William Heinemann.
22. Burston, J. (1958) Kupffer cell sarcoma. *Cancer,* **11,** 798–802.
23. Carnaghan, R.B.A. (1967) Hepatic tumours and other chronic liver changes in rats following a single oral administration of aflatoxin. *British Journal of Cancer,* **21,** 811–814.
24. Centre for Disease Control (1977) Increased risk of hepatocellular adenoma in women with long term use of oral contraception. *Morbidity and Mortality Weekly Report,* **26,** 293–294.
25. Chan, C.H. (1975) Primary carcinoma of the liver. *Medical Clinics of North America,* **59** (4), 989–994.
26. Christopherson, W.M. & Mays, E.T. (1977) Liver tumours and contraceptive steroids. *Journal of the National Cancer Institute,* **58,** 167–171.
27. Coady, A. (1976) Tropical cirrhosis and hepatoma. *Journal of the Royal College of Physicians of London,* **10,** 133–144.
28. Cochrane, A.M.G., Murray-Lyon, I.M., Brinkley, D.M. & Williams, R. (1977) Quadruple chemotherapy versus radiotherapy in treatment of primary hepatocellular carcinoma. *Cancer,* **40,** 609–614.
29. Cochrane, A.M.G. & Williams, R. (1976) Humoral effects of hepatocellular carcinoma. In *Hepatocellular Carcinoma* (Ed.) Okuda, K. & Peters, R.L. pp. 333–352. London: John Wiley and Sons.
30. Cohen, C.I. (1976) Intracytoplasmic hyaline globules in hepatocellular carcinomas. *Cancer,* **37,** 1754–1758.
31. Conn, H.O. (1972) Rational use of liver biopsy in the diagnosis of hepatic cancer. *Gastroenterology,* **62,** 142–146.
32. Conn, H.O. & Yesner, R. (1963) A re-evaluation of needle biopsy in the diagnosis of metastatic cancer of the liver. *Annals of Internal Medicine,* **59,** 53–61.
33. Creech, J.L. & Johnson, M.N. (1974) Angiosarcoma of the liver in the manufacture of polyvinyl chloride. *Journal of Occupational Medicine,* **16,** 150–151.
34. Cruickshank, A.H. & Sparshott, S.M. (1971) Malignancies in natural and experimental hepatic cysts: experiments with aflatoxin in rats and the malignant transformation of cysts in human livers. *Journal of Pathology,* **104,** 185–190.
35. Davis, M., Portmann, B., Searle, M., Wright, R. & Williams, R. (1975) Histological evidence of carcinoma in a hepatic tumour associated with oral contraceptives. *British Medical Journal,* **iv,** 496–498.
36. Desai, H.N. (1976) Clinical aspects of hepatocellular carcinoma in man. *South African Medical Journal,* **50,** 1611–1613.
37. Dixon, A.G. & Burns, W.A. (1973) Liver biopsy in patients with malignancy: a post mortem study. *Laboratory Investigation,* **28,** 405 (abstract).
38. Doll, R., Muir, C. & Waterhouse, J. (1970) Cancer incidence in five continents. *Unio Internationalis Contra Cancrum.* Vol. II. Berlin: Springer-Verlag.
39. Doll, R., Payne, P. & Waterhouse, J. (1966) Cancer incidence in five continents. *Unio Internationalis Contra Cancrum.* Vol. I. Berlin: Springer-Verlag.
40. Duck, B.W. (1975) Vinyl chloride carcinogenesis. *British Journal of Cancer,* **32,** 260.
41. Edington, G.M. & Gilles, H.M. (1976) *Pathology in the Tropics,* 2nd ed., pp. 558, 597. London: Edward Arnold.
42. Edmondson, H.A. (1958) Tumours of the liver and intrahepatic bile ducts. *Atlas of Tumour Pathology.* Section VII, Fascicle 25. Washington, D.C.: Armed Forces Institute of Pathology.
43. Edmondson, H.A. & Peters, R.L. (1971) Liver. In *Pathology* (Ed.) Anderson, W.A.D. 6th ed., p. 1243. St Louis: C.V. Mosby.
44. Edmondson, H.A., Henderson, B. & Benson, B. (1976) Liver-cell adenomas associated with use of oral contraceptives. *New England Journal of Medicine,* **294,** 470–472.
45. Eleftheriou, N., Heathcote, J., Thomas, H.C. & Sherlock, S. (1977) Serum alpha-fetoprotein levels in patients with acute and chronic liver disease. *Journal of Clinical Pathology,* **30,** 704–708.
46. Elkington, S.G., McBrien, D.J. & Spencer, H. (1963) Hepatoma in cirrhosis. *British Medical Journal,* **ii,** 1501–1503.
47. Exelby, P.R., Filler, R.M. & Grosfeld, J.L. (1975) Liver tumors in children in the particular reference to hepatoblastoma and hepatocellular carcinoma: American Academy of Pediatrics, Surgical Section Survey, 1974. *Journal of Pediatric Surgery,* **10,** 329–337.
48. Farber, E. (1976) On the pathogenesis of experimental hepatocellular carcinoma. In *Hepatocellular Carcinoma* (Ed.) Okuda, K. & Peters, R.L. pp. 3–22. London: John Wiley and Sons.
49. Fechner, R.E. (1977) Benign hepatic lesions and orally administered contraceptives. *Human Pathology,* **8,** 255–268.
50. Fechner, R.E. (1977) Hepatic tumours and oral contraceptives. *Pathology Annual, Part 1* (Ed.) Sommers, S.C. & Rosen, P.R. pp. 293–310. New York: Appleton-Century-Croft.
51. Gallagher, P.J., Millis, R.R. & Mitchison, M.J. (1972) Congenital dilatation of the intrahepatic bile ducts with cholangiocarcinoma. *Journal of Clinical Pathology,* **25,** 804–808.
52. Garancis, J.C., Tang, T., Panares, R. & Jurevics, I. (1969) Hepatic adenoma: biochemical and electron microscopic study. *Cancer,* **24,** 560–568.
53. Grabowski, M., Stenram, U. & Bergquist, A. (1975) Focal nodular hyperplasia of the liver, benign hepatomas, oral contraceptives and other drugs affecting the liver. *Acta Pathologica Microbiologica Scandinavica,* **83A,** 615–622.

54. Graivier, L., Jennings, R.L., Jones, W.A. & Rea, W.J. (1966) Liver angioma in the neonate. *American Journal of Surgery,* **112,** 777–782.

55. Grossman, E., Goldstein, M.J., Koss, L.G., Winawer, S.J. & Sherlock, P. (1972) Cytological examination as an adjunct to liver biopsy in the diagnosis of hepatic metastases. *Gastroenterology,* **62,** 56–60.

56. Hadziyannis, S.J., Guistozi, A., Moussouros, A. & Merikas, G. (1974) Hepatitis B core and surface antigens in the liver in primary liver cell carcinoma. In *Diseases of the Liver and Biliary Tract,* 5th Quadrennial Meeting of the International Association for the Study of the Liver, Acapulco, pp. 174–178. Basel: Karger, 1976.

57. Hayes, D., Lamki, H. & Hunter, I.W.E. (1977) Hepatic cell adenoma presenting with intraperitoneal haemorrhage in the puerperium. *British Medical Journal,* **iv,** 1394.

58. Higgins, G.K. (1970) The pathologic anatomy of primary hepatic tumours. In *Tumours of the Liver* (Ed.) Pack, G.T. & Islami, A.H. pp. 15–37. London: William Heinemann.

59. Higginson, J. (1956) Primary carcinoma of the liver in Africa. *British Journal of Cancer,* **10,** 609–621.

60. Higginson, J. (1970) The epidemiology of primary carcinoma of the liver. In *Tumours of the Liver* (Ed.) Pack, G.T. & Islami, A.H. pp. 38–52. London: William Heinemann.

61. Hoffman, H.S. (1942) Benign hepatoma: review of the literature and report of a case. *Annals of Internal Medicine,* **17,** 130–139.

62. Homer, L.W., White, H.J. & Read, R.C. (1968) Neoplastic transformation of Meyenburg complexes of the liver. *Journal of Pathology and Bacteriology,* **96,** 499–502.

63. Huang, S.N. (1975) Immunohistochemical demonstration of hepatitis B core and surface antigens in paraffin sections. *Laboratory Investigation,* **33,** 88–95.

64. Isaacson, C. (1978) The changing pattern of liver disease in South African Blacks. *South African Medical Journal,* **53,** 365–368.

65. Ishak, K.G. (1976) Mesenchymal tumours of the liver. In *Hepatocellular Carcinoma* (Ed.) Okuda, K. & Peters, R.L. pp. 247–307. London: John Wiley and Son.

66. Ishak, K.G. & Glunz, P.R. (1967) Hepatoblastoma and hepatocarcinoma in infancy and childhood. *Cancer,* **20,** 396–422.

67. Ishak, K.G. & Rabin, L. (1975) Benign tumours of the liver. *Medical Clinics of North America,* **59,** 995–1014.

68. Ishak, K.G., Willis, G.W., Cummins, S.D. & Bullock, A.A. (1977) Biliary cystadenoma and cystadenocarcinoma. Report of 14 cases and review of the literature. *Cancer,* **38,** 322–338.

69. Ito, J. & Johnson, W.J. (1969) Hepatoblastoma and hepatoma in infancy and childhood. *Archives of Pathology,* **87,** 259–266.

70. Johnson, F.L., Feagler, J.R., Lerner, K.G., Majerus, P.W., Siegel, M., Hartmann, J.R. & Thomas, E.D. (1972) Association of androgenic-anabolic steroid therapy with development of hepatocellular carcinoma. *Lancet,* **ii,** 1273–1276.

71. Johnson, P.J., Williams, R., Thomas, H., Sherlock, S. & Murray-Lyon, I.M. (1978) Induction of remission in hepatocellular carcinoma with doxorubicin. *Lancet,* **i,** 1006–1009.

72. Jupp, P.G., Prozesky, O.W., McElligott, S.E. & van Wyk, L.A.S. (1978) Infection of the common bedbug (*Cimex lenticularis*) with hepatitis B virus in South Africa. *South African Medical Journal,* **53,** 598–600.

73. Keeley, A.F., Iseri, O.A. & Gottlieb, L.S. (1972) Ultrastructure of hyaline cytoplasmic inclusions in a human hepatoma: relationship to Mallory's alcoholic hyaline. *Gastroenterology,* **62,** 280–293.

74. Kew, M.C. (1978) Hepatoma and the HBV. In *Viral Hepatitis* (Ed.) Vyas, G.N., Cohen, S.N. & Schmid, R. pp. 439–450. Philadelphia: Franklin Institute Press.

75. Kew, M.C., Van Coller, B., Prowse, C.M., Skikne, B., Wolfsdorf, J.I., Isdale, J., Krawitz, S., Altman, H., Levin, S.E. & Bothwell, T.H. (1976) Occurrence of primary hepatocellular carcinoma and peliosis hepatis after treatment with androgenic steroids. *South African Medical Journal,* **50,** 1233–1237.

76. Klatskin, G. (1977) Hepatic tumours: possible relationship to use of oral contraceptives. *Gastroenterology,* **73,** 386–394.

77. Knowles, D.M., Kaye, G.I. & Goodman, G.C. (1975) Nodular regenerative hyperplasia of the liver. *Gastroenterology,* **69,** 746–751.

78. Lancaster, M.C. (1968) Comparative aspects of aflatoxin-induced hepatic tumours. *Cancer Research,* **28,** 2288–2292.

79. *Lancet* (1970) Malaria and lymphoma (Editorial). *Lancet,* **ii,** 1121–1122.

80. Larouze, B., London, W.T., Saimot, G., Werner, H.G., Lustbader, E.D., Payet, M. & Blumberg, B.S. (1976) Host responses to hepatitis B infection in patients with primary hepatic carcinoma and their families. *Lancet,* **ii,** 534–538.

81. Larouze, B., Blumberg, B.S., London, W.T., Lustbader, E.D., Sankale, M. & Payet, M. (1977) Forecasting the development of primary hepatocellular carcinoma by the use of risk factors: studies in West Africa. *Journal of the National Cancer Institute,* **58,** 1557–1561.

82. Lee, F.I. (1966) Cirrhosis and hepatoma in alcoholics. *Gut,* **7,** 77–95.

83. MacDonald, R.A. (1956) Cirrhosis and primary carcinoma of the liver. *New England Journal of Medicine,* **255,** 1179–1183.

84. MacNab, G.M., Alexander, J.J., Lecatsas, G., Bey, E.M. & Urbanowitz, J.M. (1976) Hepatitis B surface antigen produced by a human hepatoma cell line. *British Journal of Cancer,* **34,** 509–515.

85. MacNab, G.M., Urbanowicz, J.M., Geddes, E.W. & Kew, M.C. (1976) Hepatitis-B surface antigen and antibody in Bantu patients with primary hepatocellular carcinoma. *British Journal of Cancer,* **33,** 544–548.

86. MacSween, R.N.M., Thomas, H.C., Tilney, N.L. & Horne, C.H.W. (1974) Cell mediated and humoral immunity in a rat experimental cirrhosis model. In *Diseases of the Liver and Biliary Tract.* 5th Quadrennial Meeting of the International Association for the Study of the Liver, Acapulco, pp. 23–26. Basel: Karger, 1976.

87. Makk, L., Delmore, F., Creech, J.L., Ogden, L.L., Fadell, E.H., Songster, C.L., Clanton, J., Johnson, M.N. & Christopherson, W.M. (1976) Clinical and morphological features of hepatic angiosarcoma in vinyl chloride workers. *Cancer,* **37,** 149–163.

88. Margolis, S. & Homcy, C. (1972) Systemic manifestations of hepatoma. *Medicine (Baltimore),* **51,** 381–391.

89. Martini, G.A. (1978) The liver in hereditary haemorrhagic telangiectasia: an inborn error of vascular structure with multiple manifestations. A reappraisal. *Gut*, **19**, 531–537.
90. Maupas, P., Werner, B., Larouze, B., Millman, I., London, W.T., O'Connell, A. & Blumberg, B.S. (1975) Antibody to hepatitis-B core antigen in patients with primary hepatic carcinoma. *Lancet*, **ii**, 9–11.
91. Maxfield, W.S., Ferrante, W.A., Shuler, S.E. & Leslie, C.L. (1973) A comparison of diagnostic accuracy of liver scans, liver function tests, and liver biopsy. *Progress in Clinical Medicine*, **5**, 55–70.
92. Mays, E.T., Christopherson, W.M. & Barrows, G.H. (1974) Focal nodular hyperplasia of the liver and possible relationship to oral contraceptives. *American Journal of Clinical Pathology*, **61**, 735–746.
93. Melnick, P.J. (1955) Polycystic liver. *Archives of Pathology*, **59**, 162–172.
94. Meyer, P., Li Volsi, V.A. & Cornog, J.L. (1974) Hepatoblastoma associated with an oral contraceptive. *Lancet*, **ii**, 1387.
95. Millward-Sadler, G.H. (1978) Personal observations.
96. Misugi, K. & Reiner, C.B. (1965) A malignant true teratoma of childhood. *Archives of Pathology*, **80**, 409–412.
97. Moesner, J., Baunsgaard, P., Starklint, H. & Thommesen, N. (1977) Focal nodular hyperplasia of the liver. *Acta Pathologica Microbiologica Scandinavica*, **85** (Sect. A), 113–121.
98. Mokhobo, K.P. (1976) Herb use and necrodegenerative hepatitis. *South African Medical Journal*, **50**, 1096–1099.
99. More, J.R.S. (1966) Cystadenocarcinoma of the liver. *Journal of Clinical Pathology*, **19**, 470–474.
100. Morris, H.P. (1965) Studies on the development, biochemistry and biology of experimental hepatomas. *Advances in Cancer Research*, **9**, 228–302.
101. Motsay, G.J. & Gamble, W.G. (1972) Clinical experience with hepatic adenoma. *Surgery, Gynecology and Obstetrics*, **134**, 415–418.
102. Nagasue, N., Inokuchi, K., Kobayashi, M. & Saku, M. (1976) Hepatic dearterialization for nonresectable primary and secondary tumours of the liver. *Cancer*, **38**, 2593–2603.
103. Nagasue, N., Inokuchi, K., Kobayashi, M. & Saku, M. (1977) Serum alpha-fetoprotein levels after hepatic artery ligation and postoperative chemotherapy. Correlation with clinical status in patients with hepatocellular carcinoma. *Cancer*, **40**, 615–618.
104. Nakashima, T., Okuda, K., Kojiro, M., Sakamoto, K., Kubo, Y. & Shimokawa, Y. (1975) Primary liver cancer coincident with *Schistosomiasis japonica*. *Cancer*, **36**, 1483–1489.
105. Napoli, V.M. & Campbell, W.G. (1977) Hepatoblastoma in infant sister and brother. *Cancer*, **39**, 2647–2650.
106. Nayak, N.C. & Sachdeva, R. (1975) Localisation of hepatitis B surface antigen in conventional paraffin sections of the liver: comparison of immunofluorescence, immunoperoxidase and orcein staining methods with regard to their specificity and reliability as antigen markers. *American Journal of Pathology*, **81**, 479–492.
107. Nayak, N.C., Chawla, V., Malaviya, A.N. & Chandra, N.K. (1972) Alpha-fetoprotein in Indian childhood cirrhosis. *Lancet*, **i**, 68–69.
108. Nayak, N.C., Dhar, A., Sachdeva, R., Mittal, A., Seth, H.N., Sudarsanam, D., Reddy, B., Wagholikar, U.L. & Reddy, C.R.R.M. (1977) Association of human hepatocellular carcinoma and cirrhosis with hepatitis B virus surface and core antigens in the liver. *International Journal of Cancer*, **20**, 643–654.
109. Neame, P.B. & Pillay, V.K. (1964) Spontaneous hypoglycaemia, hepatic and renal necrosis following the intake of herbal medicines. *South African Medical Journal*, **38**, 729–732.
110. Nissen, E.D., Kent, D.R., Nissen, S.E. & MacRae, D. (1976) Association of liver tumours with oral contraceptives. *Obstetrics and Gynecology*, **48**, 49–55.
111. Ohbayashi, A. (1976) Genetic and familial aspects of liver cirrhosis and hepatocellular carcinoma. In *Hepatocellular Carcinoma* (Ed.) Okuda, K. & Peters, R.L. pp. 43–52. London: John Wiley and Sons.
112. Okuda, K. (1976) Clinical aspects of hepatocellular carcinoma. In *Hepatocellular Carcinoma* (Ed.) Okuda, K. & Peters, R.L. pp. 387–436. London: John Wiley and Sons.
113. Okuda, K., Kubo, Y., Okazaki, N., Arishima, T., Hashimoto, M., Jinnouchi, S., Sawa, Y., Shimokawa, Y., Nakajima, Y., Noguchi, T., Nakano, M., Kojiio, M. & Nakashima, T. (1977) Clinical aspects of intrahepatic bile duct carcinoma including hilar carcinoma. A study of 57 autopsy proven cases. *Cancer*, **39**, 232–246.
114. Orloff, M.J., Chandler, J.G. & Bernstein, J.E. (1970) Transplantation of the liver. In *Tumours of the Liver* (Ed.) Pack, G.T. & Islami, A.H. pp. 213–239. London: William Heinemann.
115. O'Sullivan, J.P. (1976) Oral contraceptives and liver tumours. *Proceedings of the Royal Society of Medicine*, **69**, 351–353.
116. O'Sullivan, J.P. & Wilding, R.P. (1974) Liver hamartomas and patients on oral contraceptives. *British Medical Journal*, **iii**, 7–10.
117. Pack, G.T. & Islami, A.H. (1970) Surgical treatment of liver tumours. In *Tumours of the Liver* (Ed.) Pack, G.T. & Islami, A.H. pp. 166–186. London: William Heinemann.
118. Palmer, P.E. & Woolfe, H.J. (1976) Alpha-1-antitrypsin deposition in primary hepatic carcinomas. *Archives of Pathology and Laboratory Medicine*, **100**, 232–236.
119. Peers, F.G. & Linsell, C.A. (1973) Dietary aflatoxins and liver cancer – a population based study in Kenya. *British Journal of Cancer*, **27**, 473–484.
120. Peters, R.L. (1976) Pathology of hepatocellular carcinoma. In *Hepatocellular Carcinoma* (Ed.) Okuda, K. & Peters, R.L. pp. 107–169. London: John Wiley and Sons.
121. Peters, R.L., Afroudakis, A.P. & Tatter, D. (1977) The changing incidence of association of hepatitis B infection with hepatocellular carcinoma in California. *American Journal of Clinical Pathology*, **68**, 1–7.
122. Phillips, M.J., Langer, B., Stone, R., Fisher, M.M. & Ritchie, S. (1973) Benign liver cell tumours: classification and ultrastructural pathology. *Cancer*, **32**, 463–470.
123. Pollard, S.M. & Millward-Sadler, G.H. (1974) Malignant haemangioendothelioma involving the liver. *Journal of Clinical Pathology*, **27**, 214–221.

124. Primack, A., Vogel, C.L. & Barker, L.F. (1973) Immunological studies in Ugandan patients with hepatocellular carcinoma. *British Medical Journal,* **i,** 16–19.

125. Prince, A.M. (1970) Prevalence of serum-hepatitis-related antigen (SH) in different geographic regions. *American Journal of Tropical Medicine and Hygiene,* **19,** 872–879.

126. Prince, A.M. (1978) Risk of development of primary liver cancer PLC in hepatitis B carriers in the USA and Africa. In *Viral Hepatitis* (Ed.) Vyas, G.N., Cohen, S.N. & Schmid, R. p. 724. Philadelphia: Franklin Institute Press.

127. Prince, A.M., Metselaar, D., Kafuko, G.W., Mukwaya, L.G., Ling, C.M. & Overby, L.R. (1972) Hepatitis B antigen in wild-caught mosquitoes in Africa. *Lancet,* **ii,** 247–253.

128. Prince, A.M., Szmuness, W., Michon, J., Demaille, J., Diebolt, G., Linhard, J., Quenum, C. & Sankale, M. (1975) A case/control study of the association between primary liver cancer and hepatitis B infection in Senegal. *International Journal of Cancer,* **16,** 376–383.

129. Purtilo, D.T. (1976) Clonorchiasis and hepatic neoplasms. *Tropical and Geographical Medicine,* **28,** 21–27.

130. Purtilo, D. & Gottlieb, L.S. (1973) Cirrhosis and hepatoma occurring at Boston City Hospital. *Cancer,* **32,** 458–462.

131. Purves, L.R., Manso, C. & Torres, F.O. (1973) Serum alpha-fetoprotein levels in people susceptible to primary liver cancer in Southern Africa. *Gann Monograph,* **14,** 51–66.

132. Regelson, W., Kim, U., Ospina, J. & Holland, J.F. (1968) Haemangioendothelial sarcoma of liver from chronic arsenic intoxication by Fowler's solution. *Cancer,* **21,** 514–522.

133. Ruiter, D.J., Byck, W., Pauwels, E.J.K., Taconis, W.J. & Spaander, P.J. (1977) Correlation of scintigraphy with short interval autopsy in malignant focal liver disease. *Cancer,* **39,** 172–177.

134. Ruoslahti, E., Seppälä, M., Vuopio, P., Saksela, E. & Peltokallio, P. (1972) Radio immunoassay of alpha-fetoprotein in primary and secondary cancer of the liver. *Journal of the National Cancer Institute,* **49,** 623–630.

135. Sachdeva, R., Nayak, N.C., Sama, S.K. & Seth, H.N. (1976) Hepatitis B surface antigen in the liver – its appearance in conventional paraffin sections. *Indian Journal of Medical Research,* **64,** 1027–1034.

136. Scheuer, P.J. (1970) *Liver Biopsy Interpretation.* 2nd ed., p. 116. London: Baillière Tindall.

137. Schoental, R. (1968) Toxicology and carcinogenic action of pyrrolizidine alkaloids. *Cancer Research,* **28,** 2237–2246.

138. Sherlock, S., Feldman, C.A., Moran, B. & Scheuer, P.J. (1966) Partial nodular transformation of the liver with portal hypertension. *American Journal of Medicine,* **40,** 195–203.

139. Shikata, T. (1976) Primary liver carcinoma and cirrhosis. In *Hepatocellular Carcinoma* (Ed.) Okuda, K. & Peters, R.L. pp. 53–72. London: John Wiley and Sons.

140. Shikata, T., Uzawa, T., Yoshiwara, N., Akatsuka, T. & Yamazaki, S. (1974) Staining methods of Australia antigen in paraffin sections: detection of cytoplasmic inclusion bodies. *Japanese Journal of Experimental Medicine,* **44,** 25–36.

141. Silverman, J.F., Yao-Shi, F., McWilliams, N.B. & Kay, S. (1975) An ultrastructural study of mixed hepatoblastoma with osteoid elements. *Cancer,* **36,** 1436–1443.

142. Simmons, M.J., Yap, E.H., Yu, M., Seah, C.S., Chew, B.S., Fung, W.F., Tan, A.Y.O. & Shanmugarathnam, K. (1971) Australia antigen in Singapore Chinese patients with hepatocellular carcinoma. *Lancet,* **i,** 1149–1151.

143. Simpson, L.W. & Middlecote, B.D. (1973) The Budd-Chiari syndrome in the Bantu. In *Liver* (Ed.) Saunders, S.J. & Terblanche, J. p. 257. London: Pitman Medical Books.

144. Smith, J.B. & Blumberg, B.S. (1969) Viral hepatitis, postnecrotic cirrhosis and hepatocellular carcinoma. *Lancet,* **ii,** 953.

145. Smith, I.E., Taylor, K.J., McCready, V.R., Powles, T.J. & Bondy, P.K. (1976) Comparison of gray-scale ultrasound with other methods for the detection of liver metastases from breast carcinoma. *Clinical Oncology,* **2,** 47–53.

146. Smythe, P.M., Schonland, M.M., Brereton-Stiles, G., Coovadia, H.M., Grace, H.J., Loening, W.E.K., Mafoyane, A., Parent, M.A. & Vos, G.H. (1971) Thymolymphatic deficiency and depression of cell-mediated immunity in protein-calorie malnutrition. *Lancet,* **ii,** 939–944.

147. Steiner, P.E. & Higginson, J. (1959) Cholangiolocellular carcinoma of the liver. *Cancer,* **12,** 753–759.

148. Steyn, M. & Purchase, I.F.H. (1970) *Symposium on Mycotoxins in Human Health, Pretoria* (Ed.) Purchase, I.F.H. London: Macmillan, 1971.

149. Stocker, J.T. & Ishak, K.G. (1978) Undifferentiated (embryonal) sarcoma of the liver: a report of 31 cases. *Cancer,* **42,** 336–348.

150. Stumpf, H.H. & Liber, A.F. (1954) Hepatocellular adenomatosis. *American Journal of Medicine,* **17,** 887–890.

151. Sutton, C.A. & Eller, J.L. (1968) Mesenchymal hamartoma of the liver, *Cancer,* **22,** 29–34.

152. Tabor, E., Robert, J., Gerety, C.L., Vogel, A.C., Bayly, P.P., Anthony, C.H. & Lewethys, F.B. (1977) Hepatitis B virus infection and primary hepatocellular carcinoma. *Journal of the National Cancer Institute,* **58,** 1197–1200.

153. Tan, A.Y.O., Law, C.H. & Lee, Y.S. (1977) Hepatitis B antigen in the liver cells in cirrhosis and hepatocellular carcinoma. *Pathology,* **9,** 57–64.

154. Tate, R.C., Chacko, M.V., Singh, S. & Ogden, L. (1972) Parenchymal hamartoma of the liver in infants and children. *American Journal of Surgery,* **123,** 346–350.

155. Tesluk, H. & Nordin, W.A. (1955) Haemangioendothelioma of the liver following thorium dioxide administration. *Archives of Pathology,* **60,** 493–501.

156. Thomson, J.G. (1961) Primary carcinoma of the liver in the three ethnic groups in Capetown. *Acta Unionis Internationalis contra Cancrum,* **17,** 632–638.

157. Thomson, J.G. (1961) Cirrhosis of the liver in Europeans, Coloureds and Native Africans in Cape Town. *Acta Unionis Internationalis contra Cancrum,* **17,** 623–631.

158. Vana, J., Murphy, G.P., Aronoff, B.L. & Baker, H.W. (1977) Primary liver tumours and oral contraceptives. Results of a survey. *Journal of the American Medical Association,* **238,** 2154–2158.

159. Visfeldt, J. & Poulsen, H. (1972) On the histopathology of liver and liver tumours in thorium-dioxide patients. *Acta Pathologica et Microbiologica, Scandinavica,* **80A,** 97–108.

160. Vogel, C.L., Anthony, P.P., Mody, N. & Barker, L.F. (1970) Hepatitis-associated antigen in Ugandan patients with hepatocellular carcinoma. *Lancet,* **ii,** 621–624.
161. Vogel, C.L., Anthony, P.P., Sadikali, F., Barker, L.F. & Peterson, M.R. (1972) Hepatitis-associated antigen and antibody in hepatocellular carcinoma: results of a continuing study. *Journal of the National Cancer Institute,* **48,** 1583–1588.
162. Wainwright, J. & Schonland, M.M. (1977) Unpublished data.
163. Wainwright, J., Schonland, M.M. & Candy, H.A. (1977) Toxicity of *Callilepis laureola. South African Medical Journal,* **52,** 313–315.
164. Warren, K.S., Rosenthal, M.S. & Domingo, E.O. (1969) Mouse hepatitis virus (MHV3) infection in chronic murine *Schistosomiasis mansoni. Bulletin of the New York Academy of Medicine,* **45,** 211–224.
165. Warren, S. & Drake, W.L. (1951) Primary carcinoma of the liver in hemochromatosis. *American Journal of Pathology,* **27,** 573–609.
166. Whelton, M.J., Petrelli, M., George, P., Young, W.B. & Sherlock, S. (1969) Carcinoma at the junction of the main hepatic ducts. *Quarterly Journal of Medicine,* **38,** 211–230.
167. Wilkins, L. & Ravitch, M.M. (1952) Adrenocortical tumour arising in the liver of a 3 year old boy with signs of virilism and Cushing's syndrome. *Pediatrics,* **9,** 671–681.
168. Williams, A.O. (1975) Hepatitis B surface antigen and liver cell carcinoma. *American Journal of the Medical Sciences,* **270,** 53–56.
169. Willis, R.A. (1973) *The Spread of Tumours in the Human Body.* 3rd ed. London: Butterworths.
170. Wogan, G.N. (1976) Aflatoxins and their relationship to hepatocellular carcinoma. In *Hepatocellular Carcinoma* (Ed.) Okuda, K. & Peters, R.L. London: John Wiley and Sons.
171. Zelman, N.S. (1962) Liver fibrosis in hereditary haemorrhagic telangiectasia. *Archives of Pathology,* **74,** 66–72.

Chapter 39

Involvement of the Liver by Lymphoreticular Disease

D.H. WRIGHT

The Kupffer cells with their important phagocytic activity may be regarded as part of the lymphoreticular system; lymphoid tissue, however, is not a normal component of the liver. Primary lymphomas of the liver are extremely rare and their primary nature is difficult to establish without a full autopsy. In contradistinction, the liver is probably the commonest site at which deposits or infiltrates of leukaemic and lymphomatous cells are found outside the lymph nodes, spleen and bone marrow. Liver infiltration is a characteristic feature of many of the leukaemias and lymphocytic lymphomas and does not materially alter the therapy or prognosis of these neoplasms. Involvement of the liver by Hodgkin's disease, on the other hand, is of serious import and has considerable therapeutic and prognostic consequences. Malignant lymphomas may cause solitary or multiple tumour masses in the liver in much the same way as metastatic carcinoma and sarcoma. More frequently, they produce diffuse and often subtle infiltrates in the portal triads or the sinusoids, or in both, in a pattern that is often characteristic of a certain type of leukaemia or lymphoma. The identification of lymphoreticular neoplasms and their separation from inflammatory infiltrates will, however, ultimately depend upon the cytological characteristics of the infiltrating cells.

HODGKIN'S DISEASE

The liver is the second most common extranodal site of Hodgkin's disease after the spleen. In autopsy series the incidence of liver involvement by Hodgkin's tissue ranges from 36 to 63 per cent,[19,28,34,51,57] occurring both as diffuse infiltrates and as bulky tumour masses. The high percentage of patients with liver involvement in autopsy series reflects the poor prognosis of this form of the disease as well as the natural progression of the disease, the incidence of hepatic involvement at laparotomy being in the region of 5 to 10 per cent.[4,21,30,31]

Jaundice has long been recognized as a manifestation of Hodgkin's disease and may have several causes. In two large series of cases described by Levitan, Diamond and Craver[35] and Bouroncle, Old and Vazques,[8] infiltration of the liver was the usual cause of the jaundice, with haemolytic anaemia second in frequency. Bouroncle, Old and Vazques described two patients with cholestasis in whom bile duct obstruction was excluded by laparotomy and cholangiogram and hepatotoxic drugs had not been administered. They suggest that Hodgkin's disease may sometimes cause cholestasis other than by obstruction. If this is so, it must be extremely rare and it cannot be overlooked that one of their cases had 'terminal liver involvement' at autopsy.

Liver biopsy is rarely the primary means of diagnosis of Hodgkin's disease and even in those patients in whom this is the first positive tissue diagnosis this should be confirmed whenever possible by subsequent lymph node biopsy. An exception to this rule may be lymphocyte-depleted Hodgkin's disease which sometimes presents with fever, pancytopenia, lymphocytopenia and abnormalities of liver function without overt peripheral lymphadenopathy. In such cases, without lymph nodes available for biopsy, a tissue diagnosis of Hodgkin's disease is often provided by bone marrow or liver biopsy. In a series of 13 cases of lymphocyte-depleted Hodgkin's disease, Neiman, Rosen, and Lukes[41] found positive evidence of tumour in two of three liver biopsies and in the livers of eight of nine patients that came to autopsy.

The presence of liver infiltration is of considerable importance in the management of patients with Hodgkin's disease, dictating systemic therapy rather than any form of localized treatment. The management and therapy of Hodgkin's disease is well reviewed by Kaplan.[31] Liver function tests are of little value in predicting liver involvement and, when compared with laparotomy and biopsy findings, are seen to be insensitive and unreliable.[4,19,20,31] The only two laboratory tests of liver function that may be rewarding are the serum alkaline phosphatase and the bromsulphthalein retention test.[31] Others have found that an elevated serum alkaline phosphatase is frequently associated with non-specific lesions and with normal liver biopsies, and is therefore of little use in the diagnosis of hepatic Hodgkin's disease.[1] Similarly, liver scintigraphy appears to be too insensitive to detect early hepatic involvement and cannot discriminate between abnormalities due to Hodgkin's tissue and those associated with non-specific lesions.[36]

From the discussion above, it is apparent that an accurate assessment of liver involvement can be obtained only from histological examination. Despite the fact that Hodgkin's tissue is often diffusely distributed in the liver, blind percutaneous needle biopsy, when compared with open biopsy at laparotomy, identifies only half the patients with hepatic involvement.[4] Visualization of the liver through a peritoneoscope improves the yield of positive biopsies to the same level as that obtained at laparotomy.[5] Since it is the usual procedure when staging patients with Hodgkin's disease to perform a laparotomy and splenectomy, however, both needle and wedge biopsies of the liver can be obtained at this operation. Clearly, the likelihood of obtaining a positive biopsy will be greatest in those patients with visible macroscopic deposits that can be directly sampled, but the majority of patients have no visible tumour on the capsular surface of the liver. Most surgeons take a wedge biopsy of liver together with one or more needle biopsies from each lobe. The wedge biopsy, even when taken blindly, appears to be superior to needle biopsies in revealing tumour deposits, presumably because of the larger area sampled.[19,21,34] Glees et al[21] performed four quadrant Menghini needle biopsies and one wedge biopsy specimen from the liver edge on 203 patients with Hodgkin's disease with macroscopically normal livers. There was evidence of liver involvement in 15 patients (7.4 per cent); the wedge biopsy was positive in 14 whereas the needle biopsies were positive in only 8. In only one patient was the wedge biopsy negative while the needle biopsies were positive.

Some guidance as to the likelihood of liver involvement in Hodgkin's disease can be obtained from other clinical and pathological features. Hepatic infiltrates are more common in patients with lymphocyte depleted forms of the disease[41] and those with systemic (B) symptoms.[31] Liver infiltrates never occur in the absence of spleen involvement, with the possible exception of the extremely rare cases of Hodgkin's disease of the intestine.[31] Kim, Dorfman and Rosenberg,[34] reporting a series of 400 cases of Hodgkin's disease subjected to laparotomy, found that liver involvement was always associated with spleen involvement and that if the spleen was involved and over 900 g in weight the liver was invariably involved. In addition to this high incidence of concurrent spleen and liver involvement, Kaplan et al[32] reported subsequent involvement of the liver after intervals ranging from two to 69 months in over 30 patients (in a series of 285 patients) who initially presented with positive spleens and negative livers, as judged by liver function tests, liver scans, needle biopsies and/or open biopsies. The association of liver infiltrates with splenic involvement and the difficulties of excluding liver involvement with certainty by any of the techniques available have led a number of therapists to give radioactive gold colloid or quadruple combination chemotherapy to all patients with stage III disease.[31,32]

Histology

Hodgkin's disease infiltrates in the liver always involve the portal triads though extension from the portal areas and fusion of adjacent tumour deposits may form larger nodules (Figures 39.1 and 39.2). Occasionally, biopsies show tumour deposits that appear to be within the hepatic lobule, but serial sections will usually demonstrate that these connect with an adjacent portal area. With the widespread adoption of staging

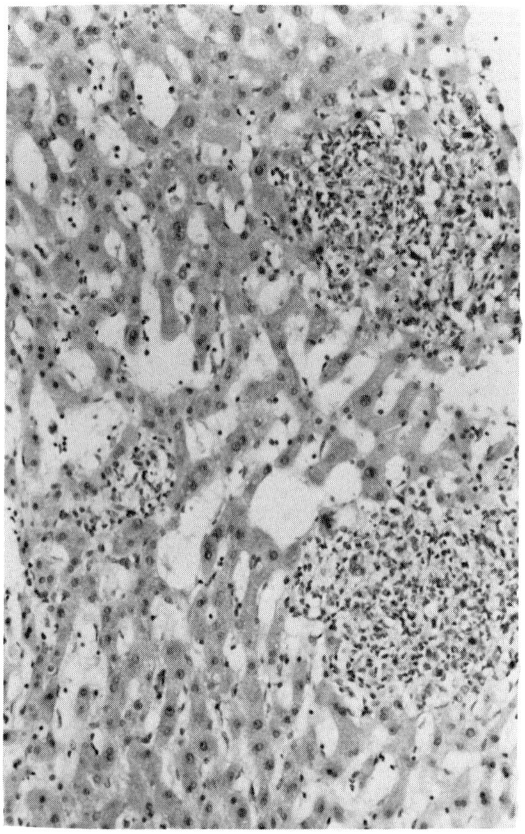

Figure 39.1. Hodgkin's disease. Note distribution of tumour in portal areas. Needle biopsy. Haematoxylin and eosin ×120.

procedures, including liver biopsy, it soon became apparent that a large proportion of patients with Hodgkin's disease had hepatic portal infiltrates. Even when Reed–Sternberg cells could not be demonstrated in these infiltrates, it was often assumed that they represented Hodgkin's disease, especially if the patient also had splenic involvement, and that a larger sample of tissue would have demonstrated more typical Hodgkin's tissue. This assumption is, however, erroneous and would lead to the categorization of a large proportion of patients with stage II or III disease as having stage IV disease. Since the criteria used to diagnose Hodgkin's disease in lymph node biopsies cannot be generally applied to liver biopsies, mainly because of the small quantity of tissue available for study, minimum criteria were established for the diagnosis of hepatic Hodgkin's disease. In the absence of Reed–Sternberg cells these are: *the recognition of mononuclear cells with the nuclear features of Reed–Sternberg cells in one of the characteristic cellular environments of Hodgkin's disease.*[43] It is mandatory in such cases to section through the biopsy serially to look for unequivocal Reed–Sternberg cells (Figure 39.2). The presence of atypical histiocytes in the infiltrate is regarded as suggestive of Hodgkin's disease and, in such cases, if a more definitive histological diagnosis cannot be obtained, the clinician should use all the other available data in determining the stage.[43] This should not be a common problem; it hinges to a considerable extent on what the pathologist regards as atypical histiocytes. If the atypicality relates to nuclear pleomorphism, coarse nuclear chromatin and prominent nucleoli and is not merely irregularity induced by traction artefact it is likely that the infiltration is due to Hodgkin's disease and that serial sections or examination of other biopsies will provide supportive evidence.

Non-specific triaditis occurs in about one-third of patients with Hodgkin's disease.[1,34] This varies from the accumulation of occasional lymphocytes, plasma cells, histiocytes and granulocytes, to prominent infiltrates expanding

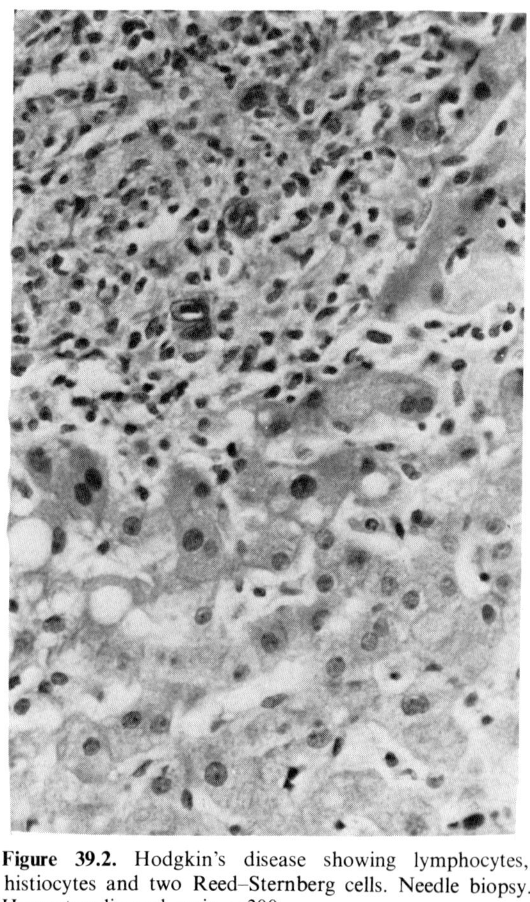

Figure 39.2. Hodgkin's disease showing lymphocytes, histiocytes and two Reed–Sternberg cells. Needle biopsy. Haematoxylin and eosin ×300.

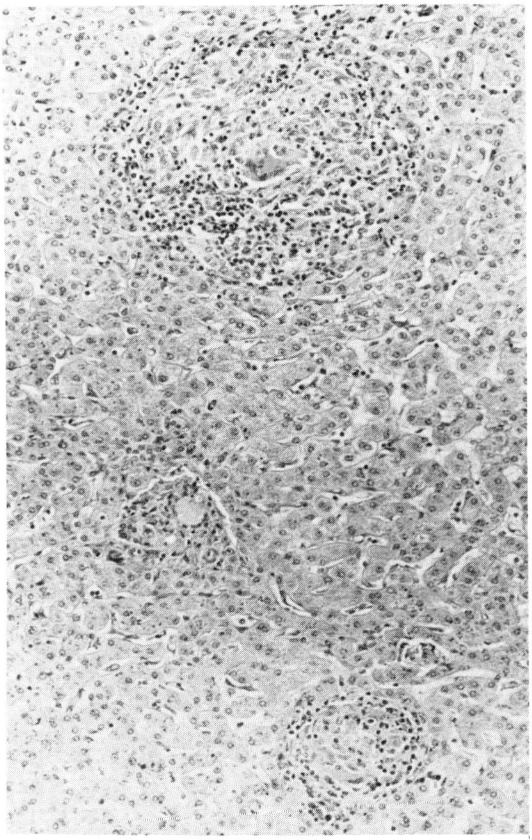

Figure 39.3. Hodgkin's disease showing epithelioid cell and giant cell granulomas in portal areas without evidence of Hodgkin's tissue. Wedge biopsy. Haematoxylin and eosin ×120.

the triad. A few patients may exhibit features of chronic active hepatitis.[1] Isolated epithelial cells and giant cell granulomas have been reported in approximately 10 per cent of liver biopsies from patients with Hodgkin's disease[1,34] (Figures 39.3 and 39.4). These appear to be more common in patients with nodular sclerosing Hodgkin's disease than with the other subtypes.[29] Granulomas in the liver are usually, but not invariably, associated with similar lesions in the spleen. They do not indicate involvement of the liver by Hodgkin's disease but since they may accompany Hodgkin's tissue, serial sectioning should be performed, particularly if the spleen is involved by Hodgkin's tissue. The cause of the granulomas is uncertain. Immune complexes are capable of inducing granulomas,[47] but, if they are responsible for this manifestation of Hodgkin's disease, it is curious that in the spleen they are localized primarily to the periarteriolar T cell area.

Finally, in analysing portal infiltrates in patients with Hodgkin's disease, totally unrelated causes should be borne in mind. The author recently saw an immigrant child with mixed cellularity Hodgkin's disease, thought to be stage IV because the liver showed marked portal infiltrates of lymphoid cells, eosinophils and histiocytes. However, atypical cells were not seen and serial sections revealed granulomas surrounding ova of *Schistosoma mansoni*.

NON-HODGKIN'S LYMPHOMAS

Liver biopsy is not usually the primary means of diagnosis of malignant lymphoma and even if a biopsy indicates lymphomatous disease this should be substantiated by a lymph node biopsy whenever possible. There are occasions when the diagnosis of lymphoma must rest on the histology of the liver biopsy or when the liver biopsy plays a major role in supporting a diagnosis of malignant lymphoma. Lympho-

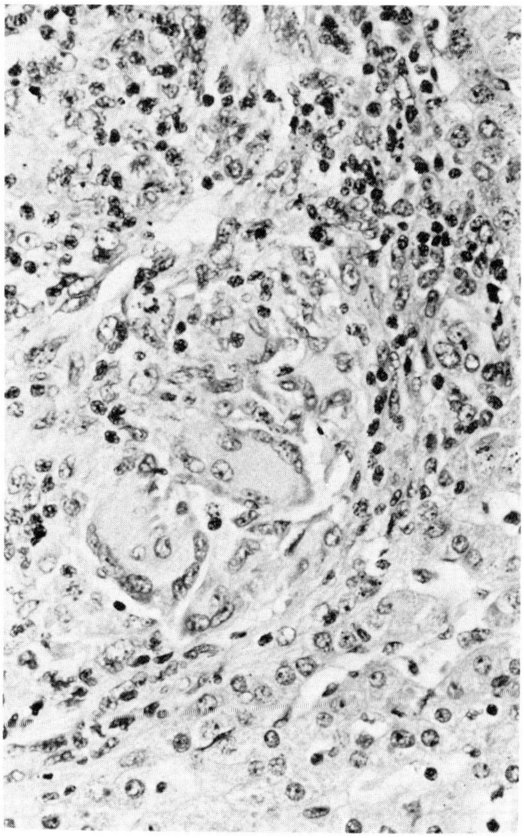

Figure 39.4. Hodgkin's disease showing epithelioid cell and giant cell granuloma in a portal area. No Hodgkin's cells or atypical histiocytes present. This lesion does not indicate involvement of the liver by Hodgkin's tissue. Wedge biopsy. Haematoxylin and eosin ×300.

Table 39.1. *Cytological Types and Patterns of Infiltration of Leukaemias and Lymphomas in the Liver.*

Cell type	Description of cell	Rappaport classification	Pattern of liver involvement
Well-differentiated lymphocytic	Small lymphocyte	DLWD	Portal
Lymphoplasmacytoid	Lymphocytes with varying degrees of plasma cell differentiation	DLWD	Portal
Follicular centre cell lymphoma–diffuse	(a) Predominantly small centrocytes	DLPD	Portal or large tumour masses
	(b) Predominantly large centrocytes and centroblasts	DH	
	(c) Mixed	DMHL	
Follicular centre cell lymphoma–follicular	(a) Predominantly small centrocytes	NLPD	Portal or large tumour masses
	(b) Predominantly large centrocytes and centroblasts	NH	
	(c) Mixed	NMHL	
Immunoblastic sarcoma	Immunoblasts (large open nucleus, single large nucleolus, well-defined pyroninophilic cytoplasm)	DU	Tumour masses
Poorly-differentiated lymphocytic lymphoma (lymphoblastic lymphoma)	Heterogeneous group including the convoluted T-cell lymphoma	DLPD	Tumour masses, more diffuse portal and sinusoidal infiltrates in cases that become leukaemic
Burkitt's lymphoma	Burkitt lymphoma cells	DUBL	Tumour masses
Histiocytic lymphoma	'True histiocytes'. Reniform or folded nuclei, abundant cytoplasm, may exhibit phagocytosis	DH	Tumour masses
Malignant histiocytosis (histiocytic medullary reticulosis)	Cells vary from well-differentiated histiocytes to pleomorphic multinucleated cells. Phagocytosis, including erythrophagocytosis, prominent	MH	Subtle portal and sinusoidal infiltrates
Cutaneous T-cell lymphoma (Sezary's syndrome, mycosis fungoides)	Cerebriform cells		Portal
Hairy cell leukaemia (leukaemic reticulo-endotheliosis)	Hairy cells		Portal and sinusoidal (angiomatous lesions)
Monocytic leukaemia	Monocytes. May exhibit phagocytosis but are less pleomorphic than in malignant histiocytosis		Portal and sinusoidal
Granulocytic leukaemia	Cells of the granulocyte series from myeloblasts to granulocytes		Sinusoidal

Rappaport classification: DLWD = diffuse lymphocytic well differentiated; DLPD = diffuse lymphocytic poorly differentiated; DH = diffuse histiocytic; DMHL = diffuse mixed histiocytic lymphocytic; NLPD = nodular lymphoma poorly differentiated; NH = nodular histiocytic; NMHL = nodular mixed histiocytic lymphocytic; DU = diffuse undifferentiated; DUBL = diffuse undifferentiated (Burkitt's lymphoma); MH = malignant histiocytosis.

reticular neoplasms are more commonly diffusely spread throughout the liver than metastatic carcinoma and the chances of obtaining a positive biopsy are correspondingly greater.[23] The small size of the biopsy may be a constraining factor in arriving at a definitive diagnosis and even when lymphoma cells can be unequivocally identified it may not be possible to determine whether they are forming follicles or are diffuse. Lymphomatous and leukaemic cells are particularly vulnerable to traction artefact and this may be considerable in needle biopsies, especially from patients with large cell lymphomas.

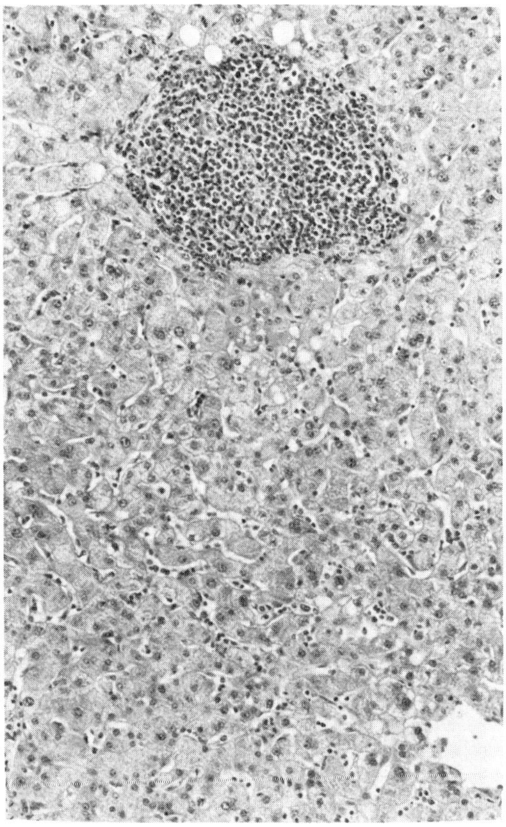

Figure 39.5. Follicular centre cell lymphoma, small centrocytic type (lymphocytic lymphoma poorly differentiated). Note that tumour cells are confined to expanded portal area. Limiting cell plate remains intact. Wedge biopsy. Haematoxylin and eosin × 120.

Considerable confusion has existed in the diagnosis and classification of non-Hodgkin's lymphomas during the past decade. This confusion is partly semantic but owes much to the enormous range of histological artefacts to which lymphoma biopsies are subjected. Happily for the hepatologist fixation of liver biopsies is usually an order of magnitude better than that of lymph nodes and spleen and the preservation of cytological detail is correspondingly better. The diagnosis and classification of the non-Hodgkin's lymphomas rests essentially on their cytological characteristics together with the presence or absence of a follicular structure. In the liver this may be supported by characteristic patterns of infiltration (Table 39.1).

The concept of follicular centre cell lymphomas that may be either nodular or diffuse in their overall pattern has done much to clarify the classification of lymphomas. A simplified classification of the non-Hodgkin's lymphomas is shown in Table 39.1 together with a brief description of the cytology of each category. The corresponding designation in the Rappaport classification[42] is shown since this is probably still the most widely used classification and forms the basis of many of the studies of lymphoma of the liver.

The incidence of liver involvement by non-Hodgkin's lymphoma in an autopsy series reported by Kim, Dorfman and Rosenberg[34] was 45 out of 86 (52 per cent). The reported incidence of hepatic involvement detected by biopsy has varied widely: 12 per cent;[54] 16 per cent;[33] 22 per cent;[15] 56 per cent.[38] As with Hodgkin's lymphoma, wedge biopsies taken at laparotomy are more frequently positive than are percutaneous needle biopsies,[34,38] hepatic involvement is very rare in the absence of splenic involvement,[34,38,54] and both liver function tests and liver scans are unreliable indications of hepatic involvement. Chabner et al[10] found biochemical and scintigraphic evidence of liver disease in only 22 of 41 patients with biopsy-proven hepatic lymphoma.

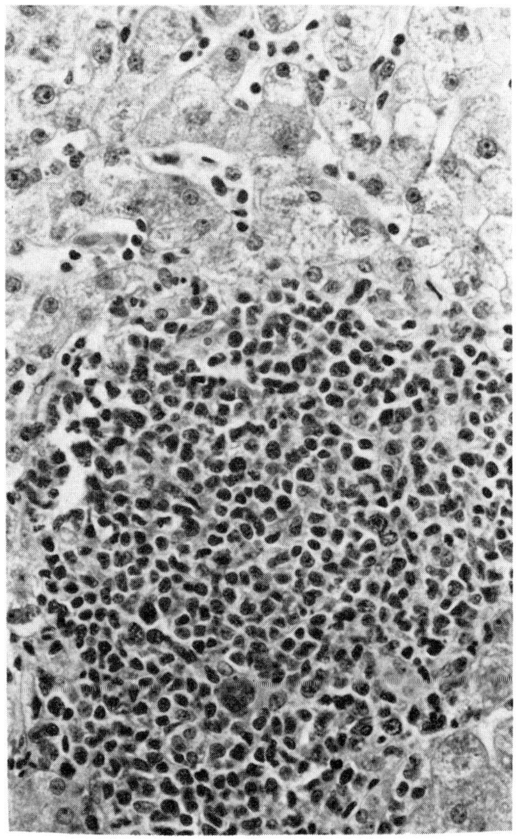

Figure 39.6. Follicular centre cell lymphoma, small centrocytic type. Note irregularity of lymphoid cells compared with small lymphocytes. Wedge biopsy. Haematoxylin and eosin × 300.

Lotz et al[38] found a higher incidence of liver involvement in patients with diffuse lymphomas than in patients with nodular lymphomas whereas Kim, Dorfman and Rosenberg[34] found the reverse of this. In both of these groups, however, it was the lymphocytic poorly differentiated category, both nodular and diffuse, that most frequently involved the liver (Figures 39.5 and 39.6). Most of these cases would probably fall into the centrocytic category of follicular centre cell lymphomas. A follicular pattern may not be discernible in the liver except in those cases showing large tumour nodules even when the tumour shows follicularity elsewhere. In needle biopsies this is in part due to the small sample available for study but is also due to the fact that dissemination in the liver frequently consists of small collections of centrocytes throughout the portal areas. It is recognized that centrocytic lymphomas frequently show widespread dissemination to liver, bone marrow and spleen, even at presentation. While laparotomy and liver biopsy may significantly alter the staging of patients with non-Hodgkin's lymphoma,[10] this is of much less consequence than in Hodgkin's disease and in many instances will not alter the treatment schedule.

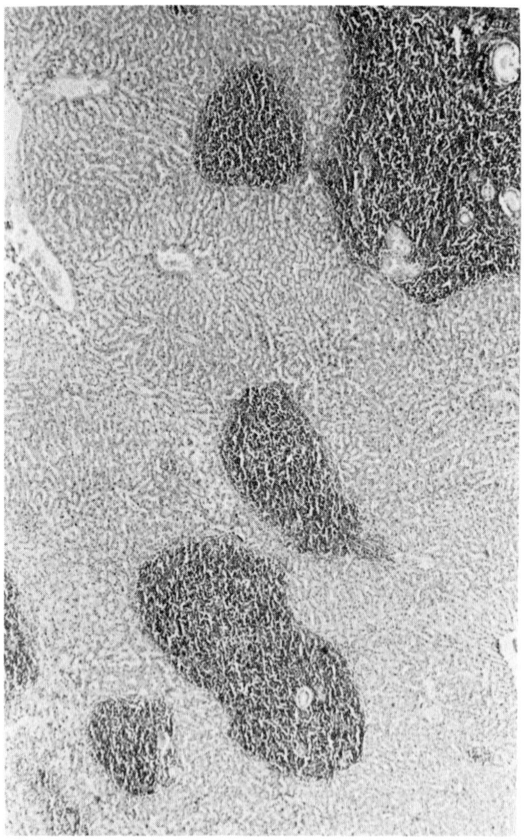

Figure 39.7. Well-differentiated lymphocytic lymphoma/chronic lymphocytic leukaemia. Tumour cells confined to the portal areas. Post-mortem section. Haematoxylin and eosin ×30.

Well-differentiated lymphocytic lymphoma shows a high incidence of hepatic involvement (Figure 39.7) but since a large proportion of these patients show blood and bone marrow involvement liver biopsy is not usually indicated. It is probable that in any lymphoma that shows leukaemic manifestations tumour cells will be found in the liver. Thus, in a series of 13 patients with mycosis fungoides subjected to staging laparotomy Variakojis, Rosas-Uribe and Rappaport[53] found splenic involvement only in the four patients with mycosis cells in the peripheral blood. One of these patients showed tumour cells in the portal triads of the liver.

Non-neoplastic and non-specific portal infiltrates appear to be less common in the non-Hodgkin's lymphomas than in Hodgkin's disease though Lotz et al[38] point out that it may be difficult to separate early infiltrations with lymphocytic lymphomas from reactive lymphoid infiltrates since they do not show the cytological atypia of the large cell lymphomas. Epithelioid cell granulomas may be found in the liver in patients with non-Hodgkin's lymphomas but with less frequency (2 per cent) than in Hodgkin's disease (12 per cent).[34]

A few patients present with apparent primary lymphomas of the liver causing a solitary tumour mass. On investigation these will usually prove to be part of a more widely disseminated process, but a small number of authenticated primary lymphomas of the liver have been recorded.[11,17,49,50]

Malignant Histiocytosis (Histiocytosis Medullary Reticulosis)

Scott and Robb-Smith[45] described ten patients, four of their own and six from the literature, with a disease characterized by 'fever, wasting and generalised lymphadenopathy associated with splenic and hepatic enlargement and in the final stages jaundice purpura and anaemia with profound leukopenia'. They designated this condition 'histiocytic medullary reticulosis' although the term 'malignant histiocytosis' introduced by Rappaport[42] is now more widely used. The liver is frequently involved[9,46,56] and exhibits both a sinusoidal and a portal pattern of infiltration, either one or both of which may be present. In an autopsy series of 14 cases

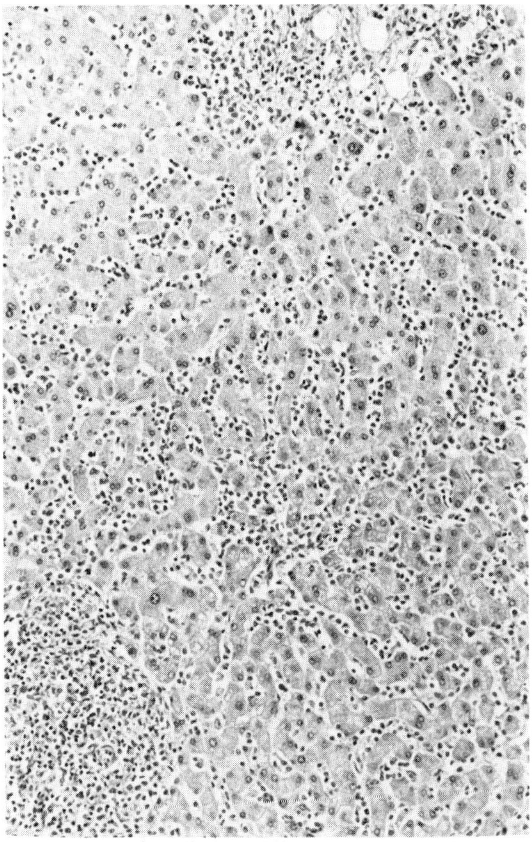

Figure 39.8. Monocytic leukaemia. Diffuse infiltration of portal areas and sinusoids by leukaemic cells. Post-mortem section. Haematoxylin and eosin × 120.

Warnke, Kim and Dorfman found liver involvement in 12. The organ was usually grossly enlarged and showed a diffuse mottled pattern of infiltration without discrete tumour masses. Phagocytosis and, in particular, erythrophagocytosis by tumour cells and morphologically normal histiocytes is a characteristic of this tumour. The neoplastic histiocytes may show extreme degrees of pleomorphism with giant cell forms though in some patients the degree of cytological atypia may be minimal.[9,42] The presence of erythrophagocytosis in apparently normal Kupffer cells or sinusoidal and portal histiocytes should alert the pathologist to the possibility of malignant histiocytosis and a careful search should be made for histiocytes exhibiting cytological atypia. The appearances of malignant histiocytosis in the liver are characteristic though Hodgkin's disease and monocytic leukaemia may be considered in the differential diagnosis. However, any resemblance between the giant cells seen in malignant histiocytosis and Reed–Sternberg cells is superficial. The atypical histiocytes in malignant histiocytosis are often accompanied by plasma cells which may be highlighted by the methyl green-pyronine stain whereas plasma cells are not a prominent feature of Hodgkin's infiltrates. Infiltration of the sinusoids in a diffuse fashion by atypical cells and erythrophagocytosis by tumour cells which are characteristic features of malignant histiocytosis are not seen in Hodgkin's disease.

Monocytic leukaemia characteristically shows diffuse portal and perisinusoidal infiltrates of leukaemic cells, some of which may exhibit erythrophagocytosis (Figures 39.8 and 39.9). This condition can be differentiated histologically from malignant histiocytosis by the lack of tumour cell pleomorphism and the delicate nuclear chromatin of the leukaemic cells, and clinically by the presence of a leukaemic blood picture.

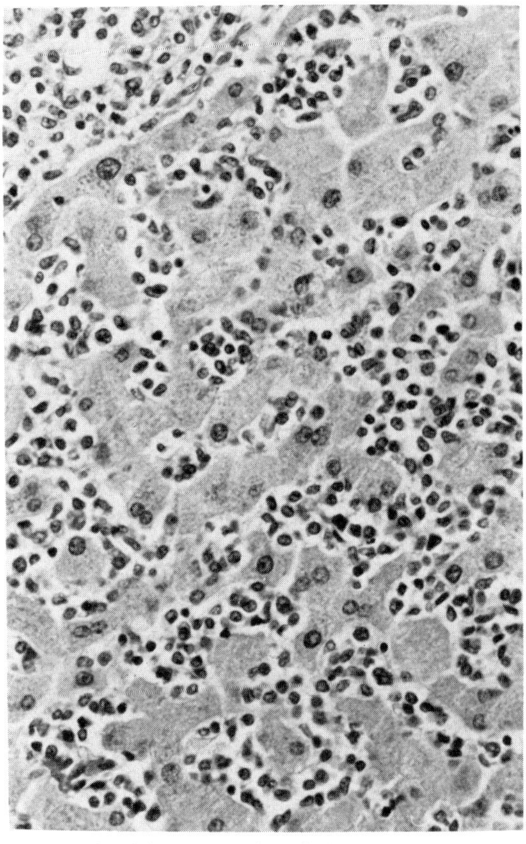

Figure 39.9. Higher power view of Figure 39.8 to show oval or reniform nuclei of leukaemic cells. These cells are more regular and more abundant than those seen in malignant histiocytosis. × 300.

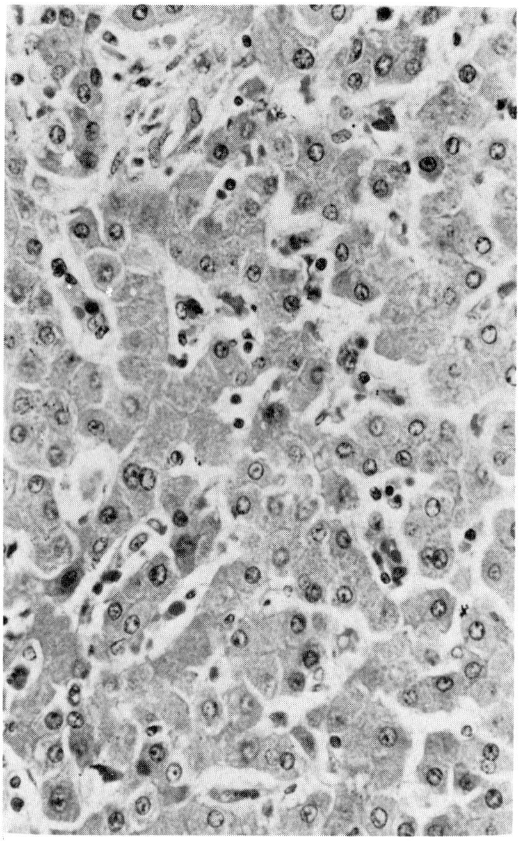

Figure 39.10. Malignant histiocytosis of intestine. Several cells in sinusoids show erythrophagocytosis but the degree of cytological atypia of these cells is minimal. Post-mortem section. Haematoxylin and eosin × 300.

Malignant Histiocytosis of the Intestine

Isaacson and Wright[27] have recently described a form of intestinal malignant histiocytosis associated with malabsorption and ulcerative jejunitis. They designated this condition 'malignant histiocytosis' rather than 'histiocytic lymphoma' in view of the diffuse and often grossly inconspicuous nature of the tumour infiltrates in the bowel and the subtle diffuse infiltrates of tumour cells seen in the lymph nodes, spleen, liver and bone marrow. The appearance of this tumour in many organs, including the liver (which was involved in 50 per cent of their patients), is indistinguishable from malignant histiocytosis (histiocytic medullary reticulosis). This condition should be borne in mind when examining liver biopsies from patients with suspected intestinal lymphoma. The infiltrates in the liver (Figure 39.10) are often inconspicuous and a careful search should be made for evidence of erythrophagocytosis and for sinusoidal or portal histiocytes exhibiting cytological atypia.

Hairy Cell Leukaemia

Hairy cell leukaemia (leukaemic reticuloendotheliosis) frequently presents as pancytopenia with splenomegaly and the patients may well be subjected to diagnostic needle biopsy of the liver. The leukaemic cells infiltrate both the portal triads and the sinusoids and might be confused with chronic lymphocytic leukaemia. Whereas the latter gives a predominantly portal infiltration sinusoidal infiltrates are usually the major feature in hairy cell leukaemia (Figure 39.11). In addition, the cells in hairy cell leukaemia have a more open and finer nuclear chromatin than chronic lymphocytic leukaemia cells and they are more widely spaced in the tissues, often with an apparent clear zone around them which presumably corresponds to the halo of villous processes that surrounds each cell. In a recent elegant study, Nanba et al[40] have described splenic pseudosinuses and hepatic angiomatous lesions (Figures 39.11 and 39.12) that appear to be pathognomonic for this

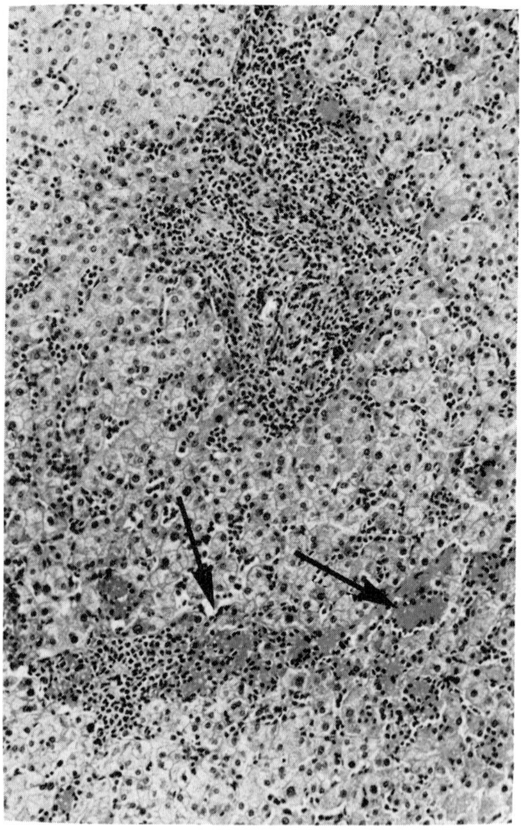

Figure 39.11. Hairy cell leukaemia (leukaemic reticuloendotheliosis). Note distribution of leukaemic cells in portal areas and sinusoids and presence of angiomatous lesions (arrows). Wedge biopsy. Haematoxylin and eosin × 120.

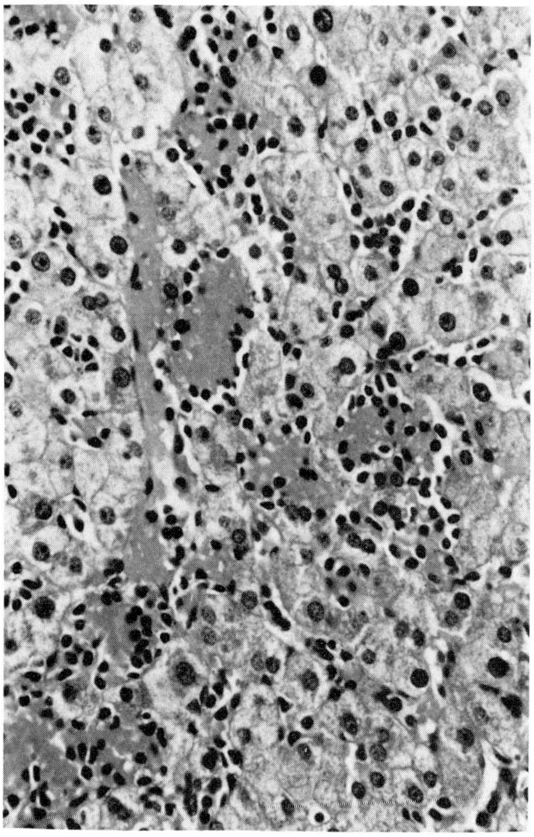

Figure 39.12. Higher power view of Figure 39.11 to show angiomatous lesions lined by hairy cells. ×300.

condition. The hepatic angiomatous lesions were seen in three of five wedge biopsies of liver taken at the time of splenectomy; presumably they would be seen with lower frequency in needle biopsies. These lesions consist of dilated blood filled spaces lined by a layer of hairy cells occurring most frequently in the portal areas, and when they connect with adjacent portal areas they give the liver a gross nutmeg pattern. They are also seen in the lobules where they are often surrounded by thick reticulum fibres which are often continuous with the reticulin framework of adjacent sinusoids.

Fabre et al[13] noted that hairy cells attach to sinusoidal walls in vivo, anchoring themselves by extending cytoplasmic processes through endothelial pores into the space of Disse in a similar manner to the normal attachment of Kupffer cells. Nanba et al[40] postulate that attachment of hairy cells leads to degeneration of endothelial cells and their associated basement membrane with subsequent dilatation of the sinusoid to form an angiomatous lesion lined by hairy cells.

NON-NEOPLASTIC DISEASES SIMULATING MALIGNANT LYMPHOMA AND LEUKAEMIA

Angioimmunoblastic Lymphadenopathy

Angioimmunoblastic lymphadenopathy (AIL) is a recently described condition[18,39] that often clinically and histologically resembles Hodgkin's disease. The stricter criteria generally applied to the diagnosis of Hodgkin's disease probably account for the increased awareness of AIL as an entity though there may be an actual increase in incidence of this condition, possibly associated with certain therapeutic agents.[39] Patients with AIL present with fever, anaemia, joint pains, skin rashes, lymphadenopathy that is usually generalized and often massive, and hepatosplenomegaly. Examination of the blood frequently reveals anaemia, lymphopenia and varying degrees of dysproteinaemia. Clinically, the patients are usually thought to have malignant lymphoma and the diagnosis is customarily established by lymph node biopsy. The nodal architecture is grossly distorted or totally obliterated by a proliferation of arborizing small blood vessels, plasmablasts and plasma cells, often accompanied by deposits of amorphous eosinophilic interstitial material. Frankly malignant cells are not seen nor are tumour infiltrates found at autopsy, death frequently being due to intercurrent infection associated with immunological deficiency, though a small number of cases of AIL terminating with unequivocal malignant lymphoma have been recorded.

The nature of AIL is uncertain. It has been described as a non-neoplastic hyperimmune proliferation of the B-cell system involving an exaggeration of lymphocyte transformation to immunoblasts and plasma cells that may be triggered by a hypersensitivity reaction to therapeutic agents[39] and an autoimmune disorder in which a deficiency of the T-cell regulatory functions probably predisposes to an abnormal proliferation and autoaggressive reaction of the B-cell system.[18]

Studies in the author's laboratory suggest that AIL may consist of two entities, one with a poor prognosis in which a marked T-cell proliferation is found and one with a better prognosis in which B-cells predominate. Involvement of the liver has been found in a high proportion of patients with AIL both in biopsy and autopsy material. It consists mainly of a portal infiltrate of lymphocytes, blast cells and plasma cells with variable numbers of histiocytes and eosinophils. The angiomatous proliferation that is often such a prominent feature in the lymph nodes is inconspicuous in the liver, possibly because of the small size of the infiltrates. In most patients the limiting cell plate is intact though varying degrees of liver cell necrosis, sometimes extensive, may be present.[39] AIL can usually be easily distinguished from malignant lymphoma by the pleomorphic nature of the infiltrate. It does not show atypical histiocytes, Hodgkin's cells or Reed–Sternberg cells and in any event the infiltrate is usually too plasmacytoid for Hodgkin's disease. Confusion with infectious mononucleosis or the lesions of benign idiopathic splenomegaly[37] might occur though these should be separable by clinical features and on lymph node biopsy.

Infectious Mononucleosis

Infectious mononucleosis (IM) follows infection with the Epstein–Barr virus (EBV) in adolescents and young adults; infection in childhood is usually asymptomatic or trivial and escapes recognition. The virus probably enters the body through the nasopharynx and rapidly colonizes the B-lymphocytes, which bear EBV receptors, throughout the body. This elicits a vigorous T-cell and antibody response which terminates with elimination of most of the infected cells and is responsible for much of the symptomatology of the disease. The atypical glandular fever cells seen in the peripheral blood are EBV-infected B-lymphoblasts, which predominate in the early stage of the disease, and reactive T-lymphoblasts, which predominate in the later stages. Hepatitis and jaundice have long been recognized as manifestations of IM. Since, however, the infectivity of EBV appears to be restricted to B-lymphocytes and nasopharyngeal epithelial cells, the liver changes are presumably mediated by immunological mechanisms and not by direct infection of hepatocytes.

Infectious mononucleosis is usually diagnosed by a combination of clinical and haematological features and confirmed by a positive heterophile antibody test. Liver biopsy is rarely indicated and like lymph node biopsy may be regarded as an iatrogenic complication of the disease. However, the corollary of this is that it is the atypical case, possibly one with clinical features suggestive of lymphoma, that is most likely to be biopsied.

In a study of 10 Paul–Bunnell positive cases of IM Wadsworth and Keil[55] noted portal

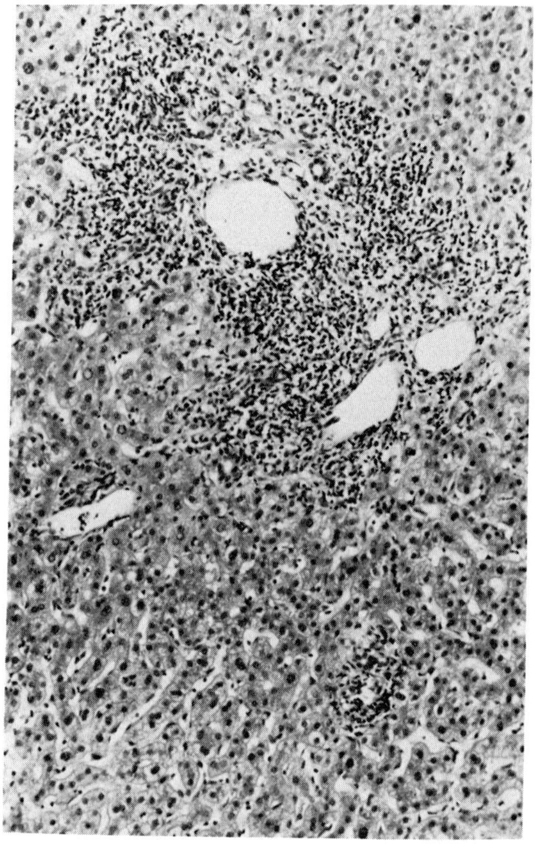

Figure 39.13. Infectious mononucleosis. Expansion of portal areas by lymphoid cells and plasma cells with some spillage into the surrounding sinusoids. Needle biopsy. Haematoxylin and eosin × 120.

infiltrates of lymphocytes and polymorphs to be the earliest manifestation of the disease, occurring within five days of onset. The maximum changes are seen between 10 and 30 days and consist of portal, sinusoidal and focal lobular infiltrates of lymphoid cells (Figures 39.13 and 39.14).[22] These lymphoid cells show a range of appearances from lymphoblastoid cells through to small lymphocytes with often a considerable plasma cell component in the later stages of the disease (Figure 39.13). Extensive liver cell necrosis has been reported in IM[2,3] but this appears to be distinctly uncommon, minimal focal liver cell necrosis being the usual finding.[25,55] Liver function tests do not appear to be well correlated with the liver histology.[55]

The differentiation of the hepatic changes of IM from leukaemia or lymphoma is likely to be most difficult in the early stages of the disease when lymphoblastoid cells predominate, perhaps not surprisingly since at this stage IM

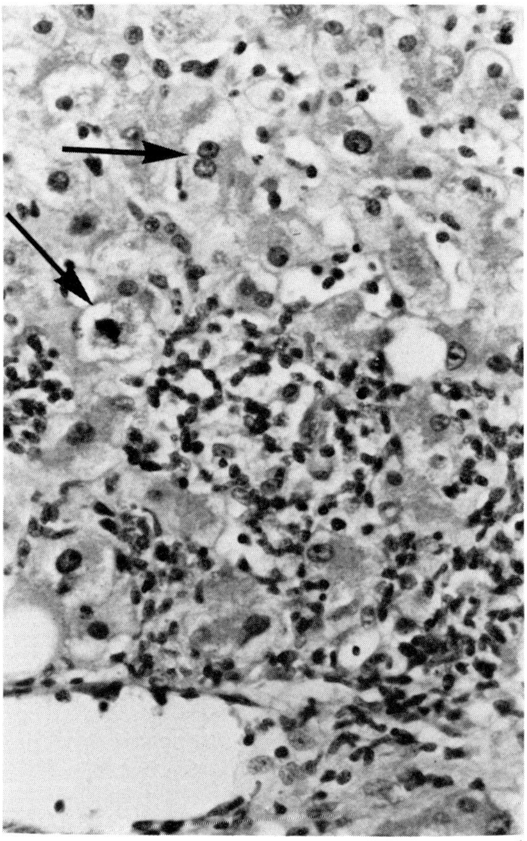

Figure 39.14. Infectious mononucleosis. Note extension of lymphoid cells into lobule. Arrows indicate twinning of liver cells and mitosis in hepatocyte. Needle biopsy. Haematoxylin and eosin ×300.

has many features of a malignant proliferation.[12] The presence of focal liver cell necrosis, Kupffer cell hyperplasia and polymorph infiltrates would favour IM.

Late IM might be confused with lymphocytic or lymphoplasmacytoid lymphomas, a separation that might not be possible on cytology alone. This group of lymphomas in general does not extend into the lobules and is often sharply demarcated by the limiting cell plate.

Infection with cytomegalovirus may cause a hepatitis similar to that seen in IM.[48] As in IM this appears to be related to hypersensitivity reactions rather than direct infection of hepatocytes,[7] although 13 cases of putative postnatal cytomegalovirus hepatitis, in whom viral inclusions were seen in hepatocytes, were described by Henson, Grimley and Strano.[24] Eleven of these patients died during disseminated cytomegalovirus infection and two had liver biopsies for suspected hepatitis.

Tropical Splenomegaly Syndrome

Splenomegaly is a common clinical problem in the tropics and when portal hypertension, visceral leishmaniasis and other recognized causes have been excluded, there remains a group with no obvious aetiology. This was labelled by earlier workers in East Africa as 'idiopathic tropical splenomegaly'. The patients with this syndrome characteristically exhibit a marked sinusoidal lymphocytosis in liver biopsies[26] (Figures 39.15 and 39.16) and the reason for including this condition here is the similarity of the infiltrate to leukaemia or lymphoma. Antibody studies and the response to antimalarial drugs provide evidence that the tropical splenomegaly syndrome is an unusual reaction to malaria, specifically to *Plasmodium malariae*, possibly due to a defect in suppressor T-cell activity,[14] and almost certainly has a genetic basis. The massive splenomegaly is due in part to follicular hyperplasia but due mainly to infiltration of the splenic cords with lymphocytes and plasma cells. Patients often

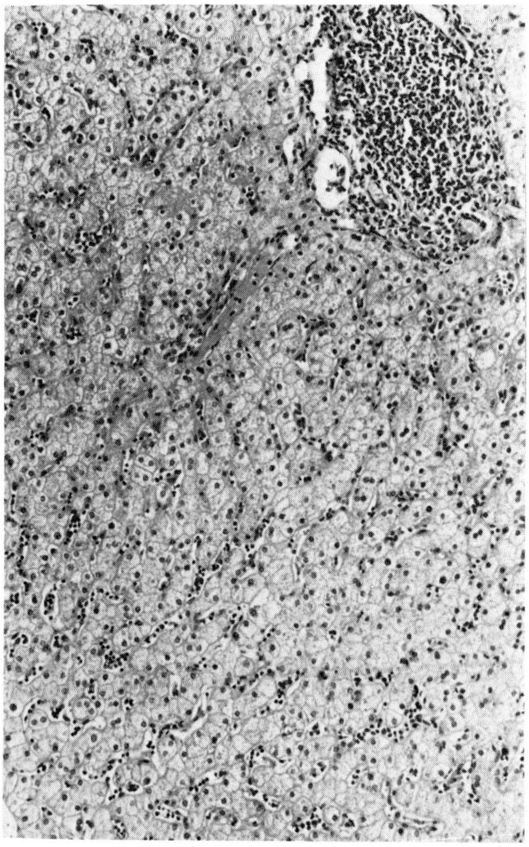

Figure 39.15. Tropical splenomegaly syndrome. Infiltration of portal areas and sinusoids by small lymphocytes. Wedge biopsy. Haematoxylin and eosin × 120.

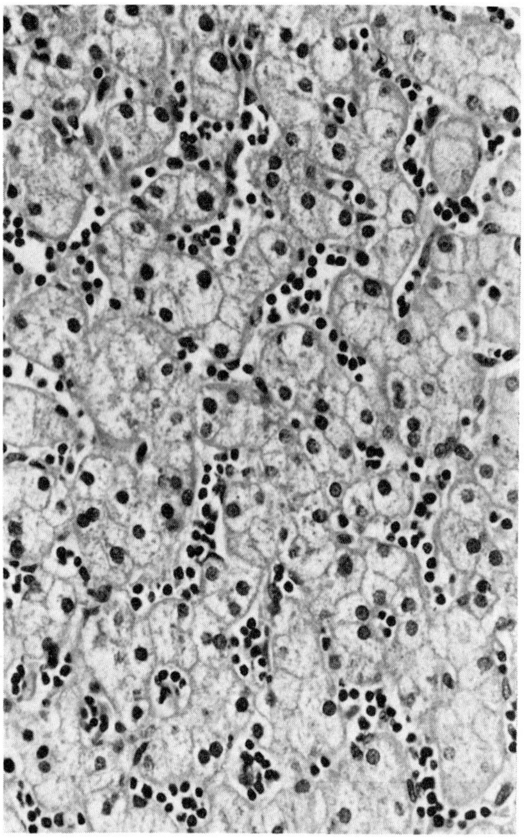

Figure 39.16. Higher power view of Figure 39.15 showing that the intrasinusoidal cells are predominantly small lymphocytes. ×300.

exhibit signs of hypersplenism and anaemia may be profound, particularly during pregnancy. Serum IgM levels are markedly elevated. Liver biopsy is often used both to exclude other causes of splenomegaly and to provide positive evidence of tropical splenomegaly syndrome. The liver biopsy shows Kupffer cell hyperplasia, a common feature in many African liver biopsies, and marked sinusoidal lymphocytosis (Figure 39.16). The cells in the sinusoids consist mainly of small lymphocytes though there may be some evidence of activation on electron microscopy,[16] and occasional plasma cells are usually present. Expansion of the portal triads by lymphoid cells may be found but this is usually little more than that seen in the normal indigenous African population. Sagoe[44] stressed the value of the raised serum IgM and the reaction to anti-malarial drugs in the differentiation of tropical splenomegaly syndrome from malignant lymphoma. However, this differentiation is equally possible by careful examination of the liver biopsy. The only malignancy that gives rise to an infiltration composed of small lymphoid cells or lymphoplasmacytoid cells is well-differentiated lymphocytic lymphoma (chronic lymphocytic leukaemia). Nevertheless, in this disease the infiltrate is predominantly in the portal triads rather than the sinusoids (Figure 39.7). Hairy cell leukaemia gives a sinusoidal infiltrate but can be differentiated from the tropical splenomegaly syndrome by the characteristics of the lymphoid cells and sometimes by the presence of angiomatous lesions (see above; Figures 39.9 and 39.10).

Although tropical splenomegaly syndrome is thought to be an unusual reaction to malarial infection it should be stressed that malarial pigmentation of the Kupffer cells and histiocytes in the portal triads, which is such a prominent feature of acute malarial infection, is not seen in this condition.

Felty's Syndrome

Sinusoidal lymphocytosis similar to that described in the tropical splenomegaly syndrome has been reported in Felty's syndrome.[6]

ACKNOWLEDGEMENTS

I am grateful to Dr J. Fawcett for providing the tissue from which Figures 39.11 and 39.12 were prepared, and to Professor M.S.R. Hutt for providing the tissue from which Figures 39.15 and 39.16 were prepared.

REFERENCES

1. Abt, A.G., Kirschner, R.H., Belliveau, R., O'Connell, M.J., Slansky, B.D., Greene, W.H. & Wiernik, P.H. (1974) Hepatic pathology associated with Hodgkin's disease. *Cancer,* **33,** 1564–1571.
2. Ainley, N.H. (1949) A fatal case of infectious mononucleosis with extensive zonal necrosis of the liver. *Ulster Medical Journal,* **18,** 219–224.
3. Allen, U.R. & Bass, B.H. (1963) Fatal hepatic necrosis in glandular fever. *Journal of Clinical Pathology,* **16,** 339–341.
4. Bagley, C.M., Roth, J.A., Thomas, L.B. & DeVita, V.T. (1972) Clinicopathological correlation of liver biopsies in 127 patients with Hodgkin's disease. *Annals of Internal Medicine,* **76,** 219–225.
5. Bagley, C.M. Jr, Thomas, L.B., Johnson, R.E., Chretien, P.B. & DeVita, V.T. (1973) Diagnosis of liver involvement by lymphoma: results in 96 consecutive peritoneoscopies. *Cancer,* **31,** 840–847.
6. Blendis, L.M., Ansell, I.D., Lloyd Jones, K., Hamilton, C. & Williams, R. (1970) Liver in Felty's syndrome. *British Medical Journal,* **i,** 131–134.

7. Boukowsky, H.L., Lee, R.V. & Klatskin, G. (1975) Acute granulomatous hepatitis. Occurrence in cytomegalovirus mononucleosis. *Journal of the American Medical Association,* **233,** 1284–1288.
8. Bouroncle, B.A., Old, J.W. & Vazques, A.G. (1962) Pathogenesis of jaundice in Hodgkin's disease. *Archives of Internal Medicine,* **110,** 872–883.
9. Byrne, G.E. & Rappaport, H. (1973) Malignant histiocytosis. In *Gann Monograph on Cancer Research,* **15,** 145–162.
10. Chabner, B.A., Johnson, R.E., Chretien, P.B., Schein, P.S., Young, R.C., Canellos, G.P., Hubbard, S.H., Anderson, T., Rosenhoff, S.H. & DeVita, V.T. (1975) Percutaneous liver biopsy, peritoneoscopy and laparotomy: an assessment of relative merits in the lymphomata. *British Journal of Cancer,* **31** (Suppl. 2), 242–247.
11. Chambers, T.J., O'Donoghue, D.P. & Stansfeld, A.G. (1976) A case of primary lymphoma of the liver. *Journal of Clinical Pathology,* **29,** 967–970.
12. Dameshek, W. (1969) Speculations on the nature of infectious mononucleosis. In *Infectious Mononucleosis* (Ed.) Carter, R.L. & Penman, H.G. pp. 225–240. Oxford: Blackwell Scientific Publications.
13. Fabre, J., Delsol, G. & Fédou, R. (1974) Étude de lésions hépatique de la 'hairy cell leukemia'. *Virchows Archives Abt. B. Zellpathology,* **15,** 139–156.
14. Fakunle, Y.M. & Greenwood, B.M. (1976) A suppressor T-cell defect in tropical splenomegaly syndrome. *Lancet,* **ii,** 608–609.
15. Ferguson, D.J., Allen, L.W., Griem, M.L., Moran, E.M., Rappaport, H. & Ultman, J.E. (1973) Surgical experience with staging laparotomies in 125 patients with lymphoma. *Archives of Internal Medicine,* **131,** 356–361.
16. Fluck, D.J., Hutt, M.S.R., Fluck, D.M. & Stuiver, P.C. (1973) Ultrastructure of the hepatic sinusoids in the tropical splenomegaly syndrome. *Transactions of the Royal Society of Tropical Medicine and Hygiene,* **67,** 638–645.
17. Freeman, C., Berg, J.W. & Cutler, S.J. (1972) Occurrence and prognosis of extranodal lymphomas. *Cancer,* **29,** 252–260.
18. Frizzera, G., Moran, E.M. & Rappaport, H. (1975) Angioimmunoblastic lymphadenopathy. Diagnosis and clinical course. *American Journal of Medicine,* **59,** 803–818.
19. Givler, R.L., Brunk, S.F., Hass, C.A. & Guleserian, H.P. (1971) Problems of interpretation of liver biopsy in Hodgkin's disease. *Cancer,* **28,** 1335–1342.
20. Glatstein, E., Guernsey, J.M., Rosenberg, S.A. & Kaplan, H.S. (1969) The value of laparatomy and splenectomy in the staging of Hodgkin's disease. *Cancer,* **24,** 709–718.
21. Glees, J.P., Thomas, M., Redding, W.H., Hefney, M. & Gazet, J.C. (1978) Liver biopsy at lymphoma laparotomy. *Lancet,* **i,** 210–211.
22. Gowing, N.F.C. (1975) Infectious mononucleosis: histopathological aspects. *Hematologic and Lymphoid Pathology Decennial, 1966–1975* (Ed.) Sommers, S.C. pp. 261–280. New York: Appleton Century-Crofts.
23. Grossman, E., Goldstein, M.J., Koss, L.G., Winawer, S.J. & Sherlock, P. (1972) Cytological examination as an adjunct to liver biopsy in the diagnosis of hepatic metastases. *Gastroenterology,* **62,** 56–60.
24. Henson, D.E., Grimley, P.M. & Strano, A.J. (1974) Post natal cytomegalic hepatitis. *Human Pathology,* **5,** 93–103.
25. Hoagland, R.J. & McCluskey, R.T. (1955) Hepatitis in mononucleosis. *Annals of Internal Medicine,* **43,** 1019–1030.
26. Hutt, M.S.R. (1975) Idiopathic tropical splenomegaly in Uganda (big spleen disease). In *Hematologic and Lymphoid Pathology Decennial, 1966–1975* (Ed.) Sommers, S.C. pp. 31–44. New York: Appleton Century-Crofts.
27. Isaacson, P. & Wright, D.H. (1978) Intestinal lymphoma associated with malabsorption. *Lancet,* **i,** 67–70.
28. Jackson, H. & Parker, F. (1947) *Hodgkin's Disease and Allied Disorders.* New York: Oxford University Press.
29. Kadin, M.E., Donaldson, S.S. & Dorfman, R.F. (1970) Isolated granulomas in Hodgkin's disease. *New England Journal of Medicine,* **283,** 859–861.
30. Kadin, M.E., Glatstein, E. & Dorfman, R.F. (1971) Clinicopathological studies of 117 untreated patients subjected to laparotomy for the staging of Hodgkin's disease. *Cancer,* **27,** 1277–1294.
31. Kaplan, H.S. (1972) *Hodgkin's Disease.* Cambridge, Mass.: Harvard University Press.
32. Kaplan, H.S., Dorfman, R.F., Nelsen, T.S. & Rosenberg, S.A. (1973) Staging laparotomy and splenectomy in Hodgkin's disease: analysis of indications and patterns of involvement in 285 consecutive unselected patients. In *National Cancer Institute Monograph,* **36,** 291–301.
33. Kim, H. & Dorfman, R.F. (1974) Morphological studies of 84 untreated patients subjected to laparotomy for the staging of non-Hodgkin's lymphomas. *Cancer,* **33,** 657–674.
34. Kim, H., Dorfman, R.F. & Rosenberg, S.A. (1976) Pathology of malignant lymphomas in the liver: application in staging. *Progress in Liver Disease,* **5,** 683–698.
35. Levitan, R., Diamond, H.D. & Craver, L.F. (1961) Jaundice in Hodgkin's disease. *American Journal of Medicine,* **30,** 99–111.
36. Lipton, M.J., DeNardo, G.L., Silverman, S. & Glatstein, E. (1972) Evaluation of the liver and spleen in Hodgkin's disease. 1. The value of hepatic scintigraphy. *American Journal of Medicine,* **52,** 356–366.
37. Long, J.C. & Aisenberg, A.C. (1974) Malignant lymphoma diagnosed at splenectomy and idiopathic splenomegaly. *Cancer,* **33,** 1054–1061.
38. Lotz, M.J., Chabner, B., DeVita, V.T., Johnson, R.E. & Berard, C.W. (1976) Pathological staging of 100 consecutive untreated patients with non-Hodgkin's lymphomas: extramedullary sites of disease. *Cancer,* **37,** 266–270.
39. Lukes, R.J. & Tindle, B.H. (1975) Immunoblastic lymphadenopathy: a hyperimmune entity resembling Hodgkin's disease. *New England Journal of Medicine,* **292,** 1–8.
40. Nanba, K., Soban, E.J., Bowling, M.C. & Berard, C.W. (1977) Splenic pseudosinuses and hepatic angiomatous lesions. Distinctive features of hairy cell leukaemia. *American Journal of Clinical Pathology,* **67,** 415–426.
41. Neiman, R.S., Rosen, P.J. & Lukes, R.J. (1973) Lymphocyte depletion Hodgkin's disease: a clinicopathological entity. *New England Journal of Medicine,* **288,** 751–755.
42. Rappaport, H. (1966) Tumors of the hematopoietic system. In *Atlas of Tumor Pathology.* Washington D.C.: Armed Forces Institute of Pathology.

43. Rappaport, H., Berard, C.W., Butler, J.J., Lukes, R.J. & Thomas, C.B. (1971) Report of the Committee on Histopathological Criteria Contributing to Staging of Hodgkin's Disease. *Cancer Research,* **31,** 1864–1865.
44. Sagoe, A.S. (1970) Tropical splenomegaly syndrome. Long term prognanil therapy correlated with spleen size, serum IgM and lymphocytic transformation. *British Medical Journal,* **iii,** 378–380.
45. Scott, R.B. & Robb-Smith, A.H.T. (1939) Histiocytic medullary reticulosis. *Lancet,* **ii,** 194–198.
46. Serk-Hanssen, A. & Purohit, G.P. (1968) Histiocytic medullary reticulosis. Report of 14 cases from Uganda. *British Journal of Cancer,* **22,** 506–516.
47. Spector, W.G. & Heesom, N. (1969) The production of granulomata by antigen–antibody complexes. *Journal of Pathology,* **98,** 31–39.
48. Stern, H. (1972) Cytomegalovirus and E.B. virus infections of the liver. *British Medical Bulletin,* **28,** 180–185.
49. Torres, A. (1969) Primary lymphocytic follicular lymphoma of liver. *Cancer,* **23,** 1185–1189.
50. Torres, A. & Bollozos, G.D. (1971) Primary reticulum cell sarcoma of the liver. *Cancer,* **27,** 1489–1492.
51. Uddströmer, M. (1934) On the occurrence of lymphogranulomatosis (Sternberg) in Sweden, 1915–1931 and some considerations as to its relation to tuberculosis. *Acta Tuberculosis Scandinavica Supplement,* **1,** 1–225.
52. Vardiman, J.W., Byrne, G.E. & Rappaport, H. (1975) Malignant histiocytosis with massive splenomegaly in asymptomatic patients. A possible chronic form of the disease. *Cancer,* **36,** 419–427.
53. Variakojis, D., Rosas-Uribe, A. & Rappaport, H. (1974) Mycosis fungoides: pathologic findings in staging laparotomies. *Cancer,* **33,** 1589–1600.
54. Veronesi, U., Musumeci, R., Pizzetti, F., Gennari, L. & Bonadonna, G. (1974) The value of staging laparotomy in non-Hodgkin's lymphomas (with emphasis on the histiocytic type). *Cancer,* **33,** 446–459.
55. Wadsworth, R.C. & Keil, P.G. (1952) Biopsy of the liver in infectious mononucleosis. *American Journal of Pathology,* **28,** 1003–1025.
56. Warnke, R.A., Kim, H. & Dorfman, R.F. (1975) Malignant histiocytosis (histiocytic medullary reticulosis). 1. Clinicopathological study of 29 cases. *Cancer,* **35,** 215–230.
57. Westling, P. (1965) Studies of the prognosis in Hodgkin's disease. *Acta Radiologica* (Suppl. 245), 5–125.

Chapter 40

Paediatric Liver Disease: Medical Aspects

ALEX P. MOWAT

JAUNDICE IN INFANCY

Jaundice occurs in up to 90 per cent of healthy newborn infants. In the majority the cause will be a temporary inefficiency of hepatic excretion of bilirubin, usually referred to as physiological jaundice. Jaundice may thus imprudently be disregarded although it is an important clinical sign which can be the first indication of serious treatable underlying liver disease such as galactosaemia or choledochal cyst. It may also allow the identification of infants at risk of developing brain damage due to bilirubin encephalopathy. As in all age groups, the diagnosis of jaundice in infancy is simplified if classified into unconjugated and conjugated hyperbilirubinaemia. Although physiological jaundice is, strictly speaking, not a disease of the liver, consideration must be given to it as it modifies the clinical, pharmacological and biochemical features of all types of liver disease in the first two to three weeks of life.

UNCONJUGATED HYPERBILIRUBINAEMIA

Physiological Jaundice

Physiological jaundice can be defined as a temporary inefficient hepatic excretion of bilirubin which results in jaundice in full-term infants between the second and eighth day of life. Maximum serum bilirubin concentrations occur on the second to fourth day of life and rarely exceed 100 μmol/l (6 mg/dl). In premature infants, jaundice starts on the second day of life and persists until the tenth, with maximum serum bilirubins of 200 to 250 μmol/l (12 to 15 mg/dl) occurring between the fifth and seventh day of life.

Pathophysiology

The physiology of bilirubin formation and excretion is discussed elsewhere (Chapters 11, 13 and 14). Our knowledge of the causes of physiological jaundice is imperfect since this disorder cannot ethically be studied in individual infants. It is currently considered that physiological jaundice results from a combination of three factors affecting bilirubin metabolism, namely:

1. Increased bilirubin production.
2. Impaired hepatic uptake and excretion of bilirubin.
3. Enteric reabsorption of bilirubin.

There is good evidence of increased bilirubin production from reduced red blood cell survival in the human infant. The red cell life is approximately 90 days in the newborn. Bilirubin production from non-haemoglobin sources, if expressed by unit weight, is more than twice that of the adult.[37]

In man the plasma clearance of bilirubin is impaired but the exact reason for this is uncertain. Lower ligandin levels have been demonstrated in human neonatal livers.[5] Deficient glucuronyl transferase activity has been shown but the increase to adult levels was not complete until the seventieth day.[24] In the

Table 40.1. *Post-natal Causes of Pathological Unconjugated Hyperbilirubinaemia.*

1. Haemolytic disease
2. Bacterial infection
3. Hypoxia
4. Hypoglycaemia
5. Galactosaemia
6. Fructosaemia
7. Intestinal obstruction
8. Drugs sharing excretory pathways with bilirubin
9. Hypothyroidism

rhesus monkey in which a biphasic physiological jaundice occurs, deficient glucuronyl transferase activity is thought to contribute to high serum bilirubin levels in the first 24 hours of life, but the lower serum bilirubin levels on the second, third and fourth day of life are due to defective hepatic uptake. In this animal model enteric reabsorption of bilirubin adds to the bilirubin load on the liver.[29] In the human infant, the serum bilirubin is inversely related to the amount of bilirubin in the stool.[48]

Pathological Neonatal Unconjugated Hyperbilirubinaemia

Any degree of clinical jaundice in the first 24 hours of life is pathological. If the pattern of jaundice deviates from that described above for physiological jaundice, either in time or severity, underlying disease must be suspected. Early identification and treatment of those causes which operate post-natally (Table 40.1), and measures to prevent kernicterus, are essential.

It would be inappropriate in this textbook to consider in detail the investigation and treatment of each of these aggravating factors, or the precise indications for measures to control hyperbilirubinaemia. Exchange transfusion remains the most effective way of immediately reducing the risk of kernicterus. Phototherapy, in which the jaundiced infant is exposed to artificial light of a wavelength of between 400 and 500 nm, is effective in controlling hyperbilirubinaemia provided severe haemolysis is not present. No serious short-term complications from its use have as yet been recorded. The main danger in its use is that it masks jaundice and may cause a delay in diagnosing such disorders as septicaemia. Phenobarbitone has no place in the management of established hyperbilirubinaemia in infancy.

Prolonged Neonatal Unconjugated Hyperbilirubinaemia

If jaundice persists beyond 10 to 14 days of age, it is important that haemolysis, e.g. due to glucose-6-phosphate dehydrogenase deficiency or microspherocytosis, be excluded by finding a reticulocyte count of less than 2 per cent. Hypothyroidism, evidenced by a low T_4 and high thyroid-stimulating hormone concentration, must also be excluded. The most common cause of such jaundice is that associated with breast feeding. Serum bilirubin concentration rises to between 250 and 340 μmol/l (15 and 20 mg/dl) in the second or third week of life in infants who are entirely well. Jaundice may persist for as long as four months. If breast feeding is discontinued, however, the jaundice will resolve within six days and, surprisingly, may not recur if breast feeding is recommenced.[6] The aetiology of this syndrome is not known.[46] Seventy-five per cent of siblings of affected infants are similarly affected. Two agents in breast milk have been considered to be responsible, 3-alpha 20-beta pregnanediol and free fatty acids, but the evidence for either of these is not conclusive. Kernicterus has not complicated this condition, but breast feeding should be discontinued for a period of 24 to 48 hours if the serum bilirubin levels rise to 290 μmol/l (17 mg/dl). Very rarely, prolonged jaundice may be due to Gilbert's syndrome or to the Crigler–Najjar syndrome.

CONJUGATED HYPERBILIRUBINAEMIA IN INFANCY

Conjugated hyperbilirubinaemia in infancy is always pathological. It may arise from disorders of the hepatocyte or from lesions of the biliary tree. Clinical features and standard laboratory tests of liver function frequently do not distinguish whether the disease arises primarily in the hepatocyte or in the biliary tree. Very rarely, conjugated hyperbilirubinaemia may be caused by a genetically-determined abnormality in the excretion of bilirubin glucuronide.

Hepatitis Syndrome in Infancy

Clinical features

Jaundice with dark bile-containing urine and, in most instances, pale or clay-coloured stools, is the most usual presentation. Jaundice is often continuous with physiological jaundice but may present as late as four months. Rarely, the presenting feature is malabsorption.

Hepatomegaly is usually found and 50 per cent of cases show splenomegaly. Failure to thrive and haemolytic anaemia may also occur.[2,21,41]

Laboratory investigations

The serum bilirubin ranges from 70 to 850 μmol/l (4 to 50 mg/dl) with between 40 and 80 per cent direct reacting. Standard tests of liver function show an elevation of the aspartate transaminase to levels of between two and six times normal with similar elevations of the alkaline phosphatase. The prothrombin time may be prolonged. The serum albumin may be low. Thrombocytopenia may be found.

Diagnosis and Management of the Infant with Conjugated Hyperbilirubinaemia

Conjugated hyperbilirubinaemia in infancy has many causes (Table 40.2). Rarely, the clinical history or examination will identify the cause. In the majority of infants a systematic scheme of investigation is required (Table 40.3). The priorities in investigation are the recognition of those causes which are amenable to specific therapy, the recognition of genetically-determined disorders and the identification of patients who require surgical intervention.

Table 40.2. *Causes of Conjugated Hyperbilirubinaemia in Infancy.*

Hepatocellular lesions
- Metabolic defects
- Infection
- Post-haemolytic disorders
- Toxic or deficiency disorders,
  - e.g. intravenous nutrition and drugs
- Familial syndromes
- Idiopathic

Structural defects
- Bile duct abnormalities,
  - e.g. Biliary atresia
  - Spontaneous perforation of the bile duct
  - Choledochal cyst
- Infantile polycystic disease of the liver and kidney
- Vascular lesions,
  - e.g. Veno-occlusive disease
  - Haemangio-endothelioma
- Chromosomal abnormalities

Table 40.3. *Outline of Scheme of Investigation in Infants with Conjugated Hyperbilirubinaemia.*

Stage I. Initiate immediately

1 (a) Bacterial culture of blood, urine and stools
(b) WR or VDRL
(c) Toxoplasma complement fixation antibody in serum
(d) Listeria antibody
(e) Viral culture of urine and stool
(f) Hepatitis B surface antigen in serum
(g) Viral antibody test

2 (a) Urinanalysis for non-glucose reducing substances
(b) Red blood cell galactose-1-phosphate uridyl Transferase
(c) Blood sugar
(d) Alpha-1-antitrypsin phenotype
(e) Serum and urinary amino acids
(f) Sweat electrolyte determination

3 (a) Peripheral blood count including reticulocyte count
(b) Blood group
(c) Coombs' test

4 Prothrombin time

5 Serum bilirubin, albumin, transaminase and alkaline phosphatase

6 (a) Blood urea
(b) Serum sodium, potassium, chloride, bicarbonate, calcium and phosphate

Stage II

1 Ultrasonic scan of abdomen for choledochal cyst
2 Barium meal to show duodenal displacement by choledochal cyst
3 Chest x-ray to demonstrate cardiac lesions
X-ray of long bones for evidence of intra-uterine infection
5 Diagnostic paracentesis of abdomen if appropriate

Stage III

Percutaneous liver biopsy. Tissue for histological examination, enzymatic studies, bacterial or viral culture

Stage IV

^{131}I rose bengal faecal excretion test

Stage V

Laparotomy and operative cholangiogram

Complete as soon as possible but ALWAYS by the time an infant is 60 days old

Infections

Conjugated hyperbilirubinaemia with hepatocellular damage complicates many bacterial infections, particularly urinary *E. coli* infections, septicaemia and enteritis. Urinalysis and blood and stool cultures are necessary investigations in every case. Syphilis and toxoplasmosis must be excluded since specific treatment is available. It must be remembered that bacterial infection can complicate other primary causes of liver damage such as galactosaemia or biliary atresia.

Generalized infections acquired in utero, during delivery or early in the newborn period, by viruses such as rubella, cytomegalovirus, herpes simplex virus, coxsackie B and adenovirus, may cause hepatitis. Often, other organs such as the brain, eyes, heart and haemopoietic system may be affected to an even greater extent than the liver.[25] Listeria, cytomegalovirus, rubella virus and hepatitis B virus have all been associated with extrahepatic biliary atresia as well as hepatitis. Cytomegalovirus has been recovered from the urine of infants with a wide range of hepatobiliary disorders, as well as from the urine of infants who have no liver disease.[17] Thus, although the infant may have evidence of contact with pathogens, a more serious underlying disorder requiring urgent identification may be present.

Viral hepatitis B. Hepatitis B surface antigen has been found in a small number of infants with hepatitis, in some cases leading to cirrhosis. More commonly the hepatitis is anicteric and causes no symptoms. Infection is derived either from an asymptomatic carrier mother or a mother who has had hepatitis in the last trimester of pregnancy, or early in the puerperium, and also from hepatitis B surface antigen positive blood or serum. The risk of infection appears greatest when the mother's blood contains the e antigen or when hepatitis occurs in the last trimester of pregnancy or early in the puerperium. In most instances, the liver disease is mild.[30] Fulminant hepatitis may occur.[26]

Genetically-determined metabolic disorders

Of the metabolic disorders causing hepatocellular damage, in infancy it is important to identify immediately galactosaemia, fructosaemia and tyrosinosis since they are amenable to dietary treatment.

The clinical features are indistinguishable from those described above except that in both galactosaemia and fructosaemia hypoglycaemia may occur. The diagnosis of these two conditions should be suspected when a non-glucose reducing substance is found in the urine when it is tested with Clinitest tablets or Benedict's solution and when the glucose oxidase test for glucose is negative. It must be emphasized that urinary tests will be abnormal only if the offending monosaccharide has been ingested shortly before the time of testing. Some patients with galactosaemia do not have galactosuria.[39] The diagnosis in such patients can be made only by determining the activity of galactose-1-phosphate uridyl transferase activity in red blood cells.

Similarly, fructosaemia may not be complicated by fructosuria. The diagnosis in this case will be suspected from the relationship between the time of introduction of fructose into the diet and the onset of symptoms or by the finding of hypoglycaemia. It may also be suspected when the liver biopsy shows distended hepatocytes with moderate fatty infiltration. The diagnosis can be confirmed only by showing a low or absent hepatic fructose-1-phosphatase in the liver biopsy. These two conditions must be identified since the effect of not treating the patient is devastating, while with appropriate treatment the prognosis is excellent.

Tyrosinosis presents diagnostic difficulties. It usually presents in the first four weeks of life with failure to thrive, hepatocellular failure, bleeding diathesis and renal tubular dysfunction, while later vitamin D-resistant rickets emerges. The diagnosis may be suspected when the urine contains high concentrations of amino acids, particularly tyrosine and phenylalanine, and also shows a high excretion of parahydroxyphenyl lactic acid and parahydroxyphenyl acetic acid.[55] These may be found in infants with hepatocellular necrosis for other reasons. A diagnosis of tyrosinaemia must be initially tentative but may be revised when the biochemical features resolve as the liver disease improves.[65] Where the diagnosis is suspected a low phenylalanine, low tyrosine diet should be instituted. Unfortunately, the response is not satisfactory in many cases.

Cystic fibrosis, Niemann–Pick disease, neurovisceral sphingomyelin storage disease with ophthalmoplegia, Gaucher's disease, Wolman's disease, Dubin–Johnson syndrome and trihydroxy stannic acidaemia are all rare causes of hepatocellular damage in infancy.[40] By far the most common genetically determined cause in South-east England is alpha-1-antitrypsin deficiency.[51]

Alpha-1-antitrypsin deficiency. Hepatic disease found in association with this genetic deficiency of serum glycoprotein is considered in detail elsewhere (see Chapter 35). Between 10 and 20 per cent of infants presenting with the hepatitis syndrome in infancy have alpha-1-antitrypsin deficiency, phenotype Z. It is important that this be identified for the following reasons:

1. The hepatitis is frequently severe and the

stools completely acholic. It is thus indistinguishable from biliary atresia. The findings on percutaneous liver biopsy are frequently identical with those found in biliary atresia. The PAS-positive magenta-coloured inclusions which are characteristic of the disease in later life may not be found in the first 12 weeks of life (see Chapter 35).[60]

2. The prognosis for liver disease associated with this deficiency is much more serious than that found in the idiopathic variety. Of 33 infants with alpha-1-antitrypsin deficiency and hepatitis in infancy, only seven, aged between three and seven years, had no clinical abnormality and normal liver function tests.[42] In contrast, only one of 27 survivors from 29 cases of idiopathic hepatitis in infancy had any evidence of severe liver disease.[49]

Hepatocellular Causes of Jaundice in Infancy

Post-haemolytic cholestasis

When unconjugated hyperbilirubinaemia due to severe haemolysis has been protracted, or if there has been marked anaemia at birth, the urine may contain bilirubin and the stools may become acholic. Laboratory investigations show typical features of the hepatitis syndrome. Liver biopsy shows hepatocellular necrosis and giant cell transformation, with hepatocellular and bile canalicular cholestasis. Jaundice usually resolves spontaneously over a period of four to ten weeks. The long-term prognosis is good.[62]

Conjugated hyperbilirubinaemia associated with parenteral nutrition

Intravenous alimentation, using solutions of amino acids, dextrose and lipids with added vitamins and electrolytes, is a commonly employed procedure in paediatrics, particularly for premature infants with gastrointestinal disorders such as necrotizing enterocolitis. Conjugated hyperbilirubinaemia frequently follows. The aetiology of this is unknown but, since the frequency of the disorder increases with the duration of intravenous feeding, it is thought that the intravenous feeding, rather than associated harmful factors such as sepsis, hypoxia, intra-abdominal surgery and drugs, may be important. It is uncertain whether the intravenous lipids or the amino acids are responsible. A further possibility is that lack of essential nutrients and trace elements, or even single amino acids, may contribute to the disorder. Lack of gastrointestinal stimulation of bile secretion has also been suggested as a possible factor.

As well as showing features of cholestasis and hepatocellular damage, there is marked hyperplasia of Kupffer cells, widening of portal tracts and increased portal fibrosis.

The clinical and biochemical features are indistinguishable from those of other forms of hepatitis in infancy. When intravenous nutrition is withdrawn, the jaundice gradually settles over a period of some weeks and liver function tests gradually return to normal. The long-term prognosis is uncertain.[7]

Chromosomal abnormalities

In trisomy 13 and 18, between 20 and 30 per cent of patients have hepatitis. The diagnosis of these trisomies is suspected from the marked abnormalities found on physical examination and is confirmed by analysis of the chromosomal karyotype.[61] They thus present no problem in differential diagnosis.

Familial syndromes

Several distinct syndromes of unknown cause but with an increased incidence within families have been described. In a group of patients with common ancestry in South-west Norway, obstructive jaundice in infancy has been followed by recurrent episodes of jaundice throughout childhood and later life. Towards puberty, affected children develop oedema of the limbs due to hypoplasia of lymph vessels. It has been suggested that deficiency of intrahepatic lymphatics may contribute to the cholestasis.[1]

Congenital hypoplasia and stenosis of the pulmonary arteries, sometimes associated with other cardiovascular malformations, have been found in association with a very heterogeneous pattern of liver disease usually described under the term 'arterio-hepatic dysplasia'.[32,64] Alagille and co-workers[3] describe a syndrome in infants who subsequently developed intrahepatic bile duct hypoplasia and a characteristic facial appearance: prominent forehead, deeply set eyes with mild hyperteleorism and a nose which in profile is in the same plane as the forehead. They frequently have harsh systolic murmurs maximal at the left sternal border and, in some, pulmonary arterial stenosis has been demonstrated. Vertebral arch defects, growth retardation and mental retardation may be found.

Progressive familial cholestasis

Progressive intrahepatic cholestasis proceeding to early death, often in the first decade, has been described in a number of reports such as those in the Amish Byler family, as well as in a number of smaller sibships. In most families, jaundice occurs intermittently initially, often being provoked by intercurrent infection, but remission is never complete. Hepatomegaly persists and eventually progresses to hepatic fibrosis, cirrhosis and its complications.[35,47]

Idiopathic hepatitis in infancy

In the majority of infants no cause can be identified. Such cases frequently occur in children who have been born prematurely with low birthweight and who often require medical attention because of complications of prematurity. In many instances jaundice is continuous with physiological jaundice but in some cases it may start as late as four months. It persists for up to six months. It may frequently be sufficiently severe to cause completely acholic stools. Undoubtedly, some of these infants have an unrecognized genetic disorder and the prognosis for this group is not homogeneous. It may be better than early reports suggest; for example, of 29 such cases, identified between 1971 and 1973, 27 are alive and well, although one has cirrhosis.[49]

Intrahepatic bile duct hypoplasia

This is an ill-understood disorder which is defined pathologically by the absence or diminution of the number and size of intralobular intrahepatic bile ducts seen on a wedge liver biopsy obtained at laparotomy. The disorder may arise in association with extrahepatic biliary atresia but also complicates many other forms of hepatocellular disease starting in infancy, such as alpha-1-antitrypsin deficiency and the arteriohepatic dysplasia syndromes.

Symptoms may occur in the first three months of life or be delayed to beyond three years. In the former case there are usually typical features of the hepatitis syndrome, but these progress to pruritus without jaundice or with only moderate elevation of the serum bilirubin. A liver biopsy in the first six months of life frequently shows bile duct reduplication as the principal pathological feature in the portal tracts. Gradually, biliary hypoplasia develops.

In the late onset cases pruritus and hepatomegaly with elevated alkaline phosphatase and serum bile salts are followed by elevation in the serum bilirubin. Liver biopsy in such cases frequently shows varying degrees of fibrosis. Portal hypertension and cirrhosis gradually follow. Pruritus and xanthelasma develop. In some patients, jaundice may clear completely but tests of liver function remain abnormal.[36]

In the individual case, the diagnosis of such rare progressive conditions cannot be made in the newborn period in the absence of a positive family history. Only the subsequent evolution of the disease allows an eventual diagnosis to be made.

Differential Diagnosis of Surgically Correctable Causes of Conjugated Hyperbilirubinaemia and Severe Cholestasis due to Hepatocellular Disease

Three surgically correctable disorders must be excluded: extrahepatic biliary atresia, choledochal cyst and spontaneous perforation of the bile duct. All three may present with a cholestatic syndrome identical to that described above.

In choledochal cyst, clinical examination may show a mass extending down from the liver margin towards the umbilicus. This will be palpable only if the cyst is large and contains fluid at the time of examination. Careful palpation below the edge of the liver is always worth while in such infants.

Spontaneous perforation of the bile duct produces ascites which is relatively rare in hepatocellular disorders, unless these are very severe as, for example, in tyrosinosis or galactosaemia. It may be complicated by bile-stained herniae which are almost pathognomonic.

In the majority of cases however, there will be no clinical features which will distinguish those cases requiring surgery. Standard tests of liver function are equally unhelpful unless they show a progressive fall in serum bilirubin towards normal, which will exclude extrahepatic biliary atresia. Over the years, many tests on blood and serum have been advocated to help distinguish between extrahepatic biliary atresia and hepatitis, e.g. alpha-fetoprotein, lipoprotein-X, 5′-nucleotidase and red cell haemolysis in the presence of peroxidase. None is 100 per cent reliable and, in an individual case, may give misleading results.[34]

If jaundice and other features of hepatocellular necrosis persist, and no metabolic cause for the liver disease has been determined, two further investigations are of value.

If the platelet count is greater than 40 $\times 10^9$/l and the prothrombin time is prolonged by fewer than five seconds, a *percutaneous liver biopsy*, using a Menghini needle, provides valuable help in differentiating hepatocellular causes for the jaundice from extrahepatic biliary atresia or bile duct obstruction complicating choledochal cyst. Unfortunately, there is no single histological feature which is specific for either condition. The most valuable feature is the finding of widening of all portal tracts in biliary atresia. They show prominent distorted elongated and angulated bile ducts, increased fibrosis and inflammatory cell infiltrate. The hepatic architecture is preserved in the early stages and there is little hepatocellular necrosis. In contrast, in hepatitis, hepatocellular necrosis, disorganization of liver cords, and inflammatory cell infiltrate in the hepatic parenchyma and portal tracts are frequently seen. This investigation gives good separation of the two groups but it is likely to be less than the 100 per cent which is claimed by Brough and Bernstein.[12]

The other test of value is the intravenous radioactive *rose bengal faecal excretion test*. Excretion of less than 10 per cent of the isotope in a 72-hour period is indicative of complete obstruction to bile flow. It does not distinguish whether this is due to hepatobiliary tract disease or to hepatocellular disease. If the excretion is less than 10 per cent and the biopsy features are of extrahepatic biliary atresia, immediate laparotomy is indicated. If the histological features are those of hepatitis, it is reasonable to postpone surgery for a further three weeks, during which time the infant is given cholestyramine in a dose of 1 g four times per day. If atresia is not present excretion may rise to above 10 per cent.[14] This does not occur invariably, however.[41]

By combining these two investigations, liver biopsy and rose bengal faecal excretion test, it is possible to avoid laparotomy in patients with hepatocellular disease and yet proceed to laparotomy by 60 days of age in patients with biliary atresia.

Treatment

Bacterial infection, listeria, syphilis and toxoplasmosis can all be treated by specific agents. No therapy which is shown to modify the course of idiopathic hepatitis or that due to viral cause is available. Careful, supportive management, particularly the correction of haemorrhagic diathesis by infusions of fresh frozen plasma or platelets, correction of fluid and electrolyte abnormalities, and albumin infusions to correct the hypoalbuminaemia complicated by peripheral oedema and ascites, may be required in individual cases. Secondary bacterial or monilial infection will require treatment.

Nutrition can be improved by a diet low in natural fats and supplemented with medium chain triglycerides. Proprietary milks so constituted are available. Fat-soluble vitamins A, D and K should be given by mouth in amounts between two and three times those required by healthy infants of the same age. It may be necessary to give these by parenteral injection if steatorrhoea is severe. It should be noted that vitamin D requirements in this syndrome are very variable. In part, this may be due to ineffective hepatic metabolism of cholecalciferol. Close biochemical monitoring is needed, to avoid rickets on the one hand and hypercalcaemia on the other.

Cholestyramine is particularly helpful as a symptomatic measure if pruritus is a problem, provided there is some bile flow. Where cholestasis is complete, as in biliary atresia, its effect is less marked. Cholestyramine has the additional advantage of improving liver function in some patients.

Corticosteroids are of no proven value in this syndrome and predispose the patient to the risks of overwhelming infection. Phenobarbitone, by its effect on microsomal function, by which it possibly increases bile flow, may cause some lessening of the degree of jaundice in a minority of patients. There is no evidence that this has any effect on the long-term prognosis.

REYE'S SYNDROME

Reye's syndrome is an acute disorder characterized by a severe encephalopathy with marked cerebral oedema, but without cellular infiltration or demyelination and with diffuse fatty infiltration of the viscera. Typically, it occurs in a child who is recovering from what appears to be a mild, unremarkable respiratory tract infection or exanthomatous illness, such as chicken-pox. Over 800 cases have been reported since the condition was first highlighted by Reye and his colleagues in 1963.[52]

It is predominantly a disease of childhood of world-wide distribution. It occurs in minor epidemics but direct case-to-case spread is unusual. Two epidemiological patterns of disease have been described. One occurs in a young age group (median six years) and is associated with a variety of preceding viral infections, including varicella.[19] The other occurs in an older age group (median 11 years) and is related to epidemics of influenza B.[19,20] Electron microscopy of the liver and brain shows abnormal mitochondria which are swollen and pleomorphic. Many biochemical abnormalities found in this syndrome reflect changes in mitochondrial function.[11] What combination of genetic, infective or toxic influences cause this acute reversible abnormality of mitochondrial structure and function is unknown. The effects of the mitochondrial abnormality are exaggerated by tissue destruction and lipolysis.

The principal pathological changes occur in the liver, but lesser degrees of changes may be found in the kidney and other organs. In the first 24 hours after the onset of symptoms hepatic glycogen is depleted. Thereafter lipid within the hepatocyte cytoplasm shows a progressive accumulation which gradually displaces other cytoplasmic constituents. Hepatic necrosis is absent or inconspicuous. Cerebral oedema is marked, with no significant inflammatory cell reaction in the brain or meninges. Secondary changes due to cerebral oedema and hypoxia may occur.

Clinical Features

The disorder is usually found in a patient aged from six months to 15 years who is apparently recovering from a mild, unremarkable prodromal illness such as influenza B infection or chicken-pox. Vomiting develops and becomes persistent and profuse. This may coincide with, or be rapidly followed by, a change in the mental state which shows a rapid escalation from irrational behaviour through delirium to lethargy and coma with eventual decerebrate rigidity. Convulsions occur in 30 per cent of cases. Hyperpnoea often develops during the progression of the encephalopathy. The rate of progression varies from three to 60 hours. The condition may stabilize, improve and recover completely at any stage short of brain death. Usually, no clinical features indicate hepatic involvement, although the liver may be palpable, even enlarged, in 40 per cent of cases and liver function tests are very deranged. Characteristic features are elevation of the serum transaminase, prolongation of the prothrombin time, and hyperammonaemia. Jaundice is rarely present. Acidosis, hypoxia, dehydration, electrolyte disturbances and hypoglycaemia may complicate the picture.

Therapy is far from satisfactory. Approximately 40 per cent of recognized cases still die. Thirty per cent of those who develop seizures or decerebrate posturing develop long-term neurological sequelae.[18]

Treatment

Treatment aims at preventing the metabolic complications and cerebral oedema. Early diagnosis and intravenous 10 or 15 per cent glucose at a rate of 1.2 $l/m^2/24$ hr may correct hypoglycaemia, minimize protein breakdown and lipolysis and stop the accumulation of ammonia and fatty acids. Hypoxia must be prevented by intubation and positive pressure respiration. Intensive monitoring and supportive care, with rapid correction of the many biochemical abnormalities which may occur, are also thought to be of value. To try to minimize the chances of cerebral oedema, the serum osmolality should be maintained at more than 320 mosmol/l. Mannitol, in a dose of 1 to 2 g/kg over a 20-minute period, may also help. Continuous monitoring of intracranial pressure has also been advocated.[56] Exchange transfusion and peritoneal dialysis, although occasionally giving very satisfactory results,[9] have not been shown to be of value.[18]

LESIONS OF THE LIVER AND BILIARY SYSTEM IN CYSTIC FIBROSIS

Over 70 per cent of children with cystic fibrosis diagnosed in infancy now survive beyond the age of 12 years. Fifty per cent of these have minimal or no respiratory insufficiency. As many as 20 per cent of adolescents with this condition may have cirrhosis and its complications.[54] Cirrhosis has been documented histologically as early as four years of age.[10]

In infancy, prolonged conjugated hyperbilirubinaemia may occur from obstruction of the extrahepatic bile ducts by inspissated or even solid bile. Intrahepatic pathological changes range from a reversible increase in portal tract inflammation and cholestasis to an obstructive biliary type of cirrhosis.[23]

Gallbladder abnormalities are particularly common in cystic fibrosis and take the form of small gallbladders which are unable to concentrate bile. They occur more frequently in patients who have cirrhosis, but the significance of the association is uncertain.[27] Gallstones are found in up to 8 per cent of cases.[63] Cholecystitis may occur.

In the majority of patients with liver involvement this is totally asymptomatic and the incidental finding of splenomegaly is usually the first indication of liver disease. When tests of liver function are carried out prospectively in patients with cystic fibrosis, up to 40 per cent have abnormalities in childhood.[50] Such is the variability of cystic fibrosis that in some patients the diagnosis of cystic fibrosis is made only when alimentary bleeding complicates cirrhosis.

Management of Hepatobiliary Lesions

If cholestasis in infancy is prolonged, lavage of the biliary tree may relieve it. If cholecystitis complicates the abnormalities of the gallbladder and gallstone formation, cholecystectomy should be performed.

Cirrhosis complicating cystic fibrosis appears to progress rather slowly. The main danger is therefore that of alimentary bleeding due to portal hypertension. As in other forms of cirrhosis the place of portal decompression in the management of bleeding varices is unresolved. Schuster and co-workers[54] have reported their experience of surgery in the management of 35 of 43 patients with portal hypertension complicating cystic fibrosis. In eight, pulmonary disease was considered too advanced to merit surgery, nine patients died within six months of surgery, and 11 died nine months to $11\frac{1}{2}$ years following surgery. The remaining patients are well one month to 15 years following surgery. The authors conclude that, in patients with portal hypertension and good pulmonary status, prophylactic shunting should be undertaken before pulmonary disease is too severe. Intensive medical therapy, physiotherapy and adequate psychological preparation, plus careful postoperative follow-up, are essential. Hypersplenism is not reversed by successful portasystemic shunting. Splenectomy is required.

Other complications of cirrhosis occur relatively infrequently. Hypoprothrombinaemia may be reversed by large doses of vitamin K given by mouth.

INDIAN CHILDHOOD CIRRHOSIS

Indian childhood cirrhosis is the end product of an idiopathic form of liver disease with unique histological, clinical and biochemical features. It is a significant cause of mortality in the preschool child in India and is considered to be the fourth most common cause of death in large paediatric centres in that country. It is limited to India, Pakistan, Sri Lanka, Burma and Malaysia. It is rare in ex-patriates in the United Kingdom.

Pathologically, the disorder is characterized by the accumulation of hyaline within the hepatocytes, marked fibrous tissue deposition extending throughout the hepatic parenchyma and a distinct lack of regeneration nodules. Early in the disease hepatocellular necrosis occurs with focal inflammatory cell infiltrate. There is little infiltration or inflammation of the portal tract. The final picture is that of a 'micro micronodular' cirrhosis[44] with excess copper.[67]

Two clinical forms are recognized. In the majority of cases the disease progresses through three stages. The first is characterized by irritability, anorexia, low-grade fever and abdominal distension with hepatomegaly. This may start at any time between two weeks and 10 years of age, with the maximum incidence at one to three years. Over the course of one to eight months, cirrhosis becomes established with a hard, large liver, splenomegaly and evidence of portal hypertension. Persistent jaundice develops. In the final stage there is a small liver, repeated gastrointestinal bleeding, pulmonary infection and hepatic encephalopathy. In approximately a quarter of cases the whole course is that of a hepatitis terminating in death three to four months after the onset.[53]

Standard tests of liver function show changes compatible with hepatocellular necrosis. Serum immunoglobulins are elevated and smooth muscle antibodies are present in up to 45 per cent of cases. Serum complement component beta-1-c is often low. Cell mediated immunity is depressed and there may be a higher incidence of hepatitis B surface antigen in the serum than in control populations for the same area.[16]

No community or class is exempt from this disorder. It is not associated with malnutrition. A positive family history is found in 30 per cent of cases. Several successive siblings may be affected, or unaffected siblings may intervene. No specific treatment exists. The complications of hepatitis and cirrhosis may require symptomatic treatment.

POLYCYSTIC DISEASE OF THE LIVER AND KIDNEY

Two main forms are recognized. The 'adult' variety is inherited in an autosomal dominant fashion, usually with a high degree of penetrance. The predominant features are renal enlargement and renal failure. The condition may present in infancy or as an incidental finding at autopsy in the elderly. Hepatic involvement is rare, but occasionally hepatomegaly and portal hypertension have been reported.

Infantile Polycystic Disease of the Kidneys and Liver

This disorder is inherited in an autosomal recessive fashion. The most severely affected patients present in the perinatal period with massively enlarged kidneys sometimes causing dystocia, and rapidly die from renal failure. Such cases have minimal hepatic involvement, as do those who present in the neonatal period with progressive renal failure usually leading to death by 12 months of age. Less severely affected infants are noted to have large kidneys at birth, but only at the age of three to six months are features of renal failure first apparent. This tends to be slowly progressive throughout childhood. Such patients show a moderate degree of hepatic fibrosis and ultimately develop portal hypertension. The least severely affected patients have little clinical evidence of renal involvement and present with hepatomegaly, or features of portal hypertension, usually between the age of three months and five years.

Diagnosis may be suspected on the basis of the clinical findings of hepatomegaly and palpably enlarged kidneys. Laboratory investigations show features of renal impairment with normal liver function tests, other than the alkaline phosphatase which may be elevated. The nephrogram may be diagnostic. In the adult form it shows large kidneys with wide separation of the calices. In the infantile form it shows enlargement of the kidneys with typically alternating radio-dense and radio-translucent streaks in the renal cortex and medulla. The nephrogram picture may persist for hours or days. Sometimes the calices are seen to be blunted, shortened or indistinct. Rarely, the appearances may be indistinguishable from those of medullary sponge kidney.

Ultrasonic scanning may demonstrate cysts in the kidney but those in the liver are usually too small to be demonstrated. The diagnosis is confirmed by liver biopsy which shows that the portal tracts contain a vast increase in fibrous tissue with abundance of dilated channels lined by biliary epithelium. The hepatic parenchyma is normal.

The treatment is that of renal failure. If alimentary bleeding complicates portal hypertension, portacaval anastomosis is often well tolerated by those patients.[4,8]

Congenital Hepatic Fibrosis

In congenital hepatic fibrosis bands of fibrous tissue containing linear or circular spaces lined by bile duct epithelial cells join all portal tracts. There is no increase in cellular infiltration. Hepatocellular function is almost always normal. It rarely occurs as a single entity but is frequently associated with abnormalities in the kidneys or pancreas.[43]

The main clinical features are abdominal distension, hepatomegaly and those due to portal hypertension. Abdominal pain may be prominent in some cases. Cholangitis is occasionally a cause. Presentation is usually at one or two years of age but the disorder may present with alimentary bleeding as late as 60 years.

Liver function tests are normal in most cases, but the serum alkaline phosphatase may be elevated. The diagnosis is confirmed by percutaneous liver biopsy using a Trucut needle.

The main problem in clinical management is alimentary bleeding secondary to portal hypertension. Hepatic encephalopathy rarely complicates the bleeding. Early portacaval anastomosis has been advised since these patients tolerate such surgery more satisfactorily than do patients with cirrhosis.[57] Many patients will remain free from alimentary bleeding if they avoid aspirin, however. Liver function tests are frequently more abnormal after shunting than before. Long-term follow-up of 18 patients with portacaval anastomosis has recently been reported. It would seem reasonable to reserve surgery for those patients who have marked alimentary bleeding without aspirin administration and where other causes of alimentary bleeding have been excluded by endoscopy.

GLYCOGEN STORAGE DISEASES

Glycogen storage diseases are inherited metabolic disorders in which the concentration or molecular structure of glycogen in tissues is abnormal. In the majority, there is excessive glycogen storage and defective breakdown. Liver, heart, skeletal muscle, kidney, bone and brain may be affected. The clinical features depend not only on which organs are involved, but also on the action of the particular enzyme which is deficient in each of the 10 different types of glycogen storage disease.[38] In most series, a proportion of cases have the clinical features of a particular form of glycogen storage disease but have no demonstrable enzymatic deficiency.[33,58] A wide spectrum of clinical severity may occur in each category.

Clinical Features

The majority of cases present in infancy with hypoglycaemia which may be complicated by convulsions and mental retardation, particularly in types I, III and VI. Acidosis, vomiting and diarrhoea occur frequently.

Hepatomegaly due to glycogen and fat deposition occurs as an early feature in all types. The liver may extend to the right iliac crest. It is typically soft. Splenomegaly is unusual, except in type IV glycogen storage disease in which an abnormal glycogen is stored and cirrhosis develops by one year of age. Cirrhosis may occur as a later complication in type III glycogen storage disease. Serum aspartate transaminase levels are elevated in types VI, IX and X, in which increased hepatic fibrosis also occurs.

Malabsorption and diarrhoea may be troublesome complications. Short stature and adiposity are usual. Xanthoma and gouty tophi develop in late childhood or early adult life.

Biochemical features

Hypoglycaemia on fasting is an almost constant feature. Intravenous glucagon in a dose of 0.7 mg/m^2 produces a rise of blood glucose of less than 1.94 mmol/l (35 mg/dl). Hyperlipidaemia and acidosis are frequent features. Hyperuricacidaemia also occurs commonly.

Diagnosis

The diagnosis is suspected on the basis of the clinical features, hypoglycaemia on fasting and a diminished rise of blood sugar following intravenous glucagon. Precise classification is dependent on demonstrating the enzyme deficiency (Table 40.4) in leucocyte, liver or muscle biopsy.

Table 40.4. *Enzymatic Classification of Glycogen Storage Diseases.*

Type	Enzymatic activity absent	Affected tissue	Tissue required for diagnosis
I	Glucose-6-phosphatase	Liver, kidney, intestine	Liver
II	Lysosomal α-1,4 and α-1,6 glucosidase	All tissues	Leucocytes, liver or muscle
III	Amylo-1-6 glucosidase (± phosphorylase kinase deficiency)	Liver, muscle, heart, in various combinations	Leucocytes, liver or muscle
IV	Amylo-1-4 → 1-6 transferase	Generalized (abnormal glycogen)	Leucocytes, liver
V	Phosphorylase	Muscle only	Muscle
VI	Liver phosphorylase *deficiency* (not complete absence)	Liver	Leucocytes, liver
VII	Phosphofructokinase	Muscle and erythrocytes	Erythrocytes and muscle
VIII	? Inactive liver phosphorylase (normal activating system)	Liver, brain	Liver
IX	Liver phosphorylase kinase	Liver	Erythrocytes, leucocytes, liver
X	Cyclic 3′,5′-AMP-dependent kinase	Liver, muscle	Liver, muscle

Table 40.5. *Lipid Storage Disorders.*

Disorder	Enzyme deficient	Principal clinical features
Tay–Sachs' disease	Ganglioside GM_2 hexosaminidase (hexosaminidase A)	Dementia, tetraplegia, cherry-red spot in macula
GM_1 gangliosidosis (type I)	β-galactosidases	Motor and mental retardation
Gaucher's disease	Glucosyl ceramide β-glucosidase	Skin pigmentation, bone and lung involvement, hypersplenism
Niemann–Pick's disease	Sphingomyelinase	Convulsions, blindness, tetraplegia, pulmonary infiltration
Fucosidosis	α-fucosidase	Dementia, spasticity, cardiomyopathy
Wolman's disease	Acid esterase	Vomiting, diarrhoea, developmental delay, calcified adrenals
Cholesterol ester storage disease	Acid esterase	Malabsorption
Familial hyperlipoproteinaemia		
Type I	Lipoprotein lipase	Xanthoma, abdominal pain, lipaemia retinalis
Type IV	Unknown	Xanthoma and premature atherosclerosis
Type V	Unknown	Xanthoma and severe abdominal pain

Treatment

Hypoglycaemia may be prevented by frequent feeding of carbohydrate rich meals. Acidosis is controlled by bicarbonate. Gradual improvement occurs over the first few years of life. Growth retardation is a continuing problem for many patients. Continuous feeding by nasogastric tube may remedy this.[31] In a few patients, growth has been stimulated and the metabolic effects considerably improved by portacaval shunt (see Chapter 45).[59]

LIPID STORAGE DISORDERS

Fatty acids, cholesterol or complex lipids are abnormally stored in the lipid storage disorders. All are inherited in an autosomal recessive fashion with the possible exception of some cases of Gaucher's disease, which can be inherited in an autosomal dominant fashion. The diagnosis may be confirmed by showing a deficiency of the specific enzyme in peripheral blood leucocytes (Table 40.5), with the exception of the familial hyperlipoproteinaemias. Within each abnormality there is considerable heterogeneity. Tay–Sachs' disease, for example, has three variants. It most commonly starts in the first year of life but the onset may be between five and 10 years, or may be after 10 years.

Although hepatomegaly is a constant feature in all of these disorders, the principal clinical features are those due to central nervous system involvement. Gaucher's disease can cause severe derangement of liver architecture, however, and be complicated by portal hypertension. Hypersplenism may be sufficiently severe to merit splenectomy.[28]

In the Niemann–Pick disorders, disruption of liver architecture is frequent, particularly in type D variant and in that associated with progressive neurological deterioration which presents initially as a defect in conjugate upward gaze.[45] No treatment is available for any of these disorders, although in familial lipoproteinaemia efforts may be made to lower the hyperlipaemia by dietary changes or cholestyramine.

Table 40.6. *Mucopolysaccharidosis.*

Disorder	Material stored	Enzyme deficient	Diagnostic investigations
Mucopolysaccharidosis I (Hurler)	Heparin and dermatan sulphates	α-L-iduronidase	Dermatan and heparin sulphate in urine or enzyme deficiency in leucocytes
II (Hunter)	Heparin and dermatan sulphates	Sulpho-iduronate sulphatase	Dermatan and heparin sulphate in urine
III (San Filippo)	Heparin sulphate	Heparin-sulpho-glucosamine sulphatase or *N*-acetyl α-glucosaminidase	Heparin sulphate in urine
IV (Maroteaux–Lamy)	Dermatan sulphate	Arylsulphatase B	Dermatan sulphate in urine
Mannosidosis	Mannose-rich oligosaccharides	Acid α-mannosidase	Deficient enzymatic activity in leucocytes

MUCOPOLYSACCHARIDOSIS

The mucopolysaccharidoses are a group of related disorders in which progressive skeletal changes, mental deterioration, visceral enlargement and corneal clouding are manifest to varying degrees. These arise because abnormal polysaccharides, complex structures containing amino acids, amino sugars, uronic acids, and sulphates, are deposited in the tissues and excreted in the urine. Hepatomegaly, splenomegaly, progressive mental deterioration, corneal clouding and coarse facies are the main features. Symptoms start at the age of six months and usually lead to death by the end of the first decade. These disorders are inherited in an autosomal recessive fashion, except for Hunter's syndrome, which is believed to be inherited in an X-linked fashion. Principal biochemical and diagnostic features are given in Table 40.6. There is no effective treatment.[22]

REFERENCES

1. Aagenaes, O. (1974) Hereditary recurrent cholestasis with lymphoedema – two new families. *Acta Paediatrica Scandinavica,* **63,** 465–471.
2. Alagille, D. (1972) Clinical aspects of neonatal hepatitis. *American Journal of Diseases of Children,* **123,** 287–291.
3. Alagille, D., Odievre, M., Gautier, M. & Domergues, J.P. (1975) Hepatic ductular hypoplasia associated with characteristic facies, vertebral malformations, retarded physical, mental and skeletal development and cardiac murmur. *Journal of Pediatrics,* **86,** 63–71.
4. Annand, S.K., Chan, J.C. & Lieberman, E. (1975) Polycystic disease and hepatic fibrosis in children. *American Journal of Diseases of Children,* **129,** 810–825.
5. Arias, I.M. (1976) Extracellular and intracellular transport of bilirubin. In *Liver Diseases in Infancy and Childhood* (Ed.) Berenberg, S.R. pp. 1–17. The Hague: Martinus Nijhoff, Medical Division.
6. Arias, I.M., Gartner, L.M., Seifter, S. & Furman, M. (1964) Prolonged neonatal unconjugated hyperbilirubinaemia associated with breast feeding, and a steroid. Pregnane-3(alpha), 20(beta)-diol, in maternal milk that inhibits glucuronide formation in vitro. *Journal of Clinical Investigation,* **43,** 2037–2047.
7. Bernstein, J., Chang, C.-H., Brough, A.J. & Heidelberger, K.P. (1977) Conjugated hyperbilirubinaemia in infancy associated with parenteral alimentation. *Journal of Pediatrics,* **90,** 361–367.
8. Blyth, H. & Ockenden, B.G. (1971) Polycystic disease of the kidneys and liver presenting in childhood. *Journal of Medical Genetics,* **8,** 257–279.
9. Bobbo, R.C., Schubert, W.K., Partin, J.C. & Partin, J.S. (1975) Reye's syndrome: treatment by exchange transfusion with special reference to the 1974 epidemic in Cincinnati, Ohio. *Journal of Pediatrics,* **87,** 881–889.
10. Bodian, D.M. (1953) *Fibrocystic Disease of the Pancreas.* p. 104. London and New York: Grune & Stratton.
11. Bove, K.E., McAdams, K.J., Partin, J.C., Partin, J.S., Hug, G. & Schubert, W.K. (1975) The hepatic lesion in Reye's syndrome. *Gastroenterology,* **69,** 685–697.
12. Brough, A.J. & Bernstein, J. (1974) Conjugated hyperbilirubinaemia in early infancy: a re-assessment of liver biopsy. *Human Pathology,* **5,** 507–516.
13. Brown, T., Hug, G., Jansky, L., Bove, K., Scheve, A., Ryana, M., Brown, H., Schubert, W.K., Partin, J.C. & Lloyd-Still, J. (1976) Transiently reduced activity of carbamyl phosphate synthetase and ornithine transcarbamylase in liver of children with Reye's syndrome. *New England Journal of Medicine,* **294,** 861–866.
14. Campbell, D.P., Poley, J.R., Alavpavic, P. & Smith, E.I. (1974) The differential diagnosis of neonatal hepatitis and biliary atresia. *Journal of Pediatric Surgery,* **9,** 699–708.
15. Chandra, R.K. (1974) Indian childhood cirrhosis – clinical, biochemical, geneological, histomorphological and immunological observations. *Medica Chirurgica Digest,* **3,** 63–68.
16. Chandra, R.K. (1975) Lymphocyte response to hepatitis B surface antigen. Findings in hepatitis and Indian childhood cirrhosis. *Archives of Diseases in Childhood,* **50,** 559–561.
17. Chiba, S., Hori, S., Kawamura, N. & Nakao, T. (1975) Primary cytomegalovirus infection and liver involvement in early infancy. *Tohoku Journal of Experimental Medicine,* **117,** 143–147.
18. Corey, L., Rubin, R.J. & Hattwick, M.A.W. (1977) Reye's syndrome: clinical progression and evaluation of therapy. *Pediatrics,* **60,** 708–714.
19. Corey, L., Rubin, R.J., Hattwick, M.A.W., Noble, G.R. & Cassidy, E. (1976) A nationwide outbreak of Reye's syndrome. Its epidemiological relationship to influenza B. *American Journal of Medicine,* **61,** 615–625.
20. Corey, L., Rubin, R.J., Thompson, T.R., Noble, G.R., Cassidy, E., Hattwick, M.A.W., Gregg, M.B. & Eddins, D. (1977) Influenza B-associated Reye's syndrome: incidence in Michigan and potential for prevention. *Journal of Infectious Diseases,* **135,** 398–407.
21. Danks, D.M., Campbell, P.E., Jack, I., Rogers, J. & Smith, A.L. (1977) Studies of the aetiology of neonatal hepatitis and biliary atresia. *Archives of Diseases in Childhood,* **52,** 360–367.
22. Dekaban, A.S., Holden, K.R. & Constantopoulos, G. (1972) The effect of plasma or whole blood transfusion on patients with various types of mucopolysaccharidoses. *Pediatrics,* **50,** 688–692.
23. di Sant Agnese, P.A. & Blanc, W.A. (1956) A distinctive type of biliary cirrhosis of the liver. *Pediatrics,* **18,** 387–409.
24. Di Tori, R., Luapi, L. & Ansenelli, V. (1968) Glucuronation of the liver of premature babies. *Nature,* **212,** 265–269.
25. Dommergues, J.P. (1973) Hépatites infectieuses non virales du nourrisson. *La Revue du Praticien,* **23,** 4941–4954.
26. Dupuy, J.M., Frommel, D. & Alagille, D. (1975) Viral hepatitis type B in infancy. *Lancet,* **i,** 191–193.
27. Feigelson, J., Pecau, Y., Cathelineau, L. & Navarro, J. (1975) Additional data on hepatic function tests in cystic fibrosis. *Acta Paediatrica Scandinavica,* **64,** 337–344.

28. Fredrickson, D.S. & Sloan, S.R. (1972) Lipid storage disorders. In *The Metabolic Basis of Inherited Disease* (Ed.) Stanbury, J.B., Wyngaarden, J.P. & Fredrickson, D.S. 3rd ed., pp. 783–795. New York: McGraw-Hill.

29. Gartner, L.M., Lee, T.-S., Vaisman, S., Lane, D. & Zarafu, I. (1977) Development of bilirubin transport and metabolism in the newborn rhesus monkey. *Journal of Pediatrics*, **90**, 513–527.

30. Geraty, R.J. & Schweitzer, I.L. (1977) Viral hepatitis B during pregnancy, the newborn period and infancy. *Journal of Pediatrics*, **90**, 368–374.

31. Greene, H.L., Slonim, A.E., O'Neil, J.A. & Barr, R.M. (1976) Continuous nocturnal naso-gastric feeding for management of type I glycogen storage disease. *New England Journal of Medicine*, **294**, 423–427.

32. Greenwood, R.D., Rosenthal, A., Crocker, A.D. & Nadas, A.S. (1976) Syndrome of intrahepatic biliary dysgenesis and cardiovascular malformations. *Pediatrics*, **58**, 243–254.

33. Hug, G. (1976) Glycogen storage disease. In *Birth Defects, Original Article series*, **12**(6), 145–175.

34. Johnston, D.I., Mowat, A.P., Orr, H. & Kohn, J. (1976) Serum alphafetoprotein levels in extrahepatic biliary atresia, idiopathic neonatal hepatitis and alpha-1 antitrypsin deficiency (PiZ). *Acta Paediatrica Scandinavica*, **65**, 623–629.

35. Linarelli, L.G., Williams, C.N. & Phillips, M.J. (1972) Byler's disease: fatal intrahepatic cholestasis. *Journal of Pediatrics*, **81**, 484–492.

36. Luders, D. (1974) Hypoplasia of intrahepatic bile ducts and other forms of intrahepatic cholestasis in infancy. *Monatsschrift für Kinderheilkunde*, **122**, 207–216.

37. Maisels, M.J. (1972) Bilirubin: on understanding and influencing its metabolism in the newborn infant. *Pediatric Clinics of North America*, **19**, 447–501.

38. McAdams, A.J., Hug, G. & Bove, K.E. (1974) Glycogen storage disease, types I–X. Criteria for morphologic diagnosis. *Human Pathology*, **5**, 463–486.

39. Monk, E.M., Mitchell, A.J.H., Milligan, D.W.A. & Holten, J.B. (1977) Diagnosis of classical galactosaemia. *Archives of Diseases in Childhood*, **52**, 943–946.

40. Mowat, A.P. (1977) Persistent neonatal jaundice. In *Essentials of Paediatric Gastroenterology* (Ed.) Harries, J.T. pp. 266–285. Edinburgh, New York and London: Churchill Livingstone.

41. Mowat, A.P., Psacharopoulos, H.T. & Williams, R. (1976) Extrahepatic biliary atresia versus neonatal hepatitis. Review of 137 prospectively investigated infants. *Archives of Diseases in Childhood*, **51**, 763–770.

42. Mowat, A.P., Psacharopoulos, H.T., Williams, R., Portman, B. & Tait, R.A.J. (1977) Prognosis in childhood of liver disease associated with alpha-1-antitrypsin deficiency, type PiZ. *Gut*, **18**, A978.

43. Murray-Lyon, I.M., Ockenden, B.G. & Williams, R. (1973) Congenital hepatic fibrosis – is it a single clinical entity? *Gastroenterology*, **64**, 653–656.

44. Nayak, L.C. & Ramalingaswami, V. (1975) Indian childhood cirrhosis. *Clinics in Gastroenterology*, **4**, 333–349.

45. Neville, B.G.R., Lake D.D., Stephens, R. & Sanders, M.V. (1973) Neuro-visceral storage disorder with vertical supranuclear ophthalmoplegia and its relationship to Neimann–Pick Disease. *Brain*, **96**, 97–120.

46. Odièvre, M. (1976) Breast feeding and neonatal hyperbilirubinaemia. In *Liver Diseases in Infancy and Childhood* (Ed.) Berenberg, S.R. pp. 34–40. The Hague: Martinus Nijhoff, Medical Division.

47. Odièvre, M., Gautier, M., Hadchouel, L. & Alagille, D. (1973) Severe familial intrahepatic cholestasis. *Archives of Diseases in Childhood*, **48**, 806–812.

48. Poland, R.A. & Odell, J.B. (1971) Physiologic jaundice: intrahepatic circulation of bilirubin. *New England Journal of Medicine*, **284**, 1–4.

49. Psacharopoulos, H.T. & Mowat, A.P. (1978) Epidemiological study of hepatitis in infancy, aetiology and prognosis. *Proceedings of an International Workshop on neonatal hepatitis and biliary atresia*. Washington, D.C., 1977. In press.

50. Psacharopoulos, H.T. & Mowat, A.P. (1978) Unpublished observations.

51. Psacharopoulos, H.T., Mowat, A.P. & Williams, R. (1977) *Gut*, **18**, A977.

52. Reye, R.D.K., Morgan, G. & Baral, J. (1963) Encephalopathy and fatty degeneration of the viscera. *Lancet*, **ii**, 749–752.

53. Scharma, U., Saxena, S., Mahta, J.A.B. & Scharma, M.L. (1975) Indian childhood cirrhosis, a clinical-pathological study of 50 cases. *Archives of Child Health (Calcutta)*, **17**, 56–64.

54. Schuster, S.R., Schwachman, H., Toyama, W.M., Rubino, A. & Taik-khaw, K. (1977) The management of portal hypertension in cystic fibrosis. *Journal of Paediatric Surgery*, **12**, 201–206.

55. Scriver, C.R. & Rosenberg, L.E. (1973) Tyrosine in amino acid metabolism and its disorders, Ch. 6, pp. 338–362, Vol. 10, *Major Problems in Clinical Paediatrics*. Philadelphia: W.B. Saunders.

56. Shaywitz, B.A., Leventhal, J.M., Kramer, M.S. & Vañes, J.A.L. (1977) Long continuous monitoring of intracranial pressure in severe Reye's syndrome. *Pediatrics*, **59**, 595–599.

57. Sokhi, J.S., Morice, G.J.E., McGee, J. & Blumgart, L.M. (1975) Congenital hepatic fibrosis: aspects of diagnosis and surgical management. *British Journal of Surgery*, **62**, 621–623.

58. Spencer-Peat, J., Norman, M.E., Lake, B.D., McNamara, J. & Patrick, A.D. (1971) Hepatic glycogen storage disease: clinical and laboratory findings in 23 cases. *Quarterly Journal of Medicine*, **40**, 95–114.

59. Starzl, T.E., Putnam, C.W., Porter, K.A., Halgrimson, C.G., Corman, J., Brown, B.I., Gotlin, R.W., Rodgerson, D.O. & Greene, H.L. (1973) Portal diversion for the treatment of glycogen storage disease in humans. *Annals of Surgery*, **178**, 525–538.

60. Talbot, I.C. & Mowat, A.P. (1975) Liver disease in infancy: histological features and relationship to α_1-antitrypsin phenotype. *Journal of Clinical Pathology*, **28**, 559–563.

61. Taylor, A. (1968) Autosomal trisomy hepatitis syndromes. *Journal of Medical Genetics*, **5**, 2227–2235.

62. Walker, W. (1971) Haemolytic disease of the newborn. In *Recent Advances in Paediatrics* (Ed.) Bairdner, D. & Hull, D. 4th ed., pp. 119–170. London: J.A. Churchill.

63. Warwick, W.J., L'Heureux, P.R., Sharp, H.L. & Isenberg, T.L. (1976) Gallstones and cystic fibrosis. *Proceedings of the Seventh International Cystic Fibrosis Congress*, p. 100. Paris, 1976.

64. Watson, G.H. & Miller, V. (1973) Arterio-hepatic dysplasia. *Archives of Diseases in Childhood*, **48**, 459–466.

65. Yu, J.S., Walker-Smith, J.A. & Borhard, E.N.A. (1971) Neonatal hepatitis and premature infant simulating hereditary tyrosinosis. *Archives of Diseases in Childhood,* **46,** 306–309.
66. Kerr, D.N.S., Okonkwo, S. & Choa, R.G. (1978) Congenital hepatic fibrosis: the long-term prognosis. *Gut,* **19,** 514–520.
67. Tanner, M.S., Portmann, B., Mowat, A.P., Williams, R., Pandit, A.M., Mills, C.F. & Bremner, I. (1979) Increased hepatic copper concentration in Indian childhood cirrhosis. *Lancet,* **i,** 1203–1205.

Chapter 41

Paediatric Liver Disease: Surgical Aspects

H. HOMEWOOD NIXON

GALLBLADDER AND BILIARY TREE

Obstructive Jaundice in Infancy

The important practical problems in this condition are the differentiation of 'neonatal hepatitis' from biliary atresia and the determination of whether there is an anatomical obstruction sufficiently complete to justify an attempt at surgical relief.

The typical histological features of neonatal hepatitis are areas of parenchymatous necrosis with disruption of the sinusoidal reticulin architecture of the lobule, a tendency to form giant multinucleate hepatocytes and an inflammatory reaction. There is a multifactorial aetiology (see Chapter 28): some cases are associated with Australia (hepatitis) antigen, some with an alpha-1-antitrypsin deficiency and other familial types also occur. Cytomegalovirus, toxoplasmosis, rubella, herpes simplex and syphilis have to be considered and a similar clinical picture of obstructive jaundice can result from such varied conditions as galactosaemia, pyruvic kinase deficiency, hypothyroidism or urinary tract infection. It is necessary to exclude such 'medical' causes before considering the diagnosis to rest between idiopathic neonatal hepatitis and potentially operable conditions, of which the commonest is extrahepatic biliary atresia. However, viruses have been isolated from cases of atresia as well as hepatitis, so the presence of a virus does not in itself distinguish the two conditions.[11, 12]

In biliary atresia the main histological features in the liver are cholestasis, perilobular fibrosis, inflammatory cells and proliferating new bile ductules. At least 20 per cent of cases will show the same kind of hepatocyte giant cells as are seen in hepatitis and these are no longer considered to be specific for the one or the other condition. In only 10 per cent of cases of biliary atresia is the atresia restricted to the distal part of the biliary tract, so that orthodox anastomosis to the alimentary tract is seldom practicable. In the great majority, the extrahepatic atresia extends back to involve intrahepatic bile ducts but it may be patchy in distribution. Histologically the extrahepatic bile ducts may show evidence of previous inflammation and occasionally the duct may show features of acute inflammation, being swollen with the lumen blocked by recent inflammatory tissue. The picture is one of reaction in ducts which have already formed, and not of primary agenesis or hypoplasia. In a few cases the common bile duct may be so dilated as to be called a choledochal cyst. The writer prefers to call this group 'cystic dilatation of the common bile duct', because the presentation and symptomatology are so different from choledochal cysts seen in later infancy or childhood as to suggest that there may be aetiological differences. These cases present in the neonatal period with the typical picture of complete obstruction, just like other cases of biliary atresia from which they cannot be differentiated clinically since the cystic mass is usually not large enough to be palpable.

It might be expected that biliary atresia would

present with a progressive rise in the level of bilirubin in contrast with a fluctuating level in neonatal hepatitis, but in fact this is not found. Serial observations are therefore valueless in individual cases. Furthermore, bile may pass into the stools of a baby who later proves to have complete atresia, suggesting that obstruction has developed post-natally. Other liver function tests have also been used in an attempt to differentiate the two conditions. Turbidity tests, transaminase levels, lipoprotein-X, alpha-fetoprotein, bile acid patterns and their response to cholestyramine and the response of the bilirubin level to a course of corticosteroids have been shown to give an accuracy of around 80 per cent.[52,53,58,74] No single test has proved entirely reliable.

Landing suggests the existence of a condition which he calls infantile sclerosing cholangitis.[39,68] This is a spectrum of disease ranging from neonatal hepatitis in the form that principally affects the parenchyma to either frank atresia or else a choledochal cyst in the form which principally attacks the ducts. This would explain overlapping test results and the fact that ducts may be present in a biopsy on one occasion but absent on another. Landing suggests that a virus may be the aetiological agent. Jenner and Howard,[31] however, have suggested that an enzyme deficiency may be present in the liver, allowing accumulation of toxic monohydroxy bile acids. On epidemiological grounds Danks[12] believes that the aetiological agents for hepatitis and atresia are likely to be distinct.

Occasionally a complete set of extremely fine ducts is found. This condition has been called hypoplasia of the bile ducts.[43] Clinically such cases may relent but, after remission, later cirrhotic changes sometimes supervene. This condition may well represent another part of Landing's spectrum of disease, but the appearance of hypoplasia may also be simply due to collapse of under-used ducts in the presence of cholestasis.

There is also a condition known as intrahepatic biliary atresia in which investigation reveals completely normal extrahepatic ducts but the smaller (interlobular) intrahepatic ducts appear to be absent. The usual classification of biliary atresia into extrahepatic and intrahepatic is imprecise because extrahepatic atresia usually also involves the larger intrahepatic ducts. Intrahepatic atresia, on the other hand, involves only the smallest interlobular bile ducts.

Some cases of intrahepatic atresia diagnosed by biopsy have later recovered completely. It has been suggested that the condition is one in which the ducts collapse because parenchymal changes limit the secretion of bile so that the collapsed ducts are not visible. However, the presence of a familial incidence, and of a syndrome associating such intrahepatic atresia with cardiac lesions, commonly pulmonary atresia, suggests that this is in fact a distinct entity.[25]

Wood and Blalock[72] reported an association of situs inversus with extrahepatic biliary atresia and in reviewing cases from his hospital the author has observed this association on four occasions. However, in general, cases of extrahepatic atresia, as observed by Danks,[12] are remarkably free from other anomalies, whereas cases of neonatal hepatitis have a high proportion of apparently unassociated but perhaps predisposing conditions.

Management

There is no single test which will differentiate hepatitis from atresia, yet it is important that there should be no undue delay in the diagnosis of cases where surgical relief can be effective. Such delay will result in progressive and irreversible cirrhosis.[36,51] In a series of atresias from Great Ormond Street Hospital, London, severe cirrhosis was much more frequent in cases over three months of age (Tables 41.1 and 41.2). This coincides with Kasai's more recent observation that his technique of porto-enterostomy has been of little value unless performed before that age.[34] The warning of Gellis against early investigation lest unnecessary damage be inflicted on a potentially recoverable hepatitis no longer applies; his opinion was reached before the heterogeneity of neonatal hepatitis, including the more severe familial types, was recognized. With the

Table 41.1. *Obstructive Jaundice.*

Estimated severity of cirrhosis			
Age at operation	No. of cases	Cirrhosis	
Under 3 months	27	Mild or absent	9
		Moderate or severe	18
Over 3 months	18	Moderate or severe	18
Total	45		

Data from The Hospital for Sick Children, Great Ormond Street, London, 1958–1963.

Table 41.2. *Forty-five Cases of Obstructive Jaundice in Infancy.*

Diagnostic open biopsy and cholangiogram	
Extrahepatic biliary atresia	30
Neonatal hepatitis	9
Cystic dilatation of bile ducts	5
Intrahepatic atresia	1
Total	45
(No mortality or important complications)	

Data from The Hospital for Sick Children, Great Ormond Street, London, 1958–1963.

methods of investigation now available laparotomy may usually be avoided in the absence of atresia.[22]

Any infant whose conjugated hyperbilirubinaemia persists for more than two weeks should be considered not to have physiological jaundice. The writer's present practice is to exclude the more common specific causes of 'neonatal hepatitis' and then to perform a needle biopsy under brief general anaesthesia using a Trucut needle and to use radioactive rose bengal excretion and imaging. 1 μCi/kg (3.7×10^4 Bq/kg) of ^{131}I rose bengal is injected and then the faeces are collected, with care taken that they are uncontaminated by urine. If less than 10 per cent of the activity appears in the stool complete anatomical obstruction may be assumed. If more than 20 per cent is excreted patent ducts may be assumed. In the intermediate range repetition of the test after a two-week trial of cholestyramine may clarify the diagnosis.[46, 58]

Imaging, particularly using new hepatobiliary agents such as hydroxyindole diacetic acid (HIDA) may also be helpful (see Chapter 26). Apart from the demonstration of dye entering the small intestine, perhaps the most valuable finding is the golf-ball-like shadow which may be seen below the liver in the rare cystic dilatation of the common bile duct. This condition is readily amenable to surgery. If imaging suggests patency of the ducts and supports the biopsy findings, surgery is contraindicated. If both imaging and biopsy suggest atresia, exploration should be performed. There is a group of cases in which, even with the aid of expert pathology, doubt remains. In these cases it is still advisable to operate.[70] A small transverse upper abdominal incision is made just above the liver margin and an operative cholangiogram performed. A large wedge biopsy can be taken for histology at the same time. Biopsy from both lobes of the liver should be performed since the findings in the two lobes may differ, possibly because of the differential streaming of the portal blood between the two lobes.[23] Should exploration reveal a frankly atretic gallbladder exploration should be continued. If the gallbladder has a lumen a cholangiogram is undertaken. If doubt remains a decision to carry out full exploration should await the biopsy report. This policy is preferable to relying on frozen section as this is frequently difficult to assess.

In performing operative cholangiography it is helpful to mobilize the fundus of the gallbladder which is sometimes buried in the enlarged liver and to place three stay sutures near its apex. The tip is then cut off to demonstrate whether a lumen is present or not. If present, a fine rubber catheter is inserted and tied in place with a thread ligature. A rubber catheter is preferable to a plastic catheter because it is less likely to slip out or leak during the injection of the dye. If the gallbladder is very small, however, it may be necessary to use a fine plastic tube. Although this may seem to be an elaborate way of injecting the dye into the gallbladder, attempts to introduce it by needle may be difficult unless its lumen is quite large. If a poor picture results it may be doubtful whether, for example, the needle is placed correctly in the wall of the gallbladder. Once the catheter is introduced, the biliary system is flushed with saline. Forty per cent Hypaque is then injected from a 10 ml syringe and the radiograph is taken during injection. The dye will pass into the duodenum and proximally into the liver if the whole duct is patent. If dye enters the duodenum but does not extend towards the liver, this usually means that the proximal (i.e. hepatic) ducts are atretic. This condition may also be suspected if the gallbladder is found to contain colourless mucoid bile.

In extrahepatic atresia the most common finding is atresia of all the ducts with perhaps a narrow lumen in the gallbladder itself. The next most common finding is a patent gallbladder, cystic duct and common bile duct but atretic common hepatic, right and left hepatic ducts (Figure 41.1). Unfortunately, obstruction limited to the lower end of the duct and cystic dilatation of the duct are less common (Figure 41.2). In a series of 40 cases there were only four cases of the latter type in which anastomosis to the alimentary tract was practicable.[54] Furthermore, although two of these four were technically operable, a long delay in establishing the diagnosis had resulted in severe irreversible cirrhosis.

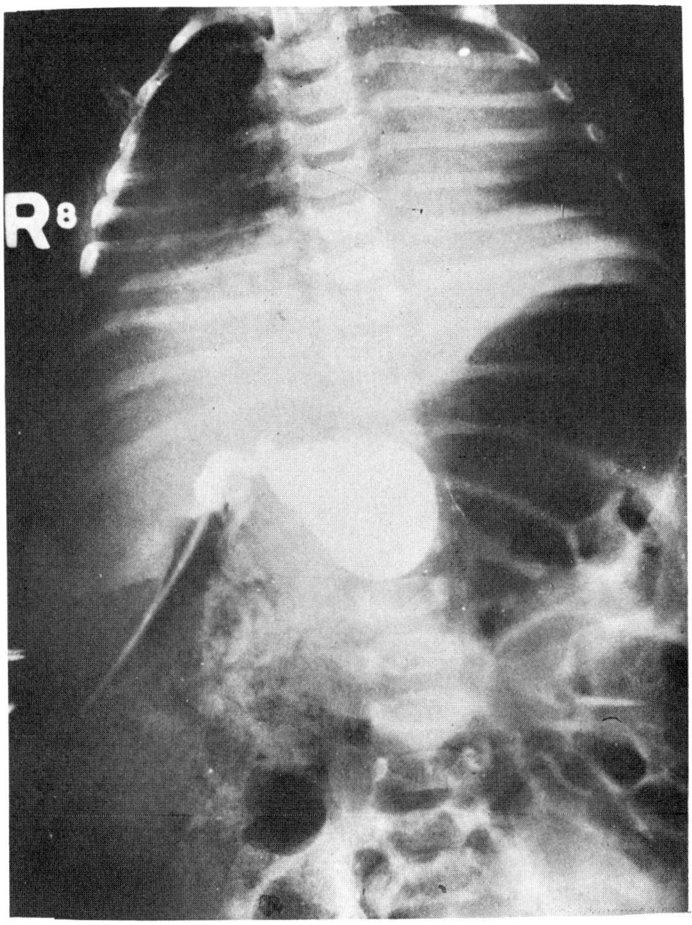

Figure 41.1. Cystic dilatation of bile duct. Presenting as neonatal obstructive jaundice it is clinically indistinguishable from other forms of biliary atresia but eminently operable by orthodox techniques. By courtesy of Butterworths Ltd.

Operative procedures

Patent extrahepatic duct. A Roux-en-Y procedure is the operation of choice. The duct is anastomosed to the jejunum, making the Y arm 15 to 25 cm long, to minimize reflux of intestinal contents and consequent ascending cholangitis. If the duct is cystically dilated, it is preferable to excise it subtotally, to trim it down as far as seems safe in order to reduce the hazard of stasis and infection. An anastomosis 2 cm wide is made to the oblique end of the divided jejunum. The writer's preference is to use chromic catgut to join the duct to the jejunum, with a few 4/0 silk sutures placed as a second row and to support the anastomosis by attaching it if possible to the capsule of the liver. The intestinal anastomosis is performed with an invaginating mattress suture layer of 4/0 or 3/0 silk. The junction of the proximal divided end of the jejunum and the side of the Roux arm is attached to the hole in the mesentery of the transverse colon so that the side arm is retained in the supracolic compartment and the risk of internal herniation is thus minimized. A drain is placed in Morison's pouch and brought out through a separate stab wound in the right flank.

No recognizable patent extrahepatic duct. There has been great interest in the use of various operations described by Japanese surgeons for such cases. The most widely used procedure is Kasai's operation.[33, 34] This is, in essence, a Roux-en-Y portoenterostomy, the end of the Roux arm being anastomosed to the raw surface left in the porta hepatis after dissecting the atretic ducts as far as the liver and then dividing and excising them at this level. The rationale for this procedure is the presence of microscopic ducts in the upper end of the tissue excised from such cases and evidence that good bile flow may be achieved by their drainage. Kasai has reported the best long-term follow-up of cases treated by such portoenterostomies and stresses that benefits have been much less when the procedure is performed over the age of three months.[34]

The gallbladder or its atretic remnant is mobilized as a guide to the site of the atretic

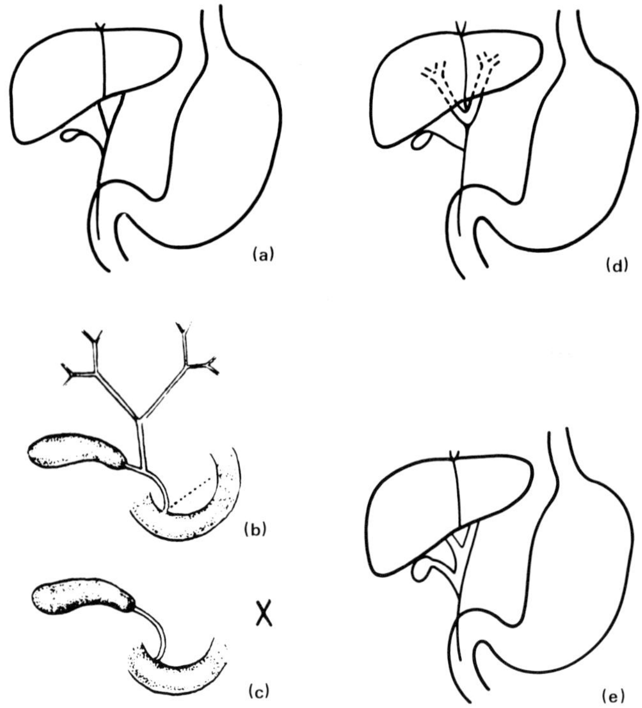

Figure 41.2.(a) Complete extrahepatic atresia; commonest finding. (b) Complete filling of main ducts in neonatal hepatitis (the pancreatic duct usually also fills as shown). (c) No retrograde filling above junction of cystic and common bile duct. Second commonest form of atresia. By courtesy of Butterworth Ltd. (d) and (e) Rarer forms of extrahepatic atresia suitable for orthodox surgery.

common bile duct. Dissection of the tissue from the cystic duct junction into the porta hepatis is then performed. To facilitate this dissection it is often necessary to open up the fissure by dividing the bridge of liver stretching across from the right to the left lobe. Sometimes a partial excision of the quadrate lobe improves exposure when this is particularly prominent and overhangs the porta. The use of diathermy in the porta hepatis itself should be eschewed because it would encourage scarring and sealing of the microscopic ducts on the patency of which this operation relies. The end of the Roux arm may be sutured directly over the raw surface around the porta hepatis. It may be more convenient to close the end of the loop and then to make a separate incision near its end in the antimesenteric border and to suture this over the raw surface of the porta hepatis. The anastomosis is carried out with fine catgut and supported with silk sutures to the undersurface of the liver.

In Kasai's original operation he recommended dissection up to the porta hepatis and division of the tissue at this level. Kimura carried out a similar operation but recommended incising through the capsule of the liver for 1 or 2 mm before making the anastomosis. Lilly[41] has suggested that frozen sections of the transected tissue should be examined and that the incision should be continued into the porta hepatis until patent ductules are found. Although this will not ensure bile drainage because areas of patent duct may be present between areas of atresia,[21] it has the prognostic advantage of identifying cases that would otherwise be blindly anastomosed to non-duct bearing portions of porta hepatis.

In spite of good postoperative bile flow in a reasonable proportion of cases, the development of progressive cirrhosis, portal hypertension and eventual death may yet ensue.[50] (Possible mechanisms for this are discussed in Chapter 14.) Nevertheless, it has been shown that in some cases milder fibrotic changes in the liver may regress.[6, 34] Japanese workers have attributed the late failure of some operations to ascending cholangitis.[37] Various modifications have therefore been performed in the hope of reducing this tendency in the belief that treatment with antibiotics alone had proved insufficient to relieve cholangitis. Sawaguchi and Suruga formed a temporary external biliary fistula. Considerable problems of electrolyte management resulted and these procedures seemed merely to delay the onset of cholangitis until the fistula was closed. Kasai then developed the double-Y hepatic portojejunostomy (Figure 41.3) and has achieved better results with this technique. Of 12 patients

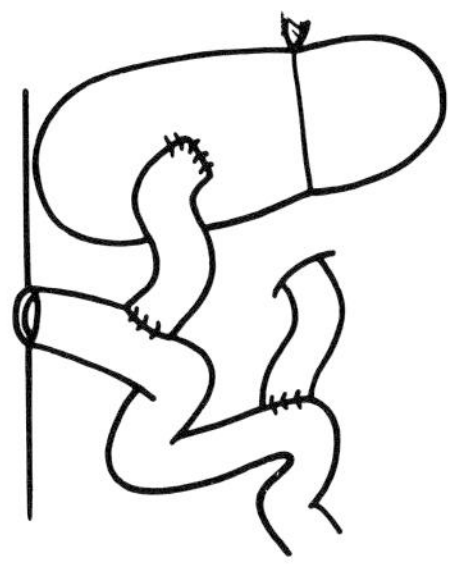

Figure 41.3. Kasai's modified 'double Y' operation intended to reduce the hazard of postoperative cholangitis.

who underwent this modified operation from January 1971 to July 1972, seven showed excellent or fair postoperative bile excretion and in 1974, when their cases were reported, six of them had continued well without jaundice.

Ikeda[30] has used a gastric tube to drain bile from the porta hepatis but experience of this procedure is limited and the long-term results are not known. In neonates who have an atretic common hepatic duct but a patent mucus-containing gallbladder and patent common bile duct, it is tempting to anastomose the porta hepatis to the gallbladder and retain the ampulla of Vater to prevent reflux cholangitis. The common duct in these cases, however, is so narrow that it easily becomes blocked with mucus or blood after the operation. This may jeopardize the end result even if a good immediate flow of bile is obtained, and re-operation may be necessary.

Other methods of treatment

All attempts to produce artificial bile ducts by thrusting metallic or plastic tubes into the liver have failed. Lymphatico-intestinal anastomoses, based on the observation that in bile duct obstruction there is a massive flow of bile in the lymph, have also been unsuccessful. In one of the writer's own cases following anastomosis of the thoracic duct to the oesophagus, the bilirubin level was reduced from 200 to 100 μmol/l (12 to 6 mg/dl) overnight and the ascites disappeared.[54] The loss of fluid, electrolytes and protein, however, was so great that the child became gravely ill and recovered only when the anastomosis clotted a few days later. There do not appear to have been any successes from such techniques.

Children with biliary atresia may have large 'bile lakes' seen in their liver biopsies.[19] It has therefore been suggested that it may be rational to wait or even to carry out a second operation in such cases. However, these lakes drain a limited amount of adjacent parenchyma and no long-term successes have been reported.

The course of the untreated or unsuccessfully treated case

It is surprising how long a child with biliary atresia, with a hard liver and enlarging spleen, may continue to lead an apparently normal life. The abdomen is commonly protuberant because of gaseous distension, which is not readily explained, rather than because of the ascites which develops later. The degree of jaundice may fluctuate considerably, often in association with apparently unrelated incidents such as upper respiratory tract infections. Pruritus may be an early symptom and the response to cholestyramine has been variable. Antihistamines may help but may also cause troublesome drowsiness. Parents will usually notice that the child is tired and easily fatigued before more specific symptoms occur. Frank ascites causing respiratory distress is often late in onset. A low fat diet is beneficial in the presence of this liver failure but absorption of calcium and magnesium is reduced. Parenteral vitamin D may help. Ascites may be improved with a low salt diet, Lasix and spironolactone, reducing the need for paracentesis to relieve the respiratory distress. The presence of frank ascites, however, appears to presage an early onset of fatal liver failure with drowsiness and increasing jaundice. The related portal hypertension sometimes causes haematemesis from oesophageal varices. The resultant hypovolaemia, anaemia and absorption of breakdown products from the blood in the intestine add to the load on the inefficient liver and may produce serious deterioration in the child's general condition. Although in these patients operations such as portasystemic shunts or transection of the varices (e.g. the Milnes–Walker operation) may be performed, in many cases only conservative management with transfusion, antibiotics such as neomycin, and enemas to evacuate the bowel may be considered justified, depending on the quality of life remaining for the child.

Children who have been treated by portoenterostomy will often survive for some time with passage of bile in the stool. However, they usually have either advancing or persisting liver disease. Their fluctuant course sometimes appears to benefit from long-term administration of antibiotics. Such a response supports the view that some late problems of these operations are due to cholangitis. The hope that microscopic ducts will unite with the apposed intestine without formal mucosa-to-mucosa anastomosis and thus give a permanent free channel without a tendency to stricture formation seems to the writer unduly optimistic. This is particularly so when the care needed to avoid producing a stricture following suture of the relatively healthy common bile duct in the adult is considered.

Unfortunately, the group of children with obstructive jaundice in early infancy most likely to benefit from surgery is still that minority with a patent extrahepatic duct suitable for orthodox anastomosis, and presenting when liver changes are minimal. Nevertheless, portoenterostomy, although only partially successful in many hands, seems to be associated with more long-term survivors than has previously been reported. In these tragic cases, where the outcome is often so uncertain or so long delayed, such procedures may lead to further advances in their management.

Rare causes of obstructive jaundice in infancy amenable to operation

Hyperfixation. The author has observed an instance of persistent obstructive jaundice, commencing in the first days of life, which appeared to be caused by extrinsic obstruction of the common bile duct by cholecystocolic and choledochoduodenal bands. Liver biopsy was 'compatible with extrahepatic obstruction'. The bands were divided, the jaundice cleared and the child is well five years later.

Fibromatosis. Amann and Klingenberg[3] described a case of neonatal jaundice resulting from 'localized congenital fibromatosis of the head of the pancreas'. Louhimo[44] described a rather similar finding in a 2½-year-old child but stressed that the fibrous mass was almost entirely extrapancreatic. As in Amann's case the lesion was localized, though a relationship to retroperitoneal fibrosis was considered. The portal vein was slightly involved and reference was made to a case of Eiseman and Yeoh[16] in which portal hypertension was associated with retroperitoneal fibrosis.

Neonatal spontaneous perforation of the common bile duct. A rare cause of non-haemolytic neonatal jaundice is an apparently spontaneous perforation of the common bile duct. The clinical presentation is similar to that of 'hepatitis/atresia' although a palpable collection in the right hypochondrium may arise early in the disease, and the baby may become acutely ill with increasing abdominal distension from biliary peritonitis. Tiny pigment calculi have been found as a possible cause of the perforation in some instances. Simple drainage has proved adequate treatment although cholecyst-enterostomy-en-Y has also been employed.[40,42]

Some of the cystic dilatations of the common bile duct seen in early infancy are similar to those seen later, but in others there may be a complete absence of an epithelial lining. The shaggy lining suggests the formation of a pseudocyst. These dilatations may result from such a localized perforation of the bile duct – certainly it seems very early for the loss of lining to be attributable to pressure atrophy as found in other cysts.[9,32]

Hydrops of the Gallbladder

This condition usually presents in a child with acute abdominal pain and tenderness over the gallbladder which may be palpable. Laparotomy reveals a tensely dilated organ containing sterile bile. Less commonly, hydrops may be a cause of recurrent rather than acute abdominal pain.

Cholecystectomy has been carried out on suspicion of stenosis of the cystic duct but a simple cholecystostomy has also sufficed. An instance of hydrops of the gallbladder has also been reported in a newborn.[63]

Cholecystitis

Acute cholecystitis

Acute cholecystitis is rare in childhood and is usually misdiagnosed as high appendicitis. Ternberg, Jessie and Keating,[71] reviewing 74 instances of acute acalculous cholecystitis, found that the condition commonly occurred as a complication of other illness. Although cholecystectomy has been employed, cholecystostomy has also proved adequate.

Chronic cholecystitis

The clinical syndrome is similar to that seen in the adult and is usually found in older girls. Even in teenagers, pregnancy seems to be a predisposing factor and use of the oestrogen 'pill' may result in an increased incidence.

Chronic cholecystitis with calculi

Calculi may develop in children with cholecystitis, and an increased tendency to cholelithiasis has also been reported in patients with ileal pathology.[57] Attacks of pain and fever are encountered as in the adult but radiation to the shoulder blade and fatty dyspepsia occur less frequently. Jaundice is occasionally present although common duct stones are rarely found. Plain radiography and a cholecystogram should therefore be considered in children with obscure recurrent abdominal pain. In the majority of cases pigment stones are responsible. Preoperative liver function tests, a blood count and fragility curve should be performed. A cholangiogram may be required to reveal radiolucent calculi,[45] and ultrasonography may be diagnostic.

At operation a cholangiogram should be performed. Cholecystectomy is commonly undertaken but O'Donnell and Puri[56] have found cholecystostomy to suffice and have not observed any recurrent stones in their series.

Haemolytic Anaemia

When splenectomy is performed during childhood for hereditary spherocytosis, it is rare to find pigment stones in the gallbladder. This contrasts with adults with this condition in whom splenectomy has been delayed. If present, these calculi may safely be removed at the time of splenectomy and, since the cause of their formation is removed, cholecystectomy is superfluous.

Pancreatitis

Pancreatitis in childhood may be traumatic, familial or 'idiopathic' but in some cases it is related to biliary tract disease. Cholangiography is therefore indicated. A morphine provocative test to elicit the pain has been suggested.[27]

A personal case with a history of several years of recurrent pancreatitis, yet with no apparent evidence of biliary tract disease, was nevertheless found to have a dilated common bile duct. Following trans-duodenal sphincteroplasty she has been symptom-free for three years.

Choledochal Cyst

Neonatal cystic dilatation of the duct has already been discussed with biliary atresia. It may have an identical course.

Cysts which present later in childhood or even in adult life are said to have a classical triad of pain, jaundice and a mass in the right upper quadrant of the abdomen. In most series, however, only a minority of cases have all three. In particular it should be realized that a considerable proportion, 18 per cent in Saito and Ishida's series,[61] may be entirely free of jaundice. Vomiting may also be a symptom, and about three-quarters of the children are female. Alonso-Lej, Rever and Pessagno[1] classified the pathology of these cases into three groups – cystic, diverticular and choledochocoele. The great majority are of the cystic type. There may be similar cystic dilatations within the liver (Caroli syndrome[8]) or a fusiform dilatation of the intrahepatic ducts. Saito and Ishida's list of 16 proposed aetiological factors of congenital choledochal cyst reveals our ignorance of the cause. Their preference is for a weakness of the proximal wall of the choledochus with obstruction to the distal portion, possibly resulting from viral cholangitis.

The liver parenchyma is commonly only mildly involved, with inflammatory infiltrate, cholestasis and slight fibrosis.

The condition appears to be much more common in Japanese than in Europeans and North Americans. A similar impression has been obtained in biliary atresia but Shim's study[65] in the Hawaiian population revealed no significant difference between the incidence in caucasians and Japanese, although there was a higher rate in Filipinos and a fivefold increase in Chinese.

Investigations should include liver function tests and a plain abdominal radiograph which will usually reveal displacement of bowel shadows. A barium meal demonstrates typical widening of the duodenal loop (Figure 41.4). Preoperative cholangiography is unlikely to show the cyst because of dilution of the dye. Ultrasound scanning is now proving an invaluable alternative method to demonstrate such cysts and major ducts.

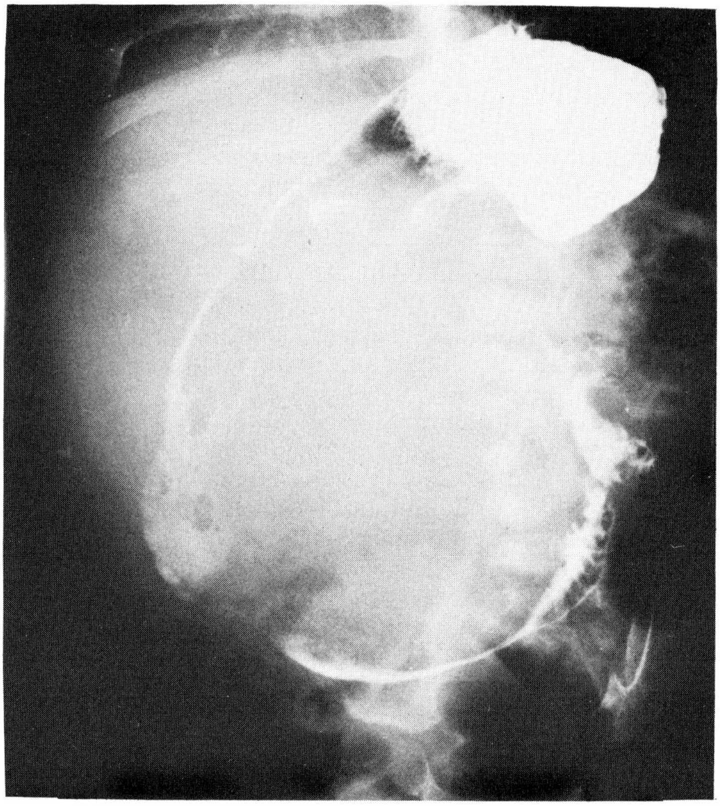

Figure 41.4. Gross displacement of stomach and duodenum by a choledochal cyst. Diagnosis was delayed probably because this was one of the cases with no jaundice. (Ultrasound scanning may replace this form of examination.)

Classical treatment is to anastomose the cyst either directly side to side to the duodenum or to a Roux-en-Y arm of jejunum. However, with the latter procedure, even including a long side arm, bouts of cholangitis, presumably due to stasis in the cyst, have occurred and may cause progressive liver damage. With direct anastomosis to the duodenum, direct contamination of the cyst with food occurs.

It is therefore advisable, whenever possible, to excise most of the cyst and perform a Roux-en-Y anastomosis to a remnant of the upper end of the cyst, leaving only sufficient of the cyst to allow a 2 to 3 cm anastomosis.[4,73] It is important to leave a small remnant of choledochus at the lower end to avoid damage to the pancreatic duct. If cystectomy appears hazardous because of adhesions causing undue bleeding or masking the anatomy, it is wiser to desist and merely trim down the cyst to as small a size as is consistent with safety. The anastomosis should be wide because considerable contraction of the residuum of the cyst occurs after operation.

With such management of the uncomplicated case, life expectancy is normal.

LIVER DISEASE

The child's liver may be the site of primary or secondary malignant tumours, benign and hamartomatous tumours, and also non-neoplastic enlargements from which these tumours need to be differentiated.

For non-neoplastic enlargements the surgeon is likely to be involved only if biopsy is required to diagnose metabolic disorders involving the liver. A punch biopsy instrument such as the 'Trucut' needle obtains good specimens reliably so that open biopsy is not often required. Open biopsy may, however, be helpful in providing a larger bulk of tissue for special examinations. The orthodox wedge biopsy technique is satisfactory. Catgut sutures are placed to encircle the liver on either side of the proposed excision for haemostasis. The wedge is then excised; residual bleeding points are coagulated and the gap is closed by catgut sutures placed around the original haemostatic sutures. It may be helpful to biopsy both lobes of the liver, for in certain circumstances streaming of portal blood may differentially affect the lobes.[23]

Open biopsy may be a part of laparotomy to determine whether hepatomegaly is diffuse or results from a localized lesion displacing the margin downwards. Biopsies guided by the macroscopic findings may be required to determine the nature of a tumour and its treatment. This may help decide, for example, whether right hemihepatectomy is justified for malignancy, or even whether no resection at all is required for some benign hamartomas.

A rare non-neoplastic cause of liver enlargement in the newborn has been encountered on one occasion. The baby was admitted following a stressful asphyxial delivery because of functional intestinal obstruction. As the obstruction settled the left lobe of the liver enlarged. At operation it was found to be totally infarcted and was easily resected from the healthy right lobe. It is uncertain whether the infarction was related to the vascular effects complicating asphyxial delivery or to the umbilical catheter used to monitor the child's progress after delivery.

Liver Tumours (See Chapter 38)

Primary malignant tumours

Hepatoblastoma. This embryoma generally develops from a single focus in an otherwise normal liver and is the commonest malignant hepatic tumour of childhood. It commonly arises in the first two years of life and usually occurs in the right lobe of the liver. There is a slight male preponderance. The degree of maturation of hepatocytes and heterotopia of stromal tissues varies widely from case to case.

Symptoms are rare. Usually the mother notices a swelling when handling the baby, or perhaps it is recognized during a routine medical examination for vague malaise or abdominal discomfort. Serious symptoms are absent because there is an ample reserve of surrounding normal liver. Precocious puberty has been described very occasionally and generalized osteoporosis is a rare and bizarre occurrence. The tumour may perhaps produce steroid hormones.

Adenocarcinoma. Adenocarcinoma may present in the same fashion as hepatoblastoma but the child is usually older – about seven or eight years of age.

Rhabdomyosarcoma. Rhabdomyosarcoma of the bile ducts may present as a symptomless mass when it arises from the smaller ducts within the liver. It may, however, affect the main ducts within or outside the liver when it causes obstructive jaundice which may be demonstrable by cholangiography. The tumour may also first obstruct either the right or the left hepatic ducts. Infection arising behind the obstruction may lead to an unusual presentation with jaundice and multiple abscesses in one lobe of the liver. The tumour may be of an infiltrating type presenting only as a symptomless mass.

Secondary malignant tumours

Secondary deposits in the liver are not uncommon: the most frequent primary tumours are nephroblastomas and neuroblastomas. The latter are important because they may cause hepatomegaly in the absence of a demonstrable primary and so be confused with primary liver tumours. The enlargement may be diffuse or multilobular. The vascularity may resemble an angioma at laparotomy.

Benign liver tumours

Most are hamartomas and may be solid or cystic, single or multiple, intrahepatic or pedunculated. Clinically, they present as a symptomless diffuse or localized swelling of the liver, except in the event of haemorrhage from an angioma, torsion of a pedunculated tumour or infection of a cystic lesion.

Angioma. The angioma may be mainly solid or may contain large cavernous spaces. Its nature may be suspected from the presence of associated cutaneous angiomas, but these do not always occur.

Hepatic angiomas have the same tendency to spontaneous resolution as those in other sites[5] but complications such as high output cardiac failure, consumption thrombocytopenia, or intraperitoneal haemorrhage may preclude this happy outcome. In a group of angiomas from our hospital two children succumbed to haemorrhage from oesophageal varices caused by portal hypertension.[15]

Hamartomatous cysts. These may present with symptomless liver enlargement or with secondary infection producing local tenderness, fever, malaise and possibly jaundice. The cysts may be single or multiple. These larger cysts are quite distinct from the condition of so-called 'congenital cystic disease of the liver' (or 'congenital hepatic fibrosis') in which there are usually cystic changes also in the kidneys. The liver cysts in this latter condition are only microscopically recognizable.

There is also an uncommon association of macroscopic liver cysts with renal cystic disease.

Benign cystic mesenchymoma. These are commonly pedunculated and hence may be mobile on examination. Occasionally they undergo torsion to cause an acute abdominal emergency with pain and peritonism with reflex vomiting.

Investigation of liver tumour

Clinical examination may identify a tumour within the organ but further investigation may be necessary to distinguish this from displacement of the border of the liver by a tumour behind or above it.

Routine investigations may reveal leucocytosis in the presence of infection in cysts, or a leucoerythroblastic anaemia with marrow involvement by malignant tumour such as neuroblastoma. Lymphocytosis may also be found with neuroblastoma. It has been suggested that this is evidence of an immune reaction to the tumour and that such cases fare better. The usual liver function tests are unlikely to be affected except very late in the spread of malignant disease through the organ. Nevertheless these, and particularly serum protein and prothrombin levels, should be determined before any operation.

Specific investigations may be indicated: the VMA level will be raised in neuroblastoma, and alpha-fetoprotein is raised in the majority of hepatoblastomas.[35, 69] Further estimations during treatment may be of prognostic value and sometimes give early warning of recurrence.

Plain radiography of the abdomen will outline the extent of the lesion and may reveal calcification in hamartomas or, rarely, in the wall of a persistently infected cyst. Chest x-ray and skeletal survey are mandatory for possible malignant tumours. The relatively common hepatoblastoma usually recurs locally and metastasizes to the lungs. Skeletal metastases are more important in neuroblastomas as bony lesions (not merely marrow involvement) are associated with a very bad prognosis. IV-S tumours, on the other hand (those presenting with liver, skin and marrow involvement), do astonishingly well even without treatment. Recent techniques of bone imaging are more sensitive than standard radiological surveys as indicators of bony metastases.

Localization of the tumour in one or both lobes of the liver is obviously of great importance in considering resection. The most accurate method for detecting small lesions and localizing the distorted vascular tree is angiography but this is not without risk, especially in these children who are usually small. Ultrasonography, however, now gives much information without risk and may be repeated to assess response to treatment. Technetium imaging has proved a safe repeatable investigation. Venography via the inferior vena cava has also been used and may be helpful in demonstrating distortion of its course or obstruction of its lumen with consequent development of collateral channels.

Finally, if a malignant tumour is suspected, needle or, more usually, open biopsy is required for confirmation of the diagnosis before embarking on treatment which has considerable risks.

Treatment

Primary malignant tumour. Resection remains the mainstay of treatment of primary malignant tumours. Resection of the left lobe is straightforward. Unfortunately, the vast majority of malignant tumours occur in the right lobe. Resection of the right half of the liver, the functional right lobe, is a major undertaking[28] (see Chapter 49). This is principally because the hepatic veins drain the liver from three segments, unlike the Glissonian triad which joins or bifurcates at the porta hepatis and divides the liver into two halves about the 'gallbladder plane'. If the tumour is more extensive, necessitating resection up to the falciform ligament, technical problems are further increased.[55, 67]

Specific points relevant to hepatic resection in the writer's paediatric practice are worthy of emphasis:

1. Right hepatectomies in children may be performed through an oblique abdomino-thoracic incision. More recently, however, a midline incision extended upwards by sternotomy of the lower half of the bone has been used. This gives a good exposure of the confluence of the hepatic veins and vena cava without the somewhat drastic rotation of the

liver sometimes required with the other approach. It is not necessary to open the chest so that postoperative recovery is more straightforward.

2. However straightforward the procedure may appear, it is necessary to place controlling slings around the inferior vena cava above and below the liver before beginning to divide the latter. Apart from the possibility of severe blood loss which cannot be adequately replaced, problems of postoperative haemostasis may occur after massive bleeding.
3. The 'finger fracture' technique of Lin, in the author's experience, has not reduced blood loss and a stormy postoperative course may occur. This may be the result of multiple small areas of necrotic tissue left by the technique.

   When diathermy excision is used the postoperative course is usually uneventful and biliary leakage is not a problem. Great caution when approaching the region of the main hepatic veins is essential, however, for these can be opened by the diathermy without any feeling of resistance. A change to blunt dissection at this point is advisable.
4. The common recommendation to cover the raw surface of the remaining liver with the falciform ligament is unsatisfactory as this may be too small. Omentum is therefore preferable.
5. As mentioned above, biliary leakage from the raw surface has not proved to be a problem. Drainage of the extrahepatic bile ducts has been used in the writer's experience only on one occasion, when possible damage to the duct wall during dissection was suspected.

Postoperatively, careful observation for bilirubinaemia, hypoglycaemia or hypoproteinaemia as a result of failure of the residual liver should be kept. Despite extensive resections performed for these tumours, which sometimes involve removing the right lobe plus part of the left lobe, if the residual liver is normal no serious effects of reduced liver function should materialize.

The results of operative treatment alone for hepatoblastomas, adenocarcinomas and rhabdomyosarcomas have been poor, although better than with radiotherapy.[10,18] The poor results of palliative radiotherapy alone have led to a belief that it was ineffective against hepatoblastoma. However, in the writer's experience, preoperative radiotherapy has enabled resection to be performed in three children whose tumours involved both lobes. Although two died of recurrence, the third is well and free of tumour eight years later.

The American Academy survey in 1974[18] reported that 33 per cent of hepatoblastomas were bilobar and inoperable. There was 60 per cent survival in the 78 cases where the tumour was apparently completely excised. Adjuvant chemotherapy appeared to confer no significant benefit, but more recently a response to chemotherapy with vincristine and other drugs has been observed. Prophylactic use of chemotherapy may produce an improvement in survival similar to that seen with rhabdomyosarcoma. The best regimen has not been determined but vincristine, cyclophosphamide and adriamycin, in courses over a two year period according to tolerance, seem reasonable.

Neuroblastoma. The primary site may not be identifiable or may be recognizable as an old calcified focus. In the absence of bony metastases, 'IVS' patients do well without treatment when neuroblastomas arise in the first year of life. When they arise later it appears that at least 80 per cent of patients do well, but this assessment is based on smaller numbers. Chemotherapy should be considered in older patients but more experience is necessary and radiotherapy for the diffusely involved liver is not recommended. A problem may arise in infants when life is jeopardized because the size of the tumour restricts diaphragmatic movement. Schnaufer and Koop[62] have shown that temporary insertion of a silastic-covered Dacron patch to enlarge the abdominal wall may successfully tide over such a period.

Benign tumours. *Angioma.* Haemorrhage is surprisingly rare in these tumours and can often be managed conservatively. A large angioma in the left lobe can be safely removed by left hepatectomy. In the right lobe the risks of operation are greater and, in the case of angioma involving both lobes, resection is impracticable. Conservative management may include the use of steroids, with a dose of 30 mg of prednisone on alternate days.[24] As with angiomas in other sites, the response is uncertain but may be dramatic.

Cardiac failure may respond to usual conservative management with additional use of steroids.[5,24] An inadequate response, however, may justify surgery. Ligation of the right hepatic artery[14] and even of the main arterial trunk[49] may be performed without ill effects, presumably because of adequate collaterals.

Radiotherapy may also expedite healing of the angioma but its hazards in the growing child must be recognized. In this otherwise benign condition it should be considered only as a last resort if all else fails to control cardiac failure.

Cystic hamartoma. These intrahepatic cysts are usually recognized only when they become infected. They may then be localized, however, by imaging. Blood cultures may identify responsible organisms and determine antibiotic treatment. Adequate drainage of the cyst or cysts usually involves open laparotomy to place the drains correctly. Large tube drains should be used and they should be left in situ until sinograms demonstrate collapse of the cyst, sometimes as long as three weeks later. Collapse does not always occur and recurrence of infection may necessitate excision of the cyst. Sometimes segmental resection of the part of the liver containing the cyst is more convenient (see Chapter 49). Resection of the cyst may leave a cavity which cannot be closed by suture and it should be drained by suction using a large diameter soft tube. If suitably placed it may be packed with omentum.

Extrahepatic hamartomas are usually cystic and are easily removed by clamping and transfixing the pedicle.

Surgical Aspects of Infections of the Liver

Granulomatous disease of childhood is a condition in which the leucocytes cannot form endogenous hydrogen peroxide, as recognized by the nitroblue tetrazolium (NBT) test, so that resistance to certain organisms, including staphylococci, is diminished. Repeated infections and generalized malaise ensue with widespread lymphadenitis and, in many cases, liver abscesses. Antibiotic treatment may be complicated by further opportunistic infections. The defect is responsive to immunosuppressive agents such as cyclophosphamide in combination with antibiotic therapy.

Liver abscesses are accompanied by a swinging temperature and severe malaise (see also Chapter 51). Surgical drainage may become necessary if conservative treatment fails. Imaging is invaluable in directing surgery if drainage is required and also in assessing the response. The cavity contains necrotic debris more than frank pus. Nevertheless, surgical intervention may successfully terminate an exacerbation of the disease and repeated drainage is sometimes necessary.

If repeated courses of antibiotics have been used it is particularly important to culture for anaerobic organisms such as Bacteroides and for opportunist infections.

Hydatid cyst. The Casoni test may confirm this diagnosis. Calcification on the radiograph indicates death of the parasite. Carcassonne et al[7] recommend excision of the cyst or cysts and consider hepatectomy to be usually unnecessary. Wide exposure is obtained and the area isolated by packs soaked in 2 per cent formalin. Half the cyst content is then aspirated and replaced with 2 per cent formalin. After five minutes the cyst is emptied, opened and its daughter cysts removed. 'Controlled pericystectomy' is then performed by blunt pledget dissection between the pericyst and the liver parenchyma. Vessels and bile ducts are ligatured or diathermied as necessary. The cavity is left open with a suction drain.

Marsupialization is the simplest treatment but is condemned as a definitive measure. In the treatment of ruptured hydatid cysts it may, however, be a practicable primary measure to be followed some weeks later by a definitive resection. Such rupture into the peritoneal cavity may cause acute abdominal pain with peritonism and there may be a severe allergic reaction including a skin rash. In addition to dealing with the cyst cavity, by resection if possible, it is important to clear the abdominal cavity of free scolices, using swabs moistened with saline and dilute formalin. Dilute silver nitrate solution is an alternative scolicide. An unusual and less virulent form of hydatidosis affecting Eskimos has been described. Spontaneous regression may occur without surgical excision in these cases.

The surgical management of this disease is more fully discussed in Chapter 56.

Amoebic hepatitis. This condition is treated primarily by chemotherapy. A frank abscess may require surgical drainage, but without accompanying chemotherapy this may prove disastrous. The new drug tinidazole may minimize the need for surgery in the future[64] (see Chapter 51).

Portal Hypertension

Most cases of portal hypertension in childhood are of extrahepatic origin, the so-called cavernomatous transformation of the portal vein. The usual cause is the development of a collateral circulation around the thrombosed portal vein. It is uncommon to obtain a clear story of umbilical infection or other cause for the thrombosis.

Occasionally, however, one sees an infant with a mild fever and ascites which may be found to be encysted on exploration to exclude an infective cause of the 'sub-acute abdomen'. The spleen is usually moderately enlarged. The condition settles to be followed by the development of portal hypertension. A lateral radiograph in the acute stage of thrombosis shows anterior displacement of the duodenum. This finding is a contra-indication to operation at that time.[13]

Portal hypertension may be recognized following the investigation of symptomless splenomegaly or of anaemia due to blood loss. If the portal hypertension is untreated there is a risk of recurrent haemorrhage from oesophageal varices. Liver function remains good although mild changes may occur, presumably as a result of lack of portal blood supply.[17]

In the United Kingdom, an hepatic aetiology of portal hypertension does not often occur in childhood, but cirrhosis is more common in some other countries. Congenital hepatic fibrosis ('congenital cystic disease of the liver') is an important cause because liver function is maintained in spite of the maldevelopment of small bile ducts. The 'cysts' are microscopic and grossly the liver appears to be normal. It is a familial condition and there is associated cystic disease of the kidneys which may be recognized on intravenous pyelography although there may be no functional disturbance during childhood.

Cystic fibrosis causes portal hypertension with increasing frequency as better management of pulmonary lesions achieves longer survival. Haemorrhage from oesophageal varices and liver failure also may occur.

The uncommon long-term survivor of biliary atresia is also a candidate for portal hypertension.

Portal hypertension may occur in histiocytosis X[26] and may develop as a rare complication of diffuse hepatic haemangiomatosis.

Posthepatic obstruction of the hepatic veins or congenital stenosis of the inferior vena cava are other rare causes (Budd–Chiari syndrome). Veno-occlusive disease attributed to native herbal medication may occur in endemic areas. With a post-sinusoidal block, hepatomegaly and ascites are early features and jaundice is likely. When the vena cava is obstructed, superficial varices appear on the abdominal wall.

Management

Barium swallow and oesophagoscopy will confirm the presence of oesophageal varices. Liver function tests are normal. Early investigation of the portal venous anatomy is probably not indicated, though transcutaneous splenic portography and punch liver biopsy are often advocated at this stage. These investigations are not without some risk, however, and the author prefers to leave them until specific problems such as haematemesis arise.

The primary treatment should be conservative with sedation and transfusion as necessary. Pitressin is given to produce contraction of the vessels, and should preferably be administered by intramuscular injection. The hazards of intravenous Pitressin in children may be considered too great. A plastic nasogastric tube should be passed to keep the stomach empty to avoid vomiting and also to assess whether bleeding has ceased. If bleeding persists a Sengstaken tube should be used (some consider this too hazardous because displacement of the balloon into the oesophagus may compress the trachea with serious or even fatal results. With careful nursing supervision the writer has never encountered this complication) (see Chapter 44).

With conservative management virtually every bleed in childhood can be controlled.[20] This approach has two benefits. Firstly, with the usual extrahepatic obstruction, haematemesis may occur as early as the first year of life. Later development of collateral vessels may either render surgery unnecessary or at least delay it until late childhood and often adult life. Secondly, if a shunt should become necessary, its success will depend on the actual diameter of the anastomosis and not on its size relative to the patient. Hence the longer a shunt can be postponed, the better the chance of success.

For these reasons, if haemorrhage fails to respond to the conservative measures outlined, a 'palliative' operation on the varices is advised rather than a shunt. The Milnes–Walker procedure is suitable and a thoracic approach is to be preferred. There is no evidence that abdominal procedures give better results. They may, in addition, be followed by vascular adhesions which complicate a later shunt operation. Sclerotherapy may also be of value[29] (see Chapter 44). Some would consider a mesocaval shunt of the Clatworthy type or the use of a jump graft of jugular vein a preferable course in these uncommon cases where conservatism has failed.

Portasystemic shunts

Should haemorrhage recur after a palliative operation shunt surgery may be required. In the commoner extrahepatic cases the portal vein is not patent so that end-to-side portacaval shunting is not feasible. The choice therefore lies between a central splenorenal and a mesocaval shunt. The latter is probably more successful,[38] but neither is entirely reliable in children. For a shunt to be successful it should have a diameter of at least 1 cm but it is not always possible to achieve this in childhood. Although dacron jump grafts have been unsatisfactory in children success has recently been achieved using autogenous jugular vein.[2]

Lester Martin[47] has pointed out that even in cavernomatous transformation of the portal vein, if the duodenum is mobilized a short but adequate length of proximal portal vein may be found to make a shunt. This manoeuvre should, however, be reserved for children in whom other methods have failed.

If shunting is not successful excision of the lower oesophagus and upper part of the stomach with colonic interposition may be used as a last resort, but even this major operative procedure is really palliative and hypertensive vessels may redevelop after an interval of some years.

When the cause of portal hypertension is intrahepatic, such as with congenital hepatic fibrosis, the choice of operation is simpler because an orthodox portacaval shunt can be performed. With normal liver function significant side-effects should not occur. If future liver function is at risk when conditions such as cyctic fibrosis are present an alternative form of shunt may be indicated if a suitably large vein is available.

Postoperative assessment

Since any shunt operation has a significant failure rate, patency may need to be assessed postoperatively. After a mesocaval or portacaval shunt a splenoportogram is practicable but it carries a small risk of haemorrhage and may even necessitate splenectomy. Angiography also carries a small risk. An oral fructose load test is entirely safe and may be helpful. If the shunt is patent the sugar will short circuit the liver to give a prompt rise in the plasma level.[48,59] Smith and MacPherson[66] have similarly used D-xylose. Barium swallow may demonstrate collapse of the oesophageal varices but the simplest procedure is to determine the haemoglobin concentration on repeated occasions and check the stool for occult blood. If bleeding persists more elaborate investigations may be indicated (see Chapter 44).

REFERENCES

1. Alonso-Lej, F., Rever, W.B. & Pessagno, D. (1959) Congenital choledochus cyst with a report of two and an analysis of 94 cases. *International Abstracts of Surgery,* **108,** 1.
2. Altman, R.P. (1976) Portal decompression by interposition mesocaval shunt in patients with biliary atresia. *Journal of Pediatric Surgery,* **11,** 809.
3. Amann, F.W. & Klingenberg, A. (1974) Localised congenital fibromatosis of the head of the pancreas – as a cause of neonatal icterus. *Zeitschrift für Kinderchirurgie,* **14,** 399.
4. Babut, J.M., Feuilly, J. & Germain, M. (1973) Surgical removal or internal by-pass, a therapeutic alternative in surgery of cystic dilatations of the common bile duct. *Annales de Chirurgie Infantile,* **14,** 379.
5. Braun, P., Ducharme, J.C., Riopelle, J.L. & Davignon, A. (1975) Haemangiomatosis of the liver in infants. *Journal of Pediatric Surgery,* **10,** 121.
6. Cameron, Sir R. & Bunton, G.L. (1960) Congenital biliary atresia. *British Medical Journal,* **ii,** 1253.
7. Carcassonne, M., Aubrespy, P., Dor, V. & Choux, M. (1973) Hydatid cysts in childhood. In *Progress in Pediatric Surgery,* vol. 5, pp. 1–36. Baltimore, London and Tokyo: University Park Press.
8. Caroli, J., Soupalt, R., Kossakowski, J., Plocker, L. & Paradowska, T. (1958) La dilatation polycystique congénitale des voies biliaires intrahépatiques. Essai de classification. *Semaines des Hôpitaux de Paris,* **34,** 488.
9. Caulfield, E. (1936) Bile peritonitis in infancy. *American Journal of Disease in Childhood,* **52,** 1348.
10. Clatworthy, H.W. Jr, Schiller, M. & Grosfeld, J.L. (1974) Primary liver tumours in infancy and childhood. *Archives of Surgery,* **109,** 143.
11. Danks, D.M., Campbell, P.E. & Connelly, J.F. (1965) An aetiological study of neonatal jaundice in a children's hospital. *Australian Paediatric Journal,* **1,** 193.
12. Danks, D.M., Campbell, P.E., Jack, I., Rogers, J. & Smith, A.L. (1977) Studies of the aetiology of neonatal hepatitis and biliary atresia. *Archives of Disease in Childhood,* **52,** 360.
13. Daves, M.L. (1966) Clatworthy's sign. *Radiology,* **86,** 480.
14. de Lorimer, A.A., Simpson, E.B., Baum, R.S. & Carlsson, E. (1967) Hepatic artery ligation for hepatic haemangiomatosis. *New England Journal of Medicine,* **277,** 333.
15. Easton (1978) Unpublished observations.
16. Eiseman, B. & Yeoh, K.S. (1962) Portal hypertension associated with idiopathic retroperitoneal fibrosis. *British Journal of Surgery,* **50,** 225.
17. Engert, J., Meister, P., Hecker, W.Ch. & Strassburg, R. (1973) Portal hypertension in childhood. *Zeitschrift für Kinderchirurgie,* **14,** 233.

18. Exelby, P.R., Filler, R.M. & Grosfeld, J.L. (1975) Liver tumours in children in the particular reference to Hepatoblastoma and Hepatocellular Carcinoma: American Academy of Pediatrics Surgical Section Survey – 1974. *Journal of Pediatric Surgery,* **10,** 329.
19. Fonkalsrud, E.W. & Arima, D. Bile lakes in congenital biliary atresia. *Zeitschrift für Kinderchirurgie,* **17,** 295.
20. Fonkalsrud, E.W., Myers, N.A. & Robinson, M.J. (1974) Management of extrahepatic portal hypertension in children. *Annals of Surgery,* **180,** 487.
21. Gautier, M., Jehan, P., Odievre, M. & Hugon, R.N. (1976) Histologic study of biliary fibrous remnants in 45 cases of extrahepatic biliary atresia: correlation with post-operative bile flow restoration. *Journal of Pediatrics,* **89,** 704.
22. Gellis, S.S. (1975) Biliary atresia. *Pediatrics,* **55,** 8.
23. Ghosh, M.L. & Emery, J.L. (1973) Hypoxia and asymmetrical fibrosis of the liver in children. *Gut,* **14,** 209.
24. Goldberg, S.J. & Fonkalsrud, E.W. (1969) Successful treatment of hepatic haemangioma with corticosteroids. *Journal of the American Medical Association,* **208,** 2473.
25. Greenwood, R.D. Rosenthal, A., Crocker, A.C. & Nadas, A.S. (1976) Syndrome of intrahepatic biliary dysgenesis and cardiovascular malformations. *Pediatrics,* **58,** 243.
26. Grosfeld, J.L., Fitzgerald, J.F., Wagner, W.M., Newton, W.A. & Baehner, R.L. (1976) Portal hypertension in infants and children with histiocytosis X. *American Journal of Surgery,* **131,** 108.
27. Hendren, W.H., Greep, J.M. & Patton, A.S. (1965) Pancreatitis in childhood: experience with 15 cases. *Archives of Disease in Childhood,* **40,** 132.
28. Hobsley, M. (1958) Intrahepatic anatomy, a surgical evaluation. *British Journal of Surgery,* **45,** 635.
29. Hunt, P.S., Johnston, G.W. & Rodgers, H.W. (1969) The emergency management of bleeding oesophageal varices with sclerosing injections. *British Journal of Surgery,* **56,** 305.
30. Ikeda, K. & Suita, S. (1975) Hepatic portogastrostomy using a gastric tube for the treatment of congenital biliary atresia. *Zeitschrift für Kinderchirurgie,* **17,** 360.
31. Jenner, R.E. & Howard, E.R. (1975) Unsaturated monohydroxy bile acids as a cause of idiopathic obstructive cholangiopathy. *Lancet,* **ii,** 1073.
32. Johnston, J.H. (1961) Spontaneous perforation of the common bile duct in infancy. *British Journal of Surgery,* **48,** 532.
33. Kasai, M. (1974) Treatment of biliary atresia with special reference to hepatic portoenterostomy and its modifications. In *Progress in Pediatric Surgery,* vol. 6. Munich, Berlin and Vienna: Urban & Schwarzenberg.
34. Kasai, M., Watanabe, I. & Ryoji, O. (1975) Follow up studies of longterm survivors after hepatic portoenterostomy for 'non-correctable' biliary atresia. *Journal of Pediatric Surgery,* **10,** 173.
35. Kew, M. (1974) Progress report: alphafetoprotein in primary liver cancer and other diseases. *Gut,* **15,** 814.
36. Kimura, S. (1974) The early diagnosis of biliary atresia. In *Progress in Pediatric Surgery,* vol. 6. Munich, Berlin and Vienna: Urban & Schwarzenberg.
37. Kobayashi, A., Uysunomiua, T., Ohbe, Y. & Shimizu, K. (1973) Ascending cholangitis after successful surgical repair of biliary atresia. *Archives of Disease in Childhood,* **48,** 697.
38. Lambert, M.J., Tank, E.S. & Turcotte, J.G. (1974) Late sequelae of mesocaval shunts in children. *American Journal of Surgery,* **127,** 19.
39. Landing, B.H. (1974) Considerations of the pathogenesis of neonatal hepatitis, biliary atresia and choledochus cyst – the concept of infantile obstructive cholangiopathy. In *Progress in Pediatric Surgery,* vol. 6. Munich, Berlin and Vienna: Urban & Schwarzenberg.
40. Lees, W. & Mitchell, J.E. (1966) Bile peritonitis in infancy. *Archives of Disease in Childhood,* **41,** 188.
41. Lilly, J.R. & Altman, R.P. (1975) Hepatic portenterostomy (the Kasai operation) for biliary atresia. *Surgery,* **78,** 76.
42. Lilly, J.R., Weintraub, W.H. & Altman, R.P. (1974) Spontaneous perforation of the extrahepatic bile ducts and bile peritonitis in infancy. *Surgery,* **75,** 664.
43. Longmire, W.S. Jr (1964) Congenital biliary hypoplasia. *Annals of Surgery,* **159,** 335.
44. Louhimo, I. (1967) Obstructive jaundice due to retroperitoneal fibrosis in a child. *Journal of Pediatric Surgery,* **2,** 164.
45. MacMillan, R.W., Schullinger, J.N. & Santulli, T.V. (1974) Cholelithiasis in childhood. *American Journal of Surgery,* **127,** 689.
46. Maksoud, J.G., Thorn, A.F., Kieffer, J. & Carvalho-Pinto, V.A. (1971) Faecal excretion of rose bengal I^{131} in the diagnosis of jaundice in infancy with special reference to biliary atresia. *Pediatrics,* **48,** 966.
47. Martin, L.W. (1967) A retropancreatic portal systemic shunt for portal hypertension in children. *Archives of Surgery,* **95,** 332.
48. Martin, L.W. & Bryant, L.R. (1962) Use of fructose to determine the patency of portal systemic shunts. *Archives of Surgery,* **85,** 783.
49. Mattioli, L., Lee, K.R. & Holder, T.M. (1974) Hepatic artery ligation for cardiac failure due to hepatic haemangioma in the newborn. *Journal of Pediatric Surgery,* **9,** 859.
50. Miyata, M., Santani, M., Ueda, J. & Okamoto, E. (1974) Longterm results of hepatic portoenterostomy for biliary atresia: special reference to postoperative portal hypertension. *Surgery,* **76,** 234.
51. Moore, T.C. (1953) Congenital atresia of the extrahepatic bile ducts. Report of 31 proved cases. *Surgery, Gynecology and Obstetrics,* **96,** 215.
52. Morrissey, K.P. & Javitt, N.B. (1973) Extrahepatic biliary atresia: diagnosis by serum bile acid patterns and response to cholestyramine. *Surgery,* **74,** 116.
53. Mowat, A.P., Psacharopoulos, H.T. & Williams, R. (1976) Extrahepatic biliary atresia versus neonatal hepatitis. Review of 137 prospectively investigated infants. *Archives of Disease in Childhood,* **51,** 763.
54. Nixon, H.H. (1964) Leberchirurgie im Sauglings und Kindesalter. *Zeitschrift für Kinderchirurgie,* **1,** 83.
55. Nixon, H.H. (1965) Hepatic tumours in childhood and their treatment by major hepatic resection. *Archives of Disease in Childhood,* **40,** 169.
56. O'Donnell, B. & Puri, P. (1977) Longterm results of simple removal of pigment gallstones in childhood. In *Progress in Pediatric Surgery,* vol. 10. Munich, Berlin and Vienna: Urban & Schwarzenberg.
57. Pellerin, D., Bertin, P., Nihoul-Fekete, A. & Ricour, A. (1975) Cholelithiasis and ileal pathology in childhood. *Journal of Pediatric Surgery,* **10,** 35.
58. Poley, J.R., Ide Smith, E., Boon, D.J., Bhatia, M., Smith, C.W. & Thompson, J.B. (1972) Lipoprotein X and the double 131-rose bengal test in the diagnosis of prolonged infantile jaundice. *Journal of Pediatric Surgery,* **7,** 660.
59. Rohrer, G.V. & Welsh, J.D. (1968) Urinary fructose excretion after fructose loading before and after portal shunting. *Archives of Surgery,* **96,** 979.

60. Saidi, F. (1976) *Surgery of Hydatid Disease*. London, Philadelphia and Toronto: W.B. Saunders.
61. Saito, S. & Ishida, M. (1974) Congenital choledochus cyst (cystic dilatation of the common bile duct). In *Progress in Pediatric Surgery,* vol. 6. Munich, Berlin and Vienna: Urban & Schwarzenberg.
62. Schnaufer, L. & Koop, C.E. (1975) Silastic abdominal patch for temporary hepatomegaly in stage IV–S neuroblastoma. *Journal of Pediatric Surgery,* **10,** 73.
63. Scobie, W.G. & Bentley, J.F.R. (1969) Hydrops of the gallbladder in a newborn infant. *Journal of Pediatric Surgery,* **4,** 457.
64. Scragg, J.N. & Proctor, E.M. (1977) Tinidazole in treatment of amoebic liver abscess in children. *Archives of Disease in Childhood,* **52,** 408.
65. Shim, W.K.T., Kasai, M. & Spence, M.A. (1974) Racial influence on the incidence of biliary atresia. In *Progress in Pediatric Surgery,* vol. 6. Munich, Berlin and Vienna: Urban & Schwarzenberg.
66. Smith, R.C. & Macpherson, A.I.S. (1976) Assessment of portasystemic shunt patency by estimation of D-xylose excretion. *British Journal of Surgery,* **63,** 435.
67. Stone, H.H. (1975) Major hepatic resections in children. *Journal of Pediatric Surgery,* **10,** 127.
68. Strauss, L., Valderrama, E. & Alpert, Ll. (1972) Biliary tract anomalies: the relationship of biliary atresia to neonatal hepatitis. In *Birth Defects: Original Article Series,* vol. 8. Baltimore: Wilhaw-Wilkins.
69. Sugahara, K., Kashii, A., Kogure, H., Manoka, J., Shirakura, T. & Mitani, S. (1973) Serum alpha fetoprotein and resection of primary hepatic cancer. *Archives of Surgery,* **106,** 63.
70. Swenson, O. & Fisher, J.A. (1952) Utilization of cholangiogram during exploration for biliary atresia. *New England Journal of Medicine,* **247,** 247.
71. Ternberg, Jessie L. & Keating, J.P. (1975) Acute acalculous cholecystitis. *Archives of Surgery,* **110,** 543.
72. Wood, G.O. & Blalock, A. (1940) Situs inversus totalis and diseases of the biliary tract. Survey of the literature and report of a case. *Archives of Surgery,* **40,** 885.
73. Yue, P.C.K. (1974) Choledochal cyst: a review of 18 cases. *British Journal of Surgery,* **61,** 896.
74. Zelter, P.M., Neerhout, R.C., Fonkalsrud, E.W. & Stiehm, E.R. (1974) Differentiation between neonatal hepatitis and biliary atresia by measuring serum alpha fetoprotein. *Lancet,* **i,** 373.

Chapter 42

Portasystemic Encephalopathy

JOSEF E. FISCHER

Syndromes of neuropsychiatric disturbance in liver disease are varied and range from subtle alterations in a patient's behaviour, including mild personality change, loss of drive, irritability and disturbance in sleep rhythm, to confusion, drowsiness, stupor and, finally, deep coma. In general, syndromes segregate into those accompanying acute fulminant hepatitis, where onset is rapid, the patient passing through drowsiness, delirium, convulsions, decerebrate rigidity, unresponsiveness and deep coma within a comparatively short period (often less than 24 hours), and chronic liver disease, in which hepatic encephalopathy more often manifests as acute exacerbations precipitated by generally reversible causes; between exacerbations, the patient's neurological status may be entirely normal. Acute fulminant hepatitis may present as a psychiatric disturbance.[210] Chronic encephalopathy may occasionally be found as progressive and irreversible neurological symptomatology as in 'acquired hepatocerebral degeneration', with dementia, parkinsonism or other extrapyramidal signs suggesting involvement of the cerebellum or basal ganglia.[148] In other patients, spastic paraplegia, indistinguishable from a neoplasm of the spinal cord, is secondary to demyelination.[135] The underlying hepatic disease may be minimal.

Other symptoms of hepatic encephalopathy are not unique for liver disease. Asterixis, common in hepatic encephalopathy, is more common in uraemia, and is seen in patients with respiratory insufficiency, hypokalaemia, congestive heart failure and even during hypoglycaemia.[34,179] It is generally thought of as cerebral in origin, although it may represent disruption of integration of proprioceptive information at various levels of the neuroaxis, resulting in periodic lapses in posture. Conn has suggested that asterixis may be a lesion associated with crossing corticospinal tracts, as it has been observed on the contralateral side of developing cerebral thrombosis.[35]

The severity of both acute and chronic hepatic encephalopathy and the response to treatment can be graded on the basis of clinical signs and tests of cerebral function (see also Chapters 27, 43 and 44).

Cerebral function may be assessed by simple tests for constructional apraxia such as the ability to draw a five-pointed star and to copy a short sentence, and by electroencephalogram. Although the change in the pattern of the electroencephalogram is not specific for hepatic encephalopathy, it provides a useful adjunct to diagnosis and assessment of therapy.[137]

In the absence of pre-existing liver disease, coma accompanies fulminant hepatic failure generally of viral[31,114,154] or toxic origin such as poisoning with paracetamol, halothane[104,139] or tetracycline.[171] Whether the encephalopathy associated with Reye's syndrome is secondary to a viral encephalitis or toxic metabolic products of hepatic failure is not clear at the present time.[151]

Against the background of chronic liver disease, a variety of clinical events, such as gastrointestinal bleeding, infection and overdiuresis, may provoke hepatic encephalopathy. Depression occurring with liver disease may be secondary to overdosage with sedatives, but this is not properly considered to be hepatic encephalopathy.

The pathophysiological mechanisms in acute vs chronic liver disease may not be similar.

Clinical presentations, variations in subtlety, and the chronic nature of the encephalopathy associated with chronic liver disease suggest that it may be of different origin from the acute toxic insult seen with acute fulminant hepatitis. The author will assume for the purpose of argument, however, that the two are related.

Attention has invariably focused on toxins in the production of hepatic encephalopathy. Presumably, these toxins, arising in the gut, are normally metabolized by the liver, and when they are either physiologically or anatomically shunted around the liver they accumulate in the circulation and 'poison' the brain. Another view, proposed by Geiger, is that the liver may normally provide factors required for CNS function.

In isolated perfused brain preparations, electrical activity was prolonged when the liver was included in the circuit. With the liver removed, both provision of cytidine and uridine in the perfusate and frequent changes in the perfusion medium were instrumental in prolonging electrical activity.[82] Thus both a positive and detoxifying mechanism were presumed. Cytidine and uridine do not presumably traverse the blood–brain barrier unchanged, and their metabolism was unchanged in a small series of patients with coma.[166] It is nonetheless possible that whereas chronic hepatic encephalopathy results from the accumulation of toxins, in acute fulminant hepatitis an 'active' substance secreted by the liver may not be present. Since Geiger's experiments have not been enlarged upon, most of the discussion which follows will focus on toxins.

HISTOLOGY

Most notable in the brain pathology of patients dying in hepatic coma is the absence of striking findings. Cerebral oedema is blamed for an increasing percentage of deaths in hepatic coma; it does not respond to steroids, mannitol, urea or other usual therapeutic measures.[112,202,204] A fairly constant finding is hyperplasia of protoplasmic type II astrocytes, most prominent in the cortex but also found in other parts of the brain.[197] The pseudopods of these cells may contribute to the control of the passage of materials across the blood–brain barrier. In cerebral oedema, it is possible that oedema of the pseudopods disrupts the tight junctions and opens up abnormal passages through which toxic materials may enter the brain.

The meaning of these astroglial changes is not clear. It is increasingly thought that the astroglia are the cells which govern the extracellular environment of the brain; as such, their dysfunction may contribute to disruption in neurological function. As discussed elsewhere, glutamine may be a glial metabolite.[14,205] Elevation of cerebrospinal fluid glutamine is one of the most reliable biochemical correlates of hepatic encephalopathy,[83,93] and thus an anatomical–biochemical correlation may be implicit. Whether the astrocytic protoplasmic hyperplasia observed is an attempt on the part of the glia to maintain neuronal homeostasis or is a pathological response to toxins and even contributes to the mechanism of hepatic encephalopathy is not known.

Finally, in hepatocerebral degeneration, irreversible neuronal damage and degeneration as well as demyelination may occur. If demyelination does occur, spinal cord symptoms may be present with lesions involving lateral and ventral corticospinal tracts. While chronic encephalopathy is generally considered to be irreversible, Conn followed two patients treated with lactulose who showed improvement from seemingly irreversible neurological deficits, and the author has observed one such case, treated with an oral amino acid supplement rich in branched chain amino acids.

CHEMICAL PATHOLOGY

There are no 'hepatic function tests' or plasma electrolyte disturbances invariably associated with hepatic encephalopathy. Indeed, in chronic liver disease, severe encephalopathy, including the 'irreversible' hepatocerebral and spinal cord degeneration, may even be associated with normal values for hepatic function tests. Clotting factor deficiencies reflect only the severity of hepatic dysfunction, and are not related to the degree of encephalopathy. Hypoglycaemia generally presages a fatal outcome as it is usually encountered in greatly advanced hepatic failure when glucose homeostasis cannot be maintained, but it has been reported in non-comatose patients with severe viral hepatitis.[59] While hypokalaemia and alkalosis are common in hepatic disease, they are not invariable in encephalopathy although they may aggravate it.

Elevated creatinine and blood urea concentrations, with a disparate elevation in the latter, are common in the early 'hepatorenal syndrome' but again are not necessarily part of hepatic encephalopathy. A raised blood urea level may reflect gastrointestinal bleeding, which certainly contributes to hepatic encephalopathy.

In the clinical setting, blood ammonia determination of venous blood, drawn in a heparinized tube, is the most widely performed test for hepatic encephalopathy. The correlation between clinical status and blood ammonia is approximate, and numerous patients with clinical encephalopathy may have normal blood ammonia levels. While arterial ammonia concentration is better correlated with clinical status, 10 per cent of patients with hepatic coma have normal arterial ammonia levels.[183] Cerebrospinal fluid ammonia and glutamine are more often elevated than peripheral blood ammonia.

Pathological findings in the cerebrospinal fluid are not characteristic. CSF is clear and colourless, except when hyperbilirubinaemia is present. No characteristic pattern of cells, glucose, protein and electrolytes has been discerned, while CSF glutamine is usually elevated. It should be pointed out, however, that there are at least three distinctive cerebrospinal fluid circulations, and lumbar CSF, so easily available, probably does not reflect brain stem or cortical cerebrospinal fluid values.[186]

PATHOGENESIS OF HEPATIC ENCEPHALOPATHY

The final disturbance in hepatic encephalopathy must involve derangements in neurotransmission. This is certainly true in the more subtle grades of non-comatose encephalopathy, in which derangements of sleep pattern, euphoria, subtle changes in personality, etc., are present. Whether the hepatic coma seen in acute fulminant hepatitis is merely toxic is not clear, but cases of fulminant hepatitis presenting as psychiatric disorders have been reported. Thus it is likely that whatever the mechanism of hepatic encephalopathy, it involves subtle changes in neurotransmission, whether secondary to energy changes, alterations in synthesis or metabolism of the neurotransmitters themselves. These will be discussed in turn.

Cerebral Energy Metabolism

Most of the available data in this area are the result of animal experiments. In man, data concerning only total brain consumption of glucose and oxygen are available. The results are variable. Cerebral blood flow and cerebral oxygen consumption are impaired and brain glucose utilization is decreased in hepatic coma, but these changes follow hepatic coma and do not precede loss of consciousness. In one study, glucose consumption, cerebral blood flow and cerebral oxygen consumption were unchanged for the first 24 hours of acute coma after which they decreased.[143] Another study showed decreases prior to coma[58] and two studies were equivocal.[54,145] The weight of evidence suggests that decreased oxygen consumption in hepatic encephalopathy follows the onset of coma and is probably due to decreased cerebral activity. Oxygen consumption may not be the proper parameter to measure, however. In Wernicke's encephalopathy, for example, depressed cerebral oxygen consumption is not associated with unconsciousness.[172] In animals with hepatic encephalopathy following acute ammonia poisoning, adenosine triphosphate and creatine phosphate were normal in the cortex but decreased in the brain stem.[168] Other investigators report brain stem and cerebellar creatine phosphate decreased with unchanged levels of ATP.[90] Methodological problems have hampered the interpretation of these results since it is known that these labile intermediates change while the brain is being removed, dissected and frozen. An additional problem in these experiments is the induction of anaesthesia prior to sacrifice.

More recently, a rapid freezing technique, using a freeze blow apparatus, has been introduced.[196] When anaesthesia was not utilized and the metabolic status of the animal was monitored with maintenance of normal blood gases, blood glucose and body temperature, cerebral high-energy sources or labile metabolic intermediates were unchanged unless hypoglycaemia supervened, in which case ATP all but disappeared and cyclic AMP greatly increased.[19] In other studies using an in-situ freezing technique changes in high-energy intermediates were found after induction of coma.[91] This study also utilized anaesthesia, however, thus complicating interpretation. Glutamate and aspartate excitatory neurotransmitters were decreased, confirming previous work.[19] Thus, energy changes in causation of hepatic coma do not seem tenable at present.

Clinical Axioms

Any hypothesis about the pathogenesis of hepatic coma must satisfy several clinical observations:

1. Hepatic function is usually diminished in hepatic coma.
2. Shunting of portal blood around the liver parenchyma, spontaneously or on a surgical basis, is present.
3. The substance(s) involved in the production of symptoms of hepatic encephalopathy arise in the gut.
4. Gut bacteria play a role in that altering gut bacterial flora ameliorates hepatic encephalopathy.
5. Those substances involved in hepatic coma may be of nitrogenous origin, as coma is most commonly provoked by increased dietary protein or gastrointestinal bleeding.
6. While ammonia may not be *the* aetiological agent, serum ammonia generally reflects the presence of hepatic encephalopathy, although a correlation is not exact.

Ammonia

Ammonia has traditionally been the leading villain in the pathogenesis of hepatic encephalopathy. While it is clear that patients with hepatic damage are especially sensitive to the cerebral toxic effects of ammonia,[141] this does not necessarily imply that in spontaneously-occurring encephalopathy ammonia is the principal aetiological agent. Meat intoxication in animals with hepatic damage following Eck's fistula was recognized before the turn of the century. An understanding of protein intoxication was developed, and it was shown that ammonia intoxication in such animals mimics spontaneous hepatic encephalopathy. Finally, increased blood ammonia is found in many patients with hepatic encephalopathy[122] and blood ammonia determinations are still the most widely performed biochemical tests for hepatic encephalopathy.

Several hypotheses have been put forward to explain the toxic action of ammonia. It was initially hypothesized that ammonia blocked energy production by depletion of the cerebral Krebs cycle of 2-oxoglutarate, utilized in the synthesis of glutamine.[17] This is no longer tenable, as the depletion of 2-oxoglutarate has not been demonstrated in experimental animals.[173] Furthermore, brain glutamine is derived from the synthesis of ammonia with a rapidly turning-over pool of glutamic acid rather than from 2-oxoglutarate.[16]

Other possible toxic effects of ammonia have been proposed, including the accumulation of the inhibitory neurotransmitter, γ-aminobutyric acid (GABA).[84] However, the concentration of GABA in the brains of rats with hepatic coma[19] or after ammonia intoxication is not increased.[170] The inhibitory effects of ammonia on the synthesis of acetylcholine by inhibition of pyruvate decarboxylase have not been confirmed because normal levels of acetylcholine are present in the cortex and brain stem of ammonia-intoxicated animals.[199] It is possible, however, that synthesis and turnover are altered as these have not been examined.

Disruptions in energy production continue to occupy an important place in the ammonia hypotheses. These studies have been afflicted by the methodological problems outlined above. However, using the recently developed ultra-rapid freeze blow technique, slight decreases in phosphocreatine were found in ammonia-intoxicated animals.[89] In a more recent study, after 60 minutes of massive ammonia intoxication in animals with portacaval shunts ATP decreased in all regions of the brain, but the reduction in total high-energy phosphate was most marked in the brain stem. The authors of the latter paper concluded that the cerebral dysfunction in chronic relapsing ammonia intoxication is not primarily due to energy failure.[91]

The author's own studies utilized an experimental model in which anaesthesia was not used, animals were intubated when they became comatose, and blood glucose and arterial blood gases, as well as normal rectal temperature, were maintained carefully. Following hepatic artery ligation 48 hours after portacaval shunt, blood ammonia concentrations in excess of 705 μmol/l (1200 μg/dl) were found. Brain was obtained by a freeze blow technique. Cerebral high-energy phosphate compounds and Krebs cycle intermediates were unchanged.[19] The brain stem was not sampled by this technique. Thus, despite much discussion, it would appear that ammonia does not significantly alter brain energy content.

Even if one were to accept the toxic effects of ammonia on the brain of animals with hepatic encephalopathy, many difficulties remain with the ammonia hypothesis. In vivo toxicity of ammonia may be dissociated from venous ammonia levels by monoamine oxidase inhibitors in man[44] and by inhibitors of glutamine synthetase in experimental animals.[203] Arterial ammonia concentrations, while correlating better with encephalopathy than venous ammonia, may still be normal with grade 4 hepatic encephalopathy.[183] Cerebral uptake of ammonia has not been demonstrated in severe coma. More recent neurophysiological evidence, moreover, indicates that ammonia cannot be the sole cause of hepatic encephalopathy, as the site of ammonia toxicity is localized to the cortex and perhaps the amygdala, but the arousal response of the reticular activating system, which is thought to be severely involved in hepatic encephalopathy, is not affected.[92] This further suggests that ammonia is not toxic to the brain stem, nor to some of the lower centres involved in hepatic coma. Therefore, even if ammonia has a role in the pathogenesis of hepatic coma, it cannot explain all the neuropsychiatric signs and symptoms in hepatic coma.

Moreover, not all the changes in neurotransmitters seen in hepatic encephalopathy are induced by ammonia intoxication. These include strikingly elevated tryptophan and serotonin levels,[10,42,63,106] alterations in brain phenylalanine, tyrosine and their derivative amines[63,64] and alterations in metabolites of dopamine and serotonin.[105] Furthermore, ammonia given to experimental animals in amounts far in excess of levels found in man failed to change cerebral serotonin, and this again suggests that ammonia intoxication is not a useful model for human hepatic encephalopathy.[199]

Another alternative to the classical ammonia hypothesis incriminates an intermediate metabolite, 2-oxogluteraminate, which is elevated in the CSF of patients with hepatic coma. Infusion of 10 μmol of 2-oxogluteraminate, 20 times the highest recorded value in man, into the lateral ventricles of rats produces EEG changes similar to those found in human hepatic coma.[52] The specific role of this latest alternative to the classical ammonia theory requires further investigation.

Short Chain Fatty Acids

Several investigators have noted an increase in short chain fatty acid levels in the peripheral circulation of patients with hepatic encephalopathy. Butyrate, valerate, and octonoate are increased in the blood and CSF of patients with hepatic encephalopathy.[30,187] Precedent exists in another form of coma: that found with the Jamaican vomiting sickness which is induced by hypoglycin A and results in isovaleric acidaemia.[188] Finally, intraperitoneal injection of butyrate, valerate and octonoate can apparently produce a rapidly reversible coma lasting for up to one hour in experimental animals.[198]

The liver is presumably active in the catabolism of such fatty acids absorbed from the gut. It is not clear whether such excesses of fatty acids originate from protein, over-diuresis, sepsis or some of the other stimuli which are known to provoke hepatic encephalopathy. Moreover, the clinical status of encephalopathy in patients with cirrhosis correlates poorly with the levels of any of the short chain fatty acids.[198] Indeed, short chain fatty acids have been administered without any undue toxic effect to patients with cirrhosis.[125] On balance, therefore, short chain fatty acids are unlikely to be solely responsible for hepatic encephalopathy.

Unhappiness with the ammonia and the short chain fatty acid theories alone has led Zieve to propose that a synergism exists between ammonia and fatty acids.[211] Normal animals have been rendered comatose by ammonia salts supplemented with short chain fatty acids. However, the concentrations of ammonia achieved in these experiments range from 590 to 1470 μmol/l (1000 to 2500 μg/dl), values almost never seen in patients except, occasionally, in Reye's syndrome. An attempt to implicate long chain fatty acids, displaced from a decreased serum albumin,[121] is not tenable as non-esterified fatty acids are seen in much higher concentrations in the post-traumatic state as well as following starvation.

Short chain fatty acids increase to a very minor extent after a prolonged fast.

Derangement in Neurotransmitters

From the variety of derangements which are associated with hepatic encephalopathy in both acute and chronic circumstances, it becomes apparent that there are major disturbances in neurotransmission. The many candidates for neurotransmitter function in the central nervous system include amines, such as acetylcholine, norepinephrine (noradrenaline), dopamine, serotonin and histamine; the entire range of excitatory amino acids such as glutamate and aspartate; inhibitory amino acids including glycine, serine and GABA; the prostaglandins; substance P; and more recently the peptide neurotransmitters.[11] The physiology of many central neurotransmitters has been extensively studied, particularly the neuropharmacology of the adrenergic neurotransmitters, norepinephrine and dopamine. The structural requirements of the peripheral adrenergic system appear to be a phenolic ring and a short carbon side chain with a hydroxyl group on the β position of the side chain.[71] Structural requirements appear to hold true for the central nervous system with the exception that a non-β-hydroxylated configuration appears to be preferred for the striatum.[7] The concept of 'false' neurotransmitters evolved from evidence that the peripheral adrenergic neurone would take up compounds less active than the putative neurotransmitters in response to electrical stimulation.[71,107] These would accumulate under toxic or pharmacological conditions or in response to accumulation of exogenous precursors.[41,128] Such substances appear to be taken up by central nervous system synaptosomes and in brain slices or isolated synaptosomes can be released in response to ionic or electrical depolarizing stimulation.[7,12]

Catecholamines

Both the peripheral adrenergic system and the brain can control the entry of neurotransmitter material into the neurones. Surprisingly, however, other variables such as exogenous intake, and particularly the liver and its metabolism of amino acids and amines, control the concentrations of materials available for synthesis within the neurone. Amino acids and amines derived from gut bacterial action absorbed into the portal circulation are generally inactivated by the liver and their plasma concentrations kept within a narrow range despite a wide range of intake. The blood–brain barrier contributes to the control of neurotransmitter material by selectively allowing precursor amino acids to penetrate and excluding most circulating amines. However, the blood-brain barrier operates on a series of competitive principles by which decreased plasma concentrations of certain amino acids may result in the increased uptake of other amino acids of that group.[132] Thus with failure of hepatic function, both the peripheral and the central nervous system can be 'fooled' into accepting and synthesizing other precursor amino acids or incorrect amounts of these precursors, leading to altered neurotransmitter synthesis and derangements in neurotransmission.

In hepatic encephalopathy, the accumulation of inactive or false neurochemical transmitters is suggested by several circumstances: firstly, blood is shunted around the liver and hepatic function is usually decreased; secondly, nitrogenous compounds, amines and amino acids are present in abundance and those absorbed from the portal circulation escape metabolism and clearance by the liver, flooding the central and peripheral nervous systems.[66,68] In the periphery, depletion of norepinephrine might result in a state of high cardiac output and low vascular resistance often seen in hepatic failure.[119] When norepinephrine depletion occurs, those vascular beds with a normally high resting sympathetic tone dilate and increased blood flow follows in skin, muscle and splanchnic bed, as is seen in hepatic failure. The kidney, normally reasonably vasodilated, thus tends to lose flow, and its resistance, while initially unchanged, increases relative to the other non-vital areas with a decreased fraction of the elevated cardiac output while total flow initially remains the same.[193] Cardiac output then increases reflexly to maintain perfusion to vital organs. The decreased renal perfusion pressure triggers the release of renin, renal vasoconstriction occurs, renal blood flow decreases and redistribution of flow between cortex and medulla takes place, resulting in the high output, low peripheral resistance 'type 2' hepatorenal syndrome.[50]

Octopamine

Since the initial neurotransmitter hypothesis was proposed, the findings of accumulation of octopamine in the brain and blood of experimental animals and in the blood and urine of patients with hepatic encephalopathy have been confirmed with an excellent correlation between octopamine and the grade of encephalopathy.[110,118,161] Phenylethanolamine, another amine capable of acting as a false neurochemical transmitter, increases as well.[163] In more recent experiments in which CSF has been measured simultaneously with blood, CSF levels of these inactive or 'false' neurochemical transmitters increase even before the elevation of blood octopamine and phenylethanolamine, reaching maximal levels with grade 3 to 4 coma and decreasing rapidly when appropriate therapy is undertaken.[178]

Other amines

Within the central nervous system, disturbances in serotonin, dopamine and norepinephrine metabolism have been documented. Serotonin, which may replace norepinephrine or dopamine in the adrenergic system, is markedly increased in both chronic encephalopathy and acute hepatic failure.[42,43,105,106] Increased 5-hydroxyindoleacetic acid has long been known to be present in the CSF and brain of animals and CSF of patients with experimental hepatic failure.[105] In both dogs and primates when appropriate therapy for hepatic encephalopathy is undertaken, 5-hydroxyindoleacetic acid promptly returns to normal as the animal recovers.[178]

On the basis of accumulated evidence, it would appear likely that there is little or no disturbance in overall dopamine metabolism and that synthesis proceeds normally until quite late in hepatic coma. It is likely, however, that some block exists at the step in synthesis by which norepinephrine is synthesized from dopamine, thus resulting in an accumulation of homovanillic acid within the CSF.[105] Inhibitory influences on the synthesis of norepinephrine, by inhibition by dopamine beta oxidase, include the accumulation of other inactive neurochemical transmitters[51] and other neutral amino acids as well as the ability of excessive phenylalanine and tyrosine to result in an accumulation of octopamine rather than increased synthesis of norepinephrine within the brain.

Changes in Other Neurotransmitters in Hepatic Encephalopathy

With the recognition that amino acids may serve as neurotransmitters, it became of interest to investigate changes in excitatory neurotransmitters. Using the freeze blow technique a decrease in the excitatory amino acids, glutamate and aspartate, was observed in hepatic coma in rats.[19] These findings have subsequently been confirmed.[91] Whether these antedate, are a contributor to or are the result of hepatic encephalopathy is not clear.

Elevated glutamine concentrations are consistently found in the brain and CSF of animals and man with hepatic coma.[19,83,93] The normal function of glutamine is not clear, and it may merely be a metabolite of ammonia within the brain. Recent work suggests that glutamine may be taken up into nerve terminals in competition with glutamate and released by depolarizing stimuli.[13] Since glutamine is neuropharmacologically inert, it may function as an inactive transmitter in the place of glutamate, an excitatory neurotransmitter.

Levels of the inhibitory neurotransmitter γ-aminobutyric acid (GABA) are normal in advanced experimental hepatic coma.[19]

Taurine, a ubiquitous inhibitory neurotransmitter, is increased both in the brains of animals with experimental encephalopathy[177] and in the CSF of primates with encephalopathy secondary to end-to-side portacaval shunt. It could thus be involved in hepatic encephalopathy. The suggestion is supported by the finding that plasma levels of taurine correlated well with the grade of encephalopathy in a series of 60 patients.[160] Studies of serine and glycine, other inhibitory amino acid neurotransmitter candidates, are not available as yet.

AMINO ACIDS IN HEPATIC ENCEPHALOPATHY

Derangements in plasma amino acids in patients and animals with hepatic encephalopathy are well-established findings. The pattern consists of increased phenylalanine, tyrosine, free but not necessarily total tryptophan, methionine, histidine, glutamate and aspartate, together with decreased or normal levels of the branched chain amino acids, leucine, isoleucine and valine.[4,21,73,94,95,96,120,153,185,208] These findings assumed increased significance when it was realized that certain neutral amino acids served as precursors for CNS neurotransmitters. This group of competing neutral amino acids includes tryptophan, tyrosine, phenylalanine, methionine and histidine and the branched chain amino acids. Subsequent investigations have revealed that in addition to the classical amino acid pattern, namely increased phenylalanine, tyrosine, free tryptophan and decreased branched chain amino acids, leucine, isoleucine and valine, associated with hepatic encephalopathy, two other distinct amino acid patterns exist.[158] In the patient with chronic cirrhosis and acute exacerbation, increased phenylalanine, tyrosine and methionine, free tryptophan and decreased branched chain amino acids appear to be associated with hepatic encephalopathy (Figure 42.1). Others claim that it is associated with severe liver disease, but not specifically with encephalopathy.[124] Other investigators agree that it indicates the presence of encephalopathy, but not necessarily its grade as initially proposed.[162] In acute fulminant hepatitis, however, severe hyperamino-

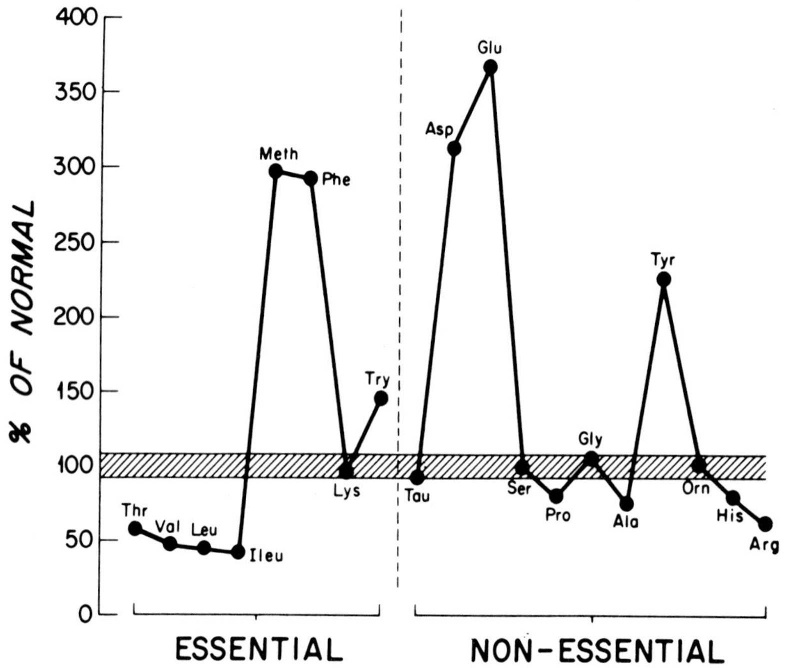

Figure 42.1. Mean plasma levels of amino acids (plasma aminogram) represented as percentage of normal in 13 patients with chronic liver disease and acute decompensation and encephalopathy. This pattern should be contrasted with that shown in Figure 42.2. (Thr = threonine; Val = valine; Leu = leucine; Ileu = isoleucine; Meth = methionine; Phe = phenylalanine; Lys = lysine; Try = tryptophan; Tau = taurine; Asp = aspartate; Glu = glutamate; Ser = serine; Pro = proline; Gly = glycine; Ala = alanine; Tyr = tyrosine; Orn = ornithine; His = histidine; Arg = arginine.) From Rosen et al[158] with kind permission of the authors and the editor of *Gastroenterology*.

acidaemia of all amino acids is present. Its source appears to be the necrotic liver. Among all the amino acids only the branched chain amino acids leucine, isoleucine and valine do not appear elevated and levels may even by slightly decreased (Figure 42.2). The concentrations of phenylalanine, tyrosine and methionine may be as high as 700 to 800 per cent of normal, and in a series of 15 patients no patient with a tyrosine level higher than 60 μg/ml (or 600 per cent of normal) survived acute fulminant hepatitis, regardless of therapy, which seems to indicate that hepatic necrosis was so severe as to be beyond retrieval.[158] These different amino acid patterns influence the form of therapy used in these various forms of encephalopathy.

Following portacaval shunt, survival in experimental animals has been related to various diets. Those resulting in the shortest survival were rich in the aromatic amino acids, phenylalanine, tyrosine and tryptophan.[32] In patients, little data are available. Blood is 'more toxic' than an equinitrogenous amount of casein,[18] and milk and cheese are apparently better tolerated than diets containing equal amounts of protein given as meat.[60] Perhaps the reason for this is that casein contains more branched chain amino acids and fewer aromatic amino acids as compared with meat. More recently, vegetable protein, which shares these properties to a lesser extent, has been proposed as a diet for patients with hepatic encephalopathy.[86] A defined amino acid diet with these properties may soon be available for patients with chronic encephalopathy. In preliminary experiments it appears to be better tolerated than natural protein.

Tryptophan is thought to be toxic in liver disease. Plasma total tryptophan is slightly elevated in hepatic encephalopathy while free tryptophan is markedly increased.[43,106] Free tryptophan levels, which may be five to 10 times normal, are influenced by the ratio of free plasma tryptophan to protein-bound tryptophan, by plasma non-esterified fatty acids[138] and by the distribution of the branched chain amino acids.[61] As a result, CSF tryptophan is greatly increased in man[106] and in animals with experimental hepatic encephalopathy, compared with plasma tryptophan, as is brain 5-hydroxyindoleacetic acid. Therapy results in decreased 5-hydroxyindoleacetic acid.[74,178] Brain tryptophan is increased both because of

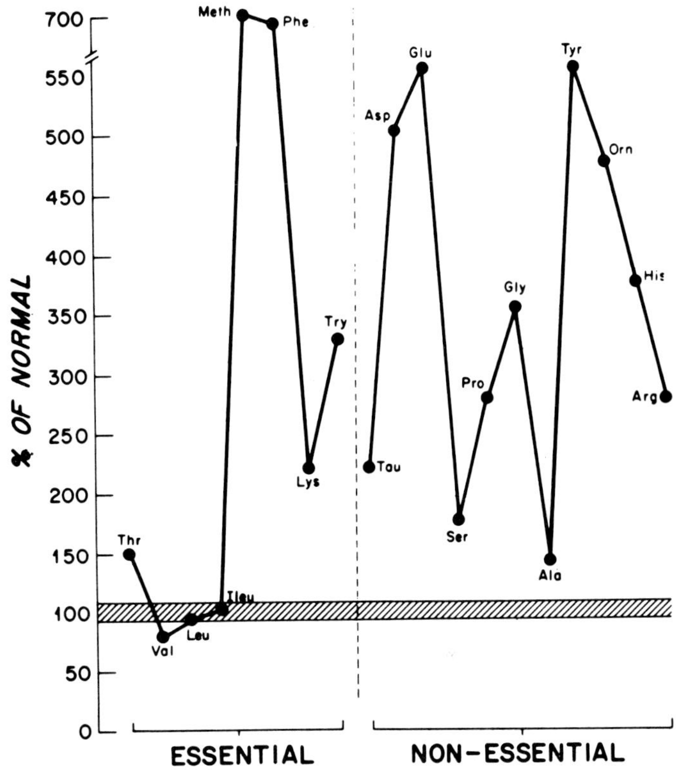

Figure 42.2. Mean plasma levels of amino acids (plasma aminogram) represented as percentage of normal in five patients with acute hepatic necrosis with associated hepatic encephalopathy. Two of the five patients represented here had tyrosine and phenylalanine levels greater than 800 per cent normal. (Abbreviations as in legend to Figure 42.1.) From Rosen et al[158] with kind permission of the authors and the editor of *Gastroenterology*.

the decreased levels of the branched chain amino acids[43, 61, 101] and because of increased plasma free tryptophan. Serotonin, an inhibitory neurotransmitter amine, is greatly increased in the experimental animal with acute hepatic coma.[43, 63]

Methionine is another amino acid thought to be toxic in hepatic encephalopathy. Administered intravenously, it is well tolerated. Intracarotid arterial injections of large amounts of methionine into normal dogs failed to produce coma.[163] Oral tolerance of methionine may be increased by oral antibiotics,[140] suggesting that the toxic factor is not methionine but a metabolic product. While some investigators have suggested that methionine may decrease brain ATP levels by the formation of *S*-adenosylmethionine,[88] normal levels of brain ATP have been found in rats with elevated blood and brain methionine.[19] *S*-adenosylmethionine has been proposed as therapy for hepatic encephalopathy. Exogenously administered methionine is probably of less importance to the brain as the brain synthesizes its own methionine when deprived of other sources.[134]

Phenylalanine, however, is the amino acid whose concentration is highest in brain as well as in blood. One factor is the decreased conversion of phenylalanine to tyrosine by hepatic phenylalanine-4-hydroxylase, whose activity is decreased early in hepatic impairment. An additional factor in both man and experimental animals is the decreased concentration of the branched chain amino acids, both on a relative basis, as in acute fulminant hepatitis, in which they remain normal despite tremendous increases in other amino acids, and as an absolute decrease, as is seen in chronic liver disease with acute exacerbation. These branched chain amino acids are unique in that they are not only incorporated into protein but can be catabolized into ketone bodies by brain, muscle and kidney, undergoing deamination to an α-oxo-analogue with net production of ammonia, and subsequently forming acetyl-coenzyme A.

More recent investigations reveal that the low plasma concentrations of branched chain amino acids are the result of decreased release from muscle (where branched chain amino acids are utilized for energy) as well as of increased oxidation by fat.[180] As other energy sources, such as glucose and ketone bodies, are decreased in hepatic failure, the branched chain amino acids are the sole remaining form of energy which may be available without the intervention of the liver, and without passing through glucose by gluconeogenesis. Thus, muscle and other visceral organs will utilize branched chain amino acids selectively. This has important ramifications both for the brain and the periphery. In addition to the liver, the kidney is the one organ which may catabolize the branched chain amino acids into glucose, thus providing glucose to the periphery instead of a failing liver. This also, incidentally, results in increased renal vein ammonia. In this case, the activity or concentration of the initial catabolic enzyme active in the breakdown of these amino acids, branched chain amino acid transaminase, should be increased, and this is what we have found in animals following portacaval shunt.[181]

HORMONAL BACKGROUND

Insulin, glucagon and presumably other hormones influence the plasma concentrations of various amino acids. Insulin promotes the catabolism of the branched chain amino acids by both muscle and fat and it has been suggested that the decreased branch chain concentrations within the circulation are secondary to oxidation of these amino acids by muscle under the influence of insulin.[126,180] The role of glucagon, however, appears to have been neglected until recently.

In recent experiments with animals, following end-to-side portacaval shunt, both insulin and glucagon increased modestly, retaining a normal insulin/glucagon ratio. As the animal enters hepatic encephalopathy, there is a dramatic rise in the plasma concentration of glucagon while insulin either remains stable or decreases.[180,182] The result is a reverse insulin/glucagon ratio which some have associated with catabolism. While it is difficult to implicate glucagon as a catabolic hormone in the periphery, since direct infusion of glucagon into forearms fails to release muscle amino acids,[27] increased plasma glucagon is characteristically associated with an increase in catabolic substances such as steroids or epinephrine.

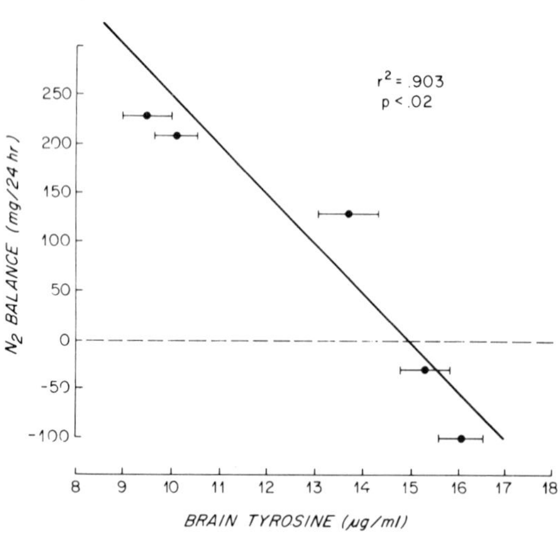

Figure 42.3. Inverse relationship of brain tyrosine with nitrogen balance. Groups of rats with end-to-side portacaval shunts were infused with an amino acid mixture containing 35 per cent branched chain amino acids, and isocaloric hypertonic dextrose of 25 cal/100 g body weight/24 hr. Amino acids infused ranged between 0 and 1.0 g/100 g body weight/24 hr. Note the inversely proportional relationship between brain tyrosine and nitrogen balance, with lower brain tyrosine being recorded as nitrogen balance becomes positive.

INFLUENCES ON PLASMA AROMATIC AMINO ACID CONCENTRATIONS

Plasma concentration of plasma aromatic amino acid is independent of exogenous intake with normal hepatic function.[159] With impaired hepatic function, however, exogenous intake is extremely important in determining plasma levels of amino acids, independent of route of administration.[159] In rats with impaired hepatic function following end-to-side portacaval shunts, exogenous intake influenced plasma and brain aromatic amino acid concentrations, as well as brain octopamine.[159]

Even more interesting is the association between nitrogen balance and plasma and brain levels of aromatic amino acids. In rats with end-to-side portacaval shunts, increasing amounts of amino acids were given at an isocaloric level of hypertonic dextrose sufficient to promote nitrogen retention at 0.40 g amino acid/100 g rat bodyweight/24 hr. Plasma and brain aromatic amino acids and brain octopamine varied inversely with the presence or absence of positive nitrogen balance (Figure 42.3). In the catabolic animal, plasma aromatic amino acids were increased, whereas in the anabolic animal, plasma phenylalanine and tyrosine and brain tyrosine and octopamine were decreased despite the fact that increased amounts of phenylalanine and tryptophan were being given with increased protein intake.[159] These results suggest that the fate of the administered aromatic amino acids was intracellular protein synthesis, and that in the presence of positive nitrogen balance, plasma aromatic amino acids and brain aromatic amino acid will be decreased. Similarly in patients, those with hepatic encephalopathy were in negative nitrogen balance.[159] Thus, a second influence on plasma aromatic amino acids and brain dysfunction is anabolism.

A third influence on plasma and brain aromatic amino acids is the plasma concentration of the branched chain amino acids. These amino acids are an important determinant of the efflux of various other amino acids from muscle.[79, 131] The administration of small doses of equimolar concentrations of the branched chain amino acids, valine, leucine and isoleucine, to rats with portacaval shunts decreased the level of plasma tyrosine. Brain tyrosine was also decreased, but to a greater extent than plasma tyrosine.[56] The results were interpreted as showing that (a) branched chain amino acids decrease breakdown of muscle, decreasing release of endogenous aromatic amino acids, and (b) the plasma tyrosine/brain tyrosine ratio is reduced to normal, presumably because of competition of the branched chain amino acids at the blood-brain barrier.

Thus, in the presence of impaired hepatic function, exogenous intake, the plasma concentrations of the branched chain amino acids and the presence of anabolism or catabolism all help to determine the plasma levels of aromatic amino acids. In addition, the branched chain amino acids have further influence by competing with the aromatic amino acids for entry into brain across the blood barrier.

These influences also help explain the 'sensitivity hypothesis'. This, as originally enunciated by Schenker,[167] states that the brain of the patient with liver disease is more sensitive to various noxious stimuli which will render that patient comatose, whereas in the normal individual no such effect will be observed. The various stimuli include gastrointestinal bleeding, over-diuresis, sepsis or intercurrent stress. The brain of the experimental animal with liver disease is abnormal in that thc blood-brain barrier cannot protect the brain from excessive uptake of aromatic amino acids for reasons to be discussed. The various noxious stimuli previously referred to, including sepsis, increase the catabolic rate and this results in decreased plasma branched chain amino acids and increased aromatic amino acids secondary to lean tissue mass breakdown. The same may be said for any other intercurrent stress, over-diuresis and gastrointestinal bleeding. Thus, the common thread of all of these factors is an alteration in the plasma amino acid pattern in the direction of aggravation of a pattern already present. When this is combined with alterations of the blood-brain barrier, hepatic encephalopathy is more likely to result.

THE BLOOD-BRAIN BARRIER

Previous investigations have assumed that the blood-brain barrier is qualitatively normal in the animal with chronic liver disease and in the patient with severe cirrhosis, and that the observed CNS effects are based on alterations in plasma amino acid pattern alone. Recent experimental evidence from this and other laboratories has suggested that this is not the case. The blood-brain barrier is altered in a subtle way in chronic liver disease[100] and completely disrupted in the late stages of acute hepatic coma.[112]

In experiments in which plasma and CSF amino acids were simultaneously determined in animals with hepatic encephalopathy, animals were treated with infusions of an amino acid mixture rich in branched chain amino acids. It was observed that whereas CSF concentrations of the other neutral amino acids varied to a considerable extent, the CSF concentration of the branched chain amino acids remained within narrow (normal) limits over a wide range of plasma concentrations.[178] This phenomenon had previously been observed in rats, both in brain[100] and in CSF.[178] It was suggested that the brain preferred, as it were, to maintain a normal concentration of the branched chain amino acids. In subsequent experiments using the Oldendorf technique[132] it was determined that the brain uptake index (BUI) of the large neutral amino acids was increased within 24 hours after end-to-side portacaval shunt. This was a specific increase in the neutral amino acid group, as the BUI of arginine was decreased, and the BUI of other substances such as glucose or inulin was unchanged.[55, 100] Administration of small doses of branched chain amino acids to these animals returned the BUI of the neutral amino acids to normal.[55] This suggests that the primary regulating factor of the neutral amino acid group may be the concentrations of the branched chain amino acids, particularly leu-

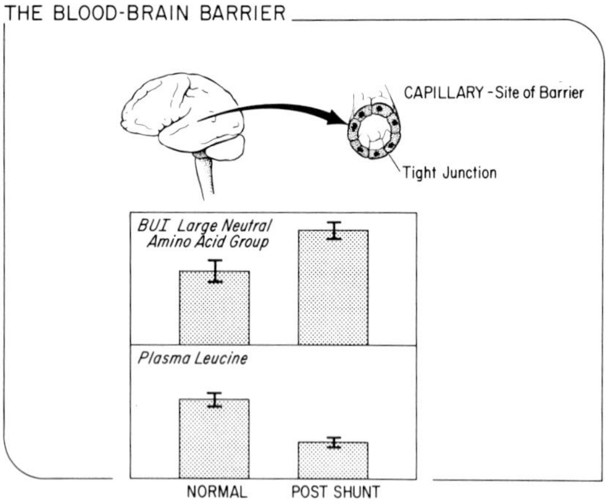

Figure 42.4. The blood-brain barrier in chronic liver disease. The capillaries of the brain, the site of the blood-brain barrier, differ from all other capillaries in that tight junctions rather than pores are present. The flow of all substances is controlled by active transport. Brain uptake index (BUI) was determined by the method of Oldendorf[132] as described in the text. Under normal circumstances, plasma leucine which appears to be the controlling amino acid of the 'large' amino acid group is normal and is represented by a normal BUI for 'large' neutral amino acids. Post shunt, when plasma leucine drops, the brain in an attempt to maintain a normal concentration of brain leucine increases its uptake of the neutral amino acid group and increased aromatic amino acid penetration occurs.

cine. This has previously been alluded to as the 'large' neutral amino acid uptake system and appears to be a leucine-preferred system. In severe liver disease, when the plasma concentration of the branched chain amino acids is decreased, the blood-brain barrier attempts to increase its active transport of these critical branched chain amino acids to maintain a normal concentration of the branched chain amino acids within the brain, for protein synthesis, energy or lipid synthesis, etc. The uptake index of such branched chain amino acids is increased and the uptake index of the aromatic amino acids, utilizing the same system, is increased at the same rate (Figure 42.4). Conversely, the administration of branched chain amino acids apparently restores the blood-brain barrier to normal.[43,55]

Under stressful circumstances or in sepsis with sudden decreases in the branched chain amino acids and increases in the aromatic amino acids, an even greater increase in BUI of the 'large' neutral amino acid group may be expected. However, since the plasma concentrations of the branched chain amino acids are even lower, increases in uptake of the toxic aromatic amino acids may be expected. Thus sepsis, intercurrent stress, diuresis or any other alteration in plasma aromatic amino acids will worsen the situation and increase brain uptake of aromatic amino acids. These findings may explain, in part, Schenker's sensitivity hypothesis in which a number of seemingly unrelated noxious stimuli such as sepsis, overdiuresis, etc., may provoke hepatic coma.[167]

Another phenomenon which appears to be independent of the competition phenomenon is a direct relationship between CSF and, presumably, brain aromatic amino acids and the plasma concentration. This is shown in Figure 42.5 in which the CSF concentrations of phenylalanine, tyrosine and other amino acids appear directly related to plasma concentrations. This suggests that in acute fulminant hepatitis, when branched chain amino acids may be normal, the extremely elevated plasma aromatic amino acids will result in flooding of the brain with, for example, phenylalanine and tyrosine. Conversely, therapy of acute hepatic encephalopathy in fulminant hepatic necrosis would involve a plasma laundering technique, such as the Rhone–Poulenc dialyser using a polyacrilonitrile membrane. This has recently been used in an effort to decrease the plasma concentrations of these aromatic amino acids,[45,133,175] as has administration of large amounts of branched chain amino acids to prevent the aromatic amino acids from traversing the blood-brain barrier (Figure 42.6). The latter therapy has been applied clinically by Delafosse and his co-workers who report excellent results in waking up a majority of their patients by administering 60 g of branched chain amino acids per day, in addition to polyacrilonitrile membrane dialysis, as opposed to the 30 to 40 per cent awakening usually reported.[45]

In the later stages of acute hepatic necrosis, however, there is complete disruption of the blood-brain barrier with associated cerebral oedema.[112,133,175] Whether the cerebral oedema precedes or follows the disruption of the blood-brain barrier is not clear, but it is not responsive to the usual modes of therapy and may be responsible for as much as 40 per cent of deaths.[202] It should be pointed out, however, that in acute hepatic necrosis inulin, sucrose and all other materials appear to penetrate with ease as if the barrier is completely disrupted,[112] in contrast to the very distinct alterations of the blood-brain barrier in chronic hepatic disease.[100]

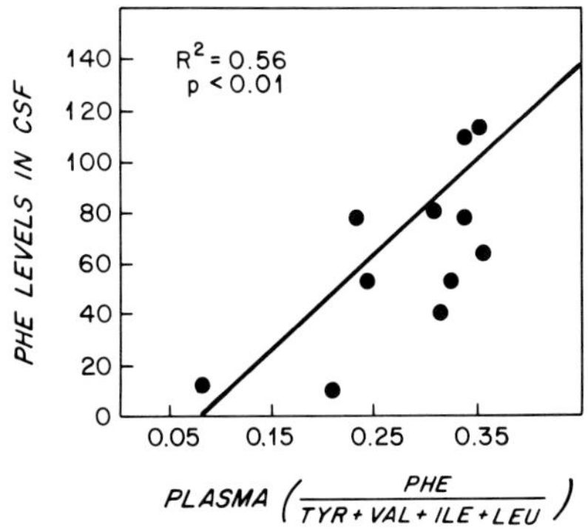

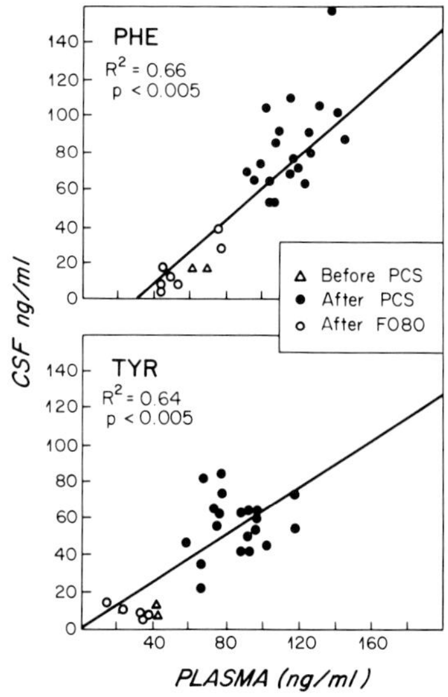

Figure 42.5. Regression coefficients representing penetration of aromatic amino acids across the blood-brain barrier. On the left, the phenylalanine levels in the cerebrospinal fluid appear to correlate with the concentration of phenylalanine in the plasma in competition with the other 'large' neutral amino acids including tyrosine, valine, isoleucine, leucine and tryptophan. On the right, the behaviour of CSF phenylalanine and tyrosine (presumably reflecting brain phenylalanine and tyrosine), suggesting that the plasma and brain concentrations of these aromatic amino acids are directly related. The findings have application in fulminant hepatitis when high plasma concentrations of aromatic amino acids are present. (PCS = portacaval shunt; FO80 = high branched chain/low aromatic amino acid solution.)

PRECIPITATING CAUSES OF HEPATIC ENCEPHALOPATHY

From what has been discussed above, a final pathophysiological mechanism would explain:

1. The alterations in plasma and brain aromatic amino acids.
2. The depletion of norepinephrine, and increased serotonin and β-hydroxyphenolethanolamines.
3. A widespread derangement in neurotransmission.
4. The relationship between 1, 2 and 3.

It has long been known that the aminergic system makes up only 5 per cent of the total neurones within the brain. Recently, startling information has been forthcoming concerning the neuroanatomy of the aminergic system, in which only approximately 5 per cent of the axonal varicosities (from which neurotransmitter is released) are associated with postsynaptic neurones; the remainder lack close cellular apposition and other characteristics associated with classical synapses.[49] By implication, neurotransmitters released from other nerve endings diffuse into the surrounding medium. Other studies suggest that no cell in the cerebral cortex is further than 30 μm away from an aminergic nerve ending.[48] Similar findings apparently apply for the traditional opposition of norepinephrine and serotonin.[47] All of these suggest a neuromodulator role.

Hepatic coma may therefore be a widespread disturbance in cerebral neurotransmission resulting from altered synthesis and an imbalance in the norepinephrine/β-phenylethanolamine serotonin modulating system secondary to disturbed peripheral metabolism of the amino acid precursors, the aromatic amino acids.

Further disturbances may involve the recently described possible feedback loop to the locus caeruleus, also noradrenergic. Correction of the peripheral amino acid abnormalities may enable normal modulation to resume, resulting in clearing of hepatic encephalopathy.

A variety of events may cause unconsciousness in patients with pre-existing liver disease, including infection, gastrointestinal haemorrhage, overdose of sedatives, tranquillizers, electrolyte imbalance and overdiuresis. In a recent study of 100 episodes of hepatic coma the principal causes were, in order of occurrence: azotaemia, either spontaneous or diuretic induced, the injudicious

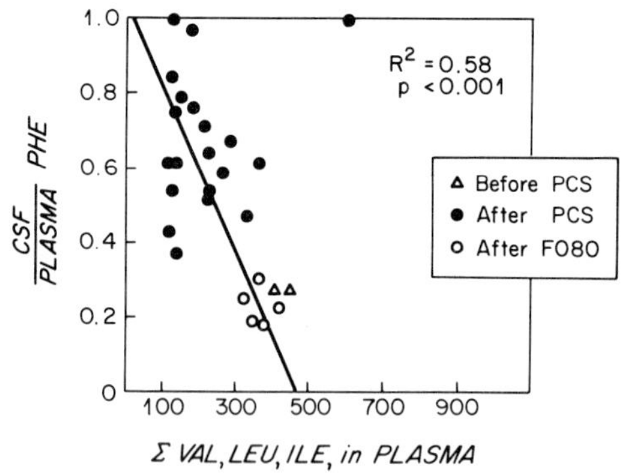

Figure 42.6. The relationship between CSF and plasma phenylalanine, and the sum of the molar concentrations of plasma branched chain amino acids, valine, leucine and isoleucine. These findings suggest that despite the high plasma concentrations of phenylalanine an excess of plasma branched chain amino acids far in excess of physiological concentrations will result in decreased permeability of the blood-brain barrier to aromatic amino acids.

use of sedatives, tranquillizers or analgesics, gastrointestinal haemorrhage, hypokalaemia, alkalosis and protein intoxication.[62]

The Use of Sedatives in Patients with Compromised Hepatic Function

There is probably no safe sedative in hepatic encephalopathy, despite recent evidence that some sedatives may be safer than others. Because of limitations of space, a long list of problems in the metabolism or excretion of sedatives is not included.[67,169] While it is doubtful that overdoses of sedatives cause hepatic coma, nonetheless this diagnosis is an important consideration in patients with known hepatic disease who manifest altered consciousness. Abuse of chlordiazepoxide accounted for about half of the episodes of oversedation in a recent study.[62] Clearance of chlordiazepoxide, diazepam and related drugs is reduced in such patients.[127] The same may be true for chlorpromazine, morphine and other opiate derivatives such as methadone, meperidine and codeine, all of which are metabolized in part by the liver, [22,98,109] and barbiturates, the excretion of some of which, especially those with short actions, is dependent on the liver.[26] Other factors besides hepatic metabolism which contribute to the prolonged persistence of opiates are protein binding and transport by serum albumin, which is of course decreased in most patients with chronic liver disease.

Gastrointestinal Haemorrhage

Gastrointestinal haemorrhage, even if slight, may be life-threatening to these patients as it adds to the protein load of an already overburdened liver. In addition, the hypotension which is associated with gastrointestinal haemorrhage decreases perfusion of the compromised liver. It is the author's impression that bleeding oesophageal varices are responsible for greater injury to the liver of a patient with cirrhosis compared with bleeding gastritis, as the liver appears to depend on the increased portal perfusion pressure to maintain viability. This portal hypertension is obviously compromised when variceal bleeding ensues. Blood is particularly poorly tolerated as it contains large amounts of aromatic amino acids, and is more toxic than an equinitrogenous amount of casein given orally.[18]

Rapid diagnosis of gastrointestinal bleeding is essential. Peripheral intravenous Pitressin infusion appears to be the preferred treatment as few advantages have been demonstrated with Pitressin infused into the superior mesenteric artery. Initial cessation of bleeding with Pitressin infusion is rapid, but the rebleeding rate is high.[38] The Sengstaken–Blakemore tube may be used as a temporary measure, but even in expert hands it rarely serves as definitive therapy.[37] Other temporary measures include the embolization of either endogenous clot or Gelfoam into varices, which may serve until the patient can tolerate a definitive portal hypertension-relieving procedure.

Gastritis appears to respond better than bleeding oesophageal varices to Pitressin infusion.[5] Surgery, poorly tolerated in such patients, may be necessary to control haemorrhage from gastritis.[206] Emergency shunts tend to be poorly tolerated, with a high mortality, and therapeutic trials of end-to-side portacaval shunts have revealed only equivocal evidence of life extension, although the mode of death is altered from bleeding to hepatic failure.[97,150] This may be secondary to further impairment of hepatic function because of decreased provision of substrate-rich portal blood.[9]

DIURETIC THERAPY

Although hepatic encephalopathy has been widely associated with the diazides which cause hypokalaemia and alkalosis, any form of over-diuresis can precipitate the condition. The proposed mechanism by which such encephalopathy occurs has traditionally been related to the ammonia theory of hepatic encephalopathy because the kidney is an important source of ammonia and hypokalaemia increases ammonia production in the renal vein. It is not clear whether this increased output represents increased production or diversion of ammonia from urine into the circulation.[6] With the development of metabolic alkalosis, freely diffusible ammonia rises very rapidly and diffusion of ammonia into the brain is facilitated, whereas a lower pH will convert ammonia largely into the non-diffusible NH_4^+ form.[29] The same may be true for amines. Toxicity of diuretics, however, may not in itself be dependent on the ammonia hypothesis. Apart from the liver, the kidney is the only organ capable of manufacturing glucose from amino acids. With a failing liver, the kidney may augment glucose production in an attempt to maintain peripheral energy supply, thus resulting in decreased branched chain amino acids facilitating the entry of the toxic aromatic amino acids into the brain.[75,101] Evidence of this has been forthcoming in several of our patients in hepatic coma following over-diuresis.[69] In addition, one major source of renal vein ammonia may be the deamination of branched chain and other amino acids for glucose production, a process which may be increased by hypokalaemia and alkalosis.[142]

That over-diuresis may decrease plasma volume, thus decreasing hepatic perfusion and function, should not be overlooked.

SEPSIS AND OTHER STRESS

Sepsis or even minor degrees of infection result in hepatic encephalopathy in patients with chronic hepatic impairment. Spontaneous bacterial peritonitis with ascites and recurrent encephalopathy has been re-emphasized recently.[36] Clinical signs may not exist, and only suspicion leading to paracentesis will make the diagnosis possible. Patients with cirrhosis and malnutrition are susceptible to infections. In addition to simple malnutrition, alcohol has an adverse affect on leucocyte migration,[25] and serum bacteriocidal activity[102] depresses white cell mobilization and impairs phagocytosis (in mice).[113] An active serum inhibitor has been recently proposed.[46] All stresses, including infection and pneumonitis, increase metabolic demands, resulting in increased lysis of lean body mass to utilize the branched chain amino acids which decrease even further with infection.[77,201] The increased release of aromatic amino acids in infection results in increased plasma concentrations of these toxic metabolites. Therapy of any but the most trivial infection in patients with hepatic decompensation should probably include proper nutritional support.

ROUTINE THERAPEUTIC MEASURES IN PATIENTS WITH HEPATIC ENCEPHALOPATHY

General support

The usual clinical clichés apply. Maintenance of adequate oxygenation (which may be measured by 'arterial blood gases'); the provision of vitamins, especially of the B group; careful attention to fluid and electrolyte balance to avoid over-hydration and hyponatraemia; the administration of 'salt poor' 25 per cent albumin will treat low concentrations of serum albumin, which arise from either decreased synthesis or increased catabolism, and will maintain intravascular volume and urinary output. The measurement of urinary sodium in these patients gives an excellent guide to the requirement for administered sodium. Parenteral nutrition may be necessary in patients in whom oral intake is interrupted for more than a few days. These patients have notoriously poor oral intake, and many patients with alcoholic liver disease are so anorectic that they eat only a thousand calories daily and then with difficulty. Steroids, useful in chronic active hepatitis,[184] are catabolic and may contribute to the deterioration of such patients. Finally, when confronted with a patient in apparent hepatic encephalopathy, other causes of coma should not be overlooked, particularly since trivial trauma may give rise to subdural haematomas or intracranial haemorrhage in patients with deficient clotting mechanisms. Meningitis may occur and should be ruled out with lumbar puncture.

ESTABLISHED EFFECTIVE THERAPY

Decreasing the Role of Toxins Originating from the Gut

Most established therapies concentrate on altering the contents of the gut. This includes decreasing the gut protein load, altering intestinal flora, or altering the rate of absorption of protein, amino acids, amines or ammonia. Increasing intestinal transit by the use of laxatives to rid the gut of accumulated blood or protein is part of every regimen for hepatic encephalopathy. Protein restriction in patients capable of oral intake is a cornerstone of therapy and usually includes restriction to 40 g protein/24 hr, which is the minimal intake of protein on which one can expect a patient to survive indefinitely. Oral intake of fewer than 20 g protein/24 hr is not compatible with prolonged survival. The imminent availability of chemically defined diets using large amounts of branched chain amino acids and deficient in aromatic amino acids, the clinical use of which in a few patients has had a beneficial effect (unpublished observation), may ameliorate the problem of protein intolerance. In one particularly well-studied patient it was possible to increase oral intake from fewer than 20 g protein/24 hr to 55 g protein/24 hr while improving hepatic and cerebral function with the disappearance of seemingly irreversible choreoathetotic movements, explosive speech and other symptoms.[157]

Bowel Sterilization

Non-absorbable antibiotics, such as neomycin, kanamycin or paramomycin have been used for years in an attempt to alter bowel flora by the suppression of urease-producing organisms. According to the 'ammonia hypothesis', this will result in decreased absorption of ammonia. Approximately 1 per cent of oral or rectal neomycin is absorbed[108] with some risk of chronic nephrotoxic or ototoxic effects.[15] As renal function fails, continued administration of neomycin is risky as its urinary concentration may reach as high as 10 μg/ml, which is generally considered to be a bactericidal level.

There are few data on the minimal effective dose, and starting doses range from 6 to 8 g/24 hr, with maintenance doses varying between 1 and 4 g/24 hr. In addition to preventing absorption of ammonia, other effects of these antibiotics may be selective malabsorption of the aromatic amino acids[57,72] as well as the presumably decreased ammonia flux. A similar mechanism has been suggested in germ-free animals treated with non-absorbable antibiotics.[129]

Lactulose

Lactulose has recently appeared as another mainstay in chronic encephalopathy in addition, or as an alternative, to neomycin. A non-absorbable synthetic disaccharide (β1,4-galactoside fructose),[20] it has been shown to be effective in three controlled studies.[39,53,176] An additional study has demonstrated that it may be as effective as neomycin, and that the additive effects of lactulose and neomycin may be superior to those of neomycin or lactulose alone.[39] It is not completely metabolized in the small intestine, but is hydrolysed by bacterial action in the colon, producing acidic diarrhoea when amounts of up to 60 to 160 g/24 hr are utilized. Stool frequency is increased. The clinical effects may be mediated by reduction in colonic pH with resulting decreased ammonia absorption, or it may decrease the absorption of aromatic amino acids, and decrease brain octopamine.[80] Its effects, however, are not simply due to those of increased stool frequency as other agents, such as sorbitol, do not consistently alter pH and are not as effective. The effects of lactulose on bacterial and stool counts are unimpressive. An alternative explanation is that lactulose decreases the time in which a stool is in contact with bacteria, and thus decreases ammonia production.[3] Lactulose is of potential benefit in patients with renal impairment in whom neomycin may be toxic, or it may be useful as a synergistic drug in patients resistant to either form of therapy alone.

Colon Bypass

An early development in the therapy of hepatic encephalopathy, colon bypass, anecdotally and in one controlled study,[123,150] may indeed ameliorate chronic portasystemic encephalopathy. The operative morbidity and mortality, however, have made this a rare procedure. Ileostomy appears superior to ileorectal anastomosis as colonization of the small intestine above the ileorectal anastomosis decreases the effectiveness of the procedure with time.

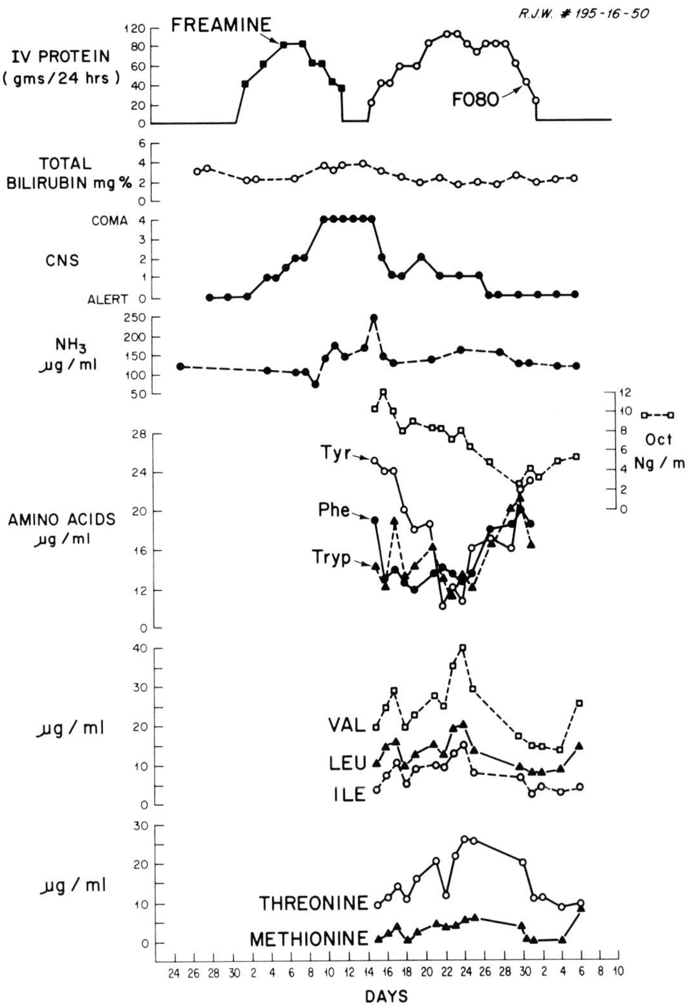

Figure 42.7. Therapy of a patient with an oesophageal fistula, empyema, sepsis, hepatic failure and encephalopathy with a solution enriched with branched chain amino acids and decreased aromatic amino acids (FO80). The patient underwent variceal ligation for bleeding oesophageal varices, developed an oesophageal leak, and had drainage of the empyema. Parenteral nutrition with a standard solution rich in aromatic amino acids (Freamine) was undertaken. This resulted in hepatic encephalopathy. The patient was in grade 4 coma and placed on a respirator. Therapy with FO80 was begun. Up to 120 g amino acids/24 hr with hypertonic dextrose was achieved and during this time the patient awoke, was weaned from the respirator and the oesophageal fistula closed. (Oct = octopamine; other abbreviations as in legend to Figure 42.1.)

PROCEDURES LACKING ESTABLISHED EFFICACY

L-Dopa Therapy

Numerous investigators have confirmed the apparent awakening of patients with acute or chronic hepatic encephalopathy with L-dopa therapy.[2, 66, 70, 115, 137, 144, 164] An initial report suggested that patients with fulminant hepatic necrosis may awake following extremely large doses of L-dopa, but this practice appears to have been abandoned.[137] While most studies have been uncontrolled, in cross-over studies L-dopa apparently increases cerebral oxygen consumption and decreases response time.[115]

The mode of action of L-dopa may be secondary to a number of mechanisms including replenishment of the normal transmitters, dopamine and norepinephrine,[66, 68] release of competing neurotransmitters such as serotonin[130] or β-hydroxyphenylethanolamines,[24, 99] or the absorption of methyl groups, thus preventing the synthesis of potentially toxic methylated amines.[209] In addition, L-dopa may prevent the gastrointestinal absorption of phenylalanine and tyrosine which is thought to be important in the pathogenesis of hepatic encephalopathy.[195]

Several problems prevent the widespread use of L-dopa in patients with chronic encephalopathy who are usually treatment failures with

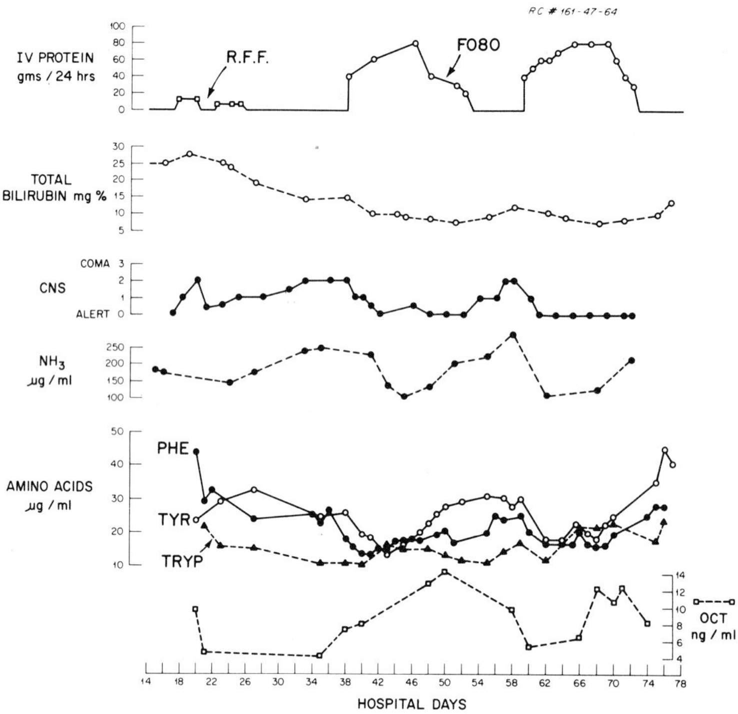

Figure 42.8. Therapy of a patient with severe alcoholic hepatitis with FO80. The patient with known cirrhosis of the liver was admitted with severe alcoholic hepatitis, a blood urea nitrogen level of 35.7 mmol/l (100 mg/dl) and a bilirubin level of approximately 510 µmol/l (30 mg/dl). The patient would not tolerate an infusion of essential amino acids (RFF), even up to amounts of 15 g/24 hr. The patient went into encephalopathy with an elevated plasma ammonia level, clouding of consciousness, and elevated aromatic amino acid levels. Two periods of treatment with FO80 were undertaken, associated with decreased bilirubin, clearing of encephalopathy, decrease in ammonia and decreasing aromatic amino acids. A trial of oral nutrition was undertaken without success, and during this time bilirubin rose, ammonia became elevated again and the patient went back into hepatic encephalopathy. These findings were once again reversed with reinstitution of parenteral nutrition. (Abbreviations as in previous legends.)

neomycin and lactulose. Gastrointestinal tolerance decreases with time and the incidence of gastritis, nausea and anorexia increases. This may be partially overcome by the use of decarboxylase inhibitors, which decrease the destruction of L-dopa in the periphery, enabling more L-dopa to avoid destruction and reach the brain.

Up to 30 per cent of patients may not absorb L-dopa even when antacid is added to aid absorption in the duodenum.[156] Even if L-dopa were absorbed, recent evidence suggests that patients pass from a stage of reversible to irreversible hepatic coma, and if therapy is initiated following this no significant response may be expected.[70]

Corticosteroids

Few patients dying with acute fulminant hepatitis die ‘without benefit’ of massive doses of steroids. Although apparently valuable in the treatment of chronic active hepatitis,[184] their value in fulminant hepatitis has never been adequately documented. The initial report[103] has never been confirmed either in uncontrolled studies[40, 154] or in two preliminary controlled trials.[169] The side-effects of steroids, including catabolism, have recently been the subject of some interest, and the pendulum appears to be swinging away from steroids in the treatment of fulminant hepatic failure.

PERFUSION TECHNIQUES

With the exception of ‘artificial hepatic support’ which will be subsequently discussed, other forms of perfusion including exchange transfusion, plasmapheresis, cross-circulation and

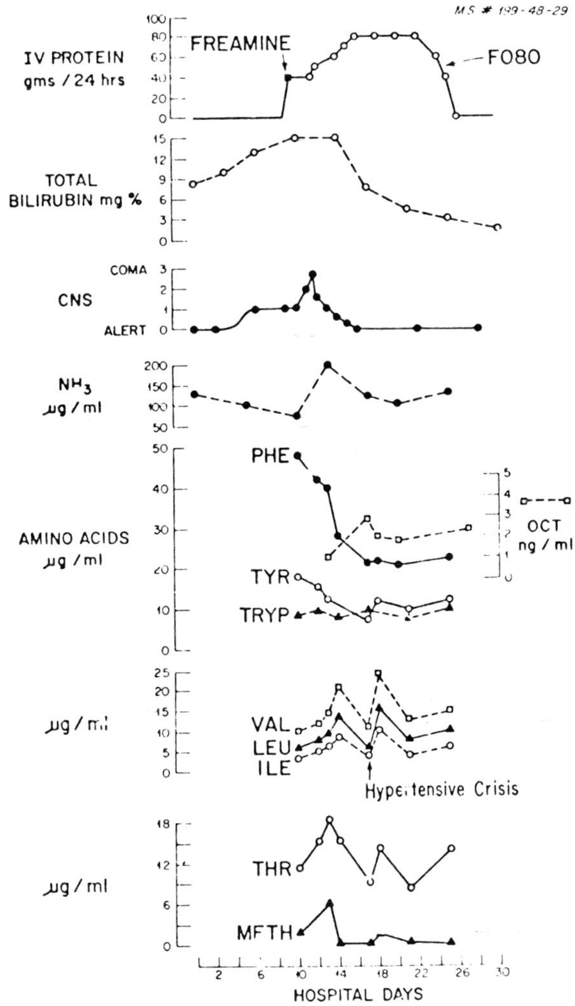

Figure 42.9. Therapy of acute viral hepatitis with FO80. Patient would not take oral nutrition, and an attempt was made to treat with a standard amino acid solution following which encephalopathy became marked. Note that shortly after the onset of proper nutrition with FO80, encephalopathy cleared, ammonia decreased, aromatic amino acids decreased and branched chain amino acids increased. A temporal relationship (which has been seen in many other patients) appears in which provision of adequate nutrition is associated with a return of bilirubin towards normal. Note also that a hypertensive crisis is associated with a decrease in the branched chain amino acids. (Abbreviations as in previous legends.)

perfusion with isolated porcine, bovine or baboon livers may be considered under one heading.[1, 23, 33, 111, 136, 146, 152, 155, 192] Perfusion using healthy livers has a theoretical advantage if the liver secretes a substance necessary for brain metabolism. Dramatic awakening from hepatic coma has been reported by several investigators, but increased survival has not resulted. In a recent prospective controlled trial using a small number of patients, exchange transfusion did not provide any benefit.[149] In the largest series reported, the results have been disappointing to the extent that this group has abandoned exchange transfusions.[165] Haemodialysis may provide temporary relief from renal failure but survival from the hepatorenal syndrome is rare. Hyperbaric oxygenation has also been employed without convincing effect.[85]

MISCELLANEOUS FORMS OF THERAPY

Acetohydroxamic acid has not been totally evaluated.[76] It is effective only when given systemically, and reduces ammonia levels when given orally but not rectally. It is rapidly absorbed from the upper gastrointestinal tract.[207] Side-effects have not been reported. Decreased venous blood ammonia has been recorded but little sustained clinical improvement was found.

A double lumen tube with large volumes of saline to perform colonic lavage has been used.[207] It is not clear whether this potentially hazardous technique has anything to offer compared with the usual cleansing enemas. In addition, fluid is rapidly absorbed from the colon and fluid overload becomes a hazard.

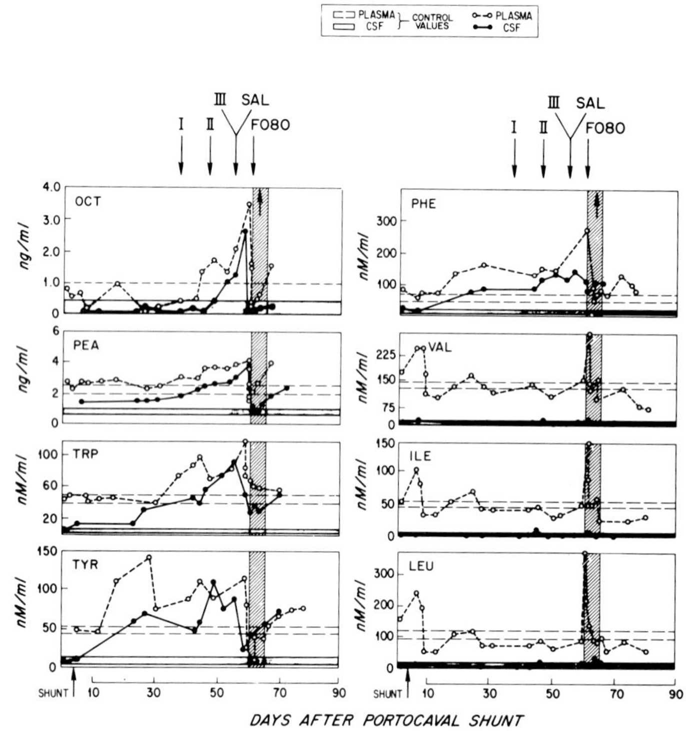

Figure 42.10. Plasma and CSF concentrations of octopamine, phenylethanolamine, tryptophan, tyrosine, phenylalanine and the three branched chain amino acids in a normal dog following end-to-side portacaval shunt and the development of hepatic encephalopathy. As the animal developed encephalopathy, octopamine, phenylethanolamine and the aromatic amino acids increased in the plasma and CSF. After the animal developed stage 3 encephalopathy, saline was administered for three days without improvement. The administration of FO80 decreased all levels of aromatic amino acids both in CSF and in the plasma to within normal limits, associated with the animal's prompt awakening. Note that the CSF concentrations of the branched chain amino acids remain unchanged. (Abbreviations as in previous legends.)

Feeding pure cultures of non-urease-producing lactobacilli to alter bowel flora and decrease production of ammonia has not been successful. Patient acceptance of lactobacillus colonization is poor and to date the clinical results are variable.[116, 147]

Another approach has been to immunize patients against urease, thereby decreasing the tolerance of the body for urease-producing bacteria. Jack–Bean urease has been administered in this attempt, and has been reported to decrease blood ammonia levels and increase ^{14}C-labelled urea in the urine. Severe reactions to this immunization have been reported, however, and the hazards of the treatment generally preclude its widespread use.[190, 191]

Manipulation of Plasma (and Presumably Brain) Amino Acids

With the recent emphasis on derangements of plasma amino acid patterns and their potential effects on the brain in hepatic encephalopathy, it seems inevitable that attempts should be made to alter plasma amino acid patterns to ameliorate hepatic encephalopathy. In general, these fall into two categories, infusional and 'laundering' techniques, which will be discussed in turn.

Infusional techniques

This form of therapy is being carried out on an experimental basis in several centres, generally in patients with chronic hepatic disease with acute decompensation. The theoretical purpose of this form of therapy is to provide comparatively large amounts of branched chain amino acids to decrease muscle catabolism, decrease the release of aromatic amino acids from muscle and promote their utilization, and to compete with the aromatic amino acids at the blood-brain barrier. Following the initial report of improvement in hepatic encephalopathy in patients with chronic liver disease given large amounts of protein in the form of special amino acid mixtures[75] (Figures 42.7, 42.8 and 42.9), other centres have confirmed the efficacy of this solution for nutritional support which is also associated with improvement in hepatic encephalopathy.[87] A randomized controlled trial is under way.

Further investigations in experimental

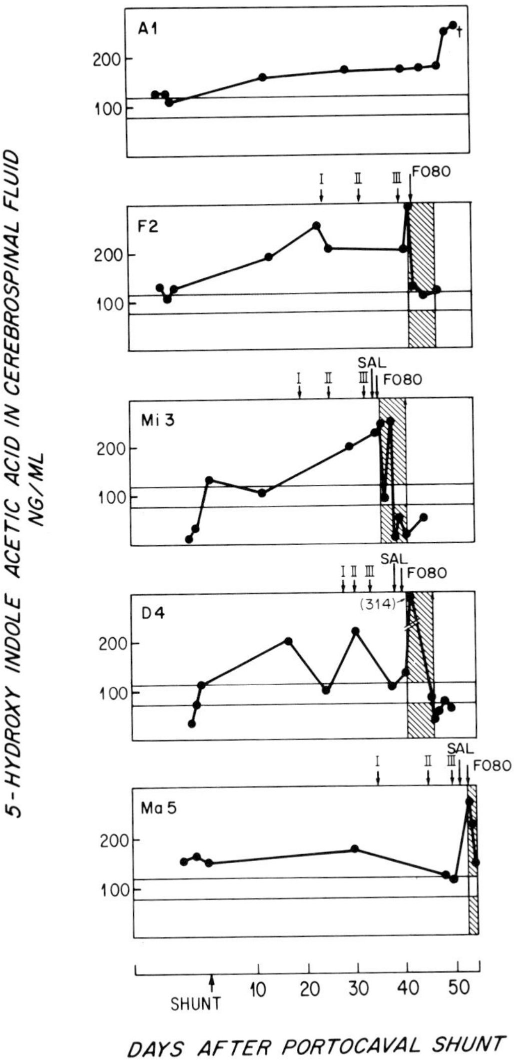

Figure 42.11. 5-Hydroxyindoleacetic acid in five monkeys with chronic indwelling lateral ventricular CSF cannulas, following end-to-side portacaval shunt. Note that (A1) when the animal remains untreated 5-hydroxyindoleacetic acid continues to rise and the animal dies in hepatic encephalopathy. The other four animals are allowed to pass through stages 1, 2 and 3 of encephalopathy, at which point an internal jugular cannula is placed and saline is infused. No improvement is noted. After three days of saline infusion, FO80, an amino acid mixture with 23 per cent dextrose rich in branched chain amino acids and poor in aromatic amino acids, is infused. Within 24 hours the animals awake from encephalopathy. A profound and rapid decrease in CSF 5-hydroxyindoleacetic acid is associated with infusion, indicating correction of abnormal indole metabolism.

animals with chronic indwelling catheters in their lateral ventricles, as well as in large and small animals in which brain and sagittal sinus blood amino acids have been measured, have revealed the following: as animals go into hepatic encephalopathy, concentrations of the aromatic amino acids, the sulphur-containing amino acids, tryptophan, and their amine derivatives including octopamine, phenylethanolamine, serotonin and the sulphur-containing inhibitory neurotransmitter, taurine, rise precipitously.[177,178] When amino acid infusions are given, the animal's neurological state improves. Simultaneously, CSF and, presumably, brain concentrations of the aromatic amino acids and their amine derivatives decrease precipitously as do the sulphur-containing amino acids in both dogs and monkeys[178] (Figures 42.10 and 42.11). With the later discovery that the blood-brain barrier is altered in chronic liver disease, perhaps secondary to decreased plasma leucine in a leucine-preferred system,[100] administration of leucine and the other branched chain amino acids will have a beneficial effect on restoring the blood-brain barrier towards normal, particularly in regard to the apparently isolated abnormality in the transport of 'large' neutral amino acids.[55,100]

With this form of therapy, up to 120 g protein equivalent in the form of amino acids have been administered to patients with protein intolerance in chronic hepatic encephalopathy with beneficial effects, including the clearing of encephalopathy and in some cases apparent improvement in hepatic function. Oral synthetic diets consisting of large amounts of branched chain amino acids and decreased aromatic amino acids appear to hold similar promise, as previously noted.[65] These findings may have distinct value in a group of patients with chronic post-shunt encephalopathy in whom inadequate protein and nutrition presumably contribute to the late deaths from hepatic failure.

The alpha-keto acids

Another approach to nutritional supplementation as well as to the improvement of encephalopathy uses the keto-analogues of the essential amino acids.[200]

In a series of patients with chronic hepatic encephalopathy, protein intolerance was apparently increased for long periods of time in patients given a mixture of the keto-analogues of five essential amino acids and four amino acids. The ammonia donor in this series appears to be glutamine, which was decreased.[117] Improved nutrition and clearing of hepatic encephalopathy were observed in some patients in unpredictable fashion, although caloric

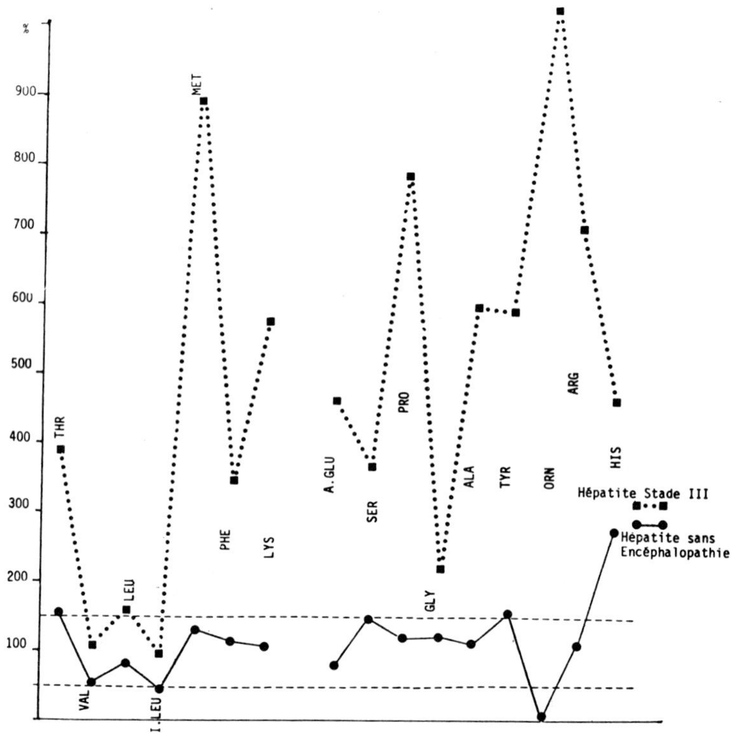

Figure 42.12. Amino acid patterns in patients with fulminant hepatitis, stage 3 coma and after perfusion with Rhone–Poulenc 6 from the data of Delafosse et al (personal communication). Note that in patients with hepatitis and encephalopathy stage 3, extremely high levels of methionine and phenylalanine and other amino acids are seen although the levels of the branched chain amino acids are normal (■ . . ■). The similarity between these data and those of Rosen et al[158] (Figure 42.2) is striking. After perfusion (●——●), amino acids return to normal levels and the patient awakens. (Abbreviations as in previous legends.)

intake was largely uncontrolled.[64] One beneficial effect of the alpha-keto analogues appears to be decreased muscle catabolism, as decreased plasma levels of tyrosine and glycine were observed in these patients despite the fact that tyrosine and glycine were not given. It is the author's belief that the use of alpha-keto analogues, either intravenously or orally, constitutes the most appropriate form of therapy for patients who are intolerant of nitrogen because of hepatorenal impairment, such as a hepatorenal syndrome. However, the amount of calcium and sodium with which these acids must be given (as salts) has so far prevented the widespread application of such nutritional therapy.

The artificial liver

It is becoming increasingly clear that in fulminant hepatitis, the hyperaminoacidaemia is so severe as to preclude the effectiveness of infusional techniques. Artificial haemo-perfusion techniques have greater promise. The first of these was a charcoal haemo-perfusion technique which was initially successful[81] but was abandoned when manufacturing problems and platelet clumping made hypotension an irremedial problem in such patients. Nonetheless, the increased percentage of patients waking up and surviving acute fulminant hepatitis, compared with prior experience, made this a promising form of therapy. A new form of therapy, which has received favourable comments, utilizes a polyacrilonitrile membrane with a pore size considerably larger than that of the standard artificial kidney cellophane membrane. With the polyacrilonitrile membrane, clearance of amino acids is extremely rapid, with up to 50 g cleared in four hours. Restoration of consciousness of patients with acute fulminant hepatitis has been considerably greater than that of associated controlled groups, although they were neither temporally matched nor observed simultaneously.[133]

Survival from acute fulminant hepatitis in one group,[45, 175] though not in another,[133] appears to be greater than that previously observed.

While it has generally been supposed by at least one author that the branched chain amino acids are not cleared by this form of therapy[133] this does not appear to be the case.[45, 175] Delafosse and his co-workers have used theoretical considerations in protecting the brain by adding large amounts (up to 60 g/24 hr), of branched chain amino acids in association with polyacrilonitrile membrane perfusion.[45] In their early experience, they report a 100 per cent restoration of consciousness for patients with acute fulminant hepatitis (Figure 42.12). This may be secondary to the observed effect of large doses of branched chain amino acids in protecting the blood-brain barrier against the large amounts of aromatic amino acids (Figure 42.6). The beneficial effects of polyacrilonitrile membrane haemodialysis may be secondary to clearance of amino acids or, as recently proposed, of 'middle' molecules.[133] The amino acid clearance data of Opolon,[133] however, appear to be at variance with those of other investigators and the results can be explained on the basis of amino acid changes alone, without resorting to data on peptides. One particular problem which remains to be resolved with polyacrilonitrile haemodialysis is the myopathy which follows the clearance of such large amounts of amino acids, and which takes up to a year to improve.[174] This may be partially ameliorated by providing optimal nutrition in the form of selected amino acids and/or hypertonic glucose in such patients.

Amino acid ratios

It has been proposed that the relationship between the molar ratios of the various neutral amino acids of the large neutral amino acid group may be helpful in correlating plasma aromatic amino acids with hepatic encephalopathy.[74] While all workers may agree that an abnormally low ratio of branched chain amino acids to aromatic amino acids occurs either in the presence of severe liver disease or indicates hepatic encephalopathy, many investigators do not agree that the ratio is useful in determining the grade of encephalopathy. As stated previously, the behaviour of the blood-brain barrier indicates that two forces are at work in the uptake of the toxic aromatic amino acids in hepatic encephalopathy: the first is the chronically low concentration of branched chain amino acids in the plasma which alters the blood-brain barrier, a leucine-preferred system, and allows increased uptake of aromatic amino acids at the same rate as the brain attempts to maintain normal concentrations of leucine; the second, as shown in Figure 42.5, is the absolute concentrations of the aromatic amino acids. Proper therapy of hepatic encephalopathy involves a decrease in the concentration of aromatic amino acids, either by infusional or by 'plasma laundering' techniques.

The results presented here may suggest a unifying relationship between many metabolic comas. The disorders in nitrogen metabolism are present in uraemia with abnormalities in plasma amino acids, as well as in the metabolic coma accompanying sepsis in which a plasma amino acid pattern remarkably similar to that shown in hepatic failure exists, and which includes decreased branched chain amino acids and markedly increased aromatic amino acids.[77] Understanding the behaviour of the blood-brain barrier as well as peripheral metabolism in these various disorders may enable the proper diagnosis and therapy of these metabolic dysfunctions of the brain to be given.

REFERENCES

1. Abouna, G.M. (1972) Improved technique of exchange transfusion for hepatic coma. *Surgery, Gynecology and Obstetrics*, **134**, 658–662.
2. Abramsky, O. & Goldschmidt, Z. (1972) Treatment and prevention of acute hepatic encephalopathy by intravenous levodopa. *Surgery*, **75**, 188–193.
3. Agostini, L., Down, P.F., Murison, J. & Wrong, O.M. (1972) Faecal ammonia with pH during lactulose administration in man: a comparison with other cathartics. *Gut*, **13**, 829–866.
4. Aguirre, A., Yoshimura, M., Westman, T. & Fischer, J.E. (1974) Plasma amino acids in dogs with two experimental forms of liver damage. *Journal of Surgical Research*, **16**, 339–345.
5. Athanasoulis, C.A., Baum, S.A., Waltman, A., Ring, E.J., Imbembo, A. & Vander Salm, T.J. (1974) Control of acute gastric mucosal hemorrhage. *New England Journal of Medicine*, **290**, 597–603.
6. Baertl, J.M., Sancetta, S.M. & Gabuzda, G.J. (1963) Relation of acute potassium depletion to renal ammonium metabolism in patient with cirrhosis. *Journal of Clinical Investigation*, **42**, 696–707.
7. Baldessarini, R.J. (1971) Release of aromatic amines from brain tissues of the rat in vitro. *Journal of Neurochemistry*, **18**, 2509–2518.
8. Baldessarini, R.J. (1978) Biological transmethylation of *S*-adenosylmethionine. Development of assay methods and implications for neuropsychiatry. *International Review of Neurobiology*. In press.

9. Baldessarini, R.J. & Fischer, J.E. (1967) *S*-adenosylmethionine following portacaval anastomoses. *Surgery,* **62,** 311–318.
10. Baldessarini, R.J. & Fischer, J.E. (1973) Serotonin metabolism in rat brain after surgical diversion of the portal venous circulation. *Nature* (*New Biology*), **254,** 272–275.
11. Baldessarini, R.J. & Karobath, M. (1973) Biochemical physiology of central synapses. *Annual Review of Physiology,* **35,** 273–304.
12. Baldessarini, R.J. & Vogt, M. (1971) The uptake and subcellular distribution of aromatic amines in the brain of the rat. *Journal of Neurochemistry,* **18,** 2519–2533.
13. Baldessarini, R.J. & Yorke, C. (1974) Uptake and release of possible false transmitter amino acids by rat brain tissue. *Journal of Neurochemistry,* **23,** 839–848.
14. Benjamin, A.M. & Quastel, J.H. (1972) Location of amino acids in brain slices from the rat. *Biochemical Journal,* **128,** 631–646.
15. Berk, D.P. & Chalmers, T. (1970) Deafness complicating antibiotic therapy of hepatic encephalopathy. *Annals of Internal Medicine,* **73,** 393–396.
16. Berl, S., Takajaki, G., Clarke, D.D. & Waelsch, H. (1962) Metabolic compartments in vivo: ammonia and glutamine acid metabolism in brain and liver. *Journal of Biology and Chemistry,* **237,** 2562–2569.
17. Bessman, S.P. & Bessman, A.W. (1955) The cerebral and peripheral uptake of ammonia in liver disease with a hypothesis for the mechanism of hepatic coma. *Journal of Clinical Investigation,* **34,** 622–628.
18. Bessman, A.N. & Mirick, G.S. (1958) Blood ammonia levels following the ingestion of casein and whole blood. *Journal of Clinical Investigation,* **37,** 990–998.
19. Biebuyck, J., Funovics, J., Dedrick, D.F., Scherer, Y.D. & Fischer, J.E. (1975) Neurochemistry of hepatic coma. Alterations in putative neurotransmitter amino acids. In *Artificial Liver Support* (Ed.) Williams, R. & Murray-Lyon, I.M. pp. 51–60. London: Pitman Medical.
20. Bircher, J., Muller, J., Guggenheim, P. & Haemmerli, U.P. (1966) Treatment of chronic portal–systemic encephalopathy with lactulose. *Lancet,* **i,** 890–892.
21. Bollman, J.R., Flock, E.V., Grindlay, J.H., Bickford, R.G. & Lichtenheld, F.R. (1957) Coma with increased amino acids of brain in dogs with Eck's fistula. *Archives of Surgery,* **75,** 405–411.
22. Bonnycastel, D.D. & Delia, C.W. (1950) Effect of hepatectomy upon the analgesic action of L-methadone. *Proceedings of the Society for Experimental Biology and Medicine,* **74,** 589–591.
23. Bosman, S.C.W., Terblanche, J., Saunders, G.G., Harrison, G.G. & Barnard, C.N. (1968) Cross-circulation between man and baboon. *Lancet,* **ii,** 583–585.
24. Brandau, K. & Axelrod, J. (1972) The biosynthesis of octopamine. *Naunyn Schmiedebergs Archives of Pharmacology,* **273,** 123–133.
25. Brayton, R.G., Stokes, P.E., Schwartz, M.S. & Louria, D.B. (1970) Effect of alcohol and various diseases on leukocyte mobilization, phagocytosis and intracellular bacterial killing. *New England Journal of Medicine,* **282,** 123–128.
26. Breen, K.J., Shaw, J., Alvin, J., Henderson, G.I., Hoyumpa, A.M. & Schenker, S. (1973) The effect of experimental hepatic injury on the clearance of phenobarbital and paraldehyde. *Gastroenterology,* **64,** 992–1004.
27. Brennan, M.F., Aoki, T.T., Muller, W.A. & Cahill, G.F. Jr (1974) The role of glucagon as a catabolic hormone. *Surgical Forum,* **25,** 72–74.
28. Budd, M., Tanaka, K., Holmes, L.B., Efron, M.L., Crawford, J.D. & Isselbacher, K.J. (1967) Isovaleric acidemia: clinical features of a new genetic defect of leucine metabolism. *New England Journal of Medicine,* **277,** 321–327.
29. Carter, C.C., Lifton, J.F. & Welch, M.J. (1973) Organ uptake and blood pH and concentration effects of ammonia in dogs determined with ammonia labelled with 10 minutes half-lived nitrogen 13. *Neurology,* **23,** 204–213.
30. Chen, S., Mahadevan, V. & Zieve, L. (1970) Volatile fatty acids in the breath of patients with cirrhosis of the liver. *Journal of Laboratory and Clinical Medicine,* **75,** 622–627.
31. Clark, R., Borirakchanyavat, V., Davidson, A.R., Thompson, R.P.H., Widdop, B., Goulding, R. & Williams, R. (1973) Hepatic damage and death from overdose of paracetamol. *Lancet,* **i,** 66–70.
32. Condon, R.E. (1971) Effect of dietary protein on symptoms and survival in dogs with an Eck fistula. *American Journal of Surgery,* **121,** 107–114.
33. Condon, R.E., Bombeck, D.T. & Steigmann, P. (1970) Heterologous bovine liver perfusion therapy of acute hepatic failure. *American Journal of Surgery,* **119,** 147–154.
34. Conn, H.O. (1960) Asterixis in non-hepatic disorders. *American Journal of Medicine,* **29,** 647–661.
35. Conn, H.O. (1973) Current diagnosis and treatment of hepatic coma. *Hospital Practice,* **8,** 65–72.
36. Conn, H.O. & Fessel, J.M. (1971) Spontaneous bacterial peritonitis in cirrhosis: variation on a theme. *Medicine,* **50,** 161–197.
37. Conn, H.O. & Simpson, J.A. (1967) Excessive mortality with balloon tamponade. *Journal of the American Medical Association,* **202,** 587–592.
38. Conn, H.O., Ramsley, G.R. & Storer, E.H. (1972) Selective intraarterial vasopressin in the treatment of upper gastrointestinal tract hemorrhage. *Gastroenterology,* **63,** 634–645.
39. Conn, H.O., Leevy, C.M., Maddrey, W.C., Rodgers, J.B., Seeff, L. & Vlachevic, Z.R. (1974) Lactulose in the treatment of chronic portal systemic encephalopathy. A prospective double-blind cooperative comparison of lactulose with neomycin. *Gastroenterology,* **67,** 784 (abstract).
40. Cook, G.C. & Sherlock, S. (1965) Jaundice and its relation to therapeutic agents. *Lancet,* **i,** 175–179.
41. Crout, J.F., Alpers, H.S., Tatum, E.L. & Shore, P.A. (1964) Release of metaraminol (Aramine) from the heart by sympathetic nerve stimulation. *Science,* **145,** 828–829.
42. Cummings, M.G., Soeters, P.B., James, J.H., Keane, J.M. & Fischer, J.E. (1976) Regional brain indoleamine metabolism following chronic portacaval anastomosis in the rat. *Journal of Neurochemistry,* **27,** 501–509.
43. Cummings, M.G., James, J.H., Soeters, P.B., Keane, J.M., Foster, J. & Fischer, J.E. (1976) Regional brain study of indoleamine metabolism in the rat in acute hepatic failure. *Journal of Neurochemistry,* **27,** 741–746.
44. Dawson, A.M. & Sherlock, S. (1957) Effect of an amine oxidase inhibitor on arterial ammonium levels in liver disease. *Lancet,* **i,** 1332–1333.

45. Delafosse, B., Bouletreau, P. & Motin, J. (1977) Variation des acides amines plasmatiques au cours des hépatites graves avec encephalopathie. *La Nouvelle Presse Médicale,* **6,** 1207–1211.
46. DeMeo, A.N. & Andersen, B.R. (1972) Defective chemotaxis associated with a serum inhibition in cirrhotic patients. *New England Journal of Medicine,* **286,** 735–740.
47. Descarries, L., Beaudet, A. & Watkins, K.C. (1975) Serotonin nerve terminals in adult rat neocortex. *Brain Research,* **100,** 563–588.
48. Descarries, L., Watkins, K.C. & Lapierre, Y. (1977) Noradrenergic axon terminals in the cerebral cortex of rat. III. Topometric ultrastructural analysis. *Brain Research,* **133,** 197–222.
49. Dismukes, K. (1977) New look at the aminergic nervous system. *Nature,* **269,** 557–558.
50. Dodsworth, J.M., James, J.H., Cummings, M.G. & Fischer, J.E. (1973) Diagnosis and therapy of hepatorenal syndrome: a tentative classification. *Surgical Forum,* **24,** 396–398.
51. Dodsworth, J.M., James, J.H., Cummings, M.G. & Fischer, J.E. (1974) Depletion of brain norepinephrine in acute hepatic coma. *Surgery,* **75,** 811–820.
52. Duffy, T.E., Vergara, F. & Plum, F. (1974) α-Ketoglutaramate in hepatic encephalopathy. *Research Publications, Association for Research in Nervous and Mental Disease,* **53,** 39–52.
53. Elkington, S.G., Floch, M.H. & Conn, H.O. (1969) Lactulose in the treatment of chronic portal–systemic encephalopathy. A double-blind clinical trial. *New England Journal of Medicine,* **281,** 408–413.
54. Erbsloh, F. (1963) Comments on liver brain correlations in systemic hypoxaemia. In *Selective Vulnerability of the Brain in Hypoxaemia* (Ed.) Schade, J.P. & McMenamy, W.H. pp. 305–308. Philadelphia: F.A. Davis.
55. Escourrou, J., James, J.H. & Fischer, J.E. (1978) Effects of portacaval anastomosis on blood barrier: neutral amino acid transport. *Journal of Neurochemistry.* In press.
56. Escourrou, J., James, J.H., Hodgman, J.M. & Fischer, J.E. (1976) Effect of branched chain amino acids on plasma and brain amino acids and brain neurotransmitters. *Gastroenterology,* **71,** 904 (abstract).
57. Faloon, W.W., Pase, I., Woodfolk, C., Nankin, H., Wallace, K. & Haro, E.N. (1965) Effect of neomycin and kanamycin upon intestinal absorption. *Annals of the New York Academy of Sciences,* **132,** 879–887.
58. Fazekas, J.F., Ticktin, H.E., Ehrmantraut, W.R. & Alman, R.W. (1956) Cerebral metabolism in hepatic insufficiency. *American Journal of Medicine,* **21,** 843–849.
59. Felig, P., Brown, W.V., Levine, R.A. & Klatskin, G. (1970) Glucose homeostasis in viral hepatitis. *New England Journal of Medicine,* **283,** 1436–1440.
60. Fenton, J.C.B., Knight, E.J. & Humpherson, P.L. (1966) Milk and cheese diet in portal–systemic encephalopathy. *Lancet,* **i,** 164–165.
61. Fernstrom, J.D. & Wurtman, R.J. (1971) Brain serotonin content: physiological dependence on plasma tryptophan levels. *Science,* **173,** 149–151.
62. Fessel, J.M. & Conn, H.O. (1972) An analysis of the causes and prevention of hepatic coma. *Gastroenterology,* **62,** 191 (abstract).
63. Fischer, J.E. (1974) False neurotransmitter and hepatic coma. *Research Publications, Association for Research in Nervous and Mental Disease,* **53,** 53–73.
64. Fischer, J.E. (1976) Non-amino acids: non-toxic or antitoxic. *Gastroenterology,* **71,** 329 (editorial).
65. Fischer, J.E. (1977) Unpublished observations.
66. Fischer, J.E. & Baldessarini, R.J. (1971) False neurotransmitters and hepatic failure. *Lancet,* **ii,** 75–79.
67. Fischer, J.E. & Baldessarini, R.J. (1976) Pathogenesis and therapy of hepatic coma. In *Progress in Liver Disease* (Ed.) Popper, H. & Schaffner, F. pp. 363–397. New York: Grune & Stratton.
68. Fischer, J.E. & James, J.H. (1972) Treatment of hepatic coma and hepatorenal syndrome: mechanism of action of L-dopa and aramine. *American Journal of Surgery,* **123,** 222–230.
69. Fischer, J.E., Freund, H. & Rosen, H.M. (1977) Changes in plasma amino acid patterns following diuresis in patients with cirrhosis. Unpublished observations.
70. Fischer, J.E., Funovics, J.M. & Falcao, H.A. (1976) L-dopa in hepatic coma. *Annals of Surgery,* **183,** 386–391.
71. Fischer, J.E., Horst, W.D. & Kopin, I.J. (1965) β-hydroxylated sympathomimetic amines as false neurotransmitters. *British Journal of Pharmacology,* **24,** 477–484.
72. Fischer, J.E., James, J.H., Keane, J.M., Shuman, L., Dodsworth, J. & Funovics, J.M. (1974) An alternative mechanism for beneficial effects of intestinal sterilization in hepatic encephalopathy. *Surgical Forum,* **25,** 369–372.
73. Fischer, J.E., Yoshimura, N., James, J.H., Cummings, M.G., Abel, R.M. & Deindoerfer, F. (1974) Plasma amino acids in patients with hepatic encephalopathy: effects of amino acid infusions. *American Journal of Surgery,* **127,** 40–47.
74. Fischer, J.E., Funovics, J.M., Aguirre, A., James, J.H., Keane, J.M., Wesdorp, R.I.C., Yoshimura, N. & Westman, T. (1975) The role of plasma amino acids in hepatic encephalopathy. *Surgery,* **38,** 276–290.
75. Fischer, J.E., Rosen, H.M., Ebeid, A.M., James, J.H., Keane, J.M. & Soeters, P.B. (1976) The effect of normalization of plasma amino acids on hepatic encephalopathy in man. *Surgery,* **80,** 77–91.
76. Fishbein, W.M., Carbone, P.P. & Hochstein, H.D. (1965) Acetohydroxamate: bacterial urease inhibitor with therapeutic potential in hyperammonaemic states. *Nature,* **208,** 46–48.
77. Freund, H., Ryan, J.A. & Fischer, J.E. (1979) Amino acid derangements in patients with overwhelming sepsis: treatment with branched chain amino acid rich infusions. *Annals of Surgery.* In press.
78. Freund, H., Smith, A.R., Rossi-Fanelli, K., Krause, R. & Fischer, J.E. (1978) Metabolic encephalopathy and coma produced by phenylalanine and tryptophan. Submitted for publication.
79. Fulkes, R.M., Li, J.B. & Goldberg, A.L. (1975) Effect of insulin, glucose and amino acids on protein turnover in rat diaphragm. *Journal of Biological Chemistry,* **250,** 280–298.
80. Funovics, J.M. & Soeters, P.B. (1976) Unpublished observations.
81. Gazzard, B., Weston, M.J., Murray-Lyon, I.M., Flax, H., Record, C.O., Portman, B., Langley, P.G., Dunlop, E.H., Mellon, P.J., Ward, M.B. & Williams, R. (1974) Charcoal hemoperfusion in the treatment of fulminant hepatic failure. *Lancet,* **i,** 1301–1307.
82. Geiger, A. & Yamasaki, S. (1956) Cytidine and uridine requirements of the brain. *Journal of Neurochemistry,* **1,** 93–100.

83. Gilon, E., Szeinberg, A., Tauman, G. & Bodonyi, E. (1959) Glutamine estimation in cerebrospinal fluid in cases of liver cirrhosis and hepatic coma. *Journal of Laboratory and Clinical Medicine,* **53,** 714–719.
84. Goetchus, J.S. & Webster, L.T. (1965) γ-aminobutyrate and hepatic coma. *Journal of Laboratory and Clinical Medicine,* **65,** 257–267.
85. Goulon, M., Rapin, M., Barois, A., Got, C., Grobuis, S., Gajdos, P. & Azizi, P.P. (1971) Essai de traitement des hépatites virales graves par l'oxygen-hyperbare. *Annals de Médecine Interne (Paris),* **122,** 93–98.
86. Greenberger, N.J., Carley, J.E. & Schenker, S. (1976) Diet therapy of chronic hepatic encephalopathy (CHE): role of vegetable protein and carbohydrate loading. *Gastroenterology,* **69,** 825 (abstract).
87. Haalberg, D. (1977) Personal communication.
88. Hardwick, D.F., Applegarth, D.A., Cockcroft, D.M., Ross, P.M. & Calder, R.J. (1970) Pathogenesis of methionine induced toxicity. *Metabolism,* **19,** 381–391.
89. Hawkins, J., Miller, A.L., Nielsen, R.C. & Veech, R.L. (1973) The acute action of ammonia on rat brain metabolism in vivo. *Biochemistry Journal,* **134,** 1001–1008.
90. Hindfeldt, B. & Siesjo, B.K. (1970) The effect of ammonia on the energy metabolism of the rat brain. *Life Sciences,* **9,** 1021–1028.
91. Hindfeldt, B., Plum, F. & Duffy, T.E. (1977) Effect of acute ammonia intoxication on cerebral metabolism in rats with portacaval shunts. *Journal of Clinical Investigation,* **59,** 386–396.
92. Holm, E. (1975) *Ammoniak und hepatische Enzephalopathie.* Stuttgart: Gustav Fischer Verlag.
93. Hourani, B.T., Hamlin, E.M. & Reynolds, T.B. (1971) Cerebrospinal fluid glutamine as a measure of hepatic encephalopathy. *Archives of Internal Medicine,* **127,** 1033–1036.
94. Iber, F.L., Rosen, H., Levenson, S.M. & Chalmers, T.C. (1957) The plasma amino acids in patients with liver failure. *Journal of Laboratory and Clinical Medicine,* **50,** 417–425.
95. Iob, V., Coon, W.W. & Sloan, M. (1966) Altered clearance of free amino acids from plasma of patients with cirrhosis of the liver. *Journal of Surgical Research,* **6,** 233–239.
96. Iob, V., Mattson, W.J. Jr, Sloan, M., Coon, W.W., Turcotte, J.G. & Child, C.G. III (1970) Alterations in plasma-free amino acids in dogs with hepatic insufficiency. *Surgery, Gynecology and Obstetrics,* **130,** 794–801.
97. Jackson, F.C., Perrin, E.B., Feux, W.R. & Smith, A.G. (1971) A clinical investigation of the portacaval shunt. V. Survival analysis of the therapeutic operation. *Annals of Surgery,* **174,** 672–698.
98. Jaffe, J.H. (1970) Narcotic analgesics. In *The Pharmacologic Basis of Therapeutics* (Ed.) Goodman, L.S. & Gilman, A. pp. 237–275. New York: Macmillan.
99. James, J.H. & Fischer, J.E. (1975) Release of octopamine and α-methyloctopamine by L-dopa. *Biochemical Pharmacology,* **24,** 1099–1101.
100. James, J.H., Escourrou, J. & Fischer, J.E. (1978) Portacaval anastomosis increases the activity of blood brain neutral amino acid transport. *Science.* In press.
101. James, J.H., Hodgman, J.M., Funovics, J.M., Yoshimura, N. & Fischer, J.E. (1976) Brain tryptophan, plasma free tryptophan and distribution of plasma neutral amino acids. *Metabolism,* **25,** 471–476.
102. Johnson, W.D., Stokes, P. & Kaye, D. (1969) The effect of intravenous ethanol on the bactericidal activity of human serum. *Yale Journal of Biology and Medicine,* **42,** 71–85.
103. Katz, R., Velasco, M., Klinger, J. & Alessandri, H. (1962) Corticosteroids in the treatment of acute hepatitis in coma. *Gastroenterology,* **42,** 258–266.
104. Klion, F.M., Schaffner, R. & Popper, H. (1969) Hepatitis after exposure to halothane. *Annals of Internal Medicine,* **71,** 467–477.
105. Knell, A.J., Davidson, A.R., Williams, R., Kantamaneni, B.D. & Curzon, G. (1974) Dopamine and serotonin metabolism in hepatic encephalopathy. *British Medical Journal,* **ii,** 549–551.
106. Knott, P.J. & Curzon, G. (1974) Effect of increased rat brain tryptophan on 5-hydroxytryptamine and 5-hydroxyindolyl acetic acid in the hypothalamus and other brain regions. *Journal of Neurochemistry,* **22,** 1065–1071.
107. Kopin, I.J. (1968) False adrenergic transmitters. *Annual Review of Pharmacology,* **8,** 377–394.
108. Kunin, C.M., Chalmers, T.C., Leevy, C.M., Sebastyen, S.C., Lieber, C.S. & Finland, M. (1960) Absorption of orally-administered neomycin and kanamycin. *New England Journal of Medicine,* **262,** 380–385.
109. Laidlaw, J., Read, A.E. & Sherlock, S. (1961) Morphine tolerance with hepatic cirrhosis. *Gastroenterology,* **40,** 389–397.
110. Lam, K.C., Tall, A.R., Goldstein, G.B. & Mistillis, S.P. (1973) Role of a false neurotransmitter, octopamine, in the pathogenesis of hepatic and renal encephalopathy. *Scandinavian Journal of Gastroenterology,* **8,** 465–472.
111. Lepore, M.J. & Martel, A.J. (1970) Plasmapheresis with plasma exchange in hepatic coma. *Annals of Internal Medicine,* **72,** 165–174.
112. Livingstone, A.S., Potvin, M., Goresky, C.A., Finlayson, M.K. & Hinchey, E.J. (1977) Changes in the blood brain barrier in hepatic coma after hepatectomy in the rat. *Gastroenterology,* **73,** 697–704.
113. Louria, D.B. (1963) Susceptibility to infection during experimental alcohol intoxication. *Transactions of the Association of American Physicians,* **76,** 102–112.
114. Lucke, B. & Mallory, T. (1946) The fulminant form of epidemic hepatitis. *American Journal of Pathology,* **22,** 867–945.
115. Lunzer, M., James, I.M., Weisman, J. & Sherlock, S. (1974) Treatment of chronic hepatic encephalopathy with levodopa. *Gut,* **15,** 555–562.
116. MacBeth, W.A.A.G., Kass, E.H. & McDermott, W.V. (1965) Treatment of hepatic encephalopathy by alteration of intestinal flora with *Lactobacillus acidophilus. Lancet,* **i,** 399–403.
117. Maddrey, W.C., Weber, F.L., Coulter, A.W. & Walser, M. (1976) Effects of ketoanalogues of essential amino acids in portal systemic encephalopathy. *Gastroenterology,* **71,** 190–195.
118. Manghani, K.K., Lunzer, M.R., Billing, B.H. & Sherlock, S. (1975) Urinary and serum octopamine in patients with portal systemic encephalopathy. *Lancet,* **ii,** 943–946.
119. Mashford, M.L., Mahon, W.A. & Chalmers, T.C. (1962) Studies of the cardiovascular system in the hypotension of liver failure. *New England Journal of Medicine,* **267,** 1071–1074.

120. Mattson, W.J. Jr, Iob, V., Sloan, M., Coon, W.W., Turcotte, J.G. & Child, C.G. III (1970) Alterations of individual free amino acids in brain during acute hepatic coma. *Surgery, Gynecology and Obstetrics*, **130,** 263–266.

121. Mays, E.T. (1972) Encephalopathy and fatty acid toxicity. *Surgical Forum*, **23,** 352–354.

122. McDermott, W.V. & Adams, R.D. (1954) Episodic stupor associated with Eck fistula in the human with particular reference to the metabolism of ammonia. *Journal of Clinical Investigation*, **33,** 1–9.

123. McDermott, W.V., Victor, M. & Point, W.W. (1962) Exclusion of the colon in the treatment of hepatic encephalopathy. *New England Journal of Medicine*, **267,** 850–854.

124. Morgan, M. & Sherlock, S. (1977) Presented in discussion at conference on *Fulminant Hepatic Failure*, Washington, D.C. February 7–8, 1977.

125. Morgan, M.H., Bolton, C.H., Morris, J.S. & Read, E.A. (1974) Medium chain triglycerides and hepatic encephalopathy. *Gut*, **15,** 180–184.

126. Munro, H.N., Fernstrom, T.D. & Wurtman, R.T. (1975) Insulin plasma amino acid imbalance and hepatic coma. *Lancet*, **i,** 722–724.

127. Murray-Lyon, I.M., Young, J., Parkes, J.D., Knill-Jones, R.P. & Williams, R. (1971) Clinical and electroencephalographic assessment of diazepam in liver disease. *British Medical Journal*, **iv,** 265–266.

128. Muscholl, E. & Maitre, L. (1963) Release by sympathetic stimulation of α-methylnoradrenaline stored in the heart after administration of α-methyldopa. *Experientia*, **19,** 658–670.

129. Nance, F.C., Batson, R.C. & Kline, D.G. (1971) Ammonia production in germ-free Eck fistula dogs. *Surgery*, **70,** 169–174.

130. Ng, K.Y., Chase, T.N., Colburn, R.W. & Kopin, I.J. (1970) L-dopa induced release of cerebral monoamines. *Science*, **170,** 76–78.

131. Oddessey, R. & Goldberg, A.L. (1972) Oxidation of leucine by rat skeletal muscle. *American Journal of Physiology*, **223,** 1376–1383.

132. Oldendorf, W.K. (1971) Brain uptake of radiolabelled amino acids, amines, and hexoses after arterial injection. *American Journal of Physiology*, **221,** 1629–1639.

133. Opolon, P., Rapin, J.R., Huguet, C., Granger, A., Delorine, M.L., Boschat, M. & Sausse, A. (1976) Hepatic failure coma (HFC) treated by polyacrilonitrile membrane (PAN) hemodialysis (HD). *Transactions of the American Society of Artificial Internal Organs*, **22,** 701–708.

134. Ordonez, L.A. & Wurtman, R.J. (1973) Enzymes catalyzing the de novo synthesis of methyl groups in the brain and other tissues of the rat. *Journal of Neurochemistry*, **21,** 1447–1455.

135. Pant, S.S., Ribeiz, J. & Richardson, E.P. (1968) Spastic paraparesis following portacaval shunt. *Neurology*, **18,** 134–141.

136. Parbhoo, S.P., Kennedy, J., James, I.M., Chalstrey, L.J., Ajdukiewicz, A., Brock, P.J., Xanalatos, C., Sayer, P. & Sherlock, S. (1971) Extracorporeal pig liver perfusion in treatment of hepatic coma due to fulminant hepatitis. *Lancet*, **i,** 659–665.

137. Parkes, J.D., Sharpstone, P. & Williams, R. (1970) Levodopa in hepatic coma. *Lancet*, **ii,** 1341–1343.

138. Perez Cruet, J., Chase, T.N. & Murphy, D.L. (1973) Dietary regulation of brain tryptophan and neutral amino acids in human. *Nature*, **248,** 693–695.

139. Peters, R.L., Edmondson, H.A., Reynolds, T.B., Meister, J.C. & Curphey, T.J. (1969) Hepatic necrosis associated with halothane anesthesia. *American Journal of Medicine*, **47,** 748–764.

140. Phear, E.A., Ruebner, B., Sherlock, S. & Summerskill, W.H.J. (1956) Methionine toxicity in liver disease and its prevention by chlortetracycline. *Clinical Science*, **15,** 93–117.

141. Phillips, G.B., Schwartz, R., Gabuzda, G.J. & Davidson, C.S. (1952) The syndrome of impending hepatic coma in patients with cirrhosis of liver given nitrogenous substances. *New England Journal of Medicine*, **247,** 239–246.

142. Pitts, R.F. (1971) The role of ammonia production and excretion in regulation of acid base balance. *New England Journal of Medicine*, **284,** 32–41.

143. Polli, E., Bianchi-Porro, G. & Maiolo, A.T. (1969) Cerebral metabolism after portacaval shunt. *Lancet*, **i,** 153–156.

144. Posado, J.G., Penicha, J.H. & Tirado-Arroyava, S. (1972) Effect of 3,4-dihydroxyphenylalanine (L-dopa) in hepatic coma. *Archivos de Investigacion Medica*, **3,** 1–8.

145. Posner, J.B. & Plum, F. (1960) The toxic effects of carbon dioxide and acetazolamide in hepatic encephalopathy. *Journal of Clinical Investigation*, **39,** 1246–1258.

146. Ranek, L., Hansen, R.I., Hilden, M., Ramsoe, K., Schmidt, A., Winkler, K. & Tygstrup, N. (1971) Pig liver perfusion in the treatment of acute hepatic failure. *Scandinavian Journal of Gastroenterology*, **9,** 161–169 (supplement).

147. Read, A.E., McCarthy, C.F., Heaton, K.W. & Laidlaw, J. (1966) *Lactobacillus acidophilus* (Enpac) in the treatment of hepatic encephalopathy. *British Medical Journal*, **i,** 1267–1270.

148. Read, A.E., Sherlock, S., Laidlaw, J. & Walker, J.G. (1967) The neuropsychiatric syndromes associated with chronic liver disease and an extensive portalsystemic collateral circulation. *Quarterly Journal of Medicine*, **36,** 135–150.

149. Redeker, A.G. & Yamahiro, H.S. (1973) Controlled trial of exchange transfusion therapy in fulminant hepatitis. *Lancet*, **i,** 3–6.

150. Resnick, R.H., Iber, F.L., Isihara, A.M., Chalmers, T.C., Zimmerman, H. & the Boston Inter-hospital Liver Group (1974) A controlled study of the therapeutic portacaval shunt. *Gastroenterology*, **67,** 843–857.

151. Reye, R.D.K., Morgan, G. & Baral, J. (1963) Encephalopathy and fatty degeneration of the viscera. A disease entity in childhood. *Lancet*, **ii,** 749–752.

152. Reynolds, T.B. (1969) Exchange transfusion in fulminant hepatic failure. *Gastroenterology*, **56,** 170–172.

153. Richmond, J. & Girdwood, R.H. (1962) Observations on amino acid absorption. *Clinical Science*, **22,** 301–314.

154. Ritt, D.J., Whelan, G., Werner, D.J., Eigenbrodt, E.H., Schenker, S. & Combes, B. (1969) Acute hepatic necrosis with stupor or coma. *Medicine*, **48,** 151–172.

155. Rivera, R.A., Slaughter, R.L. & Boyce, H.W. (1970) Exchange transfusion in the treatment of patients with acute hepatitis in coma. *American Journal of Digestive Diseases*, **15,** 580–602.

156. Rivera-Calimlim, L., Dujovne, C.A., Morgan, J.P., Lasagna, L. & Bianchine, J.R. (1970) L-dopa treatment failure: explanation and correction. *British Medical Journal,* **iv,** 93–94.
157. Rosen, H.M., Freund, H. & Fischer, J.E. (1977) Unpublished observations.
158. Rosen, H.M., Yoshimura, N., Hodgman, J.M. & Fischer, J.E. (1977) Plasma amino acid patterns in hepatic encephalopathy of differing etiology. *Gastroenterology,* **72,** 483–487.
159. Rosen, H.M., Soeters, P.B., James, J.H., Hodgman, J.M. & Fischer, J.E. (1978) Influences of exogenous intake and nitrogen balance on plasma and brain aromatic amino acids metabolism. *Metabolism,* **27,** 393–404.
160. Rossi-Fanelli, F., Capocaccia, R.L. & Fischer, J.E. (1977) Correlation of plasma taurine levels with grades of hepatic encephalopathy (HE) in man. *Gastroenterology,* **72,** 1181 (abstract).
161. Rossi-Fanelli, F., Cangiano, C., Attili, A., Angelico, M., Casano, A., Capocaccia, L., Strom, L. & Crito, C. (1976) Octopamine plasma levels and hepatic encephalopathy: a reappraisal of the problem. *Clinica Chimica Acta,* **67,** 255–261.
162. Rossi-Fanelli, F., Cangiano, C., Attili, A. & Capocaccia, L. (1978) Amino acids in hepatic encephalopathy. *American Journal of Digestive Disease.* In press.
163. Rossi-Fanelli, F., Smith, A.R., Cangiano, C., Bozzi, A., James, J.H., Kay, L.A., Perelle, B.A., Capocaccia, L. & Fischer, J.E. (1978) Simultaneous determination of phenylethanolamine and octopamine in plasma and cerebro-spinal fluid. In *Biochemistry of Phenylethylamines* (Ed.) Moosmaim, A. New York: Raven. In press.
164. Sarrazen, A., Emerit, J., Oliver, L., Reblo, F. & Bousquet, O. (1971) Traitement du coma hèpatique par la L-dopa, premiers resultats. *Presse Médicale,* **79,** 2226–2227.
165. Saunders, S.J., Hickman, R., MacDonald, R. & Terblanche, J. (1972) The treatment of acute liver failure. In *Progress in Liver Disease* (Ed.) Popper, H. & Schaffner, F. pp. 333–334. New York: Grune & Stratton.
166. Schafer, W.H. & Isselbacher, K.J. (1961) Uridine metabolism in chronic liver disease. *Gastroenterology,* **40,** 782–786.
167. Schenker, S. (1970) Hepatic coma: current concepts of pathogenesis. *Viewpoints of Digestive Disease,* **2,** 1–4.
168. Schenker, S. & Mendelson, J.H. (1964) Cerebral adenosine triphosphate in rats with ammonia-induced coma. *American Journal of Physiology,* **206,** 1173–1176.
169. Schenker, S., Breen, K.J. & Hoyumpa, A.A. Jr (1974) Hepatic encephalopathy: current status. *Gastroenterology,* **66,** 121–151.
170. Schenker, S., McCandless, D.W., Brophy, E. & Lewis, M.S. (1967) Studies on the intracerebral toxicity of ammonia. *Journal of Clinical Investigation,* **46,** 838–848.
171. Schultz, J.C., Adamson, J.S. Jr, Workman, W.W. & Norman, T.D. (1963) Fatal liver disease after intravenous administration of tetracycline in high doses. *New England Journal of Medicine,* **268,** 999–1004.
172. Shimogyo, S., Scheinberg, P. & Reimouth, O. (1967) Cerebral blood flow and metabolism in the Wernicke Korsakoff syndrome. *Journal of Clinical Investigation,* **46,** 849–854.
173. Shorey, J., McCandless, D.W. & Schenker, S. (1967) Cerebral alphaketogluterate in ammonia intoxication. *Gastroenterology,* **53,** 706–711.
174. Silk, D.B.A. (1977) Personal communication.
175. Silk, D.B.A., Trewby, P.N., Chase, R.A., Mellon, P.J., Hand, M.A., Davies, M., Langley, P.G., Wheller, P.G. & Williams, R. (1977) Treatment of fulminant hepatic failure by polyacrilonitrile membrane hemodialysis. *Lancet,* **ii,** 1–3.
176. Simmons, F., Goldstein, H. & Boyle, J.D. (1970) A controlled clinical trial of lactulose in hepatic encephalopathy. *Gastroenterology,* **59,** 827–832.
177. Smith, A.R., Rossi-Fanelli, F. & Fischer, J.E. (1978) Sulfur containing amino acids in hepatic coma in plasma and CSF of dog and monkey. Submitted for publication.
178. Smith, A.R., Rossi-Fanelli, F., Ziparo, V., James, J.H., Perelle, B.A. & Fischer, J.E. (1978) Serial alterations in CSF and plasma metabolites, amino acids and 5-hydroxyindole acetic acid in hepatic coma in the dog. *Annals of Surgery,* **187,** 343–350.
179. Smythe, C.M. & Baroody, N.B. (1957) Hepatic type 'flapping tremor' occurring in patients without hepatic disease. *Journal of the American Medical Association,* **165,** 31–34.
180. Soeters, P.B. & Fischer, J.E. (1976) Insulin, glucagon, amino acid imbalance and hepatic encephalopathy. *Lancet,* **ii,** 880–882.
181. Soeters, P.B. & Fischer, J.E. (1978) Fat of the branch chain of the amino acids in rats with experimental hepatic damage. Submitted for publication.
182. Soeters, P.B., Weir, G.C., Ebeid, A.M. & Fischer, J.E. (1977) Insulin, glucagon, portasystemic shunting and hepatic failure in the dog. *Journal of Surgical Research,* **23,** 183–188.
183. Summerskill, W.H.J. & Wolfe, S.J. (1957) The metabolism of ammonia and α-keto acids in liver disease and hepatic coma. *Journal of Clinical Investigation,* **36,** 361–372.
184. Summerskill, W.H.J., Ammon, H.V. & Baggenstoss, A.H. (1974) Treatment of chronic hepatitis. In *The Liver and Its Diseases* (Ed.) Schaffner, F., Sherlock, S. & Leevy, C.M. pp. 218–226. New York: Intercontinental Medical Book Corporation.
185. Svec, M.H. & Freeman, S. (1949) Effect of impaired hepatic circulation on plasma free amino acids of dogs. *American Journal of Physiology,* **159,** 357–364.
186. Sweet, W.H. & Locksley, H. (1954) Formation, flow and reabsorption of cerebrospinal fluid in man. *Journal of Nervous and Mental Diseases,* **119,** 457–461.
187. Takahashi, Y. (1963) Serum lipids in liver disease. Liver disease and the relationship of serum lipids and hepatic coma. *Japanese Journal of Gastroenterology,* **60,** 571–579.
188. Tanaka, K., Isselbacher, K.F. & Shih, V. (1972) Isovaleric and α-methylbutyric acidemias induced by hypoglycin A: mechanism of Jamaican vomiting sickness. *Science,* **175,** 69–71.
189. Thompson, L. (1978) Personal communication.
190. Thompson, A. & Holmes, A.W. (1967) Immune inhibition of urea breakdown in patients with cirrhosis. *Gastroenterology,* **52,** 14–17.
191. Thompson, A. & Visek, W.J. (1963) Some effects of induction of urease immunity in patients with hepatic insufficiency. *American Journal of Medicine,* **35,** 804–812.
192. Trey, C., Burns, D. & Saunders, S. (1966) Treatment of hepatic coma by exchange blood transfusions. *New England Journal of Medicine,* **274,** 473–481.

193. Tristani, F.E. & Cohn, J.J. (1967) Systematic and renal hemodynamics in oliguric hepatic failure: effect of volume expansion. *Journal of Clinical Investigation,* **46,** 1894–1906.

194. Unger, R.H. (1971) Glucagon and the insulin/glucagon ratio in diabetes and other catabolic illnesses. *Diabetes,* **20,** 834–843.

195. van Woert, H.M. (1971) Phenylalanine and tyrosine metabolism in Parkinson's disease treated with levodopa. *Clinical and Pharmacology Therapy,* **12,** 368–375.

196. Veech, R.L., Harris, R.L., Veloso, D. & Veech, E.H. (1973) Freeze blowing: a new technique for the study of brain in vivo. *Journal of Neurochemistry,* **20,** 183–188.

197. Waggoner, R.W. & Malamud, N. (1942) Wilson's disease in the light of cerebral changes following ordinary acquired liver disorders. *Journal of Nervous and Mental Diseases,* **96,** 410–423.

198. Walker, C.O., McCandless, D.W., McCarry, J.D. & Schenker, S. (1970) Cerebral metabolism in short chain fatty acid-induced coma. *Journal of Laboratory and Clinical Medicine,* **76,** 569–583.

199. Walker, C.O., Speeg, K.V. Jr, Levinson, J.D. & Schenker, S. (1971) Cerebral acetylcholine, serotonin and norepinephrine in acute ammonia intoxication. *Proceedings of the Society for Experimental Biology and Medicine,* **136,** 668–671.

200. Walser, M., Lund, P., Ruderman, N.B. & Coulter, A.W. (1973) Synthesis of essential amino acids from their alpha keto analogues by perfused rat liver and muscle. *Journal of Clinical Investigation,* **52,** 2865–2877.

201. Wannemacher, R.W. Jr & Dinterman, R.E. (1977) Total body catabolism in starved and infected rats. *American Journal of Clinical Nutrition,* **30,** 1510–1512.

202. Ware, A.J., D'Agostino, A.N. & Combes, B. (1971) Cerebral edema: a major complication of massive hepatic necrosis. *Gastroenterology,* **61,** 877–884.

203. Warren, K.S. & Schenker, S. (1964) Effect of an inhibitor of glutamine synthesis (methionine sulfoxamine) on ammonia toxicity and metabolism. *Journal of Laboratory and Clinical Medicine,* **64,** 442–449.

204. Williams, R. (1973) Hepatic encephalopathy. *Journal of the Royal College of Physicians of London,* **8,** 63–74.

205. Williams, A.H., Ma Hta Kyu, Fenton, J.C.B. & Cavanagh, J.B. (1972) The glutamate and glutamine content of rat brain after portacaval anastomosis. *Journal of Neurochemistry,* **19,** 1073–1077.

206. Wirthlin, L.S., van Urk, H., Malt, R.B. & Malt, R.A. (1974) Predictions of surgical mortality in patients with cirrhosis and non-variceal gastroduodenal bleeding. *Surgery, Gynecology and Obstetrics,* **139,** 65–68.

207. Wolpers, E., Phillips, S.F. & Summerskill, W.H.J. (1970) Ammonia production in the human colon. Effects of cleansing, neomycin, and acetohydroxamic acid. *New England Journal of Medicine,* **283,** 159–164.

208. Wu, C.J., Gollman, G. & Butt, H.R. (1955) Changes in free amino acids in the plasma during hepatic coma. *Journal of Clinical Investigation,* **34,** 845–849.

209. Wurtman, R.J., Rose, C.M., Mathysse, S., Stephenson, J. & Baldessarini, R. (1970) L-dihydroxyphenylalanine: effect on *S*-adenosylmethionine in brain. *Science,* **169,** 395–397.

210. Zacharski, L.R., Litin, E.M., Mulder, D.W. & Cain, J.C. (1970) Acute fatal hepatic failure presenting with psychiatric symptoms. *American Journal of Psychiatry,* **127,** 158–162.

211. Zieve, F.J., Zieve, L., Doizaki, W.M. & Gilsdorf, R.B. (1974) Synergism between ammonia and fatty acids in the production of coma: implications for hepatic coma. *Journal of Pharmacology and Experimental Therapeutics,* **191,** 10–16.

Chapter 43

Portal Hypertension

D.B.A. SILK
ROGER WILLIAMS

ANATOMY OF THE PORTAL VENOUS SYSTEM

The portal system includes all veins which collect blood from the abdominal part of the alimentary tract, the spleen, pancreas and gall bladder. The portal vein (Figure 43.1) begins at the level of the second lumbar vertebra just posterior to the head of the pancreas at the junction of the splenic and superior mesenteric veins. It is about 6 to 8 cm long, 1.2 cm in diameter and contains no valves.[67] The splenic veins originate at the splenic hilum and join near the tail of the pancreas with the short gastric vessels to form the main splenic vein. This proceeds in a transverse direction in the body and head of the pancreas and receives numerous tributaries from the head of the pancreas, and the left gastroepiploic vein enters it near the spleen. The inferior mesenteric vein draining blood from the left part of the colon and rectum usually enters its middle third, although occasionally it enters the junction of the superior mesenteric and splenic veins.

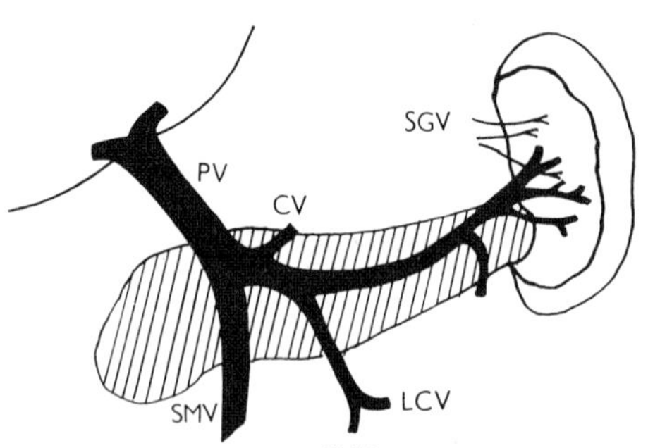

Figure 43.1. The extrahepatic portal venous system. Anterior aspect. PV portal vein, CV coronary vein, SGV superior gastric veins, LCV left colic vein, SHV superior haemorrhoidal vein, SMV superior mesenteric vein. The pancreas is represented by the shaded area.

Usually the coronary vein (left gastric vein) joins the portal vein at its origin, although sometimes it joins the splenic instead of the portal vein.

The best available estimates indicate that about two-thirds of total hepatic blood flow and about half the oxygen consumption are supplied by the portal vein, the remainder being supplied by the hepatic artery.[279]

Collateral Circulation

Normally the pressure in the portal vein ranges between 5 and 10 mmHg, and this pressure will rise if there is an increased resistance to blood flow in the portal vein, liver or hepatic vein. When the portal pressure rises above 10 mmHg, a collateral circulation begins to develop between the high pressure portal system and neighbouring low pressure veins, so permitting a diversion of portal blood into the systemic veins. The actual sites for the development of portal collateral vessels are those areas where veins draining into the portal system are in immediate juxtaposition to veins draining into the superior and inferior vena cavae. These areas are the submucosa of the oesophagus and stomach, the submucosa of the rectum, the anterior abdominal wall and the left renal vein.

Submucosa of the oesophagus and stomach

Anastomoses form between tributaries of the coronary vein (portal system) and azygos vein (superior vena cava) and result in submucosal varices of the oesophagus and upper stomach. Anastomoses may also form between the perisplenic vessels (portal system) and the short gastric vessels (superior vena cava) and contribute to the submucosal plexus of the stomach.

Submucosa of the rectum

Anastomoses form between the superior and middle haemorrhoidal veins (portal system) and inferior haemorrhoidal veins (inferior vena cava) and result in haemorrhoids.

Anterior abdominal wall

The umbilical vein remnant of the fetal circulation, although normally non-functional, can serve as an anastomosis between the main left portal vein and the epigastric veins of the anterior abdominal wall that drain into the superior and inferior vena cavae. These umbilical vein–epigastric vein connections result in dilated veins in the anterior abdominal wall (caput medusae).

Left renal vein

Portal venous blood may be carried to the left renal vein, either directly from the splenic vein or via diaphragmatic, pancreatic or gastric veins.

Extrahepatic Obstruction

When the cause of the portal obstruction is within the vein itself (extrahepatic portal vein obstruction), additional collaterals are formed as the blood is endeavouring to bypass the obstruction and so return towards the liver. Collaterals, which are seen to varying degrees according to how far along the portal vein the block extends, re-enter the portal vein in the porta hepatis beyond the block, and include veins in the hilum of the liver, venae comitantes of the portal vein and hepatic artery, veins in the suspensory ligaments of the liver and para-umbilical veins.

Collaterals and Portal Hypertension

The effect of the collateral circulation is to transmit the high pressure within the portal venous system to the systemic venous system. Very occasionally this may be so successful that portal pressures fall to normal or near normal levels.[278,300] In general, there is no relationship between the degree of portasystemic shunting and portal pressure.[92]

CLINICAL FEATURES OF PORTAL HYPERTENSION

History

Hepatic cirrhosis is the commonest cause of portal hypertension. Possible aetiological factors such as alcohol ingestion or past episodes of jaundice may provide clues to its presence. Haematemesis is the commonest presentation of portal hypertension, and the number and severity of previous haemorrhages should be noted together with their immediate effects, and particularly whether there was associated confusion, coma or development of ascites. Melaena with haematemesis may also result from bleeding varices and, perhaps less frequently, melaena alone.

Physical Examination

The stigmata of chronic liver disease should be looked for. These include jaundice, ascites, vascular spiders, palmar erythema, testicular atrophy, gynaecomastia and loss of body hair. Muscle wasting is commonly associated with cirrhosis, especially that due to alcohol ingestion.[194] In cases of intrahepatic portal hypertension, when blood is shunted from the left branch of the portal vein into the para-umbilical veins, prominent anterior abdominal wall veins may be apparent (caput medusae). These veins can be better visualized by infra-red photography. Blood flow is directed away from the umbilicus, whereas in inferior vena caval obstruction the collateral channels carry blood upwards to reach the superior vena caval system.

Although splenomegaly is an important indicator of portal hypertension, Sherlock[245] and others have felt for some time that the spleen size bears no relationship to the height of the portal venous pressure.[68,132] In a recent study we have observed patients with grade IV oesophageal varices who have a normal spleen size, and patients with enlarged spleens who had no evidence of varices on barium swallow.[299] The reliability of splenomegaly as a physical sign of portal hypertension is thus open to criticism.

INVESTIGATION OF PORTAL HYPERTENSION

Visualization of Oesophageal Varices

Of the various methods for assessing the collateral circulation, examination of the oesophagus for varices is the simplest. This can be done by direct visualization at oesophagoscopy or by a barium swallow.

Ghahremani and colleagues[86] were the first to report that the administration of anticholinergic drugs enhanced the radiological demonstration of varices. We have confirmed this by clearly showing apparent normality of the oesophagus using standard techniques, whereas on a number of occasions examination with Buscopan (hyoscine-*N*-butyl bromide) revealed the presence of varices.[290] With the increased availability of flexible fibreoptic endoscopes, oesophagoscopy is being used more and more as a means of visualizing varices. It is impossible to say in general whether endoscopy is superior to radiology with respect to the routine visualization of varices as comparisons of the techniques are so dependent upon the expertise available. Thus, at the University of Southern California about half the patients with varices seen at endoscopy had normal barium swallows,[221] whereas in other studies there was very close agreement between the incidence of varices seen at endoscopy and on barium examination using Buscopan.[289,290]

Visualization of the Portal Venous System

The portal vein can be visualized via a number of routes. At laparotomy a catheter can be threaded into a branch of the superior mesenteric vein in the mesentery. This was the preoperative technique extensively practised by Hunt.[108] The technique has the disadvantage, however, of prolonging operating time as well as anaesthetic time. Moreover, it is now appreciated that knowledge of the venography appearance is more helpful beforehand so the correct preoperative approach can be planned.

Percutaneous portography

For many years the most widely practised method for visualizing the portal venous system has been percutaneous splenoportography. The technique affords not only an excellent opportunity to visualize the portal venous system, but also allows measurement of the pressure at the same time. Full technical details of the method have been reviewed in detail in several publications.[6,130,229] Because of the risk of haemorrhage, the use of the technique is contraindicated if the patient is deeply jaundiced, has a prothrombin time more than two seconds prolonged or has ascites. Provided, however, that these criteria are adhered to, the technique in skilled hands is very safe, with a failure rate of less than 5 per cent.[229]

Percutaneous splenoportography has in the past been extensively used during the investigation of patients being considered for surgical decompression of portal hypertension. The technique can also be combined with hepatic vein catheterization when extrahepatic obstruction of the portal vein is suspected.[5] As a result of the widespread use of the technique, it has been possible to document in detail the distribution of collateral systems in patients with portal hypertension, and the findings of one large series of 848 technically successful examinations in patients with cirrhosis are summarized in Figure 43.2.[229] There are two limitations of splenoportography: non-visualization of major veins and lack of reproducibility.

Non-visualization of major veins. In up to 6 per cent of cases of cirrhosis the portal vein may not be visualized.[13,39,229] This is thought to occur when contrast medium enters a major collateral circulation proximal to the junction of the splenic and superior mesenteric veins, for example splenorenal collaterals,[278] a situation that may be compounded by the flow of 'unstained' mesenteric blood either directly into the coronary–gastro-oesophageal–azygos system or back along the splenic vein into splenorenal collaterals. It has also been suggested that non-visualization of the portal vein or portal and splenic veins occurs because a true reverse flow of hepatic arterial blood either perfuses the sinusoids or bypasses them via

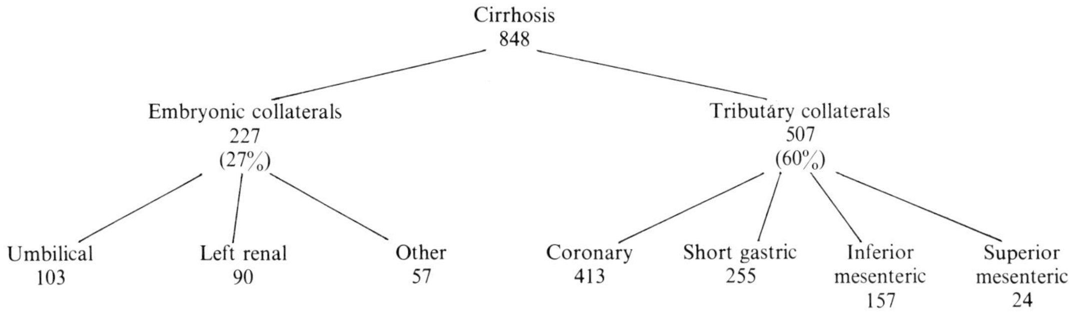

Figure 43.2. Distribution of collateral systems in technically successful percutaneous splenoportograms.[229]

arteriovenous intrahepatic shunts, back down the portal vein.[297,300] Results of direct electromagnetic flow meter determinations of direction and volume of portal venous flow argue somewhat against such an explanation, however, as true reverse flow has only rarely been recorded.[39, 253]

In patients with extrahepatic portal hypertension due to splenic and portal vein block, it is important to visualize the superior mesenteric vein so that the feasibility of a mesenterico-caval shunt can be ascertained. Splenoportography is not the investigation of choice in these patients even when the portal block occurs proximal to the junction of the superior mesenteric vein. Coeliac axis or superior mesenteric arterio-portography provides a better means of visualizing the superior mesenteric vein.[303]

Lack of reproducibility. If inadequate material is injected into the spleen or too few films are taken, the true state of the portal venous system may not be revealed. Moreover, whether or not this is the explanation, bleeding varices have been observed with a normal portogram[70] and, in one patient, the first examination revealed almost complete non-visualization of the portal vein due to diversion of contrast medium down splenorenal collaterals, whereas at the second examination there was prompt visualization of the splenoportal axis with demonstration of gastro-oesophageal varices.[229]

Splenoportography and Shunting

For 25 years, elective or therapeutic portacaval shunting was a widely practised operation for patients who were thought to have bled from oesophageal varices. There is little doubt that percutaneous splenoportography became widely acclaimed during this period. This was so not least because it was the group of patients with moderately- to well-preserved liver function who were selected for surgery, in whom it was possible to visualize the portal venous system preoperatively by splenoportography.[295] Since 1971, however, the concept of elective portocaval shunting has been questioned, and today the operation is not as widely practised because the accumulative analysis of three controlled clinical trials of elective portacaval shunting[113, 219, 230] shows that survival following surgery is not significantly different from that of patients receiving control therapy alone.[54] For this reason, as well as the development of new techniques for visualizing the portal venous system, fewer percutaneous splenoportograms are being performed now compared to the number undertaken in the heyday of elective portacaval shunting.

Additional Techniques for Visualizing the Portal System

Umbilical portography has been preferred to splenoportography by some.[28, 153, 202, 298] To a large extent the technique has been superseded since the introduction of safe percutaneous transhepatic catheterization of the portal vein. Umbilical portography provides good detail of the portal system in most cases although difficulties can arise in cirrhotic patients because of kinking of the vein. Portal manometry can be performed, and the technique has been of value after the spleen has been removed. Umbilical venography has been combined with transhepatic venography, transhepatic cholangiography, and needle biopsy – the so-called 'minilap' performed under local anaesthesia through a small vertical incision made halfway between the xiphisternum and umbilicus.[260, 301]

As mentioned above, safe techniques for visualizing the portal venous system via a percutaneous transhepatic approach have now been developed. Based upon the methods originally described by Bierman and colleagues,[17, 18] Lunderqvist and coworkers[147, 148] were the first successfully to cannulate routinely the portal venous system of patients with portal hypertension. Using this technique more recently, Okuda et al[191] obtained adequate portograms in 67 per cent of 30 cases. Portal manometry can also be performed, and technically satisfactory results were obtained by Reynolds and his colleagues in 84 per cent of 126 cases.[27]

Coeliac axis and superior mesenteric arterioportography

Arterial portography has also superseded splenic portography as a most widely used technique for investigating patients with suspected portal hypertension.[24, 33, 129, 185, 231] There are several reasons for this. Firstly, unlike splenoportography, the technique can be performed on deeply jaundiced patients with ascites and prolonged prothrombin time. Secondly, its detection of hepatoma is far superior to that of splenoportography. It also provides a valuable means of demonstrating a splenic arteriovenous fistula,[304] showing the patency of the portal vein in patients who have previously had a splenectomy for portal hypertension,[224] determining whether the superior mesenteric vein is patent in a patient with a known splenic and portal vein block,[303] and investigating the patency of portacaval, mesocaval and splenorenal shunts.

Pressure Measurements

The most widely used technique is splenic puncture during percutaneous splenoportography. The intrasplenic pressure is normally slightly higher than the portal venous pressure, as would be expected from the direction of flow in the portal system. The portal pressure can be measured directly at operation, but the pressure so recorded may be affected by the lack of intra-abdominal pressure and by anaesthesia. In one series the operative pressure was on average 50 mm of saline lower than the splenic pressure recorded with the patient awake.[45] Portal pressure can be measured directly in the unanaesthetized patient during umbilical vein catheterization, either alone or during the 'minilap' described previously.[123,124,202,260,301]

Another technique for measuring portal pressure is the measurement of intrahepatic parenchymal pressure. Initially, pressure recordings were made via a Vim Silverman needle or a fluid-filled catheter introduced into the liver substance,[282] but with the advent of the thin Chiba needle and percutaneous transhepatic cholangiography the technique has been greatly refined.[27] Using the Chiba needle under close radiological control Boyer et al[27] have safely obtained valid portal venous pressure recordings in 84 per cent of 123 patients.

Finally, several groups have measured the portal pressure indirectly via a catheter wedged in a small hepatic vein (wedged hepatic vein pressure, WHVP).[81, 160, 200, 220] Such recordings have been regarded as representing sinusoidal venous pressure, results usually being expressed as the pressure recorded above inferior vena caval pressure. WHVP measurements will not of course provide any information about the portal venous pressure in cases in which there is a block of the hepatic veins or inferior vena cava (Budd–Chiari syndrome) nor in cases in which there is an extrahepatic block in the portal venous system. Until very recently, no systematic comparisons were made between WHVP and direct simultaneous measurements of portal venous pressure in other causes of portal hypertension. The timely arrival of such a study allows one to draw firmer conclusions of the overall value of WHVP measurements as a means of accurately predicting portal venous pressure in such cases.[27] Only in alcoholic liver disease was there an almost exact correlation between the two measurements ($r = 0.96$ and 0.91 for alcoholic liver disease without and with evidence of active hepatic inflammation). In chronic active hepatitis and primary biliary cirrhosis, as well as in a number of other miscellaneous cases of hepatic disorder, the relationship was far less pronounced. The relative inexactness of this relationship confirms that to localize the site of increased vascular resistance either to 'pre-sinusoidal' or 'post-sinusoidal' regions of the liver is to oversimplify the pathophysiology of the haemodynamic changes in portal hypertension.[221] Therefore, if precise knowledge of pressure measurements is required, hepatic vein catheterization and direct portal measurement are best regarded as complementary procedures and should be performed together.

Clinically, the techniques delineated above for measuring portal pressure have proved useful, not only in confirming the diagnosis of portal hypertension but also in distinguishing between suprahepatic, intrahepatic, and extrahepatic causes. Beyond this, however, portal pressure measurements have proved of limited clinical usefulness. Thus, measurements of portal pressure by intrasplenic manometry do not correlate with the size of oesophageal varices assessed radiologically,[299] and it is not possible to predict from pressure measurements whether or not or when a patient will bleed from oesophageal varices.[221] A recent study, however, has demonstrated that the severity and duration of active haemorrhage from oesophageal varices is directly proportional to the degree of portal hypertension.[2] All those patients in the study with proven haemorrhagic varices stopped bleeding when the portal pressure was less than 34 cm of saline solution, whereas the bleeding could not be controlled in any of those whose portal pressure exceeded 46 cm saline.

BLOOD FLOW MEASUREMENTS

Quantification of Shunting in the Portal Venous System

Early attempts to quantify portal blood flow were based upon a grading system applied to the radiological filling of the portal venous system at splenoportography.[296] Later methods for more precisely quantifying the fractional shunting of splenic venous blood flow were based upon the monitoring of the appearance of intrasplenically injected radioactive indicators in hepatic venous[42] or branchial artery blood.[183] Such techniques had the disadvantage that fractional sampling of venous or arterial blood was required and no distinction could be made between intra- and extrahepatic sites of portasystemic shunting.[240] With the advent of scintiscanning techniques, semi-quantitative determinations of the degree of shunted blood flow were performed by measuring total counts over the lung and liver areas following intrasplenic injection of ^{131}I-macroaggregated albumin.[280] Though this method was simple to perform, it provided at best only an estimation of the total of intra- and extrahepatic shunting.

Recently, however, two methods have been described for accurately quantifying intra- and extrahepatic portasystemic shunting.[191, 264] In the first, the total percentage of shunted splenic venous flow was determined by scintillation splenoportography following intravenous and later intrasplenic injection of ^{99}Tc^{m} albumin microspheres, the fraction of hepatic blood flow passing via intrahepatic shunts being determined from the characteristic of the hepatic activity versus time curve after intrasplenic injection of microspheres.[264] In the second, total percentage of shunted splenic venous flow, as well as its intra- and extrahepatic components, was determined by scintillation splenoportography following transhepatic catheterization of the portal venous system and injection of ^{99}Tc^{m}-macroaggregated albumin (splenic hilum) and ^{131}I-macroaggregated albumin (porta hepatis).[191]

Neither method would appear to take into account mesenterico-caval communications[191, 264] although, at least in patients with alcoholic liver disease, the contribution of this route towards total extrahepatic shunting of splenic venous flow was found to be minimal.[92] This was not, however, the view of Lebrec and colleagues[138] who have separately determined the percentage of shunting of superior mesenteric and splenic venous blood using an indicator dilution technique based on selective catheterization of the splenic and superior mesenteric arteries and hepatic vein. All 20 patients studied had a long history of alcoholic intake and, of these, mesenteric shunting was essentially complete in 25 per cent. For the entire group mesenteric shunting averaged 59 per cent.

Measurement of Portal Vein and Total Hepatic Blood Flow

Hepatic blood flow was originally measured by constant infusions of the dyes bromsulphthalein (BSP) or indocyanine green (IG) and catheterization of the hepatic vein.[29, 41] Multiple indicator dilution techniques involving the rapid injection of ^{51}Cr-labelled red blood cells and ^{125}I-albumin microaggregates into the superior mesenteric artery and subsequent rapid serial sampling of blood from the portal and hepatic veins[105, 106] have confirmed that the above methods[29, 41] provide an estimate of *functional* rather than *total* hepatic blood flow. The differences between values of total hepatic blood flow, estimated by analysis of portal and hepatic indicator dilution curves after injection of ^{51}Cr-labelled red blood cells,[106] and functional hepatic blood flow, are thought to be due to the presence of abnormal intrahepatic intervascular communications.[191, 264] In the light of these studies the techniques of assessing hepatic blood flow in which measurements are made of the rates of disappearance from peripheral blood of radioactively labelled colloidal gold[296] and ^{131}I-macroaggregated albumin,[240] substances presumed to be completely extracted by Kupffer cells during one passage through the liver, will provide at best only an indirect estimate of hepatic blood flow because no account is taken of intrahepatic shunting.

Recently, techniques for selectively measuring portal vein blood flow in the unanaesthetized patient have also been described. Most of the methods depend upon portal blood sampling by the umbilical approach. Stone et al[258] calculated portal vein flow from comparisons of portal and hepatic venous xenon concentrations after administration of xenon into the duodenum. Alternatively, it has been possible to estimate portal venous flow by infusing xenon continuously in a peripheral portion of the portal bed or the splenic artery and measuring its concentration in the portal vein adjacent to the liver.[261] A more indirect method of assessing portal vein flow is by measuring splenoportal venous flow velocity during scintillation splenoportography following the intrasplenic injection of ^{99}Tc^{m}-labelled albumin microspheres.[264] Splenoportal venous flow velocity has also been assessed following injection of lipiodol droplets into a distal branch of the portal system via an umbilical approach and, when combined with measurements of the anteroposterior and lateral diameters of the portal vein on high-speed cinefluorography, direct estimations of portal vein flow rates have been derived.[217]

At operation, the rate of portal venous blood flow is best assessed by using electromagnetic flow meters.[40] Indirect estimates of the direction and magnitude of portal flow can be obtained either by the method of difference between free portal and hepatic-occluded pressures[156] or by the method of difference between splanchnic-occluded and hepatic-occluded pressures.[252]

Splenic Blood Flow

Splenic blood flow has been assessed by determining the splenic clearance of radiolabelled xenon injected through a coeliac axis catheter,[307] together with an estimate of spleen size determined radiologically. Total spleen blood flow is increased in patients with cirrhosis and portal hypertension,[21, 307] although in some of these patients blood flow/100 g tissue was reduced. The highest flows have been recorded in patients with tropical splenomegaly.[306] Splenic aneurysms have been demonstrated by coeliac axis arterioportography in a third of patients with established cirrhosis and portal hypertension.[304] Their occurrence is related to spleen size, and particularly to the length of history, as well as the rate of splenic blood flow.[303, 304] The clinical significance of splenic aneurysms is related to the fact that they occasionally rupture and this leads to haemoperitoneum and death.

The Value of Blood Flow Measurements in Portal Hypertension

Recurrent bleeding from oesophageal varices continues to present a very serious clinical problem for which the portasystemic shunt still remains the most effective means of controlling haemorrhage.[220] The portasystemic shunt will never be an ideal surgical operation, however, because it is unphysiological in two major ways. Firstly, it increases shunting of blood from the bowel to the systemic circulation, bypassing the detoxifying action of the liver. Secondly, it removes some or all of the portal inflow to the liver. The relative contributions of these physiological alterations to the two major complications of shunting, namely hepatic failure and recurrent hepatic encephalopathy, are uncertain.

Warren and colleagues[295] have always adhered strongly to the view that patients with normal or increased hepatic blood flow should respond poorly to portacaval shunting because of sudden removal of large quantities of portal blood from the liver. In line with this concept, Maillard and co-workers found a higher operative death rate in patients whose pre-shunt portal blood flow, measured at surgery by flowmeter, was over 800 ml/min.[151] A logical corollary is that it might be anticipated that a portacaval shunt would be well tolerated in those patients with a high degree of spontaneous portasystemic shunting, because it would merely replace fragile spontaneous shunts with a surgical shunt.[77] Available data indicate, however, that only 5 to 15 per cent of patients with portal hypertension have a marked decrease in portal flow.[163, 173, 213, 297] Moreover, these are often patients in whom major surgery is contraindicated on account of their poor liver function. In the hope that some critical level of portal flow could be defined, below which the portacaval shunt would be well tolerated, the development of increasingly refined techniques for characterizing the splanchnic haemodynamics has continued. Hand in hand with this has been the development of surgical procedures that provide the least diversion of portal flow and yet enough reduction in collateral flow to stop variceal bleeding. The distal splenorenal shunt[294] or one of its modifications,[293] the splenocaval shunt,[269] and arterialization of the portal vein in conjunction with portacaval shunt[1, 152] are examples of this approach.

Preliminary experiences with the distal splenorenal shunt have produced conflicting results. Thus, on the one hand, the findings of a controlled clinical trial, in which patients who had bled from varices were randomized to receive a *total* portacaval anastomosis or a selective splenorenal shunt, showed that the incidence of encephalopathy in patients who received the selective splenorenal shunt (1/22, 4.5 per cent) was significantly less than that after total portacaval anastomosis (10/24, 41.7 per cent, $P < 0.005$).[83] On the other hand, in a more recent controlled study, in which a modified distal splenorenal shunt was performed on 25 patients, the mortality was higher (60 per cent) (mean follow-up 43 months) and seven of the survivors showed evidence of encephalopathy.[281]

In deference to Warren's postulate, several other authors have recently published evidence showing a lack of relationship between portal blood flow and incidence of encephalopathy, hospital mortality or long-term survival following elective portacaval shunt.[40, 156, 253] The most impressive of these studies is by Burchell and co-workers, who measured portal flow directly at operation using an electromagnetic flowmeter.[40]

To add to the controversy, Smith[252] has questioned the validity of any preoperative assessment of portal blood flow, for he has shown statistically insignificant correlations between pre- and peroperative assessments of portal pressure, degree of portasystemic shunting and portal blood flow velocity.

One important reason why it has so far been difficult to predict morbidity and mortality following portasystemic shunting is that investigations have been predominantly directed towards portal vein blood flow rather than hepatic artery flow. It is now known that hepatic artery blood flow increases after portal vein clamping or completion of a portacaval shunt.[38, 76, 198, 213, 241] Moreover, this adaptation of hepatic artery blood flow is variable.[38, 76, 198, 213, 241] Burchell and his colleagues were the first to draw attention to a possible relationship between the extent of increases in hepatic artery flow after portasystemic shunting and outcome following surgery,[38] and the later studies of Zimmon and Kessler[314] support a conclusion that prognosis after portacaval anastomosis is influenced by the ability of hepatic blood flow to sustain hepatic sinusoidal pressure.

Further work is clearly needed to define the practical value of preoperative haemodynamic measurements as a means of selecting patients for portasystemic shunting. One looks forward in the future to a wider prospective application of some of the newer, more sophisticated techniques that provide precise measurements of both total hepatic and portal venous flow.

CLASSIFICATION OF PORTAL HYPERTENSION

Several authors have classified portal hypertension according to the presumed anatomical location of the obstruction, namely presinusoidal, sinusoidal, or post-sinusoidal.[20, 244] Such a classification is dependent largely upon the wedged hepatic vein pressure. As mentioned previously, the recent study of Boyer et al[27] showing an inexact relationship between WHVP and portal pressure in patients with presumed 'post-sinusoidal' portal hypertension confirms that there is insufficient haemodynamic data available to define precisely the location of the increased vascular resistance.[221] A more satisfactory classification would be to divide portal hypertension caused by increased resistance into three major types – suprahepatic, intrahepatic and extrahepatic – broadly based on the location of the presumed increase in vascular resistance (Table 43.1).

SUPRAHEPATIC PORTAL HYPERTENSION

Budd–Chiari Syndrome

Hepatic venous outflow obstruction, known as the Budd–Chiari syndrome after the physicians describing it, is histologically characterized by severe centrizonal and sinusoidal congestion. The syndrome may arise from obstruction at any site from the efferent vein of the lobule to

Table 43.1. *Portal Hypertension.*

Increased resistance to flow		
	Suprahepatic:	Budd–Chiari syndrome
		Right-sided heart failure
		Constrictive pericarditis
	Intrahepatic:	Alcoholic hepatitis
		Alcoholic cirrhosis
		Cryptogenic cirrhosis
		Chronic active hepatitis
		Chronic active hepatitis with cirrhosis
		Primary biliary cirrhosis
		Secondary biliary cirrhosis
		Haemochromatosis
		Wilson's disease
		Alpha-1-antitrypsin deficiency
		Blood dyscrasias
		Granulomatous liver disease
		Congenital hepatic fibrosis
		Partial nodular transformation of the liver
		Schistosomiasis
		Idiopathic non-cirrhotic portal hypertension
		Veno-occlusive disease
	Extrahepatic:	Portal vein thrombosis
Increased hepatic blood flow		
		Tropical splenomegaly syndrome
		Blood dyscrasias
		Cirrhosis with congestive splenomegaly
		Hepatoportal arteriovenous fistulae

the entry of the inferior vena cava into the right atrium. A similar picture may be produced by constrictive pericarditis or right-sided heart failure and these must be distinguished.

There are several known causes of the Budd–Chiari syndrome. Thrombosis of the hepatic vein may be associated with myeloproliferative disease, especially primary and secondary polycythaemia.[199, 268, 271] Thrombosis of the hepatic veins has been reported in paroxysmal nocturnal haemoglobinuria,[74, 102] and in association with oral contraceptives,[103, 135, 256] and possibly pregnancy.[227] Tumours may obstruct the hepatic veins and inferior vena cava directly or in company with blood clot.[135, 199]

An important cause of the syndrome, especially from the therapeutic standpoint, is a fibrous diaphragm or web across the upper vena cava at, or just above, the entrance of the left and middle hepatic veins.[232, 265] In many instances the cause remains unknown.[48, 199]

Clinically, patients usually present with a painful, tender liver and gross ascites resistant to diuretic therapy. Portal hypertension and rupture of varices tend to occur late in the course of the illness. The prognosis is poor, approximately one-third of patients surviving for a year or less from the time of presentation.[268] Prognosis is best when surgical correction of a proximal web by trans-atrial membranotomy is possible.[99]

Liver scanning with $^{99}Tc^{m}$ sulphur colloid has been shown to be the most useful screening test.[268] Characteristically, the anteroposterior scan shows central uptake of radiocolloid in the caudate lobe together with reduced uptake in the right lobe. The site and extent of the outflow obstruction can be determined by radiological techniques which include inferior venacavography, hepatic venography, coeliac axis arteriography and, much less reliably, by splenoportography.[32, 34, 131, 208]

Various portasystemic shunting procedures have been advocated for the treatment of the Budd–Chiari syndrome, including side-to-side portacaval, splenorenal and mesocaval shunt.[210] Suffice to say, the outcome has been extremely variable, at least half the patients dying in the immediate postoperative period. In the acute form, orthotopic liver transplantation may offer the best hope of survival.[43]

Right-sided Heart Failure and Constrictive Pericarditis

Severe right-sided heart failure is associated with centrizonal congestion and liver cell necrosis on liver biopsy. The degenerating cells are often packed with a brown, presumably lipochrome, pigment.[242] In some cases of chronic heart failure centrizonal reticulin condensation occurs followed by centrizonal reticulin proliferation and phlebosclerosis.[44] As the condition progresses, fibrous tissue bands pass from central vein to central vein and a fully developed cardiac cirrhosis results. Only minimal fibrosis is seen in the portal tracts.[69] A true cardiac cirrhosis is rare and is usually associated with mitral valve disease complicated by tricuspid incompetence and constrictive pericarditis. Features of portal hypertension are thought to be rare and usually absent except in very severe cardiac cirrhosis associated with constrictive pericarditis.[233] However, in one autopsy series oesophageal varices were present in 6.7 per cent of 74 patients with congestive cardiac failure, some of whom had no evidence of cirrhosis.[146]

INTRAHEPATIC PORTAL HYPERTENSION

Cirrhosis

The common types of cirrhosis associated with portal hypertension and of clinical significance include cryptogenic cirrhosis, cirrhosis complicating chronic active hepatitis, alcoholic cirrhosis and primary biliary cirrhosis. Less common are haemochromatosis, Wilson's disease, secondary biliary cirrhosis and cirrhosis associated with alpha-1-antitrypsin deficiency.

Alcoholic Liver Disease (see also Chapter 32)

Changing patterns

In America, the frequency of alcoholism in patients with cirrhosis is high, with figures varying between 64 and 84 per cent,[66, 84] and appears to be reflected in the fact that 61.1 per cent of 247 patients undergoing portacaval shunts in a recent series had underlying alcoholic cirrhosis.[277] Reports in the literature suggest that up to 1964 the frequency of alcoholism in patients with cirrhosis in Britain was much lower – 24 per cent[243] and 33 per cent[259] and this again appeared to be reflected in the fact that of 249 patients who had undergone portal decompression for intrahepatic portal hypertension between 1948 and 1967, only 35 (14.1 per cent) had underlying alcoholic cirrhosis, the vast majority having cryptogenic cirrhosis.[313]

The consumption of alcohol in Britain has, however, been steadily increasing over the last 20 years,[65] and more recent studies show that the frequency of alcoholism in all patients with cirrhosis is now much higher, values ranging from 51 to 65 per cent.[99, 100, 114] This increase is particularly marked in the female population.[128, 174]

As yet we do not know with certainty whether these increases will be reflected in changes of aetiological frequencies in patients with cirrhosis seen with portal hypertension and bleeding varices. There is every reason to believe that this will occur, however, as a similar proportion of those patients with alcoholic and cryptogenic cirrhosis followed up for between three and eight years bled from their varices.[259]

Pressure studies in patients with established alcoholic cirrhosis show that WHVP correlates almost exactly with portal vein pressure,[27, 222] which suggests that the increased vascular resistance is sinusoidal or post-sinusoidal, rather than pre-sinusoidal.

Alcoholic hepatitis

In our unit at King's College Hospital, London, the incidence of alcoholic hepatitis, especially in women, has increased markedly over the past five years.[128] The characteristic histological features include fatty infiltration, hepatocyte necrosis and 'ballooning', alcoholic hyaline and polymorphonuclear infiltration. These changes are often localized to the centrilobular zone and may be accompanied by collagen formation.[145] In our experience, as well as that of others, a number of these patients develop portal hypertension which is reversible if the histological features improve.[90, 139, 197, 218] Haemodynamic data support these conclusions. Transient elevations in WHVP,[139] transient portal venous stasis[166] and increased hepatic artery blood flow[50] have been documented in alcoholic hepatitis. As in alcoholic cirrhosis, most of the increased vascular resistance appears to be either sinusoidal or post-sinusoidal.[27] In a few patients with obliteration of the central veins[72] the site of the block may be predominantly post-sinusoidal, and spontaneous reversal of portal venous blood flow has been observed in at least one case.[27]

Cryptogenic Cirrhosis

In Britain, cryptogenic cirrhosis has been regarded as an important cause of portal hypertension.[108, 313] By definition, these patients form a heterogeneous group, and there is the possibility that, with improved diagnostic techniques, including the ready availability of markers of autoimmunity and HB_sAg infection, patients diagnosed 10 years ago as having cryptogenic cirrhosis might now be considered as having chronic active hepatitis.[244]

Chronic Active Hepatitis

Chronic active hepatitis (CAH) (see also Chapter 29) must now be regarded as an important cause of portal hypertension.

The problem of portal hypertension in CAH is exemplified by the fact that during the follow-up of 82 patients with the disease 42 per cent and 31 per cent of the patients had oesophageal varices and presented with haematemesis, respectively.[168, 170] In a more recent study, gastrointestinal haemorrhage was a presenting factor in 32 per cent of 42 patients with CAH admitted to a specialist referral unit.[299]

With respect to portal haemodynamics, WHVP is raised, indicating increased sinusoidal or post-sinusoidal resistance.[27] In addition, however, there is clearly a pre-sinusoidal component as portal pressure in some patients exceeds WHVP.[27]

Signs of portal hypertension may be transient and reversible early on in the disease.[168] As adhered to above, this is not a situation unique to CAH, for transient portal hypertension may occur in other forms of acute hepatic injury such as viral hepatitis[249] and alcoholic hepatitis.[90, 139, 197, 218] Prednisone therapy in CAH may delay the development of portal hypertension.[177]

Primary Biliary Cirrhosis (see also Chapter 31)

During a survey at St Bartholomew's Hospital, London, of the liver microscopy of 250 patients who had undergone portal decompression for intrahepatic portal hypertension, 23 (9.2 per cent) were found to have primary biliary cirrhosis.[313] Of these, rupture of oesophageal varices was the presenting symptom in 15 (65.2 per cent).[312] Such a high incidence of haemorrhage as the presenting symptom of the disease is not in accord with the experience of the Royal Free Group, London,[246] and in their experience portal hypertension is common as a later complication.[125] This difference may well be due to the fact that patients referred to the former centre tend to have gastrointestinal haemorrhage as the predominant problem, whereas many of those referred to the latter have jaundice as the major presenting symptom.

In the study of Zeegan and colleagues[312] it was of interest that only 26 per cent of their 23 cases had nodular regeneration on liver biopsy, despite the fact that their portal pressures were markedly raised at operation. This suggests that the portal hypertension in the non-cirrhotic group was due to an increase in pre-sinusoidal resistance produced by the portal tract lesions. In patients who have established cirrhosis, WHVP is raised,[27] suggesting increased sinusoidal or post-sinusoidal resistance. Even in these patients, however, there is also the likelihood of increased pre-sinusoidal resistance, for in three of eight patients studied portal vein pressure exceeded WHVP.[27]

Blood Dyscrasias (see also Chapter 8)

Portal hypertension occasionally develops in the myeloproliferative disorders.[7, 63, 98, 143, 190, 226, 238, 250, 263, 311] It may also occur, rarely, in acute leukaemia,[136] chronic leukaemia,[64] Hodgkin's disease,[142] Gaucher's disease,[111, 115] or histiocytosis X.[91]

Blendis and colleagues[19, 21] have investigated in some detail the pathophysiology of the portal hypertension associated with blood dyscrasias. A prominent feature was the close relationship in many patients between the degree of portal hypertension and the extent of splenic enlargement and associated increases in spleen and liver blood flow. In nine of 16 patients this increased liver blood flow was associated with a concomitant paralleled increase in pre-sinusoidal resistance. In other patients, however, the WHVP was disproportionately raised in relationship to intrasplenic pressure and spleen and liver blood flow. It appeared, therefore, that in some patients with blood dyscrasias portal hypertension develops primarily on account of increased portal flow secondary to splenomegaly, a situation analogous to 'tropical splenomegaly' (see below), whereas in others the increase in portal pressure could be attributed to a primary elevation of intrahepatic portal resistance, which in turn is contributed to by an increased flow.

Granulomatous Liver Disease
(see also Chapter 37)

Most authors agree that tuberculosis and sarcoidosis are implicated in about two-thirds of cases[93, 107] and in about 20 per cent the cause is unknown.[36, 93, 107]

Patients with granulomatous liver disease rarely develop portal hypertension.[87, 150, 209, 285] Why portal hypertension should occur only in a minority of cases is unclear, but the intensity of granulomatous infiltration and the position of the granulomas within the portal tracts may be significant factors.

The pathophysiology of the portal hypertension is not well understood; there is some evidence that pre-sinusoidal resistance is increased in relation to massive granulomatous deposits in the portal tracts.[169] However, elevations of WHVP have been recorded,[150] which suggests obstruction at sinusoidal or post-sinusoidal level.

Congenital Hepatic Fibrosis

The term 'congenital hepatic fibrosis' was introduced in 1961 by Kerr and colleagues[122] to describe a fibrotic change in the liver, distinct from cirrhosis, occurring in children and young adults who commonly presented with hepatosplenomegaly and portal hypertension. In some cases the disease appeared to be inherited in an autosomal recessive manner, especially in those with polycystic disease of the kidney which in a later study bore resemblance to medullary sponge kidney.[121] Murray-Lyon, Ockenden and Williams[176] have questioned whether congenital hepatic fibrosis can be considered as a distinct entity, because the characteristic changes in the liver have in fact been found in at least four genetically and clinically distinct renal syndromes,[23] as well as in patients who appear to have entirely normal kidneys at post-mortem.[178, 305] Other cases have been shown to have dysplastic kidneys,[112] Meckel's syndrome[80] or, very rarely, autosomal dominant adult type polycystic disease.[101] Murray-Lyon et al[176] therefore conclude that congenital hepatic fibrosis is best considered as a manifestation of several different diseases and not as a single clinical entity.

The clinical details of 75 cases in the literature have recently been reviewed.[255] Haematemesis, presumed to be variceal in origin, was a presenting symptom in 37 per cent of these cases and a total of 50 per cent bled from their varices at some time during the course of the illness. Portal hypertension in most of the patients was presumed to be due to an increased intrahepatic pre-sinusoidal resistance, although a raised WHVP has been observed in some patients.[14]

Partial Nodular Transformation of the Liver

In 1966, Sherlock and co-workers described four patients with non-cirrhotic nodules of liver parenchyma in the hilar region obstructing the circulation within the liver.[247] Patients with this disorder characteristically have a better prognosis than do those with cirrhosis, and the disorder is difficult to diagnose except at post-mortem. Haemodynamic studies suggested an increase in intrahepatic post-sinusoidal resistance.

Schistosomiasis

Hepatic schistosomiasis (see also Chapter 56) occurs as a complication of infection with the three common species: *S. japonicum*, *S. mansoni* and *S. haematobium*. In Africa, *S. mansoni* and *S. haematobium* predominate, while *S. japonicum* infection is endemic in Asia and the Far East. Liver involvement may occur early after infestation with *S. mansoni,* but it usually occurs only after multiple exposures to *S. haematobium*. In the liver, the ova penetrate and obstruct the portal branches and are deposited either in the large radicles, producing the coarser type of bilharzial hepatic fibrosis, or in the small portal tracts, producing the fine diffuse form. Portal hypertension commonly develops, and in countries where schistosomiasis is prevalent, such as Japan, China, the Philippines, Africa, Egypt, West Indies, Puerto Rico and northern parts of South America, this is an important cause of portal hypertension.

Characteristically, the intrasplenic pressure is raised while the WHVP is normal, indicating that portal hypertension is pre-sinusoidal in origin and presumably related to the portal zone reaction.

In the countries where hepatic schistosomiasis is common, patients usually present with ruptured varices late in the course of the illness and, contrary to what is usually believed, liver function may be severely impaired and ascites may often be present. The incidence of portasystemic encephalopathy is high following portasystemic shunting in these patients.[292] This is likely to be due both to impairment of liver function and the cut-off of a high portal blood flow, and nowadays shunt operations have been abandoned in areas such as Egypt where the disease is prevalent.

Idiopathic Non-cirrhotic Intrahepatic Portal Hypertension

Reports have appeared in the literature from both tropical and temperate areas of a heterogeneous group of patients with intrahepatic portal hypertension without cirrhosis but with a variety of minor hepatic abnormalities. In some of the early cases from America, the liver was considered to be histologically normal.[167,207] Subsequently, mild portal fibrosis was described either alone[248] or in combination with sinusoidal dilatation[274] and cellular infiltration.[110, 215] In addition, in Indian and American patients vascular and lobular abnormalities have been described, including thickened and dilated portal vein radicles, focal nodulation, and more subtle disturbances of hepatic architecture.[11, 26, 164, 184, 286]

Zeegan et al[313] have recently described 44 patients with non-cirrhotic portal hypertension. The histological features comprised minor portal tract abnormalities together with a subtle distortion of lobular architecture, with no evidence of liver cell necrosis, bile ductular proliferation, cellular infiltration or intimal thickening of portal venous radicles. Often, mild portal tract fibrosis was seen, sometimes with thin septa radiating into the parenchyma and areas of portal tracts linked together by these septa.

Hunt[108] originally noted that some of these patients had a previous history of chronic arsenic ingestion, and more recently other workers have drawn attention to other such cases.[175, 283, 302]

The implication of arsenic ingestion as a possible aetiological factor in the development of this syndrome is of interest, for similar histological features have been noted in patients exposed to vinyl chloride[270, 286] and in vineyard sprayers exposed to Bordeaux mixture which consists of a complex series of copper salts.[203] It is interesting to speculate, therefore, whether idiopathic non-cirrhotic portal hypertension represents a variant of veno-occlusive disease (see below).

With regard to the aetiology of the portal hypertension in these cases, there is some evidence from portal venography of narrowing and blockage or shrinking of small intrahepatic branches of the portal vein.[11, 26, 266, 286, 313] This would accord with the fact that increases in intrahepatic pre-sinusoidal resistance have also been demonstrated.[22, 110, 164, 207] Increased splenic blood flow could also be a contributing, rather than the sole, factor involved as patients have presented with a bleed but may have had varices for years.[22]

To illustrate the complexity of this syndrome, however, Basu et al[11] have demonstrated a raised WHVP in some of their patients who had normal or reduced liver blood flow, all indicative of post-sinusoidal obstruction.

Survival following portasystemic shunting

The group of Zeegan's patients with idiopathic non-cirrhotic portal hypertension is notable because those who underwent portasystemic shunting did particularly well compared with those with cirrhosis[313] (Figure 43. 3). The cumulative survival of 44 such patients for 10 years following portasystemic shunting was 77 per cent, compared with 22 per cent of 201 patients with cirrhosis.[313]

Veno-occlusive Disease

This is a condition in which hepatic damage is severe, and histologically there is an occlusion of medium as well as small hepatic veins which leads to the development, in the actue stage, of massive hepatic necrosis and, in the chronic form, to non-portal cirrhosis and portal hypertension.[31] There is good evidence that development of the disease is related to ingestion of pyrrolizidine alkaloids found in a large number of widely distributed plants, of which the best-known genera are *Senecio*, *Crotalaria* and *Heliotropium*.[35, 157] Classically, patients are afflicted because they ingest contaminated grain (and subsequently bread) or herbal teas brewed as folk remedies from the plants containing pyrrolizidine alkaloids.

Originally described in South Africa,[309] veno-occlusive disease is now endemic in Jamaica.[262] Massive outbreaks have now been recorded in Afghanistan[172] and India[267] and, recently, cases originating from Ecuador[149] and America[257] have been described.

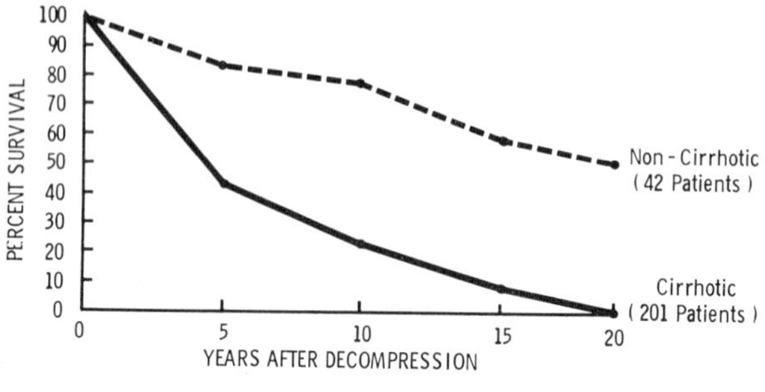

Figure 43.3. Survival of patients with portal hypertension following portasystemic shunting. 201 patients with cirrhosis and 42 patients with non-cirrhotic portal hypertension.

EXTRAHEPATIC PORTAL HYPERTENSION

Portal Vein Thrombosis

Obstruction of the main portal vein may arise at any point in its course. In response to obstruction the venae comitantes enlarge and assume a leash-like cavernous appearance.[89] The aetiological factors in 81 non-cirrhotic patients with portal vein thrombosis are shown in Table 43.2.[88] In agreement with two other large series, no aetiological factor could be identified in over half the cases, and a definite history of sepsis was obtained in less than a third.[78, 272]

Biochemical tests of liver function have in general been shown to be normal, with the possible exception of the alkaline phosphatase which, even in some adult patients, is raised.[88,273] The major clinical problem is bleeding from varices, and this often occurs repeatedly. In contrast to the situation in cirrhosis, the prognosis of individual bleeding episodes in extrahepatic portal hypertension is excellent.[78,88] Despite this, the final cause of death is usually bleeding varices.[104,162,276] If the splenic vein is patent, the treatment of choice in these patients is a splenorenal shunt. Operation should be delayed until the patient is an adequate size, for if it is undertaken in childhood, stoma size is inadequate and the shunt will subsequently block.[78,95] Contrary to the early encouraging experience of Pemberton and Kierman,[201] recent reports indicate that a high rebleeding rate follows splenectomy.[78,88] It thus seems clear that this particular operation should be avoided, especially since the splenic vein should be preserved for a later shunt procedure. The only type of shunt that can be undertaken if the splenic vein is thrombosed is a mesocaval shunt. However, in some patients, even the superior mesenteric vein is thrombosed.

Table 43.2. *Aetiological Factors in 81 Non-cirrhotic Patients with Portal Vein Thrombosis.*[88]

	No.	%
Sepsis		
Umbilical	7	8.6
Portal pyaemia	10	12.3
Other	1	1.2
Trauma	1	1.2
Neoplasm	1	1.2
Unknown	61	75.3

Proximal gastric resection appears to be one of the most effective temporary means of controlling haemorrhage, although haemostasis is achieved at the expense of a high incidence of gastrointestinal complications.[88] Johnson and Rodgers[118] have reported extremely favourable results of oesophageal sclerotherapy in patients with extrahepatic portal hypertension who have bled from varices; 29 of their patients received a total of 82 injections, with an average period of 30 months' freedom from haemorrhage. Because of these results, patients with extrahepatic portal hypertension who are referred to our unit on account of variceal haemorrhage are being offered this form of therapy.[308]

INCREASED HEPATIC BLOOD FLOW

In several conditions an increased hepatic blood flow is an important, if not exclusive, factor involved in the pathogenesis of the portal hypertension.

Idiopathic Tropical Splenomegaly

Idiopathic tropical splenomegaly (see also Chapter 39) is common in East Africa and is probably widely distributed throughout the tropics. Portal hypertension, as shown by a raised intrasplenic pressure, is common in these patients,[137] some of whom bleed from varices.[153] Haemodynamic studies have shown that increased spleen and liver blood flow is an important factor concerned in the rise of portal pressure.[306]

Cases have also been described in which portal hypertension has resulted from increased splenic venous blood flow caused by splenic arteriovenous fistulae[117] and capillary haemangiomatosis of the spleen.[205]

Finally, as has already been mentioned above, detailed haemodynamic studies have shown that increases in total spleen blood flow leading to increased hepatic blood flow are an important contributory factor in the portal hypertension that develops in the blood dyscrasias.[19, 21]

Cirrhosis

Although in cirrhosis portal hypertension is mainly due to increases in intrahepatic resistance consequent upon the development of regeneration nodules, in a few patients total spleen blood flow is markedly increased, especially in those with large spleens.[19, 21, 307] The effect this has on total hepatic blood flow is uncertain because part of the spleen blood flow is diverted into collateral circulation before reaching the liver. Nonetheless, increased spleen blood flow in cirrhosis may in part account for the raised pre-sinusoidal resistance seen in some patients.[27, 140]

Hepatoportal Arteriovenous Fistulae

These are a rare cause of portal hypertension, and are usually associated with a previous history of trauma or develop in association with primary hepatocellular carcinoma.[182] In the latter series, eight of 80 patients with hepatocarcinoma had portal hypertension in association with a hepatoportal fistula. Presumably, although this was not specifically mentioned, at least some of these patients did not have an underlying cirrhosis. The diagnosis is made by arteriography.

MANAGEMENT OF ACTIVELY BLEEDING VARICES

Problems of Diagnosis

The recent advent of upper gastrointestinal fibreoptic panendoscopy and its increasing use in patients with portal hypertension suspected to be bleeding from varices have resulted in a reappraisal of the actual sites of bleeding. In the first two published series, a remarkably low proportion of patients (18 per cent and 39 per cent) was actually observed to be actively bleeding from varices.[62, 155] This was attributed to the fact that almost all the patients examined were alcoholics, and acute alcohol ingestion was thought to be the cause of the high incidence of bleeding from erosive gastric lesions (31 per cent in one series,[62] 59 per cent in the other[155]). In a later study, 60 per cent of 50 patients were found to be actually bleeding from varices.[289] The proportion of those with variceal bleeding was equally distributed between the alcoholic and non-alcoholic groups, and it was notable that the later investigation showed a much higher incidence of bleeding from gastric varices (22 per cent) than was found in the previous studies (12 per cent[62] and 0 per cent[155]). The reasons for the higher incidence of bleeding gastric varices in the later study[289] is not entirely clear. It is possible that more sophisticated endoscopists participated in the study. Alternatively, it is possible that the patients were endoscoped at an earlier stage after the bleeding episode. This explanation seems quite likely, for in the most recently published study, in which patients were endoscoped shortly after initial resuscitation, 66 per cent of 84 episodes of bleeding were diagnosed as being due to varices.[186]

We have recently been concerned about what effect delaying endoscopy has on the diagnosis of bleeding sites in patients with portal hypertension. Consequently, we are currently involved in a study of patients referred to our unit in whom a presumptive diagnosis of bleeding varices has been made. Upper gastrointestinal endoscopy is performed as soon as the patients are admitted, and to date only 18.6 per cent of these 70 patients have been shown to be actively bleeding from varices (Table 43.3).

However, a high proportion (65.5 per cent) of the patients subsequently rebleed while under our care, and when re-endoscoped within two hours a much higher proportion (75 per cent) show evidence of active variceal haemorrhage (Figure 43.4). We believe it is significant that some of these patients who were finally found to be bleeding from varices also had clear evidence of oesophageal and gastric erosions which in other studies had been implicated as a major source of bleeding.[62, 155, 196] In our opinion, therefore, evidence is accruing to support the view that the majority of patients with portal hypertension who present with upper gastrointestinal haemorrhage are in fact bleeding from ruptured varices.

Pathogenesis of Variceal Haemorrhage

Despite extensive study the mechanism leading to the onset of variceal haemorrhage remains

Table 43.3. *Results of Initial Endoscopy in 70 Patients with Suspected Variceal Haemorrhage.*

	No.	%	Time of endoscopy (median)
Active bleeding			
Varices, visible	13	18.6	5 hr
Varices, presumed	1	1.4	12 hr
Erosion, visible	4	5.7	5 hr
No active bleeding	52	74.3	4 hr

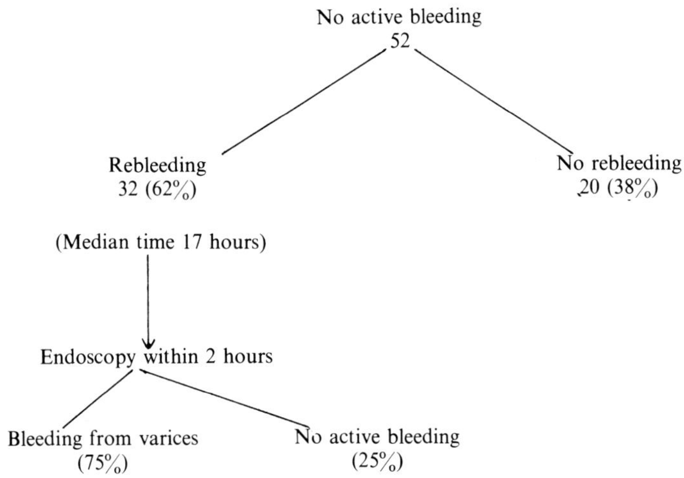

Figure 43.4. Outcome of 52 of 70 patients admitted to the Liver Unit, King's College Hospital, with a suspected diagnosis of variceal haemorrhage in whom initial endoscopy was negative.

unclear. Initially, it was felt that bleeding was precipitated mainly by the height of the portal pressure.[141, 193] This now seems less likely, because the magnitude of raised intrasplenic pressures measured shortly after bleeding is extremely variable.[2] Other authors have suggested that acid-pepsin regurgitation and erosion of the oesophageal mucosa contribute to the rupture.[206, 288] Certainly, pathological studies in patients who died of variceal haemorrhage have revealed erosion of the oesophageal mucosa in a high proportion of cases.[47, 206, 288] If peptic oesophagitis plays an important role in the rupture of oesophageal varices, it would be reasonable to assume that gastro-oesophageal reflux would be a common occurrence in these patients. However, a recent study has shown that the lower oesophageal pressure measurement in patients with cirrhosis a few weeks before they bled from varices was normal.[71] Although it can be argued that isolated measurements, performed several weeks before bleeding occurs, are meaningless in these patients, other evidence suggests that a competent sphincter retains this ability at least over a period of several months.[310]

Our own view is that a significant proportion of our patients with endoscopically proven active variceal haemorrhage has concomitant gastric and/or oesophageal erosions.[171] In the hope of defining the possible role of acid in more detail, a controlled clinical trial is in progress to determine whether prophylactic cimetidine therapy has any beneficial effect with respect to reducing the frequency of variceal haemorrhage in patients with portal hypertension and demonstrable oesophageal varices.

Prognosis of a Variceal Bleeding Episode

It comes with no surprise that mortality associated with bleeding varices varies considerably from series to series, with recent mortality figures ranging from 36 per cent[204] to 60 per cent.[186] Of the factors that affect survival, types of treatment offered, severity of hepatocellular dysfunction, general clinical condition and the severity of haemorrhage are all obviously crucial. A separate and additionally important factor has to be considered when comparing survival figures of different groups, however. Many reported series come from referral centres. By definition these results will be biased, for an unknown number of patients in whom referral was initially contemplated will have failed to survive long enough for referral to have taken place.

EMERGENCY MEDICAL TREATMENT

Sengstaken–Blakemore Tube

The triple lumen Sengstaken–Blakemore tube (SBT) was introduced in 1950 as a means of controlling variceal haemorrhage.[236] The original tube, with an oesophageal and a gastric balloon, was later modified by having a hypopharyngeal aspiration tube taped to it[25] (Figure 43.5), and more recently a fourth lumen has actually been incorporated into the tube to aspirate secretions above the oesophageal balloon (Figure 43.6).

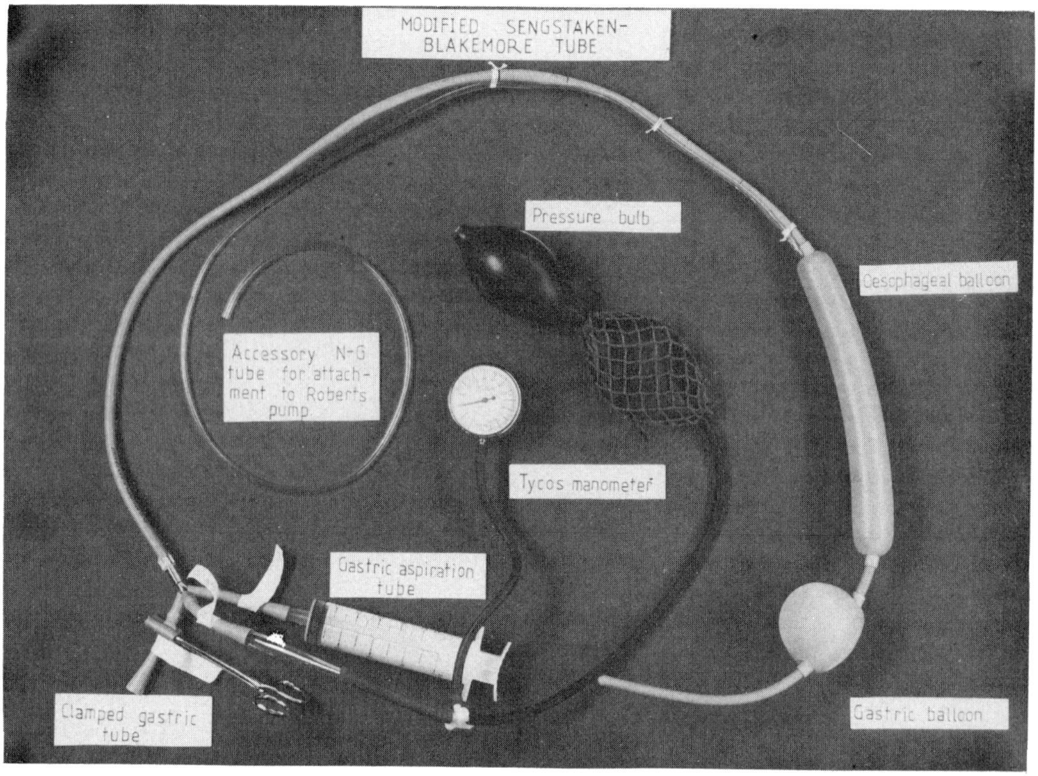

Figure 43.5. The modified three lumen Sengstaken–Blakemore tube.

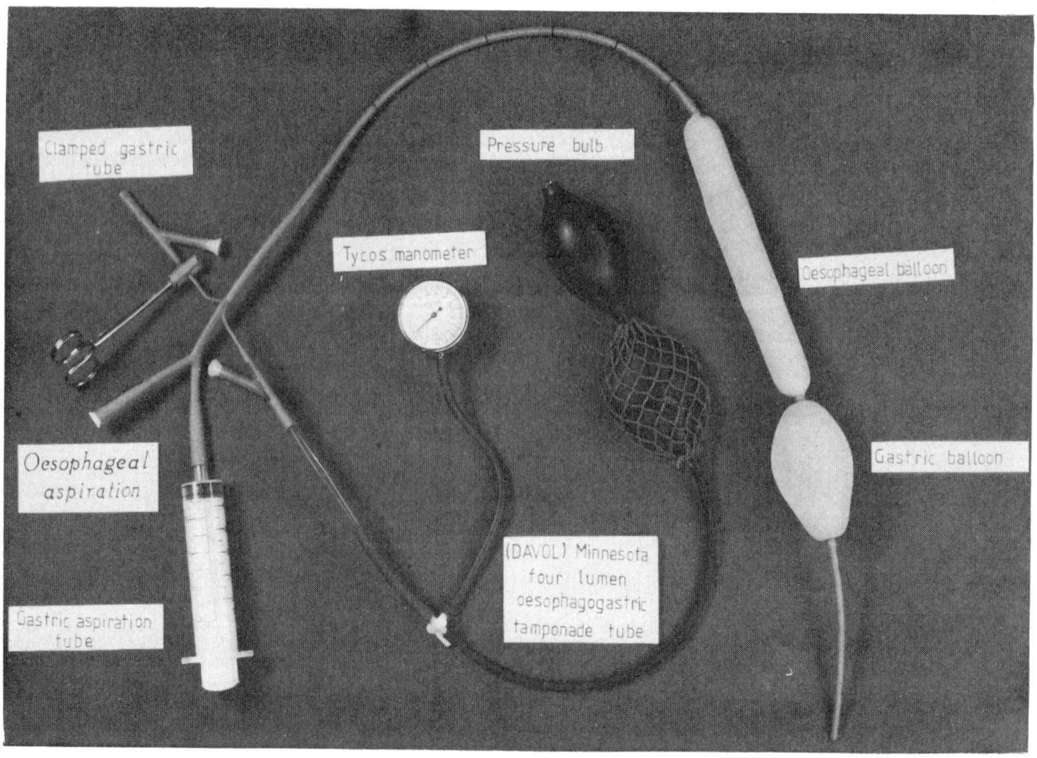

Figure 43.6. The Minnesota four lumen oesophagogastric tamponade tube.

The SBT with its varied modifications has been widely used as a temporary means of controlling variceal haemorrhage. Initially, traction was applied to the tube[73, 133, 291] but this has now generally been abandoned because of the high incidence of oesophageal laceration and rupture.[51, 55]

The results of therapy using the SBT are conflicting. The best results have been reported by Hermann and Traul,[97] Pitcher[204] and Johansen and Baden.[116] These authors achieved primary haemostasis in 88 to 92 per cent of their patients. At least one of these series [204] has been criticized[53] on the grounds that a high proportion (60 per cent) of the patients who were selected for the study were considered to be 'good risk' patients, and that the author either personally administered or supervised therapy. The report of Johansen and Baden[116] is also open to some criticism because details of the clinical condition of the patients were not given and because, although primary haemostasis was achieved in 88 per cent of 91 patients, rebleeding was common, with the result that *permanent* haemostasis after one to three tube treatments was achieved in only 45 per cent of the cases. The complication rate was, however, low in all of these studies.

Poor results were reported by Conn and Simpson[55] who, over a nine-year period, observed primary haemostasis in only 56 per cent of their patients, and a treatment mortality of 22 per cent. Their complications included regurgitation of gastric contents, rupture of the oesophagus, oesophageal laceration, respiratory obstruction and regurgitation of the tube.

In the most recently published prospective study, the value of tamponade by the SBT as a primary measure to stop variceal haemorrhage was again demonstrated, because bleeding was stopped as soon as tamponade was effected in 85 per cent of 45 bleeding episodes.[186] However, the haemorrhage restarted after removal of the tube in 60 per cent of these, and final control of bleeding by the SBT was achieved in only 46 per cent of the episodes in which the tube was inserted. The final overall mortality in the series was 60 per cent. Thus, as in other studies, successful tamponade using the SBT was followed by rebleeding and subsequent mortality in a high proportion of cases.

It seems reasonable to conclude from the above representative studies that the use of the SBT represents a valuable primary therapy for controlling active variceal haemorrhage. It is apparent, firstly, however, that variable proportions of those patients successfully treated rebleed, and secondly that the rebleeding is most likely to occur in those patients with severe hepatic dysfunction and poor general clinical condition and who bled torrentially in the first instance.[55, 57, 94, 186, 216]

Linton–Nachlas Tube

The Linton–Nachlas tube was introduced by Linton[144] and further developed by Nachlas.[180] The triple lumen tube differs from the SBT in that only a single gastric balloon has been incorporated. This gastric ballon has a larger capacity (300 to 600 ml) than the gastric balloon of the SBT, and the tube is thought to work through compression of the cardio-oesophageal junction, cutting off the blood flow to the oesophageal varices. Traction on the tube is required, and investigators have achieved this by attaching weights of between 200 and 1000 g to the distal end of the tube. Initial results were encouraging. Nachlas[181] found the tube to be effective in 10 of 13 patients, and Bertrand and Michell[15, 161] reported haemostasis in all of 58 treatment episodes in 32 patients. In the eight patients with the tube in position for more than 36 hours, ulcerations developed at the cardio-oesophageal junction but no other complications were seen.[15, 161] Because of these encouraging results, Burcharth and Malmstrøm[37] undertook a study to compare the effectiveness of the Linton–Nachlas and Sengstaken–Blakemore tubes. The trial had to be terminated because on three occasions the gastric balloon of the Linton–Nachlas tube was inflated when it was situated in the distal oesophagus, with the result that two of the patients died from a ruptured oesophagus.

Both types of tamponade tube have the disadvantage that intubation of critically ill patients requires considerable expertise. While this is not necessarily a problem in specialized units, it is in regional and district centres, especially since it is to these centres that most patients with actively bleeding varices are initially referred. An alternative primary form of therapy in these situations is vasopressin (Pitressin).

Vasopressin (Pitressin)

It has been known for many years that posterior pituitary extract lowers the portal pressure in animals.[49, 119, 158] A similar effect was later observed in man,[234, 237] and in initial studies, when vasopressin was given systemically to patients bleeding from varices, effective control of variceal haemorrhage was observed.[52, 234, 237] In all these reports, however, the incidence of rebleeding was high, a finding that was confirmed in a larger controlled investigation.[159]

Vasopressin is thought to lower portal venous pressure principally by constricting the splanchnic arteriolar bed, causing an increase in resistance to inflow of blood to the gut.[60, 240] In addition, a recent study suggests that vasopressin causes a constriction of smooth muscle in the oesophageal wall which could shut off the inflow of blood from the coronary vein to the varices.[4] The constrictor effect on the smooth muscle of arterioles is generalized, and use of the systemic dose required to lower portal pressure (20 u) has been associated with potentially serious side-effects, including decrease of cardiac output, vasoconstriction of the coronary arteries, tachyphylaxis and its known antidiuretic effect.[58, 251]

In the light of these side-effects, Nusbaum and colleagues[187, 188, 189] suggested that variceal bleeding could be controlled by a continuous infusion of a minimal amount of vasopressin into the superior mesenteric artery. These and other investigators reported encouraging results from this form of therapy.[16,30,225] We, as well as others, noted less impressive results especially in regard to recurrence of haemorrhage after initial control,[56, 154, 179] development of side-effects related to catheter insertion[179] and spontaneous bacterial peritonitis related to vasoconstriction of the splanchnic vascular bed.[9]

Conn and his colleagues[57] have subsequently performed a prospective controlled clinical trial comparing conventional treatment (SBT not used) with conventional therapy plus selective intra-arterial vasopressin in patients with acute variceal haemorrhage.

Vasopressin was significantly more effective than conventional therapy in controlling haemorrhage from varices. Paradoxically, however, survival was not affected. The failure of initial cessation of haemorrhage to improve survival is reminiscent of the situation with the Sengstaken–Blakemore tube, and systemic vasopressin, in that many of those who died had severe underlying hepatocellular dysfunction and there was a high frequency of recurrent haemorrhage.

In the light of the results of the controlled trial referred to above,[57] selective intra-arterial infusion of vasopressin can no longer be advocated as a primary form of emergency therapy for bleeding varices. Indeed, subsequent upon publication of Conn's results, selective infusion of vasopressin (0.2 u/min) into the superior mesenteric artery of patients with portal hypertension was found to cause only a small decrease (mean 9.6 per cent) in free portal pressure.[165] Moreover, significant systemic side-effects (fall in cardiac output, increase in arterial blood pressure and decrease in femoral arterial Po_2) were also noted.[165] The lack of reduction of systemic side-effects by selective intra-arterial infusion compared to systemic administration of vasopressin has now been confirmed in a careful haemodynamic study performed in dogs.[10]

Synthetic Vasopressin Derivatives

Octapressin (2-phenylalanine-5-lysine-vasopressin) is a chemically related peptide that has the same mode of action as vasopressin[4, 46, 60] and, when administered systemically in the same dose as vasopressin, has been shown to lower portal pressure in patients with portal hypertension.[275]

Recently, a new compound, triglycyl-lysine-vasopressin (t-GLVP) has been synthesized.[287] It is practically inactive per se on smooth muscle, but serves as a chemical depot form of vasopressin, because the added amino terminal glycine residues are slowly cleaved off in vivo by membrane bound amino oligopeptidases,[3, 120, 126] resulting in a slow release of active nonapeptide hormone.[59, 60, 134] Thus, although efficiency of release is low, necessitating higher dosages,[60] it is possible to achieve smooth muscle pharmacological activity for up to 10 hours after a single dose as compared to 20 to 40 minutes after an equipotent dose of vasopressin.[59, 60, 134] Initial clinical experience with t-GLVP was encouraging, as variceal haemorrhage was controlled in 88 per cent of 15 patients treated.[287] Potentially, use of the compound has added advantages over the high potency, short-acting forms of the hormone[287] in that cardiotoxic side-effects are avoided, and there appears to be practically complete suppression of the potential thrombolytic action of the short-acting forms.[82]

EMERGENCY MEDICAL MANAGEMENT OF VARICEAL HAEMORRHAGE (KING'S COLLEGE HOSPITAL, LONDON)

In our experience, the Boyce modifications[25] and four lumen modifications of the Sengstaken–Blakemore tube, as well as systemic vasopressin, have proved an effective means of initially controlling active variceal haemorrhage. Currently, a trial is in progress to compare the efficacy of tamponade alone, systemic t-GLVP alone and the two in combination. In our past experience, the incidence of rebleeding after deflation of the Sengstaken–Blakemore tube or after systemic or intra-arterial vasopressin is high. Consequently, the use of the Sengstaken–Blakemore tube and t-GLVP represents the first link in a chain of therapy which, in addition, includes oesophageal and percutaneous transhepatic sclerotherapy.

OTHER FORMS OF EMERGENCY MANAGEMENT

Surgery

If variceal bleeding cannot be controlled by medical measures alone, most groups have resorted to some form of surgical intervention. In addition, surgery has been considered by some as a primary therapy for bleeding varices.[195] Surgical aspects of therapy are covered in detail in this book (see Chapter 44) and elsewhere.[96] In brief, emergency portacaval anastomosis (for review of overall results see Prandi et al[211]) has been widely advocated, with an overall mean operative mortality of 40 per cent. However, Prandi et al[211] have emphasized the extremely poor outlook (approaching 100 per cent mortality) of those patients with poor hepatic reserve who bleed torrentially. Emergency mesocaval shunts have attracted interest but, again, operative mortality is high.[254] Oesophageal or high gastric transection or trans-thoracic–trans-oesophageal ligation of the varices have all received consideration. The operative mortality of all these procedures is high, approaching 50 per cent in most hands for emergency oesophageal transection, for example.[85, 214, 228] The unsatisfactory nature of the results of emergency surgery for variceal haemorrhage has resulted in a resurgence of interest in sclerotherapy as a primary means of controlling variceal haemorrhage.

Oesophageal Sclerotherapy

Injection of a sclerosing agent through an oesophagoscope was introduced by Crafoord and Frenckner in 1939.[61] Later, the method was used by Fearon and Sass-Kortsak,[75] Orloff[192] and Hunt and colleagues.[109] Recently, Johnston and Rodgers[118] have reviewed their experience of 217 injections performed in 117 unselected patients. The results appeared to be excellent as not only was bleeding controlled in 177 of the cases but a single injection was sufficient in 158 of these. It is notable, however, that 25 per cent of patients included in their series had extrahepatic portal hypertension with well-preserved hepatic function. Full clinical details of the other patients treated were not included in the paper, so it is impossible to determine in what way the results were influenced by such factors as hepatic reserve, general clinical condition and severity of haemorrhage. In these early sclerotherapy series, the old rigid oesophagoscope was used.

Encouraged by the results of Johnston and Rodgers,[118] we embarked upon a pilot study to determine its efficacy as an adjunct to medical therapy in the treatment of our patients who had active variceal haemorrhage. The plan was to inject the varices via an oesophagoscope once initial haemostasis had been achieved by the use of the Sengstaken–Blakemore tube, usually in combination with at least one systemic injection of vasopressin. Our immediate results were not nearly as impressive as those of Johnston and Rodgers, since only 13 of the first 25 patients survived to leave hospital. However, the clinical condition of many of the patients, including some of those who survived, was extremely poor and most had suffered torrential variceal haemorrhage. To start with, a specially modified rigid oesophagoscope was used.[8] Two of the deaths early on in the series were caused by a ruptured oesophagus, and consequently we now use an oblique viewing fibreoptic endoscope, which is surrounded by a plastic sleeve to steady the varices and compress them once the sclerosant material has been injected.

Clearly, the significance of these preliminary results cannot be determined. In view of the fact that a number of 'poor risk' patients survived to leave hospital, we have now embarked upon a prospective, randomized controlled clinical trial comparing conventional treatment with conventional therapy plus oesophageal sclerotherapy. All patients admitted with endoscopically proven active variceal bleeding (extrahepatic portal hypertension excluded) are considered for entry into the trial. Once primary haemostasis has been achieved with systemic t-GLVP or the Sengstaken–Blakemore tube, or a combination of the two, patients are randomized to receive standardized conventional care or oesophageal sclerotherapy. Patients in the sclerotherapy group are discharged after the first injection and are readmitted at 2 to 3 weekly periods for further injections which are continued either until the patient is withdrawn from the trial or until the oesophageal varices are too small to inject. Results to date are preliminary as only 10 patients have been randomized to sclerotherapy and 10 to conservative therapy. The results are of interest, however, because the proportion of patients dying or withdrawn from the trial (on account of further variceal haemorrhage or complications of sclerotherapy) is so far similar in the two groups.

Percutaneous Transhepatic Sclerotherapy
(see also Chapter 44)

Recently, the technique of percutaneous transhepatic venography has been modified by Lunderqvist and co-workers.[147, 148, 284] They have elegantly demonstrated that it is possible to stop oesophageal variceal bleedings by injection of sclerosing agents through transhepatic selective catheterization of the left gastric coronary vein. Their latest published figures show that the procedure has successfully stopped variceal bleeding in all 20 patients so far treated.[12] This is the approach currently being adopted by Sherlock and colleagues.[235] At the time of their initial report, 11 cases of active bleeding varices had been treated with initial cessation of bleeding in 10 of these. So far, follow-up times have been too short to allow a proper assessment of the efficacy of percutaneous transhepatic sclerotherapy as a means of preventing further episodes of variceal haemorrhage from occurring.

CONCLUSION

In 1971, Conn[53] pointed out that dramatic changes were taking place in the field of portal hypertension. He postulated then that the solution to the problem of bleeding varices would most likely be achieved by the invention of a completely new 'mousetrap' and not by minor revisions of an old one. He suggested that the revolutionary new mousetrap might be the local arterial infusion of vasopressin. This does not appear to have been the case. Possibly, it might be oesophageal or percutaneous transhepatic sclerotherapy but we shall have to await events.

REFERENCES

1. Adamsons, R.J., Kinkhabwala, M., Moskowitz, H., Himmelfarb, E., Minkowitz, S. & Lerner, B. (1972) Portacaval shunt with arterialization of the hepatic portion of the portal vein. *Surgery, Gynecology and Obstetrics*, **135**, 529–535.
2. Adamsons, R.J., Butt, K., Dennis, C.R., Kinkhabwala, M., Moskowitz, H., Gordon, D. & Babich, A. (1977) Prognostic significance of portal pressure in patients with bleeding oesophageal varices. *Surgery, Gynecology and Obstetrics*, **145**, 353–368.
3. Adibi, S.A. (1977) Clearance of dipeptides from plasma: role of kidney and intestine. In *Peptide Transport and Hydrolysis*, pp. 265–286. Amsterdam: Elsevier Scientific.
4. Aronsen, K.F., Bjorkman, I. & Londstrom, K. (1975) The mechanism of vasopressin's haemostatic effect in bleeding oesophageal varices. Abstracts, *10th Congress of the European Society of Experimental Surgery, Paris*, p. 97.
5. Atkinson, M. & Sherlock, S. (1954) Intrasplenic pressure as an index of the portal venous pressure. *Lancet*, **i**, 1325–1328.
6. Atkinson, M., Barnett, E., Sherlock, S. & Steiner, R.E. (1955) The clinical investigation of the portal circulation with special reference to portal venography. *Quarterly Journal of Medicine*, **24**, 77–93.
7. Aufses, A.H. (1960) Bleeding varices associated with haematologic disorders. *Archives of Surgery*, **80**, 655–659.
8. Bailey, M.E. & Dawson, J.L. (1975) Modified oesophagoscope for injecting oesophageal varices. *British Medical Journal*, **ii**, 540–541.
9. Bar-Meir, S. & Conn, H.O. (1976) Spontaneous bacterial peritonitis induced by intra-arterial vasopressin therapy. *Gastroenterology*, **70**, 418–421.
10. Barr, J.W., Lakin, R.C. & Rösch, J. (1975) Similarity of arterial and intravenous vasopressin on portal and systemic haemodynamics. *Gastroenterology*, **69**, 13–19.
11. Basu Mallick, K.C., Sen Gupta, K.P., Basu, A.K., Biswas, S.K., Pal, N.C. & Boyer, J. (1967) Non cirrhotic portal fibrosis with portal hypertension. A new syndrome. Part II. Histopathological studies. *Indian Journal of Medical Research*, **55**, 351–359.
12. Bengmark, S. (1975) Surgical management of portal hypertension. *Clinics in Gastroenterology*, **4**, 395–423.
13. Benhamou, J.P., Maillard, J.N., Rueff, B. & Michon, H. (1963) Les fausses thromboses portale essentialle. *Presse Médicale*, **70**, 2397–2402

14. Benhamou, J.P., Antoine, B., Debray, Ch., Nezelof, Ch., Roux, M., Watchi, J.M. & Pequignot, H. (1969) La fibrose hépatique congénitale. *Presse Médicale*, **77**, 167–174.
15. Bertrand, L. & Michel, H. (1969) La sonde de Linton–Nichlas. *Archives Francaises des Maladies Appareil Digestif*, **58**, 797–804.
16. Bhatia, C.K., Nidiry, J., Harrell, J., Mock, J. & Danovitch, S.H. (1973) Selective splanchnic perfusion of vasopressin in the management of torrential gastrointestinal haemorrhage. *Annals of Internal Medicine*, **78**, 818.
17. Bierman, H.R., Kelly, K.H. & White, L.P. (1955) Transhepatic venous catheterization and venography. *Journal of the American Medical Association*, **158**, 1331–1334.
18. Bierman, H.R., Steinbach, H.L., White, L.P. & Kelly, K.H. (1952) Portal venepuncture. A percutaneous, transhepatic approach. *Proceedings of the Society of Experimental Biological Medicine*, **79**, 550–552.
19. Blendis, L.M. (1969) *The Spleen and Haemodilution Anaemia*. MD Thesis, University of London.
20. Blendis, L.M. (1974) Certain consequences of cirrhosis. *Medicine*, **8**, 563–577.
21. Blendis, L.M., Banks, D.C., Ramboer, C. & Williams, R. (1970) Splenic blood flow and splanchnic haemodynamics in blood dyscrasia and other splenomegalies. *Clinical Science*, **38**, 73–84.
22. Blendis, L.M., Smith, P.M., Lawrie, B.W., Stephens, M.R. & Evans, W.D. (1977) Haemodynamic studies in vinyl chloride monomer workers with portal hypertension. *Gut*, **18**, 400–401.
23. Blyth, H. & Ockenden, B.G. (1971) Polycystic disease of the kidneys and liver presenting in childhood. *Journal of Medical Genetics*, **8**, 257–284.
24. Boijsen, E., Ekman, C.A. & Olin, T. (1963) Coeliac and superior mesenteric angiography in portal hypertension. *Acta Chirurgica Scandinavica*, **126**, 315–322.
25. Boyce, H.W. Jr (1962) Modification of the Sengstaken–Blakemore tube. *New England Journal of Medicine*, **267**, 195–196.
26. Boyer, J.L., Sen Gupta, K.P., Biswas, S.K., Pal, N.C., Basu Mallick, K.C., Iber, F.L. & Basu, A.K. (1967) Idiopathic portal hypertension. Comparison with the portal hypertension of cirrhosis and extrahepatic portal vein obstruction. *Annals of Internal Medicine*, **66**, 41–68.
27. Boyer, T.D., Triger, D.R., Horisawa, M., Redeker, A.G. & Reynolds, T.B. (1977) Direct transhepatic measurement of portal vein pressure using a thin needle. Comparison with wedged hepatic vein pressure. *Gastroenterology*, **72**, 584–589.
28. Braasted, F.W., Wukarsch, D.C. & Jordan, P.H. Jr (1970) The practicability of umbilical vein cannulation in patients with and without portal hypertension. *Archives of Surgery*, **101**, 32–35.
29. Bradley, S.E., Ingelfinger, F.J., Bradley, G.P. & Curry, J.J. (1945) The estimation of hepatic blood flow in man. *Journal of Clinical Investigation*, **24**, 890–897.
30. Brand, B., Rosch, J. & Krippaehne, W.W. (1972) Experiences with angiography in diagnosis and treatment of acute gastrointestinal bleeding of various etiologies: preliminary report. *Annals of Surgery*, **176**, 419–434.
31. Bras, G., Brooks, S.E.H. & Watler, D.C. (1961) Cirrhosis of the liver in Jamaica. *Journal of Pathology and Bacteriology*, **82**, 503–512.
32. Brink, A.J. & Botha, D. (1955) Budd–Chiari syndrome: diagnosis by hepatic venography. *British Journal of Radiology*, **28**, 330–331.
33. Bron, K.M. & Fisher, B. (1967) Arterial portography: indications and technique. *Surgery*, **61**, 137–152.
34. Bronte-Stewart, B. & Goetz, R.H. (1952) Budd–Chiari syndrome. High inferior vena caval obstruction demonstrated by venography. *Angiology*, **3**, 167–178.
35. Bull, L.G., Culvenor, C.C.J. & Dick, A.T. (1968) *The Pyrrolizidine Alkaloids*. pp. 1–293. Amsterdam: North Holland.
36. Bunim, J.J., Kimberl, D.V., Thomas, L.B., Van Scott, G.J. & Klatskin, G. (1962) The syndrome of sarcoidosis, psoriasis, and gout. *Annals of Internal Medicine*, **57**, 1018–1040.
37. Burcharth, F. & Malmstrøm, J. (1976) Experiences with the Linton–Nachlas and the Sengstaken–Blakemore tubes for bleeding oesophageal varices. *Surgery, Gynecology and Obstetrics*, **142**, 529–531.
38. Burchell, A.R., Rousselot, L.M. & Panke, W.F. (1968) A seven year experience with side to side portacaval shunt for cirrhotic ascites. *Annals of Surgery*, **168**, 655–670.
39. Burchell, A.R., Moreno, A.H., Panke, W.F. & Rousselot, L.M. (1965) Some limitations of splenic portography. 1. Incidences, haemodynamics and surgical implications of the nonvisualised portal vein. *Annals of Surgery*, **162**, 981–995.
40. Burchell, A.R., Moreno, A.H., Panke, W.F. & Nealon, T.F. (1974) Hemodynamic variables and prognosis following portal caval shunts. *Surgery, Gynecology and Obstetrics*, **138**, 359–369.
41. Caesar, J., Shaldon, S., Chiandussi, L., Guevara, L. & Sherlock, S. (1961) The use of indocyanine green in the measurement of hepatic blood flow and as a test of hepatic function. *Clinical Science*, **21**, 43–57.
42. Caesar, J., Barber, K.M., Baraona, E. & Sherlock, S. (1962) The estimation of portal–systemic collateral flow in man using splenic injection of radio-active indicator. *Clinical Science*, **23**, 77.
43. Calne, R.Y. & Williams, R. (1977) Orthotopic liver transplantation: the first 60 patients. *British Medical Journal*, **i**, 471–476.
44. Castberg, T. (1952) Vascular changes in chronic passive congestion of the liver. *Acta Pathologica et Microbiologica Scandinavica*, **30**, 358–370.
45. Castro Silva, L., Do Goffi, F.S. & Da Silva Bastos, E. (1966) An appraisal and comparative study of the measurement of portal pressure by transparietal intrasplenic manometries and laparotomy. *Surgery*, **60**, 1137–1140.
46. Cerletti, A., Weber, H. & Weidmann, H. (1963) Zur Wirkung von Phenylalanine Z lysine-Vasopressin (Octapressin) auf den Arteriellen und Venosen Anteil eines Peripheren Gefassgebiets. *Helvetica Physiologica et Pharmacologica Acta*, **21**, 394–401.
47. Chiles, N.H., Baggenstoss, A.H. & Olsen, A.M. (1953) Oesophageal varices: comparative incidence of ulceration and spontaneous rupture as a cause of fatal haemorrhage, *Gastroenterology*, **25**, 565–573.
48. Clain, D., Freston, J., Kreel, L. & Sherlock, S. (1967) Clinical diagnosis of the Budd–Chiari syndrome. A report of six cases. *American Journal of Medicine*, **43**, 544–554.
49. Clark, J.A. (1928) A comparison of the effects of adrenaline and pituitrin on the portal circulation. *Journal of Physiology*, **66**, 274–280.

50. Cohn, J.N., Khatri, I.M. & Groszmann, R.J. (1972) Hepatic blood flow in alcoholic liver disease measured by an indicator dilution technique. *American Journal of Medicine*, **53**, 704–714.

51. Conn, H.O. (1958) Hazards attending the use of oesophageal tamponade. *Journal of the American Medical Association*, **259**, 701–707.

52. Conn, H.O. (1970) The prognosis and management of bleeding oesophageal varices. *Annals of the New York Academy of Science*, **170**, 345–357.

53. Conn, H.O. (1971) Sengstaken–Blakemore tube revisited. *Gastroenterology*, **61**, 398–400.

54. Conn, H.O. (1974) Therapeutic portacaval anastomosis: to shunt or not to shunt. *Gastroenterology*, **67**, 1065–1073.

55. Conn, H.O. & Simpson, J.A. (1967) Excessive mortality with balloon tamponade. *Journal of the American Medical Association*, **202**, 587–591.

56. Conn, H.O., Ramsby, G.R. & Storer, E.H. (1972) Selective intra-arterial vasopressin in the treatment of upper gastrointestinal haemorrhage. *Gastroenterology*, **63**, 634–645.

57. Conn, H.O., Ramsby, G.R., Storer, E.H., Mutchnick, M.G., Joshi, P.H., Phillips, M.M., Cohen, G.A., Fields, G.N. & Petroski, D. (1975) Intra-arterial vasopressin in the treatment of upper gastrointestinal haemorrhage. A prospective, controlled clinical trial. *Gastroenterology*, **68**, 211–221.

58. Corliss, R.J., McKenna, D.H., Sialer, S., O'Brien, G.S. & Rowe, G.G. (1968) Systemic and coronary haemodynamic effects of vasopressin. *American Journal of Medical Science*, **256**, 293–299.

59. Cort, J.H., Jeanjean, M.F., Thomson, A.E. & Nickerson, M. (1968) Effect of 'hormonogen' forms of neurohypophysial peptides in haemorrhagic shock in dogs. *American Journal of Physiology*, **214**, 455–462.

60. Cort, J.H., Albrecht, I., Novakova, J., Muller, J.L. & Jost, K. (1975) Regional and systemic haemodynamic effects of some vasopressins: structural features of the hormone which prolong activity. *European Journal of Clinical Investigation*, **5**, 165–175.

61. Crafoord, C. & Frenckner, P. (1939) New surgical treatment of varicose veins of the oesophagus. *Acta Oto-Laryngologica*, **27**, 422–429.

62. Dagradi, A.E., Mehler, R. & Ton, D.T. (1970) Sources of upper gastrointestinal bleeding in patients with liver cirrhosis and large esophagogastric varices. *American Journal of Gastroenterology*, **54**, 458–463.

63. Dagradi, A.E., Siemsen, J. & Brook, J. (1967) Bleeding esophageal varices in myelofibrosis. *American Journal of Gastroenterology*, **44**, 536–544.

64. Dal Palu, C., Ruol, A. & Belloni, G. (1963) Postsinusoidal portal hypertension in a patient with chronic lymphatic leukaemia. *American Journal of Digestive Diseases*, **8**, 845–851.

65. Davis, M. & Williams, R. (1977) Alcoholic liver disease – a suitable case for transplantation? *British Journal of Alcohol and Alcoholism*, **12**, 91–94.

66. Douglass, B.E. & Snell, A.M. (1950) Portal cirrhosis: an analysis of 444 cases with notes on modern methods of treatment. *Gastroenterology*, **15**, 407–425.

67. Douglass, B.E., Baggenstoss, A.H. & Hollinshead, W.H. (1950) Variations in the portal system of veins. *Proceedings of the Mayo Clinic*, **25**, 26–31.

68. Dumont, A.E., Amorosi, E. & Stahl, W.M. (1970) Significance of splenomegaly in patients with hepatic cirrhosis and bleeding oesophageal varices. *Annals of Surgery*, **171**, 522–526.

69. Dunn, G.D., Hayes, P., Breen, K.J. & Schenker, S. (1973) The liver in congestive failure: a review. *American Journal of Medical Science*, **265**, 174–189.

70. Duppmann, J.L. & Shapiro, R. (1961) Bleeding esophageal varices in the presence of normal splenoportogram, a case report. *American Journal of Roentgenology*, **86**, 1103–1107.

71. Eckardt, V.F., Grace, N.D. & Kantrowitz, P.A. (1976) Does lower oesophageal sphincter incompetency contribute to oesophageal variceal bleeding? *Gastroenterology*, **71**, 185–189.

72. Edmondson, H.A., Peters, R.L., Reynolds, T.D. & Kuzma, O.T. (1963) Sclerosing hyaline necrosis of the liver in the chronic alcoholic. *Annals of Internal Medicine*, **59**, 646–673.

73. Eichhorn, R. (1964) A device to simplify the application of the Sengstaken tube. *Gastroenterology*, **47**, 600–601.

74. Falchuk, Z.M. & Leventhal, B.G. (1973) Budd–Chiari syndrome in a patient with paroxysmal nocturnal hemoglobinuria. *American Journal of Digestive Diseases*, **18**, 900–904.

75. Fearon, B. & Sass-Kortsak, A. (1959) The management of oesophageal varices in children by injection of sclerosing agents. *Annals of Otology, Rhinology and Laryngology*, **78**, 908–915.

76. Ferguson, D.J. (1963) Hemodynamics in surgery for portal hypertension. *Annals of Surgery*, **158**, 383–386.

77. Fomon, J.H. & Warren, W.D. (1969) Hemodynamic studies in portal hypertension. *Annual Review of Medicine*, **20**, 277–290.

78. Fonkalstrud, E.W., Myers, N.A. & Robinson, M.J. (1974) Management of extrahepatic portal hypertension in children. *Annals of Surgery*, **180**, 487–493.

79. Forshaw, J. (1972) Alcoholic cirrhosis of the liver. *British Medical Journal*, **iv**, 608–609.

80. Fried, K., Liban, E. & Lurie, M. (1971) Polycystic kidneys associated with malformations of the brain, polydactyly and other birth defects in new born sibs. *Journal of Medical Genetics*, **8**, 285–290.

81. Friedman, E.W. & Weiner, R.S. (1951) Estimation of hepatic sinusoid pressure by means of venous catheters and estimation of portal pressure by hepatic vein catheterization. *American Journal of Physiology*, **165**, 527–531.

82. Gader, A.M.A., Da Costa, J. & Cash, J.D. (1973) A new vasopressin analogue and fibrinolysis. *Lancet*, **ii**, 1417–1418.

83. Galambos, J.T., Warren, W.D., Rudman, D., Smith, R.B. & Salem, A.A. (1976) Selective and total shunts in the treatment of bleeding varices. *New England Journal of Medicine*, **295**, 1089–1095.

84. Garceau, A.J. & Chalmers, T.C. (1963) The natural history of cirrhosis. Survival with esophageal varices. *New England Journal of Medicine*, **268**, 469–473.

85. George, P., Brown, C., Ridgway, G., Crofts, B. & Sherlock, S. (1973) Emergency oesophageal transection in uncontrolled variceal haemorrhage. *British Journal of Surgery*, **60**, 635–640.

86. Ghahremani, G.G., Port, R.B., Winans, C.J. & Williams, J.R. (1972) Esophageal varices. Enhanced radiologic visualisation by anticholinergic drugs. *American Journal of Digestive Diseases*, **17**, 703–712.

87. Gibson, J.A. (1973) Granulomatous liver disease and portal hypertension. *Proceedings of the Royal Society of Medicine*, **66**, 502–503.
88. Gibson, J.A., White, H., Fairclough, P.D., Farthing, M.J., Clark, M.L. & Dawson, A.M. (1979) Experience of 82 patients with extrahepatic portal hypertension. In preparation.
89. Gibson, J.B., Johnston, G.W., Fulton, T.T. & Rodgers, H.W. (1965) Extrahepatic portal venous obstruction. *British Journal of Surgery*, **52**, 129–139.
90. Green, J., Mistilis, S. & Schiff, L. (1963) Acute alcoholic hepatitis; a clinical study of 50 cases. *Archives of Internal Medicine*, **112**, 67–78.
91. Grosfeld, J.L., Fitzgerald, J.F., Wagner, V.M., Newton, W.A. & Baehner, R.L. (1976) Portal hypertension in infants and children with histiocytosis X. *American Journal of Surgery*, **131**, 108–113.
92. Groszmann, R., Kotelanski, B., Cohn, J. & Khatsi, A.M. (1972) Quantitation of portasystemic shunting from the splenic and mesenteric beds in alcoholic liver disease. *American Journal of Medicine*, **53**, 715–722.
93. Guckian, J.C. & Perry, J.E. (1966) Granulomatous hepatitis: an analysis of 63 cases and review of the literature. *Annals of Internal Medicine*, **65**, 1081–1100.
94. Hallenbeck, G.A., Comess, M.S., Wollaeger, E.E. & Gage, R.P. (1959) Bleeding varices due to cirrhosis; survival after (1) non-surgical treatment, (2) splenectomy with or without omentopexy, and (3) portacaval and splenorenal shunts. *Archives of Surgery*, **78**, 774–785.
95. Hamilton, D.W. & Hunt, A.H. (1970) Extrahepatic portal obstruction. *Medical Journal of Australia*, **1**, 493–499.
96. Hermann, R.E. (1975) Shunt operations for portal hypertension. *Surgical Clinics of North America*, **55**, 1073–1087.
97. Hermann, R.E. & Traul, D. (1970) Experience with the Sengstaken–Blakemore tube for bleeding esophageal varices. *Surgery, Gynecology and Obstetrics*, **130**, 879–885.
98. Hickling, R.A. (1937) Chronic non-leukaemic myelosis. *Quarterly Journal of Medicine*, **6**, 253–275.
99. Hirooka, M. & Kimura, C. (1970) Membranous obstruction of the hepatic portion of the inferior vena cava: surgical correction and etiological study. *Archives of Surgery*, **100**, 656–663.
100. Hodgson, H.J.F. & Thompson, R.P.H. (1976) Cirrhosis in South London. *Lancet*, **ii**, 118–121.
101. Hoeffel, J.C., Jacottin, G. & Bourgeois, J.M. (1971) A propos d'une famille associant des cas de polylkystose rénale de type juvenile et de type adulte. *Annals of Radiology*, **14**, 204–209.
102. Horler, A.R., Shaw, M.T. & Thompson, R.B. (1970) Budd–Chiari syndrome as a complication of paroxysmal nocturnal hemoglobinuria. *Postgraduate Medical Journal*, **46**, 618–634.
103. Hoyumpa, A.M. Jr, Schiff, L. & Helfman, E.L. (1971) Budd–Chiari syndrome in women taking oral contraceptives. *American Journal of Medicine*, **50**, 137–140.
104. Hsia, D.Y. & Gellis, S.S. (1955) Portal hypertension in infants and children. *American Journal of Digestive Diseases*, **90**, 290–298.
105. Huet, P.M., Lavoie, P. & Viallet, A. (1973) Simultaneous estimation of hepatic and portal blood flows by an indicator dilution technique. *Journal of Laboratory and Clinical Medicine*, **83**, 836–846.
106. Huet, P.M., Marleau, D., Lavoie, P. & Viallet, A. (1976) Extraction of ^{125}I-albumin microaggregates from portal blood. An index of functional blood supply in cirrhotics. *Gastroenterology*, **70**, 74–81.
107. Hughes, M. & Fox, H. (1972) A histological analysis of granulomatous hepatitis. *Journal of Clinical Pathology*, **25**, 817–820.
108. Hunt, A.H. (1965) An analysis of 584 cases of portal hypertension seen between 1947–1963, with particular reference to surgical treatment. *St Bartholomew's Hospital Journal of Clinical Research* (Suppl.) **11**, LXIX, i–xv.
109. Hunt, P.S., Johnston, G.W. & Rodgers, H.W. (1969) The emergency management of bleeding oesophageal varices with sclerosing injection. *British Journal of Surgery*, **56**, 305–307.
110. Imanaga, H., Yamamoto, S. & Kuroyanagi, Y. (1962) Surgical treatment of portal hypertension according to state of intrahepatic circulation. *Annals of Surgery*, **155**, 42–50.
111. Imperato, A.M. (1960) Gaucher's disease with ascites; response to portacaval shunt. *Annals of Surgery*, **151**, 431–436.
112. Ivemark, B.I., Oldfelt, V. & Zetterstrom, R.I. (1959) Familial dysplasia of kidneys, liver and pancreas. A probably genetically determined syndrome. *Acta Paediatrica Scandinavica*, **48**, 1–11.
113. Jackson, F.C., Perrin, E.D., Felix, R. & Smith, W.R. (1971) A clinical investigation of the portacaval shunt. V. Survival analysis of the therapeutic operation. *Annals of Surgery*, **174**, 672–701.
114. Jain, S., Paton, A. & Wansbrough-Jones, M.H. (1973) Cirrhosis in Birmingham. *Midlands Medical Review*, **9**, 13–16.
115. Jarett, S.N., Kew, M.C. & Litnaitsky, D. (1966) Gaucher's disease with portal hypertension. Case report. *Journal of Paediatrics*, **68**, 810–812.
116. Johansen, T.S. & Baden, H. (1973) Re-appraisal of the Sengstaken–Blakemore balloon tamponade for bleeding oesophageal varices; results in 91 patients. *Scandinavian Journal of Gastroenterology*, **8**, 181–183.
117. Johnston, G.W. & Gibson, J.B. (1965) Portal hypertension resulting from splenic arteriovenous fistulae. *Gut*, **6**, 500–502.
118. Johnston, G.W. & Rodgers, H.W. (1973) A review of 15 years' experience in the use of sclerotherapy in the control of acute haemorrhage from oesophageal varices. *British Journal of Surgery*, **60**, 797–800.
119. Katz, L.N. & Rodbard, S. (1939) The integration of the vasomotor responses in the liver with those in other systemic vessels. *Journal of Pharmacology and Experimental Therapeutics*, **67**, 407–422.
120. Kenny, A.J. (1977) Endopeptidases in the brush border of the kidney proximal tubule. In *Peptide Transport and Hydrolysis*. pp. 209–220. Ciba Foundation Symposium 50 (New Series). Amsterdam: Elsevier Scientific.
121. Kerr, D.N.S., Warrick, C.K. & Hart-Mercer, J. (1962) A lesion resembling medullary sponge in patients with congenital hepatic fibrosis. *Clinical Radiology*, **13**, 85–91.

122. Kerr, D.N.S., Harrison, C.V., Sherlock, S. & Walker, R.M. (1961) Congenital hepatic fibrosis. *Quarterly Journal of Medicine,* **30,** 91–117.

123. Kessler, R.E. & Zimmon, D.S. (1967) Umbilical vein catheterization in man. *Surgery, Gynecology and Obstetrics,* **124,** 594–597.

124. Kessler, R.E., Tice, D.A. & Zimmon, D.S. (1973) Value, complications and limitations of umbilical vein catheterization. *Surgery, Gynecology and Obstetrics,* **136,** 529–535.

125. Kew, M.C., Varma, R.R., Santos, H.A., Scheuer, P.J. & Sherlock, S. (1971) Portal hypertension in primary biliary cirrhosis. *Gut,* **12,** 496.

126. Kim, Y.S. (1977) Intestinal mucosal hydrolysis of proteins and peptides. In *Peptide Transport and Hydrolysis.* pp. 151–176. Ciba Foundation Symposium 50 (New Series). Amsterdam: Elsevier Scientific Publishing.

127. King, H. & Shumacker, H.B. Jr (1968) Splenic studies. II. Portal hypertension in children associated with gastroesophageal hemorrhage. *Archives of Surgery,* **65,** 499–510.

128. Krasner, N., Davis, M., Portmann, B. & Williams, R. (1977) The changing pattern of alcoholic liver disease in Great Britain – relationship to sex and manifestations of autoimmunity. *British Medical Journal,* **i,** 1497–1500.

129. Kreel, K. & Williams, R. (1964) Arteriovenography of the portal system. *British Medical Journal,* **ii,** 1500–1503.

130. Kreel, L. (1970) Radiology of the portal system. *Gut,* **11,** 620–626.

131. Kreel, L., Freston, J.W. & Clain, D. (1967) Vascular radiology in the Budd–Chiari syndrome. *British Journal of Radiology,* **40,** 755–759.

132. Krook, H. (1957) Circulatory studies in liver cirrhosis. *Acta Medica Scandinavica* (Suppl.), **318**.

133. Kulick, G. & Rousselot, L.M. (1959) Combined pressure control and signal apparatus for safer emergency management of bleeding esophagogastric varices. *Gastroenterology,* **36,** 756–759.

134. Kyncl, J., Rezabek, K., Rasafirek, E., Pliska, V. & Rudinger, J. (1974) Hormonogen analogues of lysine-vasopressin: rat pressor and antidiuretic activities. *European Journal of Pharmacology,* **28,** 294–301.

135. Langer, B., Stone, R.M., Colapinto, R.F., Meindok, H., Phillips, M.J. & Fisher, M.M. (1975) Clinical spectrum of the Budd–Chiari syndrome and its surgical management. *American Journal of Surgery,* **129,** 137–145.

136. Lascavi, A.D., Girter, R.L., Soper, R.T. & Hill, L.F. (1968) Portal hypertension in a case of acute leukaemia treated with antimetabolites for ten years. *New England Journal of Medicine,* **279,** 303–306.

137. Leather, H.M. (1961) Portal hypertension and gross splenomegaly in Uganda. *British Medical Journal,* **i,** 15–18.

138. Lebrec, D., Kotelanski, B. & Cohn, J.N. (1976) Splanchnic hemodynamics in cirrhotic patients with oesophageal varices and gastrointestinal bleeding. *Gastroenterology,* **70,** 1108–1111.

139. Leevy, C.M., Zinke, M., Baber, J. & Chey, W.Y. (1958) Observations on the influence of medical therapy on portal hypertension in hepatic cirrhosis. *Annals of Internal Medicine,* **49,** 837–851.

140. Leevy, C.M., Meadenhall, C.L., Lesko, W. & Howard, M.M. (1962) Estimation of hepatic blood flow with indocyanine green. *Journal of Clinical Investigation,* **41,** 1169–1179.

141. Liebowitz, H.R. (1961) Pathogenesis of oesophageal varix rupture. *Journal of the American Medical Association,* **175,** 875–879.

142. Lima, J.P., Voneye, G., De Lima, C.P. & Ludwig, O.K. (1962) Portal venous pressure in Hodgkin's disease with hepatic involvement and esophageal varices. *American Journal of Medicine,* **32,** 618–620.

143. Linman, J.N. & Bethell, F.H. (1957) Agnogenic myeloid metaplasia. *American Journal of Medicine,* **22,** 107–122.

144. Linton, R.R. (1953) The emergency and definitive treatment of bleeding oesophageal varices. *Gastroenterology,* **24,** 1–9.

145. Lischner, M.W., Alexander, J.F. & Galambos, J.T. (1971) Natural history of alcoholic hepatitis. 1. The acute disease. *American Journal of Digestive Diseases,* **16,** 481–494.

146. Luna, A., Meister, H.P. & Szanto, P.B. (1968) Esophageal varices in the absence of cirrhosis. Incidence and characteristics in congestive heart failure and neoplasm of the liver. *American Journal of Clinical Pathology,* **49,** 710–717.

147. Lunderqvist, A. & Vang, J. (1974) Transhepatic catheterization and obliteration of the coronary vein in patients with portal hypertension and esophageal varices. *New England Journal of Medicine,* **291,** 646–649.

148. Lunderqvist, A. & Vang, J. (1974) Sclerosing injection of esophageal varices through transhepatic selective catheterization of the gastric coronary vein. A preliminary report. *Acta Radiologica,* **15,** 546–552.

149. Lyford, C.L., Vergara, G.G. & Moeller, D.D. (1976) Hepatic veno-occlusive disease originating in Ecuador. *Gastroenterology,* **70,** 105–108.

150. Maddrey, W.C., Johns, C.J., Bointnott, J.K. & Iber, F.L. (1970) Sarcoidosis and chronic hepatic disease: a clinical and pathologic study of 20 patients. *Medicine,* **49,** 375–395.

151. Maillard, J.N., Benhamou, J.P. & Rueff, B. (1966) Valeur pronostique de la mesure peropératoire de débit porte dans l'hypertension portale par cirrhose. In *Presses Universitaires de France.* Congrès Francais de Chirurgie, edn 68, pp. 593–601. Paris: Presses Universitaires de France.

152. Maillard, J.N., Benhamou, J.P. & Rueff, B. (1970) Arterialization of the liver with portacaval shunt in the treatment of portal hypertension due to intrahepatic block. *Surgery,* **67,** 883–890.

153. Marsden, P.D., Hutt, M.R.S. & Banwell, J.G. (1964) Abnormal splenovenograms in non-cirrhotic patients with portal hypertension and marked splenomegaly. *Journal of Tropical Medicine and Hygiene,* **67,** 239–245.

154. Marubbio, A.T. Jr, Lombardo, R.P. & Holt, P.R. (1973) Control of variceal bleeding by superior mesenteric artery pitressin perfusions – complications and indications. *American Journal of Digestive Diseases,* **18,** 239–243.

155. McCray, R.S., Martin, F., Amir-Ahmadi,, H., Sheaken, D.G. & Zamcheck, N. (1969) Erroneous diagnosis of haemorrhage from esophageal varices. *American Journal of Digestive Diseases,* **14,** 755–760.

156. McDermott, W.V. Jr (1972) Evaluation of the hemodynamics of portal hypertension in the selection of patients for shunt surgery. *Annals of Surgery,* **176,** 449–456.

157. McLean, E.K. (1970) The toxic actions of pyrrolizidine (*Senecio*) alkaloids. *Pharmacological Review*, **22**, 429–483.
158. McMichael, J. (1932) The portal circulation. 1. The action of adrenaline and pituitary pressor extract. *Journal of Physiology*, **75**, 241–263.
159. Merigan, T.C. Jr, Plotkin, G.R. & Davidson, C.S. (1962) Effect of intravenously administered posterior pituitary extract on hemorrhage from bleeding esophageal varices. *New England Journal of Medicine*, **266**, 134–135.
160. Meyers, J.D. & Taylor, W.J. (1951) An estimation of portal venous pressure by occlusive catheterization of an hepatic venule. *Journal of Clinical Investigation*, **30**, 662–663.
161. Michel, H. & Bertrand, L. (1972) La sonde de Linton–Nachlas dans le traitement des ruptures de varices oesophagiennes cirrhotique; supériorité sur celle de Sengstaken–Blakemore. *Biologie et Gastro-enterologie (Paris)*, **5**, 611–620.
162. Mikkelson, W.P. (1966) Extrahepatic portal hypertension in children. *American Journal of Surgery*, **111**, 333–340.
163. Mikkelson, W.P., Turrill, F.L., & Pattison, A.C. (1962) Portacaval shunt in cirrhosis of the liver: clinical and haemodynamic aspects. *American Journal of Surgery*, **104**, 204–215.
164. Mikkelson, W.P., Edmondson, H.A., Peters, R.L., Redeker, A.G. & Reynolds, T.B. (1965) Extra and intrahepatic portal hypertension without cirrhosis (hepato portal sclerosis). *Annals of Surgery*, **162**, 602–620.
165. Milette, B., Huet, P.M., Lavoie, P. & Viallet, A. (1975) Portal and systemic effects of selective infusion of vasopressin into the superior mesenteric artery in cirrhotic patients. *Gastroenterology*, **66**, 6–12.
166. Miller, F.J. Jr, Maddrey, W.C., Sheff, R.N., Harrington, D.P. & White, R.I. Jr (1975) Hepatic venography and hemodynamics in patients with alcoholic hepatitis. *Radiology*, **115**, 313–317.
167. Miller, M.C. & Brandt, J.L. (1962) Portal hypertension in the absence of both liver disease and vascular obstruction. *American Journal of Digestive Diseases*, **7**, 442–448.
168. Mistilis, S.P. (1975) Chronic active hepatitis. In *Diseases of the Liver* (Ed.) Schiff, L. pp. 787–814. Philadelphia: J.B. Lippincott.
169. Mistilis, S.P., Green, J.R. & Schiff, L. (1964) Hepatic sarcoidosis with portal hypertension. *American Journal of Medicine*, **36**, 470–475.
170. Mistilis, S.P., Skyring, A.P. & Blackburn, C.R. (1968) Natural history of active chronic hepatitis. 1. Clinical features, course, diagnostic criteria, morbidity, mortality, and survival. *Australian Annals of Medicine*, **17**, 214–223.
171. Mitchell, K.J., Macdougall, B.R.D., Silk, D.B.A. & Williams, R. (1979) A reappraisal of endoscopy findings in patients with portal hypertension suspected of bleeding from gastro-oesophageal varices. In preparation.
172. Mohabbat, O., Younos, M.S., Merzad, A.A., Srivastova, R.N., Sedig, G.G. & Aram, G.N. (1976) An outbreak of hepatic veno-occlusive disease in North Western Afghanistan. *Lancet*, **ii**, 269–271.
173. Moreno, A.H., Burchell, A.R., Rousselot, L.M., Panke, W.F. & Shapsky, S.F. (1967) Portal blood flow in cirrhosis of the liver. *Journal of Clinical Investigation*, **46**, 436–445.
174. Morgan, M. & Sherlock, S. (1977) Sex related differences among 100 patients with alcoholic liver disease. *British Medical Journal*, **i**, 939–941.
175. Morris, J.S., Schmid, M., Newman, S., Scheuer, P.J. & Sherlock, S. (1974) Arsenic and non-cirrhotic portal hypertension. *Gastroenterology*, **64**, 86–94.
176. Murray-Lyon, I.M., Ockenden, B.G. & Williams, R. (1973) Congenital hepatic fibrosis – is it a single clinical entity? *Gastroenterology*, **64**, 653–656.
177. Murray-Lyon, I.M., Stern, R.B. & Williams, R. (1973) Controlled trial of prednisone and azathioprine in active chronic hepatitis. *Lancet*, **i**, 735–737.
178. Murray-Lyon, I.M., Shilkin, K.B., Laws, J.W., Illing, R.C. & Williams, R. (1972) Non-obstructive dilatation of the intrahepatic biliary tree with cholangitis. *Quarterly Journal of Medicine*, **41**, 477–489.
179. Murray-Lyon, I.M., Pugh, R.N.H., Nunnerley, H.B., Laws, J.W., Dawson, J.L. & Williams, R. (1973) Treatment of bleeding oesophageal varices by infusion of vasopressin into the superior mesenteric artery. *Gut*, **14**, 59–63.
180. Nachlas, M.M. (1955) A new triple-lumen tube for the diagnosis and treatment of upper gastrointestinal haemorrhage. *New England Journal of Medicine*, **252**, 720–721.
181. Nachlas, M.M. (1956) Experiences with triple-lumen single-balloon tube in massive upper gastro-intestinal hemorrhage. *Gastroenterology*, **30**, 913–928.
182. Nagasue, N., Inokuchi, K., Kobayashi, M. & Saku, M. (1977) Hepatoportal arteriovenous fistula in primary carcinoma of the liver. *Surgery, Gynecology and Obstetrics*, **145**, 504–508.
183. Nakamura, T., Nakamura, S., Kaneko, T., Suzuki, T., Tokita, K. & Abe, S. (1962) Measurement of extrahepatic shunted blood in liver cirrhosis. *Journal of Laboratory and Clinical Medicine*, **6**, 889–901.
184. Nayak, N.C. & Ramalingaswami, V. (1969) Obliterative portal venography of the liver. *Archives of Pathology*, **87**, 359–369.
185. Nebesar, R.A. & Pollard, J.J. (1966) Portal venography by selective arterial catheterization. *American Journal of Roentgenology*, **97**, 477–487.
186. Novis, B.H., Duys, P., Barbezat, G.O., Clain, J., Bank, S. & Terblanche, J. (1976) Fibreoptic endoscopy and the use of the Sengstaken tube in acute gastrointestinal haemorrhage in patients with portal hypertension and varices. *Gut*, **17**, 258–263.
187. Nusbaum, M., Younis, M.T. & Baum, S. (1974) Control of portal hypertension. Selective mesenteric arterial infusion of vasopressin. *Archives of Surgery*, **108**, 342–347.
188. Nusbaum, M., Baum, S., Sakiyalak, P. & Blakemore, W.S. (1967) Pharmacologic control of portal hypertension. *Surgery*, **62**, 299–310.
189. Nusbaum, M., Baum, S., Kuroda, K. & Blakemore, W.S. (1968) Control of portal hypertension by selective mesenteric arterial drug infusion. *Archives of Surgery*, **97**, 1005–1012.
190. Oishi, N., Swisher, S.N., Stormont, J.M. & Schwartz, S.I. (1960) Portal hypertension in myeloid metaplasia. *Archives of Surgery*, **81**, 80–86.
191. Okuda, K., Suzuki, K., Musha, H. & Arimizu, N. (1977) Percutaneous transhepatic catheterization of the portal vein for the study of portal hemodynamics and shunts. *Gastroenterology*, **73**, 279–284.

192. Orloff, M.J. (1967) Emergency portacaval shunt: a comparative study of shunt, varix ligation and non-surgical treatment of bleeding esophageal varices in unselected patients with cirrhosis. *Annals of Surgery*, **166,** 456–478.
193. Orloff, M.J. & Thomas, H.S. (1963) Pathogenesis of esophageal varix rupture. A study based on gross and microscopic examination of the esophagus at the time of bleeding. *Archives of Surgery*, **87,** 301–307.
194. Orloff, M.J., Dugvary, L.R. & Kosta, L.D. (1977) Criteria for selection of patients for emergency portacaval shunt. *American Journal of Surgery*, **134,** 146–152.
195. Orloff, M.J., Charters, A.C., Chandler, J.G., Condon, J.K., Grambort, D.E., Modafferi, T.R., Levin, S.E., Brown, N.B., Sviokla, S.C. & Knox, D.G. (1975) Portacaval shunt as emergency procedure in unselected patients with alcoholic cirrhosis. *Surgery, Gynecology and Obstetrics*, **141,** 59–68.
196. Palmer, E.D. (1969) The vigorous diagnostic approach to upper gastrointestinal tract haemorrhage. *Journal of the American Medical Association*, **207,** 1477–1480.
197. Palmer, E.D. & Brick, I.B. (1954) Esophageal varices in non-cirrhotic patients. *American Journal of Medicine*, **17,** 641–644.
198. Panke, W.F., Rousselot, L.M. & Burchell, A.R. (1968) A 16 year experience with end-to-side portacaval shunt for variceal haemorrhage. *Annals of Surgery*, **168,** 957–965.
199. Parker, R.G.F. (1959) Occlusion of the hepatic veins in man. *Medicine (Baltimore)*, **38,** 369–402.
200. Paton, A., Reynolds, T.B. & Sherlock, S. (1953) Assessment of portal venous hypertension by catheterization of hepatic vein. *Lancet*, **i,** 918–921.
201. Pemberton, J.J. & Kierman, P. (1945) Surgery of the spleen. *Surgical Clinics of North America*, **25,** 880–890.
202. Piccone, V.A., Le Veen, H.H., White, J.J., Skinner, G.B. & MacLean, L.D. (1967) Transumbilical portal hepatography – a significant adjunct in the investigation of liver disease. *Surgery*, **61,** 333–346.
203. Pimentel, J.C. & Menezes, A.P. (1977) Liver disease in vineyard sprayers. *Gastroenterology*, **72,** 275–283.
204. Pitcher, J.L. (1971) Safety and effectiveness of the modified Sengstaken–Blakemore tube: a prospective study. *Gastroenterology*, **61,** 291–298.
205. Pitlik, S., Cohen, L., Hadar, H., Srulijes, C. & Rosenfield, J.B. (1977) Portal hypertension and esophageal varices in hemangiomatosis of the spleen. *Gastroenterology*, **72,** 937–940.
206. Polish, E. & Sullivan, B.G. (1961) Esophagitis associated with haemorrhage from esophageal varices. *Annals of Internal Medicine*, **54,** 908–911.
207. Polish, E., Christie, J., Cohen, A. & Sullivan, B. Jr (1962) Idiopathic presinusoidal portal hypertension (Banti's syndrome). *Annals of Internal Medicine*, **56,** 624–627.
208. Pollard, J.J. & Nebesar, R.A. (1967) Altered hemodynamics in Budd–Chiari syndrome demonstrated by selective hepatic and selective splenic angiography. *Radiology*, **89,** 236–243.
209. Porter, G.H. (1961) Hepatic sarcoidosis – a cause of portal hypertension and liver failure. *Archives of Internal Medicine*, **108,** 482–495.
210. Prandi, D., Rueff, B. & Benhamou, J.P. (1975) Side-to-side portacaval shunt in the treatment of Budd–Chiari syndrome. *Gastroenterology*, **68,** 137–141.
211. Prandi, D., Rueff, B., Roche-Sicot, J., Sicot, C., Maillard, J.N., Benhamou, J.P. & Fauvert, F. (1976) Life-threatening haemorrhage of the digestive tract in cirrhotic patients. *American Journal of Surgery*, **131,** 204–209.
212. Preisig, R., Bircher, J. & Paumgartner, G. (1972) Physiologic and pathophysiologic aspects of the hepatic hemodynamics. In *Progress in Liver Disease*, Vol. IV (Ed.) Popper, H. & Schaffner, F. pp. 201–216. New York and London: Grune and Stratton.
213. Price, J.B., Voorhees, A.B. Jr & Britton, R.C. (1967) Operative hemodynamic studies in portal hypertension. *Archives of Surgery*, **95,** 843–852.
214. Pugh, R.N.H., Murray-Lyon, I.M., Dawson, J.L., Pietroni, M.C. & Williams, R. (1973) Transection of the oesophagus for bleeding oesophageal varices. *British Journal of Surgery*, **60,** 646–649.
215. Ramalingaswami, V., Wig, K.L. & Sama, S.K. (1962) Cirrhosis of the liver in Northern India: a clinicopathological study. *Archives of Internal Medicine*, **110,** 350–358.
216. Ratnoff, O.D. & Patek, A.J. Jr (1942) The natural history of Laennec's cirrhosis of the liver. *Medicine (Baltimore)*, **21,** 207–268.
217. Reichle, F.A., Sovak, M., Soulen, L. & Rosemond, G.P. (1972) A method of portal vein flow determination in the unanesthetized patient. *Gastroenterology*, **62,** 185.
218. Reichman, S. & Davis, W.D. Jr (1957) The splenic approach to the portal circulation, intrasplenic and intrahepatic pressure measurements in acute and convalescent hepatitis. *Gastroenterology*, **33,** 609–615.
219. Resnick, R.H., Iber, F.L. & Ishihara, A.M. (1974) A controlled study of the therapeutic portocaval shunt. *Gastroenterology*, **67,** 843–857.
220. Reynolds, T.B. (1974) The role of hemodynamic measurements in portosystemic shunt surgery. *Archives of Surgery*, **108,** 276–281.
221. Reynolds, T.B. (1975) Portal hypertension. In *Diseases of the Liver* (Ed.) Schiff, L. pp. 330–367. Philadelphia: J.B. Lippincott.
222. Reynolds, T.B., Ito, S. & Iwatsuki, S. (1970) Measurement of portal pressure and its clinical application. *American Journal of Medicine*, **49,** 649–657.
223. Reynolds, T.B., Geller, H.M., Kuzma, O.T. & Redeker, A.G. (1960) Spontaneous decrease in portal pressure with clinical improvement in cirrhosis. *New England Journal of Medicine*, **263,** 734–739.
224. Rosch, J. & Dotter, C.T. (1971) Extrahepatic portal obstruction in childhood and its angiographic diagnosis. *American Journal of Roentgenology*, **112,** 143–149.
225. Rosch, J., Dotter, C.T. & Rose, R.W. (1971) Selective arterial infusions of vasoconstrictors in acute gastrointestinal bleeding. *Radiology*, **99,** 27–36.
226. Rosenbaum, D.L., Murphy, G.W. & Swisher, S.N. (1966) Hemodynamic studies on the portal circulation in myeloid metaplasia. *American Journal of Medicine*, **41,** 360–368.

227. Rosenthal, T., Shani, M., Deutsch, V. & Samra, H. (1972) The Budd–Chiari syndrome after pregnancy. Report of two cases and a review of the literature. *American Journal of Obstetrics and Gynecology*, **113,** 789–792.
228. Rothwell-Jackson, R.L. & Hunt, A.H. (1971) The results obtained with emergency surgery in the treatment of persistent haemorrhage from gastro-oesophageal varices in the cirrhotic patient. *British Journal of Surgery*, **58,** 205.
229. Rousselot, L.M. & Burchell, A.R. (1975) In *Diseases of the Liver* (Ed) Schiff, L. pp. 368–423. Philadelphia: J.B. Lippincott.
230. Rueff, B., Degos, F., Degos, J.D., Maillard, J.N., Prandi, D., Sicot, J., Sicot, C. & Fauvert, F. (1976) A controlled study of therapeutic portacaval shunt in alcoholic cirrhosis. *Lancet*, **i,** 655–659.
231. Ruzicka, F.F. Jr & Rossi, P. (1969) Arterial portography. Patterns of venous flow. *Radiology*, **92,** 777–787.
232. Schaffner, F., Gadboys, H.L., Safran, A.P., Baron, M.G. & Aufses, A.H. (1967) Budd–Chiari syndrome caused by a web in the inferior vena cava. *American Journal of Medicine*, **42,** 838–843.
233. Schubert, W.K. (1975) Liver disease in infancy and childhood. In *Diseases of the Liver*, pp. 1173–1245. (Ed.) Schiff, L. Philadelphia: J.B. Lippincott.
234. Schwartz, S.I., Bales, H.W., Emerson, G.L., Mahoney, E.B. & Rochester, N.Y. (1959) The use of intravenous Pituitrin in treatment of bleeding esophageal varices. *Surgery*, **45,** 72–80.
235. Scott, J., Long, R., Dick, R. & Sherlock, S. (1976) Percutaneous transhepatic catheterization and sclerosis of bleeding varices. *Gut*, **17,** 390.
236. Sengstaken, R.W. & Blakemore, A.H. (1950) Balloon tamponade for the control of haemorrhage from oesophageal varices. *Annals of Surgery*, **131,** 781–789.
237. Shaldon, S. & Sherlock, S. (1960) The use of vasopressin ('Pitressin') in the control of bleeding from oesophageal varices. *Lancet*, **ii,** 222–225.
238. Shaldon, S. & Sherlock, S. (1962) Portal hypertension in the myeloproliferative syndrome and the reticuloses. *American Journal of Medicine*, **32,** 758–764.
239. Shaldon, S., Chiandussi, L., Guevara, L., Caesar, J. & Sherlock, S. (1961) The measurement of hepatic blood flow and intrahepatic shunted blood flow by colloidal heat-denatured human serum albumin labelled with I^{131}. *Journal of Clinical Investigation*, **40,** 1346–1354.
240. Shaldon, S., Dolle, W., Guevara, L., Iber, F.L. & Sherlock, S. (1961) Effect of pitressin on the splanchnic circulation in man. *Circulation*, **24,** 797–807.
241. Shenk, W.G., McDonald, J.C., McDonald, K. & Drapanas, T. (1962) Direct measurement of hepatic blood flow in surgical patients. *Annals of Surgery*, **156,** 463–471.
242. Sherlock, S. (1951) The liver in heart failure; relation of anatomical functional and circulatory changes. *British Heart Journal*, **13,** 273–293.
243. Sherlock, S. (1966) Waldenstrom's chronic active hepatitis. *Acta Medica Scandinavica* (Suppl.), **445,** 426–434.
244. Sherlock, S. (1974) Chronic hepatitis. *Gut*, **15,** 573–580.
245. Sherlock, S. (1975) The portal venous system and portal hypertension. In *Diseases of the Liver and Biliary System*, pp. 150–216. London: Blackwell Scientific Publications.
246. Sherlock, S. & Scheuer, P.J. (1973) The presentation and diagnosis of 100 patients with primary biliary cirrhosis. *New England Journal of Medicine*, **289,** 674–678.
247. Sherlock, S., Feldman, C.A., Moran, B. & Scheuer, P.J. (1966) Portal nodular transformation of the liver with portal hypertension. *American Journal of Medicine*, **40,** 195–203.
248. Siderys, H. & Vellios, F. (1964) Portal hypertension without cirrhosis or extrahepatic obstruction – report of a case. *American Journal of Surgery*, **108,** 785–789.
249. Silk, D.B.A., Hanid, M.A., Trewby, P.N., Davies, M., Chase, R.A., Langley, P.G., Mellon, P.J., Wheeler, P.G. & Williams, R. (1977) Treatment of fulminant hepatic failure by polyacrylonitrile membrane haemodialysis. *Lancet*, **ii,** 1–3.
250. Silverstein, M.N., Wollaeger, E.E. & Baggenstoss, A.H. (1973) Gastrointestinal and abdominal manifestations of agnogenic myeloid metaplasia. *Archives of Internal Medicine*, **131,** 532–537.
251. Slotnick, I.L. & Teigland, J.D. (1951) Cardiac accidents following vasopressin injection (Pitressin). *Journal of the American Medical Association*, **146,** 1126–1129.
252. Smith, G.W. (1973) An assessment of the validity of preoperative hemodynamic studies in portal hypertension. *Surgery*, **74,** 130–138.
253. Smith, G.W., Westgaard, T. & Bjorn-Hansen, R. (1971) Hepatic venous angiography in the evaluation of cirrhosis of the liver. *Annals of Surgery*, **173,** 469–480.
254. Smith, M.G.M., Cruft, R.J., Davidson, A.R., Laws, J.W., Dawson, J.L. & Williams R. (1974) Mesentericocaval jump graft in the management of portal hypertension. Experience with 24 cases. *British Medical Journal*, **iii,** 705–708.
255. Sommerschild, H.C., Langmark, F. & Maurseth, K. (1973) Congenital hepatic fibrosis. Report of two new cases and review of the literature. *Surgery*, **73,** 53–58.
256. Sterup, K. & Mosbech, J. (1967) Budd–Chiari syndrome after taking oral contraceptives. *British Medical Journal*, **iv,** 660.
257. Stillman, A.E., Huxtable, R., Consroe, P., Kohnen, P. & Smith, S. (1977) Hepatic veno-occlusive disease due to pyrrolizidine (*Senecio*) poisoning in Arizona. *Gastroenterology*, **73,** 349–352.
258. Stone, R., Tentove, W., Effros, R. & Leevy, C.M. (1972) Portal venous blood flow. Its estimation and significance. *Gastroenterology*, **62,** 126.
259. Stone, W.D., Islam, N.R.K. & Paton, A. (1968) The natural history of cirrhosis. *Quarterly Journal of Medicine*, **37,** 119–132.
260. Strack, P.R., Newman, H.K., Lerner, A.G., Green, S.H., Meng, C.H., Del Guercio, L.R.M. & State, D. (1971) An integrated procedure for the rapid diagnosis of biliary obstruction, portal hypertension and liver disease of uncertain etiology. *New England Journal of Medicine*, **285,** 1225–1231.
261. Strandell, T., Erwald, R., Kulling, K.G., Lundbergh, P., Marion, S.O. & Wiechel, K.L. (1972) Simultaneous determinations of portal vein and hepatic artery blood flow by indicator dilution technique in awake man. *Acta Medica Scandinavica*, **191,** 139–140.

262. Stuart, K.L. & Bras, G. (1957) Veno-occlusive disease of the liver. *Quarterly Journal of Medicine*, **26**, 291–317.

263. Sullivan, A., Rheinlander, H. & Weintramb, L.R. (1974) Esophageal varices in agnogenic myeloid metaplasia: disappearance after splenectomy. *Gastroenterology*, **66**, 429–432.

264. Syrota, A., Vinot, J.M., Paraf, A. & Roucayrol, J.C. (1976) Scintillation splenoportography: hemodynamic and morphological study of the portal circulation. *Gastroenterology*, **71**, 652–659.

265. Takenchi, J., Takada, A., Hasamura, Y., Matsuda, Y. & Ikegami, F. (1971) Budd–Chiari syndrome associated with obstruction of the inferior vena cava. *American Journal of Medicine*, **51**, 11–70.

266. Talner, L.B., Boyer, J.L. & Clemett, A.R. (1969) Intrahepatic portal vein occlusion: a cause of portal hypertension. *Radiology*, **92**, 1265–1270.

267. Tandon, B.N., Tandon, H.D., Tandon, R.K., Nardrassathan, M. & Joshi, Y.K. (1976) An epidemic of veno-occlusive disease of liver in central India. *Lancet*, **ii**, 271–272.

268. Tavill, A.S., Wood, E.J., Kreel, L., Jones, E.A., Gregny, M. & Sherlock, S. (1975) The Budd–Chiari syndrome: correlation between hepatic scintigraphy and the clinical, radiological, and pathological findings in nineteen cases of hepatic venous outflow obstruction. *Gastroenterology*, **68**, 509–518.

269. Texeira, E.D., Yu, H. & Bergan, J.J. (1968) Selective decompression of oesophago-gastric varices. *Archives of Surgery*, **96**, 4–8.

270. Thomas, L.B., Popper, H., Berk, P.D., Selikoff, I. & Falk, H. (1975) Vinyl-chloride-induced liver disease. *New England Journal of Medicine*, **292**, 17–22.

271. Thomas, M. & Caroli, J. (1971) Polycythenine et syndrome de Budd–Chiari. À propos de 17 observations. *Annales de Médecine Interne*, **122**, 1175–1186.

272. Thompson, E.N. & Sherlock, S. (1964) The aetiology of portal vein thrombosis with particular reference to the role of infection and exchange transfusion. *Quarterly Journal of Medicine*, **33**, 465–480.

273. Thompson, E.N., Williams, R. & Sherlock, S. (1964) Liver function in extrahepatic portal hypertension. *Lancet*, **ii**, 1352–1356.

274. Tisdale, W.A., Klatskin, G. & Glenn, W.W.L. (1959) Portal hypertension and bleeding varices. Their occurrence in the absence of both intrahepatic and extrahepatic obstruction of the portal vein. *New England Journal of Medicine*, **261**, 209–218.

275. Tsakiris, A., Haemmerli, U.P. & Bulmann, A. (1964) Reduction of portal venous pressure in cirrhotic patients with bleeding with oesophageal varices, by administration of a vasopressin derivative phenylalanine^2-lysine^8-vasopressin. *American Journal of Medicine*, **36**, 852–861.

276. Turcotte, J.G. & Child, C.G. (1972) Idiopathic extrahepatic portal hypertension in adults. *American Journal of Surgery*, **123**, 35–42.

277. Turcotte, J.G. & Lambert, M.J. (1973) Variceal haemorrhage, hepatic cirrhosis, and portacaval shunts. *Surgery*, **73**, 810–817.

278. Turner, M.D., Sherlock, S. & Steiner, R.E. (1957) Intrasplenic pressure measurement and splenic venography in the clinical investigation of the portal circulation. *American Journal of Medicine*, **23**, 846–859.

279. Tygstrup, N., Winkler, K., Mellemgaard, K. & Andreassen, M. (1962) Determination of the hepatic arterial blood flow and oxygen supply in man by clamping the hepatic artery during surgery. *Journal of Clinical Investigation*, **41**, 447–454.

280. Ueda, H., Kitani, K., Kameda, H., Yamada, H. & Iio, M. (1967) Detection of hepatic shunts by the use of ^{131}I-macroaggregated albumin. *Gastroenterology*, **52**, 480–487.

281. Vang, J., Simert, G., Hansson, J.A., Thylen, U. & Bengmark, T.S. (1977) Results of a modified distal splenorenal shunt for portal hypertension. *Annals of Surgery*, **185**, 224–228.

282. Venness, J.A. (1966) Intrahepatic pressure: an accurate reflection of portal pressure. *Medicine*, **45**, 445–452.

283. Viallet, A., Guillaume, E., Cote, J., Legare, A. & Lavole, P. (1972) Presinusoidal portal hypertension following chronic arsenic intoxication. *Gastroenterology*, **62**, 177.

284. Viamonte, M. Jr, Le Page, J., Lunderqvist, A., Pereiras, R., Russell, E., Viamonte, M. & Camacho, M. (1975) Selective catheterization of portal vein and its tributaries. *Radiology*, **114**, 457–460.

285. Vilinskas, J., Joyeuse, R. & Serlin, O. (1970) Hepatic sarcoidosis with portal hypertension. *American Journal of Surgery*, **120**, 393–396.

286. Villeneuve, J.P., Huet, P.M., Joly, J.G., Marleau, D., Cote, J., Legare, A., Lafortune, M., Lovoie, P. & Viallet, A. (1976) Idiopathic portal hypertension. *American Journal of Medicine*, **61**, 459–464.

287. Vosmik, J., Jedlicka, K., Mulder, J.L. & Cort, J.H. (1977) Action of the triglycyl hormonogen of vasopressin (Glypressin) in patients with liver cirrhosis and bleeding esophageal varices. *Gastroenterology*, **72**, 605–609.

288. Wagenknecht, T.W., Noble, J.F. & Baronofsky, J.D. (1953) Nature of bleeding in esophageal varices. *Surgery*, **33**, 869–874.

289. Waldram, R., Davis, M., Nunnerley, H. & Williams, R. (1974) Emergency endoscopy after gastrointestinal haemorrhage in 50 patients with portal hypertension. *British Medical Journal*, **iv**, 94–96.

290. Waldram, R., Nunnerley, H., Davis, M., Laws, J.W. & Williams, R. (1977) Detection and grading of oesophageal varices by fibre-optic endoscopy and barium swallow with and without Buscopan. *Clinical Radiology*, **28**, 137–141.

291. Wallace, A. III, Wallace, W.B. & Balfour, D.C. Jr (1953) Use of head mask to aid oesophageal tamponade. *Gastroenterology*, **24**, 20–22.

292. Warren, K.S. & Reboucas, G. (1964) Blood ammonia during bleeding from esophageal varices in patients with hepatosplenic schistosomiasis. *New England Journal of Medicine*, **271**, 921–926.

293. Warren, M.D., Atef, A., Salam, A., Taralder, D. & Hutson, R.B. (1972) End renal vein-to-splenic shunts for total or selective portal decompression. *Surgery*, **72**, 995–1006.

294. Warren, W.D., Fomon, J.J. & Zeppa, R. (1969) Further evaluation of the selective decompression of varices by distal splenorenal shunt. *Annals of Surgery*, **169**, 652–660.

295. Warren, W.D., Restrepo, J.E., Respress, J.C. & Muller, W.H. (1963) The importance of haemodynamic studies in management of portal hypertension. *Annals of Surgery*, **158**, 387–404.

296. Warren, W.D., Foman, J.J., Viamonte, M. & Zeppa, R. (1967) Preoperative assessment of portal hypertension. *Annals of Surgery,* **165,** 999–1012.
297. Warren, W.D., Fomon, J.J., Viamonte, M., Martiney, L.O. & Kalser, M. (1968) Spontaneous reversal of portal venous flow in cirrhosis. *Surgery, Gynecology and Obstetrics,* **126,** 315–323.
298. Watts, J. & Douglas, M.C. (1971) Clinical applications and complications of umbilical vein cannulation. *British Journal of Surgery,* **58,** 61–66.
299. Westaby, S., Wilkinson, S.P., Warren, R. & Williams, R. (1978) Spleen size and portal hypertension. *Digestion,* **17,** 63–68.
300. Wexler, M.J. & Maclean, L.D. (1975) Massive spontaneous portal-systemic shunting without varices. *Archives of Surgery,* **110,** 995–1003.
301. Wexler, M.J., McLean, A.P.H., Skinner, G.B. & Maclean, L.D. (1973) 'Minilap': an accurate, rapid and safe approach to the diagnosis of liver disease and jaundice. *Annals of Surgery,* **178,** 736–744.
302. Williams, R. (1971) Clinicopathological conference. Chronic arsenical poisoning and non-cirrhotic portal hypertension – a case for diagnosis. *British Medical Journal,* **iv,** 725–730.
303. Williams, R. (1976) Assessment and management of portal hypertension. *Rendiconti Gastroenterologica,* **8,** 33–45.
304. Williams, R., Kreel, L. & Blendis, L.M. (1967) Coeliac catheterization: uses and values in portal hypertension. In *The Liver* (Ed.) Read, A.E. pp. 125–135. London: Butterworth Publications.
305. Williams, R., Scheuer, P.J. & Heard, B.E. (1964) Congenital hepatic fibrosis with an unusual pulmonary lesion. *Journal of Clinical Pathology,* **17,** 135–142.
306. Williams, R., Parsonson, A., Somers, K. & Hamilton, P.J.S. (1966) Portal hypertension in idiopathic tropical splenomegaly. *Lancet,* **i,** 329–333.
307. Williams, R., Condon, R.E., Williams, H.S., Blendis, L.M. & Kreel, L. (1968) Splenic blood flow in cirrhosis and portal hypertension. *Clinical Science,* **34,** 441–452.
308. Williams, R., Mitchell, K.J., Macdougall, B.R.D. & Wilkinson, S.P. (1978) Emergencies in liver disease. In *The Management of Medical Emergencies.* Tunbridge Wells: Pitman Medical.
309. Willmot, F.C. & Robertson, G.W. (1920) Senecio disease or cirrhosis of the liver due to senecio poisoning. *Lancet,* **ii,** 848–849.
310. Winans, C.S. & Harris, L.D. (1967) Quantitation of lower esophageal sphincter competence. *Gastroenterology,* **52,** 773–778.
311. Wyatt, J.B. & Sommers, S.C. (1950) Chronic marrow failure, myelosclerosis and extra medullary hematopoiesis. *Blood,* **5,** 329–347.
312. Zeegan, R., Stansfeld, A.G., Dawson, A.M. & Hunt, A.H. (1969) Bleeding oesophageal varices as the presenting feature in primary biliary cirrhosis. *Lancet,* **ii,** 9–13.
313. Zeegan, R., Stansfeld, A.G., Dawson, A.M. & Hunt, A.H. (1970) Prolonged survival after portal decompression of patients with non-cirrhotic intrahepatic portal hypertension. *Gut,* **11,** 610–617.
314. Zimmon, D.S. & Kessler, R.E. (1973) Hepatic hemodynamic factors reflect prognosis after portacaval shunt. *Gastroenterology,* **64,** 166.

Chapter 44

The Surgery of Portal Hypertension

K.E.F. HOBBS

The complications of portal hypertension, especially haemorrhage from oesophageal varices, frequently require surgical treatment. There are several different approaches to this, but most of the operations carry a high morbidity and an overall mortality similar to, or sometimes worse than conservative management. In this chapter the aetiology and complications of portal hypertension will be considered, as well as the value of the various diagnostic tests and the alternative methods of surgical treatment in current use.

THE PORTAL CIRCULATION

The portal vein in the adult is about 8 cm long. It arises from the junction of the splenic and superior mesenteric veins at the level of the second lumbar vertebra behind the neck of the pancreas and in front of the inferior vena cava. It ascends towards the porta hepatis in the edge of the lesser omentum, passing behind the duodenum and common bile duct. At the porta hepatis it divides into right and left branches, one for each of the two main lobes of the liver. These branches are then bound with those of the hepatic artery and bile duct by a loose perivascular fibrous capsule of Glisson and enter the liver. They all divide into smaller branches which in the periphery of the hepatic lobules form the portal triads.

The portal blood passes into the sinusoids which lie between the liver cell plates where it mixes with arterial blood. The sinusoids drain into the central veins and these join together to form the hepatic veins which drain into the vena cava.

Between the portal and systemic venous systems are anastomotic channels which normally carry very little blood. They may dilate and assume clinical importance in portal hypertension. They are in the submucosa of the oesophagus and rectum, in the retroperitoneal tissues and in the ligamentum teres.

The normal portal blood flow contributes about 75 per cent of the total oxygen entering the liver.[43] The flow rate is about 1 to 1.2 l/min at a pressure of between 6 and 12 cm of water. These flow characteristics may change markedly during digestion, under anaesthesia and in portal hypertension.

Techniques for Demonstrating the Portal Venous System and Measuring the Haemodynamic Status

Haemodynamic studies

Total blood flow. Total blood flow can be estimated by a variety of techniques. It can be calculated using the Fick principle, when a dye which is removed only by the liver is infused at a constant rate. Bromsulphthalein, indocyanine green, ^{131}I rose bengal, galactose and ethanol have all been used as indicators.[73] However, extraction of each of these compounds by the liver is not total during a single passage, so there are errors in these techniques. Another useful indicator is a ^{131}I-labelled colloid albumin which has the best removal during a single passage through the liver with minimal extrahepatic uptake. Liver blood flow can also be calculated by measuring the rate of removal of dye from the circulation after a bolus has been injected intravenously.[49]

Other techniques include recording the loss of radioactivity over the liver following the injection of a suitable radio-isotope such as radioactive argon[60] or krypton,[45] square wave electromagnetic flow meters applied to the afferent vessels and intraluminal flow meters.[16] The use of implantable flow meters allows estimation of differential flow in each vessel and these last two techniques have been used in the experimental animal, but are impractical in unanaesthetized man.

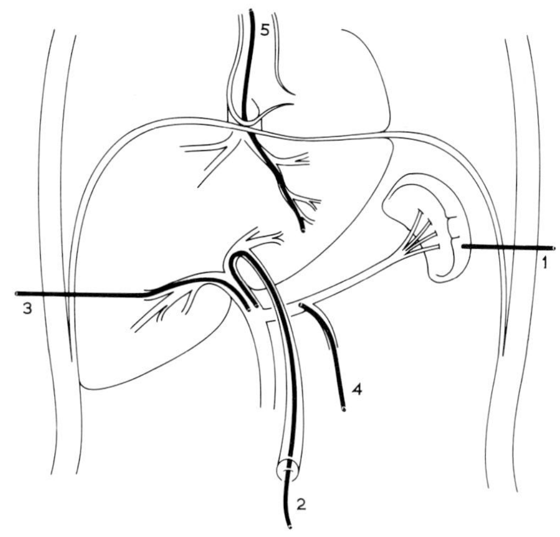

Figure 44.1. Catheterization of the portal and hepatic veins: 1. Percutaneous trans-splenic; 2. Via dilated umbilical vein; 3. Percutaneous transhepatic; 4. Directly through a branch at laparotomy; 5. Wedged hepatic vein via subclavian.

Portal pressure. Portal pressure can be measured by inserting a manometer into the portal circulation. The most commonly used approach is percutaneous needle puncture of the splenic pulp. Since there is free communication between the splenic pulp and the portal vein tributaries, any pressure recording made in the pulp will be equivalent to the portal pressure (Figure 44.1).

Another means of access to the portal venous system is through the obliterated umbilical vein. This can be exposed in the epigastrium under local anaesthesia and dilated with a bougie. It communicates with the left branch of the portal vein in the liver, so that with the help of radiographic image intensification a cannula can be passed through the umbilical vein and manipulated into the main portal vein (Figure 44.1 (2)). The third approach is percutaneous puncture of a branch of the portal vein within the liver. A thin needle is inserted directly into the liver and radiopaque contrast slowly injected as it is withdrawn. With radiographic image intensification it is possible to see when the contrast enters a branch of the portal vein. A guide wire is then passed down the needle into the vessel and a catheter introduced over this directly into the portal vein (Figure 44.1 (3)). All of these three commonly-used techniques of access to the portal venous system can be performed with the patient fully conscious but sedated. Portal angiography can be carried out at the same time as the pressure measurements are made (see Chapter 22).

At laparotomy, portal pressure can be measured by inserting a manometer into the vein or one of its tributaries (Figure 44.1 (4)). This reading may be different from the portal pressure measured by other techniques in the conscious subject due to the effect of positive pressure ventilation, the open peritoneal cavity and the difficulty in fixing a comparable zero reference point.[44, 69]

There are reports in the literature of pressure recordings made in various parts of the portal system after clamping the portal vein during surgery. Pressure readings made on either side of an occlusion clamp on the main portal vein have been called 'hepatic occluded portal pressure' and 'splanchnic occluded portal pressure'. By subtracting the first of these from the second, the 'maximum perfusion pressure' is obtained. This is said to represent the hydrostatic gradient for flow to the liver within the portal vein.[56] In some types of liver disease the portal vein acts as a venous drainage channel for the liver, so the flow in the portal vein is reversed. Under these circumstances the 'maximum perfusion pressure' becomes negative. It must be appreciated, however, that any pressure measurement made after total occlusion of the flow in a vessel is of doubtful value since this represents a non-physiological situation. The significance of these recordings and calculations will be discussed later.

Hepatic vein pressure. A catheter can be advanced from an arm vein through the vena cava into one of the hepatic veins under radiographic control. If it is further advanced until it is wedged in one of the branches of the hepatic vein, stopping the flow, the pressure recording is called the 'wedged hepatic vein pressure' (Figure 44.1 (5)). Since these hepatic veins are in direct communication with the hepatic sinusoids, this value is the same as the pressure within the sinusoids. Furthermore, in the normal liver, due to the absence of any sphincters, it is said to be identical to the portal pressure.[44] When the catheter is withdrawn slightly into the hepatic tree, the 'free hepatic vein pressure' is obtained.

Interpretation of pressure studies. The measurements of portal, wedged hepatic vein and free hepatic vein pressures are of value in confirming the diagnosis of portal hypertension and identifying the site of the obstruction. A rise in portal pressure above 12 cm of water confirms the diagnosis of portal hypertension. There appears to be no relationship, however, between the pressure in the portal vein, the flow in the portal vein and the severity of either the liver disease or its complications.[17] Patients with high portal pressures may be free from clinical problems, while low pressures may be associated with gross hepatocellular disease and bleeding from oesophageal varices. This may be explained by the development of portasystemic shunts; these may lower the portal pressure by reducing the resistance to flow, while at the same time reducing the portal blood flow into an already sick liver.

Comparison of the portal venous pressure with the wedged hepatic vein pressure may allow the site of any block to be localized. A rise in portal pressure in the presence of a normal wedged hepatic vein pressure suggests blockage of the portal vein or the presinusoidal portal tract region. A rise in both pressures suggests direct communication between the portal vein and central vein via abnormal intrahepatic shunts which develop around the nodules in cirrhosis. In patients with veno-occlusive disease, the wedged hepatic vein pressure is low. Catheterization of the hepatic veins is impossible when they are thrombosed or when there is thrombosis of the inferior vena cava.

Attempts have been made to correlate various pressure readings, including the 'maximum perfusion pressure', and flow measurements with the prognosis and management of the disease.[33] Unfortunately, no correlation has been found and prognosis seems to be related much more to the type and severity of liver cell disease than the haemodynamic status.[8,54] It may be argued that there is no place for carrying out the measurements, which are expensive and often uncomfortable and dangerous for the patient.[54]

As new approaches to portal hypertension are investigated in the future, however, it may be shown that retrospective analysis of these pressures and flow rates will correlate with results. Certainly, some patients fare well and others badly after treatment for portal hypertension, but so far no way has been found for predicting the outcome. Recently it has been suggested that there may be a relationship between a good hepatic arterial flow rate and success from certain surgical shunt procedures.[9] However, this suggestion has yet to be confirmed. In the investigation of patients with clinical portal hypertension, visualization of the portal system is probably of greater value than haemodynamic studies.

Visualization of portal circulation

The portal circulation can be well demonstrated radiographically following intravascular injection of radiopaque contrast media. There are several techniques for achieving this:

1. Percutaneous intrasplenic injection
2. Umbilical vein catheterization
3. Percutaneous transhepatic catheterization of the portal vein
4. Observation of the venous phase of the superior mesenteric and coeliac arteriograms. See Chapter 22 for further details.

Ultrasound scanning of the abdomen is now proving a useful, non-invasive technique by which patency of the main branches of the portal system may be assessed. The splenic, superior mesenteric and the portal vein can often be seen and patency determined.[70] Great expertise is required before reliable results can be obtained, however, and further development in this field is anticipated (see Chapter 21).

Pathophysiology of the Portal Circulation

Portal hypertension is produced as a result of increased resistance to normal portal blood flow. In rare circumstances it can result from an increase in the volume of portal blood flowing into the liver from a grossly enlarged spleen, or one in which there are arteriovenous fistulae.[36] Obstruction to portal flow can occur at several levels and not all of these are within the liver,

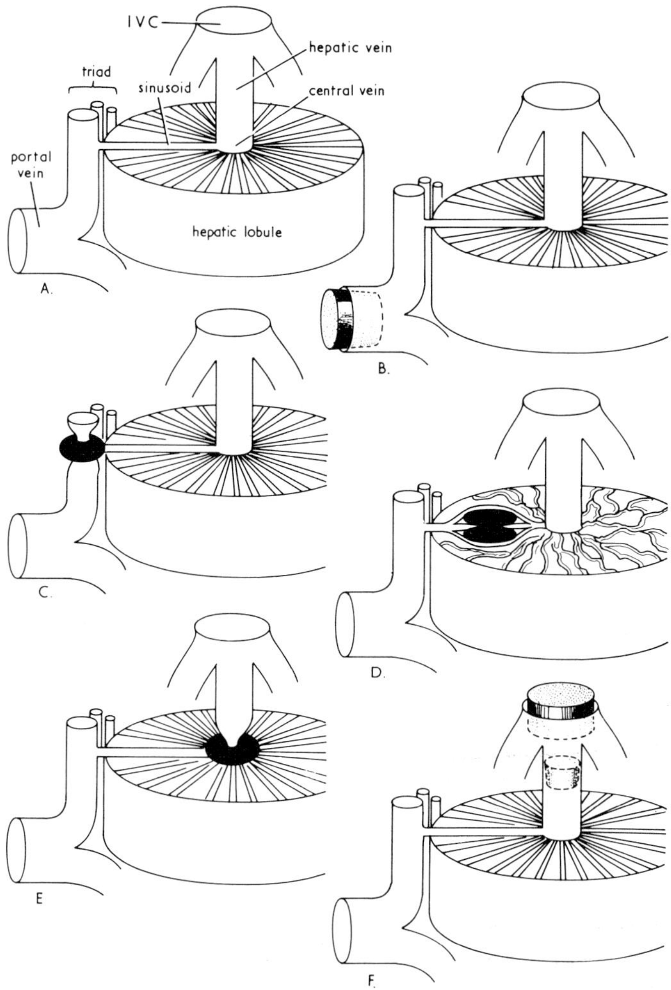

Figure 44.2. Diagrammatic representation of the different sites of resistance to flow in portal hypertension: A. Normal; B. Portal vein block, e.g. portal vein thrombosis or tumour at the liver hilum; C. Cellular proliferation in the region of the portal triads, e.g. schistosomiasis; D. Sinusoidal occlusion, e.g. cirrhosis; E. Centrizonal congestion and fibrosis due to 'bush teas'; F. Occlusion of the central vein or hepatic vein, e.g. Budd–Chiari syndrome or renal tumour in the inferior vena cava.

nor are they necessarily associated with liver disease. These are illustrated diagrammatically in Figure 44.2. They can be divided into pre-hepatic, hepatic and post-hepatic, or pre-sinusoidal, sinusoidal and post-sinusoidal. The narrowing or obstruction may lie in the portal vein or its branches (Figure 44.2 (B)), in the region of the portal triad (Figure 44.2 (C)), in the sinusoids (Figure 44.2 (D)), around the central vein (Figure 44.2 (E)) or within the lumen of the hepatic veins and vena cava (Figure 44.2(F)). In all cases increased resistance to portal venous drainage from the gut and resulting portal hypertension cause the portal systemic anastomotic channels to open, allowing the portal blood to return to the systemic venous system, usually bypassing the liver.

Clinical problems resulting from portal hypertension are related to four factors:

1. Rupture of pathologically dilated portal systemic anastomotic channels, especially in the submucosa of the oesophagus
2. Portasystemic encephalopathy resulting from portal blood entering the systemic circulation without prior detoxification in the liver
3. Splenomegaly
4. Ascites

In all cases these problems are complicated by the severity of any hepatocellular disease.

Pathological anastomotic channels

Oesophageal varices. The development of oesophageal varices is a major clinical problem associated with portal hypertension. These varices are dilated submucosal veins in the fundus of the stomach and the lower half of the oesophagus. The dilatation is due to increased blood flow through the vessels which form part of the anastomotic pathway between the portal venous system and the azygos veins in the chest. Due to their size and the volume of blood passing through them they are in danger of rupturing. It is uncertain what causes them to rupture, but sudden changes in portal pressure,[38] the large size of the varices[44] and damage by gastro-oesophageal reflux of gastric acid have all been suggested although evidence against each hypothesis has also been produced.[55] In children there may be an association between a mild upper respiratory tract infection and the onset of bleeding. Haemorrhage from varices is sometimes massive and repeated, and management is discussed later in the chapter.

Rectal varices. Very rarely the portasystemic anastomoses in the wall of the rectum dilate and rupture, producing massive bleeding. Although this anastomotic network is in the region of haemorrhoidal plexus and the pile-bearing area, the dilatation of the vessels which occurs in portal hypertension seems to be different from true haemorrhoids.

Other anastomotic channels. Other anastomotic collaterals develop between the portal vein and diaphragmatic, intercostal, pulmonary, lumbar and renal veins, but these rarely bleed. However, these anastomoses may contribute to portasystemic encephalopathy by producing routes for portal blood to bypass the liver. Another collateral anastomosis is that between a patent umbilical vein branch of the portal vein and the veins of the anterior abdominal wall around the umbilicus. This dilatation of subcutaneous veins radiating away from the umbilicus produces the 'caput medusae', a striking but uncommon physical sign which causes no significant clinical problem.

Portasystemic encephalopathy

The relationship between liver disease and abnormal mental activity has been appreciated for centuries and Hippocrates is credited with its first description. Two main types of encephalopathy are found in liver disease: firstly, an acute, rapidly progressive state leading to coma, which is associated with acute severe liver disease and is reversible in only a few cases[61] (see Chapter 27); and secondly, the encephalopathy associated with portasystemic shunting and chronic liver disease[20] (see Chapter 42). Although initially reversible, this second type may progress to a stage of hepatocerebral degeneration,[64] which may represent a third type of encephalopathy.

There is much controversy regarding the aetiology of portasystemic encephalopathy, but it seems to be related both to increased cerebral sensitivity to circulating toxins and to higher concentrations of such toxins in the systemic circulation. The concentration of these compounds in the systemic circulation is related not only to the degree of hepatocellular disease but also to the degree of portasystemic shunting, whether it has developed spontaneously or has been created surgically.

Splenomegaly

Splenomegaly is very common in portal hypertension. The simple explanation that it is secondary to increased venous drainage pressure is probably inadequate.[62] There appears to be no marked correlation between splenic size and the degree of portal hypertension. Very occasionally the size of the spleen contributes to the portal hypertension because of an associated increase in blood flow.[36] Splenectomy alone, however, rarely provides a permanent cure for haemorrhage from oesophageal varices secondary to portal hypertension. At one time this was practised, but rebleeding usually occurred. More recently it has been carried out in conjunction with coronary vein ligation, with reasonable success in selected cases.[53]

The main problem of the splenomegaly, apart from the physical size of the spleen, is that it is commonly physiologically overactive. This results in a pancytopenia and the lowered number of circulating platelets in particular may exacerbate any haemorrhagic tendency resulting from impaired hepatocellular function.

Ascites (see Chapters 43 and 46)

Some degree of ascites is common in patients with portal hypertension. Several factors contribute to this, including increased portal pressure, a low serum albumin concentration and impaired aldosterone metabolism as a result of hepatocellular disease, and increased hepatic lymph production associated with cirrhosis.[29] Surgical portal decompression has been used for the relief of 'intractable ascites' associated with portal hypertension.[7] With modern medical therapy, however, simple ascites is rarely an indication for decompression surgery today, although its development in a patient with poor liver cell function is a very grave sign. A peritoneo-jugular shunt has recently been developed[28,67] and has given initially promising results.

MANAGEMENT OF PATIENTS ADMITTED WITH BLEEDING OESOPHAGEAL VARICES

Oesophageal varices are the cause of haemorrhage in about 2 per cent of patients with upper gastrointestinal bleeding admitted to an average district general hospital in the United Kingdom;[47] in other countries the incidence varies from 1 to 16 per cent.[71]

The first two priorities in the management of such a patient are resuscitation and diagnosis. The most efficient way of achieving both is to begin with immediate consultation between medical and surgical teams. Although the initial management is usually medical, a surgical presence at an early stage is a valuable asset. Apart from the psychological value to the patient of meeting all the doctors involved in his care, the timing of any surgical procedure is of vital importance in such sick patients. Emergency major surgery carried out in the middle of the night by an inexperienced team carries a much higher mortality and morbidity than planned urgent surgery by an experienced team. Early consultation results in a more carefully planned approach to emergency procedures.

Resuscitation

This follows the general lines of resuscitation for major haemorrhage. Colloid-containing fluids and cross-matched blood are required. If whole blood is given it should be as fresh as possible. The amount is estimated by observing the pulse, blood pressure, central venous pressure and haemoglobin levels. Haemorrhage from oesophageal varices may be severe, especially if they are secondary to cirrhosis, and five to ten litres of fluid are sometimes needed. Since impaired clotting is frequent, calcium, platelets and fresh frozen plasma containing other clotting factors are frequently required. Throughout the period of resuscitation it is essential to monitor electrolyte levels, as these can become severely deranged following massive transfusions in the presence of liver disease with impaired aldosterone metabolism.

Confirmation of Diagnosis

Patients admitted to hospital with upper gastrointestinal bleeding need to have the cause established urgently. Since gastric erosions and peptic ulcers are much more common than ruptured oesophageal varices, it is dangerous to assume that patients with proven cirrhosis, portal hypertension and oesophageal varices are bleeding from these causes. There is a higher incidence of peptic ulcer and gastric lesions in cirrhotic patients than in the normal population. Massive upper gastrointestinal bleeding in 30 per cent of patients with known cirrhosis is due to causes other than the varices.[37,40]

There are two main ways of establishing the site of bleeding. The oesophagus and stomach can be visualized radiographically with radio-paque contrast media or, preferably, by oesophagogastric endoscopy. Endoscopy is undoubtedly the most reliable diagnostic method in centres with appropriate equipment and expertise.[58] However, radiological examination allows adequate diagnosis to permit safe management of such patients. It has been suggested that the additional diagnostic advantages of endoscopy do not necessarily justify provision of such services where they do not already exist.[18] In some centres, selective coeliac angiography is used in an attempt to demonstrate the site of upper gastrointestinal haemorrhage. Although reports have shown the success of this approach when there is active bleeding, it is not in general use nor are the necessary facilities and expertise universally available.

Assessment of Liver Function and Clinical State

Once the patient has been resuscitated and the diagnosis of haemorrhage from oesophageal varices confirmed, it is necessary to establish both the cause of the varices and the degree of hepatocellular disease.

History and clinical examination

There may be a history suggesting liver disease. The patient may be an alcoholic or have a past history of hepatitis or jaundice from other causes; he may have come from a part of the world where schistosomiasis or the drinking of 'bush tea' containing hepatotoxic alkaloids is common. In a child, a history of umbilical sepsis at birth suggests portal thrombosis whilst jaundice present at birth or soon afterwards may indicate congenital liver disease.

Clinical examination may reveal jaundice, palmar erythema, spider naevi, flapping tremor, fetor or other signs of hepatocellular dysfunction. Encephalopathy, hepatosplenomegaly and ascites may be present. A peri-umbilical caput medusae or rectal varices are rare accompaniments of portal hypertension. A venous hum over the liver sometimes indicates the presence of abnormal collateral vessels.

Initial tests

Venous blood should be taken as soon as possible, before any transfusion is given, to obtain a baseline and to assess the severity of the haemorrhage and of the liver disease. The initial tests should include a haemoglobin and haematocrit, platelet count, prothrombin and partial thromboplastin times, liver function tests, plasma proteins and electrolytes, including calcium. Since malignant hepatomas occur in patients with long-standing cirrhosis,[27,50] these must be excluded in any patients having haemorrhage from oesophageal varices. Measurement of the serum alpha fetoprotein level which is often raised in patients with malignant hepatomas may be valuable.

A chest x-ray and an electrocardiogram should be performed. An electroencephalogram is valuable in patients who have bled since this may indicate the presence and severity of encephalopathy or the susceptibility of the patient to this complication if shunt surgery is being considered.

Specific tests to determine the causes of portal hypertension

The successful management of portal hypertension sometimes depends on the cause. Patients with extrahepatic portal obstruction without liver cell damage have a better prognosis than patients with cirrhosis.[63] Some types of cirrhosis, such as primary biliary cirrhosis, carry a better prognosis after surgical treatment of bleeding varices than others; in older patients with alcoholic cirrhosis who continue drinking the prognosis is very poor.[2] It is thus important to establish the cause of the portal hypertension before proceeding to any definitive treatment.

Needle biopsy of the liver will provide histological evidence of the hepatic pathology. With care, this is a relatively safe procedure. It is discussed in Chapter 18. A technetium liver scintiscan may be of value in demonstrating space-occupying lesions suggesting malignant change (see Chapter 20). The anatomy and patency of the portal circulation should be assessed by angiography and ultrasonography (see Chapters 21 and 22).

Management of Oesophageal Varices

Management can be discussed under three headings:

1. Acute control of bleeding
2. Management of oesophageal varices after major haemorrhage
3. Prophylaxis against bleeding when oesophageal varices have been diagnosed

Acute control of bleeding

By the time the patient has been admitted to hospital, resuscitated, and the cause of the haemorrhage confirmed as being due to ruptured oesophageal varices, the bleeding may have stopped spontaneously. This is due to a combination of a fall in the portal pressure secondary to the haemorrhage and normal haemostasis. If bleeding continues two techniques are available in the immediate management: treatment with vasopressin or insertion into the stomach and oesophagus of a Sengstaken tube.

The smooth muscle stimulant vasopressin or Pitressin causes the arterioles of the gut to constrict, thus reducing blood flow into the gut with a slight increase in the systolic arterial pressure. The resulting fall in volume of venous drainage from the gut produces a fall in portal pressure which may allow spontaneous haemostasis within the ruptured veins. The disadvantages of this preparation are that cardiac and renal perfusion are also reduced and this may complicate management.

Pitressin is usually given intravenously in a dosage of 20 u diluted in 100 ml of 5 per cent dextrose over 20 minutes. Due to its smooth muscle stimulant effect there is great gastro-intestinal activity, and violent defaecation occurs. If this does not occur it suggests that an inadequate dosage has been given. A maximum of three doses over a one-hour period can be given. Usually it is found that the bleeding stops during the treatment, but often recurs shortly afterwards. Subsequent injections have less effect than the initial one.[51]

Some authorities have advocated slow intra-arterial infusion of Pitressin via a catheter positioned in the superior mesenteric artery; this allows the drug to have its maximum effect where it is most needed on the arterioles of the intestine. Although theoretically of greater value than intravenous administration, there is no evidence from clinical studies to confirm that this is any more effective.[13] Since radiological control is necessary to ensure that the catheter is correctly placed, this technique does not enjoy widespread use.

Tamponade is an alternative or additional treatment in the acute situation. This is achieved by passing a Blakemore–Sengstaken tube into the stomach. The most recent design (Sengstaken Model D WSP, Warne Surgical Products Ltd; Figure 44.3) consists of a four-lumen tube. One lumen communicates with a balloon which can be inflated in the stomach. Traction of two or three pounds is applied to the tube and this forces the inflated balloon to press the oesophagogastric junction of the stomach against the diaphragm at the oesophageal hiatus. This occludes the vessels in the wall of the stomach and oesophagus which fill the oesophageal varices from below. Sometimes this manoeuvre alone will control the bleeding. If it is unsuccessful, the second balloon in the oesophageal part of the balloon can be inflated;

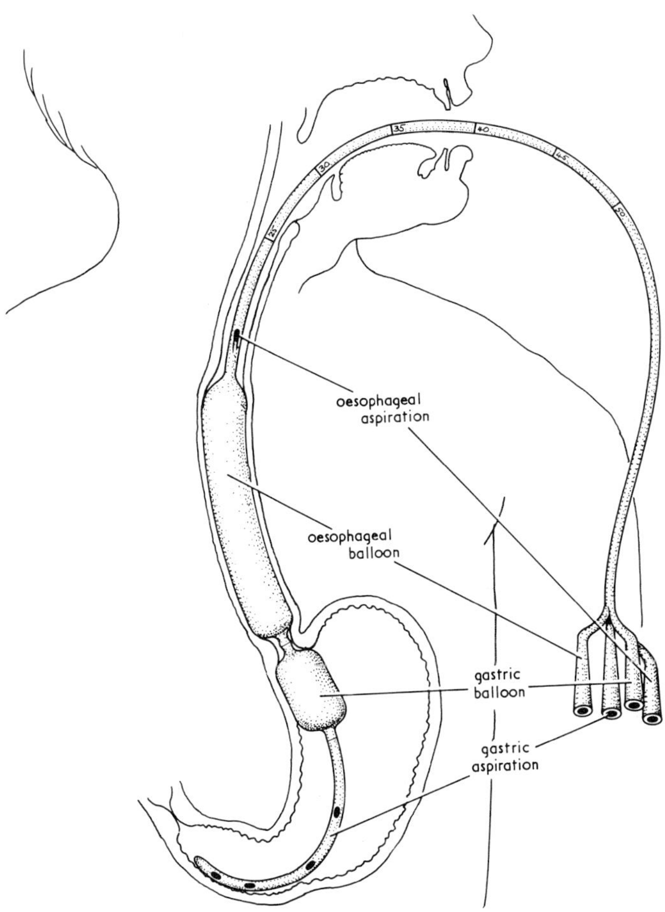

Figure 44.3. Blakemore–Sengstaken tube (Model D WSP).

direct pressure is thus applied to the varices. A pressure of 2.5 to 4.0 kPa (20 to 30 mmHg) is required. There are two other lumens in the tube. One is used to aspirate the stomach below the inflated balloons and the other aspirates saliva which collects in the oesophagus above the inflated oesophageal balloon.

The advantage of this tube is that immediate control of the bleeding can usually be achieved. However, the tube is difficult to pass, very uncomfortable for the patient, and needs to be supervised by a nurse or clinician experienced in the management of such patients. No balloon should be inflated for more than 24 hours, otherwise avascular necrosis of the oesophagus will occur. Unfortunately, there may be some rebleeding when the balloons are deflated. Other problems may also arise with this tube.[12] One of the balloons may fail to deflate, making removal difficult. Sometimes bleeding continues despite the tamponade and the unwary clinician may be lulled into a false sense of security. Oesophageal obstruction is produced by the inflated balloons and the saliva which collects may be aspirated into the lungs. Aspiration through the proximal lumen is designed to prevent this, but its function must be watched closely as it can readily become blocked. Laryngeal obstruction may be caused by the inflated oesophageal balloon if the gastric balloon should burst or become deflated and the tube becomes displaced.

Although the Sengstaken tube is a life-saving instrument its hazards must be appreciated. It certainly has a place in management, either while definitive surgery is awaited or during transport of the patient to a specialist centre. It is sometimes the only treatment necessary for children with oesophageal varices secondary to portal vein thrombosis without liver disease because their clotting ability is unimpaired.[63]

These techniques will usually control the acute bleeding. However, they sometimes fail and rebleeding occurs; the second phase of management then has to be employed.

Management of oesophageal varices after major haemorrhage

There are three main approaches to the problem:

1. Sclerosis of the varices
2. Ligation or occlusion of the varices
3. Decompression of the portal system

Sclerosis of the varices. It is possible to stop haemorrhage from a ruptured oesophageal varix by inducing thrombosis and sclerosis within it. This can be achieved by injecting a sclerosant or clotting agent either directly into the dilated vein or through a catheter introduced from below through the portal vein.

Direct injection of oesophageal varices is performed through a rigid oesophagoscope using a long needle attached to a syringe. Although in theory this is a simple technique, some expertise is required to perfect it. Modifications to a rigid oesophagoscope have been described which make the procedure fairly simple.[1] An additional slit is made in the wall of the distal end of the instrument (Figure 44.4A). The 'scope is introduced into the oesophagus and rotated until the dilated varix bulges into the slit (Figure 44.4B); a sclerosant such as ethanolamine oleate is injected into the varix and the instrument is again rotated. The wall of the instrument than applies pressure to the treated varix and allows a second, parallel varix to appear in the slit (Figure 44.4C). Later, a Sengstaken tube is passed and the oesophageal balloon inflated.

Some clinicians have achieved excellent results using this approach, but it has not received universal acclaim. Rebleeding may occur since the local sclerosis does nothing to relieve the cause of the portal hypertension and the thrombosis does not affect the large feeding vessels below. However, any rebleeding can be treated by repeating the procedure. The most serious problem with this technique is that sclerosant can be injected into the wall of the oesophagus, outside the lumen of the vein, causing local necrosis and subsequent mediastinitis which may be fatal. However, the overall morbidity and mortality of this operation compares very favourably with other techniques for treating bleeding oesophageal varices[26] and it deserves wider consideration than it enjoys at present. Some workers are investigating the use of the flexible endoscope for this purpose.

An alternative technique for inducing thrombosis within the oesophageal varices is by injecting thrombotic agents from below through a catheter introduced into the portal vein.[48] Percutaneous, transhepatic cannulation of the portal vein is carried out as described previously. Under radiological screening the catheter is advanced into the coronary vein and radiopaque dye injected. This usually demonstrates clearly that the coronary vein is supplying a leash of oesophageal varices. When the catheter tip is suitably placed the thrombotic agent is introduced. Various materials have been used and newer ones are being investigated. These include 50 per cent dextrose, the thrombus-inducing agents thrombin and Gelfoam and, more recently, compounds such as cyanoacrylate which set into a hard mass on contact with blood.

The effect of the procedure is then investigated immediately by the injection of more radiopaque contrast. Following this the catheter is withdrawn and an attempt made to reposition it at the splenic end of the splenic vein. This allows any branches to be demonstrated and thrombosed. Finally, the catheter is withdrawn into the main portal vein and a 'free flush' of radiopaque contrast is injected to check the effectiveness of the procedure. The catheter is then slowly withdrawn and more Gelfoam injected to block the track made by the catheter through the liver.

The technique has produced good results. In experienced hands the varices can be demonstrated and thrombosed in approximately 70 per cent of cases. Some complications have been encountered. Bleeding from the liver puncture into the pleural and peritoneal cavities and biliary peritonitis were problems initially encountered; these have been overcome by ensuring that the catheter track is occluded by injecting Gelfoam as the catheter is withdrawn. Extensive portal vein thrombosis has sometimes been observed, and on one occasion when the new cyanoacrylate was being used the catheter became 'frozen' in the sclerosed vessel; however, removal was possible at laparotomy. Reports of controlled trials of this technique in major centres, and especially of the long-term follow-up of these patients, are awaited.

Ligation of the varices. Direct ligation of the columns of oesophageal varices (Boerema–Crile operation) and transection with re-suture of the lower end of the oesophagus have been techniques used to control acute haemorrhage. These operations are carried out through a left lateral thoracotomy. They are major surgical procedures for a very sick patient, however. This type of surgery in patients with cirrhosis carries an overall 30 per cent mortality[22] and rebleeding is common.[14] In patients with oesophageal varices secondary to extrahepatic portal vein occlusion without liver cell damage results are somewhat better. Some surgeons have stopped flow in the oesophageal varices by transecting the oesophagogastric junction at laparotomy[59] while Hassab[23] has described a technique of ligating all the collaterals from the abdomen coursing up to the oesophagus. Results of these procedures vary according to different reports, but they seem somewhat better than for thoracic operations. Nevertheless, all such operations have a high mortality.

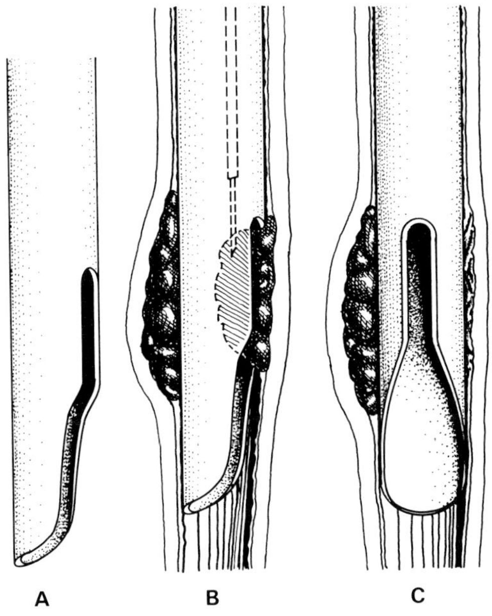

Figure 44.4. A. Modified oesophagoscope. B. Injection of varix. C. Pressure on thrombosed varix by rotation of scope.

Occlusion of the varices. An ingenious approach to the management of oesophageal variceal haemorrhage has been reported[6] and recently modified.[25] This consists of introducing a capsule or 'button' into the lower oesophagus via a gastrotomy (Figure 44.5). A tight ligature is then placed around the oesophagus circumferentially, ligating all vessels in the wall against the capsule. The second part of the capsule is then inserted into the lumen of the oesophagus and approximated to the first, enclosing the ligated portion of the wall; it is held tightly against the first piece by a spring clip. The circumferentially ligated wall and the enclosed vessels feeding the varices undergo necrosis and slough into the lumen of the oesophagus, while healing occurs at the approximated edges of the occlusion capsule. The necrosis releases the capsule which is passed eventually through the anus. This technique has not been widely used but has been reported to be simple to use, and early accounts suggest it is valuable. Oesophageal stricture may occur, however.

Decompression of the portal system. Theoretically, the ideal way to stop the bleeding caused by portal hypertension is to relieve it by decompression. Certainly, if an adequate pathway is provided for portal blood to reach the systemic circulation haemorrhage from oesophageal varices will stop. Nevertheless, there are serious side-effects to this type of surgery, and increased liver cell dysfunction and porta-systemic encephalopathy are common. It is necessary to consider traditional techniques for decompressing the portal venous system before discussing newer ones.

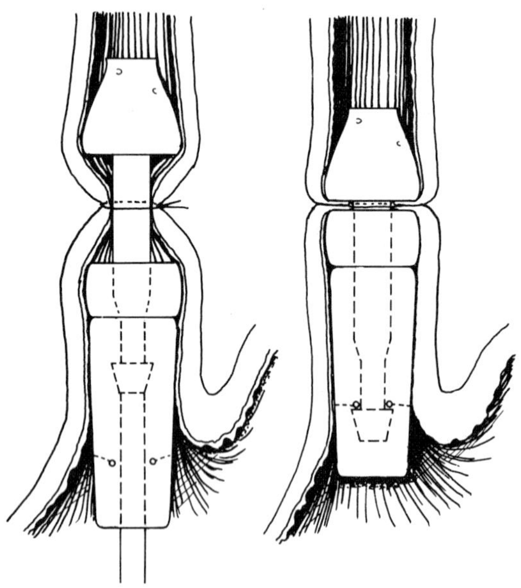

Figure 44.5. A. Boerema button with ligation of the oesophagus on the open instrument. B. Closure of the capsule encompassing the ligated oesophageal wall.

History. Eck in 1877[19] found it was possible to produce a 'fistula' between the portal vein and the inferior vena cava in dogs without all of the animals dying. He suggested that this procedure might have some value in patients with portal hypertension. Although various portasystemic shunts were tried clinically for the relief of ascites, only Vidal in 1910[65] reported the success of shunting for portal hypertension. Then in 1928 McIndoe[35] reported his studies on the vascular pathophysiology in cirrhosis. However, the operation was only rarely used before the late 1930s and early 1940s. At this time Blakemore[4] started to carry out portacaval shunts in an attempt to treat patients bleeding to death from oesophageal varices. He was largely encouraged by the work of doctors George and Alan Whipple[72] but the results were very disappointing; although the patients survived the operation they suffered a very high incidence of hepatic failure and problems of the central nervous system. In 1952 Blakemore concluded: 'the late failures are attributed to the normal progression of the cirrhotic process which has been unchanged by the shunt'.[5]

Current practice. Surprisingly little progress in the management of portal hypertension by decompression surgery has been made in the past 25 years. The problem is probably better understood now, however, and some conclusions can be made.

Although a complete portacaval end-to-side shunt (Figure 44.6B) undoubtedly decompresses the entire portal system and stops acute oesophageal variceal bleeding, such a shunt is associated with a very high incidence of portasystemic encephalopathy.[52] In addition, the liver cells, already damaged by the cirrhotic process, may be deprived of part of their blood supply and any 'hepatotrophic factors' which may come from the pancreas.[57] Unfortunately, many studies have now shown that survival following shunt surgery for bleeding oesophageal varices is hardly any better than that following conservative management, while the incidence of encephalopathy may be worse.[42,66] Other reports, however, suggest that the incidence of encephalopathy may be just as high in patients treated conservatively.[32]

It has been shown that in some cirrhotic processes part of the venous drainage of the liver may be through the portal vein. Thus, in these patients, an end-to-side portacaval shunt would theoretically reduce the venous drainage of the liver and so increase sinusoidal pressure. Certainly this group of patients seems to fare better with a side-to-side shunt.[46] A series of shunts having these characteristics, including splenorenal (Figure 44.6C), inferior vena caval–mesenteric and mesocaval anastomoses (Figure 44.6D), has been described.

True comparison of the results of these different shunts is difficult because of the poorly-controlled trials that have been attempted. However it seems that in cirrhotic patients with portal hypertension an adequate shunt, whether it is portacaval, splenorenal or mesocaval, will provide adequate decompression of the portal system and stop haemorrhage. If the shunt remains patent, rebleeding is unlikely, but the incidence of portasystemic encephalopathy and liver failure is high. If the shunt is inadequate or becomes blocked, portasystemic encephalopathy and liver failure are less of a problem and rebleeding is common.[30,51]

As a result of these observations the operation of choice in the acute situation can be related to the preference and expertise of the individual surgeon. The easiest and quickest procedure is the safest and is associated with the shortest anaesthetic time and lowest post-operative complications. I believe the mesocaval jump graft[15] fulfils these criteria and it is my shunt operation of choice at the moment.

Unfortunately, none of these surgical shunt procedures significantly affects the overall

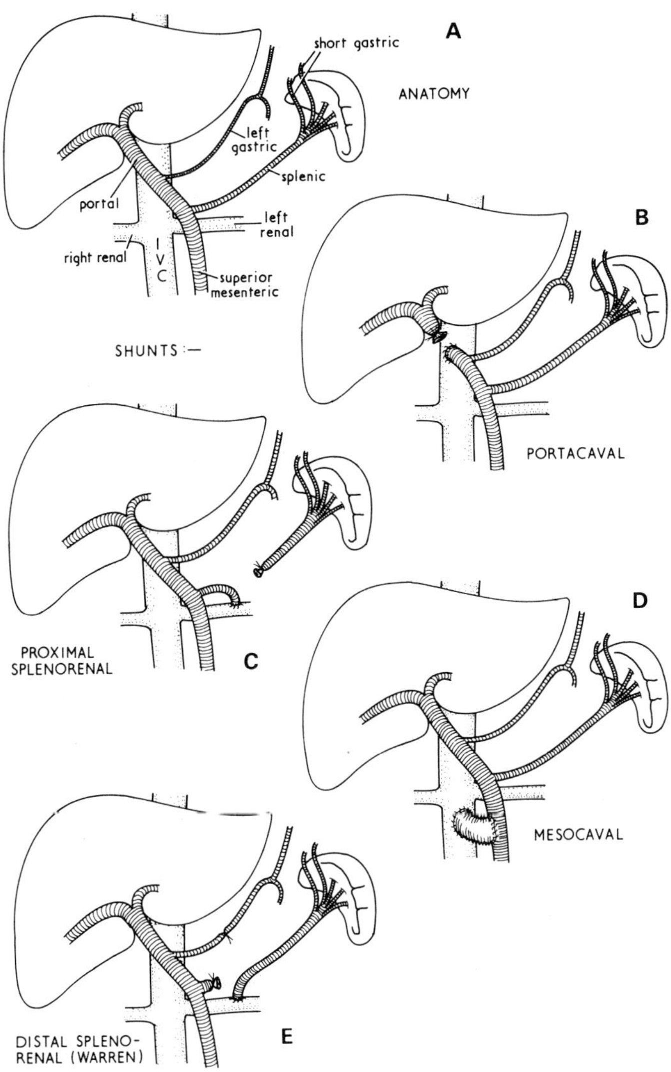

Figure 44.6. A. Diagrammatic representation of the portal system. B. Portacaval shunt. C. Proximal splenorenal (Linton) shunt. D. Mesocaval (Drapanas) shunt. E. Distal splenorenal (Warren) shunt.

mortality of the disease. Figures vary in different centres, but there is an overall mortality rate of about 15 per cent following acute shunt surgery. Of those surviving, 12 per cent have further haemorrhage. Of the 50 per cent of patients who survive five years, between 15 and 44 per cent are reported to develop portasystemic encephalopathy.[3,32] The acute mortality of the surgical procedure is related partly to the state of liver function and partly to the length of conservative treatment before surgery. By operating early on all alcoholic cirrhotic patients who are bleeding from oesophageal varices an operative survival rate of 51 per cent has been reported.[39] It must be appreciated, however, that the series inevitably included patients with good liver function who may have survived with purely conservative therapy.

In order to attempt to quantify liver function, Child and Turcotte[10] have described a method of assessing hepatic functional reserve. Since this description, several attempts have been made to modify it by adding a scoring system.[41] The concept is to identify certain measurable aspects of liver function which are known to compare with the severity of the liver disease. By adding these together it is possible to construct a category of liver disease. Child and Turcotte describe three of these, A, B and C; category A includes those patients with the best hepatic functional reserve while category C patients have the worst reserve. Comparison of early mortality from portal hypertension with their grading shows that best survival is associated with best hepatic functional reserve. The five-year survival rate for patients in category A is about 50 per cent, for those in category B it falls to almost 15 per cent and for those in category C it is only 8 per cent.[56] (See also Chapter 48 and Table 48.8.)

The best results of all are in patients with extrahepatic portal vein thrombosis and no hepatocellular dysfunction; they rarely require surgery to control haemorrhage. If they do, splenectomy and splenorenal shunt is probably the operation of choice if the splenic vein is patent, and this procedure has a low complication rate.[11] The best prognosis following shunt surgery for the complications of cirrhosis is seen in patients with primary biliary cirrhosis.[2] The next group, with fair results, is comprised of alcoholics who have really stopped drinking.[39] The worst results are seen in patients with chronic active hepatitis and alcoholics who continue drinking.[2] One conclusion that can be drawn from these results is that the aim of surgery in portal hypertension should be to decompress the oesophageal venous plexus without diverting the high-pressure portal flow away from the liver. None of the procedures mentioned so far meets these aims.

Recently, a new shunt which permits oesophageal vein decompression while theoretically maintaining the portal hypertension and liver blood flow has been described; this is the proximal splenorenal, reversed splenorenal or Warren shunt[68] (Figure 44.6E). The technique consists of dividing the portal end of the splenic vein and dissecting sufficient of the vein off the pancreas to allow the splenic end of the division to be anastomosed to the side of the left renal vein. The portal side is ligated as are the coronary vein and any other major veins arising from the portal vein which communicate with the decompressed splenic vein. The superior mesenteric venous flow from the intestine continues into the liver while the spleen is decompressed, together with any veins which drain into it from the oesophageal plexus through the short gastric veins. Thus a state of selective decompression of the oesophageal varices is produced while maintaining liver blood flow.

It is too soon to assess the long-term effects of this interesting procedure. The results are mixed and, although initially encouraging, the complication rate does not now seem to be very different from other shunt procedures.[21] The main problem with the operation is that it takes longer to perform and is more complicated than the other shunt techniques, so it is probably not indicated in the emergency situation. Theoretically, it is difficult to believe that anastomotic vessels between the high-pressure venous system and the low-pressure splenic venous drainage system which will follow shunting will not dilate to produce major shunts and thus encephalopathy. Furthermore, since part of the venous drainage of the pancreas is now into the systemic system, any hepatotrophic factors which may be produced there and which may be of value in encouraging liver regeneration[57] are still lost to portal inflow to the liver as in any other shunt procedure.

Another newly-described procedure is arterialization of the hepatic venous stump after portacaval end-to-side shunt.[31] In theory, the portal system is thereby decompressed but liver blood supply through the portal vein is maintained. The initial results are not encouraging but investigations of this technique are continuing.

Other shunting procedures such as that between the left gastric vein and vena cava have been described.[24] A high success rate in controlling haemorrhage with no complicating portasystemic encephalopathy is claimed but other workers have not reported similar success.

Re-introduction of the technique of transposition of abdominal organs has been described recently.[3] Originally the omentum was transposed subcutaneously and more recently the spleen has been placed in the anterior abdominal wall or in the chest. The procedure is designed to stimulate the development of an adequate collateral circulation to decompress the portal system. Some reports of these techniques, which are not widely used, are encouraging and perhaps the concept deserves wider investigation.

Factors affecting a decision to carry out shunt surgery

Consideration has to be given to further active treatment in all patients who have had a life-threatening haemorrhage, but for whom initial conservative treatment was successful. Any decision will be affected by the cause of the portal hypertension and the patient's social circumstances.

No totally satisfactory treatment is available yet for patients with portal hypertension. Portasystemic shunt should not be undertaken lightly in a patient whose agile mental activity is necessary for his work. However, a patient living in a part of the world remote from good medical care may require a shunt, since the risks attending his return home may be less than the risk of rebleeding following conservative management.

Prophylaxis against bleeding when oesophageal varices have been diagnosed

Since decompression of the portal system is technically fairly easy, it is inevitable that this has been assessed in many centres as a technique for prophylaxis against bleeding before any haemorrhagic complications of portal hypertension develop.[32] The studies suggest that surgery is not indicated in these patients; although bleeding ceases to be a problem after a prophylactic shunt the prognosis is no better than with conservative management. This concept, however, may require review when a shunt which carries a well-proven low mortality and morbidity is developed. Furthermore, the success of prophylactic sclerosis, either through an oesophagoscope or by the percutaneous transhepatic route, has not been reported yet although trials of these techniques are under way.

CONCLUSIONS

The management of a patient with haemorrhage from bleeding oesophageal varices complicating portal hypertension remains unsatisfactory. The outcome of treatment for active bleeding is probably dependent more upon the state of liver function at the time of the bleed than on the treatment given. Conservative measures include oesophageal tamponade or parenteral Pitressin and often these will stop an acute bleed. Frequently, however, bleeding recurs and more active treatment is required.

The choice must then be between sclerosis, compression, ligation of the varices or their feeding collaterals and portal decompression by a portasystemic shunt. Each method carries a significant mortality and morbidity. At present, the most promising techniques are sclerosis, either through an oesophagoscope or through the liver, and the Warren distal splenorenal shunt. Although there are occasional reports of successful therapy using less conventional methods, none of the results is so good as to contraindicate more traditional shunting procedures.

No method has yet been found for improving prognosis once portal hypertension has been diagnosed. Research in this field is active, nonetheless, and hopefully as a result of this the care of these unfortunate patients will be improved. Even liver transplantation may play a part in their management in the future.

REFERENCES

1. Bailey, M.E. & Dawson, J.L. (1975) Modified oesophagoscope for injecting oesophageal varices. *British Medical Journal*, **ii**, 540.
2. Bauer, J.J., Gelernt, I.M. & Kreel, I. (1976) Portosystemic shunting in patients with primary biliary cirrhosis: a good risk disease. *Annals of Surgery*, **183**, 324.
3. Bengmark, S. (1975) Surgical management of portal hypertension. In *Clinics in Gastroenterology*, **4** (2) (Ed.) Popper, H. pp. 395–423. London: W.B. Saunders.

4. Blakemore, A.H. (1946) Portacaval anastomosis: a report on fourteen cases. *Bulletin of the New York Academy of Medicine*, **22,** 254.
5. Blakemore, A.H. (1952) Portacaval shunting for portal hypertension. *Surgery, Gynecology and Obstetrics*, **94,** 443–454.
6. Boerema, I., Klopper, P.J. & Holscher, A.A. (1970) Transabdominal ligation-resection of the oesophagus in cases of bleeding oesophageal varices. *Surgery*, **67,** 409.
7. Burchell, A.R., Rousselot, L.M. & Panke, W.F. (1968) A seven year experience with side-to-side portacaval shunt for cirrhotic ascites. *Annals of Surgery*, **168,** 655.
8. Burchell, A.R., Moreno, A.H., Panke, W.F. & Nealon, T.F. (1974) Haemodynamic variables and progress following portacaval shunts. *Surgery, Gynecology and Obstetrics*, **138,** 359.
9. Burchell, A.R., Moreno, A.H., Panke, W.F. & Nealon, T.F. (1976) Hepatic artery flow improvement after portacaval shunt. *Annals of Surgery*, **184,** 289.
10. Child, C.G. & Turcotte, J.G. (1964) Surgery in portal hypertension. In *Major Problems in Clinical Surgery: The Liver and Portal Hypertension* (Ed.) Child, C.G. pp. 1–85. Philadelphia: W.B. Saunders.
11. Clatworthy, H.W. Jr (1974) Extrahepatic portal hypertension. In *Major Problems in Clinical Surgery: Portal Hypertension* (Ed.) Child, C.G. pp. 243–266. Philadelphia: W.B. Saunders.
12. Conn, H.O. (1958) Hazards attending the use of oesophageal tamponade. *New England Journal of Medicine*, **259,** 701.
13. Conn, H.O., Ramsby, G.R., Storer, E.H., Mutchnick, M.G., Joshi, P.H., Phillips, M.M., Cohen, G.A., Fields, G.N. & Petroski, D. (1975) Intraarterial vasopressin in the treatment of upper gastrointestinal haemorrhage: a prospective, controlled clinical trial. *Gastroenterology*, **68,** 211.
14. Cooperman, A.M. & Hermann, R.E. (1977) Ligation procedures in the management of portal hypertension. *Surgery*, **81,** 382.
15. Drapanas, T. (1975) Interposition mesocaval shunt. In *Practice of Surgery, Current Review* (Ed.) Ballinger, W.F. & Drapanas, T. p. 463. Vol. II. St Louis: C.V. Mosby.
16. Drapanas, T., Kluge, D.N. & Schenk, W.G. Jr (1960) Measurement of hepatic blood flow by BSP and by the electromagnetic flowmeter. *Surgery*, **48,** 1017.
17. Drapanas, T., LoCicero, J. III & Dowling, J.B. (1975) Haemodynamics of the interposition mesocaval shunt. *Annals of Surgery*, **181,** 523.
18. Dronfield, M.W., McIllmurray, M.B., Ferguson, R., Atkinson, M. & Langman, M.J.S. (1977) A prospective randomised study of endoscopy and radiology in acute upper gastrointestinal tract bleeding. *Lancet*, **i,** 1167.
19. Eck, N.V. (1877) On the question of ligature of the portal vein. *Voyenno Medical Journal*, **130,** 1. (Trans. *Surgery, Gynecology and Obstetrics* (1953)), **96,** 375.
20. Faloon, W. & Evans, G.L. (1970) Precipitating factors in genesis of hepatic coma. *New York State Journal of Medicine*, **70,** 2891.
21. Galambos, J.T., Warren, W.D., Rudman, D., Smith, R.B. & Salam, A.A. (1976) Selective and total shunts in the treatment of bleeding varices. *New England Journal of Medicine*, **295,** 1089.
22. George, P., Brown, C., Ridgway, G., Crofts, B. & Sherlock, S. (1973) Emergency oesophageal transection in uncontrolled variceal haemorrhage. *British Journal of Surgery*, **60,** 635.
23. Hassab, M.A. (1967) Gastroesophageal decongestion and splenectomy in the treatment of oesophageal varices in bilharzial cirrhosis: further studies with a report of 355 operations. *Surgery*, **61,** 169.
24. Inokuchi, K., Kobayashi, M., Ogawa, Y., Saku, M., Nagasue, N. & Iwaki, A. (1975) Results of left gastric vena caval shunt for oesophageal varices: analysis of one hundred clinical cases. *Surgery*, **78,** 628.
25. Johnston, G.W. & Kelly, J.M. (1976) Early experience with the Boerema button for bleeding oesophageal varices. *British Journal of Surgery*, **63,** 117.
26. Johnston, G.W. & Rodgers, H.W. (1973) A review of 15 years experience in the use of sclerotherapy in the control of acute haemorrhage from oesophageal varices. *British Journal of Surgery*, **60,** 797.
27. Kobayashi, M., Inokuchi, K., Hagasue, N., Saku, M. & Iwaki, A. (1977) Successful treatment of early cancer of the liver and portal hypertension in patients presenting with bleeding oesophageal varices. *British Journal of Surgery*, **64,** 542.
28. LeVeen, H.H., Christoudias, G., Ip, M., Luft, R., Falk, G. & Grosberg, S. (1974) Peritoneo-venous shunting for ascites. *Annals of Surgery*, **180,** 580–591.
29. Lieberman, F.L., Denison, C.K. & Reynolds, T.B. (1970) The relationship of plasma volume, portal hypertension, ascites and renal sodium retention in cirrhosis. *Annals of the New York Academy of Sciences*, **170,** 202.
30. Linton, R.R. (1974) Portal hypertension as I see it in 1973: the treatment of bleeding oesophageal varices secondary to portal cirrhosis of the liver. In *Major Problems in Clinical Surgery. Vol. xiv: Portal Hypertension* (Ed.) Child, C.G. pp. 196–232. Philadelphia: W.B. Saunders.
31. Maillard, J.N., Rueff, B., Prandi, D. & Sicot, C. (1974) Hepatic arterialization and portocaval shunt in hepatic cirrhosis: an assessment. *Archives of Surgery*, **108,** 315.
32. Malt, R.A. (1976) Portasystemic venous shunts. *New England Journal of Medicine*, **295,** 24.
33. McDermott, W.F. Jr (1972) Evaluation of the haemodynamics of portal hypertension in the selection of patients for shunt surgery. *Annals of Surgery*, **176,** 449.
34. McDermott, W.V., Barnes, B.A., Nardi, G.L. & Ackroyd, F.W. (1968) Post shunt encephalopathy. *Surgery, Gynecology and Obstetrics*, **126,** 585.
35. McIndoe, A.H. (1928) Vascular lesions of portal cirrhosis. *Archives of Pathology*, **5,** 23.
36. Nissan, S. & Bar-Maor, J. A. (1971) Bleeding oesophageal varices due to splenic arteriovenous fistula. *American Journal of Gastroenterology*, **55,** 379.
37. Novis, B.H., Duys, S.P., Barbezat, G.O., Clain, J., Bank, S. & Terblanche, J. (1976) Fibreoptic endoscopy and the use of the Sengstaken tube in acute gastrointestinal haemorrhage in patients with portal hypertension and varices. *Gut*, **17,** 258.
38. Orloff, M.J. & Thomas, H.S. (1963) Pathogenesis of oesophageal varix rupture. *Archives of Surgery*, **87,** 301.
39. Orloff, M.J., Charters, A.C., Chandler, J.G., Condon, J.K., Grambort, D.E., Modafferi, T.R., Levin, S.E., Brown, N.B., Sviokla, S.C. & Knox, D.G. (1975) Portacaval shunt as emergency procedure in unselected patients with alcoholic cirrhosis. *Surgery, Gynecology and Obstetrics*, **141,** 59.
40. Palmer, E.D. (1969) The vigorous diagnostic approach to upper gastrointestinal haemorrhage. *Journal of the American Medical Association*, **207,** 1477.

41. Pugh, R.N.H., Murray-Lyon, I.M., Dawson, J.L., Pietroni, M.C. & Williams, R. (1973) Transection of the oesophagus for bleeding oesophageal varices. *British Journal of Surgery*, **60,** 646.
42. Resnick, R.H., Iber, F.L., Ishihara, A.M., Chalmers, T.C., Zimmerman, H. & the Boston Inter-Hospital Liver Group (1974) A controlled study of the therapeutic portocaval shunt. *Gastroenterology*, **67,** 843.
43. Reynolds, T.B. & Redeker, A.G. (1965) Hepatic haemodynamics and portal hypertension. In *Progress in Liver Disease*. Vol. 2 (Ed.) Popper, H. & Schaffner, F. pp. 457–473. New York: Grune & Stratton.
44. Reynolds, T.B., Ito, E. & Iwatsuki, S. (1970) Measurement of portal pressure and its clinical application. *American Journal of Medicine*, **49,** 649.
45. Rice, G.C., Ryan, C.J., Leiberman, D.P., Mathie, R.T., McGhee, E., Harper, A.M. & Blumgart, L.H. (1977) Measurement of liver blood flow in the rat using an ^{85}Krypton clearance technique. *British Journal of Experimental Pathology*, **58,** 236.
46. Riddell, A.G., Bloor, K., Hobbs, K.E.F. & Jacquet, N. (1972) Elective splenorenal anastomosis. *British Medical Journal*, **i,** 731.
47. Schiller, K.F.R., Truelove, S.C. & Williams, G.D. (1970) Haematemesis and melaena with special reference to factors influencing the outcome. *British Medical Journal*, **ii,** 7.
48. Scott, J., Dick, R., Long, R.G. & Sherlock, S. (1976) Percutaneous transhepatic obliteration of gastro-oesophageal varices. *Lancet*, **ii,** 53.
49. Shaldon, S., Chandussi, L., Guevara, L., Caesar, J. & Sherlock, S. (1961) The measurement of hepatic blood flow and intrahepatic shunted blood flow by colloidal heat-denatured human serum albumen labelled with I^{131}. *Journal of Clinical Investigation*, **40,** 1346.
50. Sherlock, S. (1968) Hepatic tumours. In *Diseases of the Liver and Biliary System*, 4th ed., Ch. 25, pp. 651–680. Philadelphia: F.A. Davis.
51. Sherlock, S. (1968) Portal venous system and portal hypertension. In *Diseases of the Liver and Biliary System*, 4th ed., Ch. 8, pp. 212–236. Philadelphia: F.A. Davis.
52. Sherlock, S., Hoorigan, K. & George, P. (1970) Medical complications of shunt surgery for portal hypertension. *Annals of the New York Academy of Sciences*, **170,** 392.
53. Smith, G.W. (1970) Splenectomy and coronary vein ligation for the control of bleeding esophageal varices. *American Journal of Surgery*, **119,** 122.
54. Smith, G.W. (1974) Use of haemodynamic selection criteria in the management of cirrhotic patients with portal hypertension. *Annals of Surgery*, **179,** 782.
55. Smith, G.W. & Edwards, O.E. (1966) Haemorrhage from varices in patients with achlorhydria. *Gastroenterology*, **51,** 1054.
56. Smith, G.W., Maddrey, W.C. & Zuidema, G.D. (1974) Portal hypertension as we see it. In *Major Problems in Clinical Surgery: Portal Hypertension* (Ed.) Child, C.G. pp. 1 35. Philadelphia: W.B. Saunders.
57. Starzl, T.E., Porter, K.A., Kashiwagi, N. & Putnam, C.W. (1975) Portal hepatotrophic factors, diabetes mellitus and acute liver atrophy, hypertrophy and regeneration. *Surgery, Gynecology and Obstetrics*, **141,** 843.
58. Stevenson, G.W., Cox, P.R., & Roberts, C.J.C. (1976) Prospective comparison of double contrast barium meal examination and fibreoptic endoscopy in acute upper gastrointestinal haemorrhage. *British Medical Journal*, **ii,** 723.
59. Tanner, N.C. (1954) In Discussion on portal hypertension. *Proceedings of the Royal Society of Medicine*, **47,** 475.
60. Torrance, H.B. & Gowenlock, A.H. (1962) Radioactive colloid clearance techniques to measure liver blood flow in man. *Clinical Science*, **22,** 413.
61. Trey, S., Lipworth, L., Chalmers, T.C., Davidson, C.S., Gottlieb, L.S., Popper, H. & Saunders, S.J. (1968) Fulminant hepatic failure. *New England Journal of Medicine*, **279,** 798.
62. Tumen, H.L. (1970) Hypersplenism and portal hypertension. *Annals of the New York Academy of Sciences*, **170,** 332.
63. Turcotte, J.G. (1974) Portal hypertension as I see it. In *Major Problems in Clinical Surgery: Portal Hypertension* (Ed.) Child, C.G. pp. 78–120. Philadelphia: W.B. Saunders.
64. Victor, M., Adams, R.D. & Cole, M. (1965) The acquired (non-Wilsonian) type of chronic hepatocerebral degeneration. *Medicine*, **44,** 345.
65. Vidal, M. (1910) Discussion of the Eck operation. *Revue de Chirurgie*, **42,** 1181.
66. Voorhees, A.B. Jr, Price, J.B. & Britton, R.C. (1970) Portal systemic shunting procedures for portal hypertension: 26 years experience in adults with cirrhosis of the liver. *American Journal of Surgery*, **119,** 501.
67. Wapnick, S., Grosberg, S., Kinney, M. & LeVeen, H.H. (1977) LeVeen continuous peritoneal-jugular shunt. *Journal of the American Medical Association*, **237,** 131–133.
68. Warren, W.D. & Salam, A.A. (1974) Surgery for the portal hypertension of cirrhosis: the need for change. In *Major Problems in Clinical Surgery. Vol. xiv: Portal Hypertension* (Ed.) Child, C.G. pp. 127–164. Philadelphia: W.B. Saunders.
69. Warren, W.D., Fomon, J.J., Viamonte, M. & Zeppa, R. (1967) Pre-operative assessment of portal hypertension. *Annals of Surgery*, **165,** 999.
70. Webb, L.J., Berger, L.A. & Sherlock, S. (1977) Grey-scale ultrasonography of portal vein. *Lancet*, **ii,** 675.
71. Welch, C.E. & Hedberg, S. (1973) Gastrointestinal haemorrhage. 1: General considerations of diagnosis and the therapy. *Advances in Surgery*, **7,** 95.
72. Whipple, G.H. (1945) The problem of portal hypertension in relation to hepatosplenopathies. Personal communication to A.O. Whipple. *Annals of Surgery*, **122,** 449.
73. Winkler, K., Larsen, J.A., Munkner, T. & Tygstrup, N. (1965) Determination of the hepatic blood flow in man by simultaneous use of five test substances measured in two parts of the liver. *Scandinavian Journal of Clinical and Laboratory Investigation*, **17,** 473.

Chapter 45

Portasystemic Shunting for Metabolic Disease

THOMAS E. STARZL
JOSEPH BENICHOU

For many years portal venous diversion has been used for the haemodynamic objectives of stopping or preventing haemorrhage from oesophageal varices or, less commonly, to treat intractable ascites. Since 1963, a new dimension has been added to the old operation of portacaval shunt by employing this procedure to alter favourably the course of patients with two inborn errors of metabolism, glycogen storage disease and hyperlipoproteinaemia. In this chapter we will discuss the results and the potential postoperative risks of portal diversion for these new indications, as well as the possible mechanisms of benefit.

GLYCOGEN STORAGE DISEASE

Portal diversion was first performed for glycogen storage disease almost 14 years ago.[34] Then the rationale for the procedure was naive by today's standards. It was hoped that by short-circuiting splanchnic venous blood around the liver, glucose would be made more readily available to peripheral tissues with relief of hypoglycaemia, and that the liver would be coincidentally deglycogenated. As will be discussed later, it has since been learned from animal experimentation that the consequences of portacaval shunt are far more subtle and wide-ranging than that simple view.

That first patient, who had Type III glycogen storage disease, is still alive almost 14 years after portacaval transposition. The by-passed portal venous blood is replaced with blood returning from the inferior vena cava with this operation, which was first described in animals by Child et al[6] (Figure 45.1). The transposition was used in order to avoid the potential hazards of Eck fistula. It was appreciated then and amply confirmed since[24] that most animals, including subhuman primates, develop wasting and encephalopathy after portal diversion, but it was not appreciated that humans would be an exception to this generalization.

Our first patient had a remarkably untroubled convalescence and was discharged from the hospital nine days postoperatively. Before and after operation, there were elevations in the transaminases which a decade later were still slightly increased. She had a splenectomy 43 months after transposition for thrombocytopenia at which time the portacaval anastomosis draining the splanchnic bed was proved to be open. There has been no evidence of portal hypertension, indicating that the portacaval anastomosis draining the splanchnic bed is still open. An inferior vena cavagram almost 10 years postoperatively revealed flow of systemic venous blood from the distal vena cava to the liver but with a major by-pass around the liver through azygous and hemiazygous collaterals (Figure 45.2). The degree of azygous by-passing was similar to that observed with a

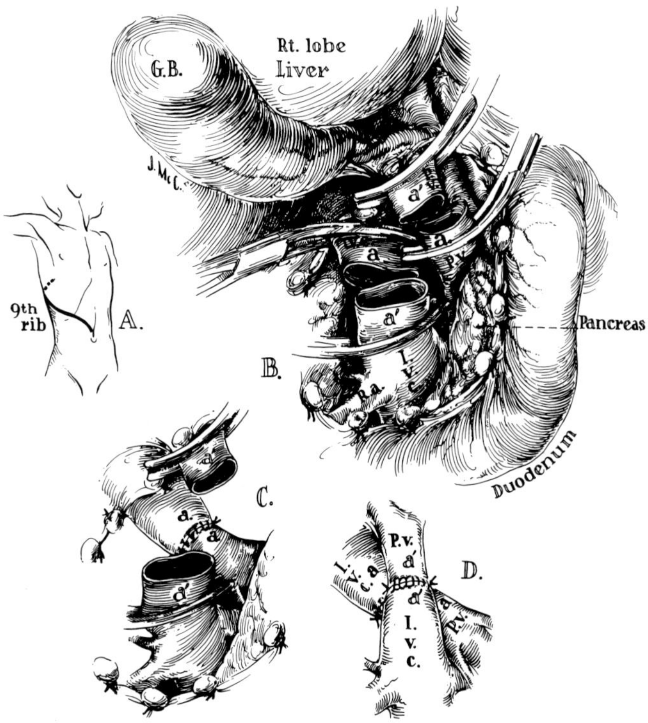

Figure 45.1. The operation of portacaval transposition that was used for the first two patients with glycogen storage disease who were treated with portal diversion. Note that the central portal vein is revascularized with vena caval blood. From Starzl et al,[34] with the kind permission of the editor of *Surgery*.

comparable angiographic study more than nine years earlier when the patient was three-months postoperative.

A patient similarly treated by Riddell et al[25] in Bristol, England, also survived for a long time. Riddell's patient moved to Canada and was temporarily lost to follow-up. Eventually he was traced through the Immigration Department. Angiographic studies were carried out in Calgary, Alberta, in December 1971, and confirmed by us in January 1973. The vena cava was obstructed (Figure 45.3, left), a complication which had probably occurred a long time previously since collateral venous channels were highly developed and lower limb oedema was minimal. The anastomosis draining the splanchnic venous bed was shown to be open (Figure 45.3, right).

One more portacaval transposition was performed. The attempt cost the life of our second patient, when the liver was unable to transmit the rerouted vena caval flow, causing hepatic swelling and uncontrollable acidosis. This seven-year-old child died two days later. We[27] and Hermann and Mercer[16] subsequently recommended that the simpler procedure of portacaval shunt be used. To our knowledge this approach has been followed in all later cases. By the spring of 1973[35] our own series of patients had reached seven, and six more had been formally reported in the literature from other centres. Since then our cases have increased to 10 and it is upon this personal experience (Table 45.1) that most of the opinions in this report will be based. We have had no operative deaths or technical failures after end-to-side portacaval shunt.

Our original patient with transposition is still living after 14 years, as are seven of the eight patients treated with simple portacaval shunts. These last seven patients now have follow-ups of one to $5\frac{1}{3}$ years (mean 50 months). The ages of all of our 10 patients, types of disease and symptoms are summarized in Table 45.1. Type I disease (glucose-6-phosphatase deficiency) has been the most common indication for treatment, with Type III disease (amylo-1,6-glucosidase deficiency) being a distant second.

Metabolic effects

After portal diversion, most of the children who had pre-existing hypoglycaemia did not have relief of this problem or the relief was not complete. Thus, night feedings usually had to be

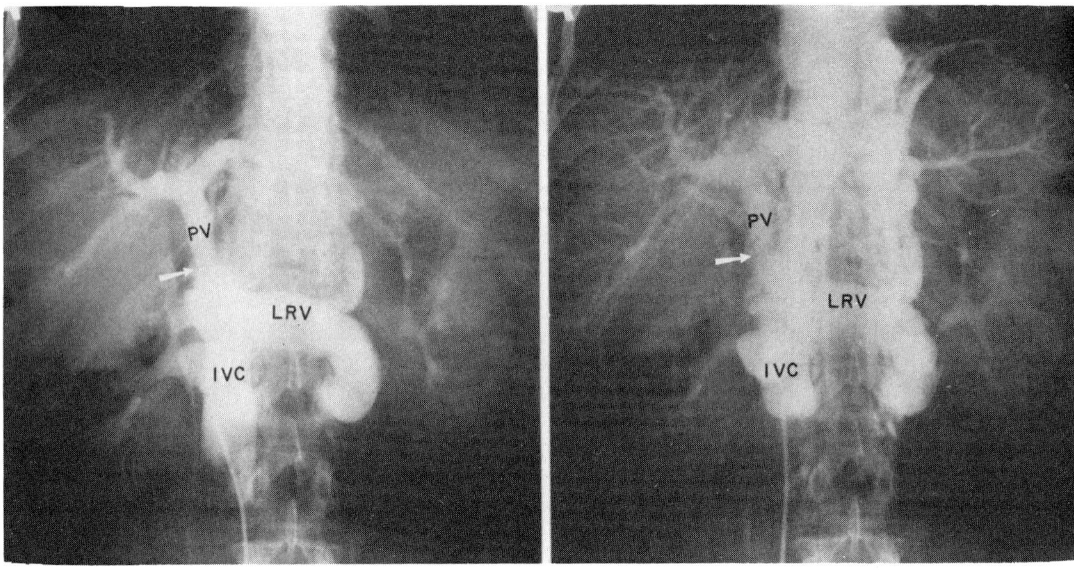

Figure 45.2. Inferior vena cavagram in March 1973, 9½ years postoperatively in Colorado Case 1 showing a patent caval–portal anastomosis (arrow) under two conditions of dye injection. Significant flow through the liver, as well as around it by the azygous and other collaterals, was well seen at fluoroscopy. IVC – distal inferior vena cava; LRV – left renal vein; PV – portal vein. From Starzl et al,[35] with the kind permission of the editor of *Annals of Surgery*.

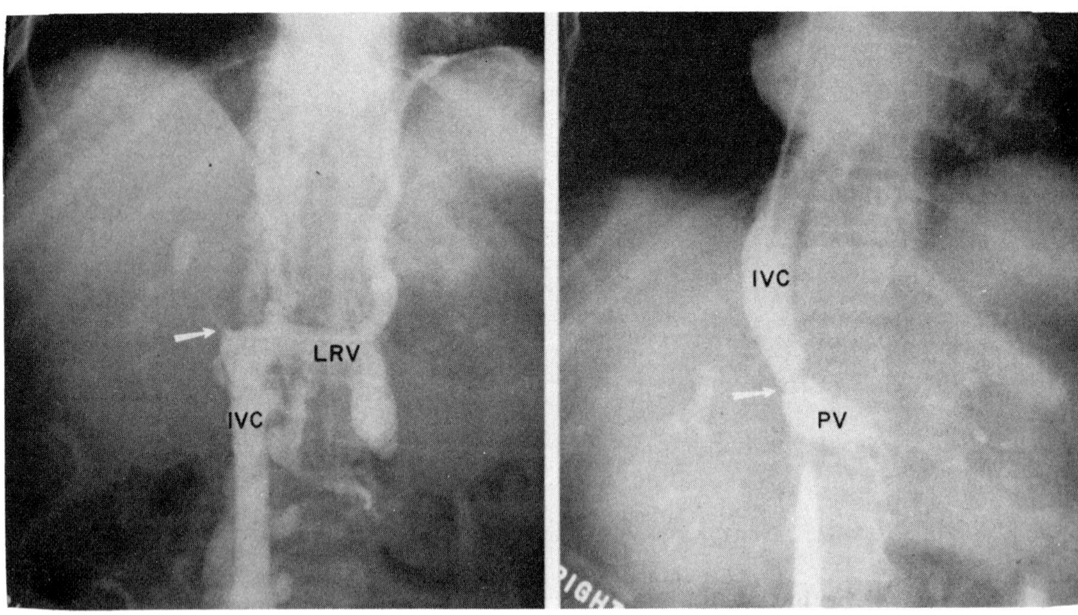

Figure 45.3. Studies of the Bristol case of portacaval transposition. The original operation was on 5 May 1965, and the examination depicted, which was in December 1971, was performed by Dr R.J. Sommerville at the Foothills Hospital, Calgary, Alberta. (Left) Inferior vena cavagram showing obstruction at the anastomotic site (arrow). IVC – distal inferior vena cava; LRV – left renal vein. Note the extensive collaterals via the azygous system. (Right) Demonstration of a patent portacaval anastomosis (arrow) by means of a retrograde catheterization. IVC – proximal inferior vena cava; PV – portal vein. From Starzl et al,[35] with the kind permission of the editor of *Annals of Surgery*.

Table 45.1. *Patients with Glycogen Storage Disease Treated by Portal Diversion at the University of Colorado.*

Case No.	Age	Glycogen storage disease type	Date of operation	Symptoms preoperatively			Persistent hypoglycaemia postoperatively	Survival post-shunt
				Hypo-glycaemia	Acidosis	Growth retardation		
1[a]	8	III	10.15.63	×	×	×	No	Alive 14 years
2[a]	7	I	6.26.68	×	×	×	–	Died 2 days
3	7	I	5.2.72	×	×	×	Yes[b]	Alive 5 years
4	11	I	5.17.72	×	×	×	No	Died $4\frac{3}{4}$ years
5	10	VI	8.2.72			×	–	Alive $4\frac{3}{4}$ years
6	5	III	11.7.72	×	×	×	No	Alive $4\frac{1}{2}$ years
7	3	III	11.8.72	×	×	×	Yes	Alive $4\frac{1}{2}$ years
8	8	I	8.13.73	×	×	×	Yes[b]	Alive $3\frac{3}{4}$ years
9	12	I	12.14.73	×	×	×	Yes[b]	Alive $3\frac{1}{2}$ years
10	1	I	9.2.76	×	×	×	Yes	Alive 8 months

[a] Operation was portacaval transposition. The last eight patients had simple portacaval shunt.
[b] Overnight feeding via nasogastric tube started $2\frac{1}{2}$ to 4 years after portacaval shunt.

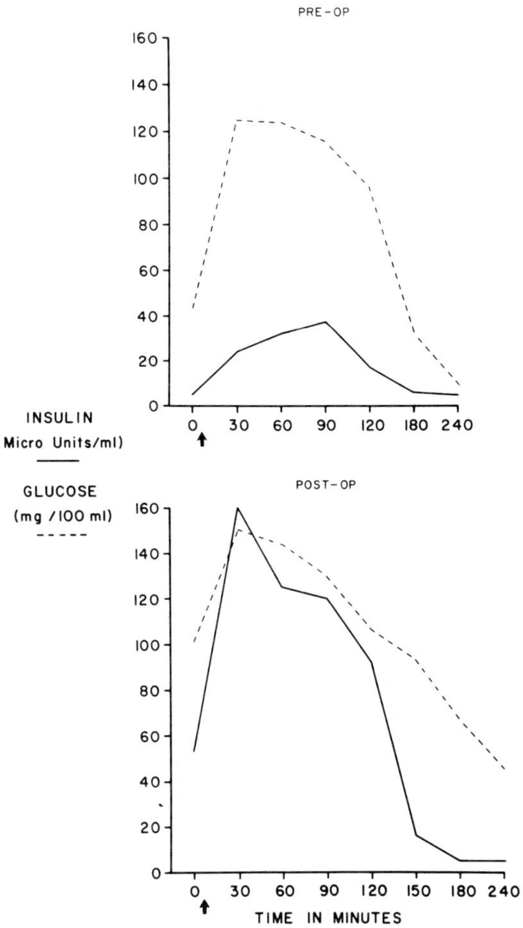

Figure 45.4. Plasma insulin and glucose concentrations before and after portacaval shunt in a child (Case 8, Table 45.1) with Type I glycogen storage disease. Oral glucose tolerance test.

continued. Studies of plasma insulin and glucagon in several of these patients have revealed changes (Figure 45.4). The flat peripheral insulin curves typical of Type I glycogen disease[22] became significantly elevated after portacaval shunt, and there were smaller increases in glucagon. The glucose tolerance curves were a little different before and after operation.

Liver glycogen concentrations in all the patients later biopsied were not changed. In spite of this, the liver size in several of our patients and those reported by others underwent a very obvious reduction as measured with liver scan planimetry. Even if obvious shrinkage did not occur, postoperative biopsies always showed a diminution in individual hepatocyte size similar to that produced in animals by portacaval shunt.[35]

In contrast to the incomplete relief of hypoglycaemia, all components of the hyperlipidaemia which is a characteristic of the Type I disease had profound and permanent relief (Figure 45.5), as was first observed by Hermann and Mercer[16] and confirmed by Folkman et al[12] and in our own cases.[35] Correction of other metabolic defects was observed, including abnormal bleeding, uric acid elevations and abnormal calcium metabolism.[35]

Growth

All 10 of our patients had growth retardation before portacaval shunt. Afterwards, height

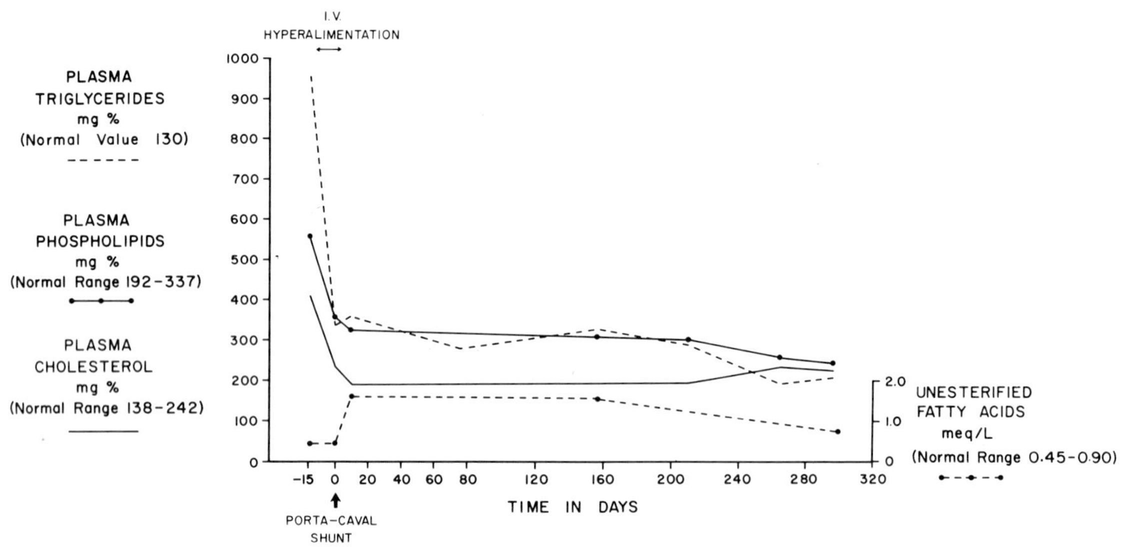

Figure 45.5. Effect of parenteral hyperalimentation and end-to-side portacaval shunt on the plasma lipids of Patient 4 whose diagnosis was Type I glycogen storage disease. Note the rapid and relatively complete reversal of all abnormalities. From Starzl et al,[35] with the kind permission of the editor of *Annals of Surgery*.

increases, which in most cases had virtually ceased, have occurred at the rates listed in Table 45.2, that is, approximately 0.5 cm per month.

Quantitative measures of growth were obtained with radiographic techniques.[35] An example of the results is shown in Figure 45.6. Comparison of the wrist and hands in this seven-year-old stunted child before and $11\frac{1}{2}$ months after operation showed the phenomenal effects of bone age doubling. In addition to the size change, mineralization occurred, as did the appearance of new wrist bones. Circulating somatotrophin in these patients was normal. The growth spurts may have been at least partially attributable to the increased insulin distribution to the periphery mentioned earlier (see Figure 45.4) since, in recent years, insulin has been recognized to be a major growth hormone comparable in potency to somatotrophin. The simpler possibility that better nutrition was responsible must also be considered.

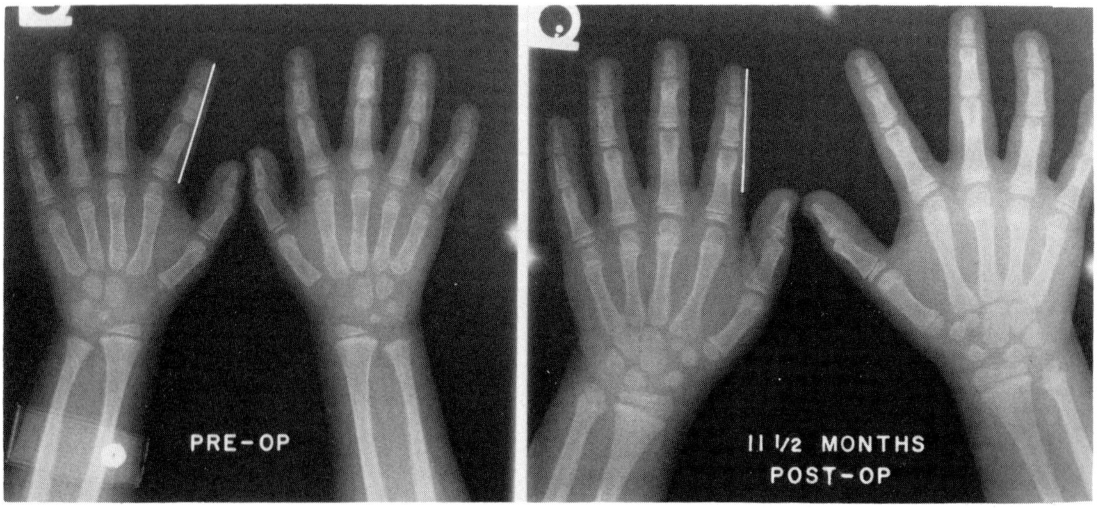

Figure 45.6. The dramatic wrist and hand bone growth and mineralization in Case 3 in the first $11\frac{1}{2}$ postoperative months. The bracket on the left index finger is 5 cm in length. From Starzl et al,[35] with the kind permission of the editor of *Annals of Surgery*.

Table 45.2. *Growth Rate and Complications Following Portal Diversion for Glycogen Storage Disease.*

Case No.	Growth rate (cm/month over 9 to 120 months)	Complications
1	0.49	
2	Op. Death	
3	0.50	Macroadenomatosis
4	0.28	Died $4\frac{3}{4}$ years post-shunt. Primary pulmonary hypertension, $NH_3 = 85$ µg/100 ml; macroadenomatosis
5	0.53	Renal artery stenosis surgically corrected 32 months post-shunt
6	0.62	
7	0.50	
8	0.49	
9	0.88	Renal stone two months post-shunt. Mild arterial hypertension; macroadenomatosis
10	0.22	
Mean	0.47	

Encephalopathy and other risks

None of our patients has developed hepatic encephalopathy. The highest blood ammonia recorded was 49.3 µmol/l (84 µg/per cent) in a child who died almost five years after portacaval shunt during an attempt at transcaval radiographic visualization of the portacaval anastomosis. This patient (Case 4) had not achieved the full expected growth after operation (Table 45.2), had mild systemic hypertension, and had unexplained transient bouts of cyanosis, hyperventilation and unconsciousness. Except for the slightly elevated blood ammonia, liver function was normal.

At autopsy, the liver had macroadenomatosis. Very minor protoplasmic astrocytosis was present in the brain. A finding that had not been suspected during life was advanced right ventricular hypertrophy and dilatation. The smaller pulmonary arteries and arterioles had medial muscle hypertrophy, medial and intimal fibrosis, scattered fibrinoid necrosis and numerous plexiform lesions. In retrospect, the patient died from a cardiopulmonary complication of the kind that has been documented in patients with Type I glycogen storage disease or other liver disease.[21]

This complication has been termed 'vasoconstrictive pulmonary hypertension'. It has been speculated that a humoral vasoconstrictive agent, which normally is completely detoxified by the liver, is responsible for the hypertrophic lesions in the pulmonary vasculature. It is conceivable, although unlikely, that the development of a renal artery stenosis in Patient No. 5 (Table 45.2) could have been caused by the same mechanism.

Three of our 10 patients developed the hepatic lesions which have been termed both macroadenomatosis and nodular hyperplasia. Filling defects were noted by liver scan with some waxing and waning of size. This complication is common in patients with Type I glycogen storage disease, particularly with advancing age, and was recently reported in seven of eight patients who were three to 28 years old.[18]

The value of enteral or parenteral feeding

Seven years ago, Folkman et al[12] of Boston Children's Hospital added an important therapeutic dimension by showing how preoperative parenteral hyperalimentation would reduce the risk of portacaval shunt by normalizing preexisting hepatomegaly, acidosis and other abnormalities, including hyperlipidaemia. The Harvard group as well as the Vanderbilt team[3,14] have greatly extended these original observations.

Greene et al,[14] for example, showed that continuous night feeding through a gastrostomy or gastric tube resulted in many of the same benefits as the parenteral hyperalimentation or as the portacaval shunt. Apparently, the night feeding was originally tried to control the nocturnal hypoglycaemia which, as mentioned earlier, was not relieved by portal diversion. It was soon observed that the night feedings contributed to, or were primarily responsible for, the same kinds of growth spurts and relief of metabolic abnormalities (including hyperlipidaemia) which are ameliorated by portacaval shunt. Greene et al[14] have shown that systemic plasma insulin levels are more than doubled by such treatment and that glucagon is decreased, leading them to speculate that the hormone changes were responsible for the benefits. Whatever the explanation, this kind of treatment is an alternative to portal diversion as the primary treatment of children with glycogen storage disease, and even after portacaval shunt it has an additional value as has been evident in three of our patients (Table 45.1) who had hypoglycaemia, retardation of growth, or both. Glucose and amino acid mixtures have both been effective for the gastric feeding.

HYPERLIPIDAEMIA

The observations about lipid lowering after portacaval shunt in patients with Type I glycogen storage disease (see Figure 45.5) were responsible for our suggesting the same operation to treat hyperlipidaemia.[31] It has been 4½ years since a completely diverting portacaval shunt was first performed clinically for the purpose of lowering the serum concentration of cholesterol and low density lipoproteins (LDL). Since then, we have treated two more patients by this method. As of May 1977, an additional nine patients had the same procedure in other centres and were documented in the literature.[8,11,20,26,36,37]

These 12 cases represent less than half of the true total. Through an informal registry that has been kept at the National Institutes of Health, Bethesda, U.S.A., it is known that more than 30 portacaval shunts have been carried out for the treatment of hyperlipidaemia with results that are in general agreement with the smaller sample which is accessible through the formal literature and upon which we will comment in this chapter. All three of our patients had homozygous Type II hyperlipidaemia.

In Type II hyperlipidaemia, Goldstein and Brown[13] have suggested that there may be an absence of or defect in the cell surface receptor sites which normally bind and transport LDL cholesterol into the cell. Because cholesterol does not enter the cell, they proposed that there is an absence of the normal feedback suppression of cholesterol synthesis.

The homozygous form of Type II hyperlipoproteinaemia has a shockingly poor prognosis if, as is usually the case, there is not a good response to medical therapy. Lipid-rich deposits are laid down in widely separated superficial and deep parts of the body, including blood vessels where premature atherosclerosis is the consequence. Cardiac valves are similarly affected, with aortic stenosis being particularly common. The patients usually die of cardiovascular complications before the age of 20 years despite all conventional therapy. The gravity of the situation seemed to justify the trial of a new approach.

Colorado cases

Our first patient, an 11-year-old girl, had suffered a major myocardial infarction about two months before the portacaval shunt. After the portal diversion, her serum cholesterol values fell from about 20 mmol/l (800 mg/dl) to levels that were consistently below 10 mmol/l (400 mg/dl) (Figure 45.7). Unsightly xanthomas began to resorb from visible subcutaneous and tendinous locations (Figure 45.8). Attacks of pre-existing angina pectoris became less frequent and finally stopped. By cardiac catheterization 16 months after the end-to-side portacaval shunt was performed, there was good evidence that reversal of aortic stenosis had occurred, with a diminution of the aortic valve gradient from 7.45 to 1.33 kPa (56 to 10 mmHg).[28] The coronary arteries were also thought to be less diseased than before, although three stenoses were still present. More than 1½ years after portacaval shunt, the girl died suddenly while coming home from school.

At autopsy, the residual coronary artery disease was confirmed. There was a large ventricular aneurysm. The conclusion was that death was probably caused by an acute cardiac arrhythmia.[33] She should have been submitted to a coronary revascularization procedure as was done in Case 2 (see below). The decision against this was taken with the hope that the coronary artery stenoses would regress spontaneously.

The portacaval shunt was widely patent. The liver, which weighed 618 g, was grossly normal, and microscopically it was unchanged from the biopsy specimen that was obtained six months postoperatively. On light and electron microscopy, the most prominent findings were shrinkage of the hepatocyte size, depletion of rough endoplasmic reticulum, and the accumulation of intracytoplasmic lipid deposits. These changes are typical of those caused in the liver

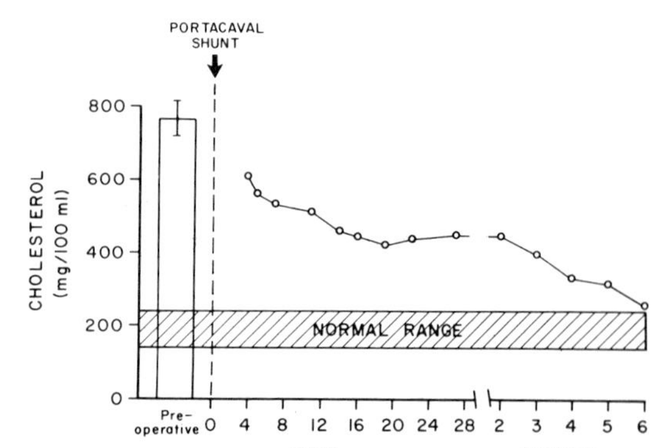

Figure 45.7. Serum cholesterol concentrations after portacaval shunt in Patient 1, Table 45.3.

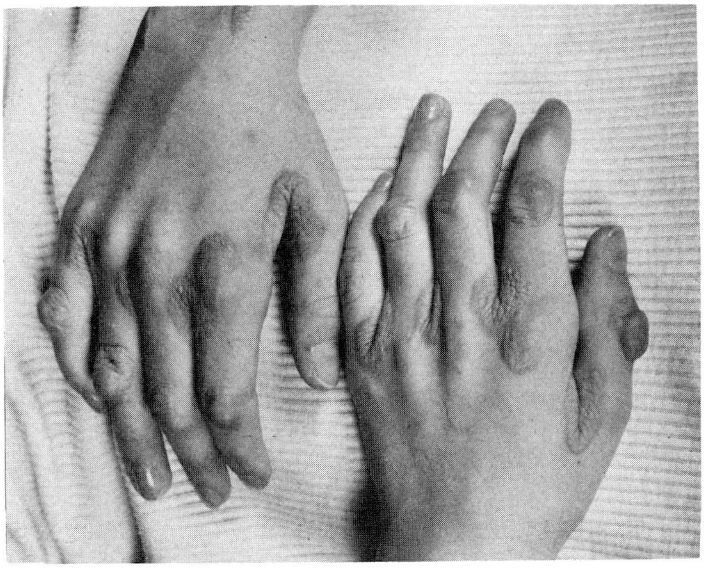

(a)

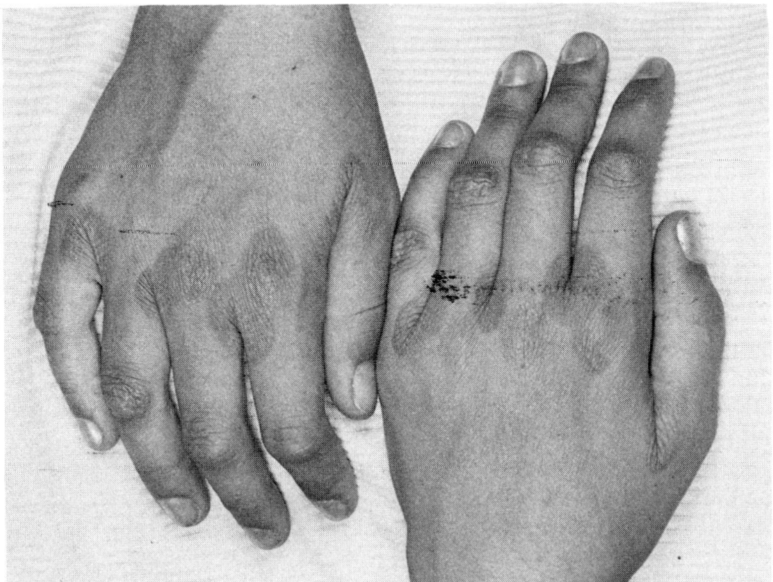

(b)

Figure 45.8. The hands of Patient 1 of the hyperlipidaemia series two weeks before (a) and 16 months after (b) portacaval shunt.

by portacaval shunt in all species studied so far.[24] Hepatic function had not been changed by portacaval shunt as judged by standard liver function tests.

We have performed a portacaval shunt on two more patients with the same diagnosis (Cases 2 and 3, Table 45.3). Patient No. 2 was a seven-year-old girl at the time of operation. She had preoperative serum cholesterol values that averaged 25.82 ± 1.22 (s.d.) mmol/l (997 ± 47 [s.d.] mg/100 ml) while she was on a very low cholesterol diet. Six months after the shunt, the cholesterol level measured in the same laboratory was 15.54 mmol/l (600 mg/100 ml) (a 40 per cent reduction), despite a relaxation of the diet. These values have continued to fall under careful medical management by Dr David Bilheimer of Southwestern University Medical Center. The cholesterol concentrations during the last year have been 11.66 ± 1.73 mmol/l (450 ± 67 mg per cent). The xanthomas on her heels, elbows and hands either have resorbed

Table 45.3. *Patients with Type II Hyperlipidaemia Treated at the University of Colorado.*

Case No.	Age	Date of operation	Serum cholesterol mmol/l (mg/100 ml)			Clinical result	Comments
			Pre-shunt	Post-shunt	Final % reduction		
1	12	3.1.73	19.92(769)	7.51(290)	62	Died 18½ months; cardiac arrest	Old myocardial infarct with ventricular aneurysm; residual stenoses of coronary arteries; xanthomas had disappeared
2	7	10.4.74	25.82(997)	11.66(450)	55	Good	Had aortic and mitral valve replacement plus double coronary artery by-pass 25 months after shunt; xanthomas nearly completely disappeared
3	8	8.5.75	25.90(1000)	15.54(600)	40	Good	Xanthomas slowly disappearing

completely or have greatly diminished in size.

This child also had aortic stenosis and angina pectoris. Because of persistence of her cardiac disease, she was treated with aortic and mitral valve replacement plus double coronary artery by-pass two years after portacaval shunt. The operation was carried out by Dr Robert McGehee and his associates at the Fort Worth Children's Hospital. The patient has returned to school with essentially unlimited activities.

Dr Bilheimer has written us: 'Our therapeutic approach continues to be one of trying to get Mary's cholesterol as low as possible with medication. I am totally convinced that the portacaval shunt was tremendously helpful to her. I doubt that we would have proceeded with the cardiac surgery if her cholesterol were still in the 23 to 25 mmol/l (900 to 1000 mg per cent) range. Her present cardiac difficulties are an extension of those already present before the shunt surgery. Our main job now is to try and retard the development of atherosclerosis in her coronary by-pass grafts.'

A third patient had a portacaval shunt performed 24 months ago. The child was from France and has been managed through a collaborative effort with Professor Jean Rey and Dr J. Schmitz of the Hôpital des Enfants Malades and Professor J.-L. deGennes of the Hôpitaux de Paris (Clinique Endocrinologique de la Pitié). The patient was eight years old at the time of operation on 5 August 1975. Preoperatively, typical xanthomas were prominent on the feet, knees, elbows, buttocks and popliteal fossa. The serum cholesterol concentration averaged 25.90 mmol/l (1000 mg per cent) with very little variation despite a low cholesterol diet and maximal treatment with cholestyramine, nicotinic acid and clofibrate. Skin culture results[13] were diagnostic of homozygous Type II hyperlipidaemia. Aortic angiography in April 1975 showed severe atheromatous disease of the aorta with supra-aortic narrowing. The coronary, mesenteric and renal arteries were patent. There was mild aortic insufficiency.

After portal diversion the serum cholesterol value fell to 14.3 to 16.8 mmol/l (550 to 650 mg per cent) (40 per cent fall). The visible xanthomas slowly resorbed. The patient was asymptomatic before operation and remained so afterwards with good growth and development. His working electrocardiogram was normal in June 1977. At that time, mesenteric arteriography was performed at the Hôpital de la Pitié in Paris. Late phase venography showed the portacaval shunt to be patent.

The patient was seen in Denver during the first week of August 1977. The cholesterol concentrations ranged from 15 to 16 mmol/l (580 to 616 mg per cent). Liver function tests were normal except for a blood ammonia of 93 μmol/l (158 μg per cent) (normal less than 35 μmol/l [less than 60 μg per cent]).

Changes in peripheral insulin and glucagon content in two of our three patients have been noted. Preoperative values were normal. Postoperatively, systemic venous insulin and glucagon values were both increased, especially the former (Figure 45.9).

None of our three patients with hyperlipidaemia has had any signs of hepatic encephalopathy, although one (Patient 3) has an elevated blood ammonia value. Nevertheless,

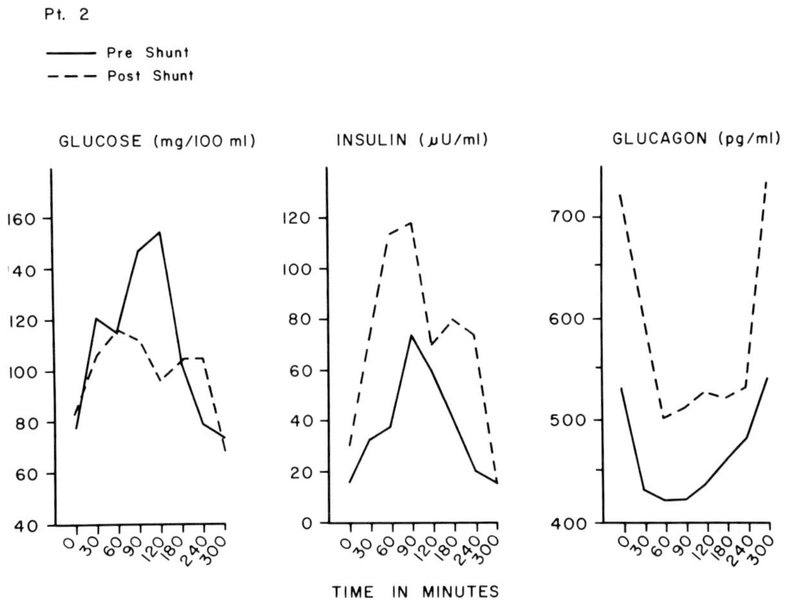

Figure 45.9. Systemic venous plasma glucose, insulin and glucagon concentrations in Patient 2 with hyperlipidaemia before and after portacaval shunt. Oral glucose tolerance test.

the use of portacaval shunt to ameliorate hyperlipidaemia accepts a trade-off of sub-optimal conditions of liver perfusion in return for metabolic improvements (see 'Mechanism of Portal Diversion Effects', below). Realization of this fact has prompted us to recommend portacaval shunt for this inborn error only if the patient was homozygous. However, the freedom from encephalopathy in our cases suggests that symptomatic heterozygotes who are refractory to medical therapy should also be considered for portal diversion. The patient of Weglicki et al[37] probably had the heterozygous trait.

Other reports

In the nine cases reported in the literature by others,[8,11,20,26,36,37] the decreases in serum cholesterol have been variable from patient to patient, as in our three cases. A significant fall was usually obtained if the shunt was patent. Cardiac symptoms were often relieved and resorption of xanthomas proceeded even if the falls in serum cholesterol concentration were not great. The latter finding has raised the possibility that cholesterol depots may keep the serum cholesterol concentrations high until the resorption is nearly complete. Failure to observe an antilipidaemic effect has been associated with thrombosis of the shunt.[8,11]

Weglicki et al[37] have used portacaval shunt and coronary artery by-pass together in a young patient suffering from premature athero-sclerosis. This kind of combined therapy will probably be used more frequently in the future, as was illustrated also by the management of our Patient 2.

MECHANISM OF PORTAL DIVERSION EFFECTS

It has been increasingly appreciated during the last decade that venous blood from the splanchnic viscera has liver-supporting qualities not found to the same degree in other kinds of arterial or venous blood.[29,30,32] The so-called hepatotrophic effects of portal blood have been noted under several experimental conditions to include hypertrophy, glycogen storage, hyper-plasia and increase of several synthetic func-tions. The main splanchnic venous hepato-trophic factors are almost certainly endogenous hormones of which the single most important seems to be insulin. The high concentrations of nutrients from the intestine probably play a significant contributory role.

With portacaval shunt these humoral and non-humoral portal factors are lost to the liver on first pass. Subtle but fundamental changes in hepatocyte structure and function result. As suggested earlier, changes in the hormone environment of the liver and the rest of the body caused by portacaval shunt could explain the palliation of patients with glycogen storage disease.

The loss of portal hepatotrophic factors may also explain the amelioration of hyperlipidaemia. The antilipidaemic effect of portacaval shunt can be demonstrated with a normal starting level of serum cholesterol just as easily as with a pathologically high concentration. This was first observed by Winter et al[38] in normal dogs and confirmed in that species by us[32] and by others.[7,15,17] The same has been seen in rats,[10,23] pigs[4,5] and baboons.[29]

Our studies in the dog[29] and investigations in the rat,[19,23] pig[4,5] and human[2] have shown or suggested that a reduction in hepatic cholesterol and/or LDL synthesis is responsible, at least in part, for the cholesterol falls. Only the report of Coyle et al in dogs has denied this.[7] Other factors may contribute to the antilipidaemic effect of portal diversion as Ahrens and we have speculated.[1,29]

Our experiments in dogs have suggested that the main reason for decreased hepatic cholesterol synthesis is deprivation in the liver of insulin.[29] One consequence is a moderately severe liver injury of the kind described earlier in the autopsy findings of Patient 2.

Eaton[9] has recently proposed that the changes in glucagon metabolism may be important in the antilipidaemic effect of portal diversion. Further clarification of these mechanisms will be important if treatment alternatives to portacaval shunt are to be evolved.

SUMMARY

Complete portacaval shunt was used to treat 10 patients with glycogen storage disease. A favourable effect was noted on body growth and a number of metabolic abnormalities. More recently, continuous night feedings with an intermittently-placed gastric tube or through a gastrostomy has been shown to be helpful either before or after portacaval shunts. Such alimentation techniques may eliminate the need for shunts in some patients and be of adjuvant benefit in others.

Three patients with homozygous Type II hyperlipidaemia were submitted to complete portacaval shunt. There was a substantial fall in serum cholesterol in each case, resorption of xanthomatous deposits on the skin and tendons, and possibly a partial reversal of some cardiovascular complications. One patient died, 18 months after portacaval shunt, apparently from a cardiac arrhythmia. The other two patients are in good health, one after subsequent double heart valve replacement and double coronary artery by-pass. Portal diversion seems capable of markedly altering the outlook of patients with homozygous Type II hyperlipidaemia.

Experience with portal diversion to treat patients with glycogen storage disease and hyperlipidaemia has also been accumulated in other centres with generally confirmatory results. If the desired corrections are not realized, thrombosis of the portacaval shunt must be suspected.

ACKNOWLEDGEMENTS

The work was supported by research grants MRIS 8818–01 and 7227–01 from the Veterans Administration; by Grant Numbers AM–17260 and AM–07772 from the National Institutes of Health; and by Grant Numbers RR–00051 and RR–00069 from the General Clinical Research Centers Program of the Division of Research Resources, National Institutes of Health; Faculty Scholar, Josiah Macy, Jr Foundation.

REFERENCES

1. Ahrens, E.J. Jr (1974) Homozygous hypercholesteraemia and the portacaval shunt: the need for a concerted attack by surgeons and clinical researchers. *Lancet*, **ii**, 449–451.
2. Bilheimer, D.W., Goldstein, J.L., Grundy, S.M. & Brown, M.S. (1975) Reduction in cholesterol and low density lipoprotein synthesis in a patient with homozygous familial hypercholesterolemia. *Journal of Clinical Investigation*, **56**, 1420–1430.
3. Burr, I.M., O'Neill, J.A., Karzou, D.T., Howard, L.J. & Greene, H.L. (1974) Comparison of the effect of total parenteral nutrition, continuous intragastric feeding and portacaval shunt in a patient with Type I glycogen storage disease. *Journal of Pediatrics*, **85**(6), 792–795.
4. Carew, T.E., Saik, R.P., Johansen, K.H., Dennis, C.A. & Steinberg, D. (1976) Low density and high density lipoprotein turnover following portacaval shunt in swine. *Journal of Lipid Research*, **17**, 441–450.
5. Chase, H.P. & Morris, T. (1976) Cholesterol metabolism following portacaval shunt in the pig. *Atherosclerosis*, **24**, 141–148.

6. Child, C.G., Barr, D., Holswade, G.R. & Harrison, C.S. (1953) Liver regeneration following portacaval transposition in dogs. *Annals of Surgery*, **138**, 600.
7. Coyle, J.J., Schwartz, M.Z., Marubbio, A.T., Varco, R.L. & Buchwald, H. (1976) The effect of portacaval shunt on plasma lipids and tissue cholesterol synthesis in the dog. *Surgery*, **80**, 54–60.
8. Cywes, S., Davies, M.R.Q., Louw, J.H., Berger, G.M.B., Bonnici, F. & Joffe, H.S. (1976) Portacaval shunt in two patients with homozygous Type II. *South African Medical Journal*, **50**, 239–242.
9. Eaton, R.P. (1976) Glucagon and lipoprotein. *Metabolism*, **25**(Suppl. 11), 1415–1418.
10. Edwards, K.D.G., Herz, R., Sealey, J.E. & Bradley, S.E. (1976) Lowering of blood pressure, plasma renin substrate, cholesterol and triglyceride by portacaval anastomosis in rats fed on a 60% sucrose/5% lard diet. *Clinical Science and Molecular Medicine*, **51**, 1455–1465.
11. Farriaux, J.-P., Ribet, M., Lebecq, M.-F. & Lemaitre, L. (1976) Traitement de l'hypercholestérolémie familiale de type II par anastomose portocave. *La Nouvelle Presse Médicale*, **5**(No. 34), 2219–2221.
12. Folkman, J., Philippart, A., Tze, W.-J. & Crigler, J. Jr (1972) Portacaval shunt for glycogen storage disease: value of prolonged intravenous hyperalimentation before surgery. *Surgery*, **72**, 306–314.
13. Goldstein, J.L. & Brown, M.S. (1973) Familial hypercholesterolemia: identification of a defect in the regulation of 3-hydroxy-3-methyl-glutaryl coenzyme A reductase activity associated with overproduction of cholesterol. *Proceedings of the National Academy of Science*, **70**, 2804–2808.
14. Greene, H.L., Slonim, A.E., O'Neill, J.A. Jr & Burr, I.M. (1976) Continuous nocturnal intragastric feeding for management of Type I glycogen storage disease. *New England Journal of Medicine*, **294**, 1125–1129.
15. Guzman, I.J., Coyle, J.J., Schneider, P.D., Varco, R.L. & Buchwald, H. (1977) The effect of selective visceral caval shunt on plasma lipids and cholesterol. *Surgery*, **82**, 42–50.
16. Hermann, R.E. & Mercer, R.D. (1969) Portacaval shunt in the treatment of glycogen storage disease: report of a case. *Surgery*, **65**, 499–503.
17. Horak, W., Gangl, A., Funovics, J. & Brabner, G. (1975) Effect of portacaval shunt and arterialization of the liver on bile acid metabolism. *Gastroenterology*, **69**, 338–341.
18. Howell, R.R., Stevenson, R.E., Ben-Menachem, Y., Phyliky, R.L. & Berry, D.H. (1976) Hepatic adenomata with Type I glycogen storage disease. *Journal of the American Medical Association*, **236**, 1481–1484.
19. James, J., Soeters, P.B. & Fischer, J.E. (1977) *In vivo* demonstration of impaired cholesterol and fatty acid synthesis following portacaval shunt (PCS). (Abstract) *Gastroenterology*, **72** (No. 5, Part 2), 1075.
20. Krogh, L. & Wickens, J.T. (1974) Letter: Portacaval shunt for hypercholesterolaemia. *South African Medical Journal*, **48**(56), 2302.
21. Levine, O.R., Harris, R.C., Blanc, W.A. & Wellins, R.B. (1973) Progressive pulmonary hypertension in children with portal hypertension. *Journal of Pediatrics*, **83**, 964–972.
22. Lockwood, D.H., Merimee, T.J., Edgar, P.J., Greene, M.L., Fujimoto, W.Y., Seegmiller, J.E. & Howell, R.R. (1969) Insulin secretion in Type I glycogen storage disease. *Diabetes*, **18**, 755–758.
23. Magide, A.A., Press, C.M., Myant, N.B., Mitropoulos, K.A. & Balasubramaniam, S. (1976) The effect of portacaval anastomosis on plasma lipoprotein metabolism in rats. *Biochimica et Biophysica Acta*, **441**, 303–307.
24. Putnam, C.W., Porter, K.A. & Starzl, T.E. (1976) Hepatic encephalopathy and light and electron micrographic changes of the baboon liver after portal diversion. *Annals of Surgery*, **184**, 155–161.
25. Riddell, A.G., Davies, R.P. & Clark, A.D. (1966) Portacaval transposition in the treatment of glycogen storage disease. *Lancet*, **ii**, 1146–1148.
26. Russell, D., Heimann, K.W., Levin, S.E., Mendelsohn, D., Mega de Andrade, A., Lieberthal, S., Mieny, C., Dinner, M., Joffe, B.I. & Seftel, H.C. (1976) Portacaval shunt for homozygous hypercholesterolaemia. *Lancet*, **ii**, 1205 (Letter to the Editor).
27. Starzl, T.E., Brown, B.I., Blanchard, H. & Brettschneider, L. (1969) Portal diversion in glycogen storage disease. *Surgery*, **65**, 504–506.
28. Starzl, T.E., Chase, H.P., Putnam, C.W. & Nora, J.J. (1974a) Letter to the Editor. Follow-up of patient with portacaval shunt for the treatment of hyperlipidemia. *Lancet*, **ii**, 714–715.
29. Starzl, T.E., Lee, I.Y., Porter, K.A. & Putnam, C.W. (1975a) The influence of portal blood upon lipid metabolism in normal and diabetic dogs and baboons. *Surgery, Gynecology and Obstetrics*, **140**, 381–396.
30. Starzl, T.E., Porter, K.A., Watanabe, K. & Putnam, C.W. (1976) Effects of insulin, glucagon, and insulin/glucagon infusions on liver morphology and cell division after complete portacaval shunt in dogs. *Lancet*, **i**, 821–825.
31. Starzl, T.E., Putnam, C.W., Chase, H.P. & Porter, K.A. (1973) Portacaval shunt in hyperlipoproteinaemia. *Lancet*, **ii**, 940–944.
32. Starzl, T.E., Porter, K.A., Kashiwagi, N., Lee, I.Y., Russell, W.J.I. & Putnam, C.W. (1975b) The effect of diabetes mellitus on portal blood hepatotrophic factors in dogs. *Surgery, Gynecology and Obstetrics*, **140**, 549–562.
33. Starzl, T.E., Chase, H.P., Putnam, C.W., Nora, J.J., Fennell, R.H. Jr & Porter, K.A. (1974b) Letter to the Editor. Portacaval shunt in hyperlipidemia. *Lancet*, **ii**, 1263.
34. Starzl, T.E., Marchioro, T.L., Sexton, A.W., Illingworth, B., Waddell, W.R., Faris, T.D. & Herrmann, T.J. (1965) The effect of portacaval transposition on carbohydrate metabolism: experimental and clinical observations. *Surgery*, **57**, 687–697.
35. Starzl, T.E., Putnam, C.W., Porter, K.A., Halgrimson, C.G., Corman, J., Brown, B.I., Gotlin, R.W., Rodgerson, D.O. & Greene, H.L. (1973) Portal diversion for the treatment of glycogen storage disease in humans. *Annals of Surgery*, **178**, 525–539.
36. Stein, E.A., Mieny, C., Spitz, L., Saaron, I., Pettifor, J., Heimann, K.W., Bersohn, I. & Dinner, M. (1975) Portacaval shunt in four patients with homozygous hypercholesterolemia. *Lancet*, **i**, 832–835.
37. Weglicki, W.B., Ganda, O.P., Soeldner, J.S., Murawski, B.J., Cohn, L.H. & Couch, N.P. (1977) Portacaval diversion for severe hypercholesterolemia. *Archives of Surgery*, **112**, 634–640.
38. Winter, I.C., van Dolah, H.E. & Crandell, L.A. (1941) Lowered serum lipid levels in the Eck fistula dog. *American Journal of Physiology*, **133**, 566–571.

Chapter 46

Ascites, Electrolyte Disorders and Renal Failure

S.P. WILKINSON
ROGER WILLIAMS

ASCITES IN CIRRHOSIS

Although cirrhosis is the commonest cause of ascites,[27,38] it may also be found with other liver diseases, especially Budd–Chiari syndrome and subacute hepatic necrosis, and is a rare complication of fulminant viral hepatitis, obstructive jaundice and portal vein thrombosis. Other relatively common causes include abdominal malignancies, cardiac failure, constrictive pericarditis, nephrotic syndrome, malnutrition and tuberculosis. It is particularly important to recognize constrictive pericarditis since this is surgically curable, and many such patients are misdiagnosed as having cirrhosis and given a poor prognosis. It should be suspected when there is a very high jugular venous pressure without cardiac enlargement, pulsus paradoxus, a characteristic loud added heart sound, pericardial calcification, and absence of the other usual cutaneous stigmata of chronic liver disease; but cardiac catheterization is often necessary for confirmation of the diagnosis.

Ascites may occur as a manifestation of acute pancreatitis or with chronic pancreatic disease, especially in association with a pseudocyst or ruptured pancreatic duct. The latter is usually referred to as 'pancreatic ascites'. It occurs predominantly in alcoholics and bears no close temporal relationship to bouts of acute pancreatitis.[62]

Rare causes of ascites include hypothyroidism and systemic lupus erythematosus. A massive ovarian cyst is often mistaken for ascites.

Ascites in cirrhosis implies a poor prognosis, with 25 to 50 per cent of patients not surviving more than one year.[8,169,195] It is often, though not necessarily, associated with other manifestations of advanced cirrhosis, including oesophageal varices and encephalopathy. It may arise spontaneously or be precipitated by any acute event associated with impairment of liver function, such as gastrointestinal haemorrhage, infections or surgery, or be the first clinical manifestation of a hepatoma.

In the most severe cases, more than 50 litres of fluid may be present in the abdominal cavity. With the patient supine the flanks appear full and are dull to percussion, but the upper flank becomes resonant when a lateral position is adopted ('shifting dullness'). About 2 litres of fluid can be detected in this way. By careful percussion with the patient kneeling on 'all fours' it has been claimed that as little as 120 ml can be detected.[118] In the obese patient, the clinical detection of ascites may be difficult and aspiration, by introducing a 21 gauge needle into the flank, may be required to confirm its presence, local anaesthetic not being necessary.

Associated Findings

Ascites is associated with a number of other clinical findings. Peripheral oedema is usually present, but much less marked than the degree of ascites. Ten per cent of patients also have a pleural effusion, usually confined to the right side. Postulated mechanisms include movement of fluid through lymphatics in the diaphragm,[105] acquired anatomical defects in the diaphragm,[129] and the effect of a high portal pressure transmitted to the azygous and hemiazygous venous systems.[201] Umbilical, inguinal, femoral, or incisional herniae may be found. Prominent venous collaterals may radiate away from the umbilicus (due to portal hypertension), or from the groin to the costal margin (due to compression of the vena cava). If tense, ascites may cause basal pulmonary atelectasis and impair function of the gastro-oesophageal sphincter,[196] the latter potentially exposing the patient to oesophageal erosions.

Spontaneous bacterial peritonitis

A complication of ascites that is extremely important to recognize is a spontaneous bacterial peritonitis. Nearly 10 per cent of all cases of ascites due to cirrhosis admitted to hospital have been reported to have this complication.[40,51,55] Characteristically, the patient has fever, abdominal pain, reduced or absent bowel sounds, and encephalopathy. Rebound tenderness is less common and sometimes the only clinical manifestation is an otherwise unexplained deterioration in liver function. A diagnostic ascitic tap (10 ml) is necessary for diagnosis. The fluid is usually, though not necessarily, turbid, with a leucocyte count, predominantly polymorphs, above 1.0×10^9/l (1000/cu mm). The responsible organism can often be identified from a Gram stain of the centrifugal deposit and will be a gram-negative bacillus in two-thirds of cases and a pneumococcus in one-quarter. Other unusual organisms have also been implicated. The protein content of the ascitic fluid is invariably low (<25 g/l). The prognosis is poor with a hospital mortality of about 90 per cent. Often, however, it is possible to treat the bacterial infection effectively with suitable antibiotics, the patient dying from other manifestations of cirrhosis that have been precipitated by the peritonitis, such as haemorrhage, renal failure or coma.

Diagnostic Ascitic Tap

All patients admitted to hospital with ascites should have a 10 to 20 ml aspiration for diagnostic purposes. This is most often useful for the diagnosis of spontaneous bacterial peritonitis, but is also of value in the diagnosis of tuberculous peritonitis, malignancy and 'pancreatic ascites'.

Macroscopic abnormalities include turbidity, blood staining and chylous ascites. A turbid fluid usually implies bacterial infection. Bloody ascites is associated with malignancy, including hepatoma. Chylous ascites is caused by lymphatic obstruction and is usually due to a lymphoma or other malignancies, but may occasionally be found in cirrhosis.[107,154]

Microscopic and bacteriological examination is of value for the diagnosis of infection: with a spontaneous bacterial peritonitis, excessive polymorphs and the offending organism are often found; and with tuberculous infection, an excess of lymphocytes is seen. Only rarely are malignant cells found in patients with hepatoma.

Biochemical determinations on ascitic fluid are of limited value. In uncomplicated cirrhosis the protein concentration is usually <25 g/l, but may be as high as 43 g/l.[183] The mechanism for high and low protein concentrations is discussed later. Without underlying liver disease the protein concentration of ascitic fluid in abdominal tuberculosis is almost invariably >25 g/l,[197] but is usually lower than this when superimposed on cirrhosis.[34] Low values are found with spontaneous bacterial peritonitis, and high or low values with malignancy.[159] 'Pancreatic ascites' is also associated with a high protein concentration, but a more important diagnostic investigation is the ascitic amylase which is invariably extremely high.[62]

A recent report suggests that an increased γ-glutamyl transpeptidase concentration in the ascitic fluid is diagnostic of the presence of hepatoma in cirrhosis.[165]

Mechanism of Ascites Formation

Both local factors and changes in renal function have to be considered.

Local factors

A raised pressure at the venous end of the splanchnic capillaries, consequent to portal hypertension, and a reduced plasma albumin concentration will both favour transudation of fluid into the peritoneal cavity by altering the Starling equilibrium. In one study, the measured changes in portal pressure and plasma albumin concentration alone were sufficient to account for ascites formation,[11] but others have found the correlation to be less close.[46,242] Furthermore, if these were the only factors, the ascitic fluid should have the characteristic of a transudate with a very low protein concentration. This is by no means always so and, in one series, in 20 per cent of patients with ascites not complicated by infection or malignancy the values were greater than 25 g/l.[183] The protein present in ascites may be derived largely from hepatic lymph. Characteristic of cirrhosis is a partial block to hepatic venous outflow ('post-sinusoidal portal hypertension') and in some cases this may be so marked that blood flows retrogradely from the liver into the portal vein.[222] Secondary to the venous outflow block increased quantities of hepatic lymph are formed and, because the hepatic sinusoids are extremely permeable to proteins,[148] this is a protein-rich fluid. Evidence for an increased production of hepatic lymph in cirrhosis includes reports that the lymphatics in the hilum of the liver are characteristically distended[14] and the flow of lymph within the thoracic duct markedly increased.[64,242] Presumably, the capacity of the thoracic duct is exceeded and the additional lymph exudes from the surface of the liver since external drainage of the thoracic duct has resulted in amelioration of ascites.[65]

Patients with 'early' cirrhosis have been reported to have a much higher ascitic fluid protein concentration than those with 'late' cirrhosis.[242] It was suggested that the post-sinusoidal area was the earliest site of vascular obstruction, resulting in increased hepatic lymph formation; and that as the cirrhosis progressed the pressure was transmitted back through the portal venous system, resulting in an increasing contribution of splanchnic interstitial fluid to the ascites.

Changes in renal function

For ascites to accumulate, the renal excretion of sodium and water must be less than the amounts ingested. The virtual absence of sodium from the urine in patients accumulating ascites on a normal diet was demonstrated 30 years ago.[75]

There are two theories to explain how the formation of ascites and retention of sodium by the kidney are related. The first is that, because of loss of fluid into the peritoneal compartment and pooling of blood in the splanchnic circulation, the 'effective' extracellular fluid (ECF) and blood volumes are reduced. Renal perfusion therefore falls and the kidneys retain sodium both as a result of activation of the renin–angiotensin–aldosterone system and through other less clearly defined mechanisms. The sodium retention is thus *secondary* to ascites formation. There are, however, a number of findings that are difficult to fit into this concept: (a) renal perfusion, as assessed from measurements of the glomerular filtration rate and renal plasma flow, is often normal or even increased at a time when ascites is forming;[71,110,241] (b) total exchangeable sodium is often increased by up to 25 per cent in patients who have never had ascites; thus sodium retention must have occurred *independently* of ascites formation;[176] and (c) a spontaneous loss of ascites with an increased renal excretion of sodium can occur without any changes in plasma volume or portal pressure, two measurements which taken together give some indication of the extent of splanchnic pooling.[127]

The alternative concept ('overflow' theory) was proposed by Lieberman and colleagues.[128] They have suggested that the renal retention of sodium (and water) is the *primary* abnormality and that expanded ECF 'overflow' to the peritoneal cavity results if the local factors (plasma oncotic pressure, portal pressure, hepatic lymph drainage) are sufficiently altered to favour fluid transudation. In support of this view is the observation that ascites can be induced in cirrhosis by administration of the sodium-retaining mineralocorticoid 9α-fluoro-hydrocortisone.[58] Furthermore, when a porta-caval shunt reduces the portal pressure, which is one of the essential local factors, ascites may be replaced by peripheral oedema,[26,46] i.e. sodium is still being retained but is no longer preferentially localized to the peritoneal compartment.

These two concepts are by no means mutually exclusive and both may be simultaneously operative.

Mechanism of sodium retention

Glomerular filtration rate, renal plasma flow and renal blood flow range from twice normal to almost zero in patients with ascites.[71,73,110,241] When these are markedly reduced (functional renal failure; see section on renal failure) this alone is sufficient to account for the reduced rate of renal sodium excretion. In the others, the increased sodium reabsorption in the nephron occurs at both proximal[185] and distal sites,[240] the latter being quantitatively more important.

Role of aldosterone. When renal function is

unimpaired, hyperaldosteronism is likely to be of major importance in mediating the renal retention of sodium. Evidence for this includes: (a) patients forming ascites characteristically have an increased plasma concentration and an increased rate of renal excretion of aldosterone;[44, 135, 244] (b) the aldosterone antagonist, spironolactone, will almost invariably reverse the sodium retention if given in sufficient dosage,[67, 213, 240] as will adrenalectomy;[90, 138] and (c) in a study into the effects of β-adrenergic blockade on the renin-aldosterone system and sodium excretion, the changes in the latter were exactly as would have been predicted from the changes in aldosterone.[238] In addition to its well-known effect on the distal tubule of the nephron, hyperaldosteronism might also be responsible for the increased proximal sodium reabsorption described in cirrhosis, since micropuncture studies have also shown an effect of this hormone on the proximal convoluted tubule.[98]

Despite the evidence for the importance of hyperaldosteronism, two recent studies have shown that the plasma aldosterone concentration may be normal in some patients forming ascites.[224, 240] There may therefore be an increased sensitivity of the renal tubule to aldosterone in cirrhosis, as has been described in dogs with constriction of the thoracic segment of the inferior vena cava,[56] an experimental model with many similarities to the cirrhotic patient with ascites.

The importance of aldosterone in mediating the abnormal sodium retention by the kidney has been questioned. In one study, aminoglutethimide, a drug that interferes with steroid synthesis, was given to patients with 'long-standing diuretic-resistant ascites', and although plasma aldosterone concentrations fell the renal sodium excretion did not increase.[180] Such patients, however, invariably have a markedly reduced renal perfusion,[8] so factors other than aldosterone would be expected to have mediated the sodium retention. In another study, it was found that isothermic water immersion to the neck, a procedure that is followed by a redistribution of the blood volume to the thoracic region and is therefore similar to the effect of an acute saline load, increased sodium excretion when endogenous aldosterone was either blocked with spironolactone or enhanced with deoxycorticosterone acetate (DOCA).[72] Although this study demonstrates that the natriuresis of acute volume expansion is independent of suppression of aldosterone, a fact well-established by others,[61, 124] there seems little reason to presume that the mechanism for the induction of a natriuresis in response to an acute volume load is related to that responsible for chronic sodium retention in cirrhosis.

The normal response to exogenously administered aldosterone is to 'escape' from its sodium-retaining effect and to return to sodium balance at an increased extracellular fluid (ECF) volume, expansion of the latter being the stimulus to the natriuresis.[12] If aldosterone is to be implicated in the pathogenesis of the sodium retention of cirrhosis, there must be some derangement in this 'escape' mechanism. There is good evidence that this may be so in that, when the mineralocorticoid 9α-fluorohydrocortisone was given to a group of patients with cirrhosis without ascites, 'escape' occurred in only 10 of 15 studies, and those who continued to retain sodium formed ascites.[58] Presumably, the retained fluid is localized to the peritoneal cavity ('overflow ascites') so that the 'effective' ECF is never expanded.

Mechanism for hyperaldosteronism and increased plasma renin activity. The increased levels of aldosterone in cirrhosis are due to both increased secretion and impaired hepatic metabolism,[54, 180, 207, 211] but the former is quantitatively far more important. The increased secretion is often assumed to be secondary to increased activity of the renin–angiotensin system since many groups have reported increases in plasma renin activity

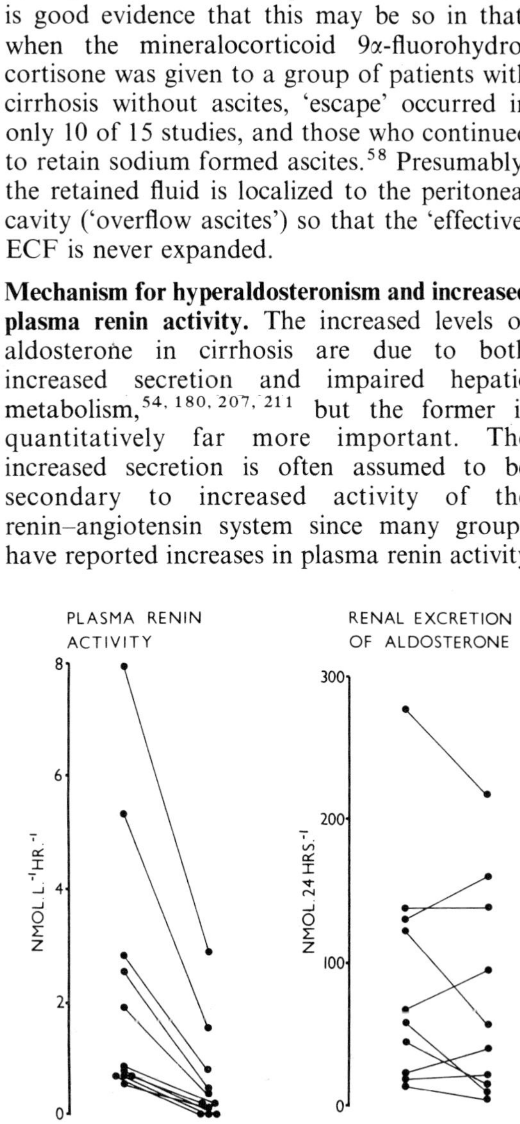

Figure 46.1. Illustrating the dissociation between the effects of β-adrenergic blockade on plasma renin activity and the rate of renal excretion of aldosterone in cirrhosis with ascites (from Wilkinson et al,[238] with kind permission of the editor of *Gastroenterology*).

(PRA)[32,76] and plasma angiotensin concentrations.[87,141] This cannot be the only factor, however, since when PRA was reduced by β-adrenergic blockade, values for aldosterone did not necessarily follow[238] (Figure 46.1).

The increased PRA in cirrhosis is also likely to be the result of several factors, including: (a) increased renin secretion by the kidney; (b) impaired hepatic metabolism; and (c) a postulated splanchnic source of renin. When renal blood flow is reduced, renin secretion by the kidney will be increased because of a reduced pressure in the afferent arterioles, where the baroreceptors that mediate renin release are located. When total renal blood flow is normal or increased, the mechanism may be related to changes in the distribution of flow within the kidney. Renin secretion is largely confined to the afferent arterioles of the short outer cortical nephrons,[53] and a redistribution of plasma flow from this nephron group to the longer juxtamedullary nephrons, without necessarily any change in total renal plasma flow, has been shown to be associated with an increased PRA[241] (Figure 46.2). This intrarenal redistribution of plasma flow is not to be confused with the generalized vasoconstriction responsible for the development of functional renal failure, and its mechanism is obscure.

Hyponatraemia may be another important factor, probably by reducing the sodium load at the macula densa, an area of the distal convoluted tubule of the nephron that is immediately adjacent to the renin-secreting juxtaglomerular cells. In cirrhosis, PRA has been shown to be inversely related to the plasma sodium concentration[241] and hypertrophy of the macula densa has been related to the occurrence of hyponatraemia.[171]

The liver is an important site for metabolism of renin.[96] An increased PRA in cirrhosis might therefore be partly due to impaired liver function. This has been investigated by determining PRA in both peripheral venous and hepatic venous blood.[21] In control subjects the highest values were found in peripheral blood, but in cirrhosis PRA was highest in hepatic venous blood. These results were interpreted to indicate that not only does the liver inadequately metabolize renin in cirrhosis, but that a splanchnic source of renin might also contribute to the increased PRA. Evidence for a splanchnic source of renin was found in control subjects, in that portal venous blood was found to have a higher PRA than was peripheral blood, but the PRA of portal venous blood in cirrhosis was not determined.

The relative quantitative importance of each of the factors involved in the pathogenesis of an increased PRA is unknown.

Other factors involved in sodium retention. (i) *Natriuretic hormone*. There is increasing evidence for the existence of a natriuretic hormone(s) that may be of major importance in the regulation of sodium excretion.[60] Some studies point to the liver as its source.[149,189] An impaired production by the cirrhotic liver might therefore contribute towards the sodium retention and could also explain the apparently increased 'sensitivity' of the kidney to aldosterone. (ii) *Intrarenal redistribution of blood flow*. The juxtamedullary nephrons of the kidney, because of their greater length, might be relatively 'sodium retaining'.[92] Thus the redistribution of blood or plasma flow from outer cortical to juxtamedullary nephrons, that has already been described in relation to an increased PRA, could also be a factor responsible for renal sodium retention. However, recent evidence from micropuncture studies in the rat now suggest that the juxtamedullary nephrons may actually be relatively 'salt losing'.[200] In cirrhosis, it has not been possible to relate changes in sodium excretion to those in the intrarenal distribution of plasma flow.[238] (iii) *Sodium receptors in the portal venous system*. There is evidence from both animal and human studies for the existence of specific sodium receptors in the portal venous bed. Thus, infusions of saline into the portal vein or oral ingestion of sodium have been shown to be associated with a more rapid natriuresis than when an identical amount of sodium is given into the systemic circulation.[121,122] Spontaneous portasystemic

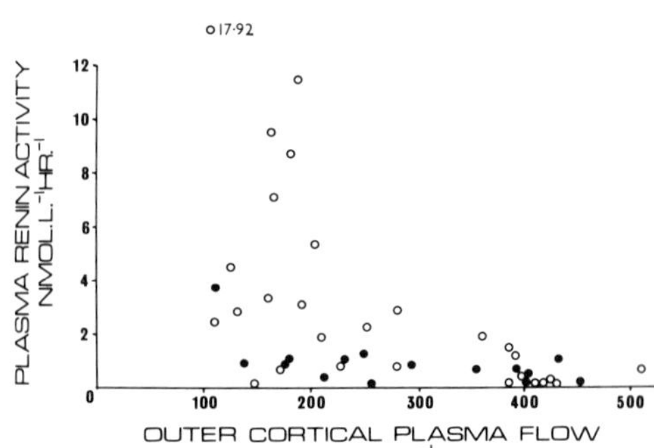

Figure 46.2. Relation of plasma renin activity to the calculated effective plasma flow to outer cortical nephrons. The latter is determined by using the technique of 'transit renography' (● no ascites; ○ ascites. From Wilkinson et al,[241] with kind permission of the editor of *Clinical Science and Molecular Medicine*).

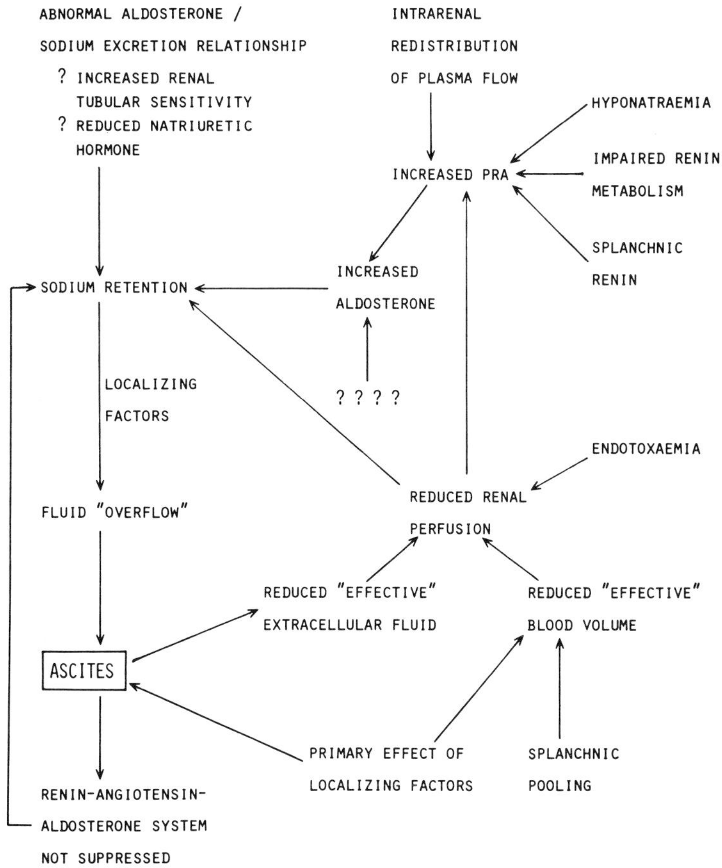

Figure 46.3. Proposed mechanism for the relationship between abnormalities of renal function and ascites formation.

shunts are characteristic of cirrhosis, and shunting of sodium absorbed from the gut away from the proposed sodium receptors could also contribute towards sodium retention.

Summary of the pathogenesis of ascites formation

A scheme incorporating both traditional and 'overflow' theories of ascites formation, together with the changes in renal function, is shown in Figure 46.3. Aldosterone, either because of an increased renal tubular 'sensitivity' or, more often, because of an increased plasma concentration, is of major importance in the initiation of sodium retention. Water retention also occurs to restore the osmotic equilibrium and the expanded ECF 'overflows' to the peritoneal cavity if the localizing factors (increased portal pressure, reduced plasma oncotic pressure and impaired lymph drainage) favour this. Since the 'effective' ECF is therefore not expanded, 'escape' from the sodium-retaining effects of aldosterone does not occur, the renin–aldosterone system is not suppressed and sodium retention continues. If the localizing factors do not favour ascites formation (not illustrated), the 'effective' ECF is expanded, 'escape' occurs and the renin–aldosterone system is suppressed with a return to sodium balance at a higher level of total body sodium. This explains the observations that in the absence of ascites total body exchangeable sodium is often increased,[176] and both PRA[241] and the plasma aldosterone concentration[240] may be reduced. The increased plasma aldosterone concentration is largely due to an increased secretion and this can only partly be explained on the basis of increased activity of the renin–angiotensin system. Factors responsible for the increased PRA include an intrarenal redistribution of blood flow, hyponatraemia, impaired hepatic metabolism and a splanchnic source of renin.

The 'overflow' mechanism may be the only way of explaining ascites formation when renal blood flow is normal or increased. However, a primary effect of the localizing factors with loss of fluid from the ECF into the peritoneal compartment may also be important in other patients, since this reduces the 'effective' ECF whilst splanchnic pooling of blood reduces the 'effective' blood volume. Renal perfusion would therefore fall, resulting in renal sodium retention both via the renin–aldosterone system and by another more direct route. Endotoxaemia might be another factor responsible for a reduced renal perfusion, especially when the latter is marked (see 'Renal Failure', below).

Treatment of ascites

The main indications for treating ascites are cosmetic and to relieve discomfort. Although ascites may increase gastro-oesophageal reflux,[196] it has not been demonstrated that its relief reduces the frequency of bleeding from oesophageal varices or erosions. When the hepatic lesion is partially reversible (e.g. chronic hepatitis after treatment with corticosteroids, alcoholic hepatitis after abstention from alcohol) ascites will often resolve with the improvement in hepatic function. Most patients, however, require specific treatment; namely, dietary sodium restriction and diuretics.

Dietary sodium restriction. A 'no added' salt diet, together with avoidance of salty foods, will reduce the daily sodium intake to 50 mmol (50 mEq). Often it is necessary to reduce intake even further, with complete avoidance of salt in the cooking, and use of special salt-free bread, butter, biscuits and cakes. It is important to ensure that sodium-containing medications are not administered; in particular, most commercially available 'antacids' contain large quantities of sodium. In this way the daily sodium intake can be reduced to 20 mmol (20 mEq). Water restriction is necessary only when hyponatraemia is present (see below).

Diuretics. Three groups of diuretics are commonly used: potassium-sparing diuretics, loop diuretics and thiazides. The potassium-sparing diuretics include the aldosterone antagonist spironolactone, amiloride, and triamterene and act at the distal part of the nephron. They inhibit both sodium reabsorption and potassium secretion. Loop diuretics are the most powerful of all diuretics and include frusemide, ethacrynic acid and bumetanide. Their action is to inhibit active chloride transport from the ascending limb of the loop of Henle (sodium reabsorption from this part of the nephron is passive and secondary to chloride reabsorption[37,177]). They also cause a marked increase in the renal excretion of potassium. Thiazides include

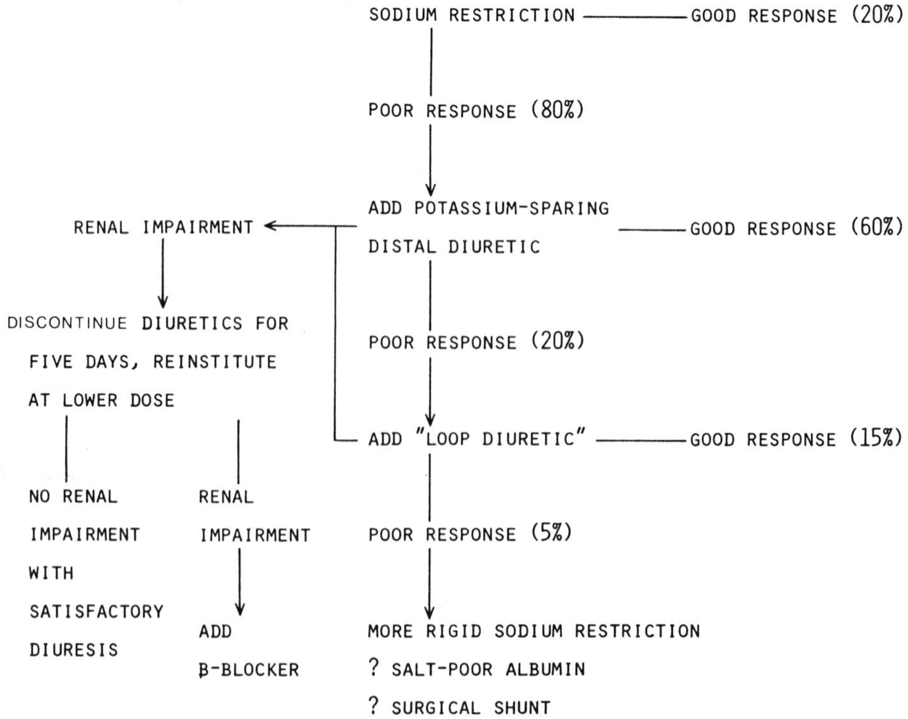

Figure 46.4. Treatment protocol for ascites (based on personal experience at King's College Hospital, 1972–1977).

chlorothiazide and bendrofluazide. Their chief site of action is the cortical segment of the ascending limb of the loop of Henle. They also promote potassium excretion.

Bed rest. The importance of bed rest has not been critically evaluated. If gross ascites is present the patient will necessarily be largely confined to bed, and if ankle oedema is marked it is wise to keep the patient in bed in order to hasten mobilization of the fluid.

Treatment regimen (Figure 46.4)

In cases of mild ascites it is reasonable to try the effect of dietary sodium restriction as an outpatient measure. If this fails or if there is marked ascites the patient should be admitted to hospital. Sodium restriction alone should also be tried for three days for inpatients. In all, about 20 per cent will satisfactorily lose ascites on a 20 to 50 mmol/day (20 to 50 mEq/day) sodium intake.

In the remainder, in whom diuretics will be necessary, careful monitoring of treatment is essential. Ideally, the renal sodium excretion should exceed intake by 50 to 100 mmol/day (50 to 100 mEq/day). Unfortunately, urine collections are cumbersome and in practice the use of daily weighing is satisfactory. Weight loss should be about 0.5 kg/day. If the rate of weight loss exceeds this there is a high risk of inducing renal impairment, unless there is also marked peripheral oedema when a more rapid weight loss (say 1 kg/day) is safe (see below). The plasma concentrations of sodium and potassium should be checked twice weekly since hyponatraemia, hyperkalaemia and hypokalaemia may all occur with diuretics.

In view of the importance of aldosterone and an enhanced distal sodium reabsorption, spironolactone, amiloride or triamterene is a logical first choice of diuretic. Spironolactone has been most extensively investigated and, providing renal impairment is not present, will almost invariably result in loss of ascites.[67, 213, 240] The starting dose should be 100 mg daily but there may be a delay of two or three days before a full effect is seen and dosage should therefore not be increased more frequently than every third day. As much as 1000 mg/day may be required. The value of both triamterene and amiloride has also been shown[184, 214] and recommended doses are 100 to 500 mg/day and 10 to 60 mg/day, respectively. These three diuretics may actually cause potassium retention, especially if used in high doses. Potassium supplements should not therefore be given and 'salt substitutes', which are largely potassium compounds, are to be avoided.

If sodium restriction and a distal diuretic are ineffective (20 per cent of all patients; Figure 46.4), a more powerful loop diuretic should be added. Frusemide is the most widely used. The starting dose should be 40 mg on alternate days, slowly increasing to 120 mg/day. In this group of patients there is the greatest risk of developing diuretic-induced renal impairment, since renal function is already moderately impaired[8] and further impairment will render the patient refractory to diuretics. Potassium supplements (up to 100 mmol/day [100 mEq/day] as a slow release or effervescent chloride) are often necessary despite the simultaneous use of a potassium-sparing diuretic.

Maintenance therapy. The aim of treatment should be to reduce the amount of ascites until it is only just detectable. If the last trace of ascites has been mobilized there is a risk of depleting the ECF. The patient should be informed of his new ideal body weight and encouraged to weigh himself at home daily. He can readily be taught to adjust the dose of diuretics and sodium intake as necessary. The maintenance regimen may be considerably less than that used initially. Once the patient is stable plasma electrolyte disorders are unusual, and determinations at one- or two-monthly intervals at outpatient attendances are sufficient.

Diuretic-resistant ascites. Lack of response to the above regimen usually indicates inadequate sodium restriction, which may be due to medications, or renal failure. The latter may have been precipitated by over-aggressive diuretic therapy in the preceding days or have arisen spontaneously. There is no specific therapy for spontaneously occurring renal failure and the prognosis is extremely poor (see below).

Diuretics for ascites with cirrhosis and hepatoma. The development of a hepatoma does not appear directly to influence the efficacy of diuretics. As with cirrhosis without hepatoma, the response to treatment depends on the renal function.[139]

Diuretic-induced renal impairment. In one study, renal impairment occurred in 26 per cent of 85 patients on diuretic therapy.[178] The prognosis is much better than for spontaneously occurring renal failure in that renal function usually returns to normal after the diuretics have been withdrawn. The mechanism may, in part, be due to ECF volume depletion. The maximum rate at which ascites can be mobilized is less than 1 litre/day and may be as little as 100 ml. A negative fluid balance in excess of these values will lead to a contraction of the ECF and a reduced renal blood flow. Oedema fluid, however, can be more rapidly mobilized.[193] Another mechanism may also be involved since in some patients renal impairment may occur without a negative fluid balance.[239] This may be due to activation of the renin–angiotensin system by the diuretic, the increased amounts of angiotensin II being responsible for a renal vasoconstriction. β-adrenergic blocking drugs prevent renin release by the kidney and, after administration of propranolol or practolol, re-introducing diuretics has not resulted in a recurrence of the renal impairment. Effective β-blockade is essential and this can be assessed by a reduction in pulse rate of at least 15 per cent. Up to 160 mg/day of propranolol has been used but this drug is metabolized by the liver and careful observation for signs of toxicity is necessary. In most cases, however, β-blockade is unnecessary and temporary withdrawal of diuretics for a few days and then re-introducing them at a lower dose is usually satisfactory (Figure 46.4).

Other complications of diuretics. Diuretics may precipitate hepatic encephalopathy.[195] The mechanism for this is multifactorial and includes hyponatraemia, hypokalaemia, a metabolic alkalosis, conversion of increased amounts of urea to ammonia when uraemia occurs, and reduced cerebral and hepatic blood flow resulting from ECF depletion.

Potassium depletion may occur with loop diuretics and thiazides. The importance of using potassium-sparing diuretics in cirrhosis has been shown by measurements of total body potassium. When ascites was controlled by spironolactone or amiloride alone total body potassium was within normal limits,[227] but when frusemide or thiazides were used markedly reduced values were often found.[198] The more potent loop diuretics should therefore be reserved for patients resistant to the effect of sodium restriction and potassium-sparing diuretics.

Several of the diuretics are associated with specific side-effects. Spironolactone may cause gastric ulceration,[137] but whether it increases the frequency of gastric haemorrhage in cirrhosis has, surprisingly, never been evaluated in a controlled trial. All of the potassium-sparing diuretics increase bicarbonate excretion and may therefore result in a metabolic acidosis.[36] A metabolic alkalosis may occur secondary to potassium depletion with any of the loop diuretics or thiazides and ethacrynic acid also has a specific effect to increase hydrogen ion excretion.[39]

Albumin infusions, ascites reinfusion and shunt procedures. Although rarely used now, salt-poor albumin infusions are a logical approach to treatment. By increasing the plasma oncotic pressure, one of the 'local' factors involved in the formation of ascites is corrected. Furthermore, the expanded plasma volume may induce a natriuresis. The increase in plasma albumin concentration is often associated with an improvement in the patient's well-being. Unfortunately, the benefits are only short-lived, and it may precipitate variceal haemorrhage.[229]

Complete paracentesis should never be used as a means of treating ascites in a patient with cirrhosis since it carries a risk of precipitating hepatic and renal impairment,[97] hyponatraemia[153] and infection.[108] However, in a patient with very tense ascites that is causing respiratory embarrassment, removal of a small quantity, say 2 litres, to alleviate symptoms is quite safe.

Paracentesis with reinfusion of the fluid has been advocated but large quantities of fluid are necessarily circulated with risk of pulmonary oedema. A reinfusion with frusemide to prevent this complication has been reported to be successful.[68] Another means of helping to prevent circulatory overload is by concentrating the ascitic fluid by ultrafiltration.[31] A machine is now commercially available for this ('Rhodiascit'), in which the ascitic fluid is concentrated two- to threefold by pressure ultrafiltration, the protein concentrate is then reinfused and the ultrafiltrate which contains substances of molecular weight of $<15\,000$ is discarded. This procedure has been widely used, especially in Europe.[9, 125, 150, 202, 209, 210, 232] It is not free of potentially serious complications, including pulmonary oedema, peritonitis, intravascular coagulation and gastrointestinal haemorrhage. Less severe complications include fever, hyponatraemia and prolongation of the prothrombin time. The great advantage of this technique is that it is a *relatively* safe means of removing large quantities of ascites in a short period of time, the main indication therefore being to shorten hospitalization for patients with genuine socio-economic reasons for this. There has been much discussion as to whether it should be used for treating patients with spontaneous functional renal failure, i.e. those with true diuretic-resistant ascites. The procedure does not improve renal function in these patients[125,232] and since a diuresis is unlikely to occur the risk of pulmonary oedema is high. It has been our experience that ascites reinfusion hastens demise in such patients.

Various surgical procedures have been devised for the relief of ascites, but the indications for their use have not been established. The ascitic fluid can be directly infused into the circulation by connecting a suitable cannula between the peritoneal compartment and a jugular vein, via a subcutaneous route at the front of the thorax. A valve is interposed to prevent reflux ('Leveen Shunt').[123]

The cribriform plate at the junction of the thoracic duct and left subclavian vein often becomes clotted. Since hepatic lymph is an important source of ascitic fluid, adequate drainage is necessary and a logical treatment for ascites is to re-implant the thoracic duct away from the cribriform plate.[190]

Portacaval shunts have also been used to relieve ascites[35,144] but, because of the associated high mortality and risk of encephalopathy, are rarely done today. Preferably, a side-to-side shunt should be performed since this will relieve both pre- and post-sinusoidal portal hypertension. An end-to-side shunt in a patient with post-sinusoidal portal hypertension may result in intractable ascites.

ELECTROLYTE DISORDERS

Abnormalities in the plasma concentrations of sodium and potassium are almost invariable in advanced cirrhosis and fulminant hepatic failure (see Chapter 27). The most common are hyponatraemia and hypokalaemia and the underlying mechanism for each is multifactorial.

Hyponatraemia

Hyponatraemia may be profound and, not infrequently, the plasma sodium concentration is below 110 mmol/l (110 mEq/l) in terminal liver failure. Neurological changes strikingly similar to those of hepatic encephalopathy, including confusion, convulsions, stupor and coma, may occur as a direct consequence of the hyponatraemia. Indeed, the EEG changes of hyponatraemia are said to be indistinguishable from those of hepatic encephalopathy.[161] The hyponatraemia is paradoxical in that it is associated with a marked increase in the total body exchangeable sodium. Pathogenic mechanisms to be considered include dilution of the ECF, potassium depletion, use of powerful diuretic regimens and a shift of sodium from the ECF to the intracellular compartment.

Dilution

In most chronic disease states, and cirrhosis is no exception, hyponatraemia is due to a relative inability of the kidneys to excrete water so that the ECF becomes diluted. In cirrhosis and fulminant hepatic failure this is largely due to the increased reabsorption of sodium by the proximal part of the nephron,[185] so that insufficient is available for the diluting segment (ascending limb of the loop of Henle) to generate 'free water'. An increase in circulating antidiuretic hormone (ADH) may also be a factor, but the published data are conflicting.[120,152,168,243] The very profound hyponatraemia often seen terminally may be largely iatrogenic. There is always reluctance to administer sodium-containing fluids to these patients for fear of increasing ascites. Consequently, they are maintained on intravenous 5 per cent dextrose which, in a patient with an impaired ability to excrete the water load, will invariably result in progressive hyponatraemia.

Potassium depletion

The majority of the total body exchangeable potassium resides in the intracellular compartment and depletion is characteristic of cirrhosis, especially when ascites is present (see above). Loss of potassium will therefore lead to intracellular hypo-osmolality and thus water will migrate from cells to restore osmotic equilibrium between the ECF and intracellular compartment, leading to hyponatraemia. Administration of potassium chloride alone has resulted in correction of hyponatraemia without any change in sodium balance.[116]

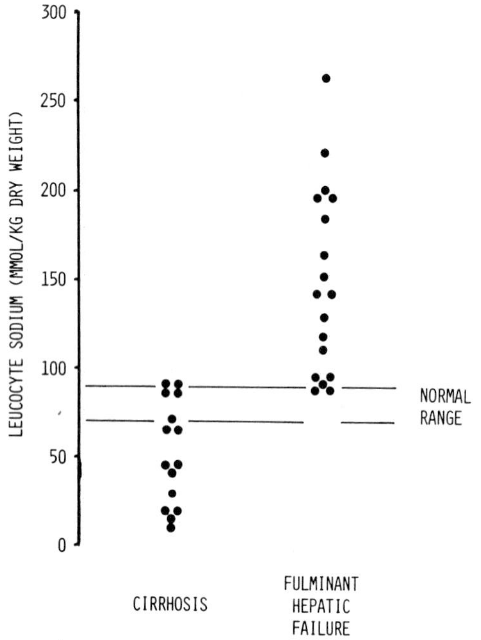

Figure 46.5. Contrasting values for intracellular sodium content, as measured in peripheral blood leucocytes, associated with hyponatraemia in cirrhosis and fulminant hepatic failure (plasma sodium concentration 120 mmol/l [120 mEq/l] ±s.e. 2 and 122 mmol/l [122 mEq/l] ±s.e. 2, for cirrhosis and fulminant hepatic failure, respectively. By kind permission of Dr A.N. Alam).

Diuretic therapy

Diuretics not infrequently result in a lowering of the plasma sodium concentration. This may be partly due to a true sodium depletion. In addition, the ensuing hypovolaemia stimulates ADH release and sodium reabsorption by the proximal part of the nephron. With 'loop' diuretics and thiazides potassium depletion may also be involved.[77]

Shift of sodium into cells

Impairment of the membrane sodium pump mechanism with a consequent increase in intracellular sodium content has long been thought of as a mechanism for hyponatraemia in severely ill patients. This is most unlikely to be important in cirrhosis since even in terminal disease with profound hyponatraemia the intracellular sodium content has been found to be *reduced*[3] (Figure 46.5). In fulminant hepatic failure, however, the intracellular sodium content has been reported to be high and to show an inverse correlation with the plasma sodium concentration.[1] This has been attributed to a circulating toxin suppressing the membrane Na–K–ATPase activity.[2]

Treatment of hyponatraemia

With so many factors contributing to the development of hyponatraemia there are no rigid rules for treatment. However, if it has clearly developed following the use of diuretics, these should be discontinued until the plasma sodium concentration has returned to normal and then re-introduced at a lower dose, although spontaneous hyponatraemia should not be considered as a contraindication to initiating diuretic therapy.[10] If associated with hypokalaemia, it is worth trying the effect of intravenous potassium supplementation, and up to 200 mmol (200 mEq) daily may be required. The only logical treatment in most cases is water restriction, and this may have to be very rigid with avoidance of intravenous dextrose solutions if progressive hyponatraemia is to be prevented. If encephalopathy has been precipitated by the development of hyponatraemia it is reasonable to administer hypertonic saline, but this will be at the expense of increasing the amounts of ascites present. Hyponatraemia can be corrected by peritoneal dialysis, but this does not appear to prolong survival.[174]

Hypokalaemia

Although the plasma potassium concentration does not always correlate closely with total exchangeable potassium in cirrhosis,[41] hypokalaemia usually implies total body depletion. Measurements of either total body potassium or total exchangeable potassium may be somewhat misleading since much of the exchangeable potassium resides in muscle and muscle mass is characteristically reduced in cirrhosis. However, measurements of intracellular potassium have shown reduced values, especially in patients accumulating ascites.[3] With renal failure, both total exchangeable[41] and intracellular potassium[3] return to normal, probably because of the potassium retention associated with this complication. Potassium depletion may precipitate hepatic encephalopathy through two mechanisms: (a) it increases renal ammonia production;[84] and (b) since there is a reduced quantity available for Na^+–K^+ exchange in the distal convoluted tubule of the nephron a Na^+–H^+ exchange occurs with a resulting metabolic alkalosis and the latter facilitates uptake of ammonia into brain cells.[221]

Two important factors responsible for potassium depletion are hyperaldosteronism, and 'loop' and thiazide diuretics. Other factors include renal tubular acidosis, respiratory alkalosis and magnesium depletion.

Renal tubular acidosis

Renal tubular acidosis (RTA) has been described in association with several types of cirrhosis, including alcoholic,[158] chronic active hepatitis and primary biliary cirrhosis.[91] It is a distal (type II) RTA and has been attributed to both an autoimmune reaction directed against the distal tubular acidification site[206] and an abnormal renal handling of the sodium ion.[158] Usually it is a subclinical entity but, if overt, the acidosis and the hypokalaemia which is so characteristically found can precipitate encephalopathy[192] and nephrocalcinosis.[91] The mechanism for potassium depletion is related to the ion exchange mechanism in the distal convoluted tubule. Because it is unable to secrete H^+ in exchange for Na^+, excessive K^+ is secreted.

Respiratory alkalosis

A respiratory alkalosis is characteristic of advanced liver disease. Less H^+ will be available to the distal tubular ion exchange site and so increased amounts of K^+ will be lost.

Magnesium depletion

Magnesium depletion results in potassium depletion and hypokalaemia.[181,225,226] The mechanism is not clear but it is impossible to correct the potassium deficit until the magnesium depletion is first corrected. Magnesium depletion has been described in cirrhosis.[132] The mechanisms for it include hyperaldosteronism,[95] diuretic therapy[133] and, in those with an alcoholic aetiology, an effect of alcohol per se.[143] Evidence for magnesium depletion could not be found in patients with ascites which was controlled by spironolactone alone.[227] The quantitative importance of magnesium depletion in the pathogenesis of hypokalaemia in cirrhosis is unknown, but if the latter is resistant to oral and intravenous potassium supplements additional magnesium should be given (up to 200 mmol [400 mEq] daily of magnesium sulphate intravenously is best, oral preparations being relatively poorly absorbed).

RENAL FAILURE

Renal failure may occur in association with a variety of liver diseases including hepatocellular disease, obstructive jaundice, shock, and septicaemia, or when a pathological, toxic, or infectious condition simultaneously affects both organs (Table 46.1).

Cirrhosis

Flint[83] was the first to draw attention to the occurrence of renal failure in patients dying with cirrhosis. He also made important observations relating to the nature of the renal failure, in that albuminuria was unusual and in half of the cases the kidneys appeared normal at autopsy but in the other cases a variety of pathological changes was found. Hecker and Sherlock[97] gave the first more recent description of the features of the renal failure and noted that, in most patients, the urine sodium concentration was negligible, proteinuria absent, and renal histology normal; findings of a 'prerenal' type of uraemia. Others have confirmed these findings[20,162,191,212] and Vesin suggested the term 'functional renal failure',[212] but the typical biochemical (high urine sodium concentration, isomolar urine) and histological changes of acute tubular necrosis may also occur.[191] Other evidence that the renal failure of cirrhosis may occur either

Table 46.1. *Renal Failure with Liver Disease.*

1. Hepatocellular disease
   - Cirrhosis
   - Fulminant hepatic failure
   - Acute viral hepatitis
2. Obstructive jaundice
3. Shock and sepsis
4. Pathological condition affecting both organs
   - Polycystic disease
   - Congenital hepatic fibrosis
   - Amyloid
   - Sickle-cell disease
   - Reye's syndrome
5. Toxin or drug affecting both organs
   - Carbon tetrachloride
   - Tetracyclines
   - Methoxyflurane
   - Rifampicin; many others
6. Specific infections
   - Some leptospiral infections
   - Hepatitis B
   - Yellow fever
   - Malaria

with or without tubular necrosis includes measurements of urinary lysozyme, a sensitive marker of renal tubular damage, which may be elevated or normal.[235] Whether these two types of renal failure are really distinct entities or represent the ends of a single spectrum is a subject of debate but, in support of the latter, functional renal failure can progress to acute tubular necrosis,[191] and 'intermediate' forms exist.[17]

The incidence of renal failure in patients dying with cirrhosis has been variously reported as being between 44 and 84 per cent.[179,191] In one study, its severity was said to be out of proportion to the degree of hepatic impairment and the primary cause of death in 11 per cent.[85]

In the absence of pre-existing renal disease, the renal failure may be precipitated by events that impair hepatic and/or renal function, such as gastrointestinal haemorrhage, intercurrent infections or paracentesis, but in at least one-third of cases it arises spontaneously.[18,191] Invariably, the patient has advanced cirrhosis, though not all have encephalopathy at the time. Ascites is usually present and refractory to diuretic therapy. In many cases, the clinical course is rapidly progressive and the patient dies with encephalopathy and other manifestations of liver failure within a week of admission to hospital. In these cases there has often been a major precipitating factor.[178] In one-third of cases, the course is much more slowly progressive over several weeks or even months. These patients are generally unwell with nausea, anorexia, thirst and mild encephalopathy. Finally they succumb, often from a gastrointestinal haemorrhage or infection. There is little published information about the chances of recovery from renal failure in cirrhosis. Reynolds[172] reported that this was only 13 per cent in his series of 62 patients, but he also included cases of subacute liver disease. The most favourable prognosis is seen when the renal failure has been precipitated by a potentially reversible factor, such as an infection.

Pathophysiology and pathogenesis

Although the biochemical features of functional renal failure are of a prerenal uraemia, the failure cannot be explained on the basis of total plasma or blood volume depletion or a reduced cardiac output since these are all usually normal or increased.[115,126,142] Neither is it due to systemic hypotension since, although this may be found, it usually has developed after the onset of renal failure.[97] The most consistent finding is a reduced renal blood flow. This has been demonstrated using several techniques, including para-aminohippurate clearance,[20] dye dilution,[205] inert gas washout and radiography.[73] In the most severely affected patients, values may be reduced to only one-tenth of normal. The reduced blood flow is secondary to an increased renal vascular resistance.[19] The renal vasoconstriction involves not only the intrarenal vessels, but also the primary branches of the main renal artery and interlobar arteries.[73]

The vasoconstriction associated with functional renal failure is at least potentially reversible since the vessels again become fully patent after death.[73] Also widely quoted as evidence for the reversibility of the renal lesion are observations from renal and hepatic transplantation. Transplantation of kidneys from patients dying of cirrhosis with functional renal failure into seven human recipients resulted in a diuresis in six after one to two weeks, and values for creatinine clearance of >40 ml/min were attained in three patients.[112] More recently, in three patients with cirrhosis and renal failure who underwent liver transplantation there was a slow improvement in renal function over the following three months, but two of these patients had a high urine sodium concentration, suggestive of acute tubular necrosis.[102] Although these observations demonstrate the potential reversibility of the functional renal failure, if the vasoconstriction had been the only underlying mechanism one might have expected a more rapid return to normal of renal function in both situations. Whether other factors are involved in the pathogenesis of functional renal failure must therefore remain an open question.

There have been several theories to explain the renal vasoconstriction, including splanchnic 'pooling' of blood, a neurogenic vasoconstriction, accumulation of false neurotransmitter substances, changes in the renin–angiotensin system and a circulating renal vasoconstrictor substance.

Splanchnic pooling. Probably the most widely quoted explanation for the reduced renal perfusion is that it is secondary to pooling of blood in the splanchnic circulation, as a result of portal hypertension, so that the systemic arterial or 'effective' blood volume is reduced, even though total blood volume may be raised. In support of this concept, a dramatic improvement in renal function following a portacaval anastomosis has been reported in a patient with alcoholic cirrhosis.[186]

Although the total plasma or blood volume may be increased, it has been suggested that there might be relative deficits, the values being lower than those found in cirrhosis without renal failure.[164] A subgroup of patients with reduced values for both blood volume and cardiac output has been described, and in them renal function improved with infusion of dextran.[205] It is not clear whether these proposed deficits in blood or plasma volume were secondary to diuretic administration, which causes a quite different type of renal impairment (see above).

On the other hand, there is evidence against the concept that a reduced 'effective' or total blood or plasma volume may account for the reduced renal perfusion. In some patients, renal failure has been precipitated by a portacaval anastomosis;[35,86] Ring-Larsen, Hesse and Stigsby[175] were unable to demonstrate any change in renal blood flow after successful shunt operations in 12 patients. Intravenous reinfusion of concentrated ascitic fluid, a procedure that would be expected to correct a deficit in 'effective' blood volume, does not usually improve renal function when renal failure has developed spontaneously.[125,232] In general, only minor and inconsistent improvements in renal function have been found following intravenous administration of plasma.[173] Spontaneous improvements in glomerular filtration rate have not been associated with any changes in portal pressure or blood volume, the latter two measurements together being taken as an indirect measure of the degree of splanchnic pooling.[127]

Neurogenic vasoconstriction; false neurotransmitters. The α-adrenergic innervation of the kidney is vasoconstrictor and the role of an increased activity in the pathogenesis of renal failure has been investigated. In one study, infusions of the α-blocking drug phentolamine did not improve renal blood flow[73] but, in another, phenoxybenzamine resulted in a slight improvement in renal plasma flow if systemic hypotension was prevented by a simultaneous albumin infusion.[16] It seems unlikely, therefore, that an increased renal sympathetic tone is of major pathogenic importance. Indeed, there is now evidence for reduced sympathetic nervous activity in cirrhosis in that the pressor response to tyramine (a substance that releases noradrenaline from sympathetic nerve terminals) may be reduced,[140] as may be sympathetic reflexes.[136]

Reflexes between the splanchnic and renal circulations have also been implicated in the pathogenesis of functional renal failure. In dogs, a constriction applied to the portal vein results in a moderate reduction in renal blood flow, a reflex abolished by sympathectomy or local nerve blocks.[157] The relevance of these acute studies to the chronic elevation of portal pressure in cirrhosis is difficult to establish. With portal vein thrombosis renal function may be normal or reduced by up to 50 per cent, but not to the low values seen in functional renal failure.[109] The studies of Ring-Larsen and colleagues already referred to, in which effective reduction of a raised portal pressure was established by portacaval shunts without improving renal blood flow, show that it is unlikely that porto-renal reflexes are of major importance in mediating the reduced renal blood flow in cirrhosis.

It has been suggested that replacement of noradrenaline and other sympathetic transmitter substances from nerve terminals by poorly effective 'false transmitters' derived from gut bacteria could account for the cerebral, circulatory and renal changes seen in hepatic failure.[79] However, as pointed out above, the sympathetic nerve fibres to the kidney are vasoconstrictor so replacement with false transmitters would be expected to cause renal vasodilatation.

Renin–angiotensin system. In recent years there has been much interest in the possible role of the renin–angiotensin system in the pathogenesis of acute renal failure. It has been proposed that, as a result of some insult to the kidney, e.g. haemorrhage or shock, more renin is secreted. Angiotensin II is then formed within the kidney and 'shuts down' the renal circulation because of its vasoconstrictor action.[33] There is considerable experimental evidence both for and against such a concept.[33,78,82,155,203] Plasma renin concentration has been reported to be very high in cirrhosis when renal failure is present[188] and the renal vasoconstriction could therefore be mediated by increased amounts of angiotensin II. However, it is equally possible that the increased renin secretion is the *result* of the renal vasoconstriction. Angiotensin is unlikely to be of major pathogenic importance since the renal circulation has been reported to be refractory to its vasoconstrictor properties in cirrhosis,[94,117] and because it has no effect on the interlobular and arcuate arteries which are characteristically constricted.[69] This does not exclude a secondary role for angiotensin. The vasoconstriction may be primarily mediated by another factor, resulting in an increased secretion of renin and formation of angiotensin II, the latter perpetuating the renal vasoconstriction. The renin–angiotensin system may also be of importance in the pathogenesis of diuretic-induced renal impairment, as has already been discussed.

Circulating renal vasoconstrictor: possible role for endotoxins. Increased amounts of a circulating vasoactive substance could account for the renal vasoconstriction that underlies the renal failure of cirrhosis. One group of substances to be investigated are endotoxins. These are lipopolysaccharide components of the cell wall of gram-negative bacilli and are thought to be responsible for many of the manifestations of gram-negative septicaemia in man. A specific reversible renal vasoconstrictor effect has been demonstrated in dogs[89] and baboons.[43] The importance of endotoxins in the pathogenesis of acute renal failure in other clinical situations has been demonstrated.[216] The nature of the renal failure in the latter has not been clearly defined, though undoubtedly oliguria with a low urine sodium concentration may occur (possibly identical to the 'functional renal failure' of liver disease).[134] Acute tubular necrosis appears to be more common, however.[216]

Gram-negative organisms constitute a major part of the normal flora of the bowel. After bacterial death the free endotoxins are absorbed into the portal venous system and filtered by the reticuloendothelial cells of the liver.[166,170] Colloid liver scans, which effectively measure reticuloendothelial activity, characteristically show a reduced uptake in cirrhosis and this has been attributed to the spontaneous development of a portasystemic collateral circulation.[42] In cirrhosis one might therefore expect free endotoxins, in the absence of true gram-negative infection, to escape into the systemic circulation. Four studies have now reported that endotoxaemia, as detected by the Limulus assay, has occurred in cirrhosis without other evidence for gram-negative infection, and in each there was a close relationship with renal failure.[47,131,166,237] In one of these,[237] endotoxaemia was related to both functional renal failure and acute tubular necrosis, and this supports the concept that the two types of renal failure are part of a single spectrum.

If endotoxaemia does have a pathogenic role, the relative rarity of acute tubular necrosis must be explained. Experimentally, endotoxins appear to have two effects on the kidney: a rapidly reversible renal vasoconstriction,[43,89] and deposition of fibrin in the glomerular and peritubular capillaries[24,218] (Figure 46.6). To some extent these are interrelated in that the degree of fibrin deposition increases if the kidney is already vasoconstricted[160] and the products of intravascular coagulation, such as thrombin, are themselves renal vasoconstrictors.[167] The significance of fibrin deposits is apparent from both animal and human studies. The severity of renal structural damage is closely related to the extent of the fibrin deposits. When these are very marked, renal cortical necrosis is found, acute tubular necrosis being associated with less severe fibrin deposition. The activity of the fibrinolytic system is an important determinant to the deposition of fibrin. In the rabbit, endotoxins do not induce fibrinolysis[146] and the result is renal cortical necrosis,[88] a 'Shwartzman reaction' that can be prevented by stimulation of fibrinolysis with streptokinase.[50] In other animal models of acute renal failure, inhibition of fibrinolysis with ε-aminocaproic acid also results in renal cortical necrosis, e.g. glycerol-induced acute renal failure[219] and surgical damage to the placenta.[220] In contrast, in experimental pancreatitis in the rat, in which fibrinolysis is enhanced, intrarenal fibrin deposits have not been found.[215] The one human situation in which endotoxin-induced renal failure is commonly associated with renal cortical necrosis is pregnancy,[100] in which fibrinolysis is characteristically impaired.[145] The fibrin deposits, together with the accompanying renal structural damage, need not necessarily be of major functional significance. In the baboon, administration of endotoxins has been reported to result in

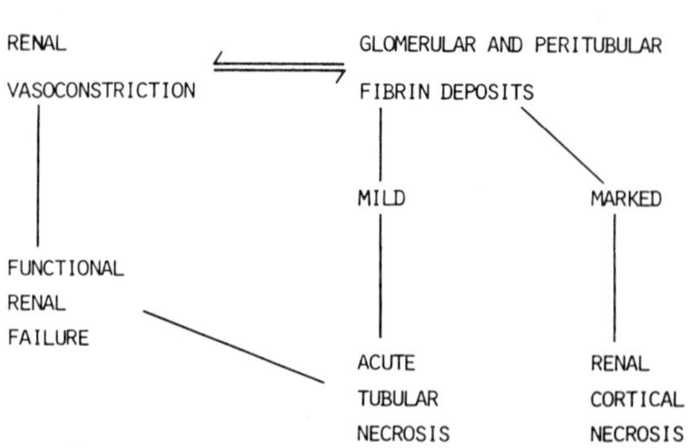

Figure 46.6. The effects of endotoxins on the kidney.

marked intrarenal fibrin deposition and severe tubular necrosis.[99] When heparin was also given, neither fibrin deposits nor renal structural damage could be found, but the severity of renal failure, as assessed by measurements of the plasma urea and creatinine concentrations, was the same in both groups of animals. The patient with cirrhosis might be uniquely protected from intrarenal fibrin deposition. The number of heparin-producing mast cells within the renal glomerulus may be markedly increased,[59] as may plasma fibrinolytic activity.[114] Braude, Douglas and Davis[30] have demonstrated in rabbits that administration of serum from animals immunized against endotoxin prevents endotoxin-induced renal cortical necrosis, and in cirrhosis circulating titres of antibodies to endotoxins are characteristically high.[28,204] Thus, if the effects of endotoxin were restricted to the vasoconstrictor effects alone, 'functional renal failure' would be expected (Figure 46.6). If the vasoconstriction is very severe, tubular necrosis could occur from tissue anoxia as well as from the effects of fibrinovascular occlusion.

Since no change in renal blood flow was found after portacaval shunt operations in one study, it was argued that toxins of intestinal origin are unlikely to be the cause of the renal failure in cirrhosis.[175] This view may be an over-simplification, however, since a *spontaneous* portasystemic shunt of 70 to 100 per cent is quite common in patients with cirrhosis in whom there has been no surgical intervention.[93,119] Furthermore, surgical relief of a raised portal pressure is likely to *reduce* endotoxin absorption.[156] It is not surprising, therefore, that a surgical shunt operation has a variable or no effect on renal function.

The possible role of other potential renal vasoconstrictors must also be considered. Catecholamines and serotonin have both been excluded.[22] A role for ferritin in the haemodynamic changes found in cirrhosis has been proposed[13] and abnormal deposits of ferritin have been found in the renal glomeruli.[81] However, the highest plasma levels occur in haemochromatosis[103] in which renal failure is unusual.

Other factors that may contribute to renal failure. Numerous glomerular lesions have been described in cirrhosis, including proliferative glomerulonephritis,[29] thickening of the basement membrane and mesangium,[80] glomerulosclerosis,[101] and immunoglobulin deposits within the mesangium[147] with a frequency of 25 to 75 per cent. The clinical significance of these changes is uncertain; in most series there is no correlation with renal function and the immunoglobulin deposits have not been associated with proteinuria. Clinical glomerulonephritis, however, has been described in 14 of 200 cases of cirrhosis.[163]

Other renal structural changes found in the kidney in cirrhosis include papillary necrosis,[66] pyelonephritis,[130] interstitial nephritis, and diabetic nephropathy.[178] The long-term use of oral neomycin in the treatment of hepatic encephalopathy may also result in blood levels sufficient to cause renal impairment.[113]

Consequences of renal failure in cirrhosis

The consequences of renal failure in cirrhosis will be similar to those of acute renal failure in other clinical situations, including retention of nitrogenous toxins, fluid overload with dilutional hyponatraemia, and potassium retention. However, hyperkalaemia is usually less severe in the patient with cirrhosis since there may have been previous potassium depletion.

Accumulation of urea is likely to result in increased production of ammonia from the increased amounts of urea that diffuse into the gut.[223] This is likely to accentuate the already high circulating levels of ammonia characteristic of liver failure and may be of particular importance in relation to the hepatic encephalopathy so often present.

Uraemia has been shown to inhibit hepatocyte regeneration in the rat.[45] If this also applies to man, the development of renal failure might prejudice recovery of the liver if there has been a potentially reversible deterioration in function as, for example, ischaemic damage to the liver after severe haemorrhage.

The commonest causes of death in acute renal failure are infection and gastrointestinal haemorrhage, both of which are also common in cirrhosis without renal failure. The combination of liver failure and renal failure is therefore likely to be one in which these complications will be particularly manifest.

Differential diagnosis of renal failure in cirrhosis

The majority of cases will fall into the categories of functional renal failure or acute tubular necrosis. Simple biochemical tests on the urine often distinguish between these (Table 46.2), but the use of casts in the urine sediment has not been of value.[235] In functional renal failure the

Table 46.2. *Differential Diagnosis of Renal Failure in Cirrhosis.*

	Urine sodium concentration (mmol/l [mEq/l])	Urine:plasma osmolality ratio
Dehydration	<12	>1.15
Functional renal failure and incipient acute tubular necrosis	<12	1.10–1.15
Acute tubular necrosis	>12 (usually >20)	<1.10

urine sodium concentration is <12 mmol/l (12 mEq/l) and the urine:plasma osmolality ratio 1.10 to 1.15. In acute tubular necrosis these values are >12 mmol/l (12 mEq/l) and <1.10 respectively. In other clinical situations acute tubular necrosis is associated with a much higher urine sodium concentration. This is possibly due to the fact that, in cirrhosis, 'intact nephrons' will be subject to the effect of very high circulating levels of aldosterone. Simple dehydration must also be considered, since the urine sodium then will again be low but the urine:plasma osmolality ratio will be higher than in functional renal failure. In practice, the biochemical changes associated with dehydration merge into those of functional renal failure and those of the latter into acute tubular necrosis. Furthermore, functional renal failure is biochemically indistinguishable from incipient acute tubular necrosis. Consequently, the nature of the renal impairment cannot always be determined on the basis of a single urine sample: it may be determined only on the course of events with sequential tests.

A small percentage of cases will be due to the other specific renal structural lesions listed above. Chronic glomerulonephritis should be suspected if there is heavy proteinuria, and diabetic nephropathy if there is underlying diabetes, but renal biopsy will be necessary for a definitive diagnosis. Urine cultures and microscopy of a fresh urine sediment should be carried out for the diagnosis of chronic pyelonephritis, but these may be normal and an intravenous pyelogram or biopsy may be required.

Renal impairment precipitated by diuretics has already been discussed.

Treatment

If a specific precipitating cause can be identified, e.g. dehydration or pyelonephritis, treatment must be directed at correcting this. Unfortunately, this is not usually the case, and there have been many attempts to reverse the vasoconstriction of functional renal failure but none have been of any real value. These include plasma expansion[173] and agents such as noradrenaline,[97] phentolamine,[73] metaraminol,[172] aminophylline,[172] mannitol,[18] angiotensin,[187] isoprenaline,[48] dopamine[25] and corticosteroids,[172] many of these being infused directly into the renal artery.

Table 46.3. *Results of Dialysis in Treating Renal Failure with Liver Disease, King's College Hospital, 1970–1975.*

	Number of patients	Haemodialysis	Peritoneal dialysis	Haemodialysis and peritoneal dialysis	Survival
Cirrhosis	25	5	18	2	0 (0%)
Fulminant hepatic failure	50	4	39	7	6 (12%)
Obstructive jaundice	6	4	1	1	4 (67%)
Prolonged hypotension	3	2	1	0	3 (100%)
Carbon tetrachloride	3	0	3	0	3 (100%)
Leptospirosis	3	1	2	0	3 (100%)

From Wilkinson,[228] with kind permission of the editor of *Medicine* (London).

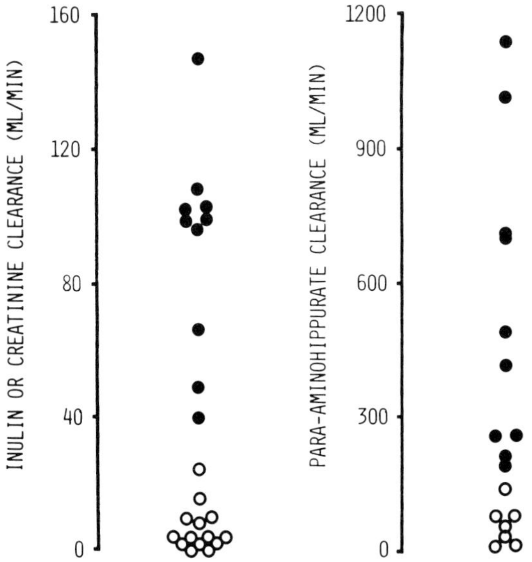

Figure 46.7. Relation of renal function to endotoxaemia, as detected by the *Limulus* assay, in fulminant hepatic failure (● *Limulus*-negative; ○ *Limulus*-positive. From Wilkinson et al,[236] with kind permission of the editor of *The Lancet*).

In our hands, the use of dialysis, either peritoneal or haemodialysis, has not improved survival in either functional renal failure or acute tubular necrosis (Table 46.3), and in many cases may have precipitated severe gastrointestinal haemorrhage.[234] Treatment is therefore based on the usual conservative management of acute renal failure, namely, restriction of fluid, sodium, potassium and protein, and withdrawal of potentially nephrotoxic drugs such as neomycin. Calcium resonium may be required to reverse hyperkalaemia.

Fulminant Hepatic Failure and Acute Viral Hepatitis (see also Chapter 27)

Up to 80 per cent of patients with fulminant hepatic failure from any cause develop renal failure and this is associated with a particularly poor prognosis.[231] Both functional renal failure and acute tubular necrosis have been described and, as in cirrhosis, may be related to endotoxaemia[236] (Figure 46.7). Renal failure is often thought of as a late complication of fulminant hepatic failure but this has not necessarily been our experience, 35 per cent of patients developing renal failure before there was severe hepatic encephalopathy.[233] The results of treating these patients with dialysis have been more favourable than for cirrhosis[234] (Table 46.3), and since complete recovery of the liver may occur it is important to persevere with treatment even in the most severely ill patients.

Renal failure has also been reported in association with otherwise uncomplicated viral hepatitis, and again both functional renal failure and acute tubular necrosis may occur.[230] The severity of the renal failure is grossly out of proportion to that of the hepatitis and specific treatment is directed more to the renal failure, the prognosis being relatively good with dialysis. Glomerulonephritis[182] and non-specific parenchymal changes[52] have also been described in acute viral hepatitis.

Obstructive Jaundice

Renal failure may occur in association with any pathology causing obstruction to the biliary tract, including calculi, carcinoma and chronic pancreatitis, either preoperatively or during the days immediately following surgery. Endotoxaemia has also been implicated in its pathogenesis and this is usually due to associated gram-negative sepsis, but cases without evidence for infection have also been described.[15, 237] In 'aseptic' cases the mechanism for the endotoxaemia may be twofold: (a) bile salts have been shown to prevent absorption of endotoxins from the gut,[111] and deficiency within the bowel lumen is to be expected with biliary obstruction; and (b) reticuloendothelial function may be depressed[63] and the clearance of endotoxins absorbed from the bowel may therefore be impaired. Histologically, the kidneys usually show fibrin deposits and tubular necrosis,[217] which might be predicted since plasma fibrinolytic activity is characteristically reduced.[104] Additional pathogenic factors are that both conjugated bilirubin[23] and bile salts[6] sensitize the renal parenchyma to the adverse effects of anoxia.

Management of cases developing renal failure preoperatively

Early relief of the biliary obstruction is essential. In one series, 13 of 15 patients treated by radical surgery survived, compared with only one of 14 who had palliative or no surgery.[5] In another series, 18 of 26 patients treated by radical surgery survived, compared with none of 16 patients treated by palliative or without surgery.[199] In both series, however, the two groups were not always comparable, radical

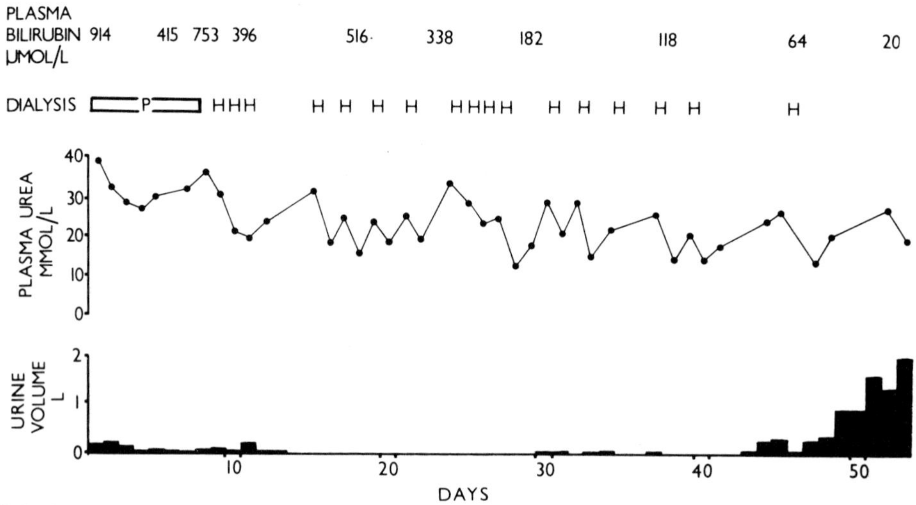

Figure 46.8. Prolonged clinical course in a patient who developed severe cholestasis and renal failure following a period of prolonged hypotension (from Wilkinson et al,[234] with kind permission of the editor of *Clinical Nephrology*).

surgery not being possible in many of those otherwise treated because of the underlying pathology (e.g. inoperable carcinoma, haemorrhagic pancreatitis). Of 11 cases with renal failure associated with biliary calculi, eight recovered after early radical surgery.[4] Dialysis is often necessary in these patients and it is our policy to treat with one four-to-six-hour period of haemodialysis as soon after admission as possible, before surgery is undertaken.

Prevention of postoperative renal failure

In the prevention of postoperative renal failure, adequate hydration at the time of surgery is of utmost importance. Three litres of dextrose-saline should be given intravenously during the preceding 24 hours. Mannitol might also be of protective value.[57] 200 ml of a 10 per cent solution should be given immediately before induction of anaesthesia and provided as necessary during the operation and for 48 hours thereafter to maintain a urine flow rate of 1 to 2 ml/min. It is essential to ensure that mannitol is not given to a dehydrated patient, and to replace the additional fluid losses with intravenous saline; otherwise depletion of the extracellular fluid will occur, making renal failure *more* likely.

Shock and Sepsis

Shock from any cause (especially haemorrhagic or cardiogenic) or severe sepsis (especially if prolonged and not adequately controlled by antibiotics) may be associated with jaundice and renal failure. Those most prone to develop this syndrome are patients who have undergone long and difficult major abdominal or thoracic operations.

Histologically, the liver may show only cholestasis without significant necrosis,[74] but centrilobular necrosis may occur if shock has been prolonged.[70] Occasionally, the only abnormality of standard liver function tests is a hyperbilirubinaemia, although the alkaline phosphatase is often raised. If hepatocellular necrosis is also present the transaminases will rise. Although the jaundice may be marked these patients rarely, if ever, progress to severe hepatic failure. The mechanism for the jaundice is multifactorial. The hepatocellular necrosis may be one factor and the increased bilirubin load, resulting from transfusions of large quantities of stored blood, another. Endotoxins specifically inhibit transport processes from liver cells to bile canaliculi,[208] but jaundice may also occur with severe pneumococcal infections,[245] organisms that do not contain endotoxins. In some series the occurrence of renal failure has been associated with a very poor prognosis[106] but dialysis has often not been used. However, three consecutive patients treated by intensive dialysis survived[234] (Table 46.3) and treatment was necessary for nearly seven weeks in one case (Figure 46.8).

Leptospirosis (see Chapter 51)

Some leptospiral infections (*L. icterohaemorrhagica*, *L. hebdomadis*) are associated with jaundice and renal failure. Leptospirosis should be suspected if there has been a typically biphasic illness. The first stage is characterized by high fever, severe headache, meningism, muscle pain and pneumonitis. As these subside jaundice and renal failure occur, often associated with conjunctional haemorrhages and bruising. Jaundice may be very marked but the serum transaminases and alkaline phosphatase are usually only minimally deranged. Liver histology shows only minimal or no necrosis.[7,194] Hepatic failure does not occur. Renal failure is the most important clinical manifestation and prognosis appears to be good with dialysis (Table 46.3).

Other Conditions

The occurrence of renal and hepatic dysfunction in the other conditions listed in Table 46.1 is largely self-explanatory. Detailed studies have been carried out in polycystic disease and congenital hepatic fibrosis, and there are several diagnostic subgroups; in some instances the liver lesion is the most severe but in others renal failure is the most important prognostic factor.[151] An immune complex type of glomerulonephritis has been described as a complication of hepatitis B infection with chronic hepatitis[49] (see Chapter 29).

REFERENCES

1. Alam, A.N., Wilkinson, S.P., Poston, L., Moodie, H. & Williams, R. (1977) Intracellular electrolyte abnormalities in fulminant hepatic failure. *Gastroenterology*, **72,** 914–917.
2. Alam, A.N., Poston, L., Wilkinson, S.P., Golindano, C. & Williams, R. (1978) A study *in vitro* of the sodium pump in fulminant hepatic failure. *Clinical Science and Molecular Medicine*, **55,** 355–363.
3. Alam, A.N., Wheeler, P., Wilkinson, S.P., Poston, L., Golindano, C. & Williams, R. (1978) Changes in the electrolyte content of leucocytes at different clinical stages of cirrhosis. *Gut*, **19,** 650–654.
4. Andersen, J.B., Sorensen, F.H. & Skjoldborg, H. (1971) Acute renal failure in association with choledocholithiasis. *Acta Chirurgica Scandinavica*, **137,** 81–86.
5. Andreassen, M., Thaysen, J.H., Engell, H.C., Madsen, C.M. & Lindenberg, J. (1961) Surgical management of biliary tract disease complicated by acute renal failure. *Acta Chirurgica Scandinavica* (Supplement) **283,** 207–220.
6. Aoyagi, T. & Lowenstein, L.M. (1968) The effect of bile acids and renal ischaemia on renal failure. *Journal of Laboratory and Clinical Medicine*, **71,** 686–692.
7. Arean, V.M. (1962) The pathologic anatomy and pathogenesis of fatal human leptospirosis (Weil's disease). *American Journal of Pathology*, **40,** 393–423.
8. Arroyo, V. & Rodes, J. (1975) A rational approach to the treatment of ascites. *Postgraduate Medical Journal*, **51,** 558–563.
9. Arroyo, V., Mas, A. & Vilardell, F. (1975) Clinical experience with the Rhone–Poulenc ascites reinfusion apparatus. *Postgraduate Medical Journal*, **51,** 571–573.
10. Arroyo, V., Rodes, J., Gutierrez-Lizarraga, M.A. & Revert, L. (1976) Prognostic value of spontaneous hyponatraemia in cirrhosis with ascites. *American Journal of Digestive Diseases*, **21,** 249–256.
11. Atkinson, M. & Losowsky, M.S. (1961) The mechanism of ascites formation in chronic liver disease. *Quarterly Journal of Medicine*, **30,** 153–166.
12. August, J.T., Nelson, D.H. & Thorn, G.W. (1958) Response of normal subjects to large amounts of aldosterone. *Journal of Clinical Investigation*, **37,** 1549–1555.
13. Baez, S., Mazur, A. & Schorr, E. (1950) Hepatorenal factors in circulatory homeostatis. XX Antidiuretic action of hepatic vasodepressor, VDM (ferritin). *American Journal of Physiology*, **162,** 198–212.
14. Bagenstoss, A.H. & Cain, J.C. (1957) Further studies on the lymphatic vessels at the hilus of the liver of man: their relation to ascites. *Proceedings of Staff Meetings at the Mayo Clinic*, **32,** 615–628.
15. Bailey, M.E. (1976) Endotoxin, bile salts and renal function in obstructive jaundice. *British Journal of Surgery*, **63,** 774–778.
16. Baldus, W.P. (1970) Etiology and management of renal failure in cirrhosis and portal hypertension. *Annals of the New York Academy of Science*, **170,** 267–276.
17. Baldus, W.P. (1973) Renal failure in advanced liver disease. In *Progress in Liver Disease*, Vol. IV (Ed.) Popper, H. & Schaffner, F., pp. 251–267. New York: Grune & Stratton.
18. Baldus, W.P., Feichter, R.N. & Summerskill, W.H.J. (1964) The kidney in cirrhosis – I. Clinical and biochemical features of azotaemia in hepatic failure. *Annals of Internal Medicine*, **60,** 353–365.
19. Baldus, W.P., Summerskill, W.H.J., Hunt, J.C. & Maher, F.T. (1964) Renal circulation in cirrhosis: observations based on catheterisation of the renal vein. *Journal of Clinical Investigation*, **43,** 1090–1097.
20. Baldus, W.P., Feichter, R.N., Summerskill, W.H.J., Hunt, J.C. & Wakim, K.G. (1964) The kidney in cirrhosis – II. Disorders of renal function. *Annals of Internal Medicine*, **60,** 366–377.
21. Barnardo, D.E., Strong, C.G. & Baldus, W.P. (1969) Failure of cirrhotic livers to inactivate renin: evidence for a splanchnic source of renin-like activity. *Journal of Laboratory and Clinical Medicine*, **74,** 495–506.
22. Barnardo, D.E., Summerskill, W.H.J., Strong, C.S. & Baldus, W.P. (1970) Renal function, renin activity and endogenous vasoactive substances in cirrhosis. *American Journal of Digestive Diseases*, **15,** 419–425.
23. Baum, M., Stirling, G.A. & Dawson, J.L. (1969) A further study into obstructive jaundice and ischaemic renal damage. *British Medical Journal*, **ii,** 229–231.
24. Beller, F.K. & Graeff, H. (1967) Deposition of glomerular fibrin in the rabbit after infusion with endotoxin. *Nature*, **215,** 295–296.

25. Bennett, W.M., Keefe, E., Melnyk, C., Mahler, D., Rosch, J. & Porter, G.A. (1975) Response to dopamine hydrochloride in the hepatorenal syndrome. *Archives of Internal Medicine,* **135,** 964–971.
26. Bergstrand, I., Ekman, C. & Kohler, R. (1964) Inferior vena caval obstruction in hepatic cirrhosis. *Acta Radiologica,* **2,** 1–8.
27. Berner, C., Fred, H.L., Riggs, S. & Davis, J.S. (1964) Diagnostic probabilities in patients with conspicuous ascites. *Archives of Internal Medicine,* **113,** 687–690.
28. Bjørneboe, M., Prytz, H. & Ørskov, F. (1972) Antibodies to intestinal microbes in serum of patients with cirrhosis of the liver. *Lancet,* **i,** 58–60.
29. Bloodworth, J.M.B. & Sommers, S.C. (1959) Cirrhotic glomerulosclerosis, a renal lesion associated with hepatic cirrhosis. *Laboratory Investigation,* **8,** 962–978.
30. Braude, A.I., Douglas, H. & Davis, C.E. (1973) Treatment and prevention of intravascular coagulation with antiserum to endotoxin. *Journal of Infectious Diseases,* **128,** S157–164.
31. Britton, R.C. (1961) A new technique for rapid control of cirrhotic ascites. *Archives of Surgery,* **83,** 52–57.
32. Brown, J.J., Davis, D.L., Lever, A.F. & Robertson, J.I.S. (1964) Variations in plasma renin concentration in several physiological and pathological states. *Journal of the Canadian Medical Association,* **90,** 201–206.
33. Brown, J.J., Gleadle, R.I., Lawson, D.H., Lever, A.F., Linton, A.L., Macadam, R.F., Prentice, E., Robertson, J.I.S. & Tree, M. (1970) Renin and acute renal failure: studies in man. *British Medical Journal,* **i,** 253–258.
34. Burack, W.R. & Hollister, R.M. (1960) Tuberculous peritonitis: a study of forty-seven proved cases encountered by a general medical unit in twenty-five years. *American Journal of Medicine,* **28,** 510–523.
35. Burchell, A.R., Rousselot, L.M. & Panke, W.F. (1968) A seven year experience with side-to-side portacaval shunt in cirrhotic ascites. *Annals of Surgery,* **168,** 655–670.
36. Burg, M.B. (1976) Mechanisms of action of diuretic drugs. In *The Kidney* (Ed.) Brenner, B.M. & Rector, F.C., pp. 737–762. Philadelphia, London and Toronto: W.B. Saunders.
37. Burg, M.B. & Green, N. (1973) Function of the thick ascending limb of Henle's loop. *American Journal of Physiology,* **224,** 659–668.
38. Cabot, R.C. (1912) The causes of ascites: a study of five thousand cases. *American Journal of Medical Science,* **143,** 1–29.
39. Cannon, P.J., Heinemann, H.O., Albert, M.S., Laragh, J.H. & Wintners, R.W. (1965) 'Contraction' alkalosis after diuresis of edematous patients with ethacrynic acid. *Annals of Internal Medicine,* **62,** 979–990.
40. Caroli, J. & Platteborse, R. (1958) Septicemie portocave. Cirrhoses du foie et septicemie à colibacille. *Semaine des Hôpitaux de Paris,* **34,** 472–487.
41. Casey, T.H., Summerskill, W.H.J., & Orvis, A.L. (1965) Body and serum potassium in liver disease. I. Relationship to hepatic function and associated factors. *Gastroenterology,* **48,** 198–207.
42. Castell, D.O. & Johnson, R.B. (1966) The ^{198}Au liver scan. An index of portal-systemic collateral circulation in chronic liver disease. *New England Journal of Medicine,* **275,** 188–192.
43. Cavanagh, D., Rao, P.S., Sutton, D.M.C., Bhagat, B.D. & Bacjmann, F. (1970) The pathophysiology of endotoxin shock in the primate. *American Journal of Obstetrics and Gynecology,* **108,** 705–722.
44. Chart, J.J. & Shipley, E.S. (1953) The mechanism of sodium retention in cirrhosis of the liver. *Journal of Clinical Investigation,* **32,** 560 (abstract).
45. Chen, T.S.M. & Leevy, C.M. (1973) Liver regeneration and uraemia. *British Journal of Experimental Pathology,* **54,** 591–596.
46. Cherrick, G.R., Kerr, D.N.S., Read, A.E. & Sherlock, S. (1960) Colloid osmotic pressure and hydrostatic pressure relationships in the formation of ascites in hepatic cirrhosis. *Clinical Science,* **19,** 361–375.
47. Clemente, C., Bosch, J., Rodes, J., Arroyo, V., Mas, A. & Maragall, S. (1977) Functional renal failure and haemorrhagic gastritis associated with endotoxaemia in cirrhosis. *Gut,* **18,** 556–560.
48. Cohn, J.N., Tristani, F.E. & Khatri, I.M. (1970) Renal vasodilator therapy in the hepatorenal syndrome. *Medical Annals of the District of Columbia,* **39,** 1–7.
49. Combes, B., Stastny, P., Shorey, J., Eigenbrodt, E.H., Barrera, A., Hull, A.R. & Carter, N.W. (1971) Glomerulonephritis with deposition of Australia antigen–antibody complexes in glomerular basement membrane. *Lancet,* **ii,** 234–237.
50. Condie, R.M., Hong, C.Y. & Good, R.A. (1957) Reversal of the lesions of the generalised Shwartzman phenomenon by treatment of rabbits with streptokinase. *Journal of Laboratory and Clinical Medicine,* **50,** 803–804.
51. Conn, H.O. & Fessel, J.M. (1971) Spontaneous bacterial peritonitis in cirrhosis: variations on a theme. *Medicine* (Baltimore), **50,** 161–197.
52. Conrad, M.E., Schwartz, F.D. & Young, M.A. (1964) Infectious hepatitis – a generalised disease. *American Journal of Medicine,* **37,** 789–801.
53. Cook, W. & Pickering, G. (1958) Location of renin within kidney. *Journal of Physiology,* **143,** 78P–79P (abstract).
54. Coppage, W.S., Island, D.P., Cooner, A.E. & Liddle, G.W. (1962) The metabolism of aldosterone in normal subjects and in patients with hepatic cirrhosis. *Journal of Clinical Investigation,* **41,** 1672–1680.
55. Curry, N., McCallum, R.W. & Guth, P.H. (1974) Spontaneous peritonitis in cirrhotic ascites. A decade of experience. *American Journal of Digestive Diseases,* **19,** 685–692.
56. Davis, J.O., Holman, J.E., Carpenter, C.C., Urquart, J. & Higgins, J.T. (1964) An extra-adrenal factor essential for chronic renal sodium retention in presence of increased sodium retaining hormone. *Circulation Research,* **14,** 17–31.
57. Dawson, J.L. (1965) Post-operative renal function in obstructive jaundice: effect of a mannitol diuresis. *British Medical Journal,* **i,** 82–86.
58. Denison, E.K., Lieberman, F.L. & Reynolds, T.B. (1971) 9-α-fluorohydrocortisone induced ascites in alcoholic liver disease. *Gastroenterology,* **61,** 497–503.
59. Devenyi, I., Szucs, L., Tessman, D. & Schill, H. (1968) Renale mastocytose und sekundarer aldosteronismus. *Virchows Archiv für Pathologische Anatomie,* **345,** 238–244.
60. de Wardener, H.E. (1977) Natriuretic hormone. *Clinical Science and Molecular Medicine,* **53,** 1–8.

61. de Wardener, H.E., Mills, I.H., Clapham, W.F. & Hayter, C.J. (1961) Studies on the efferent mechanisms of the sodium diuresis which follows the administration of intravenous saline in the dog. *Clinical Science*, **21**, 249–258.
62. Donowitz, M., Kerstein, M.D. & Spiro, H.M. (1974) Pancreatic ascites. *Medicine* (Baltimore), **53**, 183–195.
63. Drivas, G., James, O. & Wardle, N. (1976) Study of reticuloendothelial phagocytic capacity in patients with cholestasis. *British Medical Journal*, **i**, 1568–1569.
64. Dumont, A.E. & Mulholland, J.H. (1960) Flow rate and composition of thoracic duct lymph in patients with cirrhosis. *New England Journal of Medicine*, **263**, 471–474.
65. Dumont, A.E. & Witte, M.H. (1966) Contrasting patterns of thoracic duct lymph formation in hepatic cirrhosis. *Surgery, Gynecology and Obstetrics*, **122**, 524–528.
66. Edmonson, H.A., Reynolds, T.B. & Jacobson, H.G. (1966) Renal papillary necrosis with special reference to chronic alcoholism. *Archives of Internal Medicine*, **118**, 255–264.
67. Eggert, R.C. (1970) Spironolactone diuresis in patients with cirrhosis and ascites. *British Medical Journal*, **iv**, 401–403.
68. Eknoyan, G., Martinez-Maldanado, M., Yium, J.J. & Suki, W.N. (1970) Combined ascitic fluid and furosemide infusion in management of ascites. *New England Journal of Medicine*, **282**, 713–717.
69. Elkin, M. & Meng, C.H. (1966) The effects of angiotensin on renal vascularity in dogs. *American Journal of Roentgenology*, **98**, 927–930.
70. Ellenberg, M. & Osserman, K.E. (1951) The role of shock in the production of central liver cell necrosis. *American Journal of Medicine*, **11**, 170–178.
71. Epstein, F.H., Lesser, G.T. & Berger, E.Y. (1950) Renal function in decompensated cirrhosis of the liver. *Proceedings of the Society of Experimental and Biological Medicine*, **75**, 822–824.
72. Epstein, M., Pins, D.S., Schneider, N. & Levinson, R. (1976) Determinants of deranged sodium and water homeostasis in decompensated cirrhosis. *Journal of Laboratory and Clinical Medicine*, **87**, 822–839.
73. Epstein, M., Berk, D.P., Hollenberg, N.K., Adams, D.F., Chalmers, T.C., Abrams, H.L. & Merrill, J.P. (1970) Renal failure in the patient with cirrhosis. The role of active vasoconstriction. *American Journal of Medicine*, **49**, 175–185.
74. Fahrlander, H., Huber, F. & Gloor, F. (1964) Intrahepatic retention of bile in severe bacterial infections. *Gastroenterology*, **47**, 590–599.
75. Farnsworth, E.B. & Krakusin, J.S. (1948) Electrolyte partition in patients with edema of various origins: qualitative and quantitative definition of cations and anions in hepatic cirrhosis. *Journal of Laboratory and Clinical Medicine*, **33**, 1545–1554.
76. Fasciolo, J.C., de Vito, E., Romero, J.C. & Cucchi, J.N. (1964) The renin content of the blood of humans and dogs under several conditions. *Journal of the Canadian Medical Association*, **90**, 206–209.
77. Fichman, M.P., Vorherr, H., Kleeman, C.R. & Telfer, N. (1971) Diuretic induced hyponatraemia. *Annals of Internal Medicine*, **75**, 853–863.
78. Finn, W.F., Arendshorst, W.J. & Gottschalk, C.W. (1975) Pathogenesis of oliguria in acute renal failure. *Circulation Research*, **36**, 675–681.
79. Fischer, J.E. & Baldessarini, R.J. (1971) False neurotransmitters and hepatic failure. *Lancet*, **ii**, 75–79.
80. Fisher, E.R. & Hellstrom, H.R. (1959) The membranous and proliferative glomerulonephritis of hepatic cirrhosis. *American Journal of Clinical Pathology*, **32**, 48–55.
81. Fisher, E.R. & Perez-Stable, E. (1968) Cirrhotic (hepatic) lobular glomerulonephritis. *American Journal of Clinical Pathology*, **52**, 869–881.
82. Flamenbaum, W., Kotchen, T.A. & Oken, D.E. (1972) Effect of renin immunization on mercuric chloride and glycerol-induced renal failure. *Kidney International*, **1**, 406–412.
83. Flint, A. (1863) Clinical report on hydroperitoneum, based on an analysis of 46 cases. *American Journal of Medical Science*, **45**, 306–339.
84. Gabuzda, G.J. & Hall, P.W. (1966) Relation of potassium depletion to renal ammonium metabolism and hepatic coma. *Medicine*, **45**, 481–490.
85. Garceau, A.J. & Chalmers, T.C. (1963) The natural history of cirrhosis. I. Survival with esophageal varices. *New England Journal of Medicine*, **268**, 469–473.
86. Garrett, J.C., Voorhees, A.B. & Sommers, S.C. (1970) Renal failure following portasystemic shunt in patients with cirrhosis of the liver. *Annals of Surgery*, **172**, 218–225.
87. Genest, J., Boucher, R., de Champlain, J., Veyrat, R., Chretien, M. & Biron, P. (1963) Arterial angiotensin blood levels in hypertensive and oedematous diseases. *Excerpta Medica International Congress Series*, **67**, 129–137.
88. Gerber, I.E. (1936) Shwartzman reaction in kidneys of rabbits. *Archives of Pathology*, **21**, 776–796.
89. Gillenwater, J.Y., Dooley, E.S. & Frohlich, E.D. (1963) Effects of endotoxin on renal function and haemodynamics. *American Journal of Physiology*, **205**, 293–297.
90. Giuseffi, J., Werk, E.E., Larson, P.U., Schiff, L. & Elliott, D.W. (1957) Effect of bilateral adrenalectomy in a patient with massive ascites and postnecrotic cirrhosis. *New England Journal of Medicine*, **257**, 796–803.
91. Golding, P.L. (1975) Renal tubular acidosis in chronic liver disease. *Postgraduate Medical Journal*, **51**, 550–556.
92. Goodyer, A.V.N. & Jaeger, C.A. (1955) Renal response to non-shocking haemorrhage: role of autonomic system and the renal circulation. *American Journal of Physiology*, **180**, 69–74.
93. Groszmann, R., Kotelanski, B., Cohn, J.N. & Khatri, I.M. (1972) Quantitation of portasystemic shunting from the splenic and mesenteric beds in alcoholic liver disease. *American Journal of Medicine*, **53**, 715–722.
94. Gutman, R.A., Forrey, A.W., Fleet, W.P. & Cutler, R.E. (1973) Vasopressor-induced natriuresis and altered intrarenal haemodynamics in cirrhotic man. *Clinical Science and Molecular Medicine*, **45**, 19–34.
95. Hanna, S. & MacIntyre, I. (1960) The influence of aldosterone on magnesium metabolism. *Lancet*, **ii**, 348–350.
96. Heacox, R., Harvey, A.M. & Vander, A.J. (1976) Hepatic inactivation of renin. *Circulation Research*, **21**, 149–152.
97. Hecker, R. & Sherlock, S. (1956) Electrolyte and circulatory changes in terminal liver failure. *Lancet*, **ii**, 1121–1125.

98. Hierholzer, K. & Stolte, H. (1969) The proximal and distal tubular action of adrenal steroids on sodium reabsorption. *Nephron,* **6,** 188–204.
99. Hinshaw, L.B., Benjamin, B., Holmes, D.D., Beller, B., Archer, L.T., Coalson, J.J. & Whitsett, T. (1977) Response of the baboon to live *Escherichia coli* organisms and endotoxin. *Surgery, Gynecology and Obstetrics,* **145,** 1–11.
100. Hjort, P.F. & Rapaport, S.I. (1965) The Shwartzman reaction: pathogenetic mechanisms and clinical manifestations. *Annual Review of Medicine,* **16,** 135–168.
101. Horn, R.C. & Smetana, H. (1942) Intercapillary glomerulosclerosis. *American Journal of Pathology,* **18,** 93–100.
102. Iwatsuki, S., Popovtzer, M.M., Corman, J.L., Ishikawa, M., Putman, C.W., Katz, F.H. & Starzl, T.E. (1973) Recovery from 'hepatorenal syndrome' after orthotopic liver transplantation. *New England Journal of Medicine,* **289,** 1155–1159.
103. Jacobs, A., Miller, F., Wormwood, M., Beamish, M.R. & Wardrop, C.A. (1972) Ferritin in the serum of normal subjects and patients with iron deficiency and iron overload. *British Medical Journal,* **iv,** 206–208.
104. Jedrychowski, A., Hillenbrand, P., Ajdukiewiez, A.B., Parbhoo, S.P. & Sherlock, S. (1973) Fibrinolysis in cholestatic jaundice. *British Medical Journal,* **i,** 640–642.
105. Johnston, R.F. & Loo, R.V. (1964) Hepatic hydrothorax: studies to determine the source of the fluid and a report of thirteen cases. *Annals of Internal Medicine,* **61,** 385–401.
106. Kantrowitz, P.A., Jones, W.A., Greenberger, N.J. & Isselbacher, K.J. (1967) Severe post-operative hyperbilirubinaemia simulating obstructive jaundice. *New England Journal of Medicine,* **276,** 591–598.
107. Kelley, M.L. & Butt, H.R. (1960) Chylous ascites: an analysis of its etiology. *Gastroenterology,* **39,** 161–170.
108. Kerr, D.N.S., Pearson, D.T. & Read, A.E. (1963) Infection of ascitic fluid in patients with hepatic cirrhosis. *Gut,* **4,** 394–398.
109. Kew, M.C., Limbrick, C., Varma, R.R. & Sherlock, S. (1972) Renal and intrarenal blood flow in non-cirrhotic portal hypertension. *Gut,* **13,** 763–767.
110. Klinger, E.L., Vaamonde, C.A., Vaamonde, L.S., Lancestremere, R.G., Morosi, H.J., Frisch, E. & Papper, S. (1970) Renal function changes in cirrhosis of the liver: a prospective study. *Archives of Internal Medicine,* **125,** 1010–1015.
111. Kocsar, L.T., Bertok, L. & Varteresz, V. (1969) Effect of bile acids on the intestinal absorption of endotoxin in rats. *Journal of Bacteriology,* **100,** 220–223.
112. Koppel, M.H., Coburn, J.W., Mims, M.M., Goldstein, H., Boyle, J.D. & Rubini, M.E. (1969) Transplantation of cadaveric kidneys from patients with hepatorenal syndrome. Evidence for the functional nature of renal failure in advanced liver disease. *New England Journal of Medicine,* **280,** 1367–1371.
113. Kunin, C.M., Chalmers, T.C., Leevy, C.M., Sebastyen, S.C., Lieber, C.S. & Finland, M. (1960) Absorption of orally administered neomycin and kanamycin: with special reference to patients with severe hepatic and renal disease. *New England Journal of Medicine,* **262,** 380–385.
114. Kwaan, H.C., McFadzean, A.J.S. & Cook, J. (1956) Plasma fibrinolytic activity in cirrhosis of the liver. *Lancet,* **i,** 132–136.
115. Lancestremere, R.G., Davidson, P.L., Earley, L.E., O'Brien, F.J. & Papper, S. (1962) Renal failure in Laennec's cirrhosis. II. Simultaneous determination of cardiac output and renal haemodynamics. *Journal of Clinical Investigation,* **41,** 1922–1927.
116. Laragh, J.H. (1954) The effect of potassium chloride on hyponatraemia. *Journal of Clinical Investigation,* **33,** 807–818.
117. Laragh, J.H., Cannon, P.J., Bentzel, C.J., Sicinski, A.M. & Meltzer, J.I. (1963) Angiotensin II, norepinephrine, and renal transport of electrolytes and water in normal man and in cirrhosis with ascites. *Journal of Clinical Investigation,* **42,** 1179–1192.
118. Lawson, J.D. & Weissbein, A.S. (1959) The puddle sign: an aid in the early diagnosis of minimal ascites. *New England Journal of Medicine,* **260,** 652–654.
119. Lebrec, D., Kotelanski, B. & Cohn, J. (1976) Splanchnic haemodynamics in cirrhotic patients with esophageal varices and gastrointestinal bleeding. *Gastroenterology,* **70,** 1108–1111.
120. Lee, J. & Kerr, D.N.S. (1963) The concentration of vasopressin in the blood and the rate of urinary excretion of the hormone by patients with cirrhosis of the liver. *Clinical Science,* **25,** 375–384.
121. Lennane, R.J., Carey, R.M., Goodwin, T.J. & Peart, W.S. (1975) A comparison of natriuresis after oral and intravenous sodium loading in sodium-depleted man: evidence for a gastrointestinal or portal monitor of sodium intake. *Clinical Science and Molecular Medicine,* **49,** 437–440.
122. Lennane, R.J., Peart, W.S., Carey, R.M. & Shaw, J. (1975) A comparison of natriuresis after oral and intravenous sodium loading in sodium-depleted rabbits: evidence for a gastrointestinal or portal monitor of sodium intake. *Clinical Science and Molecular Medicine,* **49,** 433–436.
123. Leveen, H.H., Christoudias, G., Moon, I., Luft, R., Falk, G. & Grosberg, S. (1974) Peritoneo-venous shunting for ascites. *Annals of Surgery,* **180,** 580–590.
124. Levinsky, N.G. & Lalone, R.C. (1963) The mechanism of sodium diuresis after saline infusion in the dog. *Journal of Clinical Investigation,* **42,** 1261–1276.
125. Levy, V.G., Opolon, P., Pauleau, N. & Caroli, J. (1975) Treatment of ascites by reinfusion of concentrated peritoneal fluid – review of 318 procedures in 210 patients. *Postgraduate Medical Journal,* **51,** 564–566.
126. Lieberman, F.L. & Reynolds, T.B. (1967) Plasma volume in cirrhosis of the liver: its relation to portal hypertension, ascites and renal failure. *Journal of Clinical Investigation,* **46,** 1297–1308.
127. Lieberman, F.L., Ito, S. & Reynolds, T.B. (1969) Effective plasma volume in cirrhosis with ascites. Evidence that a decreased value does not account for renal sodium retention, a spontaneous reduction in glomerular filtration rate (GFR), and a fall in GFR during drug-induced diuresis. *Journal of Clinical Investigation,* **48,** 975–981.
128. Lieberman, F.L., Denison, E.K. & Reynolds, T.B. (1970) The relationship of plasma volume, portal hypertension, ascites, and renal sodium retention in cirrhosis. The overflow theory of ascites formation. *Annals of the New York Academy of Science,* **170,** 202–206.

129. Lieberman, F.L., Hidemura, R., Peters, R.L. & Reynolds, T.B. (1966) Pathogenesis and treatment of hydrothorax complicating cirrhosis with ascites. *Annals of Internal Medicine,* **64,** 341–351.
130. Liebowitz, H.R. (1965) Primary kidney disease in patients with cirrhosis of the liver. *New York State Journal of Medicine,* **65,** 535–541.
131. Liehr, H., Grün, M., Brunswig, D. & Sautter, Th. (1976) Endotoxinämie bei leberzirrhose. *Zeitschrift für gastroenterologie,* **14,** 14–26.
132. Lim, P. & Jacob, E. (1972) Magnesium deficiency in liver cirrhosis. *Quarterly Journal of Medicine,* **41,** 291–300.
133. Lim, P. & Jacob, E. (1972) Magnesium deficiency in patients on long-term diuretic therapy for heart failure. *British Medical Journal,* **iii,** 620–622.
134. Lucas, C.E., Rector, F.E., Werner, M. & Rosenberk, J.K. (1973) Altered renal homeostasis with acute sepsis: clinical significance. *Archives of Surgery,* **106,** 444–449.
135. Luetscher, J.A. & Johnson, B.B. (1954) Observations on the sodium retaining corticoid (aldosterone) in the urine of children and adults in relation to sodium balance and edema. *Journal of Clinical Investigation,* **33,** 1441–1446.
136. Lunzer, M., Newman, S.P. & Sherlock, S. (1973) Skeletal muscle blood flow and neurovascular reactivity in liver disease. *Gut,* **14,** 354–359.
137. Mackay, A. & Stevenson, R.D. (1977) Gastric ulceration induced by spironolactone. *Lancet,* **i,** 481 (correspondence).
138. Marson, F.G.W. (1954) Total adrenalectomy in hepatic cirrhosis with ascites. *Lancet,* **ii,** 847–848.
139. Mas, A., Arroyo, V., Rodes, J. & Bosch, J. (1975) Ascites and renal failure in primary liver cell carcinoma. *British Medical Journal,* **iii,** 629.
140. Mashford, M.L., Mahon, W.A. & Chalmers, T.C. (1962) Studies of the cardiovascular system in the hypotension of liver failure. *New England Journal of Medicine,* **267,** 1071–1074.
141. Massani, Z.M., Finkelman, S., Worcel, M., Agrest, A. & Paladini, A.C. (1966) Angiotensin blood levels in hypertensive and non-hypertensive disease. *Clinical Science,* **30,** 473–483.
142. McCloy, R.M., Baldus, W.P., Tauxe, W.N. & Summerskill, W.H.J. (1967) Plasma volume and renal circulatory function in cirrhosis. *Annals of Internal Medicine,* **66,** 307–311.
143. McCollister, R., Prasad, A.S., Doe, R.P. & Flink, E.B. (1958) Normal renal magnesium clearance and effect of water loading, chlorothiazide and ethanol on magnesium excretion. *Journal of Laboratory and Clinical Medicine,* **52,** 928 (abstract).
144. McDermott, W.V. (1958) The treatment of cirrhotic ascites by combined hepatic and portal decompression. *New England Journal of Medicine,* **259,** 897–901.
145. McKay, D.G. (1963) A partial synthesis of the generalised Shwartzman reaction. *Federation Proceedings,* **22,** 1373 1379.
146. McKay, D.G. & Shapiro, S.S. (1958) Alterations in the blood coagulation system induced by bacterial endotoxin. I. In vivo (generalised Shwartzman reaction). *Journal of Experimental Medicine,* **107,** 353–367.
147. Menigand, G., Morel-Maroger, L., Simon, J. & Deparis, M. (1970) Lésions rénales glomérulaires et cirrhose du foie. Note préliminaire sur les lésions histologiques du rein au cours des cirrhoses hépatiques d'après 20 prélèvements biopsiques. *Revue d'Études Cliniques et Biologiques,* **15,** 989–996.
148. Meyerson, H.S., Wolfram, C.G., Shirley, H.H. & Wasserman, K. (1960) Regional differences in capillary permeability. *American Journal of Physiology,* **198,** 155–160.
149. Milies, E. (1960) A new diuretic factor of hepatic origin. *Acta Physiologica Latinoamericana,* **10,** 178–193.
150. Moult, P.J.A., Parbhoo, S.P. & Sherlock, S. (1975) Clinical experience with the Rhone–Poulenc ascites reinfusion apparatus. *Postgraduate Medical Journal,* **51,** 574–576.
151. Murray-Lyon, I.M., Ockenden, B.G. & Williams, R. (1973) Congenital hepatic fibrosis – is it a single clinical entity? *Gastroenterology,* **64,** 653–656.
152. Nelson, W.P. & Welt, L.G. (1952) The effects of Pitressin on the metabolism and excretion of water and electrolytes in normal subjects and patients with cirrhosis and ascites. *Journal of Clinical Investigation,* **31,** 392–400.
153. Nelson, W.P., Rosenbaum, J.D. & Strauss, M.B. (1951) Hyponatraemia in hepatic cirrhosis following paracentesis. *Journal of Clinical Investigation,* **30,** 738–744.
154. Nix, J.T., Albert, M., Dugas, J.E. & Wendt, D.L. (1957) Chylothorax and chylous ascites; a study of 302 selected cases. *American Journal of Gastroenterology,* **28,** 40–53.
155. Oken, D.E., Mende, C.W., Taraba, I. & Flamenbaum, W. (1975) Resistance to acute renal failure accorded by prior renal failure: examination of the role of renal renin content. *Nephron,* **15,** 131–142.
156. Olcay, I., Kitahama, A., Miller, R.H., Drapanas, T., Trejo, R.A. & di Luzio, N.R. (1974 Reticulo-endothelial dysfunction and endotoxaemia following portal vein occlusion. *Surgery,* **75,** 64–70.
157. Onnis, M., Shumacker, H.B. & Bounous, G. (1962) Response to occlusion of the portal vein: blood pressure and renal blood flow. *Archives of Surgery,* **85,** 897–900.
158. Oster, J.R., Hotchkiss, J.L., Carbon, M. & Vaamonde, C.A. (1975) Abnormal renal acidification in alcoholic liver disease. *Journal of Laboratory and Clinical Medicine,* **85,** 987–1000.
159. Paddock, F.K. (1940) The diagnostic significance of serous fluids in disease. *New England Journal of Medicine,* **223,** 1010–1015.
160. Palmerio, C., Ming, S.C., Frank, E. & Fine, J. (1962) The role of the sympathetic nervous system in the generalised Shwartzmann reaction. *Journal of Experimental Medicine,* **115,** 609–612.
161. Pampligionie, G. (1973) The effect of metabolic disorders on brain activity. *Journal of the Royal College of Physicians of London,* **7,** 347–364.
162. Papper, S., Belsky, J.L. & Bleifer, K.H. (1959) Renal failure in Laennec's cirrhosis of the liver. I. Description of clinical and laboratory features. *Annals of Internal Medicine,* **51,** 759–773.
163. Patek, A.J., Seegal, D. & Bevans, M. (1951) The coexistence of cirrhosis of the liver and glomerulonephritis: report of 14 cases. *American Journal of Medical Science,* **221,** 77–85.
164. Péquingnot, G.E., Viallet, A., Combrisson, A. & Caroli, J. (1962) L'hypovolhémie relative des cirrhotiques hyperazotémiques. Circonstances d'apparition. In *Aktuelle Probleme der Hepatologie* (Ed.) Martini, G.A. & Sherlock, S., pp. 110–119. Stuttgart: Georg Thiene Verlag.

165. Peters, T.J., Seymour, C.A., Wells, G., Fakunle, F. & Neale, G. (1977) Gamma-glutamyltransferase levels in ascitic fluid and liver tissue from patients with primary hepatoma. *British Medical Journal*, **i**, 1576.

166. Prytz, H., Holst-Christensen, J., Korner, B. & Liehr, H. (1976) Portal venous and systemic endotoxaemia in patients without liver disease and systemic endotoxaemia in patients with cirrhosis. *Scandinavian Journal of Gastroenterology*, **11**, 857–863.

167. Radegran, K., Cronestrand, R. & Olsson, P. (1970) The effect of regional thrombin infusions on the renal vascular resistance. *European Journal of Surgical Research*, **2**, 460–472.

168. Ralli, E.P., Leslie, S.H., Stueck, G.H. & Laken, B. (1951) Studies of the serum and urine constituents in patients with cirrhosis of the liver during water tolerance tests. *American Journal of Medicine*, **11**, 157–169.

169. Ratnoff, O.D. & Patek, A.J. (1942) The natural history of Laennec's cirrhosis of the liver: an analysis of 386 cases. *Medicine* (Baltimore), **21**, 207–268.

170. Ravin, H., Rowley, D., Jenkins, C. & Fine, J. (1960) On the absorption of bacterial endotoxin from the gastrointestinal tract of the normal and shocked animal. *Journal of Experimental Medicine*, **112**, 783–792.

171. Reeves, G., Lowenstein, L.M. & Sommers, S.C. (1963) The macula densa and juxtaglomerular body in cirrhosis. *Archives of Internal Medicine*, **112**, 122–129.

172. Reynolds, T.B. (1974) The hepatorenal syndrome. In *The Liver and Its Diseases* (Ed.) Schaffner, F., Sherlock, S. & Leevy, C., pp. 307–313. New York: International Medical Book.

173. Reynolds, T.B., Lieberman, F.L. & Redeker, A.G. (1967) Functional renal failure with cirrhosis. The effect of plasma expansion therapy. *Medicine*, **46**, 191–196.

174. Ring-Larsen, H., Clausen, E. & Ranek, L. (1972) Peritoneal dialysis in hyponatraemia due to liver failure. *Scandinavian Journal of Gastroenterology*, **8**, 33–40.

175. Ring-Larsen, H., Hesse, B. & Stigsby, B. (1976) Effect of portal-systemic anastomosis on renal haemodynamics in cirrhosis. *Gut*, **17**, 856–860.

176. Roberti, A., Traverso, H., Vesin, P., Viguié, R. & Blanchon, P. (1966) Étude du Na et du K échangeables et des liquides extracellulaires dans les cirrhoses éthyliques. *Semaine des Hôpitaux de Paris*, **42**, 1714–1718.

177. Rocha, A.S. & Kokko, J.P. (1973) Sodium chloride and water transport in the medullary thick ascending limb of Henle. Evidence for active chloride transport. *Journal of Clinical Investigation*, **52**, 612–623.

178. Rodes, J., Bosch, J. & Arroyo, V. (1975) Clinical types and drug therapy of renal impairment in cirrhosis. *Postgraduate Medical Journal*, **51**, 492–498.

179. Rodes, J., Bruguera, M., Teres, J. & Bordas, J.M. (1970) La insufficiencia renal functional terminal de la cirrhosis hepatica con ascites. *Revista Clinica Espanola*, **117**, 475–482.

180. Rosoff, L., Zia, P., Reynolds, T. & Horton, R. (1975) Studies of renin and aldosterone in cirrhotic patients with ascites. *Gastroenterology*, **69**, 698–705.

181. Ryan, M.P., Whang, R. & Yamalis, W. (1973) Effect of magnesium deficiency on cardiac and skeletal muscle potassium during dietary potassium restriction. *Proceedings of the Society for Experimental Biology and Medicine*, **142**, 1045–1047.

182. Salomon, M.I., Sakaguchi, H., Churg, J., Dachs, S., Grishman, E., Mauntner, W., Paronetto, F. & Rosenthal, W.S. (1965) Renal lesions in hepatic disease: a study based on kidney biopsy. *Archives of Internal Medicine*, **115**, 704–709.

183. Sampliner, R.E. & Iber, F.L. (1974) High protein ascites in patients with uncomplicated hepatic cirrhosis. *American Journal of Medical Science*, **267**, 275–279.

184. Sanchez- Tapias, J.M. (1973) Estudio comparativo de la espirolactona y del triamterene en el tratamiento de la ascites en la cirrhosis hepatica. In *Fisiopatologia y tratamiento de la ascites* (Ed.) Rodes, J., Bosch, J. & Arroyo, V., pp. 105–114. Jorba: Spain.

185. Schedl, H.P. & Bartter, F.C. (1960) An explanation for and experimental correction of the abnormal water diuresis in cirrhosis. *Journal of Clinical Investigation*, **39**, 248–261.

186. Schroeder, E.T., Numann, L.J. & Chamberlain, B.E. (1970) Functional renal failure in cirrhosis: recovery after portacaval shunt. *Annals of Internal Medicine*, **72**, 923–928.

187. Schroeder, E.T., Shear, L., Sancetta, S.M. & Gabuzda, G.J. (1967) Renal failure in patients with cirrhosis of the liver. III. Evaluation of intrarenal blood flow by para-aminohippurate extraction and response to angiotensin. *American Journal of Medicine*, **43**, 887–896.

188. Schroeder, E.T., Eich, R.H., Smulyan, N., Gould, A.B. & Gabuzda, G.J. (1970) Plasma renin level in hepatic cirrhosis. *American Journal of Medicine*, **49**, 186–191.

189. Sealey, J.E. & Laragh, J.H. (1971) Further studies of a natriuretic substance occurring in human urine and plasma. *Circulation Research*, **28** (Suppl. II). 32–43.

190. Sein, M.M. (1973) Cervical lymphovenous shunt in intractable ascites – a clinical study. *British Journal of Surgery*, **60**, 900 (abstract).

191. Shear, L., Kleinerman, J. & Gabuzda, G.J. (1965) Renal failure in patients with cirrhosis of the liver. I. Clinical and pathologic characteristics. *American Journal of Medicine*, **39**, 184–198.

192. Shear, L., Bonkowsky, H.L. & Gabuzda, G.J. (1969) Renal tubular acidosis in cirrhosis: a determinant of susceptibility to recurrent hepatic precoma. *New England Journal of Medicine*, **280**, 1–7.

193. Shear, L., Ching, S. & Gabuzda, G.J. (1970) Compartmentalisation of ascites and edema in patients with hepatic cirrhosis. *New England Journal of Medicine*, **282**, 1391–1396.

194. Sheehan, H.L. (1946) Outbreak of Weil's disease in the British Army in Italy. I. Post-mortem and histological findings. *British Medical Journal*, **i**, 81–83.

195. Sherlock, S., Senewiratne, B., Scott, A. & Walker, J.G. (1966) Complications of diuretic therapy in hepatic cirrhosis. *Lancet*, **i**, 1049–1053.

196. Simpson, J.A. & Conn, H.O. (1968) The role of ascites in gastroesophageal reflux. With comments on the pathogenesis of bleeding esophageal varices. *Gastroenterology*, **55**, 17–25.

197. Sochocky, S. (1967) Tuberculous peritonitis: a review of 100 cases. *American Review of Respiratory Diseases*, **95**, 398–401.

198. Soler, N.G., Jain, S., James, H. & Paton, A. (1976) Potassium status of patients with cirrhosis. *Gut*, **17**, 152–157.

199. Sorensen, F.H., Andersen, J.B., Ornsholt, J. & Skjoldborg, H. (1971) Acute renal failure complicating biliary tract disorders. *Acta Chirurgica Scandinavica*, **137**, 87–91.

200. Stein, J.H., Osgood, R.W. & Kunau, R.T. (1976) Direct measurement of papillary collecting duct sodium transport in the rat. Evidence for heterogeneity of nephron function during Ringer loading. *Journal of Clinical Investigation*, **58**, 767–773.

201. Summerskill, W.H.J. & Baldus, W.P. (1975) Ascites. In *Diseases of the Liver*, 4th ed. (Ed.) Schiff, L., pp. 424–444. Philadelphia: Lippincott.

202. Thaler, H. & Fous, G. (1975) Experiences and problems in the management of ascites with the Rhodiascit machine. *Postgraduate Medical Journal*, **51**, 581–582.

203. Thiel, G., McDonald, F.D. & Oken, D.E. (1970) Micropuncture studies of the basis for protection of renin depleted rats from glycerol induced acute renal failure. *Nephron*, **7**, 67–79.

204. Triger, D.R., Alp, M.H. & Wright, R. (1972) Bacterial and dietary antibodies in liver disease. *Lancet*, **i**, 60–63.

205. Tristani, F.E. & Cohn, J.N. (1967) Systemic and renal haemodynamics in oliguric hepatic failure: effect of volume expansion. *Journal of Clinical Investigation*, **46**, 1894–1906.

206. Tsantoulas, D.C., McFarlane, I.G., Portmann, B., Eddleston, A.L.W.F. & Williams, R. (1974) Cell-mediated immunity to human Tamm-Horsfall glycoprotein in autoimmune liver disease with renal tubular acidosis. *British Medical Journal*, **iv**, 491–494.

207. Ulick, S., Laragh, J.H. & Lieberman, S. (1958) The isolation of a urinary metabolite of aldosterone and its use to measure the rate of secretion of aldosterone by the adrenal cortex of man. *Transactions of the Association of American Physicians*, **71**, 225–235.

208. Utili, R. Abernathy, C.O. & Zimmerman, H.J. (1976) Cholestatic effects of *Escherichia coli* endotoxin on the isolated perfused rat liver. *Gastroenterology*, **70**, 248–253.

209. van Waes, G., Schurgers, M. & Demeulenaere, L. (1975) The Rhodiascit system – individual response to reinfusion possibly related to angiotensin sensitivity. Preliminary results. *Postgraduate Medical Journal*, **51**, 567–570.

210. Ventura, E. & Zeneroli, M.L. (1975) Concentration-reinfusion (CR) of ascitic fluid in the treatment of decompensated liver cirrhosis with diuretic-resistant ascites. *Postgraduate Medical Journal*, **51**, 577–580.

211. Vecsei, P., Dusterdieck, G., Jahnecke, J., Lommer, D. & Wolff, H.P. (1969) Secretion and turnover of aldosterone in various pathological states. *Clinical Science*, **36**, 241–256.

212. Vesin, P. (1962) Late functional renal failure in cirrhosis with ascites: pathophysiology, diagnosis and treatment. In *Aktuelle Probleme der Hepatologie* (Ed.) Martini, G.A. & Sherlock, S., pp. 98–109. Stuttgart: Georg Thieme Verlag.

213. Vesin, P. (1975) In discussion. *Postgraduate Medical Journal*, **51**, 549.

214. Vesin, P., Roberti, A. & Viguie, R. (1969) Actions de l'amiloride (MK 870) sur le métabolisme hydro-électrolytique du cirrhotique ascitique. *Schweizerische Medizinische Wochenschrift*, **99**, 21–26.

215. Wardle, E.N. (1973) Fibrinogen and albumin catabolism in experimental pancreatitis in the rat. *Journal of Surgical Research*, **15**, 122–131.

216. Wardle, E.N. (1975) Endotoxinaemia and the pathogenesis of acute renal failure. *Quarterly Journal of Medicine*, **44**, 389–398.

217. Wardle, E.N. (1975) Renal failure in obstructive jaundice – pathogenic factors. *Postgraduate Medical Journal*, **51**, 512–514.

218. Wardle, E.N. & Wright, N.A. (1970) Endotoxin and acute renal failure in obstructive jaundice. *British Medical Journal*, **iv**, 472–474.

219. Wardle, E.N. & Wright, N.A. (1973a) Intravascular coagulation and glycerin hemoglobinuric acute renal failure. *Archives of Pathology*, **95**, 271–275.

220. Wardle, E.N. & Wright, N.A. (1973b) Role of fibrin in a model of pregnancy toxaemia in the rabbit. *American Journal of Obstetrics and Gynecology*, **115**, 17–26.

221. Warren, K.S., Iber, F.L., Dölle, W. & Sherlock. S. (1960) The effect of alterations in blood pH on the distribution of ammonia from blood to cerebrospinal fluid in patients with hepatic coma. *Journal of Laboratory and Clinical Medicine*, **56**, 687–694.

222. Warren, W.D., Foman, J.J., Viamonte, M., Martinez, L.O. & Kalser, M. (1968) Spontaneous reversal of portal venous blood flow in cirrhosis. *Surgery, Gynecology and Obstetrics*, **126**, 315–323.

223. Webster, L.T. & Gabuzda, G.J. (1959) Relation of azotemia to blood 'ammonium' in patients with hepatic cirrhosis. *Archives of Internal Medicine*, **103**, 15–22.

224. Wernze, H., Spech, H.J. & Müller, G. (1978) Studies on the activity of the renin–angiotensin–aldosterone system (RAAS) in patients with cirrhosis of the liver. *Klinische Wochenschrift*, **56**, 389–397.

225. Whang, R. & Welt, L.G. (1963) Observations on experimental magnesium deficiency. *Journal of Clinical Investigation*, **42**, 305–313.

226. Whang, R., Morosi, H.J., Rodgers, D. & Reyes, R. (1967) The influence of continuing magnesium deficiency on muscle potassium depletion. *Journal of Laboratory and Clinical Medicine*, **70**, 895–902.

227. Wheeler, P.G., Smith, T., Golindano, C., Alam, A.N., Wilkinson, S.P., Edmonds, C.J. & Williams, R. (1977) Potassium and magnesium depletion in patients with cirrhosis on maintenance diuretic regimes. *Gut*, **18**, 683–687.

228. Wilkinson, S.P. (1977) Liver disease and the kidney. *Medicine* (London) (2nd series), **29**, 1647–1652.

229. Wilkinson, P. & Sherlock, S. (1962) The effect of repeated albumin infusions in patients with cirrhosis. *Lancet*, **ii**, 1125–1129.

230. Wilkinson, S.P. Davies, M.H., Portmann, B. & Williams, R. (1978) Renal failure in otherwise uncomplicated acute viral hepatitis. *British Medical Journal*, **ii**, 338–341.

231. Wilkinson, S.P., Blendis, L.M. & Williams, R. (1974) Frequency and type of renal and electrolyte disorders in fulminant hepatic failure. *British Medical Journal*, **i**, 186–189.

232. Wilkinson, S.P., Davidson, A.R., Henderson, J. & Williams, R. (1975) Ascites reinfusion using the Rhodiascit apparatus – clinical experience and coagulation abnormalities. *Postgraduate Medical Journal,* **51,** 583–587.
233. Wilkinson, S.P., Moodie, H., Arroyo, V.A. & Williams, R. (1977) Frequency of renal impairment in paracetamol overdose compared with other causes of acute liver damage. *Journal of Clinical Pathology,* **30,** 141–143.
234. Wilkinson, S.P., Weston, M.J., Parsons, V. & Williams, R. (1977) Dialysis in the treatment of renal failure in patients with liver disease. *Clinical Nephrology,* **8,** 287–292.
235. Wilkinson, S.P., Hurst, D., Day, D.W. & Williams, R. (1978) The spectrum of renal tubular damage in renal failure secondary to cirrhosis and fulminant hepatic failure. *Journal of Clinical Pathology,* **31,** 101–107.
236. Wilkinson, S.P., Arroyo, V., Gazzard, B.G., Moodie, H. & Williams, R. (1974) Relation of renal impairment and haemorrhagic diathesis to endotoxaemia in fulminant hepatic failure. *Lancet,* **i,** 521–524.
237. Wilkinson, S.P., Moodie, H., Stamatakis, J.D., Kakkar, V.V. & Williams, R. (1976) Endotoxaemia and renal failure in cirrhosis and obstructive jaundice. *British Medical Journal,* **ii,** 1415–1418.
238. Wilkinson, S.P., Bernardi, M., Smith, I.K., Jowett, T.P., Slater, J.D.H. & Williams, R. (1977) Effect of β-adrenergic blocking drugs on the renin–aldosterone system, sodium excretion, and renal hemodynamics in cirrhosis with ascites. *Gastroenterology,* **73,** 659–663.
239. Wilkinson, S.P., Bernardi, M., Wheeler, P.G., Smith, I.K. & Williams, R. (1979) Diuretic-induced renal impairment without volume depletion in cirrhosis: changes in the renin-angiotensin system and the effect of β-adrenergic blockade. *Postgraduate Medical Journal,* **55,** 862–867.
240. Wilkinson, S.P., Jowett, T.P., Slater, J.D.H., Arroya, V., Moodie, H. & Williams, R. (1979) Renal sodium retention in cirrhosis: relation to aldosterone and nephron site. *Clinical Science,* **56,** 169–177.
241. Wilkinson, S.P., Smith, I.K., Clarke, M., Arroyo, V., Richardson, J., Moodie, H. & Williams, R. (1977) Intrarenal distribution of plasma flow in cirrhosis as measured by transit renography: relationship with plasma renin activity, and sodium and water excretion. *Clinical Science and Molecular Medicine,* **52,** 469–475.
242. Witte, C.L., Witte, M.H., Cole, W.R., Chung, Y.C., Bleisch, V.R. & Dumont, A.E. (1969) Dual origin of ascites in hepatic cirrhosis. *Surgery, Gynecology and Obstetrics,* **129,** 1027–1033.
243. Wolff, H.P., Koczorek, Kh.R. & Buchborn, E. (1958) Aldosterone and antidiuretic hormone (Adiuretin) in liver disease. *Acta Endocrinologica,* **27,** 45–58.
244. Wolff, H.P., Bette, L., Blaise, H., Düsterdieck, G., Jahnecke, J., Kobayashi, T., Krück, F., Lommer, D. & Schieffer, H. (1966) Role of aldosterone in edema formation. *Annals of the New York Academy of Science,* **139,** 285–294.
245. Zimmerman, H.J. & Thomas, L.J. (1950) The liver in pneumococcal pneumonia: observations in 94 cases on liver function and jaundice in pneumonia. *Journal of Laboratory and Clinical Medicine,* **35,** 556–567.

Chapter 47

Postoperative Jaundice

J. THOMAS LAMONT
KURT J. ISSELBACHER

Jaundice in the postoperative patient is a not uncommon, often perplexing and potentially serious complication of surgery and anaesthesia. The causes of postoperative jaundice vary and in most instances the exact aetiology cannot be determined. Clinical management is all the more difficult because these patients are often subject to a variety of stresses, such as hypotension, hypoxaemia, blood loss, infection, multiple drugs and anaesthetic agents, all of which are capable of damaging the liver. It is therefore important for the physician, surgeon and anaesthetist to recognize the pattern of liver injury that may occur following anaesthesia and surgery so that appropriate management can be undertaken. We will review in this chapter the hepatic complications of anaesthesia and surgery which occur in the immediate postoperative period, that is, within three weeks of surgery. Delayed postoperative liver disease which occurs more than three weeks after surgery, such as post-transfusion hepatitis (Chapter 28) or fatty liver following intestinal bypass surgery for obesity (Chapter 6), will be discussed elsewhere.

EFFECTS OF ANAESTHESIA AND SURGERY ON LIVER FUNCTION

All types of major anaesthesia, including general, spinal and epidural anaesthesia, cause a reduction in hepatic blood flow in animals and man.[8] This effect is mediated either by splanchnic vasoconstriction in the case of cyclopropane or nitrous oxide, or by decreased arterial blood pressure in the case of halothane, methoxyflurane, and spinal or epidural anaesthesia. These anaesthetic-induced changes in hepatic blood flow do not damage the normal liver. Price[40] demonstrated that ether or cyclopropane anaesthesia in healthy volunteers was not associated with a significant decrease in splanchnic oxygen consumption, although splanchnic blood flow was reduced. Similarly, methoxyflurane anaesthesia caused marked vasoconstriction of the hepatic artery and decreased hepatic blood flow although hepatic oxygen consumption was unchanged.[29] However, the effects of anaesthesia and surgery on oxygen consumption during an actual operation have not been studied.

Mild transient abnormalities of liver function tests are common after general anaesthesia and surgery. Abnormal excretion of BSP occurs within 48 hours of surgery in approximately 50 per cent of patients, and has been noted even after varicose vein stripping under spinal anaesthesia.[17] Minor elevations, usually less than 50 per cent above normal, in serum levels of transaminases, lactic dehydrogenase, alkaline phosphatase and bilirubin occur during the first postoperative week following a variety of surgical procedures.[25,32] These transient abnormalities are not associated with morphological alterations in the liver, and are usually of no clinical significance. Dawson[10] demonstrated that the incidence and degree of liver function abnormalities were not increased after halothane, compared to ether anaesthesia. Similarly, the duration of anaesthesia is not correlated with the degree of liver function abnormalities in the postoperative period.[18] Pre-existing liver disease[18] and operations in the upper abdomen[7] are associated with somewhat greater postoperative elevations of transaminases or bilirubin.[7,18] The cause of these transient and minor abnormalities of liver function is not known, but may relate to reductions in blood flow, mild systolic hypotension, transient hypoxaemia, or minor anaesthetic toxicity.

INCIDENCE AND PATHOPHYSIOLOGY OF POSTOPERATIVE JAUNDICE

The appearance of jaundice (bilirubin >2 mg per cent [34 μmol/l]) in the postoperative patient indicates a more serious derangement of liver function. The actual incidence of this complication varies with the patient population studied, and with the method used to detect jaundice. In a prospective study, Evans, Evans and Pollock[16] reported mild jaundice (serum bilirubin < 4 mg per cent [68 μmol/l]) in 17 per cent and severe jaundice (serum bilirubin > 4 mg per cent [68 μmol/l]) in 4 per cent of patients undergoing major surgery. Postoperative jaundice occurred in approximately 15 per cent of patients with acquired valvular heart disease undergoing open-heart surgery.[30,43] The incidence of postoperative jaundice following elective abdominal surgery is less than 1 per cent.[10]

A pathophysiological classification of postoperative jaundice is presented in Table 47.1. Hyperbilirubinaemia may be caused by three basic mechanisms: (a) over-production of bilirubin; (b) impaired excretion of bilirubin due to hepatocellular damage; and (c) extrahepatic obstruction. Several of these factors appear to contribute to postoperative jaundice, and in many cases it is difficult to establish a definitive diagnosis. One of the most important decisions for the clinician is to differentiate those patients who require surgical intervention for relief of mechanical obstruction from those with cholestasis due to liver injury, since re-operation in the latter group may be attended by very high morbidity and mortality. In general, most cases of postoperative jaundice are due to a combination of increased bilirubin load and hepatocellular dysfunction. Since the liver dysfunction almost always resolves spontaneously, an aggressive diagnostic and therapeutic approach is seldom indicated.

Table 47.1. *Classification of Postoperative Jaundice.*

1. Overproduction of bilirubin
   (a) Haemolytic anaemia
   (b) Haemolysis of transfused blood
   (c) Resorption of haematomas
2. Hepatocellular damage
   (a) Postoperative intrahepatic cholestasis
   (b) Circulatory failure
   (c) Halothane and methoxyflurane hepatitis
   (d) Drug-induced jaundice
   (e) Pre-existing liver disease
3. Extrahepatic obstruction
   (a) Common duct stone
   (b) Bile duct injury
   (c) Postoperative pancreatitis
4. Miscellaneous
   (a) Postoperative cholecystitis
   (b) Gilbert's syndrome

POSTOPERATIVE JAUNDICE FROM INCREASED BILIRUBIN PRODUCTION

Approximately 250 to 300 mg (427 to 513.0 μmol) of bilirubin is produced each day in the normal adult from the breakdown of senescent erythrocytes in the reticuloendothelial system. The liver is capable of conjugating and excreting at least several times this amount of bilirubin. For this reason, jaundice in patients with *haemolytic anaemia* is quite rare and seen only with massive haemolysis. Haemolytic anaemia as a cause of postoperative jaundice is unusual, but should be considered if the unconjugated bilirubin comprises[1] 90 per cent or more of total bilirubin, particularly in the presence of reticulocytosis. Patients with congenital deficiency of glucose-6-phosphate dehydrogenase may haemolyse when given certain drugs such as sulphonamides, chloramphenicol, nitrofurantoin or aspirin, or following anaesthesia and general surgery. Congenital haemolytic anaemias may also increase in severity during the postoperative period: this is particularly true of sickle cell anaemia which is worsened by the hypoxaemia, infection and trauma that may accompany surgery. Occasionally, brisk haemolysis can be accompanied by fever, severe abdominal or flank pain and tenderness ('sickle cell crisis'). This situation is easily confused with acute cholecystitis or a perforated viscus. Correct diagnosis is established by examination of the peripheral blood smear and haemoglobin electrophoresis.

Haemolysis of transfused erythrocytes is another cause of increased pigment load in the surgical patient. Approximately 10 per cent of erythrocytes in a unit of stored bank blood undergoes haemolysis within 24 hours of transfusion.[33] A 500 ml transfusion would be expected to liberate 7.5 g of haemoglobin, which in turn would be converted to 250 mg (427 μmol) of bilirubin. The normal liver can rapidly excrete this amount of extra bilirubin without an elevation of the serum bilirubin. However, multiple blood transfusions before or during surgery may result in massive pigment overload which exceeds the excretory capacity of the liver. Haemolysis would normally cause an elevation of the unconjugated bilirubin in an individual with normal liver function. In the setting of diffuse hepatocellular disease, however, or following major surgery, the liver may conjugate some of the increased bilirubin load but be unable to excrete it, with an elevation of both the unconjugated and conjugated serum bilirubin levels as a result.

Increased bilirubin production from *resorption of extravasated* blood may also contribute to postoperative jaundice in patients with severe crush injuries or ruptured aneurysms resulting in intra-abdominal or intrathoracic haematomas.[26] These patients are often in shock and in many cases show evidence of impaired renal function. The latter contributes to the severity and duration of the hyperbilirubinaemia.

POSTOPERATIVE JAUNDICE CAUSED BY HEPATOCELLULAR DAMAGE

The majority of cases of postoperative jaundice are caused by damage to the hepatocytes. This may occur before, during or after surgery. The injury may be manifested by a *hepatitis-like pattern* in which elevations of the serum transaminases and evidence of impaired synthetic function predominate; or there may be a *cholestatic pattern*, characterized by marked elevations of bilirubin and alkaline phosphatase. It should be noted that in many clinical situations a mixture of these two patterns may coexist. The pathophysiology of postoperative hepatic injury is complex and poorly understood. Although a number of aetiological factors have been suggested, including hypotension, hypoxaemia, infections and toxic or idiosyncratic effects of anaesthetic agents, the exact mechanisms of liver injury in the postoperative patient remain obscure.

Postoperative intrahepatic cholestasis. In 1950, Caroli described the occurrence of postoperative cholestatic jaundice which was attributed to an increased bilirubin load from blood transfusions.[6] Schmid described 11 similar cases of postoperative cholestasis occurring in a single hospital within an eight-month period, and felt that the jaundice resulted from transient hepatic secretory insufficiency.[45] The syndrome has also been described in burned patients,[58] following open-heart surgery[43] and after ruptured aortic aneurysm with extensive haematoma formation.[26] Although exact incidence figures are unavailable, this condition probably occurs once in every several hundred general surgical patients. The typical patient has had a major operation under general anaesthesia and has received several or more units of blood. Jaundice is first noted on the first or second postoperative day but may be delayed as long as seven to ten days following surgery. The serum bilirubin, which is predominantly conjugated, peaks on the seventh to tenth day and usually returns to normal by the second or third week. The serum levels of alkaline phosphatase and 5′-nucleotidase are elevated two- to fourfold, in contrast to transaminases, prothrombin time and albumin which are only mildly abnormal. Fever, hepatosplenomegaly or allergic manifestations such as urticaria, arthritis or eosinophilia are not observed.

Liver biopsy reveals the classical findings of cholestasis with enlargement of bile canaliculi and bile staining of the hepatocytes. Significant hepatocellular necrosis or inflammatory infiltrate are absent. These histological findings are quite non-specific: identical changes are observed in other types of cholestasis such as chlorpromazine jaundice or benign recurrent cholestasis of pregnancy. Erythrophagocytosis by Kupffer cells may be seen in massively-transfused patients and in those with large haematomas.[26]

A variety of aetiological factors have been implicated in the pathogenesis of postoperative intrahepatic cholestasis. Hypotension, hypoxaemia and blood transfusion are common elements in the majority of these patients. However, shock liver is characterized by centrilobular necrosis and elevation of transaminases,[15] features which are unusual in these patients. Sepsis may cause cholestasis, but is not a regular feature of postoperative intrahepatic cholestasis. Particularly puzzling is the occurrence of this entity in only a small fraction of surgical patients subject to similar operative stresses.

Proper recognition of postoperative intrahepatic cholestasis is most important, since the disease is self-limiting and uncomplicated in the vast majority of cases. During its initial stages, this entity cannot be distinguished on clinical grounds alone from extrahepatic bile duct obstruction due to common duct stone. Since immediate operation for common duct stone is rarely required unless sepsis is present, one is usually justified in watchful waiting. In doubtful cases or when jaundice is prolonged, ultrasound, a liver biopsy or a percutaneous, skinny needle or retrograde endoscopic cholangiogram should be performed. Obstructive jaundice after operations on the biliary tree represents a somewhat more difficult diagnostic dilemma since the common bile duct may have been inadvertently ligated or injured. The clinical picture of steadily increasing serum bilirubin to 30 mg per cent (513 μmol/l) or greater, accompanied by an enlarging liver and right upper quadrant or mid-epigastric pain should suggest the diagnosis of bile duct ligation. The presence of bile peritonitis indicates bile duct injury, and requires immediate surgical repair.

Postoperative jaundice due to circulatory failure. The liver is particularly susceptible to the effects of arterial hypotension. A fall in systemic arterial blood flow is accompanied by a drop in portal venous flow and oxygen content. In addition, there may be splanchnic vasoconstriction which further reduces blood flow to the liver from the hepatic artery. The net effect is diminished oxygen supply to the liver. This is most severe at the centre of the hepatic lobule in the hepatocytes surrounding the central vein since the oxygen tension in this area is normally lower than at the periphery of the lobule.

It is not surprising that the incidence of hepatic dysfunction and jaundice is particularly high after open-heart surgery or traumatic shock. In one large series of patients undergoing open-heart surgery for correction of valvular heart disease, the incidence of jaundice was 8.6 per cent.[43] The incidence and severity of the jaundice was related to the presence of pre-existing liver disease and the complexity of the surgery. Thus the incidence of jaundice was 8 per cent after mitral commissurotomy, 16 per cent after mitral valve replacement, 33 per cent after double valve replacement and 53 per cent after triple valve replacement. Clinically significant jaundice was reported by Nunes, Blaisdell and Margaretten[37] in 2 per cent of patients with surgical shock. The incidence of jaundice in shock is correlated with the duration of hypotension.

Postoperative jaundice after open-heart surgery or traumatic shock falls into two clinical patterns. The most common presentation is cholestatic jaundice characterized by early elevation of the bilirubin on the second or third postoperative day, with peak levels of 5 to 30 mg per cent (85 to 513.0 μmol/l) occurring on the seventh to tenth day. The alkaline phosphatase may be normal or only slightly elevated, and the transaminase is elevated two to three times above normal. This pattern is indistinguishable from postoperative intrahepatic cholestasis, and appears to be caused by a combination of increased pigment load from blood transfusions and mild hepatocellular dysfunction caused by transient hypotension and hypoxaemia. Another, more severe, pattern of postoperative jaundice occurs in patients who have prolonged shock lasting 12 hours or more. In these patients, the onset of jaundice is delayed to seven days or more following surgery, and is accompanied by laboratory evidence of severe hepatocellular necrosis with peak serum transaminase levels of 1000 or more units. Marked elevation of serum bilirubin may also occur. Death from hepatic failure is not uncommon; at autopsy the major finding is massive centrilobular necrosis with or without evidence of intrahepatic cholestasis. Patients with elevated right atrial pressures before and after open-heart surgery are particularly prone to develop centrilobular necrosis in the postoperative period.[30]

Halothane and methoxyflurane hepatitis. Soon after the introduction of halothane in England in 1956 and in the United States in 1958, scattered case reports were published of massive hepatic necrosis following its use.[4,50] In 1962, a nationwide, cooperative, retrospective study, the National Halothane Study,[48] was begun in the United States to investigate the possible association between halothane anaesthesia and postoperative hepatic necrosis. Case records from 34 hospitals covering the period 1959–1962 were scrutinized for evidence of massive liver necrosis occurring within six weeks of surgery. Of 850 500 anaesthetic administrations, only 82 cases of fatal postoperative massive liver necrosis were discovered, and of these, only nine could not be attributed to shock, hypoxia or pre-existing liver disease. Seven of these nine patients had received halothane, while in the entire series halothane was used in 30 per cent of patients. These data were interpreted as showing a possible causal relationship between halothane anaesthesia and massive liver necrosis. A second nationwide survey, the Fulminant Hepatic Failure Surveillance Study, suggested that halothane was responsible for approximately one-quarter of all cases of severe postoperative liver failure.[49]

The validity and interpretation of these studies have been challenged on several counts.[12,13] The histopathological findings in the liver in halothane hepatitis are non-specific and cannot be distinguished from acute viral hepatitis. Thus it is possible that some cases diagnosed as halothane hepatitis were in fact an exacerbation of previously undiagnosed viral hepatitis. The selection of cases for the National Halothane Study was not entirely random. Six of the seven cases of massive hepatic necrosis following halothane anaesthesia reported in the National Halothane Study were known to the participating hospital staff before the study began. The inclusion of these cases in the study might therefore have biased the data in favour of an association of massive liver necrosis and halothane.[13] Furthermore, several large retrospective studies failed to show an increased risk of hepatic complications in patients receiving halothane compared to other inhalation anaesthetics.[14,36]

Further support for the existence of halothane hepatitis as a distinct entity has come from several case reports of halothane hepatitis in anaesthetists who were chronically exposed to halothane during the course of their work. Klatskin and Kimberg[27] described a 44-year-old physician with recurrent hepatitis and cirrhosis who developed acute relapses of hepatitis upon exposure to halothane. Experimental challenge with a non-anaesthetic dose of halothane caused a relapse of the hepatitis manifested by chills, fever and liver biopsy evidence of acute hepatic necrosis. This case, as well as similar case reports of halothane hepatitis in an anaesthetist[2] and a laboratory worker[23] who developed acute hepatic necrosis upon re-challenge with halothane, supports the concept that rare individuals develop a hypersensitivity reaction to halothane manifested by hepatic necrosis. Although the existence of halothane hepatitis as a distinct clinical entity is challenged in certain quarters,[19] most hepatologists, anaesthetists and surgeons now agree that massive hepatic necrosis is a rare but definite complication of halothane anaesthesia. Because of its excellent anaesthetic properties and overall safety record, halothane continues to be widely used.

The true incidence of halothane hepatitis is unknown. The National Halothane Study discovered seven cases of fatal massive postoperative liver necrosis, presumably due to halothane, in 255 000 patients receiving halothane, an incidence of one case per 36 000. This figure is probably an underestimation, since only autopsy cases were studied and only 40 per cent of deaths were autopsied. Carney and vanDyke[5] compiled data from five retrospective studies of 146 000 administrations of halothane and found an incidence of halothane hepatitis of one in 2500, and of fatal liver necrosis of one in 11 000. Mild hepatic reactions to halothane are probably more frequent since low-grade postoperative fever and minimal transaminase elevations might not be included in retrospective studies of this type.

Multiple exposures to halothane, particularly within a short period of time, may increase the incidence and severity of the hepatitis. In a group of 360 women who underwent repetitive halothane anaesthesia during implantation of radioactive needles in the uterus, six developed postoperative hepatitis attributed to halothane.[22] The hepatic necrosis which occurs in sensitized individuals upon re-exposure to halothane appears to be specific, since exposure to other inhalation anaesthetics is not accompanied by evidence of hepatitis.[52] In several large series of halothane hepatitis, multiple exposure was noted in more than three-quarters of patients.[3,34,49] Obesity has also been noted in a large percentage of patients with halothane hepatitis.[34,39] Because of its lipid solubility, halothane is concentrated in adipose tissue. Thus, there may be delayed excretion of the drug in obese subjects. The disease is quite rare in the paediatric population and few well-documented cases have been reported, despite the fact that halothane is the most commonly used anaesthetic in the paediatric age group.[5]

In the typical case of halothane hepatitis, fever precedes jaundice by several days, and may be erroneously attributed to atelectasis or infection. The onset of jaundice is quite variable, but most often occurs within three to ten days of operation. Hepatitis which occurs more than three weeks after surgery is not likely to be related to halothane. Jaundice after a single exposure to halothane appears approximately two weeks after surgery, compared to one week after multiple exposures.[28] The patient may complain of nausea, malaise, anorexia or right upper quadrant pain. These symptoms may be quite variable and difficult to interpret in the early postoperative period following major surgery. Physical examination is unremarkable. The liver may be slightly enlarged, except in severe cases in which it is reduced in size.

The liver function tests reveal a direct hyperbilirubinaemia with peak values ranging between three and 30 mg per cent (51 to 513 μmol/l). Anicteric cases are seen and are usually associated with recovery, while bilirubin levels greater than 10 mg per cent (171.0 μmol/l) are associated with a poor prognosis. The serum transaminases are elevated to more than 500 units in the majority of cases, while the alkaline phosphatase is seldom elevated more than twofold. The most reliable indicators of the severity of halothane hepatitis are hypoprothrombinaemia and clinical or biochemical evidence of hepatic encephalopathy. Eosinophilia and a pruritic skin rash occasionally occur in patients and, in some, may be correlated with a history of multiple drug allergies. Antimitochondrial antibody, smooth muscle antibody and antinuclear antibody are sometimes detected in patients with halothane hepatitis. Recently, Walton et al[51] have reported a high incidence of liver and kidney microsomal antibodies and thyroid antibodies in patients with unexplained hepatitis following halothane.

The major histopathological findings in the liver of patients with halothane hepatitis are acute hepatocellular necrosis, often centrilobular, and mild inflammatory exudate. Ballooned hepatocytes and acidophilic bodies are frequently seen. These changes are indistinguishable from those seen in acute viral hepatitis, and therefore are of limited diagnostic value. Reticulin collapse and haemorrhage into the lobule occur in severe cases. Fatty infiltration is seen in approximately 10 to 15 per cent of cases.[28] The inflammatory exudate, composed of lymphocytes, macrophages and polymorphonuclear leucocytes, is most prominent in the portal tract, and may invade the limiting plate and extend into the lobule. Eosinophils, cholestasis and bile ductular proliferation are occasionally seen.

The clinical course of halothane hepatitis is similar to that of acute viral hepatitis except that the fatality rate is much higher. A fatal outcome is observed in 10 to 40 per cent of well-documented cases of jaundice. However, most retrospective series in the literature generally do not include cases with only febrile reactions and mild abnormalities of liver function. Death occurs within a week or two of onset. The terminal stage is characterized by deep coma, renal failure, haemorrhagic phenomena and sepsis. Since there is no specific therapy for halothane hepatitis, the management of these patients is identical to that of massive hepatic necrosis from any cause (see Chapter 27). Corticosteroids have not been beneficial, although this form of therapy has not been carefully studied. Exchange transfusion has also been tried in several cases but does not appear to improve salvage.[34] When recovery from halothane hepatitis does occur, it is usually complete; that is, chronic hepatitis or cirrhosis does not develop. The major goal of therapy in these patients is therefore to sustain life until the liver regenerates.

Halothane hepatitis must be differentiated from other causes of acute hepatic necrosis, including viral and drug hepatitis and shock liver. The interval between exposure to halothane and the onset of hepatitis is usually two weeks or less, which is much shorter than the incubation period for either hepatitis A or B virus. It is conceivable that, on a rare occasion, a patient might receive halothane anaesthesia during the incubation period of viral hepatitis; however, hepatitis B surface antigen has not been detected in cases of halothane hepatitis.[35] It is also unlikely that subclinical hepatitis A would masquerade as halothane hepatitis, since hepatitis A is most common in children and young adults, while halothane hepatitis is more common in the fourth and fifth decade. A possible role for other types of viral hepatitis (cytomegalovirus, EB viral hepatitis) as contributors to halothane hepatitis appears unlikely since these viruses rarely produce fulminant or fatal hepatitis (see Chapter 28).

Hepatic necrosis secondary to shock, hypoxaemia or acute right-sided heart failure may be difficult to differentiate from halothane hepatitis. The anaesthesia record should be carefully scrutinized for evidence of intraoperative hypotension, anoxia or heart failure. Coexistent hepatic and renal failure are sequelae of shock, but quite unusual in halothane hepatitis. Liver biopsy may be helpful in differentiating shock liver from halothane hepatitis.[1] Exposure to drugs other than halothane may cause acute hepatocellular necrosis in the postoperative patient.[49] Therefore, a careful drug history should be taken in order to rule out drug hepatitis.

Methoxyflurane (Penthrane), a halogenated anaesthetic agent related structurally to halothane, has been implicated as a cause of postoperative hepatic necrosis which resembles halothane hepatitis.[24] The usual clinical presentation is fever and jaundice occurring within three to seven days of operation, particularly following repeated exposure to the drug. Laboratory tests reveal evidence of hepatocellular damage with elevation of transaminases to 1000 units or more, prolongation of the prothrombin time and hyperbilirubinaemia (to levels of 15 mg per cent [256 μmol/l] or higher). Eosinophilia is seen in approximately 20 per cent of cases. Non-oliguric renal failure has been described after methoxyflurane anaesthesia[9] and may occur separately or in combination with hepatic necrosis. The renal tubular defect is characterized by passage of large amounts of urine of fixed specific gravity, dehydration and azotaemia in the immediate postoperative period. These abnormalities usually persist for two to three weeks and are followed by complete recovery. Apparent cross-sensitization to halothane is seen in some patients with methoxyflurane hepatitis who develop hepatic necrosis upon exposure to halothane.[24] Therefore, patients with suspected hepatic reactions to either halothane or methoxyflurane should be warned against future exposure to these agents.

The pathogenesis of halothane hepatitis is obscure. An allergic basis for halothane hepatitis is suggested by the following observations: (a) halothane hepatitis is more common, and occurs after a shorter interval in patients with multiple exposures to the agent; (b) re-challenge with small doses of halothane in patients with previous halothane hepatitis has resulted in evidence of prompt recurrence of hepatic damage;[2,27] (c) cross-sensitization to methoxyflurane, a related halogenated anaesthetic, has been reported;[24] and (d) occasionally, patients develop skin rash and eosinophilia suggestive of an acute drug hypersensitivity.

Paronetto and Popper[38] reported that halothane caused increased DNA synthesis in peripheral blood lymphocytes from 10 of 15 patients with halothane hepatitis, but not in lymphocytes from patients with various other liver diseases or from normal individuals. Antimitochondrial antibody was also present in a high proportion of patients with halothane hepatitis. These observations suggested that halothane sensitization of lymphocytes might be important in the pathogenesis of halothane hepatitis. However, abnormal lymphocyte transformation in halothane hepatitis has not been confirmed by other investigators.[31,35,51] The significance of the antimitochondrial and antimicrosomal antibodies is unclear (see Chapter 9).

The accumulation in rare individuals of toxic metabolites of halothane might also explain the hepatic necrosis in this disease. Approximately 10 to 15 per cent of halothane is metabolized to trifluoroacetic acid and bromide which are excreted in the urine and are detectable for as long as 12 days after administration of halothane.[41]

Administration of halothane to experimental animals and to the vast majority of human beings does not cause liver damage. However, it is possible that rare individuals might metabolize the compound to a toxic intermediate capable of damaging the liver. Sipes[47] reported that rats pre-treated with polychlorinated biphenyl, which enhanced the hepatic microsomal drug-metabolizing enzymes, developed massive hepatic necrosis after halothane, while control rats given halothane alone remained normal. The pre-treated rats had a significant increase in cytochrome P-450 and cytochrome *c* reductase in the liver, which may have altered the metabolism of halothane in the liver and caused accumulation of a toxic metabolite.

Drug-induced jaundice in the postoperative patient. *Drug-induced hepatitis* is often difficult to exclude as a cause of postoperative jaundice. Surgical patients usually receive several drugs before, during and after surgery which are capable of damaging the liver. In a retrospective study of fulminant postoperative hepatic failure, drugs (excluding halothane) were implicated as the primary cause of liver failure in 8 per cent of patients.[49] The offending drugs included sulfisoxazole, chloramphenicol, para-aminosalicylic acid, isoniazid and ethchlorvynol. The diagnosis of drug hepatitis is often tentative and requires careful exclusion of other causes of liver disease.

Drug-induced hepatic injury is manifested clinically by either a cholestatic pattern, or a hepatitis-like pattern. The phenothiazines are the most frequent cause of drug-induced cholestasis, and produce increases in the serum bilirubin and alkaline phosphatase levels comparable to those seen in extrahepatic biliary obstruction. Chlorothiazide, chlorthalidone, methyltestosterone and nitrofurantoin are also capable of causing drug cholestasis. A hepatitic-like presentation is the most common manifestation of drug-induced liver disease. The clinical features are similar to those of acute viral hepatitis, with striking elevations of the transaminases and, in severe cases, clinical and biochemical evidence of acute hepatic failure. Many drugs, including isoniazid, para-aminosalicylic acid, sulphonamides, tetracycline and methyldopa, are capable of causing drug hepatitis. Occasionally, features of both cholestasis and a hepatitis-like picture may be present.

The diagnosis of drug jaundice is confirmed if the abnormalities of liver function recur after re-challenge with the drug. However, deliberate re-challenge with a drug is rarely indicated or appropriate because the hepatic reaction may be serious or fatal. Careful scrutiny of the hospital record may reveal evidence of hepatic damage during previous administrations of the drug. An important diagnostic finding in drug hepatitis is the presence of fever, skin rash and eosinophilia, particularly at the onset of jaundice. Liver biopsy is of limited usefulness in drug-induced postoperative jaundice since the histological findings are seldom specific.

Postoperative jaundice in patients with pre-existing liver disease. Patients with pre-existing liver disease are generally at high risk for the development of postoperative jaundice. As might be expected, this is particularly true for patients with *cirrhosis* who undergo surgery for treatment of portal hypertension and bleeding oesophageal varices. Mild to moderate elevations of serum bilirubin, alkaline phosphatase and prothrombin time were noted more frequently in cirrhotic patients following a portacaval shunt procedure than in individuals with normal liver function undergoing cholecystectomy.[18] The postoperative course in the cirrhotic patient may be complicated by the appearance or worsening of ascites, renal failure, hepatic encephalopathy or diffuse bleeding from hypoprothrombinaemia.

The diagnosis of *acute viral hepatitis* should be considered a relatively serious contra-indication to surgery except in life-threatening situations. Surgery in patients with acute or subacute viral hepatitis is attended by an unacceptably high postoperative morbidity and mortality rate.[23] The presence of significant preoperative hypoalbuminaemia or hypo-prothrombinaemia in patients with acute viral hepatitis increases the risk of surgery. Since the majority of cases of viral hepatitis are anicteric and have only mild, non-specific symptoms, it is recommended that all patients undergoing elective surgery be screened preoperatively with measurements of serum transaminase, alkaline phosphatase and bilirubin levels. Schemel[44] found significant liver function test abnormalities in 1 in 700 patients admitted for elective surgery. These patients were asymptomatic as regards liver disease, but had significant abnormalities on liver biopsy.

When a patient with known liver disease requires surgery, special attention should be given to careful preoperative correction of anaemia, hypoprothrombinaemia, hypo-albuminaemia and electrolyte disturbances. Hypotension and hypoxaemia should be avoided because of their potential for damaging the hepatocyte. There is no evidence that halothane anaesthesia is more dangerous in the patient with pre-existing liver disease or in patients undergoing biliary tract surgery. Many physicians avoid its use in these patients, however, because of the potential difficulty in interpreting changes in liver function tests in the postoperative period.

POSTOPERATIVE JAUNDICE DUE TO BILIARY TRACT OBSTRUCTION

Blockage of the extra-hepatic biliary tree is a rare cause of postoperative jaundice, but is nonetheless important because surgical re-exploration is usually required. *Retained common bile duct stones* usually present as persistent jaundice following cholecystectomy or exploration of the common bile duct. Postoperative intrahepatic cholestasis can easily be confused with bile duct obstruction; therefore, the diagnosis of retained common duct stone should be established by cholangiography prior to re-operation.

Bile duct injury may occur during cholecystectomy, common duct exploration or other operations in the upper abdomen. The injury is often unrecognized at operation, and declares itself in the early postoperative period with jaundice, biliary fistula or bile peritonitis. If the bile duct is ligated, obstructive jaundice will appear within several days of operation and rapidly worsen. Transection of the bile duct results in a biliary fistula which may drain externally around the T-tube, or form a large collection of bile within the peritoneal cavity. The proper management of injury to the biliary collecting system is prompt surgical repair in order to prevent permanent damage to the liver (see Chapters 54 and 55).

Acute postoperative pancreatitis is an unusual complication of abdominal surgery, and is accompanied by jaundice in approximately 30 per cent of patients.[42] The cause of pancreatic inflammation after surgery unrelated to the pancreas is unknown. Direct intra-operative trauma to the gland or its ducts, or interference with the blood supply, has been implicated in its pathogenesis. Jaundice, usually low grade, results from minor obstruction to the common bile duct by inflammatory oedema at the head of the pancreas.

MISCELLANEOUS CAUSES OF POSTOPERATIVE JAUNDICE

Several rare conditions may be associated with postoperative jaundice. *Postoperative cholecystitis* may appear three to 30 days after surgery unrelated to the gallbladder or biliary tree. The typical patient is middle aged or elderly and has undergone an orthopaedic procedure. The onset of cholecystitis is heralded by anorexia, fever and right upper quadrant pain and tenderness. Liver function abnormalities include mild elevations of the serum transaminases and alkaline phosphatase, and variable elevations of the bilirubin, which rarely exceed 5 mg per cent (85 μmol/l). The mechanism of jaundice in this condition is obscure. Obstruction of the common bile duct is not observed. Acalculous cholecystitis is found in approximately half of these patients. Gangrene of the gallbladder is not uncommon, and accounted for a mortality rate of 20 per cent in a series reported by Howard and Delaney.[21]

Gilbert's syndrome is a common congenital disorder characterized by mild unconjugated hyperbilirubinaemia. These patients are asymptomatic, and other liver function tests and liver biopsy are normal. The total serum bilirubin is often less than 2 mg per cent (34.0 μmol/l); hence, the patient and physician may be unaware of the presence of Gilbert's syndrome. Fasting, infections or surgery may cause elevation of the unconjugated bilirubin to a level where jaundice becomes clinically evident. The jaundice improves as oral feedings are resumed or infections controlled, and extensive diagnostic procedures are not generally indicated. Since an increase in serum bilirubin in the postoperative period is quite likely in these patients, the importance of recognizing this condition preoperatively is obvious (see Chapter 13).

REFERENCES

1. Babior, B.M. & Davidson, C.S. (1967) Postoperative massive liver necrosis. *New England Journal of Medicine*, **276,** 645–652.
2. Belfrage, S., Ahlgren, I. & Axelson, S. (1966) Halothane hepatitis in an anaesthetist. *Lancet*, **ii,** 1466–1467.
3. Bottiger, L.E., Dalen, E. & Hallen, B. (1976) Halothane-induced liver damage: an analysis of the material reported to the Swedish adverse drug reaction committee, 1966–1973. *Acta Anaesthesiologica Scandinavica*, **20,** 40–46.
4. Burnap, T.K., Galla, S.J. & van Dam, L.D. (1958) Anesthetic, circulatory and respiratory effects of Fluothane. *Anesthesiology*, **19,** 307–310.
5. Carney, F.M.T. & vanDyke, R.A. (1972) Halothane hepatitis: a critical review. *Anesthesia and Analgesia*, **51,** 135–160.
6. Caroli, J., Paraf, A., Champeau, J. & Desvigues, M. (1950) Les ictères de la gastrectomie. *Archives de Maladies de l'Appareil Digestif*, **39,** 1057–1085.
7. Clarke, R.S.J., Doggart, J.R. & Lavery, T. (1976) Changes in liver function after different types of surgery. *British Journal of Anaesthesiology*, **48,** 119–127.
8. Cooperman, L.H., Wollman, H. & Marsh, M.L. (1977) Anesthesia and the liver. *Surgical Clinics of North America*, **57,** 421–438.
9. Crandall, W.B., Pappas, S.G. & MacDonald, A. (1966) Nephrotoxicity associated with methoxyflurane anesthesia. *Anesthesiology*, **27,** 591–607.
10. Dawson, B., Adson, M.A., Dockerty, M.B., Fleisher, G.A., Jones, R.R., Hartridge, V.B., Schnelle, N., McGuckin, W.F. & Summerskill, W.H.J. (1966) Hepatic function tests: postoperative changes with halothane or diethyl ether anesthesia. *Mayo Clinic Proceedings*, **41,** 599–607.
11. Duncan, W.A. & Raventos, J. (1959) The pharmacokinetics of halothane 'Fluothane' anaesthesia. *British Journal of Anaesthesia*, **31,** 302–313.
12. Dykes, M.H.M., Gilbert, J.P. & McPeek, B. (1972a) Halothane in the United States. *British Journal of Anaesthesia*, **44,** 925–934.
13. Dykes, M.H.M., Gilbert, J.P., Schur, P.H. & Cohen, E.N. (1972b) Halothane and the liver: a review of the epidemiologic, immunologic and metabolic aspects of the relationship. *Canadian Journal of Surgery*, **15,** 217–238.
14. Dykes, M.H.M., Wilzer, S.G., Slater, E.M., Gibson, J.M. & Ellis, D.S. (1965) Acute parenchymatous hepatic disease following general anesthesia. *Journal of the American Medical Association*, **193,** 339–344.
15. Ellenberg, M. & Osserman, K.E. (1951) Role of shock in the production of central liver cell necrosis. *American Journal of Medicine*, **11,** 170–188.
16. Evans, C., Evans, M. & Pollock, A.V. (1974) The incidence and causes of postoperative jaundice. *British Journal of Anaesthesia*, **46,** 520–525.
17. Fairlie, C.W., Barss, T.P., French, A.B., Jones, C.M. & Beecher, H.K. (1951) Metabolic effects of anesthesia in man. IV. A comparison of the effects of certain anesthetic agents on the normal liver. *New England Journal of Medicine*, **17,** 615–622.
18. French, A.B., Barss, T.P., Fairlie, C.S., Bengle, A.L., Jones, C.M., Linton, R.P. & Beecher, H.K. (1952) Metabolic effects of anesthesia in man. V. A comparison of the effects of ether and cyclopropane anesthesia on the abnormal liver. *Annals of Surgery*, **135,** 145–163.

19. Halothane and liver damage (1974) *British Medical Journal*, **ii**, 589–590.
20. Harville, D.D. & Summerskill, W.H. (1963) Surgery in acute hepatitis, causes and effects. *Journal of the American Medical Association*, **184**, 258–261.
21. Howard, R.J. & Delaney, J.P. (1972) Postoperative cholecystitis. *American Journal of Digestive Diseases*, **17**, 213–218.
22. Hughes, M. & Powell, L.W. (1970) Recurrent hepatitis in patients receiving multiple halothane anesthetics for radium treatment of carcinoma of the cervix uteri. *Gastroenterology*, **58**, 790–797.
23. Johnston, C.I. & Mendelsohn, F. (1971) Halothane hepatitis in a laboratory technician. *Australian and New Zealand Journal of Medicine*, **1**, 171–173.
24. Joshi, P.H. & Conn, H. (1974) The syndrome of methoxyflurane-associated hepatitis. *Annals of Internal Medicine*, **80**, 395–401.
25. Kalow, B., Rogoman, E. & Sims, F.H. (1976) A comparison of the effects of halothane and other anesthetic agents on hepatocellular function in patients submitted to elective operations. *Canadian Anaesthetic Society Journal*, **23**, 71–79.
26. Kantrowitz, P.A., Jones, W.A., Greenberger, N.J. & Isselbacher, K.J. (1967) Severe postoperative hyperbilirubinemia simulating obstructive jaundice. *New England Journal of Medicine*, **276**, 591–598.
27. Klatskin, G. & Kimberg, O. (1969) Recurrent hepatitis attributable to halothane sensitization in an anesthetist. *New England Journal of Medicine*, **280**, 515–522.
28. Klion, F.M., Schaffner, F. & Popper, H. (1969) Hepatitis after exposure to halothane. *Annals of Internal Medicine*, **71**, 467–477.
29. Libonati, M., Malsch, E., Price, H.L., Cooperman, L.H., Baum, S. & Harp, V.R. (1973) Splanchnic circulation in man during methoxyflurane anesthesia. *Anesthesiology*, **38**, 466–469.
30. Lockey, E., McIntyre, N., Ross, O.N., Brooks, E. & Sturridge, M.F. (1967) Early jaundice after open heart surgery. *Thorax*, **22**, 165–169.
31. Marschall, K.E., Matthieu, A. & van Dam, L.O. (1976) Recurrent B-negative hepatitis after halothane anesthesia: apparent failure to demonstrate altered sensitivity. *Anesthesiology*, **44**, 336–339.
32. McEwan, J. (1976) Liver function tests following anaesthesia. *British Journal of Anesthesia*, **48**, 1065–1070.
33. Mollison, P.L. (1962) *Blood Transfusion in Clinical Medicine*. Philadelphia: F.A. Davis.
34. Moult, P.J.A. & Sherlock, S. (1975) Halothane-related hepatitis. *Quarterly Journal of Medicine*, **44**, 99–114.
35. Moult, P.J.A., Adjukiewicz, A.B., Gaylarde, P.M., Sarkany, I. & Sherlock, S. (1975) Lymphocyte transformation in halothane-related hepatitis. *British Medical Journal*, **i**, 69–70.
36. Mushin, W.W., Rosen, M., Bowen, D.J. & Campbell, H. (1964) Halothane and liver dysfunction: a retrospective study. *British Medical Journal*, **ii**, 329–341.
37. Nunes, G., Blaisdell, F.W. & Margaretten, W. (1970) Mechanism of hepatic dysfunction following shock and trauma. *Archives of Surgery*, **100**, 546–556.
38. Paronetto, F. & Popper, H. (1970) Lymphocyte stimulation induced by halothane in patients with hepatitis following exposure to halothane. *New England Journal of Medicine*, **283**, 277–280.
39. Peters, R.L., Edmondson, H.A., Reynolds, T.B., Meister, J.C. & Curphey, T.J. (1969) Hepatic necrosis associated with halothane anesthesia. *American Journal of Medicine*, **47**, 748–764.
40. Price, H.L., Deutsch, S., Davidson, M.B., Clement, A.J., Behar, M.G. & Epstein, R.M. (1966) Can general anesthetics produce splanchnic visceral hypoxia by reducing regional blood flow? *Anesthesiology*, **27**, 24–30.
41. Rehder, K., Forbes, J., Alter, H., Hessler, O. & Stier, A. (1967) Halothane biotransformation in man: quantitative study. *Anesthesiology*, **28**, 711–715.
42. Saidi, F. & Donaldson, G.A. (1963) Acute pancreatitis following distal gastrectomy for benign ulcer. *American Journal of Surgery*, **105**, 87–96.
43. Sanderson, R.G., Ellison, J.H., Benson, J.A. & Starr, A. (1967) Jaundice following open heart surgery. *Annals of Surgery*, **165**, 217–224.
44. Schemel, W.H. (1976) Unexpected hepatic dysfunction found by multiple laboratory screening. *Anesthesia and Analgesia*, **55**, 810–812.
45. Schmid, M., Hefti, M.L., Gattiker, R., Kistler, H.J. & Senning, A. (1965) Benign postoperative intrahepatic cholestasis. *New England Journal of Medicine*, **272**, 545–550.
46. Sevitt, S. (1958) Hepatic jaundice after blood transfusion in injured and burned subjects. *British Journal of Surgery*, **46**, 68–74.
47. Sipes, I.G. & Brown, B.R. (1976) An animal model of hepatotoxicity associated with halothane anesthesia. *Anesthesiology*, **45**, 622–628.
48. Summary of the National Halothane Study (1966) *Journal of the American Medical Association*, **197**, 775–788.
49. Trey, C., Lipworth, L., Chalmers, T.C., Davidson, C.S., Gottlieb, L.S., Popper, H. & Saunders, S.J. (1968) Fulminant hepatic failure. *New England Journal of Medicine*, **279**, 798–801.
50. Virtue, R. & Payne, K.W. (1958) Postoperative death after Fluothane. *Anesthesiology*, **19**, 562–565.
51. Walton, B., Simpson, B.R., Strunin, L., Doniach, G., Perrin, J. & Appleyard, A.J. (1976) Unexplained hepatitis following halothane. *British Medical Journal*, **i**, 1171–1176.
52. Wright, R., Chisholm, M., Lloyd, B., Edwards, T., Eade, O., Hawksley, M., Moles, T. & Gardner, M. (1975) Controlled prospective study of the effect on liver function of multiple exposures to halothane. *Lancet*, **ii**, 817–820.

Chapter 48

Anaesthetic Management of Patients with Liver Disease

LEO STRUNIN

It is probable that most surgical procedures, whether carried out under a local or general anaesthetic technique, are followed by adverse changes in liver function. In the vast majority of cases these changes are of a minor nature, are rapidly reversed, and can be related to the extent of the surgical procedure.[12] In the patient with pre-existing liver disease anaesthesia and surgery may be followed by a severe deterioration in liver function and, on occasion, the development of acute liver failure. Assessment of liver function is not always straightforward and pre-existing liver disease may not be readily apparent. Nevertheless, certain presenting signs and symptoms should be looked for so that appropriate steps may be taken before, during and after anaesthesia so as to minimize any possible detrimental effects (Table 48.1).

DRUG METABOLISM

Although the exact mode and site of action of anaesthetic agents are still a matter for speculation, it is accepted that lipid solubility is a key factor. The central role of the liver in transforming lipid-soluble compounds to more water-soluble (polar) compounds is well established. This transformation is usually described as metabolism, or may be referred to as biological transformation or biotransformation. It is unlikely that such metabolism is concerned directly in producing anaesthesia but disturbance in liver function may lead to prolonged action of drugs. Furthermore, since the majority of drugs are protein bound at some stage during their passage in the body, any alteration in protein binding sites, such as may occur in certain forms of liver disease, may also affect the action of drugs. Finally, drug metabolism usually gives rise to compounds with a higher molecular weight than the original substance. Molecular size and polarity are important factors in determining the extent of biliary excretion of a compound. Compounds with a molecular weight below 310 are poorly excreted by the liver, whereas for those with a molecular weight between 500 and 1000 excretion is predominantly hepatic. Therefore, any anaesthetic drugs which rely on biliary excretion may have prolonged effects in patients with obstructive jaundice where surgical intervention is contemplated.

Premedication

It is often stated that analgesic, sedative and narcotic drugs (in particular morphine) should not be given to patients with liver disease as unwanted effects will occur. Such advice may be misleading. Patients with well-compensated liver disease will tolerate such drugs well and it is only when decompensation occurs that problems may arise. Of the liver function tests available, serum albumin may be a useful index,[8] low serum albumin levels being associated with prolonged action of drugs.

It is the author's habit to use pethidine and promethazine for premedication of patients with compensated liver disease. The response to pethidine may be helpful in determining what

Table 48.1. *Factors Relevant to the Anaesthetist in Patients with Liver Disease.*

Drug metabolism
Effects of anaesthesia on liver blood flow
Obstructive jaundice
Chronic liver disease
Major liver surgery
The HB_sAg-positive patient
Acute liver failure
Previous history of jaundice

dose of this analgesic may be used in the postoperative period. Promethazine, a phenothiazine, can cause cholestatic jaundice;[35] however, the incidence of this complication is probably less than 0.5 per cent of patients receiving the drug and is not related to the presence of pre-existing hepatic disease.

Intravenous induction agents

All the commonly used intravenous anaesthetic induction agents are metabolized by the liver. This metabolism takes place within the liver itself or as a result of enzymes produced by the liver; for example, cholinesterase is responsible for the metabolism of propanidid. In general, after single doses of intravenous induction agents, recovery from anaesthesia is a feature of redistribution of the drug rather than of its metabolism. Thiopentone metabolism proceeds at a relatively slow and fixed rate – about 15 per cent/hour.[53] Methohexitone is metabolized somewhat more rapidly and its metabolism does contribute to some extent to recovery from anaesthesia.[9]

Intravenous induction agents, such as thiopentone or Althesin, may be safely given to patients with compensated liver disease and prolonged action is unlikely.[58] Indeed, increased doses may be required because of enhanced protein binding. However, as with all sedative drugs, there may be prolonged action and depression of conscious level when intravenous anaesthetic agents are administered to patients with decompensated liver disease. If there is any doubt concerning a patient's liver function, small doses only should be given.

Non-depolarizing neuromuscular blocking drugs

Dundee and Gray[18] were the first to describe an apparent resistance of patients with liver damage to non-depolarizing muscle relaxant drugs; in this instance, *d*-tubocurarine. Similar resistance, necessitating increased doses, has also been described for pancuronium.[46,58]

The mechanism of 'curare resistance' in patients with liver disease is not entirely clear. Dundee and Gray[18] suggested that the increased requirement for *d*-tubocurarine was a result of the low pseudocholinesterase concentration sometimes found in chronic liver disease, causing an increased amount of acetylcholine at the motor end-plate to compete with *d*-tubocurarine. Since end-plate or true cholinesterase is not produced by the liver, and as patients with liver disease do not have clinical signs of end-plate sensitivity to acetylcholine, this explanation is unlikely. As an alternative, increased protein binding of muscle relaxants to the increased amount of globulin, characteristic of chronic liver disease, has been postulated.[3,6] Feldman[27] proposed that it was sequestration of *d*-tubocurarine in the enlarged liver and spleen often found in patients with chronic liver disease that led to an increased requirement for the drug. An alternative explanation relates to the volume of distribution of neuromuscular blocking drugs, which may be impaired in patients with liver disease, particularly in those with some concomitant renal disturbance.

For the various reasons quoted above, large doses of non-depolarizing muscle relaxant drugs may be given to patients with liver damage and problems may be encountered in antagonizing their effects at the end of surgery.[58] It should be noted that both *d*-tubocurarine and pancuronium are mainly excreted in the urine,[2,36] but biliary excretion may be of some relevance. It is perhaps sensible, therefore, to exercise caution in administering large doses of non-depolarizing muscle relaxant drugs to patients with chronic liver disease, particularly those with biliary obstruction.

Local anaesthetics

Ester type drugs (for example, procaine) are primarily hydrolysed, either in the plasma or in the liver, by cholinesterase. Amide type drugs (for example, lignocaine) are metabolized in the liver. In theory, therefore, patients with liver disease might have difficulty in metabolizing both types of local anaesthetic drugs. In practice, unwanted effects of local anaesthetics are almost entirely accounted for by overdosage, errors of technique or the effects of vasoconstrictors, particularly adrenaline, and rarely by allergy to individual drugs.[54] As far as metabolism is concerned the doses of local anaesthetic drugs normally employed are not likely to give rise to difficulties when used for local or regional anaesthesia. However, infusions of lignocaine are used in the treatment of cardiac dysrhythmias. In this situation, pre-existing heart failure and/or liver disease decrease the dose requirements of lignocaine.[57]

EFFECTS OF ANAESTHESIA ON LIVER BLOOD FLOW

The splanchnic organs are the gastrointestinal tract, spleen, pancreas, gallbladder, omentum and liver. The blood flowing through these organs constitutes the splanchnic blood flow (SBF). It is not usual to measure the total arterial flow, but rather the liver blood flow (LBF). Since all the arterial supply of the splanchnic organs, other than the liver, eventually drain into the liver, SBF and LBF are usually considered as interchangeable terms.[13] LBF is usually taken to mean blood flow in the hepatic artery plus that in the portal vein. LBF is related directly to perfusion pressure and inversely to splanchnic vascular resistance. The portal vein which supplies some 70 per cent of the liver blood flow is a low-pressure system and derives its supply from the splenic and superior mesenteric veins. These in turn collect blood from the spleen and gastrointestinal tract, which are supplied in their turn by high-pressure arteries, the splenic, right and left gastric, pancreaticoduodenal superior mesenteric and inferior mesenteric. If the splenic and gastrointestinal tract vascular systems increase their resistance then portal vein blood flow will fall. The hepatic artery which supplies some 30 per cent of the liver's blood supply is a direct high-pressure system. A reduction in liver blood flow could be due to a decrease either in the portal vein or hepatic artery perfusion pressures. These in turn can be due to reduced systemic arterial or increased hepatic venous pressures, the latter arising, for example, due to right-sided heart failure. During anaesthesia and surgery a number of factors may affect the complex mechanisms involved in control of liver blood flow (Table 48.2).

Table 48.2. *Factors Influencing Liver Blood Flow During Anaesthesia and Surgery.*

Cardiac output
Sympathetic nervous system activity
Ventilation
Splanchnic reflexes
Anaesthetic agents
Surgical manipulation

Sympathetic nervous activity

The splanchnic vascular bed and the hepatic artery are richly innervated by the sympathetic nervous system and contain both α- and β-adrenergic receptors.[13] Liver blood flow, therefore, is susceptible to changes in sympathetic nervous activity (Table 48.3). Hypoxia or hypercarbia increase sympathetic nervous activity and produce, among other effects, splanchnic vasoconstriction. In the experimental animal with an intact nervous system this results in a fall in liver blood flow. Following splanchnic denervation, hypercarbia causes splanchnic vasodilatation, presumably due to the direct action of carbon dioxide on blood vessels. During anaesthesia in man with nitrous oxide and suxamethonium, when carbon dioxide is added to the inspired gases, splanchnic vascular resistance increases:[22] during halothane anaesthesia hypercarbia results in vasodilatation, increased liver blood flow and diminished vascular resistance.[23] Halothane in this instance is producing a 'physiological' splanchnic denervation.

Ventilation

In the dog during inspiration, venous return from the liver is inhibited and blood flow in the vena cava comes mainly from the kidneys and lower limbs. During expiration the liver contribution to caval blood flow predominates.[45] During anaesthesia this relationship is accentuated. Intermittent positive pressure ventilation (IPPV) in man increases splanchnic vascular resistance and decreases liver blood flow, when compared with these variables during spontaneous ventilation.[23]

Splanchnic reflexes

A blow to the 'solar plexus' has ended many a contest in the boxing ring. Afferent, presumably sympathetic, fibres are stimulated and in turn excite efferents, which cause dilatation of the splanchnic capacitance vessels with resultant

Table 48.3. *Sympathetic Nervous Activity and Liver Blood Flow.*

	Splanchnic vascular resistance	Liver blood flow
Hypoxia	Increased	Reduced
Hypercarbia	Increased	Reduced
Alpha-stimulation	Increased	Reduced
Beta-blockade	Increased	Reduced
Ganglion blockade	No change	Reduced
Beta-stimulation	Reduced	Increased
N_2O, suxamethonium and hypercarbia	Increased	Reduced
Halothane and hypercarbia	Reduced	Increased

From Strunin.[56]

blood pooling and diminished venous return to the heart. The hypotension which sometimes occurs during laparotomy when abdominal viscera are subjected to traction, in the absence of any other factor, may be a similar phenomenon.

Anaesthetic agents

Although several studies have been undertaken of the effects of various anaesthetic agents on liver blood flow, most of the work has been carried out in volunteers not subjected to surgery. In addition, most subjects have had normal liver function and cardiorespiratory systems. There is very little information available on the effects of anaesthesia on liver blood flow in patients with hepatic disease. Patients with cirrhosis have decreased liver blood flow and this may be further impaired by a portacaval shunt. Intestinal obstruction with distension also decreases liver blood flow as does peritoneal infection.[32]

In general, all anaesthetic agents, including spinal and extradural anaesthetic techniques, lead to a fall in liver blood flow accompanied by a fall in oxygen uptake by the splanchnic organs. Comparison of the ratio of reduction between these two variables for various anaesthetics shows that changes in arterial carbon dioxide tension are very relevant (Table 48.4). Despite quite marked falls in oxygen uptake, no evidence of hypoxia or anaerobic metabolism has been demonstrated in fit healthy volunteers.[41,49] However, this may not be so for the patient with pre-existing liver disease or other illness.

It may be concluded from the evidence available that a spinal or extradural anaesthetic will reduce liver blood flow in proportion to the fall in mean arterial pressure produced.[39] For general anaesthesia, an oxygen/nitrous oxide relaxant sequence with intermittent positive pressure ventilation to normocapnia would seem to have the least effect on liver blood flow. Of the volatile anaesthetic agents so far studied, halothane would seem to be the least harmful. Nevertheless, the dose should be restricted, since liver blood flow will fall in proportion to the fall in arterial blood pressure produced by halothane. Both hypo- and hyperventilation seem undesirable, and methoxyflurane and cyclopropane are probably best avoided. Gelman[30] has suggested that, although anaesthetic agents do have an effect on liver blood flow, the extent of the surgical manipulation is much more relevant in decreasing liver blood flow.

Table 48.4. *Splanchnic Circulation during Anaesthesia. Ratio (R) of change in blood flow during anaesthesia to change in oxygen consumption ($R = 1$: equal reduction of both SBF and splanchnic oxygen consumption; $R < 1$: residual oxygen consumption in excess of remaining perfusion).*[a]

Anaesthetic	R	Type of ventilation
Halothane	0.85	Spontaneous
Halothane	0.82	Controlled[b]
N_2O, curare	0.82	Controlled[b]
Cyclopropane	0.79	Controlled[b]
N_2O, curare	0.59	Hyperventilation
Methoxyflurane	0.55	Controlled

[a] Modified from Libonati et al.[40]
[b] Controlled = normocarbia.

OBSTRUCTIVE JAUNDICE

It is assumed for the purposes of this section that the patient has an obstructive lesion of the biliary tree which is amenable to surgical treatment. General anaesthesia, particularly in children, may be required for certain diagnostic procedures such as needle biopsy of the liver, percutaneous cholangiography or laparoscopy. Eventually laparotomy for diagnostic and therapeutic purposes will be carried out and this presents certain anaesthetic problems.

Preoperative preparation

A prolonged prothrombin time is commonly found in the jaundiced patient and is usually due to non-absorption of vitamin K from the intestine due to the lack of bile salts. An additional factor may be hepatocellular disease and this will be suggested by the finding of a low serum albumin concentration. A course of vitamin K_1, 10 mg intramuscularly, daily for three days preoperatively, should restore the prothrombin time to normal. If the prothrombin time is persistently prolonged in excess of four seconds over the control value, it is likely that concomitant hepatocellular disease is present. In this case, fresh frozen plasma should be available and infused as necessary to reduce the risk of severe haemorrhage during surgery or diagnostic procedures.[29]

It is well recognized that there is an increased incidence of postoperative renal failure following anaesthesia and surgery in patients with obstructive jaundice (see Chapter 46).[15,63] In the past, this observation has been attributed to anoxia[14] associated with the normal fall in renal blood flow during anaesthesia and surgery, and the possible toxic effect of bilirubin.[7] More recently, Bailey[5] has suggested that postoperative renal failure may be due to excess endotoxin produced from the patient's own bowel flora, caused by the reduction in bile salts resulting from biliary obstruction. In the patients studied by Bailey[5] endotoxin was found in portal blood when serum bilirubin was in excess of 140 μmol/l (8.19 mg/100 ml). Dawson[16] showed that postoperative renal failure could be prevented by inducing a diuresis preoperatively, and maintaining it peroperatively and in the immediate postoperative period with intravenous mannitol. In the light of the findings related to endotoxin it is also sensible, in the severely jaundiced patient, to administer antibiotics preoperatively, and if there is evidence of infection in the biliary tract an additional dose should be given during the course of surgery. Table 48.5 illustrates a suitable regimen to prevent postoperative renal failure in the jaundiced patient. (See also Chapter 54.)

If the patient has been on steroid therapy for the treatment of jaundice, then 100 mg of hydrocortisone hemisuccinate should be administered with the premedication intramuscularly and continued thereafter six-hourly until steroid therapy is no longer required. Pethidine and promethazine are suitable drugs to be given as premedicants. Although it is traditionally stated that bradycardia is an accompaniment of severe jaundice, it has not been the author's experience that this is so and therefore atropine is not necessary. In the event that the patient's fluid intake has been inadequate because of illness, intravenous fluid therapy should be given preoperatively to ensure adequate hydration. A urinary catheter should be inserted, attached to a suitable volume-measuring device. Depending on the serum bilirubin concentration, mannitol therapy may be necessary (Table 48.5). If the patient has been undergoing percutaneous cholangiography, the cardiovascular state should be carefully checked; infusion of plasma expanders may be necessary before induction of anaesthesia.

Table 48.5. *Mannitol Regimen to Prevent Postoperative Renal Failure in the Jaundiced Patient.*

Serum bilirubin μmol/l (mg/100 ml)	Management
Over 20 (over 1.17)	Urinary catheter: monitor urine output. 1. If urine volume > 50 ml/h, no action. 2. If urine output < 50 ml/h, mannitol 5 or 10% i.v. until diuresis established.
Over 140 (over 8.19)	Preoperative: antibiotics and urinary catheter. Mannitol 5 to 10% i.v. to keep urine volume above 50 ml/h. Continue mannitol per-, and postoperatively (24 to 36 hours).

From Strunin.[56]

Anaesthesia

Table 48.6 shows an anaesthetic sequence which is suitable for patients with biliary obstruction undergoing laparotomy for therapeutic or diagnostic purposes.[58] Anaesthesia may be induced by an intravenous injection of a barbiturate or Althesin; increased doses may be required in patients whose plasma proteins are abnormal. For all but the most minor procedures, central venous pressure should be monitored so that circulating blood volume may be maintained at the optimum but over-transfusion with mannitol avoided. A good anaesthetic record card should be kept so that no confusion may arise in relation to the drugs administered during anaesthesia and changes in liver function postoperatively.

For rapid intubation, suxamethonium may be used and may be followed by pancuronium or fazadinium for more prolonged muscular relaxation. These drugs are preferred to *d*-tubocurarine which may cause unacceptable hypotension, thus leading to a reduction in liver blood flow (LBF). Caution should be exercised in the use of large doses of non-depolarizing muscle relaxant drugs in the severely jaundiced patient, particularly if it is thought likely that biliary obstruction will not be relieved by surgery, as there may then be difficulties in reversing the effects of these drugs. Nitrous oxide/oxygen and halothane, with or without analgesic supplements, may be safely used in the jaundiced patient. Normocapnia should be maintained during IPPV and since halothane reduces LBF the dose administered should be limited to avoid undue cardiovascular depression. Anaesthesia in the jaundiced patient, where the cause turns out to be viral in origin, is almost inevitably followed by a worsening of liver function, whatever anaesthetic agents are used (see below and Chapter 47).

Regional anaesthesia, for example extradural blockade, is also suitable for laparotomy in the jaundiced patient, and for provision of postoperative pain relief. However, a careful check of the patient's prothrombin time and clotting factors should be made as these may be abnormal and might contraindicate a regional local technique.

If a carcinoma of the head of the pancreas is found at laparotomy, splanchnic block under direct vision with 40 to 50 ml of 50 per cent ethyl alcohol should be performed. This may be carried out easily by the surgeon and may prevent intractable pain in the postoperative period.

Table 48.6. *Anaesthetic Sequence Suitable for Patients with Biliary Obstruction Undergoing Laparotomy.*

Preoperatively:	Vitamin K therapy.
Premedication:	Pethidine up to 100 mg, promethazine up to 25 mg (depending on weight and 'fitness' of patient).
Induction:	Thiopentone or Althesin. Suxamethonium for emergency intubation. Pancuronium or fazadinium for non-urgent case.
Anaesthesia:	Oxygen: nitrous oxide. IPPV to normocapnia. Incremental pethidine or synthetic analogues. Halothane permitted-control dose.
Monitoring:	Urine via catheter and volumetric device. Pulse, blood pressure and ECG. Central venous pressure (CVP). Fluid balance chart.
Infusion:	5% dextrose Blood, if necessary, via blood-warmer.
Immediate post-operative care:	Oxygen therapy – IPPV. 5 to 10% mannitol, if necessary. Antibiotics. Physiotherapy, particularly to avoid right lower lobe collapse.

From Strunin.[56]

The postoperative period

Care should be taken that any neuromuscular blocking drugs given have been adequately reversed, and if there is any doubt there should be a period of IPPV until the effects of the drugs have worn off. Oxygen should be administered to the spontaneously breathing patient until all the effects of anaesthesia have passed. Postoperative pain relief may be provided by standard analgesic drugs. If the response to the premedication is uneventful, normal dosage may be used. However, liver function may be impaired, in which case only small doses should be given and the patient's conscious level carefully monitored. Urine output should be maintained if necessary by further mannitol infusion.

Cryptogenic infantile cholestasis (see Chapter 41)

Type II cryptogenic infantile cholestasis is amenable to surgical correction by the Kasai operation.[37] This consists of laparotomy with exposure of the major intrahepatic bile ducts by resection of a cone of liver tissue from the porta hepatis, followed by direct anastomosis of the cuffed liver surface to a segment of the upper small intestine (Roux-en-Y) or to the gall-bladder. This operation is carried out within the first few months of life as soon as a diagnosis is established. From the anaesthetist's point of view, although liver cell function may be relatively normal, these are not healthy children; the surgical procedure may be lengthy, and blood loss may be marked.

No particular anaesthetic technique is recommended but all precautions which are appropriate for anaesthetizing a neonate should be taken. These include temperature control, an infant ventilator, micro-infusion apparatus for intravenous therapy, careful estimation of blood loss and skilled postoperative nursing.

CHRONIC LIVER DISEASE (CIRRHOSIS)

Patients with chronic liver disease may present for anaesthesia and surgery where their liver dysfunction is merely coincidental or as a direct result of some complication, most commonly associated with portal hypertension. In the former situation, liver dysfunction may go unnoticed preoperatively and it may be perceived only when, in the postoperative period, detrimental changes in liver function appear. It is well recognized that anaesthesia and surgery may be precipitating factors in decompensating chronic liver disease. Routine liver function tests may be of little help in detecting compensated chronic liver disease preoperatively and a careful history and examination are often more revealing. Nevertheless, attempts have been made to estimate hepatic reserve and to determine the risk of surgery, particularly portasystemic shunting. Table 48.7 illustrates the scheme devised by Child[11] which relies on two laboratory and three clinical observations in an attempt to estimate hepatic reserve. More recently, Pugh et al[50] have modified Child's system to include other tests (Table 48.8). Using this latter system, patients who score 5 to 6 points are considered to be good operative risks (Grade A); patients with 7, 8 or 9 points are moderate risks (Grade B); and those with 10 to 15 points are poor operative risks (Grade C). These gradings correlate with those of Child.[11] Allowance should be made in the grading for patients with primary biliary cirrhosis in whom the level of bilirubin is usually out of proportion to other evidence of liver damage. Where possible, only patients in the Grade A category should be considered for anaesthesia and surgery. In certain circumstances, there may be some advantage in delaying surgery so that the patient's condition may be improved; for example, after a recent gastrointestinal haemorrhage, purgation and protein restriction with restoration of blood volume may improve the patient's liver function so that subsequent anaesthesia and surgery will be less detrimental.

Preoperative preparation

Although the grading system described above may be helpful, the appearance and general demeanour of the patient may be the best guide to his suitability for anaesthesia and surgery. If the patient is jaundiced, or the prothrombin

Table 48.7. *Clinical and Laboratory Classification of Patients with Cirrhosis in Terms of Hepatic Functional Reserve.*[a]

	Group A	Group B	Group C
Serum bilirubin μmol/l (mg/100 ml)	<40 (<2.34)	40–50 (2.34–2.92)	>50 (>2.92)
Serum albumin g/l	>35	30–35	<30
Ascites	None	Easily controlled	Poorly controlled
Neurological disorder	None	Minimal	Advanced come
Nutrition	Excellent	Good	Poor – wasting
Risk of operation	Good	Moderate	Poor

[a] Data from Child.[11]

Table 48.8. *Grading of Severity of Liver Disease.*[a]

Clinical and biochemical measurement	Points scored for increasing abnormalities		
	1	2	3
Encephalopathy (grade)	None	1 and 2	3 and 4
Bilirubin µmol/l (mg/100 ml)	<25 (<1.46)	25–40 (1.46–2.34)	>40 (>2.34)
Albumin g/l	35	28–35	<28
Prothrombin time (seconds greater than control)	1–4	4–6	>6

[a] Data from Pugh et al,[50] with the kind permission of the authors and the editor of *British Journal of Surgery*.

time is prolonged, a course of vitamin K should be given before surgery and anaesthesia. If prothrombin activity is still abnormal, fresh frozen plasma should be administered just prior to anaesthesia. Cross-matched blood, as fresh as possible, should also be available in proportion to the surgical procedure planned. In patients who are HB_sAg-positive suitable precautions should be taken (see below).

In the well-compensated patient the normal premedicant drugs are well tolerated. The author prefers to use pethidine, promethazine or diazepam and, if endoscopy is contemplated, atropine may be given in addition. Patients who have been on steroid therapy for autoimmune liver disease or for the treatment of jaundice should be given additional hydrocortisone hemisuccinate at the time of the premedication. In the jaundiced patient antibiotics and intravenous mannitol may be necessary (see above).

Anaesthesia

In the ill patient oxygen should be administered during induction of anaesthesia to allow for arteriovenous shunting, which is a feature of chronic liver disease. Intravenous induction agents, such as thiopentone or Althesin, may be safely given to the patient with compensated liver disease.[58] The dose should be adjusted according to the 'fitness' of the patient, however. In the patient with porphyria these agents should be avoided and ketamine may be the drug of choice.[52] In the patient with a raised serum globulin concentration, increased doses of intravenous anaesthetic induction agents may be required as a result of increased protein binding; similarly, in the patient with a low total serum protein concentration, decreased amounts are required.

For minor surgical procedures, where intubation is not indicated, patients should be allowed to breathe spontaneously, using oxygen, nitrous oxide and halothane (see below). For more prolonged procedures, or where muscle relaxation is indicated, muscle relaxant drugs may be used with IPPV. For intubation alone, suxamethonium is suitable, and for more prolonged neuromuscular block, the non-depolarizing muscle blocking drugs, pancuronium or fazadinium, may be used. Although increased amounts of non-depolarizing neuromuscular blocking drugs may be required in patients with liver disease, care should be taken over dosage as difficulties may be encountered in reversing the effects at the end of the surgical procedure. During IPPV attempts should be made to maintain normocapnia in order to minimize the effects on liver blood flow. Similarly, if halothane is used, the dose should be limited so as not to reduce systemic arterial blood pressure and thus liver blood flow.

Patients with liver disease do not tolerate blood loss well, and this may be severe during surgery, particularly if portal hypertension is present. Central venous pressure should therefore be monitored, blood pressure and pulse measured frequently, and adequate infusion lines established for blood transfusion. Blood should be administered early in the surgical procedure to give time for the citrate anticoagulant to be adequately metabolized by the liver, and the blood should be passed through a warming coil before delivery to the patient. If blood transfusion is not required, fluids containing sodium should be avoided, and 5 per cent dextrose in water is the intravenous fluid of choice.

Use of halothane. All general, regional and spinal anaesthetic techniques will lower splanchnic blood flow. Under normal circumstances this does not seem harmful, but in patients whose liver function is already compromised further damage may occur. The basic principle, therefore, should be to ensure that splanchnic blood flow receives as little interference as possible. To this end, careful attention should be paid to oxygenation, avoidance of hypotension and the maintenance of arterial carbon dioxide tension within the normal range. Volatile anaesthetic agents which directly affect the splanchnic circulation, such as cyclopropane, diethyl ether and methoxyflurane, are best avoided. Halothane is not contraindicated; indeed many workers have advocated its use in patients with chronic liver disease. In patients with biliary tract disease, fewer postoperative complications followed when halothane anaesthesia was used than when diethyl ether anaesthesia was used.[17] In the National Halothane Study[47] cyclopropane was shown to be worst, in terms of being related to massive hepatic necrosis following surgery in patients with biliary tract disease, and halothane was associated with the fewest problems. A further interesting point emerges from this part of the National Halothane Study, in that massive hepatic necrosis appeared less frequently in patients following biliary tract surgery than after other forms of surgery. Halothane is a useful adjuvant during anaesthesia, in any event, and particularly so in patients with liver disease. Low concentrations may be easily given and, once discontinued, the time interval for elimination of the drug is relatively short. This contrasts with the administration of intravenous drugs where difficulties may be encountered in relation to metabolism and excretion in patients with liver dysfunction.

When adrenaline is used for local infiltration the use of halothane is contraindicated. Halothane, in common with some other volatile anaesthetic agents, sensitizes the myocardium to the effects of circulating catecholamines and there is therefore at least a theoretical risk that exogenously administered adrenaline may precipitate cardiac dysrhythmias in the patient anaesthetized with halothane. Local infiltration of the skin with a mixture of normal saline and adrenaline is commonly used in patients with portal hypertension to reduce bleeding from the skin and underlying structures during laparotomy.

Pseudocholinesterase. This is a non-specific esterase synthesized by the liver, and when protein synthesis is decreased, as in hepatocellular disease, pseudocholinesterase concentration falls.[28] This may be of significance if suxamethonium is administered, as pseudocholinesterase is responsible for the metabolism of suxamethonium and it is often suggested that the action of suxamethonium may be prolonged in patients with chronic liver disease. However, fresh blood and plasma concentrates contain significant quantities of pseudocholinesterase and a recent transfusion may alter the significance of pseudocholinesterase measurements. In acute liver failure, where suxamethonium may be used for emergency intubation, prolongation of its action as a result of reduced pseudocholinesterase concentration is unlikely.[60] The half-life of pseudocholinesterase is some 15 days, and most patients with acute liver failure will either have recovered in this time or have died as a result of their liver disease. By far the most important cause of failure to metabolize suxamethonium in association with pseudocholinesterase is a genetically determined abnormality of this enzyme.

Portal hypertension (see Chapters 43 and 44)

Haemorrhage, usually from the upper gastrointestinal tract, is a common complication of portal hypertension. General principles of management are directed towards resuscitation, control of haemorrhage, prevention of hepatic encephalopathy and, finally, assessment of the degree of portal hypertension with a view to elective surgery. Most patients are bleeding from oesophageal varices, but up to one-third are bleeding from lesions in other parts of the gastrointestinal tract. The precise diagnosis is made by fibreoptic endoscopy. Occasionally, a general anaesthetic may be indicated but diazepam is usually adequate although, in the severely ill patient, endoscopy may be performed without any sedation or anaesthesia. Temporary control of haemorrhage is nearly always possible with a modified Sengstaken-Blakemore tube or with the use of an infusion of vasopressin but surgical treatment may eventually be necessary. Although many different surgical procedures have been used to stop or prevent further bleeding it should be noted that most of the patients in whom operative treatment is considered are the hard core who have bled repeatedly. They often have advanced cirrhosis and it therefore seems reasonable to perform the least traumatic operation that will control bleeding. Whatever surgical procedure is used, however, the outcome largely depends on the severity of the patients' pre-existing liver disease. In patients with jaundice, ascites and encephalopathy, gastrointestinal bleeding is usually an agonal symptom. The vital importance of hepatic function is emphasized by the comparatively small risk to life in those patients with virtually normal livers who bleed from varices secondary to extrahepatic portal obstruction.

Portasystemic shunts. In general, portasystemic shunting is carried out only in patients whose liver function is relatively good, i.e. Grade A patients (see Tables 48.7 and 48.8). The major anaesthetic problem during laparotomy to perform a portasystemic shunt is haemorrhage. This arises not only as a result of deficiency in clotting factors but also because of the high venous pressure, resulting from portal hypertension, in collateral vessels within the abdomen. Various anaesthetic techniques, ranging from hypotensive spinal anaesthesia[21,31] to hypothermia,[48] have been tried in order to control bleeding, decrease hepatic metabolism and minimize the effective decreased hepatic blood flow during the surgical procedures. None of these techniques has been shown to be of any great advantage. More recently, Ward, Adu-Gyamfi and Strunin[58] have shown that a satisfactory sequence for portasystemic shunting is as follows: induction of anaesthesia with a short-acting barbiturate or Althesin; maintenance of anaesthesia with oxygen/nitrous oxide, with IPPV to maintain normocapnia; muscle relaxation by means of pancuronium bromide; and increments of analgesic agents such as pethidine or its synthetic derivatives.

Non-shunt procedures. These surgical procedures involve, in the main, a direct approach to oesophageal varices and the procedure may well be carried out in patients who are considered unfit for major portasystemic shunting. Some procedures, such as oesophageal transection, involve opening the left chest and using a double lumen endotracheal tube in order to deflate the left lung and allow access to the oesophagus. A nasogastric tube should be passed only after the chest is opened and the surgeon has access to the oesophagus so that, should haemorrhage occur, it may be controlled.

Oesophageal injection of varices may be carried out via an oesophagoscope, either of the rigid or of the fibreoptic varieties. Sclerosing material is injected, under direct vision, into the oesophageal tissue surrounding the varix. As an alternative, a catheter may be passed percutaneously into the liver and advanced via the portal vein into the major variceal supply vein.[54]

An anaesthetic technique suitable for injection of oesophageal varices via an oesophagoscope has been described by Ward, Davies and Strunin.[59] Since patients having injection of oesophageal varices may be in Grades B or C (see Tables 48.7 and 48.8) the minimum of drugs should be used for anaesthesia. Diazepam and atropine are suitable for premedication and anaesthesia is induced with a small dose of either thiopentone or Althesin. Suxamethonium is used to facilitate endotracheal intubation. The endotracheal tube should be carefully positioned so that kinking does not occur during oesophagoscopy. A large-bore infusion should be placed in a suitable peripheral vein and cross-matched blood, as fresh as possible, should always be available.

If the patient has been treated with a Sengstaken-Blakemore tube prior to injection of varices, this should be left in position until the trachea is intubated. In any event, a freshly tested Sengstaken-Blakemore tube should always be available for use in the postoperative period. At the end of the procedure, the endotracheal tube should be left in place until the patient is fully conscious, and he should then be placed in the lateral position before extubation. A further hazard which may arise is that bleeding may occur from the lower end of the oesophagus; the blood then passes into the stomach, clots and is subsequently vomited and inhaled. This may be avoided by always nursing the patient in the lateral position until it is clear that consciousness has fully returned.

Postoperative period

Following anaesthesia and surgery, patients with liver disease are particularly prone to develop chest infections. The right lower lobe is a common site for problems because of its proximity to the surgical area, in the case of liver surgery, and the effects of prolonged retraction. Nursing staff should be alerted to the presence of a chest drain which may be part of the surgical procedure since this might be unexpected in a 'liver' patient. If analgesic or sedative drugs are necessary, their initial effects should be carefully assessed; it is preferable to commence with small doses.

MAJOR LIVER SURGERY

Table 48.9 lists some of the common indications for major surgery on the liver. Liver function may be generally good, but patients should be graded, as described previously, and the presence of HB_sAg should be sought.

Since all the procedures involve laparotomy, anaesthesia should follow the lines already described for patients with chronic liver disease. Haemorrhage, particularly in patients with trauma, may be a major problem. Adequate infusion lines should be established and central venous (CVP) and arterial pressure should be monitored directly. In many instances access to the peripheral venous system may be impractical and the approach to the internal jugular vein, as described by Rao, Wong and Salem,[51] should be used to insert a central venous line and a large-bore (14 gauge) infusion line.

Hepatic tumours

Particular problems may arise in relation to hepatic tumours. During partial hepatectomy air embolus may occur due to damage to the hepatic veins; a CVP cannula should always be inserted so that any air may be aspirated. Venous obstruction by kinking of the inferior vena cava may cause hypotension during resection of large tumours. Activation of the fibrinolytic system may lead to fibrinogen depletion and increased bleeding.

In 25 per cent of patients with carcinoid tumours, the carcinoid syndrome occurs with hepatic metastases.[43] This syndrome consists of a number of symptoms which may include flushing attacks, diarrhoea, bronchospasm and valvular heart lesions. Serotonin and bradykinin are probably responsible for these symptoms and patients should be prepared preoperatively with suitable blocking drugs, such as cyproheptatine and aprotinin (Trasylol). Methotrimeprazine (Veractil) should be used to control any serotoninergic effects during surgery. These may be manifest as hypertension, increased peristalsis and a rise in blood glucose.[44] Delay in recovery from anaesthesia has been noticed in patients with carcinoid syndrome and may be related to the role of serotonin as a transmitter substance in the brain. The dose of anaesthetic drugs should therefore be minimal and caution should be exercised with postoperative sedation.

Table 48.9. *Major Liver Surgery Requiring General Anaesthesia.*

Hepatic abscess
Hepatic trauma
Liver resection for hepatic tumours
primary
secondary
Orthotopic liver transplantation

Orthotopic liver transplantation (see Chapter 52)

Anaesthesia for liver transplantation has been reviewed several times and the reader is referred to the following references for details of organization and technique: Aldrete, Levine and Gingrich;[4] Farman and Mason;[25] Farman et al[26] and Farman.[24]

Organization is important; facilities have to be available, often at night, for acid-base, serum potassium, calcium and glucose estimations. Large quantities of blood are required (the initial order should be for at least 30 units) in addition to fresh frozen plasma to provide extra clotting factors. In the event of serious haemorrhage, arrangements to provide donors for fresh blood may be necessary. If the recipient is HB_sAg-positive,[10] extra precautions (see below) will be necessary as well as a large dose of specific immunoglobulin for infusion during the anhepatic phase.

Table 48.10 outlines the anaesthetic technique employed for liver transplantation at King's College Hospital, London. It is important to keep pace with blood loss, so that the perfusion pressure of the transplanted liver is optimal. In this respect, the author has found the Bentley Autotransfuser of great help. It need not be used in its autotransfusion capacity but as an infusion device. The suction side permits rapid filling of the reservoir from either bottles or packs and is independent of gravity. All blood should be warmed before administration and the patient should be on a warming blanket; body temperature is monitored by a nasal probe.

During surgery the inferior vena cava is clamped above the liver and the venous return to the heart drastically reduced; cardiac arrest may occur.[10] Other factors may lead to cardiac arrest at other times during the procedure (Table 48.11).[1] Since many of the potential causes of cardiac arrest are reversible, for example by infusion of sodium bicarbonate, aspiration of air from the right atrium or

Table 48.10. *Anaesthesia for Orthotopic Liver Transplantation.*

Premedication:	Pethidine, promethazine or diazepam, depending on 'fitness' of patient.
Vascular lines:	(a) radial artery cannula. (b) two (2) central venous lines: one for CVP monitoring and one for drug administration. (c) two (2) intravenous infusion lines (at least 14 gauge). (d) an a-v shunt if time permits.
Monitoring:	ECG: pulse rate and rhythm. Temperature: nasal probe. Arterial blood pressure. Central venous pressure. Regular arterial blood samples for: (a) acid-base status. (b) serum potassium. (c) serum calcium. (d) blood glucose.
Anaesthesia:	(a) preoxygenation if necessary. (b) thiopentone for induction: followed by suxamethonium or pancuronium to facilitate endotracheal intubation. (c) nasogastric tube. (d) oxygen/nitrous oxide with IPPV and normocapnia. (e) increments of phenoperidine or fentanyl.

administration of calcium, direct cardiac massage should be performed by opening the chest via the diaphragm. Internal defibrillation by the same route may also be necessary.

Postoperatively, respiratory problems may occur. These may be due to excessive blood transfusion, pre-existing lung disease or related to pain from the large abdominal incision. A period of IPPV may be necessary, but should be as short as possible to reduce the risk of infection. Recently, in Cambridge,[41] a thoracic extradural block has provided good post-operative pain relief, thus avoiding the need for analgesic or sedative drugs.

THE HB_sAg-POSITIVE PATIENT (see Chapter 28)

There is a risk that patients who are HB_sAg-positive, particularly those with the e-antigen,[38] may infect theatre personnel. Precautions to be taken should begin as soon as the patient is sent for from the ward for transport to the operating theatre.[62] The patient should come straight into the operating theatre and not be dealt with in an anaesthetic room. The number of personnel in the operating theatre should be kept to a minimum and all should wear disposable caps, masks, gowns, gloves and overshoes. Unnecessary injections and blood sampling should be avoided. Where possible, disposable anaesthetic equipment should be used. Non-disposable items may be sterilized where appropriate by heating, by ethylene oxide, or by the chemical disinfectant Diversol BX (Diversey Ltd) which is a crystalline blend of chlorinated trisodium phosphate, admixed with a bromine salt.

Patients incubating viral hepatitis subjected to anaesthesia

Dykes and Bunker[20] estimated that in the United States some 200 to 300 patients per year present for anaesthesia and surgery whilst incubating viral hepatitis. Several studies after anaesthesia and surgery in such patients have suggested that liver function tends to deteriorate.[33,34,42] In general, it seems undesirable to anaesthetize such patients and the advent of immunological tests for both hepatitis A and B should reduce the incidence of these unnecessary events.

Experience of anaesthetizing patients with chronic liver disease, who are carriers of HB_sAg, does not suggest that any 'activation of virus' occurs following uneventful anaesthesia and surgery.[19]

ACUTE LIVER FAILURE (see Chapter 27)

Acute liver failure is fortunately a rare event. The anaesthetist may encounter the condition in

Table 48.11. *Factors Leading to Cardiac Arrest During Orthotopic Liver Transplantation.*

Cardiomyopathy as a result of low intracellular K^+
Hypovolaemia
Air embolism
Hypothermia due to flushing the donor liver contents into the circulation of the recipient
Delivery of acidotic blood with a high serum potassium to the heart, either from the donor liver or from the inferior extremities after revascularization of the donor liver

two situations: firstly, in the Intensive Care Unit where the most frequent cause is viral hepatitis or, secondly, as a sequel to anaesthesia and surgery. The role of the anaesthetist in the management of acute liver failure has been reviewed recently by Ward and his colleagues.[61]

Anaesthesia

On occasions the patient with acute liver failure may require a general anaesthetic. This is most commonly given so that vascular lines may be inserted, or to allow the placement of a subdural pressure transducer for the measurement of intracranial pressure. A suitable anaesthetic technique is outlined in Table 48.12. All analgesic and sedative drugs are avoided and since the patients are always semi-comatose an intravenous induction agent is unnecessary. Hyperventilation is a cardinal and probably protective feature of acute liver failure and should not be interfered with other than for the short apnoea period necessary for endotracheal intubation.[61] The short-acting depolarizing muscle relaxant suxamethonium is used to facilitate passage of the endotracheal tube. Atropine should be given concomitantly to counteract any vagal stimulation.

Spontaneous ventilation (increased minute volume supply of oxygen and nitrous oxide may be necessary) is desirable and minimal halothane may be added if nitrous oxide alone is not sufficient. Anaesthesia time should be as short as possible and the endotracheal tube should be left in situ postoperatively as the patient's conscious level may well decline temporarily and the risk of inhalation of stomach contents will therefore be increased.

Table 48.12. *Anaesthetic Technique for the Patient in Acute Liver Failure.*

Premedication:	None
Anaesthesia:	(a) preoxygenate. (b) suxamethonium and atropine i.v. (c) endotracheal intubation (Portex tube). (d) IPPV until spontaneous ventilation re-established: then O_2/N_2O 50:50, minimal halothane if necessary in addition.
Postoperatively:	(a) endotracheal tube left in situ. (b) humidification of inspired gas mixture: air/oxygen as required.

PREVIOUS HISTORY OF JAUNDICE

At the preoperative visit, if there is any suggestion from the history that liver dysfunction has occurred in the past, standard liver function tests should be carried out, including that for HB_sAg. Most patients with a history of jaundice in the past will have suffered from viral hepatitis and, provided they are HB_sAg-negative and their liver function tests are normal, are unlikely to present any major problem to the anaesthetist. A more difficult situation is where unexplained postoperative liver dysfunction has occurred recently and is linked to a specific anaesthetic drug, most commonly halothane. Under these circumstances, if a further anaesthetic is required, the patient's liver function should be required, the patient's liver function should be carefully assessed and, if there is evidence that hepatitis is still present, surgery should be delayed if possible until the hepatitis has resolved. This will obviously depend on the circumstances, but the giving of any anaesthetic to a patient with acute hepatitis will almost certainly be followed by further deterioration in liver function.

Repeated halothane anaesthesia (see Chapter 47)

In the patient in whom liver function tests are normal and the history is one of unexplained jaundice or hepatitis following a previous halothane anaesthetic, present evidence suggests that halothane should be avoided subsequently. Nevertheless, the position is sufficiently confused to make the outcome, whatever anaesthetic is administered, by no means clear. For a detailed review of this topic see Strunin.[56]

The best advice that can be given is that each case should be assessed as it arises and due attention given to the circumstances, medico-legal considerations, and the surgical procedure proposed. It should be noted that in the vast majority of patients who receive repeated halothane anaesthesia no untoward sequelae follow. Halothane is currently one of the safest and most acceptable anaesthetic agents available, and before it is discarded in favour of possibly less acceptable alternatives all the relevant circumstances should be reviewed.

REFERENCES

1. Abouna, G.N., Preshaw, R.M., Silva, J.L., Hollingsworth, W.J., Hershfield, N.B., Novak, W., Shaw, D.T. & Vettas, J.M. (1976) Liver transplantation in a patient with cholangiocarcinoma and ulcerative colitis. *Canadian Medical Association Journal,* **115,** 615.
2. Agoston, S., Vermeer, G.A., Kersten, V.W. & Meiger, D.K.F. (1973) The fate of pancuronium bromide in man. *Acta Anesthesiologica Scandinavica,* **17,** 267–275.
3. Aladjemoff, L., Dikstein, S. & Shafrir, E. (1958) Binding of tubocurarine chloride to plasma proteins. *Journal of Pharmacology and Experimental Therapeutics,* **123,** 43.
4. Aldrete, J.S., Levine, D.S. & Gingrich, T.F. (1969) Experience in anesthesia for liver transplantation. *Anesthesia and Analgesia,* **28,** 802–815.
5. Bailey, M.E. (1976) Endotoxin, bile salts and renal function in obstructive jaundice. *British Journal of Surgery,* **63,** 774–778.
6. Baraka, A. & Gabali, F. (1968) Correlation between tubocurarine requirements and plasma protein pattern. *British Journal of Anaesthesia,* **40,** 89–93.
7. Baum, M., Sterling, G.A. & Dawson, J.L. (1969) Further study into obstructive jaundice and ischaemic renal damage. *British Medical Journal,* **ii,** 229–231.
8. Branch, R.A., Morgan, M.H., James, J. & Read, A.E. (1976) Intravenous administration of diazepam in patients with chronic liver disease. *Gut,* **17,** 975–983.
9. Breimer, D.D. (1976) Pharmacokinetics of methohexitone following intravenous infusions in humans. *British Journal of Anaesthesia,* **48,** 643–649.
10. Calne, R.Y. & Williams, R. (1977) Orthotopic liver transplantation: the first 60 patients. *British Medical Journal,* **i,** 471–476.
11. Child, C.G. (1964) The liver and portal hypertension. In *Major Problems in Clinical Surgery,* Vol. 1. (Ed.) Child, C.G. Philadelphia, London and Toronto: W.B. Saunders.
12. Clarke, R.S.J., Doggart, J.R. & Lavery, T. (1976) Changes in liver function after different types of surgery. *British Journal of Anaesthesia,* **48,** 119–128.
13. Cooperman, L.H. (1972) Effects of anaesthetics on the splanchnic circulation. *British Journal of Anaesthesia,* **44,** 967–970.
14. Dawson, J.L. (1964) Jaundice and anoxic renal damage: protective effect of mannitol. *British Medical Journal,* **i,** 810–811.
15. Dawson, J.L. (1965a) The incidence of postoperative renal failure in obstructive jaundice. *British Journal of Surgery,* **52,** 663–665.
16. Dawson, J.L. (1965b) Postoperative renal function in obstructive jaundice: effect of mannitol diuresis. *British Medical Journal,* **i,** 82–86.
17. Dawson, B., Jones, R.R., Schnelle, N., Hartridge, V.B., Paulson, J.A., Adson, M.A. & Summerskill, W.H.J. (1963) Halothane and ether anesthesia in gall bladder and bile duct surgery. A retrospective study into mortality and hepatobiliary complications. *Anesthesia and Analgesia,* **42,** 759–770.
18. Dundee, J.W. & Gray, T.C. (1953) Resistance to d-tubocurarine chloride in presence of liver damage. *Lancet,* **ii,** 16–17.
19. Dykes, M.H.M. (1977) Is halothane hepatitis chronic active hepatitis? *Anesthesiology,* **46,** 233–235.
20. Dykes, M.H.M. & Bunker, J.P. (1970) Hepatotoxicity and anesthetics. *Pharmacology for Physicians,* **4,** 1–5.
21. Ebeling, W.C., Bunker, J.P., Ellis, D.S., Fromk, A.B., Linton, R.R. & Jones, C.M. (1956) Management of patients with portal hypertension undergoing venous-shunt surgery. *New England Journal of Medicine,* **254,** 141–148.
22. Epstein, R.M., Wheeler, H.O., Frumin, M.H., Habif, D.V., Papper, E.M. & Bradley, S.E. (1961) The effect of hypercapnia on estimated hepatic blood flow, circulating splanchnic blood volume, and hepatic sulfobromaphthalein clearance during anesthesia in man. *Journal of Clinical Investigation,* **40,** 592–598.
23. Epstein, R.M., Deutsch, S., Cooperman, L.H., Clement, A.H. & Price, H.L. (1966) Splanchnic circulation during halothane anesthesia and hypercapnia in normal man. *Anesthesiology,* **27,** 654–661.
24. Farman, J.V. (1976) Anaesthesia for transplant surgery. In *Recent Advances in Anaesthesia and Analgesia,* Vol. 12 (Ed.) Hewer, C.L. & Atkinson, R.S. Edinburgh, London and New York: Churchill Livingstone.
25. Farman, J.V. & Mason, S.A. (1971) Anaesthesia for liver transplantation. In *Clinical Organ Transplantation* (Ed.) Calne, R.Y. Oxford: Blackwell.
26. Farman, J.V., Lines, J.G., Williams, R., Evans, D.M., Samuel, J.R., Mason, S.A., Ashby, B.S. & Calne, R.Y. (1974) Liver transplantation in man. Anaesthetic and biochemical management. *Anaesthesia,* **29,** 17–32.
27. Feldman, S.A. (1973) *Muscle Relaxants.* London, Philadelphia and Toronto: W.B. Saunders.
28. Foldes, F.F., Rendall-Baker, L. & Birch, J.G. (1956) Causes and prevention of prolonged apnoea with succinyl choline. *Anesthesia and Analgesia,* **35,** 609.
29. Gazzard, B.G., Lewis, M.L., Ash, G., Rizza, C.R., Bidwell, E. & Williams, R. (1974) Coagulation factor concentrate in the treatment of the haemorrhagic diathesis of fulminant hepatic failure. *Gut,* **15,** 993–998.
30. Gelman, S.I. (1976) Disturbances in hepatic blood flow during anaesthesia and surgery. *Archives in Surgery,* **111,** 881–883.
31. Greene, N.M. (1952) Hypotensive spinal anesthesia. *Surgery, Gynaecology and Obstetrics,* **95,** 331–335.
32. Gump, F.E., Price, J.B. & Kinney, J.M. (1970) Whole body and splanchnic blood flow and oxygen consumption in patients with intraperitoneal infection. *Annals of Surgery,* **171,** 321–328.
33. Hardy, K.T. & Hughes, E.S.R. (1968) Laparotomy in viral hepatitis. *Medical Journal of Australia,* **1,** 710.
34. Harville, D.D. & Summerskill, W.H.J. (1963) Surgery in acute hepatitis. Causes and effects. *Journal of the American Medical Association,* **184,** 257–261.
35. Hollister, L.E. (1957) Allergy to chlorpromazine manifested by jaundice. *American Journal of Medicine,* **28,** 870.
36. Kalow, W. (1953) Urinary excretion of d-tubocurarine in man. *Journal of Pharmacology and Experimental Therapeutics,* **109,** 74–82.
37. Kasai, M., Kiman, S., Asakun, Y., Suzuki, H., Taira, Y. & Ohaski, E. (1968) Surgical treatment of biliary atresia. *Journal of Paediatric Surgery,* **3,** 615.
38. Lancet, (1976) Relation of e-antigen to infectivity of HB_sAg-positive inoculations among medical personnel. *Lancet,* **ii,** 492–493.
39. Larson, C.P. Jr, Mazze, R.I., Cooperman, L.H. & Woolman, H. (1974) Effects of anesthetics on cerebral, renal and splanchnic circulations: recent developments. *Anesthesiology,* **41,** 169–181.

40. Libonati, M., Malsch, E., Price, H.L., Cooperman, L.H., Baum, S. & Harp, Jr (1973) Splanchnic circulation during methoxyflurane anesthesia. *Anesthesiology,* **38,** 466–472.
41. Lindop, F. & Farman, J.K. (1977) Personal communication.
42. Marx, G.F., Nagayoshi, M., Shoukas, J.A. & Wollman, S.B. (1968) Unsuspected infectious hepatitis in surgical patients. *Journal of the American Medical Association,* **205,** 793–795.
43. Mason, R.A. & Steane, P.A. (1976a) Carcinoid syndrome: its relevance for the anaesthetist. *Anaesthesia,* **31,** 228–242.
44. Mason, R.A. & Steane, P.A. (1976b) Anaesthesia for a patient with carcinoid syndrome. *Anaesthesia,* **31,** 243–246.
45. Moreno, A.H., Burchell, A.R., van der Woude, R. & Burke, J.H. (1967) Respiratory regulation of splanchnic and systemic venous return. *American Journal of Physiology,* **213,** 455–465.
46. Nana, A., Cardan, E. & Leitersdorfer, T.T. (1972) Pancuronium bromide, its use in asthmatics and patients with liver disease. *Anaesthesia,* **27,** 154–158.
47. National Halothane Study (1969) *A Study of the Possible Association between Halothane Anesthesia and Postoperative Hepatic Necrosis* (Ed.) Bunker, J.P., Forrest, W.H., Mosteller, F. & Vandam, L.D. Washington: U.S. Government Printing Office.
48. Postlethwaite, R.W., Shingleton, W.W., Stephen, C.R. & Anylan, W.G. (1960) Portacaval shunt: use of hypothermia during anesthesia. *Archives of Surgery,* **80,** 125.
49. Price, H.L., Deutsch, S., Davidson, I.A., Clement, A.H., Behar, M.G. & Epstein, R.M. (1966) Can general anesthetics produce splanchnic visceral hypoxia by reducing regional blood flow. *Anesthesiology,* **27,** 24–32.
50. Pugh, R.N.H., Murray-Lyon, I.M., Dawson, J.L., Pietroni, M.C. & Williams, R. (1973) Transections of the oesophagus for bleeding varices. *British Journal of Surgery,* **60,** 646–649.
51. Rao, T.K.L., Wong, A.Y. & Salem, M.R. (1977) A new approach to percutaneous catheterisation of the internal jugular vein. *Anesthesiology,* **46,** 362–364.
52. Rizk, S.F., Jacobson, J.H. II & Silvay, G. (1977) Ketamine as an induction agent for acute intermittent porphyria. *Anesthesiology,* **46,** 305–306.
53. Saidman, L.J. & Eger, E.I. (1966) The effect of thiopental metabolism on duration of anesthesia. *Anesthesiology,* **27,** 118–126.
54. Scott, J., Long, R.G., Dick, R. & Sherlock, S. (1976) Percutaneous transhepatic obliteration of gastro-oesophageal varices. *Lancet,* **ii,** 53–55.
55. Strunin, L. (1975) Local anaesthetics. Chapter II in *Meyler's Side Effects of Drugs 1972–1975* (Ed.) Dukes, M.N.G. Philadelphia, London and Toronto: W.B. Saunders.
56. Strunin, L. (1977) *The Liver and Anaesthesia.* London, Philadelphia and Toronto: W.B. Saunders.
57. Thompson, D.D., Rowlands, M. & Melmon, K.L. (1971) The influence of heart failure, liver disease, and renal failure on the disposition of lidocaine in man. *American Heart Journal,* **22,** 417–421.
58. Ward, M.E., Adu-Gyamfi, Y. & Strunin, L. (1975) Althesin and pancuronium in chronic liver disease. *British Journal of Anaesthesia,* **47,** 1199–1204.
59. Ward, M.E., Davies, T.D.W. & Strunin, L. (1976) Anaesthesia for injection of oesophageal varices. *Annals of the Royal College of Surgeons of England,* **58,** 315–317.
60. Ward, M.E., Knights, K.M., Strunin, J.M. & Strunin, L. (1976) Serum pseudocholinesterase concentrations in fulminant hepatic failure. *British Journal of Anaesthesia,* **18,** 818.
61. Ward, M.E., Trewby, P.N., Williams, R. & Strunin, L. (1977) Acute liver failure: experience in a special unit. *Anaesthesia,* **32,** 228–239.
62. Waterson, A.P. (1976) Hepatitis B as a hazard in anaesthetic practice. *British Journal of Anaesthesia,* **48,** 21–24.
63. Zollinger, R.M. & Williams, R.D. (1956) Appraisal of progress in surgical therapy: surgical aspects of jaundice. *Surgery,* **39,** 1016.

Chapter 49

Hepatic Resection

WILLIAM V. McDERMOTT

The anatomy and blood supply of the liver, benign and malignant tumours, hepatic abscess and liver trauma are dealt with in other chapters. This chapter, therefore, will be limited to specific comments on surgical anatomy, general indications for elective hepatic resection, techniques applicable to various types of hepatic resection, and metabolic problems encountered in the immediate postoperative phase. The fascinating phenomenon of hepatic regeneration which permits the surgeon to undertake resections of up to 90 per cent of the total functioning liver mass is described in detail in Chapter 10.

Although in the history of surgery of the liver isolated instances exist in which small segments of liver tissue were removed for localized tumours, the era of planned resection of anatomically defined segments of liver began in 1952, with the work of Lortat-Jacob from France. His report[5] described a technique for resection of the right lobe of the liver and, subsequently, several similar surgical cases were reported by Quattlebaum,[12,13] Pack[9,11] and others.[6,7] During the past two decades, the operative techniques have been refined; diagnostic techniques, in terms of selective angiography, scintiscan and echograms, have evolved; the metabolic problems following major hepatic resection have been identified; and the phenomenon of hepatic regeneration has been related to these clinical problems in man. These diagnostic techniques, and the operative and postoperative management of patients following major liver surgery, now permit elective resections of intrahepatic pathology with a mortality of well under 10 per cent in most of the major centres in the world.

INDICATIONS FOR RESECTION

The indications for hepatic resection include benign and malignant tumours of the liver and, occasionally, large cysts or abscesses. Since the details of the biological potential of the various tumours and their specific clinical and histological characteristics are covered in other chapters, they will not be dealt with here.

Of the five major indications for resection, the first is for *primary malignant tumours* of the liver. These arise either from the hepatic cell and are known as hepatomas, or from the bile ducts, in which case they are known as cholangiocarcinomas. Other rare tumours of mesenchymal origin may occur, particularly those associated with exposure to vinyl chloride. All of these tumours are rare in the continental United States, although primary hepatic cell carcinoma is extremely common in the Orient and in parts of Africa. In the USA, most hepatomas are associated with cirrhosis, usually of the non-alcoholic variety, or with haemachromatosis, and ordinarily they are inoperable because of technical considerations, multicentric origins, or because the advanced degree of liver disease precludes any major operative effort. One group of primary malignant tumours of the liver occurs with an otherwise normal hepatic parenchyma, however, and is most commonly, although not invariably, found in children or young adults. These tumours tend to be slow-growing, and resection will therefore often result in either cure or long-term survival.

The second major indication for resection is for *benign tumours*; that is, any space-occupying lesion which presents a threat to life because of potential haemorrhage or which presents with symptoms relating to its size. Angiomas of the liver may become enormous and, because of their vascular nature, may bleed spontaneously or as a result of trauma. Another interesting tumour is appearing with increasing frequency among young women who have taken oral contraceptive agents. The women may present with exsanguinating intra-abdominal haemorrhage. These tumours have been referred to as 'benign hepatomas', although a more accurate pathological classification is 'focal nodular hyperplasia' and 'adenoma'.

Metastatic cancer to the liver will occasionally present as a solitary lesion amenable to an attempted curative resection. Isolated and solitary metastases are rare, however, and the surgeon should be highly selective in choosing cases which have a known primary lesion as the source of the tumour in the liver. He must first of all be reasonably certain of a cure of the primary tumour before considering hepatic resection for a metastasis. It is also essential to be certain that no distant metastases are present and that the metastatic cancer in the liver is a solitary lesion and not merely the largest of multiple deposits throughout the liver. If, at the time of a primary resection of a cancer of the gastrointestinal tract, an apparently solitary metastasis is identified and referred for consideration for resection, it is wise to wait for several weeks and then to carry out studies with arteriography, ultrasound and radio-isotope imaging prior to exploration. This period of waiting will often permit the definition of otherwise occult nests of cancer cells scattered throughout the liver and will prevent unwarranted operation. In our own experience, of nearly 100 patients who were considered for resection of an apparently solitary metastasis, only 10 were ultimately explored and the metastasis resected. Of these, only two have survived more than five years without apparent further recurrence.

The fourth indication for hepatic resection is *cancer of the gallbladder*. Except for the small cancer discovered occasionally and incidentally at cholecystectomy for gallstones, this is generally conceded to be an almost incurable disease. Not only does the tumour frequently become inoperable prior to presenting with symptoms but also primary carcinoma of the gallbladder has a tendency to early shedding of cells which appear as satellite nodules within the right lobe of the liver. If the surgeon encounters a tumour which is more than an incidental microscopic finding, the best hope for cure probably lies in concomitant right hepatic lobectomy to remove not only the gallbladder bed but also the adjacent right caudate and quadrate lobes. Cure will be rare but Brasfield[3] has reported the five-year survival of a patient in whom carcinoma of the gallbladder had already metastasized to the right lobe. Apparent cure was effected by a formal right hepatic lobectomy in this patient. In our own limited experience of five cancers of the gallbladder which ultimately proved to be resectable, no long-term cures have resulted.

Abscesses or cysts of the liver may occasionally be best treated by a formal resection which includes the adjacent hepatic parenchyma. On the other hand, abscesses or simple epithelial cysts will usually be best managed by partial excision or drainage. Echinococcal cysts of the liver present a separate entity in which consideration must be given to the infective nature of the daughter cysts within the large presenting tumour mass and to the risk of anaphylaxis from spilling contents of the cyst into the peritoneal cavity. These tumours are common in eastern Mediterranean countries, parts of South America and in Australia and New Zealand, as well as in other areas of the world where sheep farming is prevalent. The cyst must be sterilized either with 10 per cent formalin, 50 per cent saline or other suitable materials, and then evacuated with great care to avoid spillage. Once this has been completed, the endocyst can be stripped from the outer wall, which consists of an inflammatory reaction of the hepatic parenchyma to the presence of the parasite. Partial obliteration and drainage should prove curative in those cases in which total resection is not the simplest approach (see Chapter 56).

In summary, 'cures' of primary or secondary hepatic cancer are possible but infrequent after surgical resection; some palliation may be achieved by regional perfusion or by hepatic dearterialization; radiation or systemic chemotherapy has little to offer. The most successful result from elective hepatic resection is for large symptomatic benign tumours. Indications for elective hepatic resection are therefore relatively rare if the cases under scrutiny are carefully analysed and selected.

SURGICAL ANATOMY

A few comments about surgical anatomy are relevant to a description of the techniques involved in various types of resection. In Figure 49.1, the segmental anatomy of the liver is shown in a simplified drawing which relates primarily to the problems faced by the operating surgeon. If the right divisions of the hepatic arterial and portal venous inflow are divided, the line of vascular demarcation occurs, as shown in the diagram, about 4 cm lateral to the attachment of the falciform ligament. Transection of the liver along this line of demarcation, an operation which is usually referred to as right hepatic lobectomy, involves removal of the right lobe and a significant portion of the caudate and quadrate lobes. This resection can be carried out on the medial side of the attachment of the falciform ligament by added ligation of some of the proximal branches of the left hepatic artery. This procedure is referred to as an extended right hepatic lobectomy. It involves removal of the median segment of the left lobe and is a procedure compatible with survival and full regeneration but which presents formidable technical problems.

Referring again to the guidelines in Figure 49.1, a formal left hepatic lobectomy can be carried out along the appropriate demarcation lines once the left branches of the hepatic arterial and portal venous inflow are divided. Ordinarily, however, resections of a portion of the left lobe can be accomplished without a formal anatomical dissection and these details will be described in the section on techniques.

Other anatomical details which are particularly important in major hepatic resection are the locations of the ligamentous attachments to the liver; these are shown in Figure 49.2. The division of the appropriate triangular ligament is the essential initial step towards mobilization of either the right or the left lobe of the liver.

Other, more specific, details of the anatomy and the variations in the arterial inflow are dealt with in Chapter 1.

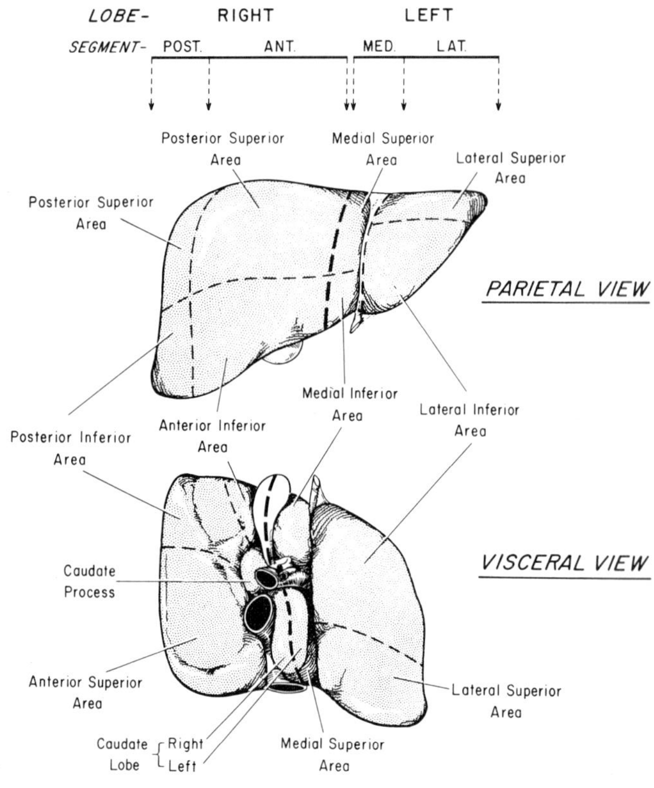

Figure 49.1. Segmental anatomy of the liver (from McDermott;[6] reprinted with the kind permission of the author and the publisher, Lea & Febiger).

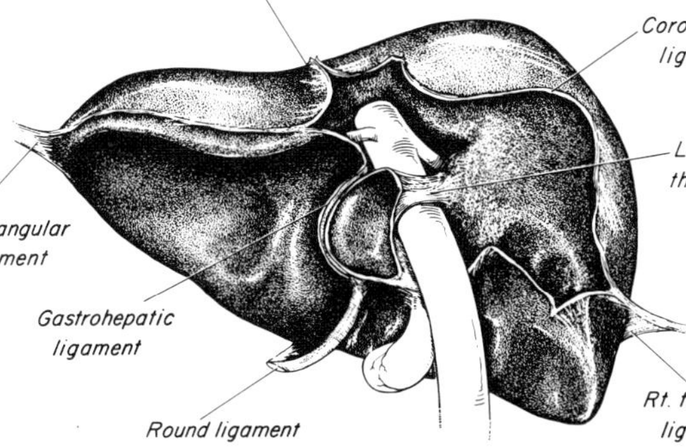

Figure 49.2. Ligamentous attachments to the liver.

TECHNIQUES OF HEPATIC RESECTION

Right hepatic lobectomy

The patient is placed at approximately 30 degrees from the supine position, with the right side elevated so that easy access to the chest may be obtained by extension of the original abdominal incision. Initial exploration is carried out through a right paramedian incision to determine the feasibility of the planned procedure. If the pathological process within the liver proves to be resectable, the incision can then be angled across the right chest wall, preferably over the fifth rib, entering the right pleural cavity by removing the rib. If the thoracic component of the incision is much lower than this, access to the vena cava as it passes through the diaphragm, and thus to the entrance of the major right and left hepatic veins, may be difficult. The diaphragm is then divided on the line of the incision, exposing the vena cava and the liver, behind which it passes in its course through the right upper quadrant. Dissection of the gastrohepatic ligament is then carried out so that the hepatic artery, portal vein and common bile duct, with their major branches (Figure 49.3a), may be identified and isolated. Preliminary arteriography is of great help in prior recognition of the frequently present anomalies of the arterial supply to the liver. These anomalies are described in Chapters 1 and 53. The most frequent (20 per cent) is the aberrant origin of the right hepatic artery from the superior mesenteric so that it crosses behind the portal vein and common bile duct instead of lying in its usual position medial to these structures. In this particular anomalous situation it is likely that the left hepatic artery will arise from the left gastric artery and enter the liver separately.

Once the anatomy of the gastrohepatic ligament has been identified and tapes have been passed around the right branches of the major structures, attention is directed to the lateral aspect of the liver. The right triangular ligament is divided, the retroperitoneal portion of the liver is exposed and the right lobe is retracted medially by the assistant. This manoeuvre will expose the retrohepatic vena cava with the multiple small venous tributaries entering it from the right caudate and quadrate lobes (Figure 49.3b). With these veins on tension, fine silk ligatures can be passed around each of them individually and the veins cut between the ligatures. The number of these small venous branches is variable, and any number between three and eight may be encountered before the major venous affluent from the liver is encountered close to the point where the vena cava passes through the diaphragm. Dissection in this area is probably the most critical part of the operation. The surgeon should be able to identify a large main right hepatic vein entering the vena cava at a slight angle, and a second vein entering from the left lobe just medial to it. If only one large vein can be identified, the right and left hepatic veins have joined in a single trunk within the liver substance, and ultimate ligation of the right hepatic vein must be deferred until the liver has been partially transected and the point of junction identified. Damage to the hepatic vein, which will be the only source of outflow from the remaining liver tissue, will

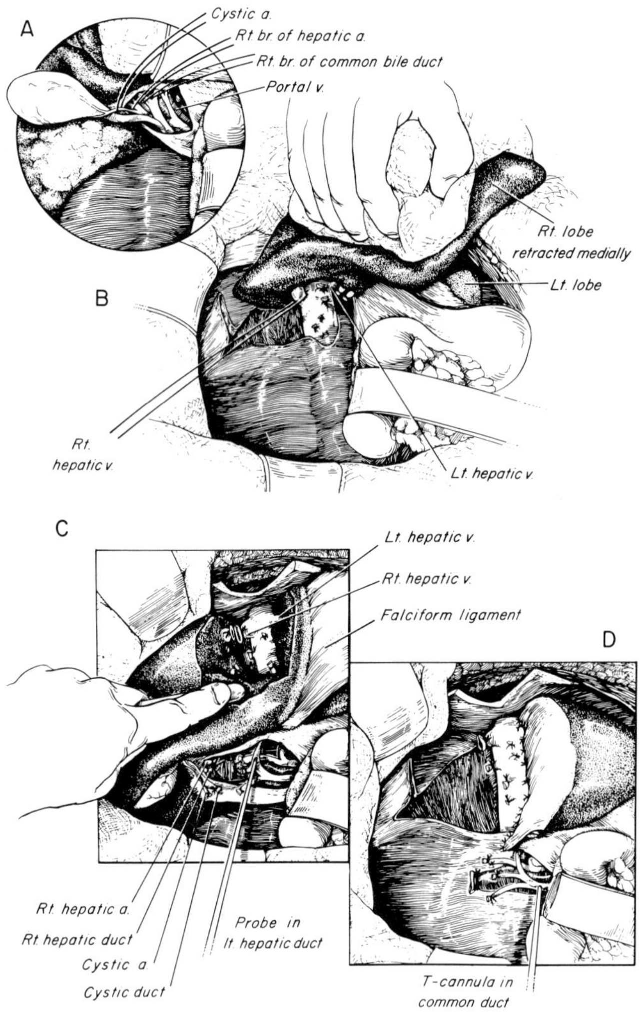

Figure 49.3. Technique of right hepatic lobectomy (from McDermott;[6] reprinted with the kind permission of the author and the publisher, Lea & Febiger).

prove catastrophic. This phase of the operative procedure is shown diagrammatically in Figure 49.3b.

At this point, attention is redirected towards the structures of the gastrohepatic ligament. The cystic duct and cystic artery are individually ligated and divided; the common duct is opened and probed in order to identify with certainty the major divisions of the biliary tract. The right hepatic duct, the right portal vein and the right hepatic artery are then securely ligated and divided (Figure 49.3c). The operator can then return to the retroperitoneal area behind the liver, and at this point ligate and divide the previously identified major right hepatic vein, presuming, as stated above, that the left hepatic vein has been satisfactorily identified and preserved. At this point, a line of demarcation will occur in the liver, identifying the devascularized portion that will include most of the right caudate and quadrate lobes. This line of vascular division between the lobes appears approximately 2 to 4 cm to the right of the attachment of the falciform ligament. Following this line of demarcation the liver capsule is then incised, and transection of the liver itself can be carried out bluntly with the handle of a knife, permitting identification, clamping and division of the various biliary, portal and arterial structures that traverse the anatomic division (Figure 49.3c). I feel that it is wise, during the transection of the liver, to have a metal probe inserted through the opening in the common bile duct into the left bile duct since this structure may in its initial course pass very close to the planned line of transection. This easy method of identification will prevent inadvertent injury to this vital structure. As mentioned before, if it has not been possible to identify the right and left hepatic veins behind the liver, one must proceed cautiously through the liver substance and identify with certainty their junction within the liver tissue before ultimate division of the right hepatic vein.

With the right lobe removed, there is relatively little bleeding from the cut surface once all the clamped structures have been ligated. Haemostasis can be easily secured by further identification of any residual bleeding points. At this point, a T-tube should be inserted in the common bile duct and the duct closed tightly around the tube. Coloured saline solution instilled into the T-tube will then identify any biliary radicles that have been overlooked during the transection of the liver. This manoeuvre should prevent a postoperative bile leak, which can be prolonged and is occasionally lethal. A satisfactory way to cover the raw surface of the liver is to detach the round ligament from the anterior abdominal wall with a section of the peritonealized attachment and suture it to the retroperitoneal tissue along the vena cava to provide a smooth haemostatic covering (Figure 49.3d).

A sump drain should be inserted into the right subphrenic area and the empty space left by removal of the large segment of liver, and an ordinary Penrose drain inserted into the hepatorenal fossa. These drains and the T-tube are brought out through appropriate small stab wounds lateral to the incision. Closure of the thoracic wound, with a chest tube for drainage, and of the abdominal incision is accomplished by standard techniques. Emphasis must be placed on the importance of using closely spaced tension sutures through all layers of the abdominal incision, since wound healing following major hepatic resection is often impaired.

Controversy exists about the use of T-tube drainage following major hepatic resection (see Chapter 50). Some surgeons have advised against this particular manoeuvre and emphasize the risk of subsequent common duct stricture. I have never found this a problem. It is probably wiser, however, to avoid a choledochotomy when an unusually small (3 mm) common duct is present. The advantages of insertion of a T-tube include the identification of residual unligated biliary radicles, as mentioned above, and the easy identification of the left hepatic duct with a metal probe during transection. Postoperatively, there are advantages of having easy access for cholangiography, and evaluation and culture of the bile if complications arise.

Left hepatic lobectomy

A technique similar to that used for identifying the left hepatic arterial, portal and biliary structures can be used for a formal left hepatic lobectomy. Unless the tumour in the left lobe is unusually large, resection can ordinarily be accomplished through an abdominal incision, but additional exposure through a median sternotomy or a right thoracotomy may occasionally be necessary.

Formal left lobectomy is usually not necessary, however, because of the anatomy of the left lobe which tapers rapidly to a thinned-out segment of liver tissue. Exposure of the left lobe can be accomplished through a median incision or through a paramedian incision with division of the falciform ligament (Figure 49.4a). Once exposure has been obtained, the left lobe can be mobilized by division of the left triangular ligament and then a wedge resection carried out as shown in Figure 49.4b. Closure of the fishmouth incision with mattress sutures will provide satisfactory haemostasis (Figure 49.4c).

Wedge resection of the liver

The techniques described above for left hepatic lobectomy may be utilized in any area of the liver if the tumour is situated peripherally. Resection may be achieved using this type of fishmouth incision without undertaking all the manoeuvres necessary with formal right or left hepatic lobectomy.

Postoperative metabolic changes

With adequate intra-operative and postoperative support and with the recognized capacity of the human liver for rapid and complete regeneration, techniques have been employed during the past two decades which involve, as in the case of formal right hepatic lobectomy, removal of approximately 80 to 85 per cent of functioning liver tissue. Several significant alterations in metabolism have been documented during the perioperative and postoperative period following major hepatic resection, and the more important of these

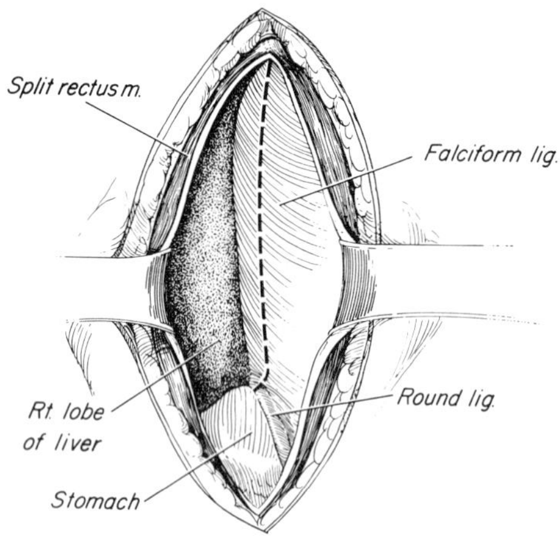

(a)

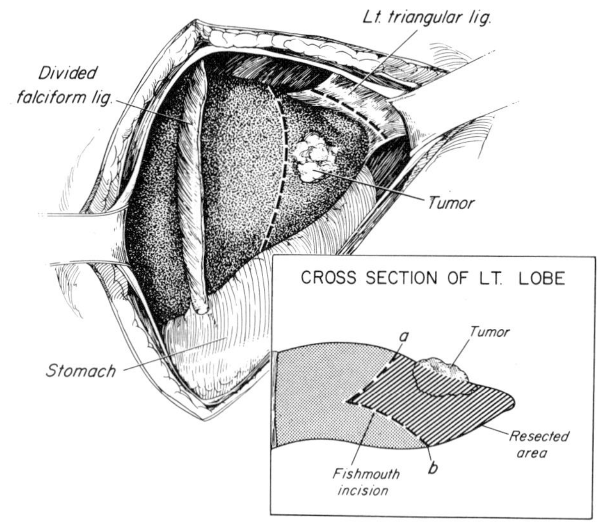

(b)

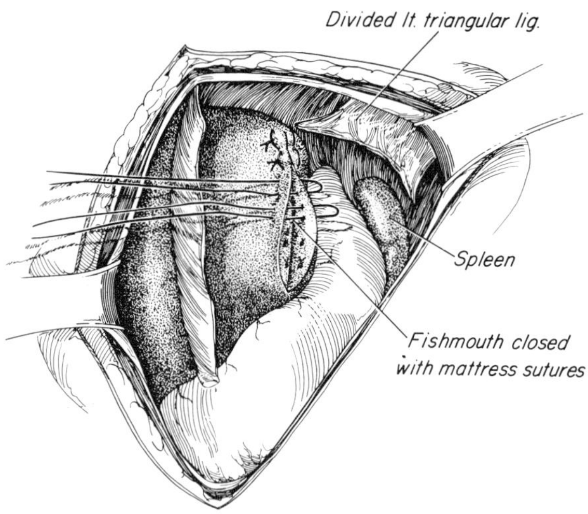

(c)

Figure 49.4. Technique of left hepatic resection.

abnormalities will be described briefly in this section.

In terms of *carbohydrate metabolism*, there is a significant risk of sudden and possibly fatal hypoglycaemia if continuous slow infusion of glucose is not administered throughout the first 48 hours. This unpredictable but very definite threat can, however, be easily controlled, and within two to three days maintenance of normal blood sugar levels is possible without the necessity of continuous parenteral support.

Disorders in *protein metabolism* are probably the most significant of the many changes which have been documented over the past decade. The liver is responsible for the synthesis of all the plasma albumin, fibrinogen and most of the globulin, and therefore considerable derangements in protein metabolism follow major hepatic resection. A consistent pattern emerges in man following right hepatic lobectomy, as noted from our own studies and those reported by Pack and Molander.[10] The most consistent and significant change is a progressive drop in serum albumin levels during the first seven to 10 days after resection. Whether this is caused by the initial inability of the small amount of residual liver to cope with the ordinary catabolic demands of the body after a major operative procedure, or whether it is caused more specifically by a tremendously increased demand for protein related to the process of regeneration within the residual liver, is not entirely clear. While individuals vary greatly in the degree of decrease in serum albumin levels, which is related to a number of factors, such as the extent of the resection, the age of the patient, the nutritional state and the general health of the individual, there is nonetheless a demonstrable need for the administration of varying amounts of human serum albumin, particularly during the first postoperative week. In contrast to this apparent defect in albumin synthesis and utilization, there has been no consistent fall in globulin levels. Electrophoretic patterns of the globulins have not shown any variation except for minor changes in the alpha-2 fraction. A consistent but varying defect in fibrinogen has been documented but has not been attended by any clinical problem.

Bilirubinaemia of varying degree has indicated an obvious defect in bilirubin metabolism. When the presence of a T-tube permits measurement of the bile output, it has been obvious that the total volume is very small during the first 24 hours and then gradually increases towards normal levels over the subsequent seven to 10 days. This increase in bile output is accompanied by a bilirubinaemia which is almost entirely in the direct component and may, on occasion, reach levels over 500 μmol/l ($\simeq$ 30 mg per cent) despite a completely patent extrahepatic biliary tract. The striking elevations in alkaline phosphatase are also consistent with an obstructive pattern. It has been postulated that sudden diversion of total portal inflow to a small residual segment of liver could cause initial hepatic congestion and compression of the bile's canaliculi; this supposition is supported by the transient portal hypertension that has been demonstrated in the immediate post-resection period. Regardless of the pathogenesis, it is reassuring that normal levels will be restored, although mild jaundice may persist for several weeks.

Reference has been made to the decreased fibrinogen level following major hepatic resection, and an increased prothrombin time is further evidence of potential defects in the underlying blood coagulation mechanism. Depressions in factors II, V, VII and X have been reported. A decrease in platelets and the occasional appearance of fibrinolysis cannot be specifically related to hepatic resection and the changes are no more pronounced than may be seen after any major surgical procedure. From the practical point of view, there are no clinically significant changes in the coagulating mechanism of blood following major hepatic resection unless serious complications such as gram-negative sepsis, gastrointestinal haemorrhage or other complications develop. Because of the measurable defects which indicate a decrease in the reserve of the clotting mechanism, it has been our practice to replace volume deficits with reasonably fresh blood transfusions and fresh frozen plasma. With these simple precautions no major problems directly related to the blood-clotting mechanism have been encountered.

Following major hepatic resection in man, there are interesting but clinically unimportant changes in lipid metabolism characterized by a fall in the level of cholesterol, with a temporary absence of esterification and a decrease in the phospholipids, triglycerides and non-esterified fatty acids. Changes in the non-esterified fatty acids relative to the triglycerides, phospholipids and cholesterol are interesting but are of no apparent clinical significance.

Variations in the *serum enzymes* are non-specific. The elevations in glutamic, oxaloacetic and pyruvic transaminases and lactic dehydrogenase are hardly surprising in view of the extent of the operative procedure and the probability of significant amounts of devitalized liver tissue left in situ following resection.

Regeneration

Extensive resection of hepatic parenchyma can be successfully undertaken as a result of the process of regeneration which occurs. This remarkable phenomenon is discussed in detail in Chapter 10. From a clinical point of view, it has been shown that the process is initiated rapidly after resection. Significant increase in the size of the remnant can be detected within a few days of operation[2] and growth is well advanced within the first few weeks. Liver function returns to normal as growth occurs[1] so that normal values may be achieved within three weeks of hemihepatectomy. More extensive resections are associated with greater degrees of impaired function but, even in these massive resections, return to normal function may be confidently expected provided no underlying hepatic pathology exists.

REFERENCES

1. Blumgart, L.H. & Vajrabukka, T. (1972) Injuries to the liver – an analysis of 20 cases with particular reference to liver resection and regeneration. *British Medical Journal*, **i**, 158.
2. Blumgart, L.H., Leach, K.G. & Karran, S.J. (1971) Observations on liver regeneration after right hemihepatectomy. *Gut*, **12**, 922–928.

3. Brasfield, R.D. (1962) Right hepatic lobectomy. *American Medical Association Archives of Surgery,* **84,** 573–581.
4. Bucher, N.L.R. (1967) Experimental aspects of hepatic regeneration. *New England Journal of Medicine,* **277,** 686–738.
5. Lortat-Jacob, J.L. & Robert, H.G. (1952) Hépatectomie droite réglée. *Presse Médicale,* **60,** 5–49.
6. McDermott, W.V. Jr (1974) *Surgery of the Liver and Portal Circulation.* Philadelphia: Lea & Febiger.
7. McDermott, W.V. Jr & Ottinger, L.W. (1966) Elective hepatic resection. *American Journal of Surgery,* **112,** 376.
8. McDermott, W.V. Jr, Greenberger, N.J., Isselbacher, K.J. & Weber, A.L. (1963) Major hepatic resection: diagnostic techniques and metabolic problems. *Surgery,* **54,** 56.
9. Pack, G.T. & Baker, H.W. (1953) Total right hepatic lobectomy: report of a case. *Annals of Surgery,* **138,** 253.
10. Pack, G.T. & Molander, D.W. (1960) Metabolism before and after hepatic lobectomy for cancer. *American Medical Association Archives of Surgery,* **80,** 685–692.
11. Pack, G.T., Miller, T.R. & Brasfield, R.D. (1955) Total right hepatic lobectomy for cancer of the gallbladder – report of three cases. *Annals of Surgery,* **142,** 6.
12. Quattlebaum, J.K. (1953) Massive resection of the liver. *Annals of Surgery,* **137,** 787.
13. Quattlebaum, J.K. & Quattlebaum, J.K. Jr (1959) Technique of hepatic lobectomy. *Annals of Surgery,* **149,** 648.

Chapter 50

Liver Trauma

ALEXANDER J. WALT

The liver, being the largest of the intra-abdominal solid organs, is the most frequently injured of these when both penetrating and blunt injuries are taken into consideration. The account which follows is based mainly on our experience at Wayne State University with 1404 hepatic injuries treated surgically at the Wayne State University Affiliated Hospitals in Detroit in the years between 1961 and 1977 (Table 50.1). The clinical picture of hepatic injury varies widely with the injuring agent. Surgical therapy has changed periodically over the past 15 years, reflecting observations made during the Vietnam conflict, introduction of new techniques and materials, re-examination of old dogmas and careful study of results.

While the liver is situated in the abdomen, it extends cephalically to the fourth right intracostal space beneath the cupola of the diaphragm and consequently may be damaged by direct blows to the thorax or by penetrating objects which enter via the thoracic cage. While most injuries reflect the severity of the blow or the nature of the missile or wounding instrument, slight or even unappreciated blows may, rarely, cause massive bleeding, especially in the pregnant woman. Rupture of hepatic adenomas, with or without a previous history of contraceptive pills, and spontaneous rupture associated with eclampsia or sickle-cell anaemia will not be further discussed, as the control of the associated haemorrhage is obtained by following the same principles to be outlined for external injury.

Injury may be penetrating or blunt in origin and the proportion of each in any series of cases reflects the social habits of the patients and the regional area (Table 50.2). Variations in this ratio markedly affect the mortality rate as the subsets have widely different outcomes. Penetrating wounds may be divided into those caused by stabs, low velocity missiles, high velocity missiles, and shotguns. Blunt injury most often results from automobile accidents affecting the driver struck by the steering wheel in the right upper quadrant, a passenger or a pedestrian; occasionally it follows falls, assaults or sports injuries. Of our last 100 consecutive blunt hepatic injuries, 77 were caused by automobiles, affecting the driver in 35, passengers in 14 and pedestrians in 23; the status of 4 patients was unknown. The other 23 victims suffered falls (5), direct blows (6) or kicks (8); in the remaining 4 patients, no history could be obtained but there was reason to believe that an assailant was being deliberately shielded. Our mortality rates are presented in Table 50.2. Shotgun wounds, blunt injury, gunshot wounds and stabs cause injuries of a decreasing order of severity. The final outcome is directly related to the number of organs injured apart from the liver. Excluding stab wounds, solitary liver injury occurs in only 5 to 10 per cent of patients. This small but favourable group has a survival rate of approximately 95 per cent. In contrast, the mortality rate rises to about 40 per cent when four organs are injured and above 50 per cent when five or more organs are damaged. A direct relationship exists between the length and depth of associated shock which in turn reflects the degree and rapidity of blood loss. In recent years, survival rates have levelled out in most major units in the United States.[1, 22, 24] On superficial review, this fact may appear to reflect lack of progress. However, many patients with injuries so severe that they would previously

Table 50.1. *Liver Injuries, Detroit General Hospital (July 1961–December 1976).*

Injury	1961–68	1969–73	1974–76	Totals	%
GSW	151	427	199	777	(55.3)
Stabs	235	153	92	480	(34.2)
Blunt	50	57	40	147	(10.5)
Totals	436	637	331	1404	(100)

GSW = gunshot wounds.
From Walt[24] with kind permission of the editor of *American Journal of Surgery*.

have died at the scene of the accident are now being so vigorously resuscitated that they reach the hospital alive although in desperate condition. With the overall improvement in pre-hospital care added to the rising rate of gunshot wounds, surgical care has in fact shown substantial improvement.

Anatomical Pathology of the Hepatic Injury

Many of the most severe hepatic crush injuries occur in victims of highway accidents who never reach the hospital alive, often because of the severity of associated injuries such as rupture of the aorta and other major vessels or because of major interference with pulmonary ventilation. In the most severely injured patients, the liver tends to be disrupted by the bursting nature of the initial force which produces compression of the liver followed by sudden release. The right lobe of the liver – and the posterosuperior surface in particular – is most likely to be smashed in such cases.[7] Under these circumstances, the nature of the damage is all too obvious at the time of operation. In other patients, however, the capsule of the liver may remain completely intact or suffer only a few stellate cracks while the central parenchyma is pulped. In this group of patients, the outer surface of the liver may be discoloured and often has a purplish appearance but the most notable change is the abnormally soft consistency of the parenchyma on palpation. Appreciation of this latter type of lesion has become more frequent since the advent of non-invasive diagnostic techniques such as sonography, isotopic scanning and invasive arteriography. The ultimate fate of this damaged tissue is variable. If not infected, the necrotic tissue may be spontaneously resorbed but in some patients it may liquefy, increase the intrahepatic pressure and lead to delayed rupture of the liver or to haemobilia. Occasionally, a patient presenting with right upper quadrant discomfort and hepatomegaly is shown to have a very large subcapsular haematoma containing up to 500 ml or more of liquefied blood which appears to have resulted from a minor blow recalled by the patient only after prompting by the physician. While these are sometimes associated with deeper parenchymal damage, we have treated a few patients who showed no sign of underlying hepatic injury and required nothing more than simple drainage of the fluid. Even more rarely, a large intrahepatic cyst containing what appears to be pure bile may develop; this clinical manifestation may not appear until many weeks after the injury.

In survivors, one or more superficial cracks in the surface of the liver are much more common than any of the above. These fissures may be deep but are usually shallow and extend for variable distances across the surface. Where the hepatic lesion appears to be due to oscillation of the liver in response to injury, the fissure not infrequently lies in juxtaposition to the suspensory falciform and coronary ligaments of the liver. Where the cracks in the liver result from direct compression, these are to be found anywhere in the parenchyma but tend to be more concentrated in the right lobe, presumably by virtue of its bulk and confined position.

Stab wounds tend to be linear and their extent depends on the type of weapon used. The force of the blow, the position of the patient at the time of impact and the left- or right-handedness of the assailant determine the situation and length of the track. Most stabs produce little serious damage except when by chance a large

Table 50.2. *Mortality: Liver Injuries.*

1961–68	46/436	10.5%
1969–73	93/637	14.6%
1974–76	40/331	12.1%

Injury	1974–76 No.	Deaths (%)
GSW	186	28 (15.1)
Stabs	91	1 (1.1)
Blunt	40	8 (20.0)
Shotgun	13	3 (23.1)
Iatrogenic	1	0 (0)
Totals	331	40 (12.1)

GSW = gunshot wounds.
From Walt[24] with kind permission of the editor of *American Journal of Surgery*.

vessel near the hilum of the liver is incised or when the weapon is long enough to pass through the liver into one of the adjacent major vessels or organs such as the aorta, the inferior vena cava, the pulmonary vein, the colon or the duodenum. The cirrhotic patient is at special risk as transected vessels in the fibrotic parenchyma may have difficulty in contracting and haemorrhage is consequently less easily controlled. Furthermore, repair of the cirrhotic liver is more difficult to effect.

Bullets impart their effects by virtue of the kinetic energy which they transmit, and this in turn is related to the muzzle velocity of the weapon which ranges from approximately 970 ft/sec in the .38 automatic pistol to 2160 ft/sec in the .303 British hunting rifle.[13] Low velocity small calibre bullets do relatively little damage unless they happen to hit a vital intrahepatic structure, especially in the vicinity of the hilum. Most often, these missiles tend to produce a neat furrow with relatively little parenchymal damage. Despite experimental evidence which shows that hepatic cells adjacent to the track are damaged by the transmitted kinetic forces and possibly by generated heat, debridement of the track is not necessary in practice. In any event, formal debridement may be virtually impossible in tracks which pass through the thick part of the liver. Attempts to achieve this in the name of theoretical considerations must be considered meddlesome. In contrast, high velocity missiles may produce tremendous destruction, leaving chunks of detached or fragmented liver tissue along the course of the missile. Bleeding in these circumstances is almost inevitably vigorous. Finally, shotgun wounds smash the liver apart and may also embed foreign material. The type and degree of anatomical derangement will naturally influence surgical decisions at the time of operation.

Specially Relevant Surgical Anatomy in Hepatic Trauma

Hepatic segments

In 1957, Goldsmith and Woodburne[5] clearly delineated the concept of the liver as an organ consisting of a right lobe with anterior and posterior segments and a left lobe with a middle and lateral segment separated by the falciform ligament. The right and left lobes in turn were demarcated by an imaginary line running between the gallbladder fossa anteriorly and the inferior vena cava posteriorly (see Chapter 1). Since then, much attention has been paid to these landmarks as guides to hepatic resection (see Chapter 49). While this anatomical contribution was invaluable for elective resections, it has had its limitations in respect of trauma. Assumptions are far too often made that portions of adjacent hepatic segments cannot be safely debrided and that a neat segmental resection is virtually mandatory. The need to ensure adequate arterial blood to the residual liver and to preserve the middle hepatic vein when the anterior segment of the right lobe is retained remains essential. As long as this is done, a superficially untidy debridement which traverses formal anatomical segmental boundaries is often the optimal therapy in hepatic trauma.

Arterial inflow[20]

The hepatic artery ordinarily supplies 35 per cent of the hepatic inflow but 40–50 per cent of its oxygen. Abnormalities of distribution abound; in about 12 per cent of patients, the superior mesenteric artery gives origin to the right hepatic artery and in about 10 to 15 per cent the left hepatic artery originates from the left gastric artery. These variations may have urgent relevance in injuries and their presence should be immediately suspected whenever the Pringle manoeuvre (occlusion of the portal triad) fails to stop hepatic bleeding.

Myths about the arterial independence of each lobe, based in part on studies of corrosive casts in the past, have abounded. These misplaced beliefs, added to poorly analysed results of hepatic ligation and extrapolation of data from canine experiments where the livers uniformly contain clostridia, led to the dogma that hepatic artery ligation in humans was likely to be lethal. In a series of studies, including serial arteriography in humans, Mays and Wheeler[15] demonstrated that an intralobar arterial network exists and this can be clearly demonstrated to be functional within about four hours of ligation of one or other hepatic artery.[8] In addition, collateral supply to the liver is available from the inferior phrenic arteries and from the pancreaticoduodenal arteries. Similar earlier scientifically untested beliefs led to the dogma that ligation of the hepatic artery, if it were to be performed, could only be done with a modicum of safety proximal to the gastroduodenal artery. In fact, the hepatic artery may be ligated with similar rates of morbidity anywhere along its course from its origin to its point of entry into the liver. When the liver is observed following ligation of the hepatic artery, the surface can often be seen to blanch and then to assume a colour darker than usual in the areas corresponding to the subtended blood supply. The implication of these observations will be discussed in greater detail later. In view of the rising popularity of hepatic artery ligation, however, it should be stressed that while the hepatic artery may usually be ligated with safety, the procedure is not always innocuous and may lead to later complications.

Venous inflow and outflow

The portal vein supplies 65 per cent of the hepatic inflow but only 50 per cent of the hepatic oxygen supply. The vein rapidly divides to supply the portal triads. Being a low pressure system, bleeding from the smaller veins can usually be stopped by direct pressure. Fortunately, when the hepatic artery has been ligated, the liver is able to increase its extraction of oxygen from the portal venous blood which helps to tide over any initial physiological crisis until the hepatic artery collaterals restore the reduced flow.[23]

The hepatic veins, three in number, right, middle and left, are large and short and enter the inferior vena cava (IVC) immediately below the diaphragm. The middle and left veins may enter separately but usually join together approximately a centimetre from the inferior vena cava to form a short common stem. Bleeding from these veins may be catastrophic and necessitates special surgical techniques. In addition, eight to 16 small veins pass directly from the liver to enter the IVC on its anterior and lateral aspects. While these may produce troublesome bleeding, they are usually spontaneously tamponaded by the weight of the overlying liver. If a formal hepatic resection is performed, careful attention must be given to haemostasis in this area.

Bile ducts

The bile ducts exit via the right and left hepatic ducts in the hilum of the liver, having followed the pattern of the portal system and hepatic arterial branches closely. Anastomoses of biliary radicles across segmental and lobar lines have been difficult to demonstrate but, clinically, interruption of a lobar duct is seldom followed by prolonged jaundice. These intrahepatic tributaries are often injured along the missile tracks but seldom cause serious difficulties. In those patients in whom a large duct is injured within the hepatic parenchyma, conservatism is still advisable as these ducts have the capacity to heal spontaneously much as the wall of the common bile duct heals following removal of a T-tube. Occasionally, however, bile may collect intrahepatically and present as a cyst which requires drainage or, rarely, resection.

Clinical Picture

In blunt injury, it is a truism that isolated hepatic injuries are uncommon, occurring in 5 to 10 per cent of any series. Consequently, it is always essential that due attention be given to concomitantly injured organs and the effects that these produce. For example, head injury with cerebral symptoms and multiple fractures of the lower limbs and/or pelvis with haemorrhage are often associated with hepatic injury and must be treated. More immediately, however, attention must be given to injury to surrounding vessels such as the aorta and its branches, the inferior vena cava (IVC) and its tributaries, and the portal vein. Haemorrhage is the leading cause of death in liver injury and its prime manifestation is hypovolaemic shock (Table 50.3). Usually, this is obvious and appropriate counter-measures, which involve the insertion of two or more intravenous cannulae and the administration of crystalloids and whole blood, can be taken. Where possible, use of the saphenous vein as a conduit for fluids is avoided where the possibility of IVC damage is suspected. Parenteral antibiotics – we favour penicillin, gentamicin and clindamycin initially in major injuries – are given during the resuscitative period whenever associated colonic damage may be present. Sepsis, next to haemorrhage, is the prime cause of complication and death, and early administration of effective antibiotics has been shown to reduce subsequent infection in the face of immediate post-injury and peritoneal contamination.

Most patients with hepatic injury present with pain in the right upper quadrant or right shoulder, some abdominal splinting and evidence of intraperitoneal blood loss. In 20 to 30 per cent of cases, however, the patient may be deceptively stable with little more than slight guarding of the upper abdomen. The colour, blood pressure, pulse and general demeanour of

Table 50.3. *Liver Injuries: Causes of Death (1974–76) in 331 Patients.*

Injury	Haemorrhage	Sepsis and/or respiratory failure	Head	Heart	Delirium tremens	Metabolic
GSW	16	3	6	1	0	1
SGW	3	0	0	0	0	0
Blunt	5	3	0	0	1	0
Stab	1	0	0	0	0	0
Total	25	6	6	1	1	1
%	62.5	15.0	15.0	2.5	2.5	2.5

GSW = gunshot wounds; SGW = shotgun wounds.
From Walt[24] with kind permission of the editor of *American Journal of Surgery*.

the patient may be relatively normal. This clinical picture may persist for hours and even days before a catastrophic deterioration, marked by acute abdominal pain and the features of gross hypovolaemic shock, occurs. This change is due to sudden haemorrhage into the peritoneal cavity where previous spontaneous tamponade of the injured liver has been disrupted. The presence of fractured ribs, especially in conjunction with fractures of the pelvis or lower limbs, should always arouse suspicion that the liver may be damaged as blunt trauma which causes this combination of injuries often damages the intra-abdominal viscera too. When clinical doubt exists, peritoneal lavage will confirm the presence or absence of intraperitoneal blood with an accuracy of about 98 per cent. Complications of this procedure are rare if the bladder is first emptied and areas of previous scarring are avoided. Special problems may be posed in the presence of concomitant pelvic fractures. In this situation where blood may track extraperitoneally, the catheter should be inserted above the umbilicus and through a small incision, with the peritoneum clearly visualized. Rarely, a negative lavage may occur in a patient who is subsequently proved to have a contained subcapsular or intraparenchymal haematoma.

At the other extreme, patients with disrupted livers may appear in the emergency department in deep hypovolaemic shock, virtually unresponsive to large, rapidly infused quantities of fluid and with a peritoneal cavity so strikingly distended by blood that a temporary tamponading effect is produced. In cases of doubt or curiosity, the use of isotopic studies or arteriography has been advocated as techniques for delineating the degree of injury. More recently, grey scale ultrasonography and computerized axial tomography (CAT) have also been advanced as valuable diagnostic adjuvants. In practice, we have seldom felt the need for these investigations. In the severely injured restless patient, these techniques are time consuming or not feasible. On the other hand, in the patient with delayed, diagnostically puzzling symptoms when haemobilia is suspected, valuable information may be obtained by delineation of an intrahepatic defect by any of these methods or by angiographic demonstration of an actively bleeding lesion.

Perspectives

The pathological effects of stab wounds, missile injuries and the disruptive force of blunt trauma vary widely. The resultant of forces playing on the liver determines the degree of damage and directly influences the outcome. Surgical skills should be directed to (a) the avoidance of unnecessary operations in patients who have ceased to bleed spontaneously and permanently, (b) control of continuing haemorrhage which is the major cause of death in 60 to 70 per cent of lethal injuries, (c) the prevention of sepsis which is responsible for about 15 to 20 per cent of the deaths after hepatic injury, (d) the repair of extrahepatic injuries and (e) prophylaxis as far as possible against delayed complications such as pulmonary and renal failure.

In the 968 patients whom we treated between 1968 and 1976 at the Wayne State University Affiliated Hospitals, we found that 492 (50.8 per cent) had stopped bleeding completely from the hepatic injury at the time of operation (Table 50.4). The majority of these patients had suffered stab wounds, and if it could have been determined that the liver alone had been injured

Table 50.4. *Liver Injuries: Methods of Treatment (1968–76) in 968 Patients.*

Procedure	No.	%
Laparotomy alone	492	50.8
Suture	367	37.9
Debridement	46	4.8
Hemi-hepatectomy	25	2.6
Hepatic artery ligation	14	1.4
IVC cannulation	8	0.8
Packs	3	0.3
Death on table or details unavailable	13	1.4
Totals	968	100

From Walt[24] with kind permission of the editor of *American Journal of Surgery*.

but had ceased to bleed no operation would have been required. Refinements of investigation may make this decision possible with confidence in the reasonable future. Another 367 patients (37.9 per cent) had suture of their hepatic wounds, but in the interests of an accurate perspective it is important to recognize that in many of these patients sutures were placed only as a form of insurance in a liver which had spontaneously ceased to bleed. In a small group of these 367 patients, however, it was sometimes necessary to extend or formally open the hepatic wound to obtain access to the bleeding area. Only 109 of our last 968 patients (11.3 per cent) operated upon required major procedures (Table 50.4).

The natural history of the total spectrum of hepatic injury has not been fully appreciated in the past as non-invasive tests were not available to give a spatial reflection of the intrahepatic damage. The introduction of new sophisticated techniques has provided this information but has also uncovered fresh problems. An increasing number of patients with blunt injury who are clinically stable and from the abdominal viewpoint virtually asymptomatic are found to have intrahepatic filling defects when non-invasive methods of investigation, such as ultrasonography or isotope scanning, are used within a few days of injury. In view of the potential hazards of rupture, haemobilia and sepsis in the presence of intrahepatic parenchymal damage, surgical intervention has been advocated as a routine in the past. Careful observation of some of these patients, however, has confirmed the fact that selected lesions may regress spontaneously and completely. In that surgical treatment of these intrahepatic lesions may lead the surgeon – sometimes unwillingly but unavoidably – into major procedures, often in patients who have other serious extra-abdominal injuries, the concept of selective conservatism is attractive. Insufficient data are available as yet on the outcome of watchful waiting or tube hepatostomy on this subset of patients.

SURGICAL MANAGEMENT

Common injuries

With a diagnosis of possible hepatic injury made and appropriate resuscitative measures instituted and aimed primarily at providing adequate intravascular volume and tissue oxygenation, the patient is anaesthetized. When fractured ribs are present, thoracostomy tubes are inserted prophylactically to avoid the possibility of a tension pneumothorax developing intra-operatively in response to positive pressure ventilation. When there has been serious blood loss or suspicion of cardiac contusion, a central venous pressure (CVP) line is invaluable. Provision is made for an adequate number of cross-matched units of blood to be available together with a blood warmer and appropriate filters. The blood should be as fresh as possible and preferably meticulously cross-matched. In massive bleeding which demands immediate operation, type-specific blood is used. O-negative blood is rarely required, and dextran should be avoided in what already promises to be a bloody procedure. Fine mesh filters, while desirable for the removal of the debris present in the multiple units to be transfused, are impractical in this setting as they limit the rapidity with which the blood may be given. A Foley catheter will have been inserted earlier and urinary flow is closely monitored as an index of visceral perfusion.

The type of incision made varies with the bias of the surgeon. We prefer a midline incision as this may be made rapidly, has great versatility, gives excellent access to all parts of the peritoneal cavity if long enough, and lends itself to ready cephalad extension when it is necessary to split the sternum to gain control of the intrapericardial inferior vena cava and the hepatic veins.[3] Alternatively, an oblique incision may be angled into the seventh or eighth right intercostal space to deal with concomitant diaphragmatic or vascular injuries. While this latter thoracico-abdominal incision was the popular approach until about 1975, it has serious limitations. This incision takes longer to make and to close, gives poorer exposure, leads to greater impairment of pulmonary function postoperatively, is often more awkward to work through, and causes the patient greater discomfort. In the face of gross peritoneal contamination, it may sometimes be wise to make a separate thoracic incision, especially if there is a need to deal with pulmonary injury anyway. Today, the rapid median sternotomy is favoured in most circumstances for control of major venous bleeding in the diaphragmatic area.

Control of bleeding is of primary importance and may usually be achieved temporarily by insertion of a large pack over the damaged area, followed by manual compression. Rapid inspection of the intestine may then be made and tissue forceps applied to any intestinal lacerations in an effort to prevent the passage of intestinal content into the peritoneal cavity. Next to haemorrhage, delayed sepsis is the most common cause of death and morbidity. On removal of the pack, one or more bleeding points may be clearly visible and controllable by haemoclips or suture ligation. In some hepatic cracks, it may be necessary to enlarge the fissure deliberately to achieve access to the bleeding site in the depths of the hepatic wound. The natural reluctance of surgeons to increase iatrogenically the size of the wound is understandable but usually misguided. Any completely or partially detached piece of liver should be removed. Widespread debridement on the sole grounds of colour change should be approached very cautiously. Viability of liver tissue is not always easy to judge, as evidenced by the favourable outcome following hepatic artery ligation. The placement of approximating sutures with 2/0 catgut swedged on a blunt-nosed 'liver needle' will usually produce a degree of pressure sufficient to promote haemostasis. These sutures, placed deeply and approximately 1.5 cm from the cut edges of the liver, are firmly tied but not so firmly as to cut through the liver tissue. While the use of baffles of Gelfoam or other materials is sometimes advocated, these are rarely required. When a fairly large wedge of liver tissue has been excised and haemostasis obtained, it is not essential to achieve meticulous approximation of the walls of the residual cavity. When this is difficult, the area may be left open. The insertion of a wad of omentum pedicled on a good supply has been recommended but is not necessary.

The low velocity missile which has traversed the liver close to the surface creates a track which may be easily opened for purposes of obtaining haemostasis. On the other hand, the track which extends deep through the central area of the thick portion of the liver, usually the right lobe, may be much more difficult to manage. Closure at the entry and exit points is undesirable as continuing bleeding within the track may cause an intrahepatic haematoma, with or without subsequent haemobilia. Tractotomy of deep lesions is likely to be extremely difficult and represents overkill in the light of the natural history of this lesion. In practice, the application of continued pressure, manually and by pack, together with what sutures may be conveniently placed in the line of injury will produce haemostasis in most cases. The insertion of a suction catheter into the track to

Table 50.5. *Liver Injuries.*[a]

	Annual No. of patients (approximate)	Hepatic artery[b] ligation	Lobectomy[b]	IVC cannulation[b] 1972–76
Baylor	130	0/1590	<2.5%	15 (7)
Dallas	110	3 (Haemobilia)/5 yrs	2 (1.8%)	4 (0)
S. Illinois	100	0	3–4 (3.5%)	3 (1)
WSU	100	14/968	25/968 (2.6%)	8 (0)
SUNY (Downstate)	75	10 (approximate)	0	0
Emory	70	7/429	7/429 (1.6%)	0
LSU	70	Seldom	4 (5.7%)	2 (0)
UCSF	70	±5%	±4/yr (5.7%)	±5/yr (10%)
Louisville	60	59/189 (31.2%)	3/189 (1.6%)	–
Colorado	40	'Extremely rarely'	Not available	9 (2)

[a] Data derived through personal communication with Jordan, Fry, Roberts, Shaftan, Stone, Cohn and Nance, Blaisdell, Polk, and Eiseman.
[b] Figures derived either from published series, work in progress, or thoughtful estimates.
() Number of survivors in parentheses.

prevent accumulation of blood has been recommended but we do not feel this to be necessary or safe. When bleeding continues to be excessive despite these conservative measures, ligation of the hepatic artery to the affected lobe will almost invariably be effective (see below).

In some patients with severe blunt injury or gunshot wounds caused by high velocity missiles, the liver substance is grossly disrupted. In such circumstances, fully or partially detached segments of liver tissue should be removed. Radical debridement of several hundreds of grams of liver tissue is preferable to formal complete lobectomy in that the survival rate with this effective although aesthetically unattractive technique of debridement is appreciably higher. Haemostasis is obtained by haemoclips or suture ligation and any residual ooze may be stopped by the direct application of microcrystalline collagen (Avitene) provided that a temporary dry field is first obtained.[17] Care must be taken to avoid spillage of the powder into the peritoneal cavity for fear of stimulating dense adhesions. Again, some surgeons advise careful suturing of omentum to the liver surface as a viable pack to provide some degree of tamponade or coverage to the damaged area but there seems little benefit to be derived from this measure. If substantial oozing continues after debridement and local haemostasis, hepatic artery ligation may be first tested for its effect by placing a vascular clamp on the appropriate artery. If this produces a satisfactory result, the artery is ligated. While this is technically easy to accomplish, this technique should not be abused and it is not a substitute for meticulous attention to the surface of the debrided area.

The enthusiasm of the last decade for formal hepatic lobectomy for trauma has disappeared (Table 50.5). The mortality rate of emergency lobectomy hovers around 50 to 60 per cent in the United States. The overall survival rate may be increased by the patient application of less aggressive measures. Resection is unavoidable, however, in those few patients who have one or other lobe completely disrupted by close-range shotgun blasts or similar high energy wounds with destruction of major veins, arteries and biliary radicles throughout the parenchyma. In these, generous exposure and early control of hepatic inflow with judicious tamponading of any bleeding outflow vessels are essential to success. Twenty-five of our last 968 patients (2.6 per cent) underwent hemi-hepatectomy; few survived.

While the high mortality rate associated with emergency hepatic lobectomy relates substantially to the associated shock, blood loss and multiple organ injury, the operation itself by the nature of the situation needs to be completed rapidly and is unusually difficult. The basic principles of lobectomy remain pertinent, such as the need to obtain early control and ligation of the appropriate hepatic artery, portal vein and hepatic bile duct at the hilum, finger fracture resection along the line of vascular demarcation and avoidance of injury to the retrohepatic IVC. A major additional problem is the safe control of the hepatic vein. As the liver is mobilized by incision of its suspensory ligaments, traction on the lacerated hepatic vein may permit entry of air, resulting in air embolism. This danger is greatly compounded when the chest is not opened and a marked differential pressure is present between the abdominal and pleural cavities. Consequently, a conscious effort must be made to obviate this debacle whether the hepatic vein is approached early in the operation or towards the end as the parenchyma is finally incised in the diaphragmatic region.

Special injuries

Central haematomas, necrotic lesions or bilious collections. Uncommonly, a central but large area deep in the parenchyma of the liver may be pulpified or be the site of a fluid collection. Some patients with these lesions will also have sustained severe concomitant cranial, thoracic or osseous injuries, making a long intra-abdominal operation especially undesirable. In these cases, the insertion of a de Pezzer or Foley catheter into the area may be highly effective.[4] The catheter is attached to low pressure suction and great care is taken to avoid the introduction of infection. Where fluid is not already present, autolysis will gradually occur and the ischaemic tissue will be evacuated over a period of two to eight weeks. Radiopaque contrast material inserted into the cavity will delineate any connection with the biliary tree and will also outline its progressive reduction in size, thereby guiding judgement as to the optimal time for removal of the catheter.

Deep crack or missile track. Rarely, these will extend horizontally across both hepatic lobes. Access to the depths of an extensive lesion with reasonable safety may be impossible. Ligation of the common hepatic artery is the most efficacious approach but in this event may occasionally fail to produce adequate haemostasis. In such cases, the time-honoured, if suspect, technique of insertion of large abdominal gauze packs in such a way as to produce considerable pressure on the liver may be life saving. The pack is left in place for five to seven days after which it is slowly removed in the operating room under direct vision. The five patients in whom we have had reason to adopt this somewhat discredited approach have all recovered well and were discharged home in about 14 days. For the occasional surgeon faced with brisk haemorrhage, who does not have the facility or facilities for major hepatic surgery, insertion of a pack and transfer of the patient to an appropriately equipped centre is recommended.

Obvious abdominal tamponade and hypovolaemic shock. The patient with obvious abdominal tamponade and hypovolaemic shock unresponsive to a large rapid infusion of fluid through multiple intravenous lines will frequently exsanguinate and die within a minute or two of release of the tamponade at operation. This clinical picture is always suggestive of major intra-abdominal vascular injury and preparations to obtain immediate and maximal control must be made before laparotomy. Ledgerwood, Kazmers and Lucas[9] have recommended a preliminary left thoracotomy and clamping of the thoracic aorta just above the diaphragm. This manoeuvre produces improved perfusion of the heart and brain and reduces blood loss when the abdomen is opened. In the unconscious patient in shock, this may be done without anaesthesia in the emergency department if necessary and is obviously preferable to an improvised laparotomy. Alternatively, control of the aorta immediately below the diaphragm may be obtained in the operating room digitally or by use of pressure via a sponge stick, a vascular clamp, an aortic compressor or by the end of a body wall retractor. Speed and effective compression are the common denominators of success. The haemostasis obtained is relative, however, for bleeding may continue through venous tears. Where bleeding remains substantial, especially after addition of temporary hepatic artery occlusion, injury to the IVC or an hepatic vein must be regarded as a likelihood.

Whether the aorta is clamped above or below the diaphragm, special precautions need to be taken on declamping, which should always be done gradually. Added fluid is given to these patients to compensate for the expanded vascular capacity distal to the released clamp. Sodium bicarbonate is infused to combat the acidosis attendant on the predictable ischaemia.

Major venous injury to the retrohepatic IVC. This remains one of the great challenges of traumatic surgery. All eight patients in whom we attempted IVC cannulation died. In a recent review of seven institutions in which IVC cannulation was performed, only 10 of 41 patients survived, seven of whom came from one unit (Table 50.5). Bleeding may be spontaneously tamponaded retroperitoneally when one or more of the smaller retrohepatic tributaries of the IVC are injured. For this reason, a non-expanding haematoma arising from that area, and usually manifesting itself in the infrahepatic region by tracking distally, should not be disturbed.

Repair of injuries to the major hepatic veins or retrohepatic IVC is extremely difficult.[12] Success depends in large measure on the quality of the surgical exposure obtained. Of the three main hepatic veins, the right is the most likely to be injured, torn by the weight of the heavy right lobe of the liver. Access is best obtained by a midline incision and median sternotomy with incision of the diaphragm anteroposteriorly down to the inferior vena cava, care being taken to avoid damage to the phrenic nerve. The liver may need to be mobilized to give optimal access and this is done by incision of the suspensory ligaments. The injured vein may be repaired when the injury is close to the junction of the hepatic vein and the IVC. In contrast, when the intrahepatic portion of the vein is injured, ligation is advisable as any attempt to dissect the vein free from the parenchyma for adequate exposure is likely to be difficult and dangerous.

When a major disruption of a portion of the wall of the IVC is present which cannot be grasped by a curved vascular clamp such as a Satinsky clamp, it is necessary to insert a stent to ensure venous return to the heart while preserving a field relatively clear of blood so that the venous injury may be repaired. Occlusion of the hepatic artery inflow and manual tamponade of the area after mobilization of the liver sufficient to permit antero-posterior compression between packs are necessary while preparations are being made. While total occlusion of venous return through the IVC for an hour or more has been reported in successful liver transplantation, this is not reproducible in the shocked hypovolaemic injured patient.

Cannulation may be achieved by the insertion of a cannula through a purse-string suture in the atrial appendage passing through the right atrium into the IVC, with appropriate holes placed for return of renal venous blood and egress of blood into the right atrium.[14] Fluids may be administered through the cannula. Alternatively, applying the same principles, one may insert the cannula through a purse-string suture directly in the abdominal IVC and position the tube so that its distal end lies at a point just above the diaphragm. Tapes are placed around the IVC at the proximal and distal portions of the cannula. Endotracheal tubes, thoracostomy tubes and specially designed cannulae with a terminal balloon have been used for this purpose. Recently, Pilcher, Harman and Moore[19] have successfully used a 28 Fr shunt, with holes appropriately situated to permit venous return, and fitted with a terminal balloon which can be inserted through the saphenous vein and so positioned as to occlude tears in the retrohepatic IVC. The advantages of this approach include ease of insertion, and the size and contour of the conduit permit venous return whilst also serving as an inlet for venous infusion. Simultaneously, defects in the vein are occluded by means of the inflated balloon. Air embolism must be avoided, adequate cardiac output ensured and free access to the damaged vein obtained as these are the main determinants of the immediate outcome.

Haemobilia. Hepatic injury may be accompanied or followed by haemobilia. Approximately 180 cases due to trauma have been reported in the world's literature but it may be assumed that the lesion is more frequent than this figure suggests.[21] Nevertheless, we are aware of only two instances in the last 1400 patients with hepatic injury whom we have treated.

Haemobilia results from the communication of an intrahepatic vessel with the biliary tree. It is a matter of some surprise that this symptom complex does not occur more often. Bleeding usually results from the accumulation under tension of blood in a parenchymal cavity either when the two ends of a track or the roof of a fissure are tightly closed by sutures or when gradual dissolution of necrotic hepatic tissue occurs. The patient may complain of epigastric discomfort or colicky pain due to the passage of clots. About half the patients are jaundiced at one time or another. In some patients, the precipitating cause may be minor, such as a gentle blow on the football field; in others, the capsule of the liver may have appeared to be intact at the original operation. Overt infection may or may not be present. Haematemesis or melaena may be the first clinical manifestation and more often than not bleeding occurs in staccato fashion rather than continuously. Anaemia with shock may occur, depending on the severity of the haemorrhage. About 50 per cent of patients develop their haemobilia more than one month after the injury and consequently all patients should be warned of this remote possibility following hepatic injury. Occurrence beyond a year after the injury is very unlikely but the rare patient may have periodic attacks over many years.

The diagnosis of haemobilia is most efficiently proven by arteriography which will delineate the site of bleeding and which may also demonstrate an arteriovenous fistula in the cavity. Ultrasonography and isotopic scanning have also been successful in demonstrating the intrahepatic filling defect. Alternatively, endoscopy may reveal the passage of blood into the duodenum through the common bile duct. Treatment depends on the nature of the lesion. Ligation of the hepatic artery is effective when no cavity is discernible. Where possible, unroofing of any cavity in the liver and direct ligation of the bleeding vessel in the wall is desirable; in this group of patients, hepatic artery ligation is added selectively. In severely ill or septic patients, embolization of the vessel by Gelfoam through an angiographic catheter has been successfully performed. If these procedures fail or are not feasible, hepatic lobectomy or segmentectomy may be unavoidable, especially in the presence of sepsis. Over 80 per cent of these patients survive if the operation can be done on a semi-elective basis.

Spontaneous and apparently permanent cessation of bleeding has been reported in fairly small peripheral hepatic lesions when conservative methods were adopted with blood replacement as the cornerstone of treatment. On the face of it, this approach appears more hazardous than operation. Nevertheless, 12 cases have been successfully followed and sequential arteriography suggests that about eight weeks are required for healing of the intrahepatic lesion.[10]

Ancillary Additions to the Hepatic Operation

Hepatic artery ligation

The classical but inappropriately discouraging

paper of Graham and Cannell in 1933,[6] reviewing the deaths of 16 of 28 patients following hepatic artery ligation (HAL) of whom only four died of hepatic failure, led to the belief that ligation of the HA was almost certain to lead to disaster. This view was reinforced by the predictable death of dogs in whom the HA was ligated. Until the work of Markowitz 15 years later, after the advent of penicillin, it was not realized that canine mortality was due to clostridial overgrowth in a hypoxic environment. In contrast, the hepatic parenchyma and bile of humans are normally sterile. On the basis of experimental and angiographic observations, Mays has shown that the case against HAL was grossly overstated. In 1977, Mays and his colleagues[2] reported ligating the HA in 59 of 189 patients with hepatic injuries. This incidence is six to ten times greater than is felt to be necessary by others working in major trauma centres but Mays's work has served to show that this manoeuvre may be performed with confidence if not with impunity (Table 50.5). Eighteen of his 59 patients died, some of later sepsis. The degree to which the relative hepatic ischaemia may promote sepsis is difficult to assess but we believe that it does predispose to this and consequently HAL should be avoided if at all possible, especially where there has been spillage of intestinal content or prolonged shock. In the Wayne State University series, HAL has been performed as a last resort in 14 of the last 968 cases (1.4 per cent) but has not been innocuous. Three patients rebled despite our conviction that the hepatic artery was ligated, and six patients eventually died. On ligation of the artery, a distinct colour demarkation can be observed in the liver. As the Po_2 of the parenchyma is already reduced, especially in shock, and reliance is placed on portal vein oxygen until collaterals develop, it is essential that optimal splanchnic circulation be ensured. This entails the elimination of hypotension, the provision of a Po_2 of approximately 13 kPa (100 mmHg), nasogastric decompression, normothermia and the cessation of enteral feeding for four to seven days to reduce metabolic demand. Broad spectrum antibiotics are given as contamination of the peritoneal cavity is usually present and residual areas of hepatic necrosis may be inadvertently left in situ.

Glucagon seems not to be of clinical value in enhancing the hepatic oxygenation as originally postulated. Recent experiments suggest that although glucagon may improve cardiac output and splanchnic circulation, these beneficial effects are at least counterbalanced by the increase in hepatic oxygen demand which is induced by the stimulation of gluconeogenesis and glycogenolysis.[25]

If the left hepatic artery is ligated, cholecystectomy need not be added as a routine, and few surgeons now advocate a second operation after 24 to 48 hours specifically to assess the state of the liver. Unless sepsis supervenes, the serum bilirubin levels peak about the fourth postoperative day at around 60 μmol/l (3 to 4 mg/dl) and the liver enzymes such as serum glutamic oxalic transaminase and lactic dehydrogenase are moderately raised for seven to ten days. In some patients, the serum alkaline phosphatase remains abnormally high for a few weeks but this level does not seem to bear a relationship to eventual outcome.

Table 50.6. *Prospective Randomized T-tube Study: Hepatic Trauma.*

Treatment	Patients	Deaths	Patients with complications	No. of complications
Drainage only	62	5	23	43
Drainage with cholecystostomy	62	5	22	39
Drainage with T-tube in CBD	65	8	38	87
Totals	189	18	83	169

From Lucas and Walt[11] with kind permission of the editor of *Journal of Trauma.*

T-tube drainage

In 1963, Merendino, Dillard and Cammock[16] postulated that biliary leakage from the liver could be reduced or eliminated by reduction of intrahepatic pressure through the insertion of a T-tube into the common bile duct. While superficially attractive, this unproved concept gained immediate popularity and the routine addition of a T-tube in patients with hepatic injury rapidly became standard practice. The presence of a T-tube in our patients seemed to increase the incidence of complications and possibly the volume of biliary drainage from perihepatic drains. The insertion of a T-tube into the common bile duct, which is often only 4 to 5 mm in diameter, frequently prolonged the operation and seemed an irrational and irrevocable step in the presence of faecal spillage, offering a ready route of access for infection into the biliary tree and, through it, into the liver. In 1972, following a prospective randomized study in 189 patients with hepatic trauma (Table 50.6), we were able to demonstrate that a T-tube increased the incidence of complications mainly through sepsis and that it should not be used except where incidental damage to the extrahepatic biliary tree was present[11] (Table 50.7). In fact, the promotion of biliary infection seemed to be confirmed and, in addition, the T-tube could be demonstrated to introduce an element of obstruction by occupying a portion of the potentially oedematous lumen of the common bile duct. In the 500 patients with liver injury whom we have treated since 1972, we have not used T-tube drainage of the common bile duct in any case and have had no reason to regret this approach. Furthermore, the T-tube is not necessary for intra-operative cholangiography, which may be performed by direct injection of the common bile duct if desired, nor for the diagnosis of haemobilia. Direct puncture of the common bile duct above a soft occluding clamp followed by the injection of radiopaque material through a No. 16 needle provides a very satisfactory radiographic pic-

Table 50.7. *Morbidity and Drainage.*[a]

Complication	Standard drainage alone	Standard plus cholecystostomy	Standard plus choledochostomy
Intra-abdominal or subphrenic abscess	5	5	12
Jaundice	3	2	11
Stress gastric bleeding	5[b]	4	7
Cholangitis	0	2	8
Biliary–cutaneous fistula	0	2	2
Bile peritonitis	0	0	1
Respiratory failure	9	8	7
Massive wound infection	6	4	9
Common bile duct obstruction	0	0	2
T-tube dislodgement	–	–	1
Inadvertent cystic duct injury	0	0	2
Haemobilia	0	0	1
Postoperative peritoneal haemorrhage	4	2	2
Miscellaneous[c]	11	10	22
Totals	43	39	87

[a] From Lucas and Walt[11] with kind permission of the editor of *Journal of Trauma*.

[b] Stress bleeding began on the fourth hospital day in one patient who was being observed after blunt abdominal injury. Surgery for stress bleeding revealed the liver injury.

[c] Includes postoperative bowel obstruction, pancreatitis, renal failure, enterocutaneous fistula, tracheal innominate artery fistula, liver abscess, and convulsions due to heroin intoxication.

ture. With regard to haemobilia, it should be stressed again that haemobilia is exceedingly rare and that, when it does occur, the temporal relationship of its appearance is such that the T-tube is likely to have been removed by the time that the bleeding begins. Few surgeons today support the use of a T-tube in hepatic trauma except when it is required as a stent for a repaired duct.

To drain or not to drain?

Extensive drainage of the perihepatic area has long been an article of surgical faith. What arguments there have been have ranged around whether to use sump drains and whether to remove the twelfth rib for purposes of dependent drainage. The need to drain has seldom been doubted because of the perceived desirability of providing egress for residual blood or the potential products of hepatic necrosis in the subphrenic space. In cases of extensive debridement or resection, excision of the twelfth rib from within the abdomen has been advocated. Alternatively, especially in the obese individual, the patient is sometimes turned on his left side at the end of the operation for the specific purpose of excision of the rib. The objective of those who support this approach is to provide posterior drainage through an incision deliberately enlarged to a size sufficient to accommodate three or four fingers. In the view of others, this usually moist dressing on which the patient lies has the potential to promote the introduction of infection from without. We have consequently preferred to use multiple Penrose and soft sump drains attached to low pressure suction placed so as not to lie in contact with a major vessel or across a hollow viscus. These drains have been brought out of the abdominal wall laterally well below the tip of the twelfth rib and have usually been left in situ with periodic shortening for 7 to 14 days, depending on the presence and quantity of drainage. Perry et al[18] have long been sceptical of this practice and state that the routine use of drains is undesirable. This group have had the courage of their iconoclastic views in their last 230 cases, among which were 158 blunt injuries and 45 patients who suffered bursting trauma. Their results suggest to them that peritoneal drains are not necessary for even major hepatic lacerations but their findings have not as yet been subjected to a prospective randomized trial. More specifically, no unusual number of complications attributable to the collection of bile – a long-standing fear of surgeons – were encountered.

Hepatic damage to a large biliary radicle

Infrequently, a major intrahepatic biliary radicle is damaged close to the hilum and the leak can be demonstrated by intra-operative cholangiography. Insertion of a stent in such a case is impossible and resection of the liver tissue in the area in an attempt to obtain exposure and to effect repair is unjustifiable. Drainage of the extrabiliary tree by a T-tube in these circumstances and sequential monitoring of the intrahepatic leak by radiopaque material shows that most of these worrisome lesions heal spontaneously without deleterious sequelae.

Associated Complications

Patients who sustain severe liver injuries are subject to all the complications that may follow major operations of any kind and reference will be made here only to lesions which are frequently, if not uniquely, associated with hepatic trauma. Apart from stab wounds, the liver is seldom injured in isolation and many serious extrahepatic complications may always be anticipated. Where possible, prophylactic or early therapeutic measures should be taken in the immediate postoperative period. A brief listing follows:

1. The right lung and pleural cavity are often injured concomitantly and, in blunt hepatic injuries, rib fractures are present in about 30 per cent of cases. If any pneumothorax is suspected – no matter how small – a chest tube is inserted before anaesthesia is begun. Gross contusion of the lung and haemothoraces of various degrees are common, impairing adequate oxygenation. Postoperatively, in serious injuries, and whenever extensive resection has been carried out, the endotracheal tube should be left in place and the patient put on a volume ventilator, with or without positive end-expiratory pressure, until it is certain that the adult respiratory distress syndrome will not occur. Ventilation and arterial blood gases are meticulously monitored. These patients have a special predisposition to pulmonary complications whenever the following factors are present: (a) age above 40 years, (b) obesity, (c) thoracico-abdominal incision with diaphragmatic restriction, (d) extensive pulmonary

contusion, (e) sustained shock, (f) massive blood transfusion, (g) associated long bone fractures possibly causing fat embolism and, above all, (h) sepsis.

2. In blunt injuries to the torso, myocardial contusion occurs more often than is generally recognized. Electrocardiographic and enzyme patterns should be carefully and sequentially studied when the cardiac output remains low in the face of an adequate intravascular volume. In such cases, a Swan–Ganz pulmonary artery catheter should be inserted.
3. Associated injuries to abdominal organs are common and the average number of organs injured in patients who suffer liver injury is about 2.5. Of these organs, the colon by virtue of the subsequent sepsis which it causes by spillage of its contents and the pancreas by virtue of its tendency to bleed or secrete corrosive pancreatic juice are most threatening.
4. When sepsis occurs, acute erosive gastritis and upper gastrointestinal bleeding are common. Consequently, nasogastric suction and the prophylactic administration of antacids or cimetidine are advisable. Neither of these measures will guarantee freedom from gastric bleeding but they seem to reduce the incidence and severity of haemorrhage. Bleeding is often heralded by the persistence or appearance of ileus and the presence of bile in the nasogastric suction, followed by streaks of altered blood. Jaundice of low degree is often present by this time and should not be attributed to re-absorption of pooled blood or the effect of massive transfusions as long as the bilirubin exceeds 70 μmol/l (4 mg/dl) or continues to rise. In these circumstances the assumption should always be made that infection is present. Antibiotics are best stopped and the patient re-examined clinically and radiographically. Subphrenic or interloop abscesses are the commonest sites of infection but the precise area may be very difficult to delineate. Ultrasonography, gallium scans and CAT scanning may help but each investigation is likely to be of assistance in only about 60 per cent of cases. When used together – an expensive undertaking – accurate localization may be achieved in about 75 per cent of patients, but false positives may also occur. Where jaundice is increasing or bleeding is substantial and unresponsive, abdominal exploration should be carried out without delay. Should signs of respiratory insufficiency develop as manifested by a low $Pa\text{O}_2$, hyperventilation with some degree of relative hypocarbia, an increasing physiological shunt and decreased lung compliance, they should be regarded as further manifestations of sepsis.
5. In that serious liver injuries require large quantities of blood, postoperative oozing immediately raises the question of whether the patient is suffering a 'washout' effect or disseminated intravascular coagulation. Coagulation studies may be helpful in that the platelets and fibrinogen are greatly reduced in DIC while the prothrombin time is prolonged, and fibrin split-products and abnormal RBCs are likely to be present. In contrast, although platelets are reduced in number, the fibrinogen level tends to remain normal and other parameters are not grossly disturbed following massive blood transfusions per se. The immediate treatment of any substantial oozing following hepatic trauma includes the administration of fresh blood if possible, together with platelets and fresh frozen plasma if marked thrombocytopenia is present. In the face of extensive trauma, there is an understandable reluctance to administer heparin which, while it may improve laboratory values, seems not to save lives very often in these circumstances and may cause short-term difficulties.

SUMMARY

Hepatic trauma is increasing in frequency in industrial society. In the United States, the mortality rate has stabilized at about 14 per cent but this incidence varies with the nature of the wounding agent, the quality of pre-hospital resuscitation and the speed with which the patient is transported to a hospital where suitable personnel and equipment are immediately available. Haemorrhage is responsible for death in 60 to 75 per cent of these patients and sepsis in about 15 to 25 per cent. Fortunately, most liver wounds either stop bleeding spontaneously (even though this may not be recognizable clinically) or are easily controlled at operation. For those patients who are bleeding briskly, local control is attempted along standard surgical principles encompassing adequate exposure and direct ligation or clipping of the offending vessels even though this may entail enlargement of the hepatic wound. Where this fails, ligation of the hepatic artery, in whichever portion of its course is appropriate to the lesion, will often be effective without causing unacceptable morbidity. Extensive debridement of liver tissue is feasible as in any soft tissue injury as long as the vascular supply to the residual tissue is adequate. The immediate cosmetic appearance of the liver is unimportant and the liver has unique regenerative capacities which permit it to compensate for loss of as much as 80 per cent of its substance (see also Chapter 10). Formal lobectomy carries a mortality rate of 50 per cent or more and should be reserved for occasions when all else has failed or where massive destruction of a lobe is present.

The most difficult problem in liver trauma is the accomplishment of successful haemostasis in retrohepatic IVC injury. Temporary devascularization of the liver by insertion of an IVC cannula and the ligation of the hepatic artery inflow may be mandatory. The mortality rate in these circumstances remains understandably high, probably exceeding 75 per cent. Occasionally, dogged persistence with manual tamponade of the retrohepatic area, following mobilization of the liver, may stop venous bleeding and preclude the need for much more elaborate surgical assault.

As it is rare for the liver to be injured in isolation in major trauma, the outcome is often determined by complications arising from associated visceral damage. The lung is at special risk and should be supported prophylactically. Renal failure has become relatively uncommon, reflecting the current appreciation of the need to protect the intravascular volume. Sepsis is an ever present risk, particularly when intestinal spillage has occurred. In such circumstances, primary colonic anastomosis should not be done.

Overall, it may be stated that the past five years have seen a distinct move towards surgical conservatism in the management of hepatic trauma. Surgical machismo has been replaced by the use of a wide variety of more mundane techniques aimed at achieving local haemostasis.

REFERENCES

1. Defore, W.W., Mattox, K.L., Jordan, G.L. & Beall, A.C. (1976) Management of 1,590 consecutive cases of liver trauma. *Archives of Surgery,* **111,** 493.
2. Flint, L.M., Mays, E.T., Aaron, W.S., Fulton, R.L. & Polk, H.C. (1977) Selectivity in the management of hepatic trauma. *Annals of Surgery,* **185,** 613.
3. Fullen, W.D., McDonough, J.J., Popp, M.J. & Altemeier, W.A. (1974) Sternal splitting approach for major hepatic or retrohepatic vena cava injury. *Journal of Trauma,* **14,** 903.
4. Gewertz, B.L. & Olsen, W. R. (1975) Hepatostomy for central hepatic hematomas. *Journal of Trauma,* **15,** 271.
5. Goldsmith, N.A. & Woodburne, R.T. (1957) The surgical anatomy pertaining to liver resection. *Surgery, Gynecology and Obstetrics,* **105,** 310.
6. Graham, R.R. & Cannell, D. (1933) Accidental ligation of the hepatic artery. *British Journal of Surgery,* **20,** 566.
7. Hardy, K.J. (1972) Patterns of liver injury after fatal blunt trauma. *Surgery, Gynecology and Obstetrics,* **134,** 39.
8. Koehler, R.E., Korobkin, M. & Lewis, F. (1975) Arteriographic demonstration of collateral arterial supply to the liver after hepatic artery ligation. *Radiology,* **117,** 49.
9. Ledgerwood, A.M., Kazmers, M. & Lucas, C.E. (1976) The role of thoracic aortic occlusion for massive hemoperitoneum. *Journal of Trauma,* **16,** 610.
10. Lockwood, T.E., Schorn, L. & Coln, D. (1977) Nonoperative management of hemobilia. *Annals of Surgery,* **185,** 335.
11. Lucas, C.E. & Walt, A.J. (1972) Analysis of randomized biliary drainage for liver trauma in 189 patients. *Journal of Trauma,* **12,** 925.
12. Madding, G.F., Lim, R.C. & Kennedy, P.A. (1977) Hepatic and vena caval injuries. *Surgical Clinics of North America,* **57,** 275.
13. Mays, E.T. (1976) Hepatic trauma. *Current Problems in Surgery,* **XIII,** 8.
14. Mays, E.T. (1976) Hepatic trauma. *Current Problems in Surgery,* **XIII,** 59–64.
15. Mays, E.T. & Wheeler, C.S. (1974) Demonstration of collateral arterial flow after interruption of hepatic arteries in man. *New England Journal of Medicine,* **290,** 993.
16. Merendino, K.A., Dillard, D.H. & Cammock, E.E. (1963) The concept of surgical biliary decompression in the management of liver trauma. *Surgery, Gynecology and Obstetrics,* **117,** 285.
17. Morgenstern, L., Michel, S.L. & Austin, E. (1977) Control of hepatic bleeding with microfibrillar collagen. *Archives of Surgery,* **112,** 941.
18. Fischer, R.P., O'Farrell, K. & Perry, J.P. (1978) The value of peritoneal drains in the treatment of liver injuries. *Journal of Trauma.* In press.
19. Pilcher, D.B., Harman, P.K. & Moore, E.E. (1977) Retrohepatic vena cava balloon shunt introduced via the sapheno-femoral junction. *Journal of Trauma,* **17,** 837.
20. Rappaport, A.M. & Schneiderman, J.H. (1976) The function of the hepatic artery. *Review of Physiology, Biochemistry, Pharmacology,* **76,** 130.
21. Sandblom, P. (1973) Hemobilia. *Surgical Clinics of North America,* **53,** 1191.
22. Trunkey, D.D., Shires, G.T. & McClelland, R. (1974) Management of liver trauma in 811 consecutive patients. *Annals of Surgery,* **179,** 722.
23. Tygstrup, N., Winkler, K., Mellemgaard, K. & Andreassen, M. (1962) Determination of the hepatic arterial blood flow and oxygen supply in man by clamping the hepatic artery during surgery. *Journal of Clinical Investigation,* **41,** 447.

24. Walt, A.J. (1978) The mythology of hepatic trauma or Babel revisited. *American Journal of Surgery,* **135,** 12–18.

25. Witte, C.L., Witte, M.H. & Kintner, K. (1978) Effect of glucagon on hepatic lymph (tissue) Po_2 after ligation of the hepatic artery: an experimental study. *Journal of Trauma,* **18,** 27.

Chapter 51

The Liver in Infection

GREG HOLDSTOCK
M. BALASEGARAM
G.H. MILLWARD-SADLER
RALPH WRIGHT

Abnormalities of structure and function of the liver occur in a wide range of infectious diseases, but the hepatic involvement is usually overshadowed by the systemic disease. Often the changes are non-specific, and factors that may be implicated in their aetiology include haematogenous or direct spread of the infection and the action of the Kupffer cells in phagocytosing and localizing the organism in the liver. Other possible factors include the action of a toxin on the liver cell after it has been released by the infecting agent. Haemolysis may also contribute to the severity of the jaundice. Although usually only a minor part of the illness, jaundice or abnormality of the liver function tests can be the main feature of the illness. In some instances they may be the only abnormality.

Many of the infectious diseases to be described are more common in the developing countries, where standards of hygiene are not as high as in western society. The early literature on jaundice occurring during a particular infectious disease should be interpreted with caution, as in many instances there may have been coincidental viral hepatitis.

Patients with chronic liver disease and cirrhosis have an increased susceptibility to infection for at least three reasons: firstly, their life-style and poor hygiene leads to a greater exposure to infectious agents; secondly, they may be malnourished; thirdly, they may well have diminished resistance to infections because of impairment of their immunological response or deficient reticuloendothelial function.

In this chapter we have concentrated on the clinical, functional and pathological changes of the liver that occur in a wide variety of infectious diseases, excluding viral infections. Special emphasis is given to those which are of the greatest clinical importance. The first part of the chapter deals with systemic infections, the second with localized intrahepatic infections.

BACTERIAL INFECTIONS

Pneumococcus

Even after the advent of antibiotics, up to a quarter of all patients with lobar pneumonia develop jaundice.[259,336] It is not clear whether the jaundice is hepatocellular or cholestatic in origin.[257,328] Haemolysis, although occasionally present, is not usually a significant factor. Early reports that jaundice was more commonly associated with specific serotypes of pneumococcus have not been confirmed.[336]

Most patients presenting with jaundice do so early in the course of their disease. There is no relationship between the development of jaundice and the severity of the disease. Jaundice is more common in patients with right lower lobe pneumonia and this has led to suggestions that a mechanical factor might be operative, but this has no scientific support.

On examination, the liver may be enlarged

and tender, but the pulmonary and systemic signs usually dominate the clinical picture. In one series of patients with lobar pneumonia, there was elevation of the bilirubin in 50 per cent of cases, of serum transaminases in 20 per cent and alkaline phosphatase in 10 per cent.[336] When haemolysis occurs, it is usually associated with underlying glucose-6-phosphate dehydrogenase deficiency.[335] Histology of the liver can show focal necrosis and an inflammatory infiltrate. The hepatocytes are usually normal but may be slightly swollen. Cholestasis can sometimes be a feature.[99] Electron microscopic studies of the liver suggest a direct toxic effect on several organelles.[99,328]

Streptococcus

Although jaundice can occur in streptococcal infections, it is not as common as in pneumococcal infections. There are a few reports of liver histology, and these have shown changes varying from a non-specific reactive hepatitis with occasional foci of parenchymal cell necrosis to multiple abscess formation.[105,173,196,270,283]

Recently, there has been a case report of a patient presenting with a prolonged pyrexia of unknown origin with a high alkaline phosphatase but normal serum transaminases, in whom *Streptococcus viridans* was cultured from liver biopsy material. Histologically, there were areas of lymphocytic infiltration and loss of hepatocytes. The patient responded to penicillin.[356]

Although specific infection of the biliary tree with *Streptococcus viridans* has been given a specific label, 'cholangitis lenta', it is doubtful whether this is a specific entity.

Staphylococcus

There are few reports of liver histology in patients with staphylococcal septicaemia. In the days prior to antibiotics, jaundice was occasionally reported.[307] In staphylococcal septicaemia, the liver may be a site of abscess formation.[58,242] We have observed one patient with a staphylococcal osteomyelitis associated with a granulomatous hepatitis (Figure 51.1).

Escherichia coli (*E. coli*)

Jaundice associated with *E. coli* infections is almost unknown in adults. However, it is not unusual in infants, when it carries a high mortality rate.[132] The mortality can be dramatically reduced if the correct therapy is instituted

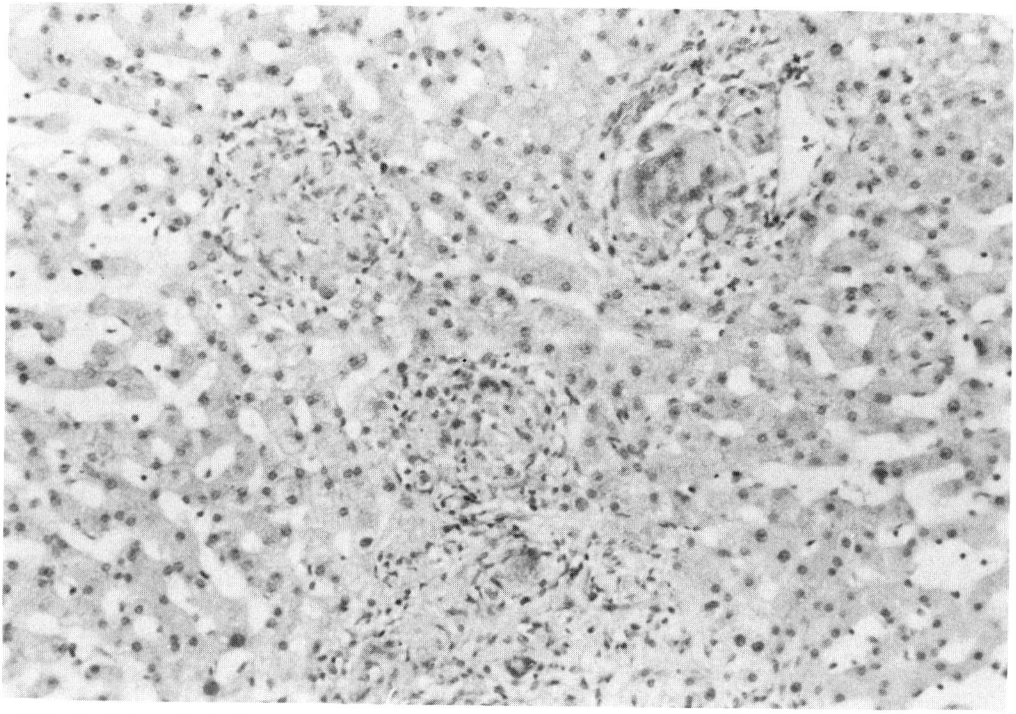

Figure 51.1. Multiple epithelioid granulomas in a patient with staphylococcal septicaemia and vertebral osteomyelitis. Haematoxylin and eosin × 500.

early in the course of the disease.[277] The liver may show areas of focal necrosis and there may be an inflammatory infiltrate.[30] In xanthogranulomatous pyelonephritis, where *E. coli* can often be the infective agent, abnormalities of the liver function tests have been reported, and histology shows a reactive hepatitis.[198]

Granuloma Inguinale

Although this infection is usually limited to the ano-genital region,[79] metastatic lesions are occasionally seen. The liver is one site affected, sometimes with multiple abscesses. Histology shows the typical Donovan bodies.[195]

Gonococcus

Perihepatitis (Fitz-Hugh–Curtis syndrome) is the best-known hepatic complication of gonococcal infections. This classically occurs in women and presents with a sudden onset of sharp pain in the right upper quadrant. The pain is so severe that it can be mistaken for pleurisy, cholelithiasis or an acute abdomen. On examination, the liver may be tender and there may be an associated friction rub.[212,334,349] Diagnosis can be further confused by the finding of a non-functioning gallbladder on cholecystography.[349] One clue to the diagnosis is that there is usually a history of prior pelvic infection, although this may have occurred several years previously. Diagnosis is supported by the isolation of gonococci from a vaginal swab. The organism can be isolated on liver biopsy.[163] A proportion of patients come to laparotomy, where the presence of a perihepatitis with adhesions and pus is confirmed. Laparoscopy may give useful diagnostic information.[269]

In long-standing cases, the so-called 'violinstring adhesions' are found between the surface of the liver and the anterior abdominal wall. If untreated, it is a self-limiting condition, but it shows a dramatic response to penicillin. This syndrome has always been attributed to direct spread of infection through the abdominal cavity, but recently the condition has been reported in men, presumably due to haematogenous spread.[112,163]

In gonococcal bacteraemia, the liver may be more commonly involved. Abnormalities of liver function tests occur in about 50 per cent of cases, the most common being elevation of the transaminases. The alkaline phosphatase and the bilirubin are only occasionally abnormal.[139,188] In gonococcal endocarditis, jaundice was a common feature, particularly before the advent of antibiotics.[35,319] The liver in these patients showed areas of focal necrosis and an inflammatory infiltrate. In many early reports, the jaundice may have been the result of therapy with acriflavine, an antiseptic which is now known to be hepatotoxic.

Typhoid Fever

Hepatomegaly is common in patients with typhoid fever (*Salmonella typhi* infection). It occurs in approximately 25 per cent of cases.[5,88,262] Jaundice is less common, being present in less than 10 per cent of patients. In early reports, coincidental viral hepatitis may have accounted for the jaundice. About 35 per cent of patients have abnormal liver function tests with mildly raised transaminase levels. The alkaline phosphatase is usually normal.

Changes on liver biopsy are non-specific, with areas of focal necrosis and a mononuclear cell inflammatory infiltrate. There may be focal nodular aggregates of Kupffer cells and macrophages in the sinusoids which may also be dilated and congested.[5,88,262] Many of these abnormalities have been reported when liver function tests have been entirely normal. Usually treatment has led to rapid improvement and the hepatomegaly has generally disappeared within three weeks.

Many examples of typhoid carrier states have been attributed to localization of infection, either in the gallbladder or in the liver. Patients may be asymptomatic or present with a clinical picture similar to that of cholecystitis, suppurative cholangitis or liver abscess. Occasionally, infection can persist in the gallbladder for long periods, and there is one report of infection persisting for 42 years.[36] Often it is best not to try to eradicate infection as this is sometimes difficult, but occasionally, for example in patients in the catering trade, it is necessary on public health grounds. It can sometimes be achieved by long courses of antibiotics, for example ampicillin, although, again, this can be difficult. Intensive attempts to eradicate infection by irrigation of the biliary tree[98] and cholecystectomy combined with antibiotics[207] have not always been successful.

Paratyphoid

In other forms of *Salmonella* infection, similar changes can occur in the liver, as in typhoid fever. In one series, 80 per cent of patients had elevation of the transaminases, 6 per cent had elevation of the alkaline phosphatase and 18 per cent of the bilirubin. The changes on liver biopsy are those of a non-specific reactive hepatitis.[213]

Shigella

Many of the early reports of jaundice complicating bacillary dysentery are possibly due to coincidental viral hepatitis. Abnormalities of the liver that have been described in *Shigella* infection include fatty change[169] and a non-specific hepatitis with focal necrosis and a marked inflammatory infiltrate. There are now several reports of *Shigella* hepatitis which are thought to be due to a direct effect of the organism.[140,320] In these patients there may be cholestasis.

In early reports, *Shigella* has been cultured from autopsy liver material.[169]

Brucellosis

This is an infectious disease caused by the genus *Brucella*, transmitted to man from domestic animals. There are three species: *B. abortus*, *B. melitensis* and *B. suis*, transmitted from cattle, sheep or goats, and pigs respectively. Brucellosis is relatively common among patients regularly coming into contact with these animals, in particular veterinary surgeons and farm-workers. The disease can run an acute, sub-acute, chronic or relapsing course, and occasionally infection can localize to a variety of organs, including the liver. On occasions, culture of liver biopsy has isolated the organism even when blood cultures have failed to do so.[69,107]

It is well known that hepatic lesions occur in brucellosis. In two series, all the patients with brucellosis who underwent a liver biopsy were found to have some abnormality[24,48] but these series were highly selected. Jaundice is rare, and in one series of 20 patients only one presented with jaundice, and this may have been due to coincidental viral hepatitis. In the same series, seven patients were found to have hepatomegaly with tenderness in the right upper quadrant, and five were found to have splenomegaly.[154]

Liver function tests are often abnormal and the alkaline phosphatase, serum transaminase and bilirubin may all be elevated.

The liver shows a granulomatous hepatitis with a marked inflammatory infiltrate and occasionally some fibrosis. Larger granulomas resemble those of sarcoidosis (Figure 51.2). There are no features to distinguish these

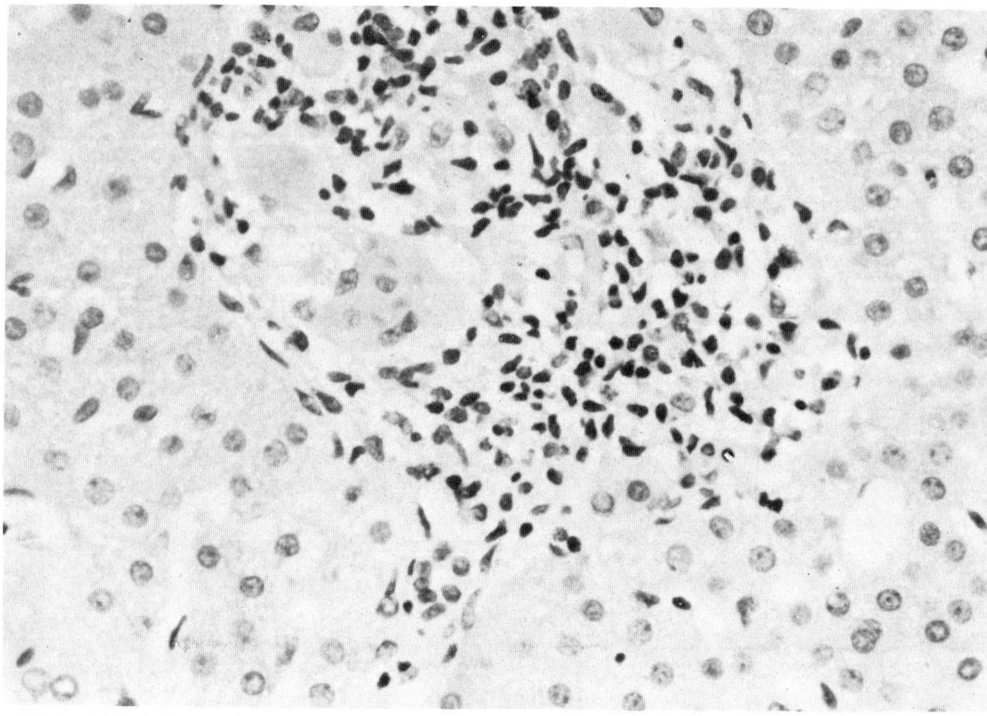

Figure 51.2. Epithelioid granuloma composed of large pale cells and a giant cell with admixed mononuclear cells. Haematoxylin and eosin × 1250.

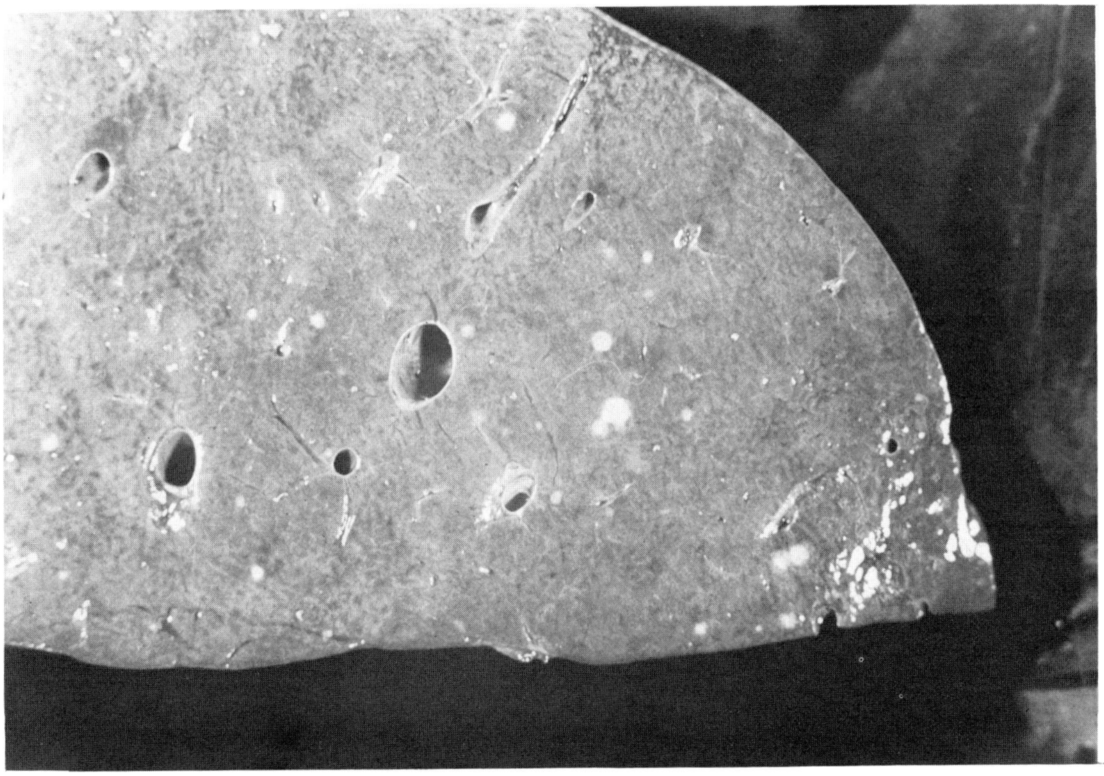

Figure 51.3. Macroscopic slice of liver containing multiple tiny necrotic abscesses due to *Listeria monocytogenes*.

changes from other conditions associated with a granulomatous hepatitis. Frequently the liver biopsy shows multiple microgranulomas scattered throughout the lobule. These are composed of a small number of histiocytes expanding and producing compression atrophy of hepatocytes.[355] Non-granulomatous foci of necrosis have been reported in infections due to *B. melitensis* or *B. suis*.[246]

Although in animal experiments these granulomas have healed without trace,[39] there are several reports in man of possible progression to cirrhosis,[154,206] but this remains unproved. Experimental studies on mice and guinea pigs show that granulomas form within five days and disappear after about six months.[39] Complete resolution was observed in the one series of patients undergoing further liver biopsy after treatment of the infection.[24]

There have been case reports of a clinical picture attributed to brucellosis indistinguishable from viral hepatitis,[226] but a coincidental viral hepatitis cannot be excluded. Less commonly, infection can produce an abscess,[316] and rarely can localize in the gallbladder.[24,48] The abscess may become calcified and have a characteristic pattern on x-ray.[11,316]

Listerosis

Listeria monocytogenes infection occasionally results in a syndrome of miliary granulomas in neonates. The liver at post-mortem may show small foci of necrosis (Figure 51.3) with a marked cellular reaction around them, as well as typical granulomas.[138,267]

Melioidosis

Infection with *Pseudomonas pseudomallei* is frequently subclinical and common in the tropics. Uncommonly it produces severe and often fatal septicaemia when the liver may be involved. Histology shows focal necrosis, inflammatory infiltrate and small discrete abscesses, and the organisms can be easily identified by Giemsa stains.[122] There may also be fatty change.[46]

Tularaemia

In fatal cases of disseminated infection with *Pasteurella tularensis*, the liver is frequently

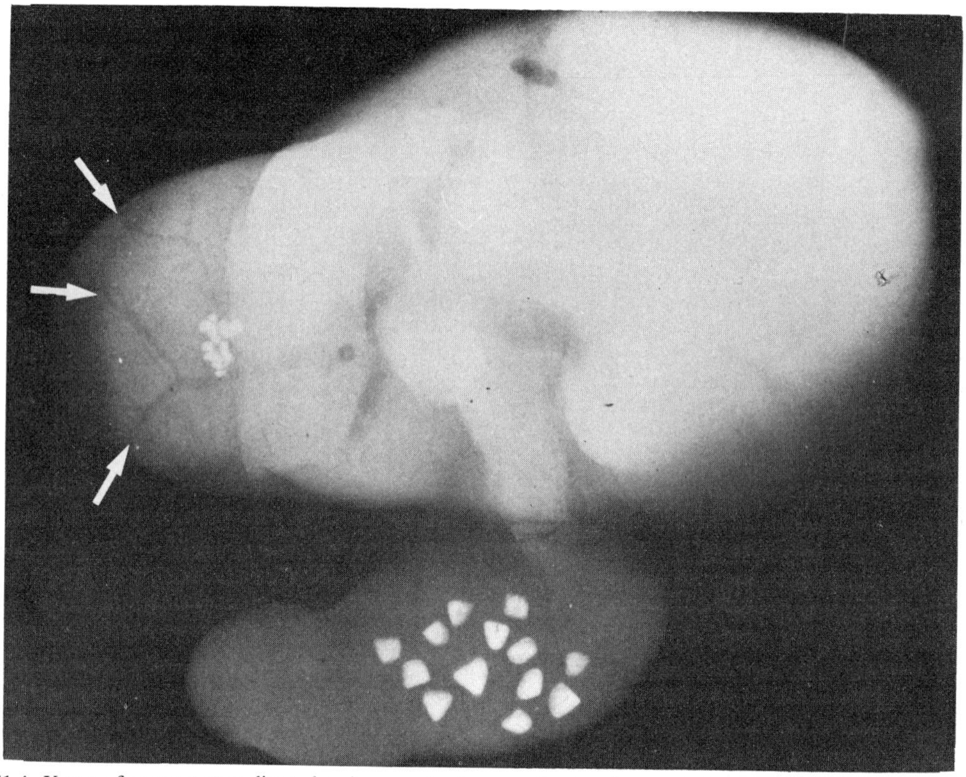

Figure 51.4. X-ray of post-mortem liver showing gas in the portal veins (arrows). Patient developed *Clostridium welchii* infection of infarcted bowel. Note the numerous gallstones and the absence of gas in the gallbladder.

involved and on occasions abnormalities of liver function tests with marked elevation of the serum transaminases suggest a hepatitis.[109,111,256] Histological changes include large foci of necrosis and, rarely, epithelioid granulomas.

Clostridium welchii (*perfringens*)

Severe jaundice occurs in up to 20 per cent of patients with gas gangrene.[76] The high bilirubin is usually explained by haemolysis resulting from release of an exotoxin. The liver may be directly involved, and plain x-ray may show collections of gas in the liver (Figure 51.4),[97] and the organism can be cultured from biopsy material.[310] There may be abscesses in the liver with areas of necrosis and gas formation.[65,97]

Clostridium welchii septicaemia can follow cholecystitis[65] or biliary tract surgery.[338] In systemic infection prognosis is poor even if specific therapy is instituted early. Although in experimental animals septicaemia can complicate massive hepatic infarction,[60] this does not seem to be the case in man.

Actinomycosis

The actinomycetales are not fungi but anaerobic or micro-aerophilic species of bacilli.[45,243] The usual species encountered clinically are *Actinomyces israelii* and *bovis*. They are common inhabitants of the normal mouth and are only rarely pathogenic. The presence of other micro-organisms may be required for them to become pathogenic.[89] Usual sites of infections are the maxillary-facial and ileocaecal regions. Infection is thought to extend by direct spread, although a haematogenous route has been postulated to explain distant involvement.[257,364] In cases of intra-abdominal actinomycosis, the liver is commonly affected, but symptoms are usually overshadowed by those of the disease elsewhere. The liver has been reported as the apparent primary site of infection in a patient with abdominal pain, anorexia, fever and abnormal liver function tests.[119] In this case report, it was presumed that there was an undetected intestinal site of infection. The liver shows a honeycomb pattern of multiloculated abscesses (Figure 51.5) which contain 'sulphur-granule' colonies within the

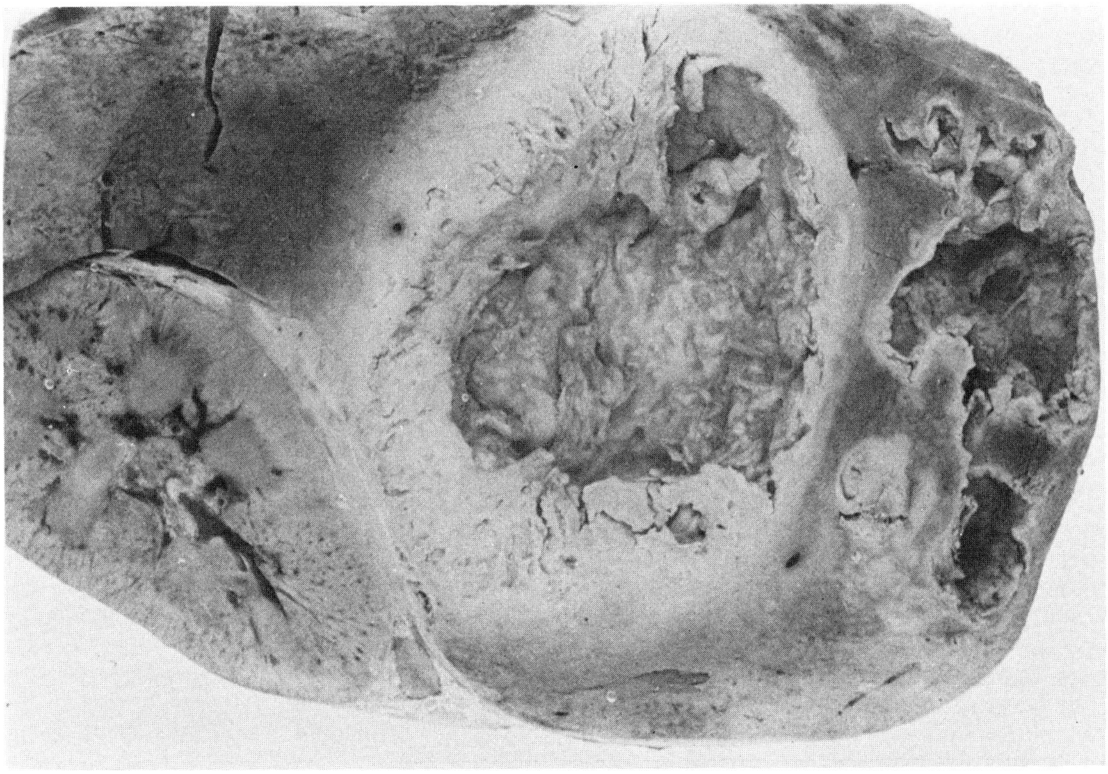

Figure 51.5. Large irregular abscess cavities lined by necrotic debris due to actinomycosis. The right kidney is bottom left. Courtesy of Professor R.C. Curran.

pus. These granules are not always present.[45,116] The wall of the abscess is hard and fibrous.

Microscopically this is not an epithelioid granulomatous disease, but there is granulation tissue in which numerous foamy macrophages, fibroblasts, plasma cells and lymphocytes can be seen. Neutrophils are present in the wall but are concentrated in the central pus. The granules are colonies of gram positive organisms. The abscesses can directly invade adjacent organs. Occasionally the gallbladder can be the primary site of infection.

Diagnosis depends on the demonstration and culture of the organism. Laparotomy is commonly required to obtain specimens for culture. Liver scan can show multiple filling defects which may be confused with metastatic liver disease.[61] Treatment with long-term penicillin is usually successful,[134] although surgical drainage is sometimes necessary.

Nocardiasis

The liver can be the site of abscess formation in the rare cases of disseminated infection with nocardiasis which usually occur in immunologically compromised hosts.[221]

MYCOBACTERIAL INFECTIONS

Tuberculosis

With modern chemotherapy and various public health programmes, the whole spectrum of tuberculosis has dramatically changed. Although tuberculosis is now relatively uncommon in western societies, it should still be considered in the differential diagnosis of many conditions.

Autopsy studies in patients dying from tuberculosis showed that the liver was frequently involved.[280,344] The reported incidence of liver involvement in tuberculosis ranges widely but may be as high as 80 per cent.[117,203,216,344] It varies with the severity of the disease state,[125] being highest in miliary tuberculosis. In patients with chronic extrahepatic tuberculosis, in particular pulmonary tuberculosis, liver involvement is now thought

Table 51.1. *The Liver and Biliary Tract in Tuberculosis.*

Hepatic granulomas
Miliary tuberculosis, including 'primary miliary tuberculosis of the liver'
Tuberculomas:
single
multiple
Tuberculous cholangitis
Tuberculosis of the gallbladder
Non-specific changes including 'fatty infiltration' and focal necrosis
Changes resulting from therapy:
Granulomatous hepatitis following BCG
Drug-induced hepatitis e.g. isoniazid rifampicin

to be unusual[104,113,167,203] unless miliary spread occurs. The liver may be involved in several ways during the course of tuberculosis, and these are summarized in Table 51.1.

There may be non-specific changes, including fatty change and reactive hepatitis related to debility rather than any specific process. Many drugs used to treat tuberculosis, including rifampicin and isoniazid, can cause a drug-induced hepatitis (see Chapter 36) and a granulomatous hepatitis can occur following bacille Calmette Guérin (BCG) injection.[59,141] The biliary tree may also be the site of infection.

Granulomatous hepatitis due to TB

Most patients present with symptoms of extrahepatic tuberculosis. Symptoms or signs of liver involvement are normally incidental findings, but occasionally patients can present with weight loss, general malaise and a pyrexia of unknown origin.[55,56]

On examination, there may be an enlarged liver or spleen. Liver function is usually well maintained, although there may be elevation of the liver enzymes, in particular the alkaline phosphatase.[172] In some patients, a liver biopsy may provide the only clue to the diagnosis.[68,72] In most patients, however, diagnosis is more obvious and a simple chest x-ray will often suffice.

The epithelioid granulomas of tuberculosis cannot be readily distinguished from other conditions, notably sarcoidosis, unless acid-fast bacilli are seen (Figure 51.6). Caseation necrosis is rare in liver biopsies (Figure 51.7), and although it is not seen in sarcoidosis, similar necrosis may occur in other infective granulomas. If the diagnosis is suspected, it is important that a liver biopsy sample be cultured.

Tuberculoma

Occasionally, solitary or multiple large caseating granulomatous nodules may form in the liver and these are called 'tuberculomas'.[14] It is important to recognize them as many of the features, including multiple filling defects on liver scans, may suggest a diagnosis of disseminated malignancy. In these cases, calcification on the plain x-ray may provide a clue, but histological confirmation must be obtained.[374]

Miliary tuberculosis

As mentioned above, most patients with miliary tuberculosis have multiple granulomas in the liver. Clinical features vary, but general malaise and weight loss are common, as is hepatomegaly. Occasionally, the liver is overwhelmingly invaded, and in these cases symptoms and signs of liver involvement may be prominent.[327] This has been called 'primary' miliary tuberculosis of the liver, but this term is misleading as, although liver abnormalities appear to be the only ones present, the infection cannot be 'primary' in the liver since there is always a primary site elsewhere, although this may be difficult to demonstrate. It is best to regard this as one end of the spectrum of miliary tuberculosis.

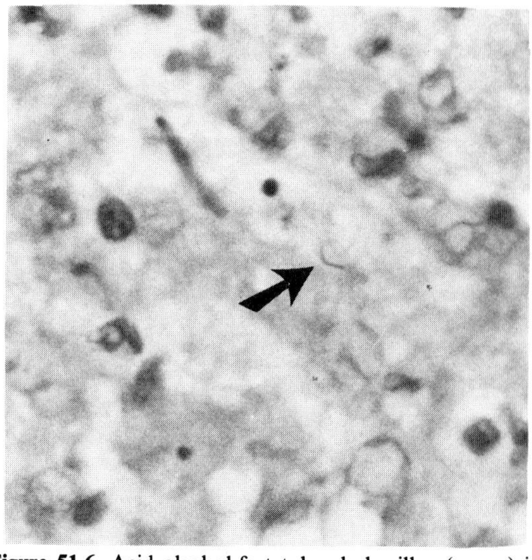

Figure 51.6. Acid alcohol-fast tubercle bacillus (arrow) in an epithelioid cell from a granuloma showing caseation necrosis. Ziehl-Neelsen × 2000.

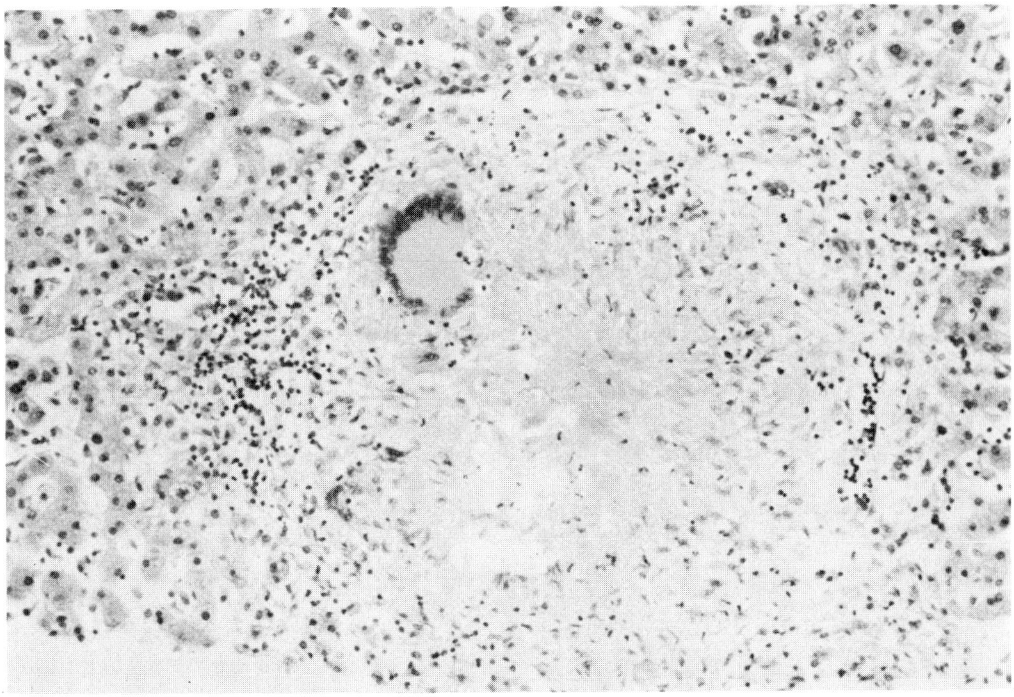

Figure 51.7. A large epithelioid granuloma with a Langhans giant cell and central caseation necrosis.

The clinical presentation is with fever, sweats and extreme malaise with prostration and weight loss. On examination, there may be hepatosplenomegaly, jaundice or ascites. Unless the condition is recognized and appropriate treatment given there is usually a particularly rapid downhill course, and if the diagnosis is missed it is usually fatal.

Tuberculosis of the biliary tract

This can take the form of tuberculous cholangitis, which is thought to be the result either of the rupture of a tuberculoma into a bile duct or to be spread from a tuberculous ulcer in the intestine.[280] Clinical features vary, but abdominal pain, general malaise and, on occasions, an obstructive jaundice can occur,[171] though it should be stressed that jaundice is rare in any form of tuberculous involvement of the liver.[67,75]

The gallbladder is another rare site of tuberculous infection. Clinical presentation is indistinguishable from that of cholecystitis, and the tuberculosis is often associated with the presence of gallstones.[182] Tuberculosis is also an unusual cause of haemobilia.[3]

Other hepatic abnormalities in tuberculosis

Apart from the granulomas, other, less specific, histological changes are occasionally found in the liver. There may be an inflammatory infiltrate, mainly of lymphocytes, with Kupffer cell proliferation and areas of focal necrosis.

Tuberculosis was once a common cause of fatty liver.[152,297] The suggested association between tuberculosis and cirrhosis is thought to be due to the life-style of the alcoholic rather than to a common pathogenic factor. The increased hepatitis B surface antigen (HB_sAg) carrier rate in patients with tuberculosis may be another cause for the hepatic abnormalities.[106] Occasionally, amyloidosis[152] and heart failure can result from long-standing infection, and both can cause abnormalities on liver biopsy (see Chapter 37).

Atypical Mycobacterial Infections

Similar changes to those in tuberculosis can be found in patients with atypical mycobacterial infections.[321]

Leprosy

In patients with leprosy, the liver is the organ most frequently involved at autopsy.[247] In life, hepatic involvement is usually asymptomatic, although sometimes there may be hepatomegaly. Similarly, the liver function tests are usually normal, although there may be elevation of the alkaline phosphatase or the serum transaminases.[63,160] There have been reports of an increased incidence of HB_sAg in patients with lepromatous leprosy,[34,63] but in some studies it has not differed from the high carrier rate in the community.[286,329] Occasionally, leprosy may progress to amyloidosis.[177]

Granulomas are the most common histological abnormalities found in the liver, occurring in 90 per cent of patients with lepromatous leprosy and 10 per cent with tuberculous leprosy. In the lepromatous variety, foam cells surround the granuloma.[4,160,296] Occasionally, Kupffer cells clump together, forming small nodules.[312] Acid-fast bacilli can be demonstrated in the granulomas and in the Kupffer cells, and their identification in the liver correlates well with that from the skin.[160] The organism cannot be cultured.

SPIROCHAETAL INFECTIONS

Syphilis

Although syphilis is relatively less common than it once was in western societies, it should still be considered in the differential diagnosis of obscure liver disease.[126] The liver may be involved in all forms of syphilis, including congenital, early and late.

Congenital syphilis

In countries where maternal screening is practised, congenital syphilis should be rarely encountered. The liver is involved in 80 per cent of cases of congenital syphilis. This high incidence is probably due to the passage of the spirochaete from the infected placenta directly into the umbilical vein and hence to the liver.[164] The liver is enlarged and firm and can account for up to one-sixth of the total body weight of the infant. Infection often results in abortion or stillbirth, and in these cases the liver can be seen macroscopically to contain small yellow dots due to multiple small gummas. Histologically, there is widespread interstitial fibrosis from the portal tracts into the lobules, separating the rather atrophic liver cells into small groups.[210] Spirochaetes are abundant throughout the liver and there may be a marked inflammatory infiltrate, occasional granulomas and an arteritis. Jaundice can be either hepatocellular or cholestatic, but is rare.

Secondary syphilis

In one large series of patients with secondary syphilis, only 1 per cent were found to have hepatitis.[129] This usually took the form of a mild and self-limiting condition presenting with tender hepatomegaly and abnormal liver function tests. More recently, there have been several reports of syphilitic hepatitis presenting with a clinical picture very similar to that of viral hepatitis.[15,41,183,236,289,300,311]

In these cases there may be considerable elevation of the serum transaminases or the alkaline phosphatase. On liver biopsy there may be focal necrosis and a widespread inflammatory infiltrate. Less common features include cholestasis, bile-duct proliferation and granulomas. Spirochaetes are difficult to see in the liver except in 'syphilitic hepatitis'[101,260] but the infection can be transmitted from the human liver into rabbit testes.[342]

Late syphilis

The liver is a common site for gummas in tertiary syphilis (Figure 51.8). They occur more often in the right lobe than in the left, and if multiple are called hepar lobatum and can be confused with metastases. There are focal lesions with central necrosis resembling caseating necrosis and surrounded by granulation tissue, and fibrosis with a marked endarteritis and a plasma cell and lymphocytic infiltration (Figure 51.9). The lesion heals by forming dense contracted scar tissue. A perihepatitis may also be present.

Usually, all these hepatic manifestations are entirely asymptomatic and are only incidental findings at laparotomy or autopsy. Occasionally, patients may complain of anorexia, weight loss, abdominal pain or fever, but, as in any syphilitic infection, symptoms and signs can be very varied. Jaundice, ascites and portal hypertension have been reported but are rare.[129,324] The presence of gummas has been reported as a rare cause of the Budd–Chiari syndrome.[91]

On examination, the liver may be large, tender, knobbly and highly suggestive of

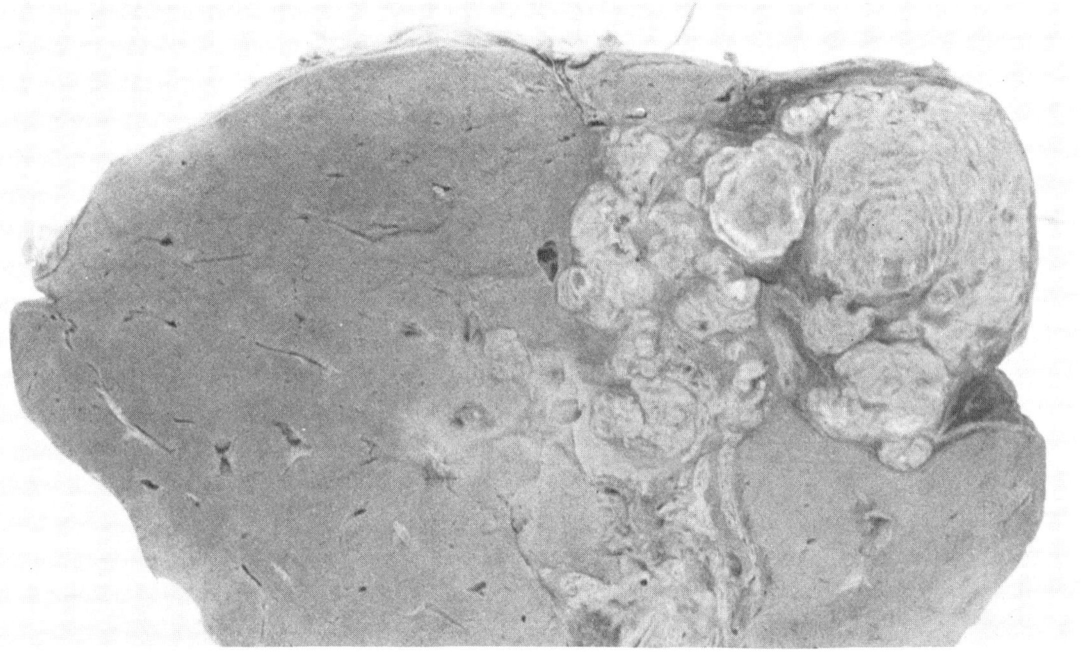

Figure 51.8. Syphilitic gumma of the liver. Gummatous necrosis is usually of firm and rubbery consistency so that cavitation is less common. Courtesy of Professor R. C. Curran.

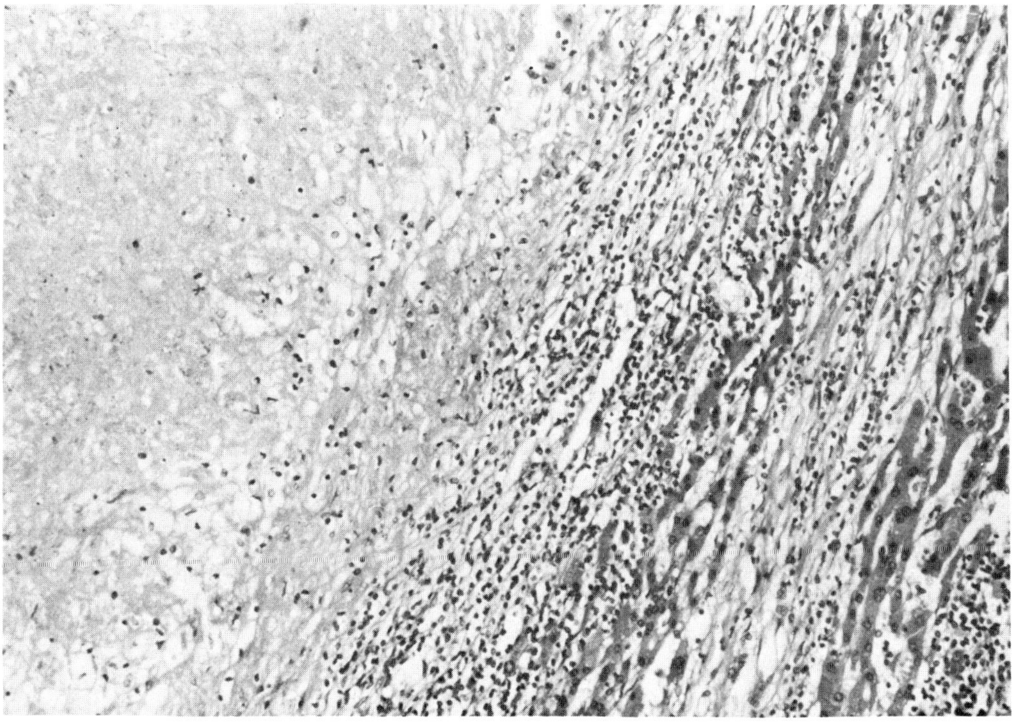

Figure 51.9. Wall of syphilitic gumma showing necrosis on the right and hepatocytes top left. The wall of the gumma between these structures is composed of compressed hepatocytes, fibrous tissue and a mixture of lymphocytes, macrophages and plasma cells. Haematoxylin and eosin × 500.

multiple tumour deposits. Occasionally, calcification may give a clue to the diagnosis.[6] Specific serological tests are available to confirm the diagnosis. It is important to be aware that some groups of patients, particularly homosexuals, have an increased incidence of syphilis. Syphilis should be considered in patients with atypical hepatitis, pyrexia of unknown origin, or in those patients presenting with unexplained abnormal liver function tests.

Syphilis and chronic liver disease

It has been suggested that there is an association between syphilis and cirrhosis.[161] In one study, 10 per cent of patients with cirrhosis also had evidence of previous syphilitic infection.[133] Similarly, there is an association between venereal disease and the HB_sAg carrier rate.[233] Both these associations may be explained on the basis of the patients' life-style and a shared source of infection. It has also been suggested that, among patients with hepatomas, a greater proportion than would be expected have evidence of previous syphilitic infection,[357] but this may in part be explained by the early use of heavy metals in the treatment of syphilis. For example, arsenic is not only carcinogenic but may cause cirrhosis. In addition, the association with hepatitis B virus infection may play a part.

Leptospirosis

This is a term used to define any disease caused by *Leptospira*. There is only one species of *Leptospira, L. interrogans*, and this can be divided into two forms, *interrogans* and *biflexa*. The former is responsible for all disease states in man: the latter is harmless. The group can be further divided, according to their antigenic status, into various serotypes, and well over 100 have now been described, forming several serogroups. The best known of these are *Leptospira icterohaemorrhagiae* and *Leptospira canicola*. The distinction between the serotypes cannot be made on the basis of morphological characteristics but depends on serological tests.

In the United States of America, at least 22 of the serotypes occur, although only about 10 regularly give rise to disease.[51,115,135] In the United Kingdom, about 15 serotypes occur,[9] although only two, *L. icterohaemorrhagiae* and *L. canicola*, commonly produce symptoms.

Terminology

Considerable confusion exists regarding the terminology of these organisms. For the sake of brevity, we will use the short but inaccurate classification, i.e. *L. icterohaemorrhagiae*, which, if written in full, becomes *Leptospira interrogans*, sub-type *icterohaemorrhagiae*. Similarly, although the term 'Weil's disease' has been used to describe an illness caused classically by *L. icterohaemorrhagiae*, it is now well established that this syndrome of jaundice and renal failure can be caused by almost any serotype of leptospirosis.

The distribution of these organisms varies greatly throughout the world, but in the United States and Britain the commonest serotypes producing symptoms are *L. icterohaemorrhagiae* (29 per cent of cases), *L. canicola* (27 per cent) and *L. autumnalis* (13 per cent).[9,135]

Epidemiology

A variety of different domestic and wild animals can act as reservoir-hosts.[271] The commonest serotypes encountered, the symptoms of the commoner syndromes, and the source of infection are summarized in Table 51.2. It is of interest that the animal host may appear ill but may still be infective even if apparently healthy. Most outbreaks of *L. icterohaemorrhagiae* result from the rat, and in some surveys up to a third of the rat population have been shown to be infected.[211,368]

The dog is the animal host in most cases of *L. canicola*, and up to one-third of the dog population may also be infected.[279] Vaccination of dogs against leptospirosis is not always successful and the animals may still act as reservoir-hosts.[102]

Infection usually results from contact with rat urine. Certain professions, such as farm-workers and refuse-collectors, are therefore particularly exposed to infection. Abroad, major outbreaks have been associated with sugar-cane cutters, ricefield workers, and soldiers, particularly during wartime. Swimming in stagnant water, dog-handling and accidental laboratory infection have all been implicated in cases of leptospirosis.[288] It has been suggested that there may also be a venereal spread. Leptospirosis is mainly a disease of young people, and both extremes of age are usually spared, although if they do become infected they fare worse. Children may be infected more commonly than is often thought.[367]

Table 51.2. *Leptospirosis.*

Serotype	Principal source of infection	Type of illness
L. icterohaemorrhagiae (Weil's disease)	Rat	Severe illness, can be fatal; jaundice frequent
L. bataviae	Field mouse	Less severe illness, rarely fatal; jaundice less common
L. autumnalis (Autumn fever; Fort Bragg fever)	?Field mouse	
Also		
L. australis		
L. pyrogenese		
L. canicola (*Canicola* fever)	Dog	Mild illness; usually anicteric
L. grippotyphosa (Mud fever)	Vole, wood mouse	
L. pomona (Swineherd's fever)	Pigs	
Also		
L. sejr		
L. ballum		
L. hebdomidis		

Outbreaks normally occur during the summer months.[13,135] About 50 serious cases a year are seen in the United Kingdom and about 100 in the United States.[115,340] It should be stressed that all these apparently distinct syndromes can be caused by almost any *Leptospira* serotype.[92,93,333]

Clinical features

The incubation period is usually between seven and 13 days, with an average of 10 days. It may be as short as two days or as long as 26. In general, the shorter the incubation period the more severe the illness. Classically, the disease runs a biphasic course: a leptospiraemic or first phase and an immune or second phase.

First phase. This is characterized by clinical manifestations of an acute systemic infection, and during this period *Leptospira* can be recovered from the blood and cerebrospinal fluid and are distributed throughout the body, accounting for the wide spectrum of clinical symptoms and signs (see Table 51.3). Typically, there is an acute onset of frontal headache associated with severe myalgic pains, particularly in the quadriceps and the spinal muscles. Abdominal pain, conjunctival suffusion and extreme prostration are occasional early features. A fluctuating fever develops and there may be associated non-specific symptoms, including anorexia, nausea, vomiting and diarrhoea. Less common presenting features include chest pain, cough and haemoptysis.[50] There may be a relative bradycardia.[49,341]

Towards the end of the first phase, *Leptospira* is removed from the blood by phagocytosis and this is associated with an increase in the levels of specific antibodies.[330] *Leptospira* remains in the kidneys, where it is found predominantly in the convoluted tubules and excreted into the urine.

Second phase. Between the first and second phase, the temperature settles, the patient recovers partially and, although weak and exhausted, often feels well. This afebrile period lasts between one and three days before fever, often associated with meningism, returns. Symptoms include skin rashes, particularly erythema nodosum,[49] iridocyclitis,[29] alopecia, endocarditis and various central nervous system manifestations. The symptoms can be mild and insignificant or extremely severe and sometimes fatal. They usually last for between one and 14 days and even after recovery there may be an occasional mild relapse. During this phase,

Table 51.3. *Manifestations of Leptospirosis.*

Common:
Fever, chills, headache, meningism, anorexia, myalgia, conjunctival suffusion.

Less common:
Nausea, vomiting, abdominal pain, jaundice, hepatomegaly, skin rash (including erythema nodosum), photophobia.

Rare:
Pneumonitis, haemoptysis, delirium, haemorrhage, diarrhoea, oedema, splenomegaly, renal failure, arthralgia, pancreatitis, peripheral neuritis, parotitis, epididymitis, haematemesis, ascites, myocarditis.

Leptospira is excreted in the urine and this may continue for several months, even after apparent recovery. There are no long-term effects on the liver or kidney.[305]

Weil's Disease

Jaundice occurs in about 30 per cent of cases due to *L. icterohaemorrhagiae*, but is less common with the other serotypes.

Weil's disease was first described in 1886,[354] and is a term employed to describe a syndrome caused by any leptospiral illness with the clinical features of extreme fever, severe jaundice, azotaemia, haemorrhage, cardiovascular collapse and an altered level of consciousness. It is often associated with a high mortality rate. The biphasic pattern described for leptospirosis in general is not so clear cut and the disease reaches a peak in the second stage. Occasionally, incomplete syndromes are seen and the presentation may be simply as an episode of afebrile jaundice[358] or as isolated renal failure. The abdominal pain can be severe[25] and can result in unnecessary laparotomy.

Jaundice and liver function

The pathogenesis of the jaundice seen in Weil's disease is unclear and has been assumed to be a hepatotoxic reaction.[12] Haemolysis may be present but does not account for the extremely high levels of bilirubin that can be observed. Serum transaminases and alkaline phosphatase levels are usually only moderately elevated,[12] although exceptionally high levels can occur.[288] The levels usually peak during the second week of the illness. Occasionally, the alkaline phosphatase can be extremely high and suggest an obstructive jaundice.[94] Bromsulphthalein excretion can be delayed even in the absence of abnormal liver function tests.[93]

Other laboratory abnormalities

Anaemia may be present, due both to haemorrhage and haemolysis. There may be a leucocytosis associated with a neutropenia; the ESR may be elevated and there may be albumin or blood in the urine.[13,275] In severe cases the urea is elevated with electrolyte imbalance associated with acute renal failure. the cerebrospinal fluid may show a pleocytosis and an excess of protein. Agglutinins appear in the second week of the illness, although diagnostic levels are rarely seen before 14 days.[331] These titres can remain elevated for several months or even years.

Pathology

At autopsy the liver is large and has a yellowish-green discoloration with subcapsular haemorrhage. On liver biopsy the cell plates are normal, centrilobular hepatocytes are swollen and there is an increase in mitosis, indicating liver regeneration.[82,292] Fat vacuoles and acidophil bodies are occasionally seen and there may be Kupffer cell proliferation or a mononuclear infiltrate. Cholestasis is sometimes a feature,[32,83] and this can persist for some time after apparent recovery. Sometimes there are small areas of focal necrosis and haemorrhage and there may be bile duct plugging of the caniculi. *Leptospira* is found in only half of the livers examined.[12] Electron microscopic studies have shown changes compatible with a toxic process to various organelle systems.[287]

All these histological changes are extremely variable and even in fatal cases the liver can be normal.[12,142] The pathological findings in other organs involved in the disease process have been reviewed elsewhere.[12,13,93,166]

Differential diagnosis

In the first phase of the illness diagnosis may be difficult as the clinical picture is vague.[340] As in most cases the disease will run a mild and benign course, a diagnosis will not usually be made, and for this reason it is difficult to assess the true incidence of leptospirosis in the general population. When jaundice and renal failure occur, diagnosis is easier and the main differential diagnosis is that of viral hepatitis. Features which may help to distinguish Weil's disease from viral hepatitis include the acute onset, the severe prostration, associated headaches and myalgias, high ESR, leucocytosis and a history of exposure to a source of infection.

Leptospira can be isolated from the blood during the first week of the illness, and although difficult to see on direct dark-field microscopy they may be demonstrated if immunofluorescent staining techniques are employed. Leptospira are usually easy to culture, and if injected into guinea pigs or hamsters cause an acute and often fatal illness. Available serological tests include specific agglutinins, complement fixation tests and lysin tests.[339] In Britain, a compound screening antigen for use in a complement fixation test is prepared and distributed by a reference laboratory. If this gives positive results, the specific serotype is then determined.[38,96,114,231,339,341]

Treatment

In vitro, various antibiotics, including penicillin and tetracycline, have been shown to be lethal to the organism.[8] They have also been shown to clear leptospira from urine,[190] and if given to guinea pigs in the first 18 hours after exposure they protect against infection.[9]

Despite these findings, most of the large studies of human infections fail to show any beneficial effect from antibiotic therapy on the course of the illness.[44,100,131,142] It is, however, generally considered that penicillin has some beneficial effect if given early in the course of the disease.[66,170,180,340,341] Conversely, there is little point in administering penicillin after the onset of jaundice.[142]

Convalescent immune serum may be effective if given early but is difficult to obtain. General measures, including careful maintenance of fluid and electrolyte balance and the management of renal failure with dialysis, are vital. Blood transfusion may be required, and in one report plasma exchange has been used successfully.[306]

Progress

Most cases of leptospirosis run a mild and uneventful course, but in Weil's disease mortality can vary from 4 to 40 per cent. In these cases, death usually occurs in the second phase of the illness and jaundice is inevitably present. Mortality is high at both extremes of age.[9,93] Weil's disease superimposed on a pre-existing cirrhosis may have a bad prognosis,[308] but patients with cirrhosis can make a full recovery.[87]

Prevention

This depends on personal and environmental hygiene, public health measures and pest control. Prophylactic vaccination for those at risk has been shown to be effective. Although it has been recommended that empirical antibiotic therapy should be given to patients known to be exposed to infection, in at least one case this has proved ineffective.[44] Precautions should be taken when nursing infected patients and care taken over disposal of urine and other body fluids.

Relapsing Fever

This is a term used to describe an acute arthropod-borne fever characterized by intermittent pyrexia and toxaemia recurring over periods of several weeks. It is caused by the spirochaetes of the genus *Borrelia*. There is an epidemic form spread by the louse (*Pediculus humanis*) and an endemic form spread by the tick, species *ornithodorus*. Most commonly associated with relapsing fever is *Borrelia recurrentis*, which is found throughout the world except in New Zealand, Australia and parts of the southwest Pacific. The disease is particularly common in areas of poor hygiene.[47]

Clinical features

The incubation period varies from three to 15 days. There is an acute onset of chills, fevers, myalgia and sometimes severe prostration. Conjunctival suffusion and episodes of bleeding may occur. There are occasional skin rashes and central nervous system abnormalities. Hepatosplenomegaly is a common feature and the liver is usually enlarged and tender in up to 60 per cent of cases. Splenomegaly is slightly more common.[314] Jaundice, in many ways similar to that seen in leptospirosis, can occur, particularly in fatal cases.[366] Although the bilirubin level may be quite high, the liver enzymes are usually normal or only mildly deranged.[156]

Pathology

Little is known of the changes that occur in the liver in relapsing fever, and most information has come from .animal work.[155] Livers are enlarged and congestive and there may be foci of necrosis. Kupffer cell proliferation, inflammatory infiltration and occasional cholestasis can occur. The spirochaetes are easily visible microscopically. As in leptospirosis, the liver can be entirely normal despite severe derangement of the liver function tests.[155]

Diagnosis is often difficult and depends on a history of exposure and demonstration of the organism, either from the site of the bite or from an aspirate of a lymph node. It is difficult to demonstrate the organism on a simple thick blood film. Agglutinins and complement fixation tests are available, although they are not in widespread use.[103]

Treatment and progress

Tetracycline, chloramphenicol and streptomycin are all effective. Penicillin is not as effective as these. Mortality is low, at about 5 per cent. There may be long-term sequelae such as uveitis.

RICKETTSIAL INFECTIONS

Q Fever

This is a self-limiting rickettsial infection caused by *Coxiella burnetii*. The organism is widely distributed in Europe, the United Kingdom and the United States. Domesticated animals, in particular cattle, sheep and goats, form the animal hosts in most cases, although occasionally wild animals are implicated. Following inhalation of the organism, patients usually present with fever, headaches and a pneumonitis. In most cases, the disease has a short, benign course and resembles influenza. Occasionally, there may be prolonged fever and toxaemia due to chronic infection.

The liver in Q fever

Liver involvement is well recognized and hepatomegaly is common. Symptoms of hepatic disease are unusual and jaundice occurs in less than 5 per cent of cases. The most common abnormality of liver function tests is an elevation of the alkaline phosphatase. Occasionally, there may be marked elevation of the serum transaminases,[248] when diagnosis can be confused with viral hepatitis. If this occurs in the absence of a pneumonitis, diagnosis can be extremely difficult.[7] Rarer manifestations of infection include symptoms suggestive of cholangitis[90] and massive hepatic necrosis.[331] The liver may be involved even if liver function tests are entirely normal.[90] Although progression to cirrhosis has been recorded,[337] it is rare and could be coincidental or due to sampling errors on liver biopsy.

Pathology of the liver. Focal hepatic necrosis, Kupffer cell proliferation, granulomas and a mononuclear cell infiltrate, particularly in the portal tracts, can be found.[151] The organisms can occasionally be isolated from the liver.[215] The close proximity of granulomas to fatty change[37] and eosinophilic necrosis of the sinusoidal wall[31] have been considered by some workers to be pathognomonic of Q fever, but have not featured in other reports. The liver is not always affected and even in fatal cases of Q fever can be entirely normal.[345]

Diagnosis and treatment

Contact with the animal host is obviously a vital clue. Because of the dangers involved, culture of the organism is rarely undertaken in the laboratory and confirmation of the diagnosis usually depends on complement fixation and agglutination tests. Treatment with tetracycline and chloramphenicol is effective. The most serious complication is endocarditis, but the disease on the whole has a low mortality, of less than 1 per cent.

MYCOPLASMAL INFECTIONS

In infections with *Mycoplasma pneumoniae*, abnormalities of the serum transaminases and the alkaline phosphatase are not unusual.[186] Manifestation of liver abnormality is unusual in *Mycoplasma* infection.[219] Reactive hepatitis has been recorded in association with *Mycoplasma pneumoniae* infection[199] and *Mycoplasma* infection has coincided with the onset of chronic active hepatitis.[148]

FUNGAL INFECTIONS

There is a wide geographical difference in the distribution of the fungi. In clinical practice today, these infections are most often seen in immunologically compromised patients, following intensive chemotherapy for various malignant diseases, in particular lymphomas and childhood leukaemia.

Treatment will not be dealt with in full. However, against the yeastlike fungi such as candida, 5-fluorocytosine and amphotericin B are often effective, while with the hyphal fungi such as aspergillus, treatment with miconazole, a new fungal agent,[85,147,209] or 5-fluorocytosine is usually successful. In general, in the severely ill patients it is preferable to commence therapy with at least two drugs, and it is important to check the agent's sensitivity to the various antibiotics.

Histoplasmosis

This is a systemic fungal infection caused by *Histoplasma capsulatum*. Although common in the United States, it is not seen in the United Kingdom. Inhalation of the organism results first in a chest infection but later, following haematogenous dissemination, almost any organ of the body can be affected.[346] Most cases are asymptomatic or present with a relatively benign acute illness, usually confined to the chest, and later chest x-rays may show calcification.

In the more serious progressive form, the disease is widely disseminated[309] and this carries a high mortality rate, especially in either extreme of age. In chronic cases, there may be fever, weight loss and lymphadenopathy; hepatosplenomegaly is common.[146,244,304] Jaundice and ascites are unusual, although there have been case reports where the liver clinically appears to be the only organ involved.[179]

Pathology

The basic change is a non-specific granulomatous hepatitis with an inflammatory infiltrate. There are no distinguishing features from granulomas seen in other conditions, in particular sarcoidosis. Sometimes the organisms can be seen both in the granulomas and in the Kupffer cells.[309] Rarely, the diagnosis of histoplasmosis can be made on liver biopsy when all other tests have been negative.[179,237]

Diagnosis

This depends on isolation and culture of the organism. Blood and bone marrow were the source of positive cultures in nearly all the cases reported by Smith and Utz.[309] Skin tests and complement fixation tests are available but their interpretation is difficult, especially in endemic areas.

Treatment and prognosis

Until recently, amphotericin B formed the basis of treatment, but newer agents are now becoming available. Treatment is not entirely satisfactory and the disease carries a high mortality. Improvement has been reported following corticosteroid therapy,[179] but this is questionable. In the long term, patients with disseminated histoplasmosis are particularly prone to adrenal failure.[290] Splenic and hepatic calcification are common sequelae.[229]

Cryptococcosis (Torulosis)

This is a systemic fungal infection caused by *Cryptococcus neoformans*. There is a world-wide distribution and all ages are affected. The common source of infection is domestic and wild animals, especially from pigeon-droppings. Cases are usually sporadic and the most common features are meningo-encephalitis[187] or granulomatous pneumonitis. Only rarely is infection disseminated to other organs and then most commonly to skin or bone. Even when the infection appears to be clinically localized, the organisms can be recovered elsewhere in the body.[189]

In the disseminated form, although hepatosplenomegaly is common, there are few symptoms attributable to hepatic dysfunction. There have been occasional reports of progressive liver failure[284] and jaundice,[120] and in these cases diagnosis can be difficult. *Cryptococcus* has been misdiagnosed as sclerosing cholangitis[184] or as an acute surgical abdomen.[254] The liver is the site of multiple granulomas which may caseate. Occasionally there may be abscess formation. Cryptococci can be seen in the biopsy material.

Diagnosis

This can be difficult, and isolation and culture of the organism are important.[128] Serological tests are available but are of limited value.

Treatment

Amphotericin B is the first line of treatment, although there are now newer anti-fungal agents. Results are often disappointing and the disease carries a mortality of about 25 per cent.

As infection is often opportunistic, the prognosis is partly influenced by the underlying disease process.

Mucormycosis

This is an acute, opportunistic, often fatal infection, usually with the *Rhizopus*, *Mucor* or *Absidia* genera of this fungus. The disease has two forms: one is localized to the nose and the paranasal sinuses, spreading into the orbit and the brain; the other is a mainly pulmonary form with features similar to many of the other fungal diseases.

Disseminated mucormycosis is rare and is usually diagnosed at post-mortem. The liver may show only non-specific features such as fatty change.[26] Occasionally, patients present with evidence of severe hepatic dysfunction.[205,325] Under these circumstances, both the bilirubin and the serum transaminases are elevated, and the clinical picture resembles that of viral hepatitis. Liver biopsy shows multifocal centrilobular hepatic necrosis,[205] with an arteritis. The organisms can sometimes be seen in the lesions. Local spread of the infection can cause massive thrombosis and hepatic necrosis.[214]

Diagnosis

This depends on demonstrating the organisms in biopsy material and is confirmed by culture.

Treatment

This is given with intravenous amphotericin B or newer anti-fungal agents, but the prognosis is poor.

Aspergillosis

Although *Aspergillus* is a common organism found in sputum and is usually of no clinical significance, aspergillosis can result in pulmonary and, rarely, systemic infection. *Aspergillus fumigatus* is the most common pathogen and has a worldwide distribution. Many infections are opportunistic.[255] The liver is an uncommon site of involvement and overt symptoms are rare. In one series of 48 cases, 12 patients were found to have hepatomegaly,[372] and liver biopsy on one patient showed discrete periportal miliary abscesses filled with aspergilli.

Two further cases have been described in which aspergillosis has been associated with the Budd–Chiari syndrome.[371] These patients presented with abdominal pain, jaundice and abnormal liver function tests. The serum transaminases, alkaline phosphatase and bilirubin were all markedly elevated.

Diagnosis

As the presence of aspergilli in the sputum usually has no clinical significance, repeated isolation of the organism is necessary if infection is to be confirmed. Biopsy and culture are necessary to confirm the diagnosis. Serological tests are available but are of little value.

Coccidioidomycosis

This is a fungal infection caused by *Coccidioides immitis*, which is endemic in western and southwestern states of the United States of America and in South America. Following inhalation of the organism, the most common presentation is with pneumonitis and this is usually benign and self-limiting. Rarely, dissemination occurs and the meninges, bones and skin are the commonly involved organs. In all these, there is a sarcoid-like reaction which can be confused with other serious conditions such as tuberculosis or a neoplasm.[303] In one early series, there was evidence of hepatic involvement in only one of 95 patients,[108] but in a more recent autopsy study about a third of cases had grossly abnormal liver function tests and widespread lesions throughout the liver. Histology showed granulomas in which the spherules of *C. immitis* can be demonstrated. There may also be a non-specific inflammatory infiltrate and areas of focal necrosis. Occasionally, solitary nodules resembling those of tuberculosis or histoplasmosis may result.

In this recent series, the liver was the organ most commonly affected, after the lungs and spleen.[27]

Diagnosis

The organisms can be seen in properly stained tissue sections and diagnosis can be confirmed by culture. Skin tests and serological tests are available but are of limited value. Diagnosis has been made solely on liver biopsy on at least four occasions.[71,73,351]

Treatment

Amphotericin B and newer anti-fungal agents are useful but the prognosis is poor. Occasionally, local surgery is required.

North American Blastomycosis

Blastomycosis is a chronic systemic fungal disease caused by *Blastomyces dermatitidis* which is most often found in North and South America. The primary infection is pulmonary and in most cases clinical features are of a mild respiratory infection. Dissemination to skin, subcutaneous tissue and other organs, especially bones, central nervous system and mucous membranes, only rarely occurs. When the disease is confined to the chest, hepatomegaly and other evidence of liver involvement are rare, but in autopsy studies of cases with disseminated disease about half have evidence of hepatic involvement.[1,52,64,201,365] Liver histology shows granulomas, an inflammatory infiltrate and occasional fibrosis.

Diagnosis

This depends on demonstrating the organism in a suitably stained tissue specimen and is confirmed by culture. Serological tests are useful.

Treatment

Treatment with anti-fungal agents is indicated but the prognosis is poor. In the disseminated form, the mortality rate is about 30 per cent.

South American Blastomycosis (Paracoccidioidomycosis)

This is a chronic systemic fungal disease caused by *Paracoccidioidomycosis brasiliensis* that occurs almost exclusively in Central and South America, particularly in Brazil. Primary infection is usually in the oral–nasal mucosa, but infection can spread to the skin, lymph glands and other organs.[220] About 20 per cent of cases with disseminated infection have hepatomegaly.[191,272,273] Histologically, there may be inflammatory infiltrate, focal necrosis or granulomas, particularly in the portal tracts. In chronic cases there may be enlargement of the portal tracts and some fibrosis.[326]

Diagnosis

This depends on demonstration, isolation and culture of the organism. Skin tests and serological tests are available. The prognosis is poor even if anti-fungal agents are employed.

Candidiasis

Candida albicans usually invades skin and mucous membranes, but occasionally, and usually opportunistically, systemic infection occurs which is often fatal. In autopsy studies, the liver contains discrete microabscesses (Figure 51.10) and granulomas in about 10 per cent of cases.[193,235] Hepatomegaly may be present and may be due to fatty change rather than local involvement with *Candida*.[57]

Diagnosis

This depends on demonstration, isolation and culture of the organism and can be aided by skin and serological tests. Treatment with 5-fluorocytosine, amphotericin B and other anti-fungal agents is indicated but the mortality rate is high, in part due to the underlying disease.

Sporotrichosis

Although usually localized to the skin and mucous membranes, systemic infection with *Sporothrix schenckii* is occasionally encountered when the liver can be the site of abscess formation.[363]

PYOGENIC LIVER ABSCESS

The wide geographical difference in the incidence of pyogenic liver abscess may in part be due to under-diagnosis of the condition. Pyogenic abscess is now the commonest cause of hepatic abscess in developed countries, accounting for about three-quarters of all cases.[80] Elsewhere, amoebic abscess is more frequent and, worldwide, is the commonest cause of liver abscess. Pyogenic liver abscess is rare and is found in about 1 per cent of post-mortems.[227]

In the past, pyogenic liver abscess was most

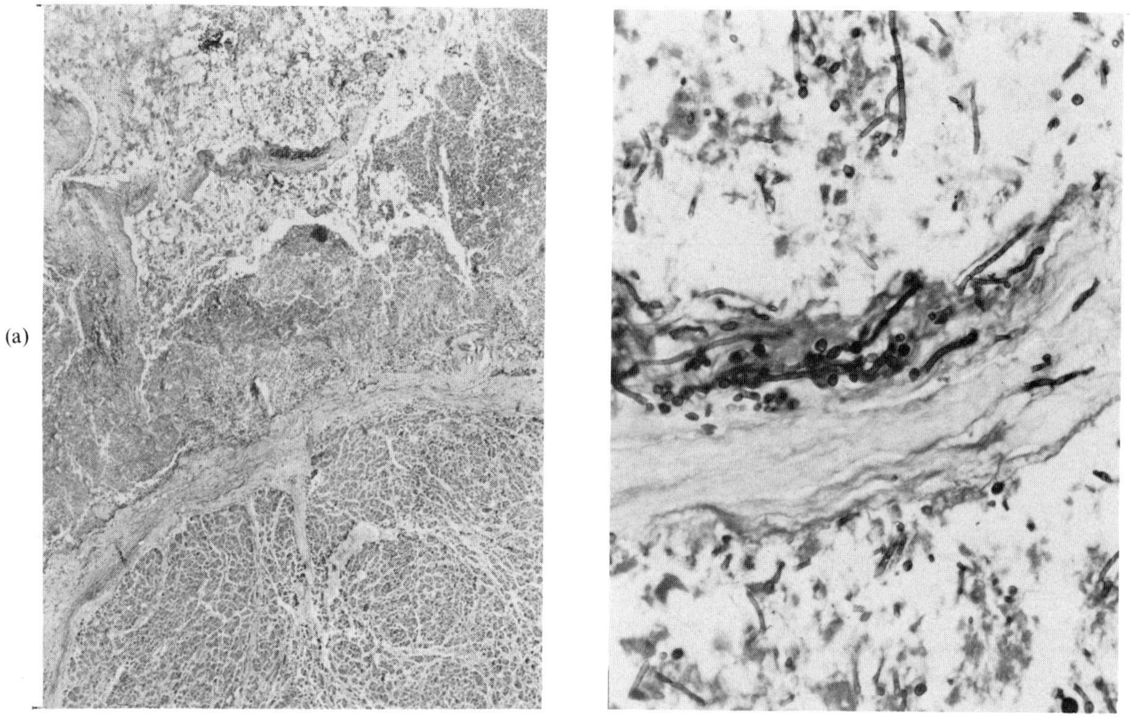

Figure 51.10. (a) Cirrhotic liver containing a fungal abscess (top). Haematoxylin and eosin × 75. (b) Hyphae and spores of *Candida albicans* are identified within the abscess. Patient died with a terminal candida septicaemia probably originating from the oesophagus. DPAS × 750.

commonly seen in children or young adults as a complication of appendicitis. These cases presented with the classic fluctuating fever. Nowadays, with the advent of antibiotics, pyogenic abscess is seen predominantly in the elderly, complicating biliary tract disease, and these cases often present with rather non-specific symptoms.[178,232]

When considering pyogenic liver abscesses, it is helpful to separate them into two groups, as the treatment is different for each. Solitary or confluent abscesses usually occur in one lobe of the liver and are amenable to surgical treatment, whilst multiple small abscesses are usually present in both lobes of the liver and cannot be treated surgically.

Pyogenic liver abscess is a serious condition and mortality may be as high as 80 per cent. This is usually due to delay in making the diagnosis. Diagnosis, employing refined investigative techniques, can now be made much earlier, and consequently the mortality rate has dropped considerably.

It is of interest that, although portal vein bacteraemia has been reported to be common in inflammatory bowel disease,[43] hepatic abscesses rarely complicate these conditions.[315,373]

Aetiology and Pathogenesis

Portal pylephlebitis

Pyogenic liver abscesses are often secondary to a distant primary focus. Before the antibiotic era, intra-abdominal sepsis, particularly appendicitis, diverticulitis and pelvic infection, was the most common cause of pyogenic liver abscess. Liver abscess may also be a complication of infected haemorrhoids, perirectal abscesses, bacillary dysentery and ulceration or perforation of a hollow viscus.

Abscess can result from infection of any site drained by the portal vein. Initially there is thrombophlebitis of the intramural vessels and this is followed by progressive involvement of the venous drainage. Small septic emboli may become detached from the thrombus and may then reach the liver via the portal vein.

Although in early reports this type of pyogenic liver abscess accounted for up to 30 per cent of all cases,[227] it is now much less common.[21,282] Abscesses are usually multiple and are most commonly found in the right lobe of the liver. This distribution has been explained on the basis of two-current blood flow in the portal vein. It is suggested that the superior mesenteric vein drains to the right lobe and the inferior mesenteric vein drains to the left lobe of the liver,[165,295,299] although recent animal studies have questioned this theory.[162]

Direct extension of infection

Abscesses can result from direct extension of infection from other adjacent sites, for example from an empyema of the gallbladder, a subphrenic abscess, pleural infection or from a perinephric abscess.[158]

Biliary tract disease

This is now the commonest cause of pyogenic liver abscess. Abscess may complicate cholelithiasis, inflammatory stricture of the duct or malignant disease of the pancreas, ampulla of Vater, gallbladder or bile ducts. Cholecystitis, ascending cholangitis and acute pancreatitis may also be associated with an hepatic abscess. Infection ascends into the intrahepatic branches of the biliary tree and may then spread through the vascular and lymphatic channels to involve the portal vein. These abscesses are usually multiple but are often confined to one lobe of the liver.

Trauma

Hepatic trauma is becoming commoner as a result of the increase in civil violence and in the number of road traffic accidents.[16,17,18] Liver abscess can result from either blunt or penetrating injuries of the liver. Trauma results in laceration, haemorrhage, tissue necrosis and extravasation of bile, all of which predispose to secondary infection. Even a simple subcapsular haematoma may become infected. This type of abscess is usually single and well localized.

Trauma accounts for up to 10 per cent of pyogenic liver abscesses,[227] but if an aggressive surgical policy is taken, then abscess should be a rare complication of trauma.[218] Necrotic tissue should be widely excised and in more serious cases resection of the involved lobe should be undertaken.

Septicaemia

Generalized septicaemia may also result in abscess formation. Bacterial seeding occurs via the hepatic artery and may complicate bacterial endocarditis or other infection. Up to 40 per cent of pyogenic liver abscesses may result from septicaemia,[228] although in most reports it accounts for only 10 per cent of cases.[302] Many reports are not comparable as some exclude cases of generalized septicaemia. The differences in the incidence of this type of liver abscess may be a reflection of the emergence of resistant organisms. The abscesses are usually small and multiple and found in both lobes of the liver.

Miscellaneous causes

Abscess may complicate both primary and secondary hepatic malignancy, and in one series this was a common cause of hepatic abscess.[276] It results from necrosis and secondary infection of the tumour. Such abscesses are usually solitary. Liver cysts may also become secondarily infected as may other abnormalities of the liver, including schistosomiasis, tuberculosis,[182] ascaris or hydatid liver disease.

Cryptogenic abscess

Table 51.4 shows the aetiological factors in 100 patients with pyogenic hepatic abscesses attending in Malaysia.[22] In most reports of hepatic pyogenic abscess, in about 10 to 15 per cent of cases no associated disease can be found, but it has been suggested that many of these cases are the result of a previous undetected bacteraemia.[322] Also, in many instances anaerobic

Table 51.4. *Aetiology of 100 Pyogenic Hepatic Abscesses in Malaysia.*[a]

Extrahepatic biliary disease:	Total 35
Cholelithiasis	25
Infective or malignant stricture	10
Intraperitoneal abdominal sepsis:	Total 20
Perforated appendicitis	8
Perforation of small intestine	2
Sepsis following gastroduodenal or pancreatic surgery	7
Penetrating gastroduodenal ulcers	3
Primary or metastatic tumours:	Total 20
Primary liver cell carcinoma	12
Secondary metastasis	8
Primary hepatic sepsis:	Total 15
Trauma	13
Infected cysts	2
Cryptogenic	5
Generalized septicaemia	5

[a] From Balasegaram.[22]

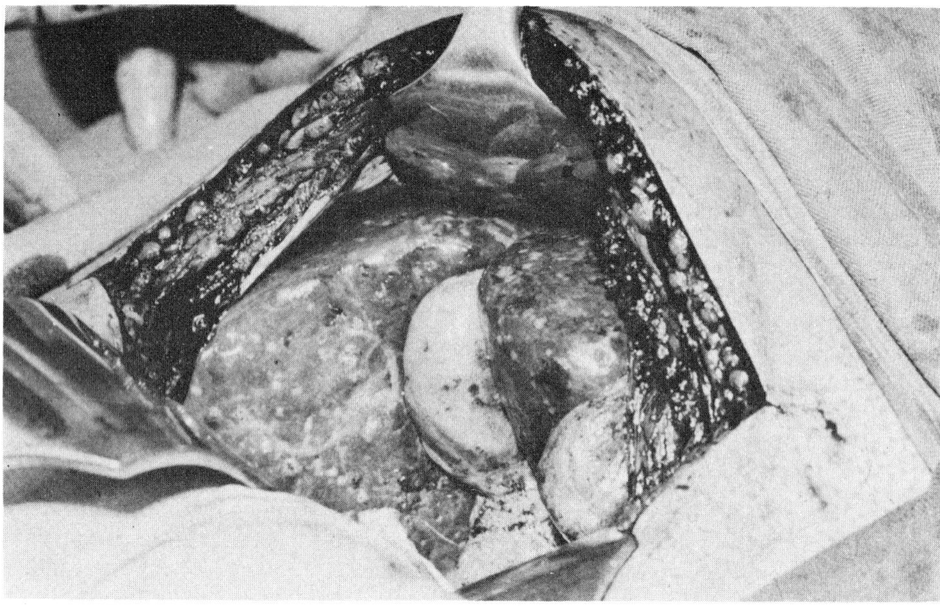

Figure 51.11. Mottled appearance of the liver due to multiple pyogenic abscesses.

bacteria have been cultured and these may have been the primary pathogen.[283] This type of abscess is usually solitary and is commonly found posteriorly in the right lobe of the liver.

Pathology

Abscesses are multiple in about 50 per cent of cases.[165,227] The liver is large and may look mottled (Figure 51.11), the area of abscess formation being pale yellow in contrast to the deep maroon colour of the adjacent hepatic tissue. The right lobe is a commoner site than the left, as discussed above, and in one series pyogenic liver abscess occurred five times more commonly in the right lobe than in the left.[281]

Multiple liver abscess

When the abscesses are associated with a pylephlebitis, they are found in relation to the portal tract. There may be considerable inflammation of the portal vein and its branches, and these are dilated and contain pus, blood clots and bacteria (Figure 51.12). Round the abscess there may be considerable hepatic necrosis and an acute inflammatory infiltrate. When abscesses complicate biliary tract disease, they are similarly closely related to the portal tracts and may contain bile-stained pus (Figure 51.13).

Solitary abscess

It is probable that many of the large solitary abscesses begin as multiple small lesions and coalesce to form one large abscess. The hepatic tissue may be extensively destroyed, and in these cases the abscesses have usually been present for a considerable time prior to the diagnosis and are surrounded by a wall of fibrous tissue.[28] The uninvolved parts of the liver may show a reactive hepatitis, severe inflammatory infiltrate, focal necrosis or other non-specific changes.

Bacteriology

Almost any organism may be implicated in an hepatic abscess, as has been described in the preceding part of this chapter. The most common pathogens cultured from the abscesses are shown in Table 51.5. In about two-thirds of patients, more than one organism is cultured.[245] Table 51.6 compares the recovery rate of anaerobic and aerobic organisms in two studies. In early reports, *E. coli* was the most common organism and accounted for 60 to 70 per cent of cases,[245,302] particularly in the presence of biliary tract disease.[295] In recent reports it is no longer the commonest pathogen and accounts for less than a quarter of cases of liver abscess.[192] Anaerobic organisms are now much more common and are cultured from up to 50 per cent of abscesses. The real incidence of anaerobic organisms may well be higher, as in

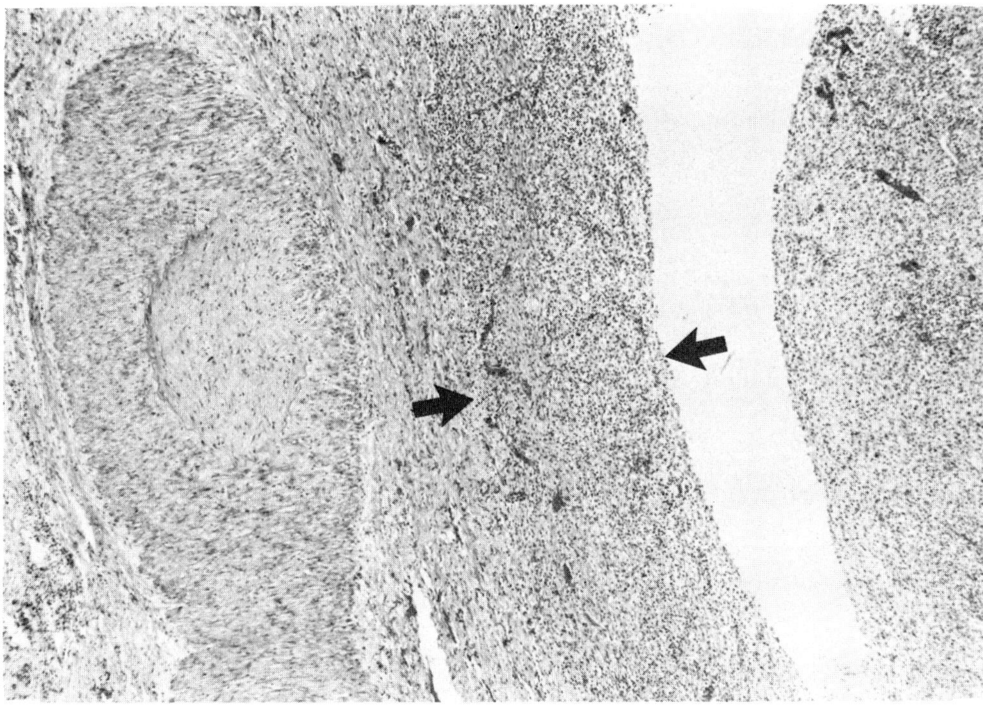

Figure 51.12. Portal pyaemia: one wall of the portal vein (between arrows) is replaced by a mixture of granulation tissue and pus. The hepatic artery cut tangentially is on the right. Haematoxylin and eosin × 600.

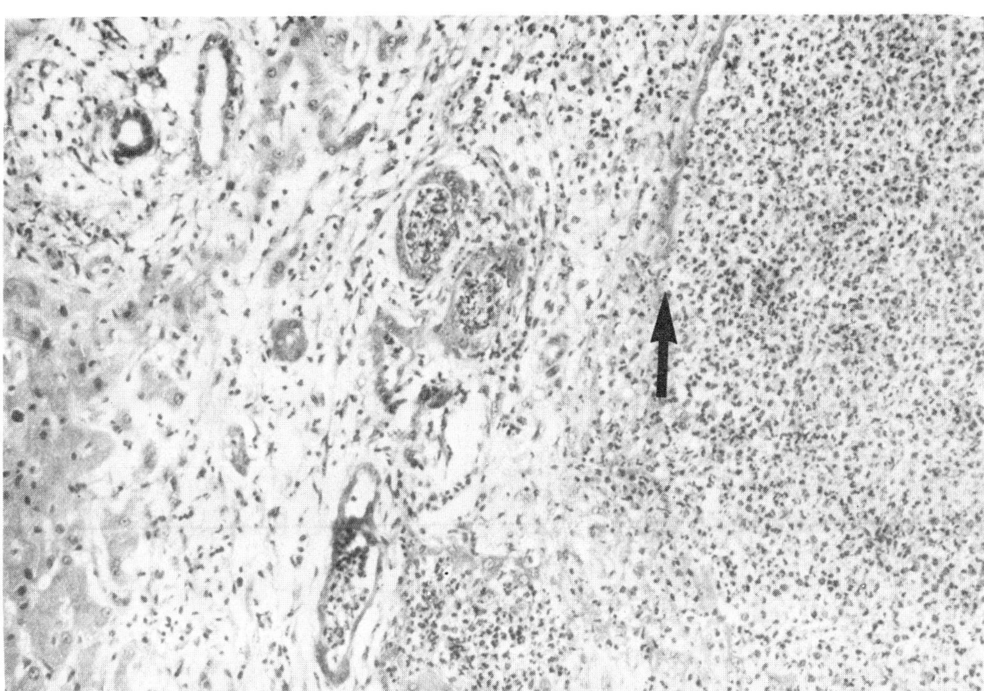

Figure 51.13. Multiple abscesses due to cholangitis. Pus (right) fills the lumen of a distended bile duct with the residual epithelium indicated by an arrow. Several smaller bile ducts are also filled with pus. Haematoxylin and eosin × 500.

Table 51.5. *Some Common Organisms Cultured from Pyogenic Liver Abscess.*[a]

Escherichia coli
Klebsiella
Streptococcal species (*S. faecalis*, *S. viridans*, anaerobic, microaerophilic)
Staphylococcal species (*S. aureus*, *S. albus*)
Proteus species
Bacteroides
Pseudomonas species
Clostridium species
Actinomyces
Pneumococcus

[a] After Pitt and Ziudema.[245]

many studies inadequate techniques for their culture were employed, and this explains why in some series up to 50 per cent of cases are sterile on culture.[281] Recovery of anaerobic organisms is also common in cryptogenic abscesses, and it has been suggested that the primary site of infection is likely to be the gastrointestinal tract in these cases.[265,283]

Features suggesting anaerobic infection include foul-smelling pus, gas in the abscess cavity and lack of aerobic growth on culture. Occasionally, there may be superimposed infection on other intrahepatic conditions, such as tuberculous abscess or ascaris infection.[222]

Clinical Features

The classic presentation is with abdominal pain, swinging pyrexia and nocturnal sweating, vomiting, anorexia, malaise and weight loss. The pain is mainly in the right lower chest or right upper quadrant of the abdomen and may be pleuritic or diaphragmatic and referred to the shoulder-tip. It is often relieved by the patient's lying on the right side, presumably due to the splinting effect of the rib cage. Any pattern of pyrexia can occur and Cronin[74] found that only a quarter of his cases had the traditional swinging fever. It has been shown that the pyrexia can be remittent, intermittent or continuous, depending on the type of abscess and the pathogenic organism involved.[227] Price and colleagues[253] have described a 'picket fence' configuration of the temperature chart. Jaundice, ascites and diarrhoea can also occur. Jaundice is present in 15 to 20 per cent of cases, particularly when complicating biliary tract disease. Jaundice usually indicates suppurative cholangitis and multiple abscess formation, and is a poor prognostic sign.

On examination, there may be hepatomegaly or tenderness over the right upper quadrant or rib cage, with intercostal oedema. Local tenderness is often present and is best detected by finger percussion.[95] If the abscess is in the left lobe of the liver, there may be a mass in the epigastrium. In advanced cases, severe debilitation and wasting can occur.

Patients may present with symptoms of complications of pyogenic liver abscess, such as rupture of the abscess into the chest, pericardium or abdomen. They may also present with septicaemia and shock. Over the years the clinical picture has changed.[178,232,294] Many of the classical symptoms may not be present and it is important to have a high index of suspicion if the diagnosis is not to be missed. Diagnosis should be considered in any patient presenting with a pyrexia of unknown origin, especially if this follows recent abdominal surgery.

Laboratory Investigations

In two-thirds of cases there will be a marked leucocytosis, but the white count can be normal. The ESR is usually raised, especially in long-standing cases, and there is often a low-grade anaemia of chronic infection. Serum B_{12} may be grossly elevated,[53] but this is non-specific and occurs in intrahepatic malignant disease and other conditions. The alkaline phosphatase may be raised and there may be hypoalbuminaemia. The serum transaminases are usually normal, but if raised are a bad prognostic sign.

Radiology

There may be elevation or alteration of the contour of the right dome of the diaphragm in about 50 per cent of cases. This can be associated with a pleural reaction or pneumonic consolidation. There may also be a right-sided pleural effusion, empyema, lung abscesses or

Table 51.6. *Organisms Cultured from Two Series of Hepatic Abscess Patients.*

	Pitt & Ziudema[245]	Sabbaj, Sutter & Finegold[283]
No.	80	49
Aerobic	67%	38%
Anaerobic	10%	34%
Aerobic and anaerobic	17%	16%
Sterile	6%	10%

The series of Pitt & Ziudema[245] spans 20 years, and if compared to the more recent series of Sabbaj, Sutter & Finegold[283] it shows the changing nature of the pathogens.

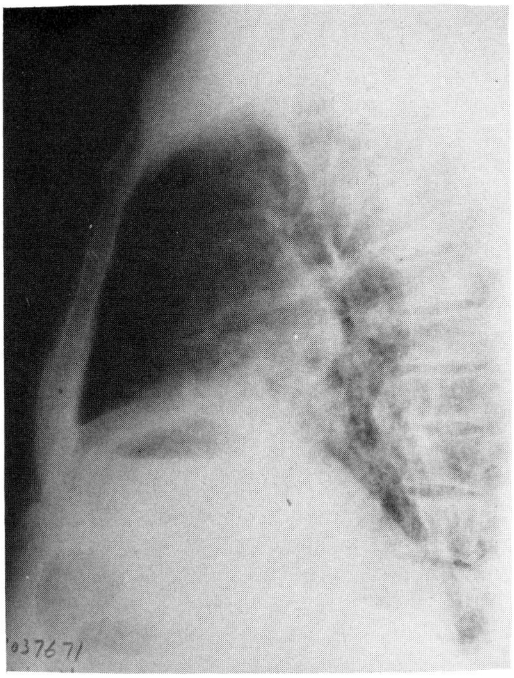

Figure 51.14. Gas-filled pyogenic liver abscess with a fluid level.

bronchopleural fistulae. In early cases screening may show reduced diaphragmatic movement. On plain abdominal film, hepatomegaly may be shown, and there may be a gas-filled fluid level in the abscess cavity (Figure 51.14).[110]

Routine cholecystogram and intravenous cholangiography are usually not helpful. Liver scanning may show the larger lesions (Figure 51.15), but ultrasound (Figure 51.16) or CAT scanning is particularly valuable and will detect lesions as small as 2 cm in diameter[181] (see Chapter 26). Angiography is helpful to confirm the diagnosis (Figure 51.17),[225,241] and very small lesions may be demonstrated by this method.[174]

Liver Biopsy and Aspiration

Although some workers feel that suspected liver abscess is a contraindication to liver biopsy,[185] this is not necessarily so provided one is prepared to aspirate the abscess, and may be helpful in confirming the diagnosis. Closed aspiration with instillation of antibiotics has been recommended by some as an alternative to surgical drainage.[208,238]

Treatment

Medical

Antibiotics are indicated, and in general their choice must be governed by the results of in vitro tests of bacterial sensitivity. If therapy has to be started before this knowledge is available, a broad-spectrum antibiotic should be prescribed to be effective against both aerobic and anaerobic organisms. A combination of gentamycin and metronidazole or clindamycin is appropriate. A further agent active against staphylococcal infections should also be added, e.g. flucloxacillin. Therapy should be continued for at least two months, except when the abscess has been totally excised, when a shorter course is adequate.[282]

Antibiotics can also be given directly into the bile ducts through a T-tube inserted at laparotomy.[20] It has also been suggested that antibiotics may be more effective if administered directly into the portal circulation via the reopened umbilical vein.[240]

Surgical

Closed drainage and instillation of antibiotics have been effective in some cases[208] but surgical drainage of pyogenic abscess is still the treatment of choice.

In early series, pleural or peritoneal contamination was a sinister complication,[227] and an extraperitoneal surgical approach was recommended. Fortunately, with the advent of broad-

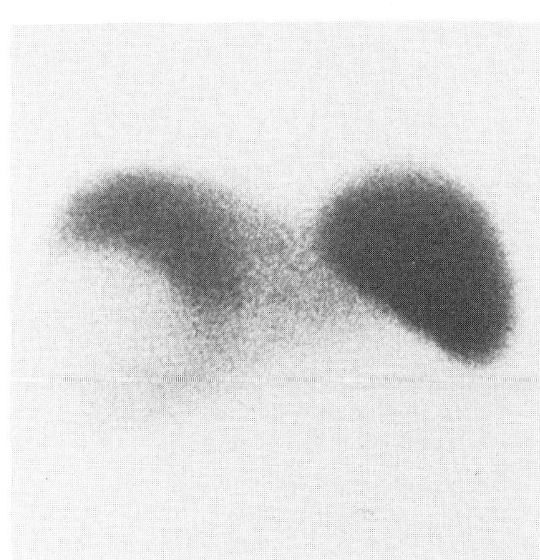

Figure 51.15. Radio imaging demonstrating a large single filling defect in the postero-lateral aspect of the right lobe.

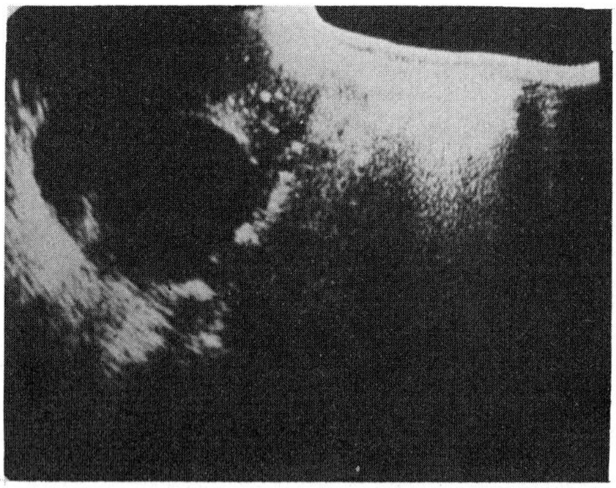

Figure 51.16. Ultrasound on the same patient as Figure 51.15 confirming the presence of a slightly irregular abscess cavity in the posterior part of the right lobe.

spectrum antibiotics this is no longer a major problem,[10,17] and transperitoneal drainage is now widely practised. The surgical approach depends on the size, location and number of the abscesses. The posterior approach is via an incision over the twelfth rib. After subperiosteal resection of the rib, a transverse excision is made through its bed at the level of the spinal process of the first lumbar vertebra. The peritoneum is then mobilized and extraperitoneal drainage can be achieved.

When the abscess is anterior or inferior, the approach is via a right subcostal incision. The involved lobe of the liver is then located and separated from the rest of the viscera and the abscess cavity can be opened and drained. Lavage with either saline or antibiotic solution is then performed. Soft pliable drains are brought out through a stab wound, and this allows for drainage, irrigation and later sinograms to monitor progress. Hard rubber catheters should be avoided as these may erode the hepatic parenchyma and cause haemorrhage.

At laparotomy there may be no visible evidence of the site of the abscess if it is deep within the liver, although there may be an altered consistency on palpation. In these cases needle aspiration will confirm the site of the abscess.

A trans-thoracic approach is indicated if there are pleural or pulmonary complications. If there are multiple small abscesses, surgery is not possible and treatment depends on prolonged antibiotic therapy.

Prognosis

Mortality and morbidity from hepatic abscess is extremely high, and usually results from delay in diagnosis. In reports as recent as 1968, the quoted mortality rate has been as high as 80 to 90 per cent.[33,258,352]

In recent years, as the diagnosis rate has improved from 20 to nearly 80 per cent,[10,80,258]

(a)

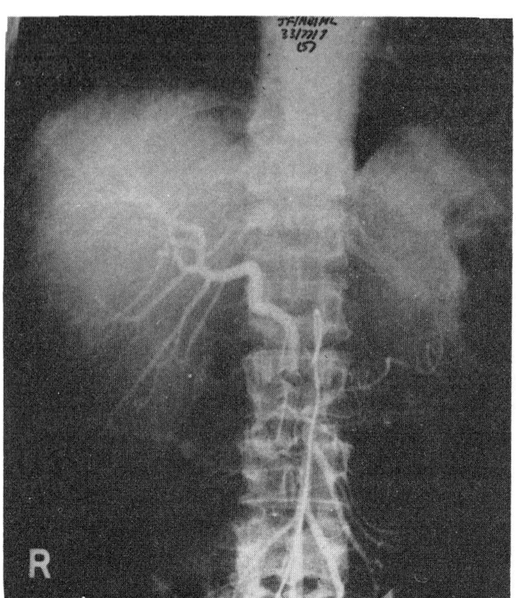

(b)

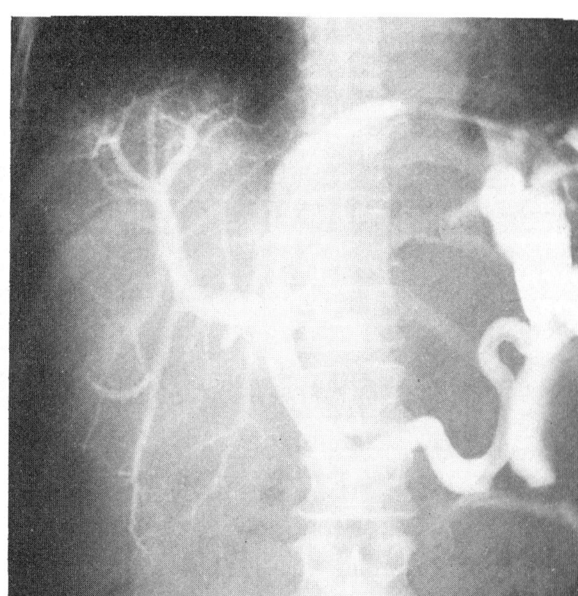

Figure 15.17 (a) Coeliac angiogram showing uniform distortion and displacement of vessels due to an abscess. (b) Splenoportogram on the same patient showing the stretching of vessels due to the abscess cavity.

so the mortality rate has dropped and is now less than 10 per cent in some series.[283]

Features associated with a poor prognosis are old age, the presence of multiple abscesses, coexistent biliary tract disease, associated malignant disease, elevated serum transaminases, hypoalbuminaemia, polymorphonucleocytosis, bacteraemia, anaerobic infection and pulmonary, peritoneal or other significant complications.[227,245,352]

Prognosis can be improved only if early diagnosis is made, and it is important to maintain a high index of suspicion of the diagnosis if cases are not to be missed.

PROTOZOAN INFECTIONS

In the tropics a number of parasites commonly infect the liver.[143]

Kala-azar (Visceral Leishmaniasis)

Leishmania donovani parasitize cells of the reticuloendothelial system, but although enlargement of the liver and spleen is a major feature of the disease, liver function is usually well maintained. Liver biopsy shows hypertrophic reticuloendothelial cells, the majority containing Leishman-Donovan bodies. Other changes encountered include an inflammatory infiltrate, fatty change and occasional portal zone fibrosis.[77,86,298]

Toxoplasmosis

Infections of *Toxoplasma gondii* are usually asymptomatic but can occasionally present with the syndrome of glandular fever, with lymphadenopathy, low-grade fever and general malaise.[54] As with infectious mononucleosis, patients have been described in whom jaundice is the predominant symptom and whose clinical picture is identical to that of viral hepatitis.[347,350] In these patients the transaminase levels can be high, and differentiation between the two may be helped by the prolonged prodromal phase and the presence of lymphadenopathy in toxoplasmosis. On liver biopsy, there may be liver-cell necrosis and an inflammatory infiltrate. *T. gondii* can rarely be demonstrated in the liver. Acquired toxoplasmosis is one cause of granulomatous hepatitis.[202]

Malaria

Both *Plasmodium falciparum* and *Plasmodium vivax* have been found in the liver. In patients with uncomplicated primary malaria, hepatomegaly is a common finding and may be associated with jaundice.[200,261] Although haemolysis may be present, it does not fully account for the jaundice. Liver function tests are abnormal in over 50 per cent of cases, commonly with elevated serum transaminases or bilirubin.[84] Transaminases can be markedly elevated and suggest a diagnosis of viral hepatitis. On histology, there may be Kupffer cell proliferation, so-called brown malarial pigment (Figure 51.18) and a mononuclear cell inflammatory infiltrate. Occasionally, granulomas and areas of focal necrosis occur. Hepatocytes may be swollen and there is evidence of cell regeneration.

Post-mortem studies on patients dying with blackwater fever showed centrilobular necrosis,[81] but this may have been in part due to post-mortem changes. Electron microscopic studies have shown distortion of the cell membrane with, among other changes, mitochondrial abnormalities.[278]

Giardiasis

Infection with *Giardia lamblia*, which has a worldwide distribution, is often asymptomatic but may result in malabsorption. Rarely, there may be symptoms suggestive of cholelithiasis[313] and the parasite has been found in the gallbladders of a few patients undergoing cholecystectomy for gallstones, although the two conditions are unlikely to be related.[118,168]

Balantidiasis

Infection with *Balantidium coli* is usually asymptomatic but may result in diarrhoea, the clinical picture resembling invasive amoebiasis.[168] There is at least one report of an hepatic abscess due to *Balantidium coli.*[353]

AMOEBIC LIVER ABSCESS

It has been estimated that amoebic abscess complicates between 3 and 9 per cent of cases of amoebiasis,[23] but this is likely to be an overestimation as non-invasive amoebiasis often goes undiagnosed.

(a) 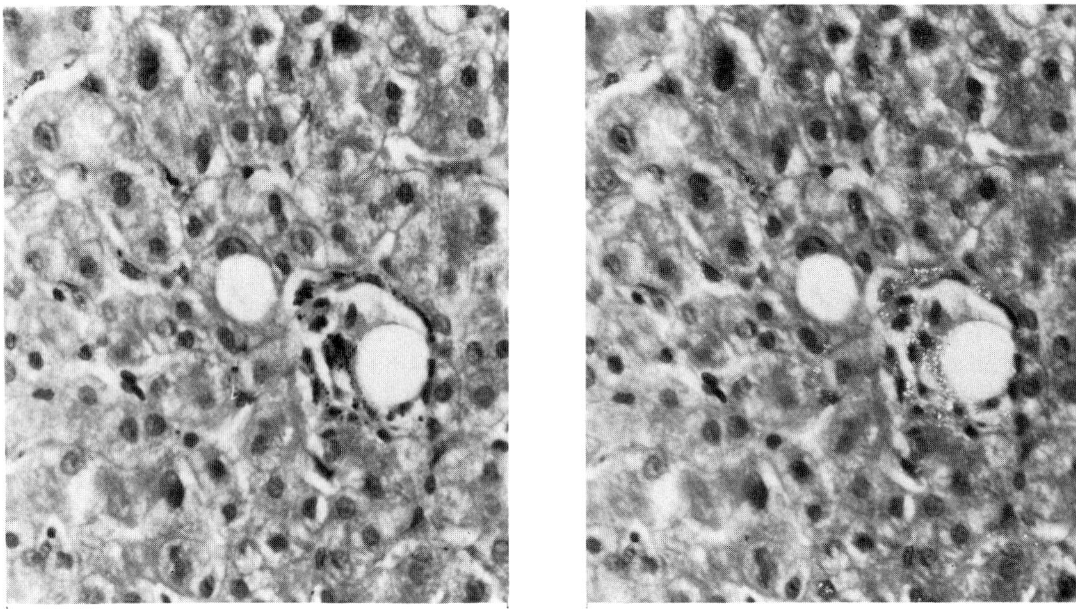 (b)

Figure 51.18. A focal collection of mononuclear cells containing finely particulate black malarial pigment (a) which is doubly refractile in polarized light (b).

Aetiology and Pathogenesis

The disease is due to an infection with a protozoan parasite, *Entamoeba histolytica*. It is one of a number of amoebae present in the colon, but with rare exceptions the remainder have not been shown to be pathogenic.

E. histolytica may occur in stools in the cystic or trophozoite form. The mature cysts are 10 to 20 μ in diameter, and are resistant to drying and an acid pH. After ingestion, they rupture in the intestine, releasing four metacystic trophozoites. The trophozoites exist in two forms, a small or 'minuta', 10 to 20 μ in diameter, which needs to be distinguished from *Entamoeba hartmanni*, which it morphologically resembles closely, and a larger trophozoite, 20 to 60 μ in diameter, present in patients with invasive disease. Characteristically, these large trophozoites are actively motile, ingest red blood cells and contain proteases, hyaluronidase[149] and mucopolysaccharidases capable of causing tissue destruction. They are destroyed by desiccation and acid pH. Trophozoites are destroyed by gastric acid, so that transmission can occur only by swallowing cysts.

The common mode of transmission is by ingestion of water or vegetables contaminated by cysts. Direct faecal–oral transmission may occur under conditions of poor personal hygiene. Most large outbreaks have been due to contamination of the water supply by sewage. A high proportion of the general population are cyst-passers in endemic areas. Even in temperate zones in the United States and the United Kingdom, surveys indicate a rate of 1 to 3 per cent, so indigenous amoebiasis can occur without foreign travel.[157] The majority of cases in Western Europe and the United States still occur in immigrants or others who have returned from an endemic area.[332] There may be a long latent period before the development of invasive amoebiasis, particularly in the case of amoebic liver abscess, and some individuals living in temperate areas may have become infected after residence in an endemic area more than 20 years previously.[369] In other words, *E. histolytica* may exist as a commensal in the intestine for many years before becoming invasive but, conversely, there may be rapid onset of invasion following infection.

The factors governing invasiveness are poorly understood, but include virulence of the parasite, diet, bacterial flora of the intestine, and host resistance, both humoral and cell-mediated immunity.[224] Strains isolated in temperate zones are often avirulent, whereas those in the tropics are often virulent. Virulence is maintained when strains are transmitted to animals.[157] Although amoebic abscesses are usually sterile, invasion of the intestine does not occur in the absence of bacteria, as is evident from the resistance to infection of germ-free guinea pigs.[239]

High titres of circulating antibodies to a number of amoebic antigens occur following

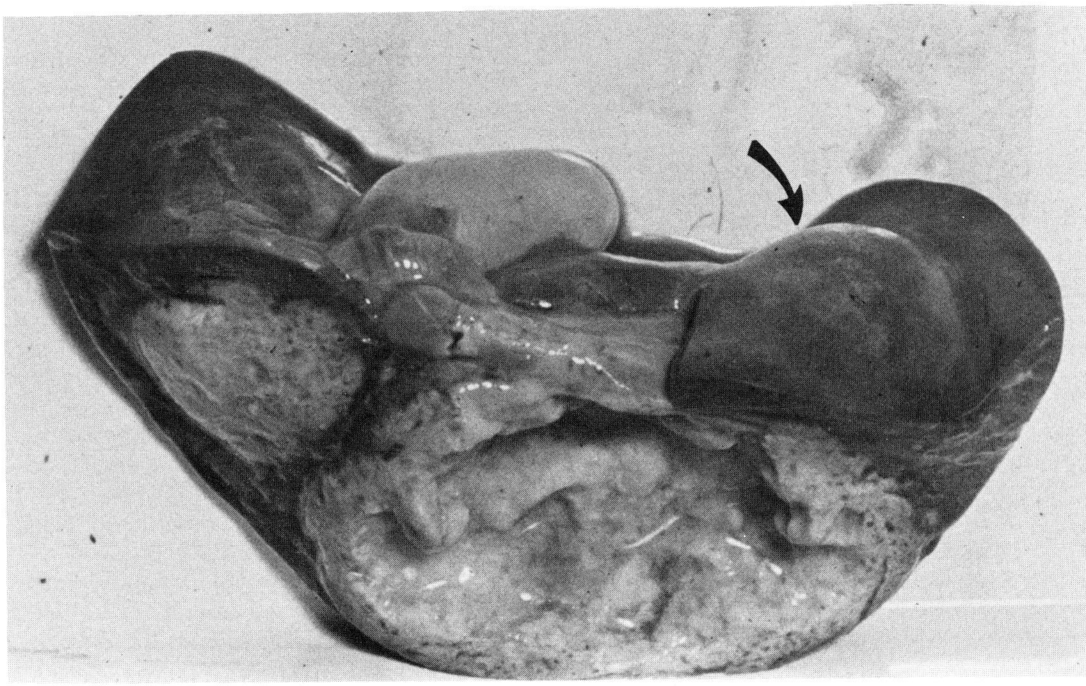

Figure 51.19. Autopsy specimen of liver showing two large amoebic abscesses. The larger abscess can also be seen as a bulge expanding the left lobe of the liver (arrow).

invasive amoebiasis and may persist for years,[176] but reinfection can still occur.[150] Persistence of precipitating antibody to a wide range of amoebic antigens is necessary to maintain immunity. Using leucocyte migration inhibition, Ortiz-Ortiz et al[230] found that cell-mediated immunity was negligible during the acute untreated phase of amoebic liver abscess, and developed only during its resolution. They postulated that the relative absence of cell-mediated immunity is reflected in the mild tissue inflammatory response provoked by the infection.

Protective cell-mediated immunity appears to develop slowly in amoebiasis and may play an important role in limiting tissue invasiveness and in aiding resolution, rather than in its prevention.[157,291]

Pathology

Amoebic liver abscesses vary in size from a few centimetres in diameter to very large abscesses containing several litres of pus (Figure 51.19). They may be single or multiple. Although amoebae reach the liver from the intestine, most patients with amoebic liver abscesses have no evidence of intestinal disease at the time of presentation, and presumably the infection can remain dormant in the intestine for many years before spreading to the liver. Once the liver is infected, the abscess usually develops rapidly over a period of weeks or months. Although tender hepatomegaly can occur during acute amoebic dysentery, there is no evidence for an amoebic hepatitis due to diffuse involvement of the liver in the absence of abscess formation.[2,157,251,360] The pus from amoebic liver abscesses may have the appearance classically described as 'anchovy sauce', but is often yellow or green. Microscopy of the pus shows few pus cells and it consists mainly of tissue debris. Tissue destruction probably results from the release of cytoplasmic enzymes, such as hyaluronidase, proteases and mucopolysaccharides by the trophozoites. The inflammatory reaction in the wall of the abscess is a low-grade response of lymphocytes, macrophages and fibroblasts, with a relative absence of neutrophils. Trophozoites can be readily demonstrated in the wall of the abscess in the area of degenerating liver cells (Figure 51.20) and with appropriate techniques can be isolated from the pus. Fibrosis develops in the wall of the abscess, but even very large abscesses can resolve completely without residual scarring. Calcification is rare.

E. histolytica can be seen in aspirated abscess

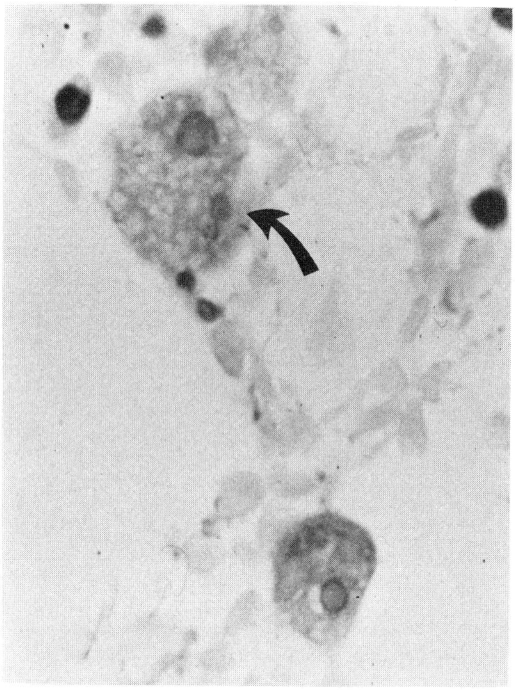

Figure 51.20. *Entamoeba histolytica;* the amoebae are usually much larger than all other accompanying inflammatory cells in the exudate, including macrophages. Erythrophagocytosis is a characteristic feature. Courtesy of Dr P. Isaacson. Haematoxylin and eosin × 1250.

fluid or the necrotic liver tissue. The trophozoites may also be shown when an immunofluorescent stain is used, a technique that can be applied to previously fixed sections.[234]

Clinical Features

There have been several recent reviews of the clinical presentation of amoebic liver abscess.[23,62,223,263,301] It occurs at any age, including childhood. It is much more common in males than in females, but the explanation for the sex difference is unknown. The onset is usually insidious, with pain in the right upper quadrant of the abdomen, malaise, feverishness and weight loss. Occasionally it is acute with rigors and severe hepatic pain. In one series, over half the patients had a history of less than two weeks,[2] but in some cases symptoms develop over many months with malaise, fever and vague abdominal pain. At presentation, virtually all patients have pain in the right upper quadrant of the abdomen or right lower chest, epigastrium or right shoulder-tip. It is a dull ache, often worse at night, but is occasionally pleuritic. Cough and symptoms of diaphragmatic irritation, such as hiccup, may occur even in the absence of rupture through the diaphragm. Anorexia, nausea, weight loss and night sweats are other common symptoms. Diarrhoea, with or without evidence of active amoebic dysentery, occurs in less than 20 per cent of patients, and jaundice is relatively uncommon. Occasionally, patients may present with acute obstructive jaundice.[130,264] Fulminant hepatic failure secondary to amoebic abscess is a very rare complication.[285]

Over 90 per cent of patients have tender hepatomegaly, and a point of maximum tenderness can often be detected, either in the intercostal space or over the enlarged liver. There may be dullness to percussion with diminished air entry at the right lung base due to a raised right diaphragm or accumulation of pleural fluid. Occasionally, this may be the predominant sign in the absence of hepatomegaly if the abscess is high under the diaphragm.[2] A fixed raised diaphragm may be demonstrated on percussion. Large abscesses may produce visible bulging of the right lower chest or a hepatic mass. The spleen is occasionally palpable.

Pyrexia may be sustained, low grade and, rarely, swinging with rigors. Large or multiple chronic abscesses may be associated with cachexia and chronic anaemia. In less than 10 per cent of patients, the abscess is confined to the left lobe of the liver, occasionally with a visible and palpable mass in the epigastrium which may be tender.[266] Their recognition is important because of the danger of rupture into the pericardium.

Complications

Complications occur either as a result of rupture of the abscess into adjacent structures or from secondary infection. Extension may occur into the chest producing an amoebic empyema, hepatobronchial fistula, lung abscess or consolidation. Pleuritic pain, cough and dyspnoea are the usual symptoms and are associated with appropriate physical signs. A right basal effusion of serous fluid or linear atelectasis may be found before frank rupture occurs. Spontaneous cure may be produced by drainage of the abscess into the bronchus with the pus being coughed up. Before adequate treatment was available, this was the best chance of cure. Rupture may be either insidious or acute, with sudden onset of tearing pleuritic pain and tachypnoea.[2,144] In one series of 2074 patients with amoebic abscess 146 cases ruptured into the chest.[2]

Other complications resulting from local rupture of the abscess are rare, but they may be difficult to diagnose and are associated with a relatively high mortality. Forty out of 2074 cases reported by Adams and Macleod[2] ruptured into the peritoneum or bowel and required diagnostic laparotomy and drainage. In the same series, 27 patients presented with rupture into the pericardium. This is the most sinister complication[2,145,159] and carries a high mortality rate. Patients may present with symptoms of a pericardial effusion or with shock. Rarely, rupture occurs either externally or into the rectus sheath. In the latter case, a 'collar-stud' abscess may be produced, communicating with the original abscess cavity in the left lobe. Haemobilia[250] and brain abscess[249] are also rare complications. Secondary bacterial infection is likewise rare, but may be introduced by aspiration.

Investigations

Laboratory investigations

A normocytic, normochromic anaemia is common, particularly in long-standing cases. Leucocytosis is present in over three-quarters of cases, especially in acute ones. The erythrocyte sedimentation rate is almost always raised. Hypoalbuminaemia is present in over half the patients, particularly those with large or chronic abscesses. Liver function tests are seldom helpful in diagnosis. The alkaline phosphatase and aspartate aminotransferase are moderately elevated, the bilirubin is usually normal and clinically overt jaundice is rare. Extrahepatic obstruction may be seen very exceptionally, caused by pressure from a large abscess on the biliary tree or from rupture into a major bile duct.

Serological tests in the diagnosis of amoebic liver abscess. Serological tests for amoebiasis are of considerable value in diagnosis. These tests are positive in over 90 per cent of cases of amoebic liver abscess.[2,157,175] Techniques include gel diffusion,[197] latex agglutination,[217] indirect haemagglutination, immunofluorescence and cellulose acetate precipitin.[42,318] The more sensitive techniques have the disadvantage of remaining positive for long periods after pre-existing invasive intestinal amoebiasis. False-positive results may also be produced in endemic areas.

Sigmoidoscopy and stool examination

These should be undertaken in all patients with amoebic liver abscess, for although the majority of patients will have no evidence of coexistent colitis, amoebae can readily be detected in rectal biopsies by appropriate staining.

Radiology

A raised right diaphragm is an important radiological sign which is present in half to three-quarters of patients, sometimes without enlargement of the liver below the right costal margin.[293] Atelectasis or pleural effusion at the right base are also common.[23] After rupture through the diaphragm, a pleural effusion, lung abscess, consolidation or, rarely, features of a bronchopleural or hepatopleural fistula may be present; in such cases a fluid level may be seen in the hepatic abscess. Radiological features of pericardial effusion are present if this complicates a left lobe abscess.

Hepatic scintiscan, ultrasound and angiography

As has been discussed fully in the section on pyogenic abscess, colloid liver scans provide valuable information about the site and number of liver abscesses.[194,348] When these are combined with ultrasound, abscesses can be distinguished from solid tumours, but it may not be possible to differentiate an abscess from a cyst.[181,204] This distinction is important because hydatid cysts may also be common in areas where amoebiasis is endemic; the needling of hydatid cysts is dangerous and may facilitate spread. Angiography, on the other hand, may be helpful. Gordon and associates[121] have claimed that combined colloid 113m-Indium ($^{113}In^{m}$) and transferrin-bound $^{113}In^{m}$ scanning, which visualizes hepatic blood flow, can be used to differentiate abscesses, cysts and tumours. Hepatic scanning is also of value in localizing the site of the abscess prior to needle aspiration.

Differential Diagnosis

The diagnosis is based on the clinical and radiological features. It is confirmed by aspiration of pus from the liver, demonstration of *E. histolytica* on microscopy and by positive serology for amoebic antigens. A raised right diaphragm, intercostal point tenderness or tenderness over the liver can all occur with both pyogenic and amoebic liver abscesses. The distinction is particularly difficult when an amoebic abscess presents acutely with swinging pyrexia. A positive serological test for amoebiasis may be helpful, but needle aspiration with culture for bacteria and the demonstration of trophozoites prior to the administration of antibiotics or amoebicidal drugs may be the only conclusive way of distinguishing between the two. As indicated earlier, a proportion of patients with amoebic liver abscesses have secondary infection. It is important to recognize that amoebic pus may not have the characteristic 'anchovy sauce' appearance and may be yellow or green, due to layering within the abscess cavity.

It can be difficult to distinguish between amoebic and pyogenic abscess. Features that favour amoebiasis are pain, diarrhoea and the presence of multiple abscesses. In both, the white blood count and the ESR may be elevated.[23]

The distinction between amoebic liver abscess and hydatid cysts of the liver is particularly important in areas where both conditions are endemic, but either condition can occur in patients who have never left the United Kingdom. Hydatid cysts are more likely to be calcified, show a characteristic echo pattern on ultrasonography and a positive Casoni skin test. In endemic areas, primary hepatoma is also often common, and distinction may be difficult clinically, particularly if the amoebic abscess is chronic and firm on palpation. Conversely, amoebic abscess may be misdiagnosed as primary hepatoma; in one series, 15 patients in whom this diagnosis was made proved to have an amoebic liver abscess at autopsy.[19] Confusion can also occur with secondary carcinomatosis.[369] The distinction between tumour and amoebic abscess should be readily made on the basis of serological tests, ultrasonography and angiography.

In areas where amoebiasis is uncommon, delay in diagnosis may occur because the disorder has not been considered.[369] A history of travel abroad to an endemic area, even many years previously, and a raised right diaphragm may first lead to a suspicion of the condition. Neither factor, however, may be present. Pain or tenderness in the right upper quadrant may lead to a suspicion of gallbladder disease, and finding a non-functioning gallbladder on cholangiography may appear to confirm this diagnosis. It is important to recognize that failure of the gallbladder and biliary tree to opacify may occur in patients with amoebiasis.[70,369]

Confusion with chronic liver disease, such as chronic active hepatitis, may be hazardous[323] as the administration of corticosteroids appears to be associated with the development of fulminant amoebic liver abscess. The importance of having a high index of suspicion for amoebiasis in non-endemic areas has been repeatedly emphasized.[42,175,369]

Treatment

Several controlled clinical trials reviewed by Adams and Macleod[2] established the effectiveness of emetine and chloroquine in the treatment of amoebic liver abscess. Emetine was preferably given as the dihydroemetine preparation in a dose of 80 mg intramuscularly daily for 10 days, with an initial 600 mg of chloroquine followed six hours later by 300 mg intramuscularly and then 150 mg twice daily by mouth for 29 days. This was found to be more effective than chloroquine alone, and was followed by a lower relapse rate.[361,362] On the other hand, both treatment failure and relapse are said to be rare if chloroquine is given for a longer period of 10 weeks in a dose of 500 mg daily.[274,343]

Both these drugs have largely been superseded by the introduction of metronidazole (Flagyl) for the treatment of amoebic liver abscess. Powell and colleagues[252] found it to be highly effective when given orally for a period of four to 10 days. They recommended using 750 mg three times daily for 10 days, with or without a loading dose of 2.4 g followed by 1.2 g six-hourly.

In a further randomized controlled trial of 36 patients with amoebic liver abscess, Cohen and Reynolds[70] compared metronidazole 750 mg three times daily for 10 days with chloroquine 0.5 g daily for 10 weeks. They showed that both drugs are highly effective in treatment, but metronidazole is associated with a shorter course of treatment and a slightly more rapid response. In addition, it is effective against intestinal amoebiasis. There is therefore no need to give additional drugs such as di-iodohydroxyquine. Nevertheless, there have been reports of failure of metronidazole to cure amoebic abscesses.[78,124,137,359] If metronidazole is ineffective, chloroquine 500 mg daily for two to 10 weeks, with or without dihydroemetine 1 to 1.5 mg per kg daily, given either intramuscularly or subcutaneously for 10 days, should be added.[175] Emetine has the disadvantage of cardiac and neurological toxicity. These side-effects appear to be less with dihydroemetine, but the drug cannot be given parenterally. Both chloroquine and metronidazole are associated with gastrointestinal side-effects. In addition, metronidazole may have an effect similar to Antabuse (disulfiram). Alcohol should therefore be avoided when this drug is given.[175]

A few patients continue to be cyst-passers after treatment with metronidazole. In these cases another luminal amoebicidal drug may be necessary.[2] A therapeutic response to metronidazole is a valuable aid to diagnosis, but should be interpreted with caution because this drug is also effective against gram negative organisms. Patients may relapse even after apparently adequate treatment.[123]

Needle aspiration

There is controversy over the indications for percutaneous needle aspiration of the abscess.[2,157,175] Small abscesses are likely to resolve with metronidazole treatment, so that the only indication for aspiration in these cases is to confirm the diagnosis if this is in doubt. Preferably, aspiration should be performed before treatment is started. If the abscess is large and there is point tenderness, Adams and Macleod[2] advocate aspiration, although there is no controlled evidence that this accelerates healing.[175] Decompression of the abscess may relieve symptoms and should be undertaken if there is evidence to suggest that rupture into adjacent structures is likely. After careful selection of the point of maximum tenderness, a medium-bore needle should be introduced following local anaesthesia of the skin and subcutaneous structures as for liver biopsy. A 50-ml syringe with a three-way stopcock should be used to permit removal of large amounts of fluid as described for pyogenic abscesses. In large or multiple abscesses without point tenderness, radiological techniques may be useful in identifying the site for aspiration. Repeated aspiration may be necessary, but an interval of a few days should be allowed to elapse between the procedures. Needle aspiration of abscesses in the left lobe is sometimes more difficult than for right lobe abscesses, particularly in the case of a collar-stud abscess.

Surgical drainage

Surgical drainage is required in only the most exceptional cases in western society, where patients present relatively early. The conservative regimen described above is usually adopted in most endemic areas.[2] Open surgical drainage should be considered under the following circumstances:

1. Patients not responding to medical treatment, in spite of repeated needle aspiration.[144]
2. Multiple abscesses.
3. Left lobe abscesses pointing below the costal margin, with signs of impending rupture into the pericardium.
4. Rupture or impending rupture into other adjacent structures, particularly into the peritoneum or a hollow viscus, or through the abdominal wall.
5. Abscesses with secondary infection not controlled by antibiotics.

One of us has adopted a more radical approach in an endemic area where patients present late and have failed to respond to medical treatment.[22] The techniques and approach are similar to those described for pyogenic abscess.

Prognosis

The prognosis of amoebic liver abscess, even in endemic areas, is extremely good unless presenting in an advanced stage or with one of the complications. Of 1859 cases of uncomplicated liver disease reported by Adams and Macleod,[2] only 13 patients (0.7 per cent) died. Of 146 patients with extension into the chest, the mortality rate was 6.2 per cent, whereas 38 patients (18.4 per cent) who developed peritonitis and 27 patients (29.6 per cent) with pericardial involvement died. The mortality rate in 271 patients treated surgically by one of us was 8 per cent[22] and could be attributed to the late presentation of patients with complications of the disease. If adequately treated, resolution of the abscess is complete but immunity is not permanent and reinfection can occur.

REFERENCES

1. Abenathy, R.S. (1959) Clinical manifestations of pulmonary blastomycosis. *Annals of Internal Medicine*, **51,** 707–739.
2. Adams, E.B. & Macleod, I.N. (1977) Invasive amebiasis. I. Amebic liver abscess and its complications. *Medicine* (*Baltimore*), **56,** 325–334.

3. Agrawal, H.S., Benson, J.W. & Major, J.J. (1967) An unusual case of hemobilia. Hepatic tuberculosis with haemorrhage. *Archives of Surgery*, **95,** 202–206.
4. Agrawal, S.C., Maheshwari, H.B. & Mittal, M.M. (1973) A histological study of liver lesions in leprosy. *Indian Journal of Medical Research*, **61,** 389–395.
5. Aksel, A., Gokaz, A., Karacadag, S. & Telatar, H. (1973) The liver in typhoid fever. *American Journal of Gastroenterology*, **60,** 141–146.
6. Alergant, C.D. (1956) Gumma of liver with calcification. *Archives of Internal Medicine*, **98,** 340–343.
7. Alkan, W.J., Evenchik, Z. & Eshchar, J. (1965) Q fever and infectious hepatitis. *American Journal of Medicine*, **38,** 54–61.
8. Alston, J.M. & Broom, J.C. (1944) The action of penicillin on leptospira and on leptospiral infections in guinea-pigs. *British Medical Journal*, **ii,** 718–719.
9. Alston, J.M. & Broom, J.C. (1958) *Leptospirosis in Man and Animals*. Edinburgh: Livingstone.
10. Altemeier, W.A., Showengerdt, C.G. & Whitley, D.H. (1970) Abscess of the liver. Surgical considerations. *Archives of Surgery*, **101,** 258–266.
11. Arcomano, J.P., Pizzolato, N.F., Singer, R. & Zucker, S.M. (1977) A unique type of calcification in chronic brucellosis. *American Journal of Roentgenology, Radium Therapy and Nuclear Medicine*, **128,** 135–137.
12. Arean, V.M. (1962) The pathologic anatomy and pathogenesis of fatal human leptospirosis (Weil's disease). *American Journal of Pathology*, **40,** 393–423.
13. Ashe, W.F., Pratt-Thomas, H.R. & Kumpe, C.W. (1941) Weil's disease; complete review of American literature and abstract of world literature; 7 case reports. *Medicine*, **20,** 145–210.
14. Ashton, N. (1946) A case of multiple tuberculomata of the liver. *Journal of Pathology and Bacteriology*, **58,** 95–97.
15. Baker, A.L., Kaplan, M.M., Wolfe, H.J. & McGowan, J.A. (1971) Liver disease associated with early syphilis. *New England Journal of Medicine*, **284,** 1422–1423.
16. Balasegaram, M. (1970) Hepatic surgery – present and future. *Annals of the Royal College of Surgeons, England*, **47,** 139–158.
17. Balasegaram, M. (1972) Hepatic surgery: a review of a personal series of 95 major resections. *Australian and New Zealand Journal of Surgery*, **42,** 1–10.
18. Balasegaram, M. (1972) Hepatic calculi. *Annals of Surgery*, **175,** 149–154.
19. Balasegaram, M. (1972) New concepts of hepatic amoebiasis. *Annals of Surgery*, **175,** 528–534.
20. Balasegaram, M. (1975) Surgical management of hepatic lesions. *Malaysian Journal of Surgery*, **2,** 117–130.
21. Balasegaram, M. (1976) Surgery of the liver. In *Recent Developments in Surgery* (Ed.) Choudhrie, A.V. pp. 262–286. Nagpur, India: Rangachari & Co., Nagpur Press.
22. Balasegaram, M. (1978) Unpublished observations.
23. Barbour, G.I. & Juniper, K. Jr (1972) A clinical comparison of amebic and pyogenic abscess of the liver in sixty-six patients. *American Journal of Medicine*, **53,** 323–334.
24. Barrett, G.M. & Rickards, A.G. (1953) Chronic brucellosis. *Quarterly Journal of Medicine*, **22,** 23–42.
25. Barton, L.C., Escobedo, M.B. & Keating, J.P. (1973) Leptospirosis with acalculous cholecystitis. *American Journal of Diseases of Children*, **126,** 350–351.
26. Bauer, H., Ajello, L., Adams, E. & Hernandez, D.U. (1955) Cerebral mucormycosis: pathogenesis of the disease. Description of the fungus, *Rhizopus orgzae*, isolated from a fatal case. *American Journal of Medicine*, **18,** 822–831.
27. Bayer, A.S., Yoshikawa, T.T., Galpin, J.E. & Guze, L.B. (1976) Unusual syndromes of coccidioidomycosis; diagnostic and therapeutic considerations. A report of 10 cases and review of the English literature *Medicine*, **55,** 131–152.
28. Beaver, D.C. (1931) Granulomatous abscess of the liver – treatment failure with metronidazole. *Journal of the American Medical Association*, **224,** 1394–1395.
29. Beeson, P.B., Hankey, D.D. & Cooper, C.F. (1951) Leptospiral iridocyclitis. Evidence of human infection with *Leptospira pomona* in the United States. *Journal of the American Medical Association*, **145,** (4), 229–230.
30. Bernstein, J. & Brown, A.K. (1962) Sepsis and jaundice in early infancy. *Pediatrics*, **28,** 873–882.
31. Bernstein, M., Edmondson, H.A. & Barbour, B.H. (1965) The liver lesion in Q fever. *Archives of Internal Medicine*, **116,** 491–498.
32. Bhamarapravati, N., Boonyapaknavig, V., Viranuvatti, V., Tuchinda, U., Boonnag, D. & Nye, S.W. (1966) Liver changes in leptospirosis: a study of needle biopsies in twenty-two cases. *American Journal of Proctology*, **17,** 480–487.
33. Block, M.A., Schuman, B.H. & Eyler, W.R. (1964) Surgery of liver abscesses. *Archives of Surgery*, **88,** 602–610.
34. Blumberg, B.S., Melartin, L., Lechat, M. & Guinto, R.S. (1967) Association between lepromatous leprosy and Australia antigen. *Lancet*, **ii,** 173–176.
35. Blumer, G. & Nesbit, R.R. (1936) A case of gonococcal septicaemia with endocarditis and hepatitis. *International Clinics*. (Philadelphia: Lippincott.) **4,** 44–48.
36. Botsford, T.W. (1941) Acute typhoidal cholecystitis and cholelithiasis occurring 43 years after typhoid fever: report of case. *New England Journal of Medicine*, **224,** 799–800.
37. Bouzakoura, C. & Cox, J.N. (1974) L'hépatite granulomateuse dans la flèvre. *Schweizerische Medizinische Wochenschrift*, **104,** 796–800.
38. Bragger, J.M. & Adler, B. (1976) A card test for the serodiagnosis of human leptospirosis. *Journal of Clinical Pathology*, **29,** 198–202.
39. Braude, A.I. (1951) Studies in the pathology and pathogenesis of experimental brucellosis. II. The formation of hepatic granuloma and its evolution. *Journal of Infectious Diseases*, **89,** 87–94.
40. *British Medical Journal* (1973) Misdiagnosis of amoebiasis (Editorial). *British Medical Journal*, **ii,** 379–380.
41. *British Medical Journal* (1975) Secondary syphilis and hepatitis (Editorial). *British Medical Journal*, **i,** 112.
42. *British Medical Journal* (1978) Misdiagnosis of amoebiasis (Editorial). *British Medical Journal*, **ii,** 379–380.
43. Brooke, B.N. & Slaney, G. (1958) Portal bacteraemia in ulcerative colitis. *Lancet*, **i,** 1206–1207.

44. Broom, J.C. & Norris, T.St M. (1957) Failure of prophylactic oral penicillin to inhibit a human laboratory case of leptospirosis. *Lancet*, **i**, 721–722.
45. Brown, J.R. (1973) Human actinomycosis: a study of 181 subjects. *Human Pathology*, **4**, 319–330.
46. Brundage, W.G., Thuss, C.J. & Walden, D.C. (1968) Four fatal cases of medioidosis in US soldiers in Vietnam. Bacteriologic and pathologic characteristics. *American Journal of Tropical Medicine and Hygiene*, **17**, 183–191.
47. Bryceson, A.D.M., Parry, E.H.O., Perine, P.L., Warrell, D.A., Vukotich, D. & Leithead, C.S. (1970) Louse-borne relapsing fever. A clinical and laboratory study of 62 cases in Ethiopia and a reconsideration of the literature. *Quarterly Journal of Medicine*, **39**, 129–170.
48. Buchanan, T.M., Faber, L.C. & Feldman, R.A. (1974) Brucellosis in the United States, 1960–1972. An abattoir-associated disease. *Medicine*, **53**, 403–413.
49. Buckler, J.M.H. (1977) Leptospirosis presenting with erythema nodosum. *Archives of Diseases in Childhood*, **52**, 418–419.
50. Burke, B.J., Searle, J.F. & Mattingly, D. (1976) Leptospirosis presenting with profuse haemoptysis. *British Medical Journal*, **ii**, 982.
51. Busch, L.A. (1970) Leptospirosis 1965–1968. *Journal of Infectious Diseases*, **121**, 458–460.
52. Busey, J.F., Baker, R., Birch, L., Buechner, M., Chick, E.W., Justice, F.K., Matthews, J.H., McDearman, S., Pickar, D.N., Sutliff, W.D., Walkup, H.E. & Zimmerman, S. (1963) Blastomycosis. 1. A review of 198 collected cases in Veterans Administration Hospitals. Blastomycosis Co-operative Study of the Veterans Administration. *American Review of Respiratory Diseases*, **89**, 659–672.
53. Butler, T.J. & McCarthy, C.F. (1969) Pyogenic liver abscess. *Gut*, **10**, 389–399.
54. Callahan, W.P., Russell, W.O. & Smith, M.G. (1946) Human toxoplasmosis. A clinicopathologic study with presentation of five cases and review of the literature. *Medicine*, **25**, 343–397.
55. Case Records of the Massachusetts General Hospital: No. 3 (1970) *New England Journal of Medicine*, **282**, 153–159.
56. Case Records of the Massachusetts General Hospital: No. 51 (1971) *New England Journal of Medicine*, **285**, 1474–1480.
57. Case Records of the Massachusetts General Hospital: No. 44 (1974) *New England Journal of Medicine*, **291**, 1021–1027.
58. Case Records of the Massachusetts General Hospital: No. 30 (1975) *New England Journal of Medicine*, **293**, 247–253.
59. Case Records of the Massachusetts General Hospital: No. 34 (1975) *New England Journal of Medicine*, **293**, 443–448.
60. Chan, A.Y.S., Goldbloom, V.C. & Gurd, F.N. (1951) Clostridial infection as a cause of death after ligation of the hepatic artery. *Archives of Surgery*, **63**, 390–402.
61. Chandarlapaty, S.K.C., Dusol, M., Edwards, R., Pereiras, R., Clark, R. & Schiff, E.R. (1975) ^{67}Gallium accumulation in hepatic actinomycosis. *Gastroenterology*, **69**, 752–755.
62. Chellappa, M. & Rangabashyam, N. (1977) Amoebic liver abscess: a review and study of 167 cases. *Medical Journal of Malaysia*, **31**, 192–197.
63. Chen, T.S.N., Drutz, D.J. & Whelan, G.E. (1976) Hepatic granulomas in leprosy: their relation to bacteremia. *Archives of Pathology*, **100**, 182–185.
64. Cherniss, E.I. & Waisbren, B.A. (1956) North American blastomycosis: a clinical study of 40 cases. *Annals of Internal Medicine*, **44**, 105–123.
65. Clancy, M.T. & O'Brian, S. (1975) Fatal *Clostridium welchii* septicaemia following acute cholecystitis. *British Journal of Surgery*, **62**, 518–519.
66. Clein, L. (1973) Penicillin in leptospirosis. *British Medical Journal*, **iii**, 354.
67. Cleve, E.A., Gibson, J.R. & Webb, W.M. (1954) Atypical tuberculosis of the liver with jaundice. *Annals of Internal Medicine*, **41**, 251–260.
68. Cohen, A.G. & Giges, B. (1951) Punch biopsy of liver in detection of haematogenous tuberculosis. *Journal of the American Medical Association*, **146**(15), 1416–1417.
69. Cohen, F.B., Robins, B. & Lipstein, W. (1957) Isolation of *Brucella abortus* by percutaneous liver biopsy. *New England Journal of Medicine*, **257**, 228–230.
70. Cohen, H.G. & Reynolds, T.B. (1975) Comparison of metronidazole and chloroquine for the treatment of amoebic liver abscess. *Gastroenterology*, **69**, 35–41.
71. Coodley, E.L. (1967) Disseminated coccidioidomycosis: diagnosis by liver biopsy. *Gastroenterology*, **53**, 947–952.
72. Craddock, C.G. & Meredith, H.C. (1949) Punch liver biopsy in the diagnosis of miliary tuberculosis. *New England Journal of Medicine*, **241**, 527–528.
73. Craig, J.R., Hillberg, R.H. & Balchum, O.J. (1975) Disseminated coccidioidomycosis. Diagnosis by needle biopsy. *Western Journal of Medicine (San Francisco)*, **122**(2), 171–174.
74. Cronin, K. (1953) Pyogenic abscess of the liver. *Gut*, **2**, 53–59.
75. Curry, F.J. & Alcott, D. (1955) Tuberculous hepatitis with jaundice: report of 2 cases. *Gastroenterology*, **28**, 1037–1042.
76. Darke, S.G., King, A.M. & Slack, W.K. (1977) Gas gangrene and related infection: classification, clinical features and aetiology, management and mortality: a report of 88 cases. *British Journal of Surgery*, **64**, 104–112.
77. Da Silva, J.R. & De Paola, D. (1961) Hepatic lesions in American kala-azar: a needle-biopsy study. *Annals of Tropical Medicine and Parasitology*, **55**, 249–255.
78. Datta, D.V., Singh, S.A.K. & Chhuttani, P.N. (1974) Treatment of amebic liver abscess with emetine hydrochloride, niridazole and metronidazole. A controlled clinical trial. *American Journal of Tropical Medicine and Hygiene*, **23**, 586–589.
79. Davis, C.M. (1970) Granuloma inguinale. A clinical, histological and ultrastructural study. *Journal of the American Medical Association*, **211**, 632–636.
80. De Bakey, M. & Jordan, G.L. (1969) Hepatic amoebiasis. In *Diseases of the Liver* (Ed.) Schiff, L. pp. 892–909. Philadelphia: Lippincott.
81. De Brito, T., Barone, A.A. & Faria, R.M. (1969) Human liver biopsy in *P. falciparum* and *P. vivax*. A light and electron microscopy study. *Virchow's Archiv für Pathologische Anatomie und Physiologie und für Klinische Medizin*, **348**, 220–229.
82. De Brito, T., Marcondes Machado, M., Monstans, S.D., Hoshimo, S. & Freg-Müller, E. (1967) Liver biopsy in human leptospirosis: a light and electron microscopic study. *Virchow's Archives: A Pathological Anatomy and Histology*, **342**, 61–69.

83. De Brito, T., Penna, D.O., Hoshino, S., Pereira, V.G., Calder, A.C.P.G. & Rothstein, W. (1970) Cholestasis in human leptospirosis: a clinical, histochemical, biochemical and electron microscopy study based on liver biopsies. *Beiträge zur Pathologischen Anatomie und Allgemeinen Pathologie*, **140**, 345–361.
84. Deller, J.J., Cifarelli, P.S. & Berque, S. (1967) Malaria hepatitis. *Military Medicine*, **132**, 614–620.
85. Deresinski, S.C., Galgiani, J.N. & Stevens, D.A. (1977) Miconazole treatment of human coccidioidomycosis: status report. In *Coccidioidomycosis, Current Clinical and Diagnostic Status* (Ed.) Ajello, L. pp. 267–292. New York: Stratton Intercontinental Medical Book Corp.
86. Dhumeaux, D., Etévé, J., Golvan, Y.S., Hecht, Y. & Carroli, J. (1970) Difficultés diagnostiques dans un cas de Leishmaniose viscérale observé à Paris. *Revue Medico-Chirurgicale des Maladies de Foie*, **45**, 241–247.
87. Diaz-Rubio, M. & Garrachon, J. (1962) Hepatitis y leptospirosis. *Revista Clinica Espanola*, **87**, 6–18.
88. Diem, L.V., My, T.Q., Chi, N.V., Nhon, N.T. & Thuc, T.K. (1976) Typhoid fever with hepatitis. *Journal of Tropical Medicine and Hygiene*, **79**, 25–27.
89. Duncan, J.A. (1965) Abdominal actinomycosis: changed concepts. *American Journal of Surgery*, **110**, 148–152.
90. Dupont, H.L., Hornick, R.B., Levin, H.S., Rapoport, M.I. & Woodward, T.E. (1971) Q fever hepatitis. *Annals of Internal Medicine*, **74**, 198–206.
91. Dykes, P.W., Ellis, H.A. & Gourevitch, A. (1963) The Budd–Chiari syndrome in a patient with hepatic gummata. *British Journal of Surgery*, **50**, 934–937.
92. Edwards, G.A. (1959) Clinical characteristics of leptospirosis: observations based on a study of 12 sporadic cases. *American Journal of Medicine*, **27**(1), 4–17.
93. Edwards, G.A. & Domm, B.M. (1960) Human leptospirosis. *Medicine*, **39**, 117–156.
94. Edwards, G.E. & Weir, T.S. (1964) Leptospiral jaundice simulating common duct obstruction. *American Surgeon*, **30**, 619–622.
95. Eliason, E.L. (1926) Pylephlebitis and liver abscess following appendicitis. *Surgery, Gynecology and Obstetrics*, **43**, 510–522.
96. Ellinghausen, H.C., Diesch, S.L. & Top, F.H. (1972) Leptospirosis. In *Communicable and Infectious Diseases* (Ed.) Top, F.H. & Wehrle, P.F. pp. 359–371. St Louis: C.V. Mosby.
97. Elson, M.W. (1960) Antemortem radiographic demonstration of gas gangrene of the liver. *Radiology*, **74**, 57–60.
98. Erlik, D. & Reitler, R. (1960) Intrahepatic typhoid infection as cause of the carrier state. *Lancet*, **i**, 1216–1218.
99. Fährlander, H., Huber, F. & Gloor, F. (1964) Intrahepatic retention of bile in severe bacterial infections. *Gastroenterology*, **47**, 590–599.
100. Fairburn, A.C. & Semple, S.J.G. (1956) Chloramphenicol and penicillin in the treatment of leptospirosis among British troops in Malaya. *Lancet*, **i**, 13–16.
101. Fehér, J., Somogyi, T., Timmer, M. & Jozsa, L. (1975) Syphilis hepatitis: clinical, immunological and morphological aspects. *Acta Medica Academiae Scientiarum Hungaricae*, **32**, 155–161.
102. Feigin, R.D., Lobes, L.A., Anderon, D. & Pickering, L. (1973) Human leptospirosis from immunized dogs. *Annals of Internal Medicine*, **79**, 777–785.
103. Felsenfeld, O. & Wolf, R.H. (1969) Immunoglobulins and antibodies in *Borrelia turicatae* infections. *Acta Tropica (Basel)*, **26**, 156–166.
104. Finckh, E.S., Baker, S.J. & Ryan, M.M. (1953) Value of liver biopsy in the diagnosis of tuberculosis and sarcoidosis. *Medical Journal of Australia*, **2**, 369.
105. Fishbein, W.N. (1962) Jaundice as an early manifestation of scarlet fever. *Annals of Internal Medicine*, **57**, 60–72.
106. Fitzgerald, G.R., Grimes, H., Reynolds, M., Hitchcock, H. & McCarthy, C.F. (1975) Hepatitis-associated antigen-positive hepatitis in a tuberculosis unit. *Gut*, **16**, 421–428.
107. Fogel, R. & Lewis, S. (1960) Diagnosis of *Brucella melitensis* infection by percutaneous needle biopsy of the liver. *Annals of Internal Medicine*, **53**, 204–215.
108. Forbus, W.D., Schackelford, P.G., Lins, R.D. & Fey, D.K. (1946) Coccidioidomycosis: a study of 95 cases of the disseminated type with special reference to the pathogenesis of the disease. *Military Surgeon*, **99**, 633–675.
109. Foshay, L. (1940) Tularemia: a summary of certain aspects of the disease including methods for early diagnosis and the results of serum treatment in 600 patients. *Medicine*, **19**, 1–83.
110. Foster, S.C., Schneider, B. & Seaman, W.B. (1970) Gas-containing pyogenic intrahepatic abscesses. *Radiology*, **94**, 613–618.
111. Francis, E. (1928) Tularemia: a summary of present-day knowledge. *Medicine*, **7**, 411–432.
112. Francis, T.I. & Osoba, A.O. (1972) Gonococcal hepatitis (Fitz-Hugh-Curtis syndrome) in a male patient. *British Journal of Venereal Disease*, **48**, 187–188.
113. Frank, B.B. & Raffensperger, E.C. (1965) Hepatic granulomata. Report of a case with jaundice improving on antituberculous therapy and review of the literature. *Archives of Internal Medicine*, **115**, 223–234.
114. Galton, M.N. (1962) Methods in the laboratory diagnosis of leptospirosis. Laboratory diagnosis of microbial disease. *Annals of the New York Academy of Sciences*, **98**, 675–680.
115. Geistfeld, J.G. (1975) Leptospirosis in the United States, 1971–1973. *Journal of Infectious Diseases*, **131**, 743–745.
116. Georg, L.K., Robertstad, G.W., Brinkman, S.A. & Hicklin, M.D. (1965) A new pathogenic anaerobic actinomyces species. *Journal of Infectious Diseases*, **115**, 88–99.
117. Gold, J., Wigderson, A., Lehman, E. & Schwartz, I.R. (1957) Tuberculous hepatitis. Report of a case with review of the literature. *Gastroenterology*, **33**, 113–120.
118. Goldstein, F., Thornton, J. & Szydlowski, T. (1978) Biliary tract dysfunction in giardiasis. *American Journal of Digestive Diseases*, **23**, 559–560.
119. Golematis, B., Hatzitheofilou, C. & Melissas, J. (1977) Liver actinomycosis. *American Journal of Gastroenterology*, **67**, 148–150.
120. Gollan, J.L., Davidson, G.P., Anderson, K., White, T.A. & Kimber, C.L. (1972) Visceral cryptococcosis without central nervous system or pulmonary involvement: presentation as hepatitis. *Medical Journal of Australia*, **1**, 469–471.

121. Gordon, F., Cuaron, A., Munoz, J.R. & Landa, L. (1973) Scanning of the hepatic blood pool in the differential diagnosis of space-occupying lesions of the liver, with emphasis on amebic abscess. *Annals of Internal Medicine*, **78,** 247–250.

122. Greenawald, K.A., Nash, G. & Foley, F.D. (1969) Acute systemic melioidosis. Autopsy findings in four patients. *American Journal of Clinical Pathology*, **52,** 188–198.

123. Gregory, P.B. (1976) A refractory case of hepatic amoebiasis. *Gastroenterology*, **70,** 585–588.

124. Griffin, F.M. (1973) Failure of metronidazole to cure hepatic amebic abscess. *New England Journal of Medicine*, **288,** 1397.

125. Guckian, J.C. & Perry, J.E. (1966) Granulomatous hepatitis. An analysis of 63 cases and review of the literature. *Annals of Internal Medicine*, **65,** 1081–1100.

126. Guthe, T. (1975) Syphilis. In *Textbook of Medicine* (Ed.) Beeson, P.B. & McDermott, W. 14th ed., pp. 416–427. Philadelphia: W.B. Saunders.

127. Guthe, T. (1975) Relapsing fever. In *Textbook of Medicine* (Ed.) Beeson, P.B. & McDermott, W. 14th ed., pp. 434–436. Philadelphia: W.B. Saunders.

128. Gutierrez, F., Fu, Y.S. & Lurie, H.I. (1975) Cryptococcus histologically resembling histoplasmosis. A light and electron microscopical study. *Archives of Pathology*, **99,** 347–352.

129. Hahn, R.D. (1943) Syphilis of the liver. *American Journal of Syphilis, Gonorrhea and Venereal Diseases*, **27,** 529–562.

130. Haider, Z., Rasul, A. & Ahmed, I. (1975) Amoebic liver abscess presenting as obstructive jaundice: a case report. *Journal of Tropical Medicine and Hygiene*, **78,** 131–132.

131. Hall, H.E., Hightower, J.A., Rivera, R.D., Byrne, R.J., Smadel, J.E. & Woodward, T.E. (1951) Evaluation of antibiotic therapy in human leptospirosis. *Annals of Internal Medicine*, **35,** 981–998.

132. Hamilton, J.R. & Sass-Kortsak, A. (1963) Jaundice associated with severe bacterial infection in young infants. *Journal of Pediatrics*, **63,** 121–132.

133. Harris, J.R.W., McCann, V.J., Mahoney, J.D.H., Kennedy, J. & Fulton, T.T. (1974) Syphilis and chronic liver disease. *British Journal of Venereal Diseases*, **50,** 267–269.

134. Harvey, J.C., Cantrell, J. & Fisher, A.M. (1957) Actinomycosis: its recognition and treatment. *Annals of Internal Medicine*, **46,** 868–885.

135. Heath, C.W., Alexander, A.D. & Galton, M.M. (1965) Leptospirosis in the United States. Analysis of 483 cases in man, 1949–1961. *New England Journal of Medicine*, **273,** 857–864; 915–922.

136. Heineman, H.S. (1972) The clinical syndrome of malaria in the United States. *Archives of Internal Medicine*, **129,** 607–616.

137. Henn, R.M. & Collin, D.B. (1973) Amebic abscess of the liver. Treatment failure with metronidazole. *Journal of the American Medical Association*, **224,** 1394.

138. Hoeprich, P.D. (1958) Infection due to *Listeria monocytogenes*. *Medicine*, **37,** 143–160.

139. Holmes, K.K., Counts, G.W. & Beaty, H.N. (1971) Disseminated gonococcal infection. *Annals of Internal Medicine*, **74,** 979–993.

140. Hornsey, J.T., Schwarzmann, S.W. & Galambos, J.T. (1976) Shigella hepatitis. *American Journal of Gastroenterology*, **66,** 146–149.

141. Hunt, J.S., Silverstein, M.J., Sparks, F.C., Haskell, C.M., Pilch, Y.H. & Morton, D.L. (1973) Granulomatous hepatitis: a complication of BCG immunotherapy. *Lancet*, **ii,** 820–821.

142. Hutchinson, J.H., Pippard, J.S., Gleeson-White, M.H. & Sheehan, H.L. (1946) Outbreak of Weil's disease in the British army in Italy. *British Medical Journal*, **i,** 81–83.

143. Hutt, M.S.R. (1971) Some aspects of liver disease in Ugandan Africans. *Transactions of the Royal Society of Tropical Medicine and Hygiene*, **65,** 273–285.

144. Ibarra-Perez, C. & Selman-Lama, M. (1977) Diagnosis and treatment of amebic 'empyema'. *American Journal of Surgery*, **134,** 283–287.

145. Ibarra-Perez, C., Green, S.L., Calvillo-Juárez, H. & De La Cruz, J.V. (1972) Diagnosis and treatment of rupture of amebic abscess of the liver into the pericardium. *Journal of Thoracic and Cardiovascular Surgery*, **64,** 11.

146. Israel, H.L., Delamater, E., Sones, M., Willis, W.D. & Mirmelstein, A. (1952) Chronic disseminated histoplasmosis. *American Journal of Medicine*, **12,** 252–260.

147. Janssen Research Foundation Symposium (1977) New possibilities in the treatment of systemic mycosis. *Proceedings of the Royal Society of Medicine*, **70** (Suppl. 1), 1–56.

148. Jansson, E., Wegelius, R. & Visakorpi, J.K. (1972) Chronic active hepatitis and concomitant mycoplasma infection. *Lancet*, **i,** 1395.

149. Jarumilinta, R. & Maegraith, B.G. (1969) Enzymes of *Entamoeba histolytica*. *Bulletin of the World Health Organization*, **41,** 269–273.

150. Jenkinson, S.G. & Hargrove, M.D. (1975) Recurrent amebic abscess of the liver. *Journal of the American Medical Association*, **232,** 277–278.

151. Johnson, J.W., McLeod, C.G., Stookey, J.L., Higbee, G.A. & Pedersen, C.E. (1977) Lesions in guinea-pigs infected with *Coxiella burnetii* strain M-44. *Journal of Infectious Diseases*, **135**(6), 995–998.

152. Jones, J.M. & Peck, W.M. (1944) Incidence of fatty liver in tuberculosis with special reference to tuberculous enteritis. *Archives of Internal Medicine*, **74,** 371–374.

153. Joseph, W.L., Kahn, A. & Longmore, W.P (1967) Pyogenic liver abscess. Changing concepts, abstracts ed. *Program of the Society for Surgery of the Alimentary Tract Incorporated*, June 1967.

154. Joske, R.A. & Finckh, E.S. (1955) hepatic changes in human brucellosis. *Medical Journal of Australasia*, **1,** 266–269.

155. Judge, D.M., La Croix, J.T. & Perine, P.L. (1974) Experimental louse-borne relapsing fever in the grivet monkey, *Cercopithecus aethiops*. II. Pathology. *American Journal of Tropical Medicine and Hygiene*, **23**(5), 962–968.

156. Judge, D.M., Samuel, I., Perine, L. & Vukotic, D. (1974) Louse-borne relapsing fever in man. *Archives of Pathology*, **97,** 136–140.

157. Juniper, K. (1978) Amoebiasis. *Clinics in Gastroenterology*, **7,** 3–29.

158. Kahan, M.G. & Tilney, N.L. (1972) Hepatic abscess produced by extension of a perinephric abscess. *American Journal of Surgery*, **124,** 687–689.

159. Kapoor, O.P. & Shah, N.A. (1972) Pericardial amoebiasis following amoebic liver abscess of the left lobe. *Journal of Tropical Medicine and Hygiene*, **75,** 7–10.

160. Karat, A.B.A., Job, C.K. & Rao, P.S.S. (1971) Liver in leprosy: histological and biochemical findings. *British Medical Journal*, **i**, 307–310.
161. Karmi, G., Thirkettle, J.L. & Read, A.E.A. (1969) The association of syphilis with hepatic cirrhosis: a report of six cases and a review of the literature. *Postgraduate Medical Journal*, **45**, 675–679.
162. Karran, S.J., Leach, K.G., Wisbey, M.L. & Blumgart, L.H. (1975) Uptake of colloid in rat liver following intravenous, intrasplenic and intramesenteric injection. *Journal of Nuclear Medicine*, **5**, 377–379.
163. Kimble, M.W. & Knee, S. (1970) Gonococcal perihepatitis in a male. The Fitz-Hugh-Curtis syndrome. *New England Journal of Medicine*, **282**, 1082–1084.
164. King, A. & Nicol, C. (1969) Congenital syphilis. In *Venereal Disease*. pp. 75–94. London: Baillière, Tindall and Cassell.
165. Kinney, T.D. & Ferrebee, J.W. (1948) Hepatic abscess. Factors determining its localization. *Archives of Pathology*, **45**, 41–47.
166. Klatskin, G. (1975) Hepatitis associated with systemic disease. In *Diseases of the Liver* (Ed.) Schiff, L. pp. 711–744. Philadelphia: Lippincott.
167. Klatskin, G. & Yesner, R. (1950) Hepatic manifestations of sarcoidosis and other granulomatous diseases. A study based on histological examination of tissue obtained by needle biopsy of the liver. *Yale Journal of Biology and Medicine*, **23**, 207–248.
168. Knight, R. (1978) Giardiasis, isosporiasis and balantidiasis. *Clinics in Gastroenterology*, **7**, 31–47.
169. Knox, J.H.N. & Schorer, E.H. (1910) A bacteriological and clinical study of a series of 74 cases of diarrhoea in children. *Johns Hopkins Hospital Report*, **14**, 1–54.
170. Kocen, R.S. (1962) Leptospirosis. A comparison of symptomatic and penicillin therapy. *British Medical Journal*, **i**, 1181–1183.
171. Kohen, M.D. & Altman, K.A. (1973) Jaundice due to a rare cause: tuberculous lymphadenitis. *American Journal of Gastroenterology*, **59**, 48–53.
172. Korn, R.J., Kellow, W.F., Hellar, P., Chomet, B. & Zimmerman, H.J. (1959) Hepatic involvement in extrapulmonary tuberculosis. *American Journal of Medicine*, **27**, 60–71.
173. Kotin, P. & Butt, F.N. (1951) Streptococcal hepatitis. *Archives of Pathology*, **52**, 288–292.
174. Kreel, L. (1972) *Angiography in the Diagnosis of Gastrointestinal Disease* (Ed.) Badenoch, J. 2nd ed., pp. 54–80. Edinburgh: Churchill-Livingstone.
175. Krogstad, D.J., Spencer, H.C. & Healy, G.R. (1978) Current concepts in parasitology. Amebiasis. *New England Journal of Medicine*, **298**, 262–265.
176. Krupp, I.M. (1974) Comparison of counterimmunoelectrophoresis with other serologic tests in the diagnosis of amebiasis. *American Journal of Tropical Medicine and Hygiene*, **23**, 27–30.
177. *Lancet* (1975) Amyloidosis and leprosy (Editorial). *Lancet*, **ii**, 589.
178. *Lancet* (1976) Pyogenic liver abscess – a continuing problem of management (Editorial). *Lancet*, **i**, 1170–1171.
179. Lanza, F.L., Nelson, R.S. & Somayaji, B.N. (1970) Acute granulomatous hepatitis due to histoplasmosis. *Gastroenterology*, **58**, 392–396.
180. Lawson, J.H. (1973) Penicillin in leptospirosis. *British Medical Journal*, **iv**, 109.
181. Lawson, T.L. (1977) Hepatic abscess – ultrasound as an aid to diagnosis. *American Journal of Digestive Diseases*, **22**, 33–37.
182. Leader, S.A. (1951) Tuberculosis of the liver and gallbladder with abscess formation: a review and case reports. *Annals of Internal Medicine*, **37**, 594–606.
183. Lee, R., Thornton, G.F. & Conn, H.Q. (1971) Liver disease associated with secondary syphilis. *New England Journal of Medicine*, **284**, 1423–1425.
184. Lefton, H.B., Farmer, R.G., Buchwald, R. & Haselby, R. (1974) Cryptococcal hepatitis mimicking primary sclerosing cholangitis. *Gastroenterology*, **67**, 511–515.
185. Lesesne, H.R., Holt, W. & Orringer, E. (1976) Is hepatic abscess a contraindication to percutaneous liver biopsy? *Gastroenterology*, **70**, 297–298.
186. Levine, D.P. & Lerner, A.M. (1978) The clinical spectrum of *Mycoplasma pneumoniae* infection. In *Symposium on Infectious Diseases* (Ed.) McHenry, N.C. & Lerner, P.I. pp. 961–978. Philadelphia: W.B. Saunders.
187. Lewis, J.L. & Rabinovich, S. (1972) The wide spectrum of cryptococcal infections. *American Journal of Medicine*, **53**, 315–321.
188. Lightfoot, R.W. & Gotschlich, E. (1974) Gonococcal disease. *American Journal of Medicine*, **56**, 347–356.
189. Littman, M.L. (1959) Cryptococcosis (torulosis), current concepts and therapy. *American Journal of Medicine*, **27**, 976–998.
190. Lloyd Hart, V. (1944) A case of Weil's disease treated with penicillin. *British Medical Journal*, **ii**, 720.
191. Londero, A.T. & Ramos, C.D. (1972) Paracoccidioidomycosis. A clinical and mycologic study of forty-one cases observed in Santa Maria, RS, Brazil. *American Journal of Medicine*, **52**, 771–775.
192. Longmore, W.P. Jr, Passaro, E.P. Jr & Joseph, W.I. (1966) The surgical treatment of hepatic lesions. *British Journal of Surgery*, **53**, 852–859.
193. Louria, D.B., Stiff, D.P. & Bennett, B. (1962) Disseminated moniliasis in the adult. *Medicine*, **41**, 307–337.
194. Lundberg, Y. (1976) A comparison of angiography and scintigraphy: a diagnostic method for amebic liver abscess. *Scandinavian Journal of Infectious Diseases*, **8**, 263–265.
195. Lyford, J., Johnson, R.W., Blackman, S. & Scott, R.B. (1946) Pathologic findings in a fatal case of disseminated granuloma inguinale with miliary bone and joint involvement. *Bulletin of the Johns Hopkins Hospital*, **79**, 349–357.
196. MacMahon, H.E. & Mallory, F.B. (1931) Streptococcus hepatitis. *American Journal of Pathology*, **7**, 299–325.
197. Maddison, S.E. (1965) Characterization of *Entamoeba histolytica* antigen-antibody reaction by gel diffusion. *Experimental Parasitology*, **16**, 224.
198. Malek, R.S., Greene, L.F., Deweerd, J.H. & Farrow, G.M. (1972) Xanthogranulomatous pyelonephritis. *British Journal of Urology*, **44**, 296–308.
199. Mardh, P.A., Skude, G. & Akerman, M. (1974) *Mycoplasma pneumoniae* infection – a cause of acute pancreatitis and non-specific reactive hepatitis in man and experimentally infected animals. In *Les mycoplasmes de l'homme, des vegetaux et des insectes* (Ed.) Bove, J.M. & Duplan, J.K. pp. 403–410. Paris: Inserm.
200. Martelo, O.J., Smoller, M. & Saladin, T.A. (1969) Malaria in American soldiers. *Archives of Internal Medicine*, **123**, 383–387.

201. Martin, D.S. & Smith, D.T. (1939) Blastomycosis (American blastomycosis, Gilchrist's disease): report of 13 new cases. *American Review of Tuberculosis*, **39,** 488–515.
202. Martinez-Vazquez, J.M., Guardia, J. & Pattiss, A. (1975) Granulomatous hepatitis in acquired toxoplasmosis in adults. *Semaine des Hôpitaux de Paris*, **51,** 963–965.
203. Mather, G., Dawson, J. & Hoyle, C. (1955) Liver biopsy in sarcoidosis. *Quarterly Journal of Medicine*, **24,** 331–350.
204. Matthews, A.W., Gough, K.R., Davies, E.R., Ross, F.G.M. & Hinchliffe, A. (1973) The use of combined ultrasonic and isotope scanning in the diagnosis of amoebic liver disease. *Gut*, **14,** 50–53.
205. McBride, R.A., Corson, J.M. & Dammin, G.J. (1960) Mucormycosis. Two cases of disseminated disease with cultural identification of *Rhizopus*; review of literature. *American Journal of Medicine*, **28,** 832–846.
206. McCullough, N.B. & Eisele, C.W. (1915) Brucella hepatitis leading to cirrhosis of the liver. *Archives of Internal Medicine*, **88,** 793–802.
207. McFadzean, A.J.S. & Ong, G.B. (1966) Intrahepatic typhoid carriers. *British Medical Journal*, **i,** 1567–1571.
208. McFadzean, A.J., Chang, K.P. & Wong, C.C. (1953) Solitary pyogenic abscess of the liver treated by closed aspiration and antibiotics. *British Journal of Surgery*, **41,** 141–152.
209. McHenry, M.C. & Ficker, D.O. (1978) Newer antibacterial and antimycotic drugs. Clinical appraisal. In *Symposium on Infectious Disease, The Medical Clinics of North America* (Ed.) McHenry, M.C. & Lerner, P.I. pp. 873–897. Philadelphia: W.B. Saunders.
210. McIntosh, J. (1909) The occurrence and distribution of *Spirochaeta pallida* in congenital syphilis. *Journal of Pathology and Bacteriology*, **13,** 239–245.
211. McKiel, J.A., Rappay, D.E. & Cousineau, J.G. (1970) Domestic rats as carriers of leptospires and salmonellae in eastern Canada. *Canadian Journal of Public Health*, **61,** 336–340.
212. McLain, L.G., Decker, M., Nye, D., Mehta, S. & London, R. (1978) Gonococcal perihepatitis. *Journal of the American Medical Association*, **239,** 339–341.
213. Meals, R.A. (1976) Paratyphoid fever. *Archives of Internal Medicine*, **136,** 1422–1428.
214. Meyer, R.D., Rosen, P. & Armstrong, D. (1972) Phycomycosis complicating leukemia and lymphoma. *Annals of Internal Medicine*, **77,** 871–879.
215. Mitchell, R., Grist, N.R., Bazaz, G. & Kenmuir, A.C. (1966) Pathological, rickettsiological and immunofluorescence studies of a case of Q fever endocarditis. *Journal of Pathology and Bacteriology*, **91,** 317–323.
216. Morris, E. (1930) Tuberculosis of the liver. *American Review of Tuberculosis*, **22,** 585; 592.
217. Morris, M.N., Powell, S.J. & Elsdon-Dew, R. (1970) Latex agglutination test for invasive amoebiasis. *Lancet*, **i,** 1362.
218. Morton, J.R., Roys, G.D. & Bricker, D.L. (1972) The treatment of liver injuries. *Surgery, Gynecology and Obstetrics*, **134,** 298–302.
219. Mufson, M.A., Manko, M.A., Kingston, J.R. & Chanak, R.M. (1961) Eaton agent pneumonia. Clinical features. *Journal of the American Medical Association*, **178,** 369–374.
220. Murray, H.W., Littman, M.L. & Roberts, R.B. (1974) Disseminated paracoccidioidomycosis (South American blastomycosis) in the United States. *American Journal of Medicine*, **56,** 209–220.
221. Murray, J.F., Finegold, S.M., Froman, S. & Will, D.W. (1961) The changing spectrum of nocardiosis. A review and presentation of nine cases. *American Review of Respiratory Diseases*, **83,** 315–330.
222. Nagarty, H.F., Hedayati, E. & Assassi, B. (1975) Liver abscess due to an ascaral in Iran. *American Journal of Tropical Medicine and Hygiene*, **24,** 371–372.
223. Naidoo, P.M., Keeton, G., Stein, L., Kottler, R. & Horwitz, M. (1974) Hepatic amoebiasis. A study of 32 cases in the Western Cape. *South African Medical Journal*, **48,** 1159–1160.
224. Neal, R.A. (1971) Pathogenesis of amebiasis. *Bulletin of the New York Academy of Medicine*, **5,** 462–468.
225. Noyy, S.B., Wallace, S., Goldman, A. & Ben-Menauchem, Y. (1974) Pyogenic liver abscess. Angiographic diagnosis and treatment by closed aspiration. *American Journal of Roentgenology, Radiotherapy and Nuclear Medicine*, **121,** 388–395.
226. Nushan, H. & Bailey, A.A. (1953) Acute hepatitis due to brucellosis. *Annals of Internal Medicine*, **39,** 915–919.
227. Ochsner, A., De Bakey, M. & Murray, S. (1938) Pyogenic abscess of the liver. An analysis of 47 cases with review of the literature. *American Journal of Surgery*, **40,** 292–319.
228. Ogden, W.W., Hunter, P.R. & Rivers, J.D. (1961) Liver abscess. *Postgraduate Medicine*, **30,** 11–19.
229. Okudaira, M., Straub, M. & Schwarz, J. (1961) The etiology of discrete splenic and hepatic calcifications in an endemic area of histoplasmosis. *American Journal of Pathology*, **39,** 599–607.
230. Ortiz-Ortiz, L., Zamacona, G., Sepulveda, B. & Capin, N.R. (1975) Cell-mediated immunity in patients with amebic abscess of the liver. *Clinical Immunology and Immunopathology*, **4,** 127–134.
231. Palit, A. & Gulasekharam, J. (1973) Genus-specific leptospiral antigen and its possible use in laboratory diagnosis. *Journal of Clinical Pathology*, **26,** 7–16.
232. Palmer, E.D. (1975) The changing manifestations of pyogenic liver abscess. *Journal of the American Medical Association*, **231,** 192.
233. Papaevangelou, G., Trichopoulous, D., Papoutsakis, G., Kremastinou, T. & Paulides, E. (1974) Hepatitis B antigen in prostitutes. *British Journal of Venereal Diseases*, **50,** 228–231.
234. Parelkar, S.N., Stamm, W.P. & Hill, K.R. (1971) Indirect immunofluorescent staining of *E. histolytica* in tissues. *Lancet*, **i,** 212.
235. Parker, J.C., McCloskey, J.J. & Knauer, K.A. (1976) Pathobiologic features of human candidiasis. A common deep mycosis of the brain, heart and kidney in the altered host. *American Journal of Clinical Pathology*, **65,** 991–1000.
236. Parker, J.D.J. (1972) Uncommon complications of early syphilis, hepatitis, periostitis, iritis with papillitis and meningitis. *British Journal of Venereal Diseases*, **48,** 32–36.
237. Partridge, B.M. & Tanser, A.R. (1966) Disseminated histoplasmosis and its treatment. *Postgraduate Medical Journal*, **42,** 568–572.
238. Patterson, H.C. (1970) Open aspiration for solitary abscess of the liver. *American Journal of Surgery*, **119,** 326–329.

239. Phillips, B.P., Wolfe, P.A. & Rees, C.W. (1955) Studies on the ameba-bacteria relationship in amebiasis: comparative results of the intracecal inoculation of germfree, monocontaminated and conventional guinea pigs with *Entamoeba histolytica*. *American Journal of Tropical and Medical Hygiene*, **4**, 675–692.
240. Piccone, V.A. (1968) In discussion of pyogenic liver abscess. Changing patterns in approach. *American Journal of Surgery*, **115**, 63–68.
241. Piccone, V.A., Ferrante, J. & Leveen, H.H. (1968) Angial retrograde hepatography versus direct transumbilical hepatography. A comparison of two new methods. *American Journal of Surgery*, **115**, 17–21.
242. Pieron, R. (1977) Miliary abscess of the liver during septicaemia caused by staphylococcus. Peritoneoscopic diagnosis. *Semaine des Hôpitaux de Paris*, **53**, 383–388.
243. Pine, L. & Georg, L. (1965) The classification and phylogenetic relationships of the actinomycetales. *International Bulletin of Bacterial Nomenclature and Taxonomy*, **15**, 143–163.
244. Pinkerton, H. & Iverson, L. (1952) Histoplasmosis: three fatal cases with disseminated sarcoid-like lesions. *Archives of Internal Medicine*, **90**, 456–467.
245. Pitt, H.A. & Ziudema, G.D. (1975) Factors influencing mortality in the treatment of pyogenic hepatic abscess. *Surgery, Gynecology and Obstetrics*, **140**, 228–234.
246. Popper, H. & Schaffner, F. (1957) In *Liver; Structure and Function*, 1 (Ed.) Popper, H. and Schaffner, F. pp. 651–681. New York: McGraw-Hill.
247. Powell, C.S. & Swan, L.L. (1955) Leprosy: pathologic changes observed in fifty consecutive necropsies. *American Journal of Pathology*, **31**, 1131–1147.
248. Powell, O.W. (1961) Liver involvement in Q fever. *Australasian Annals of Medicine*, **10**, 52–58.
249. Powell, S.J. & Neame, P.B. (1960) A case of amoebic brain abscess. *British Medical Journal*, **ii**, 1136–1137.
250. Powell, S.J., Sutton, J.B. & Lautre, G. (1973) Haemobilia in amoebic liver abscess. *South African Medical Journal*, **47**, 1555–1557.
251. Powell, S.J., Wilmot, A.J. & Elsdon-Dew, R. (1959) Hepatic amoebiasis. *Transactions of the Royal Society of Tropical Medicine and Hygiene*, **53**, 190–195.
252. Powell, S.J., Macleod, I., Wilmot, A.J. & Elsdon-Dew, R. (1966) Metronidazole in amoebic dysentery and amoebic liver abscess. *Lancet*, **ii**, 1329–1331.
253. Price, J.E., Joseph, W.L. & Mulder, D.G. (1967) Diagnosis and treatment of intrahepatic abscess. *Annals of Tropical Medicine and Parasitology*, **63**, 139–142.
254. Procknow, J.J., Benfield, J.R., Rippon, J.W., Diener, C.F. & Archer, F.L. (1965) Cryptococcal hepatitis presenting as a surgical emergency. First isolation of *Cryptococcus neoformans* from point source in Chicago. *Journal of the American Medical Association*, **191**, 269–274.
255. Prystowsky, S.D., Vogelstein, B., Ettinger, D.S., Merz, W.G., Kaizer, H., Sulica, V.I. & Zinkham, W.H. (1976) Invasive aspergillosis. *New England Journal of Medicine*, **295**, 655–658.
256. Pullen, R.L. & Stuart, B.M. (1945) Tularemia. Analysis of 225 cases. *Journal of the American Medical Association*, **129**, 495–500.
257. Putman, H.C., Dockerty, M.B. & Waugh, J.M. (1950) Abdominal actinomycosis; analysis of 122 cases. *Surgery*, **28**, 781–800.
258. Pyrtek, L.J. & Bartus, S.A. (1965) Hepatic pyemia. *New England Journal of Medicine*, **272**, 351–354.
259. Radford, A.J., Rhodes, F.A. & Matz, L.R. (1967) The association of jaundice with lobar pneumonia in the territory of Papua and New Guinea. *Medical Journal of Australia*, **2**, 678–681.
260. Rajam, R.V. & Rangiah, P.N. (1954) Early syphilitic hepatitis. *Indian Journal of Venereal Disease*, **20**, 83–94.
261. Ramachandran, S. & Perera, M.V.F. (1976) Jaundice and hepatomegaly in primary malaria. *Journal of Tropical Medicine and Hygiene*, **79**, 207–210.
262. Ramachandran, S., Godfrey, J.J. & Perera, V.F. (1974) Typhoid hepatitis. *Journal of the American Medical Association*, **230**, 236–240.
263. Ramachandran, S., Goonatillake, H.D. & Induruwa, P.A.C. (1976) Syndromes in amoebic liver abscess. *British Journal of Surgery*, **63**, 220–225.
264. Ramachandran, S., Pakianathian, V. & Aiyathurai, J.E.J. (1976) Severe obstructive jaundice due to amoebic liver abscess. *Medical Journal of Australia*, **1**, 925.
265. Rambo, W.M. & Black, H.C. (1969) Intrahepatic abscess. *American Surgeon*, **35**, 144–148.
266. Rasaretnam, R. & Wijetilaka, S.E. (1976) Left lobe amoebic liver abscess. *Postgraduate Medical Journal*, **52**, 269–274.
267. Ray, C.J. & Wedgewood, R.J. (1964) Neonatal listeriosis: six case reports and a review of the literature. *Pediatrics*, **34**, 378–392.
268. Recknagel, R.D. (1967) Carbon tetrachloride hepatotoxicity. *Pharmacological Review*, **19**, 145–208.
269. Reichert, J.A. & Valle, R.F. (1976) Fitz-Hugh-Curtis syndrome. A laparoscopic approach. *Journal of the American Medical Association*, **236**, 266–268.
270. Reid, T.M.S. & Davidson, A.I. (1976) *Streptococcus milleri* liver abscess. *Lancet*, **i**, 648–649.
271. Reinhard, K.R. (1963) Leptospirosis. In *Diseases Transmitted from Animals to Man* (Ed.) Hull, T. 5th ed., pp. 624–651. Springfield: C.C. Thomas.
272. Restrepo, A., Robledo, M., Gutiérrez, F., Sanclemente, M., Castañeda, E. & Calle, G. (1970) Paracoccidioidomycosis (South American blastomycosis). A study of 39 cases observed in Medellín, Colombia. *American Journal of Tropical Medicine and Hygiene*, **19**, 68–76.
273. Restrepo, A., Robledo, M., Giraldo, R., Hernández, H., Sierra, F., Gutierrez, F., Londoño, F., Lopez, R. & Calle, G. (1976) The gamut of paracoccidioidomycosis. *American Journal of Medicine*, **61**, 33–42.
274. Reynolds, T.B. (1971) Amoebic abscess of the liver. *Gastroenterology*, **60**, 952–954.
275. Robertson, K. (1946) Weil's disease: a rare condition? *British Medical Journal*, **ii**, 810–813.
276. Robertson, R.D., Foster, J.H. & Peterson, C.G. (1966) Pyogenic liver abscess studied by cholangiography. Case report and 25 year review. *American Surgeon*, **32**, 521–530.
277. Rooney, J.C., Hill, D.J. & Danks, D.M. (1971) Jaundice associated with bacterial infection in the newborn. *American Journal of Diseases of Children*, **122**, 39–41.

278. Rosen, S., Roycroft, D., Hano, M.J. & Barry, K.G. (1967) The liver in malaria. Electron microscopic observations on a hepatic biopsy obtained 15 minutes post-mortem. *Archives of Pathology*, **83,** 271–278.

279. Rosenberg, B.L. (1951) Canicola fever. Review, with report of two new cases. *American Journal of Medicine*, **11,** 75–91.

280. Rosenkranz, K. & Howard, L.D. (1936) Tubular tuberculosis of the liver. *Archives of Pathology*, **22,** 743–754.

281. Rothenberg, R.E. & Linder, W. (1964) The single pyogenic liver abscess. *Surgery, Gynecology and Obstetrics*, **59,** 31–40.

282. Rubin, R.H., Swartz, I. & Malt, R. (1974) Hepatic abscess: changes in clinical, bacteriological and therapeutic aspects: *American Journal of Medicine*, **57,** 601–607.

283. Sabbaj, J., Sutter, V.L. & Finegold, S.M. (1972) Anaerobic pyogenic liver abscess. *Annals of Internal Medicine*, **77,** 629–638.

284. Sabesin, S.M., Fallon, H.J. & Andride, V.T. (1963) Hepatic failure as a manifestation of cryptococcosis. *Archives of Internal Medicine*, **111,** 661–669.

285. Saltzman, D.A., Smithline, N. & Davis, J.R. (1978) Fulminant hepatic failure secondary to amebic abscess. *American Journal of Digestive Diseases*, **23,** 561–567.

286. Salzano, F.M. & Blumberg, B.S. (1970) The Australia antigen in Brazilian healthy persons and in leprosy and leukaemia patients. *Journal of Clinical Pathology*, **23,** 39–42.

287. Sandborn, E.B., Côté, M.G. & Viallet, A. (1966) Electron microscopy of a human liver in Weil's disease (*Leptospirosis icterohaemorrhagica*). *Journal of Pathological Bacteriology*, **92,** 369–374.

288. Sarasin, G., Tucker, D.N. & Arean, V.M. (1963) Accidental laboratory infection caused by *Leptospira icterohaemorrhagiae*. Report of a case. *American Journal of Clinical Pathology*, **40** (2), 146–150.

289. Sarkany, I. (1973) Pruritus and cholestatic jaundice due to secondary syphilis. *Proceedings of the Royal Society of Medicine*, **66,** 236–237.

290. Sarosi, G.A., Voth, D.W., Dahl, B.A., Doto, I.L. & Tosh, F.E. (1971) Disseminated histoplasmosis: results of long-term follow-up. A Center for Disease Control Co-operative Mycoses Study. *Annals of Internal Medicine*, **75,** 511–516.

291. Savanat, T., Viriyanond, P. & Nimitmongkol, N. (1973) Blast transformation of lymphocytes in amebiasis. *American Journal of Tropical Medicine and Hygiene*, **22,** 705–710.

292. Scheuer, P.J. (1972) In *Liver Biopsy Interpretation*. pp. 136–137. London: Baillière Tindall.

293. Schmidt, A.G. (1969) Plain film roentgen diagnosis of amebic hepatic abscess. *American Journal of Roentgenology*, **107,** 47–50.

294. Schraibman, I.G. (1974) Non-parasitic liver abscess. *British Journal of Surgery*, **61,** 709–712.

295. Schwartz, S.I. (1964). In *Surgical Diseases of the Liver*. New York: McGraw-Hill.

296. Sehgal, V.N., Tyagi, S.P. & Kumar, S. (1972) Microscopic pathology of the liver in leprosy patients. *Internal Journal of Dermatology*, **11,** 168–172.

297. Seife, M., Kessler, B.J., Hoffman, J. & Lisa, J.R. (1951) A clinical, functional and needle biopsy study of the liver in pulmonary tuberculosis. *American Review of Tuberculosis*, **63,** 202–206.

298. Sen Gupta, P.C., Chakravarty, N.K., Ray, H.N. & Das Gupta, B. (1956) The liver in kala-azar. *Annals of Tropical Medicine and Parasitology*, **50,** 252–259.

299. Serege, H.; quoted by Kinney, T.D. & Ferrebee, J.W. (1948) Hepatic abscess. Factors determining its location. *Archives of Pathology*, **45,** 41–47.

300. Sewell, J. & Ahmed, M.A. (1975) Secondary syphilis and hepatitis. *British Medical Journal*, **iii,** 42.

301. Shabot, J.M. & Patterson, M. (1978) Amebic liver abscess: 1966–1976. *Digestive Diseases*, **23,** 110–118.

302. Sherman, J.D. & Robbins, S.L. (1960) Changing trends in the casuistics of hepatic abscess. *American Journal of Medicine*, **28,** 943–950.

303. Shields, L.H. (1959) Disseminated cryptococcosis producing a sarcoid type reaction. The report of a case treated with Amphotericin B. *Archives of Internal Medicine*, **104,** 763–770.

304. Silverman, F.N., Schwarz, J., Lahey, M.E. & Carson, R.P. (1955) Histoplasmosis. *American Journal of Medicine*, **19,** 410–459.

305. Simpson, B., Cook, A.T., Dimond, A.H., Brown, M. & Thin, R.N.T. (1967) Renal function after leptospirosis. *British Medical Journal*, **iii,** 472–474.

306. Sitprija, V. & Chusilp, S. (1973) Renal failure and hyperbilirubinaemia in leptospirosis treatment with exchange transfusion. *Medical Journal of Australia*, **1,** 171–173.

307. Skinner, D. & Keefer, C.S. (1941) Significance of bacteremia caused by *Staphylococcus aureus*. A study of 122 cases and a review of the literature concerned with experimental infection in animals. *Archives of Internal Medicine*, **68,** 851–875.

308. Smith, J. (1949) Weil's disease in the northeast of Scotland. *British Journal of Industrial Medicine*, **6,** 213–220.

309. Smith, J.W. & Utz, J.P. (1972) Progressive disseminated histoplasmosis. A prospective study of 26 patients. *Annals of Internal Medicine*, **76,** 557–565.

310. Smucker, E.E., Reid, S.E. & Harding, H.B. (1960) Spontaneous fatal gas gangrene septicaemia. *Journal of the American Medical Association*, **174,** 898–900.

311. Sobel, H.J., Wolf, E.H. & Passaic, N.J. (1972) Liver involvement in early syphilis. *Archives of Pathology*, **93,** 565–568.

312. Sood, V.K. & Grueber, H.L. (1969) Correlation of histopathologic changes in the liver and bone marrow of leprosy patients. *International Journal of Leprosy*, **37,** 28–39.

313. Soto, J.M. & Dreiling, D.A. (1977) *Giardia lamblia*. A case presentation of chronic cholecystitis and duodenitis. *American Journal of Gastroenterology*, **67,** 265–269.

314. Southern, P.M. & Sanford, J.P. (1969) Relapsing fever. A clinical and microbiological review. *Medicine*, **48,** 129–149.

315. Sparberg, M., Gottschalk, A. & Kirsner, J.B. (1970) Liver abscess complicating regional enteritis. Report of two cases. *Gastroenterology*, **59,** 548–551.

316. Spink, W.W. (1957) Suppuration and calcification of the liver and spleen due to longstanding infection with *Brucella suis*. *New England Journal of Medicine*, **257,** 209–210.

317. Spink, W.W. (1964) Host-parasite relationship in human brucellosis with prolonged illness due to suppuration of the liver and spleen. *American Journal of the Medical Sciences*, **247**, 129–136.
318. Stamm, W.P., Ashley, M.J. & Parelkar, S.N. (1973) Evaluation of a latex agglutination test for amoebiasis. *Transactions of the Royal Society of Tropical Medicine and Hygiene*, **67**, 211–213.
319. Steiner, W.R. & Walton, L.C. (1938) Gonorrhoeal endocarditis with bilateral parotitis and toxic jaundice as additional complications. *Annals of Internal Medicine*, **11**, 1464–1471.
320. Stern, M.S. & Gitnick, G.L. (1976) Shigella hepatitis. *Journal of the American Medical Association*, **235**, 2628.
321. Stewart, C. & Jackson, L. (1976) Spleno-hepatic tuberculosis due to *Myobacterium kansasii*. *Medical Journal of Australia*, **2**, 99–101.
322. Stokes, J.F. (1960) Cryptogenic liver abscess. *Lancet*, **i**, 355–358.
323. Stuiver, P.C. & Goud, T.J.L.M. (1978) Corticosteroids and liver amoebiasis. *British Medical Journal*, **ii**, 394–395.
324. Symmers, D. & Spain, D. (1946) Hepar lobatum – clinical significance of the anatomic changes. *Archives of Pathology*, **42**, 64–68.
325. Symmers, W.H.C. (1962) Histopathologic aspects of the pathogens of some opportunistic fungal infections, as exemplified in the pathology of aspergillosis and the phycomycetoses. *Laboratory Investigation*, **11**, 1073–1090.
326. Teixeira, F., Gayotto, L.C. & De Brito, T. (1978) Morphological patterns of the liver in South American blastomycosis. *Histopathology*, **2**, 231–237.
327. Terry, R.B. & Gunnar, R.M. (1957) Primary miliary tuberculosis of the liver. *Journal of the American Medical Association*, **164**, 150–157.
328. Theron, J.J., Pepler, W.J. & Mekel, R.C.P.M. (1972) Ultrastructure of the liver in Bantu patients with pneumonia and jaundice. *Journal of Pathology*, **106**, 113–122.
329. Tin Shwe & Zuckerman, A.J. (1972) Australia antigen and antibody in British patients with leprosy. *Journal of Clinical Pathology*, **25**, 401–402.
330. Tong, M.J., Rosenberg, E.B., Votteri, B.A. & Che-Chung, T. (1971) Immunological response in leptospirosis. Report of three cases. *American Journal of Tropical Medicine and Hygiene*, **20**(4), 625–630.
331. Tongue, J.I. & Derrick, E.H. (1959) A fatal case of Q fever associated with hepatic necrosis. *Medical Journal of Australia*, **46**, 1(18), 594–597.
332. Triger, D.R. (1978) Amoebic liver abscess in Wessex – a retrospective survey of 24 cases. *Journal of Tropical Medicine and Hygiene*, **81**, 54–59.
333. Trimble, A.P. (1957) Clinical aspects of leptospirosis in Malaya. *Proceedings of the Royal Society of Medicine*, **50**, 125–128.
334. Trimble, C. (1970) Gonococcal perhepatitis simulating acute cholecystitis. *Surgery, Gynecology and Obstetrics*, **130**, 54–56.
335. Tugwell, P. (1973) Glucose-6-phosphate dehydrogenase deficiency in Nigerians with jaundice associated with lobar pneumonia. *Lancet*, **i**, 968–970.
336. Tugwell, P. & Williams, A.O. (1977) Jaundice associated with lobar pneumonia. *Quarterly Journal of Medicine*, **46**, 97–118.
337. Turck, W.P.G., Howitt, G., Turnberg, L.A., Fox, H., Longson, M., Matthews, M.B. & Das Gupta, R. (1976) Chronic Q fever. *Quarterly Journal of Medicine*, **45**, 193–217.
338. Turner, F.P. (1964) Fatal *Clostridium welchii* septicaemia following cholecystectomy. *American Journal of Surgery*, **108**, 3–7.
339. Turner, L.H. (1968) Leptospirosis. II. Serology. *Transactions of the Royal Society of Tropical Medicine and Hygiene*, **62**, 880–889.
340. Turner, L.H. (1969) Leptospirosis. *British Medical Journal*, **i**, 231–235.
341. Turner, L.H. (1973) Leptospirosis. *British Medical Journal*, **i**, 537–540.
342. Turner, T.B., Hardy, P.H. & Newman, B. (1969) Infectivity tests in syphilis. *British Journal of Venereal Diseases*, **45**, 183–196.
343. Turrill, F.L. & Burnham, J.R. (1966) Hepatic amebiasis. *American Journal of Surgery*, **111**, 424–430.
344. Ullom, J.T. (1909) The liver in tuberculosis. *American Journal of the Medical Sciences*, **137**, 694–702.
345. Urso, F.P. (1975) The pathologic findings in rickettsial pneumonia. *American Journal of Clinical Pathology*, **64**, 335–342.
346. Vaněk, J. & Schwarz, J. (1971) The gamut of histoplasmosis. *American Journal of Medicine*, **50**, 89–104.
347. Vethanyagam, A. & Bryceson, A.D.M. (1976) Acquired toxoplasmosis presenting as hepatitis. *Transactions of the Royal Society of Tropical Medicine and Hygiene*, **70**, 524–525.
348. Vicary, F.R., Cusick, G., Shirley, I.M. & Blackwell, R.J. (1977) Ultrasound and amoebic liver abscess. *British Journal of Surgery*, **64**, 113–114.
349. Vickers, F.N. & Maloney, P.J. (1964) Gonococcal perihepatitis. *Archives of Internal Medicine*, **114**, 120–123.
350. Vischer, T.L., Bernheim, C. & Engelbrecht, F. (1967) Two cases of hepatitis due to *Toxoplasma gondii*. *Lancet*, **ii**, 919–921.
351. Ward, J.R. & Hunter, R.C. (1958) Disseminated coccidioidomycosis demonstrated by needle biopsy of the liver. *Annals of Internal Medicine*, **48**, 157–162.
352. Warren, K.W. & Hardy, K.J. (1968) Pyogenic hepatic abscess. *Archives of Surgery*, **97**, 40–45.
353. Wegner, F. (1967) Abcesso hepatico producido por le *Balantidium coli*. *Kasmera*, **2**, 433–441.
354. Weil, A. (1886) Uber eine eigentumliche mit Mitztumour, Icterus und Nephritis ernhergehende, akute infektionkheit. *Deutsches Archiv für Klinische Medizin*, **39**, 209–232.
355. Weinbren, K. (1975) Diseases of the liver. In *Recent Advances in Pathology* (Ed.) Harrison, C.V. & Weinbren, K. pp. 120–121. Edinburgh, London and New York: Churchill Livingstone.
356. Weinstein, L. (1978) Bacterial hepatitis: a case report on an unrecognised cause of fever of unknown origin. *New England Journal of Medicine*, **299**, 1052–1054.
357. Wells, R.F. & Lundberg, G.D. (1963) Hepatoma: review of 43 cases with comments on syphilis as an etiologic factor. *Gastroenterology*, **44**, 598–601.
358. Whitmore, J.T., Cerda, J.J. & Offutt, R.G. (1971) Urban leptospirosis presenting as afebrile jaundice. *American Journal of Digestive Diseases*, **16**, 455–459.
359. Wilde, H. (1973) Hepatic amebic abscess not responding to metronidazole. *New England Journal of Medicine*, **289**, 378.

360. Wilmot, A.J. (1962) *Clinical Amoebiasis*. Oxford: Blackwell Scientific.
361. Wilmot, A.J., Powell, S.J. & Adams, E.B. (1958) The comparative value of emetine and chloroquine in amebic liver abscess. *American Journal of Tropical Medicine and Hygiene*, **7,** 197.
362. Wilmot, A.J., Powell, S.J. & Adams, E.B. (1959) Chloroquine compared with chloroquine and emetine combined in amebic liver abscess. *American Journal of Tropical Medicine and Hygiene*, **8,** 623–624.
363. Wilson, D., Mann, J.J., Bennett, J.E. & Utz, J.P. (1967) Clinical features of extracutaneous sporotrichosis. *Medicine*, **46,** 265–279.
364. Wilson, E. (1961–2) Abdominal actinomycosis, with special reference to the stomach, *British Journal of Surgery*, **49,** 266–270.
365. Witorsch, P. & Utz, J.P. (1968) North American blastomycosis: a study of 40 patients. *Medicine,* **47,** 169–200.
366. Wolff, B.P. (1946) Asiatic relapsing fever: report of 134 cases treated with mapharsen. *Annals of Internal Medicine*, **24,** 203–216.
367. Wong, M.L., Kaplan, S., Dunkle, L.M., Stechenberg, B.W. & Feigin, R.D. (1977) Leptospirosis: a childhood disease. *Journal of Pediatrics*, **90**(4), 532–537.
368. World Health Organization (1967) Current problems in leptospirosis. *Research Report of a WHO Experimental Group. WHO Teaching Report*, **380,** 5–31.
369. Wright, R. (1966) Amoebiasis – a diagnostic problem in Great Britain. *British Medical Journal,* **i,** 957–959.
370. Young, A.E. (1976) The clinical presentation of pyogenic liver abscess. *British Journal of Surgery*, **63,** 216–219.
371. Young, R.C. (1969) The Budd–Chiari syndrome caused by aspergillus. Two patients with vascular invasion of the hepatic veins. *Archives of Internal Medicine*, **124,** 754–757.
372. Young, R.C., Bennet, J.E., Vogel, C.L., Carbone, P.P. & De Vita, V.T. (1970) Aspergillosis. The spectrum of the disease in 98 patients. *Medicine*, **49,** 147–173.
373. Zarnow, H., Grant, T.H., Spellberg, M. & Levin, B. (1976) Unusual complications of regional enteritis. Duodenobiliary fistula and hepatic abscess. *Journal of the American Medical Association*, **235,** 1880–1881.
374. Zipser, R.D., Rau, J.E., Ricketts, R.R. & Bevans, L.C. (1976) Tuberculous pseudotumours of the liver. *American Journal of Medicine*, **61,** 946–951.

Chapter 52

Hepatic Transplantation

R.Y. CALNE

Clinical liver transplantation has been practised for 14 years; the first orthotopic liver graft was performed by Starzl in 1963. By July 1977 the Transplant Registry had 259 orthotopic transplants recorded. The Denver group have transplanted more than 120 livers and our own series from Cambridge and King's College Hospital, London, has reached 70 orthotopic transplants. A report on our first 60 cases has recently been published.[6]

HISTORICAL BACKGROUND

The first attempts at liver transplantation reported by Welch and colleagues were heterotopic.[15,29] Several techniques have been described but all involve some compromise compared with orthotopic grafting. Thus, with the liver in the right paracolic gutter, in order to achieve satisfactory vascular inflow to the liver and biliary drainage, the venous outflow must arise from the infrahepatic vena cava and this may be liable to obstruction and kinking. If the liver is placed in the splenic fossa, although there is more room to accommodate it, the venous outflow may again be difficult to position correctly and inflow from the splenic vein may not be sufficient.

In my opinion, a readily safe, reliable method of auxiliary liver transplantation has yet to be described. It would seem possible that in the future transplants of hepatic lobes using microvascular techniques may offer the best chance of achieving a reliable reproducible technique. A further important consideration is the nutrition of an auxiliary transplanted liver. If this organ is in competition with a normal liver, the graft is liable to rapid atrophy which can only be prevented by serious interference with the function of the blood supply of the normal liver.[16] An auxiliary transplant for parenchymatous liver disease presumably would not be so seriously affected by competitive nutritional atrophy due to the serious disease of the recipient's own liver. One would expect atrophy, however, if an auxiliary transplant were performed to provide enzymes missing in a patient whose liver function was otherwise normal.

The surgically more acceptable operation of orthotopic liver transplantation was pioneered by Dr Francis Moore and his colleagues[17,18] at the Peter Bent Brigham Hospital in 1958, and independently by Dr Starzl and his colleagues.[24,25] Although the techniques used by the two groups varied, both agreed that it was necessary to prevent portal and caval congestion during the anhepatic phase and devised shunting procedures. Fortunately, the primate species, and particularly man, do not require these external shunts which would complicate liver grafting. Both groups of workers were successful despite extreme technical difficulties, and surviving animals were shown to reject their livers quite aggressively with features similar to the rejection of canine renal allografts. The first report of successful orthotopic liver grafting in man was by Starzl et al.[26] Since then, the Denver group have been outstanding in their achievements with liver grafts. Although a number of other centres have attempted liver grafting, the only other large series of orthotopic liver allografts is our own, the Cambridge/King's College Hospital series dating back to 1968.[6] In this chapter I have concentrated on our own experience and have referred to the results from Denver. The main difference between the two series has been the predominance of young recipients, mostly cases of biliary atresia, in Denver. The results in these patients have been better than those in adults, and Starzl considers that children are the best liver recipients. I have always been reluctant to transplant kidneys in young children because of the uncertain long-term prognosis, the frequent invasive and often painful investigations that are required both pre- and postoperatively and, particularly, the side-effects of corticosteroid drugs which cause stunting of growth and cushingoid facies that can be very distressing to children. Despite full and informed discussion with parents, their emotional relationship to the child leads them to wish to try any new treatment, whereas an adult patient can understand the argument more rationally and can elect whether or not to receive a graft. As results improve and immunosuppression becomes less toxic my reservations on transplanting in children will disappear.

For patients with non-malignant parenchymatous liver disease and those suffering from deficiency of essential enzymes produced by the liver, the possibility of grafting an extra or accessory liver is attractive, since this does not require removal of the recipient's own diseased liver, which is often a difficult and hazardous procedure (see above). Forty-three such transplants have been recorded but only two recipients are living; one of them, a case of Dr Fortner's, is still alive, with good function in the transplant, more than four years after operation.

Table 52.1. *Indications for Orthotopic Liver Grafting in 70 Patients Treated 2 May 1968 to 1 July 1977.*

Primary cancer of the liver and bile ducts		35
Hepatocellular carcinoma	21	
Cholangiocarcinoma	12	
Kupffer cell sarcoma	1	
Haemangio-endothelioma	1	
Metastatic cancer of the liver		4
Cirrhosis		26
Cryptogenic	9	
Primary biliary	4	
Alcoholic	3	
Post-hepatitis	3	
Secondary biliary	3	
Subacute hepatic necrosis	1	
Sclerosing cholangitis	1	
Haemochromatosis	1	
Galactosaemia	1	
Alpha-1-antitrypsin deficiency		1
Budd–Chiari syndrome		2
Extrahepatic biliary atresia		2

In this chapter I will reserve my comments to the orthotopic operation, which is a surgically acceptable procedure with the liver lying in its natural position. For primary malignant disease of the liver the orthotopic operation is the only choice as the diseased organ must be removed. Since there is a tendency for hepatoma to develop in cirrhotic livers, this would be another point in favour of the orthotopic operation for treatment of patients with cirrhosis.

INDICATIONS FOR ORTHOTOPIC LIVER TRANSPLANTATION

In the 70 recipients of our series, the indications fell into two main categories, malignancy of the liver and parenchymatous liver disease. The details are shown in Table 52.1. Although four transplants were for metastatic cancer of the liver, we now feel that this is not a suitable indication. Recurrence has occurred in all cases shortly after operation. It would seem that the secondary deposits growing in the liver are unlikely to be the sole manifestation of the growth which usually is widely disseminated throughout the body.

Primary malignancy of the liver may be suitable for treatment by liver grafting but it is difficult to exclude the presence of metastases from the liver. All primary tumours should, if possible, be treated by partial resection. When, however, both lobes of the liver are affected or the remaining liver is severely cirrhotic this cannot be done. Cholangiocarcinoma has the reputation of being a slow-growing tumour, and palliative intubation of the duct system to relieve jaundice is the most commonly practised surgical procedure. The diagnostic procedure of opening the duct and taking biopsies may in itself be responsible for disseminating the cholangiocarcinoma. Even if the liver transplant is the first surgical procedure, without preliminary biopsy, recurrences have occurred. Thus, in one of our patients the clinical diagnosis was suspected and histology was

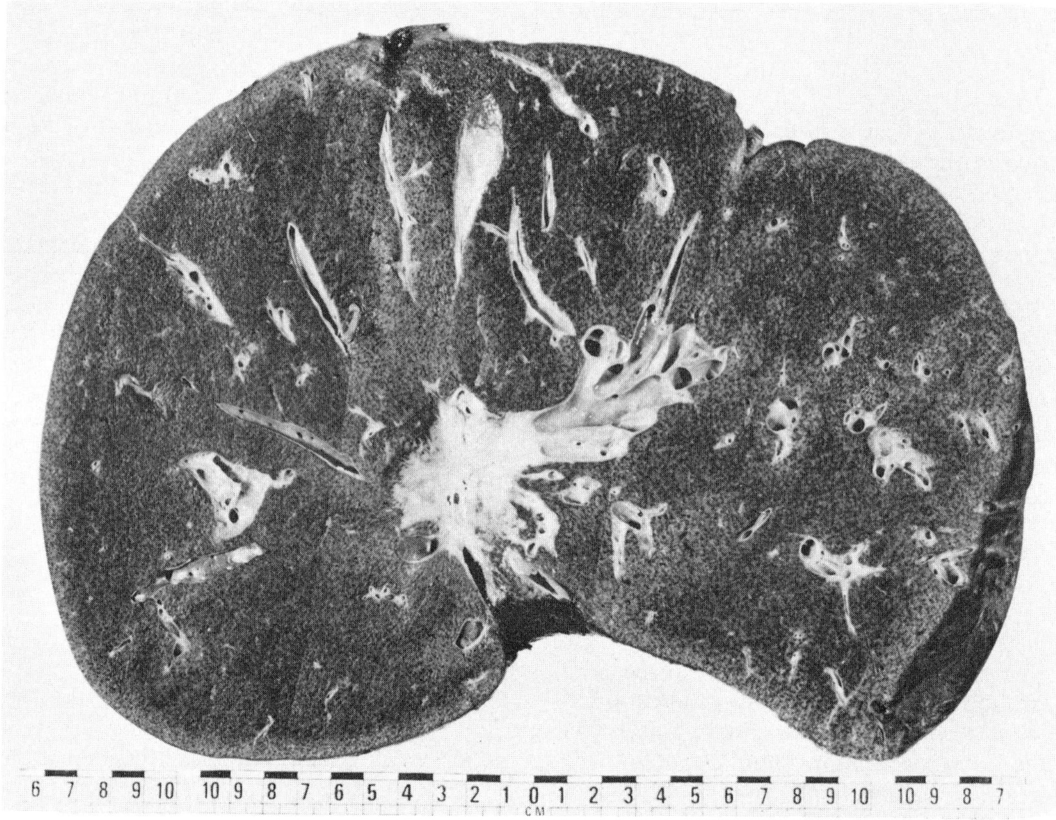

Figure 52.1. Primary cholangiocarcinoma producing jaundice when the tumour was still of small size.

obtained by needle biopsy at operation. It was felt that this was a highly favourable growth for treatment by liver grafting (Figure 52.1). There was no evidence of dissemination of growth at operation and the patient's postoperative course was uneventful. One year after surgery, however, the patient died from widespread recurrence of the cholangiocarcinoma. Starzl[23] has a patient surviving more than one year without evidence of recurrence but the experience overall has been disappointing

Primary hepatoma may occur in association with cirrhosis or on its own (see Chapter 38). This tumour is extremely common in parts of Africa and Asia. Patients usually die from metastatic growth within three to six months after diagnosis of the tumour and they often present with metastases in the lungs.

In Europe, this tumour may be much more slow-growing. Differentiation from a benign adenoma, such as that associated with taking oral contraceptives, may be difficult. Important features of malignancy are spread of the tumour into the venules of the liver and infiltration of liver tissue by malignant cells with no evidence of a capsule. Fifty per cent of the hepatomas in our series have produced alpha-fetoprotein. Although recurrence of hepatoma after transplantation has been distressingly common, some patients appear to have been cured. One of our patients survived more than five years and died from cholangitis. At autopsy there was no evidence of recurrent growth. The longest current survivor lives four years after operation. This young woman had had a partial hepatic resection for tumour. Four years later the tumour recurred in the remaining lobe. She was treated by orthotopic liver transplantation and is clinically free from growth and in excellent health (Figure 52.2).

There is a good chance of offering palliation for cholangiocarcinoma and hepatoma but only a minority of patients can expect to be cured by the elimination of all growth with removal of the liver.

Cirrhotic processes may be suitable for treatment by liver grafting if the liver disease is terminal and there is no serious disease of other organs. After the patients have been managed carefully by conventional methods, skilled assessment is necessary since an accurate prognosis of cirrhosis is notoriously difficult. If it is clear that the patient is not going to be able to leave hospital or can survive only in a severely handicapped manner, then liver transplantation may be considered. The operation should not be offered to terminal, moribund patients, since they are unlikely to survive surgery.

Alcoholic cirrhotics may be candidates for transplantation if they have given up alcohol and have reasonably stable personalities. Most alcoholics are unsuitable, however, because of their lack of cooperation and poor reliability in attending follow-up clinics and taking immunosuppressive treatment.

Patients with a positive Australia (HB_sAg) antigen are a hazard to the surgical and nursing staff and to other patients, but if suitable precautions are taken, antigenaemia per se should not exclude a patient from liver transplantation. One of our patients with a liver tumour who was HB_sAg-positive was treated with immune gamma globulin in the anhepatic phase of the operation and in the early postoperative phase. More than a year after liver transplantation he is in good health and his blood is HB_sAg-negative.

The cirrhotic who has developed intractable encephalopathy after a shunt procedure for variceal bleeding is highly suitable for liver transplantation. The lowered portal pressure is a bonus to the surgeon.

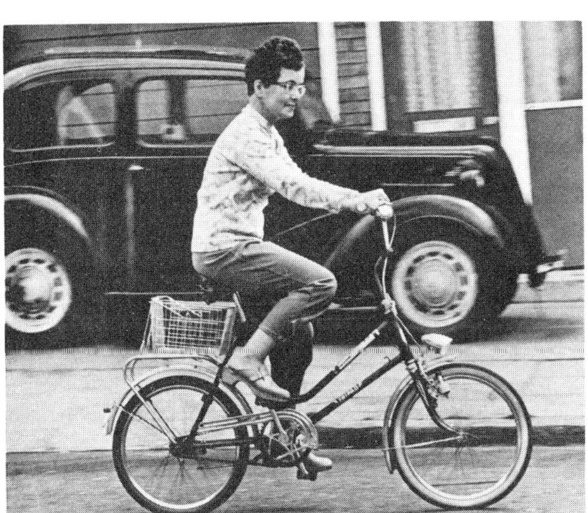

Figure 52.2. Patient cycling uphill 2½ years after transplantation. From Calne and Williams,[6] with the kind permission of the editor of *British Medical Journal*.

The Budd–Chiari syndrome may also be a suitable condition for liver transplantation since the disease often produces distressing symptoms in young people and the prognosis is grave. As discussed earlier, we have been reluctant to transplant in children and have only a small experience with patients suffering from extrahepatic biliary atresia. Starzl,[22] however, has shown that the best results are obtained in paediatric patients and believes that they should not be excluded on the grounds of age.

Acute hepatic necrosis is not at present a suitable condition for liver grafting because of the uncertain prognosis with modern intensive care, and since some patients, even those in severe hepatic coma, will recover completely. Moreover, patients in acute liver failure are serious operative risks.

PREOPERATIVE ASSESSMENT

A patient referred for consideration of a liver transplant with primary malignancy of the liver requires extensive investigation. First, it is important to confirm that the tumour is in fact a primary and not a secondary deposit from an occult source, such as a small primary cancer of the colon, kidney or pancreas. With large tumours, needle biopsies are performed. The patient's blood is screened for alpha-fetoprotein and HB_sAg. Colloid and selenomethionine scanning may show uptake of selenomethionine by a hepatoma. Chest x-ray, intravenous urography, barium meal and follow through, sigmoidoscopy, barium enema, total body bone scan and hepatic arterial and superior mesenteric angiography are routine investigations. Angiography of the inferior vena cava and abdominal lymphatics may be useful. Hepatoma is likely to spread to the lungs and hilar lymph nodes and micrometastases may be impossible to detect prior to transplantation. This defect of preoperative assessment must be accepted.

In assessing patients with parenchymatous non-malignant liver disease the most important requirement is to determine to what extent the disease is interfering with the patient's way of life. If he is developing increasingly severe encephalopathy and has repeated bleeds from varices with poor liver function, a long prothrombin time and low serum albumin, then he can be offered liver transplantation. It is useful to determine whether the portal vein is patent by splenoportography or the venous phase of mesenteric arteriography. In cases of Budd–Chiari syndrome a cavagram should be performed to make sure the main inferior vena cava is patent. In this condition the patient will need to be anticoagulated postoperatively. Failure to do this in one of our patients resulted in catastrophic thrombosis of major vessels a few weeks after a successful liver graft.

DONOR OPERATION

The donor should fulfil the requirements of a suitable kidney donor; that is, on a ventilator with brain death and an intact circulation. HLA typing is performed but only for retrospective analysis. So far there has been no correlation of rejection or acceptance of the graft and degree of HLA matching. It has generally been regarded as wise to adhere to blood group principles and avoidance of a positive leucocyte cross-match between recipient and donor, but when these rules have been transgressed, liver grafts, in marked contrast to kidney allografts, have functioned satisfactorily without evidence of acute rejection.

Removal of the liver from the donor should not jeopardize kidney removal, but if the kidneys and their vessels are removed first there may be interference with the vasculature of the liver. The procedure we adopt is to skeletonize the liver and both kidneys with the circulation intact and then insert a catheter into the aorta via the right common iliac artery and drain the vena cava via the common iliac vein. The aortic cannula is declamped and whilst exsanguination occurs, a cannula is inserted into the portal vein to start cooling the liver. This perfusion, with Hartmann's solution, continues while both kidneys are removed, taking Carrel patches of aorta and the renal veins up to the vena cava. After 1500 cc of Hartmann's solution at 4° have been infused into the portal vein, the perfusate is changed to plasma protein fraction with additives.[28] Whilst this perfusion is in progress, the liver is removed and inserted into a bowl containing iced saline. After 300 to 400 cc of perfusate have gone through the portal vein, the cannula is removed and substituted for a smaller cannula which is inserted into the hepatic artery through which 150 cc of the perfusate are infused. The liver in the bowl containing cold saline is inserted into a sterile polythene bag and this into another similar bag. This second bag is placed in a polystyrene box which contains ice and which can be easily transported by car or plane. Twenty-seven livers removed in other hospitals and brought by road or air have had total ischaemia times between two and $10\frac{1}{2}$ hours. All 27 livers have functioned satisfactorily when transplanted orthotopically, maintaining the lives of the recipients. We believe that with such a simple and effective preservation method continuous perfusion apparatus is neither desirable nor necessary.

RECIPIENT OPERATION

The technique used is based on that described originally by Starzl et al.[26] It is of great importance that anaesthesia be given by skilled and experienced anaesthetists, since the recipients may be very ill prior to surgery and the operation imposes serious physiological demands on cardiovascular and pulmonary reserves. If the patient has a reasonable coagulation profile, a high epidural anaesthetic is given together with light general inhalation anaesthesia. The epidural is continued in the postoperative phase and permits the patient to inspire deeply and to cough immediately after operation. If the patient has severe coagulation

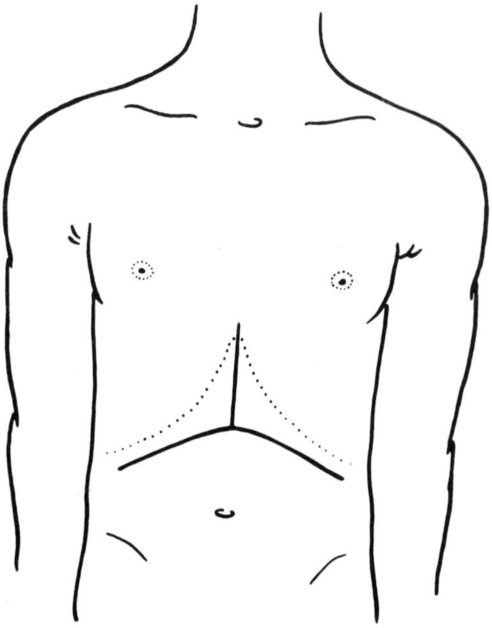

Figure 52.3. Bilateral subcostal incision with upward vertical extension for liver transplantation.

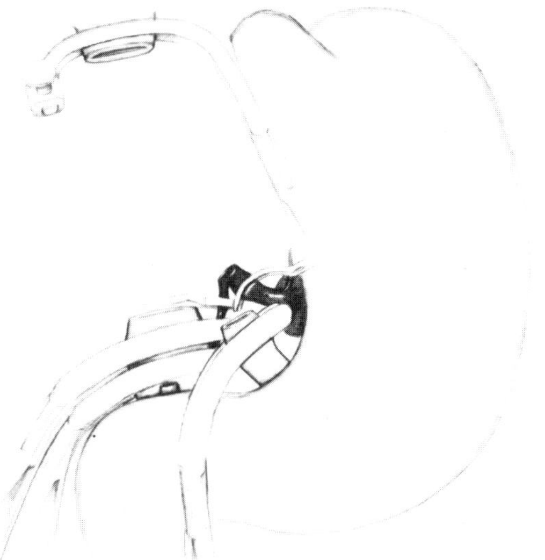

Figure 52.4. Removal of the donor liver with clamping of the hepatic artery, portal vein and inferior vena cava above and below the liver. (From Calne, R.Y. and Williams, R. (1978) Experience of 50 orthotopic liver grafts. An improvement in early post-operative survival following the introduction of a new technique of biliary drainage. *Proceedings of the Fifth Asian Pacific Congress on Gastroenterology, May 1976.*) With the kind permission of the editor of *Malaysian Journal of Surgery.*

defects, so that an epidural anaesthetic would be contraindicated, the postoperative management is more difficult but may be helped by multiple and repeated intercostal blocks. During the operation the pulse rate, ECG, arterial and central venous pressures are monitored continuously. Frequent estimations are made of the serum levels of potassium, calcium and the arterial blood gases and pH. Large cannulae are inserted into tributaries of the superior vena cava to permit rapid intravenous infusions. The incision shown in Figure 52.3 gives adequate exposure without opening the chest. If there is portal hypertension and coagulopathy, severe bleeding may occur without the severance of any large vessels and it is essential to be meticulous with the technique of haemostasis, using suture ligation wherever possible. The structures of the free edge of the lesser omentum are separated from each other and controlled. Once the donor liver is safely in the operating room, the irretraceable step of recipient hepatectomy can be taken. Dissection behind the liver should start only at this stage, since haemostasis in this area may not be possible until the liver has been removed. The structures in the lesser omentum and the infrahepatic vena cava are clamped and divided, and a special clamp with a screw clip is applied to the inferior vena cava above the liver, including a cuff of diaphragm (Figure 52.4). At this stage, the return of blood to the heart may be impaired by 50 per cent and cardiac arrest may occur. Rapid intravenous infusion into the superior vena cava is usually necessary. This must not be excessive, otherwise the circulation can be overloaded, producing pulmonary oedema. All bleeding from the posterior abdominal wall is controlled. The donor liver is now removed from ice. The upper caval anastomosis may be difficult to see, particularly if the donor liver is relatively large for the space available. 2/0 mersilene is used for this anastomosis. The donor and recipient portal veins are then anastomosed end-to-end. Just prior to completion of this, the liver is flushed out with 500 cc of plasma protein fraction at room temperature, without any additives, to remove potassium ions and acid metabolites which could be toxic if suddenly allowed to flood into the circulation. The vena cava below the liver is clamped. Clamps are removed from the portal vein and the vena cava above the liver. The donor and recipient venae cavae below the liver are anastomosed end-to-end with prolene, and a small Carrel patch of donor aorta containing the orifice of the coeliac artery is anastomosed to the recipient hepatic artery close to the gastroduodenal branch (Figure 52.5). On revascularization of the liver

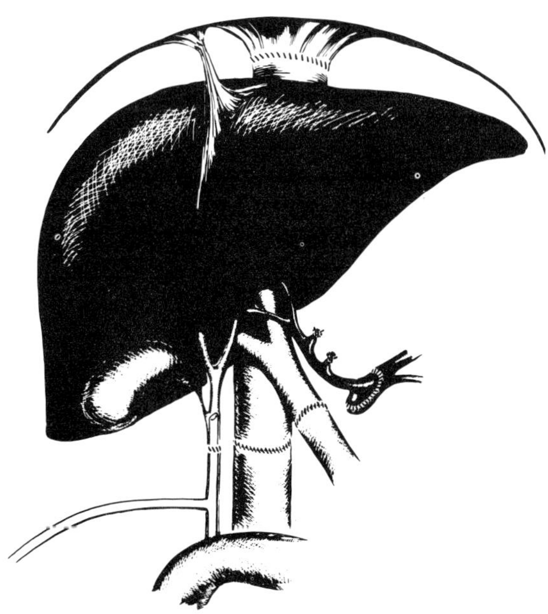

Figure 52.5. Diagram of orthotopic liver transplantation with drainage of bile via a choledochostomy over a T-tube. (From Calne, R.Y. (1969) Surgical aspects of clinical liver transplantation in 14 cases. *British Journal of Surgery*, **56**, 729–736.) With the kind permission of the editor of *British Journal of Surgery*.

the patient may require added bicarbonate and calcium to cover the outpouring of potassium ions and acidic radicals, not only from the ischaemic liver but also from the territory drained by the clamped portal vein.

The most common and serious complication following liver grafting has resulted from inadequate biliary drainage. Techniques using the cystic duct and gallbladder for anastomosis to the recipient gastrointestinal tract, usually a Roux loop, have the disadvantages of a blind sump of common duct below the cystic duct which may accumulate sludge, and a narrow cystic duct which may become blocked. Immunosuppressive drugs predispose to cholangitis when there is no protection from reflux by the sphincter of Oddi.

We have obtained good results with direct duct-to-duct anastomosis (Figure 52.5) when the donor and recipient ducts are of sufficient calibre, but normal common bile ducts can be as small as 2 mm in diameter. For a safe anastomosis microsurgical techniques are required. There must be no tension at the anastomosis, and a good blood supply is necessary, particularly to the donor duct. In the last two years more satisfactory results have been achieved using the gallbladder as a conduit between the donor and recipient ducts without relying on the cystic duct (Figure 52.6).[5] This technique has the advantage of preserving the sphincter of Oddi, eliminating tension and providing well-vascularized tissue for anastomosis. In addition, a special T-tube is used, with a narrow irrigating limb inserted into the donor main-duct system. Irrigation through this limb is instituted postoperatively with 1 litre of Hartmann's solution containing heparin each 24 hours. This is done to discourage the formation of sludge aggregates. At 10 days a cholangiogram is performed, and if this is satisfactory the T-tube is spigoted and, provided the patient's condition is good, is left undisturbed for three months, when another cholangiogram is performed. If bile drainage appears to be satisfactory, the T-tube is removed. If the recipient common duct is unsuitable for anastomosis, the gallbladder conduit can be joined to a long Roux loop (Figure 52.7).[7]

Two large tube drains are brought out from each extremity of the wound and the patient is nursed in an intensive care area. In patients with severe cirrhosis, pulmonary AV shunts may cause difficulty in achieving adequate oxygenation of the blood, and mechanical ventilation for 24 hours or more may be necessary. Respiratory infection is a common hazard after liver grafting, so it is preferable for the patient to be extubated shortly after operation so that he can sit up, fully conscious, and be able to breathe deeply and cough.

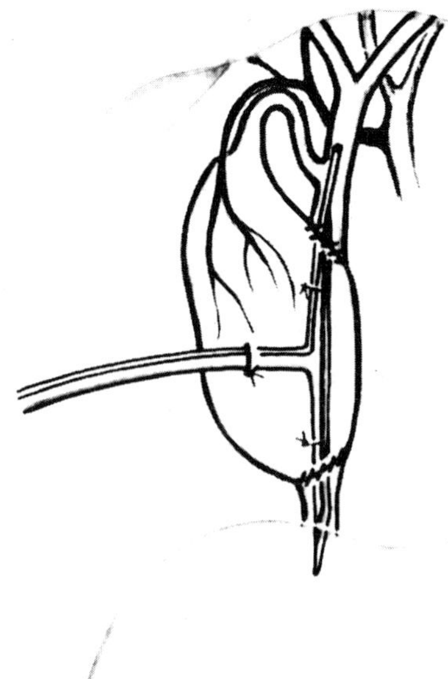

Figure 52.6. Pedicle graft conduit with donor gallbladder. Hartmann's pouch is anastomosed to donor common duct and the fundus is anastomosed to recipient common duct. Irrigating T-tube is inserted with irrigating arm through upper anastomosis. Blood supply to gallbladder is carefully preserved. From Calne and Williams,[6] with the kind permission of the editor of *British Medical Journal.*

IMMUNOSUPPRESSION

Immunosuppression consists of the same regimen used in kidney transplantation, namely azathioprine and prednisolone, although in the first three postoperative days cyclophosphamide is given instead of azathioprine because of the latter's hepatotoxic effects.

Several of our patients have been weaned completely from prednisolone, and maintenance immunosuppressive drug dosage is generally less than that required in patients with kidney grafts.

In Denver, antilymphocyte globulin is given but we do not use this agent.

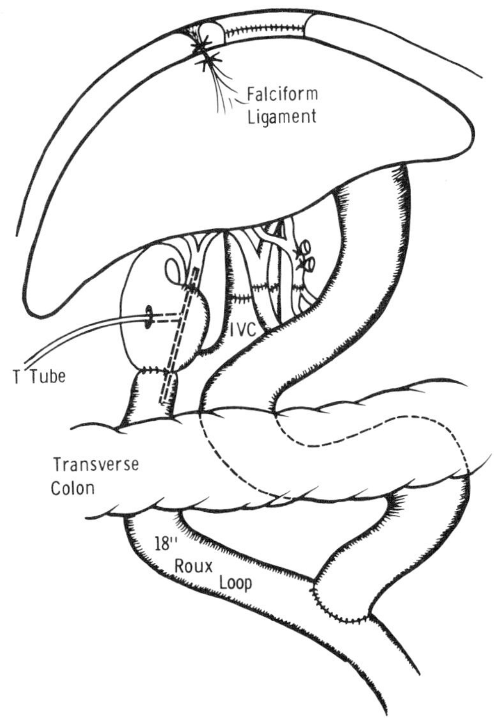

Figure 52.7. Diagram of the use of the vascularized gallbladder as a conduit between the donor common duct and a long Roux loop of jejunum in a patient whose own common duct could not be used. Hartmann's pouch is anastomosed to the common bile duct of the donor and the fundus of the gallbladder to the Roux loop. With the kind permission of the editor of *World Journal of Surgery*.

REJECTION

This can be very difficult to diagnose. Any impairment of liver function in the post-operative phase may indicate rejection. Needle biopsy of the liver is often unhelpful. We have found a positive leucocyte migration test[13] to be useful, and if the T-tube cholangiogram is normal in the presence of deteriorating liver function the steroid dose is increased for a few days, as in the treatment of renal allograft rejection crises. Rejection has been the cause of death in only four of our patients, a very much lower incidence than that observed with kidney grafts. In three of these patients, in addition to mononuclear cell infiltration of portal tracts and the presence of lipid-filled histiocytes in the walls of arterioles and in the sinusoids, there appeared to be a predilection for the small bile duct epithelium within the liver to be a special target for rejection. The appearances are not unlike those of primary biliary cirrhosis. The clinical features in these cases were relentless and progressive, intrahepatic jaundice predominating with relatively good parenchymal function, until pre-terminal liver failure ensued.

RESULTS

In our overall results, shown in Table 52.2, of 35 patients transplanted between 1968 and 1974 there were 11 deaths during or within the first postoperative week. Of the 35 patients transplanted subsequently, there were two deaths in this period. We believe that this improvement in early mortality is due to the greater experience of surgeons and anaesthetists, and to confidence in the preservation technique that has widened the pool of potential donors and has permitted transplantation before a moribund state has been reached. Eight patients lived more than a year and, of the present patients currently alive, one has survived four years after operation. Our longest survivor died after five years and three months from biliary tract infection.

Patients who have been discharged from hospital have often done extremely well, requiring fewer steroids than kidney graft patients and capable of full integration into society. One hundred and three patients from the Denver series received transplants more than a year ago.[22] Twenty-nine per cent survived a year or more. The Denver group pointed out that the mortality rate falls markedly in patients surviving beyond a year; half of their one-year survivals are still alive. Fifteen patients are alive more than two years after operation, eight more than three years and four more than five years. The longest survivor is $7\frac{1}{2}$ years post-transplantation with normal liver function. She lives at home and attends school. One female patient has had a normal pregnancy and given birth to a healthy child.

In our experience, tumour recurrence has been common in patients with primary malignancy of the liver, but since palliation can be excellent without completely eliminating the growth, there is no difference in principle between treating a patient with liver cancer by transplantation and giving similar palliative surgery to a patient with cancer of the lung, stomach or colon. I nevertheless feel that parenchymatous liver disease, rather than primary malignancy, should be the main indication for liver transplantation.

Table 52.2. *Cambridge/King's: 70 Orthotopic Liver Allografts, July 1977.*

Year	Deaths: Within 1st month	Deaths: 1 to 6 months	Deaths: 6 months to 1 year	Deaths: More than 1 year	Alive: Date of operation	Total operations
1968	4	3				7
1969	5	1	2	1 (lived 5 years 3 months)		9
1970		7				7
1971	3	1				4
1972	1					1
1973	3	1		1 (lived 2 years 1 month)		5
1974	1				1 19 Feb 74	2
1975	1	2	2	2 (lived 13 months) (lived 14 months)	1 30 Dec 75	8
1976	1	7	2	2 (lived 1 year)	5 3 Oct 76 10 Nov 76 19 Nov 76 17 Dec 76 29 Dec 76	17
1977	4				6 3 Feb 77 21 Feb 77 21 Feb 77 7 Mar 77 11 June 77 1 July 77	10
Total	23	22	6	6	13	70

EXPERIMENTAL OBSERVATIONS

Despite the rapid rejection of canine liver allografts in unimmunosuppressed animals, azathioprine treatment can result in prolonged survival.[27] Some animals have lived after cessation of immunosuppressive drug treatment. Rejection of canine liver allografts can be held in check with immunosuppressive agents more easily than is possible in animals with kidney allografts.

Garnier et al[14] and Cordier et al[9] grafted livers in unimmunosuppressed pigs and reported some long-term survivors. Similar observations were made by Peacock and Terblanche[19] and our own group.[8] We have previous experience of experimental kidney allografting in the pig and have noticed a marked difference in the pattern of rejection, which was frequently extremely mild, of liver allografts. We started a programme designed to try to determine why there was a spectrum of rejection of different tissues in the same species. Initially, empirical observations showed that skin was inexorably rejected in pigs between five and 10 days postoperatively. No long-term surviving skin grafts were observed in a large number of experiments. The first attempts at clarifying these observations depended on developing tissue typing in the pig. This was accomplished in our laboratories by Bradley, White and Edwards,[2] Bradley et al,[1,3,4] and White et al.[30] An important observation was that identity of the loci of the major histocompatibility complex (MHC) resulted in only a few days extra survival of skin grafts between siblings, whereas renal allografts between similarly MHC matched donor and recipient siblings usually survived indefinitely and, when one chromosome was matched and the other mismatched, approximately one-third of the animals survived indefinitely. Orthotopic liver allografts have survived complete MHC mismatches of donor and recipient without immunosuppressive drug treatment. We have attempted to develop in vitro correlates of the in vivo reactions by setting up cell cultures of kidney and liver cells[10] and have investigated the behaviour of lymphocytes and sera from recipient animals before and after liver transplantation with different degrees of donor and recipient mismatch. It has been shown that liver cells possess less MHC surface antigens than kidney cells[11] and hepatocytes are more resistant to killing by allogeneic lymphocytes in tissue culture than are kidney cells (unpublished observations). These may be relevant factors in the relatively privileged immunological state of the liver. The contribution of Kupffer cells and hepatic metabolites may also be important.[12] In two clinical cases it has been shown that six months after grafting, Kupffer cells became of host origin.[20,21]

Certainly the whole liver, as opposed to separated hepatocytes, has cells with full representation of MHC antigens. The Kupffer cells in particular possess both serologically defined and lymphocyte defined antigenic determinants. It may well be that the mechanism responsible for the acceptance of liver, when fully understood, could provide a tool for manipulation of recipients of other allografts, and we are now attempting to extend our studies from the pig to man. Now that the surgical results of human liver grafts have improved, it is clear that progressive and uncontrollable rejection is unusual and, in this respect, man resembles the pig.

Patients referred for new and dangerous surgical operations are usually treated too late. With increasing confidence in the operation, enabling surgery to be performed a little earlier, the results of liver grafting for non-malignant parenchymatous liver disease could well be better than those currently obtained with kidney grafts from cadaver donors.

ACKNOWLEDGEMENTS

Much of the material in this chapter results from the experience of the combined Cambridge/King's College Hospital, London, series of orthotopic liver transplants. I am indebted to my many colleagues in both hospitals concerned in this programme and particularly to Dr Roger Williams.

REFERENCES

1. Bradley, B.A., Edwards, J.M. & Franks, D. (1973) Histocompatibility phenotyping by the mixed lymphocyte reaction. *Tissue Antigens*, **3**, 340–347.
2. Bradley, B.A., White, D.J.G. & Edwards, J.M. (1974) Restriction of the polymorphisms defined by mixed lymphocyte reactions in the pig. *Tissue Antigens*, **4**, 283–290.
3. Bradley, B.A., Edwards, J.M., Dunn, D.C. & Calne, R.Y. (1972) Quantitation of mixed lymphocyte reaction by gene dosage phenomenon. *Nature New Biology*, **240**, 54–56.
4. Bradley, B.A., White, D.J.G., Calne, R.Y., Dunn, D.C., Edwards, J.M., Bitter-Suermann, H., Sampson, D. & Herbertson, B.M. (1973) Genes determining mixed lymphocyte reactions; their use in predicting renal allograft survivals. *Proceedings of the 8th Leucocyte Culture Conference* (Ed.) Osoba, D. pp. 1–7. London and New York: Academic Press.
5. Calne, R.Y. (1976) A new technique for biliary drainage in orthotopic liver transplantation utilizing the gall bladder as a pedicle graft conduit between the donor and recipient common bile ducts. *Annals of Surgery*, **184**, 605–609.
6. Calne, R.Y. & Williams, R. (1977) Orthotopic liver transplantation: the first 60 patients. *British Medical Journal*, **i**, 471–476.
7. Calne, R.Y., McMaster, P., Portmann, B., Williams, R. & Wall, W.J. (1977) Observations on preservation, bile drainage and rejection in 64 human orthotopic liver allografts. *Annals of Surgery*, **186**, 282–290.
8. Calne, R.Y., White, J.H.O., Yoffa, D.E., Binns, R.M., Maginn, R.R., Herbertson, B.M., Millard, P.R., Molina, V.P. & Davis, D.R. (1967) Observations of orthotopic liver transplantation in the pig. *British Medical Journal*, **iv**, 645–648.
9. Cordier, G., Garnier, H., Clot, J.P., Camplez, P., Gorin, J.P., Clot, P., Bassinier, J.P., Nizza, M. & Levy, R. (1966) La greffe de foie orthotopique chez le porc. Premiers resultats. *Mémoires de l'Académie de chirurgie (Paris)*, **92**, 799.
10. Daniel, M.R. & Edwards, M.J. (1975) Interaction of pig lymphocytes with allogeneic kidney cells in vitro. *British Journal of Experimental Pathology*, **56**, 349–357.
11. Davies, H.ff.S., Taylor, J.E., Daniel, M.R. & Wakerley, C. (1976) Differences between pig tissues in the expression of major transplantation antigens: possible relevance for organ allografts. *Journal of Experimental Medicine*, **143**, 987–992.
12. Davies, H.ff.S., Taylor, J., White, D.J.G. & Binns, R. (1977) Major transplantation antigens of pig kidneys and livers: comparisons between the whole organs and their parenchymal constituents. Submitted to *Transplantation (Baltimore)*.
13. Eddleston, A.L.W.F., Smith, M.G.M., Mitchell, C.G. & Williams, R. (1971) Application of the leucocyte migration test to the diagnosis of rejection after transplantation. *Transplantation*, **12**, 11–17.

14. Garnier, H., Clot, J.P., Bertrand, M., Camplez, P., Kunlin, A., Gorin, J.P., Legoaziou, F., Levey, R. & Cordier, G. (1965) Biologie expérimentale: greffe de foie chez le porc: approche chirurgicale. *Comptes rendus hebdomadaires des séance de l'Académie des science (Paris),* **260,** 5621–5623.
15. Goodrich, E.O., Welch, H.F., Nelson, J.A., Beecher, T.S. & Welch, C.S. (1956) Homotransplantation of the canine liver. *Surgery,* **39,** 244–251.
16. Marchioro, T.L., Porter, K.A., Dickinson, T.C., Faris, T.D. & Starzl, T.E. (1965) Physiologic requirements for auxiliary liver homotransplantation. *Surgery, Gynecology and Obstetrics,* **121,** 17–31.
17. Moore, F.D., Smith, L.L., Burnap, T.K., Dallenbach, F.D., Dammin, G.J., Gruber, U.F., Shoemaker, W.C., Steenburg, R.W., Ball, M.R. & Belko, J.S. (1959) One-stage homotransplantation of the liver following total heptatectomy in dogs. *Transplantation Bulletin,* **6,** 103–107.
18. Moore, F.D., Wheeler, H.B., Demissianos, H.V., Smith, L.L., Balankura, O., Abel, K., Greenberg, J.B. & Dammin, G.J. (1960) Experimental whole organ transplantation of the liver and of the spleen. *Annals of Surgery,* **152,** 374–387.
19. Peacock, J.H. & Terblanche, J. (1967) Orthotopic homotransplantation of the liver in the pig. In *The Liver* (Ed.) Read, A.E. pp. 333–336. London: Butterworth.
20. Porter, K.A. (1969) Pathology of the orthotopic homograft and heterograft. In *Experience in Hepatic Transplantation* (Ed) Starzl, T.E. pp. 422–471. Philadelphia: W.B. Saunders.
21. Portmann, B., Schindler, A.-M., Murray-Lyon, I.M. & Williams, R. (1976) Histological sexing of a reticulum cell sarcoma arising after liver transplantation. *Gastroenterology,* **70,** 82–84.
22. Putnam, C.W., Halgrimson, C.G., Koep, L. & Starzl, T.E. (1977) Hepatic transplantation. *World Journal of Surgery,* **1,** 165–175.
23. Starzl, T.E. (1977) Personal communication.
24. Starzl, T.E., Bernhard, V.M., Cortes, H. & Benvenuto, R. (1959) A technique for one-stage hepatectomy in dogs. *Surgery,* **46,** 880–886.
25. Starzl, T.E., Kaupp, H.A., Brock, D.R., Lazarus, R.E. & Johnson, R.V. (1960) Reconstructive problems in canine liver homotransplantation with special reference to the postoperative role of hepatic venous flow. *Surgery, Gynecology and Obstetrics,* **111,** 733–743.
26. Starzl, T.E., Marchioro, T.L., von Kaulla, K.N., Hermann, G., Brittain, R.S. & Waddell, W.R. (1963) Homotransplantation of the liver in humans. *Surgery, Gynecology and Obstetrics,* **117,** 659–676.
27. Starzl, T.E., Marchioro, T.L., Porter, K.A., Taylor, P.D., Faris, T.D., Hermann, T.J., Hlad, C.J. & Waddell, W.R. (1965) Factors determining short- and long-term survival after orthotopic liver homotransplantation in the dog. *Surgery,* **58,** 131–155.
28. Wall, W.J., Calne, R.Y., Herbertson, B.M., Smith, D.P., Underwood, J., Kostakis, A. & Williams, R. (1977) Simple hypothermic preservation for transporting human livers long distances for transplantation. *Transplantation,* **23,** 210–216.
29. Welch, C.S. (1955) A note on transplantation of the whole liver in dogs. *Transplantation Bulletin,* **2,** 54–55.
30. White, D.J.G., Bradley, B.A., Calne, R.Y. & Binns, R.M. (1973) The relationship of the histocompatibility locus in the pig to allograft survival. *Transplantation Proceedings,* **5,** 317–320.

Chapter 53

Calculous Disease and Cholecystitis

STEPHEN KARRAN
R.H.S. LANE

Calculous disease of the biliary tree is associated with a variety of clinical presentations although in over 50 per cent of cases it is asymptomatic. Symptoms such as biliary 'colic' and jaundice are produced by the mechanical effects of obstruction whilst stasis predisposes to ascending cholangitis and septicaemia. Obstruction to the outflow of bile from the gallbladder by a calculus in Hartmann's pouch similarly may predispose to acute cholecystitis or cause distension by mucus of the gallbladder (mucocoele). Empyema formation and septicaemia develop in some cases and the patient may present with these complications. A calculus may also perforate the gallbladder by pressure necrosis with subsequent local abscess formation, generalized peritonitis or with the formation of a fistula into adjacent bowel sometimes causing intestinal obstruction (gallstone ileus). The clinical presentation of gallstones on occasion, however, is vague and ill-defined, with symptoms such as left-sided abdominal or chest pain, so that other pathology in the chest or abdomen must be excluded.

PREVALENCE OF CALCULOUS DISEASE

The clinical presentation of calculous disease in obese fertile females in the fifth decade is well known. There is little doubt, however, that new patterns of disease are emerging in developed countries where younger women are affected more frequently than previously. This increased prevalence is almost certainly related to the widespread use of oestrogenic contraceptives, as indicated by the Boston Collaborative Studies.[9,10]

Experimental studies which provide support for this aetiological mechanism have demonstrated an alteration in the relative composition of bile in animals following the administration of pharmacological doses of oestrogens.[49] Precipitation of cholesterol from supersaturated solutions lying outside the micellar zone (see Chapter 12) is more liable to occur under these circumstances. Although in these animal studies high doses of oestrogens were given over a short period of time, it is not unreasonable to suggest that the chronic administration of lower doses might exert a similar action leading to an increased tendency to cholelithiasis.

Autopsy studies (Table 53.1) have also provided valuable information about the prevalence of calculous disease, even though published data from certain parts of the world are limited.[11] There is, for example, lack of age and sex standardization in many published reports, making interpretation of data difficult. However, large differences in the prevalence of calculous disease between industrialized and non-industrialized countries cannot be accounted for solely by lack of standardized data. Remarkably high prevalence rates have been recorded in certain communities, such as among the American Indians in Chile. In other parts of the world, particularly Australia and Panama, autopsy data suggest an increasing prevalence over the last 50 years.

A recent prospective autopsy study in nine towns in England and Wales revealed marked variations in the prevalence of multiple calculi but not of solitary stones.[5] The prevalences in men tended to be higher in more affluent towns. In women, however, the prevalences were found to be higher in the three southern towns included in the study than in those towns of similar socio-economic status in central and

Table 53.1. *World Distribution of Gallstones.*[a]

	Pre-1940 (%)	Post-1940 (%)
Africa:		
Accra	–	0
Ibadan	–	0.8
Kinshasa (Leopoldville)	–	0.7
Kampala	–	0.9
Johannesburg (Bantu)	3.9	2.4
Johannesburg (White)	15.5	14.7
Nairobi	0.1	–
Asia:		
Thailand	–	2.9
Japan	3.6	4.4
Korea	2.9	4.5
Singapore	–	6.6
Java	1.6	–
Peking	2.3	–
Tomsk	3.1	–
Calcutta	5.4	–
Australia:		
Melbourne	–	14.9
Brisbane	–	31.1
Adelaide	12.0	–
Europe:		
Leningrad	2.2	1.9
Dublin	–	4.9
Birmingham	–	8.6
London	4.1	12.1
Manchester	7.1	–
Leeds	8.4	–
Innsbruck	–	13.9
Vienna	24.6	–
Basel	10.7	–
Erfurt	–	15.8
Göttingen	4.4	–
Kiel	5.9	–
Dresden	6.3	–
Munich	7.1	–
Erlangen	7.2	–
Rostock	9.6	–
Strasbourg	12.0	–

[a]Autopsy data adapted from Brett and Barker.[11]

northern England. As a result of autopsy studies various dietary factors such as refined carbohydrates have been implicated. As yet, however, there is little convincing evidence to support such claims.

In all studies a female preponderance of between 2:1 (Australia) and 4:1 (Bantu) is reported. In addition, the composition of stones varies. Caucasians, for example, have predominantly mixed stones, whilst pigment stones are more common in Asians and the Bantu.

Surveys based on cholecystography performed in Japan also suggest an increased frequency of calculous disease in recent years.

GALLSTONES

The most commonly-found gallstones are composed of cholesterol together with calcium salts such as calcium carbonate, phosphate or bilirubinate. These components are often deposited in alternating layers (laminae) to constitute the 'mixed' stones which account for approximately 80 per cent of calculi found at operation. Such calculi are usually multiple and may be faceted as a result of lying in contiguity within the gallbladder. They are frequently associated with signs and symptoms of inflammation, and are thus often referred to as 'inflammatory' stones. Coexisting infection is important in the formation and growth of such calculi.

Less frequently, stones composed almost entirely of cholesterol are found. These tend to be solitary and are round or ovoid. They are pale yellow in colour and usually 1 to 2 cm in diameter. The formation of cholesterol gallstones is described in Chapter 12.

Approximately 10 to 20 per cent of all stones contain appreciable amounts of calcium rendering them radiopaque (Figure 53.1).

Pigment stones occur in the East in up to 40 per cent of cases, whereas they comprise approximately 5 per cent of gallstones found in western society. Bilirubinate stones are amorphous with a putty-like consistency and present a layered appearance when cut. Infection of the biliary tree is a predisposing factor, and β-

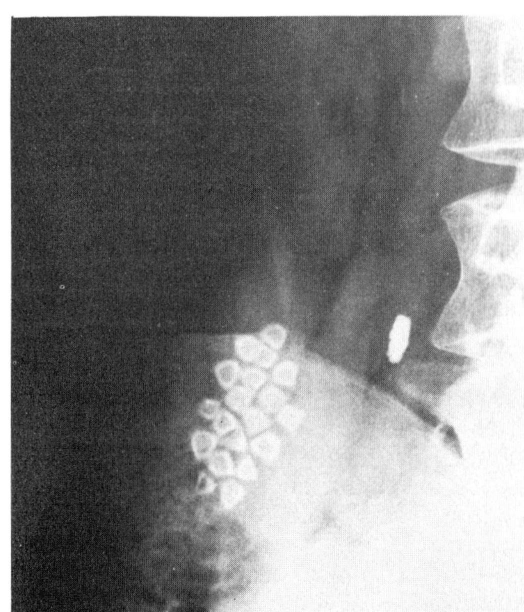

Figure 53.1. Radiopaque calculi seen on plain abdominal film.

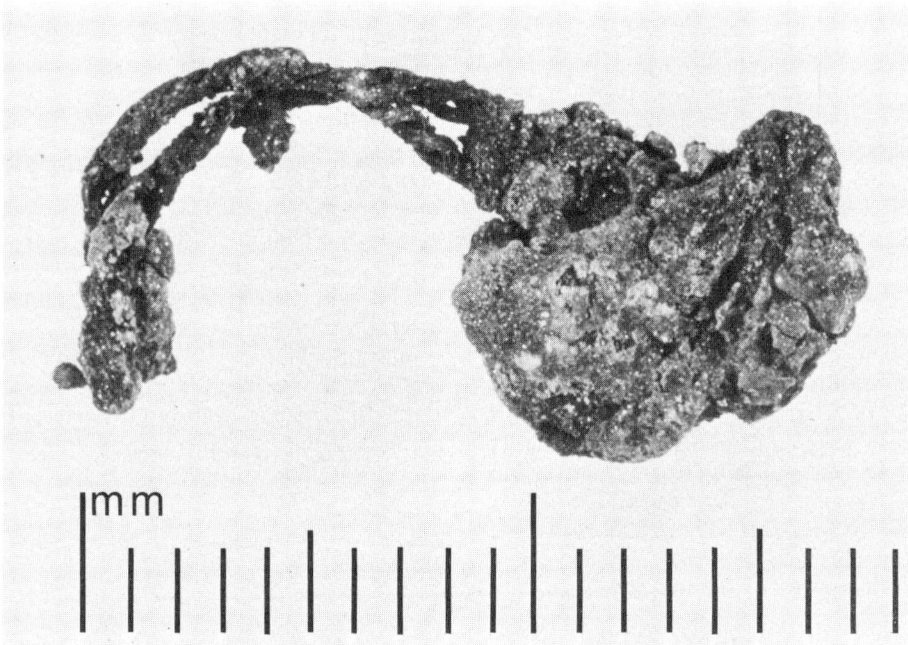

Figure 53.2. Bilirubinate calculus which caused obstructive jaundice. It had formed around two silk ligatures used five years previously to ligate the cystic duct. These had presumably ulcerated into the common bile duct to act as a nidus for stone formation.

glucuronidase, an enzyme liberated in abundance by *Escherichia coli* which occurs commonly in bile, is implicated in their formation.[52] β-glucuronidase hydrolyses soluble conjugated bilirubin to form free bilirubin and glucuronic acid and the calcium salt of free bilirubin precipitates as a pigment stone. The pH of bile is optimum for the activity of β-glucuronidase.[52] Maki[52] has demonstrated in vitro that calcium bilirubinate stones can be produced when calcium carbonate, calcium chloride and high molecular weight compounds are added to normal bile that has been incubated with *E. coli*.

The high incidence of both haemolytic disease and biliary tract infections, including anaerobic infections which are particularly common in the elderly,[74] is the probable reason why these calculi are prevalent in the Far East. The aetiological importance of infection, which may be secondary to parasitic infestation, is highlighted in countries such as Japan where pigment stones are common in farming communities, but far less so in urban society.

Bilirubinate calculi form around foreign bodies such as non-absorbable suture material within the biliary tree (Figure 53.2). Ascaris eggs similarly have been shown to form a 'nidus' for the development of these stones.[52]

Recent x-ray diffraction studies, however, by Arnaud and his colleagues from Strasbourg,[2] in which the crystalline constituents of gallstones were accurately determined, have demonstrated that there is no satisfactory system of classification in current usage. These studies show that previous macroscopic and x-ray analyses have given an erroneous picture of the composition of calculi. Semi-quantitative assay was carried out on calculi from 152 patients. Seventy-eight per cent of the stones analysed were 'mixed', consisting of cholesterol and its derivatives, bile salts, bile pigments and various minerals. It is particularly interesting that no pure cholesterol stones were found in this study and 22 per cent of the calculi were composed entirely of minerals. Four patients were found to have pure calcium phosphate stones. Five other patients had stones composed of calcium phosphate and calcite, and in a further six the calculi were formed of calcium phosphate together with vaterite and calcite. A new compound, montmorillonite ($4SiO_2$-$Al_3O_3[1 + x]H_2O$), was identified as the exclusive component of 10 other pure mineral stones.

These authors point out that the regular occurrence of both iron and aluminium in gallstones has implications with regard to the pathogenesis and management of patients. Confirmation of these findings, particularly in patients from other parts of the world and with different dietary intakes, is obviously required.

PRESENTATION OF GALLSTONES

Inflammation of the gallbladder may present as an acute episode (acute cholecystitis), necessitating emergency admission to hospital. Multiple calculi within the gallbladder often present in this way. On the other hand, many patients are referred with vague chronic symptoms suggestive of gallbladder disease (chronic cholecystitis). On occasions, complications of calculous disease, such as obstructive jaundice, acute pancreatitis or intestinal obstruction may be the cause of presentation.

Calculi may also be detected coincidentally by abdominal radiography or laparotomy for unrelated disease. Gallstones are frequently discovered at post-mortem, having caused no symptoms during life. In addition, elderly patients may be found to have carcinoma of the gallbladder in association with calculi which have been asymptomatic for many years.

ACUTE AND ACUTE-ON-CHRONIC CHOLECYSTITIS

Calculous cholecystitis

Calculi within the gallbladder commonly present as 'acute cholecystitis'. However, histological examination of most gallbladders removed surgically shows changes of chronic inflammation associated with the presence of gallstones. Acute inflammatory changes are sometimes superimposed, particularly if the gallbladder has been removed during an attack of acute cholecystitis. These acute-on-chronic changes are usually associated with gallstones and are commonly precipitated by calculous obstruction of the cystic duct. Varying degrees of chronic inflammation are found, particularly muscle hypertrophy, diverticula and fibrosis. Superimposed acute inflammatory changes include redness and patchy ulceration. The mucosa is incompletely covered by a fibrinopurulent exudate and there is intramural oedema separating the muscle and collagen bundles. Vasodilation is pronounced, with interstitial haemorrhages in the stroma. Initially, the neutrophil exudate appears small compared with these other changes, but subsequently it may become florid and form intramural abscesses.

Vessels show inflammatory changes: fibrin thrombi in capillaries and arterioles, together with reaction of vascular endothelium to the inflammatory process, are superimposed upon an endarteritis obliterans. In some cases necrosis of the wall may occur (gangrenous cholecystitis). Perforation is a common sequel of gangrenous cholecystitis, particularly in the elderly.[24] Focal areas of infarction are frequent in this condition and usually occur at the fundus of the gallbladder, the furthest point from the arterial inflow to the organ.

In rare instances fibrinoid necrosis may be found in the wall of an artery or arteriole. This latter finding has been interpreted as being the primary event by some authors.[47]

Acalculous cholecystitis

Acute cholecystitis also occurs on rare occasions when there is no preceding history of gallbladder disease; up to 10 per cent of all clinical cases of acute cholecystitis fall within this category and should be classified as acute acalculous cholecystitis.

The aetiology of this condition is multiple and the pathogenesis is often obscure.

Systemic infections may precipitate acalculous cholecystitis.[70] Streptococcal cholecystitis is a notifiable condition in children,[20] typhoid fever is complicated by cholecystitis on rare occasions[79] (see Chapter 51), and infection with gas-forming organisms, such as *Clostridium welchii*, is particularly severe.[16]

Acalculous cholecystitis may also develop as a complication of systemic disease, particularly diabetes mellitus.[53] Other disorders such as polyarteritis nodosa and sarcoidosis occasionally involve the gallbladder and present as acute cholecystitis.[48]

Acute acalculous cholecystitis has been reported following trauma,[46,70] and various operative procedures, for example, have been implicated. These include not only abdominal procedures but also hip and other orthopaedic operations.[36] Several cases of acute acalculous cholecystitis have been described following burns.[1,59]

Bacterial embolization, impaired local tissue perfusion and abnormal cellular metabolism can reasonably explain the pathogenesis of many cases. Other suggested factors of dubious significance include obstruction to the cystic duct by kinking, periductal adhesions or enlarged cystic lymph nodes,[35] and inflammation of the biliary tree caused by reflux of pancreatic secretions.[81]

On macroscopic examination the gallbladder is reddened, inflamed and has a thickened wall. A fibrinopurulent exudate may be present on the serosal surface. When the gallbladder is opened the thickened wall is usually extremely oedematous. The mucosal surface has a finely granular appearance and is both inflamed and covered with pus. Parts of the mucosa and wall may be yellow and necrotic. The contents of the gallbladder are a mixture of pus, fibrin, bile and blood. Microscopically there is little or no fibrosis. Throughout all layers there is vascular dilatation and congestion with gross oedema. Within the wall margination and emigration of polymorphs are seen with formation of abscesses of varying sizes. The mucosal surface is necrotic and ulcerated.

The acute necrotizing nature of this inflammation together with the absence of pre-existing fibrosis frequently results in perforation.

Gangrene of the gallbladder due to torsion

This very rare condition may arise if the mesentery of the gallbladder is redundant. Necrosis and gangrene of the organ with symptoms and signs of peritonitis result.[3,17,31,72]

Clinical Presentation

Acute cholecystitis is characterized by anorexia, nausea and vomiting, fever and severe pain in the right hypochondrium. On examination there is marked tenderness and guarding in the right hypochondrium, especially on deep inspiration (Murphy's sign), and a tender inflammatory mass may be palpable in this region. Occasionally a band of hyperaesthesia may be found between the right ninth and eleventh ribs posteriorly (Boas's sign). After 24 hours the inflamed gallbladder becomes less tender.

Differential diagnosis includes acute inflammation of a high retrocaecal appendix, acute pancreatitis, diverticulitis, renal infections and perforated peptic ulcer. Preliminary investigations include estimation of the haemoglobin, total white cell count, serum amylase, urinalysis and x-rays of the chest and abdomen as 10 to 20 per cent of gallstones may be visible on plain radiography (see Figure 53.1). Elevation of the serum amylase above 1000 iu is highly suggestive of acute pancreatitis. This investigation should be performed routinely because calculous disease of the biliary tree is the commonest precipitating cause of acute pancreatitis in the United Kingdom.

Conservative Management

Oral intake should initially be restricted to clear fluids. Intravenous infusion may be required if the patient is dehydrated or unable to tolerate oral fluids. Suitable analgesia (e.g. pethidine) and an anti-emetic are prescribed if required, and in severe cases the use of a wide-spectrum antibiotic is justified. The majority of attacks settle within two to three days and a fat-free diet may then be commenced. The patient is allowed home and further investigations are arranged as an outpatient.

Oral cholecystography is performed six to eight weeks later, by which time liver function, which is frequently impaired during the acute attack, has returned to normal. Non-opacification of the gallbladder at this time is strongly indicative of gallbladder disease and gallstones may be demonstrated (Figure 53.3). Ultrasonography may also be of value, particularly as it can be performed as soon as the initial severe attack has settled. Although this investigation is not as accurate in the diagnosis of cholelithiasis and gallbladder disease as conventional radiology, the advantages of achieving early diagnosis may be considerable. In certain centres the accuracy of diagnosis with ultrasound approaches that of cholecystography.[55] In our studies, however, a false negative diagnostic rate of 7 per cent occurred and more disturbingly there was a false positive rate of 3 per cent.[15] Further experience and improvements in equipment may increase the value of ultrasonography in the diagnosis of calculous cholecystitis. It is unlikely, however, to assume the prime importance in this situation that it has achieved in the diagnosis of obstructive jaundice.

When the diagnosis of cholelithiasis has been confirmed, elective cholecystectomy should be recommended, unless there are serious contraindications to surgery, as further symptoms may be anticipated in the majority of patients.

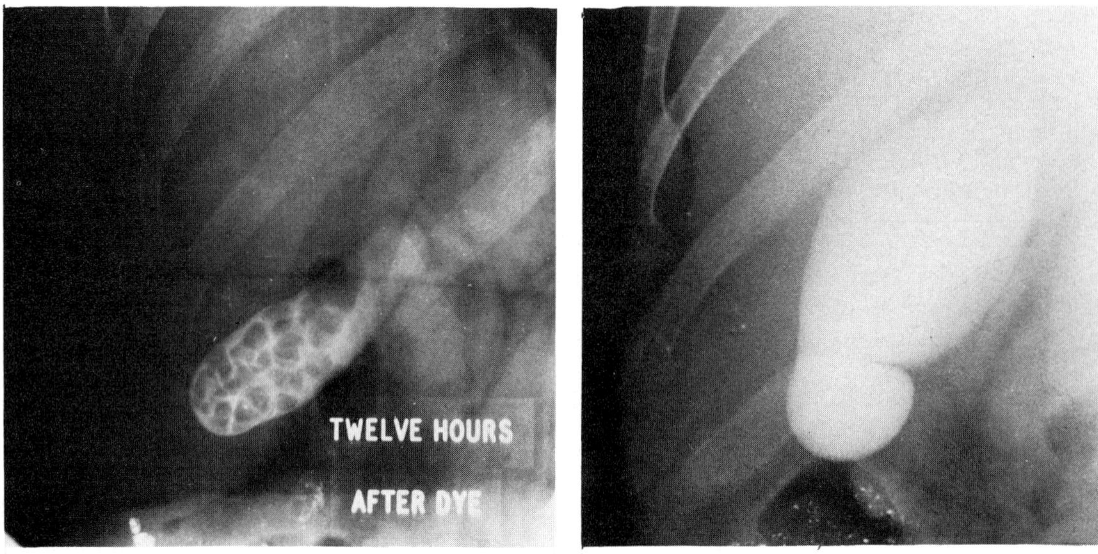

Figure 53.3. (a) Faceted gallstones seen on oral cholecystography. (b) Phygian cap. This commonest developmental abnormality of the gallbladder is associated with an increased incidence of gallstones.

Early Operation

Conservative treatment may have to be abandoned, especially in elderly patients who tolerate acute inflammation poorly, if signs and symptoms do not settle within 48 hours.

Cholecystostomy

In sick, and particularly elderly patients, simple drainage of the biliary tree by cholecystostomy (see below) may be advisable. When cholecystostomy has been performed, definitive cholecystectomy should in most cases be undertaken when the patient has fully recovered, even though dense adhesions at that time may make the procedure difficult. However, if further major surgery is deemed hazardous, an appreciable proportion of patients may remain free of further trouble. It is important, therefore, at the time of operation to clear the gallbladder completely of infected bile and calculi, particularly stones causing obstruction in Hartmann's pouch. Care should be taken to avoid forcing calculi down the cystic duct.

Early cholecystectomy

Patients with acute cholecystitis who are admitted during the initial attack can be satisfactorily treated by cholecystectomy at this time.[54,73,76,80,85] It is often easy and safe to perform cholecystectomy within the first 72 hours because of the absence of dense fibrous adhesions from previous inflammation. After the initial 72-hour period the formation of vascular adhesions makes accurate dissection more difficult so that the risk of damage to bile ducts is increased. The general condition of the patient, the experience of the surgeon, and the availability of operative cholangiography, all influence the decision to operate at this time. An additional hazard associated with early cholecystectomy is the increased risk of incorrect preoperative diagnosis.[54] Providing adequate safeguards are taken, however, early cholecystectomy offers the opportunity of reducing the overall morbidity and also the duration of hospitalization. Emergency operations on the biliary tree carry a significant risk of serious septic complications. Prophylactic antibiotic cover should therefore be used.

Complications of Acute Cholecystitis

Gangrene and perforation

These complications are particularly liable to occur in the elderly. Gangrene of the gallbladder may occur in the presence of severe inflammation and be either patchy or widespread. Occasionally the entire gallbladder is involved. Perforation and peritonitis ensue. The fundus of the gallbladder, being the point furthest from the main arterial supply, or Hartmann's pouch where an impacted calculus causes pressure necrosis, are sites particularly at risk.

Perforation of a chronically inflamed gallbladder will not infrequently produce a localized abscess rather than generalized peritonitis, due to dense adhesions and adherence of omentum. Fistulation into other organs also occurs (see below).

Mucocoele and empyema

Impaction of a calculus, which is usually large and solitary, in Hartmann's pouch causes distension of the gallbladder with mucus (mucocoele) or with a clear transudate (hydrops).

A non-tender mobile mass is palpable in the right hypochondrium. It may attain a large size and extend into the right iliac fossa. In assessing such a mass, palpation and percussion should commence in the fossa and proceed cephalad. Other masses which may be confused with a mucocoele include carcinomas of the ascending colon and hepatic flexure, cysts or tumours of the right kidney, omental masses and large intrahepatic lesions such as metastases or cysts. Necrosis and haemorrhage within hepatic lesions produce pain and local tenderness, and clinical differentiation from primary gallbladder pathology may be difficult. Specific radiological and other imaging investigations are then required (see Chapters 20, 21 and 22).

Infection of obstructed bile leads to distension of the organ with pus (empyema). This mass is extremely tender and the patient becomes toxic. Gram negative septicaemia is likely and emergency drainage of the biliary system under antibiotic cover is indicated.

Septicaemia

Patients with cholecystitis occasionally present in septicaemic shock even though there is no history of previous gallbladder disease. Faber and his colleagues[25] reported three such patients with positive blood cultures at the time of admission. *Clostridium welchii* was isolated from the blood of one patient and from the bile of another. Two of these three patients required dialysis for renal failure.

CHRONIC CHOLECYSTITIS

Chronic inflammation of the gallbladder is almost always found in association with gallstones. Although its pathogenesis is debatable, resolution of acute inflammation and recurrent mechanical irritation by calculi have been implicated.

The gallbladder is usually of normal size or somewhat smaller, though on occasion it may be very shrunken. The serosal surface has a grey-white appearance and the wall is of a similar colour and thickened. Occasionally, small yellow flecks of bile may be identified in the wall. Within the lumen gallstones are usually found and these may fill the organ or be contained in thick viscid biliary mud. The mucosal surface is finely granular or smooth and may show the impressions of the stones lying within the lumen.

Microscopically, pronounced fibrosis in the mucosa also separates the muscle bundles of the muscularis and forms a thick subserosal adventitial layer. The muscular coat is not only widely split by this fibrosis but is also hypertrophied.[32] The mucosa is flat and atrophic, having lost most of its papillary structure. Epithelial lined diverticula (Rokitansky–Aschoff sinuses) extend from the mucosa through the muscle coat and into the adventitia where they frequently become dilated. These diverticula are most commonly found in the body and fundus of the gallbladder and they may contain bile. They should not be confused with the mucus-secreting glands in the neck of the gallbladder.

Inflammatory cells are usually scanty and confined to a few lymphocytes, plasma cells and macrophages scattered through all layers. Occasionally, however, lymphoid follicles may be found and these may be a prominent feature. When inspissated bile from the diverticula escapes into the tissues a granulomatous foreign body giant cell reaction ensues. Bile is present in the midst of an inflammatory zone of foamy lipid-laden histiocytes, foreign body giant cells, lymphocytes and plasma cells. Cholesterol clefts are frequently present in the giant cells. Vessels within the wall of the gallbladder, especially in the adventitia, usually show endarteritis obliterans which is proportional to the severity of the chronic inflammatory changes.

Dystrophic calcification may occur as in any diseased organ. In the gallbladder it produces a characteristic translucent grey-white appearance and the wall is very brittle (porcelain gallbladder) (Figure 53.4).

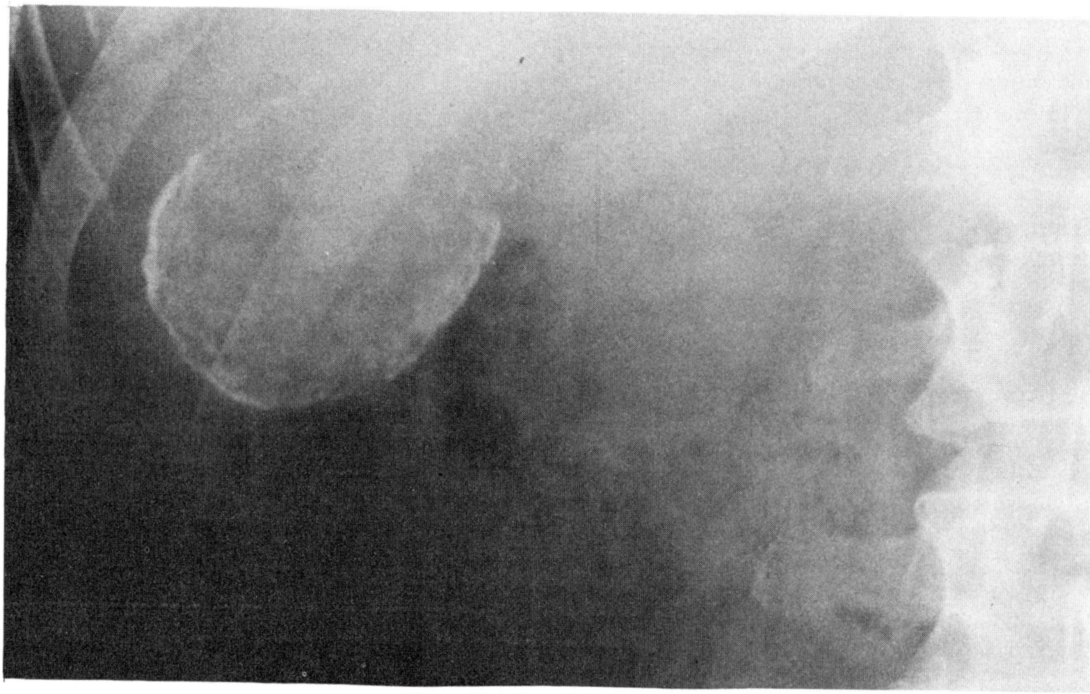

Figure 53.4. Porcelain gallbladder.

Inspissation of bile within the gallbladder follows chronic obstruction of the cystic duct or Hartmann's pouch by a stone, and can result in a mucocoele in which the contents of the organ become clear and mucoid.

Diverticular disease of the gallbladder may rarely be florid and the cystic distension great. This condition, 'cholecystitis glandularis proliferans', is particularly associated with narrow strictures of the gallbladder[7] (Figure 53.5).

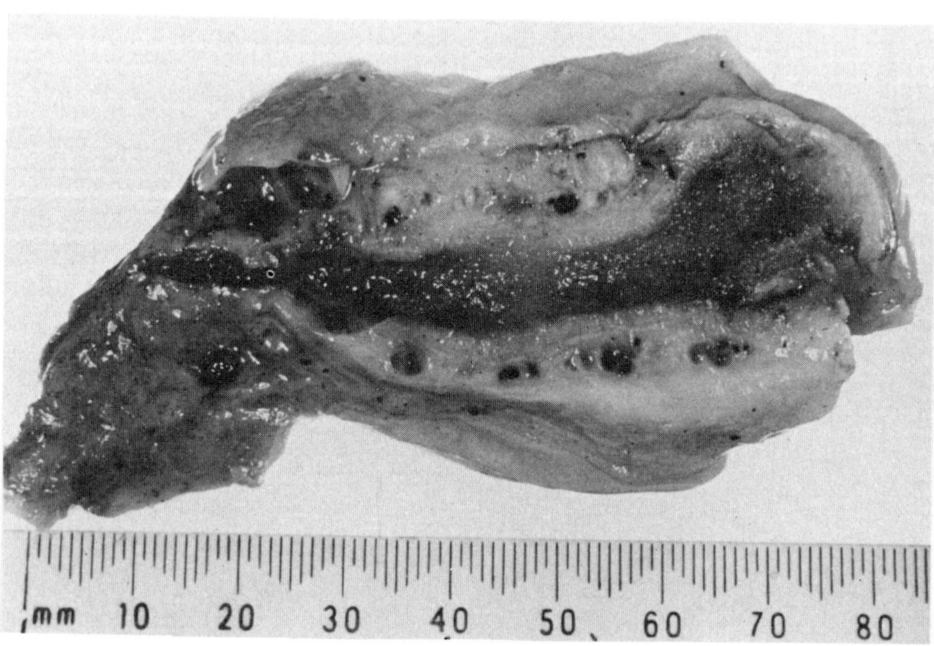

Figure 53.5. Cholecystitis glandularis proliferans.

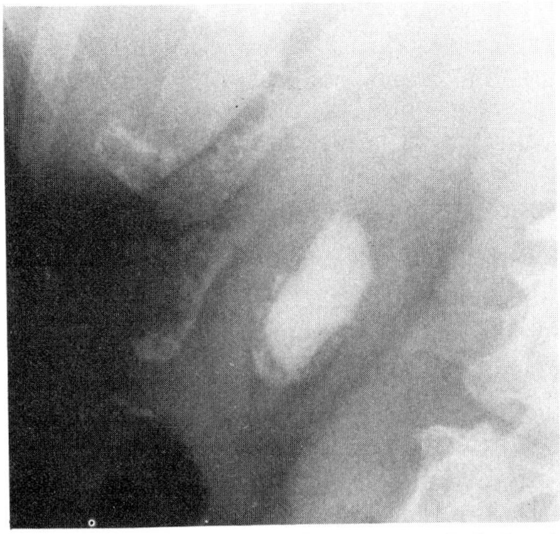

Figure 53.6. Adenomyomatosis seen on oral cholecystography after fatty meal.

A similar process localized to the fundus, in which numerous bundles of smooth muscle are intermingled, is termed adenomyoma[8] (Figure 53.6). Although this has been interpreted as a focal variant of cholecystitis glandularis proliferans, it is more probably a hamartomatous lesion.[19]

Occasionally, the gallbladder mucosa shows numerous yellow specks set against a dark green or, in the fresh state, a red background. This appearance has been likened to the outside of a strawberry and the condition termed 'strawberry gallbladder' or cholesterosis. Microscopically the tips of the papillary folds are distended and contain numerous foamy pale-staining macrophages. Using special techniques, cholesterol can be demonstrated within these cells.

Cholesterosis is associated with the presence of cholesterol stones.

Clinical Presentation

The following symptoms are the usual ways in which chronic inflammation of the gallbladder presents.

Flatulent dyspepsia

This complaint frequently occurs after meals, especially fatty ones, and is characterized by excessive belching, upper abdominal fullness and occasional heartburn. It is thus not always easily distinguished from symptoms produced by other upper gastrointestinal pathology such as peptic ulceration. In one series, sensitivity to fatty foods was found in nearly 70 per cent of patients with symptoms produced by gallstones.[22]

Nausea

This is the commonest single symptom[56] and is associated with intolerance of fatty foods. The sight or smell of such food is often sufficient to provoke an intense wave of nausea and may even produce vomiting.

Abdominal or chest pain

The patient may complain of vague abdominal or chest pain which defies accurate localization. Variations in the nature and distribution of discomfort and pain caused by gallbladder disease are manifold. This versatility of clinical presentation causes difficulties in diagnosis, and conditions such as myocardial ischaemia must be excluded. The pain may be acute in onset and severe in intensity. It is often localized in the right hypochondrium and may radiate through to the back between the shoulder blades.

This attack of pain is often associated with impaction of a stone in Hartmann's pouch and is precipitated by a heavy meal, particularly a fatty meal. The pain is not characteristically intermittent and cramplike as with intestinal colic. Rather it is of longer duration, lasting usually three or four hours, and is constant in intensity. Biliary 'spasm' is therefore a much more appropriate term than biliary 'colic'. After a few hours the stone may become dislodged and pain ceases. If the stone remains impacted acute cholecystitis is likely to supervene. In patients presenting with 'acute cholecystitis' it is not unusual to obtain a history of episodes of gallstone 'colic' which have occurred over a period of years.

Change of bowel habit

Some patients complain of a change in bowel habit, and both constipation or looseness of the motions may be noticed. The reported association of cholecystitis with diverticular disease and hiatus herniation (Saint's triad) is of doubtful validity.

Heartburn and regurgitation

In their survey, Earlam and Thomas[22] reported an incidence of heartburn in 42 per cent of patients whilst regurgitation of either bitter or acid-tasting fluid occurred in 31 per cent. The need to undertake gastrointestinal radiology and endoscopy should be remembered in such cases. Accurate preoperative diagnosis is the key to the reduction in the frequency of cases of 'post-cholecystectomy syndrome', where no convincing histological evidence is obtained to explain apparently organic symptomatology.

CALCULI IN MAJOR BILIARY DUCTS

Calculi are found in the common bile duct in approximately 10 per cent of patients with calculous disease. Though these may remain asymptomatic for many months, complications eventually develop in the majority of patients. Unrelieved obstruction leads to progressive impairment of hepatocellular function. Infection with consequent cholangitis or septicaemia invariably develops. Pressure necrosis causes perforation into the peritoneal cavity, intestinal tract and various other sites. Unless previous biliary diversion, such as choledochoduodenostomy, has been performed to allow free drainage of bile, calculi should be removed at the earliest opportunity.

Obstructive jaundice

Impaction of calculi in the common bile duct usually occurs at its lower end above the ampulla. The intensity of the jaundice may fluctuate if the calculus becomes dislodged, releasing bile into the duodenum. Partial obstruction to the flow of bile is common. If the calculus remains impacted, however, jaundice deepens with progressive hepatocellular impairment.

Physical examination is often normal apart from icterus. Residual tenderness in the right hypochondrium, however, may be present and other stigmata of hepatocellular dysfunction may develop. If the gallbladder is palpable in a jaundiced patient the cause is usually neoplastic obstruction of the biliary tree (Courvoisier's law). This is most frequently due to carcinoma of the head of the pancreas. The additional statement often made, that enlargement of the gallbladder is unlikely because of fibrosis from chronic inflammation, is patently untrue. Every experienced surgeon has seen dilated, chronically inflamed gallbladders. This point has been emphasized by Lord Smith,[75] yet the fallacy is perpetuated in clinical teaching.

Exceptions occur to this useful dictum. For example, if one calculus is impacted in the lower end of the common bile duct and a second stone obstructs the cystic duct, a mucocoele or empyema develops in addition to the obstructive jaundice. On the other hand, malignant obstruction high in the biliary tree, for example at the porta hepatis or in the common hepatic duct, produces jaundice without dilatation of the gallbladder.

In the majority of patients, a careful history and examination, urinalysis and simple blood tests will achieve diagnosis. The use of non-invasive liver imaging by ultrasound, and with the newer hepatobiliary agents such as hydroxyindole-diacetic acid (HIDA), increases the accuracy of definitive diagnosis in skilled hands to over 90 per cent of cases. Only in the remaining few patients are more invasive procedures such as endoscopic retrograde cholangiopancreatography and transhepatic cholangiography necessary. Using these techniques the level and nature of the obstruction should be revealed preoperatively in nearly all patients (see Chapter 26).

Ascending cholangitis

Fever and rigors associated with obstructive jaundice characterize 'Charcot's triad', or 'intermittent hepatic fever'. These are the sequelae of ascending infection associated with bile stasis. Elderly patients with calculous disease are particularly at risk as 70 per cent have infected bile.[18] Liver function is deranged, occasionally severely, and antibiotic therapy and relief of the biliary obstruction are urgently required to prevent septicaemia. Timing of surgical intervention is critical. With an immediate response to antibiotic therapy surgery may be delayed for a day or two. If, however, the fever continues or if the patient's condition deteriorates with progressive hepatocellular dysfunction, emergency drainage of the biliary tree is mandatory. Acute liver failure may otherwise be precipitated.

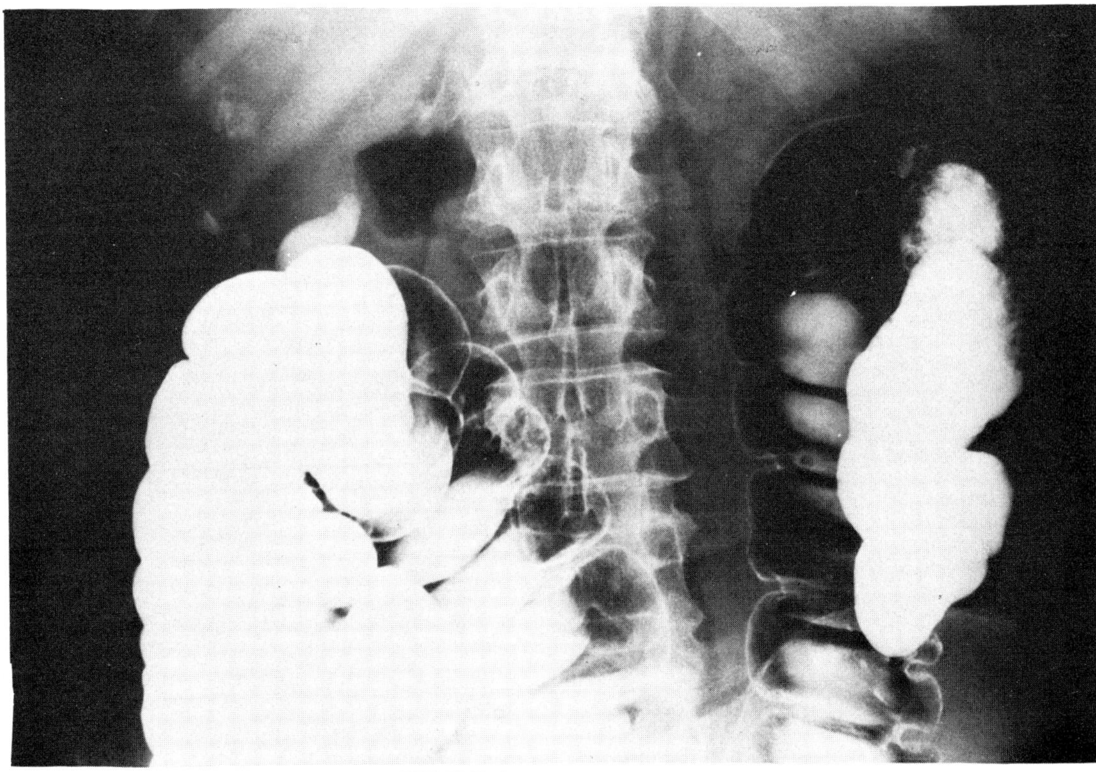

Figure 53.7. Fistula between colon and gallbladder demonstrated on barium enema.

Acute pancreatitis

Calculous disease of the biliary tree may present with acute pancreatitis. Patients presenting in this way should therefore be investigated for the presence of gallstones as soon as possible. Ultrasonography is of particular value, being non-invasive and independent of hepatocellular function. Oral cholecystography is often unhelpful for several weeks following a severe attack of acute pancreatitis due to associated impairment of hepatocellular function.

BILIARY FISTULAE

This section excludes operative fistulae, which are discussed in Chapter 54.

Biliary fistulae usually occur as a result of pressure necrosis from calculi lying within a chronically inflamed gallbladder or major bile duct. Although cases of external cutaneous fistulae have been reported the vast majority occur into other internal organs. The commonest fistula (70 to 80 per cent) is that between the gallbladder and the duodenum (cholecystoduodenal). Rarer fistulae occur between the gallbladder and the common bile duct (cholecystocholedochal), the common bile duct and the duodenum (choledochoduodenal) and the gallbladder and the colon (cholecystocolic) (Figure 53.7). Diverticular disease, carcinoma of the hepatic flexure and Crohn's disease must be suspected in the latter variety. A penetrating duodenal ulcer can form a fistula with either the gallbladder or the common bile duct (Figure 53.8). Trauma, amoebic abscess and hydatid disease may also rarely be responsible.

Cases of fistulation into the stomach, right pleural cavity and bronchial tree, pericardial cavity, portal vein, small intestine, urinary bladder and pelvis of the right kidney have been reported.[51]

GALLSTONE ILEUS

Intestinal obstruction caused by calculi (gallstone ileus) has a peak incidence at 60 years of age and rarely occurs before 50 years.

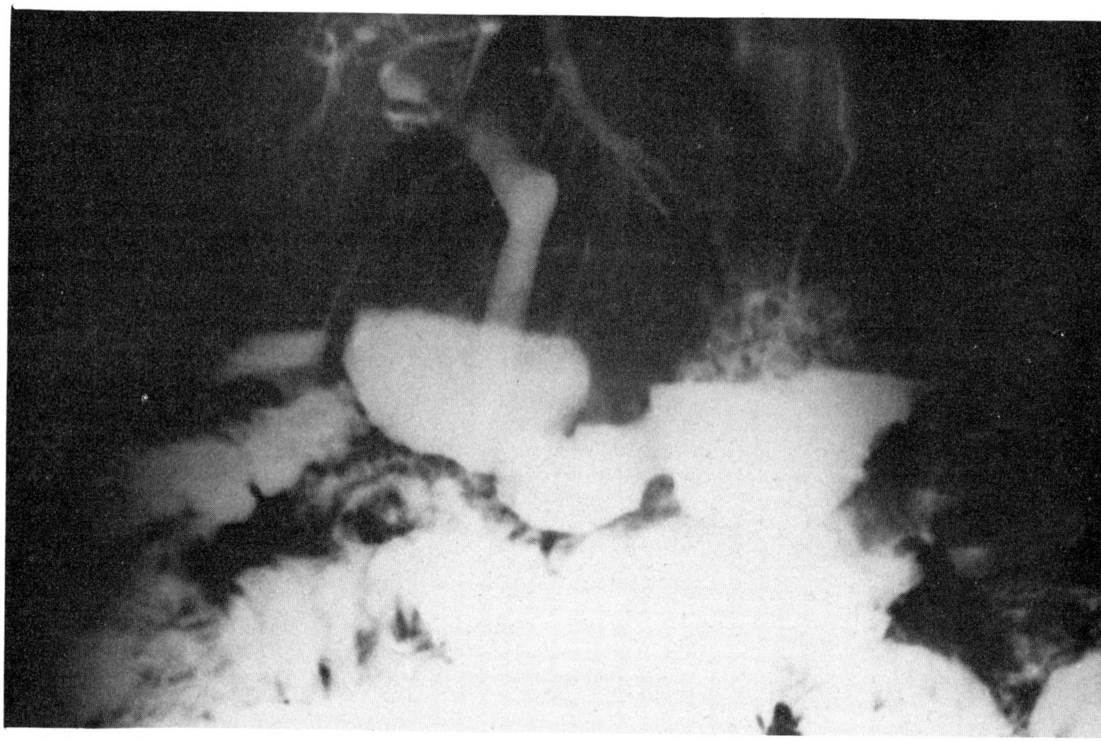

Figure 53.8. Fistula from duodenum to common bile duct.

Gallstone ileus accounts for some 2 per cent of all cases of intestinal obstruction[37] and females are affected more commonly than males (7:1). In comparison, the female preponderance for fistula formation alone is only 3:1 so that other factors, such as the relatively smaller diameter of the intestinal lumen in the female, must account for this discrepancy.

Calculi which cause intestinal obstruction are usually larger than 2.5 cm in diameter.[71] Smaller stones mixed with faeces, however, may obstruct a colon already stenosed by diverticular or other disease. Gallstone ileus is associated with a high morbidity and death has been reported in up to 35 per cent of patients.[78] The high complication rate is largely due to difficulties in achieving early diagnosis. Obstruction is intermittent and occurs at progressively lower sites in the intestine. Patients are often obese and have associated cardiorespiratory disease. Serious fluid and electrolyte disturbance are added complications.

In 40 per cent of patients there is a history of biliary tract disease, such as biliary 'colic' or right hypochondrial pain. A recent episode of severe pain due to erosion of the gallstone into the duodenum may also have occurred. Previous episodes of jaundice or ascending cholangitis, however, are not common. As already stressed, the intestinal obstruction is characteristically intermittent, and occurs at progressively lower parts of the bowel. Obstruction may occur in the duodenum, but the commonest site is the narrowest part of the ileum two feet proximal to the ileocaecal valve, the site of rotation of the gut and of a Meckel's diverticulum. In 179 cases reported by Brockis in 1957[12] obstruction occurred in the ileum in 72 per cent. It may, however, occur at almost any level, and reported sites include the pylorus, duodenum, jejunum, ileocaecal valve and sigmoid colon. The variation in signs and symptoms caused by the changing level of obstruction should, in fact, be an aid to diagnosis.[23]

The demonstration of air in the biliary tree on abdominal radiography is sufficient to warrant laparotomy (Figure 53.9). Occasionally the calculus may be visible within the lumen of the bowel (Figure 53.10). Operation should be undertaken under suitable prophylactic antibiotic cover after correction of fluid and electrolyte losses. At laparotomy it is sometimes possible to milk the stone proximally into healthy bowel and crush it without breaching the integrity of the bowel lumen. If this

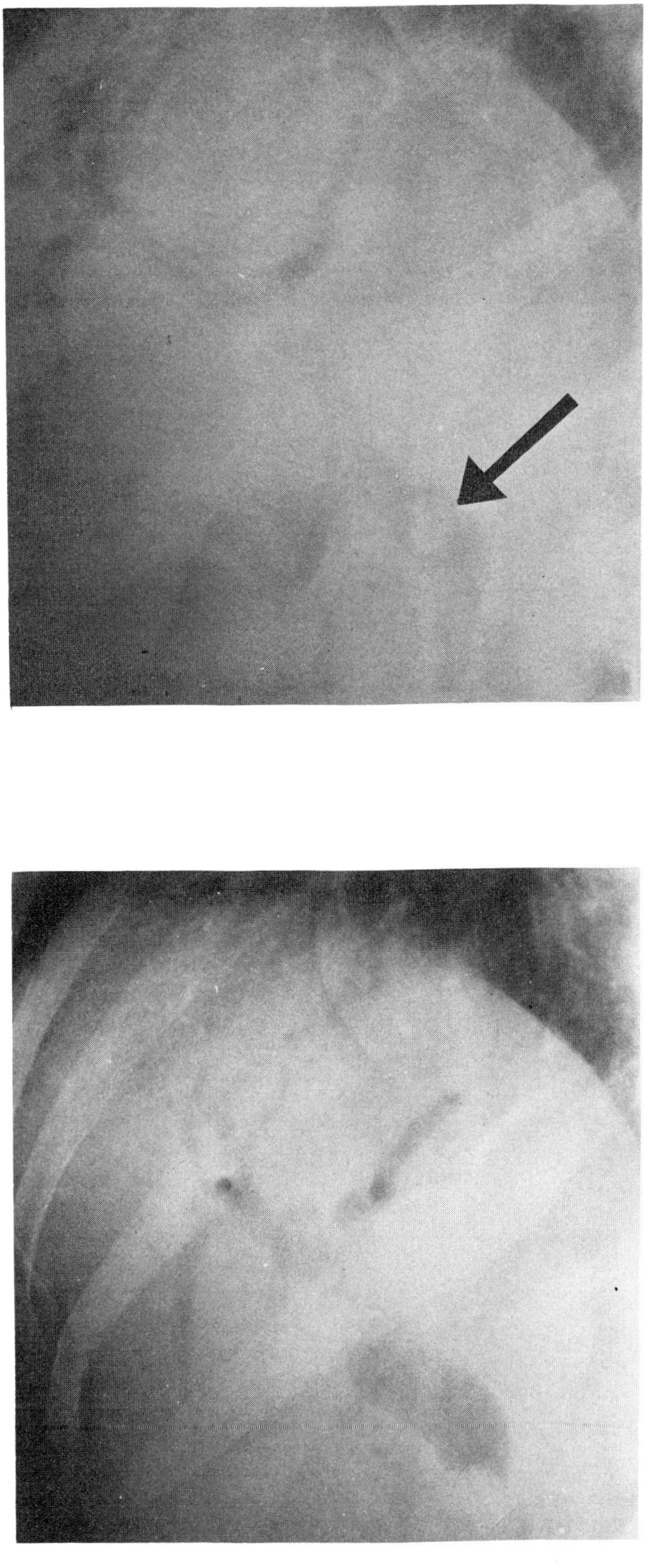

(a)

(b)

Figure 53.9. Gas in biliary tree resulting from passage of stone into bowel. An additional mobile calculus within the duct is outlined by this gas: (a) supine (calculus marked with arrow); (b) erect.

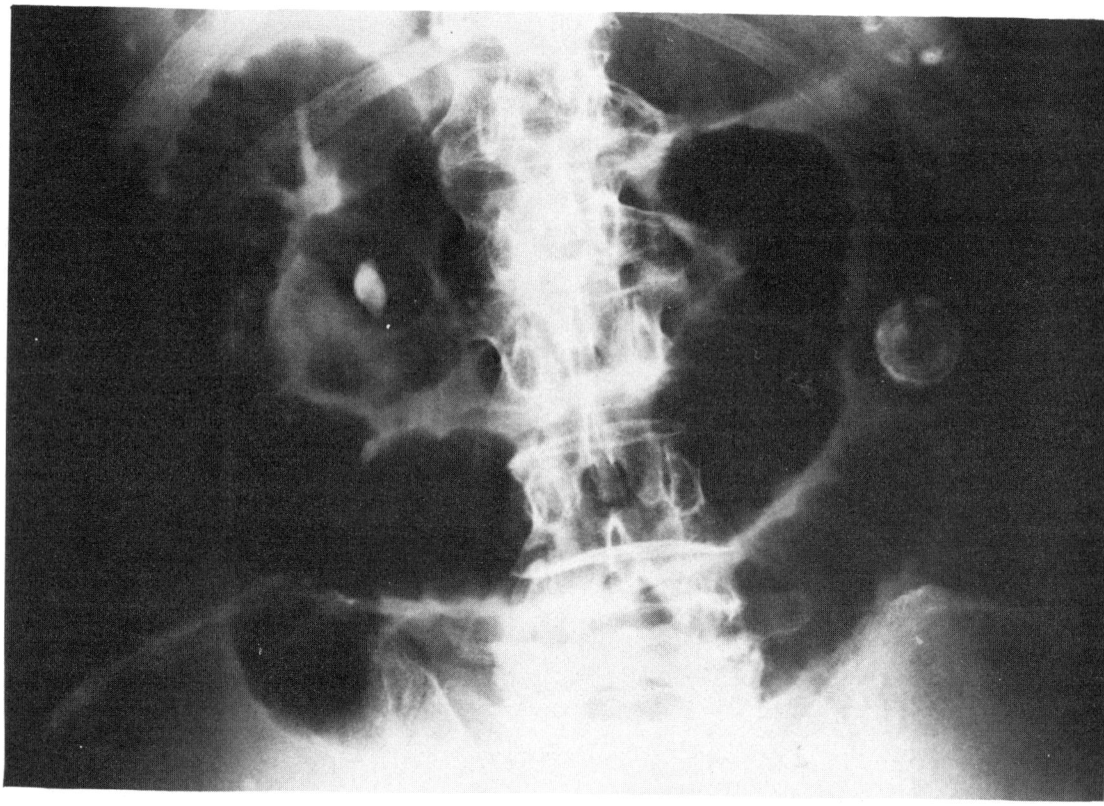

Figure 53.10. Gallstone in small bowel.

manoeuvre cannot be achieved the calculus should be removed through an enterotomy made in the antimesenteric border. Gangrenous or perforated bowel should be dealt with in the usual manner and careful examination of the rest of the bowel made to exclude further calculi. Firmly impacted calculi are more safely managed by formal resection than by extensive enterotomy. Occasional cases of multiple calculi causing either a closed loop or else recurrent intestinal obstruction have been reported.[26] Attention to the primary biliary pathology at this time is often unnecessary and may be hazardous. If after the operation the patient suffers from cholangitis or recurrent biliary 'colic', and subsequent investigations reveal calculi in the biliary tract, then cholecystectomy, exploration of the bile ducts and closure of the fistula must be advised.

ANTIBIOTIC THERAPY IN BILIARY TRACT SURGERY

Biliary tract surgery is associated with a high incidence of serious septic complications.[18,39]

Although many of these complications may be prevented or treated by appropriate antibiotic therapy, indiscriminate use of these agents should be condemned. Patients who are particularly at risk include the elderly, the obese and patients with jaundice or recent rigors. Emergency procedures, exploration of the common bile duct and procedures in which the integrity of the intestinal lumen is breached are all associated with increased risk. Most patients with uncomplicated acute cholecystitis settle satisfactorily with bed-rest, clear fluids and analgesics. During the conservative management of these patients antibiotics may be indicated if the patient fails to settle or if complications arise. When surgery is undertaken, however, there is good evidence of the value of carefully chosen antibiotic prophylaxis, particularly in these high-risk patients.[60,77]

Organisms most commonly responsible for biliary tract sepsis in western countries are those commonly found in the intestinal lumen. Anaerobic organisms such as *Bacteroides*, however, are surprisingly infrequently detected, despite the use of sensitive culture media and assay techniques.[38] In the East, however, these anaerobes appear to play a significant role in biliary tract sepsis,[74] particularly in the elderly.

This difference in the bacterial flora in the biliary tree may well arise as a result of the high incidence of parasitic infestation in eastern countries (see Chapter 56).

Antibiotics for use in the treatment of biliary tract infection must possess the relevant spectrum of activity against those organisms commonly found in bile. In particular, they should be active against *E. coli*, *Klebsiella*, *Streptococcus faecalis* and *Staphylococcus*.[38,77] Activity against less frequent but potentially serious organisms, such as *Pseudomonas* and *Proteus*, is also an advantage.

Good biliary excretion of the antibiotic is often claimed to be advantageous in hepatobiliary disease. Systemic activity, however, is more important. Protection from wound sepsis following biliary tract surgery has been shown with aminoglycosides such as gentamicin which are poorly excreted in bile.[40] Similar protection has been observed in the presence of obstructive jaundice when the biliary excretion of the chosen antibiotic, such as the cephalosporin, cephazolin, is negligible.[60] When antibiotics are used prophylactically for biliary tract procedures, positive bacterial cultures are still obtained from bile.[6,38,77] Relief of the obstruction and the careful removal of calculi and debris are basic principles which must therefore be adhered to in the management of biliary sepsis.

Chemoprophylaxis in Biliary Tract Surgery

With recognition of the risk of serious septic complications following operations on the biliary tree, considerable interest has been shown in the potential value of prophylactic antibiotic regimens. This interest has developed despite the acknowledged hazards of prophylactic chemotherapy. In addition to those patients with high-risk factors already mentioned, cases arise in which septicaemia and death may occur, even in fit young patients undergoing straightforward cholecystectomy.[6] The use of suitable chemoprophylaxis should therefore be considered in any biliary tract procedure, particularly when high-risk factors, e.g. obesity or jaundice, have been identified or are likely to arise, e.g. exploration of the biliary tree or breaching of the intestinal lumen.

What criteria, however, should apply to a prophylactic antibiotic regimen?

Firstly, the chosen antibiotic must possess the relevant spectrum of activity against those organisms which are likely to be responsible for the septic complications. Not only should it possess the appropriate spectrum of activity, however, but it must also be delivered in such a way that adequate concentrations are present in tissues for long enough to be effective. The timing of the administration of prophylactic antibiotics has been shown to be critical.[14] The chosen regimen must achieve satisfactory tissue levels before manipulation of the biliary tree is commenced as dissemination of organisms is likely to be produced at this time.

Secondly, the chosen antibiotic must be safe. Hazards which are acceptable in the therapy of life-threatening conditions are not acceptable for prophylaxis. Major hazards include oto- and nephrotoxicity and hypersensitivity reactions, and these are all avoidable.

Finally, encouragement of the emergence of resistant organisms and production of superinfections such as candidiasis give particular cause for concern. Short courses of antibiotics in adequate doses appear to reduce this risk. The ultimate extension of this philosophy is, of course, a single dosage regimen.

We have chosen, therefore, to evaluate a 2 g dose of cephazolin given intramuscularly at the time of premedication.[30,60] This cephalosporin is excreted in bile,[67] has a wide spectrum of activity against those organisms likely to cause sepsis and is of low toxicity. Furthermore, the emergence of resistant organisms against cephaloridine, an antibiotic of the same family of cephalosporins, has not been seen following the installation of this antibiotic into the wound in over 1000 cases.[64]

Following the administration of 2 g with the premedication, the average blood levels of cephazolin at induction of anaesthesia were 60 mg/l, and these levels were maintained throughout the operative procedures. Average levels in the common bile duct exceeded 30 mg/l provided there was no obstruction. Cephazolin levels in gallbladder bile were 17 mg/l.

In patients with obstructive jaundice, however, negligible levels of the antibiotic were present in the bile. Despite this fact these patients were protected against wound sepsis (see below). We therefore support Keighley's assertion that systemic levels of an antibiotic are more important than levels in the bile for the prevention of septic complications.[40,41]

The levels of cephazolin in blood were considerably in excess of the concentrations likely to be effective against most organisms. For example, 95 per cent of strains of *E. coli* are inhibited by a concentration of 6 mg/l or less of cephazolin[69] and these organisms are likely to be present in bile.[38,44] Staphylococci are the predominant organisms associated with all postoperative wound infections[65] and virtually all strains of staphylococci are inhibited at a concentration of 0.3 mg/l.[69]

Cephalosporins are associated with a very low incidence of toxic reactions. Providing blood levels are monitored they can be safely used even in renal failure.[62] Patients with a blood urea in excess of 6 mmol/l (35 mg/dl), however, were excluded from our studies. Allergic reactions to cephalosporins have been recorded and approximately 8 per cent of patients who are sensitive to penicillin are also sensitive to these antibiotics.[63] Patients with a history of allergy to penicillin were therefore excluded from these studies.

Serious postoperative septic complications were reduced from 12 to 2 per cent in patients receiving 2 g of cephazolin, including patients with obstructive jaundice.[30,60] Strachan and his colleagues[77] report similar results using the same antibiotic in a multicentre trial.

In addition, a reduction in both hospital stay and other septic complications was observed in the treated group.[61] No toxic reactions occurred and no evidence of alterations in bacterial flora was found in patients receiving prophylactic therapy.

In a further recent study, Morran and his co-workers[57] evaluated the prophylactic use of an intravenous infusion of 10 ml of co-trimoxazole (160 mg trimethoprim plus 800 mg sulphamethoxazole). A reduction in wound sepsis from 21 to 4 per cent was found and a reduction in postoperative pulmonary complications was also noted.

From these studies it is apparent that a carefully chosen prophylactic antibiotic regimen is of value, particularly in high-risk cases undergoing biliary tract surgery. Constant vigilance, however, is required for potential hazards, particularly the emergence of resistant organisms. Because of such hazards it is our belief that the use of 'first-line', life-saving, therapeutic agents such as gentamicin, is not justified for prophylaxis. These antibiotics should be reserved for the treatment of established infection.

OPERATIVE PROCEDURES

Cholecystectomy

After induction of general anaesthesia the patient is positioned on an operating table suitable for cholangiography. A 10 to 15° tilt to the right ensures that the biliary tree does not overlie the spine which might interfere with interpretation of radiographs.

Following skin preparation with Betadine or other suitable agent, towels are attached by stitching them to the skin or with an adhesive transparent dressing to avoid the use of radiopaque metal skin clips. Various incisions are suitable, including upper right paramedian, upper midline, Kocher's, Mayo Robson or transverse incisions. Oblique or transverse incisions are particularly suitable in obese patients with a wide costal arch. They are readily extended laterally to allow excellent access to the duodenum should mobilization of this be required (Kocher's manoeuvre). Extra exposure may similarly be achieved by adding a transverse limb to a paramedian incision, but this will increase the risk of wound dehiscence and herniation unless great care is taken with closure. Non-absorbable sutures such as nylon should be used, and additional deep tension sutures may be required.

Systematic careful laparotomy is performed, assessing the hiatus, stomach and duodenum. The intestinal tract is examined throughout its length, and the liver, spleen, kidneys, uterus and ovaries palpated.

Following severe inflammatory episodes dense adhesions may surround the gallbladder and the omentum may be adherent. These adhesions must be carefully dissected from the right.

A pack is placed over the duodenum and the assistant standing on the patient's left side spreads his left hand so that the common bile duct lies between the second and third fingers. He then applies traction downwards and to the left to put the bile duct on the stretch and with his right hand retracts the liver upwards with a lipless deep retractor. If access is difficult a second assistant should retract the liver.

The free edge of peritoneum containing the cystic duct is divided with scissors and this duct is exposed by blunt dissection. The peritoneal fold often contains an appreciable amount of fat which must be cleared before the anatomy can be properly displayed. Dissection is aided by lateral traction to the gallbladder using a sponge-holding or other suitable large forceps.

Ligation of the cystic artery

It is convenient to dissect the cystic artery at an early stage so that the cystic duct can be straightened prior to cholangiography. Variations in the arterial supply of the gallbladder are common (Figure 53.11). Careful dissection and display are thus important. The artery may be divided between ligatures if these can be safely applied. However, if there is difficulty in applying two ligatures it is usually safe to apply a single securely tied ligature of thread or silk to the cystic artery well away from the gallbladder, and diathermy the end on the gallbladder wall. To apply the ligature, an angled clamp (e.g. Lahey forceps) is passed around the artery and a loaded ligature carrier passed down to it. When the ligature has been securely tied the cystic artery is divided, leaving a stump on the hepatic arterial side which is long enough so that the ligature does not inadvertently slip off.

Care must be taken in the display of the cystic artery to avoid damage to the right hepatic artery. This usually runs near the superior border of the neck of the gallbladder before turning cephalad into the right lobe of the liver. Although damage can often be satisfactorily repaired with 4/0 arterial sutures, ligation may rarely be necessary to control haemorrhage. In the event of major haemorrhage the temptation to apply clamps blindly to try to stop the bleeding should be rigorously resisted. Instead, immediate control is obtained by finger and thumb compression of the main hepatic trunk as it lies in the lesser omentum (Pringle's manoeuvre). Control may be achieved from either side of the table but once achieved it is helpful if the assistant maintains it. This manoeuvre allows accurate vascular repair or time to summon help from a more experienced surgeon. With a bloodless field the area of damage can be carefully inspected. Intermittent relaxation of control readily identifies the site of the bleeding. A soft clamp applied accurately to the right hepatic artery gives additional control during repair. Repair or even ligature of the right hepatic artery usually produces no more than a moderate temporary impairment of hepatocellular function, providing this was previously normal.

Blind application of crushing clamps in an attempt to stem brisk haemorrhage will probably damage the ductal system with subsequent stenosis. Inadvertent ligature of ducts may also occur.

Dissection of biliary ducts

The area between common hepatic and cystic ducts (Calot's triangle) is then cleared so that the junction of these two ducts can be positively identified. Blunt pledget dissection displacing the leaf of peritoneum upwards is usually satisfactory. A blunt angled dissector (e.g. Lahey forceps) may be used to clear the cystic duct down to the junction, and traction on the gallbladder at this time is helpful. It is important to keep the dissection close to the cystic duct to avoid damage to vessels in this critical triangle. Care should also be taken to avoid displacing calculi from the gallbladder into the ducts.

Rare hamartomatous malformations of the portal system may prove particularly hazardous during this dissection.[28]

Various abnormalities in the ductal system are shown in Figure 53.12. Failure to display the anatomy properly leads to tragedies. When there is absolutely no doubt that the ducts have been correctly identified, a ligature is placed around the cystic duct near to the gallbladder to prevent displacement of calculi into the common bile duct.

Operative cholangiography

Most surgeons perform operative cholangiography routinely. Properly performed this procedure reduces the incidence of negative exploration of the ducts.[45] Careless application of this valuable technique, however, may result in unnecessary morbidity. Negative exploration of a narrow biliary tree, for example, may cause late stricture formation. Difficulties in interpretation of the films arise with introduction of air bubbles which cause radiolucent filling defects. The introduction of an excessive amount of contrast at the first injection also may obscure small radiopaque calculi. To avoid this latter difficulty the injection of 1 ml is usually enough for the first film.

Operative cholangiography is performed by cannulation of the cystic duct after the cystic artery has been divided and the cystic duct ligated at the neck of the gallbladder. The duct distal to this ligature is opened on its anterior surface with scissors or a fine blade. Suitable cannulae are illustrated in Figure 53.13. They should be connected to a syringe filled with saline and all air bubbles expelled from the system. At the time of cannulation the saline is gently expressed by the nurse to prevent

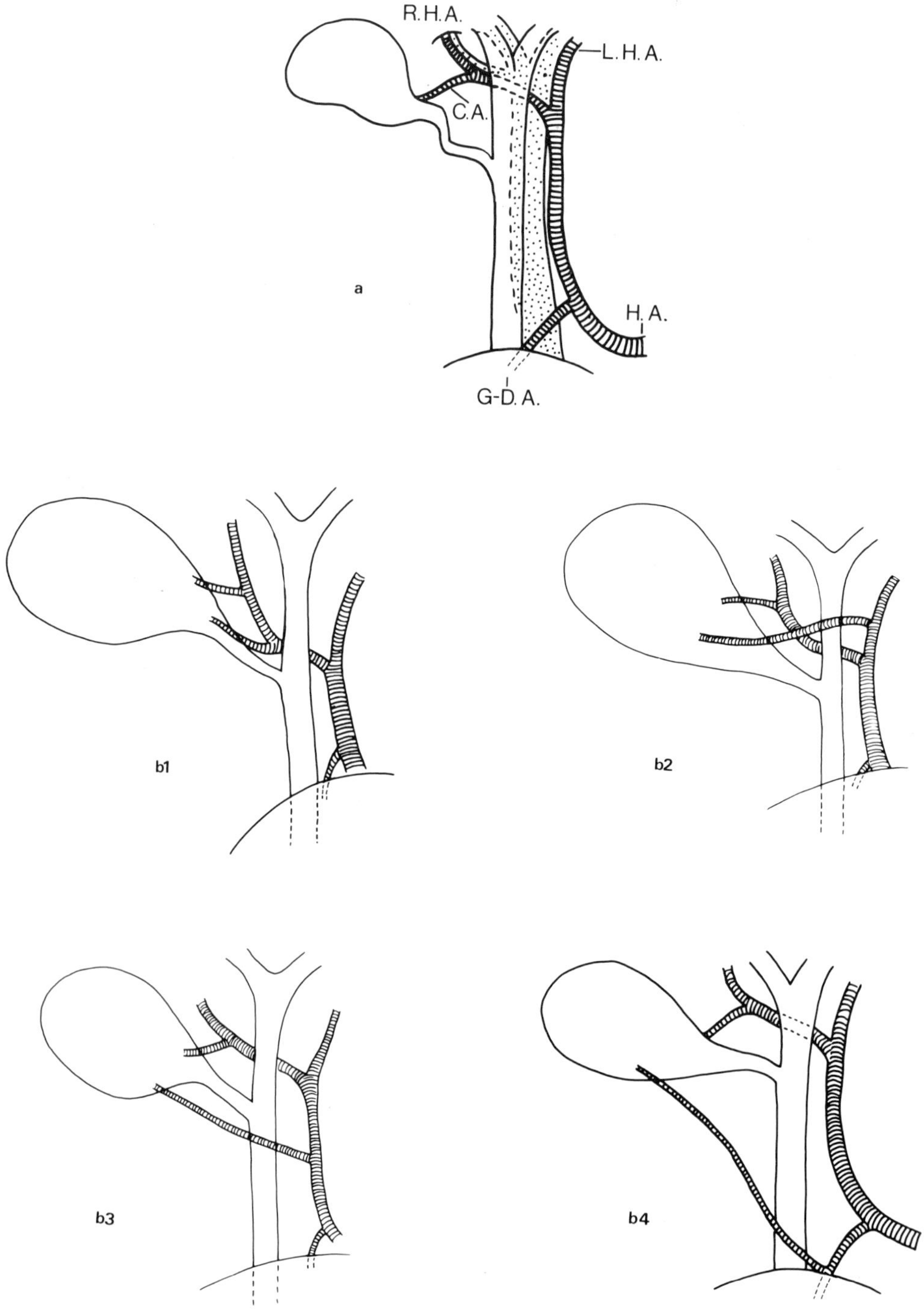

Figure 53.11. Hepatic arterial variations. (a) Normal relationship of vessels with the biliary tree. R.H.A. = right hepatic artery; L.H.A. = left hepatic artery; C.A. = cystic artery; G-D.A. = gastroduodenal artery; H.A. = hepatic artery. Portal vein is shown stippled.

(b) Accessory cystic arteries arising from (1) right hepatic artery; (2) left hepatic artery; (3) hepatic artery; (4) gastroduodenal artery.

(c) Abnormalities of main artery (1) looping in front of biliary tree; (2) bifurcating in front of ducts; (3) main trunk passing behind ducts with left hepatic artery passing in front; (4) high origin of gastroduodenal artery.

(d) Variations of right hepatic artery: (1) low bifurcation with artery lying alongside cystic duct; (2) artery looping behind gallbladder before turning to enter liver; (3) abnormal origin (e.g. from superior mesenteric artery).

It must be emphasized that although such congenital abnormalities may cause danger for the unwary, operative difficulties are far more commonly caused by distortion or obliteration of previously normal anatomy by inflammation.

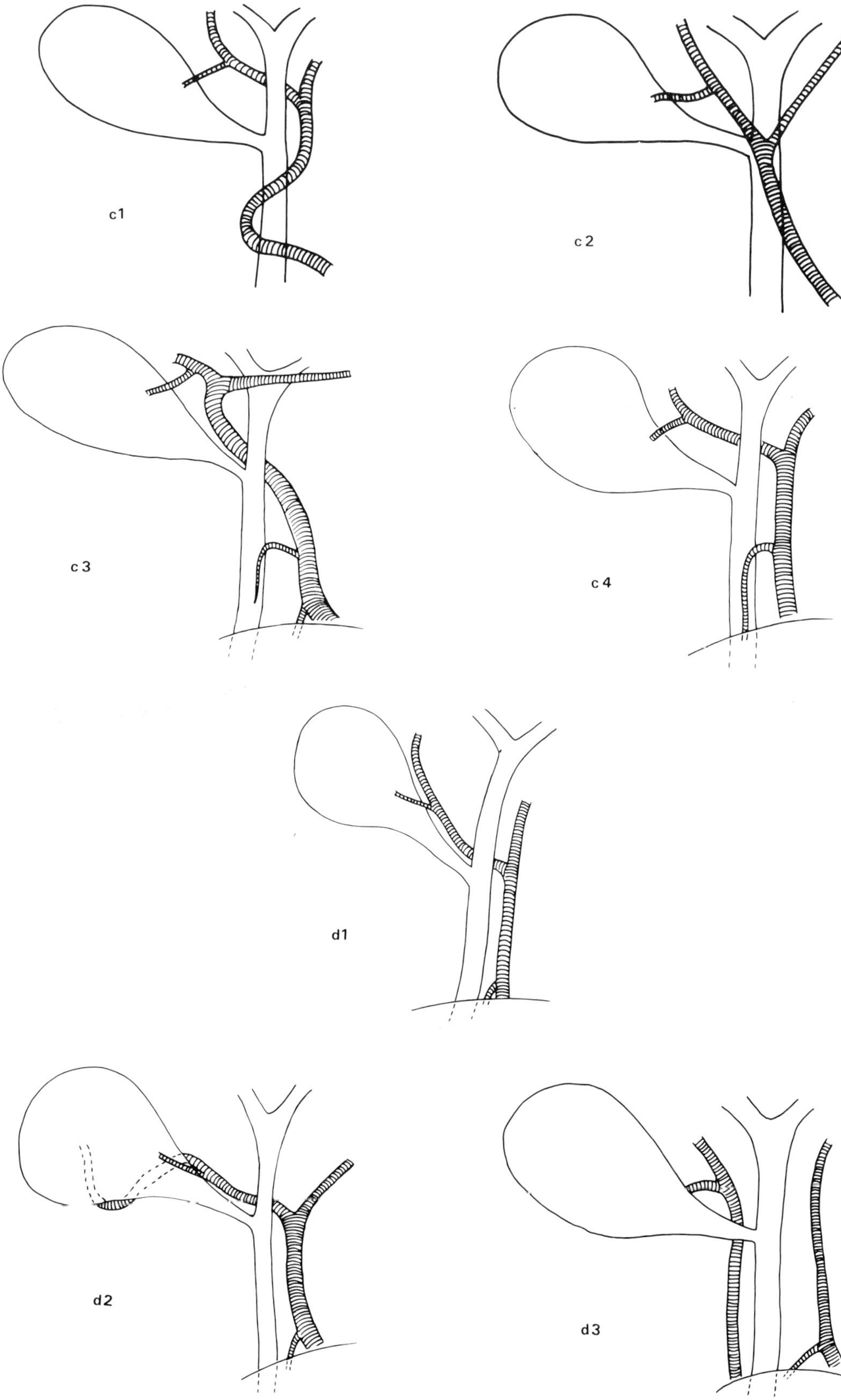
c1
c2
c3
c4
d1
d2
d3

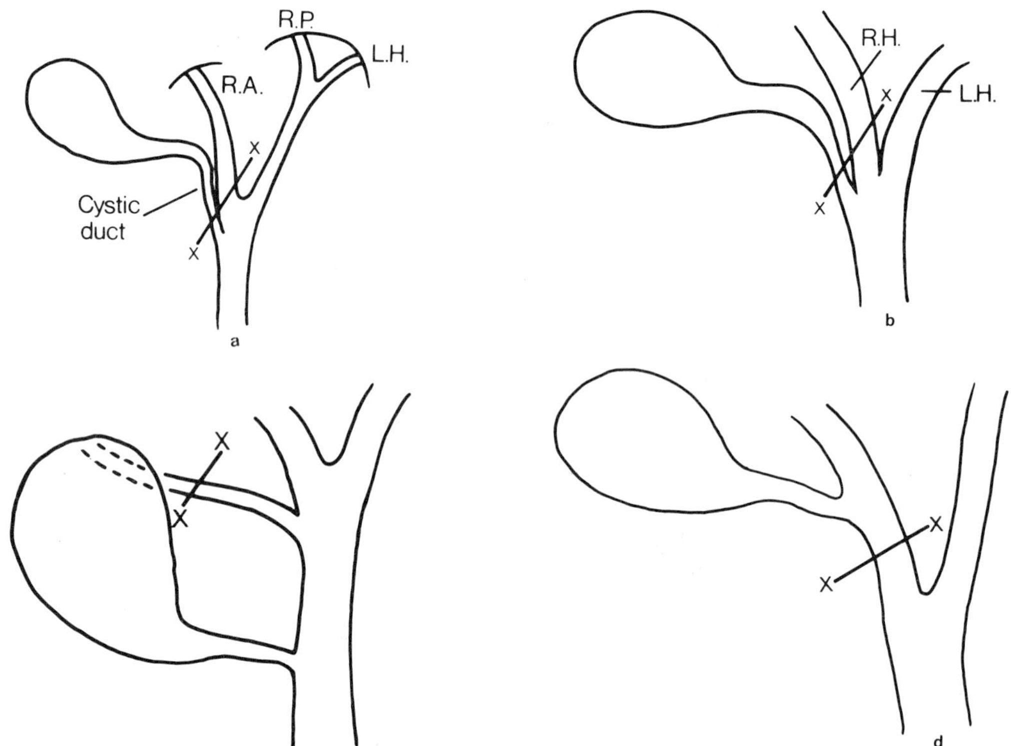

Figure 53.12. Anatomical variations in extrahepatic biliary tree. (a) Right anterior hepatic duct adjacent to cystic duct. (b) Right hepatic duct adjacent to cystic duct. (c) Subvesical duct. (d) Cystic duct joining right hepatic duct.
x—x = injury is liable at this site; R.A. = right anterior hepatic duct; R.P. = right posterior hepatic duct; R.H. = right hepatic duct; L.H. = left hepatic duct.
In addition, on very rare occasions the gallbladder may be congenitally absent or duplicated.
It must be emphasized that although such congenital abnormalities may cause danger for the unwary, operative difficulties are far more commonly caused by distortion or obliteration of previously normal anatomy by inflammation.

introduction of air bubbles into the duct. If cannulation of the cystic duct cannot be achieved, dye may be injected directly into the common duct using a fine needle. A 'butterfly' needle is useful for this purpose. Bile leakage, however, is liable to occur with this technique. Three injections of half strength Conray 280, or similar contrast medium, are performed. Following the initial 1 ml, a second injection of 2 to 3 ml and a final 5 to 10 ml will outline the biliary tree in most cases (Figure 53.14). Further amounts, however, may be required to outline a grossly dilated system. If a negative filling defect is seen and an air bubble is suspected, the biliary tree should be repeatedly flushed with saline before further contrast is injected.

Persistent filling defects suggest the presence of calculi in the ducts. If these defects are irregular and faceted, the likelihood of multiple calculi, which may occupy intrahepatic as well as extrahepatic ducts, should be borne in mind. A common duct lumen wider than 12 mm is suspicious of obstruction. It must be remembered, however, that there is a wide range in the diameter of the normal undilated common bile duct. Several studies have shown that this range extends from 4 to 17 mm.[21,50] Other features which suggest obstruction should therefore be taken into account. Irregularities of the lower end of the common duct usually result from impacted calculi (Figure 53.15). Characteristically, an impacted calculus yields a crescentic filling defect with half-shadowing caused by dye lying alongside part of the stone.

In a normal ductal system the lumen is less than 12 mm in diameter (see above) and no filling defects are seen. Rapid emptying of contrast into the duodenum also occurs. Spasm at the ampulla, however, may prevent duodenal filling and exploration of the ducts on this criterion alone will result in unnecessary morbidity. In this event the examination should be repeated and the use of amyl nitrite in the anaesthetic circuit may be helpful in relieving spasm. It must be emphasized again that careful technique and skill in interpretation of the

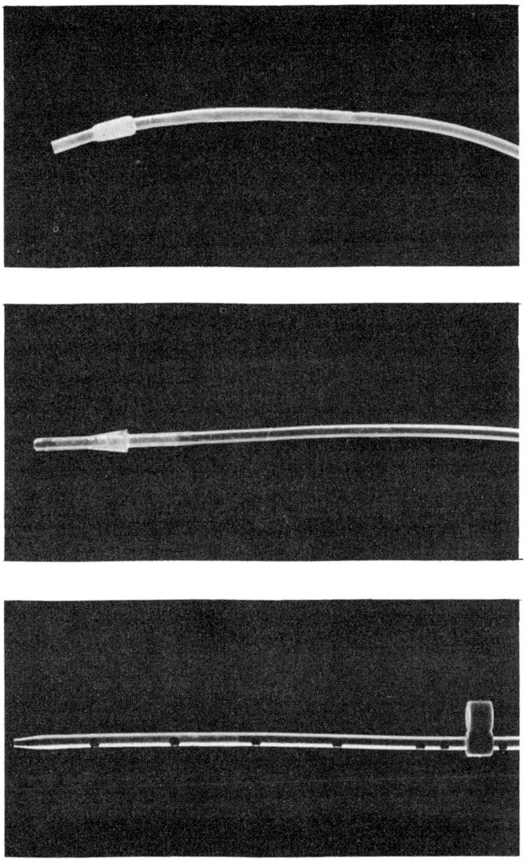

Figure 53.13. Cannulae suitable for operative cholangiography: (a) Stoke on Trent; (b) Broomé; (c) Deseret.

radiographs are essential to the value of cholangiography.

When cholangiography is deemed satisfactory the cannula is removed. The cystic duct is divided and its stump doubly ligated with catgut flush with the common duct to reduce the likelihood of further calculus formation within a duct remnant. Over-enthusiastic dissection to achieve flush ligation, however, may cause damage to the common bile duct, particularly when the terminal part of the cystic duct lies within the wall of the common duct, or runs parallel to it for some distance before joining the common hepatic duct. This anatomical variation occurs in approximately 20 per cent of patients (Figure 53.16).

Absorbable ligatures should be used to ligate the cystic duct stump. Non-absorbable ligatures may ulcerate into the lumen of the common bile duct to act as a nidus for calculus formation. Such a case, presenting with obstructive jaundice due to two impacted pigment stones, is illustrated in Figure 53.2. Particular care should be taken to avoid damage to the common duct which may occur if these are 'tented' up by this retraction (see Figure 53.17).

Following secure ligature of the cystic duct stump the gallbladder is removed. A clamp placed on the proximal divided cystic duct stump at the neck of the gallbladder serves as a useful retractor. Scissor dissection close to the gallbladder wall is usually satisfactory. Care is taken to avoid opening the gallbladder and spilling infected bile or damaging the liver. In difficult cases, injection of saline into the plane between the gallbladder and liver may be helpful in allowing the gallbladder to be 'shelled' out of its fossa.

Haemostasis is then carefully obtained. A pack left in the gallbladder fossa for a few minutes will usually control haemorrhage and diathermy is used to deal with individual bleeding points. Under-running with catgut is occasionally required. Suture of the peritoneum at the edge of the gallbladder bed adds little to the control of haemorrhage or the prevention of bile leakage from the gallbladder bed. It may, in addition, result in an undetected subcapsular collection.

A corrugated drain placed in the gallbladder bed is brought out through a separate stab incision. Failure to take this simple precaution may lead to undetected bile leakage or haemorrhage. This is particularly likely in the presence of an undetected subvesical duct which may have been damaged during the operation. Subvesical ducts have been found in 20 to 50 per cent of post-mortem dissections[33,34,42] (see Figure 53.12c). A subphrenic or subhepatic collection occurs which readily becomes infected, resulting in abscess formation, peritonitis or septicaemia.

The drain should be removed after 48 hours when it is clear that no leakage or bleeding has occurred. The morbidity of providing effective drainage in this way is negligible. The mere presence of a drain, however, must not allow a false sense of security if no drainage occurs and there is a deterioration in the general condition of the patient. The possibility of an undetected collection of bile or blood in the subhepatic or subphrenic spaces must be considered. Systemic manifestations, or even shock, are likely if infection supervenes and effective drainage is required urgently.

Secure closure with non-absorbable sutures is achieved in the standard manner.

(a)

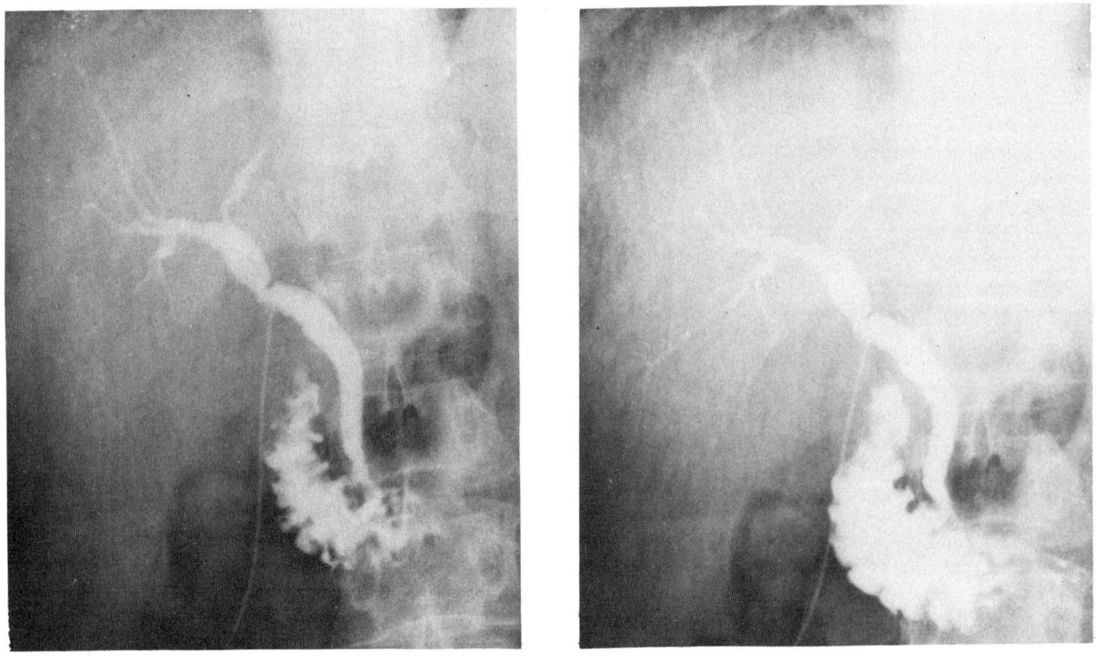

(b)

Figure 53.14. (a) and (b) Normal operative cholangiogram. (NB. artefactual 'filling defect' at level of cystic duct is caused by traction on cannula.)

Retrograde cholecystectomy

On occasion it is easier to perform cholecystectomy in a 'retrograde' manner, particularly if the cystic duct is very short or encased in dense adhesions. Accurate demonstration of the anatomy of the biliary tree is invaluable in this situation. It is often not possible to perform cholangiography by cannulation of the cystic duct, and injection of contrast directly into the common duct is therefore indicated. When retrograde cholecystectomy is undertaken, aspiration of the gallbladder allows it to be gripped more firmly for retraction although this may not be possible if the gallbladder is packed with calculi.

With downward retraction on the gallbladder the reflection of the peritoneum at the edge of the gallbladder fossa is cut with scissors. The gallbladder is dissected from the liver, proceeding from the fundus towards the neck. The cystic artery is ligated and divided. In the presence of dense inflammatory adhesions at the

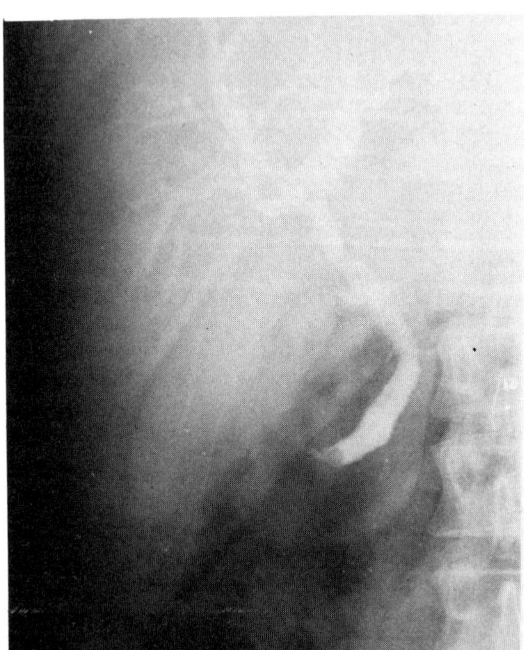

Figure 53.15. Calculus impacted at lower end of common bile duct causing obstructive jaundice.

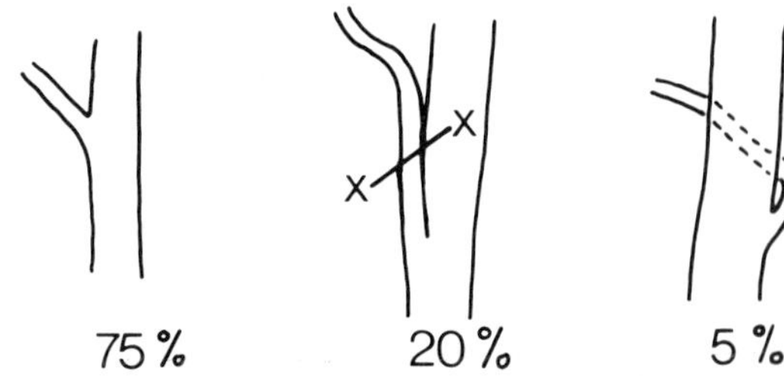

Figure 53.16. Junctional variations of the cystic and common hepatic ducts. x—x = injury is liable at this site. From Kune,[43] with kind permission of the author and the publishers Little, Brown & Co.

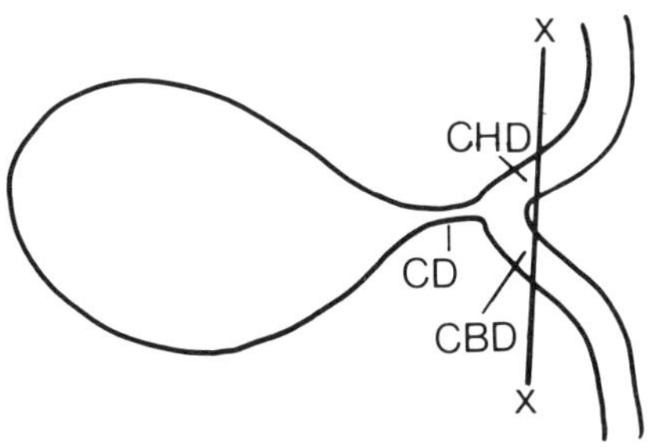

Figure 53.17. Tenting-up of the major biliary ducts. CHD = common hepatic duct; CBD = common bile duct; CD = cystic duct; x—x = injury is liable at this site.

neck of the gallbladder damage to the hepatic ducts or vessels may occur unless great care is taken.

Once the cystic artery has been ligated and the gallbladder mobilized on to the cystic duct, cholecystectomy is performed after ligature of this duct with catgut.

Cholecystostomy

Inflammation of the gallbladder may be so severe that cholecystectomy is considered hazardous. Temporary drainage of the gallbladder (cholecystostomy) to remove infected bile, pus and calculi may prove life-saving, particularly in the elderly or infirm.

A purse-string catgut suture is placed around the fundus of the inflamed gallbladder. The area is carefully packed off to prevent spillage of infected bile into the general peritoneal cavity. A trocar and cannula are inserted into the fundus and, after withdrawal of the trocar, infected bile is aspirated. Alternatively, a simple incision in the fundus may be used to introduce a metal sucker to aspirate the gallbladder. Calculi are gently extracted with forceps or scoop. Generally, there is little risk of forcing calculi down the cystic duct as this is often fibrosed and a large calculus may be impacted in Hartmann's pouch. This potential hazard should nevertheless be remembered and carefully avoided.

Once the gallbladder has been satisfactorily emptied, a wide-bore soft tube of rubber or latex is inserted in the gallbladder and the purse string tightened. A Winsbury-White catheter is particularly suitable (Figure 53.18). Additional catgut sutures are used to secure the tube which is then brought out through a separate stab incision. Drainage and closure are performed in the usual way. A full course of antibiotic therapy is indicated.

Exploration of the Common Bile Duct

Removal of calculi may be achieved either through the supraduodenal portion of the common bile duct or transduodenally through the ampulla of Vater. The former route is generally to be preferred as leakage from the duodenotomy may cause considerable morbidity and even mortality, and pancreatitis may also result from interference with the ampulla. This approach has, however, been extensively used with low morbidity. (See Chapter 54 for further discussion.)

Supraduodenal exploration

Once the common hepatic and bile ducts have been dissected and carefully palpated, two catgut stay sutures (3/0 or 4/0) are placed in the anterior wall of the duct so as to allow a vertical incision to be made between them. Exploration with scoops and stone forceps is performed followed by saline lavage.

Free passage of dilators through the ampulla into the duodenum may be reassuring but carries a small hazard of producing pancreatitis. The normal ampulla allows passage of a Bakes size 6 or 7 dilator without difficulty but spasm or stricture may prevent easy instrumentation. Following dilatation, small residual calculi will sometimes pass. Choledochoscopy (see Chapter 24), if available, will prevent the retention of residual calculi.

T-tube drainage

Following exploration of the duct it is common practice to insert a soft T-tube for biliary drainage. The edges of the choledochotomy are approximated with 4/0 plain catgut sutures

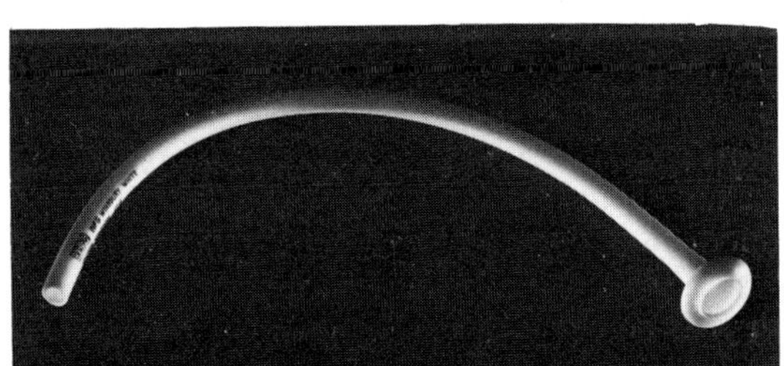

Figure 53.18. Cholecystostomy catheter.

(a) 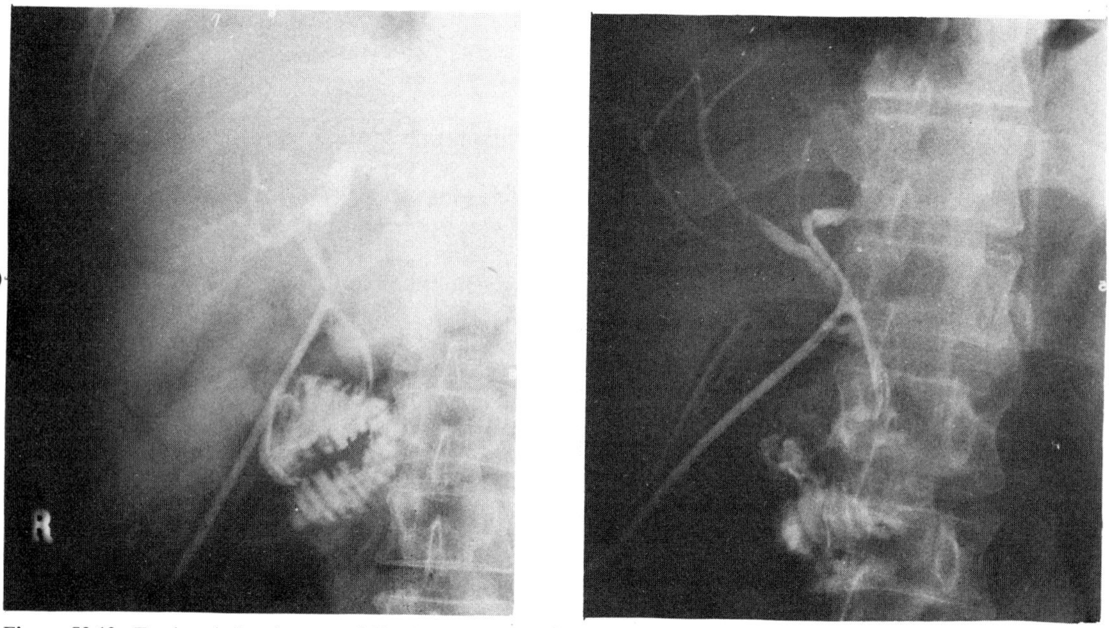 (b)

Figure 53.19. T-tube cholangiograms following removal of calculus shown in Figure 53.15. (a) post-exploratory; (b) postoperative.

around the tube, which is then led out through a separate stab incision by the shortest route and connected with aseptic precautions to a closed drainage bag.

T-tube drainage is not without morbidity. The use of soft plastic T-tubes has been abandoned as bile leeches out the plasticizer, and the tube becomes rigid and its removal hazardous.[28] The tube also may become partially or completely dislodged. Although it may be left in situ for several weeks, ulceration through the wall of the duct from pressure necrosis has occurred and ascending infection results if strict aseptic precautions are not observed. Careful primary closure of the duct using fine catgut sutures leads to no increase in morbidity, providing no calculi are missed.[84] In general, however, it is wise to leave a 14 French gauge or larger T-tube in situ following exploration. This enables operative post-exploratory and postoperative cholangiograms (Figure 53.19) to be performed. The latter are obtained seven to ten days after operation, although they may be performed safely at an earlier time if indicated. If the postoperative films are normal at ten days, with no calculi or leakage and there is free drainage into the duodenum, the tube is removed. A fistula results which seals itself within a day or two provided there is no distal biliary obstruction. The risk of biliary peritonitis is minimal at this time as the tube track has become walled off by adhesions and omentum. Clinical features which imply the absence of distal obstruction are a steadily diminishing volume of biliary drainage through the T-tube and absence of pain on intermittent and then permanent clamping of the tube. The drainage bag must not be allowed to act as a siphon and therefore should be positioned at the same level as the common bile duct.

Transduodenal exploration for the removal of impacted calculi

Mobilization of the duodenal loop by incision of the peritoneum on the lateral wall (Kocher's manoeuvre) facilitates palpation of the ampullary region so that impacted calculi may be more easily detected. Palpation is often easier from the left side of the table using the left hand. The index finger is placed behind the duodenal loop and the thumb compresses the lower end of the duct from the front. The duodenal loop is packed off and duodenotomy is performed through a transverse incision.

An impacted calculus will often present as a palpable bulge at the ampulla. The stone is exposed by cutting directly on to it with diathermy. It is then dislodged and extracted with a dissecting probe.

The patency of the lower end of the common bile duct is maintained by sphincteroplasty (see Chapter 54). Secure closure of the duodenum without stenosis can be achieved in two layers at the end of the procedure. Silk or Dexon should be used for the seromuscular layer to avert leakage.

Combined supraduodenal and transduodenal approach

The successful use of a combined approach to the removal of calculi has been reported by Aubrey and his colleagues.[4] In 40 consecutive patients they were able to achieve complete clearance of the ducts in all cases and encountered postoperative pancreatitis in only one. The possibility of achieving clearance safely in this way, particularly in difficult cases, should encourage the surgeon to persist in removing all calculi at the *first* operation. Antibiotic cover should be given. Trasylol (aprotinin) may be of benefit in the prevention of postoperative pancreatitis but the evidence in favour of its use is not convincing. With this aggressive combined approach at the initial operation the problems of retained calculi can be avoided. Choledochoscopy, however, achieves the same objective with less risk of morbidity.

Choledochoduodenostomy

Following exploration of the common bile duct this procedure is of value if there is doubt as to whether evacuation has been complete, or when ductal calculi have been removed on a previous occasion. The procedure should not be undertaken if the common duct is less than 10 mm in diameter. In addition, an adequate stoma of at least 2 cm is necessary as stenosis with ascending infection may ensue. This procedure is more fully discussed in Chapter 54.

POST-CHOLECYSTECTOMY SYNDROME

The number of patients with persistent symptoms following cholecystectomy is almost certainly diminishing with the use of more accurate diagnostic techniques. Endoscopy, in particular, has played a significant role, firstly in the avoidance of cholecystectomy for an incorrect diagnosis, and secondly in the investigation of complex postoperative biliary problems by retrograde cannulation (see Chapters 54 and 23).

NON-OPERATIVE MANAGEMENT OF RETAINED CALCULI

Re-operation on the biliary tract is associated with technical difficulties. Attention has therefore been paid to various non-operative techniques to remove retained or recurrent calculi.

Dissolution of calculi with sodium cholate infusions[82] or heparinized saline[29] has been advocated. Experience with these techniques has been reviewed by Wheeler[83] and Motson.[58] Although such agents may have some chemical effect upon calculi the disappearance of the latter from the biliary tree could in some cases be explained by simple flushing into the duodenum. An irrigation system using saline is therefore probably just as effective, and Motson[58] reported a successful outcome in 50 per cent of cases. Care should be taken to avoid performing irrigation with too high a pressure, as this may cause hepatocellular damage, and a maximum pressure of 25 cm of the solution is

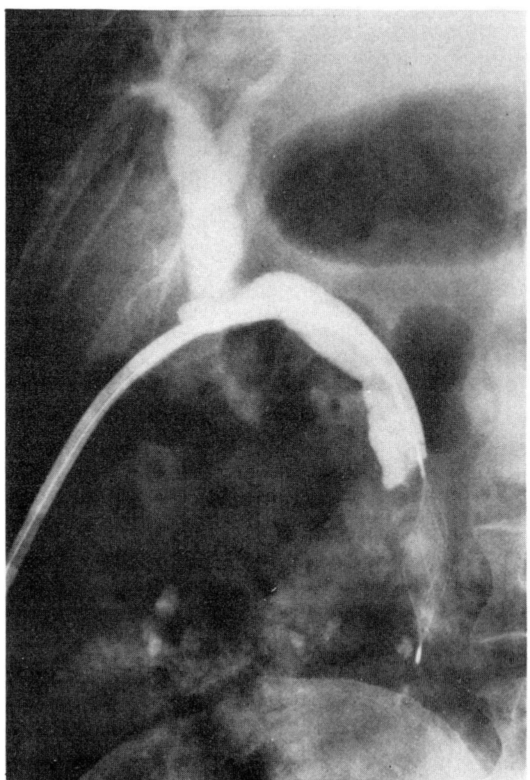

Figure 53.20. Dormia basket passed through catheter into common bile duct and opened distal to stone. From Rees and Lawrie,[68] with kind permission of the authors and the editor of *British Journal of Surgery*.

recommended. A useful way of monitoring irrigation is to insert a central venous pressure apparatus between the irrigating fluid and the T-tube. The apparatus is set so that the top of the manometer is 30 cm above the biliary tree. If the pressure should rise too rapidly the irrigating fluid will overflow from the manometer. It is important also to ensure that there is free flow within the system.

Removal of calculi through the T-tube or its track[13] or even displacement of a stone onwards into the duodenum has also been reported.[27] It should be noted that instrumentation of the T-tube or its track is facilitated firstly by the use of a tube of 14F gauge minimum size and secondly if the tube is brought out by the shortest possible route. A Dormia basket or a catheter introduced through the choledochoscope, or simply along the T-tube track, may also be successful in either withdrawing calculi retained in the lower common duct or propelling them onwards into the duodenum.

Whenever instrumentation is utilized, however, the timing of the procedure is important. Maturation of the T-tube track must be allowed to occur, otherwise serious damage may result. The patient can usually be allowed home in the meantime, providing there is free drainage of bile from the T-tube. If the bile is infected, a suitable antibiotic regimen is justified and aseptic care of the T-tube is mandatory. After six weeks the track has become fibrosed and the patient is readmitted. Following removal of the T-tube, a soft steerable catheter (e.g. medi-Tech) is guided along the fistulous track under image intensification until the site of the filling defect is reached. A Dormia basket is then passed through the catheter and opened distal to the stone (Figure 53.20). Using this technique, Rees and Lawrie[68] achieved easy removal of the retained calculus in 13 out of 16 patients with minimal morbidity. These authors stress that multiple attempts at removal of the stone can be made over a period of weeks if the first attempt is not successful. This simple technique with its low morbidity thus has much to commend it.

Endoscopic papillotomy for the removal of retained common bile duct stones is described in Chapter 23.

When retained calculi are present, in most cases it should prove possible to avoid re-exploration, using a non-operative technique. It is important to remember that all these procedures carry a risk of producing septicaemia. Whenever possible, bile should be obtained for culture and prophylactic antibiotic cover should be used.

REFERENCES

1. Alawneh, I. (1978) Acute non-calculous cholecystitis in burns. *British Journal of Surgery*, **65**, 243–245.
2. Arnaud, J.P., Aprahamian, M., Eloy, M.R. & Adloff, M. (1978) The x-ray diffraction study of gallstones: identification of pure mineral stones. *British Journal of Surgery*, **65**, 362.
3. Ashby, B.S. (1965) Acute and recurrent torsion of the gallbladder. *British Journal of Surgery*, **52**, 182–184.
4. Aubrey, D.A. & Edwards, J.L. (1978) The selective use of combined supraduodenal and transduodenal exploration of the common bile duct. *British Journal of Surgery*, **65**, 246–251.
5. Barker, D.J.P., Gardner, M.J. & Power, C. (1978) Data presented at Society for Social Medicine, Leeds (unpublished).
6. Batch, A.J.G., Amery, A.H. & Lallemand, R.C. (1978) Prophylactic cephazolin in biliary surgery. Read at 5th World Gastro-enterology Congress, Sao Paulo, Brazil.
7. Beilby, J.O.W. (1967) Structure of the gallbladder. *Journal of Pathology and Bacteriology*, **93**, 175–184.
8. Bevan, G. (1970) Acalculous adenomyomatosis of the gallbladder. *Gut*, **11**, 1029–1034.
9. Boston Collaborative Drug Surveillance Programme, Report (1973) Oral contraceptives and venous thromboembolic disease, surgically confirmed gallbladder disease and breast tumours. *Lancet*, **i**, 1399–1404.
10. Boston Collaborative Drug Surveillance Programme, Report (1974) Surgical confirmed gallbladder disease, venous thromboembolism and breast tumours in relation to postmenopausal estrogen therapy. *New England Journal of Medicine*, **290**, 15–19.
11. Brett, M. & Barker, D.J.P. (1976) The world distribution of gallstones. *International Journal of Epidemiology*, **5**, 335–341.
12. Brockis, J.G. & Gilbert, M.C. (1957) Intestinal obstruction by gallstones: a review of 179 cases. *British Journal of Surgery*, **44**, 461–466.
13. Burhenne, H.J. (1973) Non-operative retained biliary tract stone extraction. A new roentgenologic technique. *American Journal of Roentgenology, Radium Therapy and Nuclear Medicine*, **117**, 388–399.
14. Burke, J.F. (1961) The effective period of preventive antibiotic action in experimental incisions and dermal lesions. *Surgery*, **50**, 161–168.
15. Butler, M.J., Linnard, C., McGuire, P. & Dewbury, K. (1979) Evaluation of grey-scale ultrasound in acute biliary disease. In preparation.
16. Campbell, E.W. & Rogers, C.L. (1974) Submucosal gallbladder emphysema. *Journal of the American Medical Association*, **227**, 790–791.
17. Carter, R., Thompson, P.J. Jr, Brennan, L.P. & Hinshaw, D.B. (1963) Volvulus of the gallbladder. *Surgery, Gynecology and Obstetrics*, **116**, 105–108.
18. Chetlin, S.H. & Elliott, D.W. (1973) Pre-operative antibiotics in biliary surgery. *Archives of Surgery*, **107**, 319–323.
19. Christensen, A.H. & Ishak, K.G. (1970) Benign tumors and pseudotumors of the gallbladder. Report of 180 cases. *Archives of Pathology*, **90**, 423–432.
20. Crystal, R. & Fink, R.L. (1971) Acute acalculous cholecystitis in childhood. *Clinical Pediatrics (Philadelphia)*, **10**, 423–426.

21. Dowdy, G.S. Jr, Waldron, G.W. & Brown, W.G. (1962) Surgical anatomy of the pancreatobiliary ductal system. Observations. *Archives of Surgery (Chicago)*, **84**, 229–246.
22. Earlam, R.J. & Thomas, M. (1978) The clinical significance of gallstones and their radiological investigation. *British Journal of Surgery*, **65**, 164–167.
23. Edmunds, P.K.D. & Havard, C. (1961) Duodeno-colic fistula due to gallstones. *British Journal of Surgery*, **49**, 253–255.
24. Essenhigh, D.M. (1968) Perforation of the gallbladder. *British Journal of Surgery*, **55**, 175–178.
25. Faber, R.G., Ibrahim, S.Z., Thomas, D.M., Beynon, G.P.J. & Le Quesne, L. (1978) Gallstone disease presenting as septicaemic shock. *British Journal of Surgery*, **65**, 101–105.
26. Fiddian, R.V. (1959) Gallstone ileus. Recurrences and multiple stones. *Postgraduate Medical Journal*, **35**, 673–676.
27. Finnis, D. (1978) Personal communication.
28. Fraser, Sir James D. (1978) Personal communication.
29. Gardner, B. (1973) Experiences with the use of intracholedochal heparinised saline for the treatment of retained common duct stones. *Annals of Surgery*, **177**, 240–244.
30. Goh, H., Moore, L. & Karran, S.J. (1979) Double blind controlled trial of cephalosporin prophylaxis in biliary tract surgery. Unpublished data.
31. Greenwood, R.K. (1963) Torsion of the gallbladder. *Gut*, **4**, 27–29.
32. Halpert, B. (1961) Significance of the Rokitansky–Aschoff sinuses. *American Journal of Gastroenterology*, **36**, 534–539.
33. Healey, J.E. Jr, & Schroy, P.C. (1953) Anatomy of biliary ducts within human liver; analysis of prevailing pattern of branchings and major variations of biliary ducts. *American Medical Association Archives of Surgery*, **66**, 599–616.
34. Hobsley, M. (1958) Intra-hepatic anatomy; a surgical evaluation. *British Journal of Surgery*, **45**, 635–644.
35. Hoerr, S.O. & Hazard, J.B. (1966) Acute cholecystitis without gallbladder stones. *American Journal of Surgery*, **111**, 47–55.
36. Howard, R.J. & Delaney, J.P. (1972) Postoperative cholecystitis. *American Journal of Digestive Diseases*, **17**, 213–218.
37. Jenkins, H.P., Evans, R. & Kollert, W. (1961) Gallstone ileus. *Surgical Clinics of North America*, **41**, 71–81.
38. Keighley, M.R.B. (1977) Micro-organisms in the bile. A preventable cause of sepsis after biliary surgery. *Annals of the Royal College of Surgeons, England*, **59**, 329–334.
39. Keighley, M.R.B., Flinn, R. & Alexander-Williams, J. (1976) Multivariate analysis of clinical and operative findings associated with biliary sepsis. *British Journal of Surgery*, **63**, 528–531.
40. Keighley, M.R.B., Baddeley, R.M., Burdon, D.W., Edwards, J.A.C., Quoraishi, A.H., Oates, G.D., Watts, G.T. & Alexander-Williams, J. (1975) A controlled trial of parenteral prophylactic gentamicin therapy in biliary surgery. *British Journal of Surgery*, **62**, 275–279.
41. Keighley, M.R.B., Drysdale, R.B., Quoraishi, A.H., Burdon, D.W. & Alexander-Williams, J. (1976) Antibiotics in biliary disease: the relative importance of antibiotic concentrations in the bile and serum. *Gut*, **17**, 495–500.
42. Kune, G.A. (1969) The anatomical basis of liver surgery. *Australian and New Zealand Journal of Surgery*, **39**, 117–126.
43. Kune, G.A. (1972) *Current Practice of Biliary Surgery*. Boston: Little, Brown & Co.
44. Kune, G.A. & Schutz, E. (1974) Bacteria in the biliary tract. A study of their frequency and type. *Medical Journal of Australia*, **1**, 255–258.
45. Le Quesne, L.P. (1964) Operative cholangiography. In *Surgery of the Gallbladder and Bile Ducts* (Ed.) Smith, R. & Sherlock, S. pp. 131–143. London: Butterworth.
46. Lindberg, E.F., Grinnan, G.L. & Smith, L. (1970) Acalculous cholecystitis in Viet Nam casualties. *Annals of Surgery*, **171**, 152–157.
47. Lindgren, A.G. (1957) Allergic cholecystitis with vasopathia allergia (periarteritis nodosa). *Acta Pathologica et Microbiologica Scandinavica*, **41**, 281–286.
48. LiVolsi, V.A., Perzin, K.H. & Porter, M. (1973) Polyarteritis nodosa of the gallbladder, presenting as acute cholecystitis. *Gastroenterology*, **65**, 115–123.
49. Lynn, J., Williams, L., O'Brien, J., Wittenberg, J. & Egdahl, R.H. (1973) Effects of estrogen upon bile: implications with respect to gallstone formation. *Annals of Surgery*, **178**, 514–524.
50. Mahour, G.H., Wakim, K.G. & Ferris, D.O. (1967) The common bile duct in man: its diameter and circumference. *Annals of Surgery*, **165**, 415–419.
51. Maingot, R. (1964) Biliary fistulae and gallstone ileus. In *Surgery of the Gallbladder and Bile Ducts* (Ed.) Smith, R. & Sherlock, S. London: Butterworth.
52. Maki, T. (1966) Pathogenesis of calcium bilirubinate gallstone: role of *E. coli*, β-glucuronidase and coagulation by inorganic ions, polyelectrolytes and agitation. *Annals of Surgery*, **164**, 90–100.
53. Marshall, J.F. & Hartzog, D.C. (1964) Acute emphysematous cholecystitis. *Annals of Surgery*, **159**, 1011–1016.
54. McArthur, P., Cuschieri, A., Shields, R. & Sells, R.A. (1975) Controlled clinical trial comparing early with interval cholecystectomy for acute cholecystitis. *Proceedings of the Royal Society of Medicine*, **68** (11), 676–678.
55. McKay, A.J., Duncan, J.G., Imrie, C.W., Joffe, S.N. & Blumgart, L.H. (1978) A prospective study of the clinical value and accuracy of grey scale ultrasound in detecting gallstones. *British Journal of Surgery*, **65**, 330–333.
56. Moore, L., Lane, R.H.S. & Karran, S.J. (1978) Unpublished data.
57. Morran, C., McNaught, W. & McArdle, C.S. (1978) Prophylactic co-trimoxazole in biliary surgery. *British Medical Journal*, **ii**, 462–464.
58. Motson, R.W. (1977) The non-operative management of retained common duct stones. *Hospital Update*, **3**, 725–735.
59. Munster, A.M., Goodwin, M.N. & Pruitt, B.A. Jr (1971) Acalculous cholecystitis in burned patients. *American Journal of Surgery*, **122**, 591–593.
60. Papachristodoulou, A.J., Mackenzie, A., Norman, J. & Karran, S.J. (1978) Single dose cephazolin prophylaxis in biliary tract surgery. *Journal of the Royal College of Surgeons of Edinburgh*, **23**, 178–183.
61. Papachristodoulou, A.J., Mackenzie, A., Norman, J. & Karran, S.J. (1978) Single dose cephalosporin prophylaxis in major abdominal surgery. *Current Chemotherapy, American Society for Microbiology*, **2**, 856–857.
62. Parsons, R.L. (1978) Unpublished data.
63. Petz, L.D. (1971) Immunologic reactions of humans to cephalosporins. *Postgraduate Medical Journal*, **47** (Suppl.), 64–69.

64. Pollock, A.V. & Evans, M. (1975) The prophylaxis of surgical wound sepsis with cephaloridine – experiences in 2491 general surgical operations and reporting a controlled clinical trial against framycetin. *Journal of Antimicrobial Chemotherapy*, **1** (Suppl. 3), 71–83.
65. Public Health Laboratory Service, Report (1960) Incidence of surgical wound infection in England and Wales. *Lancet*, **ii**, 659–663.
66. Puestow, C.B. (1953) *Surgery of the Biliary Tract, Pancreas and Spleen*. Chicago: Year Book Medical Publishers.
67. Ram, M.D. & Watanatittan, S. (1973) Levels of cefazolin in human bile. *Journal of Infectious Diseases*, **128** (Suppl. S), 361–363.
68. Rees, B.I. & Lawrie, B.W. (1978) Non-operative removal of retained stones in the common bile duct. *British Journal of Surgery*, **65**, 334–346.
69. Ries, K., Levison, M.E. & Kaye, D. (1973) Clinical and in vitro evaluation of cefazolin, a new cephalosporin antibiotic. *Antimicrobial Agents and Chemotherapy*, **3**, 168–174.
70. Robertson, R.D. (1970) Non-calculous acute cholecystitis following surgery, trauma and illness. *American Journal of Surgery*, **36**, 610–614.
71. Rogers, F.A. & Carter, R. (1958) Gallstone intestinal obstruction. *California Medicine*, **88**, 140–143.
72. Royle, J.P. (1964) Torsion of the gallbladder. *Australian and New Zealand Journal of Surgery*, **34**, 68–70.
73. Salleh, H.B. & Balasegaram, M. (1974) Treatment of acute cholecystitis by routine urgent operation. *British Journal of Surgery*, **61**, 705–708.
74. Shimada, K., Inamatsu, T. & Yamashiro, M. (1977) Anaerobic bacteria in biliary disease in elderly patients. *Journal of Infectious Diseases*, **135**, 850–854.
75. Smith, Sir Rodney (1978) Cancer of the pancreas – Thom Bequest Lecture. *Journal of the Royal College of Surgeons of Edinburgh*, **23** (3), 133–150.
76. Sokhi, G.S. & Longland, C.J. (1973) Early and delayed operation in acute gallstone disease. *British Journal of Surgery*, **60**, 937–939.
77. Strachan, C.J.L., Black, J., Powis, S.J.A., Waterworth, T.A., Wise, R., Wilkinson, A.R., Burdon, D.W., Severn, M., Mitra, B. & Norcott, H. (1977) Prophylactic use of cephazolin against wound sepsis after cholecystectomy. *British Medical Journal*, **i**,
78. Thomas, H.S., Cherry, J.K. & Averbrook, B.D. (1962) Gallstone ileus. *Journal of the American Association*, **179**, 625–629.
79. Uthman, S.M. (1972) Acalculous acute typhoid cholecystitis. *Lebanese Medical Journal (Beirut)*, **25**, 503–505.
80. van der Linden, W. & Sunzel, H. (1970) Early versus delayed operation for acute cholecystitis: a controlled clinical trial. *American Journal of Surgery*, **120**, 7–13.
81. Wagner, D.E., Elliott, D.W., Endahl, G.L. & MacPherson, C.T. (1962) Specific pancreatic enzymes in the etiology of acute cholecystitis. *Surgery*, **52**, 259–265.
82. Way, L.W., Admirand, W.H. & Dunphy, J.E. (1972) Management of choledocholithiasis. *Annals of Surgery*, **176**, 347–359.
83. Wheeler, M.H. (1977) Dissolution of retained choledochal calculi. *Annals of the Royal College of Surgeons, England*, **59**, 153–157.
84. Wilken, B.J. (1975) Primary closure of the common bile duct. *Journal of the Royal College of Surgeons, Edinburgh*, **20**, 115–119.
85. Wright, H.K. & Holden, W.D. (1960) The risks of emergency surgery for acute cholecystitis. *American Medical Association Archives of Surgery*, **81**, 341–347.

Chapter 54

Biliary Bypass and Reconstructive Surgery

I.S. BENJAMIN
L.H. BLUMGART

Biliary bypass and reconstruction procedures are undertaken for immediate correction of trauma to the bile ducts, and for relief of biliary tract obstruction (Table 54.1). The type of short-circuiting procedure undertaken depends upon the site and pathology of the obstruction but the principles of diagnosis and the approach to surgical treatment, as well as many of the surgical techniques, are the same for both benign and malignant conditions. These broad principles and their application to treatment of benign conditions are considered in the present chapter and the management of tumours of the biliary tree and periampullary region in Chapter 55.

Table 54.1. *Indications for Biliary Bypass and Reconstruction.*

1. Trauma to bile ducts:
   - operative
   - non-operative
2. Gall stones:
   - primary
   - recurrent
3. Benign stricture:
   - congenital
   - traumatic
   - postoperative
   - stenosed biliary–enteric stoma
   - stenosed sphincter of Oddi
   - inflammatory – sclerosing cholangitis
   - post-radiotherapy
4. Malignant stricture (see Chapter 55)
5. Parasites
6. Pancreatitis causing biliary obstruction
7. Pancreatic neoplasm (see Chapter 55)
8. ? Functional disorders of biliary drainage
9. Biliary reconstruction in hepatic transplant (see Chapter 52)

Not all biliary tract obstruction is complete and it is necessary that an extended concept be adopted to take into account minor and intermittent obstruction and extensive stenotic but non-occlusive lesions of the biliary tract. Both pathological and clinical evidence for this broad view of biliary tract obstruction should be considered.

Although diagnostic approaches to jaundice are discussed in Chapter 26 it is important to recognize that many complex cases requiring biliary diversion have already been submitted to operation, perhaps on several occasions, and that very detailed preoperative information is required. Furthermore, many of these patients are severely ill, malnourished, and suffering from the pathophysiological sequelae of jaundice, infection and biliary fistula. These aspects must be taken into account in the planning and timing of surgery. There is therefore a particular diagnostic problem in such cases and the important points relating to biliary bypass and reconstruction are emphasized.

PATHOPHYSIOLOGY OF BILIARY TRACT OBSTRUCTION

While most cases of biliary obstruction present with the classical features of one or more attacks of obstructive jaundice, it is important to recognize a group of patients who have more subtle clinical symptoms. Understanding of the pathological changes and clinical features of

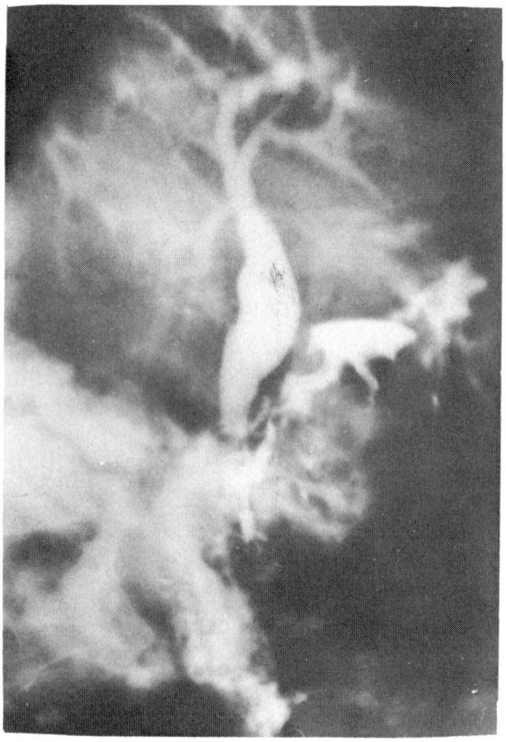

Figure 54.1. ERCP in a young woman referred after several previous operations for chronic pancreatitis. There is gross dilatation of the common bile duct in the absence of jaundice; the distorted pancreatic ductal architecture is also seen. At operation the bile duct was not only dilated but also grossly thickened, and there were histological changes of chronic ductal obstruction in the liver parenchyma (see text). Total pancreatectomy and choledochojejunostomy were performed.

incomplete or minor degrees of obstruction allows biliary tract obstruction to be considered in three main categories:

1. *Complete obstruction* producing jaundice.
2. *Intermittent obstruction* producing symptoms and typical biochemical changes with or without attacks of jaundice.
3. *Chronic incomplete obstruction* with or without symptoms or the observation of biochemical changes, leading ultimately to pathological changes in the bile ducts or liver.

Effects on Biliary Tree and Liver

There is usually some degree of ductal dilatation proximal to an obstructing lesion in the bile duct, even when this obstruction is incomplete (Figure 54.1). This is presumably due to recurrent or continuous minor degrees of obstruction which lead to a progressive increase in the diameter of the duct. The process of ductal fibrosis which occurs proximal to the obstructing lesion may, however, lead to rigidity of the duct, so that in a minority of cases even long-standing obstruction may occur without significant proximal dilatation (Figure 54.2).

Biliary tract infection plays an important role in the ductal pathology associated with obstruction. Normal bile is sterile, but in the presence of gallstones the rate of positive bile culture rises rapidly, and may be as high as 56 per cent in jaundiced patients and higher than 90 per cent in those undergoing emergency biliary decompression.[58] The incidence of infection is less when obstruction is due to tumour than in the presence of gallstones.[106] Histological examination of the bile duct shows mucosal atrophy and sometimes necrosis and squamous metaplasia,

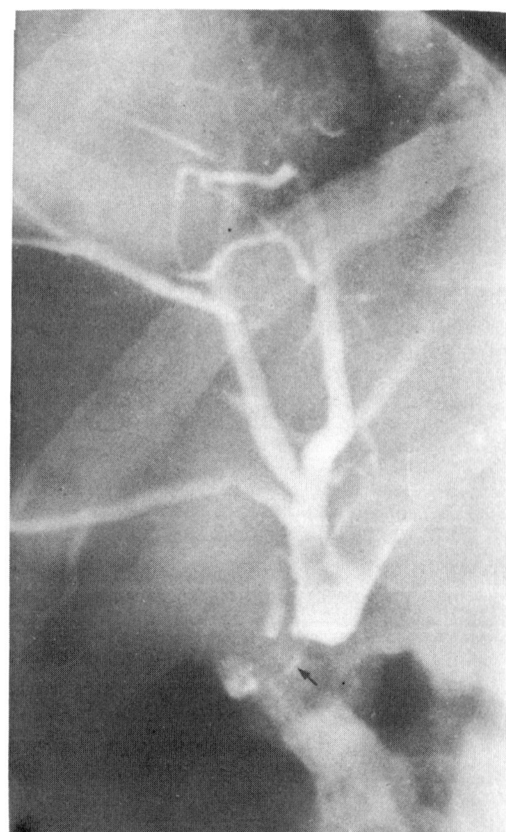

Figure 54.2. PTC in a 41-year-old man who had sustained a common bile duct injury at cholecystectomy, followed by hepaticojejunostomy Roux-en-Y. Recurrent attacks of cholangitis occurred. This examination two years later shows a strictured anastomosis (arrowed) with stones lying in the duct remnant. Despite the very narrow stricture jaundice was only intermittent and never severe. Note that the chronically fibrotic liver has not permitted significant dilatation of the intrahepatic bile ducts.

followed by inflammatory infiltration and fibrosis in the subepithelial layer.[65] These changes ultimately lead to the grossly thickened ducts familiar to the surgeon.

Proximal ductal changes are progressive and proportional to the degree and duration of obstruction, and it has been shown that progression may continue for some time following the relief of obstruction, particularly if infection has been a significant factor. This process may have an adverse effect on anastomotic healing, and this may influence judgement regarding the technique of anastomosis and the length of time for which transanastomotic tubes should be left in situ.

The chronically obstructed bile duct may become filled with mucoid aggregates of bile sludge and debris or with fibrin clots which may be mistaken for gallstones on cholangiography.[81, 96] We have observed such aggregates proximal to a stenosed choledochoduodenostomy and proximal to incomplete obstructive lesions associated with pancreatitis (Figure 54.3), and have been able to culture *E. coli* from this material.[16] It is certain that obstruction need not be severe enough to produce jaundice in order to encourage such sepsis and retention of debris with the associated pathological ductal changes, and these progressive changes may be proportional to the duration rather than to the degree of obstruction.

Distal to a severe biliary tract obstruction there is ductal collapse. The distal duct segment may be affected by inflammatory changes similar to those found in the proximal ducts, and ultimately may become completely obliterated by fibrous tissue.[65] If a duct has been subject to long-standing obstruction, this distal segment becomes unsuitable for anastomosis.

The ductal changes in long-standing biliary obstruction extend to the minor biliary radicles and portal triads of the liver, and their severity is related to the degree and duration of obstruction. Bile lakes related to the interlobar bile ducts may occur with extreme rapidity after the onset of large duct obstruction[104] and proliferation of bile ductules in the portal zones with polymorph infiltration occurs after the first week.[99] More prolonged obstruction results in marked perilobular fibrosis and progressive fibrotic changes combined with infection may produce sclerosing cholangitis. Although the progressive nature of these changes has been well documented,[24, 46, 84, 85] their regression has been less well reported. We have observed the return to near normality of liver affected by

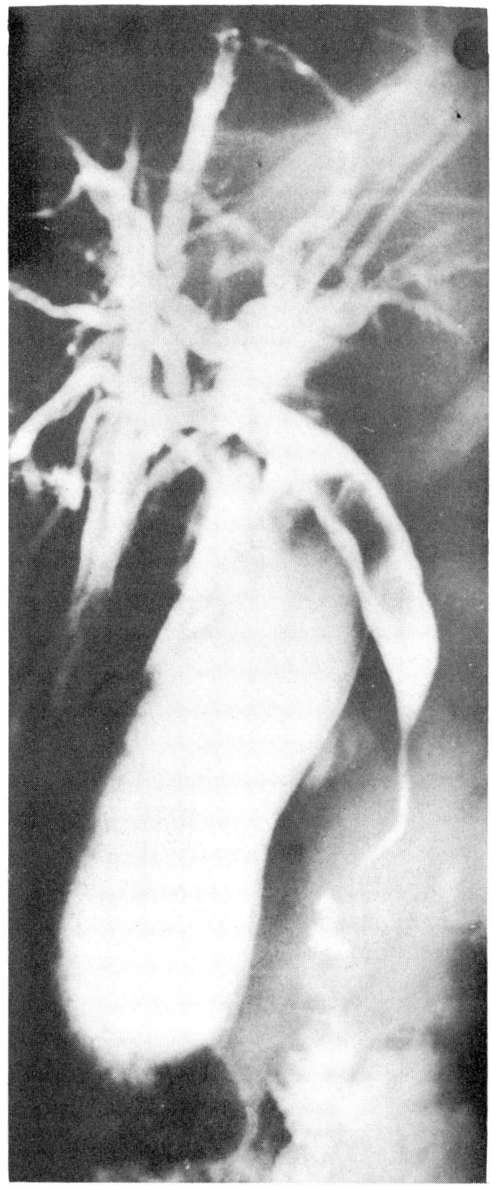

Figure 54.3. PTC in a 46-year-old woman with chronic pancreatitis. A long, smooth, narrow stricture is seen in the bile duct in its retropancreatic course, and a long filling defect lies in the dilated proximal duct. A thin ribbon-like piece of gelatinous material and a quantity of biliary 'sand' were removed from the dust at operation, and the stricture bypassed by a choledochojejunostomy Roux-en-Y.

marked fibrotic changes following relief of a long-standing biliary tract obstruction.[13]

Despite the characteristic changes which have been described, the pathologist may still have difficulty in distinguishing large duct obstruction from intrahepatic cholestasis in a needle liver biopsy. The error rate may be as high as 33 per cent even for examination of operative wedge biopsies[10, 67] but a group from the Royal

Free Hospital, London, reporting on 125 biopsies from patients with obstruction found obstruction in 83 per cent, cholestasis in 13 per cent and non-specific features in 4 per cent. In only one biopsy was a different diagnosis specifically suggested.[83] Changes in the portal triads have been shown on liver biopsy in 54 per cent of cases of uncomplicated gallstone disease and these were almost all associated with bile infection.[42] A lower incidence of such changes has been reported in malignant obstruction of the biliary tract, where infected bile is less common.[106]

Further progression of hepatic pathology leads to the development of a true secondary biliary cirrhosis, and this may be associated with portal hypertension and oesophageal varices, hypersplenism and haematological changes. Of 890 patients with biliary strictures reported from the Lahey Clinic, 169 (19 per cent) had portal hypertension of some degree,[103] and these changes may occur as early as two years from the onset of obstruction.[65] This disastrous complication of biliary tract obstruction presents particular problems in investigation and operative management.

Other Effects of Biliary Obstruction

Chronic biliary tract obstruction is associated with nutritional changes due to a combination of chronic infection, fistula formation, poor absorption of dietary fat and inadequate calorie intake. In addition, synthetic liver functions are depressed in biliary obstruction.[70] The serum albumin is frequently low and gamma globulin elevated. These changes are an index of the extent of hepatocellular damage. In some patients with obstruction at the papilla of Vater or with associated pancreatitis, pancreatic insufficiency contributes to the absorptive defect.

Anaemia may be present as a result of decreased dietary iron intake or due to intestinal bleeding from associated varices or gastric erosions. Hypersplenism may contribute to the haematological defect and platelet deficiency and both extrinsic and intrinsic coagulation defects are found.

The incidence of acute renal failure after surgery is increased in patients with obstructive jaundice, possibly due to an increased sensitivity of the kidneys to ischaemic damage.[3, 35, 60, 135] These renal changes may be related to renovascular fibrin deposition associated with endotoxaemia in jaundice,[123, 124] and this may have important implications for the management of patients with biliary tract obstruction. Changes in renal morphology and function have also been found in experimental rats with chronic biliary obstruction studied in our laboratories.[4]

DIAGNOSIS

Successful surgery in biliary tract obstruction is dependent on operative judgement and expertise and on precise preoperative pathological and anatomical diagnosis. The latter is particularly important in the complex cases which are liable to require bypass or reconstruction and in which the choice of the most appropriate operation is critical. Diagnostic techniques available in jaundice have been described earlier in this volume (see Chapter 26). However, a detailed account of the ordered application of these techniques which we have found to be of value in complex cases of biliary tract obstruction is appropriate here.

The distinction between intrahepatic and extrahepatic cholestasis should be made preoperatively in practically every case.[13] Laparotomy diagnosis is unsatisfactory not only because of the possibility of needless operation but because diagnosis on the operating table may prove impossible or be incomplete, and the surgeon may not obtain the information which will enable him to formulate a correct operative approach.

The commonest presenting symptom in patients requiring biliary bypass surgery is jaundice. However, in cases where biliary obstruction is incomplete or intermittent the presentation will be more subtle and a careful clinical history is required. Retained common bile duct stones following cholecystectomy may not produce clinical symptoms for several years, although the majority will do so. Episodes of mild jaundice and biliary colic will then ensue, or the patient may present with fever and rigors or with attacks of acute pancreatitis. The symptoms may, however, be much less distinct, amounting only to vague abdominal discomfort, weight loss, anorexia and tiredness. Occasionally, the presentation is as acute obstructive cholangitis, with rapidly developing pain and jaundice, bacteraemic shock and acute renal failure. This constitutes a dire emergency and requires early surgery.

Operative injuries to the bile duct may present

soon after surgery with jaundice or biliary fistula, and there is often a history of prolonged biliary drainage or a septic course following surgery.[66, 129] There may, however, be a delayed presentation with the late onset of jaundice and cholangitis, and many bile duct injuries have followed a cholecystectomy which the surgeon has considered to be straightforward and uneventful.[77] It is interesting to note that while the estimated incidence of such operative injuries to the bile ducts is one in 300 to 500 cholecystectomies,[65] only some 15 per cent are recognized at the time of operation.[77] The small incidence of bile duct injury during partial gastrectomy must also be considered. A careful review of the operation note and previous radiology, if available, may prove helpful.

Repeated clinical examination of the patient at frequent intervals is often helpful in difficult cases of suspected biliary tract obstruction. The constant, enlarged, non-tender gallbladder of malignant obstruction in the distal biliary tract is a well-established sign, and the intermittently palpable gallbladder sometimes associated with periampullary carcinoma may be detected.[14] Moderate hepatomegaly with tenderness will be found in extrahepatic biliary tract obstruction, but an enlarged firm liver is more suggestive of malignancy or of secondary biliary cirrhosis. The other stigmata of hepatocellular insufficiency should be sought and may be associated with secondary biliary cirrhosis. However, they should always alert the surgeon to the possibility of a non-surgical diagnosis in the jaundiced patient.

A combination of history, examination and simple laboratory tests is capable of yielding a high rate of diagnosis between intrahepatic and extrahepatic cholestasis, and indeed computer analysis of such data will yield a correct diagnostic rate of up to 90 per cent.[62] Although standard liver function tests taken on their own may be misleading or unhelpful[112] the serum alkaline phosphatase is a sensitive index of biliary tract obstruction, and is often elevated in the absence of jaundice in minor degrees of obstruction.

However, it is important to emphasize that precise diagnosis is necessary for the treatment of biliary obstruction. To achieve this, techniques for imaging of the biliary tract are indispensable (Figure 54.4). Barium studies of the upper gastrointestinal tract are of very limited value,[17] and intravenous cholangiography gives a low diagnostic yield even when the bilirubin is less than 70 μmol/l (4 mg/dl).[15] Frequently, the only information obtained relates to the size of the common bile duct and stones may be missed in up to 40 per cent of non-jaundiced patients.[89] Detailed information is obtainable by a combined use of endoscopic retrograde cholangiopancreatography, percutaneous transhepatic cholangiography and ultrasonography.

Endoscopic retrograde cholangiopancreatography (ERCP)

This technique, described in detail in Chapter 23, provides not only the ability to define the entire biliary tree even in deeply jaundiced patients but also allows upper gastrointestinal endoscopy, including inspection and, if necessary, biopsy of the ampullary region and cytology of bile and pancreatic juice.[12] In a recent personal series of 100 consecutive examinations, 58 patients had complete or partial biliary tract obstruction and a diagnosis was obtained at ERCP in 52 (90 per cent).[13] The precise indications and timing of ERCP in relation to other diagnostic tests in complex biliary cases are considered below.

Percutaneous transhepatic cholangiography (PTC)

The use of the rigid sheathed needle for this procedure has been of limited value in biliary

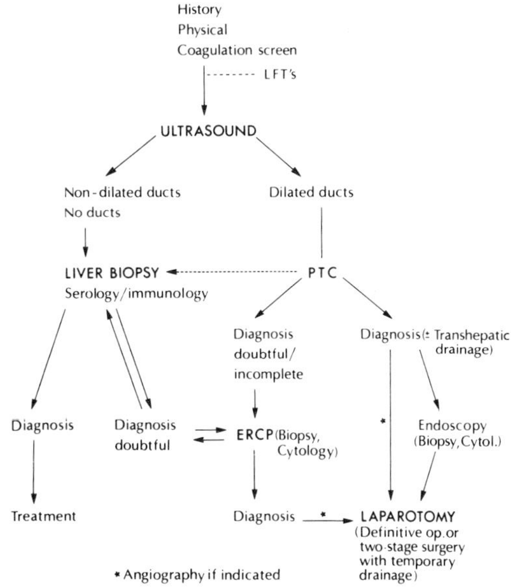

Figure 54.4. Schema for the investigation of patients with suspected biliary tract obstruction (see text).

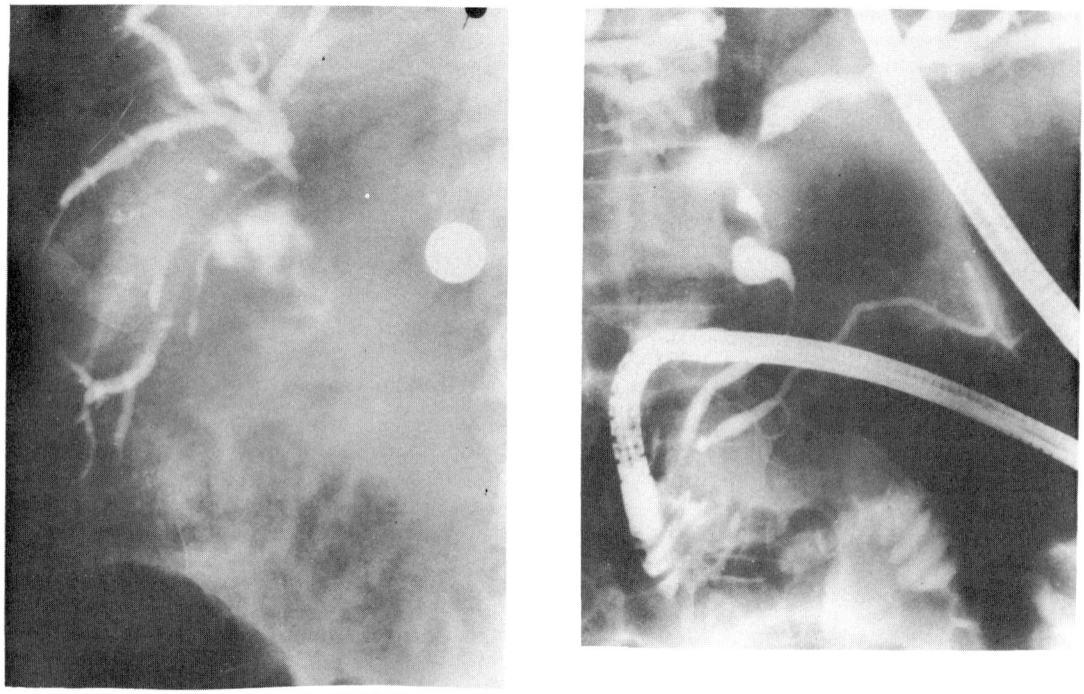

(a) (b)

Figure 54.5. (a) PTC in a 65-year-old man with obstructive jaundice. Only the right ductal system is filled, and the upper end of a high ductal stricture is outlined. (b) ERCP 24 hours later shows the extent of this stricture, involving most of the common hepatic and common bile duct, and extending into the left hepatic duct. Malignant cells were demonstrated cytologically, and the diagnosis was of an inoperable bile duct tumour. From Benjamin et al[11] with kind permission of the editors of *British Journal of Surgery*.

tract obstruction, partly because of its relatively low success rate (74 per cent) even in the dilated biliary tract[6, 50] and partly because the risk of bleeding and bile leakage necessitated preparations for an immediate laparotomy.[104] However, the introduction of the fine, flexible, 'Chiba' or 'skinny' needle has allowed a much wider use of this method of investigation in biliary tract obstruction.[41, 49, 86, 90, 119] High success rates are reported for both dilated (up to 100 per cent) and non-dilated (up to 73 per cent) ducts (Figures 54.2 and 54.10). A recent study of the value of fine needle PTC in our department has confirmed that the technique is reasonably safe. We have had a high diagnostic yield even in patients with incomplete biliary tract obstruction and without dilated bile ducts (Figure 54.2).[11]

The combination of ERCP and PTC gives precise preoperative information (Figure 54.5). This is of particular importance in complex biliary tract obstruction, especially where previous surgery has been performed. In this situation, the operative problems are frequently formidable and may render operative cholangiography difficult or impossible.

Ultrasonography

This technique (described in detail in Chapter 21), particularly when the grey scale apparatus has been used, has proved almost as accurate as fine needle PTC in the demonstration of dilated bile ducts.[69, 78, 114] It is important, however, to re-emphasize the fact that biliary tract obstruction may occur without bile duct dilatation, and that ultrasound may not always demonstrate the level and nature of an extrahepatic block.

An Integrated Diagnostic Approach

We have recently adopted a programmed approach to the investigation of the patient with suspected biliary tract obstruction (Figure 54.4). This is aimed firstly at rapid differentiation between intrahepatic and extrahepatic cholestasis, and secondly at accurate preoperative diagnosis with early planned surgery in cases with extrahepatic obstruction.[11, 13] The scheme relies on a combination of grey scale ultrasound and fine needle PTC as first-line investigations, and on ERCP in selected cases. If dilated ducts are demonstrated by grey scale ultrasound, fine needle PTC is performed under antibiotic cover. This will outline the biliary tree in the majority of cases, but if the diagnosis remains unclear or incomplete (as for example when only the upper end of a biliary stricture is outlined) ERCP may be undertaken in addition (Figure 54.5). This programmed approach is successful in demonstrating abnormalities of the biliary tree in up to 98 per cent of cases, and operative cholangiography may be unnecessary.[11, 41]

Fine needle PTC need not be followed by immediate laparotomy[11,13] (see Chapter 26) and it is possible to use the approach described above and schedule the patient for the next convenient operating list. If necessary, further investigations which may be useful or an essential adjunct to appropriate surgery may be performed. This is particularly so in cases of malignancy of the biliary tree or pancreas. Anomalies of the hepatic arterial tree are common and it is important to have information regarding these prior to major surgery. We carry out selective arteriography in almost every case of malignant disease. In addition, splenoportography (see Chapter 55, Figure 55.2) is performed, since prior knowledge of involvement of the portal vein in its retropancreatic course, or of the portal vein radicles at the hilum of the liver, is essential in the assessment of the limits of operability and in the performance of safe surgery (see also Chapter 55).

Although ultrasound followed by PTC is our usual procedure for displaying the biliary tract, ERCP is preferred in specific circumstances. The principal circumstance is in patients symptomatic after cholecystectomy. In this situation pathology unrelated to the biliary tract may be present and information available from oesophagogastroduodenoscopy and biopsy or retrograde pancreatography assumes importance.[16] Endoscopy is particularly important in patients in whom sphincteroplasty or choledochoduodenostomy has been performed. Not only is it possible to cannulate these orifices and obtain choledochography, but information regarding peristomal inflammation, patency and competence is of importance in assessing and planning operation. In a recent study, 52 patients symptomatic after cholecystectomy were submitted to ERCP. In 48 of these patients diagnostic information was obtained, and of 38 in whom biliary tract obstruction was present precise diagnosis was established by means of endoscopy and ERCP in 37.[16]

Where neoplasm of the pancreas, periampullary region or bile ducts is suspected endoscopic diagnostic techniques assume additional importance (see also Chapter 55). Thus, in an initial study of 38 patients investigated for chronic pancreatitis or pancreatic or periampullary neoplasm, pancreatic juice or bile was aspirated under direct vision from the papilla of Vater, or brush cytology or 'touch smear' cytological examination was made after biopsy.[105] Without benefit of clinical or any other information the cytologist reached a positive diagnosis of malignancy in 12 of 16 patients who proved to have malignant disease, with no false positive results.[52] These results are extremely encouraging and, when taken in conjunction with endoscopic and radiological findings, a high positive diagnostic rate for carcinoma is obtained.[12]

Other radiological investigations are occasionally of value.

Sinograms performed through a well-established fistulous track may demonstrate the nature of a distal obstruction, though the definition is seldom clear enough for precise diagnosis and PTC or ERCP may still be required.

Laparoscopy will allow direct visualization of the liver and gallbladder, and contrast medium can be injected under direct vision into the gallbladder for cholangiography. We have only rarely used this method and have reserved laparoscopy for 'target' biopsy of suspected intrahepatic tumours.

Liver biopsy has a limited place in the preoperative investigation of suspected biliary tract obstruction. The histological changes observed are not always diagnostic and may be misleading.[10, 67] In addition, in obstructive jaundice the investigation carries a significantly greater risk of haemorrhage and bile leakage than does fine needle puncture of the liver using the Chiba technique, and most experienced biliary surgeons have had to operate under emergency circumstances for these complications following needle biopsy. Despite suggestions to the contrary[32, 67, 83] there is now a strong case for restricting this procedure in suspected biliary tract obstruction to situations where a non-dilated biliary tree has been demonstrated by other means. Grey scale ultrasonography provides a useful non-invasive screening procedure for this purpose.

It cannot be too strongly emphasized that accurate preoperative diagnosis allows correct timing and choice of surgical treatment for complex disorders of the biliary tract. Few situations are so desperate that laparotomy cannot be delayed briefly in the interests of this goal, and time spent in well chosen investigation is always amply repaid at the time of surgery.

APPROACHES TO SURGERY

Once the diagnosis is established, two decisions must be made: firstly, is operation necessary, and secondly, what is the optimum time for operative interference? Not all patients with minor degrees of biliary tract obstruction, particularly after previous surgical assaults, will benefit from surgery, and the risk of progressive hepatic changes must be weighed against those of major surgery. It may be the wiser surgical decision in the very elderly and unfit patient to manage a minor degree of obstruction with courses of antibiotics.

A recent approach to some forms of biliary tract obstruction has been the use of endoscopic papillotomy.[27, 28, 33, 38, 57, 63, 93] In most instances the indication for papillotomy has been the presence of common bile duct stones, although functional conditions of the sphincter of Oddi have also been treated by this technique. High success rates for removal of stones from the common bile duct are recorded, but in some reports it is difficult to be certain of the number of cases in which the procedure was not attempted due to inability to advance the catheter into the papillary orifice. Whereas endoscopic papillotomy eliminates the hazards of anaesthesia and open operation the procedure carries a considerable morbidity rate (8.5 per cent) and mortality rate (1 to 2 per cent). Complications include haemorrhage, perforation, sepsis and pancreatitis.[28, 37] Despite claims to the contrary this may be no lower than the morbidity and mortality of operation in experienced hands, and controlled studies comparing endoscopic papillotomy with corresponding surgical operations have not been carried out. A review of common bile duct exploration in numerous centres has shown the mortality rate to be no greater than 2 to 4 per cent. In addition, open operation is required in many patients with complex problems in biliary tract obstruction in order to allow bypass or reconstructive procedures. Indeed, in a series of more than 60 cases, including many elderly patients regarded as poor anaesthetic risks and a high proportion of patients with biliary stenosis or stricture due to pancreatitis or trauma, we have encountered a mortality rate for open operation of less than 5 per cent. In 31 of these cases common bile duct stones were removed and, in addition, appropriate biliary enteric bypass surgery was performed without mortality. The late results of endoscopic papillotomy are as yet unknown and the true incidence of late stenosis, ascending cholangitis or pancreatitis remains to be determined.

There appears to be a case for endoscopic papillotomy for removal of common bile duct stones in elderly high risk patients and possibly for the temporary relief of obstructive jaundice in some situations. Similarly, in cases of true primary stenosis of the sphincter of Oddi the procedure may be considered, although there has been difficulty in the precise definition of this condition. It would seem to us unwise to treat secondary stenosis of the sphincter consequent on previous operative procedures by this method since the risks of infection, pancreatitis and re-stenosis must be high.

Preoperative Preparation

The timing of definitive surgery is determined by the general condition of the patient with particular reference to the pathophysiological disturbances associated with the biliary tract obstruction.

Impairment of *renal function* in patients with obstructive jaundice has already been described. Our own studies have shown that, preoperatively, many patients with obstructive jaundice have a significantly decreased maximal urinary concentrating ability, as well as significantly reduced serum albumin concentration and haematocrit. In a series of 16 jaundiced patients studied, nine showed a significant elevation of preoperative serum fibrin degradation products, while there was no such elevation in control subjects. Glomerular filtration rate was also reduced in five of 24 jaundiced patients preoperatively. Follow-up of these patients after surgery showed that elevated preoperative serum fibrin degradation products and a low glomerular filtration rate were important adverse factors. Hypoalbuminaemia, infection and old age also contributed to a poor prognosis.[3] The administration of mannitol as advocated by Dawson[34] resulted in a diuresis and a significant natriuresis (see also Chapter 48, Figure 48.5).

The preparation of the jaundiced patient for

surgery should ensure an adequate intake of fluid on the preoperative night by the provision of an intravenous drip of 5 per cent dextrose, and the administration of mannitol preoperatively. Urine output and fluid balance must be observed carefully in the first 24 to 48 hours after surgery, and an adequate sodium intake ensured.

The importance of guarding against *infective* complications cannot be over-emphasized. The evidence for the value of antibiotics in biliary surgery has recently been reviewed.[58] There is a high incidence of bowel organisms found in bile in patients with benign biliary tract obstruction, particularly in long-standing obstruction, in jaundiced patients, and in the elderly. While the evidence for the value of routine antibiotic prophylaxis for all biliary surgery remains unproven, its value in these specific situations must now be regarded as established.[58, 59] We have adopted a regimen of gentamicin 80 mg three times a day and carbenicillin 1 g three times a day commencing immediately before surgery, and for five days thereafter. This combination of antibiotics is also used for a period of 24 hours to cover percutaneous transhepatic cholangiography.[11] Choice of antibiotics is determined by culture and sensitivity results for a particular hospital population, and must be subjected to constant review. Careful culture of common bile duct and gallbladder bile at operation must be regularly undertaken (see also Chapter 53).

In addition to infection, *endotoxaemia* has been proposed as one of the factors responsible for the changes in renal function in obstructive jaundice.[7] Failure of the reticuloendothelial system in the liver to remove endotoxin from portal venous blood may result in peripheral endotoxaemia.[123, 124] Because of this, Bailey[7] has suggested that there may be a case for preoperative bowel preparation to reduce endotoxaemia in jaundiced patients. It has also been proposed that the feeding of bile salts to patients with obstructive jaundice might be beneficial, by reducing the anaerobic flora of the gut.[134]

Adequate *nutritional support* is essential as a preoperative measure in patients with long-standing biliary obstruction. This is particularly important in patients with an external biliary fistula, or where temporary drainage has been established prior to definitive surgery (see below). Oral nutritional supplementation with a high calorie and high protein diet may be adequate, but supplementary or total parenteral nutrition may be required. Vitamin supplementation (e.g. Multibionta Infusion: Merck, Hants, England) and vitamin K_1 should also be provided. In patients with an external fistula fluid and electrolyte losses must be carefully monitored and replaced. When the bile can be collected it is possible to return this to the patient orally, its flavour disguised in lager or stout, or by nasogastric tube.

Some of the problems described above are readily reversible and improvement is obtained by relief of biliary obstruction. A period of biliary drainage may be advisable before definitive surgery, especially where complex dissection is to be carried out in elderly, high risk cases. There are several possible approaches to this objective.

Temporary Drainage Methods

A major disadvantage of two-stage procedures is that the performance of a surgical anastomosis for temporary drainage may make subsequent definitive operation more difficult. We have frequently encountered this problem in cases referred from other centres for definitive surgery following diagnostic laparotomy and temporary decompression. There are several other methods of drainage available.

Laparotomy and drainage of the bile duct

Laparotomy allows provision of temporary drainage and, in addition, valuable diagnostic information may be obtained. Thus, where doubt still remains it is possible with the aid of lymph node biopsy, pancreatic needle biopsy or aspiration cytology to achieve further information allowing differentiation between benign and malignant disease. In addition, in cases of known malignant disease operability can be assessed by palpation of the liver for the presence of secondary deposits and by inspection and palpation of the primary lesion. No undue dissection should be carried out as this disturbs the field for later definitive surgery.

If a clearly *inoperable lesion* is encountered a simple palliative internal bypass may be performed. However, if it is considered that resection is possible then temporary drainage can be undertaken and further investigation conducted while the patient's general condition improves prior to definitive surgery. We have attempted to enjoy the benefits of decompression without its disadvantages by avoiding an anastomosis between the biliary tree and the

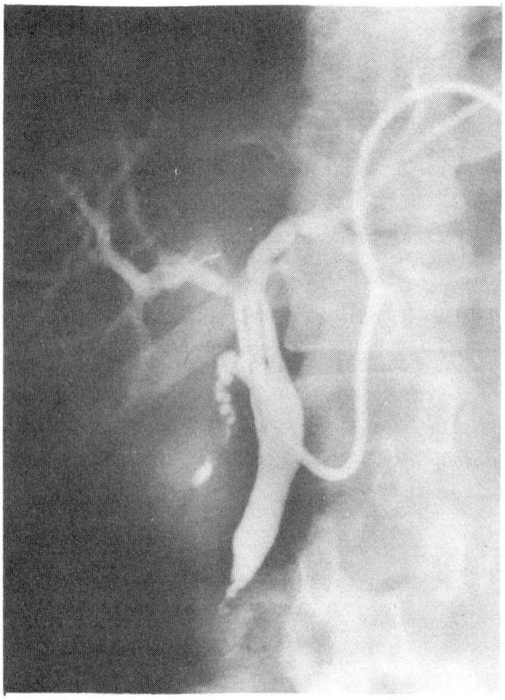

Figure 54.6. Temporary drainage of the common bile duct by means of a T-tube in a 28-year-old jaundiced man with carcinoma of the ampulla of Vater. Note that the T-tube is led to the left, away from the operative field. Jaundice subsided over a period of four weeks, during which the patient drank his own bile diluted in sweet stout. He was subsequently subjected to pancreaticoduodenectomy.

gastrointestinal tract. At operation a T-tube is inserted through a choledochotomy high in the hepatic duct. This is led out through the abdominal wall in the left subcostal region well away from the operative site (Figure 54.6). The distal limb of the T-tube is left long so that the tube may be left in situ at the time of definitive surgery, the long limb acting as a splint for a hepaticojejunostomy at that time (Figure 54.7).

Percutaneous transhepatic drainage

This recently described technique, an extension of the use of percutaneous transhepatic cholangiography, has been found particularly useful in the patient with progressive biliary tract obstruction with cholangitis, gram-negative bacteraemia and established or incipient renal failure. Various techniques have been described.[81, 82, 120] These all rely essentially upon the demonstration of a dilated biliary tract at PTC followed by the threading of a catheter over a guide wire to lie within a large dilated bile duct. This tube is then used to drain the biliary tree for several days or weeks prior to definitive surgery. Some have used this method very freely[120] and in cases of inoperable malignancy or irreparable biliary tract damage have left these catheters in situ for permanent palliation.[81]

We have treated several cases successfully by this technique (Figure 54.8), but believe that selection of cases must be careful and prior provision must be made for the establishment of drainage at the time of PTC. Ill-advised impromptu attempts to establish drainage, with improvised and inadequate equipment, may be unsuccessful and dangerous.

SURGICAL TECHNIQUES, INDICATIONS AND RESULTS

The techniques for reconstruction or bypass of the injured or obstructed biliary tract are numerous, but share many features in common. While detailed descriptions of specific operative techniques are beyond the scope of this work,

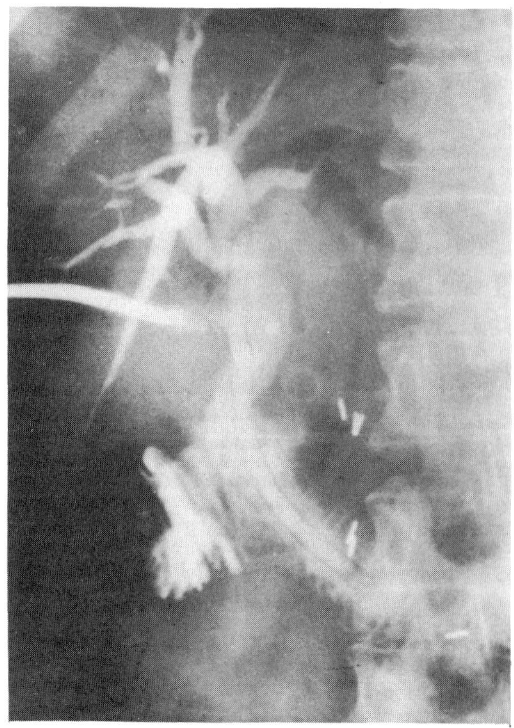

Figure 54.7. The long limb of a drainage tube used to splint a hepaticojejunostomy. In this case the tube was inserted at the time of the definitive bypass operation via a choledochotomy proximal to the anastomosis. In the case of temporary drainage the point of insertion is similar, and the tube is in situ at the time of resection.

(a) (b)

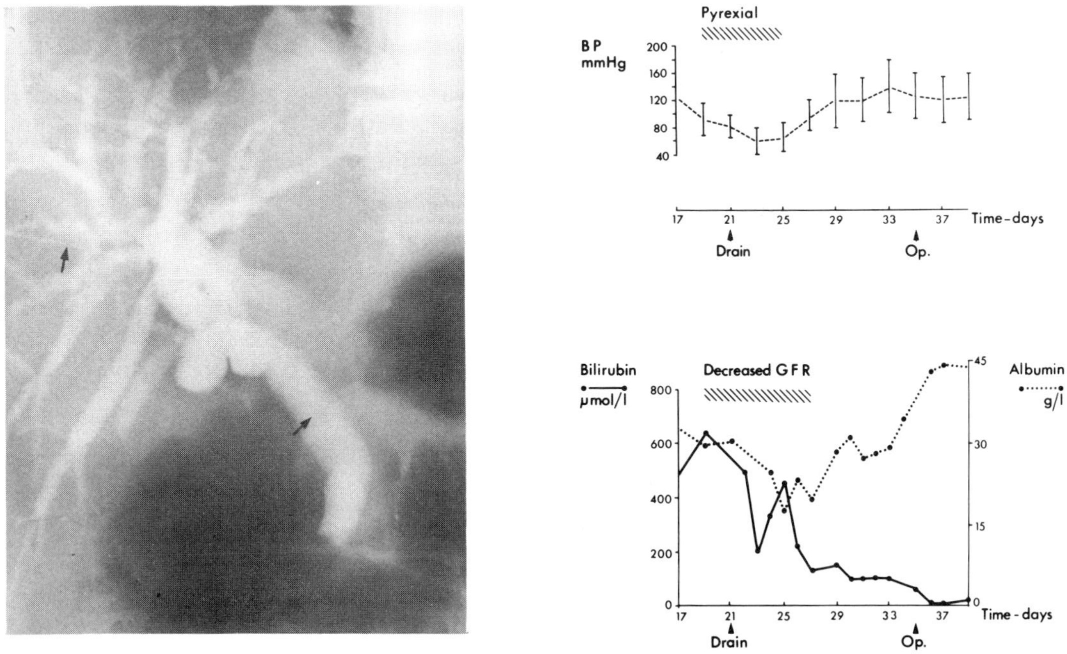

Figure 54.8. (a) PTC in a 62-year-old man referred in acute renal failure 17 days after admission with obstructive jaundice. A stone is impacted at the lower end of the common bile duct. A catheter introduced by the Seldinger technique is seen in place in the common bile duct (arrowed). (b) During a period of catheter drainage the jaundice, pyrexia, hypoalbuminaemia and renal function improved, and the patient was fit for definitive surgery two weeks later (35 days after admission). From Benjamin et al[11] with kind permission of the editors of *British Journal of Surgery*.

some important technical points in relation to the various procedures will be emphasized. Many of these techniques are equally applicable to benign and malignant disease, but features specific to the latter will be considered in Chapter 55.

Simple Repair or Reconstruction

Operative injuries to the bile ducts are not uncommon and are recognized at the time of operation in only 15 per cent of cases.[77] Non-operative trauma to the extrahepatic biliary tree is uncommon.

Non-circumferential defects in the bile duct

When there is no loss of ductal tissue these injuries may often be satisfactorily repaired by direct suture. If the duodenum is mobilized this allows approximation without tension. A single layer of interrupted sutures of fine absorbable material is inserted. The use of T-tube drainage through a separate formal choledochotomy above or below the injury rather than through the traumatic defect is recommended.[77]

Techniques for the repair of injured ducts where there has been a loss of substance of the duct wall involving the placement of venous patch grafts,[9, 79] of artificial materials[111] or of plastic procedures and subsequent instrumental dilatation[107] all result in late stenosis and have no place in the management of bile duct stricture or injury. The technique of transluminal T-tube drainage described by Smith[108] for internal decompression of an irremovable obstruction of the biliary tract may be adapted to the repair of an injured bile duct. A large bore T-tube is inserted into the duct and is then led through a jejunal Roux loop lying against the bile duct and thence brought through the abdominal wall. On removal of the T-tube an internal fistula is created. This technique is simple and safe and is a useful alternative, especially when disease and obesity have reduced access to the biliary tract or when the condition of the patient at operation gives cause for concern. Occasionally, for larger defects in the bile duct, this procedure may act as a serosal patch graft.

Complete transection of the bile duct

In this case the choice of reconstruction lies between simple end-to-end suture of the duct, and diversion of bile into the intestinal tract. The technique of end-to-end reconstruction is also applicable to repair of a short stricture after local excision[25] and has a high rate of patency if the ducts are healthy.[18] This method of repair has the theoretical advantage over biliary–enteric anastomosis of conserving the normal mechanism for biliary continence. The procedure cannot be used if there is any great disparity in size between the two ends of the bile duct, or if the ends cannot be apposed without tension. The anastomosis should be splinted by the limb of a T-tube introduced through a separate choledochotomy. In view of the limitations of end-to-end repair, it is important to consider whether the alternative of biliary–intestinal anastomosis has any significant disadvantage. Comparative studies are few, but there is no evidence that restoration of 'physiological' biliary continuity has any advantage over bile diversion.[66, 125, 127, 129]

End-to-Side Choledochoduodenostomy or Hepaticoduodenostomy

This is the simplest alternative to direct suture repair following transection of the bile duct. There must be sufficient length of duct and mobility of the duodenal loop, and the method is therefore only suitable in selected cases of low bile duct stricture. Such an anastomosis is difficult to perform in the presence of adhesions or pre-existent pancreatitis which limits the mobility of the duodenum. It should be noted that if the lower end of the bile duct cannot be identified for suture ligation it is best to abandon the search rather than undertake a hazardous dissection behind the duodenum or within the substance of the pancreas. We have never encountered a fistula from such a distal duct stump. On the other hand, biliary–duodenal fistulae, if encountered, should be closed.

The anastomosis is constructed using interrupted absorbable through-and-through sutures with careful mucosa-to-mucosa apposition. The posterior row of sutures is inserted first, held in artery forceps and only tied when all sutures are placed in satisfactory positions. A transanastomotic splint may be used or if the proximal length of duct allows, a T-tube can be inserted at a higher level, the lower limb being passed through the anastomosis into the duodenum (Figure 54.7).

It should be noted that there is a very limited place for end-to-side biliary–duodenal anastomosis since for strictures in the retropancreatic portion of the bile duct side-to-side choledochoduodenostomy is usually preferable. For more proximal strictures it is rarely possible to achieve end-to-side choledochoduodenostomy without tension.

Side-to-Side Choledochoduodenostomy

This operation has a wide range of applications and apart from its use in bile duct reconstruction[23, 44, 51, 53, 76] may be used for the relief of obstruction due to carcinoma of the ampulla or pancreatic head (see Chapter 55), chronic pancreatitis[21] or stenosis of the sphincter of Oddi.[23, 100] The role of choledochoduodenostomy in the management of functional disorders of the biliary tract is doubtful.

The *principal application* is in choledocholithiasis in two distinct situations. Firstly, in patients undergoing primary operation for gallstones in whom drainage is considered as an adjunct to exploration of the common bile duct; and secondly, in patients with residual or recurrent common duct stones following previous cholecystectomy.

There is disagreement regarding the indications for drainage procedures following duct exploration. Some authors, on the grounds of a high incidence of recurrent or residual stones, recommend drainage at primary operation,[2, 92] particularly for what are thought to be primary common duct stones.[94] Similarly, Madden[73] has recommended routine drainage after exploration of the common bile duct for recurrent or residual gallstones. Deliberate 'choledochal incontinence' has been advocated as a valuable adjunct to choledocholithotomy as prophylaxis against recurrent stones.[98]

Those who oppose the use of drainage procedures do so on the grounds of increased late morbidity from biliary sepsis consequent upon reflux of duodenal contents into the bile duct, or upon the 'sump syndrome' caused by debris remaining or accumulating within the infraduodenal bile duct after a choledochoduodenostomy in cases where there is distal ductal obstruction.[53, 107] However, it should be noted that the success of this procedure depends upon an adequate stoma.[55] Sepsis probably results from inadequate drainage from the ducts to the intestine[76] and is uncommon if the stoma remains greater than 2 cm in diameter.[36, 118] Choledochoduodenostomy is thus contra-indicated in the presence of a narrow common bile duct, and a diameter of 10 mm has been suggested as a lower limit.[23]

Our policy has been to use side-to-side choledochoduodenostomy either at primary operation or at re-exploration of the common bile duct in patients with accumulation of multiple stones where the duct diameter is at least 15 mm. We have operated on this indication extensively, particularly in elderly patients. However, in the younger patient, where the ducts are smaller and perhaps fibrosed, and particularly where obstruction is due to causes other than choledocholithiasis, we have preferred end-to-side choledocho-jejunostomy Roux-en-Y.

The incidence of anastomotic stenosis in choledochoduodenostomy may be as high as 4 to 5 per cent.[65] As elsewhere in the biliary tree stenosis is a potent cause of biliary sepsis and low-grade chronic cholangitis. We have noted infected inspissated bile aggregates in the common bile duct after ill-considered operation with anastomosis to a narrow duct, and have reported this in several patients referred because of post-cholecystectomy problems.[16] It has also been suggested that recurrent gallstones may be encouraged by deconjugation of bilirubin by β-glucuronidase liberated by *E. coli* harboured in the fenestrated biliary tract when stasis is present.[116] This is of some importance since colonic bacterial flora have been observed in the duodenum in such cases and steatorrhoea analogous to that occurring in duodenal diverticula may be present.[116]

Trans-duodenal Sphincterotomy and Sphincteroplasty

The main indications for the trans-duodenal approach to the sphincter of Oddi are for access to the distal bile duct in order to remove or allow the passage of common bile duct stones, and for the improvement of biliary drainage. The use of these operations in chronic pancreatitis unassociated with gallstones has no basis.

It is important to distinguish between sphincterotomy and sphincteroplasty. The operation of *sphincterotomy* is performed with a single cut in the wall of the duct at its lower end adjacent to the papilla of Vater. The cut divides fibres of the choledochal sphincter and does not extend outside the duodenal wall. The incision is rarely longer than 10 to 15 mm and is left unsutured. The procedure cannot be reliably expected to result in a permanent augmentation of biliary flow except when performed for organic stenosis of the sphincter of Oddi. Because of this the procedure should be used only when a stone is impacted at the lower end of the duct and cannot be removed by supraduodenal exploration.

Sphincteroplasty has been defined as 'a transduodenal method of producing a terminal choledochoduodenostomy with a stoma co-equal to that of the largest part of the common duct'.[56] The entire length of the sphincteric muscle is divided and the mucosa of the bile duct is then sutured to the duodenal mucosa to prevent narrowing. The duodenum is first mobilized and opened in the lateral wall of its second part between stay sutures of silk. The papilla of Vater is identified by vision or by palpation. This can be difficult and may be facilitated if a supraduodenal choledochotomy is made and a probe passed down into the papilla from above. This of course has disadvantages since a choledochotomy is then added to the operative procedure. In addition a false passage may be produced,[16] the probe or dilator being forced through the duodenal wall proximal to the papilla, and an anastomosis constructed in error proximal to the true papillary orifices. We now have experience of seven such patients, the common clinical presentation being recurrent acute pancreatitis or cholangitis.

Once the papilla is identified stay sutures are placed at its right upper quadrant and it is divided in an upward and lateral direction to avoid damage to the pancreatic duct which is on the medial and inferior side of the papilla. The incision should divide the full length of the choledochal sphincter. This length is variable and herein lies the risk of the operation, since if the incision is carried too far a leak may be produced at the apex of the choledochoduodenal angle. The duodenal mucosa is now sutured to that of the common duct using interrupted sutures of catgut and it is recommended that the pancreatic duct should be identified if possible before placement of the sutures. The duodenotomy is then carefully closed in two layers.

Choice of choledochoduodenostomy or sphincteroplasty

The relative merits of these operations have been argued for many years without any controlled comparative study of the two procedures. Few would debate that sphincterotomy and perhaps sphincteroplasty may be necessary when a stone is impacted at the papilla of Vater. On the other hand, there are potent criticisms against interference with the sphincter in other situations. Primary stenosis of the sphincter of Oddi for which many operate[87] is difficult to define, and while some have described a high incidence[39, 45] others deny its existence.[65] We have never encountered a case. Secondary stenotic lesions of the papilla of Vater may be treated by sphincteroplasty but the operation is then performed through scar tissue and in most instances choledochoduodenostomy or choledochojejunostomy Roux-en-Y is to be preferred.

Some have advocated the use of transduodenal sphincterotomy or sphincteroplasty for *primary* exploration of the common bile duct[56, 88] but there seems little case for this unless there is an additional indication for deliberate augmentation of biliary drainage. However, choledochoduodenostomy may equally well be used for this purpose and carries a mortality rate of less than 2 per cent, mostly in elderly patients, and not usually as a direct complication arising at or related to the site of surgery.[65] The operative mortality of sphincteroplasty is undoubtedly higher. Exploration of the common bile duct alone has a recorded mortality rate of up to 2 per cent but this has been noted to rise as high as 6 per cent with the addition of sphincteroplasty.[19, 29] Lower figures have been recorded where sphincteroplasty is a widely practised procedure.[56, 87, 88] Postoperative pancreatitis accounts for the majority of these deaths, and in 52 cases of secondary acute pancreatitis reviewed in Glasgow Royal Infirmary 10 were associated with transduodenal sphincteroplasty and two of these patients died. A very much lower incidence of acute pancreatitis was associated with other biliary surgical procedures not involving the sphincter of Oddi.[54]

No direct comparison has been made between the long-term results of the two operations, but it is likely that good results in terms of patency of the anastomosis and freedom from late complications are obtainable by either choledochoduodenostomy or sphincteroplasty in more than 75 per cent of cases with benign biliary disease.[51, 87, 91, 137] However, we have noted that, despite a widely patent sphincteroplasty, cholangitis and pancreatitis may yet occur in association with the accumulation of food debris proximal to a rigid incompetent sphincter[16] and we have seen at endoscopy debris washing to and fro through such an orifice during respiratory movement. Because of this and the risk of acute pancreatitis we prefer to avoid instrumentation of the sphincter of Oddi whenever possible and have not performed a trans-duodenal sphincteroplasty for biliary tract obstruction in five years of specialist biliary practice. Side-to-side choledochoduodenostomy can readily be added following choledochotomy in patients with multiple recurrent or residual stones and especially in the presence of biliary mud. The procedure adds little to morbidity even in high risk cases and gives added security against recurrence of stones and failure to clear the duct completely at the first operation. Provided the bile duct is 15 mm or more in diameter the results are good and we have seen no incidence of late stricture of the choledochoduodenostomy or of the 'sump syndrome' in a consecutive series of 23 patients treated by this method over a period of five years.

Cholecystojejunostomy

This method of bypass has limited application and is valueless if the obstruction approaches the site of entry of the cystic duct to the common bile duct, or in the presence of a diseased gallbladder. Even if these conditions are satisfied bile drainage may be disappointing in the presence of a narrow tortuous cystic duct. The technique is best avoided for benign obstruction of the bile ducts, and is commonly reserved for palliative treatment of obstructive jaundice due to malignancy of the distal bile duct or head of pancreas.

The anastomosis is performed side-to-side between the fundus of the gallbladder and a proximal loop of jejunum. Many surgeons add a proximal jejuno-jejunostomy, but we usually omit this step and concur with those who feel that it is unnecessary.[65]

Choledochojejunostomy and Extrahepatic Hepaticojejunostomy

The principal indications for these operations are, firstly, for the relief of biliary obstruction due to benign disease and, secondly, for

(a)

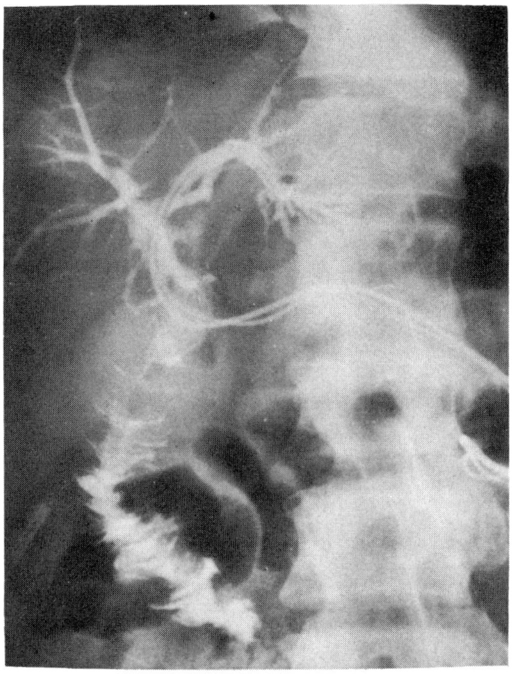

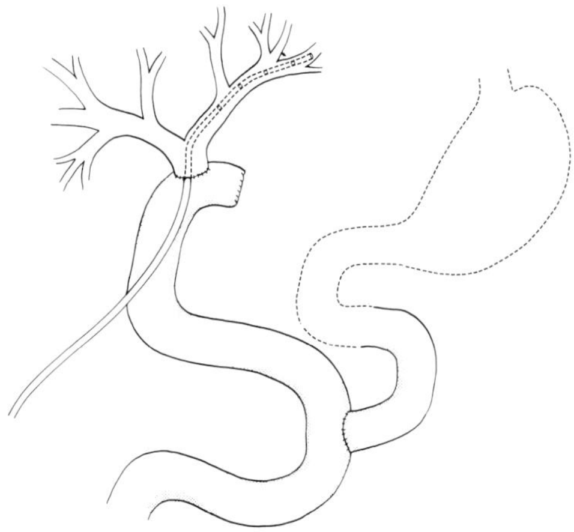

(b)

Figure 54.9. (a) Hepaticojejunostomy performed by a transhepatic approach (see text) in a 64-year-old man referred with a recurrent biliary stricture following operative bile duct injury for which there had been five previous attempts at repair. This tubogram shows two transjejunal tubes passing through a competent anastomosis: in this case both tubes lie in the left side of the intrahepatic ductal system, as intubation of the right side at operation was unsuccessful. (b) Line drawing showing the Roux-en-Y construction of the jejunal limb used for anastomosis.

reconstruction following excision of tumours of the bile duct or pancreas (see also Chapter 55).

In *benign biliary tract obstruction* the procedure may be used as an alternative method to side-to-side choledochoduodenostomy and is probably preferable in young patients with dilated ducts and multiple stones. It is especially valuable when there has been previous surgery in the distal common bile duct or at the sphincter of Oddi and in patients with chronic pancreatitis associated with biliary obstruction in whom the common bile duct is frequently narrow, thickened by inflammatory disease, of rigid texture and quite unsuitable for side-to-side anastomosis[102] (Figure 54.3). Bile duct stricture and injury to the common bile duct are less common indications and extrahepatic hepaticojejunostomy is the preferred method of reconstruction in such cases.

After division and cleaning of the duct an end-to-side anastomosis is performed to a loop of jejunum or, preferably, to a limb fashioned by the Roux-en-Y technique (Figure 54.9). This procedure produces a defunctioned limb of jejunum, thus minimizing reflux of intestinal content into the biliary tree. In addition, there is less tension at the anastomosis. A length of jejunum of 30 to 40 cm can generally be achieved quite readily without jeopardizing viability. We have found it useful to employ an automatic suturing device (GIA, Boston, Massachusetts) for division of the jejunum. This allows clean division of the jejunum, following which the row of staples at the distal end of the limb is invaginated using a Lembert suture or purse-string silk suture. This limb is brought up (usually in a retrocolic manner) to the supracolic compartment of the abdomen and the bile duct anastomosed end-to-side to the jejunum 3 to 4 cm from the blind end of the loop, the anastomosis being splinted by a transhepatic or transjejunal tube (see below) (Figure 54.10). Following completion of the anastomosis the jejunum may be stitched to the capsule of the liver or adjacent fibrous tissue in order to remove tension from the anastomosis. The Roux-en-Y jejuno-jejunostomy is now completed by anastomosis of the proximal jejunum end-to-side to the defunctioned limb in two layers of catgut and silk (Figure 54.9b). The limb is secured at its point of passage through the transverse mesocolon. External drainage from the area of the biliary–enteric anastomosis is mandatory.

A special problem exists where it is evident that the stricture in the bile duct is so high that

(a) 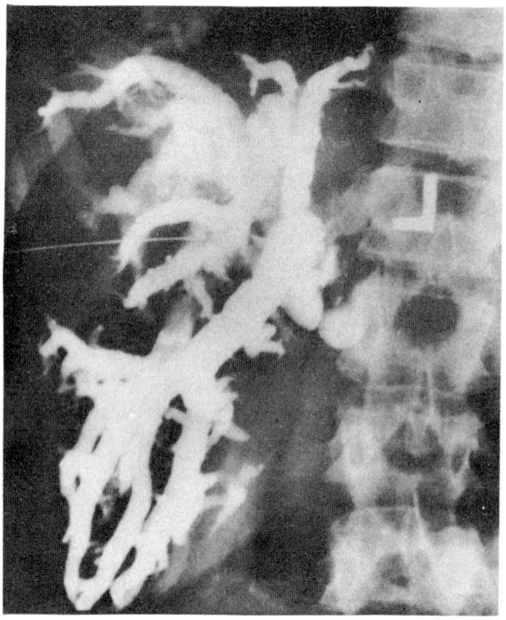

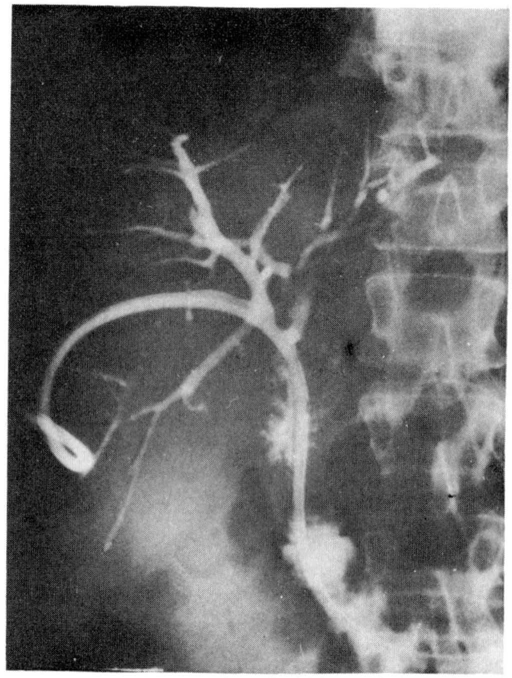 (b)

Figure 54.10. (a) PTC in a 53-year-old woman following bile duct injury at cholecystectomy. A stricture is seen high in the common hepatic duct, with grossly dilated intrahepatic ducts. (b) Tubogram in the same patient six weeks after reconstruction by hepaticojejunostomy Roux-en-Y using an infrahepatic approach with a transhepatic splintage tube. The ducts are now of normal calibre. The tube was removed at this time and the patient has remained symptom-free.

an extrahepatic duct remnant cannot be obtained. In this situation, two alternative approaches to the hilar ducts have been adopted.

Infrahepatic approach

This approach, attributed to Cole[30] and described by Cattell and Braasch,[26] consists of coring out a disc of tissue around the duct stump at the hilum of the liver with a diathermy cutting point. This is continued until the bifurcation of the ducts is identified. This dissection is accompanied by brisk bleeding from the liver substance. The hepatic artery lies deep to both right and left hepatic ducts in the majority of cases, but the operator must be watchful since in 13 per cent of patients the right hepatic artery passes anterior to its duct.[47] When the ducts have been identified, their further definition and isolation are accomplished by blunt and sharp dissection and this may be aided by the use of a fine probe, Bakes' dilator or gum-elastic bougie placed in the duct branches from below. It is not uncommon to be presented with second order ducts at this level, rather than the major right or left hepatic duct. The ducts are prepared for anastomosis, which is carried out as for extrahepatic choledocho-jejunostomy (Figure 54.10). The same principles are observed regarding the accurate apposition of mucosa, lack of tension and the use of a transanastomotic splint.

If the stricture has involved the carina of the ducts or a higher level, a separate anastomosis must be made for each major duct to the same loop of jejunum. This may be technically difficult or impossible in an area of restricted access. Such cases may be best dealt with by the transhepatic dissection described below. In either event, all ducts used for anastomosis must be probed to verify patency, and cleared of stones, debris and biliary sludge by copious washing with saline.

If accurate mucosa-to-mucosa apposition is judged to be impossible, the technique of 'mucosal graft' may be considered.[109] A seromuscular disc is excised from the wall of the jejunum leaving the mucosa intact. A fine balloon-tipped catheter is placed in the duct transhepatically (see below) and the tip passed through a small puncture wound in the jejunal mucosa. The balloon is inflated and the mucosal 'graft' is hitched up to the bile duct. While it is true that the jejunal mucosa lines the duct, it is

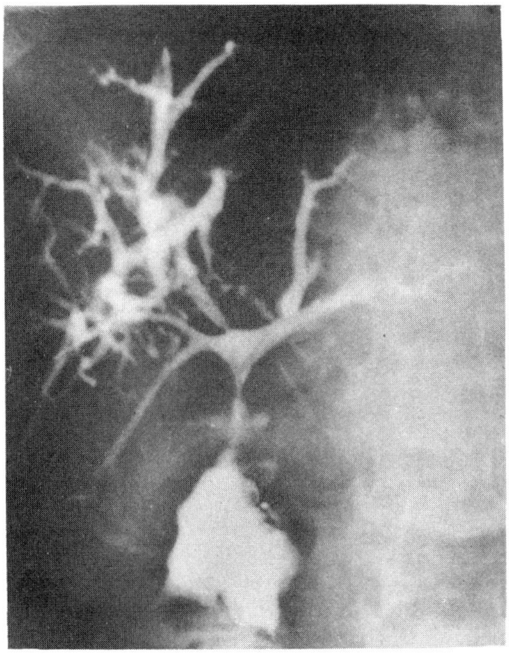

Figure 54.11. PTC showing drainage through a narrow track into the jejunum following hepatojejunostomy. This 32-year-old woman was admitted as an emergency with bleeding oesophageal varices due to secondary biliary cirrhosis, consequent upon operative bile duct injury. A mucosal graft procedure for high bile duct stricture had been performed two years previously, but re-stenosis had occurred.

At operation splenorenal shunt was performed, but no suitable duct could be found for biliary reconstruction and hepatojejunostomy was performed after coring out a cone of liver tissue at the porta. The x-ray illustrated shows considerable shrinkage of intrahepatic ducts as compared with the preoperative picture. While formal biliary reconstruction may be required at a later date, jaundice has almost completely resolved and she has now survived almost two years following operation.

important to appreciate that the outer surface of the mucosa may come into contact with and occlude side branches.[13] The tube is secured and the jejunum is suspended to the undersurface of the liver. No sutures are placed. A similar effect can be achieved without the use of a balloon catheter by securing the jejunal mucosa to a straight transhepatic tube, which is then used to pull up the mucosa into the bile duct in the manner described above.

Eighty-five per cent of patients whose records were available for analysis at two years after a mucosal graft were anicteric and without symptoms. Forty per cent had abnormal liver function tests, and one-quarter of these could be explained on the basis of adverse preoperative factors such as established biliary cirrhosis or sclerosing cholangitis.[110] Only 4 per cent developed re-stenosis when a favourable result was anticipated. Despite these promising results, failures occur (Figure 54.11) and the late outcome of the procedure remains uncertain. The technique should be reserved for cases of high stricture where mucosal suture is not possible.

Transhepatic approach

The segmental anatomy of the liver and the distribution of the bile ducts and vessels has allowed an alternative approach to the surgery of high bile duct stricture. Templeton and Dodd[115] described a case in which the hilum was approached by splitting the liver vertically in the interlobar plane into the anatomical right and left lobes, followed by a successful end-to-side anastomosis of the common hepatic duct. Waddell[121] described a further four cases. We have now adopted this approach for the treatment of high strictures, both benign and malignant (see also Chapter 55).

The plane of cleavage between the right and left lobes cannot be identified on the surface of the liver, but corresponds to a line projected backwards from the gallbladder fossa through the substance of the liver to the vena cava. The liver capsule is incised along this line and the parenchyma divided backwards by the finger fracture technique. Cirrhotic liver may require more cutting with scalpel, scissors or diathermy.[121] As the liver is divided, the two lobes are separated like the pages of a book (Figure 54.12). There is relatively little bleeding. An interlobar hepatic vein may be encountered during the dissection and tributaries of this vein may have to be ligated and divided. The middle hepatic vein is encountered posteriorly in the line of section. In most cases the major bile ducts are the first structures to be encountered in the hilum of the liver.

It is not always necessary to make a complete separation of the right and left hepatic lobes, and the position of the bile ducts, the configuration of the abdomen and costal margin, the size of the liver and the pathological condition to be dealt with influence the degree of exposure necessary. Occasionally, an abdominal incision is unsatisfactory and access may be improved by median sternotomy as described by Miller:[80] this approach avoids the disadvantage of drainage of the pleural cavity made necessary by the more conventional abdomino-thoracic incision. Once the bile ducts have been exposed by this technique, the area of the stricture (or tumour) can be excised and

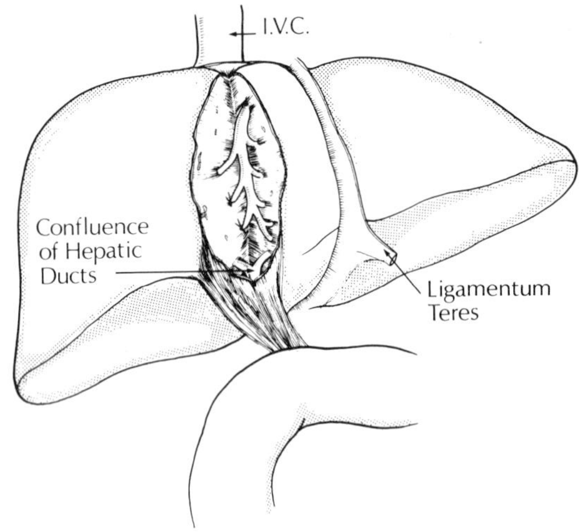

Figure 54.12. Transhepatic ('liver split') approach to the hepatic duct junction. Note that the most anterior structures encountered are hepatic ducts: the vascular structures usually lie deep to these ducts. The middle hepatic vein lies to the left of the line of section: ligation of the main trunk of this vein may produce ischaemia of the medial segment of the left lobe of the liver, drained by this vessel.

anastomosis performed to the duct or ducts thus obtained (Figure 54.9).

It is not usually necessary to suture the cut surfaces of the liver to obtain haemostasis. Suture ligation and, occasionally, the use of fibrin buffers to allow the placement of catgut sutures across the cut edges of the liver anteriorly are valuable.[136]

Choice of operation

This is finally determined at laparotomy. While the infrahepatic hilar approach may appear to be the simpler and less traumatic, this may not be so where there has been previous surgery and sepsis and where the structures of the gastrohepatic omentum have been converted to a mass of scar tissue surrounded by dilated portal radicles. In this situation, the transhepatic approach has the attraction of allowing dissection towards the bile ducts through tissues undamaged by previous surgery. We have been increasingly impressed with this 'liver split' approach to the high stricture. The technique has the additional advantage that where right or left hepatic lobectomy may be required, this can be proceeded with as a logical sequence to the initial hepatotomy (see also Chapter 55).

There are situations in which accurate mucosa-to-mucosa anastomosis cannot be achieved by any means. The use of the mucosal graft technique[109] has already been described and has an important place. However, it should be noted that in many such cases, secondary biliary cirrhosis in association with the stricture has resulted in narrow intrahepatic ducts despite the distal obstruction. In this situation a transhepatic tube cannot readily be passed.

Hepatojejunostomy

In a few instances, no identifiable structures can be found at the hilum of the liver. It is possible to perform hepatojejunostomy by suture of the open end of a Roux loop to the fibrous tissue at the hilum of the liver. In some cases the junction of the right and left hepatic ducts may be 'fishmouthed' and sewn to the thickened fibrotic capsule of the liver, and the jejunum then attached to the liver capsule to enclose the opened ducts.[61] This should be regarded as a last resort in cases where other methods are inapplicable or have failed, but in some instances prolonged palliation may be obtained by such means (Figure 54.11).

Retrograde Intrahepatic Cholangiojejunostomy (Longmire Procedure)

Longmire and his colleagues[71, 72] have described a method for dealing with an impassable obstruction at the hilum of the liver. Retrograde drainage is established through the intrahepatic portion of the dilated biliary tree within the left lobe of the liver. This operation requires partial amputation of the left lobe, the dilated stump of the left hepatic duct being then identified and anastomosed to a Roux loop of jejunum. There are several inherent limitations. Firstly, the procedure is effective in draining the entire biliary system only if there is free communication between the bile ducts of the right and left lobes of liver. However, even when this is limited, drainage of the left lobe of the liver may be an acceptable palliation in some cases.

The procedure is difficult to perform, especially in cases in which scarring due to secondary biliary cirrhosis has prevented dilatation of the intrahepatic bile ducts. Even if anastomosis is possible, drainage may be unsatisfactory through such small ducts.

Despite these reservations, the Longmire operation may prove invaluable in selected difficult cases where no other procedure is possible (Figure 54.13).

(a)

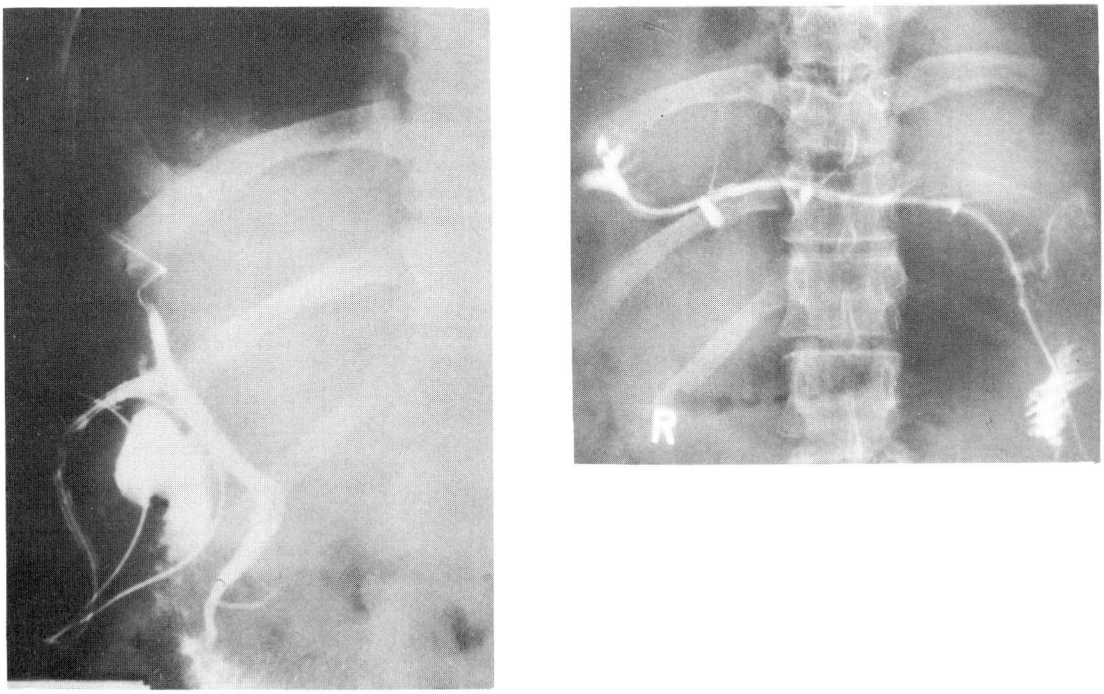

(b)

Figure 54.13. Postoperative tubogram showing retrograde intrahepatic cholangiojejunostomy (Longmire procedure). This patient had a right hepatic lobectomy performed following a road traffic accident and subsequently developed jaundice, secondary biliary cirrhosis and portal hypertension. The structures at the porta hepatis were unapproachable due to adhesions and a large collateral venous circulation and the fact that the hilum of the liver had been displaced by regeneration so that it lay almost against the right costal margin. Extensive resection of the left lobe of liver allowed anastomosis of a grossly dilated intrahepatic duct to a Roux loop of jejunum. The anastomosis was splinted using a transjejunal tube. The patient remains well and is now free of jaundice 20 months after operation. (Treated in collaboration with Mr A.G. Johnson and Dr I.M. Murray-Lyon, Charing Cross Hospital, London.)

Transanastomotic Tubes

The use of a transanastomotic tube provides several advantages in biliary bypass. Firstly, free drainage or gentle suction on such a tube may help prevent bile leakage in the early postoperative period; secondly, the presence of a tube allows postoperative radiology to be performed; and thirdly, transanastomotic splinting prevents stricture formation at the anastomosis.

It has already been noted that anastomoses performed in pathological ducts will heal with a degree of fibrosis and re-formation of stricture. The long-term splint is useful in preventing this stricture formation and is particularly important if it has been technically impossible to obtain mucosa-to-mucosa anastomosis. While the need for an internal splint is generally agreed, choice of tube and the time for which it should be left in place are open to debate. Several possible types of splintage are described here.

Short internal splints

A splint made from a short straight or Y-shaped length of tubing, passed through the anastomosis and allowed to lie free within the lumen of the bile duct and jejunum, has been used.[129] The major disadvantage is that the spontaneous passage of such tubes may take place rapidly and cannot be controlled. In addition, in a large series of patients in whom internal splints were used, 44 per cent of patients required removal of the splint because of obstruction. Use of such tubes is not recommended.

Transenteric removable tubes

A transanastomotic tube which exits through the jejunum below the biliary–enteric anastomosis and then passes through the abdominal wall obviates the necessity for a second operation to remove the splint. While specially formed Y- or T-shaped tubes have been used with enthusiasm,[130] a straight length of Latex tubing is the simplest and best form to use (Figure 54.9). Holes proximal and distal to the anastomosis encourage drainage of bile into the jejunum. These splints are simple to insert at operation, can be left in situ for prolonged periods, allow postoperative radiology and are easily removed. During operation, they tend to become dislodged and should be secured with a single fine stitch of catgut to the common bile duct during performance of the anastomosis. The point of exit from the jejunum is enclosed within a tunnel of bowel wall about 5 cm long. After exit from the bowel the tube is usually passed through omentum and then through the abdominal wall where it is secured to the skin. Light suction may be applied to the tube for several days postoperatively to minimize bile leakage, but after this free drainage under gravity is quite adequate.

Transhepatic tubes

Smith[107] described the passage of a trans-anastomotic tube through the liver parenchyma. Following operative exposure of the hepatic ducts, an instrument is passed from the hilum of the liver towards the periphery through the dilated ductal system and is pushed through the thin rim of peripheral liver tissue. The transanastomotic tube is then pulled down through the ductal system to the site of the anastomosis (Figure 54.10b). If right and left hepatic ducts are being anastomosed separately following either an infrahepatic or a trans-hepatic approach to a high bile duct lesion, bilateral tubes may be passed through separate exit points in the liver and the abdominal wall.

A variant of the transhepatic tube, the 'U-tube', has been used, and it may be easily replaced if this becomes necessary.[8,97,113] By this technique the distal end of the transhepatic tube, instead of being left free within the jejunum, is brought out through the jejunal loop, both the hepatic and jejunal ends of the tube passing through the abdominal wall. The exposed ends may then be spigoted or even joined together. Such a tube is readily washed out with saline or antibiotic solution and a new tube may easily be pulled into position under radiological control.[20] We have used this form of tubing in benign stricture, but it finds its main application in the management of patients with inoperable hilar carcinoma (see also Chapter 55, Figure 55.3).

Selection and duration of tubal splintage

A splint should be selected of such size that, when healing occurs with the formation of scar tissue, a channel of satisfactory diameter will remain on withdrawal of the tube. A fine tube may be used when a good anastomosis without tension has been achieved in a relatively healthy duct of wide calibre, since here there will be no significant anastomotic scarring. It is usually necessary, however, to recognize that a degree of re-stenosis is to be expected and the largest size of tube which will pass comfortably through the anastomosis should be used.

Latex tubes are relatively reactive and will produce a firm track of scar tissue and granulation tissue which may be considered an advantage when the tube is finally removed. If, however, the tube is being inserted for long-term palliation, non-reactivity is an advantage and a silastic tube may be employed. Such tubes may accumulate debris more slowly than latex tubes,[22] but evidence of bile salt precipitation and debris formation has been noted in chronically implanted silastic tubes in the bile ducts of dogs,[64] and the advantage of this material may not be significant.

It has been our custom to use polyethylene tubes for transhepatic splintage. The Ryle or Levin tubes used for nasogastric aspiration have a radiopaque line which makes subsequent radiographic visualization easy, particularly if the side holes are cut in this line. Their relative rigidity prevents kinking or compression during passage through the liver substance or abdominal wall, or by advancing tumour.

Some surgeons are strong proponents of long-term splintage after reconstruction of bile duct strictures.[68,130,131] There is a direct relationship between the duration of splintage and the percentage of good results following repair of bile duct injuries.[66,127] It has been recommended that splints should remain in place for six to nine months in cases of simple repair and for 12 months or longer in difficult cases where considerable fibrosis is anticipated.[65] Others, however, have felt that such long-term splinting is unnecessary. Thus, Hertzer and his colleagues[48] found no long-term advantage in continuing splintage for longer than six to 12 weeks and others have suggested that splintage for more than three to five months is unnecessary.[74,133] The decision essentially depends upon the degree of anticipated fibrosis and this will be related to the chronicity of the stricture, the degree of infection and the extent to which a surgically satisfactory anastomosis has been achieved. Smith's recommendation that a Foley catheter used in his mucosal graft technique be left for only three weeks is an exception to this general rule.[109]

It has been our practice to perform a tubogram under screening control 10 days to two weeks after surgery. If there is free flow with no significant anastomotic leakage we have rarely left temporary splintage for longer than six weeks (Figure 54.10). We would agree that, in the repair of simple recent injuries to the bile duct where a soft pliant anastomosis has been fashioned, prolonged internal splintage is contraindicated as this may excite an excessive inflammatory response.[132]

During prolonged splintage biliary debris will accumulate within and around the tube. Daily lavage with saline containing an antibiotic is probably the simplest way of preventing this complication, and has the advantage that it can be continued at home by most patients with the minimum of supervision and inconvenience. It must be emphasized that the successful usage of splintage tubes depends upon frequent follow-up with radiological control by the surgeon.

Results of Biliary Reconstruction

The overall operative mortality for the repair of benign biliary stricture ranges from 3 to 8 per cent.[26, 31, 48, 66, 122, 126] Occasionally, lower mortality rates have been reported.[20, 22] However, even in experienced hands the complexity of the operative procedures results in a high perioperative mortality. Thus, in a series of almost 1000 patients treated at the Lahey Clinic, the perioperative mortality was 13 per cent. Fifty-one per cent of the patients who died succumbed as a result of hepatic failure, renal failure, haemorrhage or severe sepsis.[127]

In the modern practice of biliary surgery, the recognition of major predisposing risk factors and appropriate preoperative preparation and postoperative prophylaxis should ensure a lower mortality rate. Thus, during a period of five years, we have performed 63 bypass or reconstructive procedures for a wide variety of benign conditions of the biliary tract with only three hospital deaths (4.8 per cent).

The long-term results of biliary bypass surgery vary widely with the indication for operation and the complexity of the reconstruction. The results for simple bypass using sphincteroplasty or choledochoduodenostomy or even choledochojejunostomy are good, and a satisfactory outcome should be obtainable in more than 80 per cent of cases. The heterogeneous population of patients contained in the larger series reporting more complex bypass procedures makes comparison difficult. However, operative survival free from evidence of further biliary tract obstruction or other major complications is obtainable in more than 60 per cent of patients and eventual success rates in some large series may be as high as 70 to 80 per cent.[110, 127] Patients with a good result at two years have greater than a 90 per cent chance of a long-term cure following biliary reconstruction,[132] and most recurrent strictures are said to occur within three years of surgery.[24] Sandblom[95] has differed from these assertions, in a report of 800 cases followed up for at least 10 years, in which there was a 20 per cent incidence of recurrent symptoms, and it may be that the usual follow-up period of three to five years is inadequate for the assessment of long-term results.

It should be emphasized that re-stenosis and recurrence, while constituting operative failure, should not be considered an ultimate therapeutic failure. It is not uncommon for patients to require several surgical procedures in order to obtain a satisfactory result.[131] By the same token it should be recognized that repair of biliary strictures is technically complicated, and even in experienced hands the failure rate may exceed 30 per cent. Such surgery should be left to surgeons accustomed to dealing with the problem. Indeed, changing concepts in the management of biliary tract obstruction have produced improvement in results, even within a single specialist centre.[20]

PORTAL HYPERTENSION SECONDARY TO BILIARY OBSTRUCTION

In a review of 890 patients referred to the Lahey Clinic for correction of a biliary stricture, 169 (19 per cent) had some degree of portal hypertension.[103] In many cases there had been one or more unsuccessful attempts at repair. Portal hypertension was found to appear on average four to five years from the onset of the stricture, but the interval could be as little as two years in neglected cases. Sedgwick and his colleagues report their experience in 18 such cases treated by splenorenal shunt, but other reports in the literature have been scanty.[1, 31, 40] A small number of cases may present with severe hypersplenism, but the majority will present in one of three ways (see also Chapter 44).

Firstly, portal hypertension (previously diagnosed or unsuspected) may produce profuse haemorrhage at the time of surgery for repair of a biliary stricture. In these circumstances the most satisfactory procedure may be immediate tube drainage of the biliary system with no attempt at a repair, and re-operation three to four weeks later to perform a splenorenal shunt. This choice of shunting procedure is dictated by the technical difficulty of portacaval shunting in the presence of previous surgical interference, and by the danger of compromising the portacaval anastomosis by a subsequent biliary operation. While impaired liver function due to biliary obstruction makes the patient a poor candidate for shunting at the first operation, the surgeon may nevertheless be compelled to undertake portal diversion at this stage in order to reduce operative bleeding. In either event formal reconstruction of the bile ducts is performed at a subsequent operation when the degree of haemorrhage will be considerably reduced.

Secondly, patients with uncorrected biliary strictures may present de novo with bleeding oesophageal varices. This emergency is managed in the conventional manner, and the patient is then considered for an urgent splenorenal shunt, followed by repair of the biliary stricture at a second operation (Figure 54.11). It should be noted that in both of these groups of patients the normal criteria for selection of patients for portasystemic shunting may have to be relaxed, since while the operative risk is considerable such a shunt may provide the only chance of achieving a subsequent satisfactory repair of the biliary stricture. Furthermore, improvement in liver function may be anticipated following repair of the stricture. Indeed, despite poor liver function, only one patient of the 18 reported by Sedgwick and his colleagues suffered from portasystemic encephalopathy after shunting and stricture repair.

The third group of patients are those who have had repair of a biliary stricture in the presence of established secondary biliary cirrhosis and have subsequently suffered a gastrointestinal bleed. If correction of the biliary stricture has been successful these patients should be considered by the usual criteria for emergency or elective splenorenal shunt.

These patients present a formidable problem in surgical management, and the decision to operate at all is rarely easy. While good results are difficult to obtain, the risks of surgery must be weighed against the near certainty of death for a patient with biliary cirrhosis and gross portal hypertension.

Sclerotherapy may be of value in these difficult cases (see Chapter 44).

BILIARY CYSTS

This term refers to a group of cystic dilatations of the biliary tree of developmental origin. These may be single or multiple, arise at any point in the extrahepatic ductal system, and take the form either of a concentric cystic dilatation or of a diverticulum originating from one of the bile ducts.

There appears to be a marked racial difference in the incidence of choledochal cyst since a large number of cases has been reported from Japan.[65] Females predominate and most patients present during childhood or early adult life.

The triad of abdominal pain, obstructive jaundice and a palpable abdominal mass is classical. A cyst may produce common bile duct obstruction by kinking or twisting or by distension and compression of the common bile duct. The most frequent site of obstruction, however, is the common duct distal to the cyst, which is usually very narrow. Debris and, occasionally, gallstones may be found within the cyst. Infrequent manifestations of biliary cysts are pancreatitis and portal hypertension due to compression of the portal vein.

Conventional contrast radiology may be helpful but is not usually diagnostic. Percutaneous transhepatic cholangiography, however, may give clear outlining of cystic malformations within the entire biliary tree, and indeed a cyst may be punctured by the cholangiogram needle. The definitive diagnosis, however, is usually established only at operation.

At operation, the precise anatomical relationships of the cyst must be determined, and operative cholangiography may be helpful. Operative management is mandatory since almost all untreated cases die of complications of the cyst.[43] Drainage of the cyst into the intestine is the treatment of choice. Careful consideration should be given at operation to the optimum route of drainage, since an operation which produces inadequate decompression or a poor anastomosis will produce a high incidence of morbidity from cholangitis. Cystojejunostomy Roux-en-Y is probably the commonest form of treatment. This is performed at the most dependent part of the cyst in the manner described for cholecystojejunostomy, and a wide anastomosis is preferred. Transanastomotic tubes are not necessary. An attractive and preferable alternative when technically possible is excision of the cyst and hepaticojejunostomy Roux-en-Y in the manner described above for the management of biliary strictures.

Multiple biliary cysts, particularly when intrahepatic, pose a difficult surgical problem, and intrahepatic choledocho-enteric anastomoses or even hepatic lobectomy may be necessary to relieve the recurrent symptoms in some cases.[43]

The prognosis of adequately drained cystic dilatation is good, and the long-term results appear to be better after cystojejunostomy than after cystoduodenostomy.[65]

SCLEROSING CHOLANGITIS

This syndrome of progressive inflammatory thickening and irregular stenosis of the extrahepatic and intrahepatic bile ducts is divided into primary and secondary forms. Secondary sclerosing cholangitis may be associated with ulcerative colitis, Crohn's disease, gallstones or biliary surgery with bile extravasation. The primary form, however, is rare and can be diagnosed only in the proven absence of biliary calculi, inflammatory bowel disease and previous surgery, and the careful exclusion of a slow growing sclerosing carcinoma of the bile ducts.[101] The aetiology of this form has not been fully defined but there is evidence of an autoimmune process and also of a widespread hypersensitivity reaction due to the entry of bacteria into the portal circulation: this latter mechanism may explain the association with inflammatory bowel disease, and the response to colectomy in ulcerative colitis.

Pathologically, there are submucosal and subserosal inflammation and fibrosis diffusely involving a variable extent of the extrahepatic and sometimes the intrahepatic bile radicles. The liver parenchyma shows the changes of cholestasis and fibrosis and may progress to a secondary biliary cirrhosis.

The presentation is usually in middle age with chronic progressive biliary tract obstruction with or without the features of cholangitis. The length of history may range from months to years. Percutaneous cholangiography or ERCP may provide a preoperative diagnosis and, when the radiological features of this condition are seen, an active search must be made for the associated primary diseases mentioned above. It is impossible, however, to distinguish with certainty the radiological appearances from those of a diffuse sclerosing cholangiocarcinoma, and laparotomy is frequently indicated (see also Chapter 55).

At operation, the bile duct is thickened diffusely or locally, and local areas of stenosis may be confirmed by use of a probe. Biopsies must be obtained of the narrowed area and of the fleshy peridochal lymph nodes which are frequently encountered, although these may show only reactive hyperplasia. Bile may also be examined cytologically but, despite all of these examinations, the ultimate differentiation from carcinoma may depend upon the course of the patient's condition or, in some cases, on autopsy findings.[5]

Management depends on the operative findings and the site of the obstruction. If there is involvement of the common duct but sparing of the intrahepatic ducts, a hepaticojejunostomy Roux-en-Y may be established. This, however, is frequently not possible. Some authors have recommended the insertion of a tube into the thickened ductal system, which may subsequently be combined with drug treatment. The use of corticosteroids may prove effective, although this is difficult to assess because of the possibility of spontaneous remission.[101] Antibiotics may also have a place. In the specific case where the disease is associated with ulcerative colitis, the response to colectomy has been impressive.[128]

The prognosis for this condition depends to some extent on the aetiology and extent of the pathological changes. While some long-term survivors have been reported, death occurs in four to ten years from the onset of symptoms in the majority of cases.[65, 101] The cause of death is usually liver failure or bleeding oesophageal varices.

THE FUTURE

Prevention

The majority of biliary strictures are avoidable. Eighty per cent occur after cholecystectomy, many go unrecognized at the time of operation, and a considerable number follow cholecystectomy which the surgeon regarded as being simple and without incident.[25] The cause and prevention of most traumatic biliary strictures have been well reviewed.[65, 77, 127] Emphasis on these principles during surgical training and frequent reminders to the trainee that 'simple cholecystectomy' is an operation not to be undertaken lightly and requiring meticulous care and constant vigilance may reduce the incidence of such injuries. It must also be remembered that 3 per cent of strictures occur after a difficult partial gastrectomy.

The second aspect of prevention lies in ensuring that any procedure undertaken for the repair of biliary stricture should be the appropriate procedure at the first attempt, since this is the single best opportunity for successful repair. Subsequent attempts become progressively more difficult and the chances of success decline.[131]

Endoscopic Papillotomy

For the few proven cases of stenosis of the sphincter of Oddi[39, 75] and for cases of retained common bile duct stones following cholecystectomy, this procedure has been used increasingly in mainland Europe[28, 37, 63, 93] (see Chapter 23) and in the United Kingdom.[33] The role of this technique in practice has yet to be fully evaluated.

New Diagnostic and Operative Techniques

The diagnostic approaches outlined at the beginning of this chapter have been made possible by the availability of sophisticated diagnostic techniques. The use of these techniques has enabled the ideal of safe, accurate, preoperative diagnosis to be approached, and there is no doubt that the planning of a correct operative procedure relies on such information. Grey scale ultrasonography is becoming increasingly available in most modern departments of radiology, and there is now no longer any place for blind diagnostic laparotomy in the management of suspected biliary tract obstruction. The use of the surgical approaches outlined allows a very aggressive attitude to be adopted in the management of the high bile duct stricture or tumour. Guided by preoperative cholangiography and arteriography, the transhepatic approach to the hilum of the liver has brought patients who would previously have been considered inoperable within the scope of resectability and adequate biliary drainage.

Liver Transplantation

There are at present few clear indications for hepatic transplantation for benign obstructive biliary disease. Several of the longest surviving patients with liver transplant, however, have had this procedure performed for congenital biliary atresia (see Chapter 52). While recurrence of tumour has hindered the progress of transplantation for hepatic malignancy, this technique may yet find a place in the radical management of the liver irretrievably damaged by chronic bile duct obstruction.

REFERENCES

1. Adson, M.A. & Wychulis, A.R. (1968) Portal hypertension in secondary biliary cirrhosis. *Archives of Surgery*, **96**, 604–612.
2. Aldrete, J. (1977) In discussion of Saharia et al. *Annals of Surgery*, **185**, 598–604.
3. Allison, M.E.M., Moss, N.G., Fraser, M., Lloyd Jones, W., Ryan, C.J., Dobbie, J.W., Kennedy, A.C. & Blumgart, L.H. (1975) Renal function in obstructive jaundice: a clinical and micropuncture study. *Proceedings of the VIth International Congress of Nephrology, Firenze, Italy: June 8–12.*
4. Allison, M.E.M., Moss, N.E., Fraser, M., Ryan, C.J., Dobbie, J.W., Kennedy, A.C. & Blumgart, L.H. (1975) Renal function before and after haemorrhage in rats with chronic bile duct obstruction: a micropuncture study. *Kidney International*, **8**, 338.
5. Altemeier, W.A. & Culbertson, W.R. (1973) Sclerosing carcinoma of the hepatic bile ducts. *Surgical Clinics of North America*, **53**, 1229–1243.
6. Arner, O., Hagberg, S. & Seldinger, S.I. (1962) Percutaneous transhepatic cholangiography: puncture of dilated and non-dilated bile ducts under roentgen television control. *Surgery*, **52**, 561–571.
7. Bailey, M.E. (1976) Endotoxin, bile salts, and renal function in obstructive jaundice. *British Journal of Surgery*, **63**, 774–778.
8. Beart, R.W. Jr, Putnam, C.W. & Starzl, T.E. (1976) Use of a U-tube in the treatment of biliary disease. *Surgery, Gynecology and Obstetrics*, **142**, 912–914.
9. Belzer, F.O., Watts, J. McK., Ross, H.B. & Dunphy, J.E. (1965) Autoreconstruction of the common bile duct after venous patch graft. *Annals of Surgery*, **162**, 346–355.

10. Benjamin, I.S., Imrie, C.W. & Blumgart, L.H. (1977) Liver biopsy in 'difficult' jaundice. *British Medical Journal*, **ii,** 578.
11. Benjamin, I.S., Allison, M.E.M., Moule, B. & Blumgart, L.H. (1978) The early use of fine needle percutaneous transhepatic cholangiography in an approach to the diagnosis of jaundice in a surgical unit. *British Journal of Surgery*, **65,** 92–98.
12. Blumgart, L.H. (1975) Endoscopy of the upper gastro-intestinal tract. In *Advances in Surgery*, Ch. 9, pp. 97–134. Chicago: Longmire.
13. Blumgart, L.H. (1978) Biliary tract obstruction – new approaches to old problems. *American Journal of Surgery*, **135,** 19–31.
14. Blumgart, L.H. & Kennedy, A. (1973) Carcinoma of the ampulla of Vater and duodenum. *British Journal of Surgery*, **60,** 33–40.
15. Blumgart, L.H., Salmon, P.R. & Cotton, P.B. (1974) Endoscopy and retrograde choledochopancreatography in the diagnosis of the patient with jaundice. *Surgery, Gynecology and Obstetrics*, **138,** 565–570.
16. Blumgart, L.H., Carachi, R., Imrie, C.W., Benjamin, I.S. & Duncan, J.G. (1977) Diagnosis and management of post-cholecystectomy symptoms: the place of endoscopy and retrograde choledochopancreatography. *British Journal of Surgery*, **64,** 809–816.
17. Bourke, J.B., Swann, J.C., Brown, C.L. & Ritchie, H.D. (1972) Exocrine pancreatic function studies, duodenal cytology and hypotonic duodenography in the diagnosis of surgical jaundice. *Lancet*, **i,** 605–608.
18. Bowers, R.M. (1964) Morbid conditions following choledochojejunostomy. *Annals of Surgery*, **159,** 424–427.
19. Braasch, J.W. & McCann, J.C. Jr (1967) Observations on single section of the sphincter of Oddi. *Surgery, Gynecology and Obstetrics*, **125,** 355–358.
20. Braasch, J.W., Warren, K.W. & Blevins, P.K. (1975) Progress in biliary stricture repair. *American Journal of Surgery*, **129,** 34–37.
21. Burgess, J.N. & Kidd, H.A. (1967) Choledochoduodenostomy in treatment of chronic pancreatitis and choledocholithiasis. *British Medical Journal*, **ii,** 607–609.
22. Cameron, J.L., Skinner, D.B. & Zuidema, G.D. (1976) Long term transhepatic intubation for hilar hepatic duct strictures. *Annals of Surgery*, **183,** 488–495.
23. Capper, W.M. (1961) External choledochoduodenostomy. An evaluation of 125 cases. *British Journal of Surgery*, **49,** 292–300.
24. Cattell, R.B. & Braasch, J.W. (1959) General considerations in the management of benign strictures of the bile duct. *New England Journal of Medicine*, **261,** 929–933.
25. Cattell, R.B. & Braasch, J.W. (1959) Primary repair of benign strictures of the bile duct. *Surgery, Gynecology and Obstetrics*, **109,** 531–538.
26. Cattell, R.B. & Braasch, J.W. (1960) Repair of benign strictures of the bile ducts involving both or single hepatic ducts. *Surgery, Gynecology and Obstetrics*, **110,** 55–60.
27. Classen, M. & Demling, L. (1974) Endoskopische Sphinkterotomie det Papilla Vateri und Steinextraktion aus dem Ductus choledochus. *Deutsche Medizinische Wochenschrift*, **99,** 469–477.
28. Classen, M. & Ossenberg, F.W. (1977) Non-surgical removal of common bile duct stones. *Gut*, **18,** 760–769.
29. Colcock, B.P. & Perey, B. (1964) Exploration of the common bile duct. *Surgery, Gynecology and Obstetrics*, **118,** 20–24.
30. Cole, W.H. (1958) Strictures of the common bile duct. *Surgery*, **43,** 320–324.
31. Cole, W.H., Ireneus, C. Jr & Reynolds, J.T. (1955) Strictures of common bile duct: studies in 122 cases. *Annals of Surgery*, **142,** 537–550.
32. Conn, H.O. (1975) Liver biopsy in extrahepatic biliary obstruction and other 'contraindicated' disorders. *Gastroenterology*, **68,** 817–821.
33. Cotton, P.B., Chapman, M., Whiteside, C.G. & Le Quesne, L.P. (1976) Duodenoscopic papillotomy and gallstone removal. *British Journal of Surgery*, **63,** 709–714.
34. Dawson, J.L. (1965) Post-operative renal function in obstructive jaundice: effect of a Mannitol diuresis. *British Medical Journal*, **i,** 82–86.
35. Dawson, J.L. (1966) The effect of haemorrhage on renal function in obstructive jaundice. *British Journal of Surgery*, **53,** 679–685.
36. Degenshein, G.A. (1974) Choledochoduodenostomy: an 18 year study of 175 consecutive cases. *Surgery*, **76,** 319–324.
37. Demling, L. (1976) International Workshop on Endoscopic Papillotomy, Munich (March 1976), *Lancet*, **i,** 1172.
38. Demling, L., Koch, H., Classen, M., Belohlavek, D., Schaffner, O., Schwamberger, K. & Stolte, M. (1974) Endoskopische Papillotomie und Gallensteinentfernung. Tierexperimentelle Untersuchungen und erste Klinische Erfahrungen. *Deutsche Medizinische Wochenschrift*, **99,** 2255–2257.
39. Drouin, J.P. (1964) Cholecystectomy with routine sphincteroplasty. *Canadian Journal of Surgery*, **7,** 367–377.
40. Ekman, C.A. & Sandblom, P. (1962) Bilio-intestinal anastomosis as a cause of liver cirrhosis with portal hypertension. *Acta Chirurgica Scandinavica*, **123,** 383–388.
41. Elias, E., Hamlyn, A.N., Jain, S., Long, R.G., Summerfield, J.A., Dick, R. & Sherlock, S. (1976) A randomized trial of percutaneous transhepatic cholangiography with the Chiba needle versus endoscopic retrograde cholangiography for bile duct visualization in jaundice. *Gastroenterology*, **71,** 439–443.
42. Flinn, W.R., Olson, D.F., Oyasu, R. & Beal, J.M. (1977) Biliary bacteria and hepatic histopathologic changes in gallstone disease. *Annals of Surgery*, **185,** 593–597.
43. Fonkalsrud, E.W. (1973) Choledochal cysts. *Surgical Clinics of North America*, **53,** 1275–1281.
44. Freund, H., Charuzi, I., Granit, G. & Berlatzky, Y. (1977) Choledochoduodenostomy in the treatment of benign biliary tract disease. *Archives of Surgery*, **112,** 1032–1034.
45. Grage, T.B., Lober, P.H., Imamoglu, K. & Wangensteen, O.H. (1960) Stenosis of the sphincter of Oddi. A clinicopathological review of 50 cases. *Surgery*, **48,** 304–317.
46. Havard, C. (1960) Non-malignant bile duct obstruction. *Annals of the Royal College of Surgeons of England*, **26,** 88–114.
47. Healey, J.E.Jr (1954) Clinical anatomic aspects of radical hepatic surgery. *Journal of the International College of Surgeons*, **22,** 542–550.

48. Hertzer, N.R., Gray, H.W., Hoerr, S.O. & Hermann, R.E. (1973) The use of T-tube splints in bile duct repairs. *Surgery, Gynecology and Obstetrics,* **137,** 413–418.
49. Hinde, G. de B., Smith, P.M. & Craven, J.L. (1977) Percutaneous cholangiography with the Okuda needle. *Gut,* **18,** 610–614.
50. Hines, C.Jr, Ferrante, W.A., Davis, W.D. & Tutton, R.A. (1972) Percutaneous transhepatic cholangiography. Experience with 102 procedures. *American Journal of Digestive Diseases,* **17,** 868–874.
51. Hoerr, S.O. & Hermann, R.E. (1973) Side-to-side choledochoduodenostomy. *Surgical Clinics of North America,* **53,** 115–1122.
52. Hughes, H. & Blumgart, L.H. (1978) Unpublished data.
53. Hurwitz, A. & Degenshein, G.A. (1964) The role of choledochoduodenostomy in common duct surgery: reappraisal. *Surgery,* **56,** 1147–1150.
54. Imrie, C.W., McKay, A.J., Benjamin, I.S. & Blumgart, L.H. (1978) Secondary acute pancreatitis: aetiology, prevention, diagnosis and management. *British Journal of Surgery,* **65,** 399–402.
55. Johnson, A.G. & Stevens, A.E. (1969) Importance of the size of the stoma in choledochoduodenostomy. *Gut,* **10,** 68–70.
56. Jones, S.A. (1973) Sphincteroplasty (not sphincterotomy) in treatment of biliary tract disease. *Surgical Clinics of North America,* **53,** 1123–1137.
57. Kawai, K., Akasaka, Y. & Murakami, K. (1974) Endoscopic sphincterotomy of the ampulla of Vater. *Gastrointestinal Endoscopy,* **20,** 148–151.
58. Keighley, M.R.B. (1977) Micro-organisms in the bile. *Annals of the Royal College of Surgeons of England,* **59,** 328–334.
59. Keighley, M.R.B., Baddeley, R.M., Burdon, D.W., Edwards, J.A.C., Quoraishi, A.H., Oates, G.D., Watts, G.T. & Alexander-Williams, J. (1975) A controlled trial of parenteral prophylactic gentamicin therapy in biliary surgery. *British Journal of Surgery,* **62,** 275–279.
60. Kennedy, A.C., Burton, J.A., Luke, R.G., Briggs, J.D., Lindsay, R.M., Allison, M.E.M., Edward, N. & Dargie, H.J. (1973) Factors affecting prognosis in acute renal failure. *Quarterly Journal of Medicine,* **42,** 73–86.
61. Kirtley, J.A.Jr (1960) Hepatocholangiojejunostomy Roux-en-Y: an alternative method of repair of bile duct strictures. *Annals of Surgery,* **151,** 123–129.
62. Knill-Jones, R.P., Cochran, K.M., Sokhi, G.S., Russell, R.I. & Blumgart, L.H. (1975) Early diagnosis of jaundice. A computer and clinical study. *British Journal of Surgery,* **62,** 654–655.
63. Koch, H. (1975) Endoscopic papillotomy. *Endoscopy,* **7,** 89–93.
64. Kolff, J. Hoeltge, G. & Hermann, R.E. (1975) Silastic T tube splints for biliary repair. *American Journal of Surgery,* **129,** 236–240.
65. Kune, G.A. (1972) *Current Practice of Biliary Surgery,* 1st ed. Boston: Little, Brown.
66. Kune, G.A., Hardy, K.J., Brown, G. & McKenzie, G. (1969) Operative injuries of the bile ducts. *Medical Journal of Australia,* **2,** 233–236.
67. Lance, P., Bevan, P.G., Hoult, J.G. & Paton, A. (1977) Liver biopsy in 'difficult' jaundice. *British Medical Journal,* **ii,** 236.
68. Lane, C.E., Sawyers, J.L., Riddell, D.H. & Scott, H.W. (1973) Long-term results of Roux-en-Y hepatocholangiojejunostomy. *Annals of Surgery,* **177,** 714–722.
69. Lawson, T.L. (1977) Evaluation of biliary tract disease by diagnostic ultrasound. *American Journal of Digestive Diseases,* **22,** 820–828.
70. Lee, E., Ross, B.D. & Haines, J.R. (1972) The effect of experimental bile-duct obstruction on critical biosynthetic function of the liver. *British Journal of Surgery,* **59,** 564–568.
71. Longmire, W.P.Jr & Lippman, H.N. (1956) Intrahepatic cholangiojejunostomy: an operation for biliary obstruction. *Surgical Clinics of North America,* **36,** 849–863.
72. Longmire, W.P.Jr & Sandford, M.C. (1949) Intrahepatic cholangiojejunostomy for biliary obstruction – further studies: report of 4 cases. *Annals of Surgery,* **130,** 455–460.
73. Madden, J.L. (1973) Common duct stones: their origin and surgical management. *Surgical Clinics of North America,* **53,** 1095–1113.
74. Madden, J.L. & McCann, W.J. (1961) Reconstruction of the common bile duct by end-to-end anastomosis without the use of an internal splint or stent support. *Surgery, Gynecology and Obstetrics,* **112,** 305–314.
75. Madden, J.L., Kandalaft, S., McCann, W.J. & Lee, B.Y. (1968) Considerations in surgery of the common duct. *Current Problems in Surgery,* May, 3–75.
76. Madden, J.L., Chun, J.Y., Kandalaft, S. & Parekh, M. (1970) Choledochoduodenostomy: an unjustly maligned surgical procedure? *American Journal of Surgery,* **119,** 45–54.
77. Maingot, R. (1964) Injuries of the biliary tract, including operative and post-operative complications. In *Surgery of the Gall Bladder and Bile Ducts* (Ed.) Smith, R. & Sherlock, S. London: Butterworth.
78. McKay, A.J., Duncan, J.G., Imrie, C.W., Joffe, S.N. & Blumgart, L.H. (1978) The clinical value and accuracy of grey-scale ultrasound in detecting gallstones. *British Journal of Surgery,* **65,** 330–333.
79. Michie, W. & Gunn, A. (1964) Bile duct injuries. A new suggestion for their repair. *British Journal of Surgery,* **51,** 96–100.
80. Miller, D.R. (1972) Median sternotomy extension of abdominal incision for hepatic lobectomy. *Annals of Surgery,* **175,** 193–196.
81. Molnar, W. & Stockum, A.E. (1974) Relief of obstructive jaundice through percutaneous transhepatic catheter – a new therapeutic method. *American Journal of Roentgenology,* **122,** 356–367.
82. Mori, K., Misumi, A., Sugiyama, M., Okabe, M., Matsuoka, T., Ishii, J. & Akago, M. (1977) Percutaneous transhepatic bile drainage. *Annals of Surgery,* **185,** 111–115.
83. Morris, J.S., Gallo, G.A., Scheuer, P.J. & Sherlock, S. (1975) Percutaneous liver biopsy in patients with large bile duct obstruction. *Gastroenterology,* **68,** 750–754.
84. Moschcowitz, E. (1952) Morphology and pathogenesis of biliary cirrhosis. *American Medical Association Archives of Pathology,* **54,** 259–275.
85. Norcross, J.W. & Dadey, J.L. (1957) Medical complications of operative bile duct injuries. *New England Journal of Medicine,* **257,** 1216–1220.
86. Okuda, K., Tanikawa, K., Emura, T., Kuratomi, S., Jinnouchi, S., Urabe, K., Sumikoshi, T., Kanda, Y., Fukuyama, Y., Musha, H., Mori, H., Shimokawa, Y., Yakushiji, F. & Matsuura, Y. (1974) Nonsurgical percutaneous transhepatic cholangio-

graphy – diagnostic significance in medical problems of the liver. *American Journal of Digestive Diseases*, **19,** 21–36.

87. Partington, P.F. (1977) 23 years of experience with sphincterotomy and sphincteroplasty for stenosis of the sphincter of Oddi. *Surgery, Gynecology and Obstetrics*, **145,** 161–168.
88. Peel, A.L.G., Hermon-Taylor, J. & Ritchie, H.D. (1974) Technique of transduodenal exploration of the common bile duct. Duodenoscopic appearances after biliary sphincterotomy. *Annals of the Royal College of Surgeons*, **55,** 236–244.
89. Le Quesne (1977) Personal communication.
90. Redeker, A.G., Karvountzis, G.G., Richman, R.H. & Horisawa, M. (1975) Percutaneous transhepatic cholangiography. An improved technique. *Journal of the American Medical Association*, **231,** 386–387.
91. Rutledge, R.H. (1976) Sphincteroplasty and choledochoduodenostomy for benign biliary obstructions. *Annals of Surgery*, **183,** 476–487.
92. Rutledge, R.H. (1977) In discussion of Saharia et al. *Annals of Surgery*, **185,** 598–604.
93. Safrany, L. (1977) Duodenoscopic sphincterotomy and gallstone removal. *Gastroenterology*, **72,** 338–343.
94. Saharia, P.C., Zuidema, G.D. & Cameron, J.L. (1977) Primary common duct stones. *Annals of Surgery*, **185,** 598–604.
95. Sandblom, J.P. (1973) In discussion of Lane et al. *Annals of Surgery*, **177,** 721.
96. Sandblom, P., Mirkovitch, V. & Saegesser, F. (1977) Formation and fate of fibrin clots in the biliary tract: a clinical and experimental study. *Annals of Surgery*, **185,** 356–366.
97. Saypol, G.M. & Kurian, G. (1969) A technique of repair of stricture of the bile duct. *Surgery, Gynecology and Obstetrics*, **128,** 1071–1076.
98. Schein, C.J. (1977) Choledochal incontinence as a purposeful adjunct to choledocholithotomy. *Surgery, Gynecology and Obstetrics*, **144,** 571.
99. Scheuer, P.J. (1973) *Liver Biopsy Interpretation*, 2nd ed. Paris: Ballière Tindall.
100. Schwartz, F., Benshimol, A. & Hurwitz, A. (1959) Choledochoduodenostomy in the treatment of stenosis of the lower portion of the common bile duct. *Surgery*, **46,** 1020–1026.
101. Schwartz, S.I. (1973) Primary sclerosing cholangitis: a disease revisited. *Surgical Clinics of North America*, **53,** 1161–1168.
102. Scott, J., Summerfield, J.A., Elias, E., Dick, R. & Sherlock, S. (1977) Chronic pancreatitis: a cause of cholestasis. *Gut*, **18,** 196–201.
103. Sedgwick, C.E., Poulantzas, J.K. & Kune, G.A. (1966) Management of portal hypertension secondary to bile duct stenosis: review of 18 cases with splenorenal shunt. *Annals of Surgery*, **163,** 949–953.
104. Sherlock, S. (1975) *Diseases of the Liver and Biliary System*, 8th ed. London: Blackwell Scientific.
105. Shida, S. (1971) Biopsy smear cytology with fibergastroscope for direct observation. In *Early Gastric Cancer* (Ed.) Murakami, T. p. 223. Tokyo: Tokyo University Press.
106. Shingleton, W.W. (1977) In discussion of Flinn et al. *Annals of Surgery*, **185,** 593–597.
107. Smith, R. (1964) Hepaticojejunostomy with transhepatic intubation. *British Journal of Surgery*, **51,** 186–194.
108. Smith, R. (1965) Transluminal T-tube drainage in pancreatobiliary surgery. *Lancet*, **ii,** 1063–1066.
109. Smith, R. (1969) Strictures of the bile ducts. *Proceedings of the Royal Society of Medicine*, **62,** 131–137.
110. Smith, R. (1978) McEwan Lecture, Glasgow 1977. *British Journal of Surgery*. In Press.
111. Stephens, F.O. & Dunphy, J.E. (1963) Grafts of the common bile duct – an historical review. *Australia and New Zealand Journal of Surgery*, **32,** 53–57.
112. Stern, R.B., Knill-Jones, R.P. & Williams, R. (1973) Pitfalls in the diagnosis of jaundice due to carcinoma of the pancreas or biliary tree. *British Medical Journal*, **i,** 533–534.
113. Stone, R.M., Cohen, Z., Taylor, B.R., Langer, B. & Tovee, E.B. (1973) Bile duct injury. Results of repair using a changeable stent. *American Journal of Surgery*, **125,** 253–256.
114. Taylor, K.J.W. & Rosenfield, A.T. (1977) Grey-scale ultrasonography in the differential diagnosis of jaundice. *Archives of Surgery*, **112,** 820–825.
115. Templeton, J.Y. III & Dodd, G.D. (1963) Anatomical separation of the right and left lobes of the liver for intrahepatic anastomosis of the biliary ducts. *Annals of Surgery*, **157,** 287–291.
116. Thomas, C.G. (1977) In discussion of Saharia et al. *Annals of Surgery*, **185,** 598–604.
117. Thomas, E., Kerr Grant, A., Holford, M., Ringwood, D., Derrington, A.W. & Magarey, J.R. (1973) Bacterial flora in the duodenum of patients after biliary fenestration. *British Journal of Surgery*, **60,** 107–111.
118. Thorbjarnarson, B. (1975) Surgery of the biliary tract. *Major Problems in Clinical Surgery*, **16,** 1–162.
119. Tsuchiya, Y. (1969) A new safer method of percutaneous transhepatic cholangiography. *Japanese Journal of Gastro-enterology*, **66,** 438–455.
120. Tylen, U., Hoevels, J. & Vang, J. (1977) Percutaneous transhepatic cholangiography (PTC) with external drainage of obstructive biliary lesions. *Surgery, Gynecology and Obstetrics*, **144,** 13–18.
121. Waddell, W.R. (1967) Exposure of intrahepatic bile ducts through interlobar fissure. *Surgery, Gynecology and Obstetrics*, **124,** 491–500.
122. Walters, W., Nixon, J.W.Jr & Hodgins, T.E. (1959) Strictures of the common bile duct. Five to 25 year follow-up of 217 operations. *Annals of Surgery*, **149,** 781–788.
123. Wardle, E.N. (1975) Endotoxaemia and the pathogenesis of acute renal failure. *Quarterly Journal of Experimental Medicine*, **174,** 389–398.
124. Wardle, E.N. & Wright, N.A. (1970) Endotoxin and acute renal failure associated with obstructive jaundice. *British Medical Journal*, **iv,** 472–474.
125. Warren, K.W. (1965) Modification of the Roux-en-Y procedure. *Surgical Clinics of North America*, **45,** 611–615.
126. Warren, K.W. & Braasch, J.W. (1964) The selection of an operative procedure for benign stricture of the bile duct. *Surgical Clinics of North America*, **44,** 717–729.
127. Warren, K.W. & Jefferson, M.F. (1973) Prevention and repair of strictures of the extrahepatic bile ducts. *Surgical Clinics of North America*, **53,** 1169–1190.
128. Warren, K.W., Athanassiades, S. & Monge, J.I. (1966) Primary sclerosing cholangitis: a study of 42 cases. *American Journal of Surgery*, **111,** 23–38.

129. Warren, K.W., McDonald, W.M. & Kune, G.A. (1966) Bile duct strictures. New concepts in the management of an old problem. In *Modern Trends in Surgery* (Ed.) Irvine, W.T. 2nd ed. London: Butterworth.
130. Warren, K.W., Mountain, S.C. & Gray, L.W. (1972) Use of the modified Y tube splint in the repair of biliary strictures. *Surgery, Gynecology and Obstetrics,* **134,** 665–668.
131. Warren, K.W., Mountain, S.C. & Midell, A.I. (1971) Management of strictures of the biliary tract. *Surgical Clinics of North America,* **51,** 711–731.
132. Way, L.W. & Dunphy, J.E. (1972) Biliary stricture. *American Journal of Surgery,* **124,** 287–295.
133. Williams, G.R. (1973) Experiences with surgical reconstruction of the hepatic ducts. *Annals of Surgery,* **179,** 540–548.
134. Williams, R.C., Showalter, R. & Kern, F.Jr (1975) In vivo effect of bile salts and cholestyramine on intestinal anaerobic bacteria. *Gastroenterology,* **69,** 483–491.
135. Williams, R.D., Elliot, D.W. & Zollinger, R.W. (1960) The effect of hypotension in obstructive jaundice. *Archives of Surgery,* **81,** 334–340.
136. Wood, C.B., Capperauld, I. & Blumgart, L.H. (1977) Bioplast fibrin buttons for the control of haemorrhage of the liver following biopsy and partial resection. *Annals of the Royal College of Surgeons of England,* **58,** 401–404.
137. Wright, N.L. (1968) Evaluation of the results of choledochoduodenostomy. *British Journal of Surgery,* **55,** 33–36.

Chapter 55

Tumours of the Biliary Tree and Pancreas

C.W. IMRIE
L.H. BLUMGART

The diagnostic techniques and many of the important points relating to the pathophysiological effects of biliary obstruction and to preoperative preparation in the jaundiced patient with benign biliary obstruction (see also Chapter 54) apply with equal force in the patient with malignant disease. Similarly, although the techniques of resection for malignant tumours differ in many respects from the procedures required for benign obstruction, the principles of reconstructive anastomosis and the use of tubal drains are similar in both situations.

BENIGN TUMOURS OF THE BILE DUCTS

Benign tumours of the biliary tree are uncommon and indeed a review of the literature up to 1970 reveals only 76 published cases. These lesions occur in all age groups and have been reported both in school children and in the very elderly, the mean age of the patients being just over 50 years.

Several different histological variants of benign tumours of the biliary ductal system have been documented.[15,21,35] The most common form is the simple *adenoma*. This may on occasion take the form of a cystadenoma or adenomyoma. *Papilloma* of the bile ducts is the next most frequent variety and rarely exceeds 2 cm in diameter. The other histological types described are leiomyoma and neurilemmoma (schwannoma).

While the clinical picture may be similar in all respects to the presentation of malignant tumours of the biliary tree with a short and progressive history of jaundice, cases have been documented with illness extending over decades. Persistent or intermittent jaundice frequently occurs and may be accompanied by pain, weight loss and, in some instances, dyspepsia. Cholangitis and haemobilia have also been reported. Percutaneous transhepatic cholangiography (PTC) and endoscopic retrograde cholangiopancreatography (ERCP) are valuable adjuncts in the localization of these lesions. It is worth noting that precise preoperative diagnosis, even with these modern advances in technique, is more difficult than in the case of malignant tumour. Cytology may be unremarkable and a negative result on material obtained at endoscopic examination does not exclude a malignant lesion. Even at operation difficulties are encountered and indeed the soft texture of some of these lesions can result in their being overlooked by the surgeon.

Peroperative choledochoscopy may be of considerable value in experienced hands but is still infrequently utilized, most surgeons relying on pre- and peroperative cholangiography. Even when the benign tumour is identified at operation, frozen section histology is difficult to interpret because of the fibrous reaction which characterizes some of these lesions. A firm histological opinion is important since local resection and end-to-end anastomosis of the extrahepatic biliary tree rather than extensive resection is justified. Although local excision of benign lesions may be followed by recurrence in up to 20 per cent of patients, this does not appear to be more frequent than after more extensive resections where the mortality is considerably higher.[21]

The prognosis for localized benign lesions is very good and indeed subsequent operations for recurrence are often successful. However, if choledochoscopy is used at the time of initial operation it may reveal the presence of additional small lesions in the biliary tree. For patients with a field change of this nature rather than recurrent lesions radical surgery may be required and the prognosis is poor.[47]

MALIGNANT TUMOURS OF THE BILE DUCT AND GALLBLADDER

Adenocarcinoma of the bile duct (cholangiocarcinoma) presents in three histological types: (a) papillary, (b) nodular and (c) diffuse. The papillary lesion tends to project into the duct and is the most easily recognized at operation. However, it is important to be aware that this tumour is occasionally associated with a field change in the biliary ductal system and further lesions may be revealed radiologically. Choledochoscopy can be valuable in this situation.[78]

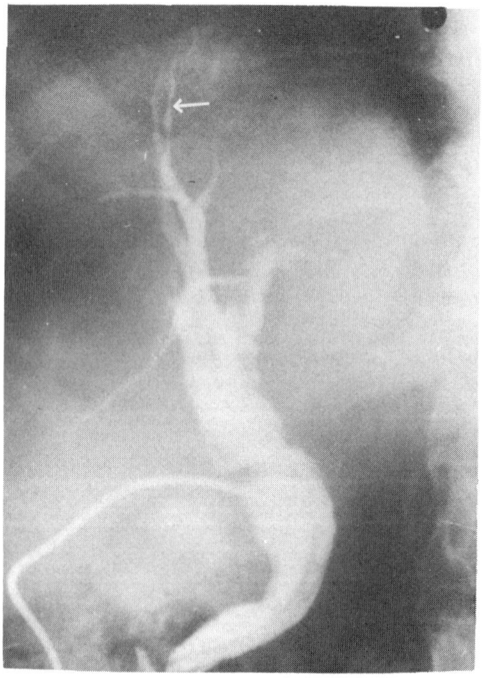

Figure 55.1. T-tube cholangiogram obtained in an elderly woman presenting with jaundice and submitted to cholecystectomy for gallstones. Exploration of the common bile duct revealed no cause for the jaundice. She was referred to our clinic for an opinion. Examination of the films revealed diffuse changes (arrowed) associated with probable sclerosing cholangitis or cholangiocarcinoma. Subsequent histology of the gallbladder revealed carcinomatous changes in the mucosal lining of the gallbladder. Cytological specimens obtained from bile aspirate through the T-tube revealed malignant cells.

The nodular type of tumour may be particularly difficult to diagnose, especially when it arises either at the confluence of the hepatic duct[43] or close to the papilla of Vater. This type of cholangiocarcinoma often presents an annular appearance with occlusion of the bile duct lumen, in contrast to the diffuse lesions which have a tendency to intramural spread and may be mistaken for sclerosing cholangitis (Figure 55.1).

The incidence of bile duct tumours in large autopsy series varies from 0.01 to 0.46 per cent[41] and while this is still a rare form of carcinoma 4500 new cases per annum may be expected in the United States, an incidence similar to that of carcinoma of the tongue.[43] The tumour has been reported in patients in their twenties and in the very aged although the majority occur in the 50 to 70 age group, males being more frequently affected than females.

The aetiology is unknown and attempts to link the presence of gallstones to bile duct cancer have been unconvincing.[56,64,67,73] This contrasts with the good association between the presence of gallstones and gallbladder carcinoma (see below).

A poorly understood relationship, however, exists between ulcerative colitis and cholangiocarcinoma. The number of documented patients with these combined conditions is small. We have a recent experience of four such cases and have seen the disease present some years after proctocolectomy, a feature also noted by Ross and Braasch.[63] In one of our patients the bile duct lesion was the presenting feature, ulcerative colitis being discovered only during subsequent investigation. Roberts-Thompson, Strickland and Mackay[62] found 29 patients with cholangiocarcinoma and ulcerative colitis and considered there was a definite consequential relationship between the two diseases but were unable to show any relationship between colitis and carcinoma of the gallbladder.

Studies from Hong Kong suggest a possible relationship between infection with *Clonorchis sinensis* and bile duct cancer,[4] but it should be noted that *Clonorchis* infection is common in Hong Kong and the association may be fortuitous. Others have suggested that infection and stasis of bile may be important. No definite relationship has been demonstrated between congenital hepatic fibrosis or polycystic disease and the presence of these tumours[23] although tumours have been reported in these conditions.[17,18]

Clinical suspicion of cholangiocarcinoma may be raised by the presentation of obstructive jaundice, weight loss and an impalpable gallbladder. However, it is desirable to obtain cytological evidence and necessary for the proper planning of therapy to demonstrate precisely the level and extent of the lesion. A suggested approach to this problem using ultrasound as the initial screening procedure has been outlined in Chapter 54 (see Figure 54.4).

Selective arteriography outlining the hepatic artery and its tributaries gives valuable preoperative information as to arterial anatomy. Percutaneous splenoportography is also important and we have come to regard it as essential in allowing full preoperative assessment of the extent of malignancy at the hilum of the liver (Figure 55.2). Indeed, it is only with such full preoperative information that the limits of resectability can be properly explored at subsequent operation.[6]

Radical resection should not be performed in the absence of a careful check for metastatic lesions. This includes preoperative liver scanning by ultrasound, isotope technique or computerized tomography. The last of these approaches has recently been combined with arteriography and has allowed detection of small metastatic lesions in the liver.[86] Finally, frozen section examination of lymph node and liver biopsy at the time of surgery may be necessary before a final decision as to the wisdom of extensive resection is taken.

Therapy is largely determined by the site and

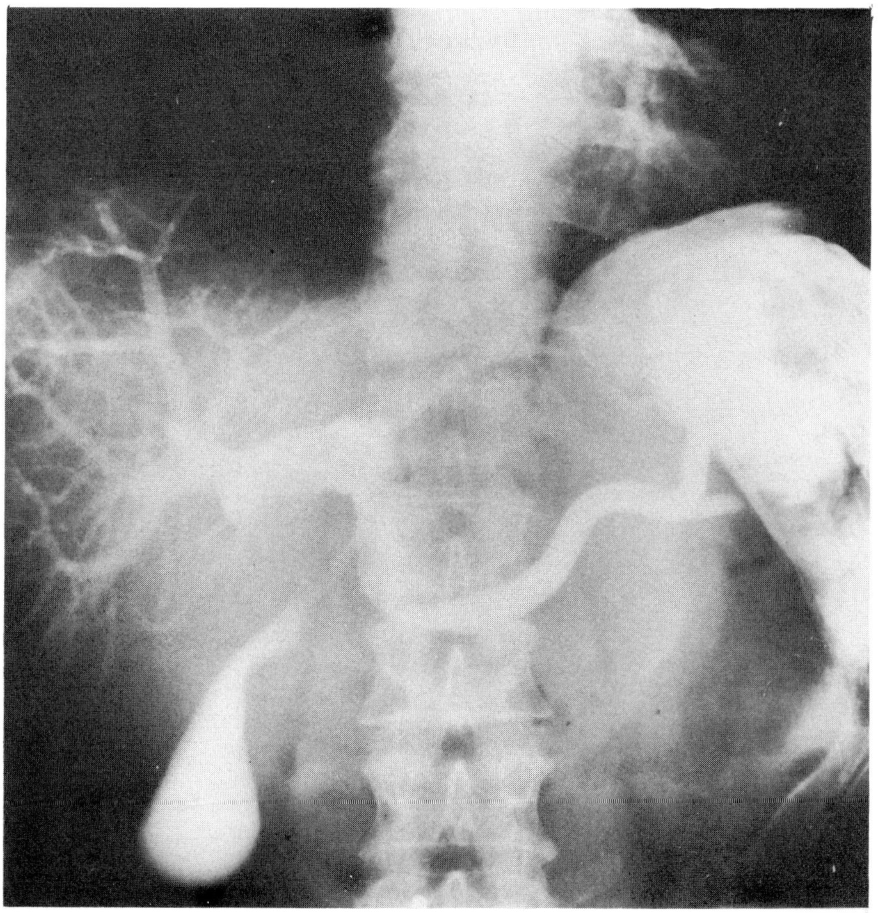

Figure 55.2. Splenoportography performed in a man with bile duct cancer at the confluence of the right and left hepatic ducts demonstrated at percutaneous cholangiography and ERCP. Note involvement of the left branch of the portal vein by tumour. Resection proved possible. Left lobectomy was performed, together with excision of the involved portion of portal vein and direct repair. Contrast from ERCP examination carried out on the same day is seen in the gallbladder.

extent of the lesion. For very extensive lesions involving wide areas of the biliary tract in the elderly, it may be both technically difficult and unwise to attempt even palliative surgery (see also Chapter 54, Figure 54.5). For lesions involving the biliary ductal apparatus below the hilum of the liver, surgical treatment involves complete wide excision including the head of the pancreas. Approximately 50 per cent of tumours, however, involve the confluence of the right and left hepatic ducts and the degree of extension into the liver substance on one or both sides governs the feasibility of resection.

Malignant tumours situated precisely at the confluence of the ducts and localized to this area can be excised and the right and left hepatic ducts separately anastomosed to a Roux loop of jejunum. An infrahepatic approach to such lesions is justified if hepatic arteriography and splenoportography reveal no involvement of major vascular structures at the hilum and, preferably, the distal extension on both sides should have been demonstrated preoperatively. In the more complex cases with some extension into the liver substance or where there is involvement of vessels at the hilum, assessment of operability is incomplete when an infrahepatic approach is made and we prefer initial hepatotomy using the liver split technique (see Chapter 54, Figure 54.12).[6,38,45] This approach permits a good view of the hilar structures, precise dissection, anastomosis of vessels at the hilum and a much better opportunity for direct mucosa-to-mucosa suture during reconstructive anastomosis. Furthermore, should the lesion extend so far into one or other hepatic lobe that hepatic lobectomy becomes necessary the resection is readily extended. It should be noted that, if the lesion extends beyond the second bifurcation of the duct system on both sides and is irresectable, nothing has been lost by the approach described above since palliative tubal drainage can still be instituted.

In patients considered inoperable on the basis of tumour extension into the liver or vascular structures, bile drainage into a Roux loop or the common bile duct is possible by inserting a tube through the area of malignant stricture. We have been impressed with the use of a 'U-tube' as advocated by Terblanche, Saunders and

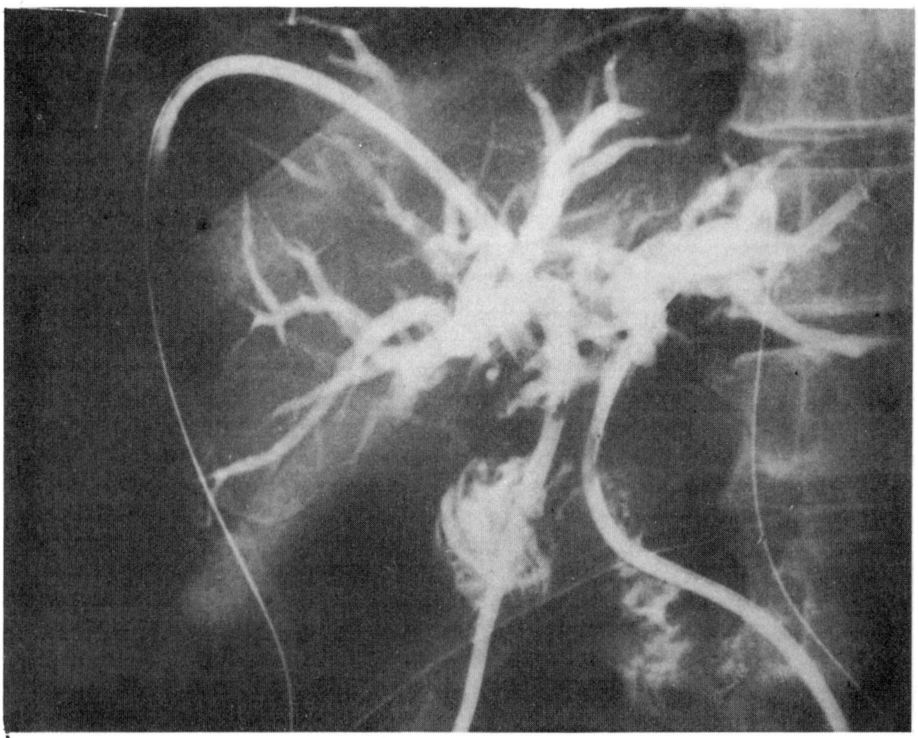

Figure 55.3. Bilateral U-tubes passed through the liver substance and into an adjacent Roux-en-Y loop of jejunum in a patient with irresectable cholangiocarcinoma involving the confluence of the hepatic ducts. Previous surgery had removed the entire length of the extrahepatic biliary ductal system. The patient was managed postoperatively with radiotherapy and regular washing of the tubes with antibiotic solution, and survived 23 months during which time he returned to work.

Louw.[76] Provided the tube is carefully placed and regularly washed out with an antibiotic solution, good results are obtainable (Figure 55.3). A template of the U-tubes should be made at the time of initial operation to enable replacement to be carried out. If necessary, the new tube can be 'railroaded' into position under radiological control. We have employed post-operative radiotherapy as advocated by Terblanche and Louw[75] and even in advanced cases a survival in years can be obtained, with a good quality of life which enables some patients to return to full employment. More recently, Japanese workers have published preliminary results of intra-operative radiotherapy for lesions of this type and initial findings are encouraging.[38] A radiation dose of up to 4000 rads, either during the operative procedure or postoperatively, does not appear to result in any serious local side-effects.

The relative success of tubal drainage combined with local radiotherapy is based on the slow growth of the malignant tumour of bile ducts, but most of these patients eventually succumb from intrahepatic extension of the primary tumour. Little is known of the susceptibility of malignant tumours of the biliary tree to single or multiple cytotoxic chemotherapy.

At the present time, despite aggressive surgical approaches, the results of surgical treatment for bile duct tumours are disappointing.[22,38,45] Useful palliation and the possibility of cure can, however, be offered to some patients. Increasing awareness of the incidence and potential resectability of these lesions, together with an increased application of modern sophisticated diagnostic techniques, may allow improvement in prognosis.

Liver transplantation has been performed in small numbers of patients with cholangiocarcinoma but the results have been disappointing[11,22] and certainly transplantation should not be considered unless the limits of resectability have been explored.[6] Indeed, should the lesion prove inoperable the palliation offered by tubal drainage and radiotherapy is comparable to the results of transplantation.[75]

Tumours of the Gallbladder

Benign papilloma of the gallbladder, occasionally single and sometimes multiple, is rarely more than a centimetre in diameter. In the neck of the gallbladder numerous glands are present and adenoma may occur. There is little evidence that malignant transformation is a frequent occurrence. Other benign tumours, e.g. fibroma, neurofibroma, leiomyoma and lipoma, have all been the subject of occasional case reports.

Carcinoma of the gallbladder has been claimed to represent almost 20 per cent of all gastrointestinal carcinoma.[11] Others have stressed the frequency of this tumour which tends to occur most commonly in the fundus and neck of the gallbladder.[2,14,34,65] The tumour is more common in women and has a peak incidence in the 70- to 75-year-old group and a female-to-male ratio of approximately 3:1.[20,25,71,74] A close association with the presence of gallstones has been noted and in some series up to 90 per cent of patients have cholelithiasis. The presence of the stone and associated inflammation with infection have been implicated as causal factors.

Histologically, 75 to 90 per cent of these lesions are well differentiated mucin-secreting adenocarcinomas, while 5 per cent are squamous cell lesions and approximately 10 per cent are anaplastic. The mode of spread of carcinoma of the gallbladder is mainly by the lymphatics along the cystic duct and thence to the common bile duct or by direct extension into the adjacent liver.

Preoperative diagnosis is uncommon although a calcified gallbladder (porcelain gallbladder) seen on x-ray may indicate carcinoma.[59] Occasionally, ERCP reveals an irregular filling defect within the gallbladder and this investigation may also suggest the presence of gallbladder carcinoma where tumour obstruction is revealed at the hilum of the liver in the presence of non-filling of the gallbladder (Figure 55.4).

Up to 50 per cent of patients may have a history of biliary disease extending for more than one year in duration.[20] In most patients this is diagnosed as an incidental finding at elective biliary surgery and the present very poor results of treatment (five-year survival approximately 3 per cent) partly reflect the age of the population affected and the limited number of patients in whom a radical surgical procedure has been attempted. It has been postulated that the liver bed becomes involved at an even earlier stage than the lymph nodes[27] so that for any younger patients hepatic resection is mandatory if the present bleak prognosis for this lesion is to be improved at all.

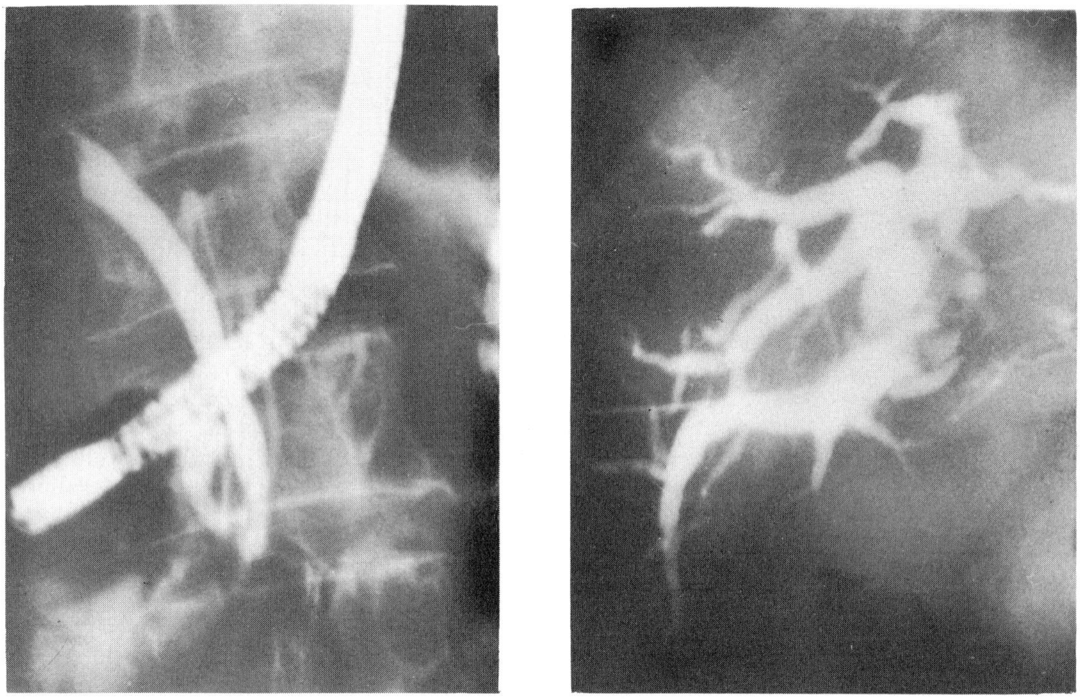

(a) (b)

Figure 55.4. (a) ERCP in a patient with carcinoma of the gallbladder involving the common hepatic duct. The common bile duct is revealed together with the cystic duct which joins the common bile duct near to the papilla of Vater. The gallbladder does not fill. Cytology obtained at ERCP confirmed the suspicion of malignancy. (b) Fine needle cholangiography obtained in the same patient reveals the right hepatic ductal system with obstruction at the hilum of the liver. Successful resection of this tumour was carried out and involved extended right hepatic lobectomy with hepaticojejunostomy to the left hepatic duct.

PERIAMPULLARY TUMOURS

A heterogeneous group of tumours occurs about the papilla of Vater and they are frequently considered together because the standard surgical therapy has been similar.[3,16,22,42,52,55,70,72,82,83] It is important, however, that these tumours be considered separately as the management and prognosis depend upon whether they arise in true periampullary tissues, the pancreas, the low common bile duct or the duodenal mucosa and upon histological variance.

Many misconceptions still exist as to the diagnosis and management of periampullary tumours. It is not clearly understood that the presentation may be with intermittent or indeed sometimes with only one attack of jaundice, that pain of a dyspeptic nature is frequently present, that the patient may present with haematemesis or melaena and that diagnosis, especially if it relies on an upper gastrointestinal barium series, is unreliable. Even experienced surgeons in a specialized unit misdiagnose periampullary lesions at operation in 10 per cent of patients.[83] Finally, there remains a belief that the mortality for resectional surgery is prohibitive and that the outcome of resection is uniformly poor. Neither of these statements is true. Pessimism is not warranted provided precise diagnosis is achieved and operation performed by an experienced surgeon.

Pancreaticoduodenectomy, originally introduced as a two-stage procedure,[84] is now frequently performed in centres specializing in this type of surgery with a mortality of less than 6 per cent.[32,44,70,81] Even in large series when the patients are drawn from multiple hospitals and not treated by specialist surgeons, the overall hospital mortality for all types of tumour is no higher than 21 per cent.[55] The resectability rate varies with the origin of the tumour, being over 70 per cent for ampullary carcinoma but falling sharply for carcinoma of the head of the pancreas to approximately 10 per cent.[52,55,82,83]

The mortality rate also varies with the origin of the tumour, ampullary carcinoma having the lowest mortality within one month of surgery

Table 55.1. *Hospital Mortality (%) of Pancreaticoduodenectomy for Periampullary Carcinomas.*

Tumour	Nakase et al[55]	Mongé et al[52]	Warren et al[82]	Smith[70]
Carcinoma of head of pancreas	25.0	21.0	11.4	20.5
Lower CBD carcinoma	22.3	16.7	19.2	18.3
Duodenal carcinoma	18.5	24.0	21.6	2.5
Ampullary carcinoma	16.4	15.6	10.8	

(Table 55.1). The fact that the operative hazard in cancer of the pancreas is much greater than that in ampullary cancer or cancer of the terminal bile duct or duodenum has led some to advocate that all patients with adenocarcinoma of pancreas should be treated only by palliative bypass surgery. Our own experiences do not support this, firstly because of difficulty in absolute diagnostic accuracy at operation and secondly because palliative bypass surgery in itself carries a mortality approaching 20 per cent.[55]

Preoperative investigations in patients with periampullary tumours include biochemical tests of liver function, upper gastrointestinal barium studies, endoscopy and biopsy/cytology and delineation of the biliary and pancreatic ductal system by means of PTC and ERCP.[6] Selective arteriography is mandatory since it facilitates assessment of resectability and allows demonstration of vascular abnormalities. In particular, the right hepatic artery frequently arises from the superior mesenteric trunk (see Chapter 1), and knowledge of this is important during radical surgery.

Despite the fact that preoperative investigations are similar it is essential that each of the four different carcinomas arising in the periampullary region be examined separately.

Duodenal Carcinoma

Primary carcinoma arising in the small bowel is uncommon but a high proportion of those found are in the duodenum. Failure to differentiate clearly between lesions arising in the duodenal mucosa and those of the ampulla itself make analysis of data from many reports impossible. Most authors who have differentiated between these tumours have regarded the lesions as being of duodenal origin only when they have been clearly separated from the ampulla. In Japan and the United Kingdom the ratio of ampullary to duodenal cancer is approximately 9:1[7,55] while in Malaysia and the United States a ratio of 3:1 has been found.[3,52,82] On the other hand, some series are small, containing less than 40 patients, and an accurate analysis of incidence is impossible.

Histologically, cancer arising in the duodenum is most frequently an adenocarcinoma. The lesion can be papillary or annular in type. Mucus secretion with signet-ring cells may also be a feature and, rarely, carcinosarcoma or leiomyosarcoma may be found.

The clinical presentation is usually with weight loss. Gastrointestinal bleeding is not uncommon and jaundice may occur where the lesion involves the papilla of Vater or common bile duct. Vomiting of pyloric type is often present and upper gastrointestinal barium studies (Figure 55.5) and endoscopy are diagnostic.

The majority of patients have resectable lesions and in specialized units the five-year survival rate is approximately 40 per cent.[52,82] If the tumours are histologically graded it is found that the better differentiated lesions are associated with improved five-year survival figures.[52]

Tumours of the Lower Common Bile Duct

These are the least frequent of the four periampullary malignancies. Histologically, the lesions are adenocarcinomatous and almost 50 per cent show a papillary form. The majority are well differentiated but local extension to the pancreas, duodenum and lymph nodes is present in almost half.[82] The lesion may be very difficult, and sometimes impossible, to differentiate from small carcinomas of the head of the pancreas, although involvement of both the pancreatic and biliary ductal system at ERCP is highly suggestive of pancreatic tumour rather than a lesion of bile duct origin.

Progressive obstructive jaundice is present in almost 100 per cent of patients with this disease.

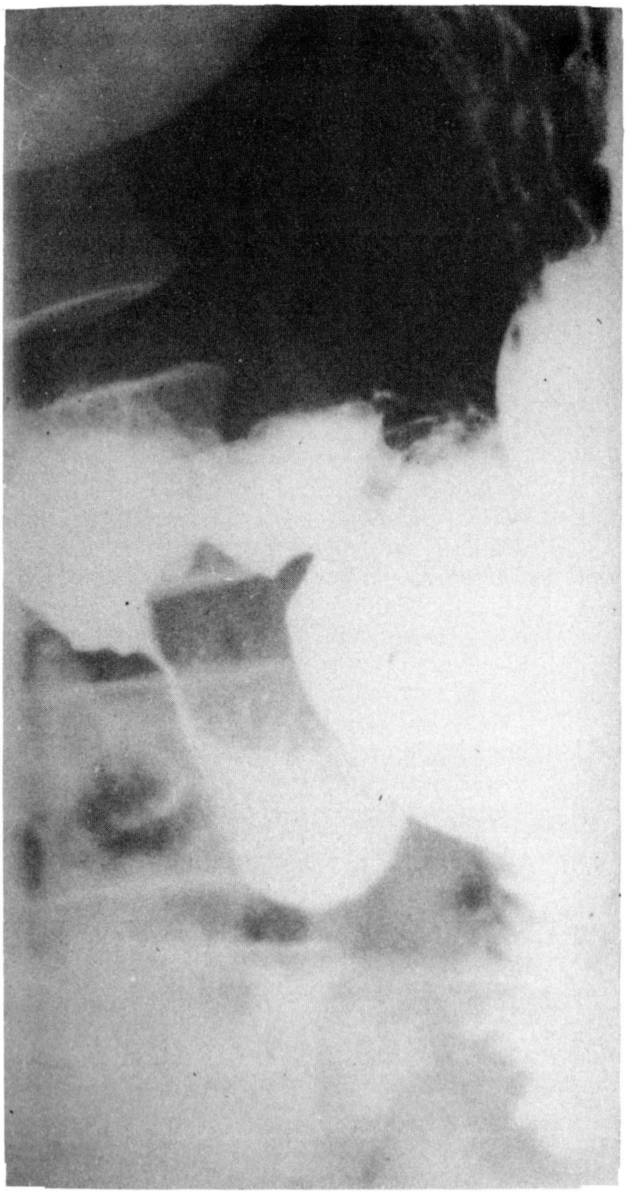

Figure 55.5. Barium meal examination in a patient with an annular carcinoma of the descending duodenum. The patient presented with vomiting of pyloric type.

The tumour growth rate may be very slow and the jaundice is occasionally intermittent. The hospital mortality for pancreaticoduodenectomy ranges from 8 to 22 per cent (Table 55.1), while the five-year survival figures of 25 per cent are less good than those for duodenal and ampullary cancer.[83] Curative surgery should usually be attempted, provided it can be carried out with an acceptable mortality rate. Occasional long-term survival is obtained.[43,83]

Ampullary Carcinoma

These lesions arise close to or at the papilla of Vater and histologically are adenocarcinomas with a varying degree of cellular differentiation. On occasion, other forms of malignant disease are found and we have encountered lymphoma and secondary tumour arising from an oat-cell carcinoma of the lung at the papilla of Vater. It is important to emphasize that benign papillomas may occur at the papilla of Vater and may be indistinguishable in presentation from the malignant lesion although endoscopy may often accurately suggest the nature of the tumour. Despite the fact that the lesions are uncommon they exceed the total number of the periampullary cancers arising in the lower common bile duct and duodenum.[52,55,82]

The clinical features have already been described but the disease, although most common in the 50 to 60 year age range, can occur in much younger patients (Figure 55.6). Endoscopy is much more reliable than hypotonic duodenography in the diagnosis of these lesions. The appearance at endoscopy together with endoscopic biopsy gives some index as to the histological variant of the disease and its prognosis.[6]

Few papers dealing with ampullary cancer detail the important aspect of histological differentiation of the individual lesions. They are roughly evenly distributed into two main histological variants.[7] Type I lesions are generally well differentiated papillary carcinomas showing a scanty stroma, clear origin from the papillary mucosa, little invasion and infrequent lymph node involvement (Figure 55.7a). Type II lesions are more invasive adenocarcinomas of intestinal type, usually with an abundant stromal reaction, local tissue infiltration and often with local nodal involvement (Figure 55.7b). It has been suggested for some years that the histology of these tumours relates to the outcome of the disease[16] but only two groups have clearly delineated the histology of these carcinomas and related this to survival. The better differentiated tumours are associated with excellent five-year survival rates in excess of 60 per cent[1] and a similar trend has been shown in a smaller British report.[7] The survival figures in patients with an intermediate degree of cellular differentiation was 58 per cent at two years and 24 per cent at five years. In contrast, no patient with a poorly differentiated tumour lived five years despite radical surgery, although

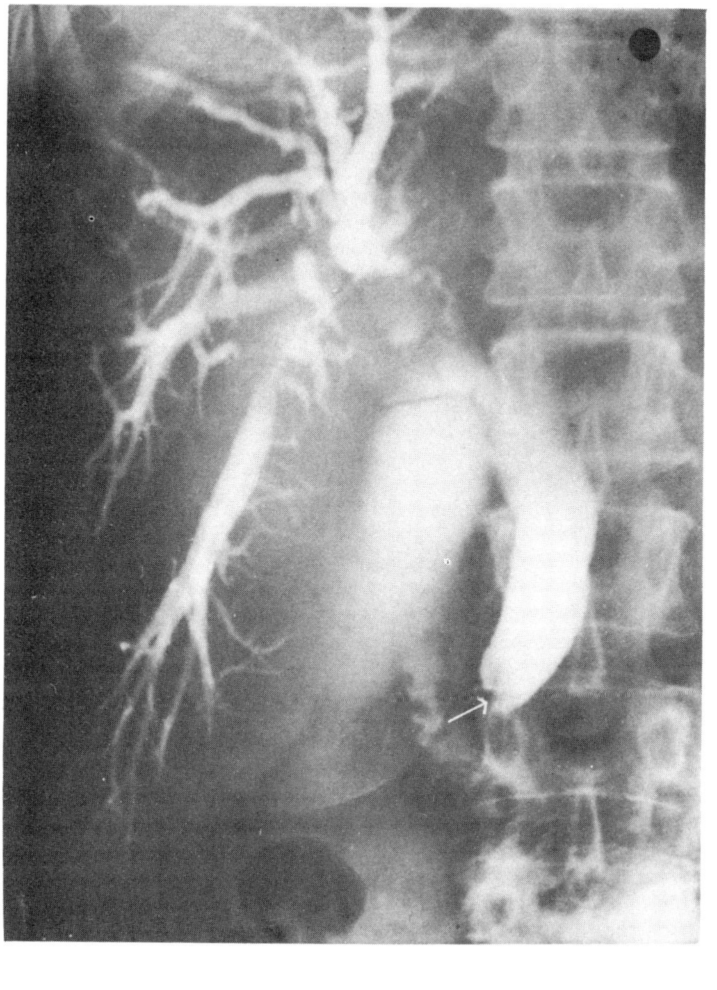

Figure 55.6. Fine needle percutaneous cholangiography in a 27-year-old man presenting with jaundice. Initial diagnosis suggested hepatitis and the patient was investigated in an infectious diseases hospital. Duodenoscopy revealed a small periampullary cancer confirmed by biopsy. The x-ray shows the dilated biliary ductal system and gallbladder and a small filling defect of a frond-like character (arrowed) at the lower end of the common bile duct. The patient was managed by initial T-tube drainage of the common hepatic duct (see also Chapter 54) and subsequent pancreaticoduodenectomy.

(a) 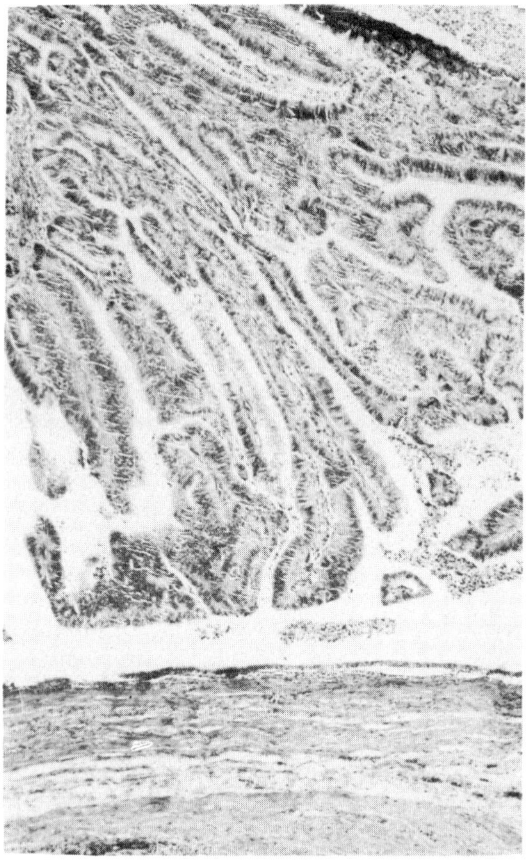 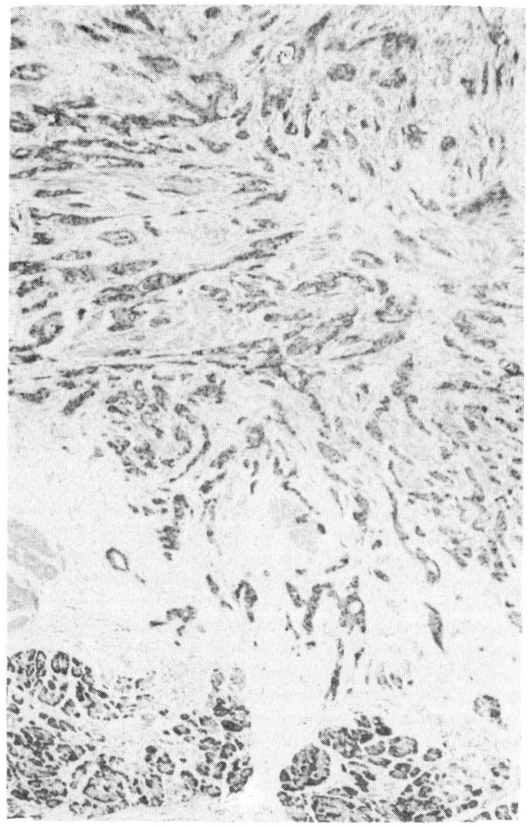 (b)

Figure 55.7. (a) Well differentiated papillary carcinoma of type I. The tumour cells are relatively tall and columnar and arranged on delicate strands of connective tissue with a scanty stromal base. There is little invasion. Haematoxylin and eosin × 35. From Blumgart,[5] with kind permission of the editors of *Journal of Surgical Oncology*. (b) A tumour of type II arising at the ampulla of Vater. This is a scirrhous adenocarcinoma which has reached the edge of the pancreas in the lower part of the field. Note the abundant stromal reaction. Such lesions are more prone to local nodal involvement. Haematoxylin and eosin × 25. From Blumgart and Kennedy,[7] with kind permission of the editors of *British Journal of Surgery*.

the two-year survival for such patients is almost 30 per cent[1] and this offers excellent palliation, especially since the mortality for palliative bypass may be as high as 20 per cent[52,55] and survival little prolonged.[83] The overall five-year survival of patients subjected to pancreaticoduodenectomy for ampullary carcinoma approaches 40 per cent in most specialized centres.[1,42,52,70] We, and several other groups of surgeons, perform pancreaticoduodenectomy for ampullary carcinoma and have a mortality of less than 10 per cent so that pessimism regarding radical surgical approaches to this lesion is unjustified.

Local resection with diathermy excision or even simple bypass may be justified in elderly unfit patients with poorly differentiated lesions and most such cases can be distinguished preoperatively using modern methods. All other patients should be submitted to radical surgery by an experienced surgeon but we believe that two-stage procedures are frequently justifiable (see also Chapter 54) and result in easier dissection, less bleeding and safer surgery.

Where surgical resection is not feasible, and in some patients where an anaplastic tumour has been resected, chemotherapy may have a place.[3] Because of the high mortality of bypass surgery, chemotherapy might be used in combination with simple transhepatic drainage methods (see also Chapter 54).

Carcinoma of the Head of Pancreas

While other malignant diseases of the head of the pancreas (e.g. islet cell tumours or cystadenocarcinoma) may arise, the most common cancer in this region is an adenocarcinoma. Squamous cell lesions are unusual and in over 90 per cent of patients with carcinoma of the pancreas the lesion arises from the duct or ductule epithelium.

The incidence of this disease has been rising in many countries and, indeed, in the last 40 years has trebled in the United States and doubled in England and Wales. Only colorectal cancer is more frequent than cancer of the pancreas among all digestive tract carcinomas. Aetiological factors which have been noted are that the disease is more frequent in males than in females. It also occurs more frequently in black than white patients and in Jewish than non-Jewish patients in the United States.[33] In most studies, the average age of patients is approximately 60 years and the sex ratio of males to females is in the region of 2:1. Cigarette smokers are at greater risk than non-smokers and tend to develop the disease at an earlier age than those who do not smoke.[33,40,54]

Several industrial chemicals, predominantly benzidine and nitrosurea compounds, have been implicated in the development of cancer of the pancreas and chemists working with these products are considered to be particularly at risk. It is now possible to induce pancreatic adenocarcinoma in several small animals by injecting nitrosurea compounds and the most useful model for the study of the disease is the Syrian hamster.[69] Irradiation, diabetes, pancreatic calcification and chronic pancreatitis do not clearly predispose to the development of this tumour.

In 60 to 65 per cent of patients suffering from adenocarcinoma of the pancreas, the primary lesion is located in the head of the gland. In the progression of the disease, the regional nodes are initially involved but spread to the liver is also very common. Next in frequency as sites of metastases are the peritoneum, adrenals and spleen. Extra-abdominal metastases are uncommon except in the lung. Occasionally, haematemesis occurs related to duodenal encroachment, and in advanced disease of the head of pancreas duodenal obstruction may be present. Pain may be particularly troublesome but this is less common than in carcinoma of the body of the gland. Often, weight loss accompanies the jaundice and both nausea and anorexia are common. Most patients have had symptoms for two or three months before presenting to a doctor and the rate of weight loss is often remarkable, amounting to ½ kg (1 lb) per week from onset of symptoms. Pruritus is very troublesome in up to 25 per cent of all patients. Rarely, patients present initially with an attack of acute pancreatitis, and this is usually associated with moderate to severe inflammation occurring distal to an obstruction in the main pancreatic duct. There is a poorly understood association with vascular thrombosis which tends to be in the venous aspect of the general circulation, although arterial thrombosis is also well recognized.

Clinical signs are most frequently those associated with obstructive jaundice and are more common the greater the duration of jaundice. A palpably enlarged liver is often found and frequently a distended gallbladder. Tenderness and ascites are less common and in only 15 per cent of patients is an abdominal mass palpable at the time of initial assessment.

The laboratory serological investigations which have been performed in the attempted diagnosis of carcinoma of the pancreas are varied and, unfortunately, no satisfactory tumour markers have yet been found. Carcinoembryonic antigen (CEA) was elevated in 85 per cent of patients with pancreatic cancer and serum alpha-fetoprotein in 24 per cent.[46,87] Neither of these fetal antigens has been found sufficiently specific to be of great clinical value, while the initial hopes that serum ribonuclease levels would be useful have proved unfounded. Oncofetal antigen (OFA), a glycoprotein which migrates in the beta region on electrophoresis, has most recently been purified from the sera of patients with pancreatic cancer.[24] The assay of this antigen which is found in fetal pancreas as well as in pancreatic cancer tissue, but not in normal adult pancreas, may prove to be useful in monitoring the course of pancreatic cancer and possibly in the diagnosis of the disease. One further recent test for the diagnosis of this troublesome disease is the micro-leucocyte adherence inhibition assay (LAI). This immunodiagnostic test appears to distinguish the blood of pancreatic cancer patients from others by the nature of their leucocyte adherence to a glass surface.[66] Of the more simple laboratory tests, hyperglycaemia is present to a variable degree and a glucose tolerance test is frequently abnormal, while diabetes has been found in almost 40 per cent of patients.[37]

In the further investigation of patients suspected of carcinoma of pancreas an upper gastrointestinal barium series may reveal abnormalities. The two most common changes are a widening of the duodenal loop and irregularities of the concave side of the duodenal mucosa.

These radiological findings result from distortion of the duodenal outline by the presence of the carcinoma. Such specific signs are present in a minority of patients but endoscopy, especially with the side-viewing instrument to obtain ERCP, is most useful. Involvement of both the pancreatic and bile ducts is highly suggestive of cancer of the pancreas and, in addition, ERCP allows cytological assessment of pancreatic juice or brush biopsy of the pancreatic duct (see also Chapter 54).[30,36] Intravenous injection of secretin may result in a diminished response in these patients due to obstruction of the duct but the stimulus may be sufficient to provoke the shedding of cells which can be successfully aspirated and subjected to cytological examination. Ultrasonically guided percutaneous needle biopsy of the pancreas is a more recent approach to the problem and in experienced hands results in a very high diagnostic rate.[28] Percutaneous transhepatic cholangiography (PTC) is less helpful than ERCP in establishing a firm diagnosis.

The great difficulty in diagnosis of carcinoma of the pancreas is well known and justifies an exploitation of all available investigation methods, including ultrasound, endoscopy with ERCP, cytology, isotope liver scan and computerized tomography (CT). Isotope pancreatic scanning has been disappointing[9] but encouraging results are now being obtained with grey scale ultrasound and CT. Even more accurate diagnostic results have been claimed with the combined use of local intra-arterial dye injection and CT scanning.[86]

The results for all forms of therapy have been particularly dismal, with most five-year survival figures in the region of 1 per cent. Surgical resection in the form of pancreaticoduodenectomy has been routinely practised by many surgeons for small lesions confined to the head of pancreas. Only 10 to 18 per cent of all patients submitted to laparotomy are found to have resectable lesions. Of these, about one-fifth succumb within the first month of surgery.[70] The most optimistic figures for pancreaticoduodenectomy as a treatment of carcinoma of the head of pancreas claim a 12 to 14 per cent survival at five years.[52,82] These figures from the Mayo and Lahey Clinics respectively specifically exclude the patients who suffered hospital mortality, and the experience of a five-year survival rate of less than 6 per cent for patients referred to a single hospital for surgical treatment probably reflects the situation more accurately.[42]

In the face of these unsatisfactory results more radical approaches have been sought. Because of the evidence of multicentricity of carcinoma arising in the head of the pancreas there has been a recent emphasis on the possible place of total pancreatectomy for patients with resectable lesions in the head of the gland.[13,31,37] Other advantages of total pancreatectomy include a better clearance of related lymph nodes, an easier reconstructive anastomosis following resection and excision of a distal part of the pancreas which is often the site of degenerative and fibrotic changes in these patients.[37] Encouraging results have been obtained by some surgeons in the United States.[10,53,58,60] In the personal series of both ReMine and Moossa over 100 patients have been submitted to total pancreatectomy for carcinoma, with a mortality rate of under 10 per cent. A recent report from Sweden, from a clinic which has practised total pancreatectomy for carcinoma of the pancreas since 1959, indicates continuing improvement in operative mortality. However, only two of 20 patients followed for five years after resection survived.[37] Longer term follow-up of more recently operated patients is necessary before full assessment of the place of total pancreatectomy will be possible. The two-year survival figures are in the region of 50 per cent and a better understanding of the metabolic problems associated with total pancreatectomy has resulted in an improved quality of life for the patient. Resectability naturally varies with the skill and determination of the operative team while non-resectability is usually determined by vascular invasion of the portal vein by hepatic or other metastases.

Some surgeons at the Sloan Kettering Institute in New York have advocated en bloc pancreatic portal vein and lymph node resection (regional pancreatectomy)[22] and have even proceeded to resection/reconstruction of the hepatic and superior mesenteric arteries when these are involved by tumour. It is argued that this approach allows a much better clearance of tumour and extends operability rates. The portal vein is reconstructed by means of end-to-end anastomosis and arterial defects made good by interposition grafts of Dacron. This aggressive approach awaits full assessment but probably has a small place, particularly for those patients in whom the portal venous wall is involved by tumour. We have used the operation in this situation and found no difficulty in approximating the transected ends of portal vein although we are much more doubtful about surgical approaches involving reconstruction of arteries in the retroperitoneum.

In patients with non-resectable lesions due to local vascular involvement the results of high dosage radiation therapy guided by the presence of metal clips placed around the lesions by the surgeon have been investigated.[29] A total of 6000 rads given in three or more courses of treatment have been usual and have yielded somewhat better results in terms of palliation when combined with systemic 5-fluorouracil. Chemotherapy with systemic 5-fluorouracil on its own has been disappointing but encouraging results have been experienced by some workers using intra-arterial 5-FU locally in the region of the tumour. In their therapeutic approach these workers have utilized intra-arterial 5-FU via a brachial catheter for 14 days at the commencement of therapy and thereafter a full course of radiotherapy (6000 rads to pancreas), including 1500 rads to the region of the liver in the hope that hepatic foci of cells may be eliminated. Although this approach is primarily intended for the treatment of patients with pancreatic lesions which are not obviously associated with hepatic metastases the same approach may be valid as a palliative procedure in advanced cases.

It has been customary for surgeons to perform bypass for obstructive jaundice by cholecystojejunostomy and to combine this with gastroenterostomy because of the problem of late duodenal obstruction. More recently, this approach has been challenged as being associated with too great a mortality and morbidity in patients with advanced disease. The more rapid procedure of inserting a temporary T-tube[3] or percutaneous transhepatic drainage[37,79] has been advocated and may be combined with chemotherapy or radiotherapy.

Experience with other chemotherapeutic agents, including mitomycin C, streptozotocin and adriamycin, has been associated with equivocal results. Recently, however, a randomized prospective control trial of chemotherapy in pancreatic cancer has reported prolongation of survival from a median of two months for the control group to a median of 11 months in the treated patients. The initial treatment consisted of a five-day course of 5-fluorouracil, cyclophosphamide, vincristine and methotrexate. Five weeks later, after physical and laboratory check-up, a further course of treatment was given. Thereafter, at six-week intervals bolus injections of 5-FU and mitomycin C were given and continued on a regular basis. In the control group no chemotherapy or placebo drugs were given but the patients were followed up and reviewed at regular intervals. The drugs were well tolerated and side-effects were comparatively mild, consisting largely of nausea. No patients were withdrawn from the trial because of drug intolerance.[49]

Carcinoma of the body and tail of the pancreas causes biliary tract obstruction only when it is very extensive or when there are secondary deposits in the porta hepatis or liver. The presentation is late and often associated with vague symptoms and, in particular, backache. Very occasionally, tumours of the body and tail of the pancreas which are diagnosed at ERCP can be treated by distal pancreatectomy, but more frequently posterior involvement of the splenic vessels and aorta is found at laparotomy, making removal impossible. Injection of phenol or similar preparations into the area of the coeliac ganglia occasionally helps to relieve the pain which is so distressing both to patient and physician. Combined local intra-arterial chemotherapy and radiotherapy offers the only real prospect of satisfactory palliation at the present time but evidence of its efficacy is still lacking as no controlled studies have been performed.

OPERATIVE CONSIDERATIONS AND SURGICAL TECHNIQUES

In patients with markedly elevated levels of serum bilirubin, a major consideration is the safety with which any operation, and especially radical excisional surgery, can be performed (see also Chapter 54). Prolonged jaundice is not only associated with deficient production of coagulation factors by the liver and significant hypoalbuminaemia but in addition there is decreased collagen synthesis and, possibly, delayed healing of wounds.[77] Most importantly, however, there is a considerable risk of postoperative acute renal failure and this is often the determinant in deciding in favour of an initial bypass procedure (see Chapter 48). This allows biliary decompression and time for correction of the pathophysiological effects of extrahepatic cholestasis before proceeding to major resectional surgery.[6,82,85]

Several methods make relief of obstructive jaundice possible (see also Chapter 54). Some workers have preferred drainage by cholecystostomy or cholecystojejunostomy. These methods have the disadvantage that biliary decompression may be inefficient due to poor bile flow

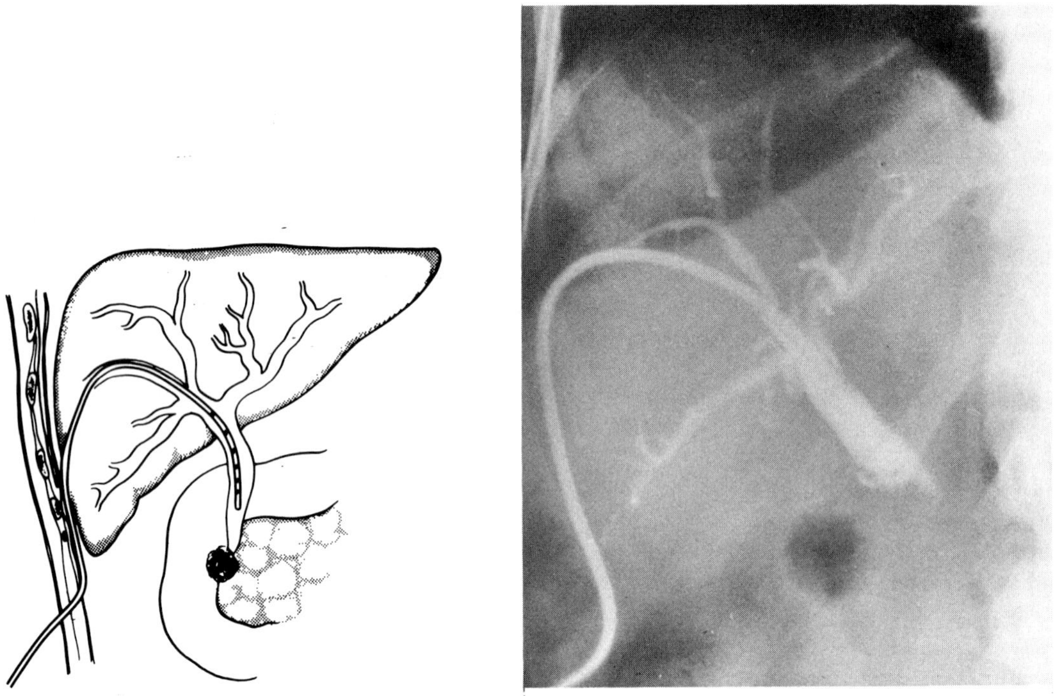

Figure 55.8. Method of transhepatic catheterization of the choledochus in carcinoma obstructing the common bile duct. Initial laparotomy is performed and choledochotomy allows a tube to be pulled through the liver substance into the common bile duct. The choledochotomy is then closed. The x-ray shows utilization of the method in a patient with a carcinoma of the head of the pancreas obstructing the lower common bile duct.

through the cystic duct, and in addition cholecystojejunostomy creates difficulty at subsequent operations since the anastomosis must first be dismantled and adhesions divided before dissection can proceed. Where the obstruction lies distally in the extrahepatic biliary tree we prefer to insert a T-tube high in the common hepatic duct (see also Chapter 54, Figure 54.6) and more recently have employed a transhepatic tube introduced after choledochotomy. The choledochotomy is then closed. This has the advantage of avoiding peritubular adhesions in the region of the hilum of the liver (Figure 55.8). An alternative method of biliary decompression in selected cases is by the percutaneous transhepatic insertion of a large bore catheter under radiological control into the dilated biliary tree (see also Chapter 54). The risk of this method is probably less than that associated with anaesthesia and surgical intervention but there are difficulties in stabilizing the catheter. In addition, it does not allow the full assessment possible at laparotomy which has the additional advantage that, should the lesion be judged inoperable, a definitive bypass may be immediately performed.

There are no good studies comparing one-stage and two-stage operations in jaundiced patients who are to be submitted to major resectional surgery. Some surgeons have been selective in their approach and reserve two-stage procedures for the more seriously ill. Thus Mongé et al,[52] in a study of over 200 patients subjected to pancreaticoduodenectomy, reported a mortality of only 11.6 per cent for seriously ill patients who were submitted to two-stage operation for periampullary carcinoma, this being lower than the overall mortality for the series. Others using a similar approach have been unable to show any difference in mortality between one- and two-stage surgery.[1] After careful preoperative assessment of nutritional and coagulation status, cardiorespiratory function and, in particular, renal function, we frequently resort to two-stage procedures. Possible disadvantages of this approach are the risk of disseminating tumour at initial operation and progression of the disease while the patient

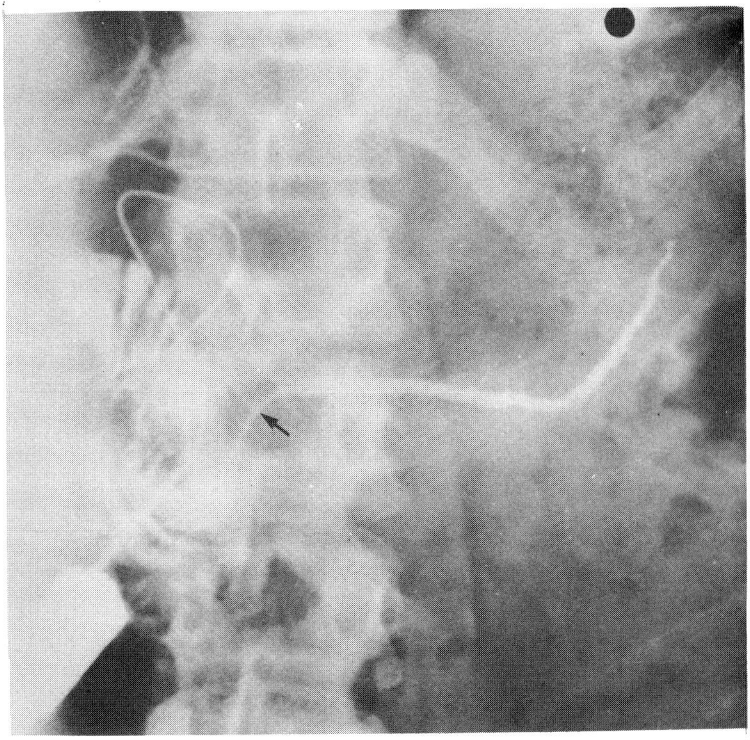

Figure 55.9. Postoperative illustration showing injection of a fine tube (arrowed) inserted in a transjejunal fashion into the pancreatic duct after end-to-side pancreaticojejunostomy. There is no leak of contrast medium. A diagrammatic representation of this procedure is shown in Figure 55.10.

awaits definitive surgery. The problem of tumour dissemination is likely to be minimized by the percutaneous transhepatic drainage method which may eventually become a standard approach.

Many surgeons are most reluctant to carry out open pancreatic biopsy because of the risk of pancreatic fistula and post-biopsy pancreatitis. When care is taken to avoid biopsy of the area of the main pancreatic duct the danger of fistula formation is minimized but we have seen pancreatic fistula formation even when the surgeon concerned has taken these precautions. We have preferred a transduodenal biopsy for lesions arising in the head of the pancreas and utilized the disposable Trucut needle system (Travenol Laboratories). This affords a good tissue sample which can, if necessary, be used for frozen section analysis. Passage of the needle across the duodenum minimizes the risk of fistula formation.

Considerable claims have also been advanced for the accuracy and safety of fine needle aspiration biopsy of the pancreas carried out at operation[39] and, indeed, a definitive diagnosis is reached in approximately 90 per cent of patients.[8] The method depends on the availability of a good cytological opinion and false positive results are uncommon. We have been employing this method more freely recently and our initial experience is encouraging. We recognize that the final decision on the presence or absence of cancer may still, in a minority of patients, rest with the surgeon's impression during operation but would emphasize that this difficult situation can be avoided in the majority of patients.

In the performance of the various anastomoses necessary in resectional surgery of the pancreas and extrahepatic ducts, it is our preference to obtain mucosa-to-mucosa apposition whenever possible. For this reason we prefer an end-to-side pancreaticojejunostomy performed across a tube left in the pancreatic duct and brought out in a transjejunal fashion through the body wall (Figure 55.9). We employ a modification of the method advocated by Warren, Veidenheimer and Pratt.[82] Buttressing mattress sutures of silk are used to effect end-to-side pancreaticojejunostomy (Figure 55.10). Using this method we have had only a single instance of fistula or leak in a series of over 25 consecutive cases. Hepaticojejunostomy is also performed by the end-to-side technique to a defunctioned loop of jejunum and the anastomosis splinted (Figure 55.11).

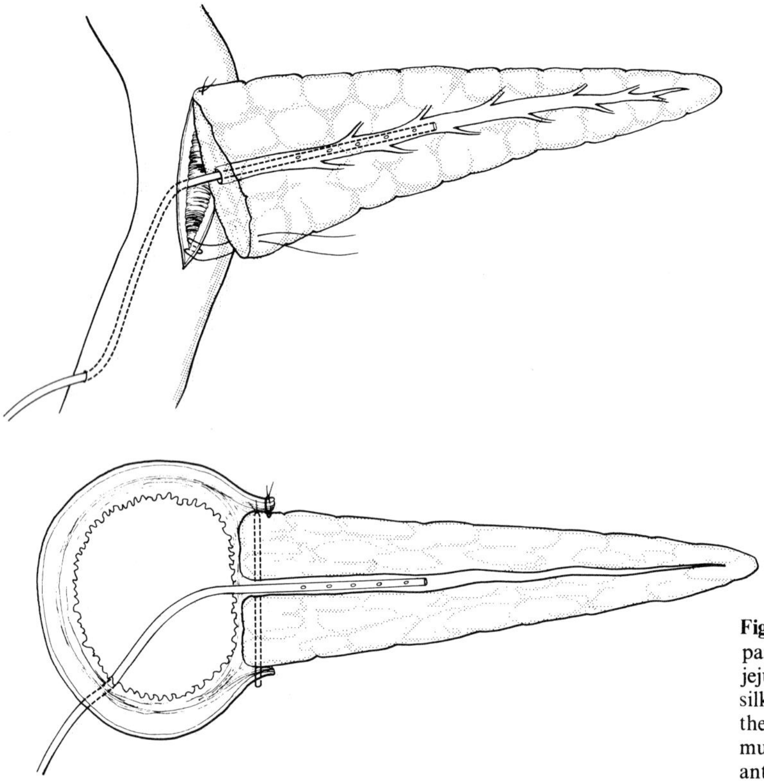

Figure 55.10. Method of end-to-side pancreaticojejunostomy over a trans-jejunal tube. Notice buttressing interrupted silk sutures to the seromuscular layer of the jejunum. The tube traverses only the mucosa and submucosa of the gut. The anterior layer of the jejunal seromuscularis is sutured so as to cover the initial transfixing layer of mattress sutures.

SURGICAL COMPLICATIONS

The most important contributory factors to the death of patients following major resectional surgery for biliary tract obstruction are renal failure, haemorrhage and fistula formation with peritonitis.[48,51,82]

The problem of renal failure associated with operative procedures in jaundiced patients has already been discussed. Pancreatic fistula formation following pancreaticoduodenectomy is a significant problem but the use of the operative approach, outlined above, is associated with a small incidence of fistula.[81] Some surgeons favour end-to-end pancreatico-jejunostomy or, alternatively, simply envelope the pancreatic neck in the open end of the Roux loop of jejunum without mucosa suture, and they have had satisfactory results.[1,42] Anastomotic breakdown may be associated with postoperative pancreatitis or simple leakage of pancreatic juice through the margins of the anastomosis. In both events haemorrhage and sepsis may occur. Late follow-up results of end-to-end anastomosis have shown that a proportion suffer stenosis and, indeed, complete separation may occur although the latter complication is more frequent after distal pancreatectomy with end-to-side anastomosis between the exposed pancreatic duct and the jejunum.

Ulcers occurring on the jejunal side of the gastrojejunal anastomosis following pancreaticoduodenectomy are invariably associated with limited gastric resections. Indeed, it has been reported that with at least 50 per cent resection of stomach, vagotomy is rarely necessary and jejunal ulcers are uncommon.[82] Our own experience agrees with this.

The incidence of diabetes following pancreaticoduodenectomy is approximately 15 per cent, while exocrine pancreatic insufficiency occurs in a slightly greater proportion of patients. Following total pancreatectomy there is always diabetes and pancreatic exocrine insufficiency, and this problem is considered below.

Where hepatic resection is necessary as part of excisional surgery related to more proximally

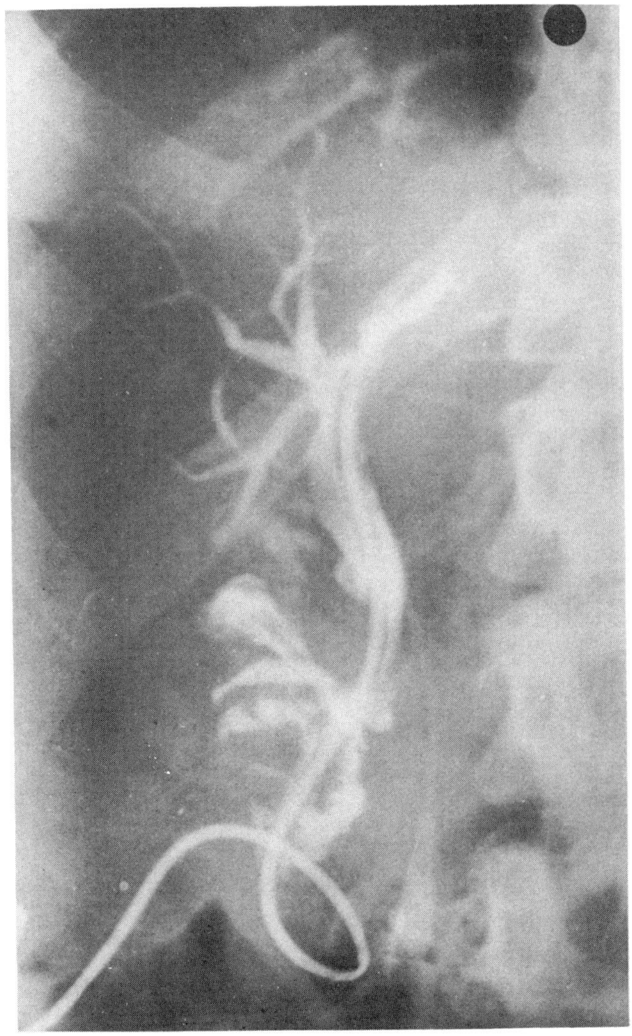

Figure 55.11. Hepaticojejunostomy performed to a Roux-en-Y loop of jejunum over a transjejunal stent. The patient had been submitted to pancreaticoduodenectomy for periampullary carcinoma.

placed cholangiocarcinomas, the well-known haematological and metabolic upsets associated with hepatic resection have to be borne in mind. The most important of these is the danger of hypoglycaemia and the need to replace labile clotting factors with fresh blood in the immediate postoperative period.[80] At a later stage it is important to ensure that hypoalbuminaemia does not reach dangerous levels.

Management of the Patient after Total Pancreatectomy

In the immediate postoperative period the management of diabetes can be difficult and abrupt falls in blood sugar levels may be life-threatening. The problem of acute hypoglycaemia following insulin injection may be a sustained potential danger in some patients after total pancreatectomy. One of our own patients died as a result of hypoglycaemia six weeks after operation and similar problems have been encountered both a number of months[37] and almost five years after surgery.[61]

The problem of the management of exocrine pancreatic insufficiency initially appears to be a straightforward matter of the patient's taking adequate oral supplements. There is great variability in the enzyme content of the different available commercial preparations.[57] To this difficulty is added the problem of digestion of the necessary enzymes by both acid and pepsin, resulting in very large numbers of tablets being required to achieve 10 per cent of the normal intraduodenal levels of lipase and trypsin. However, it has recently been shown that the addition of the H_2-receptor blocking drug cimetidine to the pancreatic enzyme supplements results in a very significant improvement in the efficacy of these drugs.[19,26,68] Although cimetidine offers the prospect of weight gain and a return to normal stools for patients following total pancreatectomy, it must be remembered that there is considerable individual patient variation in requirement of enzyme supplement. This is presumably due to the variable amount of acid and pepsin production in the gastric remnant.

REFERENCES

1. Akwari, O.E., van Heerden, J.A., Adson, M.A. & Baggenstoss, A.H. (1977) Radical pancreatoduodenectomy for cancer of the papilla of Vater. *Archives of Surgery*, **112,** 451–456.
2. Arminski, T.C. (1949) Primary carcinoma of the gall bladder. *Cancer*, **2,** 397–398.
3. Balasegaram, M. (1976) Carcinoma of the periampullary region: a review of a personal series of 87 patients. *British Journal of Surgery*, **63,** 532–537.
4. Belamaric, J. (1973) Intrahepatic bile duct carcinoma and *C. sinensis* infection in Hong Kong. *Cancer*, **31,** 468–473.
5. Blumgart, L.H. (1975) Duodenoscopy and endoscopic retrograde choledochopancreatography: Present position in relation to periampullary and pancreatic cancer. *Journal of Surgical Oncology*, **7,** 107–119.
6. Blumgart, L.H. (1978) Biliary tract obstruction. New approaches to old problems. *American Journal of Surgery*, **135,** 19–31.
7. Blumgart, L.H. & Kennedy, A.C. (1973) Carcinoma of the ampulla of Vater and duodenum. *British Journal of Surgery*, **60,** 33–40.
8. Bodner, E. (1977) The fine needle aspiration biopsy as a safe method for intra-operative differentiation of pancreatic tumour. *Irish Journal of Medical Science*, **39a** (Suppl.).
9. Bouchier, I.A.D. (1972) Difficulties in the laboratory diagnosis of pancreatic disease. *Proceedings of the Royal Society of Medicine*, **65,** 845–846.
10. Brooks, J.R. & Culebras, J.M. (1976) Cancer of the pancreas. Palliative operation, Whipple procedure or total pancreatectomy? *American Journal of Surgery*, **131,** 516–520.
11. Calne, R.Y. & Williams, R. (1977) Orthotopic liver transplantation: the first 60 patients. *British Medical Journal*, **i,** 471–476.
12. Chandler, J.G. & Fletcher, W.S. (1963) A clinical study of primary carcinoma of the gall bladder. *Surgery, Gynecology and Obstetrics*, **117,** 297–300.
13. Collins, J.J., Craighead, J.E. & Brooks, J.R. (1966) Rationale for total pancreatectomy for carcinoma of the pancreatic head. *New England Journal of Medicine*, **274,** 599–602.
14. Cooke, L., Avery-Jones, F. & Keich, M.K. (1953) Carcinoma of the gall bladder. A statistical study. *Lancet*, **ii,** 585–587.
15. Chu, P.T. (1950) Benign neoplasms of the extrahepatic biliary ducts. *Archives of Pathology*, **50,** 84–97.
16. Crile, G., Isbister, W.H. & Hawk, W.A. (1970) Carcinoma of the ampulla of Vater and the terminal bile and pancreatic ducts. *Surgery, Gynecology and Obstetrics*, **131,** 1052–1054.
17. Cruikshank, A.H. & Sparshott, S.M. (1971) Malignancy in natural and experimental hepatic cysts: experiments with aflotoxin in rats and the malignant transformation of cysts in human livers. *Journal of Pathology*, **104,** 185.
18. Daroca, P.J. Jr, Tuthill, R. & Reed, R.J. (1975) Cholangiocarcinoma arising in hepatic fibrosis. *Archives of Pathology*, **99,** 592–595.
19. Di Magno, E.P., Malagelada, G.R., Go, V.L.M. & Moertel, C.G. (1977) Fate of orally ingested enzymes in pancreatic insufficiency. Comparison of two dosage schedules. *New England Journal of Medicine*, **296,** 1318–1322.
20. Donaldson, L.A. & Busutill, A. (1975) A clinicopathological review of 68 carcinomas of the gall bladder. *British Journal of Surgery*, **62,** 26–32.
21. Dowdy, G.S., Olin, W.G., Shelton, E.L. & Waldron, G.W. (1962) Benign tumours of the extrahepatic bile ducts. *Archives of Surgery*, **85,** 503–513.
22. Fortner, J.G., Kim, D.K., Cubilla, A., Turnbull, A., Pahnke, L. & Shils, M.E. (1977) Regional pancreatectomy. *Annals of Surgery*, **186,** 42–50.
23. Gallagher, P.G., Millis, R.R. & Mitchinson, M.G. (1972) Congenital dilatation of the intrahepatic bile ducts with cholangio-carcinoma. *Journal of Clinical Pathology*, **25,** 804–808.
24. Gelder, R., Reese, C., Moossa, A.R. & Hunter, R. (1978) Purification, tissue localisation and clinical application of oncofetal antigen. *Cancer Research*, **38,** 313–324.
25. Gerst, P.H. (1961) Primary carcinoma of the gall bladder. A 30 year summary. *Annals of Surgery*, **153,** 369–372.
26. Graham, D.Y. (1977) Enzyme replacement therapy of exocrine pancreatic insufficiency in man. Relation between in vitro enzyme activities and in vivo potency in commercial pancreatic extracts. *New England Journal of Medicine*, **296,** 1314–1317.
27. Hafstrom, L., Zettergren, L. & Akesson, L.A. (1973) The natural history of primary and secondary malignant tumours of the liver. *Acta Chirurgica Scandinavica*, **139,** 264–269.
28. Hancke, S., Holm, H.H. & Koch, F. (1975) Ultrasonically guided percutaneous fine needle biopsy of the pancreas. *Surgery, Gynecology and Obstetrics*, **140,** 361–364.
29. Haslam, J.B., Cavanaugh, P.J. & Stroup, S.L. (1973) Radiation therapy of irresectable adenocarcinoma of the pancreas. *Cancer*, **32,** 1341–1345.
30. Hatfield, A.R.W. (1977) The investigation of pancreatic exocrine disorders. *British Journal of Hospital Medicine*, **18,** 528–546.
31. Hicks, R.E. & Brooks, J.R. (1971) Total pancreatectomy for ductal carcinoma. *Surgery, Gynecology and Obstetrics*, **133,** 16–20.
32. Howard, J.M. (1968) Pancreatico-duodenectomy. 41 consecutive Whipple resections without an operative mortality. *Annals of Surgery*, **168,** 629–640.
33. Howard, J.M. & Jordan, J.L. (1977) Cancer of the pancreas. In *Current Problems in Cancer*, Vol. II, No. 3. Chicago: Year Book Medical Publishers.

34. Horwitz, A. & Rosenweig, J. (1960) Carcinoma of the gall bladder – a real hazard. A summary of 20 cases. *Journal of the American Medical Association*, **173,** 234–236.
35. Hossack, K.F. & Herron, J.J. (1972) Benign tumours of the common bile duct. Report of a case and review of literature. *Australian and New Zealand Journal of Surgery*, **42,** 22–27.
36. Hughes, H. & Blumgart, L.H. (1978) Cytodiagnosis of pancreatic and periampullary cancer. Unpublished data.
37. Ihse, I., Lilja, P., Arnesjo, B. & Bengmark, S. (1977) Total pancreatectomy for cancer. *Annals of Surgery*, **186,** 675–680.
38. Iwasaki, Y., Ohto, M., Todoroki, T., Okamura, T., Nishimura, A. & Sato, H. (1977) Treatment of carcinoma of the biliary system. *Surgery, Gynecology and Obstetrics*, **144,** 219–224.
39. Koivuniemi, A., Lempinen, M. & Pantzar, P. (1972) Fine needle aspiration biopsy of pancreas. *Annales Chirurgiae et Gynaecologiae Fenniae*, **61,** 273–280.
40. Krain, L.S. (1970) The rising incidence of carcinoma of the pancreas – real or apparent? *Journal of Surgical Oncology*, **2,** 115–124.
41. Kuwayti, K., Baggenstoss, A.H., Stauffer, M.H. & Priestley, J.T. (1957) Carcinoma of the major intrahepatic and the extrahepatic bile ducts. *Surgery, Gynecology and Obstetrics*, **104,** 357–366.
42. Longmire, W.P. (1973) Periampullary tumours. *Journal of the Royal College of Surgeons of Edinburgh*, **18,** 131–136.
43. Longmire, W.P. (1976) Tumours of the extrahepatic biliary radicles. In *Current Problems in Cancer*, Vol. I, No. 2. Chicago: Year Book Medical Publishers.
44. Longmire, W.P. & Shafey, O.A. (1966) Certain factors influencing survival after pancreatico-duodenal resection for carcinoma. *American Journal of Surgery*, **111,** 8–12.
45. Longmire, W.P., McArthur, M.S., Bastounis, E.A. & Hiatt, J. (1973) Carcinoma of the extrahepatic biliary tract. *Annals of Surgery*, **178,** 333–345.
46. MacIntire, K.R., Waldmann, T.A., Moertel, C.G. & Go, V.L.W. (1975) Serum alphafoetoprotein in patients with neoplasms of the gastrointestinal tract. *Cancer Research*, **35,** 991–996.
47. Madden, J.J. & Smith, T.W. (1974) Multiple biliary papillomatosis. *Cancer*, **34,** 1316–1320.
48. Maki, T., Sato, T. & Kakizaki, G. (1966) Pancreatico-duodenectomy for periampullary carcinomas. Appraisal of the two-stage procedure. *Archives of Surgery*, **92,** 825–833.
49. Mallinson, C.N., Rake, M.O., Fox, C.A., Cyanworski, M., Cocking, B., Jackson, A. & Diffy, B. (1977) Final results of a controlled trial of chemotherapy for inoperable pancreatic cancer. *Irish Journal of Medical Science*, **146** (Suppl. 1), 19.
50. Mercadier, M.P., Clot, J.P. & Russell, T.R. (1973) Chronic recurrent pancreatitis and pancreatic pseudocysts. In *Current Problems in Surgery*. Chicago Year Book Medical Publishers.
51. Mercadier, M., Clot, J.P., Mellier, E.D. & Camplez, P. (1967) La pancréatectomie presque totale. *Annales de Chirurgie*, **21,** 681–685.
52. Mongé, J.J., Judd, E.S. & Gage, R.P. (1964) Radical pancreatoduodenectomy. A 22 year experience with the complications, mortality rate and survival rate. *Annals of Surgery*, **160,** 711–722.
53. Moossa, A.R. (1977) Personal communication.
54. Morgan, R.G.H. & Wormsley, K.G. (1977) Cancer of pancreas. Progress report. *Gut*, **18,** 580–596.
55. Nakase, A., Mautsumoto, Y., Uchida, K. & Honjo, I. (1977) Surgical treatment of cancer of the pancreas and periampullary region. *Annals of Surgery*, **185,** 52–57.
56. Neibling, H.A., Docherty, M.B. & Waugh, J.M. (1949) Carcinoma of the extrahepatic bile ducts. *Surgery, Gynecology and Obstetrics*, **89,** 429–438.
57. Pairent, F.W. & Howard, J.M. (1975) The treatment of pancreatic insufficiency. The enzyme content of commercial pancreatic supplements. *Archives of Surgery*, **110,** 739–741.
58. Pliam, M.B. & ReMine, W.H. (1975) Further evaluation of total pancreatectomy. *Archives of Surgery*, **110,** 506–512.
59. Polk, H.C. (1966) Carcinoma of the calcified gall bladder. *Gastroenterology*, **50,** 582–585.
60. ReMine, W.H. (1977) Personal communication.
61. ReMine, W.H., Priestley, J.T., Judd, E.S. & King, J.N. (1970) Total pancreatectomy. *Annals of Surgery*, **172,** 595–603.
62. Roberts-Thompson, I.C., Strickland, R.J. & Mackay, I.R. (1973) Bile duct carcinoma in chronic ulcerative colitis. *Australian and New Zealand Journal of Medicine*, **3,** 264–267.
63. Ross, A.P. & Braasch, J.W. (1973) Ulcerative colitis and carcinoma of the proximal bile ducts. *Gut*, **14,** 94–97.
64. Ross, A.P., Braasch, J.W. & Warren, K.W. (1973) Carcinoma of the proximal bile ducts. *Surgery, Gynecology and Obstetrics*, **136,** 923–928.
65. Ross, F.P. & Hickok, D.F. (1960) Hernia and gall bladder surgery in patients over 70. *New England Journal of Medicine*, **262,** 501–505.
66. Russo, A.G., Goldrosen, M.H., Douglass, H.O., Leveson, S.H., Howell, J.H., Harvey, S.R., Chu, T.M. & Holyoke, E.D. (1977) Evaluation of the micro-leucocyte adherence inhibition assay (LAI) as an immuno-diagnostic test for pancreatic cancer. *Abstracts of the American Pancreatic Association Meeting*, Chicago.
67. Sako, K., Seitzinger, G.L. & Garside, E. (1957) Carcinoma of extrahepatic bile ducts. Review of the literature and report of six cases. *Surgery*, **41,** 416–437.
68. Saunders, J.H.B., Drummond, S. & Wormsley, K.G. (1977) Inhibition of gastric secretion in treatment of pancreatic insufficiency. *British Medical Journal*, **i,** 418–419.
69. Sayers, H.G. & Orloff, M.J. (1976) Development of an animal model of pancreatic cancer. *Surgical Forum*, **27,** 456–458.
70. Smith, R. (1973) Progress in the surgical treatment of pancreatic disease. *American Journal of Surgery*, **125,** 143–153.
71. Solan, M.J. & Jackson, B.T. (1971) Carcinoma of the gall bladder – a clinical appraisal and review of 57 cases. *British Journal of Surgery*, **58,** 593–597.
72. Stephenson, L.W., Blackstone, E.H. & Aldreid, J.S. (1977) Radical resection for periampullary carcinomas. *Archives of Surgery*, **112,** 245–249.
73. Stewart, H.L., Leiber, M.M. & Morgan, D.R. (1940) Carcinoma of the extrahepatic bile ducts. *Archives of Surgery*, **41,** 662–668.
74. Strauch, G.O. (1960) Primary carcinoma of the gall bladder. *Surgery*, **47,** 368–383.
75. Terblanche, J. & Louw, J.H. (1973) 'U' tube drainage in the palliative therapy of carcinoma of the main hepatic duct system. *Surgical Clinics of North America*, **53,** 1245–1255.

76. Terblanche, J., Saunders, S.G. & Louw, J.H. (1972) Prolonged palliation in carcinoma of the main hepatic duct junction. *Surgery*, **71**, 720–731.
77. Than Than, McGee, J.O'D. & Blumgart, L.H. (1977) Prolyl hydroxylase in the skin of patients with obstructive jaundice. *Journal of Clinical Pathology*, **30**, 1044–1046.
78. Tompkins, R.K., Johnson, J., Storm, F.K. & Longmire, W.P. (1976) Operative endoscopy in the management of biliary tract neoplasms. *American Journal of Surgery*, **132**, 174–182.
79. Tylen, U., Hoevels, J. & Vang, J. (1977) Percutaneous transhepatic cholangiography (PTC) with external drainage of obstructive biliary lesions. *Surgery, Gynecology and Obstetrics*, **144**, 13–18.
80. Vajrabukka, T., Bloom, A.L., Sussman, M., Wood, C.B. & Blumgart, L.H. (1975) Postoperative problems and management after hepatic resection for blunt injury to the liver. *British Journal of Surgery*, **62**, 189–200.
81. Warren, K.W. & Jefferson, M.F. (1973) Carcinoma of the exocrine pancreas. In *The Pancreas* (Ed.) Carey, L.C. pp. 243–294. St Louis: C.V. Mosby.
82. Warren, K.W., Veidenheimer, M.C. & Pratt, H.S. (1967) Pancreato-duodenectomy for periampullary cancer. *Surgical Clinics of North America*, **47**, 639–645.
83. Warren, K.W., Choe, D.S., Plaza, J. & Relihan, M. (1975) Results of radical resection for periampullary cancer. *Annals of Surgery*, **181**, 534–540.
84. Whipple, A.O., Parsons, W.B. & Mullens, C.R. (1935) Treatment of carcinoma of ampulla of Vater. *Annals of Surgery*, **102**, 763–799.
85. White, T.T. & Harrison, C.M. (1973) *Re-operative Gastrointestinal Surgery*. pp. 109–186. Boston, Mass.: Little, Brown.
86. Wiley, A. & Wirtanen, W.I. (1978) Combined arteriography and CT scanning in the diagnosis of small hepatic metastases. Unpublished data.
87. Zamcheck, N. (1976) The present status of CEA in diagnosis, detection of recurrence, prognosis and evaluation of therapy of colonic and pancreatic cancer. *Clinics in Gastroenterology*, **5**, 625–638.

Chapter 56

Helminthic Diseases of the Liver and Biliary Tract

G.B. ONG

Helminthic infestation may affect the liver or the bile ducts either during passage of worms through these structures, or because these organs are their natural habitat. These infestations include:

1. Nematodes (roundworms)
   (a) *Ascaris lumbricoides*,
   (b) the larval stage of *Toxocara canis* or *cati*,
   (c) *Capillaria hepatica*;
2. Trematodes
   (a) *Clonorchis sinensis,* the fluke commonly found in Asia, or its relatives, *Opisthorchis felineus*, *Opisthorchis viverrini* and *Dicrocoelium dendriticum*,
   (b) *Fasciola hepatica*, the large liver fluke,
   (c) *Schistosoma japonicum* and *Schistosoma mansoni,*
   (d) the larval stage of the Cestodes, or tapeworms, e.g. *Taenia echinococcus.*

ASCARIASIS

Infestation by the roundworm, *Ascaris lumbricoides*, is possibly the earliest recorded human infestation and is referred to in texts from Mesopotamia, Greece, Rome and China.[28] It was estimated by Stoll[78] in 1947 that over 644 000 000 people throughout the world are infected with *Ascaris lumbricoides*. The greatest number of these occur in Asia, with advanced countries having the lowest rate of infestation. In Europe, the incidence is low in large cities but may be high in rural areas. In East Prussia and Silesia, for example, it has been reported to be as high as 52 per cent.[21] The incidence in Japan dropped considerably after the end of the Second World War. In the period between the Second World War and 1955 the incidence was as high as 70 to 80 per cent in some rural districts of Japan, but by 1962 the infestation rate by *Ascaris lumbricoides* was only 13 per cent.

In China, the incidence of infestation by *Ascaris* is still high, ranging from 63 to 92 per cent.[44] Infestation with *Ascaris lumbricoides* can be acquired by the ingestion of vegetables, usually as salad, but in China as pickles. In most underdeveloped countries in Asia and Africa children acquire this infestation as a result of substandard hygiene. The number of parasites harboured in children varies and as many as 2000 adult *Ascaris* have been found at autopsy.[2]

Morphology and Life Cycle

Morphology

The adult parasite lives in the small intestine. The female measures 20 to 25 cm and the male 15 to 35 cm in length. They are fusiform and creamy pink to creamy white, with two parallel streaks of white running along the whole length of the body. At the anterior end are three lips. The tail end tapers and in the male it curves ventrally. In the female the vulva is located ventrally at the junction of the anterior and middle two-thirds, at which point there is a constriction. The fragile female lays an average of over 200 000 ova daily and her life span is estimated to be between six months and one

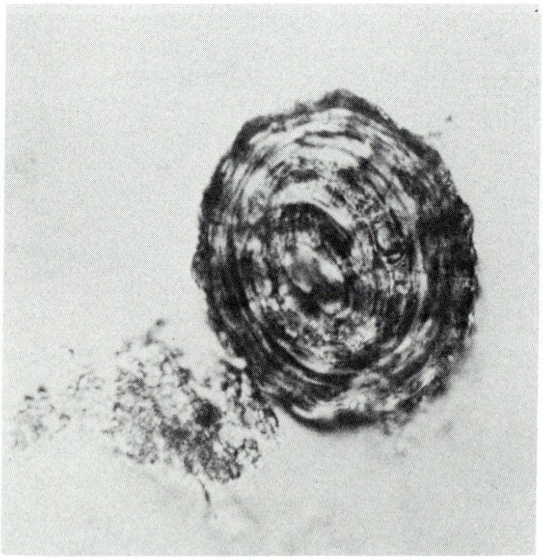

Figure 56.1. A fertilized ovum of *Ascaris lumbricoides*. × 360. Courtesy of Professor C.T. Huang.

year. The eggs which pass with the stool may be either unfertilized or fertilized.

The ovum when fertilized is oval in shape and has a double wall which appears mammillated. It is golden in colour and measures 45 to 75 μm by 35 to 50 μm (Figure 56.1). The unfertilized egg, on the other hand, is longer and irregular in shape (Figure 56.2).

Life cycle

When the ovum is passed in the stool, the embryo is not developed. Development takes place in moist shady soil. With the temperature between 23 and 30°C, it can be viable for as long as ten weeks. After the egg has been in the soil for two to three weeks, the larva will be potentially infective. Hatching of the eggs does not take place in the soil, however, but occurs in the upper part of the intestine. The shell of the egg is dissolved by the gastric juice and the larva is released into the upper part of the small intestine. The hatched larva penetrates the surface epithelium of the intestinal mucosa, enters the veins of the portal system and is carried to the liver. Some larvae may enter lymphatic vessels and are carried by the thoracic duct to the lungs.

Not all these *Ascaris* larvae reach the lungs or the liver, as many die in the intestinal mucosa. This results in focal areas of inflammation with infiltration by eosinophils and macrophages. Minute haemorrhages may occur where the parasite has penetrated the vessels.

In the liver larvae move freely in the sinusoids and some may subsequently pass through the hepatic veins to the heart and lungs.

Generally speaking, the reaction to *Ascaris lumbricoides* larval migration through the lungs is not as severe as that seen in either *Toxocara canis* or *Toxocara cati*.

Larval migration of the *Ascaris lumbricoides* may involve organs other than liver and lungs. Migration to kidneys, heart and brain has been observed. Convulsions may occur during invasion of the brain. Larvae in these organs are fairly rapidly killed and granulomas are formed. These granulomas persist but ultimately they disappear with disintegration of the larvae and there is no residual evidence of infestation. The time from larval infection to maturation and final destruction in the jejunum may be as long as four months.

Larval Migration of *Ascaris lumbricoides*

Clinical features

Clinical symptoms during the stage of larval migration vary with the severity of infection. When it is heavy there may be chills and fever, generalized body aches, malaise, anorexia and cough. Heavy infestation and larval migration to the liver may give rise to hepatomegaly, but this disappears after a few days. Examination of the blood may show eosinophilia.

There may be rhonchi over both lungs and

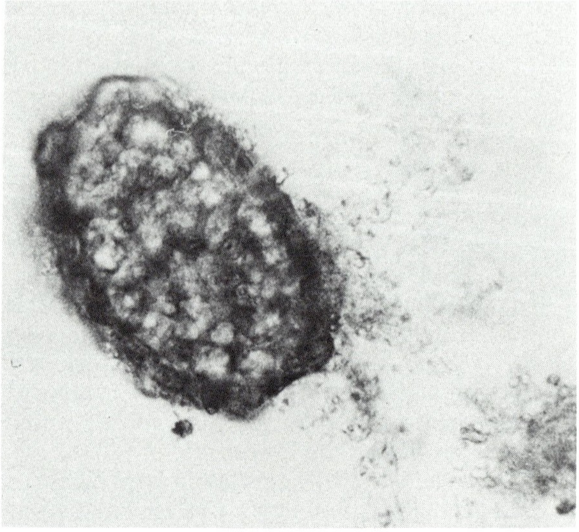

Figure 56.2. An unfertilized ovum of *Ascaris lumbricoides*. × 36. Courtesy of Professor C.T. Huang.

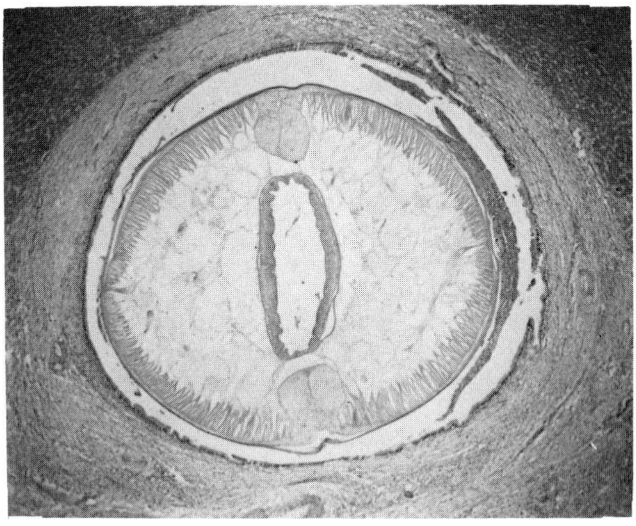

Figure 56.3. A cross-section of *Ascaris lumbricoides* in the intrahepatic duct. × 60. Courtesy of Dr T.B. Teoh.

cyanosis may occur if asthmatic attacks are severe. Occasionally congestive heart failure may supervene. The patient reported by Beaver and Danaraj[8] developed bronchial asthma and shortly after admission to hospital died of respiratory failure. Marked eosinophilia was present and at post-mortem *Ascaris* larvae were discovered in the bronchi and the right side of the heart was dilated.

Pathology

Usually there is little or no tissue reaction in the liver, but occasionally some patients show an eosinophilic reaction, probably the result of larval death. Such focal areas of inflammatory reaction will finally disappear leaving no trace of larvae. Once in the lungs, following migration through lymphatics or liver, larvae first invade the capillaries and enter the alveolar spaces. Here they consistently produce an inflammatory exudation.

The adult Indian who died of bronchial asthma reported by Beaver and Danaraj[8] had granulomas with severe inflammatory exudation in both bronchi and pulmonary alveoli.

Most of the lung changes have been described in experimental animals. However, the larval inflammatory reaction is never observed in animals sacrificed 40 days after infection. Repair of the pulmonary lesion is presumably complete by this time.

Larvae are carried from the alveoli to the pharynx where they moult and are swallowed. In the upper gastrointestinal tract they moult again before becoming mature worms.

Adult *Ascaris lumbricoides* Infestation

When there is a very heavy infestation of the worms in the intestines, hypoproteinaemia may be produced with ankle oedema and varying degrees of anaemia. There is usually loss of

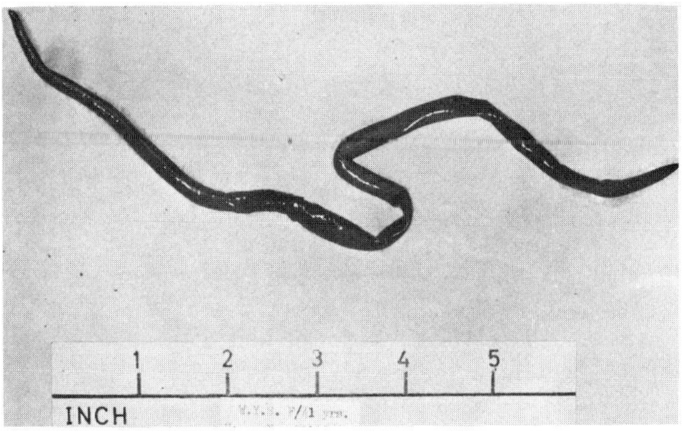

-e 56.4. Dead female *Ascaris* removed common bile duct. Bile pigments n to be deposited.

appetite and body weight. However, the principal symptoms associated with *Ascaris* infestation are produced by the migration of adult worms.

Migration

Certain factors may initiate the migration of worms in the small intestine. These include some of the vermifuges such as carbon tetrachloride formerly used in treatment.

The worms may migrate to an inflamed appendix or to a suture-line following surgery. Adult worms may also migrate to the oesophagus and then across the epiglottis to the bronchus. In a patient who is recovering from anaesthesia this migration may be fatal. The worms may also penetrate the intestines and give rise to peritonitis. Sometimes they may be found alive in the peritoneal cavity without any clinical evidence of intestinal perforation.[83]

Ascaris may invade the biliary tract and give rise to disease of the liver and the biliary system. *Ascaris* in the biliary tract has been observed by Akimoto[1] in association with reduced acid secretion in the upper gastrointestinal tract.

Having moved through the duodenum into the common bile duct *Ascaris* may lodge in the intrahepatic ducts (Figure 56.3) but is most frequently found in the common bile duct.[49]

The mechanism of *Ascaris* migration into the biliary tract has been extensively studied by Akimoto[1]. In an experiment with various sizes of tubes he showed that the *Ascaris* had a tendency to search for small openings to penetrate. External stimuli like warm or cold water or acids or alkali, as well as antihelminthics, did not influence this migration.

Infestation in the biliary tract

Ascaris may lay eggs in the intrahepatic ducts and then return to the duodenum through the ampulla of Vater. This may be achieved by its moving backwards into the duodenum, or if the ducts are dilated it may coil on itself so that the head passes back towards the duodenum.[49]

The majority of the adult worms migrating to the biliary tract live for up to one month before they die and their bodies disintegrate (Figure 56.4). Fragments drain with the bile into the duodenum, but parts are left behind. Calcium bilirubinate precipitates over these and thus forms calculi. Yasuda[87] examined such stones. After bisecting them he dissolved them, centrifuged the suspension and examined the sediment. The eggs or fragments of parasites were identified in 55 per cent of the stones. A similar result was obtained by Teoh,[80] who cut through the centres of these soft stones with a microtome. In 16 of the 40 stones examined he identified remnants of the *Ascaris lumbricoides*.

Pathological Changes in the Biliary Tract and Liver

Biliary tract

After passage of the *Ascaris* through the ampulla of Vater the duodenal papilla becomes inflamed. This is followed by spasm and may result in dilatation of the bile duct. In one series of 59 cases of *Ascaris* within the biliary tract, the worms were removed without any evidence of stone formation being found. There was dilatation of the extrahepatic biliary tract[49] and this occasionally extended into intrahepatic ducts in which *Ascaris* were lodged (Figure 56.5). In 1960 Nakamura[60] examined 22 human papillae in biliary tract diseases including 16 cases where there were no stones but there was an eosinophil infiltrate. He concluded that this could have resulted from parasitic invasion of the biliary tract.

Liver

The liver may be damaged as a result of the parasitic invasion. Eggs that are laid in the biliary tract are regurgitated in the smaller ducts and sometimes into the portal tract which is then infiltrated by eosinophils, plasma cells and macrophages (Figure 56.6). The eggs ultimately disintegrate in the granuloma which heals with a hyaline scar.

Pyogenic abscess may also complicate an *Ascaris* infestation. The organisms are most probably introduced into the biliary tract by the migrating *Ascaris*. The abscess may contain the carcasses of the lumbricoides. In some instances, live *Ascaris* may move up the biliary tract to the abscess cavity. Rupture of the abscess may lead to generalized peritonitis, or if this occurs on the superior surface of the liver penetration of the diaphragm may cause an empyema. Occasionally, migration of [illegible] *Ascaris* to the intrahepatic ducts m[illegible] rise to acute liver necrosis.

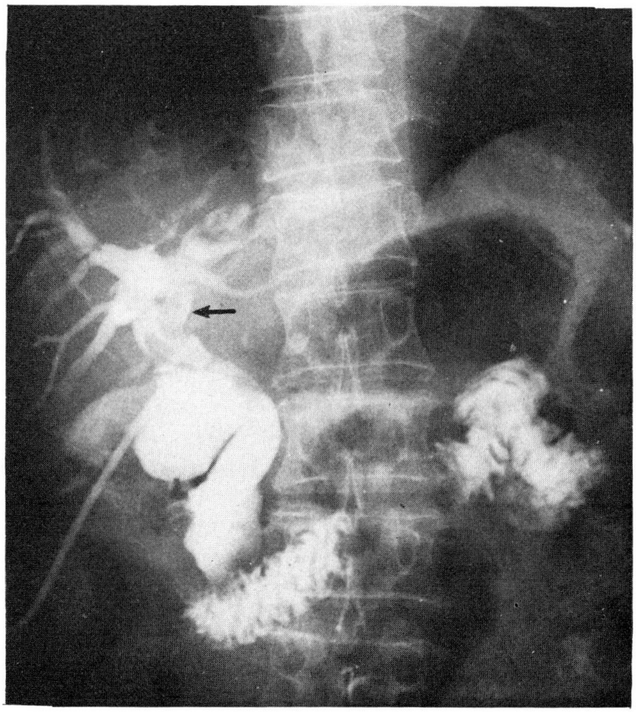

Figure 56.5. T-tube cholangiogram showing an *Ascaris* with dilated bile ducts.

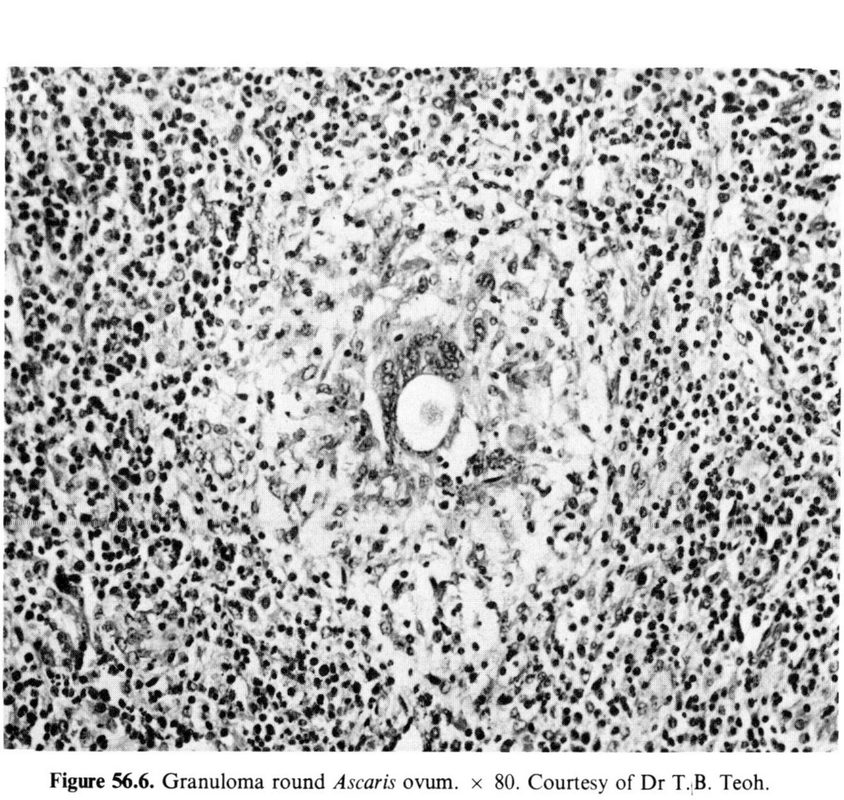

Figure 56.6. Granuloma round *Ascaris* ovum. × 80. Courtesy of Dr T.B. Teoh.

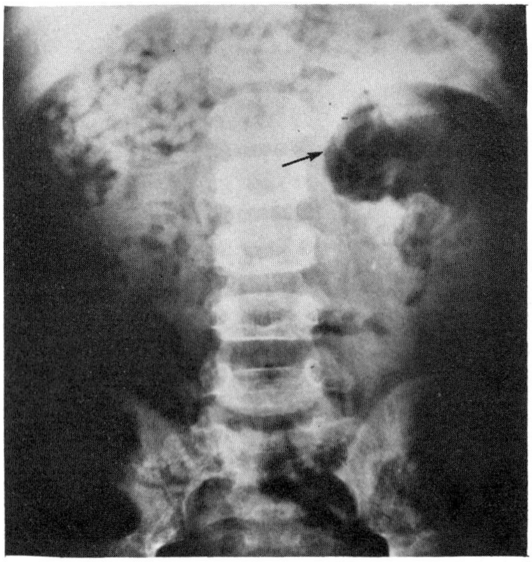

Figure 56.7. Plain x-ray of the abdomen showing an *Ascaris* in the intestine (arrow).

Pancreas

In addition to the changes occurring in the liver, the pancreas may also undergo inflammatory changes. As a result of the passage of the worm through the sphincter of Oddi, oedematous pancreatitis results. In a rare case reported by Rigby,[71] the adult *Ascaris* migrated to the pancreatic duct and caused haemorrhagic pancreatitis, ending in death of the patient.

Clinical Features of Migration into the Biliary Tract

Symptoms and signs

Severe pain, which may be acute, occurs with the migration of the worms to the biliary tract. It is localized just beneath the xiphisternum and is described as boring or lancinating. It is paroxysmal, lasting for a few minutes to a few hours. The temperature may be subnormal: pyrexia signifies severe bacterial infection. Nausea and vomiting can be persistent and severe. Jaundice is present in about 20 per cent of cases[49] but may be more frequent when there is concurrent cholelithiasis. In our experience, jaundice is usually mild and occurs a few days after the onset of pain. This is possibly due to cholangitis.

Laboratory findings

Leucocytosis is seldom present in the early stage of the disease but develops when the fever due to cholangitis occurs. In about a fifth of the patients mild eosinophilia may be present.

Diagnosis

Diagnosis of *Ascaris* migration to the biliary tract is difficult and is usually made at laparotomy. It should be suspected if pain is severe and is located just behind the xiphisternum with characteristic paroxysmal episodes. A history of vomiting of worms is helpful. Should endoscopy be performed, examination of the duodenal juice might demonstrate *Ascaris* ova.

Occasionally *Ascaris* may be demonstrated in the intestines by plain x-ray examination of the abdomen (Figure 56.7). A barium meal may outline the duodenum with the worm partially inside the common bile duct, or at the ampulla of Vater.

Treatment

As a result of extensive experience, Maki[49] believes that unless there is associated cholangitis with jaundice and high fever, operation should be initially withheld and a period of conservative treatment with antibiotics, antispasmodics and parenteral fluids should be administered. On the other hand, Reich,[69] Hosemann[29] and Miyake[58,59] advocate operative treatment including cholecystectomy.

Whenever surgical intervention is undertaken it is important to explore the whole abdomen before concentrating on the biliary tract. Adult *Ascaris* are large and can easily be palpated in the small intestine. If they are found they should be extracted by enterotomy. Failure to do so may occasion renewed migration of the *Ascaris* into the biliary tract with subsequent stone formation and cholangitis.

If worms are found in the common bile duct they are removed through a choledochotomy which may need to be high up in the common hepatic duct, and a T-tube is inserted. Should this procedure fail, the worms can be extracted through a hepatolithotomy following mobilization of the left lobe of the liver. An incision is made on its posterior aspect directly on to the duct and the worms extracted. The duct subsequently may be repaired with an intrahepatic tube in place.

Occasionally the worms may be present in an abscess cavity. The area should be packed off from the general peritoneal cavity, an incision made into the abscess and pus aspirated (Figure 56.8). An additional choledochotomy is essen-

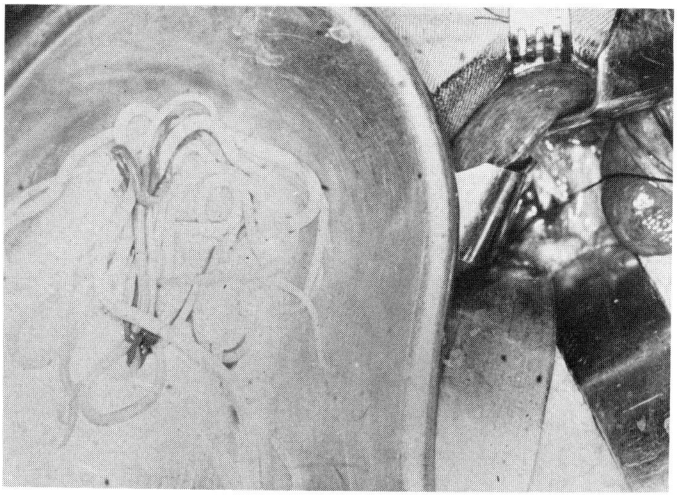

Figure 56.8. *Ascaris* removed from the common bile duct. The left hepatic duct leads to an abscess cavity.

tial, for often many of the worms are alive and require removal.

If facilities are available, operative cholangiography should also be performed and the patient treated with antibiotics and intravenous fluid replacement. When the patient has recovered sufficiently, a course of antihelminthics should be given as some worms may escape detection and give rise to fresh problems. Post-exploratory choledochoscopy will ensure complete clearance of the ducts.

TOXOCARIASIS (VISCERAL LARVA MIGRANS)

Toxocariasis is a parasitic infestation by the larvae of dog or cat roundworm, *Toxocara canis* or *Toxocara cati*. It is usually a self-limiting disease and children are more often affected than adults. It is associated with substandard hygiene and is acquired by close proximity with the infected animals.

Morphology and Life Cycle

Morphology

The adult *Toxocara canis* roundworm male measures 4 to 6 cm in length and the female 6.5 to 10 cm. The male *Toxocara cati* measures 4 to 6 cm whereas the females are 4 to 12 cm in length. *Toxocara cati* are slightly broader than the *canis* variety. The eggs are spherical and dark-brown, measuring 75 to 80 μm in the dog variety and 65 to 70 μm in *Toxocara cati* (Figure 56.9). Embryolization of the eggs takes place in the soil when conditions are suitable and they may retain their ability to infect for months or years.

Primary host infection

Dogs and cats, as well as foxes and other wild animals of the feline and canine groups, are the natural hosts. Infection of cats and dogs varies from place to place. In Great Britain, for example, dogs in rural areas are much more heavily infected than those in urban districts. Similar conditions exist in the United States. Over 80 per cent of dogs in India are infected with this parasite.

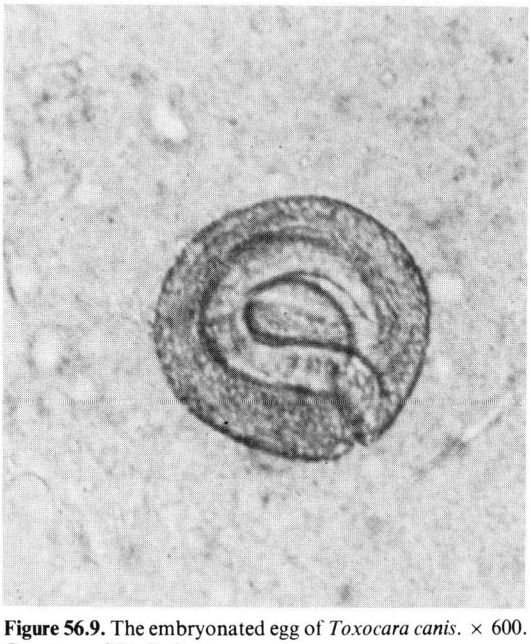

Figure 56.9. The embryonated egg of *Toxocara canis*. × 600. Courtesy of Dr P. Preston.

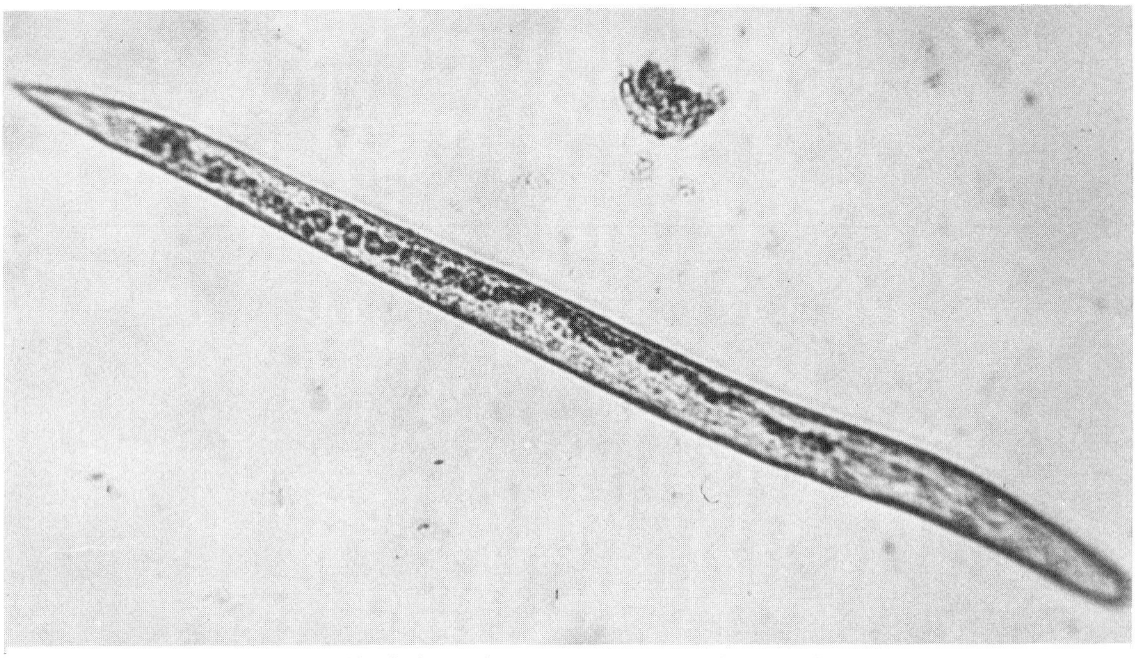

Figure 56.10. The larva of *Toxocara canis*. × 600. Courtesy of Dr P. Preston.

Life cycle

The ova are swallowed by the animals, then are digested and the larvae released (Figure 56.10). The larvae penetrate the intestines, migrate to the liver and then to the lungs. Those that enter the liver travel freely in a zigzag fashion, and wherever they move cause a local inflammatory reaction. The liver may show multiple haemorrhages. In the lungs the larvae may be found between the vascular channels and interalveolar spaces. Ultimately they enter the alveolar spaces, ascend the bronchi and trachea to the epiglottis, and are then swallowed down the oesophagus into the upper part of the gastrointestinal tract. Here they mature sexually in about three weeks.

In addition, after entering the mucosa of the stomach, instead of migrating to the lungs or liver they may invade other tissues where they grow and develop until they return to the lumen of the gut as mature worms. The parasite at the larval stage may penetrate even the placenta, and in this way infect the fetus. If infestation is heavy, some animals are born dead, but survivors have a certain degree of resistance to subsequent invasion by the parasites.

Many of the larvae may be destroyed by the host during migration. Some of them escape destruction and may lodge in a variety of tissues where they are encapsulated but viable for a long time. Some of these cysts are activated during pregnancy, become excysted and pass through the placenta to invade the fetuses. Several litters may be infected. The mechanism by which the larvae are released from the cysts is unknown. The mother may be re-infected by larvae in the faeces passed by the young. In this case the worms will mature without going through the cycle of migration.

Human infection

Human beings accidentally acquire toxocariasis by swallowing eggs in soil contaminated by infected dogs. Only at the larval stage does the parasite survive in human beings, for the larvae never grow into adult worms. Infection is usually brought about by close proximity with dogs. Thus children, by fondling pet dogs or cats, are most commonly infected.

Some of these children may form the habit of eating dirt – geophagia – and thus ingest ova of the *Toxocara*. The majority of cases recorded so far come from the southern parts of the United States, Latin America, Great Britain, France and parts of Asia, particularly India. People from the lower socio-economic strata are particularly at risk.

Toxocariasis is possibly much more prevalent than is realized, because mild infestation may be unnoticed.

Pathology

In experimental animals, the larvae penetrate the intestinal wall and produce haemorrhages and oedema in the mucosa.

The liver in some of the reported cases showed yellow nodules varying in size from 0.5 to 1 cm. Some of them may appear umbilicated and occasionally these may be mistaken for secondary tumours. Histologically, the lesions are essentially eosinophilic granulomas.[4,7] In man, it is difficult to demonstrate the offending larvae. In biopsy specimens an early granuloma is composed of epithelioid cells and multinucleate giant cells. Fibroblastic proliferation subsequently replaces the inflammatory cells until the granuloma becomes a fibrous nodule.

The lungs show an inflammatory process similar to that found in the liver.

The myocardium may also be involved. Friedman and Hervada[22] reported the case of a young child who suffered repeated attacks of heart failure and pneumonia with eosinophilia but who subsequently recovered.

The central nervous system may be infected and in children convulsions can result and the cause may not be diagnosed. Eosinophilic granulomas may be found in the brain and the leptomeninges, but demonstration of the *Toxocara* larvae is extremely difficult.

The eye is another organ subject to larval invasion. The larvae enter along the retinal vessels and produce a granulomatous lesion near the macula. Subsequently, they may enter the vitreous humour and produce an endophthalmitis. Grossly the lesion may be so severe as to be mistaken for a retinoblastoma and such eyes have been enucleated. Nichols[62] examined 27 such cases and found *Toxocara* in five of these eyes.

Clinical Features

Symptoms and signs

The disease is observed mainly in children, often toddlers, who have come into contact with domestic animals. In milder cases there may be repeated attacks of respiratory infection. Physical examination may reveal rhonchi with wheezing and the child may have asthmatic attacks with an urticarial rash and rhinorrhoea. Eosinophilia is present in over half of the cases. During this period of the illness there may be a gastrointestinal upset with anorexia and the child may fail to gain weight. Some patients may be asymptomatic when an eosinophilia and hepatomegaly are the only manifestations.

With severe infestation, there may be a fever ranging from 39 to 40°C and chest x-ray may show mottling in the lungs. Leucocytosis may be marked with an eosinophilia sometimes as high as 80 per cent. The child may have a cough with asthmatic attacks and in some cases epileptic fits. Deaths have been reported during such attacks.[11]

Ocular toxocariasis is an extremely serious complication and a child may be seen when there is ophthalmitis, or loss of visual acuity, or even blindness.

Slit-lamp examination of the eye may occasionally reveal a larva in the retina close to the macula or optic disc.[73]

Diagnosis

Any child suffering from asthmatic attacks with hepatomegaly and other signs of allergic phenomena, and living in a poor environment, should be suspected of suffering from toxocariasis.

Ocular lesions require x-ray examination. In the majority of cases, if there is no calcification present, retinoblastoma can be ruled out. A slit-lamp examination by the ophthalmologist sometimes may demonstrate the larvae in the retina. Biopsy of an enlarged liver occasionally may demonstrate the granuloma, but demonstration of the larva is difficult. Serological studies so far have not been helpful in achieving a diagnosis.

Treatment

In the majority of cases no treatment is necessary. If a severe allergic reaction occurs, steroid therapy should be given. Among the antihelminthics used is diethylcarbamazine (Hetrazan).

Prophylaxis

Children should be kept away from domestic cats and dogs and the habit of geophagia should be stopped.

CAPILLARIA HEPATICA

This is a roundworm commonly found in the liver of rats and squirrels[55] but also present in other wild animals such as pigs, beavers and some species of monkeys, and in dogs.

Morphology and Life Cycle

Morphology

The ova of *Capillaria hepatica* resemble those of *Trichuris trichiura*, but they are much larger than the latter. They are barrel-shaped and possess a double shell. At either end of the egg, the lid is pitted instead of protruding outwards like the *Trichuris trichiura* ova. Together with its size, this distinguishes the eggs from those of *Trichuris trichiura*.[56] When the eggs are discharged in the faeces they are non-infective but after exposure to the atmosphere and moisture in the soil embryolization takes place and they become infective from two to six weeks later.

Life cycle

The eggs can be swallowed by animals which prey on the host but then are not infective. Man may become infected either by ingestion of the embryonated eggs or by eating the liver of infected animals such as red squirrels or muskrats. In the latter instance the eggs are passed unchanged: abdominal colic and diarrhoea may result but the host is otherwise unharmed.

Ingestion of embryonating eggs occurs particularly in children who live in substandard conditions and who practise geophagia. Thus far, only 10 cases of human capillariasis have been reported. The eggs, after being swallowed, are hatched in the caecum. The free larvae penetrate the caecal wall, enter a vessel and are carried by the portal system to the liver. Here they mature in about three weeks and live for another four weeks when large numbers of eggs

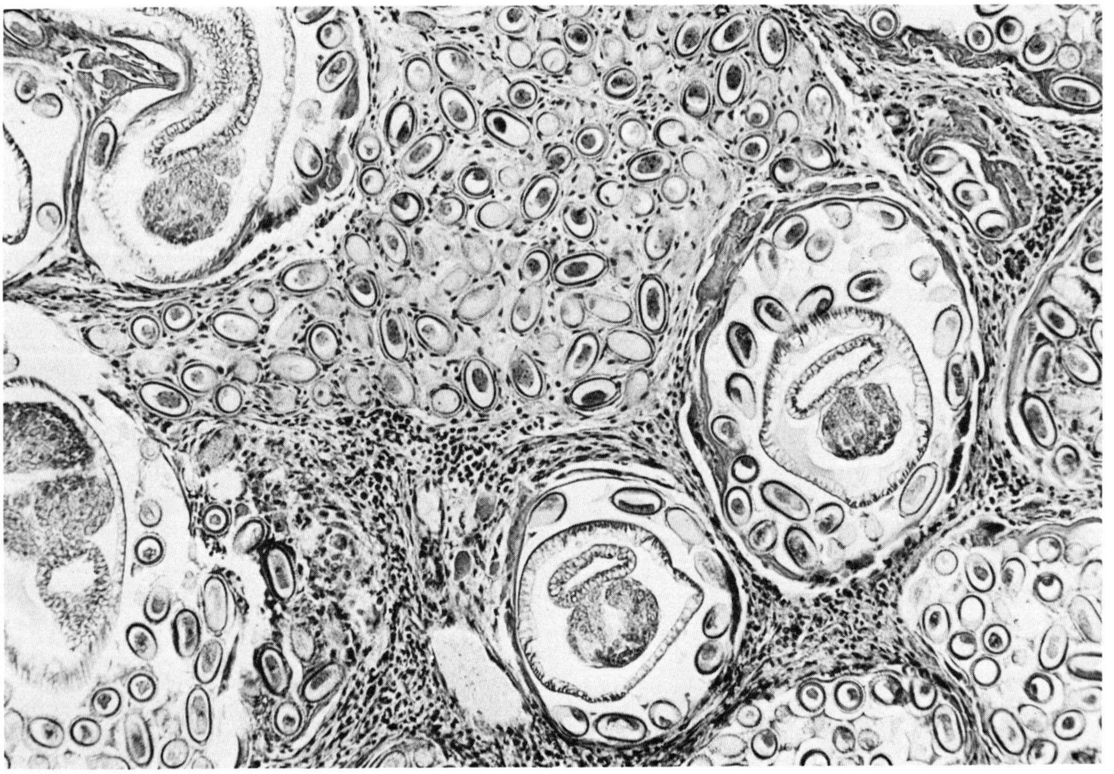

Figure 56.11. The liver of a squirrel showing many worms and eggs of *Capillaria hepatica*. × 70. Courtesy of Dr R. Ko.

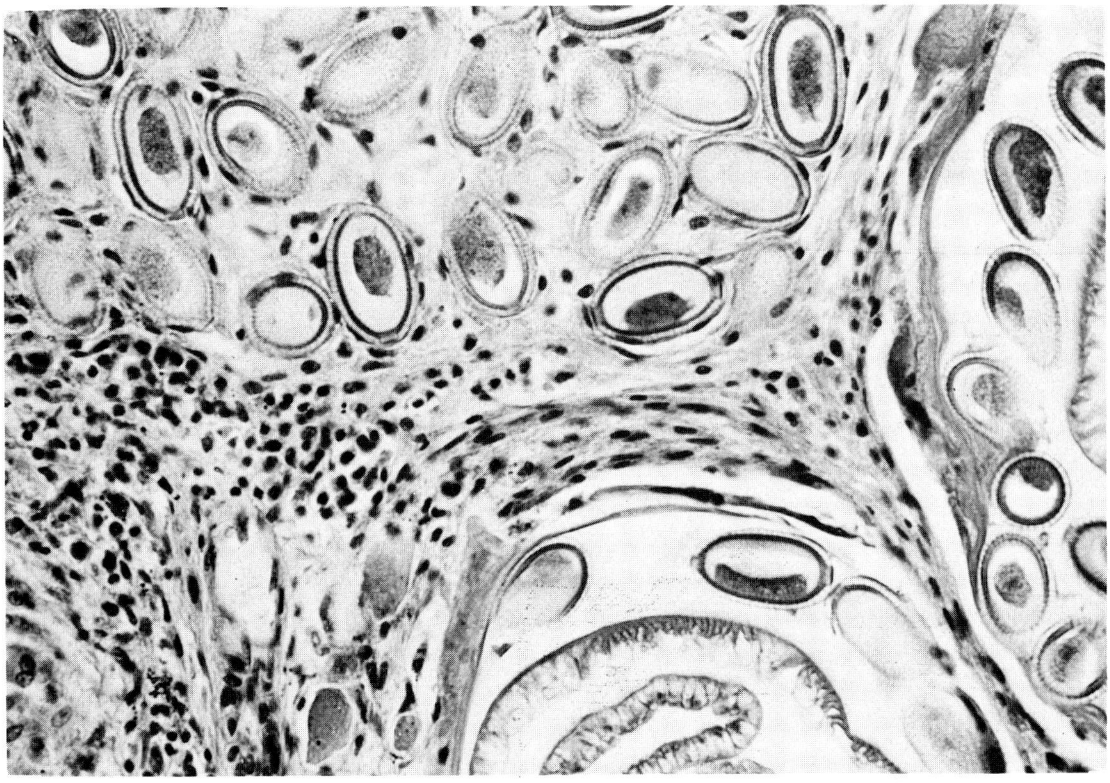

Figure 56.12. A high-power view showing the double-shelled eggs of *Capillaria hepatica* with pitted opercula. × 140. Courtesy of Dr R. Ko.

are released in the liver following the disintegration of the adult worms (Figure 56.11).

Pathology

The liver is enlarged and may be three or four times normal size. Its colour varies from pink to purple and the surface is studded with yellowish or grey nodules measuring between 0.1 and 0.2 cm in diameter, surrounded by an area of grey induration up to 3 cm in diameter.

Microscopically, the yellowish-grey area represents necrosis of the liver together with granuloma formation. Worms in varying stages of preservation and numerous eggs surrounded by eosinophils and macrophages (Figure 56.12) are found in these lesions.

Clinical Features

Infected subjects are usually acutely ill, dehydrated and undernourished. There may be a fever of 39 to 41°C, with marked loss of body weight, protruding abdomen and oedema of the extremities. The patients may suffer with night sweats together with nausea and vomiting. On examination the liver may be markedly enlarged and palpable up to 8 cm below the costal margin.

Laboratory findings

There may be an increase in leucocytes with an eosinophilia which may be as high as 85 per cent. In addition, anaemia is present. Liver function tests are usually normal, but sometimes there may be an increase of alkaline phosphatase.

Diagnosis

Diagnosis can be made from liver biopsy or at necropsy. The worms and ova are more likely to be demonstrated from the liver biopsy than in the case of toxocariasis.

Treatment

There is no known treatment.

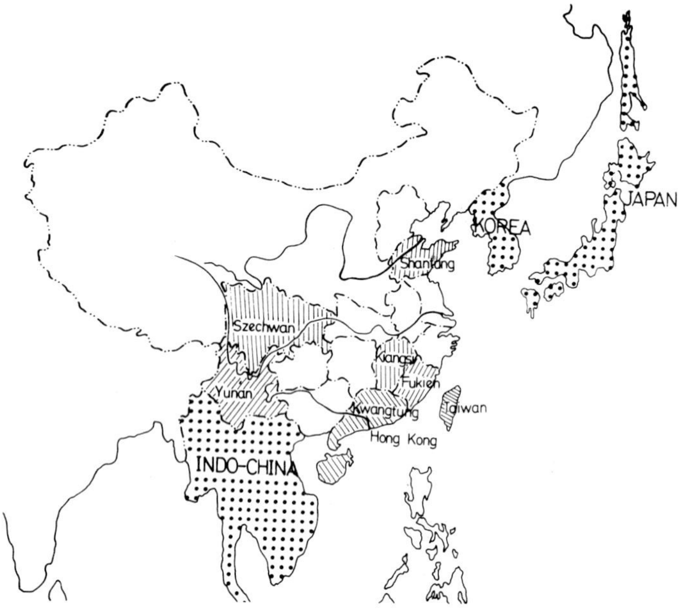

Figure 56.13. The geographical distribution of *Clonorchis sinensis*.

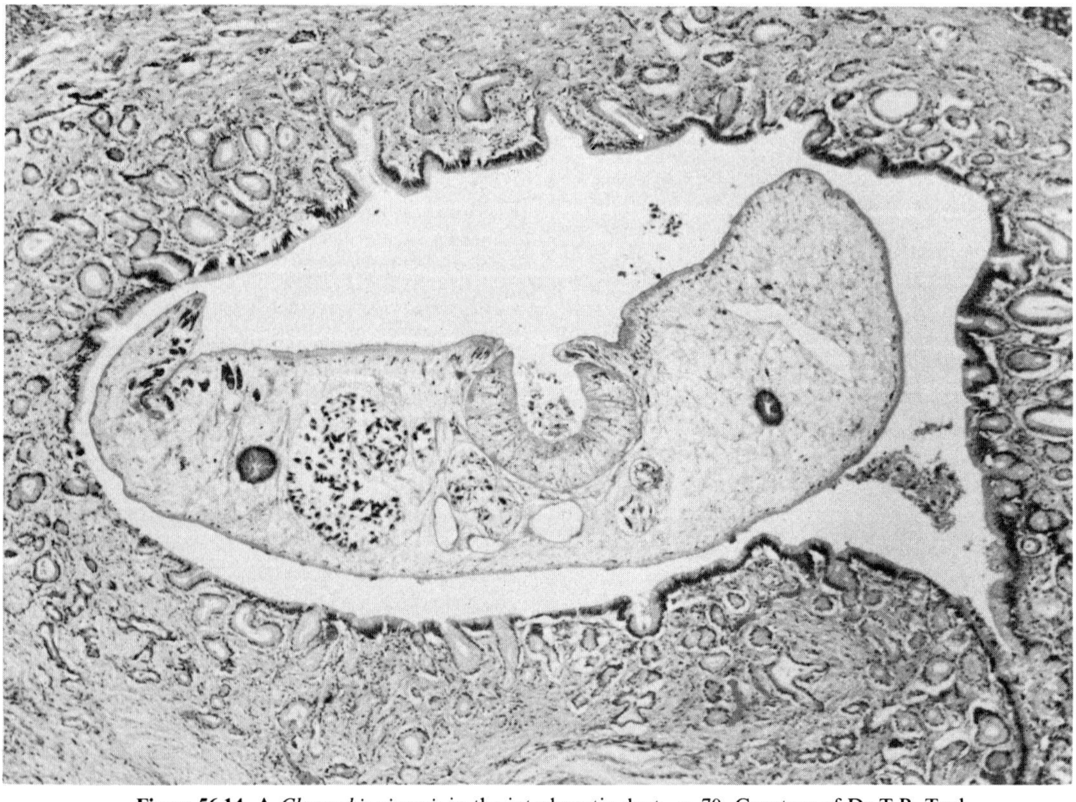

Figure 56.14. A *Clonorchis sinensis* in the intrahepatic duct. × 70. Courtesy of Dr T.B. Teoh.

Prevention

This consists of avoiding raw or partially cooked livers of squirrels. Improvement of living conditions and attention to personal hygiene are important steps in its prevention.

CLONORCHIS SINENSIS

This trematode belongs to the genus *Clonorchis*, suborder *Distomata*, of the phylum platyhelminthes. It was first described by McConnell in 1875 in the bile ducts of a Chinese carpenter in Calcutta.[53] The definitive host is man, but cats and dogs are also infested. Experimental infection can be produced in guinea pigs. There is a wide distribution of *Clonorchis sinensis* among the countries of East Asia. In Japan the infestation rate is as high as 27 per cent and the infestation rate is also high in Korea. It is widely distributed in China. Previously it was assumed that *Clonorchis* was endemic solely in the southern province of Kwangtung. It has now been discovered that an area in Hunan Province in southwest China is endemic and it is also found in Fukien and Kiangsi as well as Shangtung Provinces. Taiwan is another endemic area (Figure 56.13).

The incidence of clonorchiasis in the provinces of China varies. It is highest in Kwangtung Province, and the infestation rate in Hong Kong has been stated to be 65 per cent.[30] There is no infection known in the western hemisphere but ethnic Chinese who have emigrated to the North American continent have been known to be heavily infested. Seah,[74] in 1973, reported a rate of *Clonorchis* infestation of 15.5 per cent from examination of the stools of 400 Chinese immigrants. There was an epidemic of clonorchiasis in Shanghai in 1949 among the European population. This population, which consisted mainly of displaced Jewish stock, had taken to eating salted or pickled fresh-water fish, depicted as 'herring'.[39]

Morphology and Life Cycle

Morphology

The adult worms live in the biliary tree and occasionally in the pancreatic duct (Figures 56.14 and 56.15). The worm is flat, transparent and pinkish-white in colour when alive, but

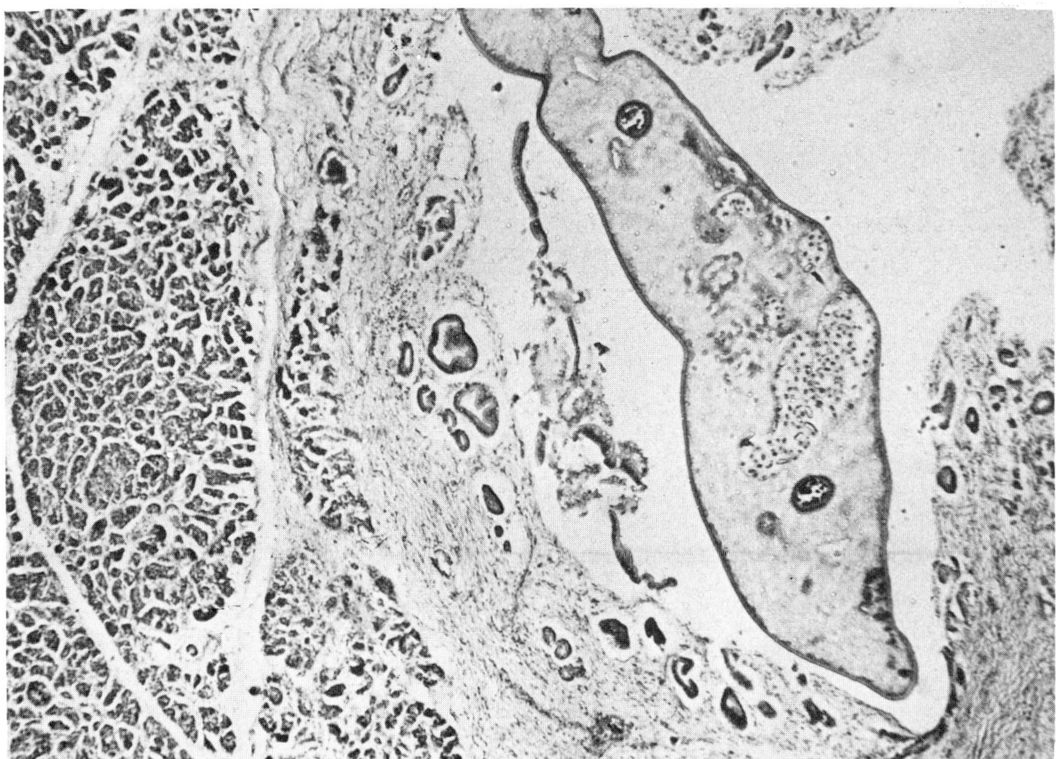

Figure 56.15. A *Clonorchis sinensis* lodged in the pancreatic duct. × 70. Courtesy of Dr T.B. Teoh.

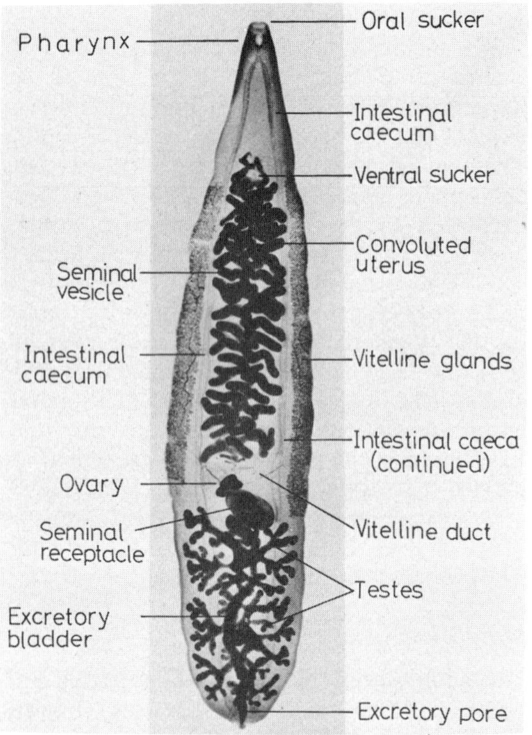

Figure 56.16. The mature *Clonorchis sinensis.* × 18. Courtesy of Professor C.T. Huang.

turns black when dead. It measures between 10 and 25 mm in length and 3 to 5 mm in breadth. The integument of the adult worm is aspinose. The oral sucker is slightly bigger than the ventral one, which is situated at the anterior fifth of the worm. The worm has a short, wide pharynx which leads into paired digestive caeca. The major part of the worm including the coiled uterus is situated about the middle third (Figure 56.16). This arises from the ootype and leads into the genital atrium which opens beside the male duct. The posterior third of the worm is occupied by branched dorsal and ventral testes. From each testis arises the vas efferens which joins with its fellow to form the vas deferens. The vas runs anteriorly and near the middle of the worm it enlarges to form the seminal vesicle before opening into the genital pore, situated just anterior to the ventral sucker (Figure 56.16).

The eggs are oval in shape and have a moderately thick yellowish-brown shell which has a distinct convex cover or operculum. This fits into a rimmed extension of the shell. At the extremity of the egg there is a short comma-shaped extension of the shell. The eggs measure between 27 and 35 microns by 11.7 to 19.5 microns and are fully embryonated when discharged into the bile ducts.

Life cycle

The eggs are released in the faeces (Figure 56.17) and in the water are swallowed by snails. The snails most commonly affected are the *Parafossarulus manchouricus* of which there are several varieties as well as the related snail *Bithynia fuchsiana.*

The miracidia are released from the operculated eggs in the snail. They penetrate the viscera of the snail and form sporocysts. A second generation of sporocysts is formed from which the redia emerge. The redia produce large numbers of cercariae which have a head, a body and a forked tail. The cercariae are free swimming organisms and on coming into contact with fresh-water fish, lose their tails, penetrate the scales of the fish and encyst in the muscles. The common fresh-water fish in south China is a variety of carp, usually known as grass carp, *Ctenopharyngodon idellus*, but other varieties of fish, like the *Pseudorasbora parva* which are found in fresh-water ponds in the northern provinces of China may be infected.

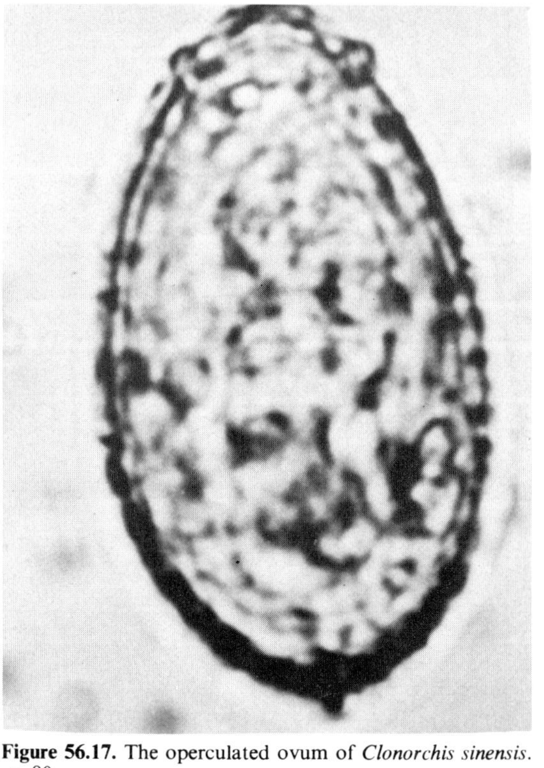

Figure 56.17. The operculated ovum of *Clonorchis sinensis.* × 80.

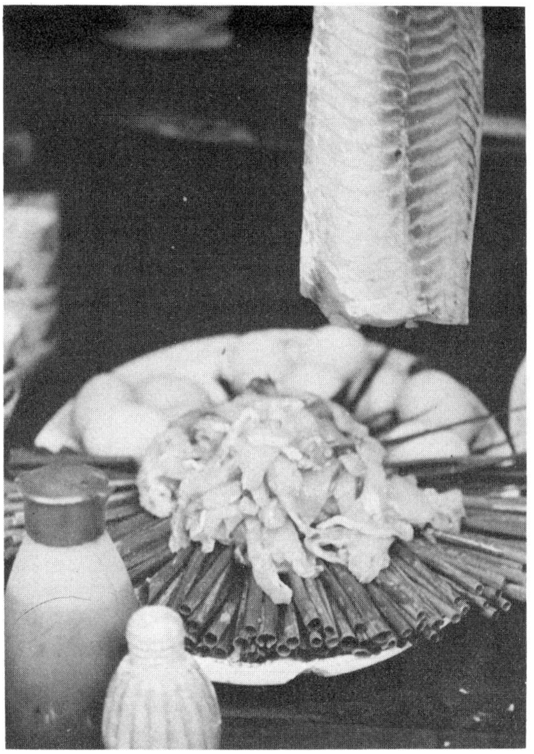

Figure 56.18. Slices of the grass carp. Hot rice porridge is poured into a bowl containing the fish.

Other second intermediate hosts may be fresh-water crayfishes, *Caridina nilotica gracilipes de Man* (Atyidae) and *Macrobrachium superbum* (Heller).[79] In southern China the fish is filleted, cut into slices (Figure 56.18) and served after pouring hot rice porridge over it.

In the other Chinese provinces, Kiangsi, Yunan and Shangtung, the fish are eaten after being roasted over an open fire. These fish are caught from streams and pools and it is mostly children who are parasitized.

In Fukien Province, the crayfish are caught, smacked between the palms until they turn red and are then eaten without cooking. This is believed to give them a medicinal quality.

The encysted metacercariae are released in the duodenum and rapidly enter the common bile duct through the ampulla of Vater. They then proceed against the bile stream to the smaller bile ducts where they mature into adult worms in about one month. Three months are required for the worms to go through the life cycle. In the bile ducts eggs are laid and are discharged in the faeces and so conclude the cycle.

The movement of the adult worm has been studied by Hou.[30] It moves against the bile stream by first attaching the oral sucker to the wall of the bile ducts. The body then undergoes contraction. The ventral sucker then attaches itself to the wall and the oral sucker is released. The worm lengthens and the oral sucker again attaches itself to the wall of the duct. In this way the worm moves against the bile stream until it reaches the smallest of the bile ducts. Here it attaches itself permanently downwards to the large bile duct before moving in order to lay the eggs.

The worm is not always successful in its movement up into the intrahepatic ducts. Occasionally desquamation of the epithelium washes the worm down with the bile stream. The presence of the worm in the duct does not as a rule cause any reaction.

The parasite draws its nutrition from protein and glucose obtained from the secretion of the epithelium. A mucoid substance that surrounds the worm is produced by the epithelium.

Pathology

The duct proximal to the worm dilates due to partial obstruction. This may show through the capsule of the liver as bluish spots. The epithelium surrounding the worm itself also undergoes changes. An adenomatous bile duct hyperplasia occurs and this is thought by Hou[30] to result from the irritation caused by the worm.

In chronic and heavy infestation with *Clonorchis sinensis*, the bile ducts become thickened with a large amount of fibrous tissue formation. This fibrosis of the duct sometimes extends into the parenchyma, but never to the extent of forming nodular cirrhosis. The liver parenchyma is otherwise normal. Cellular infiltration does not occur unless there is secondary infection. In the few cases that have cellular infiltration with eosinophilia, *Ascaris* remnants could usually also be demonstrated (Figure 56.19). The eggs laid in the bile, in the presence of obstruction, may be regurgitated into the smaller bile ducts of the portal tracts. Here an inflammatory reaction occurs and a granuloma may form.

Complications of Clonorchiasis

Development of carcinoma of the bile duct

Hou[31] has shown that hyperplasia of the epithelium, due to the chronic irritation of the bile ducts, may take place. When this persists for long enough, carcinomatous change may

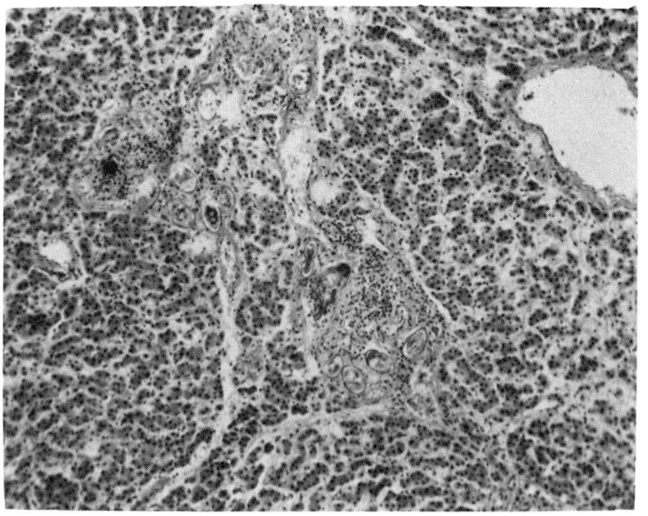

Figure 56.19. A granuloma in the portal tract with numerous *Clonorchis* ova. × 120. Courtesy of Dr T.B. Teoh.

follow. In a study of 30 cholangiocarcinomas, worms were demonstrated in 28 cases.[31]

Clonorchiasis and stone formation

When secondary infection occurs in the bile ducts, the worm usually dies and the carcass, as in *Ascaris lumbricoides*, may become the nidus of stone formation (Figure 56.20). The infection is usually with enteric organisms and may reach the bile through the portal vein or ascend in the bile. The parasite dies and as its body disintegrates calcium bilirubinate is deposited on fragments. Teoh[80] found *Clonorchis*, or its ova, in eight out of 40 stones studied. We have examined 51 such stones and found that 12 of them contained the ova of *Clonorchis sinensis*. Except for five stones removed from the

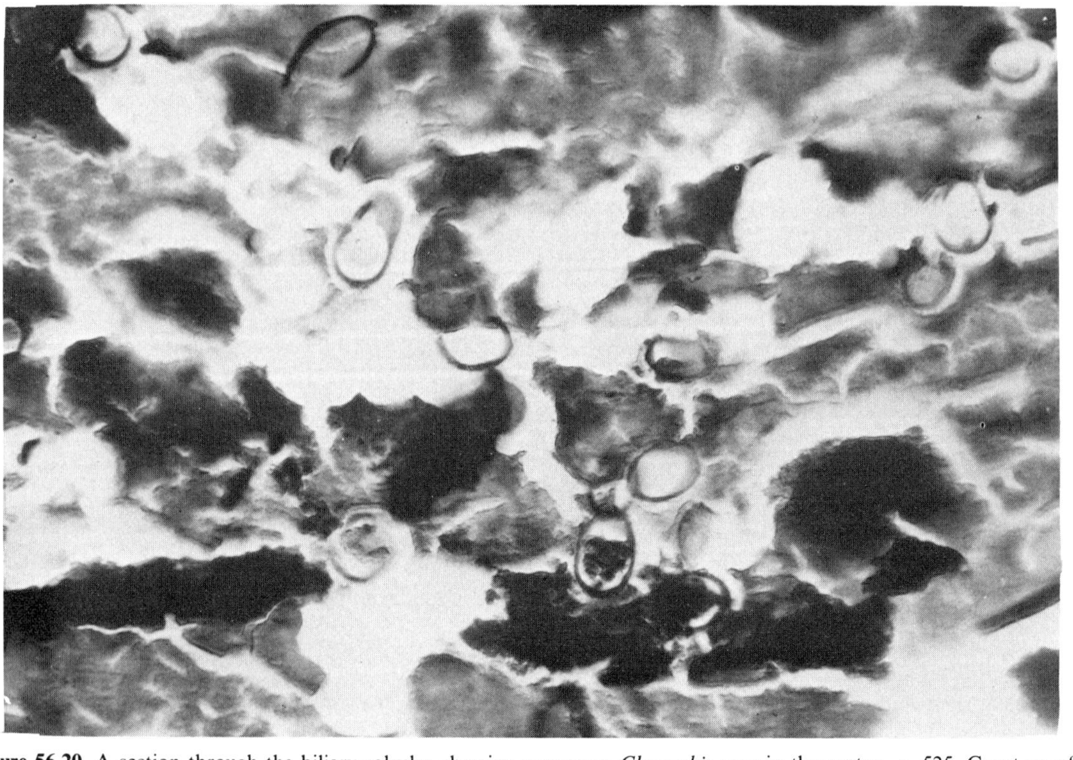

Figure 56.20. A section through the biliary calculus showing numerous *Clonorchis* eggs in the centre. × 525. Courtesy of Professor C.T. Huang.

gallbladder, the Gram stain revealed not only remnants of the parasite but also bacteria.

Hou[31] has pointed out that the parasite could not survive for any period in the gallbladder as the concentrated bile is too toxic. Thus, a gallstone may form over the dead worm without infection.

Septicaemic shock

McFadzean and Yeung[54] in 1965 reported 11 cases of fulminating bacterial infection in patients with a heavy infestation of *Clonorchis sinensis*. These patients presented with hypoglycaemia and coma. Two of the 11 patients recovered after surgical treatment; the remaining nine died.

Clinical Features

Clinical manifestation of clonorchiasis depends on the severity of the infestation. When the infestation is mild, it may not produce symptoms. Cases may be divided into three groups: mild asymptomatic infestation; moderate or heavy infestation; and mild infestation with complications.

Mild asymptomatic infestation

The number of worms may be few and may be accidentally discovered in routine stool examination. In a survey of 29 730 patients who attended the Kowloon Hospital in 1961, 1855 patients harboured *Clonorchis sinensis* – an incidence of 6.2 per cent.[65] The incidence is lower than in a report by Seah[74] who examined the stools of a group of 400 Chinese immigrants to Canada and found *Clonorchis* infestation in 62 (15.5 per cent) patients. This discrepancy in the incidence of a general population can be explained by the fact that whereas the survey conducted by Ong[65] was on a simple smear technique, Seah[74] employed a concentration method of examining the stool for ova. These worms may live for a long period and a case was reported by Seah[74] of a patient who emigrated from China more than 50 years earlier and was still harbouring ova when his stool was examined.

Moderate or heavy infestation

Patients may complain of general malaise, anorexia and epigastric discomfort, and the urine may be dark. The epigastric discomfort is constant and may be described as a feeling of distension. Jaundice without secondary infection is rare and when present is usually mild. The alkaline phosphatase and transaminase levels may be raised, but they usually subside very rapidly with the disappearance of the pain.

Intravenous cholangiography may demonstrate narrowing of the bile ducts or the intrahepatic bile ducts and occasionally the parasite may be demonstrated as a filling defect. This is best demonstrated by retrograde cholangiography which shows ectasia of the bile ducts, with multiple filling defects produced by the clumps of parasites (Figure 56.20). Scanning of the liver may show slight mottling in both lobes.

Mild infestation of Clonorchis sinensis with complications

The complications are either carcinoma, usually a cholangiocarcinoma, or biliary calculi. Cholangiocarcinoma may present with jaundice due to obstruction at the confluence of the right and left hepatic ducts, or in one of the intrahepatic ducts. The liver may be palpable and hard.

The infestation may present with biliary calculi and these patients usually have pain, chills, fever and jaundice. This Charcot's intermittent fever may completely subside after the initial attack and the patient may stay symptom-free for one or two years, but with each succeeding attack the remission becomes shorter.

Examination of these patients may reveal an enlarged liver and in a small percentage an enlarged spleen is present. The gallbladder may also be palpable. Jaundice varies in intensity, but on average the serum bilirubin is in the region of 60 to 70 mmol/l (3.5 to 4 g/dl). The alkaline phosphatase is invariably raised, up to 400 mmol/l. The serum transaminases may be raised but are seldom very high, except with obstruction to and severe infection of the bile ducts. During remission acute pancreatitis may occur.

Intravenous cholangiography may show a dilated common bile duct with filling defects, but in the majority the biliary tree is not visualized. Endoscopic retrograde cholangiopancreatography (ERCP) may show a dilated common bile duct with stones or filling defects produced by clumps of parasites. Liver scanning is of little help and shows slight mottling throughout the liver.

Diagnosis

This disease should be kept in mind if there is moderately severe pain in the epigastrium. A history of eating raw fish is helpful. The patient's general condition may be good, and the liver will be palpable but not tender. An intravenous cholangiogram may fail to visualize the biliary tract and ERCP will demonstrate the offending parasite. The diganosis is confirmed by finding the ova in the stool.

Treatment

Clonorchiasis may be discovered during routine stool examination for immigration to countries in North America and treatment may be required by the immigration authorities. So far, treatment with drugs has not been effective.

Sodium antimony tartrate was the first drug introduced by Shattuck[75] in 1924 for the treatment of clonorchiasis but it has little effect on the parasite. It is given in the same doses as for filariasis, but the results have been consistently poor with very severe side-effects. Prolonged treatment is necessary in endemic areas.

Hexachloroparaxylol has been stated to have considerable success in the treatment of clonorchiasis. Liu and his co-workers[46] reported the results of doses of 0.5 g per kg body weight given on 10 consecutive days. They claimed 100 per cent cure of all heavily infected cases three months after the completion of treatment. In mild cases half this dose for 10 consecutive days effected a complete cure. Chung et al[13] report a similar experience. However, this drug has been found to be nephrotoxic as well as neurotoxic. In dogs as well as in man its administration causes a rapid development of anaemia. It has since been withdrawn.

Chloroquine has been tried for the treatment of clonorchiasis, but is not very satisfactory in eliminating the parasites. Some cures have been reported following prolonged treatment for two months or longer. The regimen recommended is 300 mg daily for two to six months.

Surgical treatment

Surgical treatment is indicated when there is secondary infection with severe cholangitis present, especially if there is potential or actual septicaemia. Surgical intervention should be prompt and drainage of the common bile duct is often all that can be achieved. In less severe cases operative cholangiography should be done to find any stones in the intrahepatic ducts.

The removal of stones in the lower end of the common bile duct or of clumps of parasites obstructing the common bile duct requires transduodenal sphincteroplasty. This allows flukes to drain with the bile into the gastrointestinal tract. If carcinoma has developed resection or internal drainage will be required.

Prophylaxis

Infestation of this parasite can be eliminated only by education: eating raw or inadequately cooked fish in endemic areas should be discouraged.

Fish farming, which is extensive in southern China, should be carried out under hygienic conditions. Privies should not be built beside the pond.

Destruction of the snail intermediate host is much more difficult and involves great expense.

OPISTHORCHIASIS

These trematodes are very much akin to the *Clonorchis sinensis*. They are the cat liver flukes. *Opisthorchis felineus* has been found in southern, central and eastern Europe, in Siberia, Poland, India, Vietnam, Korea, Japan and the Philippines. *Opisthorchis viverrini* is found in northern Thailand and Laos.

Morphology and Life Cycle

Morphology

The adult worms of both species are similar in size and shape. They are sufficiently similar to make identification difficult.

Opisthorchis viverrini is smaller than the *Opisthorchis felineus* and has smaller oral and ventral suckers. It has an oesophagus which is longer than its pharynx and has deeply lobed testes and ovary. Its vitellaria are aggregated by a few large clusters of granular material.

When removed from the bile duct the living parasite is greyish-yellow and measures between 7 and 12 mm in length and 1.5 to 3 mm in breadth. *Opisthorchis viverrini* has oral and ventral suckers of almost equal diameter. The oral sucker is not at the terminal portion of the anterior end and the ventral sucker is situated at about one-fifth of the way along the length of the body.

Opisthorchis felineus has a small mouth and a short pharynx, with a very short oesophagus passing quickly into two blind caeca. The excretory bladder is a long tube which ends at the hind portion of the worm. The long seminal vesicle terminates in the ejaculatory duct which opens on the genital pore in front of the ventral sucker. The vitellaria are situated lateral to the caeca and are placed much more anteriorly than in the *Opisthorchis viverrini*.

The eggs measure 30 by 11 microns and are operculated. When the egg is first laid, the miracidium is not fully developed. This development takes place in the snail.

Life cycle

The eggs are passed in the stools and are swallowed by the snail which is the intermediate host, *Bithynia leachi* or *Bithynia tentaculata*. In the snail the miracidia penetrate the tissue of their intermediate host and then form sporocysts. From the sporocysts two generations of rediae develop and the daughter rediae give rise to cercariae. These mature in about two months and then leave the snails. They quickly penetrate underneath the scales of the fresh-water fish *Idus melanotus* and *Tinca tinca* and then encyst in the fish. The metacercariae, after ingestion by man, are released in the duodenum and migrate through the ampulla of Vater into the bile ducts where they mature three to four weeks after ingestion. They have also occasionally been found in the pancreatic ducts.

Pathology

In most cases of opisthorchiasis, the liver is markedly enlarged. The ducts are markedly dilated with thickened walls. The dilated ducts may be fusiform, saccular or cystic in appearance. The ductal changes in the epithelium and the ductal walls are similar to those found in *Clonorchis sinensis*. However, there does not seem to be a correlation between stone formation and opisthorchiasis.[77]

The changes that take place in the bile ducts as a result of this parasitic infestation are similar to those resulting from *Clonorchis sinensis*. The incidence of infestation in cases of cholangiocarcinoma is similar to that found by Hou[31] in his study of *Clonorchis*. It can therefore be postulated that the high incidence of cholangiocarcinoma in Thailand is directly related to this parasitic infestation.

Clinical Features, Treatment and Prognosis

These are similar to those described for *Clonorchis sinensis*.

DICROCOELIASIS

This is an infestation of the biliary tract by the trematode *Dicrocoelium dendriticum*. It is a small elongated fluke and is primarily a parasite of cattle and sheep. Goats, pigs, horses, donkeys and other herbivorous animals as well as dogs may be reservoirs. This parasite is particularly common in eastern Europe and Russia, and has been reported from Africa and North and South America. It is also found in Asiatic USSR, Java and China.

Morphology and Life Cycle

Morphology

The adult fluke is lancet-shaped and measures between 5 and 15 mm in length and 1½ to 2½ mm in breadth. It has a smooth integument and an oral sucker that is ventral in position. The ventral sucker is slightly larger than this oral sucker and is situated at about one-fifth of the way along from the anterior end of the worm. The pharynx is round and located immediately behind the oral sucker. Halfway between the two suckers the digestive tract bifurcates to form a pair of caeca. The testes and ovaries are situated more anteriorly, whereas the uterus which is coiled and forms many loops is posterior and runs to the hind portion of the worm.

The eggs are thick-shelled and dark brown in colour and measure 36 to 48 microns in length and 20 to 30 microns in breadth. The operculum is broad and has no shoulders.

Life cycle

The eggs are embryonated when passed in the faeces.

Various land snails, Helicidae, Enidae, Chrondrinidae, Vitrinidae and Ariophantidae, can act as the first intermediate host. After the ova have been ingested by one of these snails the miracidia are released.[51] They then penetrate the digestive tract of the snail to form sporocysts in the digestive gland. A second generation of sporocysts develops and these, in turn, produce cercariae. The cercariae leave the digestive gland of the snail to enter the respiratory chamber where they lose their tails and mass together to form a slime ball. As the snails crawl over vegetables this slime ball containing between 200 and 400 cercariae is released.

These balls are swallowed by a small field ant, *Formica fusca*, which is the second intermediate host.[42] The cercariae are then freed from the slime ball in the ant and penetrate the gut wall. They then develop into the infective metacercariae stage and become encysted. The fully-formed metacercariae cysts are firm and resilient. Infection occurs when an animal grazing over the field swallows the ants. Man, among other animals, may accidentally ingest the infected ants.

Pathology

Like other trematodes inhabiting the biliary tract, dicrocoeliasis produces marked changes in the portal tract. Grossly, the liver may be enlarged when there is severe infestation and there may be peripheral scarring with slight dilatation and fibrosis of the ducts. The gallbladder, especially in sheep, may occasionally contain adult flukes.

Contracture and fibrosis in the portal tract give rise to a lump in the liver. Early infection shows little microscopic changes around the large bile ducts. Later the infection may cause parenchymal degeneration and necrosis, and replacement of these areas by connective tissue – a condition similar to that caused by mature flukes in *Fasciola hepatica* infection. Lymphocytes, macrophages, plasma cells and fibroblasts surround the portal areas with occasional proliferation of the bile ducts. Sometimes infiltration by eosinophils has been observed.

Clinical Features

With mild infestation, dicrocoeliasis, like *Clonorchis sinensis* and opisthorchiasis, usually produces mild symptoms or is asymptomatic. In most cases in man the symptoms are absent or limited to flatulence and fullness of the abdomen. Diarrhoea may be observed. The disease may become severe if there is secondary infection and simulates *Clonorchis sinensis* with cholangitis.

Treatment

The treatment so far is unsatisfactory. Thymol has been tried. Fuadin has also been tried for inpatient treatment.

Prophylaxis

Vegetables and plants when taken raw should be carefully cleaned to avoid accidental swallowing of ants.

FASCIOLIASIS

This is a parasitic infestation of the biliary tract caused by the trematode, *Fasciola hepatica*. The parasite is found in sheep- and cattle-rearing countries of the world. It is common in Latin America, the United States and Mexico. In Europe, it occurs in Russia, Hungary, Germany, Spain, The Netherlands, France and the United Kingdom. In Africa, it is confined to the northern part of the continent, particularly Algeria. It is found in China, Tibet and Siberia in Asia and in Syria and other Middle Eastern countries. It is also found in Australia.

In countries where the disease is endemic, almost 100 per cent of sheep and 20 per cent of cattle are infected. Because of the extensive liver damage, this infestation has been designated as 'liver rot'. Severe infection may cause death of the animals. Man is accidentally infected by eating watercress (*Nasturtium officinale*) contaminated with the encysted metacercariae of the worm.

The number of cases reported has risen considerably and in some countries such as France, England, Germany and Cuba where the disease is endemic occasional outbreaks of almost epidemic proportions have been reported. In 1960, an outbreak of the disease took place in Hampshire, England.[18] The disease was acquired by eating the wild watercress

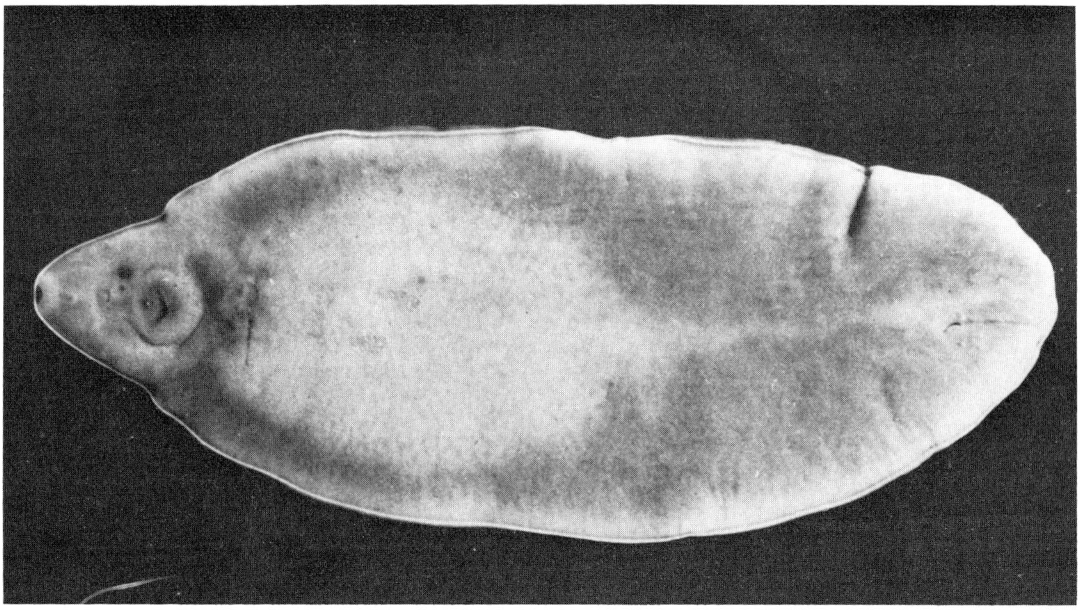

Figure 56.21. The adult *Fasciola hepatica*, ventral surface. Courtesy of Professor C.T. Huang.

(*Nasturtium officinale*). It occurred in the summer months of that year when the rainfall was extra heavy. Heavy rainfall seems to induce proliferation of the snail, *Lymnaea truncatula*, which is the intermediate host of *Fasciola hepatica*.

Morphology and Life Cycle

Morphology

The *Fasciola hepatica* is a flat, leaf-like hermaphrodite trematode (Figure 56.21).

The adult worm measures up to 30 mm in length and 13 mm in width. Its natural habitat is the bile of sheep and cattle as well as the occasional host, man. Its anterior end is conical in shape, and contains on its ventral side the oral sucker. From the anterior end the cone stretches to about a fifth of the length of the worm where it suddenly broadens out to form a shoulder at each side of the base of the cone. The worm broadens further until it comes to the broad round posterior end. The surface of the body is spiny and these spines, as well as the suckers, are used for attaching the trematode to the wall of the bile ducts (Figure 56.21).

The eggs are large, yellowish-brown, oval and operculated and measure between 130 and 150 μm by between 63 and 90 μm (Figure 56.22).

Life cycle

The eggs are laid in the biliary passages, proceed with the bile to the intestines and are evacuated in the faeces. Maturation of the eggs takes place in the water. The miracidium escapes from the eggs and is free-swimming. It soon enters into the intermediate host, a snail, *Lymnaea truncatula*. A sporocyst is formed and from it two generations of rediae are developed. The first generation of rediae develops within three weeks of penetration of the miracidium into the host. By the fourth week the second generation of rediae develops into cercariae which leave the snail as free-swimming organisms. Within a few hours the metacercariae become encysted on some aquatic plants. Cattle and sheep feeding on these plants acquire the infestation. The encysted metacercariae are released in the upper part of the intestinal tract. The metacercariae then penetrate the intestine to gain access into the peritoneal cavity. From the peritoneal cavity they penetrate the capsule of the liver into the parenchyma and become lodged in the bile ducts from where they mature (Figure 56.23).

During the time of migration, the parasite may pass through other organs such as the urinary tract and cause haematuria.[18]

Ectopic fascioliasis may also occur as a result of this migration. Cases have been reported in which the peritoneum, muscles, brain and subcutaneous tissues have been invaded. In the

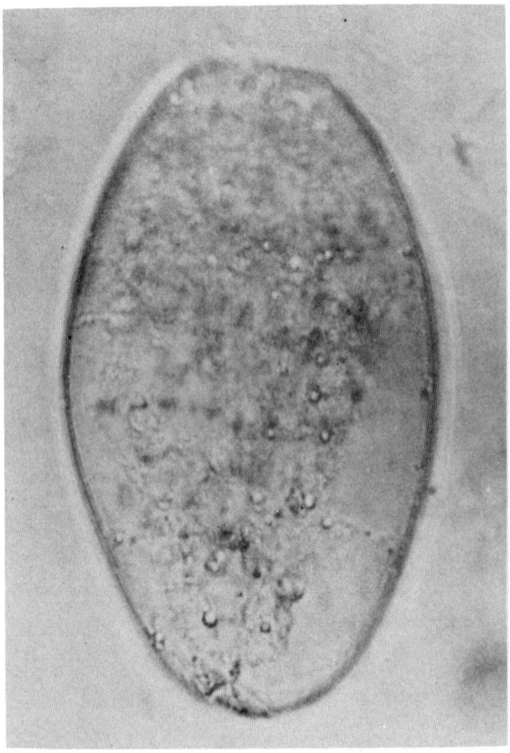

Figure 56.22. The operculated egg of *Fasciola hepatica.* × 360. Courtesy of Professor C.T. Huang.

Lebanon, where the population frequently eat infected raw sheep and goat livers, a condition called 'halzoun', first reported by Khoury in 1905,[85] occurs. In this condition, after ingestion of the infected liver there may be a swelling of the pharynx with severe desquamation. Sometimes it causes suffocation, and in severe cases death from asphyxiation may take place. This was believed by Watson and Kerim[85] to be due to the penetration of the mucosa by immature worms from the raw liver.

Pathology

During the stage of migration of young parasites in heavily infected experimental animals, haemorrhages in the liver parenchyma have been noticed.[14,41] Free blood in the peritoneal cavity occurs and section of the liver reveals tissue destruction of varying intensity. In addition to necrosis of the liver there is cellular infiltration with neutrophils, eosinophils and lymphocytes. After a period, healing takes place and evidence of tissue destruction disappears completely.

In the intrahepatic ducts the worms move to and fro and the spinous nature of the integument together with the suckers cause extensive destruction of the biliary epithelium. The worms are otherwise closely adherent to the wall of the bile ducts and are surrounded by a layer of mucin. Because of their presence, the wall of the bile ducts may show an increase of fibrosis.

Nutrition of the parasite is obtained by ingestion of the desquamated epithelium and other debris. Jennings, Mulligan and Urquhart,[32] using a radioactive isotope technique in experimental rabbit infestations, suggested that the parasites might have ingested the blood from the host. This has been challenged by Dawes,[15] who believes that it is desquamated epithelium that is ingested.

Hou[30] believes that *Clonorchis sinensis* obtains its nutrition from the periportal blood and mucin surrounding its body. This could also

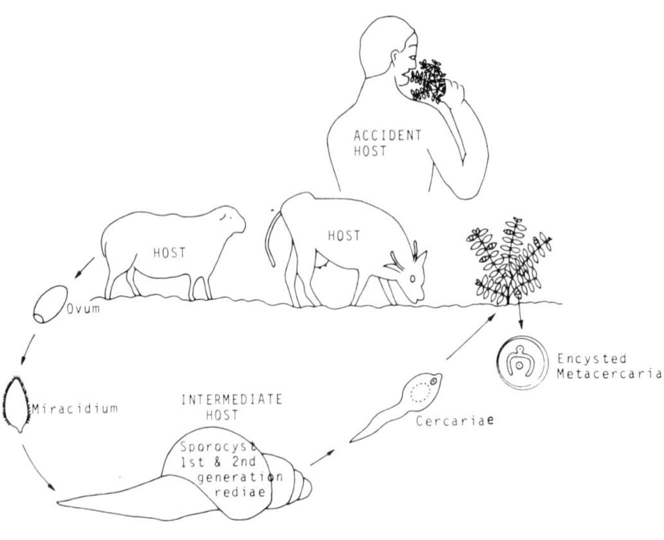

Figure 56.23. Diagram depicting the life cycle of *Fasciola hepatica.*

be the case with *Fasciola*. The complications of cholangiocarcinoma and cholangitis observed by Hou[31] in *Clonorchis sinensis* could also possibly occur in fascioliasis.

Clinical Features

Fascioliasis may produce no symptoms if the infestation is mild. If the infestation is heavy, symptoms may be severe with general malaise, anorexia, nausea, vomiting and night sweats. There may be marked loss of body weight and sometimes rapid prostration. High fever may be present in a large proportion of cases. The pain experienced is confined to the right hypochondrium or epigastrium and is of varying intensity. Jaundice may appear as may an occasional urticarial rash. Anaemia develops rapidly and may necessitate blood transfusion. Ankle oedema may be present. Examination of the abdomen may reveal hepatosplenomegaly and the enlarged liver is usually tender.

Laboratory tests

These may show an eosinophilia with raised serum alkaline phosphatase and bilirubin levels. The transaminase levels may also be elevated and there may be a reversal of the albumin:globulin ratio. There is usually haemoglobinuria.

Intravenous cholangiography may reveal a dilated bile duct due to obstruction by the adult worms.

Diagnosis

With a history of having eaten raw watercress or other aquatic plants and with symptoms of diarrhoea, prostration, fever and jaundice, together with tender hepatomegaly and an eosinophilia, the diagnosis of fascioliasis should be entertained. This is confirmed by the demonstration of ova in the stool. The concentration method may have to be used as the eggs may not be numerous. A positive serum fasciola complement fixation titre greater than 1 to 1000, together with ova in the stool, will be conclusive.

Treatment

Antihelminthic drugs have been used, but most of them, like carbon tetrachloride and emetine hydrochloride, have been abandoned because of their toxicity. Chloroquine has been used occasionally for the relief of symptoms, but it has no effect on the parasites.

Bithionol (2,2′-thio-bis(4,6 dichlorophenol)) was found to be efficacious and curative by Yoshida and his co-workers[88] in 1962. They gave two young Koreans with fascioliasis a daily dose of 50 mg for 20 days. Jones et al[33] successfully treated a patient, who had very massive infestation with *Fasciola hepatica* in the Lake District of England, with Bithionol.

Surgical treatment is limited to the complications of the diseases due to biliary obstruction and secondary infection, and to excision of ectopic flukes in the subcutaneous tissue. Occasionally a live worm may be found on exploration of the bile duct and removed.[61]

Prophylaxis

Infection by *Fasciola hepatica* is prevented by destruction of the intermediate host. Whenever possible, this can be achieved by drainage of stagnant pools in areas where the disease is endemic and where the snails *Lymnaea truncatula* abound. Public health measures should be undertaken and people should be informed of the hazards of eating raw watercress.

SCHISTOSOMIASIS (BILHARZIASIS)

This is an infestation with the flatworm of the phylum platyhelminthes. It belongs to the class of trematoda and the super family, *Schistosomatoidea*. There are three species: *Schistosoma haematobium*; *Schistosoma mansoni*; and *Schistosoma japonicum*. Of these three, *Schistosoma mansoni* and *japonicum* affect the liver. These *Schistosoma* live in the venules of the portal bed, and eggs laid within the vessels are carried by the portal blood into the portal tract of the liver where they give rise to pathological changes.

Schistosoma mansoni was first discovered by Manson[50] in a negro living in Antigua, and was described in 1902. This species produces eggs that have a sub-terminal spine. The *Schistosoma japonicum* ova were discovered by Mashima[52] in 1888 but it was Katsurada[35] who named the adult worms *Schistosoma japonicum* in 1904.

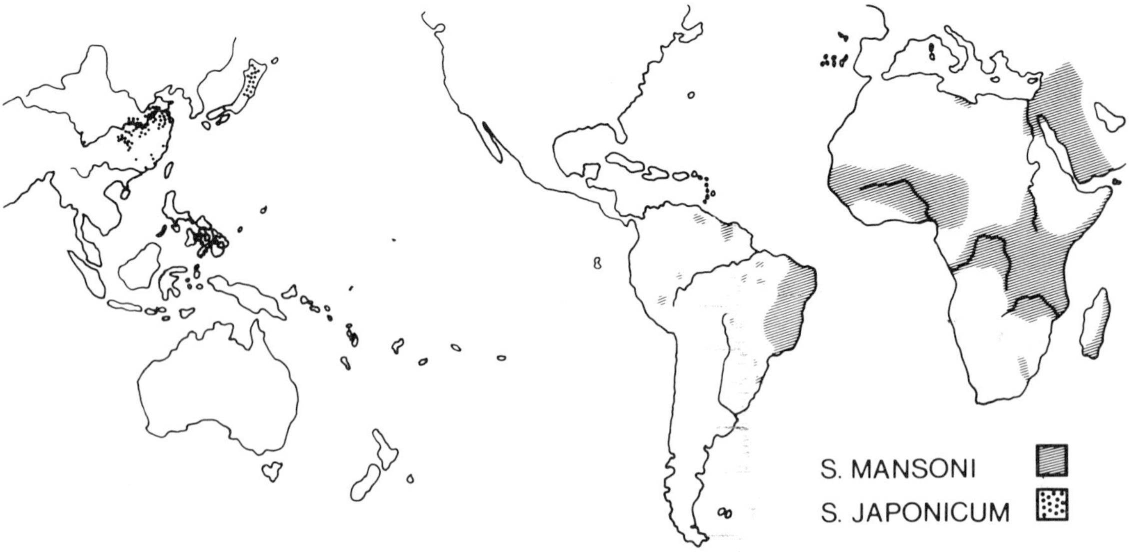

Figure 56.24. The distribution of *Schistosoma mansoni* and *japonicum*.

Distribution

Schistosoma mansoni is widely distributed in Central Africa, from Madagascar to East, Central and West Africa. It is also common in parts of the Middle East, and in the Sudan as well as in Egypt, where it has been known since ancient times. Since the building of the Aswan High Dam the disease seems to have spread more widely so that the incidence of infection encountered during the last 25 years has increased from 14 per cent in 1952 to the present rate of 80 per cent.[64] It is also widespread in Brazil and other parts of the South American continent.

Schistosoma japonicum, the Japanese variety, is confined to China, Taiwan, the Philippine islands and the Celebes (Figure 56.24). Its incidence in Japan has been reduced dramatically in recent years.

Morphology and Life Cycle

Morphology

Superficially, the three species of *Schistosoma*, the *Schistosoma mansoni*, *haematobium* and *japonicum*, appear to be similar. The adult male worm possesses a gynaecophoral canal; this harbours the female. In *Schistosoma mansoni* the male measures between 6.4 and 12 mm in length and 2 mm in width. The surface of the worm is studded with spines which are prominent in *Schistosoma mansoni* as well as in *Schistosoma haematobium*, but the surface of *Schistosoma japonicum* is fairly smooth. The female is filiform in shape and measures between 7.2 and 17 mm in length and is 1 mm in width. The male and female are usually found together and the female is lodged in the gynaecophoral canal of the male and depends on it for transport.

In Schistosoma japonicum the adult male worm is much longer, measuring between 9.5 and 19.5 mm in length and 0.9 mm in breadth. The adult female measures between 16 and 26 mm in length and 0.3 mm in its greatest width.

The schistosome has no pharynx and the oesophagus extends from the oral sucker to bifurcate into two caeca which reunite to form a single blind caecum. The bifurcation and reunification of the intestinal caeca vary with each species of worm. The intestinal caeca are short in the *Schistosoma mansoni*, but much longer in *Schistosoma japonicum* and extend almost to two-thirds of the worm's length.

The male *Schistosoma* has between six and nine testes which are connected to very short tubes to empty into the anterior portion of the gynaecophoral canal. In the female the ovary is located in the anterior half of the body. The uterus is very short and contains usually only one or two eggs in the case of *Schistosoma mansoni*, but in *Schistosoma japonicum* there may be many ova in the uterus.

The ovum with the miracidium of the *Schistosoma mansoni* has a lateral sub-terminal spine. Instead of a spine, the *Schistosoma japonicum* ovum has a notch which is situated near the front portion of the egg. It also contains a miracidium.

Life cycle

The adult worms live in pairs in the venules of the portal bed. *Schistosoma mansoni* are found in the haemorrhoidal plexus, but *Schistosoma japonicum* lives higher up in the mesenteric plexus. The female leaves the male to lay her eggs in the submucosal portion of the gut, particularly in the sigmoid colon and the rectum.

The actual mechanism by which the eggs reach the lumen of the large bowel is still not known. It is possible that the eggs might contain an enzyme which causes local necrosis of the bowel epithelium and thus allows them to penetrate the mucosa of the rectum. On the other hand, it is possible that the faeces might brush the eggs into the lumen of the bowel.

The eggs are passed in the faeces, and after coming into contact with running water and sunlight they rupture and allow the miracidium to escape. The eggs survive for only a few days if conditions are not suitable.

The miracidium penetrates the integument of the host within a few hours. For the *Schistosoma mansoni* the intermediate hosts are the aquatic snails, *Biomphalaria* and the *Australorbis* in Africa and *Tropicorbis* in South America and the Carribean Islands. The common snail, *Oncomelania nosophora*, is an intermediate host of the *Schistosoma japonicum*.

The first generation of sporocysts forms from the miracidium in the tissues of the intermediate host and contains many germ cells. After a week the germ cells begin to proliferate into a very large number of cells, and each cell subsequently becomes a new sporocyst, the daughter sporocyst, from which the cercariae develop. From one ovum between 150 000 and 300 000 cercariae may develop.

The cercariae leave the snail, usually in daylight, and in tropical countries between 2 and 3 p.m. in the afternoon when the sunlight is strongest. The cercaria swims about in the water and is infectious. It survives only a few hours and when no suitable host is available it dies. Infection takes place when the cercaria comes into contact with the bare skin of the host. It then bores through the skin with the oral sucker. At the same time hyaluronidase is secreted and this allows the softening of the integument for its boring movement. Before entering the skin the cercaria usually loses its tail but occasionally retains it as it penetrates the skin. At this point it is termed a schistosomule.

The schistosomule does not penetrate deeper than the skin before it gets into the lymphatics or a blood vessel and is then carried to the lungs. From the lungs, the worms very quickly find their way by the systemic circulation to the liver. Here, they begin to grow to maturity and pairing takes place. The couple then swim against the portal blood flow to the mesenteric veins where they finally lodge.

The whole cycle takes about 50 days from the cercarial stage to sexual maturity, but ova have been found in the stool as early as 38 days after contact with infection.[76]

Pathology

Acute phase of infection

In the acute phase of the infection, there is generalized enlargement of the lymph nodes which are discrete and of rubbery consistency. Schistosomules have been found in such lymph nodes[20] but Garcia-Palmieri and Marcial-Rojas[24] believe that the lymphadenopathy, hepatosplenomegaly and pruritus are mainly due to an allergic reaction to the ovum when it is first produced in the large intestine. Sigmoidoscopic examination shows multiple areas of hyperaemia with a yellowish necrotic centre in which may be found the ova of the schistosomes. Needle biopsy of the liver shows a marked eosinophilic infiltration mainly in the portal tract. There are also epithelioid granulomas which surround centrally located degenerating ova (Figure 56.25). However, fibrosis does not appear to be present.

Chronic phase of schistosomiasis

Pathological changes are demonstrated in the gastrointestinal tract, particularly in the large intestine at this stage. The gallbladder, duodenum and the appendix may also be involved. Many epithelioid granulomas are

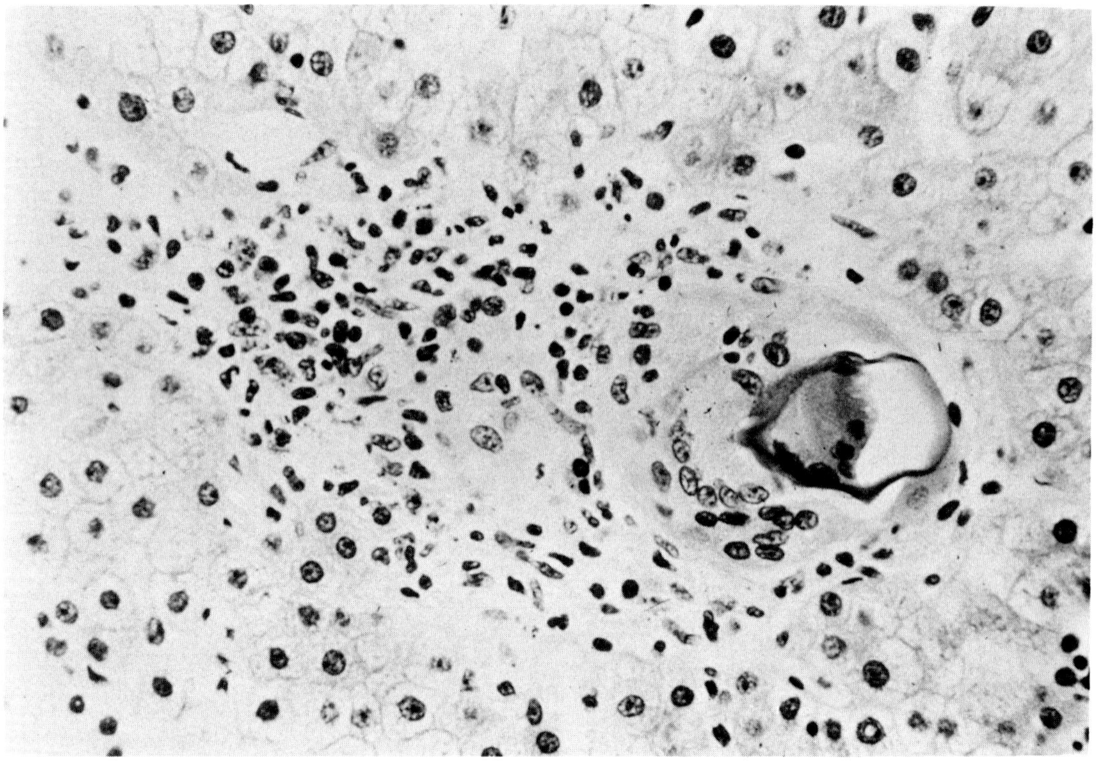

Figure 56.25. Ovum of *Schistosoma mansoni* (centre right) partially engulfed by a multinucleate giant cell.

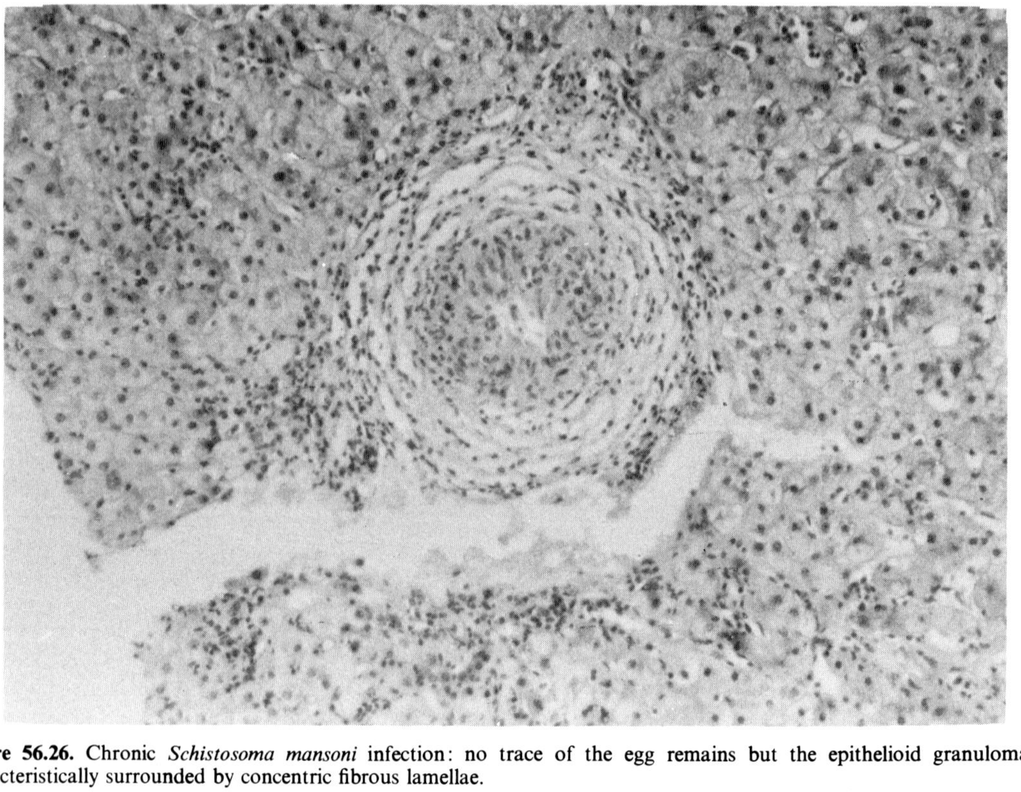

Figure 56.26. Chronic *Schistosoma mansoni* infection: no trace of the egg remains but the epithelioid granuloma is characteristically surrounded by concentric fibrous lamellae.

found with chronic inflammatory changes and fibrous proliferation.

The changes in the liver are most prominent in schistosomiasis of the *mansoni* and *japonicum* varieties. Lesions are found mainly in the portal spaces and where ova of the parasites are lodged. In the case of the *Schistosoma mansoni* the number of the ova found is very much smaller and occasionally may be absent. Granulomas are usually still present and characteristically are surrounded by concentric layers of fibrosis (Figure 56.26). The fibrosis expanding the portal tracts may be very extensive and has been described as the pipe-stem fibrosis of schistosomiasis (Figure 56.27). In *Schistosoma japonicum*, the fibrosis may be equally marked with lobulation resulting from cirrhosis (Figure 56.28). Sections of the liver show extensive periportal fibrosis around the periportal spaces, where there may be numerous ova of the *Schistosoma japonicum* (Figure 56.29). All these produce a presinusoidal obstruction to the portal blood flow and result in an enlarged spleen and oesophageal varices.

Clinical Features

These depend on the severity of infection. Many of the slightly infected patients with schistosomiasis, both of the *mansoni* and the *japonicum* varieties, may be asymptomatic. There may be a history of skin rash and diarrhoea with mild fever, but this disappears completely. Examination of the stool occasionally may demonstrate the ova and the serological tests and skin test may be positive for the parasites.

Symptomatic acute phase of the schistosomiasis

About one month after exposure to the infection the onset of symptoms may suddenly be ushered in by chills, fever and pain. There may be generalized body aches with headaches, anorexia and severe diarrhoea. The fever may be high and reach 40°C. There is usually generalized enlargement of the lymph nodes which are discrete, non-tender and of rubbery consistency. The liver may be enlarged in a proportion of cases but is soft and tender, and there is no evidence of jaundice. Eosinophilia may be absent but occasionally can be high. Liver function tests are abnormal and there is a reversed albumin:globulin ratio. Biopsy of the liver performed at this time may reveal epithelioid granulomas with an eosinophil infiltrate, but there is no fibrosis. The acute phase of this disease may last for as long as three months.

Chronic hepatosplenomegaly

The eggs of the parasites are laid in the venules of the inferior and superior mesenteric vessels, move with the blood flow and are then trapped in the portal tract. This gives rise to changes

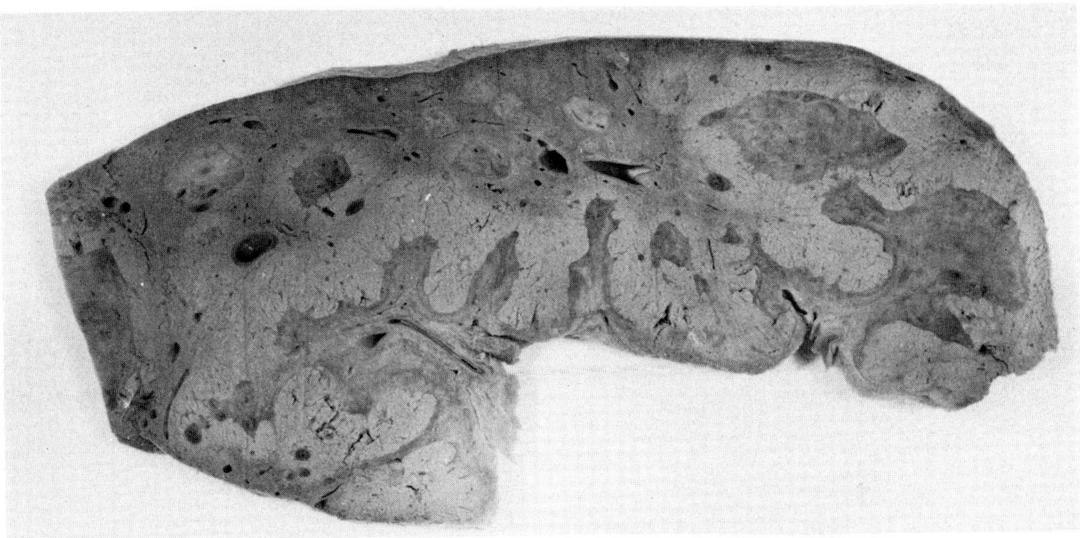

Figure 56.27. Showing periportal fibrosis (Symmers' fibrosis) in a cross-section of liver infested with *Schistosoma japonicum*. Courtesy of Dr S. Tolentino.

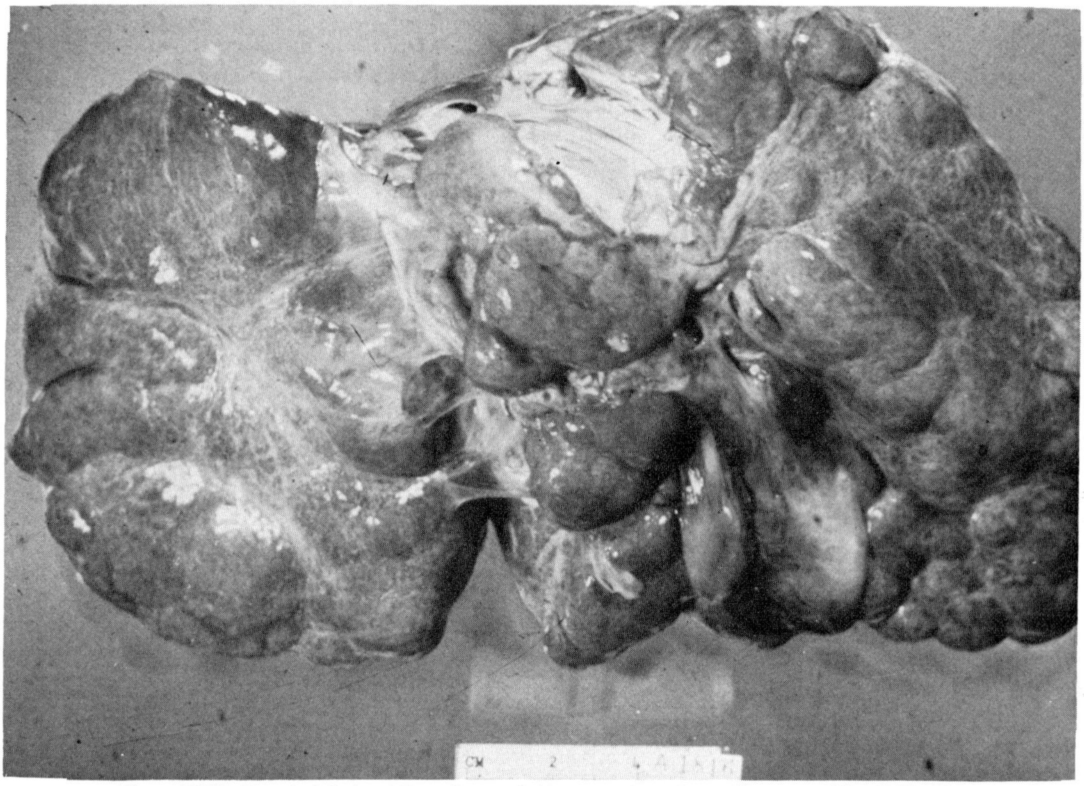

Figure 56.28. Grossly lobulated liver due to *Schistosoma japonicum*. Courtesy of Dr C.W. Chan.

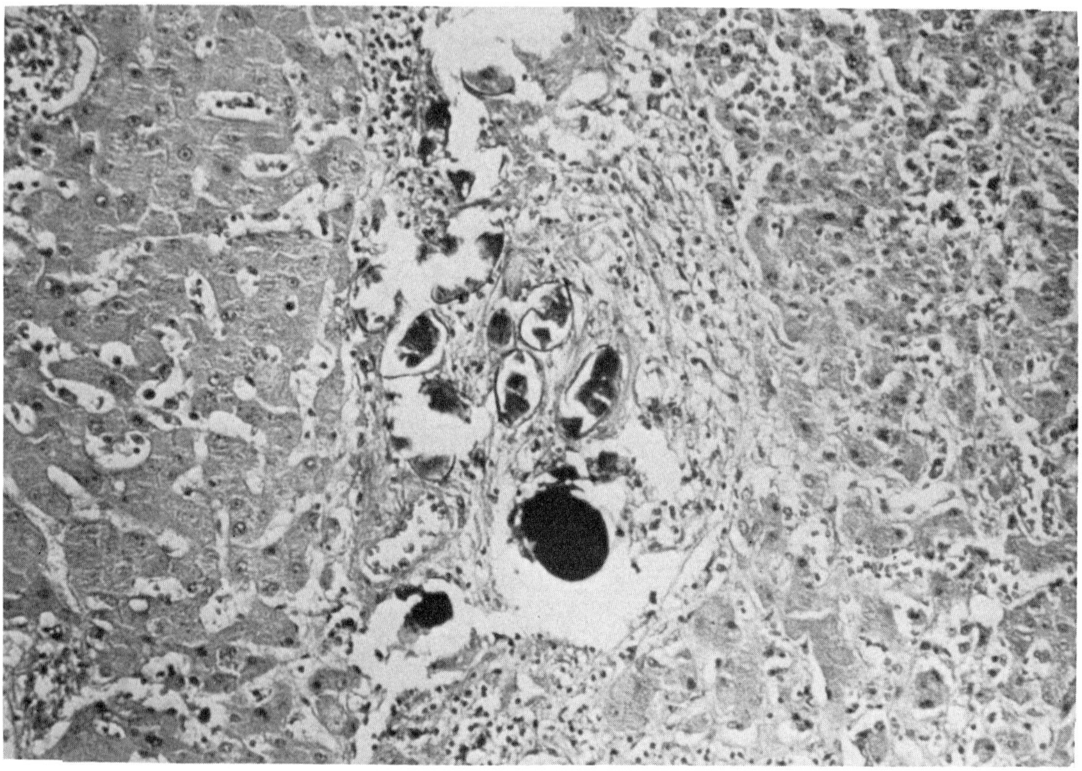

Figure 56.29. Periportal fibrosis with eggs of *Schistosoma japonicum*. × 160.

resulting in fibrosis and portal hypertension develops.

There is marked weakness and skin pallor, and because of ascites there may be shortness of breath. Patients are anorectic and in extreme cases there may be emaciation. Superficial veins may be present on the abdominal wall because of portal hypertension. There may be one or several attacks of haematemesis. Liver function is never affected to the same extent as in portal or postnecrotic cirrhosis[23] although there may be loss of axillary hair, testicular atrophy and liver palms and occasionally gynaecomastia may develop. Jaundice, however, is seldom encountered.

Hepatitis B infection. In these patients with hepatosplenic schistosomiasis there is an increased incidence of chronic hepatitis B infection and it is suggested that schistosomiasis predisposes to hepatitis B positive chronic active hepatitis. Clinically these patients with combined infections have a more rapid progression of their liver disease than with either disease alone.[3,48,68]

Diagnosis

The diagnosis in the late stages of the disease when the patient is moribund with ascites, enlarged spleen and shrunken liver poses no problems. The demonstration of ova in the stool and, if necessary, biopsy of the rectal mucosa will establish the diagnosis. Occasionally, the diagnosis can be made from needle biopsy of the liver and in the case of *Schistosoma mansoni* the typical pipe-stem fibrosis is pathognomonic even without the demonstration of ova in the periportal spaces. The bile ducts in such cases are usually normal. The diagnosis from liver biopsy tends to be more successful in *Schistosoma japonicum* because of the greater number of ova present.

Treatment

The mere demonstration of the presence of parasites is not necessarily an indication for treatment. Many patients who harbour a small number of parasites suffer no ill-effects. It is not the parasite that causes pathological changes and subsequent symptoms, but rather the number of ova laid by the worms. In such patients treatment which renders the worms infertile, even without killing the parasites, is an acceptable form of therapy. This suppressive management is particularly useful as a public health measure. Mass ambulant treatment can be instituted to control the disease. For this therapy several drugs are available, as follows.

Niridazole (Ambilhar (Ciba)) is a nitrothiazole compound with a formula of 1-(5 nitro-2-thiazolyl)-2-imidazolidinone. The drug acts on the vitelline cells of the female parasite, arresting the egg shell formation, with the eventual disappearance of its contents. Both males and females are affected, but larger doses are needed to affect the female reproductive organs. The worms become weak and ultimately are destroyed by the phagocytes, particularly in the liver. This drug, which has been found to be very useful in eradicating *Schistosoma haematobium*, is less effective but still useful against *Schistosoma mansoni* and *japonicum*.[37] Niridazole is used at a dosage of 10 to 15 mg/kg body weight per day for 10 days. In 332 patients with *Schistosoma japonicum* treated by Blas[9] in a mass screening programme in the Philippines, it was found that in six patients hallucination and other temporary psychotic behaviour occurred. The drug has toxic effects on the central nervous system as well as the liver. It should not be used when there is a portal systemic collateral circulation or in liver failure.

Lucanthone hydrochloride (Nilodin, Burroughs Wellcome; Miracil D, Bayer) is a hydrochloride of 1-(2-diethylaminoethyl) amino-4-methyl thiaxanthone. This drug acts in the same way as niridazole, by inhibiting egg-laying, and at a higher dose leads to the death of the parasite. The drug is also used in mass treatment and can be given by mouth. It is readily absorbed from the gastrointestinal tract. The drug is rapidly broken down and its metabolites act on the parasites.

Hycanthone was originally derived from lucanthone by the action of *Aspergillus sclerotiorum*. The drug was tried by Katz and his co-workers[38] in 1968 and was also used in mass treatment by Warren and his co-workers[84] on 169 patients with heavy *Schistosoma mansoni* infestation in Kenya. They found that 1.5 mg/kg body weight (half of the recommended dose) was sufficient to induce a 90 per cent reduction of egg production.

Oxamniquine, which is a tetrahydroquinoline derivative, has been recently introduced by Omer.[64] This is effective in reducing the egg count. Even when the dose given is as small as 30 mg/kg body weight, the egg count is reduced by 69 per cent and when the total dose is stepped up to a total of 60 mg/kg body weight the egg count is reduced by as much as 95 per cent.

Two antimony compounds are commonly used for the treatment of schistosomiasis. Patients undergoing treatment with antimony compounds should be hospitalized as the drug is toxic to the heart, liver and kidneys.

Tartar emetic (antimony potassium tartrate) was first used over 40 years ago and is still the most effective drug against *Schistosoma japonicum*.[37] The drug is available as a half per cent solution. The initial dose is 3 ml of the solution, given very slowly, and subsequently the doses are raised and given on alternative days from an initial dose of 3 ml to the maximum dose of 28 ml per day. The sodium salt is less toxic.

Stibophen (Fuadin) is also used and is much more effective against *Schistosoma mansoni*.[37] It is administered intramuscularly in 5 ml doses of a 6.8 per cent solution, starting with small doses of 1.5 to 3.5 ml on the first three days, and subsequently on alternative days 5 ml doses until a total dose of 18 ml is given over a period of two to three weeks. A higher total dosage has also been used.

Surgical treatment

Surgical treatment of hepatic schistosomiasis is confined to the complications of the disease. One of the serious complications is that of portal hypertension leading to haematemesis, which may occasionally be exsanguinating. Liver function is usually satisfactory until the terminal stages of the disease. However, the enlarged spleen gives rise to hypersplenism and treatment should be directed towards this complication. When the patient is weak, blood transfusion and oesophageal tamponade should be instituted.

A portacaval shunt will relieve the portal hypertension due to schistosomiasis of the liver. The patient usually withstands this operation better than does a patient with cirrhosis. The shunt may allow the eggs of the worms dislodged from the mesenteric radicles to pass through the systemic circulation to the lungs. Here they cause thrombosis of the pulmonary arterioles and give rise to pulmonary hypertension and finally cor pulmonale. During the operation the ova can be sieved from the portal blood after a dose of tartar emetic has been given and the blood then returned to the patient.

Garcia-Palmieri and his co-workers[25] performed 41 portacaval shunts on patients with schistosomiasis and in the early follow-up period found one patient who developed pulmonary hypertension from eggs shunted into the systemic circulation. They believed that a longer follow-up would demonstrate a marked increase in the number of patients with pulmonary hypertension.

Splenectomy alone has been practised for this disease. Splenectomy not only rapidly relieves the hypersplenism but also reduces the portal blood pressure. This reduction of portal hypertension is probably only temporary, for in a series of 123 operations carried out by Lan and co-workers[43] there was 14.5 per cent recurrence of haemorrhage.

Devascularization of the stomach and lower oesophagus with splenectomy was introduced by Hassab[27] in the treatment of portal hypertension resulting from schistosomiasis. Here, the spleen is removed and all the vessels supplying the proximal part of the stomach and the lower oesophagus are divided and ligated. It is difficult to evaluate the efficacy of this operation as only 38 per cent of cases were followed up for more than one year. Nevertheless, this operation cures the hypersplenism, reduces the portal pressure and avoids the shunting of the parasitic ova to the lungs. It is possibly the best procedure available for the treatment of hepatic portal hypertension caused by schistosomiasis.

Prophylaxis

Whenever possible, destruction of the snails should be carried out by draining the canals and filling them. However, this is not always possible where there is extensive irrigation, for the incidence of Bilharzial infestation has risen markedly with the building of the High Aswan Dam in Egypt.

The mass treatment of patients in endemic areas with drugs such as hycanthone for *Schistosoma mansoni* or niridazole for *Schistosoma japonicum* should be further explored.

HYDATID CYST OF THE LIVER

Hydatid cyst of the liver is caused by infestation with flatworms of the phylum platyhelminthes; of the order Cyclophyllidea and of the family *Taeniidae*. These are tapeworms and there are three species: *Echinococcus granulosus*; *Echinococcus multilocularis*; and *Echinococcus oligarthrus*. Of these three species the most common, universal and important infestation is *Echinococcus granulosus*. It has a worldwide distribution and is especially common in sheep- and cattle-rearing countries. The definitive host is the dog; cattle, sheep, pigs and man are the intermediate hosts of the larval stage of the infestation.

In the North American continent wolves and wild game such as moose, reindeer and caribou are also heavily infected. In Australia the parasite also infests the wild dog, *Canis dingo*, as well as wallabies and kangaroos. In Sri Lanka jackals and deer are often infected. In Great Britain horses have also been observed to have hydatid cysts.

Echinococcus multilocularis differs from *Echinococcus granulosus* in that the definitive hosts are various foxes, although domestic cats can also be the host. The intermediate hosts are small rodents such as tundra mice, while dogs, foxes and wolves are the definitive hosts of this type of hydatid.[67] It is found in man, most frequently in southern Germany, Switzerland, the Tyrol, and the USSR including Siberia. Cases have been reported in Canada, northern Germany, Iceland, around the Baltic, and in northern Europe as well as Alaska and the Bering Islands.

The species, *oligarthrus*, is found mainly in South America. It has been described in the liver of a Panamanian and in a few other human cases in South America.[81] Adult worms are found in pumas and jaguars in South America, while in Africa it is found in lions.

Morphology and Life Cycle

Morphology

Taenia echinococcus are small tapeworms which have four to five segments and a head, the scolex, which is pyriform in shape. It has two rows of hooks near the tip of the head, varying in number from 28 to 50. Beyond this are four suckers. A very short neck arises from the scolex, and below this are usually three segments or proglottids. The first one is a hermaphrodite, with the genital apertures alternating irregularly. The second segment is the mature segment, while the terminal proglottid is gravid and contains between 400 and 800 eggs.

The eggs, like those of all taeniae, contain the outer chitinous shell and an inner oncosphere. The spherical larva has six hooklets, a characteristic of all cestodes.

Taenia echinococcus multilocularis differs from *Echinococcus granulosus* in that it is smaller, measuring from 1.2 to 3.7 mm in length, and the number of testes is less than those of *Echinococcus granulosus*, varying from 17 to 26 with an average of 22, compared with 45 to 65 testes in the *Echinococcus granulosus*. The situation of the gonads is also different, and the uterus shows no lateral branches, in contrast to the many lateral branches present in *Echinococcus granulosus*.

Life cycle

The mature proglottid of *Echinococcus granulosus* is detached from the worm and with the eggs is passed in the stool. These eggs have a remarkable resistance to extreme temperatures and may be viable for as long as two to three months at a temperature of -16 to -18°C. They are also relatively resistant to disinfectants. For example, placed in 95 per cent alcohol, 10 per cent lysol, or 20 per cent formalin for an hour, 10 to 30 per cent of them may be still viable.[57]

When eggs are swallowed the gastric juice destroys the outer covering and the embryo is released. This larval form penetrates the intestine, enters the portal venous blood and passes to the liver where more than 70 per cent of them are arrested; 30 per cent of them may reach the systemic circulation and be carried to the lungs and to various other organs so that almost the whole body may be involved.

Once the larva has reached the liver it becomes encysted. One month after implantation it is approximately 1 mm in diameter and grows to 40 to 50 mm in about three months.[12] The cyst consists of three layers. The outer adventitial fibrous layer is formed from the tissues of the host. Inside this are two more layers, the outer one of which is the translucent chitinous laminated layer, and the innermost layer is the germinal layer (Figure 56.30).

As the cyst grows bigger the germinal layer begins to proliferate and form daughter cysts

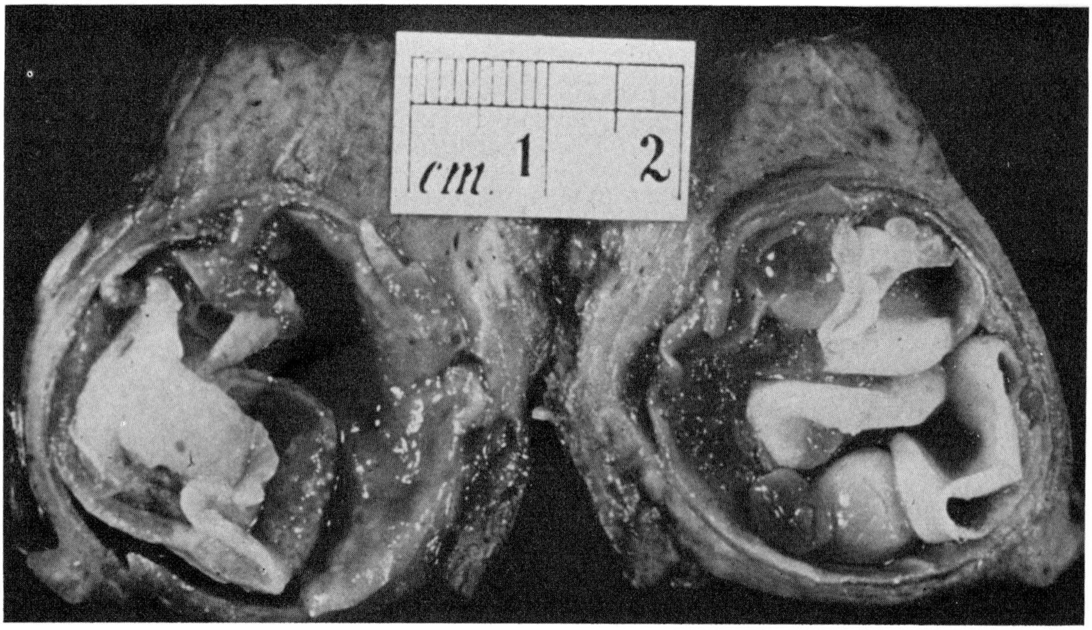

Figure 56.30. A laminated unilocular hydatid cyst with daughter cysts in the liver specimen. Courtesy of Dr C.W. Chan.

(brood capsules). A second generation of daughter cysts may be formed under certain adverse conditions. The scolices develop from the germinal layer of the daughter cysts and continue to grow in size until each acquires the ability to retract its head into its body in order to protect the hooklets. In this way the hydatid cyst from a single larva may grow into a large size with multiple daughter cysts and granddaughter cysts (Figure 56.31). The germinal layer of the cyst does not form parasites when swallowed by the host. Only the scolices develop into adult worms when swallowed by carnivorous or omnivorous animals such as dogs. In the intestines of carnivorous animals the embryos are freed from the cyst and become attached to the intestinal mucosa and grow into adult worms.

The adult worms live in the duodenum and upper part of the jejunum, and are attached by the hooklets to the mucosa between the villi. They have no digestive tract and acquire their nutrition solely by surface absorption of the intestinal content.

Pathology

In the majority of cases of *Echinococcus granulosus*, the embryo, after entering the liver through the portal circulation, is located near a central vein. A very small proportion (about 7

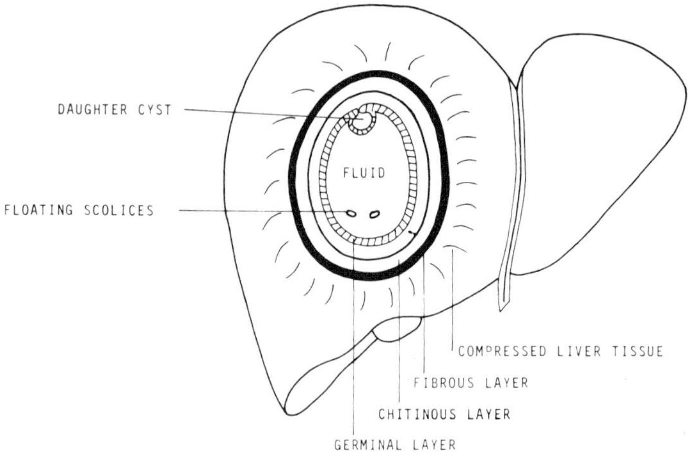

Figure 56.31. Diagrammatic representation of hydatid cyst.

per cent) are located at the portal tract. The cyst forms in the liver and may compress surrounding tissue so that there may be congestion with biliary stasis. Some are situated near Glisson's capsule but others are deeply seated. The cyst is usually tense and under great pressure.

Alveolar cyst (*Echinococcus multilocularis*)

This is characterized by multiple minute cysts embedded in fibrous tissue of the liver. Instead of containing fluid the cyst is filled with jelly-like substance. It infiltrates the surrounding liver tissue and grows centripetally. The centre of the involved liver undergoes necrosis. Study of the cyst may show the elements of the parasite and occasionally a scolex may be identified.[82] Unlike *Echinococcus granulosus*, there is no cyst wall. The disease is progressive and has been mistaken for a colloid carcinoma of the bile ducts. It is now recognized as a separate entity, but was first believed to be a variation of the larval stage of hydatid cyst.[17]

Complications

Infection

Bacterial invasion of the cyst may occur, leading to the death of the embryo. This may stimulate the formation of daughter and granddaughter cysts so that some of them may escape destruction. Ultimately the cyst may become calcified.

Rupture of the cyst

Rupture of the cyst may occur spontaneously or with minimal manipulation, as it is very tense and under high pressure. Rupture into the peritoneal cavity causes secondary cyst formation throughout the cavity.

The cyst may rupture into the intrahepatic bile ducts, and give rise to obstructive jaundice.[26,36] It may also rupture through the diaphragm into the lungs and be coughed up in the sputum. This results in bronchobiliary fistula.[70] Rupture of the cyst through the liver extraperitoneally to form a cyst between the anterior parietal peritoneum and the posterior rectus sheath has been reported.[10]

Anaphylactic shock

Rupture of the hydatid cyst either at the time of manipulation during surgery or spontaneously may give rise to anaphylactic shock.

Clinical Features

About 50 per cent of patients harbouring hydatid cysts of the liver are admitted for other reasons.[34] The most frequent presentation of hydatid cyst of the liver is an enlarged liver. Jaundice of varying degrees may be present but in the majority of these cases the cyst has ruptured into the biliary tract. There may be chills, fever and jaundice with severe pain in the right hypochondrium which may be referred to the shoulder. Examination of the blood reveals eosinophilia in about 40 per cent of patients.

Casoni test

The Casoni skin test is positive in about 70 per cent of the patients,[72] but may be as high as 87 per cent.[36] The Weinberg complement fixation test gives a positive result in over 80 per cent of cases.

Diagnosis of hepatic hydatid cyst

The appearance of a hepatic mass in an endemic area should arouse suspicion. This is even more suggestive if there is eosinophilia. Suspicion of hydatid cyst is an absolute contraindication to a needle biopsy of the liver. The lesion in the liver can be demonstrated by isotope scanning but Joske[34] demonstrated that out of 22 scans six were negative. With the introduction of computerized axial tomography, the cyst in the liver can be demonstrated more readily. However, the fluid nature of the tumour can be better demonstrated with ultrasonography (see Chapter 21). This shows a typical picture of crescentic areas within the cyst which are the edges of the daughter cysts. Selective hepatic arteriography will demonstrate the mass which is avascular and displaces the intrahepatic vessels (see Chapter 22). When the cyst has ruptured into the biliary tract, ERCP may be useful.[63]

Treatment

Treatment of the hepatic hydatid cyst is surgical. There is no drug available at the present time that can destroy the cysts. The indication for surgical treatment of a small calcified cyst possibly containing dead larvae is still debatable. Lewis and co-workers[45] argued that such cysts are inactive and should be left alone but it is now generally agreed that most hydatid cysts should be operated upon.

Operative treatment

A thoraco-abdominal approach to the hydatid of the liver either with or without thoracic complications has been suggested.[86] However, in most instances an abdominal approach is sufficient. Extreme care must be exercised whilst manipulating the liver, for occasionally the cyst that is under high tension may rupture. After the cyst is exposed, the area should be packed off completely and protected against spillage of the fluid. A small bore needle should be introduced gently and the fluid aspirated. The use of formalin that was formerly advocated[16] has been mostly abandoned because of toxicity and doubt as to its efficacy.[57] An alternative sterilization of the larvae is the introduction of hypertonic 20 per cent saline.[40] This kills the parasite very rapidly and within 10 minutes the fluid, the scolices and the cysts should be destroyed. A sucker is then introduced into the cyst shell to suck out the fluid. The cysts are then removed. The excision of the cyst shell is through the laminated chitinous or fibrous layer. The adventitial layer of the cyst should be left alone, for any excision beyond the fibrous layer will lead to much bleeding and damage of the biliary ducts.

Drainage of the diseased cavity has been practised, but this gives rise to problems with biliary fistulae as well as secondary haemorrhage. The cavity can be obliterated by filling it with omentum.[47]

Another way of closing the cavity is by 'capitonnage'. The walls of the cavity are approximated with a series of continuous or interrupted mattress sutures. The sutures are placed from the deeper to the superficial parts of the cavity. This shortens the hospital stay to 12 days.[72]

Resection

Hepatic lobectomy in certain cases has been advocated as a form of treatment.[66] It is condemned by Barros[5] as being too radical and carries a much higher mortality. However, if the cyst is localized to the lateral segment of the left lobe this is an excellent form of treatment for such a limited resection and should carry no mortality. During the process of resection, extreme care must be taken not to rupture the cyst as this may lead to a spread of the disease into the peritoneal cavity. The same precaution of injecting 20 per cent hypertonic saline must therefore be carried out before manipulation.

Resection has also a place when infection is present or when previous marsupialization has been performed. A persistent biliary fistula, or a large cavity with secondary infection, is best treated by resection. Resection is mandatory in the treatment of *Echinococcus multilocularis* as this form of echinococcal infection, simulating a malignant growth, invades the liver.

Marsupialization is condemned by most authors.[5,66,72] However, in a very sick patient with a secondary infection of the hydatid cyst, temporary marsupialization may have to be performed as a life-saving procedure. The residual discharging sinus with persistent infection causes chronic ill-health. This cavity or sinus can be dealt with by either pericystic gastrostomy[19,36] or, better still, hepatic resection.

Other procedures

When the cyst has ruptured into the bile ducts evacuation of the contents through a choledochotomy may be done. T-tube drainage is then necessary. Sphincteroplasty has also been widely used.[5]

Prognosis

A unilocular hydatid cyst of the liver, provided there are no other cysts in the body, has a fairly good prognosis. When spillage occurs at operation, 50 per cent of patients may continue to harbour the disease. When there are other associated cysts, the prognosis is grave.

Echinococcus multilocularis is serious and is progressive. Unless the disease can be eliminated by radical hepatic resection, the prognosis is hopeless.

Prophylaxis

People should be discouraged from fondling dogs or cats. Offal of dead sheep or cattle should not be fed to dogs and carcasses should be buried in deep pits or incinerated.

REFERENCES

1. Akimoto, T. (1950) On the motion of the *Ascaris lumbricoides* in a small tube. *Hirosaki Igaku* (in Japanese with English summary), **1**, 53, 131.
2. Arean, V.M. & Crandall, C. (1962) The effect of immunization fate of injected 2nd stage of *Ascaris lumbricoides* larvae in the rabbit. *American Journal of Tropical Medicine and Hygiene*, **11**, 369.
3. Barreto, V.S.T. & Rocha, N. (1978) Personal observations.
4. Barron, C.N. & Saunders, L.Z. (1966) Visceral larva migrans in the dog. *Pathologia Veterinaria (Basel)*, **3**, 315.
5. Barros, J.L. (1978) Hydatid disease of the liver. *American Journal of Surgery*, **135**, 597.
6. Beaver, P.C. (1964) Ascaris strangled in a shoe-eyelet. *American Journal of Tropical Medicine and Hygiene*, **13**, 295.
7. Beaver, P.C. (1969) The nature of visceral larva migrans. *Journal of Parasitology*, **55**, 3.
8. Beaver, P.C. & Danaraj, T.J. (1958) Pulmonary ascariasis resembling eosinophilic lung. Autopsy report with description of larvae in the bronchioles. *American Journal of Tropical Medicine and Hygiene*, **7**, 100–111.
9. Blas, B.L. (1977) Further trials with suppressive dose of Ambilhar (niridazole) for mass treatment of *Schistosoma japonicum* infection. *18th Southeast Asia Minister of Education Organisation of Tropical Medicine Seminar, Taiwan, 2–5 August 1977.*
10. Bose, S.M. & Monga, N.K. (1974) Unusual presentation of a hepatic hydatid cyst. *Australian and New Zealand Journal of Surgery*, **44**, 4, 407.
11. Brill, R, Churg, J. & Beaver, P.C. (1953) Allergic granulomatosis associated with visceral larva migrans. *American Journal of Clinical Pathology*, **23**, 1208.
12. Cameron, T.W.M. (1927) Some modern biological concepts of hydatid. *Proceedings of the Royal Society of Medicine*, **20**, 272.
13. Chung, H.L., Hsu, C.P., Ts'ao, W.L., K'o, H.Y., Yuan, C.T. & Chang, Y.C. (1965) Hexachloroparaxylol in treatment of *Clonorchis sinensis* in animal and man. *Chinese Medical Journal*, **84**, 232.
14. Dawes, B. (1962) Additional notes on the growth of *Fasciola hepatica L.* in the mouse with some remarks about recent researches in Belgium. *Journal of Helminthology*, **36**, 259.
15. Dawes, B. (1963) Hyperplasia of the bile duct in fascioliasis and its relation to the problem of nutrition in the liver fluke. *Fasciola hepatica L. Parasitology*, **53**, 123.
16. Deve, F. (1907) Des kyfes hydatiques gazeux du foie. *Revue de Chirurgie (Paris)*, **35**, 529.
17. Dew, H.R. (1958) Morphological variation in hydatid disease. *British Journal of Surgery*, **45**, 447.
18. Facey, R.V. & Marsden, P.D. (1960) Fascioliasis in man – an outbreak in Hampshire. *British Medical Journal*, **ii**, 619–625.
19. Fagarasanu, I. (1976) Pericystogastrostomy: internal drainage in the treatment of certain hydatid cysts of the liver. *British Journal of Surgery*, **63**, 624.
20. Faust, E.C. & Meleney, H.E. (1924) Studies on *Schistosomiasis japonicum*. 6. The pathology and anatomy of the disease. Monogram series. *American Journal of Hygiene*, **3**, 174.
21. Faust, E.C. & Russel, P.F. (1964) *Clinical Parasitology*. p. 419. Philadelphia: Lea & Febiger.
22. Friedman, S. & Hervada, A.R. (1960) Severe myocarditis with recovery in a child with visceral larva migrans. *Journal of Pediatrics*, **56**, 91.
23. Garcia-Palmieri, M.R. & Marcial-Rojas, R.A. (1959) Portal hypertension due to *Schistosoma mansoni*. *American Journal of Medicine*, **27**, 811.
24. Garcia-Palmieri, M.R. & Marcial-Rojas, R.A. (1962) The protean manifestations of schistosomiasis. A clinicopathological correlation. *Annals of Internal Medicine*, **57**, 763.
25. Garcia-Palmieri, M.R., Raffucci, F.L., Diaz-Bonnet, L.A. & Bernal-Rosa, J.F. (1959) Shunt surgery for portal hypertension due to *Schistosoma mansoni*. Evaluation and management in forty-one cases. *Journal of the American Medical Association*, **171**, 3, 108–268.
26. Hashimi, H.M. (1971) Intrabiliary rupture of hydatid cyst of the liver. *British Journal of Surgery*, **58**, 228.
27. Hassab, M.A. (1970) Non shunt operation in portal hypertension without cirrhosis. *Surgery, Gynecology and Obstetrics*, **131**, 168.
28. Hoeppli, R. (1959) *Parasites and Parasitic Infections in Early Medicine and Science*. Singapore: University of Malaya Press.
29. Hosemann, G. (1940) *Ascaris lumbricoides. Dire Chirugie* (2nd ed.), **2**, 276.
30. Hou, P.C. (1955) The pathology of *Clonorchis sinensis* infestation of the liver. *Journal of Pathology and Bacteriology*, **70**, 53.
31. Hou, P.C. (1956) The relationship between primary carcinoma of the liver and infestation with *Clonorchis sinensis*. *Journal of Pathology and Bacteriology*, **72**, 239.
32. Jennings, F.W., Mulligan, W. & Urquhart, G.M. (1956) Radioisotope studies on the anaemia produced by infection with *Fasciola hepatica*. *Experimental Parasitology*, **5**, 458–468.
33. Jones, E.A., Kay, J.M., Milligan, H.P. & Owens, D. (1977) Massive infection with *Fasciola hepatica* in man. *American Journal of Medicine*, **63**, 836.
34. Joske, R.A. (1974) The changing pattern of hydatid disease, with special reference to hydatid of the liver. *Medical Journal of Australia*, **1**, 129.
35. Katsurada, F. (1904) *Schistosoma japonicum* ein neuer menschichen parasit durch welchen gegenden Japan verusacht wird. *Annotationes Zoologice Japaneses*, **5**, 147.
36. Kattan, Y.B. (1975) Intrabiliary rupture of hydatid cyst of the liver. *British Journal of Surgery*, **62**, 885.
37. Katz, N. (1977) Anthelmintics – review article. *Medical Progress*, **4**, 73.
38. Katz, N., Pellegrino, J., Ferreira, M.T., Oliveira, C.A. & Dias, C.B. (1968) Preliminary clinical trials with hycanthone, a new antischistosomal agent. *American Journal of Tropical Medicine and Hygiene*, **17**, 743.
39. Koenigstein, R.P. (1949) Observations on the epidemiology of infections with *Clonorchis sinensis*. *Transactions of the Royal Society of Tropical Medicine and Hygiene*. **42**, 5, 503.
40. Koss, N., Kerstein, M.D. & Lewis, J.W. (1976) Correspondence. *American Surgeon*, **183**, 90.
41. Krull, W.H. & Jackson, K.S. (1943) Observations in the route of migration of the common liver fluke *Fasciola hepatica* in the definitive host. *Journal of the Washington Academy of Sciences*, **33**, 79.

42. Krull, W.H. & Mapes, C.R. (1953) Studies on the biology of *Dicrocoelium dendriticum* including its relation to the intermediate host, *Cidmella lubrica* (Mylleu). IX. Notes on cyst, metacercaria, and infection in the ant, *Formica fusca*. *Cornell Veterinarian*, **43,** 389.
43. Lan, H.C., K'uang, Y.L. & Chiang, Y. (1962) Surgical treatment of late schistosomiasis. *Chinese Medical Journal*, **81,** 176.
44. Leh, Y.Ch, Feng, Y.S., Chao, W.Ch & Na, H.Ch. (1953) Intestinal helminthes among farmers in the rural districts of Tsingtao. *Shantung University Bulletin*, **3,** 75.
45. Lewis, J.W., Koss, N., Kerstein, M.D. (1975) A review of echinococcal disease. *American Surgeon*, **181,** 390.
46. Liu, J., Wang, C.N., Tsang, F.J., Fan, K.C., Tu, C.C., Chang, T.F., Sun, K.J., Chiu, C.M., Cheng, S. & Tu, S.F. (1965) Hexachloroparaxylol in the treatment of *Clonorchis sinensis*. *Chinese Medical Journal*, **84,** 8.
47. Lofti, M. & Hashenian, H. (1973) Hydatid cyst disease of the liver and its treatment. *International Surgery*, **58,** 166.
48. Lyra, L.G., Rebouças, G. & Andrade, Z.A. (1976) Hepatitis B surface antigen carrier state in hepatosplenic schistosomiasis. *Gastroenterology*, **71,** 641–645.
49. Maki, T. (1972) Surgical diseases due to *Ascaris lumbricoides*. *Progress of Medical Parasitology in Japan*, **4,** 217.
50. Manson, P. (1902) Report of a case of Bilharzia from the West Indies. *British Journal of Surgery*, **2,** 1894.
51. Mapes, C.R. (1951) Studies on the biology of *Dicrocoelium dendriticum* including its relation to the intermediate host, *Cionella lubrica*. I. A study of *Dicrocoelium dendriticum* and *Dicrocoelium* infection. *Cornell Veterinarian*, **41,** 383.
52. Mashima, E. (1888) Uber warmeier in der cirrhoteschen Leber. *Tokio Medizinische Gesellschaft*, **2,** 821.
53. McConnell, J.F.P. (1875) Remarks on the anatomical and pathological revelation of a new specie of liver fluke. *Lancet*, **ii,** 271.
54. McFadzean, A.J.S. & Yeung, R.T.T. (1965) Hypoglycaemia in suppurative pancholangitis due to *Clonorchis sinensis*. *Transactions of the Royal Society of Tropical Medicine and Hygiene*, **59,** 2, 179.
55. McQuown, A.L. (1950) *Capillaria hepatica*: a report of genuine and spurious cases. *American Journal of Tropical Medicine*, **30,** 761.
56. McQuown, A.L. (1954) *Capillaria hepatica*. *American Journal of Clinical Pathology*, **24,** 448.
57. Meymarian, E. & Schwabe, C.W. (1962) Host–parasite relationships in echinococcosis. *American Journal of Tropical Medicine and Hygiene*, **11,** 360.
58. Miyake, H. (1929) *Cholelithiasis in Japan*. Tokyo: Kyorinsha.
59. Miyake, H. & Ishiyama, F. (1930) Statistische und klinische Studien auf Grund von 754 Fallen von Cholelithiasis-operationen bei Japanern. *Deutsch Zeitschrift für Chirurgie*, **225,** 187–214.
60. Nakamura, Y. (1960) Histopathological studies on the duodenal papilla in cases of biliary tract diseases with dilatation of the common bile duct. *Nippon Geka Gakkai Zaschi* (in Japanese with English summary), **61,** 1219.
61. Nicholas, J.L. (1970) Obstruction of the common bile-duct by *Fasciola hepatica*. *British Journal of Surgery*, **57,** 544.
62. Nichols, R.L. (1956) The etiology of visceral larva migrans. Diagnostic morphology of infective second-stage *Toxocara* larvae. *Journal of Parasitology*, **42,** 4, 349.
63. Nunnerley, H.B. (1978) Visualization of the liver, biliary tree and pancreas. Radiology. *Clinics in Gastroenterology*, **7,** 453–475.
64. Omer, A.H.S. (1978) Oxamniquine for treating *Schistosoma mansoni* infestation in Sudan. *British Medical Journal*, **ii,** 163.
65. Ong, G.B. (1962) A study of recurrent pyogenic cholangitis. *Archives of Surgery*, **84,** 199.
66. Pissiotis, C.A., Wander, J.V. & Condon, R.E. (1972) Surgical treatment of hydatid disease. *Archives of Surgery*, **104,** 454.
67. Rausch, R. (1956) Studies on the helminth fauna of Alaska. XXX. The occurrence of *Echinococcus multilocularis* Leuckart, 1863, on the Mainland of Alaska. *American Journal of Tropical Medicine and Hygiene*, **5,** 1086.
68. Rebouças, G. (1975) Clinical aspects of hepatosplenic schistosomiasis: a contrast with cirrhosis. *Yale Journal of Biology and Medicine*, **48,** 369–376.
69. Reich, A. (1922) Uber Spulwurmerkrankungen der Speiseröhre, der Gallenwege und der Leber. *Beiträge zur Klinischen Chirurgie*, **126,** 560–600.
70. Reventós, J., Manuel Nogueras, F., Rius, X. & Lorenzo, T. (1976) Hydatid disease of the liver with thoracic involvement. *Surgery, Gynecology and Obstetrics*, **143,** 570.
71. Rigby, H.M. (1922–3) Acute haemorrhage pancreatitis – roundworm in pancreatic duct. *British Journal of Surgery*, **10,** 419.
72. Romero-Torres, R. & Campbell, J.R. (1965) An interpretive review of the surgical treatment of hydatid diseases. *Surgery, Gynecology and Obstetrics*, **121,** 851.
73. Rubin, M., Kauffman, H.E. & Therney, J.P. (1968) An intraocular nematode. *Transactions of the American Academy of Ophthalmology and Otolaryngology*, **72,** 855.
74. Seah, S.K.K. (1973) Intestinal parasites in Chinese immigrants in a Canadian city. *Journal of Tropical Medicine and Hygiene*, **76,** 291–293.
75. Shattuck, G.C. (1924) Treatment of *Clonorchis*. *American Journal of Tropical Medicine*, **4,** 507.
76. Sotomayor, Z.R., Correa-Coronas, R. & Ramos-Morales, F. (1965) Acute Manson's schistosomiasis. *Boletín de la Asociación Médica de Puerto Rico*, **57,** 437.
77. Stitnimankarn, T. (1960) The necropsy incidence of gallstones in Thailand. *American Journal of the Medical Sciences*, **240,** 349.
78. Stoll, N.R. (1947) The worm world. *Journal of Parasitology*, **33,** 1.
79. T'ang, C.C., Liu, Y.K., Wang, P.C., Ch'en, P.H., T'ang, C.T., Ch'en, T.S., Lin, C.T., Huang, C.K., Ch'en, C.F. & Ch'en, S.H. (1963) Clonorchiasis in South Fukien with special reference to the discovery of cray fishes as second intermediate host. *Chinese Medical Journal*, **82,** 545.
80. Teoh, T.B. (1963) A study of gallstones and included worms in recurrent pyogenic cholangitis. *Journal of Pathology and Bacteriology*, **86,** 123.
81. Thatcher, V.E. & Sousa, O.F. (1966) *E. oligarthrus* in Panama and a comparison with a recent human hydatid. *American Journal of Tropical Medicine and Parasitology*, **60,** 405.
82. Walshe, J.M. (1954) *Echinococcosis alveolaris* of the liver. *Journal of Pathology and Bacteriology*, **67,** 371.
83. Wang, H.H. (1973) Migration of Ascarides into the peritoneal cavity. *Asian Journal of Medicine*, **9,** 326.

84. Warren, K.S., Ouma, J.H., Arap Siongok, T.K. & Houser, H.B. (1978) Hycanthone dose-response in *Schistosoma mansoni* infection in Kenya. *Lancet,* **i,** 352.

85. Watson, J.M. & Kerim, R.A. (1956) Observations on forms of parasitic pharyngitis known as 'halzoun' in the Middle East. *Journal of Tropical Medicine and Hygiene,* **59,** 147.

86. Yacoubian, H.D. (1976) Thoracic problems associated with hydatid cyst of the dome of the liver. *Surgery,* **79,** 544.

87. Yasuda, M. (1955) Studies on the parasitic elements in the gall stones, especially the method for detecting them. *Hirosaki Igaku* (in Japanese with English summary), **6,** 391.

88. Yoshida, Y., Miyake, T., Nakanishi, Y., Nishida, K., Yamashiki, Y., Ishikawa, T., Fujisaka, K., Tanaka, A. & Ebara, S. (1962) Two cases of human infection with *Fasciola SP* and treatments with Bithional. *Japanese Journal of Parasitology,* **11,** 411.

Index

Italic page numbers indicate illustrations, bold page numbers indicate plates, and t indicates tables.